Saunders

NURSING
DRUG
HANDBOOK
2026

Black Box Alerts advise about the increased risks of a particular drug.

Lifespan Considerations in each monograph note factors to be considered for geriatric, pediatric, pregnant, or nursing populations. Appendix G provides additional resources.

Uses section in each monograph notes the standard and off-label uses for a particular drug.

Interactions identify potential herbal, drug, and food interactions with a particular drug.

IV Incompatibilities present important information for IV drugs.

Top prescribed drugs are underlined.

PACLitaxel
HIGH ALERT

pak-li-tax-el
(Abraxane, Apo-PACLitaxel ✦)
■ **BLACK BOX ALERT** ■ Myelo-suppression is a major dose-limiting toxicity. Must be administered by certified chemotherapy personnel. Severe hypersensitivity reactions reported.
Do not confuse PACLitaxel with DOCEtaxel, PARoxetine, or Paxil.

◆ **CLASSIFICATION**

PHARMACOTHERAPEUTIC: Taxane derivative, antimitotic agent. **CLINICAL:** Antineoplastic.

USES

Conventional: Treatment of node-positive breast cancer, metastatic breast cancer after failure of combination therapy or relapse within 6 mos of adjuvant therapy; subsequent therapy for advanced ovarian cancer or as first-line therapy (in combination with CISplatin). Treatment of AIDS-related Kaposi's sarcoma; non–small-cell lung cancer (NSCLC) as first-line therapy (in combination with CISplatin). **Abraxane:** Treatment of breast cancer after failure of combination chemotherapy or relapse within 6 mos of adjuvant chemotherapy. First-line treatment of metastatic adenocarcinoma of pancreas. Treatment of locally advanced or metastatic NSCLC. **OFF-LABEL:** Bladder, cervical, small-cell lung, head and neck cancers. Treatment of adenocarcinoma. **Abraxane:** Recurrent/persistent ovarian, fallopian tube, primary peritoneal cancers.

PRECAUTIONS

Contraindications: Hypersensitivity to PACLitaxel. Hypersensitivity to drugs developed with Cremophor EL (polyoxyethylated castor oil). Treatment of solid tumors with baseline neutrophil count less than 1,500 cells/mm³; treatment of Kaposi's sarcoma with baseline neutrophil count less than 1,000 cells/mm³.

bilizes existing microtubules; inhibits their disassembly, interferes with late G mitotic phase and inhibits cell lication. **Therapeutic Effect:** Inhibits cellular mitosis; suppresses cell proliferation, and modulates immune response.

PHARMACOKINETICS

Does not readily cross blood-brain barrier. Protein binding: 89%–98%. Metabolized in liver. Excreted in feces (71%), urine (14%). Not removed by hemodialysis. **Half-life:** 3-hr infusion: 13.1–20.2 hrs; 24-hr infusion: 15.7–52.7 hrs.

LIFESPAN CONSIDERATIONS

Pregnancy/Lactation: Avoid pregnancy; may cause fetal harm. Females of reproductive potential must use effective contraception during treatment and for at least 6 mos after discontinuation. Breastfeeding not recommended during treatment and for at least 2 wks after discontinuation. May impair fertility in both females and males. **Males:** Males with female partners of reproductive potential must use effective contraception during treatment and for at least 3 mos after discontinuation. **Children:** Safety and efficacy not established. **Elderly:** May have increased risk of adverse effects.

INTERACTIONS

DRUG: **Strong CYP3A4 inhibitors** (e.g., **clarithromycin, ketoconazole, ritonavir**) may increase concentration/effect. **Strong CYP3A4 inducers** (e.g., **carBAMazepine, phenytoin, rifAMPin**) may decrease effect. **Bone marrow depressants** (e.g., **cladribine**) may increase myelosuppression. **Strong CYP2C8**

IV INCOMPATIBILITIES

◄**ALERT** ► Data for Abraxane not known; avoid mixing with other medication.
Amphotericin B complex (Abelcet, AmBisome, Amphotec), DOXOrubicin liposomal (Doxil), hydrOXYzine (Vistaril), methylPREDNISolone (SOLU-Medrol), mitoXANTRONE (Novantrone).

underlined – top prescribed drug

Side Effects section in each drug monograph specifies the frequency of particular side effects.

Adverse Reactions highlight the particularly dangerous side effects.

High Alert drugs are shaded in blue for easy identification.

Dosage in Hepatic Impairment

	Mild Impairment (AST less than 10 times upper limit of normal [ULN], bilirubin 1.25 times ULN or less)	Moderate Impairment (AST less than 10 times ULN, bilirubin 1.26–2 times ULN)	Severe Impairment (AST less than 10 times ULN, bilirubin 2.01–5 times ULN)	(AST more than 10 times ULN or bilirubin > 5 times ULN)
Breast cancer	No adjustment	Reduce dose to 200 mg/m²	Reduce dose to 130 mg/m² (may increase to 200 mg/m² in subsequent cycles)	Not recommended
NSCLC	No adjustment	Reduce dose to 75 mg/m²	Reduce dose to 50 mg/m² (may increase to 75 mg/m² in subsequent cycles)	Not recommended
Pancreatic	No adjustment	Not recommended	Not recommended	Not recommended

SIDE EFFECTS

Expected (90%–70%): Diarrhea, alopecia, nausea, vomiting. **Frequent (48%–46%):** Myalgia, arthralgia, peripheral neuropathy. **Occasional (20%–13%):** Mucositis, hypotension during infusion, pain/redness at injection site. **Rare (3%):** Bradycardia.

ADVERSE EFFECTS/TOXIC REACTIONS

Myelosuppression (anemia, neutropenia, thrombocytopenia) is an expected response to therapy, but more severe reactions including febrile neutropenia, sepsis may occur. Infections (candidiasis, respiratory tract infections, pneumonia) reported in 24% of pts. Pts with hepatic impairment may have increased risk of myelosuppression. Severe neuropathy was reported. Ocular toxicities (blurry vision, keratitis) reported in 10% of pts. Fatal interstitial lung disease (ILD), pneumonitis reported in 4% of pts. Severe hypersensitivity reactions, including anaphylaxis, may occur. Severe cardiovascular events (cardiac ischemia/infarction, chest pain, cardiac arrest, CVA, edema, hypertension, pulmonary embolism, SVT, transient ischemic attack, thrombosis) were reported.

NURSING CONSIDERATIONS

BASELINE ASSESSMENT

Obtain CBC, LFT prior to each course; pregnancy test in females of reproductive potential. Confirm compliance of effective contraception. Screen for active infection. Question history of cardiovascular disease, pulmonary disease, hepatic impairment. Receive full medication history and screen for interactions. Assess hydration status. Offer emotional support.

INTERVENTION/EVALUATION

Monitor CBC for myelosuppression; LFT for hepatotoxicity. Monitor for symptoms of hepatotoxicity (abdominal pain, jaundice, nausea, vomiting, weight loss) esp. in pts with hepatic impairment. Consider ABG, radiologic test if ILD/pneumonitis (excessive cough, dyspnea, fever, hypoxia) is suspected. Consider treatment with corticosteroids if ILD/pneumonitis is confirmed. Monitor for infections (cough, fatigue, fever). Monitor daily pattern of bowel activity, stool consistency. Monitor for ocular toxicities, hypersensitivity reactions. Monitor for symptoms of DVT (leg or arm pain/swelling), CVA (aphasia, altered mental status, headache, hemiplegia, vision loss); MI (chest

P

◆ Canadian trade name   🔖 Non-Crushable Drug   📵 High Alert drug

Saunders

NURSING DRUG HANDBOOK 2026

ROBERT J. KIZIOR, BS, RPh
Department of Pharmacy
Former Pharmacist, Alexian Brothers
   Medical Center
Elk Grove Village, Illinois
Former Adjunct Faculty Member at
   William Rainey Harper Community
   College
Palatine, Illinois

KEITH J. HODGSON, RN, BSN, CCRN
Staff Nurse, Intensive Care Unit
Former Staff Nurse, Emergency
   Department
St. Joseph's Hospital
Tampa, Florida

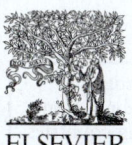

ELSEVIER

Elsevier
3251 Riverport Lane
St. Louis, Missouri 63043

SAUNDERS NURSING DRUG HANDBOOK 2026   ISBN: 978-0-443-34872-3
ISSN: 1098-8661

Previous editions copyrighted © 2025, 2024, 2023, 2022, 2021, 2020, 2019, 2018, 2017, 2016, 2015, 2014, 2013, 2012, 2011, 2010, 2009, 2008, 2007, 2006, 2005, 2004, 2003, 2002, 2001, 2000, 1999, 1998, 1997, 1996, 1995, 1994, and 1993.

International Standard Book Number: 978-0-443-4872-3

Executive Content Strategist: Sonya Seigafuse
Senior Content Development Manager: Lisa Newton
Senior Content Development Specialist: Tina Kaemmerer
Publishing Services Manager: Catherine Jackson
Senior Project Manager/Specialist: Carrie Stetz
Design Direction: Renee Duenow

Printed in China

Last digit is the print number: 9   8   7   6   5   4   3   2   1

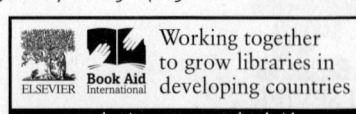

CONTENTS

AUTHOR BIOGRAPHIES

Robert J. Kizior, BS, RPh

Bob graduated from the University of Illinois School of Pharmacy and has practiced in the state of Illinois. He has worked as a hospital pharmacist for more than 40 years at Alexian Brothers Medical Center in Elk Grove Village, Illinois—a suburb of Chicago. His experience includes being the surgery satellite pharmacist, coordinating pharmacy and operating room services. He also has participated in educational programs for physicians, nurses, pharmacists, and patients, and he was formerly an adjunct faculty member at William Rainey Harper Community College in Palatine, Illinois.

An avid sports fan, Bob also has eclectic tastes in music that range from classical, big band, rock 'n' roll, and jazz to country and western. Bob spends much of his free time reviewing the professional literature to stay current on new drug information.

Keith J. Hodgson, RN, BSN, CCRN

Keith was born into a loving family in Chicago, Illinois. His mother, Barbara B. Hodgson, was an author and publisher of several medication products, and her work has been a part of his life since he was a child. By the time he was 4 years old, Keith was already helping his mother with drug cards by stacking the draft pages that were piled up throughout their home.

Because of his mother's influence, Keith contemplated becoming a nurse in college, but his mind was fully made up after he shadowed his sister in the Emergency Department. Keith received his Associates Degree in Nursing from Hillsborough Community College and his Bachelor of Science in Nursing from the University of South Florida in Tampa, Florida. Keith started his career in the Emergency Department and now works in the Trauma/Neurological/Surgical Intensive Care Unit at St. Joseph's Hospital in Tampa, Florida.

Keith's favorite interests include music, reading, Kentucky basketball, and, if he gets the chance, watching every minute of the Olympic Games.

REVIEWERS

James Graves, PharmD, MBA
Clinical Pharmacist
University of Missouri Hospital
Columbia, Missouri

Travis E. Sonnett, PharmD
VISN 20 EHRM Clinical Investigative Pharmacy
Specialist
VA Northwest Health Network—Clinical
Pharmacy Services
Washington State University College of Pharmacy
Spokane, Washington

CONSULTANTS*

Katherine B. Barbee, MSN, ANP, F-NP-C
Kaiser Permanente
Washington, District of Columbia

Marla J. DeJong, RN, MS, CCRN, CEN, Capt
Wilford Hall Medical Center
Lackland Air Force Base, Texas

Diane M. Ford, RN, MS, CCRN
Andrews University
Berrien Springs, Michigan

Denise D. Hopkins, PharmD
College of Pharmacy
University of Arkansas
Little Rock, Arkansas

Barbara D. Horton, RN, MS
Arnot Ogden Medical Center School of Nursing
Elmira, New York

Mary Beth Jenkins, RN, CCRN, CAPA
Elliott One Day Surgery Center
Manchester, New Hampshire

Kelly W. Jones, PharmD, BCPS
McLeod Family Medicine Center
McLeod Regional Medical Center
Florence, South Carolina

Linda Laskowski-Jones, RN, MS, CS, CCRN, CEN
Christiana Care Health System
Newark, Delaware

Jessica K. Leet, RN, BSN
Cardinal Glennon Children's Hospital
St. Louis, Missouri

Denise Macklin, BSN, RNC, CRNI
President, Professional Learning Systems, Inc.
Marietta, Georgia

Judith L. Myers, MSN, RN
Health Sciences Center
St. Louis University School of Nursing
St. Louis, Missouri

Kimberly R. Pugh, MSEd, RN, BS
Nurse Consultant
Baltimore, Maryland

Regina T. Schiavello, BSN, RNC
Wills Eye Hospital
Philadelphia, Pennsylvania

Gregory M. Susla, PharmD, FCCM
National Institutes of Health
Bethesda, Maryland

*The authors acknowledge the work of the consultants in previous editions.

ACKNOWLEDGMENTS

I would like to thank my co-author, Bob Kizior, for his knowledge, experience, support, and friendship. We would like to give special thanks to Sonya Seigafuse, Carrie Stetz, Tina Kaemmerer, and the entire Elsevier team for their superior dedication, hard work, and belief in us. Without this wonderful team, none of this would be possible.

Keith J. Hodgson, RN, BSN, CCRN

DEDICATION

I dedicate my work to the practicing nurse, those aspiring to become nurses, and to all health care professionals who are dedicated to the art and science of healing.

Bob Kizior, BS, RPh

I dedicate this work to my family, Jen, Brynn, and Gavin; Jen Hodgson, the love of my life; my sister, Lauren, a foundation for our family; my sister, Kathryn, for her love and support; my father, David Hodgson, the best father a son could have; my brothers-in-law, Andy and Nick, great additions to the family; the grandchildren, Paige Olivia, Logan James, Ryan James, and Dylan Boyd; and to my band of brothers, Peter, Jamie, Miguel, Ritch, George, Jon, Domingo, Ben, Craig, Pat, and Shay.

We also make a special dedication to Barbara B. Hodgson, RN, OCN. She truly was a piece of something wonderful. Barbara often gave her love and support without needing any in return and would do anything for a smile. Not only was she a colleague and a friend, she was also a small business owner, an artist, a dreamer, and an innovator. We hope the pride we offer in her honor comes close to what she always gave us. Her dedication and perseverance lives on.

Keith J. Hodgson, RN, BSN, CCRN

BIBLIOGRAPHY

American Board of Internal Medicine, Laboratory Reference Ranges, July 2023.
Drug Information Handbook for Oncology, ed 17, 2022–2023, Lexi-Comp.
Lexi-Comp's Adult Drug Information Handbook, ed 32, 2023–2024, Lexi-Comp.
Medical Letter on Drugs and Therapeutics: 2023–2024, Pharmacists Letter: 2023–2024.
Lexi-Comp's Pediatric Dosage Handbook, ed 29, ed 30, 2023–2024, Lexi-Comp.
ASHP Injectable Drug Information, 2023, American Society of Health-System Pharmacists.
US Pharmacist, 2023–2024.

NEW MEDICATIONS FOR THE 2026 EDITION

Bimekizumab-bkzx (Bimzelx)	A humanized interleukin-17A and 17F antagonist for treatment of moderate to severe plaque psoriasis in adults who are candidates for systemic therapy or phototherapy
Capivasetib (Truqap)	Kinase inhibitor, in combination with fulvestrant, for treatment of hormone receptor (HR)-positive, human epidermal growth factor receptor 2 (HER2)-negative, locally advanced or metastatic breast cancer with one or more PIK3CA/AKT1/PTEN alterations
Ceftobiprole (Zevtera)	Cephalosporin antibiotic for treatment of bacteremia, skin and skin structure infections, community acquired bacterial pneumonia
Donanemab-azbt (Kisunla)	An amyloid beta–directed antibody indicated for the treatment of early symptomatic Alzheimer's disease
Efbemalenograstim alfa-vuxw (Ryzneuta)	A leukocyte growth factor indicated to decrease the incidence of infection, as manifested by febrile neutropenia, in adults with non-myeloid malignancies receiving myelosuppressive anti-cancer drugs associated with a clinically significant incidence of febrile neutropenia
Etrasimod (Velsipity)	A sphingosine 1-phosphate receptor modulator for treatment of moderately to severely active ulcerative colitis in adults
Fruquintinib (Fruzaqla)	Kinase inhibitor for treatment of metastatic colorectal cancer (mCRC) who have been previously treated with fluoropyrimidine-, oxaliplatin-, and irinotecan-based chemotherapy, an anti-VEGF therapy, and, if RAS wild-type and medically appropriate, an anti-EGFR therapy
Gepirone (Exxua)	An azapirone antidepressant for treatment of major depressive disorder (MDD) in adults
Mirikizumab-mrkz (Omvoh)	An interleukin-23 antagonist indicated for the treatment of moderately to severely active ulcerative colitis in adults
Pirtobrutinib (Jaypirca)	Kinase inhibitor for treatment or chronic lymphocytic leukemia/small lymphocytic lymphoma (CLL/SLL); mantle cell lymphoma (MCL)
Quizartinib (Vanflyta)	Kinase inhibitor indicated for treatment of newly diagnosed acute myeloid leukemia (AML) that is FLT3 internal tandem duplication (ITD)-positive
Repotrectinib (Augtyro)	Kinase inhibitor for treatment of locally advanced or metastatic ROS1-positive non–small-cell lung cancer (NSCLC)
Tenapanor (Xphozah)	A sodium hydrogen exchanger 3 (NHE3) inhibitor indicated to reduce serum phosphorus in adults with chronic kidney disease (CKD) on dialysis

Tovorafenib (Ojemda)	A type II pan-RAF kinase inhibitor for treatment of pediatric low-grade glioma
Vonoprazan (Voquezna)	A potassium-competitive acid blocker indicated for healing and maintainance healing of all grades of erosive esophagitis and relief of heartburn associated with erosive esophagitis in adults; in combination therapy for treatment of *Helicobacter pylori* (*H. pylori*) infection in adults

PREFACE

Nurses are faced with the ever-challenging responsibility of ensuring safe and effective drug therapy for their patients. Not surprisingly, the greatest challenge for nurses is keeping up with the overwhelming amount of new drug information, including the latest FDA-approved drugs and changes to already approved drugs, such as new uses, dosage forms, warnings, and much more. Nurses must integrate this information into their patient care quickly and in an informed manner.

Saunders Nursing Drug Handbook 2026 is designed as an easy-to-use source of current drug information to help the nurse meet these challenges. What separates this book from others is that it guides the nurse through patient care to better practice and better care. This handbook contains the following:

1. **An IV compatibility chart.** This handy chart is bound into the handbook to prevent accidental loss.
2. **The Drug Classifications section.** The action and uses for some of the most common clinical and pharmacotherapeutic classes are presented. Unique to this handbook, each class provides an at-a-glance table that compares all the generic drugs within the classification according to product availability, dosages, side effects, and other characteristics. Its half-page color tab ensures you can't miss it!
3. **An alphabetical listing of drug entries by generic name.** Blue letter thumb tabs help you page through this section quickly. Information on medications that contain a Black Box Alert is an added feature of the drug entries. This alert identifies those medications for which the FDA has issued a warning that the drugs may cause serious adverse effects. Tall Man lettering, with emphasis on certain syllables to avoid confusing similar sounding/looking medications, is shown in capitalized letters (e.g., oxy**CODONE**). High Alert drugs with a color icon ⬛ are considered dangerous by The Joint Commission and the Institute for Safe Medication Practices (ISMP) because if they are administered incorrectly, they may cause life-threatening or permanent harm to the patient. The entire High Alert generic drug entry sits on a shaded background so that it's easy to spot! To make scanning pages easier, each new entry begins with a shaded box containing the generic name, pronunciation, trade name(s), fixed combination(s), and classification(s).
4. **A comprehensive reference section.** Appendixes include vital information on the correct use of oral inhalers for asthma and COPD; chronic wound care; drugs of abuse; herbals: common natural medicines; lifespan, cultural aspects, and pharmacogenomics of drug therapy; normal laboratory values; drug interactions; antidotes or reversal agents; preventing medication errors; parenteral fluid administration; and Common Terminology Criteria for Adverse Events (CTCAE). New for 2026 edition: Contraception, Hormones, and Nutrition: Enteral and Parenteral.
5. **Drugs by Disorder.** You'll find Drugs by Disorder in the front of the book for easy reference. It lists common disorders and the drugs most often used for treatment.
6. **The index.** The comprehensive index is located at the back of the book on light blue pages. Undoubtedly the best tool to help you navigate the handbook, the comprehensive index is organized by showing generic drug names in **bold**, trade names in regular type, classifications in *italics,* and the page number of the main drug entry listed first and in **bold**.

A DETAILED GUIDE TO THE SAUNDERS NURSING DRUG HANDBOOK

An intensive review by consultants and reviewers helped us to revise the **Saunders Nursing Drug Handbook** so that it is most useful in both educational and clinical practice. The main objective of the handbook is to provide essential drug information in a user-friendly format. The bulk of the handbook contains an alphabetical listing of drug entries by generic name.

To maintain the portability of this handbook and meet the challenge of keeping content current, we have also included additional information for some medications on the Evolve® Internet site. Users can also choose from 100 monographs for the most commonly used medications and customize and print drug cards. Evolve® also includes drug alerts (e.g., medications removed from the market) and drug updates (e.g., new drugs, updates on existing entries). Information is periodically added, allowing the nurse to keep abreast of current drug information.

We have incorporated the IV Incompatibilities/Compatibilities 🏵 heading. The drugs listed in this section are compatible or incompatible with the generic drug when administered directly by IV push, via a Y-site, or via IV piggyback. We have highlighted the intravenous drug administration and handling information with a special heading icon 🗐 and have broken it down by Reconstitution, Rate of Administration, and Storage.

We present entries in an order that follows the logical thought process the nurse undergoes whenever a drug is ordered for a patient:

- What is the drug?
- How is the drug classified?
- What does the drug do?
- What is the drug used for?
- Under what conditions should you **not** use the drug?
- How do you administer the drug?
- How do you store the drug?
- What is the dose of the drug?
- What should you monitor the patient for once he or she has received the drug?
- What do you assess the patient for?
- What interventions should you perform?
- What should you teach the patient?

The following are included within the drug entries:

Generic Name, Pronunciation, Trade Names. Each entry begins with the generic name and pronunciation, followed by the U.S. and Canadian trade names. Exclusively Canadian trade names are followed by a maple leaf ✦.

Black Box Alert. This feature highlights drugs that carry a significant risk of serious or life-threatening adverse effects. Black Box Alerts are ordered by the FDA.

Do Not Confuse With. Drug names that sound similar to the generic and/or trade names are listed under this heading to help you avoid potential medication errors.

Fixed-Combination Drugs. Where appropriate, fixed-combinations, or drugs made up of two or more generic medications, are listed with the generic drug.

Pharmacotherapeutic and **Clinical Classification Names.** Each entry includes both the pharmacotherapeutic and clinical classifications for the generic drug.

Action/Therapeutic Effect. This section describes how the drug is predicted to behave, with the expected therapeutic effect(s) under a separate heading.

Pharmacokinetics. This section includes the absorption, distribution, metabolism, excretion, and half-life of the medication. The half-life is bolded in blue for easy access.

Uses/Off-Label. The listing of uses for each drug includes both the FDA uses and the off-label uses. The off-label heading is shown in bold blue for emphasis.

Precautions. This heading incorporates a discussion about when the generic drug is contraindicated or should be used with caution. The cautions warn the nurse of specific situations in which a drug should be closely monitored.

Lifespan Considerations ⌛. This section includes pregnancy/lactation data and age-specific information concerning children and elderly people.

Interactions. This heading enumerates drug, food, and herbal interactions with the generic drug. As the number of medications a patient receives increases, awareness of drug interactions becomes more important. Also included is information about therapeutic and toxic blood levels in addition to effects the drug may have on lab results.

Product Availability. Each drug monograph gives the form and availability of the drug. The icon 🍂 identifies noncrushable drug forms.

Administration/Handling. Instructions for administration are given for each route of administration (e.g., IV, IM, PO, rectal). Special handling, such as refrigeration, is also included where applicable. The routes in this section are always presented in the order IV, IM, SQ, and PO, with subsequent routes in alphabetical order (e.g., Ophthalmic, Otic, Topical). **IV administration 🍂** is broken down by reconstitution, rate of administration (how fast the IV should be given), and storage (including how long the medication is stable once reconstituted).

IV Incompatibilities/IV Compatibilities ▦. These sections give the nurse the most comprehensive compatibility information possible when administering medications by direct IV push, via a Y-site, or via IV piggyback.

Indications/Routes/Dosage. Each entry provides specific dosing guidelines for adults, elderly, children, and patients with renal and/or hepatic impairment. Dose modification for toxicity has been added where applicable. Dosages are clearly indicated for each approved indication and route.

Side Effects. Side effects are defined as those responses that are usually predictable with the drug, are **not** life-threatening, and may or may not require discontinuation of the drug. Unique to this handbook, side effects are grouped by frequency listed from highest occurrence percentage to lowest so that the nurse can focus on patient care without wading through myriad signs and symptoms of side effects.

Adverse Effects/Toxic Reactions. Adverse effects and toxic reactions are very serious and often life-threatening undesirable responses that require prompt intervention from a health care provider.

Nursing Considerations. Nursing considerations are organized as care is organized:

- What needs to be assessed or done before the first dose is administered? (Baseline Assessment)
- What interventions and evaluations are needed during drug therapy? (Intervention/Evaluation)
- What teaching is needed for the patient and family? (Patient/Family Teaching)

Saunders Nursing Drug Handbook is an easy-to-use source of current drug information for nurses, students, and other health care providers. It is our hope that this handbook will help you provide quality care to your patients.

We welcome any comments to improve future editions of the handbook. Please contact us via the publisher at *http://evolve.elsevier.com/SaundersNDH*.

Robert J. Kizior, BS, RPh
Keith J. Hodgson, RN, BSN, CCRN

DRUGS BY DISORDER

Note: Not all medications appropriate for a given condition are listed, nor are those not listed inappropriate.
Generic names appear first, followed by brand names in parentheses.

Alcohol dependence
Acamprosate (Campral)
Disulfiram (Antabuse)
Gabapentin (Horizant, Neurontin)
Naltrexone (Depade, ReVia, Vivitrol)
Topiramate (Qudexy XR, Topamax, Trokendi XR)

Allergic conjunctivitis
Antihistamines
Alcaftadine (Lastacaft)
Azelastine – generic
Bepotastine (Bepreve)
Cetirizine (Zerviate)
Epinastine (Elestat)
Ketotifen (Alaway, Zaditor)
Olopatadine (Pataday, Patanol, Pazeo)
Corticosteroids
Dexamethasone (Destenza) ocular insert
Loteprednol (Alrex, Lotemax)
Prednisone (Pred Mild)
Decongestants
Naphazoline (Clear Eyes Maximum)
Naphazoline/pheniramine (Naphcon A, Opcon A)
Tetrahydrozoline (Visine AC)
Mast Cell Stabilizers
Cromolyn – generic
Lodoxamide (Alomide)
Nedocromil (Alocril)

Allergic rhinitis
Nasal spray
Antihistamines
Azelastine (Astelin, Astepro)
Azelastine/fluticasone (Dymista)
Olopatadine (Patanase)
Corticosteroids
Beclomethasone (Beconase AQ, Qnasl)
Budesonide (Rhinocort Allergy Spray)
Ciclesonide (Omnaris, Zetonna)

Flunisolide
Fluticasone (Flonase Sensimist Allergy Relief)
Mometasone (Nasonex)
Triamcinolone (Nasacort Allergy 24 HR)
Mast cell stabilizer
Cromolyn (Nasalcrom)
Anticholinergic
Ipratropium (generic)
Oral form
Antihistamines
Cetirizine (Zyrtec Allergy)
Cetirizine/pseudoephedrine (Zyrtec-D 12 hour)
Desloratadine (Clarinex)
Desloratadine/pseudoephedrine (Clarinex-D 12 hour)
Fexofenadine (Allegra)
Fexofenadine/pseudoephedrine (Allegra-D 12 hour, Allegra-D 24 hour)
Levocetirizine (Xyzal Allergy 24 hour)
Loratadine (Alavert, Claritin)
Loratadine/pseudoephedrine (Alavert-D 12 hour, Claritin-D 12 hour, Claritin-D 24 hour)
Olopatadine/mometasone (Ryaltris)
Leukotriene receptor antagonist
Montelukast (Singulair)

Alzheimer's disease
Acetylcholinesterase inhibitors
Benzgalantamine (Zunveyl)
Donepezil (Adlarity, Aricept)
Galantamine (Razadyne)
Rivastigmine (Exelon Patch)
Amyloid beta-directed monoclonal antibody
Donanemab-azbt (Kisunla)
Lecanemab (Leqembi)
NMDA receptor antagonist
Memantine (Namenda)

**NMDA receptor antagonist/
acetylcholinesterase inhibitor**
Memantine/Donepezil (Namzaric)

Angina
Amlodipine (Norvasc)
Atenolol (Tenormin)
Diltiazem (Cardizem, Dilacor)
Isosorbide (Imdur, Isordil)
Metoprolol (Lopressor)
Nadolol (Corgard)
Nicardipine (Cardene)
Nifedipine (Adalat, Procardia)
Nitroglycerin
Propranolol (Inderal)
Verapamil (Calan, Isoptin)

Ankylosing Spondylitis
NSAIDs
Diclofenac (Voltaren)
Ibuprofen (Motrin)
Naproxen (Aleve)
TNF inhibitors
Adalimumab (Humira)
Etandercept (Enbrel)
Infliximab (Remicade)
IL-17 antagonist
Ikekizumab (Taltz)
Secukinumab (Cosentyx)
Janus kinase inhibitor
Tofacitinib (Xeljanz)

Anxiety Disorders
**Selective serotonin reuptake
 inhibitors (SSRIs)**
Escitalopram (Lexapro)
Fluoxetine (Prozac)
Paroxetine (Paxil)
Sertraline (Zoloft)
**Serotonin-norepinephrine reuptake
 inhibitors (SNRIs)**
Duloxetine (Cymbalta)
Venlafaxine (Effexor XR)
Benzodiazepines
Alprazolam (Xanax)
Clonazepam (Klonopin)
Lorazepam (Ativan)
Other medications
Gabapentin (Neurontin)
Pregabalin (Lyrica)
Buspirone (generic)
Mirtazapine (Remeron)

Vilazodone (Viibryd)
Quetiapine (Seroquel)
Hydroxyzine (Vistaril)

Arrhythmias
Adenosine (Adenocard)
Amiodarone (Cordarone, Pacerone)
Digoxin (Lanoxin)
Diltiazem (Cardizem, Dilacor)
Disopyramide (Norpace)
Dofetilide (Tikosyn)
Dronedarone (Multaq)
Esmolol (Brevibloc)
Flecainide (Tambocor)
Ibutilide (Corvert)
Lidocaine
Metoprolol (Lopressor)
Mexiletine (Mexitil)
Propafenone (Rythmol)
Propranolol (Inderal)
Sotalol (Betapace)
Verapamil (Calan, Isoptin)

Arthritis, rheumatoid
Conventional DMARDs
Hydroxychloroquine (Plaquenil)
Leflunomide (Arava)
Methotrexate (Otrexup, Rasuvo, Trexall)
Sulfasalazine (Azulfidine)
Biologic agents
TNF inhibitors
Adalimumab (Humira)
Certolizumab pegol (Cimzia)
Etanercept (Enbrel)
Golimumab (Simponi, Simponi Aria)
Infliximab (Remicade, Inflectra, Renflexis)
IL-6 inhibitors
Sarilumab (Kevzara)
Tocilizumab (Actemra)
Other biologic agents
Abatacept (Orencia)
Anakinra (Kineret)
Rituximab (Rituxan)
JAK inhibitors
Baricitinib (Olumiant)
Tofacitinib (Xeljanz, Xeljanz XR)
Upadacitinib (Rinvoq)

Asthma
Short-acting beta₂ agonists (SABA)
Albuterol (ProAir HFA, Proventil HFA,
 Ventolin HFA, ProAir RespiClick)

Levalbuterol (Xopenex HFA)
Short-acting muscarinic antagonists (SAMA)
Ipratropium (Atrovent HFA)
SABA/SAMA
Albuterol/ipratropium (Combivent)
Inhaled corticosteroids (ICS)
Beclomethasone (QVAR)
Budesonide (Pulmicort)
Ciclesonide (Alvesco)
Flunisolide (Aerospan)
Fluticasone (Arnuity Ellipta, Flovent Diskus)
Mometasone (Asmanex)
Long-acting beta$_2$ agonists (LABA)
Formoterol (Perforomist)
Salmeterol (Serevent)
ICS/LABA
Budesonide/formoterol (Symbicort)
Fluticasone/vilanterol (Breo Ellipta)
Fluticasone/Salmeterol (Advair, AirDuo RespiClick, AirDuo Digihaler)
Mometasone, formoterol (Dulera)
Inhaled long-acting muscarinic antagonist (LAMA)
Tiotropium (Spiriva)
ICS/LAMA/LABA
Fluticasone/umeclidinium/vilanterol (Trelegy Ellipta)
Leukotriene modifiers
Montelukast (Singulair)
Zafirlukast (Accolate)
Zileuton (Zyflo)
Anti-immunoglobulin E antibody
Omalizumab (Xolair)
Anti-interleukin-5 (IL-5) antibodies
Benralizumab (Fasenra)
Mepolizumab (Nucala)
Reslizumab (Cinqair)
Anti-interleukin-4 (IL-4) antibody
Dupilumab (Dupixent)
TSLP blocker
Tezepelumab (Tezspire)

Atrial fibrillation
Oral anticoagulants
Vitamin K antagonist
Warfarin (Coumadin)
Direct thrombin inhibitor
Dabigatran (Pradaxa)

Direct factor Xa inhibitors
Apixaban (Eliquis)
Edoxaban (Savaysa)
Rivaroxaban (Xarelto)
Rate control
Beta-adrenergic blockers
Atenolol (Tenormin)
Bisoprolol
Carvedilol (Coreg, Coreg CR)
Metoprolol (Lopressor, Toprol XL)
Nadolol (Corgard)
Propranolol (Inderal LA, InnoPran XL)
Calcium channel blockers
Diltiazem (Cardizem CD, Cartia XT, Taztia XT, Tiazac)
Verapamil (Calan, Verelan)
Other
Digoxin (Digitek, Lanoxin)
Rhythm control
Amiodarone (Pacerone)
Dronedarone (Multaq)
Dofetilide (Tikosyn)
Flecainide
Propafenone (Rythmol SR)
Sotalol (Betapace, Sotalol AF)

Attention-deficit hyperactivity disorder (ADHD)
Amphetamine stimulants
Amphetamine (Adzenys XR-ODT, Dyanavel XR)
Dextroamphetamine (Dexedrine, ProCentra, Xelstrym, Zenzedi)
Dextroamphetamine transdermal (Xelstrym)
Lisdexamfetamine (Vyvanse)
Mixed amphetamine (dextroamphetamine and amphetamine salts) (Adderall, Adderall XR, Mydayis)
Methylphenidate stimulants
Dexmethylphenidate (Focalin, Focalin XR)
Methylphenidate (Aptensio XR, Concerta, Cotempla XR-ODT, Daytrana, Jornay PM, Metadate CD, Methylin, QuilliChew ER, Quillivant XR, Ritalin)
Serdexmethylphenidate/dexmethylphenidate (Azstarys)
Nonstimulants
Atomoxetine (Strattera)
Clonidine (Kapvay, Onyda XR)

Guanfacine (Intuniv)
Viloxazine ER (Qelbree)

Benign prostatic hypertrophy (BPH)
Alpha$_1$ adrenergic antagonists
Alfuzosin (Uroxatral)
Doxazosin (Cardura)
(Cardura XL)
Terazosin (generic)
Silodosin (Rapaflo)
Tamsulosin (Flomax)
5α-reductase inhibitors
Dutasteride (Avodart)
Finasteride (Proscar)
Phosphodiesterase-5 inhibitor
Tadalafil (Cialis)
Anticholinergic drugs
Darifenacin (generic)
Fesoterodine (Toviaz)
Oxybutynin (generic)
Solifenacin (Vesicare)
Tolterodine (Detrol, Detrol LA)
Trospium (generic)
Beta$_3$ adrenergic agonists
Mirabegron (Myrbetriq)
Vibegron (Gemtesa)

Bipolar depression
Cariprazine (Vraylar)
Lumateperone (Caplyta)
Lurasidone (Latuda)
Olanzapine/fluoxetine (Symbyax)
Quetiapine (Seroquel, Seroquel XR)

Bipolar disorder
Antimanic
Lithium (Lithobid)
Antiepileptics
Carbamazepine (Tegretol)
Lamotrigine (Lamictal)
Valproic acid (Depakote)
Antipsychotics
Aripiprazole (Abilify)
Asenapine (Saphris)
Cariprazine (Vraylar)
Iloperidone (Fanapt)
Lumateperone (Caplyta)
Lurasidone (Latuda)
Olanzapine (Zyprexa)
Olanzapine/fluoxetine (Symbyax)

Quetiapine (Seroquel)
Risperidone (Risperdal)
Ziprasidone (Geodon)

Bladder hyperactivity
Anticholinergic drugs
Darifenacin (generic)
Fesoterodine (Toviaz)
Oxybutynin (generic)
Solifenacin (Vesicare)
Tolterodine (Detrol, Detrol LA)
Trospium (generic)
Beta$_3$ adrenergic agonists
Mirabegron (Myrbetriq)
Vibegron (Gemtesa)

Bronchospasm
Albuterol (Proventil, Ventolin)
Bitolterol (Tornalate)
Levalbuterol (Xopenex)
Metaproterenol (Alupent)
Salmeterol (Serevent)
Terbutaline (Brethine)

Cerebrovascular accident (CVA)
Aspirin
Clopidogrel (Plavix)
Heparin
Nimodipine (Nimotop)
Prasugrel (Effient)
Warfarin (Coumadin)

Chronic obstructive pulmonary disease (COPD)
Inhaled short-acting antimuscarinic
Ipratropium (Atrovent HFA)
Inhaled short-acting Beta$_2$ agonists (SABA)
Albuterol (ProAir HFA, Proventil HFA, Ventolin HFA)
Levalbuterol (Xopenex HFA)
Inhaled (SABA)/(SAMA)
Albuterol/Ipratropium (Combivent Respimat)
Inhaled long-acting Beta$_2$ agonists (LABA)
Arformoterol (Brovana)
Formoterol (Perforomist)
Olodaterol (Striverdi Respimat)
Salmeterol (Serevent Diskus)

Inhaled long-acting antimuscarinic agents (LAMA)
Aclidinium (Tudorza Pressair)
Glycopyrrolate (Seebri Neohaler)
Revefenacin (Yupelri)
Tiotropium (Spiriva Respimat)
Umeclidinium (Incruse Ellipta)
Inhaled (LABA)/(LAMA)
Glycopyrrolate/formoterol (Bevespi)
Tiotropium/olodaterol (Stiolto Respimat)
Umeclidinium/vilanterol (Anoro Ellipta)
Inhaled corticosteroids (ICS)
Beclomethasone (QVAR)
Budesonide (Pulmicort)
Ciclesonide (Alvesco)
Fluticasone furoate (Arnuity Ellipta)
Fluticasone (ArmonAir RespiClick ArmonAir Digihaler, Flovent Diskus, Flovent HFA)
Mometasone (Asmanex HFA, Asmanex Twisthaler)
Inhaled ICS (LABA)
Budesonide/formoterol (Symbicort)
Fluticasone/salmeterol (Advair Diskus Advair HFA, AirDuo RespiClick, AirDuo Digihaler)
Fluticasone/vilanterol (Breo Ellipta)
ICS (LABA)/(LAMA)
Budesonide/glycopyrrolate/formoterol (Breztri)
Fluticasone/vilanterol/umeclidinium (Trelegy Ellipta)
Phosphodiesterase-4 inhibitor
Roflumilast (Daliresp)
Phospodiesterase 3 and 4 inhibitor
Ensifentrine (Ohtuvayre)

Constipation (Chronic Idiopathic)
Fiber
Methylcellulose (Citrucel)
Psyllium (Metamucil)
Osmotic Laxatives
Lactulose (Kristalose)
Polyethylene glycol (Miralax)
Stimulant Laxatives
Bisacodyl (Dulcolax)
Senna (Senokot)
Secretagogues
Linaclotide (Linzess)

Lubiprostone (Amitiza)
Plecanatide (Trulance)

Crohn's disease
Aminosalicylates (5-ASAs)
Mesalamine (Apriso, Asacol HD, Delzicol, Lialda, Pentasa)
5-ASA prodrugs
Balsalazide (Colazal)
Olsalazine (Dipentum)
Sulfasalazine (Azulfidine, Azulfidine EN-tabs)
Corticosteroids
Prednisone (Generic)
Budesonide (Ortikos, Uceris)
Immunosuppressants
Azathioprine (Azasan, Imuran)
Mercaptopurine (Purixan)
Methotrexate (Trexall)
TNF blockers
Adalimumab (Humira)
Certolizumab pegol (Cimzia)
Infliximab (Avsola, Inflectra, Remicade, Renflexis)
Integrin receptor antagonist
Vedolizumab (Entyvio)
Interleukin-12 and -23 antagonist
Risankizumab (Skyrizi)
Ustekinumab (Stelara)

Cystic fibrosis
Elexacaftor/tezacaftor/ivacaftor (Trikafta)
Ivacaftor (Kalydeco)
Lumacaftor/ivacaftor (Orkambi)
Tezacaftor/ivacaftor (Symdeco)

Deep vein thrombosis (DVT)
Dalteparin (Fragmin)
Edoxaban (Savaysa)
Enoxaparin (Lovenox)
Heparin
Tinzaparin (Innohep)
Warfarin (Coumadin)

Depression
SSRIs
Citalopram (Celexa)
Escitalopram (Lexapro)
Fluoxetine (Prozac, Prozac Weekly)

Paroxetine (Paxil, Paxil CR, Pexeva)
Sertraline (Zoloft)
SNRIs
Desvenlafaxine (Pristiq, Khedezla)
Duloxetine (Cymbalta, Drizalma
   Sprinkle)
Levomilnacipran (Fetzima)
Venlafaxine (Effexor XR)
TCAs
Amitriptyline (Elavil)
Amoxapine (generic)
Desipramine (Norpramin)
Imipramine (generic)
Nortriptyline (Pamelor)
MAOIs
Isocarboxazid (Marplan)
Phenelzine (Nardil)
Selegiline (Emsam)
Tranylcypromine (Parnate)
Other
Aripiprazole (Abilify)
Brexanolone (Zulresso)
Bupropion (Wellbutrin)
Bupropion/dextromethorphan
   (Auvelity)
Cariprazine (Vraylar)
Esketamine (Spravato)
Gepirone (Exxua)
Mirtazapine (Remeron, Remeron
   SolTab)
Olanzapine/fluoxetine (Symbyax)
Trazodone (Oleptro)
Vilazodone (Viibryd)
Vortioxetine (Trintellix)
Zuralolone (Zurzuvae)

Diabetes
Biguanides
Metformin (Glucophage, Glucophage
   XR, Glumetza, Fortamet, Riomet)
Sulfonylureas
Glimepiride (Amaryl)
Glipizide (Glucotrol, Glucotrol XL)
Glyburide (Glynase)
GLP-1 receptor agonists
Albiglutide (Tanzeum)
Dulaglutide (Trulicity)
Exenatide (Byetta, Bydureon)
Liraglutide (Victoza)
Lixisenatide (Adlyxin)

Semaglutide (Ozempic)
Tirzepatide (Mounjaro)
DDP-4 inhibitors
Alogliptin (Nesina)
Linagliptin (Tradjenta)
Saxagliptin (Onglyza)
Sitagliptin (Januvia)
SGLT2 inhibitors
Bexagliflozin (Brenzavvy)
Canagliflozin (Invokana)
Dapagliflozin (Farxiga)
Empagliflozin (Jardiance)
Ertugliflozin (Steglatro)
Meglitinides
Nateglinide (Starlix)
Repaglinide (Prandin)
Thiazolidinediones
Pioglitazone (Actos)
Alpha-glucosidase inhibitors
Acarbose (Precose)
Miglitol (Glyset)
Other
Colesevelam (Welchol)
Bromocriptine (Cycloset)
Pramlintide (Symlin)
Insulin
Rapid-acting
Insulin aspart (Fiasp, Novolog)
Insulin glulisine (Apidra)
Insulin lispro (Admelog, Humalog,
   Lyumjev)
Insulin inhalation powder (Afrezza)
Regular insulin
Humulin R
Novolin R
Intermediate insulin
NPH (Humulin N, Novolin N)
Long-acting insulin
Insulin detemir (Levemir)
Insulin glargine (Basaglar, Lantus,
   Semglee, Toujeo)
Insulin degludec (Tresiba)

Diabetic peripheral neuropathy
Amitriptyline (Elavil)
Bupropion (Wellbutrin)
Capsaicin (Trixaicin)
Carbamazepine (Tegretol)
Citalopram (Celexa)
Desipramine (Norpramin)
Duloxetine (Cymbalta)

Gabapentin (Neurontin)
Lamotrigine (Lamictal)
Lidocaine patch (Lidoderm)
Nortriptyline (Pamelor)
Oxcarbazepine (Trileptal)
Oxycodone (OxyContin)
Paroxetine (Paxil)
Pregabalin (Lyrica)
Tramadol (Ultram)
Valproic acid (Depakote)
Venlafaxine, extended-release
    (Effexor XR)

Diarrhea

Bismuth subsalicylate (Pepto-Bismol)
Diphenoxylate and atropine (Lomotil)
Fidaxomicin (Dificid)
Kaolin-pectin (Kaopectate)
Loperamide (Imodium)
Octreotide (Sandostatin)
Rifaximin (Xifaxan)

Edema

Amiloride (Midamor)
Bumetanide (Bumex)
Chlorthalidone (Hygroton)
Ethacrynic acid (Edecrin)
Furosemide (Lasix)
Hydrochlorothiazide (Hydrodiuril)
Indapamide (Lozol)
Metolazone (Zaroxolyn)
Spironolactone (Aldactone)
Torsemide (Demadex)
Triamterene (Dyrenium)

Endometriosis
Andrgenics
Danazol
Hormonal contraceptives
Ethinyl estradiol in combination
    with norethindrone, norgestrel,
    levonorgestrel, desogestrel
GnRH agonists
Goserelin
Naferelin
Leuprolide
GnRH antagonists
Elagolix
Relugolix plus estradiol 1 mg and
    norethiindone 0.5 mg
Progestins
Norethindrone

Medroxyprogesterone
Levonorgestrel IUD system

Epilepsy

Brivaracetam (Briviact)
Carbamazepine (Tegretol)
Cenobamate (Xcopri)
Clobazam (Onfi)
Clonazepam (Klonopin)
Clorazepate (Tranxene)
Diazepam (Valium)
Eslicarbazepine (Aptiom)
Ethosuximide (Zarontin)
Ezogabine (Potiga)
Fosphenytoin (Cerebyx)
Gabapentin (Neurontin)
Lacosamide (Vimpat)
Lamotrigine (Lamictal, Lamictal ODT,
    Lamictal XR)
Levetiracetam (Keppra)
Lorazepam (Ativan)
Midazolam (Versed)
Oxcarbazepine (Trileptal)
Perampanel (Fycompa)
Phenobarbital
Phenytoin (Dilantin)
Pregabalin (Lyrica)
Primidone (Mysoline)
Rufinamide (Banzel)
Tiagabine (Gabitril)
Topiramate (Qudexy XR, Topamax,
    Trokendi XR)
Valproic acid (Depakene, Depakote)
Vigabatrin (Sabril)
Zonisamide (Zonegran)

Esophageal reflux, esophagitis

Cimetidine (Tagamet)
Dexlansoprazole (Dexilant)
Esomeprazole (Nexium)
Famotidine (Pepcid)
Lansoprazole (Prevacid)
Nizatidine (Axid)
Omeprazole (Prilosec)
Pantoprazole (Protonix)
Rabeprazole (AcipHex)

Fever

Acetaminophen (Tylenol)
Aspirin
Ibuprofen (Advil, Caldolor, Motrin)
Naproxen (Aleve, Anaprox, Naprosyn)

Fibromyalgia
Acetaminophen (Tylenol)
Amitriptyline (Elavil)
Carisoprodol (Soma)
Citalopram (Celexa)
Cyclobenzaprine (Flexeril)
Duloxetine (Cymbalta)
Fluoxetine (Prozac)
Gabapentin (Neurontin)
Milnacipran (Savella)
Paroxetine (Paxil)
Pregabalin (Lyrica)
Tramadol (Ultram)
Venlafaxine (Effexor)

Febrile neutropenia
Eflapegrastim (Rolvedon)
Filgrastim (Neupogen)
Pegfilgrastim (Neulasta, Fulphla,
   Udenyca, Ziextenzo, Nyvepria,
   Stimufend)
Gastric cancer
Chemotherapy
5-Fluorouracil
Capcitabine
Carboplatin
Cisplatin
Docetaxel
Irinotecan
Oxaliplatin
Paclitaxel
Immunotherapy
Dostarlimab
Ipilimumab
Nivolumab
Pembrolizumab
Targeted therapy
Fam-trastuzumab
Ramucirumab
Trastuzumab

Gastritis
Cimetidine (Tagamet)
Famotidine (Pepcid)
Nizatidine (Axid)

Gastroesophageal reflux disease (GERD)
H_2 receptor antagonists
Cimetidine (Tagamet HB)
Famotidine (Pepcid)
Nizatidine

Proton pump inhibitors (PPIs)
Dexlansoprazole (Dexilant)
Esomeprazole (Nexium)
Lansoprazole (Prevacid)
Omeprazole (Prilosec)
Pantoprazole (Protonix)
Rabeprazole (AcipHex)
Potassium competitive acid blocker
Vonoprazan (Voquezna)

Glaucoma
Acetazolamide (Diamox)
Apraclonidine (Iopidine)
Betaxolol (Betoptic)
Bimatoprost (Lumigan)
Bimatoprost Implant (Durysta)
Brimonidine (Alphagan)
Brinzolamide (Azopt)
Carbachol
Dorzolamide (Trusopt)
Echothiophate iodide (Phospholine)
Latanoprost (Xalatan)
Levobunolol (Betagan)
Pilocarpine (Isopto Carpine)
Tafluprost (Zioptan)
Timolol (Timoptic)
Travoprost (Travatan)
Travoprost implant (iDose TR)
Unoprostone (Rescula)

Gout
Anti-inflammatory agents
Anakinra (Kineret)
Canakinumab (Ilaris)
Celecoxib (Celebrex)
Colchicine (Colcrys, Mitigare)
Ibuprofen (Motrin)
Naproxen (Naprosyn)
Prednisone
Urate-lowering agents
Allopurinol (Zyloprim)
Febuxostat (Uloric)
Probenecid
Pegloticase (Krystexxa)

Heart failure
Angiotensin-converting enzyme (ACE) inhibitors
Captopril
Enalapril (Vasotec)
Fosinopril
Lisinopril (Prinivil, Zestril)

Quinapril (Accupril)
Ramipril (Altace)
Angiotensin receptor blockers (ARBs)
Candesartan (Atacand)
Losartan (Cozaar)
Valsartan (Diovan)
Angiotensin receptor-neprilysin inhibitor
Sacubitril/valsartan (Entresto)
Beta-adrenergic blockers
Bisoprolol
Carvedilol (Coreg)
Metoprolol succinate (Toprol XL)
Soluble guanylate cyclase (sGS) inhibitor
Vericiguat (Verquvo)
Cardiac glycoside
Digoxin (Digitek, Lanoxin)
Diuretics (loop)
Bumetanide (Bumex)
Furosemide (Lasix)
Torsemide (Demadex)
HCN channel blocker
Ivabradine (Corlanor)
Mineralocorticoid receptor antagonists
Eplerenone (Inspra)
Finerenone (Kerendia)
Spironolactone (Aldactone)
SGLT2
Dapagliflozin (Farxiga)
Empagliflozin (Jardiance)
Sotagliflozin (Inpefa)
Vasodilators
Isosorbide/hydralazine (BiDil)
Hydralazine (generic)

Hepatitis B
Adefovir (Hepsera)
Entecavir (Baraclude)
Lamivudine (Epivir)
Peginterferon alpha-2a (Pegasys)
Telbivudine (Tyzeka)
Tenofovir (Viread)

Hepatitis C
Elbasvir/grazoprevir (Zepatier)
Glecaprevir/pibrentasvir (Mavyret)
Ledipasvir/sofosbuvir (Harvoni)
Ombitasvir/paritaprevir/ritonavir (Technivie)

Ombitasvir/paritaprevir/ritonavir/ dasabuvir (Viekira Pak)
Peginterferon alfa-2a (Pegasys)
Peginterferon alfa-2b (Pegintron)
Ribavirin (Copegus, Rebetol, Ribasphere)
Simeprevir (Olysio)
Sofosbuvir (Sovaldi)
Sofosbuvir/velpatasvir (Epclusa)
Sofosbuvir/velpatasvir/voxilaprevir (Vosevi)

Human immunodeficiency virus (HIV)
Nucleoside reverse transcriptase inhibitors (NRTIs)
Abacavir (Ziagen)
Emtricitabine (Emtriva)
Lamivudine (Epivir)
Tenofovir DF (Viread)
Zidovudine (Retrovir)
Non-nucleoside reverse transcriptase inhibitors (NNRTIs)
Doravirine (Pifeltro)
Efavirenz (Sustiva)
Etravirine (Intelence)
Nevirapine (Viramune)
Rilpivirine (Edurant)
Protease inhibitors (PIs)
Atazanavir (Reyataz)
Darunavir (Prezista)
Fosamprenavir (Lexiva)
Tipranavir (Aptivus)
Fusion inhibitors
Enfuvirtide (Fuzeon)
CCR5 antagonist
Maraviroc (Selzentry)
Integrase strand transfer inhibitors (INSTIs)
Cabotegravir (Vocabria)
Dolutegravir (Tivicay)
Raltegravir (Isentress)
Attachment inhibitor
Fostemsavir (Rukobia)
Post-attachment inhibitor
Ibalizumab (Trogarzo)
Capsid inhibitor
Lenacapavir (Sunlenca)
Pharmacokinetic enhancers
Cobicistat (Tybost)
Ritonavir (Norvir)

Combinations
Abacavir/lamivudine (Epzicom)
Abacavir/dolutegravir/lamivudine
   (Triumeq)
Abacavir/lamivudine/zidovudine (Trizivir)
Atazanavir/cobicistat (Evotaz)
Bictegravir/emtricitabine/tenofovir TAF
   (Biktarvy)
Cabotegravir/rilpivirine (Cabenuva)
Darunavir/cobicistat (Prezcobix)
Darunavir/cobicistat/emtricitabine/
   tenofovir TAF (Symtuza)
Dolutegravir/lamivudine (Dovato)
Dolutegravir/rilpirivine (Juluca)
Doravirine/lamivudine/tenofovir TDF
   (Delstrigo)
Efavirenz/emtricitabine/tenofovir TDF
   (Atripla)
Efavirenz/lamivudine/tenofovir TDF (Symfi,
   Symfi Lo)
Elvitegravir/cobicistat/emtricitabine/
   tenofovir TAF (Genvoya)
Elvitegravir/cobicistat/emtricitabine/
   tenofovir TDF (Stribild)
Emtricitabine/rilpivirine/tenofovir TAF
   (Odefsey)
Emtricitabine/rilpivirine/tenofovir TDF
   (Complera)
Emtricitabine/tenofovir TAF (Descovy)
Emtricitabine/tenofovir TDF (Truvada)
Lamivudine/tenofovir TDF (Cimduo)
Lamivudine/zidovudine (Combivir)
Lopinavir/ritonavir (Kaletra)

Hyperphosphatemia
Calcium acetate (Calphron)
Ferric citrate (Auryxia)
Lanthanum (Fosrenol)
Sevelamer (Renvela)
Sucroferric oxyhydroxide (Velphoro)
Tenapanor (Xphozah)

Hypertension
Thiazide diuretics
Hydrochlorothiazide
Indapamide (generic)
Metolazone (generic)
Loop diuretics
Bumetanide (Bumex)
Ethacrynic acid (Edecrin)
Furosemide (Lasix)
Torsemide (Soaanz)

Aldosterone antagonists
Eplerenone (Inspra)
Spironolactone (Aldactone)
ACE inhibitors
Benazepril (Lotensin)
Enalapril (Vasotec)
Lisinopril (Zestril, Prinivil)
Quinapril (Accupril)
Ramipril (Altace)
ARBs
Azilsartan (Edarbi)
Candesartan (Atacand)
Irbesartan (Avapro)
Losartan (Cozaar)
Valsartan (Diovan)
Calcium channel blockers
dihydropyridines
Amlodipine (Norvasc)
Nifedipine (Adalat CC, Procardia XL)
Nondihydropyridines
Diltiazem (Cardizem LA, Taztia XT)
Verapamil (Calan)
Beta-blockers
Atenolol (Tenormin)
Carvedilol (Coreg, Coreg CR)
Labetalol
Metoprolol (Lopressor, Toprol XL)
Nebivolol (Bystolic)
Central alpha-adrenergic agonists
Clonidine (Catapres)
Direct renin inhibitor
Aliskiren (Tekturna)
Direct vasodilators
Hydralazine (Apresoline)

Hypertriglyceridemia
Atorvastatin (Lipitor)
Colesevelam (Welchol)
Fenofibrate (Tricor)
Fluvastatin (Lescol)
Gemfibrozil (Lopid)
Icosapent (Vascepa)
Lovastatin (Mevacor)
Niacin (Niaspan)
Omega-3 acid ethyl esters (Lovaza)
Pravastatin (Pravachol)
Rosuvastatin (Crestor)
Simvastatin (Zocor)

Hyperuricemia
Allopurinol (Zyloprim)
Febuxostat (Uloric)

Pegloticase (Krystexxa)
Probenecid (Benemid)

Hypotension
Dobutamine (Dobutrex)
Dopamine (Intropin)
Ephedrine
Epinephrine
Norepinephrine (Levophed)
Phenylephrine (Neo-Synephrine)

Hypothyroidism
Levothyroxine (Levoxyl, Synthroid)
Liothyronine (Cytomel)
Thyroid

Idiopathic thrombocytopenic purpura (ITP)
Cyclophosphamide (Cytoxan)
Dexamethasone (Decadron)
Hydrocortisone (Solu-Cortef)
Immune globulin intravenous
Methylprednisolone (Solu-Medrol)
Prednisone
Rh$_o$(D) immune globulin (RhoGAM)
Rituximab (Rituxan)

Immunosuppressive agents
Azathioprine (Imuran)
Basiliximab (Simulect)
Belatacept (Nulijix)
Cyclosporine (Neoral, Gengraf)
Everolimus (Zortress)
Mycophenolate (CellCept, Myfortic)
Sirolimus (Rapamune)
Tacrolimus (Prograf, Envarsus XR)

Insomnia
Benzodiazepine receptor agonists
Eszopiclone (Lunesta)
Zaleplon (Sonata)
Zolpidem (Ambien, Zolpimist, Edluar, Intermezzo)
Benzodiazepines
Estazolam
Flurazepam
Lorazepam (Ativan)
Temazepam (Restoril)
Melatonin receptor agonist
Ramelteon (Rozerem)
Orexin receptor antagonist

Daridorexant (Quviviq)
Lemborexant (Dayvigo)
Suvorexant (Belsomra)
Tricyclic antidepressant
Doxepin (Silenor)

Inflammatory bowel disease
Corticosteroids
Budesonide (Ortikos)
Prednisone (generic)
Hydrocortisone (Cortenema)
Immunomodulators
Azathioprine (Imuran)
Mercaptopurine (generic)
Methotrexate (generic)
TNF inhibitors
Adalimumab (Humira)
Certolizumab (Cimzia)
Golimumab (Simponi)
Infliximab (Remicade)
Integrin receptor antagonist
Vedolizumab (Entyvio)
Interleukin (IL)-12 and -23 antagonist
Ustekinumab (Stelara)
Interleukin (IL)-23 antagonist
Risankizumab (Skyrizi)
Janus kinase (JAK) inhibitors
Tofacitinib (Xeljanz)
Upadacitinib (Rinvoq)
Sphingosine 1-phosphate (S1P) receptor modulator
Ozanimod (Zeposia)
Insert for irritable bowel disease
Corticosteroids
Budesonide (Ortikos)
Prednisone (generic)
Hydrocortisone (Cortenema)
Immunomodulators
Azathioprine (Imuran)
Mercaptopurine (generic)
Methotrexate (generic)
TNF inhibitors
Adalimumab (Humira)
Certolizumab (Cimzia)
Golimumab (Simponi)
Infliximab (Remicade)
Integrin receptor antagonist
Vedolizumab (Entyvio)
Interleukin (IL)-12 and -23 antagonist

Ustekinumab (Stelara)
Interleukin (IL)-23 antagonist
Risankizumab (Skyrizi)
Janus kinase (JAK) inhibitors
Tofacitinib (Xeljanz)
Upadacitinib (Rinvoq)
Sphingosine 1-phosphate (S1P) receptor modulator
Ozanimod (Zeposia)

Irritable bowel syndrome with constipation
Chloride channel activator
Lubiprostone (Amitiza)
Guanylate cyclase-C receptor agonist
Linaclotide (Linzess)
Plecanatide (Trulance)
Sodium hydrogen exchanger 3 inhibitor
Tenapanor (Ibsrela)

Irritable bowel syndrome with diarrhea
Antibiotic
Rifaximin (Xifaxan)
Mu-opioid receptor agonist/ delta-opioid receptor antagonist
Eluxadoline (Viberzi)
5-HT modulators
Alosetron (Lotronex)

Adenosine triphosphate-citrate lyase (ACL) inhibitor
Bempedoic acid (Nexletol)

Lipid disorders
Statins
Atorvastatin (Lipitor)
Fluvastatin (Lescol)
Lovastatin (Altoprev)
Pitavastatin (Livalo)
Pravastatin (Pravachol)
Rosuvastatin (Crestor)
Simvastatin (Zocor)
Cholesterol absorption inhibitor
Ezetimibe (Zetia)
PCSK9 inhibitors
Alirocumab (Praluent)
Evolocumab (Repatha)
PCSK9-directed siRNA

Inclisiran (Leqvio)
Bile acid sequestrants
Colesevelam (Welchol)
Colestipol (Colestid)
Cholestyramine (Questran)
Fibrates
Gemfibrozil (Lopid)
Fenofibrate (Lipofen, Lofibra, Tricor, Antara, Fibricor, Trilipix)
Fish oil
Icosapent ethyl (Vascepa)
Omega-3 acid ethyl esters (Lovaza)

Migraine prevention
Beta blockers
Metoprolol (Lopressor)
Propranolol (generic)
Antiseizure medications
Valproate (Depakote)
Topiramate (Topamax)
Serotonin-norepinephrine reuptake inhibitors
Duloxetine (Cymbalta)
Venlafaxine (Effexor)
CGRP monoclonal antibodies (oral)
Atogepant (Qulipta)
Rimegepant (Nurtec ODT)
CGRP monoclonal antibodies (parenteral)
Eptinezumab-jjmr (Vyepti)
Erenumab-aooe (Aimovig)
Fremanezumab (Ajovy)
Galcanezumab-gnlm (Emgality)

Migraine treatment
Triptans
Almotriptan (Axert)
Eletriptan (Relpax)
Frovatriptan (Frova)
Naratriptan (Amerge)
Rizatriptan (Maxalt)
Sumatriptan (Imitrex)
Zolmitriptan (Zomig, Zomig-ZMT)
Calcitonin gene-related peptide (GCRP) antagonists
Rimegepant (Nurtec)
Ubrogepant (Ubrelvy)
Zavegepant (Zavzpret)
5-HT receptor agonist
Lasmiditan (Reyvow)
Ergots

Dihydroergotamine (DHE 45, Migranal, Trudhesa)
Ergotamine (Ergomar)
Ergotamine/caffeine (Cafergot)

Multiple sclerosis (MS)
Alemtuzumab (Lemtrada)
Cladribine (Mavenclad)
Dalfampridine (Ampyra)
Dimethyl fumarate (Tecfidera)
Diroximel fumarate (Vumerity)
Fingolimod (Gilenya)
Glatiramer (Copaxone)
Interferon beta-1a (Avonex, Rebif)
Interferon beta-1b (Betaseron, Extavia)
Mitoxantrone (Novantrone)
Natalizumab (Tysabri)
Ocrelizumab (Ocrevus)
Ocrelizumab/hyaluronidase (Ocrevus Zunovo)
Ofatumumab (Kesimpta)
Ozanimod (Zeposia)
Peginterferon beta-1a (Plegridy)
Ponesimod (Ponvory)
Rituximab (Rituxan)
Siponimod (Mayzent)
Ublituximab (Briumvi)
Teriflunomide (Aubagio)

Myasthenia gravis
Cholinesterase inhibitors
Pyridostigmine (Mestanon)
Corticosteroids
Prednisone
Immunosuppressants
Azathioprine (Azasan, Imuran)
Cyclosporine (Gengraf, Neoral, Sandimmune)
Methotrexate (Trexall)
Mycophenolate (Myfortic)
Tacrolimus (Prograf)
Immunomodulating therapy
Plasmapheresis
IV Immune Globulin
Biological therapy
Efgartigimod alfa (Vyvgart)
Ravulizumab (Ultomiris)
Rozanolixizumab (Rystiggo)
Zilucoplan (Zilbrysq)

Myelodysplastic syndrome
Azacitidine (Vidaza)
Clofarabine (Clolar)
Decitabine (Dacogen)
Lenalidomide (Revlimid)

Myocardial infarction (MI)
Alteplase (Activase)
Aspirin
Atenolol (Tenormin)
Captopril (Capoten)
Clopidogrel (Plavix)
Dalteparin (Fragmin)
Diltiazem (Cardizem, Dilacor)
Enalapril (Vasotec)
Enoxaparin (Lovenox)
Heparin
Lidocaine
Lisinopril (Prinivil, Zestril)
Metoprolol (Lopressor)
Morphine
Nitroglycerin
Propranolol (Inderal)
Quinapril (Accupril)
Ramipril (Altace)
Reteplase (Retavase)
Warfarin (Coumadin)

Nausea
Aprepitant (Emend)
Chlorpromazine (Thorazine)
Dexamethasone (Decadron)
Dimenhydrinate (Dramamine)
Dronabinol (Marinol)
Droperidol (Inapsine)
Fosaprepitant (Emend)
Fosnetupitant/palonosetron (Akynzeo)
Granisetron (Kytril)
Hydroxyzine (Vistaril)
Lorazepam (Ativan)
Meclizine (Antivert)
Metoclopramide (Reglan)
Nabilone (Cesamet)
Ondansetron (Zofran)
Ozanimod (Zeposia)
Palonosetron (Aloxi)
Prochlorperazine (Compazine)
Promethazine (Phenergan)
Rolapitant (Varubi)

Obsessive-compulsive disorder (OCD)
Citalopram (Celexa)
Clomipramine (Anafranil)
Escitalopram (Lexapro)
Fluoxetine (Prozac)
Fluvoxamine (Luvox)
Paroxetine (Paxil)
Sertraline (Zoloft)

OCD (Augmentation)
Aripiprazole (Abilify)
Olanzapine (Zyprexa)
Paliperidone (Invega)
Quetiapine (Seroquel)
Risperidone (Risperdal)

Onychomycosis
Ciclopirox (Ciclodan)
Efinaconazole (Jublia)
Fluconazole (Diflucan)
Griseofulvin (Generic)
Itraconazole (Sporanox)
Tavaborole (Kerydin)
Terbinafine (Generic)

Opioid use disorder
Maintenance treatment
Buprenorphine (Brixadi, Sublocade)
Buprenorphine/Naloxone (Suboxone, Zubsolv)
Methadone (generic)
Naltrexone (Vivitrol)
Overdose reversal
Nalmefene (Opvee)
Naloxone (LifEMS Naloxone, Zimhi, ReVive, Narcan, Kloxxado)

Organ transplant, rejection prophylaxis
Azathioprine (Imuran)
Basiliximab (Simulect)
Belatacept (Nulojix)
Cyclophosphamide (Cytoxan, Neosar)
Cyclosporine (Sandimmune)
Daclizumab (Zenapax)
Everolimus (Zortress)
Mycophenolate (CellCept)
Sirolimus (Rapamune)
Tacrolimus (Prograf)

Osteoarthritis
Acetaminophen (Tylenol)
Celecoxib (Celebrex)
Diclofenac (Cataflam, Pennsaid, Voltaren)
Duloxetine (Cymbalta)
Etodolac (Lodine)
Flurbiprofen (Ansaid)
Ibuprofen (Motrin)
Ketoprofen (Orudis)
Meloxicam (Mobic)
Nabumetone (Relafen)
Naproxen (Naprosyn)
Sulindac (Clinoril)
Tramadol (Ultram)

Osteoporosis
Bisphosphonates
Alendronate (Binosto, Fosamax)
Ibandronate (Boniva)
Risedronate (Actonel, Atelvia)
Zoledronic acid (Reclast)
Anti-RANK ligand antibody
Denosumab (Prolia)
Parathyroid hormone receptor agonists
Abaloparatide (Tymlos)
Teriparatide (Forteo)
Sclerostin inhibitor
Romosozumab (Evenity)
Selective estrogen receptor modulator (SERM)
Raloxifene
Conjugated estrogens/bazedoxifene (Duavee)
Calcitonin
Miacalcin injection
Nasal spray (generic)

Overactive bladder
Anticholinergic drugs
Darifenacin (generic)
Fesoterodine (Toviaz)
Oxybutynin (generic)
Solifenacin (Vesicare)
Tolterodine (Detrol, Detrol LA)
Trospium (generic)
Beta₃ adrenergic agonists
Mirabegron (Myrbetriq)
Vibegron (Gemtesa)

Paget's disease
Alendronate (Fosamax)
Calcitonin (Miacalcin)
Etidronate (Didronel)
Pamidronate (Aredia)
Risedronate (Actonel)
Tiludronate (Skelid)
Zoledronic acid (Reclast)

Pain, mild to moderate
Acetaminophen (Tylenol)
Aspirin
Celecoxib (Celebrex)
Codeine
Diclofenac (Cataflam, Voltaren, Zipsor)
Diflunisal (Dolobid)
Etodolac (Lodine)
Flurbiprofen (Ansaid)
Ibuprofen (Advil, Caldolor, Motrin)
Ketorolac (Toradol)
Naproxen (Anaprox, Naprosyn)
Salsalate (Disalcid)
Tramadol (Ultram)

Pain, moderate to severe
Butorphanol (Stadol)
Fentanyl (Onsolis, Sublimaze)
Hydromorphone (Dilaudid)
Methadone (Dolophine)
Morphine (MS Contin)
Morphine/naltrexone (Embeda)
Nalbuphine (Nubain)
Oxycodone (OxyFast, Roxicodone)
Oxymorphone (Opana)
Ziconotide (Prialt)

Panic attack disorder
Alprazolam (Xanax)
Clonazepam (Klonopin)
Paroxetine (Paxil)
Sertraline (Zoloft)
Venlafaxine (Effexor)

Parkinson's disease
Adenosine A Receptor Antagonist
Istradefylline (Nourianz)
Carbidopa/levodopa
Immediate-release (Sinemet)
Orally disintegrating
Sustained-release (Sinemet CR)
Extended-release (Crexont, Rytary)
Intrajejunal infusion (Duopa)
Foscarbidopa/foslevodopa (Vyalev)
Dopamine agonists
Apomorphine (Apokyn, Kynmobi)
Pramipexole (Mirapex, Mirapex ER)
Ropinirole (Requip, Requip XL)
Rotigotine (Neupro)
COMT inhibitors
Entacapone (Comtan)
Opicapone (Ongentys)
Tolcapone (Tasmar)
MAO-B inhibitors
Rasagiline (Azilect)
Safinamide (Xadago)
Selegiline (Eldepryl, Zelapar)

Peptic ulcer disease
H₂ receptor antagonists
Cimetidine (Tagamet HB)
Famotidine (Pepcid)
Nizatidine
Proton pump inhibitors (PPIs)
Dexlansoprazole (Dexilant)
Esomeprazole (Nexium)
Lansoprazole (Prevacid)
Omeprazole (Prilosec)
Pantoprazole (Protonix)
Rabeprazole (AcipHex)

Peripheral neuropathy
Capsaicin
Carbamazepine
Duloxetine
Gabapentin
Lidocaine (5% patch)
Pregabalin

Pneumonia
Amoxicillin (Amoxil)
Amoxicillin/clavulanate (Augmentin)
Ampicillin (Polycillin)
Azithromycin (Zithromax)
Cefaclor (Ceclor)
Cefpodoxime (Vantin)
Ceftriaxone (Rocephin)
Cefuroxime (Kefurox, Zinacef)
Clarithromycin (Biaxin)
Co-trimoxazole (Bactrim, Septra)
Erythromycin
Gentamicin (Garamycin)
Levofloxacin (Levaquin)

Linezolid (Zyvox)
Moxifloxacin (Avelox)
Piperacillin/tazobactam (Zosyn)
Tobramycin (Nebcin)
Vancomycin (Vancocin)

Pneumonia, *Pneumocystis jirovecii*
Atovaquone (Mepron)
Clindamycin (Cleocin)
Co-trimoxazole (Bactrim, Septra)
Pentamidine (Pentam)
Trimethoprim (Proloprim)

Post-traumatic stress disorder (PTSD)
Amitriptyline (Elavil)
Aripiprazole (Abilify)
Citalopram (Celexa)
Escitalopram (Lexapro)
Fluoxetine (Prozac)
Imipramine (Tofranil)
Lamotrigine (Lamictal)
Olanzapine (Zyprexa)
Paroxetine (Paxil)
Phenelzine (Nardil)
Prazosin (Minipress)
Propranolol (Inderal)
Quetiapine (Seroquel)
Risperidone (Risperdal)
Sertraline (Zoloft)
Topiramate (Topamax)
Valproic acid (Depakote)
Venlafaxine (Effexor)
Ziprasidone (Geodon)

Postpartum depression
SSRIs
Citalopram (Celexa)
Escitalopram (Lexapro)
Fluoxetine (Prozac)
Paroxetine (Paxil)
Sertraline (Zoloft)
SNRIs
Duloxetine (Cymbalta)
Fluvoxamine (generic)
Venlafaxine (Effexor XR)
Atypical Antidepressants
Bupropion (Wellbutrin)
Mirtazapine (Remeron)
GABA Receptor Modulators
Brexanolone (Zulresso)
Zuranolone (Zurzuvae)

Prostate cancer
Luteinizing hormone–releasing hormone agonists
Leuprolide (Lupron Depot)
Goserelin (Zoladex)
Triptorelin (Trelstar)
Luteinizing hormone–releasing hormone antagonists
Degarelix (Firmagon)
Relugolix (Orgovyx)
Antiandrogens
Abiraterone (Zytiga)
Bicalutamide (Casodex)
Flutamide (Eulexin)
Nilutamide (Nilandron)
Apalutamide (Erleada)
Darolutamide (Nubeqa)
Enzalutamide (Xtandi)
Rucaparib (Rubraca)
Olaparib (Lynparza)
Immunotherapy
Pembrolizumab (Keytruda)
Sipuleucel-T (Provenge)
Chemotherapy
Docetaxel (Taxotere)
Cabazitaxel (Jevtana)
Mitoxantrone

Pruritus
Amcinonide (Cyclocort)
Cetirizine (Zyrtec)
Clemastine (Tavist)
Clobetasol (Temovate)
Cyproheptadine (Periactin)
Desloratadine (Clarinex)
Desonide (Tridesilon)
Desoximetasone (Topicort)
Diphenhydramine (Benadryl)
Fluocinolone (Synalar)
Fluocinonide (Lidex)
Halobetasol (Ultravate)
Hydrocortisone (Cort-Dome, Hytone)
Hydroxyzine (Atarax, Vistaril)
Prednisolone (Prelone)
Prednisone (Deltasone)
Promethazine (Phenergan)

Psoriasis
Vitamin D analogs
Calcipotriene (Dovonex, Sorilux)

Calcitriol (Vectical)
Retinoids
Acitretin (Soriatane)
Tazarotene (Tazorac)
Phosphodiesterase 4 (PDE4)
inhibitor
Apremilast (Otezla)
Roflumilast (Zoryve)
Immunosuppressants
Cyclosporine (Neoral)
Methotrexate (Otrexup, Rasuvo)
Steroid-free aryl hydrocarbon
    receptor agonist
Tapinarof (Vtama)
TNF inhibitors
Adalimumab (Humira)
Certolizumab pegol (Cimzia)
Etanercept (Enbrel)
Infliximab (Remicade, Inflectra,
    Renflexis)
IL 12-23 antagonist
Ustekinumab (Stelara)
IL 17A antagonists
Brodalumab (Siliq)
Ixekizumab (Taltz)
Secukinumab (Cosentyx)
IL 17A/17F
Bimekizumab (Bimzelx)
IL 23 antagonists
Guselkumab (Tremfya)
Risankizumab (Skyrizi)
Tildrakizumab (Ilumya)
Tyrosine kinase 2 inhibitor
Deucravacitinib (Sotyktu)

Psychotic disorders (see
Schizophrenia)

Pulmonary arterial hypertension
Ambrisentan (Letairis)
Bosentan (Tracleer)
Epoprostenol (Flolan)
Iloprost (Ventavis)
Macitentan (Opsumit)
Riociguat (Adempas)
Selexipag (Uptravi)
Sildenafil (Revatio)
Tadalafil (Adcirca)
Treprostinil (Remodulin, Tyvaso)

Respiratory distress syndrome (RDS)
Beractant (Survanta)

Calfactant (Infasurf)
Poractant alfa (Curosurf)

Restless legs syndrome
Cabergoline (Dostinex)
Carbamazepine (Tegretol)
Carbidopa/levodopa (Sinemet)
Clonazepam (Klonopin)
Gabapentin (Horizant, Neurontin)
Levodopa
Pramipexole (Mirapex)
Pregabalin (Lyrica)
Ropinirole (Requip)
Rotigotine (Neupro)

Schizophrenia
Aripiprazole (Abilify)
Asenapine (Saphris, Secuado)
Brexpiprazole (Rexulti)
Cariprazine (Vraylar)
Clozapine (Clozaril)
Iloperidone (Fanapt)
Lumateperone (Caplyta)
Lurasidone (Latuda)
Olanzapine/samidorphan (Lybalvi)
Olanzapine (Zyprexa, Zyprexa Zydis)
Paliperidone (Erzofri, Invega, Invega
    Hafyera, Invega Sustenna)
Quetiapine (Seroquel, Seroquel XR)
Risperidone (Risperdal, Uzedy)
Xanomeline/Trospium (Cobenfy)
Ziprasidone (Geodon)

Seasonal affective disorder
Bupropion XL (Wellbutrin XL)
Desvenlafaxine (Pristiq)
Duloxetine (Cymbalta)
Escitalopram (Lexapro)
Fluoxetine (Prozac)
Paroxetine (Paxil)
Sertraline (Zoloft)
Venlafaxine (Effexor XR)

Sickle cell disease
Crizanlizumab (Adakveo)
Exagamlogene (Casgevy)
L-glutamine (Endari)
Hydroxyurea (Droxia, Xromi)
Lovotibeglogene (Lyfgenia)
Voxelotor (Oxbryta)

Smoking cessation
Bupropion (Zyban)
Nicotine (NicoDerm, Nicotrol)
Varenicline (Chantix)

Tardive dyskinesia
Deutetrabenazine (Austedo)
Valbenazine (Ingrezza)

Thyroid disorders
Levothyroxine (Levoxyl, Synthroid)
Liothyronine (Cytomel)
Thyroid

Transient ischemic attack (TIA)
Aspirin
Clopidogrel (Plavix)
Prasugrel (Effient)
Warfarin (Coumadin)

Tremor
Atenolol (Tenormin)
Chlordiazepoxide (Librium)
Diazepam (Valium)
Lorazepam (Ativan)
Metoprolol (Lopressor)
Nadolol (Corgard)
Propranolol (Inderal)

Tuberculosis (TB)
Bedaquiline (Sirturo)
Cycloserine (Seromycin)
Ethambutol (Myambutol)
Isoniazid (INH)
Pyrazinamide
Rifabutin (Mycobutin)
Rifampin (Rifadin)
Rifapentine (Priftin)

Ulcerative colitis
Aminosalicylates (5-ASAs)
Mesalamine (Apriso, Asacol HD,
   Delzicol, Lialda, Pentasa)
5-ASA prodrugs
Balsalazide (Colazal)
Olsalazine (Dipentum)
Sulfasalazine (Azulfidine, Azulfidine
   EN-tabs)
Corticosteroids
Prednisone (Generic)
Budesonide (Uceris)

Immunosuppressants
Azathioprine (Azasan, Imuran)
Mercaptopurine (Purixan)
TNF blockers
Adalimumab (Humira)
Golimumab (Simponi)
Infliximab (Avsola, Inflectra, Remicade,
   Renflexis)
Integrin receptor antagonist
Vedolizumab (Entyvio)
Interleukin-12 and -23 antagonist
Ustekinumab (Stelara)
Interleukin-23 antagonist
Mirikizumab (Omvoh)
IL-23 antagonist
Risankizumab (Skyrizi)
Janus kinase (JAK) inhibitor
Tofacitinib (Xeljanz, Xeljanz XR)
**Sphingosine 1-phosphate receptor
   modulator**
Etrasimod (Velsipity)
Ozanimod (Zeposia)

Urticaria
Cetirizine (Quzyttir, Zyrtec)
Cimetidine (Tagamet)
Clemastine (Tavist)
Cyproheptadine (Periactin)
Diphenhydramine (Benadryl)
Hydroxyzine (Atarax, Vistaril)
Loratadine (Claritin)

Venous thromboembolism
Unfractionated heparin
Heparin
**Low-molecular-weight heparins
   (LMWHs)**
Dalteparin (Fragmin)
Enoxaparin (Lovenox)
Factor Xa inhibitor
Fondaparinux (Arixtra)
Vitamin K antagonist
Warfarin (Jantoven)
Direct thrombin inhibitor
Dabigatran (Pradaxa)
Factor Xa inhibitors
Apixaban (Eliquis)
Edoxaban (Savaysa)
Rivaroxaban (Xarelto)

Vertigo
Dimenhydrinate (Dramamine)

Diphenhydramine (Benadryl)
Meclizine (Antivert)
Scopolamine (Trans-Derm Scop)

Vomiting

Aprepitant (Emend)
Chlorpromazine (Thorazine)
Dexamethasone (Decadron)
Dimenhydrinate (Dramamine)
Dronabinol (Marinol)
Droperidol (Inapsine)
Fosaprepitant (Emend)
Granisetron (Kytril)
Hydroxyzine (Vistaril)
Lorazepam (Ativan)
Meclizine (Antivert)
Metoclopramide (Reglan)
Nabilone (Cesamet)
Ondansetron (Zofran)
Palonosetron (Aloxi)
Prochlorperazine (Compazine)
Promethazine (Phenergan)
Rolapitant (Varubi)
Scopolamine (Trans-Derm Scop)
Trimethobenzamide (Tigan)

Weight management

Sympathomimetic amines
Benzphetamine
Diethylpropion
Phendimetrazine
Phentermine (Adipex, Lomaira)
Phentermine/topiramate (Qsymia)
Hydrogel
Plenity (oral superabsorbent hydrogel)
Lipase inhibitor
Orlistat (Alli, Xenical)
Opioid antagonist/antidepressant
Naltrexone/bupropion (Contrave)
GLP-1 receptor agonist
Liraglutide (Saxenda)
Semaglutide (Wegovy)
Tirzepatide (Zepbound)
Melanocortin 4 (MC4) receptor agonist
Setmelanotide (Imcivree)

Zollinger-Ellison syndrome

Aluminum salts
Cimetidine (Tagamet)
Esomeprazole (Nexium)
Famotidine (Pepcid)
Lansoprazole (Prevacid)
Omeprazole (Prilosec)
Pantoprazole (Protonix)
Rabeprazole (AcipHex)

DRUG CLASSIFICATION CONTENTS

allergic rhinitis

Alzheimer's disease agents

angiotensin-converting enzyme (ACE) inhibitors

angiotensin II receptor antagonists

antianxiety agents

antiarrhythmics

antibiotics

antibiotic: aminoglycosides

antibiotic: carbapenems

antibiotic: cephalosporins

antibiotic: fluoroquinolones

antibiotic: macrolides

antibiotic: penicillins

anticoagulants/antiplatelets/ thrombolytics

antidepressants

antidiabetics

antidiarrheals

antifungals: systemic mycoses

antiglaucoma agents

antihistamines

antihyperlipidemics

antihypertensives

antimigraine

antipsychotics

antiseizure medications

antivirals

asthma/COPD

attention deficit/hyperactivity disorder (ADHD)

benign prostatic hyperplasia

beta-adrenergic blockers

calcium channel blockers

cancer treatment

corticosteroids

diuretics

gastroesophageal reflux disease (GERD) and peptic ulcer disease (PUD)

heart failure

hepatitis C virus infection

human immunodeficiency virus (HIV) infection

hypertension

immunosuppressive agents

insomnia

irritable bowel syndrome

laxatives

multiple sclerosis

nonsteroidal anti-inflammatory drugs (NSAIDs)

osteoporosis

Parkinson's disease treatment

rheumatoid arthritis

skeletal muscle relaxants

smoking cessation agents

weight management

Allergic Rhinitis (formerly rhinitis preparations)

USES

Relieve symptoms associated with allergic rhinitis. These symptoms include rhinorrhea, nasal congestion, pruritus, sneezing, postnasal drip, nasal pain.

Allergic rhinitis or hay fever is an inflammation of the nasal airways occurring when an allergen (e.g., pollen) is inhaled. This triggers antibody production. The antibodies bind to mast cells, which contain histamine. Histamine is released, causing symptoms of allergic rhinitis.

ACTION

Intranasal corticosteroids: Depress migration of polymorphonuclear leucocytes and fibroblasts, reverse capillary permeability, and stabilize nasal membranes to prevent/control inflammation. First-line therapy for moderate to severe symptoms or where nasal congestion is the dominant complaint.

Intranasal antihistamines: Reduce histamine-mediated symptoms of allergic rhinitis, including pruritus, sneezing, rhinorrhea, watery eyes. Second-line therapy for intermittent nasal symptoms where congestion is not dominant.

Intranasal mast cell stabilizers: Inhibit the mast cell release of histamine and other inflammatory mediators.

Intranasal anticholinergics: Block acetylcholine in the nasal mucosa. Effective in treating rhinorrhea associated with allergic rhinitis.

Intranasal decongestants: Vasoconstrict the respiratory mucosa, provide short-term relief of nasal congestion. Used only as adjuvant therapy for 3–5 days.

Oral antihistamines (second generation): First-line therapy for mild symptoms or where sneezing/itching is primary complaint (see antihistamine classification).

Oral decongestants: For primary complaint of nasal congestion.

CORTICOSTEROIDS—INTRANASAL

Generic (Brand)	Adult Dose	Pediatric Dose	Side Effects (Class)
Beclomethasone (Beconase AQ) (Qnasl) (Children's Qnasl)	Beconase AQ: 1–2 sprays in each nostril 2 times/day Qnasl: 80 mcg/spray: 2 sprays in each nostril once daily	Beconase AQ: **6–11 yrs:** 1–2 sprays in each nostril 2 times/day Qnasl: **12 yrs and older:** 2 sprays in each nostril once daily Children's Qnasl: **4–11 yrs:** 1 spray in each nostril daily	Mild dryness, irritation, burning, stinging, bleeding of nasal mucosa, throat irritation, epistaxis, headache
Budesonide (Rhinocort Allergy)	2 sprays in each nostril daily	6–11 yrs: 1–2 sprays in each nostril daily	

Generic (Brand)	Adult Dose	Pediatric Dose	Side Effects (Class)
Ciclesonide (Omnaris, Zetonna)	Omnaris: 2 sprays in each nostril daily Zetonna: 1 spray in each nostril daily	Omnaris: **6 yrs and older:** 2 sprays in each nostril once daily Zetonna: **12 yrs and older:** 1 spray in each nostril daily	
Flunisolide	2 sprays in each nostril 2 or 3 times/day	**6–14 yrs:** 2 sprays in each nostril 2 times/day or 1 spray in each nostril 3 times/day	
Fluticasone (Flonase Sensimist, Allergy Relief, Children's Flonase Sensimet Allergy Relief)	2 sprays in each nostril once daily × 7 days, then Relief, Flonase Sensimist: 1–2 sprays in each nostril once daily	**2–11 yrs:** 1 spray in each nostril daily	
Fluticasone/Azelastine (Dymista)	1 spray ir each nostril 2 times/day	**6 yrs and older:** 1 spray in each nostril 2 times/day	
Mometasone (Nasonex)	2 sprays in each nostril daily	**2–11 yrs:** 1 spray in each nostril daily	
Triamcinolone (Nasacort Allergy 24 HR, Nasacort AQ)	2 sprays in each nostril daily	**2–5 yrs:** 1 spray in each nostril once daily **6–11 yrs:** 1–2 sprays in each nostril daily	
ANTIHISTAMINES—INTRANASAL			
Azelastine 0.1%, 0.15%	0.1%: 1–2 sprays in each nostril 2 times/day 0.15%: 1–2 sprays in each nostril two times/day or 2 sprays in each nostril once daily	0.1%: **5–11 yrs:** 1 spray in each nostril 2 times/day 0.15%: **6–11 yrs:** 1 spray in each nostril 2 times/day	Nasal discomfort, epistaxis, somnolence, headache
Azelastine/Fluticasone (Dymista)	1 spray in each nostril 2 times/day	**6 yrs and older:** 1 spray in each nostril 2 times/day	
Olopatadine (Patanase)	2 sprays in each nostril 2 times/day	**6–11 yrs:** 1 spray in each nostril 2 times/day	
Olopatadine/Mometasone (Ryaltris)	2 sprays in each nostril 2 times/day	**12 yrs and older:** 2 sprays in each nostril 2 times/day	

MAST CELL STABILIZERS

Generic (Brand)	Adult Dose	Pediatric Dose	Side Effects
Cromolyn (NasalCrom)	1 spray in each nostril 3–4 times/day	**2 yrs and older:** 1 spray in each nostril 3–4 times/day	Nasal irritation, unpleasant taste

ANTICHOLINERGICS

Generic (Brand)	Adult Dose	Pediatric Dose	Side Effects
Ipratropium (Atrovent) 0.06%	2 sprays in each nostril 3–4 times/day	**5 yrs and older:** 2 sprays in each nostril 3–4 times/day	

DECONGESTANTS

Generic (Brand)	Adult Dose	Pediatric Dose	Side Effects
Oxymetazoline (Afrin, Neo-Synephrine 12 HR)	2–3 sprays in each nostril 2 times/day	**6–11 yrs:** 2–3 sprays in each nostril 2 times/day	Insomnia, tachycardia, nervousness, nausea, vomiting, transient burning, headache, rebound congestion if used longer than 72 hrs
Phenylephrine (Neo-Synephrine Cold and Sinus, Vicks Sinus)	2–3 drops/sprays in each nostril q4h as needed (0.25% or 0.5%)	**6–11 yrs:** 2–3 drops/sprays (0.25%) in each nostril q4h as needed **1–5 yrs:** 2–3 drops/sprays (0.125%) in each nostril q4h as needed	Restlessness, nervousness, headache, rebound nasal congestion, burning, stinging, dryness

Alzheimer's Disease

Alzheimer's Disease (AD) is a progressive disorder that damages/destroys nerve cells in the brain. Over time, there is a gradual loss of cognitive functions (e.g., ability to remember, use of language, ability to recognize familiar places/people). AD accounts for 60%–80% of all dementia cases. AD features include amyloid plaques and neurofibrillary tangles in the brain. A third feature is a loss of connection between nerve cells (neurons) in the brain. Although there is no cure for AD, there are efforts ongoing to find better ways to treat the disease, delay its onset, and prevent development.

Medications used to treat AD include:

Acetylcholinesterase inhibitors: Stops the breakdown of acetylcholine by delaying formation of the enzyme acetylcholinesterase. This increase of acetylcholine in the central nervous system improves cognitive deficits.

N-methyl-D-aspartate receptor antagonist: Regulates neurotransmitters and may improve thinking, memory, and speaking skills.

Amyloid beta-directed monoclonal antibodies: (Aducanumab): Reduces brain amyloid plaque (protein deposits). *(Lecanemab):* Removes a sticky protein from the brain that is thought to cause advancement of AD. It has shown to slow cognitive and functional decline in early stages of AD. *(Donanemab-azbt):* Reduces amyloid beta plaques.

ACETYLCHOLINESTERASE INHIBITORS

Name	Uses	Availability	Dose/Titration	Adverse Effects
Donepezil (Aricept, Aricept ODT)	Mild, moderate, severe AD	**T:** 5 mg, 10 mg, 23 mg **ODT:** 5 mg, 10 mg	Initially, 5 mg once daily, may increase to 10 mg once daily after 4–6 wks. After 3 months, if suboptimal response, may increase to 23 mg once daily.	Nausea, vomiting, abdominal cramping, diarrhea, bradycardia, syncope
Galantamine (Razadyne, Razadyne ER)	Mild, moderate AD	**T:** 4 mg, 8 mg, 12 mg **OS:** 4 mg/mL **ER:** 8 mg, 16 mg, 24 mg	**T, OS:** Initially, 4 mg bid; may increase to 8 mg bid after 4 wks, then to 12 mg bid after additional 4 wks **ER:** Initially, 8 mg once daily, may increase to 16 mg once daily after 4 wks, then to 24 mg once daily after additional 4 wks	Nausea, vomiting, diarrhea, weight loss, decreased appetite, syncope
Rivastigmine (Exelon, Exelon Patch)	Mild, moderate AD Patch also approved for severe AD	**C:** 1.5 mg, 3 mg, 4.5 mg, 6 mg **OS:** 2 mg/mL **PATCH:** 4.6 mg/24 hrs, 9.5 mg/24 hrs, 13.3 mg/24 hrs	**C, OS:** Initially, 1.5 mg bid, may increase in increments of 1.5 mg bid every 2 wks up to 6 mg bid **PATCH:** Initially, 4.6 mg/24h. May increase to 9 mg/24h after 4 wks, then to 13.3 mg/24h	Nausea, vomiting, abdominal cramping, diarrhea, bradycardia, syncope, loss of appetite, weight loss

Continued

Name	Uses	Availability	Dose/Titration	Adverse Effects
NMDA Receptor Antagonist				
Memantine (Namenda, Namenda XR)	Moderate, severe AD	**T:** 5 mg, 10 mg **OS:** 2 mg/mL **XR:** 7 mg, 14 mg, 21 mg, 28 mg	**T. OS:** Initially, 5 mg once daily, may increase in increments of 5 mg/wk up to 10 mg bid **XR:** Initially, 7 mg once daily. May increase by 7 mg/day every wk up to 28 mg/day	Dizziness, headache, diarrhea, constipation, confusion
NMDA Receptor Antagonist/ Acetylcholinesterase Inhibitor				
Memantine/donepezil (Namzaric)	Moderate, severe AD	**ER:** 14/10 mg, 28/10 mg	**14/10 mg:** Once daily in evening in patients previously stabilized on memantine 5 mg bid or 14 mg once daily and donepezil 10 mg once daily **28/10 mg:** Once daily in evening in patients previously stabilized on memantine 10 mg bid or 28 mg once daily and donepezil 10 mg once daily	Refer to individual agents for adverse effects
Amyloid Beta-Directed Monoclonal Antibody				
Donanemab-azbt (Kisunla)	AD	**I:** 350 mg/20 mL (17.5 mg/mL) in a single-dose vial.	700 mg as an IV infusion over 30 min q4wks for first 3 doses, then 1,400 mg q4wks	Amyloid-related imaging abnormalities (ARIA): Temporary swelling in areas of the brain; headache, confusion, dizziness, vision changes, nausea, aphasia, weakness, seizure
Lecanemab-irmb (Leqembi)	AD	**I:** 100 mg/mL (2 mL, 5 mL) vials	10 mg/kg diluted, then administered as an IV infusion over 1 hr q2wks	Infusion-related reactions, HA, amyloid-related imaging abnormalities with edema (ARIA-E)

C, Capsule; *ER,* extended-release; *I,* injection; *OS,* oral solution; *T,* tablet; *XR,* extended-release.

Angiotensin-Converting Enzyme (ACE) Inhibitors

USES

Treatment of hypertension (HTN), adjunctive therapy for heart failure (HF).

ACTION

Antihypertensive: Inhibits angiotensin-converting enzyme (ACE). ACE catalyzes conversion of angiotensin I to angiotensin II, a potent vasoconstrictor that also stimulates aldosterone secretion by adrenal cortex. Beneficial effects in HTN/HF appear to be suppression of the renin-angiotensin-aldosterone system. Reduces peripheral arterial resistance.

HF: Decreases peripheral vascular resistance (afterload), pulmonary capillary wedge pressure (preload); improves cardiac output, exercise tolerance.

ACE INHIBITORS

Name	Availability	Uses	Usual Adult Dosage	Frequent or Severe Side Effects
Benazepril (Lotensin)	**T:** 5 mg, 10 mg, 20 mg, 40 mg	HTN	**HTN:** 10–40 mg/day in 1 or 2 divided doses	**Class Effects** Cough, hypotension, rash, acute renal failure (in pts with renal artery stenosis), angioedema, hyperkalemia, mild-moderate loss of taste, hepatotoxicity, pancreatitis, blood dyscrasias, renal damage
Captopril	**T:** 12.5 mg, 25 mg, 50 mg, 100 mg	HTN HF	**HTN:** 25–150 mg/day in 2 or 3 divided doses **HF:** Initially, 6.25 mg 3 times/day. Target: 50 mg 3 times/day	
Enalapril (Vasotec)	**T:** 2.5 mg, 5 mg, 10 mg, 20 mg **IV:** 1.25 mg/mL	HTN HF	**HTN:** 5–40 mg once/day or divided bid **HF:** Initially, 2.5 mg 2 times/day. Target: 10–20 mg bid	
Fosinopril	**T:** 10 mg, 20 mg, 40 mg	HTN HF	**HTN:** 10–40 mg once daily **HF:** Initially, 5–10 mg once daily Target: 40 mg once daily	

Continued

ANGIOTENSIN-CONVERTING ENZYME (ACE) INHIBITORS—cont'd

ACE INHIBITORS

Name	Availability	Uses	Usual Adult Dosage	Frequent or Severe Side Effects
Lisinopril (Prinivil, Zestril)	**T:** 2.5 mg, 5 mg, 10 mg, 20 mg, 40 mg	HTN HF	**HTN:** 5–40 mg once daily **HF:** Initially, 2.5–5 mg once daily. Target: 40 mg once daily	
Moexipril	**T:** 7.5 mg, 15 mg	HTN	**HTN:** 7.5–30 mg/day in 1–2 divided doses	
Perindopril	**T:** 2 mg, 4 mg, 6 mg	HTN	**HTN:** 4–16 mg once daily	
Quinapril (Accupril)	**T:** 5 mg, 10 mg, 20 mg, 40 mg	HTN HF	**HTN:** 10–80 mg/day in 1 or 2 divided doses **HF:** Initially, 5 mg 2 times/day. Target: 20 mg 2 times/day.	
Ramipril (Altace)	**C:** 1.25 mg, 2.5 mg, 5 mg, 10 mg	HTN HF	**HTN:** 2.5–20 mg once daily or divided bid **HF:** Initially, 1.25–2.5 mg once daily. Target: 10 mg once daily	
Trandolapril	**T:** 1 mg, 2 mg, 4 mg	HTN HF	**HTN:** 1–4 mg once daily **HF:** Initially, 1 mg once daily. Target: 4 mg once daily	

C, Capsules; *HF,* heart failure; *HTN,* hypertension; *T,* tablets.

Angiotensin II Receptor Antagonists

USES

Treatment of hypertension (HTN) alone or in combination with other antihypertensives. Treatment of heart failure (HF).

ACTION

Angiotensin II receptor antagonists (AIIRA) block vasoconstrictor and aldosterone-secreting effects on angiotensin II by selectively blocking the binding of angiotensin II to AT₁ receptors in vascular smooth muscle and the adrenal gland, causing vasodilation and a decrease in aldosterone effects.

ANGIOTENSIN II RECEPTOR ANTAGONISTS

Name	Availability	Uses	Usual Adult Dosage	Frequent or Severe Side Effects
Azilsartan (Edarbi)	T: 40 mg, 80 mg	HTN	40–80 mg once daily	**Class Effects** Hypotension, rash, acute renal failure (in pts with renal artery stenosis), hyperkalemia, mild-moderate loss of taste, hepatotoxicity, pancreatitis, blood dyscrasias, renal damage
Candesartan (Atacand)	T: 4 mg, 8 mg, 16 mg, 32 mg	HTN HF	**HTN:** 8–32 mg once daily **HF:** Initially, 4–8 mg once daily. Target: 32 mg once daily	
Eprosartan (Teveten)	T: 400 mg, 600 mg	HTN	600–800 mg once daily	
Irbesartan (Avapro)	T: 75 mg, 150 mg, 300 mg	HTN Nephropathy	**HTN:** 150–300 mg once daily **Nephropathy:** 150–300 mg once daily	
Losartan (Cozaar)	T: 25 mg, 50 mg, 100 mg	HTN Nephropathy HF	**HTN:** 25–100 mg/day in 1 or 2 divided doses **Nephropathy:** Initially, 25–50 mg/day; may increase to 100 mg/day **HF:** Initially, 25–50 mg once daily. Target: 150 mg once daily	
Olmesartan (Benicar)	T: 5 mg, 20 mg, 40 mg	HTN	20–40 mg once daily	

Continued

ANGIOTENSIN II RECEPTOR ANTAGONISTS—cont'd

Name	Availability	Uses	Usual Adult Dosage	Frequent or Severe Side Effects
Telmisartan (Micardis)	**T:** 40 mg, 80 mg	HTN CV risk reduction	**HTN:** 20–80 mg once daily **CV risk reduction:** 80 mg once daily	
Valsartan (Diovan)	**T:** 80 mg, 160 mg	HTN HF	**HTN:** 80–320 mg once daily **HF:** Initially, 20–40 mg 2 times/day. Target: 160 mg 2 times/day	
		Post MI	**Post MI:** Initially, 20 mg 2 times/day. Titrate to target of 160 mg 2 times/day	

CV, Cardiovascular; *HF,* heart failure; *HTN,* hypertension; *MI,* myocardial infarction; *T,* tablets.

Anxiety

USES

Anxiety disorders (generalized anxiety disorder [GAD]), panic disorder, and social anxiety disorder (SAD) are the most common form of psychiatric illness. A selective serotonin reuptake inhibitor (SSRI) or a serotonin-norepinephrine reuptake inhibitor (SNRI) is generally used for initial treatment of anxiety disorders. Benzodiazepines can provide immediate relief of anxiety symptoms and are often used as adjuncts to SSRIs or SNRIs. They are for short-term relief of anxiety symptoms and are not intended to be used long term. Another medication, buspirone, a 5-HT1a receptor partial agonist, is approved as monotherapy for treatment of anxiety but is mainly used as an adjunct to other drugs.

SELECTIVE SEROTONIN REUPTAKE INHIBITORS (SSRIS)

Name	Availability	Usual Adult Dosage	Side Effects
Escitalopram (Lexapro)	**T:** 5 mg, 10 mg, 20 mg	**GAD:** 10 mg once daily	**Class:** Restlessness, sleep disturbances, nausea, diarrhea, headache, fatigue, sexual dysfunction, weight gain
Fluoxetine (Prozac)	**C:** 1C mg, 20 mg, 40 mg **T:** 10 mg, 20 mg 60 mg **S:** 20 mg/5 mL	**Panic disorder:** 20–60 mg once daily	
Paroxetine (Paxil, Paxil CR)	**T:** 10 mg, 20 mg, 30 mg, 40 mg **Susp:** 10 mg/5 mL **T:ER:** 12.5 mg, 25 mg, 37.5 mg	**GAD:** 20–50 mg once daily **Panic disorder:** 10–60 mg once daily **SAD:** 20–60 mg once daily **Panic disorder:** 12.5–75 mg once daily **SAD:** 12.5–37.5 once daily	
Sertraline (Zoloft)	**T:** 20 mg, 50 mg, 100 mg **S:** 20 mg/mL	**Panic disorder, SAD:** 25–200 mg once daily	

C, Capsules; *ER,* extended-release; *GAD,* generalized anxiety disorder; *S,* solution; *SAD,* social anxiety disorder; **Susp,** suspension; *T,* tablet.

SEROTONIN-NCREPINEPHRINE REUPTAKE INHIBITORS (SNRIS)

Name	Availability	Usual Adult Dosage	Side Effects
Duloxetine (Cymbalta)	**C, DI:** 20 mg, 30 mg, 60 mg	**GAD, panic disorder:** 60–120 mg once daily	**Class:** Restlessness, sleep disturbances, nausea, diarrhea, headache, fatigue, sexual dysfunction, weight gain, sweating, tachycardia, urinary retention, increase B/P
Venlafaxine (Effexor XR)	**C, ER** 37.5 mg, 75 mg, 150 mg	**GAD, panic disorder:** 75–225 mg once daily **SAD:** 75 mg once daily	

C, Capsules; *DR,* delayed-release; *ER,* extended-release; *GAD,* generalized anxiety disorder; *SAD,* social anxiety disorder.

Continued

ANXIETY—cont'd
BENZODIAZEPINES

Name	Availability	Usual Adult Dosage	Side Effects
Alprazolam (Xanax, Xanax XR)	**T:** 0.25 mg, 0.5 mg, 1 mg, 2 mg **ODT:** 0.25 mg, 0.5 mg, 1 mg, 2 mg **T, ER:** 0.5 mg, 1 mg, 2 mg, 3 mg	**T, ODT:** 0.5–6 mg/day in 3 divided doses **ER:** 3–6 mg once daily	**Class:** Drowsiness, lightheadedness, confusion, unsteadiness, dizziness, slurred speech, muscle weakness, memory problems
Clonazepam (Klonopin)	**T:** 0.5 mg, 1 mg, 2 mg **ODT:** 0.125 mg, 0.25 mg 0.5 mg, 1 mg, 2 mg	1–4 mg/day in 2 divided doses	
Diazepam (Valium)	**T:** 2 mg, 5 mg, 10 mg	2–10 mg/day in 2–4 divided doses	
Lorazepam (Ativan)	**T:** 0.5 mg, 1 mg, 2 mg	2–6 mg/day in 2–3 divided doses	

C, Capsules; *ER,* extended-release; *ODT,* orally disintegrating tablet; *T,* tablet.

Antiarrhythmics

USES

Prevention and treatment of cardiac arrhythmias, such as premature ventricular contractions, ventricular tachycardia, premature atrial contractions, paroxysmal atrial tachycardia, atrial fibrillation, and flutter.

ACTION

The antiarrhythmics are divided into four classes based on their effects on certain ion channels and/or receptors located on the myocardial cell membrane. Class I is further divided into three subclasses (IA, IB, IC) based on electrophysiologic effects.

Class I: Blocks cardiac sodium channels and slows conduction velocity, prolonging refractory period, and decreasing automaticity of sodium-dependent tissue.

Class IA: Blocks sodium and potassium channels.

Class IB: Shortens the repolarization phase.

Class IC: Slows conduction velocity; no effect on repolarization phase.

Class II: Slows sinus and atrioventricular (AV) nodal conduction.

Class III: Blocks cardiac potassium channels, prolonging the repolarization phase of electrical cells.

Class IV: Inhibits the influx of calcium through its channels, causing slower conduction through the sinus and AV nodes; decreases contractility.

ANTIARRHYTHMICS

Name	Availability	Uses	Dosage Range	Side Effects
Class IA				
Disopyramide (Norpace, Norpace CR)	**C:** 100 mg, 150 mg **C (ER):** 100 mg, 150 mg	AF, WPW, PSVT, PVCs, VT	**C:** 100–200 mg q6h **ER:** 200–300 mg q12h	Dry mouth, blurred vision, urinary retention, HF, proarrhythmia, heart block, nausea, vomiting, diarrhea, hypoglycemia, nervousness
Procainamide	**I:** 100 mg/mL, 500 mg/mL	AF, WPW, PVCs, VT	**Loading dose:** 15–18 mg/kg over 20–30 min. **Maintenance dose:** 1–4 mg/min as a continuous infusion	Hypotension, fever, agranulocytosis, SLE, headaches, proarrhythmia, confusion, disorientation, GI symptoms, hypotension

Continued

ANTIARRHYTMICS—cont'd

Name	Availability	Uses	Dosage Range	Side Effects
Quinidine	**T:** 200 mg, 300 mg **T (ER):** 300 mg, 324 mg	AF, WPW, PVCs, VT	**A (PO):** 400 mg q6h **(ER):** 300 mg q8–12h or 648 mg q8h	Diarrhea, hypotension, nausea, vomiting, cinchonism, fever, bitter taste, heart block, thrombocytopenia, proarrhythmia
Class IB				
Lidocaine	**I:** 300 mg for IM **IV infusion:** 2 mg/mL, 4 mg/mL	PVCs, VT, VF	**IV:** Initially, 1–1.5 mg/kg. May repeat 0.5–0.75 mg/kg q5–10 min. **Maximum cumulative dose:** 3 mg/kg, then 1–4 mg/min infusion	Drowsiness, agitation, muscle twitching, seizures, paresthesia, proarrhythmia, slurred speech, tinnitus, cardiac depression, bradycardia, asystole
Mexiletine	**C:** 150 mg, 200 mg, 250 mg	PVCs, VT, VF	**A:** Initially, 100–150 mg q8h. Adjust every 2–3 days in 50–100 mg increments. **Maximum:** 1,200 mg/day	Drowsiness, agitation, muscle twitching, seizures, paresthesia, proarrhythmia, nausea, vomiting, blood dyscrasias, hepatitis, fever
Class IC				
Flecainide	**T:** 50 mg, 100 mg, 150 mg	AF, PSVT, life-threatening ventricular arrhythmias	**A:** Initially, 50–100 mg q12h. May increase by 50 mg q12h at 4 day intervals. **Maximum:** 400 mg/day	Dizziness, tremors, bradycardia, heart block, HF, GI upset, neutropenia, flushing, blurred vision, metallic taste, proarrhythmia
Propafenone (Rythmol)	**T:** 150 mg, 225 mg, 300 mg **ER:** 225 mg, 325 mg, 425 mg	PAF, WPW, life-threatening ventricular arrhythmias	**A: T:** Initially, 150 mg q8h. May increase at 3–4 day intervals up to 300 mg q8h **ER:** Initially, 225 mg q12h. May increase at a minimum of 5 days up to 425 mg q12h	Dizziness, blurred vision, altered taste, nausea, exacerbation of asthma, proarrhythmia, bradycardia, heart block, HF, GI upset, bronchospasm, hepatotoxicity

Class II (Beta-Blockers)

Acebutolol (Sectral)	**C:** 100 mg, 200 mg, 400 mg	Ventricular arrhythmias	**A:** Initially, 200 mg 2 times/day **Maintenance:** 600–1200 mg/day in divided doses	Bradycardia, hypotension, depression, nightmares, fatigue, sexual dysfunction, SLE, arthritis, myalgia
Esmolol (Brevibloc)	**I:** 10 mg/mL	Supraventricular tachycardia	**A:** 50–200 mcg/kg/min	Hypotension, heart block, HF, bronchospasm
Propranolol (Inderal)	**T:** 10 mg, 20 mg, 40 mg	Tachyarrhythmias	**A:** Initially, 10–30 mg 3–4 times/day **Maintenance:** 10–40 mg 3–4 times/day	Bradycardia, hypotension, depression, nightmares, fatigue, sexual dysfunction, heart block, bronchospasm

Class III

Amiodarone (Cordarone, Pacerone)	**T:** 100 mg, 200 mg, 400 mg **I:** 50 mg/mL	Unstable ventricular tachycardia, life-threatening ventricular arrhythmias	**A (PO):** 800–1,600 mg/day in divided doses for 1–3 wks, then 600–800 mg/day in divided doses for 1 mo, then maintenance dose of 400 mg/day **(IV):** 150 mg bolus, then 900 mg over 18 hrs	Blurred vision, photophobia, constipation, ataxia, proarrhythmia, pulmonary fibrosis, bradycardia, heart block, hyperthyroidism or hypothyroidism, peripheral neuropathy, GI upset, blue-gray skin, optic neuritis, hypotension
Dofetilide (Tikosyn)	**C:** 125 mcg, 250 mcg, 500 mcg	AF, A flutter	**A:** Individualized	Torsades de pointes, hypotension
Dronedarone (Multaq)	**T:** 400 mg	AF, A flutter	**A (PO):** 400 mg 2 times/day	Diarrhea, nausea, abdominal pain, vomiting, asthenia
Ibutilide (Corvert)	**I:** 0.1 mg/mL	AF, A flutter	**A (60 kg or greater):** 1 mg over 10 min; **(less than 60 kg):** 0.01 mg/kg over 10 min	Torsades de pointes

Continued

ANTIARRHYTHMICS—cont'd

Name	Availability	Uses	Dosage Range	Side Effects
Sotalol (Betapace)	**T:** 80 mg, 120 mg, 160 mg	AF, PAF, PSVT, life-threatening ventricular arrhythmias	**A: (IV):** Initially, 80 mg 2 times/day. May increase at 3 day intervals of 40 mg twice daily up to 160 mg 2 times/day	Fatigue, dizziness, dyspnea, bradycardia, proarrhythmia, heart block, hypotension, bronchospasm
Class IV (Calcium Channel Blockers)				
Diltiazem (Cardizem)	**I:** 25 mg/mL vials **Infusion:** 1 mg/mL	AF, A flutter, PSVT	**A (IV):** 20–25 mg bolus, then infusion of 5–15 mg/hr	Hypotension, bradycardia, dizziness, headaches, heart block, asystole, HF
Verapamil (Calan, Isoptin)	**I:** 5 mg/2 mL	AF, A flutter, PSVT	**A (IV):** 5–10 mg. May repeat with 10 mg if no response in 10–15 min	Hypotension, bradycardia, dizziness, headaches, constipation, heart block, HF, asystole, fatigue, edema, nausea

A, Adults; *AF,* atrial fibrillation; *A flutter,* atrial flutter; *C,* capsules; *ER,* extended-release; *HF,* heart failure; *I,* injection; *PAF,* paroxysmal atrial fibrillation; *PSVT,* paroxysmal supraventricular tachycardia; *PVCs,* premature ventricular contractions; *SLE,* systemic lupus erythematosus; *SR,* sustained-release; *T,* tablets; *VT,* ventricular tachycardia; *WPW,* Wolff-Parkinson-White syndrome.

Antibiotics

USES	ACTION
Treatment of wide range of gram-positive or gram-negative bacterial infections, suppression of intestinal flora before surgery, control of acne, prophylactically to prevent rheumatic fever, prophylactically in high-risk situations (e.g., some surgical procedures or medical conditions) to prevent bacterial infection. Antibiotics should be used only if clinical or laboratory evidence suggests bacterial infection. Cultures and antibiotic susceptibility testing are essential for selecting a drug for serious infections. However, treatment must often begin before culture results are available, necessitating selection according to the most likely pathogens (empiric antibiotic selection). For empiric treatment of serious infections that may involve any one of several bacteria or that may be due to multiple pathogens, a broad spectrum of activity is desirable. Susceptibility data should be compiled into antibiograms and used to direct empiric treatment whenever possible. Antibiograms summarize regional facility-specific (or location-specific) antibiotic susceptibility patterns of common pathogens to commonly used antibiotics.	Antibiotics are natural or synthetic compounds that have the ability to kill or suppress the growth of microorganisms. One means of classifying antibiotics is by their antimicrobial spectrum. Narrow-spectrum agents are effective against few microorganisms (e.g., aminoglycosides are effective against gram-negative aerobes), whereas broad-spectrum agents are effective against a wide variety of microorganisms (e.g., fluoroquinolones are effective against gram-positive cocci and gram-negative bacilli). Antimicrobial agents may also be classified based on their mechanism of action. • Agents that inhibit cell wall synthesis or activate enzymes that disrupt the cell wall, causing a weakening in the cell, cell lysis, and death. Include penicillins, cephalosporins, vancomycin, imidazole antifungal agents. • Agents that act directly on the cell wall, affecting permeability of cell membranes, causing leakage of intracellular substances. Include antifungal agents amphotericin and nystatin, polymyxin, colistin. • Agents that bind to ribosomal subunits, altering protein synthesis and eventually causing cell death. Include aminoglycosides. • Agents that affect bacterial ribosome function, altering protein synthesis and causing slow microbial growth. Do not cause cell death. Include chloramphenicol, clindamycin, erythromycin, tetracyclines. • Agents that inhibit nucleic acid metabolism by binding to nucleic acid or interacting with enzymes necessary for nucleic acid synthesis. Inhibit DNA or RNA synthesis. Include rifampin, metronidazole, fluoroquinolones (e.g., ciprofloxacin). • Agents that inhibit specific metabolic steps necessary for microbial growth, causing a decrease in essential cell components or synthesis of nonfunctional analogues of normal metabolites. Include trimethoprim, sulfonamides.

Continued

SELECTION OF ANTIMICROBIAL AGENTS

The goal of therapy is to achieve antimicrobial action at the site of infection sufficient to inhibit the growth of the microorganism. Factors to consider in selection of an antimicrobial agent include the following:

- Sensitivity pattern of the infecting microorganism
- Location and severity of infection
- Pt's ability to eliminate the drug
- Pt's defense mechanisms
- Pt's age, pregnancy status, genetic factors, allergies, CNS disorder, preexisting medical problems

CATEGORIZATION OF ORGANISMS BY GRAM STAINING

Gram-Positive Cocci	Gram-Negative Cocci	Gram-Positive Bacilli	Gram-Negative Bacilli
Aerobic	**Aerobic**	**Aerobic**	**Aerobic**
Staphylococcus aureus	Neisseria gonorrhoeae	Listeria monocytogenes	Escherichia coli
Staphylococcus epidermidis	Neisseria meningitidis	Bacillus anthracis	Klebsiella pneumoniae
Streptococcus pneumoniae	Moraxella catarrhalis	Corynebacterium diphtheriae	Proteus mirabilis
Streptococcus pyogenes		**Anaerobic**	Serratia marcescens
Viridans streptococci		Clostridium difficile	Acinetobacter spp.
Enterococcus faecalis		Clostridium perfringens	Pseudomonas aeruginosa
Enterococcus faecium		Clostridium tetani	Enterobacter spp.
Anaerobic		Actinomyces spp.	Haemophilus influenzae
Peptostreptococcus spp.			Legionella pneumophila
Peptococcus spp.			**Anaerobic**
			Bacteroides fragilis
			Fusobacterium spp.

Antibiotic: Aminoglycosides

USES

Treatment of serious infections when other less-toxic agents are not effective, are contraindicated, or require adjunctive therapy (e.g., with penicillins or cephalosporins). Used primarily in the treatment of infections caused by gram-negative microorganisms, such as those caused by *Proteus, Klebsiella, Pseudomonas, Escherichia coli, Serratia,* and *Enterobacter.* Inactive against most gram-positive microorganisms. Not well absorbed systemically from GI tract (must be administered parenterally for systemic infections).

ACTION

Bactericidal. Transported across bacterial cell membrane; irreversibly bind to specific receptor proteins of bacterial ribosomes. Interfere with protein synthesis, preventing cell reproduction and eventually causing cell death.

ANTIBIOTIC: AMINOGLYCOSIDES

Name	Availability	Dosage Range	Class Side Effects
Amikacin	I: 50 mg/mL, 250 mg/mL	A: 5–7.5 mg/kg q8h or 15–20 mg/kg once daily CH: 5–7.5 mg/kg q8h	Nephrotoxicity, neurotoxicity, ototoxicity (both auditory and vestibular), hypersensitivity (skin itching, redness, rash, swelling) anemia, thrombocytopenia, injection site reactions (e.g., pain, irritation, redness)
Gentamicin	I: 10 mg/mL, 40 mg/mL	A: 4–7 mg/kg once daily or 1–2.5 mg/kg q8–12h CH: 2–2.5 mg/kg q8h	
Tobramycin	I: 10 mg/mL, 40 mg/mL	A: 5–7 mg/kg once daily or 1–2.5 mg/kg q8h CH: 2–2.5 mg/kg q8h	

A, Adults; *CH,* children; *I,* injection; *T,* tablets.

Antibiotic: Carbapenems

Carbapenems are a class of beta-lactam antibiotics that are used to treat severe or high-risk bacterial infections. They may be used in the treatment of intra-abdominal infections, complicated urinary tract infections, pneumonia, and sepsis. **Note:** Beta-lactamases are enzymes produced by bacteria that break open the beta-lactam ring, inactivating the beta-lactam antibiotic. Beta-lactamase inhibitors block the activity of beta-lactamase and are sometimes combined with beta-lactam antibiotics (e.g., avibactam, clavulanate, sulbactam, and tazobactam).

SPECTRUM OF ACTIVITY

Carbapenems exhibit broad spectrum activity against gram-negative bacteria including most Enterobacteriaceae (e.g., Escherichia coli, Klebsiella pneumoniae, Enterobacter, Citrobacter, Proteus mirabilis, and Serratia marcescens) and good activity against Pseudomonas aeruginosa and Acinetobacter species.

Meropenem/vaborbactam exhibits activity against Enterobacter cloacae species complex, E. coli, and K. pneumoniae.

Carbapenems exhibit narrower activity against gram-positive bacteria including methicillin-sensitive strains of Staphylococcus and Streptococcus species.

Carbapenems exhibit good activity against anaerobes (e.g., Bacteroides fragilis).

ACTION

Inhibit bacterial cell wall synthesis by binding to one or more of the penicillin-binding proteins, causing cell lysis and death.

ANTIBIOTIC: CARBAPENEMS

Name	Indications	Dosage Range	Side Effects
Doripenem (Dorbax)	Intra-abdominal infection Complicated urinary tract infection (including pyelonephritis)	500 mg q8h	Headache, diarrhea, nausea, skin rash, anemia
Ertapenem (Invanz)	Acute pelvic infections Community-acquired pneumonia Complicated intra-abdominal infections, skin and skin structure, and UTI	1 g once daily	Diarrhea, vomiting, nausea, abdominal pain, increased serum AST, ALT

Drug	Indications	Dosage	Side Effects
Imipenem (Primaxin)	Lower respiratory tract infections Urinary tract infections. Intra-abdominal infections Gynecologic infections Bacterial septicemia Bone and joint infections Skin and skin structure infections Endocarditis	500–1,000 mg q6h or 1,000 mg q8h	Decreased hematocrit, hemoglobin, eosinophilia, thrombocythemia, increased ALT, AST
Meropenem (Merrem)	Meningitis Intra-abdominal infection Pneumonia Sepsis	1.5–6 g daily divided q8h	Headache, pain, skin rash, nausea, diarrhea, constipation, vomiting, anemia
Meropenem/vaborbactam (Vabomere)	Complicated urinary tract infection (including pyelonephritis)	4 g (2 g meropenem/2 g vaborbactam) q8h	Headache, diarrhea, phlebitis/infusion site reactions

Antibiotic: Cephalosporins

USES

Cephalosporins, a class of beta-lactam antibiotics, are broad-spectrum antibiotics, which, like penicillins, may be used in a number of diseases, including respiratory diseases, skin and soft tissue infection, bone/joint infections, and genitourinary infections and prophylactically in some surgical procedures. Beta-lactamases are a diverse class of enzymes produced by bacteria that break open the beta-lactam ring, inactivating the beta-lactam antibiotic.

Beta-lactamase inhibitors are drugs that block the activity of certain beta-lactamases and are sometimes combined with beta-lactam antibiotics (e.g., avibactam, clavulanate, sulbactam, and tazobactam)

First-generation cephalosporins have activity against gram-positive organisms (e.g., streptococci and most staphylococci) and activity against some gram-negative organisms, including *Escherichia coli, Klebsiella pneumoniae,* and *Proteus mirabilis.*

ACTION

Second-generation cephalosporins have same effectiveness as first-generation and increased activity against gram-negative organisms, including *Haemophilus influenzae, Neisseria gonorrhoeae, E. coli,* and *Klebsiella.* Cefoxitin has activity against gram-negative bacilli *Bacteroides fragilis* and certain *Enterobacteriaceae.*

Third-generation cephalosporins are less active against gram-positive organisms but active against gram-negative bacteria including *Haemophilus influenzae,* and *Proteus, Citrobacter, Serratia, Enterobacteriaceae (E. coli),* and *Klebsiella* species. Ceftazidime has activity against *Pseudomonas aeruginosa.*

Fourth-generation cephalosporins have good activity against gram-positive organisms (e.g., *Staphylococcus aureus*) and gram-negative organisms (e.g., *Pseudomonas aeruginosa, E. coli, Klebsiella,* and *Proteus*). Cefepime penetrates the CNS and can be used in treating meningitis.

Fifth-generation cephalosporins have good activity against gram-positive organisms (e.g., *Staphylococcus aureus, Streptococcus* spp.) and gram-negative organisms (e.g., *E. coli, Klebsiella* spp.). Ceftaroline has activity against multidrug-resistant *Staphylococcus aureus,* including MRSA, VRSA, and VISA.

Cephalosporins inhibit cell wall synthesis or activate enzymes that disrupt the cell wall, causing cell lysis and cell death. May be bacteriostatic or bactericidal. Most effective against rapidly dividing cells.

ANTIBIOTIC: CEPHALOSPORINS

Name	Availability	Dosage Range	Side Effects
First-Generation			
Cefadroxil (Duricef)	**C:** 500 mg **T:** 1 g **S:** 125 mg/5 mL, 250 mg/5 mL, **500** mg/5 mL	**A:** 500 mg bid or 1 g once daily **CH:** 15 mg/kg q12h	Abdominal cramps/pain, fever, nausea, vomiting, diarrhea, headaches, oral/vaginal candidiasis
Cefazolin (Ancef)	**I:** 500 mg, 1 g, 2 g	**A:** 500 mg–2 g q6–8h **CH:** 25–100 mg/kg/day divided q6–8h	Fever, rash, diarrhea, nausea, pain at injection site
Cephalexin (Keflex, Keftab)	**C:** 250 mg, 500 mg **T:** 250 mg, 500 mg, 1 g	**A:** 250 mg–1 g q6–12h **CH:** 25–100 mg/kg/day divided q6–8h	Headache, abdominal pain, diarrhea, nausea, dyspepsia
Second-Generation			
Cefaclor (Ceclor)	**C:** 250 mg, 500 mg **T (ER):** 500 mg **S:** 125 mg/5 mL, 187 mg/5 mL, 250 mg/5 mL, 375 mg/5 mL	**A:** 250–500 mg q8h **ER:** 500 mg q12h **CH:** 20–40 mg/kg/day q8–12h	Rash, diarrhea, increased transaminases May have serum sickness-like reaction
Cefoxitin (Mefox.n)	**I:**1g, 2 g	**A:** 1–2 g q6–8h **CH:** 80–160 mg/kg/day divided q6h	Diarrhea
Cefprozil (Cefzil)	**T:** 250 mg, 500 mg **S:** 125 mg/5 mL, 250 mg/5 mL	**A:** 500 mg q12–24h **CH:** 7.5–15 mg/kg q12h	Dizziness, abdominal pain, diarrhea, nausea, increased AST, ALT
Cefuroxime (Ceftin, Kefurox, Zinacef)	**T:** 125 mg, 250 mg, 500 mg **I:** 750 mg, 1.5 g	**A (PO):** 125–500 mg q12h **(IM/IV):** 750 mg–1.5 g q8–12h **CH (PO):** 10–15 mg/kg q12h **(IM/IV):** 75–150 mg/kg/day divided q8h	Diarrhea, nausea, vomiting, thrombophlebitis, increased AST, ALT
Third-Generation			
Cefdinir (Omnicef)	**C:** 300 mg **S:** 125 mg/5 mL	**A:** 300 mg q12h or 600 mg once daily **CH:** 7 mg/kg q12h or 14 mg/kg once daily	Headache, hyperglycemia, abdominal pain, diarrhea, nausea

ANTIBIOTIC: CEPHALOSPORINS—cont'd

Name	Availability	Dosage Range	Side Effects
Cefotaxime	**I:** 500 mg, 1 g, 2 g	**A:** 1–2 g q4–12h **CH:** 150–180 mg/kg/day divided q4–6h	Rash, diarrhea, nausea, pain at injection site
Cefpodoxime	**T:** 100 mg, 200 mg **S:** 50 mg/5 mL, 100 mg/5 mL	**A:** 100–400 mg q12h **CH:** 5 mg/kg q12h	Rash, diarrhea, nausea
Ceftazidime (Tazicef)	**I:** 500 mg, 1 g, 2 g	**A:** 1–2 g q8–12h **CH:** 30–50 mg/kg q8h	Diarrhea, pain at injection site
Ceftriaxone (Rocephin)	**I:** 250 mg, 500 mg, 1 g, 2 g	**A:** 1–2 g q12–24h **CH:** 50–75 mg/kg/dose q24h	Rash, diarrhea, eosinophilia, increased AST, ALT
Fourth-Generation			
Cefepime	**I:** 1g, 2g	**A:** 1–2 g q8–12h **CH:** 50 mg/kg q8–12h	Rash, diarrhea, nausea, increased AST, ALT
Fifth-Generation			
Ceftaroline (Teflaro)	**I:** 400 mg, 600 mg	**A:** 600 mg q12h	Headache, insomnia, rash, pruritus, diarrhea, nausea
Ceftobiprole (Zevtera)	**I:** 667 mg of ceftobiprole medocaril sodium (equivalent to 500 mg of ceftobiprole)	**A:** 667 mg q6–8h **CH: 12–17 yrs:** 13.3 mg/kg (up to 667 mg/dose) q8h. **3 mos–11 yrs:** 20 mg/kg (up to 667 mg/dose)	Anemia, nausea, hypokalemia, vomiting, diarrhea, hypertension, leukopenia, pyrexia; increased hepatic enzymes, serum bilirubin, creatinine
Fixed-Combinations			
Ceftazidime/avibactam (Avycaz)	**I:** 2 g ceftazidime/0.5 g avibactam	**A:** 2.5 g q8h	Nausea, vomiting, constipation, anxiety
Ceftolozane/tazobactam (Zerbaxa)	**I:** 1 g ceftolozane/0.5 g tazobactam	**A:** 1.5 g q8h	Nausea, diarrhea, headache, pyrexia

A, Adults; *C,* capsules; *CH,* children; *ER,* extended-release; *I,* injection; *S,* suspension; *T,* tablets.

Antibiotic: Fluoroquinolones

USES

	ACTION
Fluoroquinolones act against a wide range of gram-negative and gram-positive organisms including *Haemophilus influenzae, Moraxella catarrhalis, Mycoplasma, Chlamydia, Legionella, Enterobacteriales* (formerly *Enterobacteriaceae*), and *Pseudomonas aeruginosa*. They are used primarily in the treatment of lower respiratory tract infections, skin/skin structure infections, urinary tract infections, and sexually transmitted diseases.	Bactericidal. Inhibit DNA gyrase in susceptible microorganisms, interfering with bacterial DNA replication and repair.

ANTIBIOTIC: FLUOROQUINOLONES

Name	Availability	Dosage Range	Side Effects, Comments
Ciprofloxacin (Cipro)	**T:** 100 mg, 250 mg, 500 mg, 750 mg **Susp:** 250 mg/5 mL, 500 mg/5 mL **I:** 200 mg, 400 mg	**A (PO):** 250–750 mg q12h **(IV):** 200–400 mg q12h	**Class:** Nausea, diarrhea, vomiting, abdominal pain/discomfort, trouble sleeping, tendinopathy including rupture of the Achilles tendon, peripheral neuropathy, central nervous system (CNS) (e.g., seizures, increased intracranial pressure), nervousness, anxiety, agitation, insomnia, nightmares, dizziness, mood alteration, confusion, tremors, depression
Levofloxacin (Levaquin)	**T:** 250 mg, 500 mg, 750 mg **I:** 250 mg, 500 mg, 750 mg **OS:** 250 mg/10 mL	**A (PO/IV):** 250–750 mg/day as single dose	
Moxifloxacin (Avelox)	**T:** 400 mg **I:** 400 mg	**A:** 400 mg/day	

A, Adults; *I,* injection; *OS,* oral solution; *PO,* oral; *Susp,* suspension; *T,* tablets.

Antibiotic: Macrolides

USES

Macrolides act primarily against most gram-positive micro-organisms and some gram-negative cocci. Azithromycin and clarithromycin appear to be more potent than erythromycin. Macrolides are used in the treatment of pharyngitis/tonsillitis, sinusitis, chronic bronchitis, pneumonia, uncomplicated skin/skin structure infections.

ACTION

Bacteriostatic or bactericidal. Reversibly binds to the P site of the 50S ribosomal subunit of susceptible organisms, inhibiting RNA-dependent protein synthesis.

ANTIBIOTIC: MACROLIDES

Name	Availability	Dosage Range	Side Effects
Azithromycin (Zithromax)	**T:** 250 mg, 600 mg **Susp:** 100 mg/5 mL, 200 mg/5 mL, 1-g packet **I:** 500 mg	**A (PO):** 500 mg once, then 250 mg once daily **(IV):** 500 mg/day **CH (PO/IV):** 10–12 mg/kg/dose on day 1, then 5–6 mg/kg/dose once daily	**PO:** Nausea, diarrhea, vomiting, abdominal pain **IV:** Pain, redness, swelling at injection site
Clarithromycin (Biaxin)	**T:** 250 mg, 500 mg **T (XL):** 500 mg **Susp:** 125 mg/5 mL	**A:** 250–500 mg q12h (or XL 1,000 mg once daily) **CH:** 7.5 mg/kg q12h	Headaches, loss of taste, nausea, vomiting, diarrhea, abdominal pain/discomfort
Erythromycin (EES, Eryc, EryPed, Ery-Tab, Erythrocin, PCE)	**T:** 200 mg, 250 mg, 333 mg, 400 mg, 500 mg **C:** 250 mg **Susp:** 100 mg/2.5 mL, 125 mg/5 mL, 200 mg/5 mL, 250 mg/5 mL, 400 mg/5 mL	**A (PO):** 250–500 mg q6–12 h **(IV):** 500 mg–1 g q6h **CH (PO):** 50 mg/kg/day in divided doses q6–8h **(IV):** 15–20 mg/kg/day in divided doses q6h	**PO:** Nausea, vomiting, diarrhea, abdominal pain **IV:** Inflammation, phlebitis at injection site

A, Adults; *C,* capsules; *CH,* children; *I,* injection; *Susp,* suspension; *T,* tablets; *XL,* long-acting.

Antibiotic: Penicillins

USES

Penicillins (also referred to as beta-lactam antibiotics) may be used to treat a large number of infections, including pneumonia and other respiratory diseases, urinary tract infections, septicemia, meningitis, intra-abdominal infections, gonorrhea and syphilis, and bone/joint infection. **Note:** Beta-lactamases are a diverse class of enzymes produced by bacteria that break open the beta-lactam ring, inactivating the beta-lactam antibiotic. Beta-lactamase inhibitors are drugs that block the activity of certain beta-lactamases and are sometimes combined with beta-lactam antibiotics (e.g., avibactam, clavulanate, sulbactam, and tazobactam).

Penicillins are classified based on an antimicrobial spectrum:

Natural penicillins are very active against gram-positive cocci but ineffective against most strains of *Staphylococcus aureus* (inactivated by enzyme penicillinase).

Penicillinase-resistant penicillins are effective against penicillinase-producing *Staphylococcus aureus* but are less effective against gram-positive cocci than the natural penicillins.

Broad-spectrum penicillins are effective against gram-positive cocci and some gram-negative bacteria (e.g., *Haemophilus influenzae, Escherichia coli, Proteus mirabilis, Salmonella,* and *Shigella*).

Extended-spectrum penicillins are effective against gram-negative organisms, including *Pseudomonas aeruginosa, Enterobacter, Proteus* spp, *Klebsiella, Serratia* spp, and *Acinetobacter* spp.

ACTION

Penicillins inhibit cell wall synthesis or activate enzymes, which disrupt the bacterial cell wall, causing cell lysis and cell death. May be bacteriostatic or bactericidal. Most effective against bacteria undergoing active growth and division.

Continued

ANTIBIOTIC: PENICILLINS—cont'd

Name	Availability	Dosage Range	Side Effects
Natural			
Penicillin G benzathine (Bicillin LA)	**I:** 600,000 units, 1.2 million units, 2.4 million units	**A:** 1.2–2.4 million units as single dose **CH:** 25,000–50,000 units/kg as single dose	Mild diarrhea, nausea, vomiting, headaches, sore mouth/tongue, vaginal itching/discharge, allergic reaction (including anaphylaxis, skin rash, urticaria, pruritus)
Penicillin G potassium (Pfizerpen)	**I:** 1, 2, 3, 5 million-unit vials	**A:** 2–4 million units q4h **CH:** 100,000–300,000 units/kg/day divided q4–6h	Rash, injection site reaction, phlebitis
Penicillin V potassium (Apo-Pen-VK)	**T:** 250 mg, 500 mg **Susp:** 125 mg/5 mL, 250 mg/5 mL	**A:** 250–500 mg q6–8h **CH:** 25–50 mg/kg/day in divided doses q6h	Diarrhea, nausea, vomiting
Penicillinase-Resistant			
Nafcillin	**I:** 500 mg, 1 g, 2 g	**A (IV):** 500 mg–2 g q4–6h **CH (IV):** 100–200 mg/kg/day in divided doses q4–6h	Inflammation, pain, phlebitis, increased risk of interstitial nephritis
Oxacillin	**I:** 250 mg, 500 mg, 1 g, 2 g	**A (IV):** 1–2 g q4–6h **CH (IV):** 25–50 mg/kg q6h	Diarrhea, nausea, vomiting, increased risk of hepatotoxicity, interstitial nephritis

Broad-Spectrum

Amoxicillin (Amoxil, Trimox)	**T:** 125 mg, 250 mg, 500 mg, 875 mg **C:** 250 mg, 500 mg **Susp:** 200 mg/5 mL, 400 mg/5 mL, 125 mg/5 mL, 250 mg/5 mL	**A:** 500 mg to 1 g q8–12h **CH:** 25–50 mg/kg/day q8h (80–90 mg/kg/day q12h for severe infections)	Diarrhea, colitis, nausea
Amoxicillin/ clavulanate (Augmentin)	**T:** 250 mg, **500 mg**, 875 mg **T (Chew):** 125 mg, 200 mg, 250 mg, 400 mg **Susp:** 125 mg/5 mL, 200 mg/5 mL, 250 mg/5 mL, 400 mg/5 mL	**A:** 875 mg q12h or 500 mg q8h **CH:** 25–90 mg/kg/day divided q12h	Diarrhea, rash, nausea, vomiting
Ampicillin	**C:** 250 mg, 500 mg **Susp:** 125 mg/5 mL, 250 mg/5 mL **I:** 125 mg, 250 mg, 500 mg, 1 g, 2 g	**A (PO):** 250–500 mg q6h **(IV):** 500 mg–2 g q6h **C (PO):** 50–100 mg/kg/day divided q6h **(IV):** 50–200 mg/kg/day divided q6h	Nausea, vomiting, diarrhea
Ampicillin/sulbactam (Unasyn)	**I:** 1.5 g, 3 g	**A:** 1.5–3 g q6h **CH:** 200–400 mg ampicillin/kg/day divided q6h	Local pain at injection site, rash, diarrhea

Extended-Spectrum

Piperacillin/tazobactam (Zosyn)	**I:** 2.25 g, 3.375 g, 4.5 g	**A:** 3.375 g q6h or 4.5 g q6–8h **CH:** 240–300 mg/kg/day divided q 6–8h	Diarrhea, insomnia, headache, fever, rash

A, Adults; *C,* capsules; *CH,* children; *I,* injection; *PO,* oral; *Susp,* suspension; *T,* tablets.

Anticoagulants/Antiplatelets/Thrombolytics

USES

Treatment and prevention of venous thromboembolism, acute MI, acute cerebral embolism; reduce risk of acute MI; reduction of total mortality in pts with unstable angina; prevent occlusion of saphenous grafts following open heart surgery; prevent embolism in select pts with atrial fibrillation, prosthetic heart valves, valvular heart disease, cardiomyopathy. Heparin also used for acute/chronic consumption coagulopathies (disseminated intravascular coagulation).

ACTION

Anticoagulants: Inhibit blood coagulation by preventing the formation of new clots and extension of existing ones *but do not dissolve formed clots.* Anticoagulants are subdivided. *Heparin* (including low molecular weight heparin). (LMWH): Combines with plasma antithrombin, forming a complex that neutralizes thrombin and factor Xa. (LMWHs inhibit factor Xa more than thrombin.) *Warfarin:* Acts indirectly to prevent synthesis in the liver of vitamin K–dependent clotting factors. *Direct thrombin inhibitors:* Bind antithrombin and indirectly inhibit factor Xa.

Antiplatelets: Interfere with platelet aggregation. Effects are irreversible for life of platelet. Medications in this group act by different mechanisms. Aspirin irreversibly inhibits cyclo-oxygenase and formation of thromboxane A_2. Clopidogrel, dipyridamole, prasugrel, and ticlopidine have similar effects as aspirin and are known as adenosine diphosphate (ADP) inhibitors. Abciximab, eptifibatide, and tirofiban block binding of fibrinogen to the glycoprotein IIb/IIIa receptor on platelet surface (known as platelet glycoprotein IIb/IIIa receptor antagonists).

Thrombolytics: Act directly or indirectly on fibrinolytic system to dissolve clots (converting plasminogen to plasmin, an enzyme that digests fibrin clot).

ANTICOAGULANTS/ANTIPLATELETS/THROMBOLYTICS

Name	Availability	Uses	Side Effects
Anticoagulants			
Direct Thrombin Inhibitors			
Argatroban	**I:** 100 mg/mL	Prevent/treat VTE in pts with HIT or at risk for HIT undergoing PCI	Bleeding, hypotension, hematuria

Bivalirudin (Angiomax)	I: 250-mg vials	Pts with unstable angina undergoing PTCA	Bleeding, hypotension, pain, headache, nausea, back pain
Dabigatran (Pradaxa)	C: 75 mg, 110 mg, 150 mg	Reduce risk for stroke/embolism with nonvalvular atrial fibrillation, prevent/treat DVT/PE, postoperative prophylaxis of DVT/ PE following hip replacement	Bleeding, gastritis, dyspepsia
Desirudin (Iprivask)	I: 15 mg	Prophylaxis of DVT following hip surgery	Bleeding, drainage from a wound, nausea, anemia, DVT, serious allergic reactions
Heparin, Low Molecular Weight Heparins			
Dalteparin (Fragmin)	I: 2,500 units, 5,000 units, 7,500 units, 10,000 units	Prevent DVT following hip surgery, abdominal surgery, or medical pts with severely restricted mobility during acute illness, unstable angina or non–Q-wave MI	Bleeding, hematoma, increased ALT, AST, pain at injection site, bruising, pruritus, fever, thrombocytopenia
Enoxaparin (Lovenox)	I: 30 mg, 40 mg, 60 mg, 80 mg, 100 mg, 120 mg, 150 mg	Prevent DVT following hip surgery, knee surgery, abdominal surgery, medical pts with severely restricted mobility during acute illness, or ischemic complications of unstable angina and non–Q-wave MI; treatment of DVT in pts with unstable angina or non–Q-wave MI	Bleeding, thrombocytopenia, hematoma, increased ALT, AST, nausea, bruising Injection site reactions, anemia, diarrhea, fever
Heparin	I: 1,000 units/mL, 2,500 units/mL, 5,000 units/mL, 7,500 units/mL, 10,000 units/mL, 20,000 units/mL	Prevent/treat VTE	Bleeding, thrombocytopenia, skin rash, itching, burning Increased hepatic transaminase
Factor Xa Inhibitor			
Apixaban (Eliquis)	T: 2.5 mg, 5 mg	Reduce risk of stroke/embolism in nonvalvular atrial fibrillation. Prevent VTE post hip/knee replacement surgery, prevent/treat recurrence following initial treatment. Treatment of DVT and PE	Bleeding, nausea, anemia Confusion, increased AST, ALT

Continued

ANTICOAGULANTS/ANTIPLATELETS/THROMBOLYTICS—cont'd

Name	Availability	Uses	Side Effects
Edoxaban (Savaysa)	T: 15 mg, 30 mg, 60 mg	Prevent thromboembolism in nonvalvular atrial fibrillation, treat DVT/PT following 5–10 days of initial therapy with a parenteral anticoagulant	Bleeding, anemia, rash, abnormal liver function tests
Fondaparinux (Arixtra)	I: 2.5 mg, 5 mg, 7.5 mg, 10 mg	Prophylaxis of DVT following hip fracture, abdominal surgery, hip surgery, knee surgery, treat DVT/PE in combination with warfarin	Bleeding, thrombocytopenia, hematoma, fever, nausea, anemia Increased AST, ALT; insomnia, dizziness, hypokalemia
Rivaroxaban (Xarelto)	T: 10 mg	Prevent DVT post knee, hip replacement or medical pts with severely restricted mobility during acute illness Prevent thromboembolism in atrial fibrillation Prevent/treat DVT/PE	Bleeding, abdominal pain, fatigue, muscle spasms, anxiety, depression, UTI, increased AST, ALT
Coumarin			
Warfarin (Coumadin)	PO: 1 mg, 2 mg, 2.5 mg, 3 mg, 4 mg, 5 mg, 6 mg, 7.5 mg, 10 mg I: 5 mg	Prevent/treat VTE in pts, prevent systemic embolism in pts with heart valve replacement, valve heart disease, MI, atrial fibrillation	Bleeding, skin necrosis, anorexia, nausea, vomiting, diarrhea, rash, abdominal cramps, purple toe syndrome, drug interactions (see individual monograph)
Antiplatelets			
Abciximab (ReoPro)	I: 2 mg/mL	Adjunct to PCI to prevent acute cardiac ischemic complications (with heparin and aspirin)	Bleeding, hypotension, nausea, vomiting, back pain, allergic reactions, thrombocytopenia
Aspirin	PO: 81 mg, 165 mg, 325 mg, 500 mg, 650 mg	TIA, acute MI, chronic stable/unstable angina, revascularization procedures, prevent reinfarction and thromboembolism post MI	Tinnitus, dizziness, hypersensitivity, dyspepsia, minor bleeding, GI ulceration
Clopidogrel (Plavix)	PO: 75 mg	Reduce risk of stroke, MI, or vascular death in pts with recent MI, noncardioembolic stroke, peripheral artery disease, reduce CV death, MI, stroke, reinfarction in pts with non-STEMI/STEMI	Bleeding, rash, pruritus, bruising, epistaxis

Cangrelor (Kengreal)	I: 50 mg	Adjunct to PCI to reduce risk of MI, repeat coronary revascularization, stent thrombosis	Bleeding
Eptifibatide (Integrilin)	I: 0.75 mg/mL, 2 mg/mL	Treat acute coronary syndrome	Bleeding, hypotension
Prasugrel (Effient)	PO: 5 mg, 10 mg	Reduce thrombotic cardiovascular events in pts with ACS to be managed with PCI (including stenting)	Bleeding, hypotension
Ticagrelor (Brilinta)	PO: 60 mg, 90 mg	Reduce thrombotic cardiovascular events in pts with ACS	Bleeding, dyspnea
Tirofiban (Aggrastat)	I: 50 mcg/mL, 250 mcg/mL	Treat acute coronary syndrome	Bleeding, thrombocytopenia, brady-cardia, pelvic pain
Vorapaxar (Zontivity)	T: 2.08 mg	Reduce thrombotic cardiovascular events (e.g., MI, stroke) in pts with history of MI or peripheral arterial disease	Bleeding
Thrombolytics			
Alteplase (Activase)	I: 50 mg, 100 mg	Acute MI, acute ischemic stroke, pulmonary embolism	Bleeding, epistaxis
Tenecteplase (TNKase)	I: 50 mg	Acute MI	Bleeding, hematuria

ACS, Acute coronary syndrome; *DVT,* deep vein thrombosis; *HIT,* heparin-induced thrombocytopenia; *I,* injection; *MI,* myocardial infarction; *PCI,* percutaneous coronary intervention; *PO,* oral; *PTCA,* percutaneous transluminal coronary angioplasty; *STEMI,* ST segment elevation MI; *T,* tablet; *TIA,* transient ischemic attack; *VTE,* venous thromboembolism.

Antidepressants

USES

Used primarily for the treatment of depression. Depression can be a chronic or recurrent mental disorder presenting with symptoms such as depressed mood, loss of interest or pleasure, guilt feelings, disturbed sleep/appetite, low energy, and difficulty in thinking. Depression can also lead to suicide.

ACTION

Antidepressants include tricyclics, monoamine oxidase inhibitors (MAOIs), selective serotonin reuptake inhibitors (SSRIs), serotonin–norepinephrine reuptake inhibitors (SNRIs), and other antidepressants. Depression may be due to reduced functioning of monoamine neurotransmitters (e.g., norepinephrine, serotonin [5-HT], dopamine) in the CNS (decreased amount and/or decreased effects at the receptor sites). Antidepressants block metabolism, increase amount/effects of monoamine neurotransmitters, and act at receptor sites (change responsiveness/sensitivities of both presynaptic and postsynaptic receptor sites).

Augmentation with a second-generation antipsychotic drug has been effective (may cause weight gain, metabolic adverse effects, akathisia). *Aripiprazole (Abilify), brexpiprazole (Rexulti), cariprazine (Vraylar), olanzapine (Zyprexa),* and *extended-release quetiapine (Seroquel XR)* are approved for adjunctive treatment of MDD.

ANTIDEPRESSANTS

Name	Availability	Dosage Range (per day)	Side Effects
Tricyclics			
Amitriptyline	**T:** 10 mg, 25 mg, 50 mg, 75 mg, 100 mg, 150 mg	Initially, 25–50 mg/day once or in divided doses, then 100–300 mg/day once or in divided doses	**Class:** Anticholinergic effects (e.g., urinary retention, constipation, dry mouth, blurred vision), orthostatic hypotension, weight gain, sedation, sexual dysfunction, QT interval prolongation, cardiac conduction delays
Amoxapine	**T:** 50 mg, 100 mg, 150 mg	Initially, 25–50 mg once a day bid to tid, then 200–300, mg/day divided bid or tid	
Desipramine (Norpramin)	**T:** 10 mg, 25 mg, 50 mg, 75 mg, 100 mg, 150 mg	Initially, 25–50 mg/day once or 2 or 3 times/day, then 100–300 mg/day once or in divided doses	

Imipramine	**T:** 10 mg, 25 mg, 50 mg **C:** 75 mg, 100 mg, 125 mg, 150 mg	**T:** Initially, 25–50 mg/day once or in divided doses, then 100–300 mg/day once or in divided doses	
Nortriptyline (Pamelor)	**C:** 10 mg, 25 mg, 50 mg, 75 mg **Susp:** 10 mg/5 mL	Initially, 25 mg once daily, then 50–200 mg/day once daily or in divided doses	Dizziness, nausea, insomnia, abdominal pain, dyspepsia
5HT1A Receptor Agonists			
Gepirone (Exxua)	**ER:** 18.2 mg, 36.3 mg, 54.5 mg, and 72.6 mg	Initially, 18.2 mg once daily with food. May increase to 36.3 mg once daily on day 4, then to 54.5 mg after day 7, and to 72.6 mg after an additional week	
Selective Serotonin Reuptake Inhibitors			
Citalopram (Celexa)	**T:** 10 mg, 20 mg, 40 mg **ODT:** 40 mg **Susp:** 10 mg/5 mL	Initially, 10 mg once daily, then 20–40 mg once daily	**Class Side Effects:** Restlessness, sleep disturbances, nausea, diarrhea, headache, fatigue, sexual dysfunction, weight gain; increased risk of bleeding; may prolong QT interval
Escitalopram (Lexapro)	**T:** 5 mg, 10 mg, 20 mg **Susp:** 5 mg/5 mL	Initially, 10 mg once daily, then 10–20 mg once daily	
Fluoxetine (Prozac)	**C:** 10 mg, 23 mg, 40 mg **C (DR):** 90 mg **T:** 10 mg, 20 mg **Susp:** 20 mg/5 mL	Initially, 20 mg once daily, then 20–60 mg once daily **DR:** 90 mg once wkly	
Paroxetine (Paxil)	**T:** 10 mg, 20 mg, 30 mg, 40 mg **Susp:** 10 mg/5 mL **ER:** 12.5 mg, 25 mg, 37.5 mg	Initially, 20 mg once daily, then 20–60 mg once daily **ER:** Initially, 12.5 mg once daily, then 25–75 mg once daily	
Sertraline (Zoloft)	**T:** 25 mg, 50 mg, 100 mg **Susp:** 20 mg/ml	Initially, 50 mg once daily, then 50–200 mg once daily	

Continued

ANTIDEPRESSANTS—cont'd

Name	Availability	Dosage Range (per day)	Side Effects
Serotonin-Norepinephrine Reuptake Inhibitors			
Desvenlafaxine (Pristiq)	**T: ER:** 25 mg, 50 mg, 100 mg	50 mg once daily	**Class Side Effects:** Similar to SSRIs. Additionally, sweating, tachycardia, urinary retention, increase in blood pressure
Duloxetine (Cymbalta)	**C: DR:** 20 mg, 30 mg, 60 mg **C: Sprinkle:** 30 mg, 40 mg, 60 mg	Initially 40–60 mg/day in 1 or 2 divided doses, then 60–120 mg/day in 1–2 divided doses	
Venlafaxine (Effexor)	**T:** 25 mg, 37.5 mg, 50 mg, 75 mg, 100 mg **T (ER):** 37.5 mg, 75 mg, 150 mg, 225 mg **C: ER:** 37.5 mg, 75 mg, 150 mg	**T:** Initially, 37.5 mg once daily, then 75–375 mg/day once daily or 2–3 doses **ER:** Initially 37.5–75 mg once daily, then 75–375 mg once daily	
Other			
Aripiprazole (Abilify)	**T:** 2 mg, 5 mg, 10 mg, 15 mg, 20 mg, 30 mg	Initially, 2–5 mg once daily, then titrate to 2–15 mg once daily	Akathesia, restlessness, tremor, extrapyramidal disorder, insomnia
Brexpiprazole (Rexulti)	**T:** 0.25 mg, 0.5 mg, 1 mg, 2 mg, 3 mg, 4 mg	Initially, 0.5–1 mg once daily, then titrate up to 3 mg once daily	Weight gain, akathisia
Bupropion (Aplenzin, Wellbutrin ER, Wellbutrin XL, Forfivo XL)	**T:** 75 mg, 100 mg **T: SR:** (12 hr): 100 mg, 150 mg, 200 mg **T: XL: (24 hr):** 150 mg, 300 mg, 450 mg **Aplenzin: (24 hr):** 174 mg, 348 mg, 522 mg	Initially, 100 mg 2 times/day. **Usual dose:** 100 mg 3 times/day **XL:** Initially, 150 mg once daily, then 300–450 mg once daily **Aplenzin:** Initially, 174 mg once daily, then 348 mg once daily **SR:** Initially, 150 mg once daily. **Usual dose:** 150 mg 2 times/day	Insomnia, irritability, agitation, tremor, headache, anxiety, HTN

Drug	Form/Strengths	Dosage	Adverse Effects
Bupropion/dextromethorphan (Auvelity)	**T (ER):** 45 mg/105 mg dextromethorphan/bupropion	Initially, 1 tablet once daily in the morning, then increase to 1 tablet twice daily separated by at least 8 hrs	Dizziness, headache, diarrhea, somnolence, dry mouth, sexual dysfunction, hyperhidrosis
Esketamine (Spravato)	**Nasal Spray:** Delivers 2 sprays containing a total of 28 mg of esketamine	**Induction Phase Wks 1–4:** Administer twice per wk day 1 (starting dose): 56 mg. **Subsequent doses:** 56 mg or 84 mg. **Maintenance Phase Wks 5–8:** Give once wkly as 56 mg or 84 mg. **Wk 9 and thereafter:** Administer q2wks or once wkly as 56 mg or 84 mg	Anxiety, dissociation, dizziness, hypertension, hypoesthesia, lethargy, nausea, sedation, vertigo, vomiting
Mirtazapine (Remeron)	**T:** 7.5 mg, 15 mg, 30 mg, 45 mg **ODT:** 15 mg, 30 mg, 45 mg	Initially, 15 mg once at bedtime, then 15–45 mg once daily	Sedation, weight gain, dizziness, dry mouth, constipation
Trazodone (Desyrel)	**T:** 50 mg, 100 mg, 150 mg, 300 mg	Initially, 75 mg 2 times/day, then 150–600 mg/day in 2 divided doses	Sedation, orthostatic hypotension, priapism dizziness, nervousness
Vilazodone (Viibryd)	**T:** 10 mg, 20 mg, 40 mg	Initially, 10 mg once daily. **Usual dose:** 20–40 mg once daily	Diarrhea, nausea, dizziness, dry mouth, insomnia, vomiting, decreased libido, weight gain
Vortioxetine (Trintellix)	**T:** 5 mg, 10 mg, 20 mg	Initially, 10 mg once daily. 20–40 mg once daily. **Usual dose:** 10–20 mg once daily	Nausea, constipation, vomiting
Zuranolone (Zurzuvae)	**T:** 20 mg, 25 mg, 30 mg	50 mg once daily for 14 days	Somnolence, dizziness, diarrhea, fatigue, nasopharyngitis, urinary tract infection

ADHD, Attention-deficit hyperactivity disorder; *C*, capsules; *DR*, delayed-release; *ER*, extended-release; *GAD*, generalized anxiety disorder; *OC*, oral concentrate; *OCD*, obsessive-compulsive disorder; *ODT*, orally disintegrating tablets; *SAD*, social anxiety disorder; *SR*, sustained-release; *Susp*, suspension; *T*, tablets.

Antidiabetics

USES

ACTION

Insulin: A hormone synthesized and secreted by beta cells of Langerhans' islet in the pancreas. Controls storage and utilization of glucose, amino acids, and fatty acids by activated transport systems/enzymes. Inhibits breakdown of glycogen, fat, protein. Insulin lowers blood glucose by inhibiting glycogenolysis and gluconeogenesis in liver; stimulates glucose uptake by muscle, adipose tissue. Activity of insulin is initiated by binding to cell surface receptors.

Alpha-glucosidase inhibitors: Work locally in small intestine, slowing carbohydrate breakdown and glucose absorption.

Metformin: Decreases hepatic glucose production, increases secretion of glucagon-like peptide-1 (GLP-1).

SGLT2 inhibitors: Decrease renal glucose reabsorption, increase urinary glucose excretion.

DPP-4: Inhibits degradation of endogenous incretins, which increases insulin secretion, decreases glucagon secretion.

Meglitinide: Stimulates pancreatic insulin secretion.

Sulfonylureas: Stimulate release of insulin from beta cells of the pancreas.

Thiazolidinediones: Enhance insulin sensitivity in muscle and fat.

SGLT2: Blocks glucose reabsorption in proximal tubule in the kidney, increases urinary glucose excretion.

ANTIDIABETICS

Note: Side effects of all insulins include hypoglycemia, weight gain, allergic reactions, injection-site reactions, lipodystrophy, pruritus, rash, edema.

INSULIN

Type	Onset	Peak	Duration	Comments
Rapid-Acting				
Apidra, glulisine	10–30 min	60 min	4–5 hrs	Refrigerate unopened vial. Do not freeze. Stable at room temperature for 28 days after opening. Can mix with NPH

Admelog, lispro	10–30 min	0.5–2 hrs	3–5 hrs	Refrigerate unopened vial. Do not freeze. Stable at room temperature for 28 days after opening.
Humalog, lispro	10–30 min	0.5–2 hrs	3–5 hrs	Refrigerate unopened vial. Do not freeze. Stable at room temperature for 28 days after opening. Can mix with NPH
Novolog, aspart	10–30 min	1–2 hrs	1–2 hrs	Refrigerate unopened vial. Do not freeze. Stable at room temperature for 28 days after opening. Can mix with NPH
Fiasp, aspart	2.5 min	60 min	3–5 hrs	Refrigerate unopened vial. Do not freeze. Stable at room temperature for 28 days after opening.
Short-Acting			
Humulin R, Novolin R, regular	30–60 min	1–5 hrs	4–12 hrs	Refrigerate unopened vial. Do not freeze. Stable at room temperature for 28 days after opening. Can mix with NPH
Intermediate-Acting			
Humulin N, Novolin N, NPH	1–2 hrs	4–12 hrs	12–24 hrs	Refrigerate unopened vial. Do not freeze. Stable at room temperature for 31 days after opening (Pen 14 days). Can mix with aspart, lispro, glulisine
Long-Acting			
Basaglar, glargine	1–4 hrs	No peak	24 hrs	Do NOT mix with other insulins. Refrigerate unopened vial. Do not freeze. Stable at room temperature for 28 days after opening.
Lantus, glargine	1–4 hrs	No peak	24 hrs	Do NOT mix with other insulins. Refrigerate unopened vial. Do not freeze. Stable at room temperature for 28 days after opening.

Continued

ANTIDIABETICS—cont'd

Type	Onset	Peak	Duration	Comments
Semglee, glargine	Not available	12 hrs	24 hrs	Do NOT mix with other insulins. Refrigerate unused vial; do not refrigerate prefilled pen. Do not freeze. Vial: Stable at room temperature for 28 days after opening vial. Pre-filled pen: Stable at room temperature per expiration date until used; then stable for 28 days.
Levemir, detemir	1–2 hrs	6–12 hrs	12–24 hrs	Do NOT mix with other insulins Refrigerate unopened vial. Do not freeze. Stable at room temperature for 42 days after opening.
Toujeo, glargine	1–6 hrs	No peak	24–36 hrs	Do NOT mix with other insulins Refrigerate unopened vial. Do not freeze. Stable at room temperature for 42 days after opening.
Tresiba, degludec	1–9 hrs	No peak	Greater than 42 hrs	Do NOT mix with other insulins Refrigerate unopened vial. Do not freeze. Stable at room temperature for 56 days after opening.

ORAL AGENTS

Name	Availability	Usual Adult Dosage	Side Effects
Sulfonylureas			
Glimepiride (Amaryl)	**T:** 1 mg, 2 mg, 4 mg	1–4 mg once daily	**Class:** Hypoglycemia, weight gain, dizziness, headache, nausea
Glipizide (Glucotrol)	**T:** 5 mg, 10 mg **T (XL):** 2.5 mg, 5 mg, 10 mg	**T:** 10–20 mg/day in 1 or 2 divided doses **XL:** 5–20 mg once daily	
Glyburide **Glynase Prestab**	**T:** 1.25 mg, 2.5 mg, 5 mg **PT:** 1.5 mg, 3 mg, 6 mg	**T:** 1.25–20 mg/day in 1 or 2 divided doses **PT:** 0.75–12 mg/day in 1 or 2 divided doses	

Alpha-Glucosidase Inhibitors

Acarbose (Precose)	**T:** 25 mg, 50 mg, 100 mg	50–100 mg 3 times/day	**Class:** Abdominal pain, diarrhea, flatulence, transaminase elevations with acarbose
Miglitol (Glyset)	**T:** 25 mg, 50 mg, 100 mg	50–100 mg 3 times/day	

Dipeptidyl Peptidase Inhibitors

Alogliptin (Nesina)	**T:** 6.25 mg, 12.5 mg, 25 mg	25 mg once daily	**Class:** Possible risk of acute pancreatitis, fatal hepatic failure, possible worsening heart failure, possible severe/disabling joint pain
Linagliptin (Tradjenta)	**T:** 5 mg	5 mg once daily	
Saxagliptin (Onglyza)	**T:** 2.5 mg, 5 mg	2.5–5 mg once daily	
Sitagliptin (Januvia)	**T:** 25 mg, 50 mg, 100 mg	100 mg once daily	

Biguanides

Metformin (Glucophage)	**T:** 500 mg, 850 mg, 1,000 mg **XR:** 500 mg, 750 mg, 1,000 mg	**T:** 1,500–2,550 mg/day in 2–3 divided doses **T: XR:** 1,500–2,000 mg once daily	GI effects (metallic taste, nausea, diarrhea, abdominal pain), vitamin B_{12} deficiency, lactic acidosis

Continued

ANTIDIABETICS—cont'd

Name	Availability	Usual Adult Dosage	Side Effects
Glucagon-Like Peptide-1 (GLP-1)			
Dulaglutide (Trulicity)	**I:** 0.75 mg/0.5 mL, 1.5 mg/0.5 mL	0.75 or 1.5 mg once wkly	**Class:** GI effects (e.g., nausea, vomiting, diarrhea), decreased appetite, renal impairment, acute renal failure, injection site reactions, risk of acute pancreatitis. Pulmonary aspiration (associated with elective procedures who had residual gastric contents)
Exenatide (Byetta)	**I:** 5 mcg, 10 mcg	5–10 mcg 2 times/day	
Exenatide extended-release (Bydureon)	**I:** 2 mg	2 mg once wkly	
Liraglutide (Victoza)	**I:** 0.6 mg, 1.2 mg, 1.8 mg (6 mg/mL)	**SQ:** 1.2 or 1.8 mg once daily	
Semaglutide (Ozempic, Rybelsus)	**I:** 2 mg/1.5 mL delivers 0.25 mg, 0.5 mg, or 1 mg per injection **T:** 3 mg, 7 mg, 14 mg	**SQ:** Initially, 0.25 mg wkly for 4 wks, then 0.5 mg/wk. May double dose q4wks up to 2 mg wkly **PO:** 7 or 14 mg once daily	
Tirzepatide (Mounjaro)	**I:** 2.5 mg, 5 mg, 7.5 mg, 10 mg, 12.5 mg, 15 mg single-dose pen	Initially, 2.5 mg wkly. After 4 wks, may increase to 5 mg wkly. After 4 wks, may further increase by 2.5 mg increments up to 15 mg once wkly	

Meglitinides

Nateglinide (Starlix)	**T:** 60 mg, 120 mg	60–120 mg 3 times/day	**Class:** Hypoglycemia, weight gain
Repaglinide (Prandin)	**T:** 0.5 mg, 1 mg, 2 mg	1–4 mg 3 times/day	

SGLT2

Bexagliflozin (Brenzavvy)	**T:** 20 mg	20 mg/day in the morning	**Class:** Genital mycotic infections, volume depletion, acute kidney injury, hypotension, ketoacidosis, fractures, increased LDL-cholesterol
Canagliflozin (Invokana)	**T:** 100 mg, 300 mg	100–300 mg/day before first meal of day	
Dapagliflozin (Farxiga)	**T:** 5 mg, 10 mg	5–10 mg/day in morning	
Empagliflozin (Jardiance)	**T:** 10 mg, 25 mg	10–25 mg/day in morning	
Ertugliflozin (Steglatro)	**T:** 5 mg, 15 mg	5–15 mg once daily	

Thiazolidinediones

Pioglitazone (Actos)	**T:** 15 mg, 30 mg, 45 mg	15–45 mg once daily	**Class:** Weight gain; HF, macular edema, possible decrease in bone mineral density/increased risk of fractures, hepatic failure

HF, Heart failure; *I,* injection; *PT,* prestab; *SQ,* subcutaneous; *T,* tablets; *XL,* extended-release; *XR,* extended-release.

Antidiarrheals

USES

Acute diarrhea, chronic diarrhea of inflammatory bowel disease, reduction of fluid from ileostomies.

ACTION

Systemic agents: Act as smooth muscle receptors (enteric) disrupting peristaltic movements, decreasing GI motility, increasing transit time of intestinal contents.

Local agents: Adsorb toxic substances and fluids to large surface areas of particles in the preparation. Some of these agents protect irritated intestinal walls. May have local anti-inflammatory action.

ANTIDIARRHEALS

Name	Availability	Type	Dosage Range
Bismuth (Pepto-Bismol)	**T:** 262 mg **C:** 262 mg **L:** 130 mg/15 mL, 262 mg/15 mL, 524 mg/15 mL	Local	**A:** 2 **T** or 30 mL **CH: (9–12 yrs):** 1 **T** or 15 mL **CH: (6–8 yrs):** 2/3 **T** or 10 mL **CH: (3–5 yrs):** 1/3 **T** or 5 mL
Diphenoxylate with atropine (Lomotil)	**T:** 2.5 mg **L:** 2.5 mg/5 mL	Systemic	**A:** 5 mg 4 times/day **CH:** 0.3–0.4 mg/kg/day in 4 divided doses **(L)**
Loperamide (Imodium)	**C:** 2 mg **T:** 2 mg **L:** 1 mg/5 mL, 1 mg/mL	Systemic	**A:** Initially, 4 mg **(Maximum:** 16 mg/day) **CH: (9–12 yrs):** 2 mg 3 times/day **CH: (6–8 yrs):** 2 mg 2 times/day **CH: (2–5 yrs):** 1 mg 3 times/day **(L)**

A, Adults; *C,* capsules; *CH,* children; *L,* liquid; *T,* tablets.

Antifungals: Systemic Mycoses

Systemic mycoses are subdivided into opportunistic infections (candidiasis, aspergillosis, cryptococcosis, and mucormycosis) that are seen primarily in debilitated or immunocompromised hosts and nonopportunistic infections (blastomycosis, histoplasmosis, and coccidioidomycosis) that occur in any host. Treatment can be difficult because these infections often resist treatment and may require prolonged therapy. Drugs for systemic antifungal treatment include amphotericin B (and its lipid formulations), azole derivatives (fluconazole, isavuconazonium, itraconazole, posaconazole, voriconazole), echinocandins (anidulafungin, caspofungin, micafungin).

ANTIFUNGALS: SYSTEMIC MYCOSES

Name	Indications	Side Effects
Amphotericin B	Potentially life-threatening fungal infections, including aspergillosis, blastomycosis, coccidioidomycosis, cryptococcosis, histoplasmosis, systemic candidiasis	Fever, chills, headache, nausea, vomiting, nephrotoxicity, hypokalemia, hypomagnesemia, hypotension, dyspnea, arrhythmias, abdominal pain, diarrhea, increased hepatic function tests
Amphotericin B lipid complex (Abelcet)	Invasive fungal infections	Chills, fever, hypotension, headache, nausea, vomiting
Amphotericin B liposomal (AmBisome)	Empiric therapy for presumed fungal infections in febrile neutropenic pts, treatment of cryptococcal meningitis in HIV-infected pts, treatment of *Aspergillus, Candida, Cryptococcus* infections, treatment of visceral leishmaniasis	Peripheral edema, tachycardia, hypotension, chills, insomnia, headache

Continued

ANTIFUNGALS: SYSTEMIC MYCOSES—cont'd

Name	Indications	Side Effects
Amphotericin colloidal dispersion (Amphotec)	Invasive *Aspergillus*	Hypotension, tachycardia, chills, fever, vomiting
Anidulafungin (Eraxis)	Candidemia, esophageal candidiasis	Diarrhea, hypokalemia, increased hepatic function tests, headache
Caspofungin (Cancidas)	Candidemia, invasive aspergillosis, empiric therapy for presumed fungal infections in febrile neutropenic pts	Headache, nausea, vomiting, diarrhea, increased hepatic function tests
Fluconazole (Diflucan)	Treatment of vaginal candidiasis; oropharyngeal, esophageal candidiasis; and cryptococcal meningitis. Prophylaxis to decrease incidence of candidiasis in pts undergoing bone marrow transplant receiving cytotoxic chemotherapy and/or radiation.	Nausea, vomiting, abdominal pain, diarrhea, dysgeusia, increased hepatic function tests, liver necrosis, hepatitis, cholestasis, headache, rash, pruritus, eosinophilia, alopecia
Isavuconazonium (Cresemba)	Treatment of invasive aspergillosis, invasive mucormycosis	Nausea, vomiting, diarrhea, increased hepatic enzymes, hypokalemia, constipation, dyspnea, cough, peripheral edema, back pain
Itraconazole (Sporanox)	Blastomycosis, histoplasmosis, aspergillosis, onychomycosis, empiric therapy of febrile neutropenic pts with suspected fungal infections, treatment of oropharyngeal and esophageal candidiasis	Congestive heart failure, peripheral edema, nausea, vomiting, abdominal pain, diarrhea, increased hepatic function tests, liver necrosis, hepatitis, cholestasis, headache, rash, pruritus, eosinophilia
Ketoconazole (Nizoral)	Candidiasis, chronic mucocutaneous candidiasis, oral thrush, candiduria, blastomycosis, coccidioidomycosis	Nausea, vomiting, abdominal pain, diarrhea, gynecomastia, increased LFTs, liver necrosis, hepatitis, cholestasis, headache, rash, pruritus, eosinophilia

Micafungin (Mycamine)	Esophageal candidiasis, *Candida* infections, prophylaxis in pts undergoing hematopoietin stem cell transplantation	Fever, chills, hypokalemia, hypomagnesemia, hypocalcemia, myelosuppression, thrombocytopenia, nausea, vomiting, abdominal pain, diarrhea, increased LFTs, dizziness, headache, rash, pruritus, pain or inflammation at injection site, fever
Posaconazole (Noxafil)	Prevent invasive aspergillosis and *Candida* infections in pts 13 yrs and older who are immunocompromised, treatment of oropharyngeal candidiasis	Fever, headaches, nausea, vomiting, diarrhea, abdominal pain, hypokalemia, cough, dyspnea
Rezafungin (Rezzayo)	Treatment of candidemia and invasive candidiasis	Diarrhea, anemia, vomiting, nausea, hypomagnesemia, abdominal pain, constipation, hypophosphatemia
Voriconazole (Vfend)	Invasive aspergillosis, candidemia, esophageal candidiasis, serious fungal infections	Visual disturbances, nausea, vomiting, abdominal pain, diarrhea, increased LFTs, liver necrosis, hepatitis, cholestasis, headache, rash, pruritus, eosinophilia

Antiglaucoma Agents

USES

Reduction of elevated intraocular pressure (IOP) in pts with open-angle glaucoma and ocular hypertension.

ACTION

Medications decrease IOP by two primary mechanisms: decreasing aqueous humor (AH) production or increasing AH outflow.

- *Alpha₂ agonists:* Activate receptors in ciliary body; inhibiting aqueous secretion and increasing uveoscleral aqueous outflow.
- *Beta blockers:* Reduce production of aqueous humor.

- *Carbonic anhydrase inhibitors:* Decrease production of AH by inhibiting enzyme carbonic anhydrase.
- *Prostaglandins:* Increase outflow of aqueous fluid through uveoscleral route.
- *Rho kinase inhibitors:* Inhibit the norepinephrine transporter. Decrease resistance in the trabecular meshwork outflow pathway, decrease aqueous humor production and increase outflow of aqueous humor.

ANTIGLAUCOMA AGENTS

Name	Availability	Dosage Range	Side Effects
Alpha₂ Agonists			
Apraclonidine (Iopidine)	**S:** 0.5%, 1%	1 drop bid or tid	Fatigue, somnolence, local allergic reaction, dry eyes, stinging
Brimonidine (Alphagan HP)	**S:** 0.1%, 0.15%, 0.2%	1 drop bid or tid	Same as apraclonidine
Prostaglandins			
Bimatoprost (Lumigan)	**S:** 0.01%, 0.03%	1 drop daily in evening	Conjunctival hyperemia; darkening of iris, eyelids; increase in length, thickness, and number of eyelashes; local irritation; itching; dryness; blurred vision
Latanoprost (Xalatan)	**S:** 0.005%	1 drop daily in evening	See bimatoprost
Latanoprostene bunod (Vyzulta)	**S:** 0.0024%	1 drop every evening	Conjunctival hyperemia, eye irritation, eye pain, iris pigmentation
Omidenepag isopropyl (Omlonti)	**S:** 0.002%	1drop daily in evening	Conjunctival hyperemia, photophobia, blurred vision, dry eye, eye pain, headache

Tafluprost (Zioptan)	S: 0.0015%	1 drop daily in evening	See bimatoprost
Travoprost (Travatan)	S: 0.004%	1 drop daily in evening	See bimatoprost
Beta Blockers			
Betaxolol (Betoptic, Betoptic-S)	Susp: (Betoptic-S): 0.25% S: (Betoptic): 0.5%	**Betoptic-S:** 1 drop 2 times/day **Betoptic:** 1–2 drops 2 times/day	Fatigue, dizziness, bradycardia, respiratory depression, mask symptoms of hypoglycemia, block effects of beta agonists in treatment of asthma
Carteolol (Ocupress)	S: 1%	1 drop 2 times/day	Same as betaxolol
Levobunolol (Betagan)	S: 0.25%, 0.5%	1 drop 1–2 times/day	Same as betaxolol
Metipranolol (OptiPranolol)	S: 0.3%	1 drop 2 times/day	Same as betaxolol
Timolol (Betimol, Istalol, Timoptic, Timoptic XE)	S: 0.25%, 0.5% G: Timoptic XE: 0.25%, 0.5%	**S:** 1 drop 2 times/day **(Istalol):** 1 drop daily **G:** 1 drop daily	Same as betaxolol
Carbonic Anhydrase Inhibitors			
Brinzolamide (Azopt)	Susp: 1%	1 drop 3 times/day	Bitter taste, stinging, redness, burning, conjunctivitis, dry eyes, blurred vision
Dorzolamide (Trusopt)	S: 2%	1 drop 3 times/day	Same as brinzolamide
Rho Kinase Inhibitors			
Netarsudii (Rhopressa)	S: 0.02%	1 drop every evening	Conjunctival hyperemia, corneal verticillata, instillation site pain, conjunctival hemorrhage, blurred vision, increased lacrimation, reduced visual acuity
Combinations			
Brimonidine/timolol (Combigan)	0.2%/0.5%	1 drop bid	See individual agents

Continued

ANTIGLAUCOMA AGENTS—cont'd

Name	Availability	Dosage Range	Side Effects
Brinzolamide/brimonidine (Simbrinza)	1%/0.2%	1 drop tid	See individual agents
Timolol/dorzolamide (Cosopt)	0.5%/2%	1 drop bid	See individual agents

C, Capsules; *G,* gel; *O,* ointment; *S,* solution; *Susp,* suspension; *T,* tablets.

Antihistamines

USES

Symptomatic relief of upper respiratory allergic disorders. Allergic reactions associated with other drugs respond to antihistamines, as do blood transfusion reactions. Effective in treatment of acute urticaria and other dermatologic conditions. May also be used for preop sedation, Parkinson's disease, and motion sickness.

ACTION

Antihistamines (H₁ antagonists) inhibit vasoconstrictor effects and vasodilator effects on endothelial cells of histamine. They block increased capillary permeability, formation of edema/wheal caused by histamine. Many antihistamines can bind to receptors in CNS, causing primarily depression (decreased alertness, slowed reaction times, drowsiness) but also stimulation (restlessness, nervousness, inability to sleep). Some may counter motion sickness.

Antihistamines are further divided into 2 classes: first-generation H₁ antihistamines, which have a central effect and are used as sedatives, and second-generation H₁ antihistamines, which have a lesser central effect and are used as antiallergic drugs.

ANTIHISTAMINES
SECOND-GENERATION H1-ANTIHISTAMINES

Name	Availability	Usual Adult Dosage	Usual Pediatric Dosage	Side Effects
Cetirizine (Zyrtec Allergy) (Children's Zyrtec Allergy)	**C:** 5 mg, 10 mg **T:** 5 mg, 10 mg **ODT:** 10 mg **Syrup:** 5 mg/5 mL	10 mg once daily	**6–17 yrs:** 5–10 mg once daily **2–5 yrs:** 2.5–5 mg once daily or 2.5 mg 2 times/day **6–23 mos:** 2.5 mg once daily	**Class:** Confusion, dizziness, headaches. Less likely to impair CNS function and cause sedation

Name	Availability	Usual Adult Dosage	Usual Pediatric Dosage	Side Effects
Desloratadine (Clarinex)	**T:** 5 mg **ODT:** 2.5 mg, 5 mg	5 mg once daily	**6–11 yrs:** 2.5 mg once daily **1–5 yrs:** 1.25 mg once daily **6–11 mos:** 1 mg once daily	**Class:** Drowsiness, dry mouth, dry eyes, blurred or double vision, dizziness, headache, difficulty urinating, constipation
Fexofenadine (Allegra Allergy, Children's Allegra Allergy)	**T:** 30 mg, 60 mg, 180 mg **ODT:** 30 mg **Susp:** 30 mg/5 mL	60 mg 2 times/day or 180 mg once daily	**2–11 yrs:** 30 mg 2 times/day **6–23 mos:** 15 mg 2 times/day	
Levocetirizine (Xyzal Allergy 24 hour, Children's Xyzal Allergy)	**T:** 5 mg **S:** 2.5 mg/5 mL	5 mg once daily	**6–11 yrs:** 2.5 mg once daily **6 mos–5 yrs:** 1.25 mg once daily	
Loratadine (Alavert, Claritin, Children's Claritin)	**C:** 10 mg **T:** 10 mg **ODT:** 10 mg **T (Chew):** 5 mg **Syrup:** 1 mg/mL	10 mg once daily	**6–11 yrs:** 10 mg once daily **2–5 yrs:** 5 mg once daily	

FIRST-GENERATION H1-ANTIHISTAMINES

Name	Availability	Usual Adult Dosage	Usual Pediatric Dosage	Side Effects
Diphenhydramine (Benadryl)	**C:** 25 mg, 50 mg **T:** 25 mg, 50 mg **I:** 50 mg/mL **Liquid:** 12.5 mg/5 mL	25–50 mg q4–6h	**12 yrs and older:** 25–50 mg q4–8h **6–11 yrs:** 12.5–25 mg q6–8h **2–5 yrs:** 6.25 mg q6–8h	
Hydroxyzine	**C:** 25 mg, 50 mg, 100 mg **T:** 10 mg, 25 mg, 50 mg **Syrup:** 10 mg/5 mL	25–50 mg q6–8h	12.5–25 mg 3–4 times/day	

C, Capsules; *Chew,* chewable; *I,* injection; *ODT,* orally disintegrating tablet; *S,* solution; *Susp,* suspension; *T,* tablet.

Continued

Antihyperlipidemics

USES

Cholesterol management.

ACTION

Bile acid sequestrants: Bind bile acids in the intestine; prevent active transport and reabsorption and enhance bile acid excretion. Depletion of hepatic bile acid results in the increased conversion of cholesterol to bile acids.

HMG-CoA reductase inhibitors (statins): Inhibit HMG-CoA reductase, the last regulated step in the synthesis of cholesterol. Cholesterol synthesis in the liver is reduced.

Niacin (nicotinic acid): Reduces hepatic synthesis of triglycerides and secretion of very low density lipoprotein (VLDL) by inhibiting the mobilization of free fatty acids from peripheral tissues.

Fibric acid: Increases the oxidation of fatty acids in the liver, resulting in reduced secretion of triglyceride-rich lipoproteins, and increases lipoprotein lipase activity and fatty acid uptake.

Cholesterol absorption inhibitor: Acts in the gut wall to prevent cholesterol absorption through the intestinal villi.

Omega fatty acids: Exact mechanism unknown. Mechanisms may include inhibition of acyl-CoA, decreased lipogenesis in liver, increased lipoprotein lipase activity.

PCSK9 inhibitors: Binds with high-affinity and specificity to LDL cholesterol receptors, promoting their degradation.

Adenosine triphosphate–citrate lyase (ACL) inhibitor: ACL is an enzyme involved in hepatic cholesterol synthesis. Increases LDL from blood.

Name	Primary Effect	Dosage	Comments/Side Effects
Bile Acid Sequestrants			
Cholestyramine (Prevalite, Questran)	Decreases LDL Increases HDL, TG	8 g once daily or 4 g two times/day	**Class Side Effects:** Constipation, heartburn, nausea, eructation, and bloating May increase triglyceride levels. Avoid use with triglyceride levels greater than 300 mg/dL.
Colesevelam (Welchol)	Decreases LDL Increases HDL, TG	3.75 g once daily or 1.875 g 2 times/day	
Cholesterol Absorption Inhibitor			
Ezetimibe (Zetia)	Decreases LDL Increases HDL Decreases TG	10 mg once daily	Administer at least 2 hrs before or 4 hrs after bile acid sequestrants **Side Effects:** Dizziness, headache, fatigue, diarrhea, abdominal pain, arthralgia, sinusitis, pharyngitis
Fibric Acid Derivatives			
Fenofibrate (Antara, Lofibra, Tricor, Triglide)	Decreases TG Decreases LDL Increases HDL	**Antara:** 43–130 mg/day **Lofibra:** 67–200 mg/day **Tricor:** 48–145 mg/day **Triglide:** 50–160 mg/day **Fenoglide:** 40–120 mg/day **Lipofen:** 50–150 mg/day	May increase levels of ezetimibe. Concomitant use of statins may increase rhabdomyolysis, elevate CPK levels, and cause myoglobinuria **Side Effects:** Abdominal pain, constipation, diarrhea, respiratory complaints, headache, fever, flulike syndrome, asthenia
Fenofibric acid (Fibricor, Trilipix)	Decreases TG, LDL Increases HDL	**Trilipix:** 45–135 mg/day **Fibricor:** 35–105 mg/day	May give without regard to meals. Concomitant use of statins may increase rhabdomyolysis **Side Effects:** Headache, upper respiratory tract infection, pain, nausea, dizziness, nasopharyngitis

Continued

ANTIHYPERLIPIDEMICS—cont'd

Name	Primary Effect	Dosage	Comments/Side Effects
Gemfibrozil (Lopid)	Decreases TG Increases HDL	600 mg 2 times/day	Give 30 min before breakfast and dinner. Concomitant use of statins may increase rhabdomyolysis, elevate CPK levels, and cause myoglobinuria **Side Effects:** Fatigue, vertigo, headache, rash, eczema, diarrhea, abdominal pain, nausea, vomiting, constipation
Niacin			
Niacin, nicotinic acid (Niacor, Niaspan)	Decreases LDL,TG Increases HDL	**Regular-release (Niacor):** 1 g tid **Extended-release (Niaspan):** 1–2 g at bedtime	Diabetics may experience a dose-related elevation in glucose **Side Effects:** Increased LFT, hyperglycemia, dyspepsia, itching, flushing, dizziness, insomnia
Statins			
Atorvastatin (Lipitor)	Decreases LDL,TG Increases HDL	Initially, 10–20 mg/day **Range:** 10–80 mg/day	May interact with CYP3A4 inhibitors (e.g., amiodarone, diltiazem, cyclosporine, grapefruit juice) increasing risk of myopathy **Side Effects:** Myalgia, myopathy, rhabdomyolysis, headache, chest pain, peripheral edema, dizziness, rash, abdominal pain, constipation, diarrhea, dyspepsia, nausea, flatulence, increased LFT, back pain, sinusitis
Fluvastatin (Lescol)	Decreases LDL,TG Increases HDL	40–80 mg/day	Primarily metabolized by CYP2C9 enzyme system. May increase levels of phenytoin, rifampin. May lower fluvastatin levels **Side Effects:** Headache, fatigue, dyspepsia, diarrhea, nausea, abdominal pain, myalgia, myopathy, rhabdomyolysis

Drug	Action	Dosage	Interactions/Side Effects
Lovastatin (Mevacor)	Decreases LDL, TG Increases HDL	Initially, 20 mg/day. Adjust at 4 wk intervals **Maximum: 80 mg/day**	May interact with CYP3A4 inhibitors (e.g., amiodarone, diltiazem, cyclosporine, grapefruit products) increasing risk of myopathy **Side Effects:** Increased CPK levels, headache, dizziness, rash, constipation, diarrhea, abdominal pain, dyspepsia, nausea, flatulence, myalgia, myopathy, rhabdomyolysis
Pitavastatin (Livalo)	Decreases LDL, TG Increases HDL	Initially, 2 mg/day. May increase at 4 wk intervals to 4 mg/day	Erythromycin, rifampin may increase concentration **Side Effects:** Myalgia, back pain, diarrhea, constipation, pain in extremities
Pravastatin (Pravachol)	Decreases LDL, TG Increases HDL	Initially, 40 mg/day. Titrate to response **Range:** 10–80 mg/day	May be less likely to be involved in drug interactions Cyclosporine may increase pravastatin levels **Side Effects:** Chest pain, headache, dizziness, rash, nausea, vomiting, diarrhea, increased LFTs, cough, flulike symptoms, myalgia, myopathy, rhabdomyolysis
Rosuvastatin (Crestor)	Decreases LDL, TG Increases HDL	Initially, 10–20 mg/day Titrate to response **Range:** 5–40 mg/day	May be less likely to be involved in drug interactions Cyclosporine may increase rosuvastatin levels **Side Effects:** Chest pain, peripheral edema, headache, rash, dizziness, vertigo, pharyngitis, diarrhea, nausea, constipation, abdominal pain, dyspepsia, sinusitis, flulike symptoms, myalgia, myopathy, rhabdomyolysis
Simvastatin (Zocor)	Decreases LDL,TG Increases HCL	Initially, 10–20 mg/day. Titrate to desired response. **Range:** 5–40 mg/day	May interact with CYP3A4 inhibitors (e.g., amiodarone, diltiazem, cyclosporine, grapefruit products) increasing risk of myopathy **Side Effects:** Constipation, flatulence, dyspepsia, increased LFTs, increased CPK, upper respiratory tract infection

Continued

ANTIHYPERLIPIDEMICS—cont'd

Name	Primary Effect	Dosage	Comments/Side Effects
ACL Inhibitor			
Bempedoic acid (Nexletol)	Decreases LDL	180 mg once daily	Back pain, extremity pain, elevated liver enzymes, hyper-uricemia, gout, tendonitis
Omega Fatty Acids			
Icosapent (Vascepa)	Decreases TG	2 g 2 times/day	**Side Effects:** Arthralgia
Lovaza	Decreases TG Increases LDL, HDL	2 g 2 times/day or 4 g once daily	Use with caution with fish or shellfish allergy **Side Effects:** Eructation, dyspepsia, taste perversion
PCSK9 Inhibitors			
Alirocumab (Praluent)	Decreases LDL	**SQ:** 75 mg q2wks or 300 mg q4wks. Maximum: 150 mg q2wks or 300 mg q4wks	**Side Effects:** Hypersensitivity reactions (e.g., rash), naso-pharyngitis, injection site reactions, influenza
Evolocumab (Repatha)	Decreases LDL	**SQ:** 140 mg q2wks or 420 mg qmo	**Side Effects:** Nasopharyngitis, upper respiratory tract infection, influenza, back pain, injection site reactions
Inclisiran (Leqvio)	Decreases LDL	**SQ:** Initially, 284 mg, repeat at 3 mos, then q6mos	Injection site reaction, arthralgia, UTI, diarrhea, bronchitis, extremity pain, dyspnea

CPK, Creatine phosphokinase; *G,* granules; *HDL,* high-density lipoprotein; *LDL,* low-density lipoprotein; *SQ,* subcutaneous; *T,* tablets; *TG,* triglycerides.

Antimigraine (Treatment/Prevention)

USES

Treatment of migraine headaches with or without aura. CGRP antibodies are used for preventive treatment of migraines.

ACTION

TRIPTANS: Selective agonists of the serotonin (5-HT) receptor in cranial arteries, which cause vasoconstriction and reduce inflammation associated with antidromic neuronal transmission correlating with relief of migraine headache.

SELECTIVE 5-HT RECEPTOR AGONIST: Selectively binds to 5-HT receptors expressed on trigeminal neurons, inhibits pain pathways in central/peripheral trigeminal system.

ERGOTS: Bind to serotonin receptors. This reduces swelling in the blood vessels. May also disrupt pain signals from the trigeminal nerves.

CGRP ANTIBODIES: A human monoclonal antibody that binds to the calcitonin gene-related peptide (CGRP) receptor, antagonizing CGRP receptor function. Used to prevent migraines, reducing the number of migraine days/month.

CGRP RECEPTOR ANTAGONISTS: CGRP is a potent endogenous vasodilator/pain signaling neuromodulator. CGRP appears to increase during migraine attacks. Used to prevent migraines, reducing the number of migraine days/month.

Continued

ANTIMIGRAINE

Name	Availability	Dosage Range	Common Side Effects
GC Receptor Antagonists			
Atogepant (Qulipta)	**T:** 10 mg, 30 mg, 60 mg	10 mg, 30 mg, or 60 mg once daily	Nausea, constipation, fatigue.
Rimegepant (Nurtec ODT)	**DT:** 75 mg	75 mg once (**Maximum:** 75 mg/day)	Nausea, somnolence
Ubrogepant (Ubrelvy)	**T:** 50 mg, 100 mg	50 or 100 mg; may repeat after 2 hrs (**Maximum:** 200 mg/day)	Nausea, somnolence
Zavegepant (Zavzpret)	**Nasal spray:** 10 mg	10 mg given as a single spray in one nostril, as needed. (**Maximum:** 10 mg in 24 hrs)	Taste disorders, nausea, nasal discomfort, vomiting
TRIPTANS			
Almotriptan (Axert)	**T:** 6.25 mg, 12.5 mg	6.25–12.5 mg; may repeat after 2 hrs (**Maximum:** 25 mg/day)	**Class:** Tingling, flushing, dizziness, drowsiness, fatigue, feeling of heaviness, tightness, pressure in the chest, somnolence, weakness. Contraindicated in pts with ischemic or vasospastic coronary artery disease, Wolff-Parkinson-White syndrome, peripheral vascular disease, ischemic bowel disease, uncontrolled HTN, or history of stroke/transient ischemic attack
Eletriptan (Relpax)	**T:** 20 mg, 40 mg	**A:** 20–40 mg; may repeat after 2 hrs (**Maximum:** 80 mg/day)	
Frovatriptan (Frova)	**T:** 2.5 mg	2.5 mg; may repeat after 2 hrs; no more than 3 T/day (**Maximum:** 7.5 mg/day)	

Name	Availability	Dosage	Side Effects
Naratriptan (Amerge)	**T:** 1 mg, 2.5 mg	1–2.5 mg; may repeat once after 4 hrs (**Maximum:** 5 mg/day)	
Rizatriptan (Maxalt, Maxalt-MLT)	**T:** 5 mg, 10 mg **DT:** 5 mg, 10 mg	5 or 10 mg; may repeat after 2 hrs (**Maximum:** 30 mg/day)	
Sumatriptan (Imitrex, Onzetra Xsail, Tos/mra, Zembrace Sym Touch)	**T:** 25 mg, 50 mg, 100 mg **NS:** 5 mg, 10 mg, 20 mg **I:** 3 mg, 4 mg, 6 mg auto-injectors **NP:** 8 pouches of 2 nose pieces each 11 mg/piece	**PO:** 25–100 mg; may repeat after 2 hrs (**Maximum:** 200 mg/day) **NS:** 5–20 mg; may repeat after 2 hrs (**Maximum:** 40 mg/day) **SQ:** 3–6 mg; may repeat after 1 hr (**Maximum:** 12 mg/day) **NP:** 22 mg; may repeat after 2 hrs (**Maximum:** 44 mg/day)	
Zolmitriptan (Zomig, Zomig-ZMT)	**T:** 2.5 mg, 5 mg **DT:** 2.5 ╷g, 5 mg **NS:** 2.5 mg/0.1 mL, 5 mg/0.1 mL	**PO:** 2.5–5 mg; may repeat after 2 hrs (**Maximum:** 10 mg/day) **NS:** 1 spray (2.5 or 5 mg) at onset of migraine headache; may repeat after 2 hrs (**Maximum:** 10 mg/day)	

ERGOTS

Name	Availability	Dosage	Side Effects
Dihydroergotamine Mesylate (D.H.E. 45) Migranal Nasal Spray Trudhesa Nasal Spray	**I:** 1 mg/mL **NS:** 4 mg/mL **NS:** 4 mg/mL	**IM/SQ:** 1 mg; may repeat at 1-hr intervals. **Maximum:** 3 mg/day; 6 mg/wk. **(Migranal):** 1 spray (0.5 mg) into each nostril repeated 15 min later (2 mg/dose). **Maximum:** 3 mg/day, 4 mg/wk **(Trudhesa):** 1 spray (0.725 mg) into each nostril; may repeat after 1 hr. **Maximum:** 2.9 mg/day, 4.35 mg/wk	**Class:** Nausea and vomiting Contraindicated in pts with arterial disease or uncontrolled HTN

Continued

ANTIMIGRAINE—cont'd

Name	Availability	Dosage Range	Side Effects
Ergotamine tartrate (Ergomar)	**SL:** 2 mg	2 mg; may repeat at 30-min intervals. **Maximum:** 6 mg/day; 10 mg/wk	
Ergotamine/caffeine (Migergot)	**T:** 1/100 mg **Supp:** 2/100 mg	2 tabs PO at attack onset, then 1 tab q30min PRN. **Maximum:** 6 tabs/attack 1 suppository at attack onset; may repeat in 1 hr if needed. **Maximum:** 2 suppositories/attack	

SELECTIVE 5-HT RECEPTOR AGONIST

Name	Availability	Dosage Range	Side Effects
Lasmiditan (Reyvow)	**T:** 50 mg, 100 mg	50 mg, 100 mg, or 200 mg (**Maximum:** 1 dose/day)	Dizziness, paresthesia, sedation, vertigo, cognitive changes, confusion

CGRP ANTIBODIES

Name	Availability	Dosage Range	Side Effects
Eptinezumab (Vyepti)	100 mg/mL single-dose vial	**IV:** 100 or 300 mg q3mos	Injection site reactions, constipation, nasopharyngitis, hypersensitivity reaction
Erenumab (Aimovig)	70 mg, 140 mg single-dose auto-injector	**SQ:** 70 or 140 mg once/mo	Injection site reactions, constipation
Fremanezumab (Ajovy)	225 mg/1.5 mL single-dose auto-injector	**SQ:** 225 mg once/mo or 675 mg q3mos	Injection site reactions
Galcanezumab (Emgality)	120 mg/mL single-use pens/syringes	**SQ:** 240 mg once, then 120 mg once/mo	Injection site reactions

A, Adults; *DT,* disintegrating tablets; *I,* injection; *IM,* intramuscular; *NP,* nasal powder; *NS,* nasal spray; *S,* solution; *SL,* sublingual; *SQ,* subcutaneous; *Supp,* suppository; *T,* tablets.

Antipsychotics

USES

Antipsychotics are primarily used in managing schizophrenia. Medications are the cornerstone of schizophrenia treatment, with atypical antipsychotic medications being the most commonly prescribed drugs. Antipsychotics control symptoms by affecting the brain neurotransmitter dopamine. They may also be used in treatment of bipolar disorder, schizoaffective disorder, and irritability associated with autism. The goals in treating schizophrenia include targeting symptoms, preventing relapse, and increasing adaptive functioning. Use of antipsychotic medications is the mainstay of schizophrenia management.

ACTION

Typical (traditional): Associated with high dopamine antagonism and low serotonin antagonism. Have frequent and potentially significant neurologic side effects, including the possibility of developing tardive dyskinesia.

Atypical: Those having moderate to high dopamine antagonism and high serotonin antagonism and those having low dopamine antagonism and high serotonin antagonism. Have a lower risk of serious side effects.

ATYPICAL ANTIPSYCHOTICS

Name	Availability	Uses/Usual Adult Dosage	Side Effects
Aripiprazole (Abilify)	**T:** 2 mg, 5 mg, 10 mg, 15 mg, 20 mg, 30 mg **ODT:** 10 mg, 15 mg **S:** 1 mg/mL **I:** 9.75 mg/1.3 mL	**Schizophrenia:** 10–30 mg/day **Bipolar I disorder (manic or mixed episodes and maintenance):** 10–30 mg/day (monotherapy or with lithium or valproate) **Major depression (adjunct):** 2–15 mg/day	Akathisia, restlessness, tremor, extrapyramidal disorder, insomnia
Aripiprazole (Abilify Maintena)	**I:** 300 mg, 400 mg	**Schizophrenia:** 400 mg once monthly Continue oral agent for 14 days after first dose.	Increased weight, akathisia, injection site pain, sedation

Continued

ANTIPSYCHOTICS —cont'd

Name	Availability	Uses/Usual Adult Dosage	Side Effects
Aripiprazole (Aristada)	**I:** 441 mg, 662 mg, 882 mg, or 1,064 mg prefilled syringe	**Schizophrenia:** 441 mg IM, 662 mg, or 882 mg monthly; 882 mg q6wks; or 1,064 mg q2mos. Continue corresponding oral aripiprazole dose for 21 days after first dose	Akathisia
Aripiprazole (Abilify Asimtufii)	**I:** 960 mg/3.2 mL, 720 mg/2.4 mL in prefilled syringes	**Schizophrenia:** 960 mg IM q2mos. **Bipolar I disorder:** 960 mg IM q2mos.	Increased weight, akathisia, injection site pain, sedation
Asenapine (Saphris)	**SL:** 2.5 mg, 5 mg, 10 mg	**Schizophrenia (acute):** 5 mg 2 times/day **Schizophrenia (maintenance):** 5–10 mg 2 times/day **Bipolar mania:** 5–10 mg 2 times/day	Somnolence, oral hypoesthesia, dizziness, extrapyramidal symptoms, akathisia
Asenapine (Secudo)	**Transdermal:** 3.8 mg/24 hrs, 5.7 mg/24 hrs, 7.6 mg/24 hrs	Initially 3.8 mg/24 hrs. May increase to 5.7 mg/24 hrs or 7.6 mg/24 hrs after 1 wk	Extrapyramidal disorder, application site reaction, weight gain
Brexipiprazole (Rexulti)	**T:** 0.25 mg, 0.5 mg, 1 mg, 2 mg, 3 mg, 4 mg	**Schizophrenia:** 2–4 mg/day **MDD:** 0.5–3 mg/day	Weight increased, akathisia
Cariprazine (Vraylar)	**C:** 1.5 mg, 3 mg, 4.5 mg, 6 mg	**Schizophrenia:** 1.5–6 mg daily **Bipolar mania:** 3–6 mg daily **Bipolar depression:** 1.5–3 mg daily	Extrapyramidal symptoms, akathisia, dyspepsia, nausea, vomiting, somnolence, restlessness
Iloperidone (Fanapt)	**T:** 1 mg, 2 mg, 4 mg, 6 mg, 8 mg, 10 mg, 12 mg	**Schizophrenia:** Target dose: 6–12 mg 2 times/day (12–24 mg/day). Initially, 1 mg 2 times/day Titrate in increments to target dose not to exceed 2 mg twice daily (4 mg/day)	Dizziness, dry mouth, fatigue, nasal congestion, orthostatic hypotension, somnolence, tachycardia, weight gain
Lumateperone (Caplyta)	**C:** 10.5 mg, 21 mg, 42 mg	**Schizophrenia:** 42 mg once daily **Depressive episodes associated with bipolar I or II disorder:** 42 mg once daily	Somnolence/sedation, dizziness, nausea, dry mouth
Lurasidone (Latuda)	**T:** 20 mg, 40 mg, 60 mg, 80 mg, 120 mg	**Schizophrenia:** 40–160 mg/day **Bipolar depression:** 20–120 mg/day	Akathisia, extrapyramidal symptoms, somnolence, nausea

Olanzapine (Zyprexa)	**T:** 2 mg, 5 mg, 7.5 mg, 10 mg, 15 mg, 20 mg **ODT:** 5 mg, 10 mg, 15 mg, 20 mg **I:** 10 mg (single-dose vial)	**Schizophrenia:** Initially, 5–10 mg once daily. Target: Up to 30 mg/day **Bipolar I disorder:** 10–15 mg once daily **Depressive episodes associated with bipolar I disorder:** 5 mg olanzapine and 20 mg fluoxetine once daily **Agitation associated with schizophrenia and bipolar I mania: IM:** 5–10 mg. May repeat 2h after initial dose and 4h after second dose	Postural hypotension, constipation, weight gain, dizziness, personality disorder, akathisia, asthenia, dry mouth, constipation, increased appetite, somnolence, dizziness, tremor
Olanzapine (Zyprexa Relprevv)	**I:** 210 mg/vial, 300 mg/vial, 405 mg/vial	Establish tolerability and target dose with oral olanzapine. May switch directly to Zyprexa Relprevv with or without taper. Zyprexa Relprevv is initiated with an 8-wk loading regimen and dosed q2wks or q4wks	Headache, sedation, weight gain, cough, diarrhea, back pain, nausea, somnolence, dry mouth, nasopharyngitis, increased appetite, vomiting
Olanzapine/samidorphan (Lybalvi)	**T:** 5 mg,10 mg, 10 mg/10 mg, 15 mg/10 mg, 20 mg/10 mg	**Schizophrenia:** Initially, 5 mg/10 mg, then up to 20 mg/10 mg **Bipolar I disorder:** Initially, 5 mg/10 mg, then up to 20 mg/10 mg	Somnolence, dry mouth, headache, constipation, increased appetite, dizziness, tremor
Paliperidone (Invega)	**T:** 1.5 mg, 3 mg, 6 mg, 9 mg	**Schizophrenia:** 3–12 mg/day **Schizoaffective disorder:** 3–12 mg/day	Extrapyramidal symptoms, somnolence, dyspepsia, constipation, weight gain, nasopharyngitis, tachycardia, akathisia
Paliperidone (Erzofri, Invega Sustenna)	**I:** 39 mg/0.25 mL, 78 mg/0.5 mL, 117 mg/0.75 mL, 156 mg/1 mL, 234 mg/1.5 mL, 351 mg/2.25 mL	**Note:** 351 mg as initial dose only. **Schizophrenia: IM:** 39–234 mg monthly **Schizoaffective disorder: IM:** 78–234 mg monthly	Injection site reactions, somnolence/sedation, dizziness, akathisia, extrapyramidal disorder
Paliperidone (Invega Trinza)	**I:** 273 mg/0.88 mL, 410 mg/1.32 mL, 546 mg/1.75 mL, 819 mg/2.63 mL	**Schizophrenia after adequate treatment with Invega Sustenna for at least 4 mos: IM:** q3mos (dose depends on previous Invega Sustenna dose)	Injection site reaction, weight gain, headache, upper respiratory tract infection, akathisia, parkinsonism

Continued

ANTIPSYCHOTICS —cont'd

Name	Availability	Uses/Usual Adult Dosage	Side Effects
Paliperidone (Invega Hafyera)	I: 1,092 mg/3.5 mL, 1,560 mg/5 mL (prefilled syringes)	**Schizophrenia after adequate treatment with Invega Sustenna for at least 4 mos or Invega Trinza for at least one 3-month cycle: IM:** q6mos (dose depends on previous Invega Sustenna or Invega Trinza dose)	Upper respiratory tract infection, injection site reaction, weight gain, headache, parkinsonism
Quetiapine (Seroquel)	**T:** 25 mg, 50 mg, 100 mg, 200 mg, 300 mg, 400 mg	**Schizophrenia:** 400–800 mg/day in divided doses **Bipolar mania:** 400–800 mg/day in divided doses **Bipolar depression:** 300 mg once daily	Somnolence, dry mouth, dizziness, constipation, asthenia, abdominal pain, postural hypotension, pharyngitis, weight gain, lethargy, increased serum ALT, dyspepsia
Quetiapine (Seroquel XR)	**T, ER:** 50 mg, 150 mg, 200 mg, 300 mg, 400 mg	**Schizophrenia:** 400–800 mg once daily **Bipolar I disorder manic or mixed (acute monotherapy or adjunct to lithium or divalproex):** 600–800 mg once daily **Bipolar disorder, depressive episodes:** 300 mg once daily	Somnolence, dry mouth, constipation, dizziness, increased appetite, dyspepsia, weight gain, fatigue, dysarthria, nasal congestion
Risperidone (Risperdal)	**T:** 0.25 mg, 0.5 mg, 1 mg, 2 mg, 3 mg, 4 mg **S:** 1 mg/mL **ODT:** 0.5 mg, 1 mg, 2 mg, 3 mg, 4 mg	**Schizophrenia:** 2–6 mg/day **Bipolar mania:** 4–6 mg/day	Parkinsonism, akathisia, dystonia, tremor, sedation, dizziness, anxiety, blurred vision, nausea, vomiting, upper abdominal pain, stomach discomfort, dyspepsia, diarrhea, salivary hypersecretion, constipation, dry mouth, increased appetite, increased weight, fatigue, rash, nasal congestion, upper respiratory tract infection, nasopharyngitis, pharynx/larynx pain

Risperidone (Perseris)	I: 90 mg, 120 mg	**Schizophrenia SubQ:** 90–120 mg once monthly	Increased weight, sedation/somnolence, musculoskeletal pain
Risperidone (Risperdal Consta)	I: 12.5 mg, 25 mg, 37.5 mg, 50 mg	**Schizophrenia: IM:** 25–50 mg q2vks **Bipolar I disorder: IM:** 25–50 mg q2vks	Headache, parkinsonism, dizziness, akathisia, fatigue, constipation, dyspepsia, sedation, weight gain, extremity pain, dry mouth
Risperidone (Uzedy)	I: 50 mg/0.14 mL, 75 mg/0.21 mL, 100 mg/0.28 mL, 125 mg/0.35 mL, 150 mg/0.42 mL, 200 mg/0.56 mL, 250 mg/0.7 mL in prefilled syringes.	**SQ:** (2 mg of oral risperidone/day): 50 mg qmos,100 mg q2mos (3 mg of oral risperidone/day): 75 mg qmos, 150 mg q2mos (4 mg of oral risperidone/day): 100 mg qmos, 200 mg q2mos (5 mg of oral risperidone/day): 125 mg qmos, 250 mg q2mos	Same as risperidone (Risperdal)
Xanomeline/Trospium (Cobenfy)	C: 50 mg/20 mg, 100 mg/20 mg, 125 mc/30 mg	**Schizophrenia:** Initially, 50 mg/20 mg twice daily for at least 2 days, then 100 mg/20 mg twice daily for at least 5 days, then 125 mg/30 mg twice daily	Nausea, dyspepsia, constipation, vomiting, hypertension, abdominal pain, diarrhea, tachycardia, elevated hepatic enzymes, decreased GI motility, angioedema, anticholinergic CNS effects
Ziprasidone (Geodon)	C: 20 mg, 40 mg, 60 mg, 80 mg I: 20 mg/mL single-dose vial	**Schizophrenia:** 40–160 mg/day in 2 divided doses **Schizophrenia (acute treatment of agitation): IM:** 10 mg q2h or 20 mg q4h **Maximum:** 40 mg/day **Bipolar I disorder (acute manic/mixed episode bipolar I disorder, maintenance treatment of bipolar I disorder as an adjunct to lithium or valproate):** 80–160 mg/day in 2 divided doses	Somnolence, extrapyramidal symptoms, dizziness, akathisia, abnormal vision, asthenia, vomiting, respiratory tract infection, headache, nausea

C, Capsules; *ER,* extended-release; *I,* injection; *IM,* intramuscular; *ODT,* orally disintegrating tablet; *S,* solution; *SL,* sublingual; *T,* tablet.

Antiseizure Medications

Epilepsy is a common, chronic neurological condition affecting the brain and nervous system. Epileptic seizure is defined as a sudden occurrence of transient signs/symptoms (e.g., loss of awareness, unresponsiveness, uncontrolled movements, or unusual behavior) caused by abnormal and excessive neuronal activity in the brain. Epilepsy is defined as at least two unprovoked seizures occurring more than 24 hrs apart; one unprovoked seizure and the probability of further seizures similar to the recurrence risk (at least 60%) after two unprovoked seizures; or the diagnosis of an epilepsy syndrome as a cluster of signs/symptoms and known etiology that tend to occur together (e.g., childhood absence epilepsy, Dravet syndrome, Lennox-Gastaut syndrome).

SEIZURE AND EPILEPSY TYPES

Seizures types are classified based on where electrical activity starts in the brain: focal, general, or unknown.

Focal (partial) onset seizures result from electrical activity in a distinct brain region. This type of seizure can occur with or without loss of consciousness. Motor symptoms may include jerking (clonic), muscles becoming limp or weak (atonic), tense or rigid muscles (tonic), brief muscle twitching (myoclonus), or epileptic spasms. There may also be repeated automatic movements (e.g., clapping or rubbing of hands, lip smacking or chewing, or running). Nonmotor symptoms may include, for example, changes in sensation, emotions, thinking, or cognition.

Generalized onset seizures involve both sides of the brain. Different types of generalized seizures include motor symptoms: sustained, rhythmical jerking movements (clonic), muscles becoming weak or limp (atonic), muscles becoming tense or rigid (tonic), brief muscle twitching (myoclonus), or epileptic spasms (body flexes and extends repeatedly). Nonmotor symptoms are usually called absence seizures. These can be typical or atypical absence seizures (staring spells) and can also have brief twitches (myoclonus) that can affect a specific part of the body or just the eyelids.

Unknown onset seizures: Motor seizures are described as either tonic-clonic or epileptic spasms. Nonmotor seizures usually include a behavior arrest. This means movement stops (e.g., person may just stare and not make any other movements).

Epilepsy types are based on the seizure types and include focal epilepsy, generalized epilepsy, combined general and focal epilepsy, and epilepsy of unknown type.

PHARMACOLOGICAL MANAGEMENT

Antiseizure drugs (ASDs) are the mainstay of treating epilepsy. The primary goal is seizure remission while minimizing adverse effects of ASDs. ASDs must be selected on the seizure and epilepsy type, the epilepsy syndrome, and adverse effects associated with the drug. ASDs should be initiated as monotherapy at a low dose with slow titration to attain an initial moderate dose that minimizes adverse events. If the seizure recurs, the dose should be increased until there are no subsequent seizures, the maximum dose is attained, or adverse events occur, whichever comes first.

ANTI-SEIZURE MEDICATIONS

Name	Indication	Usual Adult Dosage	Common Side Effects
Brivaracetam (Briviact)	Focal	50–200 mg/day in 2 divided doses	Somnolence/sedation, dizziness, fatigue, nausea/vomiting
Carbamazepine (Carbatrol, Equetro, TEGretol, TEGretol-XR)	Focal Generalized	**IR:** 800–1,600 mg/day in 2–3 divided doses **ER:** 800–1,600 mg in 2 divided doses	Dizziness, drowsiness, unsteadiness, nausea, vomiting
Cenobamate (Xcopri)	Focal	200–400 mg once/day	QT interval shortening, somnolence, dizziness, fatigue, diplopia, headache
CloBAZam (Onfi, Sympazan)	Lennox Gastaut syndrome (LGS)	**30 kg or less:** 20 mg daily **Greater than 30 kg:** 40 mg daily	Constipation, somnolence or sedation, pyrexia, lethargy, drooling
Clonazepam (KlonoPIN)	LGS Myoclonic Absence	1.5–8 mg/day in 2–3 divided doses	Ataxia, behavior disorders, drowsiness,
Eslicarbazepine (Aptiom)	Focal	800 mg once/day	Dizziness, somnolence, nausea, headache, diplopia, vomiting, fatigue, vertigo, ataxia, blurred vision, and tremor
Ethosuximide (Zarontin)	Absence	750–1,250 mg/day in 2 divided doses	Nausea, vomiting, lethargy, headache, behavioral changes

Continued

ANTI-SEIZURE MEDICATIONS—cont'd

Name	Indication	Usual Adult Dosage	Common Side Effects
Gabapentin (Neurontin)	Focal	600 mg 3 times/day	Somnolence, dizziness, ataxia, fatigue, nystagmus
Lacosamide (Vimpat)	Focal Generalized	200–400 mg/day in 2 divided doses	Diplopia, headache, dizziness, nausea, somnolence
Lamotrigine (LaMICtal, Subvenite)	Focal Generalized	**IR:** 225–375 mg/day in 2 divided doses **XR:** 200–600 mg once daily	Dizziness, ataxia, somnolence, headache, diplopia, nausea, vomiting, rash, insomnia, incoordination
Levetiracetam (Elepsia XR, Keppra	Generalized Myoclonic	**IR:** 500–1,500 mg twice daily. **XR:** 1,000–3,000 mg once/day	Somnolence, asthenia, infection, dizziness
Oxcarbazine (Oxtellar XR, Trileptal)	Focal	**IR:** 1,200–2,400 mg/day in 2–3 divided doses **XR:** 1,200–2,400 mg once/day	Dizziness, somnolence, headache, balance disorder, tremor, vomiting, diplopia, asthenia, fatigue
Perampanel (Fycompa)	Focal Generalized	8–12 mg/day at bedtime	Dizziness, somnolence, fatigue, irritability, fall, nausea, weight gain, vertigo, ataxia, headache, vomiting, contusion, abdominal pain, anxiety
Phenytoin (Dilantin, Phenytek)	Focal Generalized	300–400 mg/day in 1–3 divided doses	Nystagmus, ataxia, drowsiness, diplopia, impaired cognitive function, osteopenia
Pregabalin (Lyrica)	Focal	150–600 mg/day in 2–3 divided doses	Dizziness, somnolence, dry mouth, edema, blurred vision, weight gain, thinking abnormal (especially concentration/attention)
Rufinamide (Banzel)	LGS	3,200 mg/day in 2 divided doses	Headache, dizziness, fatigue, somnolence, nausea

Topiramate (Eprontia, Qudexy, Topamax, Trokendi)	Focal Generalized LGS	**IR:** 100–400 mg/day in 2 divided doses **ER:** 200–400 mg once/day	paresthesia, anorexia, weight loss, speech disorders/related speech problems, fatigue, dizziness, somnolence, nervousness, psychomotor slowing, abnormal vision, fever
Valproic acid (Depakote)	Focal Generalized (absence)	**IR:** 1,000–3,000 mg/day in 2–3 divided doses **ER:** 1,250–3,500 mg once/day	Alopecia, weight gain, nausea, vomiting, thrombocytopenia, decreased platelet function, drowsiness, decreased bone mineral density
Zonisamide (Zonegran)	Focal	100–400 mg once/day or in 2 divided doses	Somnolence, anorexia, dizziness, ataxia, agitation/irritability, difficulty with memory and/or concentration

ER, Extended-release; *IR*, instant-release; *XR*, extended-release.

Antivirals

USES

Treatment of HIV infection (see Human Immunodeficiency Virus [HIV] Infection classification or individual monographs). Treatment of cytomegalovirus (CMV) retinitis in pts with AIDS, acute herpes zoster (shingles) genital herpes (recurrent), mucosal and cutaneous herpes simplex virus (HSV), chickenpox, and influenza A viral illness.

ACTION

Effective antivirals must inhibit virus-specific nucleic acid/protein synthesis. Possible mechanisms of action of antivirals used for non-HIV infection may include interference with viral DNA synthesis and viral replication, inactivation of viral DNA polymerases, incorporation and termination of the growing viral DNA chain, prevention of release of viral nucleic acid into the host cell, or interference with viral penetration into cells.

Continued

ANTIVIRALS—cont'd

Name	Availability	Uses	Side Effects
Acyclovir (Zovirax)	**T:** 400 mg, 800 mg **C:** 200 mg **I:** 50 mg/mL	Mucosal/cutaneous HSV-1 and HSV-2, varicella-zoster (shingles), genital herpes, herpes simplex, encephalitis, chickenpox	Malaise, anorexia, nausea, vomiting, light-headedness
Adefovir (Hepsera)	**T:** 10 mg	Chronic hepatitis B	Asthenia, headaches, abdominal pain, nausea, diarrhea, flatulence, dyspepsia
Amantadine (Symmetrel)	**T:** 100 mg **C:** 100 mg **S:** 50 mg/5 mL	Influenza A	Anxiety, dizziness, headaches, nausea, loss of appetite
Cidofovir (Vistide)	**I:** 75 mg/mL	CMV retinitis	Decreased urination, fever, chills, diarrhea, nausea, vomiting, headaches, loss of appetite
Famciclovir (Famvir)	**T:** 125 mg, 250 mg, 500 mg	Herpes zoster, genital herpes, herpes labialis, mucosal/cutaneous herpes simplex	Headaches, nausea
Foscarnet (Foscavir)	**I:** 24 mg/mL	CMV retinitis, HSV infections	Decreased urination, abdominal pain, nausea, vomiting, dizziness, fatigue, headaches

Ganciclovir (Cytovene)	I: 500 mg	CMV retinitis, CMV disease	Sore throat, fever, unusual bleeding/bruising
Molnupiravir (Lagevrio)	C: 200 mg	COVID-19	Diarrhea, nausea, dizziness
Nirmatrelvir/ritonavir (Paxlovid)	T: Nirmatrelvir 150 mg T: Ritonavir 100 mg	COVID-19	Dysgeusia, diarrhea
Oseltamivir (Tamiflu)	C: 30 mg, 45 mg, 75 mg S: 6 mg/mL	Influenza A or B	Diarrhea, nausea, vomiting
Remdesivir (Veklury)	I: 100 mg	COVID-19	Nausea, increased serum ALT, AST
Ribavirin (Virazole)	Aerosol: 6 g OS: 40 mg/mL T: 200 mg, 400 mg, 600 mg	Lowers respiratory infections in infants, children due to respiratory syncytial virus (RSV), chronic hepatitis C	Anemia
Valacyclovir (Valtrex)	T: 500 mg, 1 g	Herpes zoster, genital herpes, herpes labialis, chickenpox	Headaches, nausea
Valganciclovir (Valcyte)	T: 450 mg OS: 50 mg/mL	CMV retinitis	Anemia, abdominal pain, diarrhea, headaches, nausea, vomiting, paresthesia
Zanamivir (Relenza)	Inhalation: 5 mg	Influenza A and B	Cough, diarrhea, dizziness, headaches, nausea, vomiting

C, Capsules; *I,* injection; *OS,* oral solution; *S,* syrup; *T,* tablet.

Asthma/COPD

USES

Asthma: Chronic lung disorder marked by recurring episodes of airway obstruction (e.g., labored breathing with wheezing and coughing) and feeling of chest constriction. Asthma is triggered by hyper-reactivity to various stimuli (e.g., pollen, dust, animal fur/feathers, exercise, viral infection, cold air). The obstruction is usually reversible with airflow good between attacks of asthma. Medication treatment includes inhaled corticosteroid (ICS), short-acting beta$_2$-agonist (SABA) as a reliever agent, inhaled antimuscarinic agent as a reliever agent, leukotriene-receptor antagonist (LTRA), inhaled long-acting beta$_2$-agonist (LABA), anti-immunoglobulin E (IgE) agent, anti-interleukin-5 (IL-5) agent, oral corticosteroids, theophylline (rarely used). Treatment guidelines recommend reliever therapies that include an anti-inflammatory component. Options include using a low-dose ICS and a SABA together or a low-dose ICS and the LABA (*formoterol*) in a single inhaler.

COPD: Disorder that persistently obstructs bronchial airflow. COPD is frequently related to cigarette smoking and mainly involves two related diseases: chronic bronchitis and emphysema. The obstruction is usually permanent with progression over time. Medication treatment includes inhaled corticosteroid (ICS), inhaled antimuscarinic agent (LAMA), and inhaled long-acting beta$_2$-agonist (LABA).

ACTION

Inhaled corticosteroids: Exact mechanism unknown. May act as anti-inflammatories, decrease mucus secretion.

Beta$_2$-adrenergic agonists: Stimulate beta receptors in lung, relax bronchial smooth muscle, increase vital capacity, decrease airway resistance.

Antimuscarinics: Inhibit cholinergic receptors on bronchial smooth muscle (block acetylcholine action).

Leukotriene modifiers: Decrease effect of leukotrienes, which increase migration of eosinophils, producing mucus/edema of airway wall, causing bronchoconstriction.

IgE: Inhibits the binding of IgE to high-affinity receptors on surface of mast cells and basophils.

IL-5: Binds to IL-5, reducing the production and survival of eosinophils.

Methylxanthines: Directly relax smooth muscle of bronchial airway, pulmonary blood vessels (relieve bronchospasm, increase vital capacity. Increase cyclic 3,5-adenosine monophosphate.

ASTHMA/COPD

SHORT-ACTING BETA₂-AGONISTS (SABAs)

Name	Availability	Usual Adult Dosage	Side Effects
Albuterol (ProAir HFA, Proventil HFA, Ventolin HFA, ProAir Respiclick, ProAir Digihaler) **Solution for nebulization**	**MDI:** 90 mcg/inh **Neb:** 0.63 mg/3 mL, 1.25 mg/3 mL, 2.5 mg/3 mL	90–180 mcg q4–6h PRN 1.25–5 mg q4–8h PRN	**Class:** Tremor, tachycardia, QT interval prolongation, hyperglycemia, hypokalemia, hypomagnesemia
Levalbuterol (Xopenex HFA)	**MDI:** 45 mcg/inh	90 mcg q4–6h PRN	

SHORT-ACTING MUSCARINIC ANTAGONIST (SAMA)

Ipratropium (Atrovent HFA) **Solution for nebulization**	**MDI:** 17 mcg/inh **Neb:** 500 mcg/2.5 mL	2 inh (34 mcg) 4 times/day PRN 500 mcg 4 times/day PRN	Dry mouth, pharyngeal irritation

SHORT-ACTING BETA₂-AGONIST/SHORT-ACTING MUSCARINIC ANTAGONIST COMBINATION

Albuterol/ipratropium (Combivent Respimat)	**MDI:** 100 mcg/20 mcg/inh	1 inh 4 times/day PRN	Upper respiratory infection, nasopharyngitis, cough, bronchitis, headache, dyspnea

Continued

Asthma/COPD—cont'd

INHALED CORTICOSTEROIDS (ICSs)

Name	Availability	Usual Adult Dosage	Side Effects
Beclomethasone (QVAR Redihaler)	**MDI:** 40 mcg/inh, 80 mcg/inh	40–320 mcg 2 times/day	**Class:** Oral candidiasis (thrush), dysphonia, reflex cough, bronchospasm
Budesonide (Pulmicort Flexhaler)	**DPI:** 90 mcg/inh, 180 mcg/inh	180–720 mcg 2 times/day	
Fluticasone furoate (Arnuity Ellipta)	**DPI:** 50 mcg/inh, 100 mcg/inh, 200 mcg/inh	100–200 mcg once daily	
Fluticasone propionate (Flovent Diskus) (Flovent HFA) (ArmonAir Digihaler)	**DPI:** 50 mcg, 100 mcg, 250 mcg **MDI:** 44 mcg/inh, 110 mcg/inh, 220 mcg/inh **DPI:** 55 mcg/inh, 113 mcg/inh, 232 mcg/inh	100–1,000 mcg 2 times/day 88–880 mcg 2 times/day 55–232 mcg 2 times/day	
Mometasone furoate (Asmanex HFA) (Asmanex Twisthaler)	**MDI:** 50 mcg/inh, 100 mcg/inh, 200 mcg/inh **DPI:** 110 mcg/inh, 220 mcg/inh	200–400 mcg 2 times/day 220–440 mcg once daily in evening or 440 mcg 2 times/day	

LONG-ACTING BETA₂-AGONISTS (LABAs)

Name	Availability	Usual Adult Dosage	Side Effects
Arformoterol (Brovana)	**Neb:** 15 mcg/2 mL	15 mcg 2 times/day	**Class:** Tremor, hyperglycemia, hypokalemia, tachycardia, QT interval prolongation
Formoterol (Perforomist)	**Neb:** 20 mcg/2 mL	20 mcg 2 times/day	
Olodaterol (Striverdi Respimat)	**MDI:** 2.5 mcg/inh	2 inh once daily	
Salmeterol (Serevent Diskus)	**DPI:** 50 mcg/blister	50 mcg 2 times/day	

INHALED CORTICOSTEROID/LONG-ACTING BETA₂-AGONIST COMBINATIONS

Budesonide/Formoterol (Symbicort)	**MDI:** 80 mcg/4.5 mcg/inh, 160 mcg/4.5 mcg/inh	2 inh 2 times/day	See individual agents
Fluticasone Furoate/Vilanterol (Breo Ellipta)	**DPI:** 100 mcg/25 mcg/inh, 200 mcg/25 mcg/inh	1 inh once daily	
Fluticasone Propionate/Salmeterol **(Advair Diskus)**[1] **(Advair HFA)**	**DPI:** 100 mcg/50 mcg, 250 mcg/50 mcg, 500 mcg/50 mcg/blister **MDI:** 45 mcg/21 mcg/inh, 115 mcg/21 mcg/inh, 230 mcg/21 mcg/inh	1 inh 2 times/day 2 inh 2 times/day	
(AirDuo Respiclick)	**DPI:** 55 mcg/14 mcg/inh, 113 mcg/14 mcg/inh, 232 mcg/14 mcg/inh	1 inh 2 times/day	
Mometasone/Formoterol (Dulera)	**MDI:** 50 mcg/5 mcg/inh, 100 mcg/5 mcg/inh, 200 mcg/5 mcg/inh	2 inh (100 mcg/5 mcg or 200 mcg/5 mcg) 2 times/day	

INHALED LONG-ACTING MUSCARINIC ANTAGONIST (LAMA)

Name	Availability	Usual Adult Dosage	Side Effects
Aclidinium (Tudorza Pressair)	**DPI:** 400 mcg/inh	1 inh 2 times/day	**Class:** Dry mouth, pharyngeal irritation, urinary retention, elevated intraocular pressure
Glycopyrrolate (Lonhala Magnair)	**Neb:** 25 mcg/mL	25 mcg 2 times/day	
Revefenacin (Yupelri)	**Neb:** 175 mcg/3 mL	175 mcg once daily	

Continued

Asthma/COPD—cont'd

Name	Availability	Usual Adult Dosage	Side Effects
Tiotropium (Spiriva Respimat) **Spiriva Handihaler)**	**MDI:** 1.25 mcg/inh **C:** 18 mcg	2 inh once/day 18 mcg once daily	
Umeclidinium (Incruse Ellipta)	**DPI:** 62.5 mcg/inh	1 inh once daily	
INHALED LONG-ACTING ANTIMUSCARINIC AGENT/LONG-ACTING BETA$_2$-AGONIST COMBINATIONS (LAMA/LABA COMBINATIONS)			
Aclidinium/Formoterol (Duaklir Pressair)	**DPI:** 400 mcg/12 mcg/inh	1 inh 2 times/day	See individual agents
Glycopyrrolate/Formoterol (Bevespi Aerosphere)	**MDI:** 9 mcg/4.8 mcg/inh	2 inh 2 times/day	
Tiotropium/Olodaterol (Stiolto Respimat)	**MDI:** 2.5 mcg/2.5 mcg/inh	2 inh once daily	
Umeclidinium/Vilanterol (Anoro Ellipta)	**DPI:** 62.5 mcg/25 mcg/inh	1 inh once daily	
INHALED CORTICOSTEROID/LONG-ACTING MUSCARINIC ANTAGONIST/LONG-ACTING BETA$_2$-AGONIST COMBINATION			
Budesonide/Glycopyrrolate/Formoterol Fumarate (Breztri Aerosphere)	**MDI:** 160 mcg/9 mcg/4.8 mcg/inh	2 inh 2 times/day	See individual agents
Fluticasone Furoate/Umeclidinium/ Vilanterol (Trelegy Ellipta)	**DPI:** 100 mcg/62.5 mcg/25 mcg/inh, 200 mcg/62.5 mcg/25 mcg/inh	1 inh once daily	

LEUKOTRIENE MODIFIERS

Name	Availability	Usual Adult Dosage	Side Effects
Montelukast (Singulair)	**T:** 10 mg **Chew:** 4 mg, 5 mg **Oral granules:** 4 mg	10 mg once daily in evening	**Class:** Neuropsychiatric events (e.g., suicidal ideation), hepatic injury
Zafirlukast (Accolate)	**T:** 10 mg, 20 mg	20 mg 2 times/day	

ANTI-IMMUNOGLOBULIN E (IGE) ANTIBODY

Name	Availability	Usual Adult Dosage	Side Effects
Omalizumab (Xolair)	**I:** 150 mg **Syringes:** 75 mg/0.5 mL, 150 mg/mL	150–300 mg SQ q4wks or 225–375 mg SQ q2wks	Injection site pain, bruising, risk of anaphylaxis

ANTI-INTERLEUKIN-5 (IL-5) AND ANTI-IL-5 RECEPTOR ALPHA ANTIBODIES

Name	Availability	Usual Adult Dosage	Side Effects
Benralizumab (Fasenra)	**I:** 30 mg/mL syringe	**SQ:** 30 mg q4wks × 3 doses, then q8wks	Headache, pyrexia, pharyngitis, hypersensitivity reactions
Mepolizumab (Nucala)	**I:** 100-mg vial, syringe	**SQ:** 100 mg q4wks	Injection site reactions, headache, back pain, fatigue, hypersensitivity reactions
Reslizumab (Cinqair)	**I:** 100 mg/10 mL syringe	**IV:** 3 mg/kg q4wks	Oropharyngeal pain, myalgia, elevated creatine phosphokinase, hypersensitivity reactions

Continued

Asthma/COPD—cont'd

ANTI-INTERLEUKIN-4 (IL-4) RECEPTOR ALPHA ANTIBODY

Name	Availability	Usual Adult Dosage	Side Effects
Dupilumab (Dupixent)	**I:** 200 mg/1.14 mL, 300 mg/2 mL syringe **Injector pen:** 300 mg/2 mL	**SQ:** 400 mg, then 200 mg q2wks OR 600 mg, then 300 mg q2wks	Injection site reactions, conjunctivitis, transient increases in blood eosinophils

THYMIC STROMAL LYMPHOPOIETIN (TSLP) BLOCKER

Name	Availability	Usual Adult Dosage	Side Effects
Tezepelumab-ekko (Tezspire)	**I:** 210 mg/1.91 mL (110 mg/mL) syringe	**SQ:** 210 mg q4wks	Pharyngitis, arthralgia, back pain

PHOSPHODIESTERASE-4 (PDE4) INHIBITOR

Name	Availability	Usual Adult Dosage	Side Effects
Roflumilast (Daliresp)	**T:** 250 mcg, 500 mcg	500 mcg once daily	Nausea, diarrhea

PHOSPHODIESTERASE (PDE) 3 AND 4 INHIBITOR

Name	Availability	Usual Adult Dosage	Side Effects
Ensifentrine (Ohtuvayre)	**Neb:** 3 mg/2.5 mL ampules	3 mg twice daily via nebulizer	Back pain, hypertension, UTI, diarrhea, insomnia, anxiety, depression, suicidal ideation

C, Capsule, inhalation; *Chew,* chewable; *DPI,* dry powder inhalation; *I,* injection; *inh,* inhalation; *IV,* intravenous; *MDI,* metered dose inhaler; *Neb,* nebulizer; *SQ,* subcutaneous.

Attention Deficit/Hyperactivity Disorder (ADHD)

ADHD is a developmental disorder associated with an ongoing pattern of inattention (difficulty paying attention), hyperactivity (having too much energy or moving and talking too much), and/or impulsivity (acting without thinking or having difficulty with self-control). The symptoms of ADHD can interfere significantly with an individual's daily activities and relationships. ADHD begins in childhood and can continue into the teen years and adulthood. Treatment for ADHD includes behavioral therapy, medication, or a combination of methods.

BEHAVIORAL THERAPY

Counseling for adult ADHD generally includes psychological counseling (psychotherapy) (e.g., cognitive behavioral therapy, marital counseling/family therapy), education about ADHD, and learning skills.

MEDICATION

Stimulants: Stimulants, which are schedule II controlled substances are the drugs of choice for treatment of ADHD in school-age children, adolescents, and adults. Use of long-acting formulations, which generally contain both immediate- and extended-release components, have become standard clinical practice. A short-acting formulation may be used in addition to improve symptom control early in the morning or to prolong the duration of action in the afternoon. Stimulants should be started at the lowest recommended dose, which may be increased q7days (or q3days in urgent cases) until a substantial improvement in symptoms is achieved. Common adverse effects include decreased appetite, abdominal pain, weight loss, headache, and sleep disturbances (e.g., delay in sleep onset). In addition, psychotic symptoms, cardiovascular events, abuse/misuse, and dependence can occur. Stimulants should be avoided in pts with serious heart problems or if increases of blood pressure or heart rate would be problematic.

Nonstimulants: Nonstimulants can be used as initial monotherapy or in combination with stimulants or if stimulants are contraindicated, ineffective, or not tolerated. Nonstimulants include atomoxetine, extended-release clonidine (oral suspension, tablets), extended-release guanfacine, and extended-release viloxazine. Atomoxetine and viloxazine are selective norepinephrine reuptake inhibitors. Common side effects may include fatigue, sleep disturbance, nausea, vomiting, headache, and decreased appetite. Extended-release clonidine and guanfacine are alpha-adrenergic agonists. Common side effects may include sleep disturbances, dizziness, drowsiness, fatigue, headache, and abdominal pain.

Continued

STIMULANTS
METHYLPHENIDATE STIMULANTS

Name	Availability	Dosage	Comments
Immediate-Release			
Ritalin	**T:** 5 mg, 10 mg, 20 mg	**CH:** Initially, 5 mg 2–3 times/day **A:** Initially, 5 mg 2–3 times/day (consider 4 times/day) or 10 mg 2 times/day **Titration:** 5–10 mg **Max/day:** 60 mg	Give in the morning, at noon, and at 4 PM, if needed; preferably 30–45 min before meals
Methylin	**T (Chew):** 2.5 mg, 5 mg, 10 mg **S (Oral):** 5 mg/5 mL, 10 mg/5 mL	Same as Ritalin	Same as Ritalin
Extended-Release			
Adhansia XR	**C:** 25 mg, 35 mg, 45 mg, 55 mg, 70 mg, 85 mg	**CH, A:** Initially, 25 mg once daily **Titration:** 10–15 mg **Max/day:** 85 mg	Give in the morning without regard to food. May give whole or sprinkled on applesauce or yogurt
Aptensio XR	**C:** 10 mg, 15 mg, 20 mg, 30 mg, 40 mg, 50 mg, 60 mg	**CH (6 yrs and older), A:** **Initially:** 10 mg **Titration:** 10 mg **Max/day:** 60 mg	Give once daily in morning (at a consistent time with regard to food). May give whole or sprinkled on applesauce
Concerta	**T (ER):** 18 mg, 27 mg, 36 mg, 54 mg	**CH (6–17 yrs): Initially:** 18 mg **A:** 18–36 mg **Titration:** 18 mg (27 mg tablet for titration between 18 and 36 mg) **Max/day: CH:** 54 mg; **Adolescents, A:** 72 mg	Give once daily in morning without regard to food. Administer whole

Cotempla XR-ODT	**ODT (ER):** 8.6 mg, 17.3 mg, 25.9 mg	**CH: Initially:** 17.3 mg **Titration:** 8.6–17.3 mg **Max/day:** 51.8 mg	Give once daily in morning at a consistent time with regard to food. Allow tablet to dissolve (with saliva [no liquid needed]) on tongue without chewing/crushing
Daytrana	**TP:** 1.1 mg/hr (10 mg/9 hr) 1.6 mg/hr (15 mg/9 hr) 2.2 mg/hr (20 mg/9 hr) 3.3 mg/hr (30 mg/9 hr)	**CH (6–17 yrs): Initially:** 10 mg **Titration:** Next highest patch strength **Max/day:** 30 mg	Wear daily for 9 hrs (apply 2 hrs before desired effect). May wear up to 16 hrs, if needed Remove at least 3 hrs before bedtime Replace once daily in the morning Apply to hip area; change site daily
Jornay PM	**C (ER):** 20 mg, 40 mg, 60 mg, 80 mg, 100 mg	**CH, A: Initially:** 20 mg **Titration:** 20 mg **Max/day:** 100 mg	Give once daily in the EVENING, between 6:30 and 9:30 PM, and at consistent time with regard to food. May give whole or sprinkled on applesauce
Metadate CD	**C (ER):** 10 mg, 20 mg, 30 mg, 40 mg, 50 mg, 60 mg	**CH, A: Initially:** 20 mg **Titration:** 10–20 mg **Max/day:** 60 mg	Give once daily in morning before breakfast. Take whole or sprinkled on applesauce. Avoid alcohol (may cause rapid release of medication)
Quillichew ER	**T (ER) Chew:** 20 mg, 30 mg, 40 mg	**CH (6 yrs and older): A: Initially:** 20 mg **Titration:** 10 mg, 15 mg, or 20 mg **Max/day:** 60 mg	Give once daily in the morning without regard to food

Continued

STIMULANTS—cont'd

Name	Availability	Dosage	Comments
Quillivant XR	**Susp (Oral):** 5 mg/mL	**CH (6 yrs and older): A: Initially:** 20 mg **Titration:** 10–20 mg **Max/day:** 60 mg	Prepared by pharmacist. Give once daily in the morning without regard to food. Shake bottle for ≥10 sec prior to use (measure dose with oral dosing dispenser provided) Store in original container at room temp for up to 4 mos
Relexxii	**T (ER):** 18 mg, 27 mg, 36 mg, 45 mg, 54 mg, 63 mg, 72 mg	**CH (6–17 yrs): Initially:** 18 mg; **A:** 18–36 mg **Titration:** 18 mg **Max/day: CH (6–12 yrs):** 54 mg; **CH (13–17 yrs), A:** 72 mg	Give once daily in morning without regard to food. Administer whole
Ritalin LA	**C (LA):** 10 mg, 20 mg, 30 mg, 40 mg, 60 mg	**CH, A: Initially:** 10–20 mg **Titration:** 10 mg **Max/day:** 60 mg	Give in morning without regard to food. May give whole or sprinkled on applesauce

DEXMETHYLPHENIDATE STIMULANTS

Name	Availability	Dosage	Comments
Immediate-Release			
Focalin	**T:** 2.5 mg, 5 mg, 10 mg	**CH, A: Initially:** 2.5 mg bid **Titration:** 2.5 mg with morning and/or noon dose **Max/day:** 20 mg	Give in the morning and/or noon at least 4 hrs apart without regard to food
Extended-Release			
Focalin XR	**C:** 5 mg, 10 mg, 15 mg, 20 mg, 25 mg, 30 mg, 35 mg, 40 mg	**CH: Initially:** 5 mg; **A:** 10 mg **Titration: CH:** 5 mg; **A:** 10 mg **Max/day: CH:** 30 mg; **A:** 40 mg	Give once daily in the morning with regard to food. Give whole or sprinkle on applesauce

SERDEXMETHYLPHENIDATE AND DEXMETHYLPHENIDATE

Name	Availability	Dosage	Comments
Azstarys	**C:** 26.1/5.2 mg, 39.2/7.8 mg, 52.3/10.4 mg	**CH (6 yrs and older), A: Initially:** 39.2/7.8 mg **Titration:** Next highest capsule strength **Max/day:** 52.3/10.4 mg	Give once daily in morning without regard to food. Give whole or sprinkled on applesauce or dissolved in 2 oz. water

AMPHETAMINE STIMULANTS

Name	Availability	Dosage	Comments
Adderall (Mixed amphetamine salts)	**T:** 5 mg, 7.5 mg, 10 mg, 12.5 mg, 15 mg, 20 mg, 30 mg	**Initially: CH (3–5 yrs):** 2.5 mg once daily; **(6 yrs and older):** 5 mg 1 or 2 times/day; **A:** 10 mg 2 times/day **Titration: CH (3–5 yrs):** 2.5 mg; **(6 yrs and older):** 5 mg 1 or 2 times/day; **A:** 10 mg 2 times/day. **Max/day:** 40 mg	Give 1–3 times/day (usual is 1 or 2 times/day) at 4- to 6-hr intervals
Adderall XR (Mixed amphetamine salts)	**C (ER):** 5 mg, 10 mg, 15 mg, 20 mg, 25 mg, 30 mg	**Initially: CH (6–12 yrs):** 5–10 mg; **(13–17 yrs):** 10 mg; **A:** 20 mg **Titration:** 5–10 mg **Max/day: CH:** 30 mg; **A:** 20 mg	Give once daily in morning without regard to food. Give whole or sprinkled on applesauce
Adzenys XR-ODT	**ODT (ER):** 3.1 mg, 6.3 mg, 9.4 mg, 12.5 mg, 15.7 mg, 18.8 mg	**CH (6–17 yrs of age): Initially:** 6.3 mg **A:** 12.5 mg **Titration:** 3.1–6.3 mg **Max/day: CH (6–12 yrs):** 18.8 mg **(13 yrs and older), A:** 12.5 mg	Give once daily in morning without regard to food. Place tablet on tongue and allow to disintegrate. Swallow whole. Do not crush or allow chewing

Continued

AMPHETAMINE STIMULANTS—cont'd

Name	Availability	Dosage	Comments
Adzenys ER	**Susp (Oral):** 1.25 mg/mL	Same as Adzenys XR-ODT	Give once daily in morning without regard to food. Shake well before use. Do not add to food or mix with other liquids
Dexedrine Spansule	**C (ER):** 5 mg, 10 mg, 15 mg	**Initially: CH:** 5 mg 1–2 times/day; **(6 yrs and older):** 5 mg 1–2 times/day or 10 mg every morning **Titration:** 5 mg **Max/day:** 40 mg	Give once daily in the morning or 2 times/day
Dyanavel XR	**Susp (Oral):** 2.5 mg/mL **T:** 5 mg, 10 mg, 15 mg, 20 mg	**A, CH: Initially:** 2.5–5 mg **Titration:** 2.5–10 mg q4–7 days **Max/day:** 20 mg	Give once daily in morning without regard to food. Shake suspension prior to dose
Evekeo	**T:** 5 mg, 10 mg	**Initially: CH (3–5 yrs):** 2.5 mg once daily; **(6 yrs and older):** 5 mg 1–2 times/day; **A:** 5–10 mg once daily **Titration: CH (3–5 yrs):** 2.5 mg; **(6 yrs and older):** 5 mg; **A:** 5–10 mg **Max/day:** 40 mg	Give 1–3 times daily (first dose upon awakening; additional doses at 4- to 6-hr intervals)
Evekeo ODT	**ODT:** 5 mg, 10 mg, 15 mg, 20 mg	**CH: Initially:** 5 mg 1–2 times/day **Titration:** 5 mg **Max/day:** 40 mg	Give once daily. May repeat after 4-6 hrs. Dissolve (with saliva; no liquid needed) on the tongue without chewing/crushing

Mydayis	**C (XR):** 12.5 mg, 25 mg, 37.5 mg, 50 mg	**Initially: CH (13–17 yrs), A:** 12.5 mg **Titration:** 12.5 mg **Max/day: CH (13–17 yrs):** 25 mg; **A:** 50 mg	Give once daily in the morning upon waking and at a consistent time with regard to food
ProCentra	**S:** 1 mg/mL	**Initially: CH (3–5 yrs):** 2.5 mg in the morning; **(6 yrs and older):** 2.5 mg 2 times/day or 5 mg in the morning or 2 times/day **Titration: CH (3–5 yrs):** 2.5 mg; **(6 yrs and older):** 2.5–5 mg **Max/day:** 40 mg	Give 2–3 times/day. First dose upon awakening; additional doses at 4- to 6-hr intervals
Vyvanse	**T, Chew:** 10 mg, 20 mg, 30 mg, 40 mg, 50 mg, 60 mg **C:** 10 mg, 20 mg, 30 mg, 40 mg, 50 mg, 60 mg, 70 mg	**Initially: CH, A:** 30 mg **Titration:** 10–20 mg **Max/day:** 70 mg	Give once daily in morning without regard to food. Take capsule whole or dissolve in water, yogurt, or orange juice and give immediately
Xelstrym	**TP:** 4.5 mg, 9 mg, 13.5 mg, 18 mg	**Initially: CH (6 yrs and older):** 4.5 mg **A:** 9 mg **Titration: CH:** 4.5 mg; **A:** Individualize **Max/day:** 18 mg	Apply 2 hrs before desired effect. Remove within 9 hrs of application
Zenzedi	**T:** 2.5 mg, 5 mg, 7.5 mg, 10 mg, 15 mg, 20 mg, 30 mg	**Initially: CH (3–5 yrs):** 2.5 mg in the morning. **(6–16 yrs):** 5 mg 1–2 times/day **Titration: CH (3–5 yrs):** 2.5 mg; **(6–16 yrs):** 5 mg **Max/day:** 40 mg	Give 2–3 times/day. First dose upon awakening; additional doses at 4- to 6-hr intervals

NONSTIMULANTS

Name	Availability	Dosage	Comments
Atomoxetine (Strattera) Contains "Black Box" warning: Increased suicidal ideation in children and adolescents	**C:** 10 mg, 18 mg, 25 mg, 40 mg, 60 mg, 80 mg, 100 mg	**Initially: 70 kg or less:** 0.5 mg/kg/day; **greater than 70 kg:** 40 mg/day **Titration: 70 kg or less:** After at least 3 days, increase to approximately 1.2 mg/kg/day. Alternatively, after 4 days, increase to 1 mg/kg/day, then further increase to 1.2 mg/kg/day after 4 more days. **Greater than 70 kg:** After at least 3 days, increase to 80 mg/day, then up to 100 mg/day after 2–4 additional wks. **Max/day: CH, A up to 70 kg:** lesser of 1.4 mg/kg or 100 mg; **CH, A over 70 kg. A:** 100 mg	Give once daily or divided 2 times/day (morning and late afternoon/early evening) without regard to food
Clonidine (Kapvay)	**T (ER):** 0.1 mg	**Initially: CH, A:** 0.1 mg at bedtime **Titration:** 0.1 mg **Max/day:** 0.4 mg	Do not break, crush, or allow chewing of tablet. Doses above 0.1 mg/day should be divided 2 times/day, with an equal or higher split dosage being given at bedtime. Discontinue in decrements of no more than 0.1 mg q3–7 days
Guanfacine (Intuniv)	**T (ER):** 1 mg, 2 mg, 3 mg, 4 mg	**Initially: CH, A:** 1 mg **Titration:** 1 mg **Max/day:** 7 mg	Give once daily at approximately the same time each day Avoid high-fat meals Do not break, crush, or allow chewing Discontinue in decrements of no more than 1 mg q3–7 days
Viloxazine (Qelbree) Contains "Black Box" warning: Increased suicidal ideation in children and adolescents	**C (ER):** 100 mg, 150 mg, 200 mg	**Initially: CH (6–11 yrs):** 100 mg; **12–17 yrs:** 200 mg **Titration: CH (6–11 yrs):** 100 mg; **(12–17 yrs):** 200 mg **Max/day:** 400 mg	Give once daily without regard to food Give whole or sprinkled on applesauce

A, Adults; *C,* capsules; *CH,* children; *Chew,* chewable; *ER,* extended-release; *LA,* long-acting; *ODT,* orally disintegrating tablets; *PO,* oral; *S,* solution; *Susp,* suspension, *T,* tablets; *TP,* transdermal patch; *XR,* extended-release.

Benign Prostatic Hyperplasia

USES

About 60% of men aged 60 yrs or older have clinically relevant prostatic enlargement due to benign prostatic hyperplasia (BPH). The goals of treatment are to decrease lower urinary tract symptoms and to prevent disease progression and complications (acute urinary retention). Mild BPH symptoms should generally be managed with surveillance and nonpharmacologic interventions. For moderate to severe BPH, medications should be added to decrease symptoms and the need for surgical intervention.

Alpha₁-adrenergic antagonists (alpha blockers): Relax smooth muscle in the prostate and bladder neck, improving urinary flow. Decrease the risk of acute urinary retention, but does not decrease prostate size or slow disease progression.

5-alpha-reductase inhibitors: Block prostatic conversion of testosterone to dihydrotestosterone, decreasing the size of the prostate over several months and, consequently, increasing the rate of urinary flow.

Phosphodiesterase type-5 inhibitors: Decrease smooth muscle tone and proliferation in the prostate, bladder neck, and urethra, which leads to improved urination.

Anticholinergics: Usually used in combination with an alpha-blocker for treatment of BPH in pts whose symptoms are mainly related to bladder irritation and urine storage (urgency, frequency, nocturia).

Beta₃-adrenergic agonists: Can be added to an alpha-blocker regimen to decrease BPH symptoms associated with storage (urgency, frequency, nocturia) and bladder irritation. Mirabegron and vibegron are FDA-approved for treatment of overactive bladder but are also used off-label in combination with an alpha-blocker for treatment of BPH in pts whose symptoms are mainly related to bladder irritation and urine storage (urgency, frequency, nocturia). Activation of beta₃-receptors in the bladder causes relaxation of detrusor smooth muscle during the storage phase of the fill-void cycle and increases bladder capacity. Beta₃-agonists do not slow disease progression or treat symptoms related to bladder outlet obstruction.

Continued

BENIGN PROSTATIC HYPERPLASIA
ALPHA₁-ADRENERGIC ANTAGONISTS

Name	Availability	Dosage	Side Effects
Alfuzosin (Uroxatral)	**T, ER:** 10 mg	10 mg once daily	**Class:** Dizziness, hypotension, ejaculation dysfunction
Doxazosin (Cardura) (Cardura XL)	**T:** 1 mg, 2 mg, 3 mg, 4 mg **T, ER:** 4 mg, 8 mg	**T:** Initially, 1 mg daily up to 8 mg daily **ER:** Initially, 4 mg once daily up to 8 mg once daily	
Terazosin (generic)	**C:** 1 mg, 2 mg, 5 mg, 10 mg	Initially, 1 mg at night up to 10–20 mg at night	
Silodosin (Rapaflo)	**C:** 4 mg, 8 mg	8 mg once daily	
Tamsulosin (Flomax)	**C:** 0.4 mg	Initially, 0.4 mg once daily up to 0.8 mg once daily	

5-ALPHA-REDUCTASE INHIBITORS

Dutasteride (Avodart)	**C:** 0.5 mg	0.5 mg once daily	**Class:** Sexual dysfunction (e.g., impotence, decreased libido, ejaculation dysfunction), breast enlargement/tenderness, rash
Finasteride (Proscar)	**T:** 5 mg	5 mg once daily	

PHOSPHODIESTERASE-5 INHIBITOR

Tadalafil (Cialis)	**T:** 5 mg	5 mg once daily	Headache, dizziness, dyspepsia, back pain, myalgia

ANTICHOLINERGIC DRUGS

Name	Availability	Dosage	Side Effects
Darifenacin (generic)	**T, ER:** 7.5 mg, 15 mg	Initially, 7.5 mg once daily up to 15 mg once daily	**Class:** Dry mouth, nausea, constipation, confusion
Fesoterodine (Toviaz)	**T, ER:** 4 mg, 8 mg	Initially, 4 mg once daily up to 8 mg once daily	
Oxybutynin (generic)	**T:** 5 mg **T, ER:** 5 mg, 10 mg, 15 mg	**T:** 5 mg 2–3 times/day up to 5 mg 2–4 times/day. **T, ER:** Initially, 5–10 mg once daily up to 5–30 mg once daily	
Solifenacin (Vesicare)	**T:** 5 mg, 10 mg	Initially, 5 mg once daily up to 10 mg once daily	
Tolterodine (Detrol, Detrol LA)	**T:** 1 mg, 2 mg **C, ER:** 2 mg, 4 mg	**T:** 1–2 mg 2 times/day **C, ER:** 2–4 mg once daily	
Trospium (generic)	**T:** 20 mg **C, ER:** 60 mg	**T:** 20 mg 2 times/day **C, ER:** 60 mg in the morning	

BETA₃-ADRENERGIC AGONISTS

Name	Availability	Dosage	Side Effects
Mirabegron (Myrbetriq)	**T, ER:** 25 mg, 50 mg	Initially, 25 mg once daily up to 50 mg once daily	Headache, dizziness, nasopharyngitis, GI upset, elevated B/P
Vibegron (Gemtesa)	**T:** 75 mg	75 mg once daily	Headache, dizziness, nasopharyngitis, GI upset

C, Capsules; *ER,* extended-release; *T,* tablet.

Beta-Adrenergic Blockers

USES

Management of hypertension, angina pectoris, arrhythmias, hypertrophic subaortic stenosis, migraine headaches, MI (prevention), glaucoma.

ACTION

Beta-adrenergic blockers competitively block beta-adrenergic receptors, located primarily in myocardium, and beta₁-adrenergic receptors, located primarily in bronchial and vascular smooth muscle. By occupying beta-receptor sites, these agents prevent naturally occurring or administered epinephrine/norepinephrine from exerting their effects. The results are basically opposite to those of sympathetic stimulation.

Effects of beta₁ blockade include slowing heart rate, decreasing cardiac output and contractility; effects of beta₂ blockade include bronchoconstriction, increased airway resistance in pts with asthma or COPD. Beta blockers can affect cardiac rhythm/automaticity (decrease sinus rate, SA/AV conduction; increase refractory period in AV node); decrease systolic and diastolic B/P; exact mechanism unknown but may block peripheral receptors, decrease sympathetic outflow from CNS, or decrease renin release from kidney. All beta blockers mask tachycardia that occurs with hypoglycemia. When applied to the eye, reduce intraocular pressure and aqueous production.

BETA-ADRENERGIC BLOCKERS

Name	Availability	Indication	Usual Adult Dosage	Frequent or Severe Side Effects
Acebutolol	**C:** 200 mg, 400 mg	HTN, ventricular arrhythmia	**HTN:** 200–800 mg/day in 2 divided doses **Arrhythmia:** Initially, 200–400 mg/day in 1 or 2 divided doses up to 1,200 mg/day in 2 divided doses	**Class:** Fatigue, depression, bradycardia, decreased exercise tolerance, erectile dysfunction, heart failure, may aggravate hypoglycemia, increase incidence of diabetes, insomnia, increase triglycerides, decrease cholesterol. Sudden withdrawal may exacerbate angina and myocardial infarction.

Atenolol (Tenormin)	T: 25 mg, 50 mg, 100 mg	HTN, MI	**HTN:** 25 mg once daily up to 100 mg/day in 1 or 2 divided doses **MI:** 12.5 mg once daily up to 100 mg/day in 1 or 2 divided doses
Bisoprolol (Zebeta)	T: 5 mg, 10 mg	HTN	**HTN:** 2.5–20 mg once daily
Carvedilol (Coreg)	T: 3.125 mg, 6.25 mg, 12.5 mg, 25 mg C (SR): 10 mg, 20 mg, 40 mg, 80 mg	HF, HTN	**HF: (Immediate-Release):** Initially, 3.25 mg 2 times/day. May increase at 2-wk intervals to 6.25 mg 2 times/day, then 12.5 mg 2 times/day, greater than 85 kg: 50 mg 2 times/day. **Extended-Release:** Initially, 10 mg once daily Titrate to 80 mg once daily **HTN: (Immediate-Release):** 12.5–50 mg/day in 2 divided doses **(Extended-Release):** 20–80 mg once daily
Labetalol (Trandate)	T: 100 mg, 200 mg, 300 mg	HTN	200–800 mg/day in 2 divided doses
Metoprolol (Lopressor [IR], Toprol XL [SRI])	T (IR): 50 mg, 100 mg T (SR): 25 mg, 50 mg	HTN, angina, HF	**IR:** **Angina:** Initially, 50 mg 2 times/day. May increase up to 400 mg/day in 2 divided doses **HTN:** 100–200 mg/day in 2 divided doses **SR:** **Angina:** 100–400 mg once daily **HF:** Initially, 12.5–25 mg once daily. Titrate up to 200 mg once daily **HTN:** 25–100 mg once daily

Continued

BETA-ADRENERGIC BLOCKERS—cont'd

Nadolol (Corgard)	**T:** 20 mg, 40 mg, 80 mg	HTN	**HTN:** 40–120 mg once daily
Nebivolol (Bystolic)	**T:** 2.5 mg, 5 mg, 10 mg, 20 mg	HTN	5–40 mg once daily
Pindolol (Visken)	**T:** 5 mg, 10 mg	HTN	10–60 mg/day in 2 divided doses
Propranolol (Inderal)	**T (IR):** 10 mg, 20 mg, 40 mg, 60 mg, 80 mg **C (SR):** 60 mg, 80 mg, 120 mg, 160 mg **S:** 4 mg/mL, 8 mg/mL **I:** 1 mg/mL	HTN, angina, arrhythmias, migraine prevention	**IR:** **Angina:** 80–320 mg/day in 2–4 divided doses **Arrhythmias:** 10–30 mg 3–4 times/day **HTN:** 80–160 mg/day in 2 divided doses **Migraine prevention:** 40–160 mg/day in 2 divided doses **SR:** **Angina:** Initially, 80 mg once daily. May increase q3–7days up to 320 mg/day. **HTN:** 80–160 mg once daily at bedtime **Migraine prevention:** 60–160 mg once daily

C, Capsules; *HF,* heart failure; *HTN,* hypertension; *I,* injection; *LVD,* left ventricular dysfunction; *MI,* acute myocardial infarction; *S,* solution; *SR,* sustained-release; *T,* tablets.

Calcium Channel Blockers

USES

Treatment of essential hypertension, treatment of and prophylaxis of angina pectoris (including vasospastic, chronic stable, unstable), prevention/control of supraventricular tachyarrhythmias, prevention of neurologic damage due to subarachnoid hemorrhage.

ACTION

Calcium channel blockers inhibit the flow of extracellular Ca^{2+} ions across cell membranes of cardiac cells, vascular tissue. They relax arterial smooth muscle, depress the rate of sinus node pacemaker, slow AV conduction, decrease heart rate, produce negative inotropic effect (rarely seen clinically due to reflex response). Calcium channel blockers decrease coronary vascular resistance, increase coronary blood flow, reduce myocardial oxygen demand. Degree of action varies with individual agent.

CALCIUM CHANNEL BLOCKERS

Name	Availability	Indications	Usual Adult Dosage	Side Effects
Amlodipine (Norvasc)	**T:** 2.5 mg, 5 mg, 10 mg	HTN, angina	**HTN:** 2.5–10 mg once daily **Angina:** 5–10 mg once daily	**Class:** Dizziness, headache, constipation, peripheral edema, flushing, tachycardia, rash, gingival hyperplasia
Diltiazem (Cardizem)	**T:** 30 mg, 60 mg, 90 mg, 120 mg **(ER):** 120 mg, 180 mg, 240 mg, 300 mg, 360 mg, 420 mg **C (SR-12HR):** 60 mg, 90 mg, 120 mg, **(ER-24HR):** 120 mg, 180 mg, 240 mg, 300 mg, 360 mg, 420 mg **I:** 5 mg/mL	**PO:** HTN, angina **IV:** Arrhythmias	**HTN:** 120–360 mg once daily **Angina: IR:** 240–360 mg/day in 3–4 divided doses. **ER:** 240–360 mg once daily **I:** 20–25 mg IV bolus, then 5–15 mg/hr infusion	
Felodipine (Plendil)	**T:** 2.5 mg, 5 mg, 10 mg	HTN	2.5–10 mg once daily	

Continued

CALCIUM CHANNEL BLOCKERS—cont'd

Name	Availability	Indications	Usual Adult Dosage	Side Effects
Isradipine	**C**: 2.5 mg, 5 mg	HTN	5–10 mg/day in 2 divided doses	
Nicardipine (Cardene)	**C (IR)**: 20 mg, 30 mg **C (ER)**: 30 mg, 45 mg, 60 mg **I**: 2.5 mg/mL	HTN, angina	**Angina/HTN**: Initially, 20–30 mg 3 times/day. May increase q3days. Usual dose: 20–40 mg 3 times/day	
Nifedipine (Adalat, Procardia)	**T (ER)**: 30 mg, 60 mg, 90 mg	HTN, angina	**HTN (ER)**: 30–90 mg once daily **Angina (ER)**: 30–90 mg once daily	
Nimodipine (Nimotop, Nymalize)	**C**: 30 mg **S**: 60 mg/20 mL	Prevent neurologic damage following subarachnoid hemorrhage	60 mg q4h for 21 days	
Verapamil (Calan, Isoptin)	**T (IR)**: 40 mg, 80 mg, 120 mg **T (SR)**: 120 mg, 180 mg, 240 mg	HTN, angina	**Angina (IR)**: Initially, 80–120 mg 3 times/day up to 480 mg/day in 3 divided doses. **(SR)**: Initially, 180 mg at HS. May increase in 1 or 2 divided doses at weekly intervals up to 480 mg/day **HTN (IR)**: 40–120 mg 3 times/day **(SR)**: 120–360 mg/day in 1 or 2 divided doses	

C, Capsules; *CR*, controlled-release; *ER*, extended-release; *HTN*, hypertension; *I*, injection; *IR*, immediate-release; *S*, solution; *SR*, sustained-release; *T*, tablets.

Cancer Treatment

CHEMOTHERAPY

Traditional chemotherapeutic agents are cytotoxic by interfering with cell division (mitosis) or inducing DNA damage. These agents target all rapidly dividing cells and are not specific only to cancer cells. They are divided into broad categories. **Alkylating agents:** Prevent cells from reproducing by damaging their DNA. **Antimetabolites:** Impede DNA/RNA synthesis by blocking the enzyme required for DNA synthesis or becoming incorporated into DNA or RNA. **Antimicrotubular agents:** Prevent assembly of microtubules (vinca alkaloids) or disassembly of microtubules (taxanes). **Topoisomerase inhibitors:** Prevent DNA replication, causing breaks of DNA strands and cell death.

Strategies in administration of traditional chemotherapy include **induction:** First-line treatment used for curative intent. **Consolidation:** Administered after remission to prolong disease-free time/survival. **Neoadjuvant:** Administered prior to local treatment (e.g., surgery) to shrink primary tumor. **Adjuvant:** Administered after local treatment when there is a risk of recurrence or to treat micrometastases (reduces relapse rates). **Maintenance:** Low dose to prolong remission.

Targeted therapy is a form of chemotherapy that blocks the growth of cancers by interfering with specific targeted molecules needed for carcinogenesis and tumor growth. Biomarkers are usually required to better determine if patients are more likely to respond to the targeted therapy. Biomarkers are genes, proteins, or other substances that are tested to provide information about cancer and help to determine treatment options. **Examples of biomarker tests: Non-small-cell lung cancer:** Changes in genes such as *KRAS, EGFR, ALK, ROS1, RET, MET,* and *BRAF.* **Breast cancer:** Estrogen receptor (ER) and progesterone receptor (PR) proteins, HER2 gene or protein status, changes in genes such as *BRCA1, BRCA2,* and *PIK3CA.*

Two common medication categories of targeted therapy are **protein kinase inhibitors:** Target protein kinases that are altered in cancer cells and account for some of their abnormal growth. **Monoclonal antibodies:** Created in a lab and designed to bind to specific targets on the cancer cell, allowing the patient's immune system to better recognize and destroy them.

HORMONAL THERAPY

Blocks ability to produce hormones or blocks access to hormones that cancer cells need to grow. Hormone therapy is primarily used in treating prostate cancer and estrogen-dependent cancers (e.g., breast, ovarian, uterine). Two main categories include **(breast cancer) selective estrogen receptor modulators (SERMs):** Blocks estrogen from connecting with breast cancer cells, reducing the cell's ability to multiply. **Estrogen receptor antagonists:** Reduce and block ER signaling in early and advanced drug-resistant cases. **Aromatase inhibitors (AIs):** Inhibit the action of the enzyme aromatase, which converts androgens into estrogens. **(Prostate cancer): Luteinizing hormone-releasing hormone (LHRH):** Initially, stimulates the production of luteinizing hormone. However, continued presence of high levels of LHRH agonists causes the pituitary gland to stop producing luteinizing hormone, thereby reducing androgens. **Anti-androgens:** Bind to androgen receptors in prostate cancer cells, starving the cancer cells of androgens.

IMMUNOTHERAPY

Stimulates the patient's own immune system to treat cancer. Types include **immune checkpoint inhibitors:** Block immune system checkpoints, allowing immune cells to better respond to the cancer. **CAR-T-cell transfer therapy:** T-cells are harvested from the patient and genetically altered to better attack cancer cells, then reintroduced back into the patient. **Monoclonal antibodies:** Created in a lab and designed to bind to specific targets on the cancer cell, allowing the patient's own immune system to better recognize and destroy them. **Immune system modulators:** Enhance the body's own immune response against cancer.

TRADITIONAL CHEMOTHERAPEUTIC AGENTS

NAME	TYPE	USES	SIDE EFFECTS
Capecitabine (Xeloda)	Antimetabolite	Breast, colorectal cancers	Nausea, vomiting, diarrhea, stomatitis, myelosuppression, palmar-plantar erythrodysesthesia syndrome, dermatitis, fatigue, anorexia
Carboplatin (Paraplatin)	Alkylating agent	Ovarian cancer	Nausea, vomiting, nephrotoxicity, myelosuppression, alopecia, peripheral neuropathy, hypersensitivity, ototoxicity, asthenia, diarrhea, constipation
Cisplatin	Alkylating agent	Bladder, ovarian, testicular cancers	Nausea, vomiting, nephrotoxicity, myelosuppression, neuropathies, ototoxicity, anaphylactic like reactions, hyperuricemia, hypomagnesemia, hypophosphatemia, hypokalemia, hypocalcemia, pain at injection site
Cyclophosphamide (Cytoxan)	Alkylating agent	ALL, AML, breast cancer, CML, Hodgkin's lymphoma, multiple myeloma, NHL, ovarian carcinoma	Nausea, vomiting, hemorrhagic cystitis, myelosuppression, alopecia, interstitial pulmonary fibrosis, amenorrhea, azoospermia, diarrhea, darkening skin/fingernails, headaches, diaphoresis
Docetaxel	Antimicrotubular (Taxane)	Breast, head and neck, NSCLC, prostate cancers, gastric adenocarcinoma	Hypotension, nausea, vomiting, diarrhea, mucositis, myelosuppression, rash, paresthesia, hypersensitivity, fluid retention, alopecia, asthenia, stomatitis, fever
Doxorubicin (Adriamycin)	Topoisomerase II inhibitor	Breast, bladder, gastric, ovarian cancers; ALL, AML, Hodgkin's lymphoma, NHL, Wilm's tumor	Cardiotoxicity, including HF; arrhythmias, nausea, vomiting, stomatitis, esophagitis, GI ulceration, diarrhea, anorexia, hematuria, myelosuppression, alopecia, hyperpigmentation of nail beds and skin, local inflammation at injection site, rash, fever, chills, urticaria, lacrimation, conjunctivitis
Etoposide (Toposar)	Topoisomerase II inhibitor	Small cell lung, testicular cancers	Nausea, vomiting, anorexia, myelosuppression, alopecia, diarrhea, drowsiness, peripheral neuropathies

Fluorouracil	Antimetabolite	Breast, colon, rectal, gastric, pancreatic cancers	Nausea, vomiting, stomatitis, GI ulceration, diarrhea, anorexia, myelosuppression, alopecia, skin hyperpigmentation, nail changes, headaches, drowsiness, blurred vision, fever
Gemcitamine (Infugem)	Antimetabolite	Breast, NSCLC, ovarian, pancreatic cancers	Nausea, vomiting, diarrhea, stomatitis, hematuria, myelosuppression, rash, mild paresthesia, dyspnea, fever, edema, flulike symptoms, constipation; increased LFT
Irinotecan (Camptosar)	Topoisomerase I inhibitor	Colorectal cancer	Diarrhea, nausea, vomiting, abdominal cramps, anorexia, stomatitis, increased AST, severe myelosuppression, alopecia, diaphoresis, rash, weight loss dehydration, headache, insomnia, dizziness, dyspnea, cough, asthenia, rhinitis, fever, back pain, chills, increased serum alkaline phosphatase,
Oxaliplatin	Alkylating agent	Colon, colorectal cancers	Fatigue, neuropathy, abdominal pain, dyspnea, diarrhea, nausea, vomiting, anorexia, fever, edema, chest pain, anemia, thrombocytopenia, thromboembolism, altered hepatic function tests
Paclitaxel	Antimicrotubular (Taxane)	Breast, NSCLC, ovarian cancers, Kaposi's sarcoma	Hypertension, bradycardia, ECG changes, nausea, vomiting, diarrhea, mucositis, myelosuppression, alopecia, peripheral neuropathies, hypersensitivity reaction, arthralgia, myalgia
Pemetrexed (Alimta, Pemfexy)	Antimetabolite	NSCLC, malignant pleural mesothelioma	Anorexia, constipation, diarrhea, neuropathy, anemia, chest pain, dyspnea, rash, fatigue
Topotecan (Hycamton)	Topoisomerase I inhibitor	Cervical, ovarian, small cell lung cancers	Nausea, vomiting, diarrhea, constipation, abdominal pain, stomatitis, anorexia, neutropenia, leukopenia, thrombocytopenia, anemia, alopecia, headache, dyspnea, paresthesia
Vincristine (Vincasar PFS)	Antimicrotubular (vinca alkaloid)	Acute lymphocytic leukemia, Hodgkin's lymphoma, NHL, Wilm's tumor, neuroblastoma, rhabdomyosarcoma	Nausea, vomiting, stomatitis, constipation, pharyngitis, polyuria, myelosuppression, alopecia, numbness, paresthesia, peripheral neuropathy, loss of deep tendon reflexes, headache, abdominal pain

PROTEIN KINASE INHIBITORS

NAME	TARGET	USES	SIDE EFFECTS
Afatanib (Gilotrif)	EGFR	NSCLC, squamous NSCLC	Diarrhea, rash/acneiform dermatitis, stomatitis, paronychia, dry skin, decreased appetite, nausea, vomiting, pruritus
Bosutinib (Bosulif)	BCR-ABL	CML	Diarrhea, abdominal pain, vomiting, nausea, rash, fatigue, hepatic dysfunction, headache, pyrexia, decreased appetite respiratory tract infection, constipation
Capmatinib (Tabrecta)	MET	NSCLC	Fatigue, pyrexia, nausea, vomiting, dyspnea, cough, pneumonia, rash dizziness
Crizotinib (Xalcori)	ALK, ROS1	NSCLC, anaplastic large cell lymphoma	Vision disorders, nausea, diarrhea, vomiting, edema, constipation, elevated transaminases, fatigue, decreased appetite, upper respiratory infection, dizziness, neuropathy
Erlotinib (Tarceva)	EGFR	NSCLC, pancreatic cancers	Rash, diarrhea, anorexia, fatigue, dyspnea, cough, nausea, vomiting
Imatinib (Gleevec)	BCR-ABL	ALL, CML, dermatofibrosarcoma protuberans, GIST, chronic eosinophilic leukemia, myelodysplastic/myeloproliferative disease	Edema, nausea, vomiting, muscle cramps, musculoskeletal pain, diarrhea, rash, fatigue, abdominal pain
Lapatinib (Tykerb)	EGFR	Breast cancer	Diarrhea, palmar-plantar erythrodysesthesia, nausea, rash, vomiting, fatigue
Larotrectinib (Vitrakvi)	TRK	Solid tumors	Fatigue, nausea, dizziness, vomiting, increased AST, cough
Regorafenib (Stivarga)	VEGF	Colorectal cancer, hepatic carcinoma, GIST	Pain (including gastrointestinal and abdominal pain), HFSR, asthenia/fatigue, decreased appetite/food intake, hypertension, infection, dysphonia, hyperbilirubinemia, fever, mucositis, weight loss, rash, nausea
Tucatinib (Tukysa)	HER2	Breast, colorectal cancers	Diarrhea, fatigue, rash, nausea, abdominal pain, infusion-related reactions, and pyrexia, palmar-plantar erythrodysesthesia, hepatotoxicity, vomiting, stomatitis, decreased appetite, anemia

MONOCLONAL ANTIBODIES

NAME	TARGET	USES	COMMON SIDE EFFECTS
Alemtuzumab (Campath)	CD52	B-cell chronic lymphocytic leukemia	Infusion-related reactions (pyrexia, chills, hypotension, urticaria, dyspnea), cytopenias (neutropenia, thrombocytopenia), infections, nausea, vomiting, abdominal pain, insomnia, anxiety
Atezolizumab (Tecentriq)	PD-L1 CI	Bladder, NSCLC, breast, small-cell lung cancers, hepatocellular carcinoma, metastatic melanoma	Fatigue/asthenia, decreased appetite, nausea, cough, dyspnea
Avelumab (Bavencio)	PD-L1 CI	Merkel cell, urothelial, renal cell carcinomas	Diarrhea, fatigue, hypertension, musculoskeletal pain, nausea, mucositis, palmar-plantar erythrodysesthesia, dysphonia, decreased appetite, hypothyroidism, rash, hepatotoxicity, cough, dyspnea, abdominal pain, headache
Bevacizumab (Avastin)	VEGF	Cervical, colorectal, NSCLC, ovarian cancers; glioblastomas; hepatocellular, renal cell carcinomas	Epistaxis, headache, hypertension, rhinitis, proteinuria, taste alteration, dry skin, hemorrhage, lacrimation disorder, back pain, exfoliative dermatitis
Durvalumab (Imfinzi)	PD-L1 CI	NSCLC, small cell lung, biliary tract cancers	Cough, fatigue, pneumonitis/radiation pneumonitis, upper respiratory tract infections, dyspnea, rash
Elotuzumab (Empliciti)	SLAMF₇	Multiple myeloma	Fatigue, diarrhea, pyrexia, constipation, cough, peripheral neuropathy, nasopharyngitis, upper respiratory tract infection, decreased appetite, pneumonia

Continued

MONOCLONAL ANTIBODIES—cont'd

NAME	TARGET	USES	COMMON SIDE EFFECTS
Ipilimumab (Yervoy)	CTLA-4 CI	Metastatic melanoma; renal, hepatocellular, esophageal carcinomas; colorectal, NSCLC cancers; malignant pleural mesothelioma	Fatigue, diarrhea, pruritus, rash, and colitis, nausea, vomiting, headache, weight loss, pyrexia, decreased appetite, insomnia
Nivolumab (Opdivo)	PD-1 CI	Metastatic melanoma; NSCLC, head and neck, colorectal, small cell lung, gastric cancers; Hodgkin's lymphoma, renal cell, urothelial hepatocellular, esophageal carcinomas; malignant pleural mesothelioma	Fatigue, rash, musculoskeletal pain, pruritus, diarrhea, nausea, asthenia, cough, dyspnea, constipation, decreased appetite, back pain, arthralgia, upper respiratory tract infection, pyrexia, headache, abdominal pain, vomiting, urinary tract infection
Ofatumumab (Arzerra)	CD20	Chronic lymphocytic leukemia	Infusion reactions, neutropenia, pneumonia, pyrexia, cough, diarrhea, anemia, fatigue, dyspnea, rash, nausea, bronchitis, upper respiratory tract infections
Pembrolizumab (Keytruda)	PD-1 CI	Metastatic melanoma; NSCLC, head and neck, gastric, cervical, small cell lung, endometrial, biliary tract cancers; urothelial, hepatocellular, Merkel cell, renal cell, esophageal, squamous cell carcinomas; Hodgkin's lymphoma	Fatigue, musculoskeletal pain, rash, diarrhea, pyrexia, cough, pruritus, dyspnea, constipation, pain, abdominal pain, nausea, hypothyroidism, decreased appetite
Trastuzumab (Herceptin)	HER2	Breast, gastric cancers	Headache, diarrhea, nausea, chills, fever, infection, CHF, insomnia, cough, rash, neutropenia, diarrhea, fatigue, anemia, stomatitis, weight loss, upper respiratory tract infections, thrombocytopenia, mucosal inflammation, nasopharyngitis, dysgeusia

HORMONAL THERAPY
BREAST CANCER

NAME	TYPE	COMMON SIDE EFFECTS
Anastrozole (Arimidex)	Aromatase inhibitor	Hot flashes, asthenia, arthritis, pain, arthralgia, pharyngitis, hypertension, depression, nausea and vomiting, rash, osteoporosis, fractures, back pain, insomnia, headache, peripheral edema lymphedema
Elacestrant (Orserdu)	Estrogen receptor antagonist	Musculoskeletal pain, nausea, fatigue, vomiting, decreased appetite, diarrhea, headache, constipation, abdominal pain, hot flush, dyspepsia; increased serum cholesterol, ALT, AST, creatinine, triglycerides; decreased serum sodium, hemoglobin
Fulvestrant (Faslodex)	Estrogen receptor antagonist	Musculoskeletal pain, nausea, fatigue, decreased hemoglobin, vomiting, decreased appetite, diarrhea, headache, constipation, abdominal pain, hot flush, dyspepsia; increased serum cholesterol, ALT, AST, creatinine, triglycerides; decreased sodium
Letrozole (Femara)	Aromatase inhibitor	Hot flashes, arthralgia, flushing, asthenia, edema, arthralgia, headache, dizziness, hypercholesterolemia, sweating increased, bone pain, musculoskeletal pain
Raloxifene (Evista)	SERM	Hot flashes, leg cramps, peripheral edema, flu syndrome, arthralgia, sweating
Tamoxifen (Soltamox)	SERM	Hot flashes, mood disturbances, vaginal discharge, vaginal bleeding, nausea, fluid retention

PROSTATE CANCER

NAME	TYPE	COMMON SIDE EFFECTS
Apalutamide (Erleada)	Antiandrogen	Fatigue, arthralgia, rash, decreased appetite, fall, weight decreased, hypertension, hot flush, diarrhea, fractures
Darolutamide (Nubeqa)	Antiandrogen	Constipation, rash, decreased appetite, hemorrhage, weight increased, hypertension, fatigue, pain in extremity
Enzalutamide (Xtandi)	Antiandrogen	Musculoskeletal pain, fatigue, hot flush, constipation, decreased appetite, diarrhea, hypertension, hemorrhage, fall, fracture, headache
Goserelin, (Zoladex)	LHRH	Hot flashes, sexual dysfunction, decreased erections, lower urinary tract symptoms
Leuprolide (Eligard)	LHRH	Malaise, fatigue, dizziness, hot flashes/sweats, gastroenteritis, testicular atrophy

CAR-T-CELL IMMUNOTHERAPY

NAME	TARGET	USES	COMMON SIDE EFFECTS
Axicabtagene ciloeucel (Yescarta)	CD-19 Autologous	Large B-cell lymphomas	CRS, fever, hypotension, encephalopathy, fatigue, tachycardia, headache, nausea, febrile neutropenia, diarrhea, musculoskeletal pain, infections with pathogen unspecified, chills, decreased appetite
Brexucabtagene autoleucel (Tecartus)	CD-19 Autologous	Acute lymphoblastic leukemia (B-cell precursor), mantle cell lymphoma	Fever, CRS, hypotension, encephalopathy, fatigue, tachycardia, arrhythmia, infection with pathogen unspecified, chills, hypoxia, cough, tremor, musculoskeletal pain, headache, nausea, edema, motor dysfunction, constipation, diarrhea, decreased appetite, dyspnea, rash, insomnia, pleural effusion, aphasia, febrile neutropenia, vomiting
Cittacabtagene autoleucel (Carvykti)	BCMA Autologous	Multiple myeloma	Pyrexia, CRS, hypogammaglobulinemia, hypotension, musculoskeletal pain, fatigue, pathogen-unspecified infections, cough, chills, diarrhea, nausea, encephalopathy, decreased appetite, upper respiratory tract infection, headache, tachycardia, dizziness, dyspnea, edema, viral infections, coagulopathy, constipation, vomiting

NAME	TARGET	USES	COMMON SIDE EFFECTS
Idecabtagene vicleucel (Abecma)	BCMA Autologous	Multiple myeloma	Pyrexia, CRS, hypogammaglobulinemia, infections unspecified, musculoskeletal pain, fatigue, febrile neutropenia, hypotension, tachycardia, diarrhea, nausea, headache, chills, upper respiratory tract infection, encephalopathy, edema, dyspnea, viral infections
Lisocabtagene maraleucel (Breyanzi)	CD-19 Autologous	Large B-cell, follicular, mantle cell lymphomas, chronic lymphocytic leukemia, small lymphocytic lymphoma (SLL)	Fever, CRS, fatigue, musculoskeletal pain, nausea, encephalopathy, edema, diarrhea
Tisagenlecleucel (Kymriah)	CD-19 Autologous	B-cell acute lymphoblastic, diffuse large B-cell, follicular lymphomas	CRS, infection, hypogammaglobulinemia, fever, decreased appetite, viral infectious disorders, headache, febrile neutropenia, hemorrhage, musculoskeletal pain, vomiting, encephalopathy, diarrhea, hypotension, cough, nausea, bacterial infectious disorders, pain, hypoxia, tachycardia, edema, fatigue, acute kidney injury

AI, Aromatase inhibitor; *ALL,* acute lymphoblastic leukemia; *AML,* acute myeloid leukemia; *CI,* checkpoint inhibitor; *CML,* chronic myeloid leukemia; *CRS,* cytokine release syndrome; *GIST,* gastrointestinal stromal tumors; *NHL,* non-Hodgkin lymphoma; *NSCLC,* non–small-cell lung cancer.

Diuretics

USES

Thiazides: Management of edema resulting from a number of causes (e.g., HF, hepatic cirrhosis), hypertension (HTN) either alone or in combination with other antihypertensives.

Loop: Management of edema associated with HF, cirrhosis of the liver, and renal disease. Furosemide used in treatment of hypertension alone or in combination with other antihypertensives.

Potassium-sparing: Adjunctive treatment with thiazides, loop diuretics in treatment of HF and hypertension.

ACTION

Increase the excretion of water/sodium and other electrolytes via the kidneys. Exact mechanism of antihypertensive effect unknown; may be due to reduced plasma volume or decreased peripheral vascular resistance. Subclassifications of diuretics are based on their mechanism and site of action.

Thiazides: Act at cortical diluting segment of nephron, block reabsorption of Na, Cl, and water; promote excretion of Na, Cl, K, and water.

Loop: Act primarily at the thick ascending limb of Henle's loop to inhibit Na, Cl, and water absorption.

Potassium-sparing: Spironolactone blocks aldosterone action on distal nephron (causes K retention, Na excretion). Triamterene, amiloride act on distal nephron, decreasing Na reuptake, reducing K secretion.

DIURETICS

Thiazide, Thiazide-related

Name	Availability	Usual Adult Dosage	Side Effects
Chlorothiazide (Diuril)	**T:** 500 mg **Susp:** 250 mg/5 mL **I:** 500 mg	**Edema:** 500–1,000 mg 1–2 times/day **HTN:** 500–1,000 mg/day in 1–2 divided doses	**CLASS** Hyperuricemia, hypokalemia, hypomagnesemia, hyperglycemia, hyponatremia, hypercalcemia, hypercholesterolemia, hypertriglyceridemia, pancreatitis, rash, photosensitivity
Chlorthalidone	**T:** 25 mg, 50 mg	**Edema:** Initially, 50–100 mg once daily or 100 mg every other day **HTN:** 12.5–25 mg once daily	
Hydrochlorothiazide	**T:** 12.5 mg, 25 mg, 50 mg **C:** 12.5 mg	**Edema:** 25–100 mg/day in 1–2 divided doses **HTN:** 25–50 mg once daily	
Indapamide (Lozol)	**T:** 1.25 mg, 2.5 mg	**Edema:** Initially, 2.5 mg/day. May increase after 1 wk to 5 mg/day. **HTN:** 1.25–2.5 mg once daily	
Metolazone (Zaroxolyn)	**T:** 2.5 mg, 5 mg, 10 mg	**Edema:** 2.5–20 mg once daily **HTN:** 2.5–5 mg once daily	

Continued

DIURETICS—cont'd

Name	Availability	Usual Adult Dosage	Side Effects
Loop			
Bumetanide (Bumex)	**T:** 0.5 mg, 1 mg, 2 mg **I:** 0.25 mg/mL	**Edema:** Initially, 0.5–2 mg/dose 1–2 times/day **Maximum:** 10 mg/day **HF:** Initially, 0.5–1 mg once daily or 2 times/day up to 10 mg/day in 1–2 divided doses	**CLASS** Dehydration, hypokalemia, hyponatremia, hypomagnesemia, hyperglycemia, metabolic alkalosis, hyperuricemia, blood dyscrasias, rash, hypercholesterolemia, hypertriglyceridemia
Furosemide (Lasix)	**T:** 20 mg, 40 mg, 80 mg **OS:** 10 mg/mL, 40 mg/5 mL **I:** 10 mg/mL	**Edema: PO:** 20–80 mg/dose. May increase by 20–40 mg/dose up to 600 mg/day. **IV:** 20–40 mg/dose. May increase by 20 mg/dose. **Maximum:** 200 mg/dose **HF:** Initially, 20–40 mg once daily or 2 times/day. Titrate up to 600 mg once daily or in divided doses.	
Torsemide (Demadex)	**T:** 5 mg, 10 mg, 20 mg, 100 mg **I:** 10 mg/mL	**Edema:** 10–200 mg/day **HTN:** 5–10 mg once daily **HF:** Initially, 10–20 mg once daily. Titrate up to 200 mg once or in divided doses.	

Name	Availability	Dosage Range	Side Effects
Potassium-sparing			
Amiloride (Midamor)	**T:** 5 mg	**Edema:** Initially, 5 mg/day. May increase to 10 mg/day. **HTN:** 5–10 mg/day in 1–2 divided doses	Hyperkalemia, nausea, abdominal pain, diarrhea, rash, headache
Eplerenone (Inspra)	**T:** 25 mg, 50 mg	**HF:** Initially, 25 mg/day, titrate to 50 mg once daily **HTN:** 50–100 mg/day in 1–2 divided doses	Hyperkalemia, hyponatremia
Spironolactone (Aldactone)	**T:** 25 mg, 50 mg, 100 mg	**Edema:** 25–200 mg/day in 1 or 2 divided doses **HTN:** 25–100 mg/day in 1 or 2 divided doses **Hypokalemia:** 25–100 mg/day **HF:** Initially, 12.5–25 mg once daily **Maximum:** 50 mg once daily	Hyperkalemia, nausea, vomiting, abdominal cramps, diarrhea, hyponatremia, gynecomastia, menstrual abnormalities, rash
Triamterene (Dyrenium)	**C:** 50 mg, 100 mg	**Edema:** 100–300 mg/day in 1–2 divided doses **HTN:** 50–100 mg/day in 1–2 divided doses	Hyperkalemia, nausea, abdominal pain, nephrolithiasis

C, Capsules; *HF,* heart failure; *HTN,* hypertension; *I,* injection; *OS,* oral solution; *Susp,* suspension; *T,* tablets.

Gastroesophageal Reflux Disease (GERD), Peptic Ulcer Disease (PUD)

GERD is the most common GI condition encountered in the outpatient setting. Symptoms include heartburn, regurgitation, dyspepsia, chest pain, belching, chronic cough. Drugs that suppress gastric acid are the standard treatment for GERD and include H_2 receptor antagonists (H_2Rts) and proton pump inhibitors (PPIs).

PUD is most commonly caused by *Helicobacter pylori* infection (other causes include use of nonsteroidal anti-inflammatory drugs [NSAIDs], including aspirin, ibuprofen, and naproxen).

H_2Rts: Inhibit histamine action at H_2 receptors on parietal cells, decreasing basal acid secretion and, to a much lesser extent, food-stimulated acid secretion. *PPIs:* Binds to activated proton pump on the apical membrane of parietal cells, resulting in inhibition of acid secretion into the gastric lumen.

H_2-RECEPTOR ANTAGONISTS (H_2RAS)

Name	Availability	Dosage	Side Effects
Cimetidine (Tagamet HB [OTC])	**T:** 200 mg, 300 mg, 400 mg, 800 mg **S:** 300 mg/5 mL	**GERD:** 400 mg 4 times/day or 800 mg 2 times/day	**Class:** Hepatic enzyme elevations, hematologic toxicity, CNS effects (e.g., headache, lethargy, depression, cognitive impairment)
Famotidine (Pepcid AC [OTC], Zantac 360 [OTC])	**T:** 10 mg, 20 mg, 40 mg **Susp:** 40 mg/5 mL	**GERD:** 10–20 mg 2 times/day	
Nizatidine (generic)	**C:** 150 mg 300 mg **S:** 15 mg/mL	**GERD:** 150 mg 2 times/day	

PROTON PUMP INHIBITORS (PPIs)

Name	Availability	Dosage	Side Effects
Dexlansoprazole (Dexilant)	**C, DR:** 30 mg, 60 mg	30–60 mg once daily	**Class:** Headache, nausea, abdominal pain, constipation, flatulence, diarrhea, gynecomastia, hepatic failure, subacute myopathy, arthralgia, severe rash, lupus erythematosus, acute interstitial nephritis
Esomeprazole (Nexium, Nexium 24HR [OTC])	**C, DR:** 20 mg, 40 mg **Susp (Pwdr):** 2.5 mg, 5 mg, 10 mg, 20 mg, 40 mg **T, DR:** 20 mg	20–40 mg once daily	
Lansoprazole (Prevacid, Prevacid 24HR [OTC])	**C, DR:** 15 mg, 30 mg **ODT:** 15 mg, 30 mg	15–30 mg once daily	
Omeprazole (Prilosec, Prilosec [OTC])	**C, DR:** 10 mg, 20 mg, 40 mg **Susp (Pwdr):** 2.5 mg, 10 mg **T, DR:** 20 mg	10–40 mg once daily	
Omeprazole/Sodium Bicarbonate (Zegerid)	20 mg/ , 680 mg, 40 mg/1,680 mg/packets for susp **C:** 20 mg/1.1 g, 40 mg/1.1 g	10–40 mg once daily	
Pantoprazole (Protonix)	**T, DR:** 20 mg, 40 mg **Granules for Susp:** 40 mg	20–40 mg once daily	
Rabeprazole (Aciphex, Aciphex Sprinkle)	**T, DR:** 23 mg **C (Sprinkle):** 5 mg, 10 mg	10–20 mg once daily	

PREFERRED REGIMENS FOR *HELICOBACTER PYLORI* INFECTION
Empiric Treatment

Drug Name	Adult Dosage	Comments
Bismuth Quadruple Therapy **Bismuth subsalicylate** + metronidazole + tetracycline + a PPI	262 or 525 mg 4 times/day 500 mg 4 times/day 500 mg 2 or 4 times/day *See footnote	**Preferred first-line option:** *Bismuth* may temporarily turn the tongue/stool black and cause tinnitus. *Metronidazole* frequently causes metallic taste; may cause a disulfiram-like reaction to alcohol. *Tetracyclines* may cause GI adverse effects, vaginal candidiasis, photosensitivity, intracranial HTN, hyperpigmentation
Rifabutin Triple Therapy **Rifabutin** + amoxicillin + esomeprazole or rabeprazole	150 mg 2 times/day 1 g 3 times/day 40 mg 2 times/day	**Alternative first-line option:** May be used in treatment-naive pts or for salvage treatment. *Rifabutin* can cause brown-orange discoloration of urine, feces, saliva, sputum, perspiration, tears, skin

Susceptibility-Based Treatment

Drug Name	Adult Dosage	Comments
Clarithromycin Triple Therapy Clarithromycin + amoxicillin + a PPI	500 mg 2 times/day 1 g 2 times/day *See footnote	*Clarithromycin* causes taste disturbances, QT-interval prolongation
Levofloxacin Triple Therapy Levofloxacin + amoxicillin + a PPI	500 mg once daily 1 g 2 times/day *See footnote	*Levofloxacin* may cause severe hypoglycemia; delirium, agitation, nervousness; disturbances in attention, memory, orientation; persistent or permanent peripheral neuropathy, tendinitis, tendon rupture, exacerbation of myasthenia gravis, *Clostridium difficile* infection, QT-interval prolongation, torsades de pointes, pseudotumor cerebri syndrome
Metronidazole Triple Therapy Metronidazole + amoxicillin + a PPI	500 mg 2 times/day 1 g 2 times/day *See footnote	*Metronidazole* frequently causes a metallic taste and may cause a disulfiram-like reaction to alcohol

*Esomeprazole 20 mg twice daily, lansoprazole 45 mg twice daily, omeprazole 40 mg twice daily, pantoprazole 40 mg twice daily, or rabeprazole 20 mg twice daily.
***C,** Capsules; **DR,** delayed-release; **Pwdr,** powder; **ODT,** orally disintegrating tablet; **S,** solution; **Susp,** suspension; **T,** tablet.

Heart Failure (HF)

HF is a complex clinical syndrome with signs and symptoms resulting from any structural or functional impairment of ventricular filling or ejection of blood. Congestive heart failure (CHF) has a range of clinical manifestations depending on the underlying pathophysiology, ejection fraction (EF), and stage of disease. HF is classified into four stages: A through D.

Stage A: Those at risk (e.g., HTN, diabetes, obesity, exposure to cardiotoxic medications, family history of cardiomyopathy) who do not have current or previous signs or symptoms of disease, structural or functional heart disease, or abnormal biomarkers indicative of HF.

Stage B (pre-HF): Pts who do not have current or previous signs or symptoms of HF but there is now evidence of one of the following: structural heart disease, increased filling pressure, and increased brain natriuretic peptide (BNP) levels or elevated cardiac troponin levels.

Stage C (symptomatic HF): Pts who demonstrate signs and/or symptoms of HF. This may be new-onset HF, resolution of symptoms, or persistent or worsening HF.

Stage D (advanced HF): Pts who have marked HF symptoms that interfere with daily living or who have experienced hospital readmissions secondary to HF.

PHARMACOTHERAPY FOR HF MANAGEMENT

Medications considered to constitute the mainstay of HF therapy include renin-angiotensin system (RAS) inhibitors (e.g., angiotensin-converting enzyme [ACE] inhibitors, angiotensin II receptor blockers [ARBs], or angiotensin receptor/neprilysin inhibitors [ARNI]), beta-adrenergic blockers (BBs), mineralocorticoid receptor antagonists (MRAs), and sodium glucose cotransporter 2 (SGLT2) inhibitors.

Other agents that are used, depending on patient-specific factors, include diuretics (pts with volume overload; loop diuretics are more effective than thiazide diuretics), hydralazine and isosorbide dinitrate (pts with African decent, esp. with persistent HF symptoms), ivabradine, digoxin, and soluble guanylyl cyclase (sGC) stimulators (vericiguat).

RAS INHIBITORS

Angiotensin Receptor-Neprilysin Inhibitors

Name	Initial Daily Dose	Target Daily Dose	Comments/Side Effects
Sacubitril/valsartan (Entresto)	49/51 mg 2 times/day	97/103 mg 2 times/day	**Initial dose:** 24/26 mg 2 times/day for pts currently taking a low-dose ACE inhibitor or ARB; for de novo therapy, and for pts with an eGFR less than 30 mL/min/1.73 m², moderate hepatic impairment, or hypotension **Side effects:** Hypotension, renal impairment, hyperkalemia, angioedema

Angiotensin-Converting Enzyme (ACE) Inhibitors

Name	Initial Daily Dose	Target Daily Dose	Comments/Side Effects
Captopril (generic)	6.25 mg 3 times/day **(CrCl 10–50 mL/min):** 75% normal dose q12–18hrs once daily **(CrCl less than 10 mL/min):** 50% normal dose q24hrs	50 mg 3 times/day	Give on empty stomach **Class side effects:** Cough, angioedema, hypotension, renal impairment, hyperkalemia **Class cautions:** Pts at risk for hypotension; serum creatinine greater than 3 mg/dL, serum potassium greater than 5 mEq/L, bilateral renal artery stenosis
Enalapril (Vasotec)	2.5 mg 2 times/day **(CrCl ≤30 mL/min):** 2.5 mg/day	10 mg 2 times/day	Increased risk of adverse effects when CrCl less than 10 mL/min
Lisinopril (Prinivil, Zestril)	2.5–5 mg once/day **(CrCl ≤30 mL/min):** 2.5 mg/day	40 mg once daily	Increased risk of adverse effects when CrCl less than 10 mL/min
Quinapril (Ramipril)	5 mg 2 times/day **(CrCl >30 mL/min):** 5 mg/day (if tolerated increase to 2 times/day); **(CrCl 10–30 mL/min):** 2.5 mg/day	20 mg 2 times/day	High-fat meal decreases absorption by 30%
Ramipril (Altace)	1.25–2.5 mg once daily **(CrCl <40 mL/min):** 25% of normal dose	10 mg once daily	Increased risk of adverse effects when CrCl less than 15 mL/min

Continued

RAS INHIBITORS—cont'd

Angiotensin Receptor Blockers (ARBs)

Name	Initial Daily Dose	Target Daily Dose	Comments/Side Effects
Candesartan (Atacand)	4–8 mg once daily	32 mg once daily	**Initial dose: 4 mg. Maximum recommended dose:** 16 mg if CrCl less than 30 mL/min **Class side effects:** Hypotension, renal impairment, hyperkalemia **Class cautions:** Monitor blood pressure, renal function, and serum potassium level after initiation and during titration
Losartan (Cozaar)	25–50 mg once daily **Hepatic impairment: (Mild to moderate):** 25 mg/day	50–150 mg once daily	No dose adjustment for mild to severe renal impairment
Valsartan (Diovan)	20–40 mg 2 times/day	160 mg 2 times/day	No dose adjustment for mild to severe renal impairment

BETA-BLOCKERS

Name	Initial Daily Dose	Target Daily Dose	Comments/Side Effects
Bisoprolol (generic)	1.25 mg once daily	10 mg once daily	*Beta1-selective agent* **Class side effects:** Fatigue, hypotension, bradycardia, asymptomatic fluid retention **Class cautions:** Transient worsening of symptoms can occur following initiation. Full clinical benefits may not occur for 3–6 mos or longer. Monitor heart rate, BP, and for signs of congestion after initiation and during titration
Carvedilol (Coreg)	3.125 mg 2 times/day	25 mg 2 times/day **(greater than 85 kg):** 50 mg 2 times/day	Beta- and alpha-blocker Take with food to decrease risk of orthostasis
Carvedilol (Coreg CR)	10 mg once daily	80 mg once daily	Beta- and alpha-blocker Take with food to decrease risk of orthostasis
Metoprolol succinate (Toprol XL)	12.5–25 mg once daily	200 mg once daily	Beta1-selective agent

MINERALOCORTICOID RECEPTOR ANTAGONISTS (MRAS)

Name	Initial Daily Dose	Target Daily Dose	Comments/Side Effects
Eplerenone (Inspra)	*Dosage based on renal function:* Serum potassium less than or equal to 5 mEq/L and eGFR greater than or equal to 50 mL/min/1.73 m². 25 mg once/day; eGFR 30–49 mL/min/1.73 m². 25 mg every other day; eGFR less than or equal to 30 mL/min/1.73 m². Not recommended. *Dose adjustment based on serum potassium:* Serum potassium greater than or equal to 6.0 mEq/L: Withhold dose and restart at 25 mg every other day when levels decrease to less than 5.5 mEq/L; 5.5–5.9 mEq/L: Withhold dose if taking 25 mg every other day, or reduce dose from 25 mg once daily to 25 mg every other day, or from 50 to 25 mg once daily; 5.0–5.4 mEq/L: No adjustment; <5.0 mEq/L: Increase dose from 25 mg every other day to once daily, or from 25 mg to 50 mg once daily	*Dosage based on renal function:* Serum potassium less than or equal to 5 mEq/L and eGFR greater than or equal to 50 mL/min/1.73 m². 50 mg once/day; eGFR 30–49 mL/min/1.73 m². 25 mg once daily; eGFR less than or equal to 30 mL/min/1.73 m². Not recommended. *Dosage adjustments based on serum potassium (see initial daily dose)*	Hyperkalemia (risk higher in pts also taking an ARNI, ACE inhibitor, ARB, or with renal impairment). **Class cautions:** Avoid initiating in pts with potassium level greater than 5 mEq/L. Use caution in renal impairment. Monitor potassium, serum creatinine levels 2–3 days after initiation, then repeat after 7 days, then monthly for 3 mos, then q3mos thereafter during treatment
Spironolactone (Aldactone)	*Dosage based on renal function:* Serum potassium less than or equal to 5 mEq/L and eGFR greater than or equal to 50 mL/min/1.73 m². 25 mg once/day; eGFR ≤30/mL/min/ 1.73 m². Not recommended. *Adjust dosage based on serum potassium:* Serum potassium is greater than or equal to 5.5 mEq/L: Withhold dose until serum potassium level is less than 5.0/ mEq/L, then consider restarting at a lower dose	*Dosage based on renal function:* Serum potassium less than or equal to 5 mEq/L and eGFR greater than or equal to 50 mL/min/1.73 m². 50 mg once/day; eGFR less than or equal to 30 mL/min/1.73 m². Not recommended. *Dosage adjustments based on serum potassium (see initial daily dose)*	Hyperkalemia, hair loss, erectile dysfunction, and gynecomastia in men; menstrual irregularities in women **Class cautions:** Avoid starting in pts with potassium level greater than 5 mEq/L. Use caution in renal impairment

Continued

SODIUM-GLUCOSE COTRANSPORTER 2 (SGLT2) INHIBITORS

Name	Initial Daily Dose	Target Daily Dose	Comments/Side Effects
Dapagliflozin (Farxiga)	10 mg once daily **Renal impairment:** Pts with HF with an eGFR greater than or equal to 30 mL/min/1.73 m^2 can take dapagliflozin to reduce risk of CV death and hospitalization for HF	10 mg once daily **Renal impairment:** See initial daily dose	**Class side effects:** UTI, mycotic infections, symptomatic hypotension, hypersensitivity reactions **Class cautions:** Assess renal function before initiation. Give in the morning to avoid nocturia. Correct volume depletion prior to initiation
Empagliflozin (Jardiance)	10 mg once daily **Renal impairment:** Pts with HF with an eGFR ≥20 mL/min/1.73 m^2 can take empagliflozin for renal and cardiac benefits	10 mg once daily **Renal impairment:** See initial daily dose	
Sotagliflozin (Inpefa)	200 mg once daily **Renal impairment:** No dose adjustment	400 mg once daily **Renal impairment:** No dose adjustment	

Hepatitis C Virus Infection

Hepatitis C virus (HCV) infection is the leading blood-borne infection in the United States. HCV is transmitted by exposure to infected blood products. Risk factors for acquiring HCV include injection drug use, receiving contaminated blood products, needle sticks, and vertical transmission. If untreated, HCV may progress to chronic HCV and long-term sequelae including cirrhosis and hepatocellular carcinoma. There are seven known genotypes of HCV (genotypes 1–7) which impact the selection of initial therapy and treatment response.

Genotype 1 is the most common and is further sub-typed into genotypes 1a and 1b. Currently, there are two indirect-acting antivirals and seven direct-acting antivirals approved for the treatment of chronic HCV

ACTION

Indirect-Acting Antivirals (IAA)

Alpha interferons (peginterferons): Induces immune response against HCV, inhibiting viral replication.

Ribavirin: Exact mechanism unknown but has activity against several RNA and DNA viruses.

Direct-Acting Antivirals (DAA)

NS3/4A protease inhibitors (PIs): Targets the serine protease NS3/NS4 that is responsible for processing HCV polyprotein and producing new viruses.

Nonstructural protein 5A (NS5A) inhibitors: Suppress the NS5A protein, which is essential for viral assembly and replication.

Nonstructural protein 5B (NS5B) inhibitors: Suppress the NS5B RNA-dependent RNA polymerase that is responsible for HCV replication.

Continued

ANTI-HEPATITIS C VIRUS PREPARATIONS

Name	Type	Genotype	Dosage	Side Effects
Elbasvir, grazoprevir (Zepatier)	DAA NS5A/NS3/4A protease inhibitor	1, 4	**Genotype 1a:** One tablet daily for 12 wks (16 wks with baseline NS5A polymorphins) **Genotype 1b:** One tablet daily for 12 wks **Genotype 4:** One tablet daily for 12 wks (16 wks peginterferon/ribavirin experienced)	Fatigue, headache, nausea
Glecaprevir, pibrentasvir (Mavyret)	DAA NS5A/NS3/4A protease inhibitor	1, 2, 3, 4, 5, 6	**Genotypes 1, 2, 3, 4, 5, 6:** Three tablets once daily. Treatment duration 8–16 wks based on patients that are mono-infected, and coinfected with compensated liver disease (with or without cirrhosis) and with or without renal impairment	Headache, fatigue, nausea, diarrhea, increased serum bilirubin
Ledipasvir, Sofosbuvir (Harvoni)	DAA (NS5A/NS5B)	1, 4, 5, 6	**Genotype 1:** One tablet (90 mg/400 mg) for 12 wks in treatment-naive pt with or without cirrhosis and treatment-experienced pt without cirrhosis; for 24 wks for treatment-experienced pts with cirrhosis **Genotypes 4, 5, 6:** One tablet daily for 12 wks	Fatigue, headache, nausea, diarrhea, insomnia; elevations in bilirubin, lipase, and creatinine kinase

Drug	Class	Genotype	Dosing	Adverse Effects
Ribavirin (Copegus, Ribasphere)	IAA (Nucleoside analogue)	1, 2, 3, 4	**Genotypes 2, 3:** 400 mg 2 times/day (with peginterferon) **Genotypes 1, 4:** <75 kg: 400 mg qam; and 600 mg qpm; 75 kg or greater: 600 mg 2 times/day	(With peginterferon): Fatigue, weakness, headache, rigors, fever, nausea, myalgia, insomnia, mood instability, hair loss
Sofosbuvir/velpatasvir (Epclusa)	DAA (NS5B/NS5A)	1, 2, 3, 4, 5, 6	One tablet daily for 12 wks	Insomnia, anemia, headache, fatigue, nausea, diarrhea
Sofosbuvir/velpatasvir/voxilaprevir (VOSEVI)	DAA (NS5B/NS5A/protease inhibitor)	1, 2, 3, 4, 5, 6	One tablet daily for 12 wks	Headache, fatigue, diarrhea, nausea

DAA, direct-acting antivirals; *IAA,* indirect-acting antivirals.

Human Immunodeficiency Virus (HIV) Infection

USES

Antiretroviral (ARV) agents are used in the treatment of HIV infection.

An ARV regimen for treatment-naïve patients generally consists of two nucleoside reverse transcriptase inhibitors (NRTIs) in combination with a third ARV medication from one of three drug classes: an integrase inhibitor (INSTI), non-nucleoside reverse transcriptase inhibitor, or a protease inhibitor (PI) with either cobicistat or ritonavir.

TREATMENT OF MDR-HIV INFECTION: Used with other antiretroviral drugs to treat multidrug-resistant HIV-1 infection (MDR-HIV) in heavily treatment-experienced adults whose current regimen is failing to decrease viral load and increase CD4+ T-cell counts.

ACTION

Nucleoside reverse transcriptase inhibitors compete with natural substrates for formation of proviral DNA by reverse transcriptase inhibiting viral replication.

Nucleotide reverse transcriptase inhibitors (NtRTIs) inhibit reverse transcriptase by competing with the natural substrate deoxyadenosine triphosphate and by DNA chain termination.

Non-nucleoside reverse transcriptase inhibitors directly bind to reverse transcriptase and block RNA-dependent and DNA-dependent DNA polymerase activities by disrupting the enzyme's catalytic site.

Protease inhibitors (PIs) bind to the active site of HIV-1 protease and prevent the processing of viral gag and gag-pol polyprotein precursors resulting in immature, noninfectious mal particles.

Fusion inhibitors interfere with the entry of HIV-1 into cells by inhibiting fusion of viral and cellular membranes.

CCR5 coreceptor antagonist selectively binds to human chemokine receptor CCR5 present on cell membrane preventing HIV-1 from entering cells.

Integrase inhibitor inhibits catalytic activity of HIV-1 integrase, an HIV-1 encoded enzyme required for viral replication.

ANTIRETROVIRAL AGENTS FOR TREATMENT OF HIV INFECTION

Name	Availability	Dosage Range	Side Effects
Nucleoside Reverse Transcriptase Inhibitors (NRTIs)			
Abacavir (Ziagen)	**T:** 300 mg **OS:** 20 mg/mL	**A:** 300 mg 2 times/day or 600 mg once daily	Nausea, vomiting, malaise, rash, fever, headaches, asthenia, fatigue, hypersensitivity reactions
Emtricitabine (Emtriva)	**C:** 200 mg **OS:** 10 mg/mL	**A:** 200 mg/day (**C**) 240 mg/day (**OS**)	Headaches, insomnia, depression, diarrhea, nausea, vomiting, rhinitis, asthenia, rash
Lamivudine (Epivir)	**T:** 100 mg, 150 mg, 300 mg **OS:** 5 mg/mL 10 mg/mL	**A:** 150 mg 2 times/day or 300 mg once daily **CH:** 4 mg/kg 2 times/day	Diarrhea, malaise, fatigue, headaches, nausea, vomiting, abdominal pain, peripheral neuropathy, arthralgia, myalgia, skin rash
Tenofovir TDF (Viread)	**T:** 300 mg	**A:** 300 mg once daily	Nausea, vomiting, diarrhea, headache, fatigue
Zidovudine (Retrovir)	**C:** 100 mg **T:** 300 mg **Syrup:** 50 mg/5 mL, 10 mg/mL	**A:** 300 mg 2 times/day	Anemia, granulocytopenia, myopathy, nausea, malaise, fatigue, insomnia

Continued

ANTIRETROVIRAL AGENTS FOR TREATMENT OF HIV INFECTION—cont'd

Non-Nucleoside Reverse Transcriptase Inhibitors (NNRTIs)

Efavirenz (Sustiva)	**C:** 50 mg, 200 mg **T:** 600 mg	**A:** 600 mg/day **CH:** 200–600 mg/day based on weight	Headaches, dizziness, insomnia, fatigue, rash, nightmares
Etravirine (Intelence)	**T:** 100 mg, 200 mg	**A:** 200 mg 2 times/day	Skin reactions (e.g., Stevens-Johnson syndrome, erythema multiforme), nausea, abdominal pain, vomiting
Nevirapine (Viramune, Viramune XR)	**T:** 200 mg **T (ER):** 400 mg **S:** 50 mg/mL	**A: (IR):** 200 mg/day for 14 days, then (if no rash) 200 mg 2 times/day **(ER):** 400 mg once daily following 14 day IR lead in.	Rash, nausea, fatigue, fever, headaches, abnormal hepatic function tests
Rilpivirine (Edurant)	**T:** 25 mg	**A:** 25 mg once daily with a meal	Depression, insomnia, headache, rash

Protease Inhibitors (PIs)

Atazanavir (Reyataz)	**C:** 100 mg, 150 mg, 200 mg, 300 mg	**A:** 400 mg/day or 300 mg (with 100 mg ritonavir) once daily	Headaches, diarrhea, abdominal pain, nausea, rash
Darunavir (Prezista)	**T:** 400 mg, 600 mg	**A:** 600 mg 2 times/day (with ritonavir 100 mg) or 800 mg once daily with ritonavir 100 mg	Diarrhea, nausea, vomiting, headaches, skin rash, constipation
Fosamprenavir (Lexiva)	**T:** 700 mg **OS:** 50 mg/mL	**A:** 1,400 mg/day with 100 mg ritonavir	Headaches, fatigue, rash, nausea, diarrhea, vomiting, abdominal pain

Ritonavir (Norvir) **C:** 100 mg **OS:** 80 mg/mL	**A:** 100–400 mg/day in 1 or 2 divided doses	Nausea, vomiting, diarrhea, altered taste, fatigue, elevated LFTs and triglyceride levels
Tipranavir (Aptivus) **C:** 250 mg **OS:** 100 mg/mL	**A:** 500 mg (with 200 mg ritonavir) 2 times/day	Diarrhea, nausea, fatigue, headaches, vomiting
Fusion Inhibitors		
Enfuvirtide (Fuzeon) **I:** 108 mg (90 mg when reconstituted)	**SQ:** 90 mg 2 times/day	Insomnia, depression, peripheral neuropathy, decreased appetite, constipation, asthenia, cough
CCR5 Antagonists		
Maraviroc (Selzentry) **T:** 150 mg, 300 mg	**A:** 300 mg 2 times/day **CYP3A4 inducers:** 600 mg 2 times/day **CYP3A4 inhibitors:** 150 mg 2 times/day	Cough, pyrexia, upper respiratory tract infections, rash, musculoskeletal symptoms, abdominal pain, dizziness
Integrase Inhibitor		
Dolutegravir (Tivicay) **T:** 50 mg	**A:** 50 mg once daily or 50 mg bid (with CYP3A inducers or resistance)	Insomnia, headache
Raltegravir (Isentress) **T:** 400 mg	**A:** 400 mg 2 times/day	Nausea, headache, diarrhea, pyrexia

Continued

ANTIRETROVIRAL AGENTS FOR TREATMENT OF HIV INFECTION—cont'd

Treatment of MDR-HIV Infection

Fostemsavir (Rukobia)	**T-XR:** 600 mg	**A:** 600 mg 2 times/day	Nausea, diarrhea, headache, dyspepsia, abdominal pain
Ibalizumab-uiyk (Trogarzo)	**I:** 200 mg	**I:** Initially, 2,000 mg as a single dose, then 800 mg q14days	Dizziness, diarrhea; decreased Hgb, leukocytes, neutrophils, platelets; increased serum bilirubin, creatinine
Lenacapavir (Sunlenca)	**T:** 300 mg **I:** 463.5 mg/1.5 mL	**Day 1: SQ:** 927 mg, **PO:** 600 mg **Day 2: PO:** 600 mg **OR** **Day 1: PO:** 600 mg **Day 2: PO:** 600 mg **Day 8: PO:** 300 mg **Day 15 SQ:** 927 mg **THEN** **SQ:** 927 mg q6mos	Nausea, injection site reactions

A, Adults; *C*, capsules; *CH*, children; *DR*, delayed-release; *ER*, extended-release; *I*, injection; *IV*, intravenous; *OS*, oral solution; *PO*, oral; *S*, suspension; *SQ*, subcutaneous; *T*, tablets; *TAF*, tenofovir alafenamide; *TDF*, tenofovir disoproxil fumarate.

FIXED-COMBINATION THERAPIES

Brand Name	Generic Name	Dosage
Atripla	Efavirenz 600 mg Emtricitabine 200 mg Tenofovir (TDF) 300 mg	1 tablet once daily
Biktarvy	Bictegravir 50 mg Emtricitabine 200 mg Tenofovir (TAF) 25 mg	1 tablet once daily
Cabenuva	Cabotegravir 400 mg, 600 mg Rilpivirine 600 mg, 900 mg	**IM:** 600/900 mg once, then 400/600 mg once/mo or 600/900 mg for 2 consecutive mos; then continue with injections q2mos starting on month 4
Cimduo	Lamivudine 300 mg Tenofovir (TDF) 300 mg	1 tablet once daily
Combivir	Lamivudine 150 mg Zidovudine 300 mg	1 tablet twice daily
Complera	Emtricitabine 200 mg Rilpivirine 27.5 mg Tenofovir (TDF) 300 mg	1 tablet once daily
Delstrigo	Doravirine 100 mg Lamivudine 300 mg Tenofovir 300 mg	1 tablet once daily
Descovy	Emtricitabine 200 mg Tenofovir (TAF) 25 mg	1 tablet once daily
Dovato	Dolutegravir 50 mg Lamivudine 300 mg	1 tablet once daily

Continued

FIXED-COMBINATION THERAPIES—cont'd

Brand Name	Generic Name	Dosage
Epzicom	Abacavir 600 mg Lamivudine 300 mg	1 tablet once daily
Evotaz	Atazanavir 300 mg Cobicistat 150 mg	1 tablet once daily
Genvoya	Cobicistat 150 mg Elvitegravir 150 mg Emtricitabine 200 mg Tenofovir (TAF) 10 mg	1 tablet once daily
Juluca	Dolutegravir 50 mg Rilpivirine 25 mg	1 tablet once daily
Odefsey	Emtricitabine 200 mg Rilpivirine 25 mg Tenofovir (TAF) 25 mg	1 tablet once daily
Prezcobix	Cobicistat 150 mg Darunavir 800 mg	1 tablet once daily
Stribild	Cobicistat 150 mg Elvitegravir 150 mg Emtricitabine 200 mg Tenofovir (TDF) 300 mg	1 tablet once daily
Symfi	Efavirenz 400 mg Lamivudine 300 mg Tenofovir (TDF) 300 mg	1 tablet once daily

Symtuza	Cobicistat 150 mg Darunavir 800 mg Emtricitabine 200 mg Tenofovir 10 mg	1 tablet once daily
Triumeq	Abacavir 600 mg Dolutegravir 50 mg Lamivudine 300 mg	1 tablet once daily
Trizivir	Abacavir 300 mg Lamivudine 150 mg Zidovudine 300 mg	1 tablet twice daily
Truvada	Emtricitabine 200 mg Tenofovir (TDF) 300 mg	1 tablet once daily

TAF, Tenofovir alafenamide; *TDF*, tenofovir disoproxil fumarate.

Hypertension (HTN) Treatment

Blood pressure is divided into 4 general categories. **Normal blood pressure:** Systolic/diastolic lower than 120/80 mm Hg. **Elevated blood pressure:** Systolic from 120–129 mm Hg and diastolic below 80 mm Hg. **Stage 1 hypertension:** Systolic from 130–139 mm Hg or diastolic 80–89 mm Hg. **Stage 2 hypertension:** Systolic is 140 mm Hg or higher or diastolic is 90 mm Hg or higher. If untreated, HTN can lead to complications, including heart attack, stroke, HF, kidney damage, and dementia. Risk factors include age, race (high BP common in pts of African descent), excess weight, lack of exercise, tobacco use, increased salt intake, low potassium levels, alcohol use, and stress.

NONPHARMACOLOGIC INTERVENTIONS

Nonpharmacologic interventions include maintaining a healthy body weight, consuming a heart-healthy diet, limiting sodium and alcohol intake, exercise, and weight loss for those who are overweight.

PHARMACOLOGIC INTERVENTIONS (DRUG THERAPY)

Drugs for initial treatment of HTN include thiazide/thiazide-like diuretics, angiotensin-converting enzyme (ACE) inhibitors, angiotensin receptor blockers (ARBs), calcium channel blockers (CCBs), and beta-adrenergic blockers (BBs).

The goal of antihypertensive drug therapy as recommended by the American College of Cardiology and American Heart Association is a BP of less than 130/80. A thiazide-like diuretic, a CCB, an ACE inhibitor, or an ARB is recommended as initial therapy (initial treatment with two antihypertensive drugs from different classes is recommended when baseline BP is greater than or equal to 20/10 mm Hg above goal). Beta blockers are recommended as initial therapy for pts with another indication for a beta blocker (e.g., myocardial infarction or HF). Many pts with HTN, especially pts of African descent, may need more than one drug to control BP. If the first drug does not achieve BP goals, adding a second drug with a different mechanism of action is generally more effective than increasing the dose of the first drug.

THIAZIDE AND THIAZIDE-LIKE DIURETICS

Name	Usual Adult Dosage	Class Comments	Class Side Effects
Chlorthalidone (generic)	12.5–25 mg once daily	*Chlorthalidone* and *indapamide* have longer durations of action than *hydrochlorothiazide* and, in some studies, have been more effective. *Metolazone* may be more effective in pts with renal impairment than other thiazide or thiazide-like diuretics.	Hypokalemia, hypomagnesemia, hyperglycemia, hyponatremia, hypercalcemia, hyperuricemia, hypercholesterolemia, hypertriglyceridemia, pancreatitis, rash, allergic reactions, photosensitivity reactions
Hydrochlorothiazide (generic)	25–50 mg once daily		
Indapamide (generic)	1.25–2.5 mg once daily		
Metolazone (generic)	2.5–5 mg once daily		

LOOP DIURETICS

Name	Usual Adult Dose	Class Comments	Class side effects
Bumetanide (Bumex)	0.5–2 mg/day once daily or in 2 divided doses	Used in pts with moderate/severe renal impairment	Hypokalemia, hypomagnesemia, hyponatremia, hyperglycemia, metabolic alkalosis, hyperuricemia, rash, hypercholesterolemia, hypertriglyceridemia, dehydration
Ethacrynic acid (Edecrin)	50–200 mg/day once daily or in 2 divided doses		
Furosemide (Lasix)	20–80 mg/day in 2 divided doses		
Torsemide (generic)	20 mg once daily		

POTASSIUM SPARING DIURETICS

Name	Usual Adult Dose	Class Comments	Side effects
Amiloride (generic)	5–10 mg/day once daily or in 2 divided doses	Used with other diuretics to prevent or correct hypokalemia	Hyperkalemia, GI disturbances, rash, headache
Triamterene (Dyrenium)	50–100 mg/day once daily or in 2 divided doses		Rash, hyperkalemia, GI disturbances, nephrolithiasis, thrombocytopenia, weakness

MINERALOCORTICOID RECEPTOR ANTAGONISTS

Name	Usual Adult Dose	Class Comments	Side effects
Eplerenone (Inspra)	50–100 mg/day once daily or in 2 divided doses	Effective as adjunctive treatment or refractory hypertension	Hyperkalemia, hyponatremia
Spironolactone (Aldactone)	25–100 mg once daily		Hyperkalemia, hyponatremia, gynecomastia, menstrual abnormalities, GI disturbances, rash, erectile dysfunction, loss of hair

ANGIOTENSIN-CONVERTING ENZYME (ACE) INHIBITORS

Name	Usual Adult Dosage	Class Comments	Class Side Effects
Benazepril (Lotensin)	10–40 mg/day in 1 or 2 divided doses	Effective for treatment of HTN. Generally well tolerated (except for cough). Less effective in pts of African descent (unless combined with a thiazide-like diuretic or a calcium channel blocker). Reduces mortality in pts without HF or left ventricular dysfunction who are at high risk for cardiovascular events. Prolongs survival in pts with HF with reduced ejection fraction (HF-rEF) and in pts with left ventricular dysfunction after an MI. Reduces proteinuria in pts with diabetic or nondiabetic nephropathy. Should not be used with ARBs.	Rash, cough, angioedema, hyperkalemia (esp. in pts with renal insufficiency or taking potassium-sparing diuretics or potassium supplements), dysgeusia, acute kidney injury (if stenosis is affecting one or both kidneys and threatening renal function), hypotension (especially with diuretic use or volume depletion), mild to moderate loss of taste, blood dyscrasias, renal damage
Captopril (generic)	25–150 mg/day in 2–3 divided doses		
Enalapril (Vasotec)	5–40 mg/day in 1 or 2 divided doses		
Fosinopril (generic)	10–40 mg once daily		
Lisinopril (Prinivil, Zestril)	10–40 mg once daily		
Quinapril (Accupril)	10–80 mg/day in 1 or 2 divided doses		
Ramipril (Altace)	2.5–20 mg/day in 1 or 2 divided doses		

ANGIOTENSIN RECEPTOR BLOCKERS (ARBS)

Name	Usual Adult Dosage	Class Comments	Class Side Effects
Azilsartan (Edarbi)	40–80 mg once daily	As effective as ACE inhibitors in reducing BP. Appears to be equally renal-protective and cardioprotective. Less effective in pts of African descent (unless combined with a thiazide-like diuretic or a calcium channel blocker). Should not be used with ACE inhibitors.	Similar to ACE inhibitors (rarely cause cough or angioedema)
Candesartan (Atacand)	8–32 mg once daily		
Eprosartan (generic)	600 mg once daily		
Irbesartan (Avapro)	150–300 mg once daily		
Losartan (Cozaar)	50–100 mg/day in 1 or 2 divided doses		
Olmesartan (Benicar)	20–40 mg once daily		
Telmisartan (Micardis)	40–80 mg once daily		
Valsartan (Diovan)	80–320 mg once daily		

DIRECT RENIN INHIBITOR

Aliskiren (Tekturna)	100–300 mg once daily	Do not use with an ACE inhibitor or ARB	Diarrhea, increased BUN, serum creatinine.

CALCIUM CHANNEL BLOCKERS (CCBS)

Name	Usual Adult Dosage	Class Comments	Class Side Effects
		Dihydropyridines	
Amlodipine (Norvasc)	2.5–10 mg once daily	CCBs are structurally and functionally heterogeneous. They all cause vasodilation and decrease total peripheral resistance. *Felodipine* and *nicardipine* cause an initial reflex tachycardia, but *isradipine, nifedipine,* and *amlodipine* have a lesser effect on HR.	Headache, dizziness, asthenia, flushing, peripheral edema (more than nondihydropyridines; more common in women), flushing, tachycardia, rash, gingival hyperplasia
Felodipine (generic)	2.5–10 mg once daily		
Isradipine (generic)	5–10 mg/day in 2 divided doses		
Nicardipine (generic)	60–120 mg/day in 3 divided doses		
Nifedipine ER (Adalat CC, Procardia XL)	30–90 mg once daily		

Nondihydropyridines

Name	Usual Adult Dosage	Class Comments	Class Side Effects
Diltiazem (Cardizem CD, Cardizem LA, Cartia XT, Dilt-XR, Matzim LA, Taztia XT, Tiadylt ER, Tiazac)	120–360 mg once daily	*Verapamil* and *diltiazem* slow HR and can slow AV conduction. Use with caution in pts also taking a beta blocker.	Headache, dizziness, AV block, constipation (especially verapamil), edema, HF; lupus-like rash with diltiazem
Verapamil (Calan SR Verelan)	120–360 mg once daily		

BETA-ADRENERGIC BLOCKERS (BBS)

Name	Usual Adult Dosage	Class Comments	Class Side Effects
Atenolol (Tenormin)	50–100 mg/day in 2 divided doses	Acceptable choice for treatment in pts with another indication for a beta blocker (e.g., migraine headache prophylaxis, cardiac arrhythmias, angina, MI, or HF). Less effective in preventing cardiovascular events.	Bronchospasm, fatigue, depression, bradycardia, erectile dysfunction, decreased exercise tolerance, insomnia, vivid dreams, hallucinations, exacerbation of HF; may mask of symptoms and delay recovery from hypoglycemia; hypertriglyceridemia, decreased high-density lipoprotein (HDL) cholesterol, worsening of peripheral arterial insufficiency; increased incidence of diabetes. Sudden discontinuation may cause exacerbation of angina/MI or precipitate thyroid storm
Bisoprolol (generic)	5–10 mg once daily		
Carvedilol extended-release (Coreg CR)	20–80 mg once daily		
Carvedilol immediate release (Coreg)	12.5–50 mg/day in 2 divided doses		
Labetalol (generic)	200–800 mg/day in 2 divided doses		
Metoprolol immediate release (Lopressor)	100–200 mg/day in 2 divided doses		
Metoprolol extended-release (Toprol-XL)	50–200 mg once daily		
Nadolol (Corgard)	40–120 mg once daily		
Nebivolol (Bystolic)	5–40 mg once daily		
Propranolol extended-release (Inderal LA, Inderal XL, InnoPran XL)	80–160 mg once daily		
Propranolol immediate release (generic)	80–160 mg/day in 2 divided doses		

Immunosuppressive Agents

CLASSIFICATION OF IMMUNOSUPPRESSIVE AGENTS

Immunosuppressive agents (IMS) are prescribed for early-stage immunosuppression, the management of late-stage immunosuppression, or the maintenance of organ rejection. In general, they are classified as induction therapies, maintenance therapies, and antirejection therapies.

Induction therapies: Therapies given immediately after transplant to prevent acute rejection. *Maintenance therapies:* Consist of all immunosuppressive medications prescribed before, during, or after trans-

plant and with the purpose of long-term use. *Antirejection immunosuppression:* Involves all immunosuppressive medications prescribed for dealing with an episode of acute rejection in the initial post-transplant period or during a specific follow-up period, typically up to 30 days after the diagnosis of acute rejection.

The major IMS agents include a combination of agents, including **calcineurin inhibitors (*tacrolimus and cyclosporine*)**, antimetabolites (*myco-*

phenolate mofetil and azathioprine), mammalian target of rapamycin inhibitors (*everolimus and sirolimus*), and corticosteroids (*IV methylprednisolone and oral prednisone*).

The primary goal in post-transplant pts is to individualize therapy to include the optimal combination of IMS, which can improve pt survival by preventing acute rejection, while also preventing or decreasing the incidence of adverse effects.

Continued

IMMUNOSUPPRESSIVE AGENTS

Name	Class	Action	Indication	Adverse effects
Azathioprine (Imuran)	Antimetabolite	Inhibition of purine synthesis and B and T cells	Prevent rejection renal transplantation	Myelosuppression, hepatitis
Basiliximab (Simulect)	IL-2 receptor antagonist	Inhibits IL-2 mediated activation of lymphocytes	Renal transplant (prophylaxis of acute rejection)	Constipation, nausea, vomiting, diarrhea, dyspepsia
Belatacept (Nulojix)	Selective T-cell co-stimulation blocker	Fusion protein blocks interaction to activate T lymphocytes	Renal transplant (prophylaxis of acute rejection)	Anemia, diarrhea, peripheral edema, UTI, constipation, cough, nausea, vomiting, leukopenia
Cyclosporine (Neoral, Gengraf)	Calcineurin inhibition	Blocks T-cell transcription	Prophylaxis of organ rejection in kidney, liver and heart transplants	Nephrotoxity, neurotoxicity, hyperlipidemia, diabetes, hepatotoxicity, refractory hypertension
Everolimus (Zortress)	mTOR kinase inhibitor	Inhibits lymphocyte response to cytokine stimulation	Prophylaxis of organ rejection in kidney (low to moderate risk), liver transplants	Peripheral edema, hypertension, hyperlipidemia, anemia, leukopenia
Mycophenlate (Cellcept, Myfortic)	Antimetabolite	Exhibits cytostatic and reversible effect on B and T lymphocytes	Prophylaxis of organ rejection in kidney, liver and heart transplants	Diarrhea, leukopenia, infection, vomiting
Sirolimus (Rapamune)	mTOR kinase inhibitor	Inhibits lymphocyte response to cytokine stimulation	Prevent rejection renal transplantation	Peripheral edema, hypertriglyceridemia, hypertension, hyperlipidemia, abdominal pair, diarrhea, fever, UTI, anemia, thrombocytopenia
Tacrolimus (Prograf)	Calcineurin inhibition	Blocks T-cell transcription	Prophylaxis of organ rejection in kidney, liver, lung and heart transplants	Hypertension, diabetes, fever, leukopenia, UTI, headache, abdominal pain, peripheral edema, hyperkalemia, hyperlipidemia

Insomnia

USES

Insomnia (primary and secondary) is one of the most common sleep disorders and is characterized by difficulty falling asleep or staying asleep. Primary insomnia is not caused by or associated with a medical condition, psychiatric problem, or medication. Secondary insomnia is due to a medical condition (e.g., depression, COPD, chronic pain). Symptoms of insomnia include daytime sleepiness, irritability, concentration difficulties, fatigue, and forgetfulness.

ACTION

Nonbenzodiazepines: Binds to inhibitory neurotransmitter GABA receptors, decreasing neuronal excitability and causing sedative and hypnotic effects.

Benzodiazepines: Binds with inhibitory neurotransmitter GABA receptors, decreasing neuronal excitability and causing sedative and hypnotic effects.

Melatonin receptor agonist: Affects melatonin receptor in the brain.

Orexin receptor antagonist: Suppresses wakefulness by inhibiting orexin A and B from binding to orexin receptors.

Continued

INSOMNIA
BENZODIAZEPINE RECEPTOR AGONISTS

Name	Availability	Usual Dosage	Side Effects
Eszopiclone (Lunesta)	**T:** 1 mg, 2 mg, 3 mg	**A:** 1–3 mg **E:** 1–2 mg	Headache, dysgeusia, dizziness
Zaleplon (generic)	**C:** 5 mg, 10 mg	**A:** 10–20 mg **E:** 5 mg	Muscle pain, dizziness, headache, nausea
Zolpidem (Ambien) (Ambien CR) (Edluar) Generic SL	**T:** 5 mg, 10 mg **T, ER:** 6.25 mg 12.5 mg **SL:** 5 mg, 10 mg **SL:** 1.75 mg, 3.5 mg	**A:** (Male): 5–10 mg (Female): 5 mg **A:** (Male): 6.25–12.5 mg (Female): 6.25 mg **E:** 6.25 mg **A:** (Male): 5–10 mg (Female): 5 mg **E:** 5 mg **A:** (Male): 3.5 mg (Female): 1.75 mg **E:** 1.75 mg	Headache, drowsiness, dizziness

BENZODIAZEPINES

Name	Availability	Usual Dosage	Side Effects
Estazolam (generic)	**T:** 1 mg, 2 mg	**A:** 1–2 mg **E:** 0.5–1 mg	**Class:** Drowsiness, sleepiness, dizziness
Flurazepam (generic)	**C:** 15 mg, 30 mg	**A:** 15–30 mg **E:** 15 mg	
Temazepam (Restoril)	**C:** 7.5 mg, 15 mg, 22.5 mg, 30 mg	**A:** 7.5–30 mg **E:** 7.5–15 mg	

MELATONIN RECEPTOR AGONIST

Name	Availability	Usual Dosage	Side Effects
Ramelteon (Rozerem)	**T:** 8 mg	**A:** 8 mg **E:** 8 mg	Dizziness, sleepiness, unusual drowsiness

OREXIN RECEPTOR ANTAGONISTS

Name	Availability	Usual Dosage	Side Effects
Daridorexant (Quviviq)	**T:** 25 mg, 50 mg	**A:** 25–50 mg **E:** 25–50 mg	Headache, somnolence, fatigue
Lemborexant (Dayvigo)	**T:** 5 mg, 10 mg	**A:** 5–10 mg **E:** 5–10 mg	Somnolence
Suvorexant (Belsomra)	**T:** 5 mg, 10 mg, 15 mg, 20 mg	**A:** 10–20 mg **E:** 10–15 mg	Somnolence

A, Adults; *C,* capsules; *E,* elderly; *ER,* extended-release; *SL,* sublingual; *T,* tablet.

Irritable Bowel Syndrome (IBS)

IBS is a highly prevalent, chronic disorder that occurs secondary to alterations in gut-brain interaction. It is characterized by symptoms of recurrent abdominal pain and changes in the consistency of bowel movements (diarrhea or constipation) and is often accompanied by bloating. IBS can be classified as diarrhea-predominant (IBS-D), constipation-predominant (IBS-C), mixed/alternating stool pattern (IBS-M), or unclassified (IBS-U). The goal of treatment is to provide symptom relief through a combination of nonpharmacologic (e.g., dietary modification, reduce stress, exercise, and psychological interventions) and medication interventions.

NONPHARMACOLOGIC TREATMENTS

DIET: A diet low in fermentable oligosaccharides, disaccharides, monosaccharides, and polyols (FODMAPs) may reduce IBS symptoms. FODMAPs are poorly absorbed, rapidly fermented, short-chain carbohydrates that may increase gas production and luminal distention, which cause bloating, flatulence, and abdominal discomfort. Examples of low-FODMAP foods include grapes, strawberries, cucumber, zucchini, dairy-free alternatives, eggs, and wheat-free grains.

SOLUBLE FIBER: Can decrease IBS symptoms (abdominal pain, stool inconsistency). Foods containing soluble fiber (e.g., oat bran, barley, beans) and supplements (e.g., psyllium) increase stool bulk and facilitate colon transit, resulting in increased stool frequency.

EXERCISE: Routine physical activity, including yoga, improves IBS symptoms (pain, discomfort, bloating). Exercise also reduces depression and anxiety and improves quality of life.

PSYCHOLOGICAL INTERVENTIONS: Psychological interventions (e.g., cognitive behavioral therapy, relaxation training, and hypnotherapy) have been effective for management of IBS symptoms (especially in pts with comorbid psychiatric disorders).

PHARMACOLOGICAL TREATMENT

DRUGS FOR IBS-C

CHLORIDE CHANNEL ACTIVATOR: Lubiprostone, a prostaglandin derivative, activates gastrointestinal chloride channels, stimulating intestinal fluid secretion.

GUANYLATE CYCLASE-C AGONISTS: Linaclotide and plecanatide target guanylate cyclase receptors on intestinal epithelium, increasing luminal intestinal secretions and accelerating intestinal transit.

NHE3 INHIBITOR: Tenapanor, a sodium-hydrogen exchanger 3 (NHE3) inhibitor, inhibits sodium absorption in the small intestine and colon, increasing fluid secretion and acceleration of intestinal transit time.

DRUGS FOR IBS-D

ANTIBIOTIC: *Rifaximin*, a minimally absorbed antibiotic, alters gut microbiota, which may reduce mucosal inflammation and visceral hypersensitivity.

OPIOID RECEPTOR AGONIST/ANTAGONIST: *Eluxadoline*, a mu-opioid receptor agonist, decreases muscle contractility, inhibits water and electrolyte secretion, and increases rectal sphincter tone. Delta-opioid receptor antagonists may reduce constipation and abdominal pain.

5-HT3 ANTAGONISTS: Antagonism of 5-HT3 receptors has been shown to decrease pain and slow intestinal transit. *Alosetron* relieves abdominal pain and discomfort, decreases bowel urgency and stool frequency, and improves stool consistency.

ADJUNCTIVE THERAPIES

ANTISPASMODICS: (e.g., *dicyclomine, hyoscyamine, peppermint oil*) may reduce abdominal spasms and cramps by decreasing smooth muscle contractions and GI motility.

ANTIDEPRESSANTS: (e.g., *tricyclic antidepressants, selective serotonin reuptake inhibitors [SSRIs]*) can reduce abdominal pain through central mechanisms and alter GI transit time through peripheral mechanisms.

ANTIDIARRHEALS: (e.g., *loperamide, diphenoxylate/atropine*) reduce stool frequency but do not reduce other IBS symptoms.

OSMOTIC LAXATIVES: (e.g., *polyethylene glycol*) can increase the frequency of bowel movements, improving symptoms or abdominal pain associated with IBS.

DRUGS FOR IBS WITH CONSTIPATION (IBS-C)

Name	Class	Usual Adult Dosage	Comments
Linaclotide (Linzess)	Guanylate cyclase-C agonist	290 mcg once daily Take at least 30 min before first meal of day	Do not crush or allow chewing. May open and sprinkle on applesauce. **Contraindications:** Less than 6 yrs of age (avoid in pts 6–18 yrs of age), mechanical bowel obstruction **Side effects:** Diarrhea, abdominal pain and distention, flatulence
Lubiprostone (Amitiza)	Chloride channel activator	8 mcg 2 times/day Take with food to minimize nausea	Do not crush, break, or allow chewing. **Contraindications:** Mechanical GI obstruction **Side effects:** Nausea, diarrhea, abdominal pain
Plecanatide (Trulance)	Guanylate cyclase-C agonist	3 mg once daily	Can be crushed and mixed with applesauce or dissolved in water **Contraindications:** Less than 6 yrs of age, mechanical bowel obstruction **Side effects:** Diarrhea, abdominal pain and distention, flatulence

Continued

Name	Class	Usual Adult Dosage	Comments
Tenapanor (Ibsrela)	Sodium-hydrogen exchanger 3 (NHE3) inhibitor	50 mg 2 times/day Take immediately before breakfast or the first meal of day and immediately before dinner	Avoid in pts 6–12 yrs of age. Do not crush, break, or chew **Contraindications:** Less than 6 yrs of age, mechanical bowel obstruction **Side effects:** Abdominal distention, diarrhea, flatulence, dizziness

DRUGS FOR IBS WITH DIARRHEA (IBS-D)

Name	Class	Usual Adult Dosage	Comments
Alosetron (Lotronex)	Selective serotonin type-3 (5-HT3) antagonist	**Initially:** 0.5 mg 2 times/day. May increase to 1 mg 2 times/day after 4 wks	For use in adult females with severe, chronic IBS-D who have failed conventional therapy. **Contraindications:** Constipation, history of GI conditions (e.g., obstruction, Crohn's disease, ulcerative colitis), severe hepatic disease (caution in mild-moderate impairment), concomitant use of fluvoxamine **Side effects:** Nausea, abdominal pain or discomfort
Eluxadoline (Viberzi)	Mu-opioid receptor agonist/delta-opioid receptor antagonist	100 mg 2 times/day (75 mg 2 times/day in pts with mild to moderate hepatic impairment; moderate to severe renal disease)	Take with food. Avoid use of medications causing constipation. **Contraindications:** Sphincter of Oddi dysfunction; known or suspected biliary duct, pancreatic duct, or GI tract obstruction; severe hepatic impairment, history of chronic or severe constipation, pancreatitis, or structural pancreatic disease, alcoholism, or daily intake of greater than 3 alcoholic beverages/day **Side effects:** Constipation, nausea, abdominal pain
Rifaximin (Xifaxan)	Antibiotic	550 mg 3 times/day for 14 days	Interacts with warfarin (monitor INR). **Contraindications:** Allergy to rifampin **Side effects:** Nausea, elevated serum ALT

ADJUNCTIVE THERAPIES
Soluble Fiber

Name	Availability	Usual Adult Dosage	Comments
Psyllium (Metamucil)	**P:** 5.8 g/teaspoon **Packet:** 5.8 g **C:** 1.8 g **Wafer:** 2 g	10–15 g/day in 2–3 divided doses	Give with 8 oz water at least 2 hrs before or after taking other medications
Methylcellulose (Citrucel)	**P:** 2 g/tablespoon **Caplet:** 500 mg	2 g 3 times/day	Give with 8 oz water
Wheat dextrin (Benefiber)	**P:** 4 g/tsp **Packet:** 4 g, 6.2 g **T (Chew):** 4 g, 6.2 g	8 g 3 times/day 8 g 3 times/day 3 tabs 3 times/day	**Powder or packets:** Give with 4–8 oz of water or sprinkled on hot or cold soft food
Calcium polycarbophil (FiberCon)	**Caplet:** 625 mg	1,250 mg 1–4 times/day	Give with 8 oz water

Osmotic Laxative

Name	Availability	Usual Adult Dosage	Comments
Polyethylene glycol (Miralax)	**P:** 17 g/scoop **Packet:** 17 g	17 g 1–2 times/day	Well tolerated and safe for long-term use

Antidiarrheals

Name	Availability	Usual Adult Dosage	Comments
Loperamide (Imodium A-D)	**Caplets:** 2 mg **S:** 1 mg/7.5 mL	2 mg as needed (max 16 mg/day)	Reduces stool frequency in pts with IBS-D but does not reduce IBS symptoms

Continued

Antispasmodics

Name	Availability	Usual Adult Dosage	Comments
Peppermint oil (Pepogest, Ibgard)	**C (EC):** 50 mg **C (EC):** 0.2 mL caps **C (SR):** 90 mg	1–3 caps 3 times/day 1 cap 3 times/day 180 mg 3 times/day	Give with water 30–90 min before or after food. Do not crush or chew. May open and sprinkle on applesauce
Dicyclomine (generic)	**C:** 10 mg **T:** 20 mg tabs **S:** 10 mg/5 mL	20–40 mg 4 times/day as needed	**Class side effects:** Visual disturbances, confusion, dry mouth, urinary retention, palpitations, constipation
Hyoscyamine (generic) Anaspaz Levsin Levsin-SL Levbid	**T, SL, ODT:** 0.125 mg **Elixir:** 0.125 mg/5 mL **S:** 0.125 mg/mL **ODT:** 0.125 mg **T:** 0.125 mg **SL tabs:** 0.125 mg **T, (ER):** 0.375 mg	**IR:** 0.125–0.25 mg 3–4 times/day as needed **ER:** 0.375–0.75 mg 2 times/day	

SELECTIVE SEROTONIN REUPTAKE INHIBITORS (SSRIS)

Name	Availability	Usual Adult Dosage	Comments
Citalopram (Celexa)	**T:** 10, 20, 40 mg	20–40 mg once daily	**Class side effects:** Agitation, sleep disturbances, nausea, weight gain, sexual dysfunction, diarrhea
Fluoxetine (Prozac)	**C:** 10, 20, 40 mg	20 mg once daily	
Paroxetine (Paxil, Paxil CR)	**T:** 10, 20, 30, 40 mg **T (ER):** 12.5, 25, 37.5	10–20 mg once daily 12.5–37.5 mg once daily	

TRICYCLIC ANTIDEPRESSANTS (TCAs)

Name	Availability	Usual Adult Dosage	Comments
Amitriptyline (generic)	**T:** 10, 25, 50, 75 mg	10–75 mg once daily	**Class side effects:** Fatigue, dizziness, weight gain, sedation, anticholinergic effects (dry mouth, urinary retention, blurred vision, confusion, constipation)
Desipramine (Norpramin)	**T:** 10, 25, 50, 75, 100 mg	10–125 mg once/day or divided 2 times/day	
Nortriptyline (Pamelor)	**C:** 10, 25, 50, 75 mg	10–125 mg once/day or divided 2 times/day	

C, Capsules; *Chew,* chewable; *EC,* enteric-coated; *ER,* extended-release; *IR,* immediate release; *ODT,* orally disintegrating tablets; *P,* powder; *S,* solution, *SL,* sublingual, *SR,* sustained-release, *T,* tablets.

Laxatives

USES	ACTION
Short-term treatment of constipation; colon evacuation before rectal/bowel examination; prevention of straining (e.g., after anorectal surgery, MI); to reduce painful elimination (e.g., episiotomy, hemorrhoids, anorectal lesions); modification of effluent from ileostomy, colostomy; prevention of fecal impaction; removal of ingested poisons.	Laxatives ease or stimulate defecation. Mechanisms by which this is accomplished include (1) attracting, retaining fluid in colonic contents due to hydrophilic or osmotic properties; (2) acting directly or indirectly on mucosa to decrease absorption of water and NaCl; or (3) increasing intestinal motility, decreasing absorption of water and NaCl by virtue of decreased transit time.

Bulk-forming: Act primarily in small/large intestine. Retain water in stool, may bind water, ions in colonic lumen (soften feces, increase bulk); may increase colonic bacteria growth (increases fecal mass). Produce soft stool in 1–3 days.

Osmotic agents: Act in colon. Similar to saline laxatives. Osmotic action may be enhanced in distal ileum/colon by bacterial metabolism to lactate, other organic acids. This decrease in pH increases motility, secretion. Produce soft stool in 1–3 days. | *Saline:* Acts in small/large intestine, colon (sodium phosphate). Poorly, slowly absorbed; causes hormone cholecystokinin release from duodenum (stimulates fluid secretion, motility); possesses osmotic properties; produces watery stool in 2–6 hrs (small doses produce semifluid stool in 6–12 hrs).

Stimulant: Acts in colon. Enhances accumulation of water/electrolytes in colonic lumen, enhances intestinal motility. May act directly on intestinal mucosa. Produces semifluid stool in 6–12 hrs.

◀**ALERT**▶ Bisacodyl suppository acts in 15–60 min.

Stool softener: Acts in small/large intestine. Hydrates and softens stools by its surfactant action, facilitating penetration of fat and water into stool. Produces soft stool in 1–3 days. |

LAXATIVES

Name	Onset of Action	Uses	Side Effects/Precautions
Bulk-forming			
Methylcellulose (Citrucel)	12–24 hrs up to 3 days	Treatment of constipation for postpartum women, elderly, pts with diverticulosis, irritable bowel syndrome, hemorrhoids	Flatulence, abdominal discomfort
Psyllium (Metamucil)	Same as methylcellulose	Treatment of chronic constipation and constipation associated with rectal disorders; management of irritable bowel syndrome	Flatulence, abdominal discomfort
Stool Softener			
Docusate (Colace, Surfak)	1–3 days	Treatment of constipation due to hard stools, in painful anorectal conditions, and for those who need to avoid straining during bowel movements	Stomachache, mild nausea, cramping, diarrhea
Saline			
Magnesium citrate (Citrate of Magnesia, Citro-Mag)	30 min–3 hrs	Bowel evacuation prior to certain surgical and diagnostic procedures	Hypotension, abdominal cramping, diarrhea, gas formation, electrolyte abnormalities
Magnesium hydroxide	30 min–3 hrs	Short-term treatment of occasional constipation	Electrolyte abnormalities can occur; use caution in pts with renal or cardiac impairment; diarrhea, abdominal cramps, hypotension

Continued

Osmotic

Lactulose (Kristalose)	24–48 hrs	Short-term relief of constipation, treatment of hyperammonemia-induced encephalopathy	Bloating, flatulence, diarrhea
Polyethylene glycol (MiraLax)	24–48 hrs	Short-term relief of constipation	Bloating, flatulence, nausea, diarrhea

Stimulant

Bisacodyl (Dulcolax)	**PO:** 6–12 hrs **Rectal:** 15–60 min	Short-term relief of constipation	Electrolyte imbalance, abdominal discomfort, gas
Senna (Senokot)	6–12 hrs	Short-term relief of constipation	Abdominal discomfort, cramps, discoloration of bowel movements

Secretagogues

Linaclotide (Linzess)	72 or 145 mcg daily at least 30 min prior to first meal of day	Use in pts not responding to other agents as replacement or adjunct	Diarrhea
Lubiprostone (Amitiza)	8–25 mcg twice daily	Same as above	Nausea (35%)
Plecanatide (Trulance)	3 mg once daily with or without food	Same as above	Diarrhea

GI, Gastrointestinal; *HF,* heart failure.

Multiple Sclerosis

USES

Multiple sclerosis (MS) is a potentially disabling disease of the brain and spinal cord. In MS, the immune system attacks the protective sheath (myelin) that covers nerve fibers, causing communication problems between the brain and the body. Symptoms of MS vary greatly depending on the amount of nerve damage and which nerves are affected (e.g., some may lose the ability to walk independently or at all, while others have long periods of remission without new symptoms). Treatments can help speed recovery from attacks, modify the course of the disease, and manage symptoms.

ACTION

Interferons: Have modulatory and anti-inflammatory effects.

Glatiramer: A mixture of synthetic homogeneous polypeptide chains containing 4 naturally occurring amino acids (glutamic acid, alanine, tyrosine, and lysine). Exhibits several immunomodulatory effects, including suppression of T-cell activation and induction and activation of suppressor T cells.

Natalizumab (humanized anti-alpha4-integrin antibody): Prevents leukocyte migration across the blood-brain barrier, which may interrupt the inflammatory cascade in MS.

Alemtuzumab (humanized anti-CD52 antibody): Causes rapid depletion of CD52-positive B and T cells.

Anti-CD20 Antibodies: (ocrelizumab, ofatumumab, rituximab): Reduces relapse rates and disability progression.

Mitoxantrone: Reduces relapse rates and slows disability progression in pts with severe MS.

S1P Receptor Modulators: (fingolimod, ozanimod, ponesimod, siponimod): Binds to S1P receptors, preventing lymphocyte egress into peripheral blood, reducing T-cell infiltration into the CNS.

Cladribine: Selectively depletes B lymphocytes, which play a major role in MS pathophysiology.

Fumarates: (dimethyl fumarate, diroximel fumarate): Antioxidants that induce expression of anti-inflammatory proteins.

Teriflunomide (pyrimidine synthesis inhibitor): Reduces T- and B-cell activation and proliferation.

MEDICATIONS FOR MULTIPLE SCLEROSIS

Name	Dosage	Side Effects
Alemtuzumab (Lemtrada)	12 mg IV once daily for 5 days; after 1 yr, give 12 mg IV once daily for 3 days	Arthralgia, malignacies, infections, pneumonitis, nasophayngitis, pyrexia, infusion reactions, malignancies nausea, vomiting, rash, fatigue, urticaria, pruritus, pain, headache, diarrhea, thrombocytopenia
Cladribine (Mavenclad)	Recommended cumulative dosage: 3.5 mg/kg body weight administered orally and divided into 2 yearly treatment courses (1.75 mg/kg/ treatment course)	Upper respiratory tract infection, headache, hypersensitivity reactions, cytopenies, malignancies, HBV reactivation, acute cardiac failure
Dimethyl fumarate (Tecfidera)	240 mg PO 2 times/day	Flushing, abdominal pain, diarrhea, nausea, lymphopenia, hepatotoxicity, progressive multifocal leukoencephalopathy (PML) infections
Diroximel fumarate (Vumerity)	**PO:** Initially, 231 mg twice daily; after 7 days, increase to maintenance dose of 462 mg twice daily	Flushing, abdominal pain, diarrhea, nausea, infection lymphopenia, hepatotoxicity, progressive multifocal leukoencephalopathy (PML)
Fingolimod (Gilenya)	0.5 mg PO once daily	Infections, hypersensitivity reactions, elevated LFTs, bradycardia, AV block, macular edema, decreased pulmonary function lymphopenia, decreased pulmonary function, malignancies, PML
Glatiramer (Copaxone, Glatopa)	**Copaxone:** 20 mg SQ once daily or 40 mg 3 times/wk **Glatopa:** 20 mg SQ once daily	Pain, erythema, inflammation, pruritus at injection site, arthralgia, transient chest pain, postinjection reactions (chest pain, palpitations, dyspnea)
Interferon beta 1a (Avonex, Rebif)	**Avonex:** 30 mcg IM wkly **Rebif:** 44 mcg 3 times/wk	Headache, flulike symptoms, myalgia, depression with suicidal ideation, generalized pain, asthenia, chills, injection site reaction, hypersensitivity reactions, anemia, hepatotoxicity seizures
Interferon beta 1b (Betaseron, Extavia)	250 mcg SQ every other day	Headache, flulike symptoms, myalgia, upper respiratory tract infection, depression with suicidal ideation, generalized pain, asthenia, chills, fever, injection site reaction, hypersensitivity reactions, anemia, hepatotoxicity, seizures lymphopenia
Mitoxantrone	12 mg/m2 IV q3mos	Nausea, vomiting, diarrhea, cough, headache, stomatitis, abdominal discomfort, fever, alopecia, cardiotoxicity (at cumulative doses greater than 100 mg/m², amenorrhea, myelosuppression, acute/chronic myeloid leukemia

Name	Dosage	Side Effects
Natalizumab (Tysabri)	300 mg IV q4wks	Headache, fatigue, depression, arthralgia, infections, hypersensitivity reactions, hepatotoxicity, thrombocytopenia, PML
Ocrelizumab (Ocrevus)	Initially, 300 mg IV then 2 wks later, 300 mg IV, then 600 mg IV q6mos; 1st 60-mg dose 6 mo after initial 300-mg dose	Infusion reactions (pruritus, rash, urticaria, erythema), decreased immunoglobulin level, HBV reactivation, malignancies, PML
Ocrelizumab Subcutaneous (Ocrevus Zunovo)	920 mg ocrelizumab and 23,000 units hyaluronidase) SQ q6 mos	Erythema, pain, swelling, pruritus, headache, nausea, PML, decreased immunoglobulin level, immune-mediated colitis; increased risk of malignancy
Ofatumumab (Kesimpta)	Initially, 20 mg administered at wks 0, 1, and 2, then 20 mg monthly starting at wk 4	Infections, systemic/local injection reactions, back pain, decreased immunoglobulin levels
Ozanimod (Zeposia)	**PO:** Initially, 0.23 mg once daily on days 1–4; then 0.46 mg once daily on days 5–7. **Maintenance:** 0.92 mg once daily starting on day 8	Infection decreased blood lymphocyte count, bradycardia, arrhythmias, macular edema, decreased pulmonary function, hypertension, increased serum ALT, AST
Pegylated interferon beta 1a (Plegridy)	125 mcg SQ q2wks	Headache, flulike symptoms, myalgia, depression with suicidal ideation, generalized pain, asthenia, chills, injection site reaction, hypersensitivity reactions, anemia, hepatotoxicity, elevated LFTs, seizures
Ponesimod (Ponvory)	**PO:** 20 mg once daily	Elevated hepatic transaminases, hypertension bradycardia, macular edema, decreased pulmonary function, cutaneous malignancies, infections
Rituximab (Rituxan)	**IV:** 1 g q2wks for 2 doses, then 500–1,000 mg q6–12 mos	Infections, infusion reactions, cytopenias cardiac arrhythmias, cough, rhinitis, angioedema, nausea, vomiting, diarrhea, myalgia, PML
Siponimod (Mayzent)	Titration required for treatment initiation Recommended maintenance dosage: 2 mg	Headache, hypertension, increased serum ALT, AST bradycardia, lymphopenia, macular edema, seizures, infections, decreased pulmonary function, cutaneous malignancies

Continued

MEDICATIONS FOR MULTIPLE SCLEROSIS—cont'd

Name	Dosage	Side Effects
Teriflunomide (Aubagio)	7 or 14 mg PO once daily	Headache, diarrhea, nausea, alopecia, paresthesia, abdominal pain, elevated LFTs, neutropenia, leukopenia, hepatic failure, acute renal failure, toxic epidermal necrolysis hypersensitivity reactions, hyperkalemia, hypophosphatemia, interstitial lung disease
Ublituximab-xiiy (Briumvi)	Initially: first infusion 150 mg IV, then 450 mg IV 2 wks after the first infusion, then 450 mg IV 24 wks after the first infusion, then q24wks thereafter	Infusion reactions, upper and lower respiratory tract infections, herpes virus–associated infections, extremity pain, insomnia, fatigue

ALT, Alanine aminotransferase; *AST,* aspartate aminotransferase; *bid,* twice daily; *IM,* intramuscular; *IV,* intravenous; *LFT,* liver function test; *PML,* progressive multifocal leukoencephalopathy; *PO,* oral; *SQ,* subcutaneous; *UTI,* urinary tract infection.

Nonsteroidal Anti-Inflammatory Drugs (NSAIDs)

USES

Nonsteroidal anti-inflammatory drugs (NSAIDs) are an FDA-approved drug class used as antipyretic, anti-inflammatory, and analgesic agents. These effects make NSAIDs useful for treating muscle pain, dysmenorrhea, arthritic conditions, pyrexia, gout, and migraines and are used as opioid-sparing agents in certain acute trauma cases. NSAIDs are most frequently used to ease the pain, inflammation, and stiffness associated with arthritis, bursitis, and tendinitis and to reduce fevers and relieve headaches.

ACTION

NSAIDs inhibit cyclooxygenase (COX) enzymes from making hormonelike chemicals called prostaglandins, one of the body's biggest contributors to inflammation.

There are 2 different kinds of cyclooxygenase: COX-1 helps protect the stomach lining, and COX-2 plays a role in inflammation. Most NSAIDs are nonspecific, interfering with both COX-1 and COX-2. While this helps relieve pain and inflammation, it also causes GI tract vulnerability to ulcers and bleeding.

A specific type of NSAID, called a selective COX-2 inhibitor, blocks the COX-2 enzyme more than the COX-1 enzyme. The only selective COX-2 NSAID currently available in the United States is celecoxib (Celebrex). Topical NSAIDs (diclofenac gel) are also available for use in acute tenosynovitis, ankle sprains, and soft tissue injuries.

Continued

NSAIDs

Name	Availability	Usual Adult Analgesic Dose	Side Effects
Celecoxib (Celebrex)	**C:** 50 mg, 100 mg, 200 mg, 400 mg	400 mg once, then 200 mg q12h	**Class: Bleeding:** May interfere with platelet function; prolong bleeding time. **GI toxicity:** May cause dyspepsia, GI ulceration, perforation, bleeding. **Renal:** May decrease renal blood flow, fluid retention, hypertension, renal failure. **Cardiovascular:** May have a prothrombotic effect (clotting), increasing risk of cardiovascular events. **Asthma:** May precipitate asthma symptoms. **Hypersensitivity reactions:** May cause anaphylaxis reactions in aspirin-sensitive pts. **CNS:** Dizziness, anxiety, drowsiness, confusion, depression, disorientation, severe headache. **Pregnancy:** Avoid use beginning at 20 wks gestation (risk of fetal renal dysfunction)
Diclofenac (Voltaren, Zipsor, Zorvolex)	**T:** 25 mg, 50 mg, 75 mg **C (Zipsor):** 25 mg **C (Zorvolex):** 18 mg, 35 mg	50 mg q8–12h **(Zipsor):** 25 mg 4 times/day **(Zorvolex):** 18–35 mg 3 times/day	
Etodolac (Lodine)	**T:** 400 mg, 500 mg **T (ER):** 400 mg, 500 mg, 600 mg **C:** 200 mg, 300 mg	**T, C:** 200–400 mg q6–8h (max: 1,000 mg/day) **T (ER):** 400–1,000 mg once daily	
Fenoprofen (Nalfon)	**C:** 200 mg, 400 mg **T:** 600 mg	200–400 mg q6–8h as needed (max: 3,200 mg/day)	

Ibuprofen (Advil, Caldolor, Motrin)	**T:** 100 mg, 200 mg, 400 mg, 600 mg, 800 mg **C:** 200 mg **Susp:** 100 mg/5 mL	**P:** 200–400 mg/dose q4–6h as needed (max: 2,400 mg/day)
Ketoprofen (Orudis KT)	**C:** 50 mg, 75 mg **C (ER):** 200 mg	**C:** 50 mg q6h or 75 mg q8h **ER:** 200 mg once daily
Ketorolac (Toradol)	**T:** 10 mg **I:** 15 mg/mL, 30 mg/mL **C: Intranasal:** 15.75 mg/spray	**PO:** 10 mg q4–6h (max: 40 mg/day); **IM/IV: less than 65 yrs old:** 30 mg IM or IV q6h (max: 120 mg/day); **65 yrs or older:** 15 mg IM or IV q6h (max: 60 mg/day); **Nasal: less than 65 yrs:** 1 spray q6–8h in each nostril (max: 126 mg/day); **65 yrs or older:** 1 spray q6–8h in one nostril (max: 63 mg/day)
Meloxicam (Mobic, Vivlodex)	**C:** 5 mg, 10 mg **T:** 7.5 mg, 15 mg **Susp:** 7.5 mg/5 mL	**C:** 5–10 mg once daily **T:** 7.5–15 mg once daily
Nabumetone (Relafen)	**T:** 500 mg, 750 mg	500–750 mg q8–12h (max: 2,000 mg/day)
Naproxen (Anaprox, Naprosyn)	**T:** 250 mg, 375 mg, 500 mg **T (CR):** 375 mg, 500 mg **Susp:** 125 mg/5 mL	250 mg q6–8h or 500 mg q12h (max: 1,250 mg on day 1, then 1,000 mg/day)

A, Adults; *C,* capsules; *CR,* controlled-release; *ER,* extended-release; *GI,* gastrointestinal; *I,* injection; *P,* pain; *Susp,* suspension; *SR,* sustained-release; *T,* tablets.

Osteoporosis

HISTORY

Osteoporosis develops when bone mineral density (BMD) and bone mass decreases or when the quality or structure of bone changes, leading to a decrease in bone strength that can increase the risk of fractures. Fractures occur most often in bones of the hip, vertebrae, and wrist.

Factors that may increase the risk for osteoporosis include: **Sex:** Chances of developing osteoporosis are greater in females. **Age:** Bone loss happens quicker, and new bone growth is slower. **Body size:** Slender, thin-boned women and men are at greater risk. **Race:** White and Asian women are at highest risk. **Family history:** Hereditary factors may increase risk. **Diet:** A diet low in calcium and vitamin D may increase risk for osteoporosis and fracture.

Diagnosis: DEXA Scan (DXA) measures the BMD at sites that are prone to fracture (e.g., hip, spine). Bone density measurement by DXA at the hip and spine is generally considered the most reliable way to diagnose osteoporosis and predict risk of fracture.

ACTION

Bisphosphonates: Nonhormonal drugs that decrease bone resorption by binding to active sites of bone remodeling and inhibit osteoclasts. Slow down bone loss, which may decrease risk of fractures.

Selective estrogen receptor modulator (SERM): Decreases bone resorption, increasing BMD and decreasing the incidence of fractures.

Conjugated estrogens and selective estrogen receptor modulator: Increases BMD in postmenopausal women.

Parathyroid hormone analogs: Increase BMD by stimulating bone formation.

RANK ligand (RANKL) inhibitor: Inhibits osteoclast formation, function, and survival, reducing bone resorption. Increases BMD and reduces the incidence of new vertebral and hip fractures.

Sclerostin inhibitor: Binds to and inhibits sclerostin, increasing bone formation and decreasing bone resorption.

BISPHOSPHONATES

Name	Availability	Dosage	Class Side Effects
Alendronate (Binosto, Fosamax)	**T:** 5 mg, 10 mg, 35 mg, 70 mg **S:** 70 mg/75 mL	**Prevention:** 5 mg/day or 35 mg/wk **Treatment:** 10 mg/day or 70 mg/wk	Hypocalcemia, may cause jaw osteonecrosis (rarely); GI (e.g., heartburn, esophageal irritation, esophagitis, abdominal pain, diarrhea); severe bone, joint, or muscle pain. **IV:** acute-phase reaction (e.g., low-grade fever, myalgia, arthralgia) within 1–3 days of the infusion
Ibandronate (Boniva)	**T:** 150 mg **I:** 1 mg/mL	**Prevention and treatment:** 150 mg/mo **IV injection: Treatment:** 3 mg/3 mos	
Risedronate (Actonel)	**T:** 5 mg, 35 mg, 150 mg **T (DR):** 35 mg	**Prevention and treatment:** 5 mg/day, 35 mg/wk, or 150 mg/mo	
Zoledronic acid (Reclast)	**I:** 5 g/100 mL	**Prevention: IV:** 5 mg every 2 yrs **Treatment: IV:** 5 mg every yr	

SERM

Name	Availability	Dosage	Side Effects
Raloxifene (Evista)	**T:** 60 mg	**Prevention and treatment:** 60 mg/day	Leg cramps, hot flashes, increased risk of thromboembolic events

Continued

PARATHYROID HORMONE

Name	Availability	Dosage	Class Side Effects
Abaloparatide (Tymlos)	I: 2,000 mcg/mL prefilled pen delivers 80 mcg/dose	**Treatment:** 80 mcg subcutaneously once daily	Muscle cramps, injection site reactions, tachycardia, hypotension, increased serum uric acid concentration, hypercalciuria, dizziness, nausea, headache, hypercalcemia
Teriparatide (Forteo)	I: 250 mcg/mL syringe delivers 20 mcg/dose	**Treatment:** 20 mcg subcutaneously once daily	

CONJUGATED ESTROGENS AND SELECTIVE ESTROGEN RECEPTOR MODULATOR

Name	Availability	Dosage	Side Effects
Conjugated estrogens and bazedoxifene (Duavee)	T: 0.45 mg/20 mg	**Prevention:** 1 tablet once daily	Muscle spasms; nausea; dyspepsia; and abdominal, neck, or oropharyngeal pain, increased risk of DVT/thromboembolism with long term use

MONOCLONAL ANTIBODY RANKL INHIBITOR

Name	Availability	Dosage	Side Effects
Denosumab (Prolia)	I: 60 mg/mL	**SQ:** 60 mg once every 6 mos	Dermatitis, rash, eczema, hypocalcemia. May cause jaw osteonecrosis (rarely).

SCLEROSTIN INHIBITOR

Name	Availability	Dosage	Side Effects
Romosozumab (Evenity)	I: 105 mg/1.17 mL syringe	**SQ:** 210 mg (2 injections) once every mo for up to 12 doses	Arthralgia, headache, increased risk of jaw osteonecrosis, atypical femoral fractures, serious cardiovascular events (e.g., MI, stroke)

DR, Delayed-release; *I,* injection; *S,* solution (oral); *SQ,* subcutaneous; *T,* tablet.

Parkinson's Disease Treatment

USES	ACTION
To slow or stop clinical progression of Parkinson's disease and to improve function and quality of life in pts with Parkinson's disease, a progressive neurodegenerative disorder.	Normal motor function is dependent on the synthesis and release of dopamine by neurons projecting from the substantia nigra to the corpus striatum. In Parkinson's disease, disruption of this pathway results in diminished levels of the neurotransmitter dopamine. Medication is aimed at providing improved function using the lowest effective dose.

TYPES OF MEDICATIONS FOR PARKINSON'S DISEASE
DOPAMINE PRECURSOR

Levodopa/carbidopa:

Levodopa: Dopamine precursor supplementation to enhance dopaminergic neurotransmission. A small amount of levodopa crosses the blood-brain barrier and is decarboxylated to dopamine, which is then available to stimulate dopaminergic receptors.

Carbidopa: Inhibits peripheral decarboxylation of levodopa, decreasing its conversion to dopamine in peripheral tissues, which results in an increased availability of levodopa for transport across the blood-brain barrier.

COMT INHIBITORS

Entacapone, tolcapone: Reversible inhibitor of catechol-*O*-methyltransferase (COMT). COMT is responsible for catalyzing levodopa. In the presence of a decarboxylase inhibitor (carbidopa), COMT becomes the major metabolizing enzyme for levodopa in the brain and periphery. By inhibiting COMT, higher plasma levels of levodopa are attained, resulting in more dopaminergic stimulation in the brain and lessening the symptoms of Parkinson's disease.

DOPAMINE RECEPTOR AGONISTS

Pramipexole: Stimulates dopamine receptors in the striatum of the CNS.

Ropinirole: Stimulates postsynaptic dopamine D2 type receptors within the caudate putamen in the brain.

Rotigotine: Action thought to be related to its ability to stimulate dopamine receptors within the caudate-putamen in the brain.

MONOAMINE OXIDASE B INHIBITORS

Rasagiline, safinamide, selegiline: Increase dopaminergic activity due to inhibition of monoamine oxidase type B (MAO B). MAO B is involved in the oxidative deamination of dopamine in the brain.

ADENOSINE A2A RECEPTOR ANTAGONIST

Istradefylline: Attenuates excessive activity of the striato-pallidal neurons in pts with Parkinson's disease. Possibly increases dopaminergic activity in the brain.

AMANTADINE:

Amantadine: A weak noncompetitive antagonist of glutamatergic (NMDA) receptors. Glutamate is thought to play a role in dyskinesia.

ANTICHOLINERGICS:

Anticholinergics (e.g., trihexyphenidyl, benztropine): Can be useful in some pts for treatment of tremor and drooling.

Parkinson's Disease Treatment

MEDICATIONS FOR TREATMENT OF PARKINSON'S DISEASE

Name	Type	Availability	Dosage	Side Effects/Comments
Amantadine Gocovri Osmolex ER		**C:** 100 mg **Syrup:** 10 mg/mL **T:** 100 mg **C (ER): (Gocovri):** 68.5 mg, 137 mg **T (ER): (Osmolex ER):** 129 mg, 193 mg, 258 mg	100 mg 2 times/day. May increase up to 400 mg/day in divided doses **ER Caps:** 274 mg once at bedtime **ER Tabs:** 129–322 mg once daily in the morning	Cognitive impairment, confusion, insomnia, hallucinations, livedo reticularis **Comments:** Added to levodopa in later disease for dyskinesias
Apomorphine (Apokyn, Kynmobi)		**I:** 10 mg/1 mL **SL:** 10 mg, 15 mg, 20 mg, 25 mg, 30 mg	**SC:** 2–6 mg 3–5×/day PRN **SL:** 10–30 mg 1–5×/day PRN	**SC:** Somnolence, dyskinesias, dizziness/postural hypotension, rhinorrhea, nausea, vomiting, confusion, edema/swelling of extremities **SL:** Nausea, oral soft tissue swelling/pain, paraesthesia, dizziness, somnolence **Comments:** For acute intermittent treatment of "off" episodes in advanced disease.
Carbidopa/ levodopa (Crexont, Rytary, Sinemet, Sinemet CR)	Dopamine precursor	**OD:** 10/100 mg, 25/100 mg, 25/250 mg **Immediate-release (Sinemet):** 10/100 mg, 25/100 mg, 25/250 mg **ER (Sinemet CR):** 25/100 mg, 50/200 mg **(Rytary):** 23.75 mg/95 mg, 36.25 mg/145 mg, 48.75 mg/ 195 mg, 61.25 mg/245 mg **(Crexont):** 35 mg/140 mg, 52.5 mg/210 mg, 70 mg/280 mg, 87.5 mg/350 mg	300–1,500 mg levodopa in divided doses **Sinemet CR:** Initially, 400 mg/day in 2 divided doses. May increase up to 1,600 mg levodopa in divided doses **Rytary:** Initially, 23.75 mg/95 mg 3 times/day May increase up to 612.5 mg/2,450 mg per day in divided doses **Crexont:** Initially, 35 mg/140 mg twice daily for first 3 days, then may increase gradually as needed up to maximum of 525 mg/2100 mg per day.	Anorexia, nausea, orthostatic hypotension initially; hallucinations, confusion, sleep disturbances with chronic use, constipation, dry mouth, headache, dyskinesia **Comments:** Most effective for Parkinson's motor symptoms. May be used first-line, especially in older pts.

Entacapone (Comtan)	COMT inhibitor	**T:** 200 mg	200 mg 3–4 times/day up to **maximum** of 8 times/day (1,600 mg)	Dyskinesias, nausea, diarrhea, urine discoloration **Comments:** Adjunct to levodopa-carbidopa for "wearing off." Prolongs the duration of action of levodopa.
Istradefylline (Nouriarz)	Adenosine A2a receptor antagonist	**T:** 20 mg, 40 mg	20–40 mg once daily	Dyskinesia, hallucinations, psychotic behavior, impulse control disorders **Comments:** Adjunct to levodopa/carbidopa for treatment of "off" episodes.
Opicapone (Ongentys)	COMT inhibitor	**C:** 25 mg, 50 mg	50 mg once daily at bedtime	Dyskinesia, constipation, increase creatine kinase, hypotension/syncope, weight loss **Comments:** Adjunct to levodopa-carbidopa for "wearing off." Prolongs the duration of action of levodopa.
Pramipexole (Mirapex, Mirapex ER)	Dopamine agonist	**T:** 0.125 mg, 0.25 mg, 0.5 mg, 0.75 mg, 1 mg, 1.5 mg **ER:** 0.375 mg, 0.75 mg, 1.5 mg, 2.25 mg, 3 mg, 3.75 mg, 4.5 mg	**T:** Initially, 0.125 mg 3 times/day May increase q5–7 days. Usual dose: 0.5–1.5 mg 3 times/day **ER:** Initially, 0.375 mg once daily. May increase q5–7 days by 0.75 mg/dose up to 4.5 mg once daily.	Side effects similar to carbidopa/levodopa. Lower risk of dyskinesias, higher risk of hallucinations, sleepiness, edema. May cause excessive daytime sleepiness, impair impulse control (e.g., gambling) **Comments:** May be used first-line in younger pts. May be added to levodopa to reduce off time, improve symptoms, or manage dyskinesias.
Rasagiline (Azilect)	MAO B inhibitor	**T:** 0.5 mg, 1 mg	0.5–1 mg once daily	Nausea, orthostatic hypotension, hallucinations, insomnia, dry mouth, constipation, vivid dreams. Many potential drug interactions. **Comments:** May be used first-line or added to levodopa to reduce off time.
Ropinirole (Requip, Requip XL)	Dopamine agonist	**T:** 0.25 mg, 0.5 mg, 1 mg, 2 mg, 3 mg, 4 mg, 5 mg **XL:** 2 mg, 4 mg, 6 mg, 8 mg, 12 mg	**T:** Initially, 0.25 mg 3 times/day. May increase at wkly intervals to 0.5 mg 3 times/day, then 0.75 mg 3 times/day, then 1 mg 3 times/day May then increase by 1.5 mg/day up to 9 mg/day, then by 3 mg/day up to total dose of 24 mg/day in divided doses. **XL:** Initially, 2 mg/day for 1–2 wks, then increase by 2 mg/day at wkly intervals	Side effects similar to carbidopa/levodopa. Lower risk of dyskinesias, higher risk of hallucinations, sleepiness, edema. May cause excessive daytime sleepiness, impair impulse control (e.g., gambling). **Comments:** May be used first-line in younger pts. May be added to levodopa to reduce off time, improve symptoms, or manage dyskinesias.

Continued

PARKINSON'S DISEASE TREATMENT —cont'd

Name	Type	Availability	Dosage	Side Effects/Comments
Rotigotine (Neupro)	Dopamine agonist	**Transdermal patch:** 1 mg/24 hrs, 2 mg/24 hrs, 3 mg/24 hrs, 4 mg/24 hrs, 6 mg/24 hrs, 8 mg/24 hrs	Early stage: Initially, 2 mg/24 hrs up to 6 mg/24 hrs Advanced stage: Initially, 4 mg/24 hrs up to 8 mg/24 hrs	Side effects similar to carbidopa/levodopa. Lower risk of dyskinesias, higher risk of hallucinations, sleepiness, edema. May cause excessive daytime sleepiness, impair impulse control (e.g., gambling). **Comments:** May be used first-line in younger pts. May be added to levodopa to reduce "off" time, improve symptoms, or manage dyskinesias.
Safinamide (Xadago)	MAO B inhibitor	**T:** 50 mg, 100 mg	Initially, 50 mg once daily. May increase after 2 wks to 100 mg once daily.	Dyskinesia, falls, hallucinations, nausea, insomnia Many potential drug interactions **Comments:** May be added to levodopa to reduce "off" time.
Selegiline (Eldepryl, Zelapar)	MAO B inhibitor	**C (Eldepryl):** 5 mg **OD (Zelapar):** 1.25 mg	**C:** 5 mg with breakfast and lunch **OD:** 1.25–2.5 mg daily in the morning	Nausea, orthostatic hypotension, hallucinations, insomnia, dry mouth, constipation, vivid dreams. Many potential drug interactions. **Comments:** May be used first-line or added to levodopa to reduce "off" time.
Tolcapone (Tasmar)	COMT inhibitor	**T:** 100 mg	Initially, 100 mg 3 times/day. May increase to 200 mg 3 times/day.	Dyskinesias, nausea, diarrhea, urine discoloration **Comments:** Adjunct to levodopa-carbidopa for "wearing off." Prolongs the duration of action of levodopa.

C, Capsules; *COMT*, catechol-*O*-methyltransferase; *CR*, controlled-release; *ER*, extended-release; *I*, Injection; *MAO B*, monoamine oxidase B; *OD*, orally disintegrating; *T*, tablets; *XL*, extended-release.

Rheumatoid Arthritis

Rheumatoid arthritis (RA) is an autoimmune disease associated with progressive disability, systemic complications, early death, and socioeconomic costs. RA affects most joints and their surrounding tissues. RA is characterized by synovial inflammation and hyperplasia, autoantibody production (e.g., rheumatoid factor), cartilage and bone destruction, and systemic features (e.g., cardiovascular, pulmonary, psychological, skeletal disorders). The clinical hallmark of RA is polyarticular synovial inflammation of peripheral joints (typically in the hands, resulting in pain, stiffness, and some degree of irreversible joint damage; deformity; and disability).

Medications used in RA include disease-modifying antirheumatic drugs (DMARDs) and biologic agents, including tumor necrosis factor (TNF) inhibitors.

Combination treatment useful in pts with a long duration of disease or clinical features indicating a poor prognosis.

DMARDS

Name	Dosage	Side Effects/Comments
Hydroxychloroquine (Plaquenil)	200–400 mg (max: 5 mg/kg actual body wt) once daily	**Side Effects:** Nausea, epigastric pain, hemolysis may occur in pts with G6PD deficiency, retinal toxicity with long-term use **Comments:** May be used alone or in combination. Life-threatening hypoglycemia, cardiomyopathy, QT interval prolongation, torsades de pointes may occur.
Leflunomide (Arava)	**Induction:** 100 mg/day for 3 days **Maintenance:** 10–20 mg/day	**Side Effects:** Diarrhea, respiratory tract infection, hypertension, headache, reversible alopecia, rash, myelosuppression, and/or elevated hepatic enzymes **Comments:** Contraindicated for use during pregnancy
Methotrexate (oral) (Rheumatrex, Trexall), Methotrexate (injectable) (Otrexup, Rasuvo)	**Induction:** 7.5–10 mg PO once wkly **Maintenance:** 7.5–25 mg PO once wkly **(Otrexup): Induction:** 7.5 IM or SQ once wkly **Maintenance:** 10–25 mg IM or SQ once wkly **(Rasuvo): Induction:** 7.5 mg IM or SQ wkly **Maintenance:** 10–30 mg IM or SQ wkly	**Side Effects:** Stomatitis, anorexia, nausea, vomiting, diarrhea, abdominal cramps, hepatic enzyme elevations, thrombocytopenia **Comments:** Not recommended in pts with CrCl <30 mL/min; should not be prescribed for women who are or may become pregnant

Continued

RHEUMATOID ARTHRITIS—cont'd

Name	Dosage	Side Effects/Comments
Sulfasalazine (Azulfidine)	**Induction:** 3–4 g/day in divided doses **Maintenance:** 2 g/day in divided doses	**Side Effects:** Headache, nausea, anorexia, rash, hemolysis may occur in pts with G6PD deficiency **Comments:** May be used alone or in combination

BIOLOGIC AGENTS

TNF INHIBITORS

Dosage	Side	Effects/Comments
Adalimumab (Humira)	40 mg SQ once wkly or q2wks	**Side Effects:** Headache, skin rash, positive ANA titer, antibody development, injection site reaction (erythema, itching, pain, swelling), upper respiratory tract infection **Comments:** Increased risk for serious infections (e.g., tuberculosis, invasive fungal infections), avoid use in pts with recent history of malignancy or preexisting demyelinating disorders
Certolizumab (Cimzia)	**Induction:** 400 mg SQ at 0, 2, 4 wks **Maintenance:** 200 mg SQ every other wk or 400 mg q4wks	**Side Effects:** Nausea, infection, upper respiratory tract infection, skin rash, injection site reactions (erythema, itching, pain, swelling) **Comments:** See adalimumab
Etanercept (Enbrel)	25 mg SQ 2 times/wk or 50 mg SQ once wkly	**Side Effects:** Headache, skin rash, diarrhea, injection site reactions (e.g., erythema, swelling), upper respiratory tract infection, rhinitis **Comments:** See adalimumab

Name	Dosage	Side Effects/Comments
Golimumab (Simponi, Simponi Aria)	**Simponi:** 50 mg SQ once monthly **Simponi Aria:** **Induction:** 2 mg/kg IV at 0 and 4 wks **Maintenance:** 2 mg/kg IV q8wks	**Side Effects:** Positive ANA titer, upper respiratory tract infection (e.g., nasopharyngitis, rhinitis), injection site reactions (erythema, itching, pain, swelling), infusion reactions (fever, urticaria, dyspnea, hypotension) **Comments:** See adalimumab
Infliximab (Remicade) Biosimilars: Inflectra, Renflexis	**Induction:** 3 mg/kg IV at 0, 2, and 6 wks **Maintenance:** 3 mg/kg IV q8wks	**Side Effects:** Nausea, diarrhea, abdominal pain, increased ANA titer, upper respiratory tract infection, sinusitis, cough, pharyngitis, infusion reactions (fever, urticaria, dyspnea, hypotension) **Comments:** See adalimumab

OTHER BIOLOGIC AGENTS

Name	Dosage	Side Effects/Comments
Abatacept (Orencia)	**IV:** 500 mg, 750 mg, or 1,000 mg IV at 0, 2, and 4 wks, then q4wks **SQ:** 125 mg SQ once wkly	**Side Effects:** Nausea, UTIs, acute exacerbation of COPD, hypertension, headache, dizziness **Comments:** May increase risk of serious infections (e.g., pneumonia, pyelonephritis, cellulitis, diverticulitis) May be used alone or in combination with a conventional DMARD.
Rituximab (Rituxan), Riabni, Ruxience, Truxima	1,000 mg IV twice, 2 wks apart	**Side Effects:** Hypotension, peripheral edema, abdominal pain anemia, arthralgia, infusion site reactions **Comments:** Pts at high risk for hepatitis B virus infection should be screened before beginning therapy. Approved for RA only in combination with methotrexate.

Continued

RHEUMATOID ARTHRITIS—cont'd

INTERLEUKIN (IL-6) INHIBITORS

Name	Dosage	Side Effects/Comments
Sarilumab (Kevzara)	**SQ:** 200 mg q2wks	Neutropenia, injection site reactions, upper respiratory tract infections, UTI, increased serum ALT **Comments:** Screening for tuberculosis recommended
Tocilizumab (Actemra) **Actemra Actpen**	**Induction: IV:** 4 mg/kg q4wks **Maintenance IV:** 8 mg/kg q4wks **Induction: SQ:** 162 mg q2wks (every wk in pts 100 kg or more) **Maintenance: SQ:** 162 mg every wk (q2wks in pts less than 100 kg)	Injection site reactions, HTN, neutropenia, increased serum ALT/AST, dyslipidemia **Comments:** Severe complications, including GI perforation and hypersensitivity with anaphylaxis, may occur

JANUS KINASE (JAK) INHIBITORS

Name	Dosage	Side Effects/Comments
Baricitinib (Olumiant)	**PO:** 2 mg once daily	**Class:** GI symptoms, nasopharyngitis, upper respiratory tract infections, headache, increased serum ALT/AST, dyslipidemia, cytopenias, infections (e.g., herpes zoster, tuberculosis) **Comments:** Risk of major cardiovascular events, malignancy, thrombosis. Should use only when TNF inhibitors are ineffective or poorly tolerated.
Tofacitinib (Xeljanz) **(Xeljanz XR)**	**PO:** 5 mg 2 times/day **PO, XR:** 11 mg once daily	
Upadacitinib (Rinvoq)	**PO, ER:** 15 mg once daily	

ALT, Alanine transaminase; *ANA,* antinuclear antibodies; *CNS,* central nervous system; *COPD,* chronic obstructive pulmonary disease; *ER,* extended-release; *GI,* gastrointestinal; *IM,* intramuscular; *IV,* intravenous; *LFT,* liver function test; *PO,* oral; *SQ,* subcutaneous; *UTI,* urinary tract infection; *PO,* oral; *XR,* extended-release.

Skeletal Muscle Relaxants

USES

Central acting muscle relaxants: Adjunct to rest, physical therapy for relief of discomfort associated with acute, painful musculoskeletal disorders (i.e., local spasms from muscle injury).

Baclofen, dantrolene, diazepam: Treatment of spasticity characterized by heightened muscle tone, spasm, loss of dexterity caused by multiple sclerosis, cerebral palsy, spinal cord lesions, CVA.

ACTION

Central acting muscle relaxants: Exact mechanism unknown. May act in CNS at various levels to depress polysynaptic reflexes; sedative effect may be responsible for relaxation of muscle spasm.

Baclofen, diazepam: May mimic actions of gamma-aminobutyric acid on spinal neurons; do not directly affect skeletal muscles.

Dantrolene: Acts directly on skeletal muscle, relieving spasticity.

SKELETAL MUSCLE RELAXANTS

Name	Indication	Dosage Range	Side Effects/Comments
Baclofen (Lioresal)	Spasticity associated with multiple sclerosis, spinal cord injury	Initially 5 mg 3 times/day Increase by 5 mg 3 times/day q3days **Maximum:** 20 mg 4 times/day	Drowsiness, dizziness, GI effects Caution with renal impairment, seizure disorders Withdrawal syndrome (e.g., hallucinations, psychosis, seizures)
Carisoprodol (Rela)	Discomfort due to acute, painful, musculoskeletal conditions	250–350 mg 4 times/day	Drowsiness, dizziness, GI effects, hypomania (at higher than recommended doses), withdrawal syndrome; hypersensitivity reaction (skin reaction, bronchospasm, weakness, burning eyes, fever) or idiosyncratic reaction (weakness, visual or motor disturbances, confusion) usually occurring within first 4 doses

SKELETAL MUSCLE RELAXANTS—cont'd

Name	Indication	Dosage Range	Side Effects/Comments
Chlorzoxazone (Lorzone)	Discomfort due to acute, painful, musculoskeletal conditions	Initially 250–500 mg 3–4 times/day **Maximum:** 750 mg 3–4 times/day	Drowsiness, dizziness, GI effects, rare hepatotoxicity Hypersensitivity reaction (urticaria, itching) Urine discoloration to orange, red, or purple
Cyclobenzaprine (Flexeril)	Muscle spasm, pain, tenderness, restricted movement due to acute, painful, musculoskeletal conditions	Initially 5–10 mg 3 times/day	Drowsiness, dizziness, GI effects Anticholinergic effects (dry mouth, urinary retention) Quinidinelike effects on heart (QT prolongation) Long half-life
Dantrolene (Dantrium)	Spasticity associated with multiple sclerosis, cerebral palsy, spinal cord injury	Initially 25 mg/day for 1 wk, then 25 mg 3 times/day for 1 wk, then 50 mg 3 times/day for 1 wk, then 100 mg 3 times/day **Maximum:** 100 mg 4 times/day	Drowsiness, dizziness, GI effects Contraindicated with hepatic disease Dose-dependent hepatotoxicity Diarrhea that is dose dependent and may be severe, requiring discontinuation
Diazepam (Valium)	Spasticity associated with cerebral palsy, spinal cord injury; reflex spasm due to muscle, joint trauma or inflammation	2–10 mg 3–4 times/day	Drowsiness, dizziness, GI effects Abuse potential
Metaxalone (Skelaxin)	Discomfort due to acute, painful, musculoskeletal conditions	800 mg 3–4 times/day	Drowsiness (low risk), dizziness, GI effects Paradoxical muscle cramps Mild withdrawal syndrome Contraindicated in serious hepatic or renal disease

Continued

Name	Indication	Dosage Range	Side Effects/Comments
Methocarbamol (Robaxin)	Discomfort due to acute, painful, musculoskeletal conditions	Initially 1,500 mg 4 times/day **Maintenance:** 1,000 mg 4 times/day	Drowsiness, dizziness, GI effects Urine discoloration to brown, brown-black, or green
Orphenadrine (Norflex)	Discomfort due to acute, painful, musculoskeletal conditions	100 mg 2 times/day	Drowsiness, dizziness, GI effects Long half-life Anticholinergic effects (dry mouth, urinary retention) Rare aplastic anemia Some products may contain sulfites
Tizanidine (Zanaflex)	Spasticity	Initially 4 mg q6–8h (**maximum** 3 times/day), may increase by 2–4 mg as needed/tolerated **Maximum:** 36 mg (limited information on doses greater than 24 mg)	Drowsiness, dizziness, GI effects Hypotension (20% decrease in B/P) Hepatotoxicity (usually reversible) Withdrawal syndrome (hypertension, tachycardia, hypertonia) Effect is short lived (3–6 hrs) Dose cautiously with creatinine clearance less than 25 mL/min

B/P, Blood pressure; *GI,* gastrointestinal.

Smoking Cessation Agents

Tobacco smoking is associated with the development of lung cancer and chronic obstructive pulmonary disease. Smoking is harmful not just to the smoker but also to family members, coworkers, and others breathing cigarette smoke.

Quitting smoking decreases the risk of developing lung cancer, other cancers, heart disease, stroke, and respiratory illnesses. Several medications have proved useful as smoking cessation aids. Nausea and lightheadedness are possible signs of overdose of nicotine warranting a reduction in dosage.

SMOKING CESSATION AGENTS

Name	Availability	Dose Duration	Cautions/Side Effects	Comments
Bupropion	**T:** 150 mg	150 mg every morning for 3 days, then 150 mg 2 times/day Start 1–2 wks before quit date **Duration:** 7–12 wks up to 6 mos for maintenance	History of seizure, eating disorder, use of MAOI within previous 14 days, bipolar disorder **Side effects:** Insomnia, dry mouth, tremor, rash	Stop smoking during second wk of treatment and use counseling support services along with medication

Continued

Name	Availability	Dose Duration	Cautions/Side Effects	Comments
Nicotine gum (Nicorette)	**Squares:** 2 mg, 4 mg	1 gum q1–2h for 6 wks, then q2–4h for 3 wks then q4–8h for 3 wks **Maximum:** 24 pieces/day **Duration:** Up to 12 wks	Recent MI (within 2 wks), serious arrhythmias, serious or worsening angina pectoris **Side effects:** Dyspepsia, mouth soreness, hiccups	2 mg recommended for pts smoking less than 25 cigarettes/day, 4 mg for pts smoking 25 or more cigarettes/day Chew until a peppery or minty taste emerges and then "park" between cheek and gums to facilitate nicotine absorption through oral mucosa Chew slowly and intermittently to avoid jaw ache and achieve maximum benefit Only water should be taken 15 min before and during chewing
Nicotine inhaler (Nicotrol)	**Cartridge:** 10 mg (delivers 4 mg nicotine)	4–16 cartridges daily; taper frequency of use over the last 6–12 wks **Duration:** up to 6 mos	Recent MI (within 2 wks), serious arrhythmias, serious or worsening angina pectoris **Side effects:** Local irritation of mouth and throat, coughing, rhinitis	Use at or above room temperature (cold temperatures decrease amount of nicotine inhaled)
Nicotine lozenge (Nicorette Lozenges)	**Lozenges:** 2 mg, 4 mg	One lozenge q1–2h for 6 wks, then q2–4h for 3 wks, then q4–8h for 3 wks **Duration:** 12 wks **Maximum:** 5 lozenges in 6 hrs; 20 lozenges in 1 day	Recent MI (within 2 wks), serious arrhythmias, serious or worsening angina pectoris **Side effects:** Local skin reaction, insomnia, nausea, sore throat	First cigarette smoked within 30 min of waking, use 4 mg; after 30 min of waking, use 2 mg Use at least 9 lozenges/day first 6 wks Only 1 lozenge at a time, 5 per 6 hrs and 20 per 24 hrs Do not chew or swallow
Nicotine nasal spray (Nicotrol NS)	10 mg/ml (delivers 0.5 mg/spray)	8–40 doses/day A dose consists of one 0.5 mg delivery to each nostril; initial dose is 1–2 sprays/hr, increasing as needed **Duration:** 3–6 mos	Recent MI (within 2 wks), serious arrhythmias, serious or worsening angina pectoris **Side effects:** Nasal irritation	Do not sniff, swallow, or inhale through nose while administering nicotine doses (may increase irritation) Tilt head back slightly for best results

SMOKING CESSATION AGENTS—cont'd

Nicotine patch (NicoDerm CQ)	**Nicoderm CQ:** 7 mg/24 hrs, 14 mg/24 hrs, 21 mg/24 hrs **Nicotrol:** 5 mg/16 hrs, 10 mg/16 hrs, 15 mg/16 hrs	Apply upon waking on quit date: **Nicoderm CQ (greater than 10 cigarettes/day):** 21 mg/24 hrs for 4 wks, then 14 mg/24 hrs for 2 wks, then 7 mg/24 hrs for 2 wks **(10 or fewer cigarettes/day):** 14 mg/24 hrs for 6 wks, then 7 mg/24 hrs for 2 wks	Recent MI (within 2 wks), serious arrhythmias, serious or worsening angina pectoris **Side Effects:** Local skin reaction, insomnia	The 16- and 24-hr patches are of comparable efficacy Begin with a lower-dose patch in pts smoking 10 or fewer cigarettes/day Place new patch on relatively hair-free location, usually between neck and waist, in the morning If insomnia occurs, remove the 24-hr patch prior to bedtime or use the 16-hr patch Rotate patch site to diminish skin irritation
Varenicline (Chantix)	**T:** 0.5 mg, 1 mg	**Days 1–3:** 0.5 mg daily; **days 4–7:** 0.5 mg 2 times/day; **day 8 to end of treatment:** 1 mg 2 times/day **Duration:** Begin 1 wk before set quit date, continue for 12 wks. May use additional 12 wks if failed to quit after first 12 wks	**Side effects:** Nausea; sleep disturbances; headaches; may impair ability to drive, operate machinery; depressed mood; altered behavior; suicidal ideation reported	Use lower dosage if not able to tolerate nausea and vomiting Use counseling support services along with medication

B/P, Blood pressure; *MAOI,* monoamine oxidase inhibitor; *MI,* myocardial infarction; *T,* tablets.

Weight Management

Adults with a body mass index (BMI) between 25 and 29.9 kg/m² are considered overweight. Those with a BMI greater than or equal to 30 are considered obese. The initial recommendation for any weight loss effort is to achieve a 5%–10% reduction in weight, which has been associated with a reduction in the risk of developing type 2 diabetes, hypertension, and dyslipidemia. Diet, exercise, and behavior modification are the preferred methods for losing weight. Several drugs and devices are FDA-approved for weight reduction and maintenance of weight loss.

SYMPATHOMIMETIC AMINES

Name	Availability	Dosage	Side Effects	Precautions
Benzphetamine	**T:** 50 mg	25–50 mg 1 to 3 times/day	**Class:** Increased HR, B/P; nervousness **Comments:** For short term use (up to 12 wks)	**Class:** *Contraindications:* Pregnancy/breast-feeding, cardiovascular disease, uncontrolled HTN, glaucoma, hyperthyroidism; history of drug abuse/agitation; use within 14 days of an MAOI
Diethylpropion Extended-Release	**T:** 25 mg **T: ER:** 75 mg	25 mg 3 times/day 75 mg once daily		
Phendimetrazine Extended-Release	**T:** 35 mg **C: ER:** 105 mg	35 mg 2–3 times/day 105 mg once daily		
Phentermine	**C:** 15 mg, 30 mg, 37.5 mg **T:** 37.5 mg	15–37.5 mg once daily		
Adipex-P **Lomaira**	**T:** 8 mg **T: C:** 37.5 mg **T:** 8 mg	8 mg 3 times/day or 15–37.5 mg once daily 8 mg 3 times/day		

SYMPATHOMIMETIC AMINE/ANTISEIZURE COMBINATION

Name	Availability	Usual Dosage	Side Effects	Precautions
Phentermine/Topiramate ER (Qsymia)	**C, ER:** 3.75 mg/23 mg, 7.5 mg/46 mg, 11.25 mg/69 mg, 15 mg/92 mg	7.5 mg/46 mg up to 15 mg/92 mg once daily	Increased B/P, nervousness, dry mouth, paresthesia, constipation, dysgeusia, insomnia, tachycardia, mood disorders/suicidal ideation, cognitive impairment, metabolic acidosis, acute closed-angle glaucoma, increased serum creatinine	*Contraindications:* Pregnancy, glaucoma, hyperthyroidism, use within 14 days of an MAOI **Caution:** Abrupt discontinuation may cause seizures

LIPASE INHIBITOR

Name	Availability	Usual Dosage	Side Effects	Precautions
Orlistat (Alli; Xenical)	**C:** 120 mg **C:** 60 mg	120 mg 3 times/day 60 mg 3 times/day	Flatulence, rectal incontinence, oily stools **Comments:** For short term use (up to 12 wks)	*Contraindications:* Pregnancy, chronic malabsorption syndrome, cholestasis

OPIOID ANTAGONIST/ANTIDEPRESSANT COMBINATION

Name	Availability	Usual Dosage	Side Effects	Precautions
Naltrexone/bupropion (Contrave)	**T, ER:** 8 mg/90 mg	16 mg/180 mg 2 times/day	Nausea, vomiting, headache, constipation, insomnia, dizziness, dry mouth, increased HR, B/P **Comments:** May cause suicidal thoughts/behavior with use of antidepressants. Can lower seizure threshold	*Contraindications:* Pregnancy, uncontrolled HTN, seizure disorder; history of seizures, bulimia, anorexia nervosa, chronic opiate use; within 14 days of an MAOI

Continued

GLUCAGON-LIKE PEPTIDE-1 (GLP-1) RECEPTOR AGONISTS

Name	Availability	Dosage	Side Effects	Precautions
Liraglutide (Saxenda)	**Prefilled pen:** 18 mg/3 mL	**SQ:** 3 mg once daily	**Class:** Nausea, vomiting, diarrhea, constipation, abdominal pain injection site reactions, headache, hypoglycemia, dyspepsia, fatigue, dizziness, gastroenteritis	**Class:** *Contraindications:* Pregnancy, family history of medullary thyroid cancer or multiple endocrine neoplasia syndrome type 2 **Precautions:** Thyroid cell tumors, cholelithiasis, hypoglycemia, acute hypersensitivity reactions, acute kidney injury, diabetic retinopathy complications, tachycardia, suicidal ideation, pulmonary aspiration (associated with elective procedures in pts who had residual gastric contents)
Semaglutide (Wegovy)	**Single-dose pen:** 0.25 mg, 0.5 mg, 1 mg/0.5 mL; 1.7 mg, 2.4 mg/0.75 mL	**SQ:** 2.4 mg once weekly		
Tirzepatide (Zepbound)	**Single-dose pens:** 2.5, 5, 7.5, 10, 12.5, 15/0.5 mL	**SQ:** 5–15 mg once wkly		

MELANOCORTIN 4 (MC4) RECEPTOR AGONIST

Name	Availability	Usual Dose	Side Effects	Precautions
Setmelanotide (Imcivree)	**I:** 10 mg/mL	**SQ: A, CH 12 yrs and older:** 2 mg once daily for 2 wks. **CH 6 to less than 12 yrs:** 1 mg once daily for 2 wks. **Target Dose:** 3 mg once daily.	Skin hyperpigmentation, injection site reactions, nausea, headache, diarrhea, abdominal pain, vomiting, depression, spontaneous penile erection.	Disturbance in sexual arousal, depression, suicidal ideation, skin pigmentation

DEVICES FOR WEIGHT MANAGEMENT

Device	Indication	Side Effects	Precautions
Orbera	BMI ≥30 kg/m² if lifestyle modification is unsuccessful	Nausea, vomiting, abdominal pain, reflux symptoms, abdominal distension/bloating	*Contraindications:* GI conditions (e.g., prior abdominal/weight reduction surgery, inflammatory bowel disease, obstructive disorders)
Obalon	BMI ≥30 kg/m² if lifestyle modification is unsuccessful	Nausea, vomiting, abdominal pain, reflux symptoms, abdominal distension/bloating	*Contraindications:* GI conditions (e.g., prior abdominal/weight reduction surgery, inflammatory bowel disease, obstructive disorders)
Plenity	BMI of 25–40 kg/m² as an adjunct to diet and exercise	Diarrhea, abdominal distension, infrequent bowel movements	*Precautions:* GI conditions (e.g., gastroesophageal reflux disease [GERD], gastric ulcers). Avoid in pts who have GI motility issues or suspected strictures (e.g., Crohn disease).

C, Capsules; *ER,* extended-release; *I,* injection; *SQ,* subcutaneous; *T,* tablet.

abacavir/ dolutegravir/ lamivudine

a-**bak**-a-veer/**doe**-loo-**teg**-ra-vir/la-**miv**-yoo-deen
(Triumeq, Triumeq PD)

■ **BLACK BOX ALERT** ■ Serious, sometimes fatal hypersensitivity reactions, lactic acidosis, severe hepatomegaly with steatosis (fatty liver) have occurred with abacavir-containing products, esp. in pts who carry the HLA-B*5701 allele. Restarting abacavir following a hypersensitivity reaction may be life-threatening. May cause hepatitis B virus reactivation.
Do not confuse abacavir with entecavir, or dolutegravir with elvitegravir or raltegravir, or lamivudine with telbivudine or lamotrigine.

FIXED-COMBINATION(S)

abacavir/dolutegravir/lamivudine (antiretrovirals): **Tablet:** 600 mg/50 mg/300 mg. **Tablet for Oral Suspension:** 60 mg/5 mg/30 mg.

◆CLASSIFICATION

PHARMACOTHERAPEUTIC: Integrase inhibitor (INSTI), reverse transcriptase inhibitor, nucleoside. **CLINICAL:** Antiretroviral.

USES

Treatment of HIV-1 infection in adults and children at least 3 mos of age and weighing at least 6 kg.

PRECAUTIONS

Contraindications: Hypersensitivity to abacavir, dolutegravir, lamivudine. Pts who test positive for the HLA-B*5701 allele. Concomitant use of dofetilide. Pts with moderate to severe hepatic impairment. **Cautions:** Diabetes, hepatic/renal impairment, coronary artery disease, history of hepatitis or tuberculosis, prior hypersensitivity reaction to INSTIs. Use in children with history of pancreatitis or risk factors for developing pancreatitis. Not recommended in pts with resistance-associated integrase substitutions or clinically suspected integrase strand transfer inhibitor resistance; creatinine clearance less than 50 mL/min; mild hepatic impairment; children weighing less than 40 kg.

ACTION

Abacavir inhibits activity of HIV-1 reverse transcriptase. Dolutegravir inhibits HIV integrase by blocking strand transfer step of retroviral DNA integration (essential for HIV replication cycle). Lamivudine inhibits reverse transcriptase by viral DNA chain termination. **Therapeutic Effect:** Interferes with HIV replication, slowing progression of HIV infection.

PHARMACOKINETICS

Abacavir, lamivudine rapidly absorbed and widely distributed. Abacavir distributes into cerebrospinal fluid (CSF) and erythrocytes. Abacavir metabolized by alcohol dehydrogenase and glucuronyl transferase. Dolutegravir metabolized in liver. Protein binding: abacavir: 50%; dolutegravir: 98.9%; lamivudine: less than 36%. Peak plasma concentration: dolutegravir: 2–3 hrs. Excretion: abacavir: urine (primary); dolutegravir: feces (53%), urine (31%); lamivudine: urine (70%). **Half-life:** abacavir: 1.5 hrs; dolutegravir: 14 hrs; lamivudine: 5–7 hrs.

⌛ LIFESPAN CONSIDERATIONS

Pregnancy/Lactation: Breastfeeding not recommended due to risk of postnatal HIV transmission. Unknown if distributed in breast milk. **Children:** Safety and efficacy not established in pts weighing less than 10 kg. **Elderly:** May have increased risk of adverse effects; worsening of hepatic, renal, cardiac function.

INTERACTIONS

DRUG: Dolutegravir may increase concentration/effect of **dofetilide** (contraindicated). **Fosphenytoin, phenytoin, nevirapine, oxcarbazepine,**

phenobarbital, primidone may decrease concentration of dolutegravir. **HERBAL: St. John's wort** may decrease effect of dolutegravir. **FOOD:** None known. **LAB VALUES:** May increase serum amylase, ALT, AST, bilirubin, cholesterol, creatine kinase (CK), creatinine, glucose, lipase, triglycerides. May decrease Hgb, Hct, neutrophils.

AVAILABILITY (Rx)

Fixed-Dose Combination Tablet: abacavir 600 mg/dolutegravir 50 mg/lamivudine 300 mg. **Fixed-Dose Combination Tablet for Oral Suspension:** abacavir 60 mg/dolutegravir 5 mg/lamivudine 30 mg.

ADMINISTRATION/HANDLING

PO
• Give without regard to food. Administer tablet whole; do not break, cut, or crush. Tablets cannot be chewed. • Administer at least 2 hrs before or at least 6 hrs after giving medications containing aluminum, calcium, iron, magnesium, sucralfate, (supplements, antacids, laxatives). • Fully disperse tablets for oral suspension in 20 mL of water. Swirl suspension until no lumps remain. Give within 30 min of mixing.

INDICATIONS/ROUTES/DOSAGE

HIV Infection
PO: ADULTS, ELDERLY, CHILDREN WEIGHING 25 KG OR MORE: 1 tablet once daily. **20–24 KG:** 6 tablets for oral suspension once daily. **14–19 KG:** 5 tablets for oral suspension once daily. **10–13 KG:** 4 tablets for oral suspension once daily. **6–9 KG:** 3 tablets for oral suspension once daily.

Dosage in Renal Impairment
Creatinine clearance less than 50 mL/ min: Not recommended.

Dosage in Hepatic Impairment
Mild impairment: Consider use of individual components. **Moderate to severe impairment:** Contraindicated.

SIDE EFFECTS

Rare (3%–1%): Insomnia, fatigue, headache, abdominal pain/distension, dyspep-

sia, flatulence, gastroesophageal reflux disease, fever, lethargy, anorexia, arthralgia, myositis, somnolence, pruritus, depression, abnormal dreams, dizziness, nausea, diarrhea, rash.

ADVERSE EFFECTS/ TOXIC REACTIONS

Serious and sometimes fatal hypersensitivity reactions including anaphylaxis, severe diarrhea, dyspnea, hypotension, intractable nausea/vomiting, multi-organ failure, pharyngitis may occur within the first 6 wks of treatment with abacavir (8% of pts). If therapy is discontinued, pts coinfected with hepatitis B or C virus have an increased risk for viral replication, worsening of hepatic function, and may experience hepatic decompensation and/ or failure. May induce immune recovery syndrome (inflammatory response to dormant opportunistic infections such as *Mycobacterium avium*, cytomegalovirus, PCP, tuberculosis, or acceleration of autoimmune disorders such as Graves' disease, polymyositis, Guillain-Barré). Fatal cases of lactic acidosis, severe hepatomegaly with steatosis have been reported. Hepatic failure occurred in 1% of pts taking dolutegravir-containing products. Abacavir-containing products may increase risk of myocardial infarction, erythema multiform, Stevens-Johnson syndrome, toxic epidermal necrolysis. May increase risk of pancreatitis.

NURSING CONSIDERATIONS

BASELINE ASSESSMENT

Obtain CBC, BMP, LFT, CD4+ count, viral load, HIV-1 RNA level. Obtain weight in kilograms. Screen for HLA-B* 5701 allele, hepatitis B or C virus infection before initiating therapy. Question for prior hypersensitivity reactions (especially to abacavir-containing products); history of diabetes, coronary artery disease, hepatic/renal impairment. Receive full medication history, including herbal products. Offer emotional support.

INTERVENTION/EVALUATION

Monitor CBC, BMP, LFT periodically. Immediately discontinue if hypersensitivity reaction is suspected, even when other diagnoses are possible (e.g., pneumonia, bronchitis, pharyngitis, influenza, gastroenteritis, reactions to other medications). Stop treatment if 3 or more of the following symptoms occur: Rash, fever, GI disturbances (diarrhea, nausea, vomiting), flu-like symptoms, respiratory distress. Assess for hepatic impairment (bruising, hematuria, jaundice, right upper abdominal pain, nausea, vomiting, weight loss). Screen for immune recovery syndrome, rhabdomyolysis (muscle weakness, myalgia, decreased urinary output). Pediatric pts should be closely monitored for symptoms of pancreatitis (severe, steady abdominal pain often radiating to the back; clammy skin, reduced B/P; nausea and vomiting accompanied by abdominal pain). Monitor daily stool pattern, consistency; I&Os. Screen for toxic skin reactions. Monitor for symptoms of MI (jaw/chest/left arm pain or pressure, dyspnea, diaphoresis, vomiting).

PATIENT/FAMILY TEACHING

• Treatment does not cure HIV infection nor reduce risk of transmission. Practice safe sex with barrier methods or abstinence. • As immune system strengthens, it may respond to dormant infections hidden within the body. Report any new fever, chills, body aches, cough, night sweats, shortness of breath. • Antiretrovirals may cause excess body fat in upper back, neck, breast, trunk; may cause decreased body fat in legs, arms, face. • Drug resistance can form if therapy is interrupted for even a short time; do not run out of supply. • Report signs of abdominal pain, darkened urine, decreased urine output, yellowing of skin or eyes, clay colored stools, weight loss. • Do not breastfeed. • Small, frequent meals may offset anorexia, nausea. • Do not take newly prescribed medications, including OTC drugs, unless approved by doctor who originally started treatment.

abaloparatide

a-**bal**-oh-**par**-a-tide
(Tymlos)

■ **BLACK BOX ALERT** ■ May cause a dose-dependent increase in the incidence of osteosarcoma. It is unknown whether abaloparatide will cause osteosarcoma in humans. Avoid use in pts at risk for osteosarcoma (e.g., pts with Paget's disease of bone or unexplained elevations of alkaline phosphatase, pediatric and young adults with open epiphyses, pts with bone metastasis or skeletal malignancies, hereditary disorders predisposing to osteosarcoma, or prior history of external beam or implant radiation involving the skeleton. Cumulative use of parathyroid analogs (e.g., teriparatide) for more than 2 yrs during a pt's lifetime is not recommended. **Do not confuse abaloparatide with teriparatide.**

◆CLASSIFICATION

PHARMACOTHERAPEUTIC: Parathyroid hormone receptor analog. **CLINICAL:** Osteoporosis agent.

USES

Treatment of postmenopausal women with osteoporosis at high risk for fracture, or who have failed or are intolerant to other osteoporosis therapy. Treatment to increase bone density in men with osteoporosis at high risk for fracture or who have failed or are intolerant of other osteoporosis therapy.

PRECAUTIONS

Contraindications: Hypersensitivity to abaloparatide. **Cautions:** Pts at risk for hypercalcemia (e.g., hyperparathyroidism, renal impairment, severe dehydration; history of hypercalciuria, urolithiasis). Avoid use in pts at increased risk for osteosarcoma (e.g., pts with Paget's disease of bone or unexplained elevations of alkaline phosphatase, open epiphyses, bone or skeletal malignancies, hereditary disorders predisposing

---

to osteosarcoma, prior radiation therapy involving the skeleton). Not recommended in pts with cumulative use of parathyroid analogs greater than 2 yrs during lifetime.

ACTION

Acts as an agonist at the parathyroid hormone (PTH) 1 receptor. **Therapeutic Effect:** Stimulates osteoblast function and increases bone mass, decreasing risk of fractures.

PHARMACOKINETICS

Widely distributed. Metabolism not specified. Degraded into small peptides via proteolytic enzymes. Protein binding: 70%. Peak plasma concentration: 0.51 hrs. Excreted primarily in urine. Not expected to be removed by dialysis. **Half-life:** 1.7 hrs.

⧗ LIFESPAN CONSIDERATIONS

Pregnancy/Lactation: Not indicated in females of reproductive potential. Unknown if distributed in breast milk or crosses the placenta. **Children:** Safety and efficacy not established. **Elderly:** No age-related precautions noted.

INTERACTIONS

DRUG: None known. **HERBAL:** None significant. **FOOD:** None known. **LAB VALUES:** May increase serum calcium, uric acid; urine calcium.

AVAILABILITY (Rx)

Prefilled Injector Pens: 3,120 mcg/1.56 mL (2,000 mcg/mL). Delivers 30 doses of 80 mcg.

ADMINISTRATION/HANDLING

SQ

• Visually inspect for particulate matter or discoloration. Solution should appear clear, colorless. • Do not use if solution is cloudy, discolored, or if visible particles are observed. • Insert needle subcutaneously into the periumbilical region of the abdomen (avoid a 2-inch area around the navel) and inject solution. • Do not inject into areas of active skin disease or injury such as sunburns, skin rashes,

inflammation, skin infections, or active psoriasis. • Do not administer IV or intramuscularly. • Rotate injection sites. **Storage** • Refrigerate unused injector pens. • After first use, store at room temperature for up to 30 days. • Do not freeze or expose to heating sources.

INDICATIONS/ROUTES/DOSAGE

Osteoporosis

SQ: ADULTS, ELDERLY: 80 mcg once daily. Give with supplemental calcium and vitamin D if dietary intake is inadequate.

Dosage in Renal Impairment

No dose adjustment.

Dosage in Hepatic Impairment

Not specified; use caution.

SIDE EFFECTS

Frequent (58%): Injection site reactions (edema, pain, redness). **Occasional (10%–5%):** Dizziness, nausea, headache, palpitations. **Rare (3%–2%):** Fatigue, upper abdominal pain, vertigo.

ADVERSE EFFECTS/TOXIC REACTIONS

May increase risk of osteosarcoma. Hypercalcemia reported in 3% of pts. Tachycardia occurred in 2% of pts (usually within 15 min after injection). Orthostatic hypotension reported in 4% of pts (usually within 4 hrs after injection). Hypercalciuria and urolithiasis reported in 20% and 2% of pts, respectively.

NURSING CONSIDERATIONS

BASELINE ASSESSMENT

Obtain PTH level. Screen for risk of osteosarcoma, hypercalcemia (as listed in Precautions); prior use of parathyroid analogs. Assess pt's willingness to self-inject medication.

INTERVENTION/EVALUATION

Monitor bone mineral density, parathyroid hormone level; serum calcium. Monitor urinary calcium levels, esp. in pts with preexisting hypercalciuria or active urolithiasis. Due to risk of orthostatic hypotension, administer the first several doses with the pt in the lying or sitting position. Monitor for orthostatic hypotension (dizziness, palpitations, tachycardia, nausea, syncope). If orthostatic hypotension occurs, place pt in supine position. Assess need for calcium, vitamin D supplementation.

PATIENT/FAMILY TEACHING

• Receive the first several injections while lying or sitting down. Slowly go from lying to standing to avoid an unusual drop in blood pressure. Immediately sit or lie down if dizziness, near-fainting, palpitations occur. • Report symptoms of high calcium levels (e.g., constipation, lethargy, nausea, vomiting, weakness); severe bone pain. • An increased heart rate may occur after injection and will usually subside within 6 hrs. • A healthcare provider will show you how to properly prepare and inject your medication. You must demonstrate correct preparation and injection techniques before using medication at home. • Vitamin D and calcium supplementation may be required if dietary intake is inadequate.

---

abatacept

a-**bay**-ta-sept
(Orencia, Orencia ClickJect)
Do not confuse Orencia with Orencia ClickJect

◆CLASSIFICATION

PHARMACOTHERAPEUTIC: Selective T-cell co-stimulation modulator. **CLINICAL:** Antirheumatic: Disease modifying.

USES

Rheumatoid arthritis: Treatment of adults with active moderate to severe RA alone or with disease-modifying antirheumatic drugs (DMARDs) other than JAK inhibitors or biologic DMARDs (e.g., TNF antagonists). **Psoriatic arthritis (PsA):** Treatment of active PsA in adults and pts 2 yrs and older. **Polyarticular juvenile idiopathic arthritis:** Treatment of moderate to severe active pJIA in pts 2 yrs and older (SQ) and 6 yrs and older (IV). **Acute graft versus host disease (aGVHD):** Prophylaxis of aGVHD, in combination with a calcineurin inhibitor and methotrexate, in adults and pts 2 yrs of age and older undergoing hematopoietic stem cell transplantation (HSCT). **Note:** Do not use with anakinra or tumor necrosis factor [TNF] antagonists.

PRECAUTIONS

Contraindications: Hypersensitivity to abatacept. **Cautions:** Chronic, latent, or localized infection; conditions predisposing to infections (diabetes, indwelling catheters, renal failure, open wounds); COPD (higher incidence of adverse effects); elderly, hx recurrent infections.

ACTION

Inhibits T-cell (T-lymphocyte) activation (binds to CD80 and CD86 on antigen-presenting cells (APCs); blocks CD28 interaction between APCs and T cells). Activated T cells are found in synovium of rheumatoid arthritic patients. **Therapeutic Effect:** Induces positive clinical response in adult pts with moderate to severely active RA or juvenile idiopathic arthritis.

PHARMACOKINETICS

Higher clearance with increasing body weight. Age, gender do not affect clearance. **Half-life:** 8–25 days.

⧗ LIFESPAN CONSIDERATIONS

Pregnancy/Lactation: Crosses placenta; unknown if distributed in breast milk. **Children:** Safety and efficacy not established in pts younger than 6 yrs. **Elderly:** May have increased risk of serious infection and malignancy.

 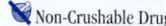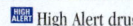

INTERACTIONS

DRUG: Anti-TNF agents, baricitinib, pimecrolimus, tacrolimus (topical), may increase adverse effects. May decrease therapeutic effect of **BCG (intravesical), vaccines (live).** May increase concentration/effects of **tofacitinib, vaccines (live). HERBAL: Echinacea** may decrease concentration/effect. **FOOD:** None known. **LAB VALUES:** None significant.

AVAILABILITY (Rx)

IV Injection, Powder for Reconstitution: 250 mg. **SQ Injection, Solution:** 50 mg/0.4 mL, 87.5 mg/0.7 mL, 125 mg/mL single-dose prefilled syringe. **Autoinjector, Solution (ClickJect):** 125 mg/mL.

ADMINISTRATION/HANDLING

 IV

Reconstitution • Reconstitute each vial with 10 mL Sterile Water for Injection using the silicone-free syringe provided with each vial and an 18- to 21-gauge needle. • Rotate solution gently to prevent foaming until powder is completely dissolved. • From a 100-mL 0.9% NaCl infusion bag, withdraw and discard an amount equal to the volume of the reconstituted vials (for 2 vials remove 20 mL, for 3 vials remove 30 mL, for 4 vials remove 40 mL), resulting in final volume of 100 mL. • Slowly add the reconstituted solution from each vial into the infusion bag using the same syringe provided with each vial. • Concentration in the infusion bag will be 10 mg/mL or less abatacept.
Rate of administration • Infuse over 30 min (60 min for aGVHD prophylaxis) using a 0.2 to 1.2 micron low protein-binding filter.
Storage • Store vials, prefilled syringes in refrigerator. • Any reconstitution that has been prepared by using siliconized syringes will develop translucent particles and must be discarded. • Solution should appear clear and colorless to pale yellow. Discard if solution is discolored or contains precipitate. • Solution is stable for up to

24 hrs after reconstitution. • Reconstituted solution may be stored at room temperature or refrigerated.

SQ
• Allow syringe to warm to room temperature (30–60 min). • Inject in front of thigh, outer areas of upper arms, or abdomen. • Avoid areas that are tender, bruised, red, scaly, or hard. • Do not rub injection site. • Rotate injection sites.

✳ IV INCOMPATIBILITIES

Do not infuse concurrently in same IV line as other agents.

INDICATIONS/ROUTES/DOSAGE

Note: Discontinue in pts developing serious infection.

Rheumatoid Arthritis (RA)
IV: ADULTS, ELDERLY WEIGHING 101 KG OR MORE: 1 g (4 vials) given as a 30-min infusion. Following initial therapy, give at 2 wks and 4 wks after first infusion, then q4wks thereafter. **WEIGHING 60–100 KG:** 750 mg (3 vials) given as a 30-min infusion. Following initial therapy, give at 2 wks and 4 wks after first infusion, then q4wks thereafter. **WEIGHING 59 KG OR LESS:** 500 mg (2 vials) given as a 30-min infusion. Following initial therapy, give at 2 wks and 4 wks after first infusion, then q4wks thereafter.
SQ: (RA): Following a single IV infusion, 125 mg given within 24 hrs of infusion, then 125 mg once a week (SQ administration may be initiated without an IV loading dose). **(PsA):** Give without an IV loading dose. 125 mg once weekly. **Transitioning from IV to SQ:** Give 1st SQ dose instead of next scheduled IV dose.

Psoriatic Arthritis (PsA)
IV: ADULTS, ELDERLY WEIGHING 101 KG OR MORE: 1 g (4 vials) given as a 30-min infusion. Following initial therapy, give at 2 wks and 4 wks after first infusion, then q4wks thereafter. **WEIGHING 60–100 KG:** 750 mg (3 vials) given as a 30-min infusion. Following initial therapy, give at 2 wks and 4 wks after first infusion, then q4wks thereafter. **WEIGHING 59 KG OR LESS:** 500 mg (2 vials) given as a 30-min infusion.

Following initial therapy, give at 2 wks and 4 wks after first infusion, then q4wks thereafter. **SQ: ADULTS, ELDERLY, CHILDREN 2 YRS AND OLDER, ADOLESCENTS WEIGHING 50 KG OR MORE:** 125 mg once weekly. **WEIGHING 25–49 KG:** 87.5 mg once weekly. **WEIGHING 10–24 KG:** 50 mg once weekly.

Juvenile Idiopathic Arthritis
Note: Dose based on body weight at each administration.
IV: CHILDREN 6 YRS AND OLDER, WEIGHING LESS THAN 75 KG: 10 mg/kg. **CHILDREN WEIGHING 75–100 KG:** 750 mg. **WEIGHING MORE THAN 100 KG:** 1,000 mg. Following initial therapy, give 2 wks and 4 wks after first infusion, then q4wks thereafter.
SQ: CHILDREN 2 YRS AND OLDER, ADOLESCENTS WEIGHING 50 KG OR MORE: 125 mg once weekly. **WEIGHING 25–49 KG:** 87.5 mg once weekly. **WEIGHING 10–24 KG:** 50 mg once weekly.

aGVHD
IV: ADULTS, CHILDREN 6 YRS AND OLDER: 10 mg/kg (maximum: 1,000 mg) on day before transplant, then on days 5, 14, and 28 after transplant. **CHILDREN 2–5 YRS:** 15 mg/kg on day before transplant, then 12 mg/kg on days 5, 14, and 28 after transplant.

Dosage Adjustment for Toxicity
Discontinue in pts developing a serious infection.

Dosage in Renal/Hepatic Impairment
No dose adjustment.

SIDE EFFECTS

Frequent (18%): Headache. **Occasional (9%–6%):** Dizziness, cough, back pain, hypertension, nausea.

ADVERSE EFFECTS/TOXIC REACTIONS

Upper respiratory tract infection, nasopharyngitis, sinusitis, UTI, influenza, bronchitis occur in 5% of pts. Serious infections, including pneumonia, cellulitis, diverticulitis, acute pyelonephritis, occur in 3% of pts. Life-threatening hypersensitivity reactions including anphylaxis, angioedema were reported.

Other reactions, including hypotension, rash, urticaria, may occur. May cause exacerbation of COPD (cough, dyspnea, wheezing). May increase risk of malignancies.

NURSING CONSIDERATIONS

BASELINE ASSESSMENT
Assess onset, type, location, duration of pain/inflammation. Inspect appearance of affected joint for immobility, deformities, skin condition. Screen for latent TB infection prior to initiating therapy.

INTERVENTION/EVALUATION
Assess for therapeutic response: Relief of pain, stiffness, swelling; increased joint mobility; reduced joint tenderness; improved grip strength. Monitor for hypersensitivity reaction. Diligently screen for infection.

PATIENT/FAMILY TEACHING
• Notify physician if infection, hypersensitivity reaction, infusion-related reaction occurs. • Do not receive live vaccines during treatment or within 3 mos of its discontinuation. • COPD pts must report worsening of respiratory symptoms.

abemaciclib

a-**bem**-a-**sye**-klib
(Verzenio)
Do not confuse abemaciclib with palbociclib or ribociclib.

◆CLASSIFICATION

PHARMACOTHERAPEUTIC: Cyclin-dependent kinase inhibitor. **CLINICAL:** Antineoplastic.

USES

Advanced or metastatic breast cancer: Used in combination with an aromatase inhibitor as initial endocrine-based therapy for treatment of adults with hormone receptor (HR)-positive, human epidermal growth factor receptor 2 (HER2)-negative advanced or metastatic breast cancer. Used

 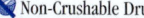

in combination with fulvestrant for treatment of adults with HR-positive, HER2-negative advanced or metastatic breast cancer with disease progression following endocrine therapy. Used as monotherapy for treatment of adults with HR-positive, HER2-negative advanced or metastatic breast cancer with disease progression following endocrine therapy and prior chemotherapy in the metastatic setting. **Early breast cancer:** Used in combination with endocrine therapy (tamoxifen or an aromatase inhibitor) for adjuvant treatment of adults with hormone receptor (HR)-positive, human epidermal growth factor receptor 2 (HER2)-negative, node-positive, early breast cancer at high risk of recurrence.

PRECAUTIONS

Contraindications: Hypersensitivity to abemaciclib. **Cautions:** Baseline cytopenias; hepatic/renal impairment, conditions predisposing to infection (e.g., diabetes, immunocompromised pts, open wounds), history of venous thromboembolism. Avoid concomitant use of strong CYP3A inhibitors, strong CYP3A inducers.

ACTION

Blocks retinoblastoma tumor suppressor protein phosphorylation and prevents progression through cell cycle, resulting in arrest of G1 phase. **Therapeutic Effect:** Inhibits tumor cell growth and decreases tumor size.

PHARMACOKINETICS

Widely distributed. Metabolized in liver. Protein binding: 96.3%. Peak plasma concentration: 8 hrs. Steady-state reached in 5 days. Excreted in feces (81%), urine (3%). **Half-life:** 18.3 hrs.

⌛ LIFESPAN CONSIDERATIONS

Pregnancy/Lactation: Avoid pregnancy; may cause fetal harm/malformations. Females of reproductive potential should use effective contraception during treatment and up to 3 wks after discontinuation. Unknown if distributed in breast milk. Breastfeeding not recommended during treatment and up to 3 wks after discontinuation. May

impair fertility in males. **Children:** Safety and efficacy not established. **Elderly:** No age-related precautions noted.

INTERACTIONS

DRUG: **Strong CYP3A4 inducers (e.g., carbamazepine, phenytoin, rifampin), moderate CYP3A4 inducers (e.g., dexamethasone, modafinil, nafcillin)** may decrease concentration/effect. May decrease effect of **BCG (intravesical), vaccines (live).** May enhance adverse/toxic effects of **natalizumab, vaccines (live). Pimecrolimus, tacrolimus** may enhance adverse/toxic effects. **HERBAL:** **Echinacea** may decrease therapeutic effect. **St. Johns wort** may decrease concentration/effect. **FOOD: Grapefruit products** may increase concentration/effect. **LAB VALUES:** May increase serum ALT, AST, bilirubin, creatinine. May decrease ANC, Hgb, Hct, lymphocytes, leukocytes, neutrophils, platelets.

AVAILABILITY (Rx)

Tablets: 50 mg, 100 mg, 150 mg, 200 mg.

ADMINISTRATION/HANDLING

PO
• Give without regard to food. • Administer whole; do not crush, cut, or divide tablets. Do not give broken or cracked tablets. • If a dose is missed or vomiting occurs, do not give extra dose. Administer next dose at regularly scheduled time.

INDICATIONS/ROUTES/DOSAGE

Breast Cancer (Advanced or Metastatic)

PO: ADULTS, ELDERLY: Monotherapy: 200 mg twice daily. **In combination with fulvestrant (and a gonadotropin-releasing hormone agonist if pre- or perimenopausal) or an aromatase inhibitor:** 150 mg twice daily. Continue until disease progression or unacceptable toxicity. Recommended dose of fulvestrant is 500 mg once on days 1, 15, 29, then monthly thereafter.

Early Breast Cancer (Adjuvant Therapy)

PO: ADULTS, ELDERLY: 150 mg twice daily (in combination with endocrine therapy [e.g., an aromatase inhibitor or tamoxifen]). Continue until completion of 2 yrs of treatment or until disease recurrence or unacceptable toxicity.

Dose Reduction for Adverse Events

Monotherapy: Starting dose: 200 mg twice daily. **FIRST DOSE REDUCTION:** 150 mg twice daily. **SECOND DOSE REDUCTION:** 100 mg twice daily. **THIRD DOSE REDUCTION:** 50 mg twice daily. **In combination with fulvestrant or an aromatase inhibitor: STARTING DOSE:** 150 mg twice daily. **FIRST DOSE REDUCTION:** 100 mg twice daily. **SECOND DOSE REDUCTION:** 50 mg twice daily.

Dose Modification

Based on Common Terminology Criteria for Adverse Events (CTCAE).

Diarrhea
Note: At first sign of loose stools, recommend treatment with antidiarrheal agents and hydration.
Grade 1 diarrhea: No dose adjustment. **Grade 2 diarrhea:** If toxicity does not resolve to Grade 1 or less within 24 hrs, withhold treatment until resolved. Then resume at same dose level. **Recurrent or persistent Grade 2 diarrhea at same dose level despite supportive measures:** Withhold treatment until recovery to Grade 1 or less, then resume at reduced dose level. **Grade 3 or 4 diarrhea or required hospitalization:** Withhold treatment until recovery to Grade 1 or less, then resume at reduced dose level.

Hematologic Toxicity
Grade 1 or 2 hematologic toxicity: No dose adjustment. **Grade 3 hematologic toxicity:** Withhold treatment until recovery to Grade 2 or less, then resume at same dose level. **Grade 3 (recurrent) or Grade 4 hematologic toxicity:** Withhold treatment until recovery to Grade 2 or less, then resume at reduced dose level.

Hepatotoxicity
Grade 1 or 2 hepatotoxicity without serum bilirubin elevation greater than 2 times ULN: No dose adjustment. **Recurrent or persistent Grade 2 hepa-**totoxicity; **Grade 3 hepatotoxicity without serum bilirubin elevation greater than 2 times ULN:** Withhold treatment until recovery to Grade 1 or less, then resume at reduced dose level. **Serum ALT, AST elevation greater than 3 times ULN with serum bilirubin elevation greater than 2 times ULN (in the absence of cholestasis); Grade 4 hepatotoxicity:** Permanently discontinue.

Other Toxicities
Any other Grade 1 or 2 toxicities: No dose adjustment. **Recurrent or persistent Grade 2 toxicity that does not resolve to Grade 1 (or baseline) within 7 days despite supportive measures:** Withhold treatment until recovery to Grade 1 or less, then resume at reduced dose level. **Any other Grade 3 or 4 toxicities:** Withhold treatment until resolved to Grade 1 or less, then resume at reduced dose level.

Concomitant Use of Strong CYP3A Inhibitors
If strong CYP3A inhibitor cannot be discontinued, reduce initial dose to 100 mg twice daily if pt taking 200 mg or 150 mg twice daily regimen. If dose was already reduced to 100 mg twice daily due to adverse effects, reduce dose to 50 mg twice daily. If CYP3A inhibitor is discontinued, increase dose (after 3–5 half-lives of CYP3A inhibitor have elapsed) to the dose used prior to initiating strong CYP3A inhibitor.

Dosage in Renal Impairment

Mild to moderate impairment: No dose adjustment. **Severe impairment, ESRD:** Not specified.

Dosage in Hepatic Impairment

Mild to moderate impairment: No dose adjustment. **Severe impairment:** Reduce dose frequency to once daily.

SIDE EFFECTS

Note: Side effects may vary if pt treated concomitantly with an aromatase inhibitor. **Frequent (90%–35%):** Diarrhea, fatigue, asthenia, nausea, decreased appetite, ab-

---

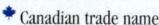 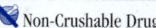

dominal pain, vomiting. **Occasional (20%–10%):** Headache, cough, constipation, arthralgia, dry mouth, decreased weight, stomatitis, dysgeusia, alopecia, dizziness, pyrexia, dehydration.

ADVERSE EFFECTS/TOXIC REACTIONS

Myelosuppression (anemia, leukopenia, neutropenia, thrombocytopenia) is an expected response to therapy. Diarrhea occurred in 81%–90% of pts. Grade 3 diarrhea occurred in 9%–20% of pts. Diarrhea may increase risk of dehydration and infection. Neutropenia reported in 37%–41% of pts. Grade 3 or 4 hepatotoxicity occurred in up to 4% of pts. Venous thromboembolism including cerebral venous thrombosis, subclavian and axillary vein thrombosis, inferior vena cava thrombosis, DVT, PE, pelvic venous thrombosis reported in 5% of pts taking concomitant aromatase inhibitor therapy. Infections including upper respiratory infection, UTI, pulmonary infection occurred in 39% of pts taking concomitant aromatase inhibitor therapy.

NURSING CONSIDERATIONS

BASELINE ASSESSMENT

Obtain ANC, CBC, BMP, LFT; pregnancy test in females of reproductive potential. Confirm HR-positive, HER2-negative status. Stress importance of antidiarrheal if diarrhea occurs. Question history of hepatic impairment, venous thromboembolism. Question usual bowel movement patterns, stool characteristics. Receive full medication history and screen for interactions. Screen for active infection. Assess hydration status. Offer emotional support.

INTERVENTION/EVALUATION

Monitor CBC for myelosuppression; LFT for hepatotoxicity q2wks for first 2 mos, then monthly for 2 mos, then as clinically indicated. Monitor for hepatotoxicity (abdominal pain, ascites, confusion, dark-colored urine, jaundice). Monitor daily pattern of bowel activity, stool consistency. Ensure compliance of antidiarrheal therapy if diarrhea occurs. If treatment-related toxicities occur, consider referral to specialist. Be alert for serious infection, opportunistic infection, sepsis. Monitor for venous thromboembolism (arm/leg pain, swelling; chest pain, dyspnea, hypoxia, tachycardia). Ensure adequate hydration, nutrition. Monitor weight, I&Os.

PATIENT/FAMILY TEACHING

• Treatment may depress your immune system and reduce your ability to fight infection. Report symptoms of infection such as body aches, burning with urination, chills, cough, fatigue, fever. Avoid those with active infection. • Report symptoms of bone marrow depression such as bruising, fatigue, fever, shortness of breath, weight loss; bleeding easily, bloody urine or stool. • Therapy may cause severe diarrhea, which may lead to dehydration and infection. Drink plenty of fluids. Take antidiarrheal medication as prescribed at the first sign of loose stools. • Use effective contraception to avoid pregnancy. Do not breastfeed. • Report symptoms of DVT (swelling, pain, hot feeling in the arms or legs), lung embolism (difficulty breathing, chest pain, rapid heart rate); liver problems (bruising, contusion; amber, dark, orange-colored urine; right upper abdominal pain, yellowing of the skin or eyes). • Do not take newly prescribed medications unless approved by the prescriber who originally started treatment. • Do not ingest grapefruit products.

abiraterone

a-bir-**a**-ter-one
(Yonsa, Zytiga)
Do not confuse Zytiga with Zetia or ZyrTEC.

◆CLASSIFICATION

PHARMACOTHERAPEUTIC: Antiandrogen. **CLINICAL:** Antineoplastic.

USES

Treatment of metastatic castration-resistant prostate cancer in combination with prednisone *(Zytiga)* or methylprednisolone *(Yousa)*. Zytiga: Treatment of metastatic, high-risk castration-sensitive prostate cancer (in combination with prednisone).

PRECAUTIONS

Contraindications: Hypersensitivity to abiraterone. Use in women who are pregnant or may become pregnant. **Cautions:** History of cardiovascular disease (especially HF, recent MI, or ventricular arrhythmia) due to potential for hypertension, hypokalemia, fluid retention; moderate hepatic impairment; adrenal insufficiency. Avoid use with strong CYP3A4 inducers.

ACTION

Selectively and irreversibly inhibits CYP17, an enzyme needed for androgen biosynthesis (expressed in testicular, adrenal, or prostatic tumor tissue). Inhibits formation of testosterone precursors DHEA and androstenedione. **Therapeutic Effect:** Lowers serum testosterone to castrate levels.

PHARMACOKINETICS

Widely distributed. Protein binding: 99%. Primarily excreted in feces. Peak plasma concentration: 2 hrs. **Half-life:** 12 hrs (up to 19 hrs with hepatic impairment).

⏳ LIFESPAN CONSIDERATIONS

Pregnancy/Lactation: Contraindicated in women who are or may become pregnant. **Children:** Safety and efficacy not established. **Elderly:** No age-related precautions noted.

INTERACTIONS

DRUG: May increase concentration/effects of **doxorubicin** (conventional), **thioridazine.** May decrease concentration/effect of **tamoxifen. Strong CYP3A4 Inducers (e.g., car-**bamazepine, phenytoin, rifampin), **dabrafenib, enzalutamide, lorlatinib** may decrease concentration/effect. **HERBAL:** None significant. **FOOD:** Do not give with **food** (no **food** should be consumed for at least 2 hrs before or 1 hr after dose). **LAB VALUES:** May increase serum ALT, AST, bilirubin, triglycerides. May decrease serum potassium, phosphate.

AVAILABILITY (Rx)

🔖 **Tablets:** *(Yonsa):* 125 mg. *(Zytiga):* 250 mg, 500 mg.

ADMINISTRATION/HANDLING

PO
• *(Yonsa):* May give without regard to food. • Do not break, crush, dissolve, or divide tablets. Give whole with water. • *(Zytiga):* Give on empty stomach only (at least 1 hr before or 2 hrs after food). • Give with water. • Administer whole. Do not break, crush, dissolve, or divide tablets. Women who are or may become pregnant should wear gloves if handling the tablets.

INDICATIONS/ROUTES/DOSAGE

◀**ALERT**▶ Consider increased dosage of predniSONE during unusual stress or infection. Interrupting predniSONE therapy may induce adrenocorticoid insufficiency. **Note:** Pts should also receive a gonadotropin-releasing hormone (GnRH) analog concurrently or should have had bilateral orchiectomy.

Metastatic Castration-Resistant Prostate Cancer
PO: ADULTS, ELDERLY: *(Yonsa):* 500 mg once daily (with methylPREDNISolone 4 mg 2 times/day). *(Zytiga):* 1,000 mg once daily (with predniSONE 5 mg 2 times/day).

Metastatic Castration-Sensitive Prostate Cancer
PO: ADULTS, ELDERLY: *(Zytiga):* 1,000 mg once daily (with prednisone 5 mg once daily).

Dosage Modification

Hepatic Enzymes Greater Than Upper Limit of Normal (ULN) (During Treatment)

Lab Values	Recommendation
ALT, AST elevations greater than 5 × ULN or bilirubin greater than 3 × ULN with 1,000 mg	Interrupt treatment and restart at 750 mg once ALT, AST less than 2.5 × ULN or bilirubin less than 1.5 × ULN.
ALT, AST elevations greater than 5 × ULN or bilirubin greater than 3 × ULN with 750 mg	Interrupt treatment and restart at 500 mg once ALT, AST less than 2.5 × ULN or bilirubin less than 1.5 × ULN.

If hepatotoxicity occurs at reduced dose of 500 mg daily, discontinue treatment.

Dosage Adjustment for Concomitant Strong CYP3A4 Inducers
Increase abiraterone dose to 1,000 mg twice daily.

Dosage in Renal Impairment
No dose adjustment.

Dosage in Hepatic Impairment
Mild impairment: No dosage adjustment necessary. **Moderate impairment:** Reduce dose to 250 mg daily. Discontinue if serum ALT, AST greater than 5 times ULN or serum bilirubin greater than 3 times ULN. **Severe impairment:** Avoid use.

SIDE EFFECTS
Frequent (30%–26%): Joint swelling/discomfort, peripheral edema, muscle spasm, musculoskeletal pain, hypokalemia. **Occasional (19%–6%):** Hot flashes, diarrhea, UTI, cough, hypertension, urinary frequency, nocturia. **Rare (less than 6%):** Heartburn, upper respiratory tract infection.

ADVERSE EFFECTS/ TOXIC REACTIONS
Mineralocorticoid excess (severe fluid retention, hypokalemia, hypertension) may compromise pts with prior cardiovascular history. Safety not established in pts with left ventricular ejection fraction less than 50%. Tachycardia, atrial fibrillation, supraventricular tachycardia, atrial flutter, complete AV block, bradyarrhythmia reported in 7% of pts. Chest pain, unstable angina, HF reported in less than 4% of pts. Stress, infection, or interruption of daily steroids may cause adrenocortical insufficiency. Hepatotoxicity (serum ALT, AST greater than 5 times ULN) reported in 2% of pts. Pts with hepatic impairment are more likely to develop hepatotoxicity.

NURSING CONSIDERATIONS

BASELINE ASSESSMENT
Obtain BMP, LFT. Question history of HF, myocardial infarction, arrhythmias, angina pectoris, peripheral edema, hepatic impairment, adrenal or pituitary abnormalities, left ventricular ejection fraction (if applicable). Question history of corticosteroid intolerance if applicable.

INTERVENTION/EVALUATION
Monitor BMP as clinically indicated. Monitor for mineralocorticoid excess (hypokalemia, hypertension, fluid retention) at least once monthly. Assess for cardiac arrhythmia if hypokalemia occurs. Obtain ECG for palpitations, dyspnea, dizziness. Monitor for symptoms of adrenocortical insufficiency during predniSONE interruption, periods of stress, infection. Measure serum ALT, AST, alkaline phosphatase, bilirubin every 2 wks for 3 mos, then monthly. If hepatotoxicity occurs, dosage modification will be necessary. Pts with moderate hepatic impairment must have LFT every wk for first month, then every 2 wks for 2 mos, then monthly. If serum ALT, AST above 5 times ULN or serum bilirubin above 3 times ULN, treatment should be discontinued.

PATIENT/FAMILY TEACHING
• Must be taken on empty stomach (no food 2 hrs before and 1 hr after dose). • If taken with food, toxic levels may result. • Sexually active men must wear condoms during treatment and for 1 wk after treatment. • Women who are pregnant or are planning pregnancy may not touch medication without gloves. • Dizziness, palpitations, headache, confusion, muscle weakness, leg swelling/discomfort

may become more apparent during periods of unusual stress, infection, or interruption of predniSONE therapy. • Report liver problems (yellowing of skin, bruising, light-colored stool, right upper quadrant pain), chest pain, palpitations. • An increase in urinary frequency or nocturia is expected as treatment becomes therapeutic. • Do not chew, crush, dissolve, or divide tablets.

---

acalabrutinib

a-**kal**-a-**broo**-ti-nib
(Calquence)
Do not confuse acalabrutinib with afatinib, cabozantinib, ibrutinib, or lenvatinib.

◆CLASSIFICATION

PHARMACOTHERAPEUTIC: Bruton tyrosine kinase inhibitor. **CLINICAL:** Antineoplastic.

USES

Treatment of adults with mantle cell lymphoma (MCL) who have received at least one prior therapy. Treatment of adults with chronic lymphocytic leukemia or small lymphocytic lymphoma. **OFF-LABEL:** Waldenström macroglobulinemia.

PRECAUTIONS

Contraindications: Hypersensitivity to acalabrutinib. **Cautions:** Baseline cytopenias; active infection, conditions predisposing to infection (e.g., diabetes, renal failure, immunocompromised pts, open wounds); history of atrial fibrillation, atrial flutter; pts at risk for hemorrhage (e.g., history of intracranial/GI bleeding, coagulation disorders, recent trauma; concomitant use of anticoagulants, antiplatelets, NSAIDS).

ACTION

Inhibits enzymatic activity of Bruton tyrosine kinase (BTK); a signaling molecule that activates the pathways necessary for B-cell proliferation. **Therapeutic Ef-** fect: Decreases malignant B-cell proliferation and tumor growth.

PHARMACOKINETICS

Widely distributed. Metabolized in liver. Protein binding: 97.5%. Peak plasma concentration: 0.75 hrs. Steady-state maintained over 12 hrs. Excreted in feces (84%), urine (12%). **Half-life:** 0.9 hrs (metabolite: 6.9 hrs).

⧗ LIFESPAN CONSIDERATIONS

Pregnancy/Lactation: Avoid pregnancy; may cause fetal harm. Unknown if distributed in breast milk. Breastfeeding not recommended during treatment and for at least 2 wks after discontinuation. **Children:** Safety and efficacy not established. **Elderly:** No age-related precautions noted.

INTERACTIONS

DRUG: **Strong CYP3A4 inhibitors (e.g., clarithromycin, ketoconazole, ritonavir), moderate CYP3A inhibitors (e.g., erythromycin, diltiazem, fluconazole, verapamil)** may increase concentration/effect. **Strong CYP3A4 inducers (e.g., carbamazepine, phenytoin, rifampin)** may decrease concentration/effect. May decrease effect of **BCG (intravesical), vaccines (live).** May enhance adverse/toxic effects of **natalizumab, vaccines (live). Pimecrolimus, tacrolimus** may enhance adverse/toxic effects. **HERBAL:** Echinacea may decrease concentration/effect. **FOOD:** None known. **LAB VALUES:** May decrease Hgb, platelets, neutrophils.

AVAILABILITY (Rx)

Tablets: 100 mg.

ADMINISTRATION/HANDLING
PO

• Give without regard to food. • Administer tablet whole with a glass of water; do not cut, crush, or dissolve. Tablets cannot be chewed. • If a dose is missed, may administer dose up to 3 hrs after regularly scheduled time. If more than 3 hrs have

---

elapsed, do not give dose. Administer next dose at regularly scheduled time.

INDICATIONS/ROUTES/DOSAGE

Mantle Cell Lymphoma

PO: ADULTS, ELDERLY: 100 mg approximately q12h. Continue until disease progression or unacceptable toxicity.

Chronic Lymphocytic Leukemia or Small Lymphocytic Lymphoma

PO: ADULTS, ELDERLY: (Single-agent therapy): 100 mg q12h. Continue until disease progression or unacceptable toxicity. **(Combination therapy with obinutuzumab):** 100 mg q12h. Continue until disease progression or unacceptable toxicity. Begin acalabrutinib at cycle 1 (28-day cycle); obinutuzumab given for 6 cycles beginning at cycle 2. Administer prior to obinutuzumab when given on the same day.

Dose Modification

Based on Common Terminology Criteria for Adverse Events (CTCAE).

Grade 3 or 4 nonhematologic toxicities; Grade 3 thrombocytopenia with bleeding; Grade 4 thrombocytopenia; Grade 4 neutropenia lasting longer than 7 days: First and second occurrence: Withhold treatment until recovery to Grade 1 or baseline, then resume at 100 mg twice daily. **Third occurrence:** Withhold treatment until recovery to Grade 1 or baseline, then resume at 100 mg once daily. **Fourth occurrence:** Permanently discontinue.

Concomitant Use of Strong CYP3A Inhibitors

Avoid use. If short-term treatment with CYP3A inhibitor is unavoidable (e.g., anti-infectives for up to 7 days), withhold acalabrutinib until strong CYP3A inhibitor is discontinued.

Concomitant Use of Moderate CYP3A Inhibitors

Decrease frequency to 100 mg once daily.

Concomitant Use of Strong CYP3A Inducers

If strong CYP3A inducer cannot be discontinued, increase acalabrutinib dose to 200 mg twice daily.

Dosage in Renal/Hepatic Impairment

Mild to moderate impairment: No dose adjustment. **Severe impairment:** Not specified; use caution.

SIDE EFFECTS

Frequent (39%–18%): Headache, diarrhea, fatigue, myalgia, bruising, nausea, rash. **Occasional (15%–13%):** Abdominal pain, constipation, vomiting.

ADVERSE EFFECTS/TOXIC REACTIONS

Myelosuppresion (anemia, neutropenia, thrombocytopenia) is an expected response to therapy. Serious and sometimes fatal hemorrhagic events including intracranial hemorrhage, GI bleeding, epistaxis occurred in 2% of pts. Petechiae, bruising reported in 50% of pts. Serious bacterial, viral, fungal infections occurred in 18% of pts. Infections due to hepatitis B virus reactivation was reported. New primary malignancies including skin cancer (7% of pts), nonskin carcinomas (11% of pts) have occurred. Progressive multifocal leukoencephalopathy (PML), an opportunistic viral infection of the brain caused by the JC virus, may result in progressive permanent disability and death. Atrial fibrillation/atrial flutter reported in 3% of pts.

NURSING CONSIDERATIONS

BASELINE ASSESSMENT

Obtain ANC, CBC; pregnancy test in females of reproductive potential. Screen for active infection. Question history of atrial fibrillation, atrial flutter; intracranial/GI bleeding, coagulation disorders, recent trauma; previous skin cancers. Conduct baseline dermatological exam and assess skin for open/unhealed wounds, lesions, moles. Receive full medication history and screen for interactions. Offer emotional support.

INTERVENTION/EVALUATION

Monitor CBC periodically for cytopenias. Closely monitor for HBV reactivation; symptoms of PML (altered mental status, seizures, visual disturbances, generalized or unilateral weakness). Obtain ECG if chest pain, dyspnea, palpitations occur. Be alert for serious infection, opportunistic infection, sepsis; nonskin carcinomas. Monitor for hemorrhagic events including intracranial hemorrhage (altered mental status, aphasia, blindness, hemiparesis, unequal pupils, seizures), GI bleeding (hematemesis, melena, rectal bleeding), epistaxis. Assess skin for new lesions, moles. Ensure adequate hydration.

PATIENT/FAMILY TEACHING

• Treatment may depress your immune system and reduce your ability to fight infection. Report symptoms of infection such as body aches, burning with urination, chills, cough, fatigue, fever. Avoid those with active infection. • Report symptoms of bone marrow depression such as bruising, fatigue, fever, shortness of breath, weight loss; bleeding easily, bloody urine or stool. • Use effective contraception to avoid pregnancy. Do not breastfeed. • PML, an opportunistic viral infection of the brain, may cause progressive, permanent disabilities and death. Report symptoms of PML, brain hemorrhage such as confusion, memory loss, paralysis, trouble speaking, vision loss, seizures, weakness • Treatment may cause new cancers, heart arrhythmias (chest pain, dizziness, fainting, palpitations, slow or rapid heart rate, irregular heart rate), reactivation of HBV. • Immediately report bleeding of any kind. • Do not take newly prescribed medications unless approved by the prescriber who originally started treatment. • Do not ingest grapefruit products.

---

acetaminophen   TOP 100

a-**seet**-a-**min**-oh-fen
(Feverall, Mapap, Ofirmev, Tylenol, Tylenol 8HR Arthritis Pain, Tylenol Children's, Tylenol Infants, Tylenol Extra Strength)

■ BLACK BOX ALERT ■ Potential for severe liver injury. Acetaminophen injection associated with acute liver failure.

Do not confuse Acephen with Aciphex, Feverall with Fiberall, Fioricet with Fiorinal, Percocet with Percodan, Tylenol with atenolol, timolol, Tylenol PM, or Tylox, or Vicodin with Hycodan.

FIXED-COMBINATION(S)

Codeine: Tablet: acetaminophen/codeine 300 mg/15 mg, 300 mg/30 mg, 300 mg/60 mg. **Hydrocodone: Elixir:** acetaminophen/hydrocodone 300 mg/10 mg/15 mL. **Tablet:** acetaminophen/hydrocodone 300 mg/5 mg, 300 mg/7.5 mg, 300 mg/10 mg. **Ibuprofen: Tablet:** acetaminophen/ibuprofen 325 mg/97.5 mg. **Injection:** acetaminophen/ibuprofen 1000 mg/300 mg.

◆ CLASSIFICATION

PHARMACOTHERAPEUTIC: Central analgesic. **CLINICAL:** Nonnarcotic analgesic, antipyretic.

USES

Fever: Temporary reduction of fever. **Pain: Injection:** Management of mild to moderate pain in pts greater than or equal to 2 yrs of age; management of moderate to severe pain when combined with an opioid in pts greater than or equal to 2 yrs. **Oral, rectal:** Temporary relief of mild to moderate pain and headache.

PRECAUTIONS

Contraindications: Hypersensitivity to acetaminophen, severe hepatic impairment or severe active liver disease. **Cautions:** Sensitivity to acetaminophen; severe renal impairment; alcohol dependency, hepatic impairment, or active hepatic disease; chronic malnutrition and hypovolemia (Ofirmev); G6PD deficiency (hemolysis may occur). Limit dose to less than 4 g/day.

ACTION

Analgesic: Activates descending serotonergic inhibitory pathways in CNS. Antipyretic: Inhibits hypothalamic heat-regulating center. **Therapeutic Effect:** Results in antipyresis. Produces analgesic effect.

PHARMACOKINETICS

Route	Onset	Peak	Duration
PO	Less than 60 min	1–3 hrs	4–6 hrs

Rapidly, completely absorbed from GI tract; rectal absorption variable. Protein binding: 20%–50%. Widely distributed to most body tissues. Metabolized in liver. Excreted in urine. Removed by hemodialysis. **Half-life:** 1–4 hrs (increased in pts with hepatic disease, elderly, neonates; decreased in children).

⌛ LIFESPAN CONSIDERATIONS

Pregnancy/Lactation: Crosses placenta; distributed in breast milk. Routinely used in all stages of pregnancy; appears safe for short-term use. **Children/Elderly:** No age-related precautions noted.

INTERACTIONS

DRUG: Alcohol (chronic use), **hepatotoxic medications** (e.g., **phenytoin**) may increase risk of hepatotoxicity with prolonged high dose or single toxic dose. **HERBAL:** None significant. **FOOD:** May decrease rate of absorption. **LAB VALUES:** May increase serum ALT, AST, bilirubin; prothrombin levels (may indicate hepatotoxicity).

AVAILABILITY (OTC)

Capsules: 325 mg, 500 mg. **Elixir:** 160 mg/5 mL. **Injection, Solution:** *(Ofirmev):* 1,000 mg/100 mL glass vial. **Liquid (Oral):** 160 mg/5 mL. **Solution (Oral Drops):** 80 mg/0.8 mL. **Suppository:** 80 mg, 120 mg, 325 mg, 650 mg. **Suspension:** 160 mg/5 mL. **Syrup:** 160 mg/5 mL. **Tablets:** 325 mg, 500 mg. **Tablets (Chewable):** 80 mg.

 Tablets (Extended-Release): 650 mg.

ADMINISTRATION/HANDLING

💉 IV

Reconstitution • Does not require further dilution. • Store at room temperature. • Withdraw doses less than 1,000 mg. • Place in separate empty, sterile container.
Rate of administration • Infuse over 15 min.

Stability • Once opened or transferred, stable for 6 hrs at room temperature.

PO

• Give without regard to food. • Do not crush or chew extended-release caplets. • Suspension: Shake well before use. • Take with full glass of water.

Rectal

• Moisten suppository with cold water before inserting well up into rectum. • Do not freeze suppositories.

INDICATIONS/ROUTES/DOSAGE

Note: Over-the-counter (OTC) use of acetaminophen should be limited to 3,000 mg/day.

Analgesia and Antipyresis

IV: ADULTS, ELDERLY, ADOLESCENTS WEIGHING 50 KG OR MORE: 1,000 mg q6h or 650 mg q4h. **Maximum single dose:** 1,000 mg; **maximum total daily dose:** 4,000 mg. **ADULTS, ADOLESCENTS WEIGHING LESS THAN 50 KG:** 15 mg/kg q6h or 12.5 mg/kg q4h. **Maximum single dose:** 750 mg; **maximum total daily dose:** 75 mg/kg/day (3,750 mg). **CHILDREN 2–12 YRS:** 15 mg/kg q6h or 12.5 mg/kg q4h. **Maximum single dose:** 750 mg. **Maximum:** 75 mg/kg/day, not to exceed 3,750 mg/day. **INFANTS AND CHILDREN LESS THAN 2 YRS (FEVER ONLY):** 15 mg/kg q6h. **Maximum:** 60 mg/kg/day. **NEONATES (FEVER ONLY):** 12.5 mg/kg q6h. **Maximum:** 50 mg/kg/day.
PO: ADULTS, ELDERLY, CHILDREN 13 YRS AND OLDER: (Regular Strength) 325–650 mg q4–6h. **Maximum:** 3,250 mg/day unless directed by healthcare provider. **Extra Strength:** 1,000 mg q6h. **Maximum:** 3,000 mg/day unless directed by healthcare provider. **Extended-Release:** 1,300 mg q8h. **Maximum:** 3,900 mg/day. **CHILDREN 12 YRS AND YOUNGER:** (Weight dosing preferred; if not available, use age. Doses may be repeated q4h. **Maximum:** 5 doses/day.)

Age	Weight (Kg)	Dose
11–12 yrs	32.7–43.2	480 mg
9–10 yrs	27.3–32.6	325–400 mg
6–8 yrs	21.8–27.2	320 mg
4–5 yrs	16.4–21.7	240 mg
2–3 yrs	10.9–16.3	160 mg
1–<2 yrs	8.2–10.8	120 mg
4–11 mos	5.4–8.1	80 mg
0–3 mos	2.7–5.3	40 mg

NEONATES: Term: 10–15 mg/kg/dose q4–6h. **Maximum:** 75 mg/kg/day.

Rectal: ADULTS, ELDERLY, CHILDREN 12 YRS AND OLDER: 325–650 mg q4–6h. **Maximum:** 3.9 g/24 hrs. **CHILDREN LESS THAN 12 YRS:** 10–20 mg/kg/dose. **Maximum daily dose:** 75 mg/kg/day.

Dosage in Renal Impairment

Creatinine Clearance	Frequency
Oral	
10–50 mL/min	q6h
Less than 10 mL/min	q8h
Continuous renal replacement therapy	q6h
IV	
30 mL/min or less (use caution, decrease daily dose, extend dosing interval)	

Dosage in Hepatic Impairment

Use with caution. IV contraindicated in pts with severe impairment.

SIDE EFFECTS

Rare: Hypersensitivity reaction.

ADVERSE EFFECTS/TOXIC REACTIONS

Early Signs of Acetaminophen Toxicity: Anorexia, nausea, diaphoresis, fatigue within first 12–24 hrs. **Later Signs of Toxicity:** Vomiting, right upper quadrant tenderness, elevated LFTs within 48–72 hrs after ingestion. **Antidote:** Acetylcysteine (see Appendix H for dosage).

NURSING CONSIDERATIONS

BASELINE ASSESSMENT

If given for analgesia, assess onset, type, location, duration of pain. Effect of medication is reduced if full pain response recurs prior to next dose. Assess for fever. Assess LFT in pts with chronic usage or history of hepatic impairment, alcohol abuse.

INTERVENTION/EVALUATION

Assess for clinical improvement and relief of pain, fever. **Therapeutic serum level:** 10–30 mcg/mL; **toxic serum level:** greater than 200 mcg/mL. Do not exceed maximum daily recommended dose: 4 g/day.

PATIENT/FAMILY TEACHING

• Consult physician for use in children younger than 2 yrs, oral use longer than 5 days (children) or longer than 10 days (adults), or fever lasting longer than 3 days. • Severe/recurrent pain or high/continuous fever may indicate serious illness. • Do not take more than 4 g/day (3 g/day if using OTC [over-the-counter]). Actual OTC dosing recommendations may vary by product and/or manufacturer. Many nonprescription combination products contain acetaminophen. Avoid alcohol.

acetylcysteine

a-**seet**-il-**sis**-teen
(Acetadote)
Do not confuse acetylcysteine with acetylcholine.

◆CLASSIFICATION

PHARMACOTHERAPEUTIC: Respiratory inhalant, intratracheal. **CLINICAL:** Mucolytic, antidote.

USES

Inhalation: Adjunctive treatment for abnormally viscid mucous secretions present in acute and chronic bronchopulmonary disease (e.g., emphysema, chronic asthmatic bronchitis, tuberculosis, bronchiectasis), acute bronchopulmonary disease (e.g., pneumonia, bronchitis, tracheobronchitis), pulmonary complications of cystic fibrosis. **Injection, PO:** Antidote in acute acetaminophen toxicity.

PRECAUTIONS

Contraindications: Hypersensitivity to acetylcysteine. **Cautions:** History of bronchial asthma; debilitated pts with severe respiratory insufficiency (increases risk of anaphylactoid reaction).

ACTION

Mucolytic splits linkage of mucoproteins, reducing viscosity of pulmonary secretions. Acetaminophen toxicity: Hepatoprotective by restoring hepatic glutathione and enhancing nontoxic sulfate conjugation of acetaminophen. **Therapeutic Effect:** Facilitates removal of pulmonary secretions by coughing, postural drainage, mechanical means. Protects against acetaminophen overdose-induced hepatotoxicity.

⌛ LIFESPAN CONSIDERATIONS

Pregnancy/Lactation: Unknown if distributed in breast milk. **Children/Elderly:** No age-related precautions noted.

INTERACTIONS

DRUG: None significant. **HERBAL:** None significant. **FOOD:** None known. **LAB VALUES:** None significant.

AVAILABILITY (Rx)

Inhalation Solution: 10% (100 mg/mL), 20% (200 mg/mL). **Injection Solution:** *(Acetadote):* 20% (200 mg/mL).

ADMINISTRATION/HANDLING

 IV

The total dose is 300 mg/kg administered over 21 hrs. Dose preparation is based on pt weight. Total volume administered should be adjusted for pts less than 40 kg and for pts requiring fluid restriction. Store unopened vials at room temperature. Following dilution in D_5W, solution is stable for 24 hrs at room temperature. Color change of opened vials may occur (does not affect potency).

Note: Newly FDA approved dosing regimen simplifies the administration by combining the first two bags of the standard regimen into a single, slower infusion.

Three-Bag Method (as Antidote): Loading, Second, and Third Doses, Pts Weighing 40 kg or More
Loading dose: 150 mg/kg in 200 mL of diluent administered over 60 min.
Second dose: 50 mg/kg in 500 mL of diluent administered over 4 hrs.
Third dose: 100 mg/kg in 1,000 mL of diluent administered over 16 hrs.

Pts Weighing More Than 20 kg but Less Than 40 kg
Loading dose: 150 mg/kg in 100 mL of diluent administered over 60 min.
Second dose: 50 mg/kg in 250 mL of diluent administered over 4 hrs.
Third dose: 100 mg/kg in 500 mL of diluent administered over 16 hrs.

Pts Weighing Less Than or Equal to 20 kg
Loading dose: 150 mg/kg in 3 mL/kg of body weight of diluent administered over 60 min.
Second dose: 50 mg/kg in 7 mL/kg of body weight of diluent administered over 4 hrs.
Third dose: 100 mg/kg in 14 mL/kg of body weight of diluent administered over 16 hrs.

PO
• For treatment of acetaminophen overdose. • Give as 5% solution. • Dilute 20% solution 1:3 with cola, orange juice, other soft drink. • Give within 1 hr of preparation.

Inhalation, Nebulization
• 20% solution may be diluted with 0.9% NaCl or sterile water; 10% solution may be used undiluted.

INDICATIONS/ROUTES/DOSAGE

Bronchopulmonary Disease
Inhalation, Nebulization
◄**ALERT**► Bronchodilators should be given 10–15 min before acetylcysteine. **ADULTS, ELDERLY, CHILDREN:** 3–5 mL (20% solution) 3–4 times/day or 6–10

mL (10% solution) 3–4 times/day.
Range: 1–10 mL (20% solution)
q2–6h or 2–20 mL (10% solution)
q2–6h. **INFANTS:** 1–2 mL (20%) or
2–4 mL (10%) 3–4 times/day.
Intratracheal: ADULTS, CHILDREN: 1–2
mL of 10% or 20% solution instilled into
tracheostomy q1–4h.

Acetaminophen Overdose

◄**ALERT►** Treatment should begin
within 8 hrs of ingestion or as soon as
possible after ingestion.
PO: *(Oral Solution 5%):* **ADULTS, EL-
DERLY, CHILDREN:** Loading dose of 140
mg/kg, followed in 4 hrs by maintenance
dose of 70 mg/kg q4h for 17 additional
doses (or until acetaminophen assay re-
veals nontoxic level). Repeat dose if emesis occurs within 1 hr of administration.
Note: Newly FDA approved dosing regimen simplifies the administration by combining the first two bags of the standard
regimen into a single, slower infusion.
IV: ADULTS, ELDERLY, CHILDREN: (Consists of 3 doses. **Total dose:** 300 mg/
kg.) 150 mg/kg (maximum 15 g) infused over 60 min, then 50 mg/kg
(maximum 5 g) infused over 4 hrs,
then 100 mg/kg (maximum 10 g) infused over 16 hrs (see Administration/
Handling for dilution). **WEIGHING MORE
THAN 100 KG:** (Consists of 3 doses. **Total
dose:** 30 g.) 15 g over 60 min; 5 g over
4 hrs; 10 g over 16 hrs. Duration of administration may vary depending on acetaminophen levels and LFTs obtained
during treatment. Pts who still have
detectable levels of acetaminophen or
elevated LFT results continue to benefit
from additional acetylcysteine administration beyond 24 hrs.

Diagnostic Bronchial Studies
Inhalation, Nebulization: ADULTS: 1–2
mL of 20% solution or 2–4 mL of 10% solution 2–3 times before the procedure.

SIDE EFFECTS

IV: (10%): Nausea, vomiting. **(7%–6%):**
Acute flushing, erythema. **(4%):** Pruri-

tus. **Frequent: Inhalation:** Stickiness
on face, transient unpleasant odor.
Occasional: Inhalation: Increased bronchial secretions, throat irritation, nausea,
vomiting, rhinorrhea. **Rare: Inhalation:** Rash. **PO:** Facial edema, bronchospasm, wheezing, nausea, vomiting.

ADVERSE EFFECTS/TOXIC REACTIONS

Large doses may produce severe nausea/
vomiting. **(Less than 2%):** Serious anaphylactoid reactions including cough,
wheezing, stridor, respiratory distress,
bronchospasm, hypotension, and death
have been known to occur with IV administration.

NURSING CONSIDERATIONS

BASELINE ASSESSMENT

Mucolytic: Assess pretreatment respirations for rate, depth, rhythm. **IV
antidote:** Obtain baseline LFT, PT/INR,
and drug screen. For use as antidote,
obtain acetaminophen level to determine need for treatment with acetylcysteine.

INTERVENTION/EVALUATION

If bronchospasm occurs, discontinue
treatment, notify physician; bronchodilator may be added to therapy. Monitor
rate, depth, rhythm, type of respiration (abdominal, thoracic). Observe
sputum for color, consistency, amount.
Auscultate lung sounds. **IV antidote:**
Administer within 8 hrs of acetaminophen ingestion for maximal hepatic
protection; ideally, within 4 hrs after
immediate-release and 2 hrs after liquid
acetaminophen formulations.

PATIENT/FAMILY TEACHING

• Sulfuric odor may be noticed during
initial administration but disappears
quickly. • Drink plenty of fluids. Adequate hydration is important part of
therapy. • Follow guidelines for
proper coughing and deep breathing
techniques.

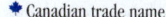 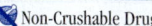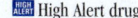

acyclovir

a-**sye**-klo-veer
(Apo-Acyclovir ✿)
Do not confuse acyclovir with ganciclovir, Retrovir, or valACYclovir, or Zovirax with Doribax, Valtrex, Zithromax, Zostrix, Zyloprim, or Zyvox.

FIXED-COMBINATION(S)

Lipsovir: acyclovir/hydrocortisone (a steroid): 5%/1%.

◆CLASSIFICATION

PHARMACOTHERAPEUTIC: Synthetic nucleoside. **CLINICAL:** Antiviral.

USES

IV: Treatment of initial and prophylaxis of recurrent mucosal and cutaneous herpes simplex virus (HSV-1 and HSV-2) in immunocompromised pts. Treatment of severe initial episodes of herpes genitalis in adults and children aged 12 yrs and older who are immunocompetent. Treatment of herpes simplex encephalitis. Treatment of neonatal herpes infections. Treatment of herpes zoster (shingles) in immunocompromised pts. **PO:** Treatment of initial episodes and prophylaxis of recurrent herpes simplex (HSV-2 genital herpes) in adults. Treatment of chickenpox (varicella) in adults and children aged 2 yrs and older who are immunocompetent. Acute treatment of herpes zoster (shingles) in adults.
Topical: (Cream): Treatment of recurrent herpes labialis (cold sores) in adults and children aged 12 yrs and older who are immunocompetent. **(Ointment):** Management of initial genital herpes and treatment of mucocutaneous HSV in adults who are immunocompromised.
OFF-LABEL: Bell's palsy, cytomegalovirus prevention in allogenic HCT recipients, herpes simplex virus prevention in immunocompromised pts, varicella virus prevention in immunocompromised pts, encephalitis, acute retinal necrosis.

PRECAUTIONS

Contraindications: Use in neonates when acyclovir is reconstituted with Bacteriostatic Water for Injection containing benzyl alcohol. Hypersensitivity to acyclovir, valACYclovir. **Cautions:** Immunocompromised pts (thrombocytopenic purpura/hemolytic uremic syndrome reported); elderly, renal impairment, use of other nephrotoxic medications. **IV use:** Underlying neurologic abnormalities, serious hepatic/electrolyte abnormalities, substantial hypoxia.

ACTION

Acyclovir is converted to acyclovir triphosphate, which competes for viral DNA polymerase, becoming part of DNA chain. **Therapeutic Effect:** Inhibits DNA synthesis and viral replication. Virustatic.

PHARMACOKINETICS

Widely distributed. Topical application not systemically absorbed. Metabolized intracellularly in viral-infected cells. Protein binding: 9%–33%. Excreted primarily in urine. Removed by hemodialysis. **Half-life:** 2.5–3.3 hrs (increased in renal impairment).

⧖ LIFESPAN CONSIDERATIONS

Pregnancy/Lactation: Crosses placenta; distributed in breast milk. **Children:** Safety and efficacy not established in pts younger than 2 yrs (younger than 1 yr for IV use). **Elderly:** Age-related renal impairment may require decreased dosage. May experience more neurologic effects (e.g., agitation, confusion, hallucinations).

INTERACTIONS

DRUG: Foscarnet may increase nephrotoxic effect. May increase adverse effects of **tizanidine.** May decrease therapeutic effect of **varicella virus vaccine, zoster vaccine.** **HERBAL:** None significant. **FOOD:** None known. **LAB VALUES:** May increase serum ALT, AST, BUN, creatinine.

AVAILABILITY (Rx)

Cream: 5%. **Injection, Solution:** 50 mg/mL. **Ointment:** 5%. **Oral Suspension:** 200 mg/5 mL. **Tablets:** 400 mg, 800 mg.

 Capsules: 200 mg.

ADMINISTRATION/HANDLING

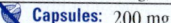 **IV**

Reconstitution • Dilute with at least 100 mL D₅W or 0.9 NaCl. Final concentration should be 7 mg/mL or less. (Concentrations greater than 10 mg/mL increase risk of phlebitis.)
Rate of administration • Infuse over at least 1 hr (nephrotoxicity due to crystalluria and renal tubular damage may occur with too-rapid rate). • Maintain adequate hydration during infusion and for 2 hrs following IV administration.
Storage • Store vials at room temperature. • IV infusion (piggyback) stable for 24 hrs at room temperature.

PO
• May give without regard to food. • Do not crush/break capsules. • Store capsules at room temperature.

Topical
Ointment • Avoid contact with eyes. • Use finger cot/rubber glove to prevent autoinoculation.
Cream • Apply to cover only cold sores or area with symptoms. • Rub until it disappears.

🔷 IV INCOMPATIBILITIES

Acetaminophen, aztreonam, levofloxacin, piperacillin/tazobactam.

🔷 IV COMPATIBILITIES

Amikacin, ampicillin, cefazolin, cefotaxime, ceftazidime, ceftriaxone, fluconazole, gen-

tamicin, linezolid, metronidazole, tobramycin, trimethoprim/sulfamethoxazole.

INDICATIONS/ROUTES/DOSAGE

Genital Herpes (Initial Episode)
IV: ADULTS, ELDERLY, CHILDREN 12 YRS AND OLDER: 5–10 mg/kg q8h. Followed with oral therapy to complete at least 10 days of therapy.
PO: ADULTS, ELDERLY, CHILDREN 12 YRS AND OLDER: 400 mg 3 times/day or 200 mg 5 times/day for 7–10 days. **CHILDREN YOUNGER THAN 12 YRS:** 40–80 mg/kg/day in 3–4 divided doses for 7–10 days. **Maximum:** 1,200 mg/day.

Genital Herpes (Recurrent)
Intermittent Therapy
PO: ADULTS, ELDERLY, CHILDREN 12 YRS AND OLDER: 800 mg 2 times/day for 5 days or 800 mg 3 times/day for 2 days or 400 mg 3 times/day for 5 days. **CHILDREN YOUNGER THAN 12 YRS:** 20 mg/kg 3 times/day for 5 days. **Maximum:** 400 mg/dose.
Chronic Suppressive Therapy
PO: ADULTS, ELDERLY, CHILDREN 12 YRS AND OLDER: 400 mg 2 times/day. **CHILDREN YOUNGER THAN 12 YRS:** 20 mg/kg twice daily. **Maximum:** 400 mg/dose.

Herpes Simplex Mucocutaneous
PO: ADULTS, ELDERLY: (Immunocompetent): 400 mg 3 times/day or 200 mg 5 times/day for 7–10 days. **(Immunocompromised):** 400 mg 5 times/day for 14–21 days. **CHILDREN:** 20 mg/kg 4 times/day for 5–7 days. **Maximum:** 800 mg/dose.
IV: ADULTS, ELDERLY, CHILDREN: 5 mg/kg/dose q8h for 7–14 days.
Topical: ADULTS: *(Ointment):* 0.5 inch for 4-inch square surface q3h (6 times/day) for 7 days.

Herpes Simplex Encephalitis
IV: ADULTS, ELDERLY, CHILDREN 12 YRS AND OLDER: 10 mg/kg q8h for 14–21 days (encephalitis) or 10–14 days (meningitis). **CHILDREN 3 MOS–YOUNGER THAN 12 YRS:** 10–15 mg/kg q8h for 14–21 days.

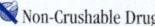 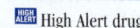

Herpes Zoster (Shingles)

IV: ADULTS, CHILDREN 12 YRS AND OLDER: 10 mg/kg/dose q8h for 7–10 days. **CHILDREN YOUNGER THAN 12 YRS:** 10 mg/kg/dose q8h for 7–10 days.
PO: ADULTS, ELDERLY, CHILDREN 12 YRS AND OLDER: 800 mg q4h 5 times/day for 7–10 days.

Herpes Labialis (Cold Sores)

Topical: ADULTS, ELDERLY, CHILDREN 12 YRS AND OLDER: Apply to affected area 5 times/day for 4 days.

Varicella-Zoster (Chickenpox)

◀**ALERT**▶ Begin treatment within 24 hrs of onset of rash.
PO: ADULTS, ELDERLY, CHILDREN OLDER THAN 12 YRS AND CHILDREN 2–12 YRS, WEIGHING 40 KG OR MORE: 800 mg 5 times/day for 5–7 days and until all lesions have crusted. **CHILDREN 2–12 YRS, WEIGHING LESS THAN 40 KG:** 20 mg/kg 4 times/day for 5 days. **Maximum:** 800 mg/dose.

Usual Neonatal Dosage

HSV (Treatment) (IV): 20 mg/kg/dose q8–12h for 14–21 days.
HSV (Chronic suppression) (PO): 300 mg/m²/dose q8h –(after completing a 14–21 day course of IV therapy) for 6 mos.
Varicella-Zoster (IV): 10–20 mg/kg/dose q8h for 7–10 days.

Dosage in Renal Impairment

Dosage and frequency are modified based on severity of infection and degree of renal impairment.
PO: Normal dose 200 mg q4h, 200 mg q8h, or 400 mg q12h. **Creatinine clearance 10 mL/min and less:** 200 mg q12h.
PO: Normal dose 800 mg q4h. **Creatinine clearance greater than 25 mL/min:** Give usual dose and at normal interval, 800 mg q4h. **Creatinine clearance 10–25 mL/min:** 800 mg q8h. **Creatinine clearance less than 10 mL/min:** 800 mg q12h.
IV:

Creatinine Clearance	Dosage
Greater than 50 mL/min	100% of normal q8h
25–50 mL/min	100% of normal q12h
10–24 mL/min	100% of normal q24h
Less than 10 mL/min	50% of normal q24h
Hemodialysis (HD)	2.5–5 mg/kg q24h (give after HD)
Peritoneal dialysis (PD)	50% normal dose q24h
Continuous renal replacement therapy (CRRT)	5–10 mg/kg q12–24h (q12h for viral meningoencephalitis/ VZV infection)

Dosage in Hepatic Impairment

Mild to moderate impairment: No dose adjustment. **Severe impairment:** Use caution.

SIDE EFFECTS

Frequent: Parenteral (9%–7%): Phlebitis or inflammation at IV site, nausea, vomiting. **Topical (28%):** Burning, stinging. **Occasional: Parenteral (3%):** Pruritus, rash, urticaria. **PO (12%–6%):** Malaise, nausea. **Topical (4%):** Pruritus. **Rare: PO (3%–1%):** Vomiting, rash, diarrhea, headache. **Parenteral (2%–1%):** Confusion, hallucinations, seizures, tremors. **Topical (less than 1%):** Rash.

ADVERSE EFFECTS/TOXIC REACTIONS

Rapid parenteral administration, excessively high doses, or fluid and electrolyte imbalance may produce renal failure. Toxicity not reported with oral or topical use.

NURSING CONSIDERATIONS

BASELINE ASSESSMENT

Question for history of allergies, esp. to acyclovir. Assess herpes simplex lesions before treatment to compare baseline with treatment effect.

INTERVENTION/EVALUATION

Assess IV site for phlebitis (heat, pain, red streaking over vein). Evaluate cutaneous lesions. Ensure adequate ventilation. Manage chickenpox and disseminated herpes zoster with strict isolation. Encourage fluid intake.

PATIENT/FAMILY TEACHING

• Drink adequate fluids. • Do not touch lesions with bare fingers to prevent spreading infection to new site. • Continue therapy for full length of treatment. • Space doses evenly. • Use finger cot/rubber glove to apply topical ointment. • Avoid sexual intercourse during duration of lesions to prevent infecting partner. • Acyclovir does not cure herpes infections. • Pap smear should be done at least annually due to increased risk of cervical cancer in women with genital herpes.

---

adagrasib

a-**da**-gra-sib
(Krazati)
Do not confuse adagrasib with alpelisib or idelalisib.

◆CLASSIFICATION

PHARMACOTHERAPEUTIC: RAS GTPase inhibitor. **CLINICAL:** Antineoplastic.

USES

Metastatic non–small-cell lung cancer (NSCLC): As a single agent for the treatment of adults with *KRAS G12C*-mutated locally advanced or metastatic non–small-cell lung cancer (NSCLC) who have received at least one prior systemic therapy. **Colorectal cancer (CRC):** In combination with cetuximab, for the treatment of adults with KRAS G12C-mutated, locally advanced or metastatic CRC, who have received prior treatment with fluoropyrimidine-, oxaliplatin-, and irinotecan-based chemotherapy.

PRECAUTIONS

Contraindications: Hypersensitivity to adagrasib. **Cautions:** Baseline cytopenias, hepatic impairment, pts at risk for interstitial lung disease (e.g., COPD, sarcoidosis, connective disease disease), pts at risk for QT interval prolongation or torsades de pointes (congenital long QT syndrome, QT interval–prolonging medications, hypokalemia, hypomagnesemia). Avoid concomitant use of strong CYP3A inducers, strong CYP3A inhibitors, sensitive CYP3A4 substrates, CYP2C9 substrates, P-glycoprotein (P-gp) substrates, QT interval–prolonging medications.

ACTION

Irreversibly binds to and inhibits *KRAS G12C* mutant forms of the RAS GTPase family, preventing downstream signaling without affecting wild-type KRAS protein. Promotes cellular death of *KRAS G12C* tumor cell lines. **Therapeutic Effect:** Causes apoptosis (cellular death) of tumor cells.

PHARMACOKINETICS

Widely distributed. Metabolized in liver. Protein binding: 98%. Peak plasma concentration: 6 hrs. Steady state reached in 8 days. Excreted in feces (75%), urine (4.5%). **Half-life:** 23 hrs.

⏳ LIFESPAN CONSIDERATIONS

Pregnancy/Lactation: Unknown if distributed in breast milk. Breastfeeding not recommend during treatment and for at least 1 wk after discontinuation. May impair fertility in both females and males. **Children:** Safety and efficacy not established. **Elderly:** No age-related precautions noted.

INTERACTIONS

DRUG: QT interval–prolonging medications (e.g., **amiodarone, azithromycin, ciprofloxacin, haloperidol, sotalol**) may increase risk of QT interval prolongation, torsades de pointes.

Strong CYP3A4 inhibitors (e.g., clarithromycin, ketoconazole, ribociclib) may increase concentration/effect. **Strong CYP3A4 inducers (e.g., carBAMazepine, PHENytoin, riFAMPin)** may decrease concentration/effect. May increase adverse/toxic effects of **CYP2D6 substrates (e.g., metoprolol, mirtazapine, risperidone), CYP3A4 substrates (e.g., busPIRone, simvastatin, tacrolimus), CYP2C9 substrates (e.g., losartan, phenytoin, warfarin), P-gp substrates (e.g., digoxin, dexamethasone, tacrolimus).** **HERBAL:** St. John's wort may decrease concentration/effect. **FOOD:** None known. **LAB VALUES:** May increase serum ALT, AST, creatinine, lipase. May decrease Hgb, lymphocytes, platelets; serum albumin, magnesium, potassium, sodium.

AVAILABILITY (Rx)
Tablets: 200 mg.

ADMINISTRATION/HANDLING
PO
• Give without regard to food. • Administer tablet whole; do not break, cut, or crush. Tablets cannot be chewed. • If a dose is missed by more than 4 hrs, skip the dose and give at next regularly scheduled time. • If vomiting occurs after administration, give the next dose at regularly scheduled time (do not give additional dose).

INDICATIONS/ROUTES/DOSAGE
CRC, NSCLC (Locally Advanced or Metastatic)
PO: ADULTS, ELDERLY: 600 mg twice daily until disease progression or unacceptable toxicity.

Dose Reduction Schedule
First reduction: 400 mg twice daily. **Second reduction:** 600 mg once daily. **Unable to tolerate 600 mg daily dose:** Permanently discontinue.

Dose Modification
Based on Common Terminology Criteria for Adverse Events (CTCAE).

GI Toxicity
Grade 3 or 4 nausea, vomiting, or diarrhea (despite supportive therapy): Withhold treatment until improved to Grade 1 or baseline, then resume at a reduced dose.

Hepatotoxicity
Grade 2 serum ALT/AST elevation: Reduce dose. **Grade 3 or 4 serum ALT/AST elevation:** Withhold treatment until improved to Grade 1 or baseline, then resume at a reduced dose. **Serum ALT/AST elevation greater than 3 times upper limit of normal (ULN) with total bilirubin greater than 2 times ULN (in absence of other causes):** Permanently discontinue.

Pulmonary Toxicity
Any grade ILD/Pneumonitis: Withhold treatment if ILD/pneumonitis is suspected. Permanently discontinue if ILD/pneumonitis is confirmed.

Other Adverse Reactions
Any other Grade 3 or 4 reaction: Withhold treatment until improved to Grade 1 or baseline, then resume at a reduced dose.

Dosage in Renal/Hepatic Impairment
No dose adjustment.

SIDE EFFECTS
Frequent (70%–35%): Diarrhea, nausea, vomiting, fatigue, musculoskeletal pain, edema, decreased appetite, dyspnea. **Occasional (24%–21%):** Cough, dizziness, constipation, abdominal pain.

ADVERSE EFFECTS/TOXIC REACTIONS
Myelosuppression (anemia, lymphopenia, thrombocytopenia) is an expected response to therapy. Life-threatening QT interval prolongation, torsades de pointes may occur. QTc interval prolongation greater than 60 msec from base-

line reported in 11% of pts; greater than 501 msec reported in 6% of pts. Severe GI reactions including GI obstruction, colitis, ileus, stenosis was reported in less than 2% of pts. Grade 3 nausea, vomiting, diarrhea occurred in 9% of pts. GI bleeding occurred in 4% of pts. Serum ALT/AST elevation reported in 32% of pts. Hepatotoxicity may lead to liver injury and hepatitis. Life-threatening ILD/pneumonitis reported in 4% of pts. Pneumonia reported in 24% of pts.

NURSING CONSIDERATIONS

BASELINE ASSESSMENT

Obtain CBC, BMP, LFT, serum magnesium; pregnancy test in females of reproductive potential. Verify presence of *KRAS G12C* mutation in plasma or tumor specimens. Question history of hepatic impairment, pulmonary disease, congenital long QT syndrome. Assess hydration status. Obtain full medication history and screen for interactions. Offer emotional support.

INTERVENTION/EVALUATION

Monitor CBC, serum electrolytes as clinically indicated. Monitor LFT for hepatotoxicity (bruising, hematuria, jaundice, right upper abdominal pain, nausea, vomiting, weight loss) monthly for the first 3 mos, then as clinically indicated. Monitor for symptoms of QT interval prolongation (chest pain, dizziness, dyspnea, palpitations, syncope), esp. in pts taking concomitant QT interval–prolonging medications. If QT interval–prolonging medications cannot be withheld, diligently monitor ECG for QT interval prolongation, cardiac arrhythmias. Monitor daily pattern of bowel activity, stool consistency. Offer antiemetics for nausea; antidiarrheals for diarrhea. Severe diarrhea or vomiting may cause dehydration, electrolyte imbalance. Consider ABG, radiologic test if pneumonitis (excessive cough, dyspnea, fever, hypoxia) is suspected. Consider treatment with corticosteroids if pneumonitis is confirmed. Monitor for symptoms

of GI bleeding (melena, hypotension), GI tract obstruction (severe, persistent, or worsening of abdominal pain), pneumonia (cough, fatigue, fever).

PATIENT/FAMILY TEACHING

• Report liver problems (abdominal pain, bruising, clay-colored stool, amber or dark-colored urine, yellowing of the skin or eyes), inflammation of the lung (excessive cough, difficulty breathing, chest pain), symptoms of cardiac arrhythmia (chest pain, dizziness, fainting, fatigue, palpitations, shortness of breath), rectal bleeding or bloody stools, symptoms of pneumonia (cough, fatigue, fever). • Immediately report severe, persistent abdominal pain; may indicate blockage in GI tract. • Treatment may affect the electrical conduction of the heart, which may lead to arrhythmias; report chest pain, dizziness, fainting, palpitations. • There is a high risk of interactions with other medications. Do not take newly prescribed medications unless approved by prescriber who originally started treatment. • Severe diarrhea or vomiting may cause dehydration, electrolyte imbalance. Report diarrhea or vomiting that does not improve with medical management. Drink plenty of fluids. • Do not breastfeed.

adalimumab

a-da-**lim**-ue-mab
(Abrilada, Cyltezo, Hadlima, <u>Humira</u>, Humira Pen, Hyrimoz, Yusimry)

■ **BLACK BOX ALERT** ■ Increased risk for serious infections. Tuberculosis, invasive fungal infections, bacterial and viral opportunistic infections have occurred. Test for tuberculosis prior to and during treatment. Lymphoma, other malignancies reported in children/adolescents. Hepatosplenic T-cell lymphoma reported primarily in pts with Crohn's disease or ulcerative colitis and concomitant azaTHIOprine or mercaptopurine.

Do not confuse Humira with HumaLOG or HumuLIN, or adalimumab with sarilumab.

◆**CLASSIFICATION**

PHARMACOTHERAPEUTIC: Monoclonal antibody. **CLINICAL:** Antirheumatic, disease modifying; GI agent; TNF blocking agent.

USES

Ankylosing spondylitis (AS): Reduces signs/symptoms in adults with active AS. **Crohn's disease:** Treatment of moderate to severe active Crohn's disease in adults and pts 6 yrs and older. **Hyrdradentis suppurativa:** Treatment of moderate to severe hyrdradentis suppurativa in adults and pts 12 yrs and older. **Juvenile idiopathic arthritis:** Reduce signs/symptoms of moderate to severe active polyarticular juvenile arthritis in pts 2 yrs and older either alone or in combination with methotrexate. **Plaque psoriasis:** Treatment of adults with moderate to severe chronic plaque psoriasis who are candidates for systemic therapy or phototherapy and when other systemic therapies are less appropriate. **Psoriatic arthritis (PsA):** Reduce signs and symptoms; inhibit progression of structural damage; improve physical function in adults with active PsA (may be used alone or in combination with non-biologic DMARDs). **Rheumatoid arthritis (RA):** Reduces signs/symptoms, inhibits progression of structural damage, and improves physical function in adults with moderate to severe active RA. **Ulcerative colitis (UC):** Treatment of moderately to severely active ulcerative colitis in adults and pts 5 yrs and older. **Uveitis (UV):** Treatment of noninfectious intermediate uveitis, posterior uveitis, and panuveitis in adults and pts 2 yrs of age and older. **OFF-LABEL:** Nonradiographic axial spondyloarthritis, peripheral spondyloarthritis (nonpsoriatic), sarcoidosis.

PRECAUTIONS

Contraindications: Hypersensitivity to adalimumab. Severe infections (e.g., sepsis, TB).

Cautions: Pts with chronic infections or pts at risk for infections (e.g., diabetes, indwelling catheters, renal failure, open wounds), elderly, decreased left ventricular function, HF, demyelinating disorders, invasive fungal infections, history of malignancies.

ACTION

Binds specifically to tumor necrosis factor (TNF) alpha cell, blocking its interaction with cell surface TNF receptors and cytokine-driven inflammatory processes. **Therapeutic Effect:** Decreases signs/symptoms of RA, psoriatic arthritis, ankylosing spondylitis, Crohn's disease, ulcerative colitis. Inhibits progression of rheumatoid and psoriatic arthritis. Reduces epidermal thickness, inflammation of plaque psoriasis.

PHARMACOKINETICS

Metabolism not specified. Elimination not specified. **Half-life:** 10–20 days.

⧗ LIFESPAN CONSIDERATIONS

Pregnancy/Lactation: Unknown if distributed in breast milk. **Children:** Safety and efficacy not established. **Elderly:** Cautious use due to increased risk of serious infection and malignancy.

INTERACTIONS

DRUG: May increase the adverse effects of **abatacept, anakinra, belimumab, canakinumab, natalizumab, tofacitinib, vaccines (live), vedolizumab.** May decrease the therapeutic effect of **BCG (intravesical), vaccines (live).** May increase the immunosuppressive effects of **certolizumab. Tocilizumab** may increase immunosuppressive effect. **HERBAL:** Echinacea may decrease effects. **FOOD:** None known. **LAB VALUES:** May increase serum cholesterol, other lipids, alkaline phosphatase.

AVAILABILITY (Rx)

Single-dose prefilled pen: 80 mg/0.8 mL, 40 mg/0.8 mL, 40 mg/0.4 mL. **Single-dose prefilled glass syringe:** 80 mg/0.8 mL, 40 mg/0.8 mL, 40 mg/0.4 mL, 20 mg/0.4 mL, 20 mg/0.2 mL, 10 mg/0.2 mL, 10 mg/0.1 mL.

ADMINISTRATION/HANDLING
SQ
• Refrigerate; do not freeze. • Discard unused portion. • Rotate injection sites. Give new injection at least 1 inch from an old site and never into area where skin is tender, bruised, red, or hard. • Give in thigh or lower abdomen. • Avoid areas within 2 inches of navel.

INDICATIONS/ROUTES/DOSAGE
Rheumatoid Arthritis (RA)
SQ: ADULTS, ELDERLY: 40 mg every other wk. Dose may be increased to 40 mg/wk or 80 mg every other wk in pts not taking methotrexate.

Ankylosing Spondylitis, Psoriatic Arthritis
SQ: ADULTS, ELDERLY: 40 mg every other wk (may continue methotrexate, other nonbiologic DMARDS, corticosteroids, NSAIDS, and/or analgesics).

Crohn's Disease
SQ: ADULTS, ELDERLY, CHILDREN 6 YRS AND OLDER WEIGHING 40 KG OR MORE: Initially, 160 mg given on day 1 or 2 injections/day over 2 days, then 80 mg 2 wks later (day 15). **Maintenance:** 40 mg every other wk beginning at day 29. **CHILDREN 6 YRS AND OLDER WEIGHING 17–39 KG:** 80 mg, then 40 mg 2 wks later. **Maintenance:** 20 mg every other wk beginning at day 29.

Plaque Psoriasis, Adult Uveitis
SQ: ADULTS, ELDERLY: Initially, 80 mg as a single dose, then 40 mg every other wk starting 1 wk after initial dose.

Juvenile Rheumatoid Arthritis, Pediatric Uveitis
SQ: CHILDREN 2 YRS AND OLDER, WEIGHING 10–14 KG: 10 mg every other wk. **WEIGHING 15–29 KG:** 20 mg every other wk. **WEIGHING 30 KG OR MORE:** 40 mg every other wk.

Ulcerative Colitis
SQ: ADULTS, ELDERLY, CHILDREN 5 YRS AND OLDER WEIGHING 40 KG OR MORE: Initially, 160 mg (1 day or 2 injections split over 2 consecutive days), then 80 mg 2 wks later (day 15), then 40 mg every other wk beginning on day 29. **CHILDREN 5 YRS AND OLDER WEIGHING 20–39 KG:** Initially, 80 mg on day 1, then 40 mg given wkly for 2 wks (a dose on day 8 and day 15). **Maintenance (beginning day 29):** 40 mg q2wks or 20 mg every wk.

Hidradenitis Suppurativa
SQ: ADULTS, ELDERLY, CHILDREN 12 YRS AND OLDER WEIGHING 60 KG OR GREATER: Initially, 160 mg (day 1) or 80 mg (days 1 and 2), then 80 mg 2 wks later (day 15), then 40 mg weekly or 80 mg every other wk beginning day 29. **CHILDREN 12 YRS AND OLDER WEIGHING 30-59 KG:** Initially, 80 mg on day 1, then 40 mg every other wk (beginning day 8).

Dosage in Renal/Hepatic Impairment
No dose adjustment.

SIDE EFFECTS
Frequent (20%): Injection site erythema, pruritus, pain, swelling. **Occasional (12%–9%):** Headache, rash, sinusitis, nausea. **Rare (7%–5%):** Abdominal or back pain, hypertension.

ADVERSE EFFECTS/TOXIC REACTIONS
Hypersensitivity reactions (rash, urticaria, hypotension, dyspnea), infections (primarily upper respiratory tract, bronchitis, urinary tract) occur rarely. May increase risk of serious infections (pneumonia, tuberculosis, cellulitis, pyelonephritis, septic arthritis). May increase risk of reactivation of hepatitis B virus in pts who are chronic carriers. May cause new onset or exacerbation of central nervous demyelinating disease; worsening and new-onset HF. May increase risk of malignancies.

NURSING CONSIDERATIONS
BASELINE ASSESSMENT
Assess onset, type, location, duration of pain or inflammation. Inspect appearance of affected joints for immobility, deformities, skin condition. Review immunization status/

 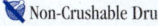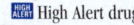

screening for TB. If pt is to self-administer, instruct on SQ injection technique, including areas of the body acceptable for injection sites.

INTERVENTION/EVALUATION

Monitor lab values, particularly CBC. Assess for therapeutic response: Relief of pain, stiffness, swelling; increased joint mobility; reduced joint tenderness; improved grip strength.

PATIENT/FAMILY TEACHING

• Injection site reaction generally occurs in first month of treatment and decreases in frequency during continued therapy. • Do not receive live vaccines during treatment. • Report rash, nausea. • A healthcare provider will show you how to properly prepare and inject your medication. You must demonstrate correct preparation and injection techniques before using medication.

---

ado-trastuzumab emtansine

ado-tras-**tooz**-oo-mab
(Kadcyla)

■ **BLACK BOX ALERT** ■ Do not substitute ado-trastuzumab for trastuzumab. Hepatotoxicity, hepatic failure may lead to death. Monitor hepatic function prior to each dose. May decrease left ventricular ejection fraction (LVEF). Embryo-fetal toxicity may result in birth defects and/or fetal demise.
Do not confuse ado-trastuzumab with trastuzumab.

◆CLASSIFICATION

PHARMACOTHERAPEUTIC: Anti-HER2. Antibody drug conjugate. Anti-microtubular. Monoclonal antibody. **CLINICAL:** Antineoplastic.

USES

Treatment of HER2-positive, metastatic breast cancer in pts who have previously received trastuzumab and a taxane agent separately or in combination (pts should have either received prior therapy for met-astatic disease or developed disease recurrence during or within 6 mos of completing adjuvant therapy). Adjuvant treatment of human epidermal growth factor receptor 2 (HER2)–positive early breast cancer in pts with residual invasive disease after taxane and trastuzumab-based treatment.

PRECAUTIONS

Contraindications: Hypersensitivity to trastuzumab. **Cautions:** History of cardiomyopathy, HF, MI, arrhythmias, hepatic disease, thrombocytopenia, pulmonary disease, peripheral neuropathy, pregnancy.

ACTION

Binds to HER2 receptor and undergoes receptor-mediated lysosomal degradation, resulting in intracellular release of DM1-containing cytotoxic catabolites. Binding of DM1 to tubulin disrupts microtubule networks in the cell. **Therapeutic Effect:** Inhibits tumor cell survival in HER2-positive breast cancer.

PHARMACOKINETICS

Metabolized in liver. Protein binding: 93%. Peak plasma concentration: 30–90 min. **Half-life:** 4 days.

⧖ LIFESPAN CONSIDERATIONS

Pregnancy/Lactation: Avoid pregnancy; may cause fetal harm. Females of reproductive potential should use effective contraception during treatment and for at least 6 mos after discontinuation. Unknown if distributed in breast milk. **Children:** Safety and efficacy not established. **Elderly:** No age-related precautions noted.

INTERACTIONS

DRUG: May decrease the therapeutic effect of **BCG (intravesical), vaccines (live).** May increase adverse effects of **vaccines (live). Strong CYP3A4 inhibitors (e.g., clarithromycin, ketoconazole, ritonavir)** may increase concentration/effect. **HERBAL: Echinacea** may decrease therapeutic effect.

FOOD: None known. **LAB VALUES:** May increase serum ALT, AST, bilirubin. May decrease platelets, serum potassium.

AVAILABILITY (Rx)

Lyophilized Powder for Injection: 100-mg vial, 160-mg vial.

ADMINISTRATION/HANDLING

◄ **ALERT** ► Use 0.22-micron in-line filter. Do not administer IV push or bolus.

 IV

Reconstitution • Must be prepared by personnel trained in aseptic manipulations and admixing of cytotoxic drugs. • Slowly inject 5 mL of Sterile Water for Injection into 100-mg vial or 8 mL Sterile Water for Injection for 160-mg vial. • Final concentration: 20 mg/mL. • Gently swirl until completely dissolved. Do not shake. • Inspect for particulate matter/discoloration. • Calculate dose from 20 mg/mL vial. • Further dilute in 250 mL of 0.9% NaCl only. • Invert bag to mix (do not shake).

Rate of administration • Infuse using 0.22-micron in-line filter. • Infuse initial dose over 90 min. • Infuse subsequent doses over 30 min. • Slow or interrupt infusion rate if hypersensitivity reaction occurs.

Storage • Refrigerate unused vials. • Reconstituted vials, diluted solutions should be used immediately (may be refrigerated for up to 24 hrs).

⚛ IV INCOMPATIBILITIES

Do not use dextrose-containing solutions.

INDICATIONS/ROUTES/DOSAGE

Note: Do not substitute with conventional trastuzumab (Herceptin).

Metastatic Breast Cancer

IV infusion: **ADULTS/ELDERLY:** 3.6 mg/kg every 3 wks until disease progression or unacceptable toxicity. **Maximum:** 3.6 mg/kg.

Breast Cancer, Early, HER2 Positive, Adjuvant Therapy

IV infusion: **ADULTS/ELDERLY:** 3.6 mg/kg q3wks for 14 cycles (in the absence of disease recurrence or unacceptable toxicity). **Maximum:** 3.6 mg/kg.

Dose Modification

Reduction Schedule for Adverse Effects
Initial dose: 3.6 mg/kg. **First reduction:** 3 mg/kg. **Second reduction:** 2.4 mg/kg.

Hepatotoxicity
Elevated serum ALT, AST: If less than 5 times upper limit of normal (ULN), continue same dose. If 5–20 times ULN, hold until less than 5 times ULN and reduce by one dose level. If greater than 20 times ULN, discontinue. **Elevated serum bilirubin:** Hold until less than 1.5 times ULN, then continue same dose. If 3–10 times ULN, hold until less than 1.5 times ULN, then reduce by one dose level. If greater than 10 times ULN, discontinue.

Cardiotoxicity
Left ventricular dysfunction: If LVEF greater than 45%, continue same dose. If LVEF 40%–45% with a decrease less than 10% from baseline, continue dose (or reduce) and repeat LVEF in 3 wks. If LVEF 40%–45% with decrease greater than 10% from baseline, hold and repeat assessment in 3 wks. Discontinue therapy if no recovery within 10% of baseline, LVEF less than 40%, or symptomatic HF.

Thrombocytopenia
Platelet count 25,000–50,000 cells/mm³: Withhold treatment until improved to 75,000 cells/mm³, then continue same dose. **Platelet count less than 25,000 cells/mm³:** Withhold treatment until improved to 75,000 cells/mm³, then reduce dose level.

Dosage in Renal/Hepatic Impairment

No dose adjustment.

SIDE EFFECTS

Frequent (40%–21%): Nausea, fatigue, musculoskeletal pain, headache, con-

 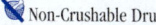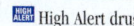

stipation, diarrhea. **Occasional (19%–7%):** Abdominal pain, vomiting, pyrexia, arthralgia, asthenia, cough, dry mouth, stomatitis, myalgia, insomnia, rash, dizziness, dyspepsia, chills, dysgeusia, peripheral edema. **Rare (6%–3%):** Pruritus, blurry vision, dry eye, conjunctivitis, lacrimation.

ADVERSE EFFECTS/TOXIC REACTIONS

Hepatotoxicity may include elevated transaminase, nodular regenerative hyperplasia, portal hypertension. Left ventricular dysfunction reported in 1.8% of pts. Interstitial lung disease (ILD), including pneumonitis, may lead to ARDS. Hypersensitivity reactions reported in 1.4% of pts. Thrombocytopenia (34% of pts) may increase risk of bleeding. Peripheral neuropathy observed rarely.

NURSING CONSIDERATIONS

BASELINE ASSESSMENT

Obtain CBC, BMP. Confirm HER2-positive status. Screen for baseline HF, hepatic impairment, peripheral edema, pulmonary disease, thrombocytopenia. Obtain negative pregnancy test before initiating treatment. Question current breastfeeding status. Obtain baseline echocardiogram for LVEF status.

INTERVENTION/EVALUATION

Monitor LFT, potassium levels before initiation and during treatment. Obtain LVEF q3mos or with any dose reduction regarding LVEF status. Observe for hypersensitivity reactions during infusion. Assess for bruising, jaundice, right upper quadrant (RUQ) abdominal pain. Obtain stat ECG for palpitations or irregular pulse, chest X-ray for difficulty breathing, cough, fever. Monitor for neurotoxicity (peripheral neuropathy).

PATIENT/FAMILY TEACHING

• Report black/tarry stools, RUQ abdominal pain, nausea, bruising, yellowing of skin or eyes, difficulty breathing, palpitations, bleeding. • Avoid alcohol. • Treatment may reduce the heart's ability to pump effectively; expect routine echocardiograms. • Report bleeding of any kind or extremity numbness, tingling, weakness, pain. • Use effective contraception to avoid pregnancy. Do not breastfeed.

afatinib

a-**fa**-ti-nib
(Gilotrif)
Do not confuse afatinib with ibrutinib, dasatinib, gefitinib, or SUNItinib.

◆CLASSIFICATION

PHARMACOTHERAPEUTIC: Epidermal growth factor receptor (EGFR) inhibitor. Tyrosine kinase inhibitor. **CLINICAL:** Antineoplastic.

USES

First-line treatment of metastatic non–small-cell lung cancer (NSCLC) in pts with epidermal growth factor (EDGF) exon 19 deletions or exon 21 (L858R) substitution mutations. Treatment of metastatic, squamous NSCLC progressing after platinum-based chemotherapy.

PRECAUTIONS

Contraindications: Hypersensitivity to afatinib. **Cautions:** Hepatic impairment; severe renal impairment; pts with hx of keratitis, severe dry eye, ulcerative keratitis, or use of contact lenses; hypovolemia; pulmonary disease; ulcerative lesions. Patients with GI disorders associated with diarrhea (e.g., Crohn's disease), cardiac risk factors, and/or decreased left ventricular ejection fraction.

ACTION

Highly selective blocker of ErbB family (e.g., EGFR, HER2); irreversibly binds to intracellular tyrosine kinase domain. **Therapeutic Effect:** Inhibits tumor growth, causes tumor regression.

PHARMACOKINETICS

Widely distributed. Enzymatic metabolism is minimal. Protein binding: 95%. Peak plasma concentration: 2–5 hrs. Excreted in feces (85%), urine (4%). **Half-life:** 37 hrs.

⧗ LIFESPAN CONSIDERATIONS

Pregnancy/Lactation: Avoid pregnancy; may cause fetal harm. Females of reproductive potential should use effective contraception during treatment and for at least 2 wks after discontinuation. Unknown if distributed in breast milk. May cause infertility in both females and males. **Children:** Safety and efficacy not established. **Elderly:** No age-related precautions noted.

INTERACTIONS

DRUG: P-glycoprotein inhibitors **(e.g., amiodarone, cycloSPORINE, ketoconazole)** may increase concentration/effect. **P-glycoprotein inducers (e.g., carBAMazepine, rifAMPin)** may decrease concentration/effect. **HERBAL:** None significant. **FOOD:** High-fat meals may decrease absorption. **LAB VALUES:** May increase serum ALT, AST. May decrease serum potassium.

AVAILABILITY (Rx)

Tablets: 20 mg, 30 mg, 40 mg.

ADMINISTRATION/HANDLING

PO

• Give at least 1 hr before or 2 hrs after meal. Do not take missed dose within 12 hrs of next dose.

INDICATIONS/ROUTES/DOSAGE

Metastatic NSCLC, Metastatic Squamous NSCLC

PO: ADULTS/ELDERLY: Initially, 40 mg once daily until disease progression or no longer tolerated. Do not take missed dose within 12 hrs of next dose.

Dose Modification

Chronic use of P-glycoprotein (P-gp) inhibitors: Reduce daily dose by 10 mg. Resume previous dose after discontinuation of inhibitor if tolerated. **Chronic use of P-glycoprotein inducers:** Increase daily dose by 10 mg if tolerated. May resume initial dose 2–3 days after discontinuation of P-gp inducer. **Moderate to severe diarrhea (more than 48 hrs):** Withhold dose until resolution to mild diarrhea. **Moderate cutaneous skin reaction (more than 7 days):** Withhold dose until reaction resolves, then reduce dose appropriately. **Suspected keratitis:** Withhold until appropriately ruled out. If keratitis confirmed, continue only if benefits outweigh risks.

Permanent Discontinuation

Discontinue if persistent severe diarrhea, respiratory distress, severe dry eye, or life-threatening bullous, blistering, exfoliating lesions, persistent ulcerative keratitis, interstitial lung disease, symptomatic left ventricular dysfunction occurs.

Dosage in Renal Impairment

Mild to moderate impairment: No dose adjustment. **Severe impairment (eGFR 15–29 mL/min):** Decrease starting dose to 30 mg once daily.

Dosage in Hepatic Impairment

Mild to moderate impairment: No dose adjustment. **Severe impairment:** Not specified; use caution.

SIDE EFFECTS

Frequent (96%–58%): Diarrhea, rash, dermatitis, stomatitis, paronychia (nail infection). **Occasional (31%–11%):** Dry skin, decreased appetite, pruritus, epistaxis, weight loss, cystitis, pyrexia, cheilitis (lip inflammation), rhinorrhea, conjunctivitis.

ADVERSE EFFECTS/TOXIC REACTIONS

Diarrhea may lead to severe, sometimes fatal, dehydration or renal impairment. Bullous and exfoliative skin lesions occur rarely. Rash, erythema, acneiform lesions occur in 90% of pts. Palmar-plantar erythrodysesthesia syndrome (PPES), a chemotherapy-induced skin condition that presents with redness, swelling, numbness, skin sloughing of the hands and feet, has been reported. Interstitial lung disease (ILD), including pulmonary infiltration, pneumonitis, ARDS, allergic alveolitis, reported in 2% of pts. Hepatotoxicity reported in 10% of pts. Keratitis symptoms, such as eye inflammation, lacrimation, light sensitivity, blurred vision, red eye, occurred in 1% of pts.

NURSING CONSIDERATIONS

BASELINE ASSESSMENT

Obtain CBC, BMP, visual acuity. Obtain negative pregnancy test before initiating therapy. Question current breastfeeding status. Screen for history/comorbidities, contact lens use. Receive full medication history, including herbal products. Assess skin for lesions, ulcers, open wounds.

INTERVENTION/EVALUATION

Monitor renal/hepatic function tests, urine output. Encourage PO intake. Assess for hydration status. Offer antidiarrheal medication for loose stool. Report oliguria, dark or concentrated urine. Immediately report skin lesions, vision changes, dry eye, severe diarrhea. Consider ABG, radiologic test if ILD/pneumonitis (excessive cough, dyspnea, fever, hypoxia) is suspected. Consider treatment with corticosteroids if ILD/pneumonitis is confirmed. Assess skin for dermal changes, toxicities.

PATIENT/FAMILY TEACHING

• Most pts experience diarrhea, and severe cases may lead to dehydration or kidney failure; maintain adequate hydration. • Use effective contraception to avoid pregnancy. Do not breastfeed. • Report any yellowing of skin or eyes, abdominal pain, bruising, black/tarry stools, dark urine, decreased urine output. • Minimize exposure to sunlight. • Immediately report eye problems (pain, swelling, blurred vision, vision changes) or skin blistering/redness. • Do not wear contact lenses (may increase risk of keratitis).

albumin

al-**bue**-min
(Albuked-5, Albuked-25, AlbuRx, Albutein, Flexbumin, Kedbumin, Plasbumin-5, Plasbumin-25)
Do not confuse albumin or Albutein with albuterol, or Buminate with bumetanide.

◆**CLASSIFICATION**

PHARMACOTHERAPEUTIC: Plasma protein fraction. **CLINICAL:** Blood derivative.

USES

Treatment of hypovolemia (with or without shock), hypoalbuminemia. To maintain cardiovascular function following the removal of large volumes of ascitic fluid after paracentesis due to cirrhotic ascites. Plasma expander in fluid management relating to severe forms of ovarian hyperstimulation syndrome (OHSS). Used in conjunction with diuretics to correct the fluid volume overload associated with ARDS, acute nephrosis. **OFF-LABEL:** Heptaorenal syndrome or acute kidney injury in cirrhosis.

PRECAUTIONS

Contraindications: Hypersensitivity to albumin. Pts at risk for volume overload (e.g., severe anemia, HF, renal insufficiency). Dilution with Sterile Water for Injection may cause hemolysis or acute renal failure. **Cautions:** Pts for whom sodium restriction is necessary, hepatic/renal failure (added protein load). Avoid 25% concentration in preterm infants (risk of intraventricular hemorrhage).

ACTION

Blood volume expander. **Therapeutic Effect:** Provides increase in intravascular oncotic pressure, mobilizes fluids into intravascular space.

PHARMACOKINETICS

Route	Onset	Peak	Duration
IV	15 min (in well-hydrated pt)	N/A	Dependent on initial blood volume

Distributed throughout extracellular fluid. **Half-life:** 15–20 days.

⌛ LIFESPAN CONSIDERATIONS

Pregnancy/Lactation: Unknown if drug crosses placenta or is distributed in breast milk. **Children/Elderly:** No age-related precautions noted.

INTERACTIONS

DRUG: None significant. **HERBAL:** None significant. **FOOD:** None known. **LAB VALUES:** May increase serum alkaline phosphatase.

AVAILABILITY (Rx)

Injection Solution: (5%): 50 mL, 250 mL, 500 mL. **(25%):** 20 mL, 50 mL, 100 mL.

ADMINISTRATION/HANDLING
🖐 IV

Reconstitution • A 5% solution may be made from 25% solution by adding 1 volume 25% to 4 volumes 0.9% NaCl (NaCl preferred). Do not use Sterile Water for Injection (life-threatening hemolysis, acute renal failure can result). **Rate of administration** • Infusion rate is variable, depending on use, blood volume, concentration of solute. **5%:** Do not exceed 2–4 mL/min in pts with normal plasma volume, 5–10 mL/min in pts with hypoproteinemia. **25%:** Do not exceed 1 mL/min in pts with normal plasma volume, 2–3 mL/min in pts with hypoproteinemia. 5% is administered undiluted; 25% may be administered undiluted or diluted in 0.9% NaCl. • May give without regard to pt blood group or Rh factor.
Storage • Store at room temperature. Appears as clear brownish, odorless, moderately viscous fluid. • Do not use if solution has been frozen, appears turbid, contains sediment, or if not used within 4 hrs of opening vial.

🔳 IV INCOMPATIBILITIES

Fat emulsion.

🔳 IV COMPATIBILITIES

Diltiazem, hydrocortisone, labetalol, lorazepam, midazolam, verapamil.

INDICATIONS/ROUTES/DOSAGE

◀ **ALERT** ▶ 5% should be used in hypovolemic or intravascularly depleted pts. 25% should be used in pts in whom fluid and sodium intake must be minimized.

Usual Dosage
IV: **ADULTS, ELDERLY:** Initially, 25 g; may repeat in 15–30 min if response is inadequate.

Dosage in Renal/Hepatic Impairment
No dose adjustment.

SIDE EFFECTS

Occasional: Hypotension. **Rare:** High dose in repeated therapy: Altered vital signs, chills, fever, increased salivation, nausea, vomiting, urticaria, tachycardia.

ADVERSE EFFECTS/TOXIC REACTIONS

Fluid overload may occur, marked by increased B/P, distended neck veins. Pulmonary edema may occur, evidenced by labored respirations, dyspnea, rales, wheezing, coughing. Neurologic changes, including headache, weakness, blurred vision, behavioral changes, incoordination, isolated muscle twitching, may occur.

NURSING CONSIDERATIONS

BASELINE ASSESSMENT
Obtain vital signs. Adequate hydration is required before albumin is administered.

INTERVENTION/EVALUATION
Monitor B/P for hypotension/hypertension. Assess frequently for evidence of fluid overload, pulmonary edema (see **Adverse Effects/Toxic Reactions**). Check skin for flushing, urticaria. Monitor I&O ratio (watch for decreased output). Assess for therapeutic response (increased B/P, decreased edema).

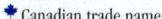 Canadian trade name   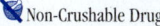 Non-Crushable Drug   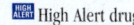 High Alert drug

albuterol

al-**bue**-ter-ol

(Airomir ✦, ProAir RespiClick, Proventil HFA, Ventolin HFA)

Do not confuse albuterol with albumin or atenolol, Proventil with Bentyl, PriLOSEC, or Prinivil, or Ventolin with Benylin or Vantin.

FIXED-COMBINATION(S)

Airsupra: albuterol/budesonide (a corticosteroid) 90 mcg/80 mcg per actuation. **Combivent Respimat:** albuterol/ipratropium (a bronchodilator): 100 mcg/20 mcg per actuation. **DuoNeb:** albuterol/ipratropium 3 mg/0.5 mg.

◆CLASSIFICATION

PHARMACOTHERAPEUTIC: Sympathomimetic (adrenergic beta$_2$-agonist). **CLINICAL:** Bronchodilator.

USES

Inhalation: Treatment or prevention of bronchospasm due to reversible obstructive airway disease in adults and pts 4 yrs and older. Prevention of exercise-induced bronchospasm in adults and pts 4 yrs and older. **Nebulization:** Treatment of bronchospasm in pts with COPD; acute attacks of bronchospasm in adults and pts aged 2 yrs and older. **OFF-LABEL:** Hyperkalemia.

PRECAUTIONS

ConInhalation: dications: Hypersensitivity to albuterol. Severe hypersensitivity to milk protein (dry powder inhalation). **Cautions:** Hypertension, cardiovascular disease, hyperthyroidism, diabetes, HF, convulsive disorders, glaucoma, hypokalemia, history of cardiac arrhythmias.

ACTION

Stimulates beta$_2$-adrenergic receptors in lungs, resulting in relaxation of bronchial smooth muscle (little effect on HR). **Therapeutic Effect:** Relieves bronchospasm and reduces airway resistance.

PHARMACOKINETICS

Route	Onset	Peak	Duration
PO	15–30 min	2–3 hrs	4–6 hrs
PO (extended-release)	30 min	2–4 hrs	12 hrs
Inhalation	5–15 min	0.5–2 hrs	2–5 hrs

Rapidly, well absorbed from GI tract; rapidly absorbed from bronchi after inhalation. Metabolized in liver. Primarily excreted in urine. **Half-life:** 3.8–6 hrs.

⧗ LIFESPAN CONSIDERATIONS

Pregnancy/Lactation: Appears to cross placenta; unknown if distributed in breast milk. May inhibit uterine contractility. **Children:** Safety and efficacy not established in pts younger than 2 yrs (syrup) or younger than 6 yrs (tablets). **Elderly:** May be more sensitive to tremor or tachycardia due to age-related increased sympathetic sensitivity.

INTERACTIONS

DRUG: Beta-blockers (e.g., **carvedilol, labetalol, metoprolol**) may decrease concentration/effect. **MAOIs** (e.g., **phenelzine, selegiline**), **linezolid, sympathomimetics** (e.g., **dopamine, norepinephrine**) may increase concentration/effect. May increase concentration/effect of **sympathomimetics** (e.g., **norepinephrine**). **HERBAL:** None significant. **FOOD:** None known. **LAB VALUES:** May increase blood glucose. May decrease serum potassium.

AVAILABILITY (Rx)

Powder Breath Activated Inhalation Aerosol: *(ProAir RespiClick):* 90 mcg/actuation. **Inhalation Aerosol Solution:** *(Proventil HFA, Ventolin HFA):* 90 mcg/spray. **Solution for Nebulization:** 0.63 mg/3 mL (0.021%), 1.25 mg/3 mL (0.042%), 2.5 mg/3 mL (0.084%), 5 mg/mL (0.5%). **Syrup:** 2 mg/5 mL. **Tablets:** 2 mg, 4 mg.

ADMINISTRATION/HANDLING

Inhalation Aerosol

• Shake container well before inhalation. • Prime prior to first use. A spacer is recommended for use with MDI. • Wait 2 min before inhaling second dose (allows for deeper bronchial penetration). • Rinse mouth with water immediately after inhalation (prevents mouth/throat dryness).

Inhalation Powder

• Device is breath activated. • Do not use with spacer. • Do not wash or put any part of inhaler in water.

Nebulization

• Administer over 5–15 min.

INDICATIONS/ROUTES/DOSAGE

Bronchspasm

Inhalation: ADULTS, ELDERLY, CHILDREN 4 YRS AND OLDER: 2 inhalations repeated q4–6h (1 inhalation q4h may be sufficient). **Nebulization: ADULTS, ELDERLY, CHILDREN OLDER THAN 12 YRS:** 2.5 mg q4–6hr prn. **CHILDREN 2–11 YRS:** 0.63–1.25 mg 3–4 times/day.

Exercise-Induced Bronchospasm

Inhalation: ADULTS, ELDERLY, CHILDREN 4 YRS AND OLDER: 2 inhalations 15–30 min before exercise.

Dosage in Renal/Hepatic Impairment

No dose adjustment.

SIDE EFFECTS

Frequent (27%–4%): Headache, restlessness, nervousness, tremors, nausea, dizziness, throat dryness and irritation, pharyngitis, B/P changes including hypertension, heartburn, transient wheezing. **Occasional (3%–2%):** Insomnia, asthenia, altered taste. **Inhalation:** Dry, irritated mouth or throat; cough, bronchial irritation. **Rare:** Drowsiness, diarrhea, dry mouth, flushing, diaphoresis, anorexia.

ADVERSE EFFECTS/TOXIC REACTIONS

Excessive sympathomimetic stimulation may produce palpitations, ectopy, tachycardia, chest pain, slight increase in B/P followed by substantial decrease, chills, diaphoresis, blanching of skin. Too-frequent or excessive use may lead to decreased bronchodilating effectiveness and severe, paradoxical bronchoconstriction.

NURSING CONSIDERATIONS

BASELINE ASSESSMENT

Assess lung sounds, pulse, B/P, characteristics of sputum. Offer emotional support (high incidence of anxiety due to difficulty in breathing and sympathomimetic response to drug).

INTERVENTION/EVALUATION

Monitor rate, depth, rhythm, type of respiration; quality and rate of pulse; ECG; serum potassium, glucose; ABG determinations. Assess lung sounds for wheezing (bronchoconstriction), rales.

PATIENT/FAMILY TEACHING

• Follow guidelines for proper use of inhaler. • Increase fluid intake (decreases lung secretion viscosity). • Do not take more than 2 inhalations at any one time (excessive use may produce paradoxical bronchoconstriction or decreased bronchodilating effect). • Rinsing mouth with water immediately after inhalation may prevent mouth/throat dryness. • Avoid excessive use of caffeine derivatives (chocolate, coffee, tea, cola, cocoa).

alectinib

al-**ek**-ti-nib
(Alecensa, Alecensaro ♦)
Do not confuse alectinib with afatinib, ibrutinib, imatinib, or gefitinib.

◆CLASSIFICATION

PHARMACOTHERAPEUTIC: Tyrosine kinase inhibitor. Anaplastic lymphoma kinase (ALK) inhibitor. **CLINICAL:** Antineoplastic.

 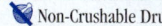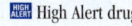

USES

Treatment of pts with anaplastic lymphoma kinase (ALK)—positive metastatic non—small-cell lung cancer (NSCLC). Adjuvant treatment in pts following tumor resection of (ALK)-positive NSCLC (tumors 4 cm or greater or node positive).

PRECAUTIONS

Contraindications: Hypersensitivity to alectinib. **Cautions:** Baseline cytopenias; bradycardia, bradyarrhythmias, chronic edema, diabetes, dehydration, electrolyte imbalance, hepatic/renal impairment, HF, ocular disease, pulmonary disease, history of thromboembolism.

ACTION

Inhibits ALK. ALK gene abnormalities may result in expression of oncogenic fusion proteins, which alter signaling and result in increased cellular proliferation/survival in tumors. **Therapeutic Effect:** Inhibition of ALK decreases tumor cell viability.

PHARMACOKINETICS

Metabolized in liver. Protein binding: Greater than 99%. Peak plasma concentration: 4 hrs. Steady state reached in 7 days. Excreted in feces (98%), urine (less than 0.5%). **Half-life:** 33 hrs.

⧖ LIFESPAN CONSIDERATIONS

Pregnancy/Lactation: Avoid pregnancy; may cause fetal harm. Females of reproductive potential should use effective contraception during treatment and for at least 1 wk after discontinuation. Unknown if distributed in breast milk. Breastfeeding not recommended during treatment and for at least 1 wk after discontinuation. **Males:** Males with female partners of reproductive potential must use barrier methods during treatment and up to 3 mos after discontinuation.

Children/Elderly: Safety and efficacy not established.

INTERACTIONS

DRUG: None significant. **HERBAL:** None significant. **FOOD: High-fat, high-calorie meals** increase absorption/exposure. **LAB VALUES:** May increase serum alkaline phosphatase, ALT, AST, bilirubin, CPK, creatinine, glucose. May decrease serum calcium, potassium, phosphate, sodium; Hgb, Hct, lymphocytes, RBCs.

AVAILABILITY (Rx)

◥ **Capsules:** 150 mg.

ADMINISTRATION/HANDLING

PO

• Give with food. • Administer whole; do not break, crush, cut, or open capsules. • If a dose is missed or vomiting occurs during administration, give next dose at regularly scheduled time.

INDICATIONS/ROUTES/DOSAGE

Non–Small-Cell Lung Cancer (Treatment/ Adjuvant Treatment)

PO: ADULTS, ELDERLY: 600 mg twice daily until disease progression or unacceptable toxicity.

Dose Reduction Schedule

First dose reduction: 450 mg twice daily. **Second dose reduction:** 300 mg twice daily. Permanently discontinue if unable to tolerate 300 mg twice daily.

Dose Modification

Bradycardia

Symptomatic bradycardia: Withhold treatment until recovery to asymptomatic bradycardia or to a heart rate of 60 bpm or greater, then resume at reduced dose level (if pt not taking concomitant medications known to cause bradycardia). **Symptomatic bradycardia in pts taking concomitant medications known to cause bradycardia:** Withhold treatment until recovery to asymptomatic bradycardia or heart rate of 60 bpm or greater. If concomitant medication can be adjusted or discontinued, then resume at same dose. If concomitant medication cannot be adjusted or discontinued, then resume at reduced dose level. **Life-threatening bradycardia in pts who are not taking concomitant medications known to cause bradycardia:** Permanently discontinue. **Life-threatening bradycardia in pts who are taking concomitant medications known to cause bradycardia:** Withhold treatment until recovery to asymptomatic bradycardia or heart rate of 60 bpm or greater. If concomitant medication can be adjusted or discontinued, then resume at reduced dose level with frequent monitoring. Permanently discontinue if bradycardia recurs despite dose reduction.

CPK Elevation
CPK elevation greater than 5 times upper limit of normal (ULN): Withhold treatment until recovery to baseline or less than or equal to 2.5 times ULN, then resume at same dose. **CPK elevation greater than 10 times ULN or second occurrence of CPK elevation greater than 5 times ULN:** Withhold treatment until recovery to baseline or less than or equal to 2.5 times ULN, then resume at reduced dose level.

Hepatotoxicity
Serum ALT or AST elevation greater than 5 times ULN with total bilirubin less than or equal to 2 times ULN: Withhold treatment until serum ALT or AST recovers to baseline or less than or equal to 3 times ULN, then resume at reduced dose level. **Serum ALT or AST elevation greater than 3 times ULN with total serum bilirubin greater than 2 times ULN in the absence of cholestasis or hemolysis:** Permanently discontinue. **Total bilirubin elevation greater than 3 times ULN:** Withhold treatment until recovery to baseline or less than or equal to 1.5 times ULN, then resume at reduced dose level.

Pulmonary Toxicity
Any grade treatment-related interstitial lung disease/pneumonitis: Permanently discontinue.

Dosage in Renal Impairment
Mild to moderate impairment: No dose adjustment. **Severe impairment:** Not specified; use caution.

Dosage in Hepatic Impairment
Mild impairment: No dose adjustment. **Moderate to severe impairment:** Not specified; use caution.

SIDE EFFECTS
Frequent (41%–19%): Fatigue, asthenia, constipation, edema (peripheral, generalized, eyelid, periorbital), myalgia, musculoskeletal pain, cough, generalized rash, papular rash, pruritus, macular rash, maculopapular rash, acneiform dermatitis, erythema, nausea. **Occasional (18%–10%):** Headache, diarrhea, dyspnea, back pain, vomiting, increased weight, blurred vision, vitreous floaters, visual impairment, reduced visual acuity, asthenopia, diplopia, photosensitivity.

ADVERSE EFFECTS/TOXIC REACTIONS
Approx. 23% of pts required at least one dose reduction. Median time to first dose reduction was 48 days. Decreased Hgb levels were reported in 56% of pts. Drug-induced hepatotoxicity with elevations of serum ALT/AST greater than 5 times ULN reported in 4%–5% of pts. Most reported cases of hepatotoxicity occurred during first 2 mos of therapy. Grade 3 interstitial lung disease occurred in less than 1% of pts. Symptomatic bradycardia reported in 7.5% of pts. Severe myalgia, musculoskeletal pain occurred in 29% of pts. CPK elevation occurred in 43% of pts. Other serious adverse effects may include endocarditis, hemorrhage (unspecified), intestinal perforation, pulmonary embolism.

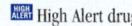

NURSING CONSIDERATIONS

BASELINE ASSESSMENT

Obtain CBC, BMP, LFT; pregnancy test in females of reproductive potential. Obtain baseline ECG in pts with history of arrhythmias, HF, concurrent use of medications known to cause bradycardia. Question history of hepatic/renal impairment, pulmonary embolism, diabetes, cardiac/pulmonary disease. Screen for medications known to cause bradycardia. Assess visual acuity. Verify ALK-positive NSCLC test prior to initiation.

INTERVENTION/EVALUATION

Monitor CBC routinely; LFTs q2wks during first 2 mos of treatment, then periodically thereafter (or more frequently in pts with hepatic impairment). Obtain BMP, serum ionized calcium, magnesium if arrhythmia or severe dehydration occurs. Monitor vital signs (esp. heart rate). Obtain ECG for bradycardia, chest pain, dyspnea. Consider ABG, radiologic test if ILD/pneumonitis (excessive cough, dyspnea, fever, hypoxia) is suspected. Consider treatment with corticosteroids if ILD/pneumonitis is confirmed. Monitor for hepatotoxicity, hyperglycemia, vision changes, myalgia, musculoskeletal pain.

PATIENT/FAMILY TEACHING

• Report history of heart problems including extremity swelling, HF, slow heart rate. Therapy may decrease your heart rate; report dizziness, chest pain, palpitations, or fainting. • Worsening cough, fever, or shortness of breath may indicate severe lung inflammation. • Use effective contraception to avoid pregnancy. Do not breastfeed. • Blurry vision, confusion, frequent urination, increased thirst, fruity breath may indicate high blood sugar levels. • Report any yellowing of skin or eyes, upper abdominal pain, bruising, black/tarry stools, dark urine. • Do not take newly prescribed medication unless approved by doctor who originally started treatment. • Avoid prolonged sun exposure/tanning beds. Use high SPF sunscreen and lip balm to protect against sunburn. • Take with food. • Avoid alcohol.

alendronate

a-**len**-dro-nate
(Binosto, Fosamax)
Do not confuse alendronate with risedronate, or Fosamax with Flomax.

FIXED-COMBINATION(S)

Fosamax Plus D: alendronate/cholecalciferol (vitamin D analogue): 70 mg/2,800 international units, 70 mg/5,600 international units.

◆CLASSIFICATION

PHARMACOTHERAPEUTIC: Bisphosphonate. **CLINICAL:** Bone resorption inhibitor, calcium regulator.

USES

Fosamax: Osteoporosis in postmenopausal females: Treatment of osteoporosis in postmenopausal females (increases bone mass, reduces incidence of fractures) and prevention of postmenopausal osteoporosis. **Increase bone mass in males with osteoporosis:** Treatment to increase bone mass in males with osteoporosis. **Glucocorticoid-induced osteoporosis:** Treatment of glucocorticoid-induced osteoporosis in men and women receiving glucocorticoids in a daily dosage equivalent to 7.5 mg or greater of prednisone and who have low bone mineral density. **Paget disease of bone:** Indicated in males and female pts with Paget disease of bone having alkaline phosphatase at least two times the upper limit of normal, or are symptomatic, or at risk for future complications from their disease. **Binosto:** Treatment of osteoporosis in males and postmenopausal women. **OFF-LABEL:** Prostate cancer (bone loss associated with androgen deprivation therapy).

PRECAUTIONS

Contraindications: Hypocalcemia, abnormalities of the esophagus, inability to stand or sit upright for at least 30 min, sensitivity to alendronate or other bisphosphonates; oral solution or effervescent tablet should not be used in pts at risk for aspiration. **Cautions:** Renal impairment, dysphagia, esophageal disease, gastritis, ulcers, or duodenitis.

ACTION

Inhibits bone resorption via actions on osteoclasts or osteoclast precursors. **Therapeutic Effect:** Leads to indirect increase in bone mineral density. **Paget's disease:** Inhibits bone resorption, leading to an indirect decrease in bone formation, but bone has a more normal architecture.

PHARMACOKINETICS

Widely distributed. Protein binding: 78%. After PO administration, rapidly taken into bone, with uptake greatest at sites of active bone turnover. Excreted in urine (as unabsorbed drug). **Terminal half-life:** Greater than 10 yrs (reflects release from bone).

⌛ LIFESPAN CONSIDERATIONS

Pregnancy/Lactation: Possible incomplete fetal ossification, decreased maternal weight gain, delay in delivery. Unknown if distributed in breast milk. Breastfeeding not recommended. **Children:** Safety and efficacy not established. **Elderly:** No age-related precautions noted.

INTERACTIONS

DRUG: **Antacids, calcium, iron, magnesium salts** may decrease the concentration/effect. **Aspirin, NSAIDs (e.g., ibuprofen, ketorolac, naproxen)** may increase adverse effects (e.g., increased risk of ulcer). **HERBAL:** None significant. **FOOD:** Concurrent **beverages, dietary supplements, food** may interfere with absorption. **Caffeine** may reduce efficacy. **LAB VALUES:** Reduces serum calcium, phosphate. Significant decrease in serum alkaline phosphatase noted in pts with Paget's disease.

AVAILABILITY (Rx)

Oral Solution: 70 mg/75 mL. **Tablets:** 5 mg, 10 mg, 35 mg, 70 mg. **Effervescent Tablets:** *(Binosto):* 70 mg.

ADMINISTRATION/HANDLING

PO
• **Tablets:** Give at least 30 min before first food, beverage, or medication of the day (except 6–8 oz plain water). Administer whole (do not allow chewing or sucking of tablet). **Tablets, effervescent:** Dissolve in 4 oz water. Wait at least 5 min after effervescence stops. Stir for 10 sec and drink. **Oral solution:** Follow with at least 2 oz of water.

INDICATIONS/ROUTES/DOSAGE

Note: Consider discontinuing after 3–5 yrs for osteoporosis in pts at low risk for fractures.

Osteoporosis
PO: **ADULTS, ELDERLY: Treatment:** 10 mg once daily in the morning or 70 mg weekly. **ADULTS, ELDERLY: Prevention:** 5 mg once daily in the morning or 35 mg weekly.

Paget's Disease
PO: **ADULTS, ELDERLY:** 40 mg once daily in the morning for 6 mos. A second course may be considered following a 6-mos posttreatment evaluation.

Dosage in Renal Impairment
Not recommended in pts with creatinine clearance less than 35 mL/min.

Dosage in Hepatic Impairment
No dose adjustment.

SIDE EFFECTS

Frequent (8%–7%): Back pain, abdominal pain. **Occasional (3%–2%):** Nausea, abdominal distention, constipation, diarrhea, flatulence. **Rare (less than 2%):** Rash; severe bone, joint, muscle pain.

ADVERSE EFFECTS/TOXIC REACTIONS

Overdose produces hypocalcemia, hypophosphatemia, significant GI disturbances.

 ✦ Canadian trade name   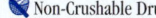 Non-Crushable Drug   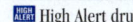 High Alert drug

Esophageal irritation occurs if not given with 6–8 oz of plain water or if pt lies down within 30 min of administration. May increase risk of osteonecrosis of the jaw.

NURSING CONSIDERATIONS

BASELINE ASSESSMENT
Obtain serum calcium, phosphate, alkaline phosphatase. Hypocalcemia, vitamin D deficiency must be corrected before beginning therapy. Assess pt's ability to remain upright for at least 30 minutes.

INTERVENTION/EVALUATION
Monitor chemistries (esp. serum calcium, phosphorus, alkaline phosphatase levels).

PATIENT/FAMILY TEACHING
• Expected benefits occur only when medication is taken with full glass (6–8 oz) of plain water, first thing in the morning and at least 30 min before first food, beverage, or medication of the day is taken. Any other beverage (mineral water, orange juice, coffee) significantly reduces absorption of medication. • Do not lie down for at least 30 min after taking medication (potentiates delivery to stomach, reducing risk of esophageal irritation). • Report new swallowing difficulties, pain when swallowing, chest pain, new/worsening heartburn. • Consider weight-bearing exercises, modify behavioral factors (e.g., cigarette smoking, alcohol consumption). • Supplemental calcium and vitamin D should be taken if dietary intake inadequate.

allopurinol

al-oh-**pure**-i-nol
(Aloprim, Zyloprim)
Do not confuse allopurinol with Apresoline or haloperidol, or Zyloprim with Zorprin or Zovirax.

Duzallo: allopurinol/lesinurad (uric acid transporter-1 inhibitor): 200 mg/200 mg, 300 mg/200 mg.

◆CLASSIFICATION

PHARMACOTHERAPEUTIC: Xanthine oxidase inhibitor. **CLINICAL:** Antigout agent.

USES

Gout: Management of primary or secondary gout (e.g., acute attack, nephropathy). **Nephrolithiasis:** Management of recurrent uric acid and calcium oxalate calculi in pts whose daily uric acid excretion >800 mg/day (males) or >750 mg/day (females). **Tumor lysis syndrome:** Management of elevated uric acid in cancer treatment for leukemia, lymphoma, or solid tumor malignancies.

PRECAUTIONS

Contraindications: Severe hypersensitivity to allopurinol. **Cautions:** Renal/hepatic impairment; pts taking diuretics, mercaptopurine or azaTHIOprine, other drugs causing myelosuppression. Do not use in asymptomatic hyperuricemia.

ACTION

Decreases uric acid production by inhibiting xanthine oxidase, an enzyme responsible for converting xanthine to uric acid. **Therapeutic Effect:** Reduces uric acid concentrations in serum and urine.

PHARMACOKINETICS

Route	Onset	Peak	Duration
PO, IV	2–3 days	1–3 wks	1–2 wks

Widely distributed. Protein binding: Less than 1%. Metabolized in liver. Excreted primarily in urine. Removed by hemodialysis. **Half-life:** 1–3 hrs; metabolite, 12–30 hrs.

⧗ LIFESPAN CONSIDERATIONS

Pregnancy/Lactation: Unknown if drug crosses placenta or is distributed in breast milk. **Children/Elderly:** No age-related precautions noted.

INTERACTIONS

DRUG: Angiotensin-converting enzyme (ACE) inhibitors (e.g., **enalapril, lisinopril**) may increase potential for hypersensitivity reactions. **Antacids** may decrease absorption. May increase concentration/effects of **azaTHIOprine, didanosine, mercaptopurine.** May increase adverse effects of **pegloticase.** May increase anticoagulant effect of **vitamin K antagonists (e.g., warfarin).** **HERBAL:** None significant. **FOOD:** None known. **LAB VALUES:** May increase serum BUN, alkaline phosphatase, ALT, AST, creatinine.

AVAILABILITY (Rx)

Injection, Powder for Reconstitution: *(Aloprim):* 500 mg. **Tablets:** *(Zyloprim):* 100 mg, 300 mg.

ADMINISTRATION/HANDLING

 IV

Reconstitution • Reconstitute 500-mg vial with 25 mL Sterile Water for Injection (concentration of 20 mg/mL). • Further dilute with 0.9% NaCl or D_5W (50–100 mL) to a concentration of 6 mg/mL or less. • Solution should appear clear and colorless.

Rate of administration • Infuse over 15–60 min. Daily doses can be given as a single infusion or in equally divided doses at 6-, 8-, or 12-hr intervals.

Storage • Store unreconstituted vials at room temperature. • Do not refrigerate reconstituted and/or diluted solution. Must administer within 10 hrs of preparation. • Do not use if precipitate forms or solution is discolored.

PO

• Give after meals with plenty of fluid. • Fluid intake should yield slightly alkaline urine and output of approximately 2 L in adults. • Dosages greater than 300 mg/day to be administered in divided doses.

IV INCOMPATIBILITIES

Cefotaxime, cytarabine, dacarbazine, diphenhydramine, gentamicin, methyl-PREDnisone, metoclopromide, ondansetron, tobramycin.

IV COMPATIBILITIES

Bumetanide (Bumex), calcium gluconate, furosemide (Lasix), heparin, HYDROmorphone (Dilaudid), LORazepam (Ativan), morphine, potassium chloride.

INDICATIONS/ROUTES/DOSAGE

◀**ALERT**▶ Doses greater than 300 mg should be given in divided doses.

Gout

PO: ADULTS, ELDERLY: Initially, 100 mg/day. Increase by 100 mg at 2–4 wk intervals needed to achieve desired serum uric acid level. **Maximum:** 800 mg/day.

Secondary Hyperuricemia Associated With Chemotherapy

Note: Begin 1–2 days before initiating induction of chemotherapy. May continue for 3–7 days after chemotherapy. **PO: ADULTS, CHILDREN OLDER THAN 10 YRS:** 600–800 mg/day in 2–3 divided doses. **CHILDREN 6–10 YRS:** 300 mg/day in 2–3 divided doses (50–100 mg/m² q8 hrs or 100 mg/m² q12 hrs). **CHILDREN YOUNGER THAN 6 YRS:** 150 mg/day in 3 divided doses. ◀**ALERT**▶ **IV:** Daily dose can be given as single infusion or at 6-, 8-, or 12-hr intervals. **IV: ADULTS, ELDERLY, CHILDREN 10 YRS OR OLDER:** 200–400 mg/m²/day. **Maximum:** 600 mg/day. **CHILDREN YOUNGER THAN 10 YRS:** 200 mg/m²/day. **Maximum:** 600 mg/day.

Recurrent Uric Acid Calcium Oxalate Calculi

PO: ADULTS: 300 mg/day in single or 2–3 divided doses.

Dosage in Renal Impairment

Dosage is modified based on creatinine clearance. **PO:** Removed by hemodialysis. Administer dose following hemodialysis or administer 50% supplemental dose.

 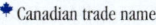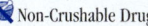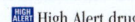

IV/PO

Creatinine Clearance	Dosage
10–20 mL/min	200 mg/day
3–9 mL/min	100 mg/day
Less than 3 mL/min	100 mg at extended intervals
HD	100 mg q48h (increase cautiously to 300 mg)

Dosage in Hepatic Impairment

No dose adjustment.

SIDE EFFECTS

Occasional: PO: Drowsiness, unusual hair loss. IV: Rash, nausea, vomiting. **Rare:** Diarrhea, headache.

ADVERSE EFFECTS/TOXIC REACTIONS

Pruritic maculopapular rash, possibly accompanied by malaise, fever, chills, joint pain, nausea, vomiting should be considered a toxic reaction. Severe hypersensitivity reaction may follow appearance of rash. Bone marrow depression, hepatotoxicity, peripheral neuritis, acute renal failure occur rarely.

NURSING CONSIDERATIONS

BASELINE ASSESSMENT

Obtain serum uric acid level, BMP; LFT in pts with hepatic impairment. Instruct pt to drink minimum of 2,500–3,000 mL of fluid daily while taking medication.

INTERVENTION/EVALUATION

Discontinue immediately if rash or allergic reaction occurs. Monitor I&O (output should be at least 2,000 mL/day). Assess serum chemistries, uric acid, hepatic function. Assess urine for cloudiness, unusual color, odor. **Gout:** Assess for therapeutic response: Relief of pain, stiffness, swelling; increased joint mobility; reduced joint tenderness; improved grip strength.

PATIENT/FAMILY TEACHING

• May take 1 wk or longer for full therapeutic effect. • Maintain adequate hydration; drink 2,500–3,000 mL of fluid daily while taking medication. • Avoid tasks that require alertness, motor skills until response to drug is established. • Avoid alcohol (may increase uric acid).

almotriptan

al-moe-**trip**-tan
Apo-Almotriptin ✦
Do not confuse almotriptan with alvimopan.

◆ CLASSIFICATION

PHARMACOTHERAPEUTIC: Serotonin receptor agonist (5-HT$_{1B}$). **CLINICAL:** Antimigraine.

USES

Acute treatment of migraine headache with or without aura in adults. Acute treatment of migraine headache in adolescents 12–17 yrs with history of migraine with or without aura and having attacks usually lasting 4 or more hrs when left untreated.

PRECAUTIONS

Contraindications: Hypersensitivity to almotriptan. Cerebrovascular disease (e.g., recent stroke, transient ischemic attacks), peripheral vascular disease, hemiplegic or basilar migraine, ischemic heart disease (including angina pectoris, history of MI, silent ischemia, and Prinzmetal's angina), uncontrolled hypertension, use within 24 hrs of ergotamine-containing preparations or another 5-HT$_{1B}$ agonist. **Cautions:** Mild to moderate renal or hepatic impairment, pt profile suggesting cardiovascular risks, controlled hypertension; history of CVA, sulfonamide allergy.

ACTION

Binds selectively to serotonin receptors in cranial arteries producing a vasoconstrictive effect. Decreases inflammation associated with relief of migraine. **Therapeutic Effect:** Produces relief of migraine headache.

PHARMACOKINETICS

Widely distributed. Protein binding: 35%. Metabolized by liver. Primarily excreted in urine. **Half-life:** 3–4 hrs.

⏳ LIFESPAN CONSIDERATIONS

Pregnancy/Lactation: Unknown if distributed in breast milk. **Children:** Safety and efficacy not established in pts younger than 12 yrs. **Elderly:** No age-related precautions noted.

INTERACTIONS

DRUG: May increase concentration/effects of **ergot derivatives (e.g., dihydroergotamine, ergotamine)**. **Strong CYP3A4 inhibitors (e.g., clarithromycin, ketoconazole, ritonavir)** may increase concentration/effect. **MAOIs (e.g., phenelzine, selegiline)** may increase concentration/effect. **HERBAL:** None significant. **FOOD:** None known. **LAB VALUES:** None significant.

AVAILABILITY (Rx)

 Tablets: 6.5 mg, 12.5 mg.

ADMINISTRATION/HANDLING

PO

• Administer whole; do not break, crush, dissolve, or divide tablets. • Take with full glass of water. • May give without regard to food.

INDICATIONS/ROUTES/DOSAGE

Migraine Headache

PO: ADULTS, ELDERLY, ADOLESCENTS 12–17 YRS: Initially, 6.25–12.5 mg as a single dose. If headache returns, dose may be repeated after 2 hrs. **Maximum:** 2 doses/24 hrs (25 mg).

Concurrent Use of CYP3A4 Inhibitors

ADULTS, ELDERLY: Recommended initial dose is 6.25 mg, maximum daily dose is 12.5 mg. Avoid use in pts with renal or

hepatic impairment AND use of CYP3A4 inhibitors.

Dosage in Renal Impairment

Creatinine clearance 30 mL/min or less: Initially, 6.25 mg in a single dose. **Maximum:** 12.5 mg/day.

Dosage in Hepatic Impairment

Initially, 6.25 mg in a single dose. **Maximum:** 12.5 mg/day.

SIDE EFFECTS

Rare (2%–1%): Nausea, dry mouth, headache, dizziness, somnolence, paresthesia, flushing.

ADVERSE EFFECTS/TOXIC REACTIONS

Excessive dosage may produce tremor, redness of extremities, decreased respirations, cyanosis, seizures, chest pain. Serious arrhythmias occur rarely but particularly in pts with hypertension, diabetes, obesity, smokers, and those with strong family history of coronary artery disease.

NURSING CONSIDERATIONS

BASELINE ASSESSMENT

Question history of peripheral vascular disease, cardiac conduction disorders, CVA. Assess onset, location, duration of migraine, and possible precipitating factors.

INTERVENTION/EVALUATION

Evaluate for relief of migraine headache and associated photophobia, phonophobia (sound sensitivity), nausea, vomiting.

PATIENT/FAMILY TEACHING

• Take a single dose as soon as symptoms of an actual migraine attack appear. • Medication is intended to relieve migraine, not to prevent or reduce number of attacks. • Lie down in quiet, dark room for additional benefit after taking medication. • Avoid tasks that require alertness, motor skills until response to drug is established. • Report immediately if palpitations, pain or tightness in chest or throat, or pain or weakness of extremities occurs.

  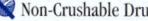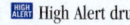

alpelisib

al-pe-lis-ib
(Piqray, Vijoice)
Do not confuse alpelisib with duvelisib, copanlisib, or idelalisib.

◆ **CLASSIFICATION**

PHARMACOTHERAPEUTIC: Phosphatidylinositol 3-kinase (P13K) inhibitor. **CLINICAL:** Antineoplastic.

USES

Piqray: Used (in combination with fulvestrant) for the treatment of men and postmenopausal women and with hormone receptor (HR)–positive, human epidermal growth factor receptor 2 (HER2)–negative, PIK3CA-mutated, advanced or metastatic breast cancer following progression on or after an endocrine-based regimen. **Vijoice:** Treatment of adults and pediatric pts 2 yrs of age and older with severe manifestations of PIK3CA Related Overgrowth Spectrum (PROS) requiring systemic therapy.

PRECAUTIONS

Contraindications: Hypersensitivity to alpelisib. **Cautions:** Baseline cytopenias; history of diabetes, dermatologic disease, pulmonary disease; pts at risk for hyperglycemia (e.g., diabetes, chronic use of corticosteroids); concomitant use of strong CYP3A inducers, BCRP inhibitors, CYP2C9 substrates. Not recommended in pts with history of Stevens-Johnson syndrome, erythema multiforme, toxic epidermal necrolysis.

ACTION

Alpelisib has selective activity against P13Ka. Mutations in the catalytic a-subunit of P13K (P13KCA) leads to P13Ka and Akt signaling, cellular transformation and tumor generation. By inhibiting phosphorylation of P13K downstream, alpelisib shows activity in cell lines with PIK3CA mutation. **Therapeutic Effect:** Inhibits tumor cell proliferation and survival.

PHARMACOKINETICS

Widely distributed. Metabolized by enzymatic hydrolysis. Protein binding: 89%. Peak plasma concentration: 2–4 hrs. Steady state reached in 3 days. Excreted in feces (81%), urine (14%). **Half-life:** 8–9 hrs.

⧗ LIFESPAN CONSIDERATIONS

Pregnancy/Lactation: Avoid pregnancy; may cause fetal harm. Females of reproductive potential must use effective contraception during treatment and for at least 7 days after discontinuation. Unknown if distributed in breast milk. Breastfeeding not recommended during treatment and for at least 7 days after discontinuation. May impair fertility in both females and males. **Males:** Males with female partners of reproductive potential must use barrier methods during treatment and for at least 7 days after discontinuation. **Children:** Safety and efficacy not established. **Elderly:** No age-related precautions noted.

INTERACTIONS

DRUG: **BCRP inhibitors (e.g., methotrexate, imatinib, rosuvastatin, topotecan)** may increase concentration/effect. **Strong CYP3A4 inducers (e.g., carbamazepine, phenytoin, rifampin)** may decrease concentration/effect. **HERBAL:** None significant. **FOOD:** None known. **LAB VALUES:** May increase serum ALT, creatinine, GGT, lipase. May decrease lymphocytes, Hgb, platelets; serum albumin, calcium, magnesium, potassium. May increase or decrease serum glucose. May prolong aPTT.

AVAILABILITY (Rx)

Tablets: *(Piqray):* 50 mg, 150 mg, 200 mg. *(Vijoice):* 50 mg, 125 mg, 200 mg.

ADMINISTRATION/HANDLING

PO

• **(Piqray):** Give with food. • Administer tablets whole; do not break, crush, or divide. Tablets cannot be chewed. Do not give if tablet is broken, cracked, or not intact. • If vomiting occurs after administration, give next dose at regularly scheduled time (do not give additional dose). • If a dose is missed, may give within 9 hrs of regularly scheduled time. After more than 9 hrs, skip dose and give next regularly scheduled time. • **(Vijoice):** Give with food. • Administer tablets whole; do not cut or divide. Tablets cannot be chewed. Do not give if tablet is broken, cracked, or not intact. • For pts unable to swallow tablets, administer as an oral suspension with food. Place tablets in a glass containing 2–4 oz of water and let it stand for approximately 5 min. Crush tablets and stir until an oral suspension is obtained. Give immediately after preparation. Discard if not within 60 min after preparation. • If a dose is missed, may give within 9 hrs of regularly scheduled time. After more than 9 hrs, skip dose and give at the next regularly scheduled time.

INDICATIONS/ROUTES/DOSAGE

Breast Cancer

PO: ADULTS, ELDERLY: **(Piqray):** 300 mg once daily (in combination with 500 mg of fulvestrant on days 1, 15, 29, then monthly). Continue until disease progression or unacceptable toxicity.

PIK3CA PROS

PO: ADULTS, ELDERLY: **(Vijoice):** 250 mg once daily. **CHILDREN 2–17 YRS OF AGE:** 50 mg once daily. May increase to 125 mg once daily in pts 6 yrs and older after 24 wks of treatment with 50 mg once daily.

Dose Reduction Schedule for Adverse Events

First dose reduction: 250 mg once daily. **Second dose reduction:** 200 mg once daily.

Dose Modification

Based on Common Terminology Criteria for Adverse Events (CTCAE).

Diarrhea

Grade 1 diarrhea: No dose adjustment. **Grade 2 diarrhea:** Withhold treatment until improved to Grade 1 or 0, then resume at same dose level. **Grade 3 or 4 diarrhea:** Withhold treatment until improved to Grade 1 or 0, then resume at reduced dose level.

Dermatologic Toxicity

Grade 1 or 2 rash: No dose adjustment. **Grade 3 rash:** Withhold treatment until improved to Grade 1 or 0, then resume at same dose level for first occurrence or reduced dose level for second occurrence. **Grade 4 rash (severe bullous, blistering, or exfoliating skin):** Permanently discontinue.

Hyperglycemia

Grade 1: No dose adjustment. **Grade 2:** No dose adjustment. If fasting plasma glucose (FPG) does not decrease to less than or equal to 160 mg/dL or 8.9 mmol/L within 21 days, reduce dose level. **Grade 3:** Withhold treatment. If FPG decreases to less than or equal to 160 mg/dL or 8.9 mmol/L within 3–5 days, resume at reduced dose level. If FPG does not decrease within 3–5 days, consider referral to specialist to manage hyperglycemia. If FPG does not decrease within 21 days with specialized therapy, permanently discontinue. **Grade 4:** Withhold treatment. Recheck FPG after 24 hrs of hyperglycemic treatment. If FPG decreases to less than 500 mg/dL or 27.8 mmol/L, follow guidelines for Grade 3 hyperglycemia. If FPG is remains greater than 500 mg/dL or 27.8 mmol/L, permanently discontinue.

Other Toxicities

Any other Grade 1 or 2 toxicities: No dose adjustment. **Any other Grade 3 toxicities:** Withhold treatment until im-

---

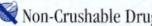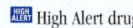

proved to Grade 1 or 0, then resume at reduced dose level. **Any other Grade 4 toxicities:** Permanently discontinue.

Dosage in Renal Impairment
Mild to moderate impairment: No dose adjustment. **Severe impairment:** Not specified; use caution.

Dosage in Hepatic Impairment
Mild to severe impairment: Not specified; use caution.

SIDE EFFECTS
Frequent (52%–19%): Diarrhea, rash, nausea, fatigue, asthenia, decreased appetite, stomatitis, mouth ulceration, vomiting, decreased weight, alopecia, mucosal inflammation. **Occasional (18%–11%):** Dry skin, xerosis, xeroderma, pruritus, dysgeusia, headache, abdominal pain, peripheral edema, pyrexia, mucosal dryness, dyspepsia.

ADVERSE EFFECTS/TOXIC REACTIONS
Anemia, lymphopenia, thrombocytopenia are expected responses to therapy. Severe hypersensitivity reactions, including anaphylaxis, may occur. Grade 3 or 4 hypersensitivity reactions reported in less than 1% of pts. Severe cutaneous reactions, including Stevens-Johnson syndrome and erythema multiforme, reported in 0.4% and 1% of pts, respectively. Hyperglycemia reported in 65% of pts. Grade 3 hyperglycemia and Grade 4 hyperglycemia reported in 33% and 4% of pts, respectively. Ketoacidosis reported in less than 1% of pts. Pneumonitis, interstitial lung disease reported in 2% of pts. Diarrhea reported in 58% of pts. Severe diarrhea may cause dehydration, acute kidney injury. UTI reported in 10% of pts.

NURSING CONSIDERATIONS

BASELINE ASSESSMENT
Obtain CBC, serum glucose level; pregnancy test in female pts of reproductive potential. Question history of diabetes, pulmonary disease, dermatologic diseases. Recommend adequate glycemic control before initiation. Assess usual bowel movement patterns, stool characteristics. Assess hydration status. Receive full medication history and screen for interactions. Offer emotional support.

INTERVENTION/EVALUATION
Monitor serum blood glucose levels as clinically indicated. Consider ABG, radiologic test if ILD/pneumonitis (excessive cough, dyspnea, fever, hypoxia) is suspected. Monitor for hyperglycemia (blurred vision, confusion, excessive thirst, Kussmaul respirations, polyuria). Monitor for skin toxicities, cutaneous reactions; hypersensitivity reactions, anaphylaxis (dyspnea, fever, hypotension, rash, tachycardia). If treatment-related toxicities occur, consider referral to specialist. Monitor daily pattern of bowel activity, stool consistency; I&Os, hydration status. If dermatologic toxicities occur, consider topical corticosteroid; addition of oral antihistamine. If hyperglycemia occurs, start or adjust antidiabetic/hyperglycemic treatment as appropriate.

PATIENT/FAMILY TEACHING
• Severe allergic reactions such as dizziness, hives, palpitations, rash, shortness of breath, tongue swelling may occur. • Treatment may cause severe rashes, peeling, or blistering of the skin. • Severe diarrhea may cause dehydration, kidney injuries. Drink plenty of fluids. • Report symptoms of high blood sugar levels (blurred vision, excessive thirst/hunger, headache, frequent urination); lung inflammation (excessive coughing, difficulty breathing, chest pain); toxic skin reactions (itching, peeling, rash, redness, swelling); UTI (fever, urinary frequency, burning during urination, foul-smelling urine). • Use effective contraception to avoid pregnancy. Do not breastfeed. • Do not take newly prescribed medications unless approved by the prescriber who originally started treatment.

ALPRAZolam

al-**praz**-oh-lam
(ALPRAZolam Intensol, ALPRAZolam XR, Apo-Alpraz ✚, Xanax, Xanax XR)

■ BLACK BOX ALERT ■ Concomitant use of benzodiazepines and opioids may result in profound sedation, respiratory depression, coma, and death. Reserve concomitant of these drugs for use in pts for whom alternative treatment options are inadequate. Limit dosages and durations to the minimum required. Follow pts for signs and symptoms of respiratory depression and sedation. Potential to be abused/misused. May cause addiction/physical dependence. Abrupt discontinuation or rapid dosage reduction may cause acute withdrawal reactions, which can be life-threatening. Use a gradual taper to discontinue.

Do not confuse ALPRAZolam with LORazepam, or Xanax with Tenex, Tylox, Xopenex, or ZyrTEC.

◆**CLASSIFICATION**

PHARMACOTHERAPEUTIC: Benzodiazepine (Schedule IV). **CLINICAL:** Antianxiety.

USES

Management of generalized anxiety disorders (GAD) in adults. Treatment of panic disorder (PD), with or without agoraphobia in adults. **OFF-LABEL:** Treatment of acute episodes of vertigo, procedural anxiety (premedication).

PRECAUTIONS

Contraindications: Hypersensitivity to ALPRAZolam. Acute narrow angle-closure glaucoma, concurrent use with ketoconazole or itraconazole or other strong CYP3A4 inhibitors. **Cautions:** Renal/hepatic impairment, predisposition to urate nephropathy, obesity. Concurrent use of CYP3A4 inhibitors/inducers and major CYP3A4 substrates; debilitated pts, respiratory disease, pts at high risk for suicide and ideation; history of drug abuse and misuse, drug-seeking behavior, dependency; elderly (increased risk of severe toxicity).

ACTION

Enhances the inhibitory effects of the neurotransmitter gamma-aminobutyric acid in the brain. **Therapeutic Effect:** Produces anxiolytic effect due to CNS depressant action.

PHARMACOKINETICS

Widely distributed. Protein binding: 80%. Metabolized in liver. Primarily excreted in urine. Minimal removal by hemodialysis. **Half-life:** 6–27 hrs.

⊠ LIFESPAN CONSIDERATIONS

Pregnancy/Lactation: Crosses placenta; distributed in breast milk. Chronic ingestion during pregnancy may produce withdrawal symptoms, CNS depression in neonates. **Children:** Safety and efficacy not established. **Elderly:** Use small initial doses with gradual increase to avoid ataxia (muscular incoordination) or excessive sedation. May have increased risk of falls, delirium.

INTERACTIONS

DRUG: CNS depressants (e.g., **alcohol, morphine, zolpidem**) may increase CNS depression. **Strong CYP3A4 inhibitors (e.g., clarithromycin, ketoconazole, ritonavir)** may increase concentration/effect. **Strong CYP3A4 inducers (e.g., carbamazepine, phenytoin, rifampin)** may decrease concentration/effect. **HERBAL: Herbals with sedative properties (e.g., chamomile, kava kava, valerian)** may increase CNS depression. **FOOD:** None significant. **LAB VALUES:** None significant.

AVAILABILITY (Rx)

Oral Solution: *(Alprazolam Intensol):* 1 mg/mL. **Tablets (Orally Disintegrating):** 0.25 mg, 0.5 mg, 1 mg, 2 mg. **Tablets (Immediate-Release): *(Xanax):*** 0.25 mg, 0.5 mg, 1 mg, 2 mg.

 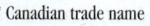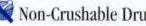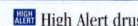

Tablets (Extended-Release): *(Xanax XR):* 0.5 mg, 1 mg, 2 mg, 3 mg.

ADMINISTRATION/HANDLING

PO, Immediate-Release
• May give without regard to food. • If oral intake is not possible, may be given sublingually.

PO, Extended-Release
• Administer once daily. • Do not break, crush, dissolve, or divide extended-release tablets. Swallow whole.

PO, Orally Disintegrating
• Place tablet on tongue, allow to dissolve. • Swallow with saliva. • Administration with water not necessary. • If using ½ tab, discard remaining ½ tab.

INDICATIONS/ROUTES/DOSAGE

Anxiety Disorders
PO: *(Immediate-Release, Oral Concentrate, ODT):* **ADULTS:** Initially, 0.25–0.5 mg 3 times/day. May titrate q3–4days. **Maximum:** 4 mg/day in divided doses. **ELDERLY:** Initially, 0.25 mg 2–3 times/day. Gradually increase to optimum therapeutic response.

Panic Disorder
PO: *(Immediate-Release, Oral Concentrate, ODT):* **ADULTS:** Initially, 0.5 mg 3 times/day. May increase at 3- to 4-day intervals in increments of 1 mg or less a day. Range: 2–6 mg/day. **Maximum:** 10 mg/day. **ELDERLY:** Initially, 0.125–0.25 mg twice daily. May increase in 0.125-mg increments until desired effect attained.
PO: *(Extended-Release):*
◄**ALERT**► To switch from immediate-release to extended-release form, give total daily dose (immediate-release) as a single daily dose of extended-release form.
ADULTS: Initially, 0.5–1 mg once daily. May titrate at 3- to 4-day intervals. **Range:** 2–6 mg/day. **Maximum:** 10 mg/day. **ELDERLY:** Initially, 0.5 mg once daily.

Dosage in Renal Impairment
No dose adjustment.

Dosage in Hepatic Impairment
Severe disease: *(Immediate-Release):* 0.25 mg 2–3 mg times/day. *(Extended-Release):* 0.5 mg once daily.

SIDE EFFECTS
Frequent (41%–20%): Ataxia, light-headedness, drowsiness, slurred speech (particularly in elderly or debilitated pts). **Occasional (15%–5%):** Confusion, depression, blurred vision, constipation, diarrhea, dry mouth, headache, nausea. **Rare (4% or less):** Behavioral problems such as anger, impaired memory; paradoxical reactions (insomnia, nervousness, irritability).

ADVERSE EFFECTS/TOXIC REACTIONS
Concomitant use with opioids may result in profound sedation, respiratory depression, coma, and death. Abrupt or too-rapid withdrawal may result in restlessness, irritability, insomnia, hand tremors, abdominal/muscle cramps, diaphoresis, vomiting, seizures. Overdose results in drowsiness, confusion, diminished reflexes, coma. Blood dyscrasias noted rarely. **Antidote:** Flumazenil (see Appendix H for dosage).

NURSING CONSIDERATIONS

BASELINE ASSESSMENT
Assess degree of anxiety; assess for drowsiness, dizziness, light-headedness. Assess motor responses (agitation, trembling, tension), autonomic responses (cold/clammy hands, diaphoresis). Initiate fall precautions. Assess for potential of abuse/misuse (e.g., drug-seeking behavior, mental health conditions, history of substance abuse).

INTERVENTION/EVALUATION
For pts on long-term therapy, perform hepatic/renal function tests, CBC periodically. Evaluate for therapeutic response: Calm facial expression, decreased restlessness, insomnia. Monitor respiratory and cardiovascular status. Diligently screen for suicidal ideation and behavior; new-onset or worsening of anxiety, depression, mood disorder.

PATIENT/FAMILY TEACHING

• If dizziness occurs, change positions slowly from recumbent to sitting position before standing. • Avoid tasks that require alertness, motor skills until response to drug is established. • Smoking reduces drug effectiveness. • Seek immediate medical attention if thoughts of suicide, new-onset or worsening of anxiety, depression, or changes in mood occur. • Seizures, acute withdrawal syndrome may occur if treatment is abruptly stopped after long-term therapy. • Avoid alcohol. • Do not take other medications without consulting prescriber.

---

alteplase ℮

al-te-plase
(<u>Activase</u>, Cathflo Activase)
Do not confuse alteplase or Activase with Altace, or Activase with Cathflo Activase or TNKase.

◆CLASSIFICATION

PHARMACOTHERAPEUTIC: Tissue plasminogen activator (tPA). **CLINICAL:** Thrombolytic.

USES

Treatment of acute ischemic stroke (AIS), acute myocardial infarction (AMI) to reduce mortality and incidence of HF; acute massive pulmonary embolism (PE) for lysis; occluded central venous catheters. **OFF-LABEL:** Acute peripheral occlusive disease, prosthetic valve thrombosis, frostbite, hemodialysis, peritoneal catheter clearance.

PRECAUTIONS

Contraindications: Hypersensitivity to alteplase. Active internal bleeding, AV malformation or aneurysm, bleeding diathesis CVA, intracranial neoplasm, intracranial or intraspinal surgery or trauma, recent (within past 2 mos), severe uncontrolled hypertension, suspected aortic dissection. **Cautions:** Recent (within 10 days) major surgery or GI bleeding, OB delivery, organ biopsy, recent trauma or CPR, left heart thrombus, endocarditis, severe hepatic disease, pregnancy, elderly, cerebrovascular disease, diabetic retinopathy, thrombophlebitis, occluded AV cannula at infected site.

ACTION

Binds to fibrin in a thrombus and converts entrapped plasminogen to plasmin, initiating local fibrinolysis. **Therapeutic Effect:** Degrades fibrin clots, fibrinogen, other plasma proteins.

PHARMACOKINETICS

Rapidly metabolized in liver. Primarily excreted in urine. **Half-life:** 35 min.

🕲 LIFESPAN CONSIDERATIONS

Pregnancy/Lactation: Use only when benefit outweighs potential risk to fetus. Unknown if drug crosses placenta or is distributed in breast milk. **Children:** Safety and efficacy not established. **Elderly:** May have increased risk of bleeding; monitor closely.

INTERACTIONS

DRUG: Heparin, low molecular weight heparins, **medications altering platelet function (e.g., clopidogrel, NSAIDs), oral anticoagulants (e.g., warfarin)** increase risk of bleeding. **HERBAL: Herbals with anticoagulant/antiplatelet properties (e.g., garlic, ginger, ginkgo biloba)** may increase adverse effects. **FOOD:** None known. **LAB VALUES:** Decreases plasminogen, fibrinogen levels during infusion, decreases clotting time (confirms the presence of lysis). May decrease Hgb, Hct.

AVAILABILITY (Rx)

Injection, Powder for Reconstitution: *(Cathflo Activase):* 2 mg, *(Activase):* 50 mg, 100 mg.

ADMINISTRATION/HANDLING

 IV

Reconstitution • *(Activase):* Reconstitute immediately before use with Sterile Water for Injection. • Reconstitute 100-mg vial with 100 mL Sterile Water for Injection (50-mg vial with 50 mL sterile water) without preservative to provide a concentration of 1 mg/mL. • *(Activase Cathflo):* Add 2.2 mL Sterile Water for Injection to provide concentration of 1 mg/mL. • Avoid excessive agitation; gently swirl or slowly invert vial to reconstitute.

Rate of administration • *(Activase):* Give by IV infusion via infusion pump (see Indications/Routes/Dosage). • If minor bleeding occurs at puncture sites, apply pressure for 30 sec; if unrelieved, apply pressure dressing. • If uncontrolled hemorrhage occurs, discontinue infusion immediately (slowing rate of infusion may produce worsening hemorrhage). • Avoid undue pressure when drug is injected into catheter (can rupture catheter or expel clot into circulation). • Instill dose into occluded catheter. • After 30 min, assess catheter function by attempting to aspirate blood. • If still occluded, let dose dwell an additional 90 min. • If function not restored, a second dose may be instilled.

Storage • *(Activase):* Store vials at room temperature. • After reconstitution, solution appears colorless to pale yellow. • Solution is stable for 8 hrs after reconstitution. Discard unused portions.

INDICATIONS/ROUTES/DOSAGE

Acute MI

IV infusion: ADULTS WEIGHING MORE THAN 67 KG: Total dose: 100 mg over 90 min, starting with 15-mg bolus over 1–2 min, then 50 mg over 30 min, then 35 mg over 60 min. **ADULTS WEIGHING 67 KG OR LESS: Total dose:** Start with 15-mg bolus over 1–2 min, then 0.75 mg/kg over 30 min (**maximum:** 50 mg), then 0.5 mg/kg over 60 min (**maximum:** 35 mg). **Maximum total dose:** 100 mg.

Acute Pulmonary Emboli

IV infusion: ADULTS: 100 mg over 2 hrs. Institute or reinstitute heparin near end or immediately after infusion when activated partial thromboplastin time (aPTT) or thrombin time (TT) returns to twice normal or less.

Acute Ischemic Stroke

◄ALERT► Dose should be given within the first 3 hrs of the onset of symptoms. **Recommended total dose:** 0.9 mg/kg. **Maximum:** 90 mg.

IV infusion: ADULTS WEIGHING 100 KG OR LESS: 0.09 mg/kg as IV bolus over 1 min, then 0.81 mg/kg as continuous infusion over 60 min. **WEIGHING MORE THAN 100 KG:** 9 mg bolus over 1 min, then 81 mg as continuous infusion over 60 min.

Central Venous Catheter Clearance

IV: ADULTS, ELDERLY: Up to 2 mg; may repeat after 2 hrs. If catheter functional, withdraw 4–5 mL blood to remove drug and residual clot.

Usual Neonatal Dosage

Occluded IV catheter: Use 1 mg/mL conc (**maximum:** 2 mg/2 mL), leave in lumen up to 2 hrs, then aspirate.

Systemic thrombosis: 0.1–0.6 mg/kg/hr for 6 hrs. Usual dose: 0.5 mg/kg/hr.

Dosage in Renal/Hepatic Impairment

No dose adjustment.

SIDE EFFECTS

Frequent: Superficial bleeding at puncture sites, decreased B/P. **Occasional:** Allergic reaction (rash, wheezing, bruising).

ADVERSE EFFECTS/TOXIC REACTIONS

Severe internal hemorrhage, intracranial hemorrhage may occur. Lysis of coronary thrombi may produce atrial or ventricular arrhythmias or stroke.

NURSING CONSIDERATIONS

BASELINE ASSESSMENT

Assess for contraindications to therapy. Obtain B/P, apical pulse. Record weight.

Evaluate 12-lead ECG, cardiac enzymes, serum electrolytes. Assess Hct, platelet count, prothrombin time (PT), activated partial thromboplastin time (aPTT), fibrinogen level before therapy is instituted. Type and screen blood.

INTERVENTION/EVALUATION

Perform continuous cardiac monitoring for arrhythmias. Check B/P, pulse, respirations q15min until stable, then hourly. Check peripheral pulses, heart and lung sounds. Monitor for chest pain relief and notify physician of continuation or recurrence (note location, type, intensity). Assess for bleeding: overt blood, occult blood in any body substance. Monitor aPTT per protocol. Maintain B/P; avoid any trauma that might increase risk of bleeding (e.g., injections, shaving). Assess neurologic status frequently.

amikacin

am-i-**kay**-sin

■ **BLACK BOX ALERT** ■ May cause neurotoxicity, nephrotoxicity, and/or neuromuscular blockade and respiratory paralysis. Ototoxicity usually is irreversible; nephrotoxicity usually is reversible.
Do not confuse amikacin with Amicar, or anakinra.

◆CLASSIFICATION

PHARMACOTHERAPEUTIC: Aminoglycoside. **CLINICAL:** Antibiotic.

USES

Treatment of serious infections including bacterial septicemia, respiratory tract, bones and joints, central nervous system (including meningitis), skin and soft tissue, intra-abdominal (including peritonitis), burns, postoperative infections; complicated and recurrent UTIs due to susceptible strains of gram-negative bacteria, including *Pseudomonas* species, *Escherichia coli,* species of indole-positive and indole-

negative *Proteus, Providencia* species, *Klebsiella-Enterobacter-Serratia* species, and *Acinetobacter* species. **OFF-LABEL:** Cystic fibrosis (acute exacerbation), drug-resistant tuberculosis.

PRECAUTIONS

Contraindications: Hypersensitivity to amikacin, other aminoglycosides. **Cautions:** Preexisting renal impairment, auditory or vestibular impairment, hypocalcemia, elderly, neuromuscular disorder, dehydration, concomitant use of neurotoxic or nephrotoxic medications.

ACTION

Inhibits protein synthesis in susceptible bacteria by binding to 30S ribosomal unit. **Therapeutic Effect:** Interferes with protein synthesis of susceptible microorganisms.

PHARMACOKINETICS

Rapid, complete absorption after IM administration. Protein binding: 0%–10%. Widely distributed (penetrates blood-brain barrier when meninges are inflamed). Excreted unchanged in urine. Removed by hemodialysis. **Half-life:** 2–4 hrs (increased in renal impairment, neonates; decreased in cystic fibrosis, burn pts, febrile pts).

⊠ LIFESPAN CONSIDERATIONS

Pregnancy/Lactation: Readily crosses placenta; small amounts distributed in breast milk. May produce fetal nephrotoxicity. **Children:** Neonates, premature infants may be more susceptible to toxicity due to immature renal function. **Elderly:** Higher risk of toxicity due to age-related renal impairment, increased risk of hearing loss.

INTERACTIONS

DRUG: Foscarnet, mannitol may increase nephrotoxic effect. **Cephalosporins (e.g., cefazolin, ceftriaxone), loop diuretics (e.g., bumetanide, furosemide), vancomycin** may increase concentration/effect. **Penicillin** may decrease concentration/effect. **HERBAL:**

None significant. **FOOD:** None known. **LAB VALUES:** May increase serum creatinine, BUN, ALT, AST, bilirubin, LDH. May decrease serum calcium, magnesium, potassium, sodium. **Therapeutic levels:** Peak: life-threatening infections: 25–40 mcg/mL; serious infections: 20–25 mcg/mL; urinary tract infections: 15–20 mcg/mL. **Trough:** Less than 8 mcg/mL. **Toxic levels:** Peak: Greater than 40 mcg/mL; **trough:** Greater than 10 mcg/mL.

AVAILABILITY (Rx)

Injection Solution: 250 mg/mL.

ADMINISTRATION/HANDLING

 IV

Reconstitution • Dilute to concentration of 0.25–5 mg/mL in 0.9% NaCl or D₅W. **Rate of administration** • Infuse over 30–60 min. **Storage** • Store vials at room temperature. • Solution appears clear but may become pale yellow (does not affect potency). • Intermittent IV infusion (piggyback) is stable for 24 hrs at room temperature, 2 days if refrigerated. • Discard if precipitate forms or dark discoloration occurs.

IM

• To minimize discomfort, give deep IM slowly. • Less painful if injected into gluteus maximus rather than in lateral aspect of thigh.

▓ IV INCOMPATIBILITIES

Ibuprofen, propofol.

▓ IV COMPATIBILITIES

Amiodarone (Cordarone), aztreonam, dexmedetomidine, magnesium sulfate, ondansetron (Zofran), potassium chloride, ranitidine is off the market vancomycin.

INDICATIONS/ROUTES/DOSAGE

Usual Parenteral Dosage
Note: Individualization of dose is critical due to low therapeutic index. Initial and periodic peak and trough levels should be determined.

IV, IM: ADULTS, ELDERLY: 15 mg/kg/day divided q8–12h. **CHILDREN, INFANTS:** 15–22.5 mg/kg/day divided q8–12h. **NEONATES:** 15 mg/kg/dose (interval based on disease, age, weight).

Dosage in Renal Impairment
Dosage and frequency are modified based on degree of renal impairment and serum drug concentration. After a loading dose of 5–7.5 mg/kg, maintenance dose and frequency are based on serum creatinine levels and creatinine clearance.

Adults

Creatinine Clearance	Dosing Interval
50 mL/min or greater	No dose adjustment
10–50 mL/min	q24–72h
Less than 10 mL/min	q48–72h
Hemodialysis	q48–72h (give after HD on dialysis days)
Continuous renal replacement therapy (CRRT)	Initially, 10 mg/kg, then 7.5 mg/kg q24–48h

Dosage in Hepatic Impairment
No dose adjustment.

SIDE EFFECTS

Frequent: Phlebitis, thrombophlebitis. **Occasional:** Rash, fever, urticaria, pruritus. **Rare:** Neuromuscular blockade (difficulty breathing, drowsiness, weakness).

ADVERSE EFFECTS/TOXIC REACTIONS

Serious reactions include nephrotoxicity (increased thirst, decreased appetite, nausea, vomiting, increased BUN and serum creatinine levels, decreased creatinine clearance); neurotoxicity (muscle twitching, visual disturbances, seizures, paresthesia); ototoxicity (tinnitus, dizziness, loss of hearing).

NURSING CONSIDERATIONS

BASELINE ASSESSMENT

Obtain BUN, serum creatinine. Dehydration must be treated prior to aminoglycoside therapy. Establish baseline hearing acuity before initiation. Question for history of allergies, esp. to aminoglycosides and sulfite. Obtain specimen for culture, sensitivity before giving first dose (therapy may begin before results are known).

INTERVENTION/EVALUATION

Monitor I&O (maintain hydration), urinalysis. Monitor results of serum peak/trough levels. Be alert to ototoxic, neurotoxic, nephrotoxic symptoms (see Adverse Effects/Toxic Reactions). Check IM injection site for pain, induration. Evaluate IV site for phlebitis. Assess for skin rash, diarrhea, superinfection (particularly genital/anal pruritus), changes of oral mucosa. When treating pts with neuromuscular disorders, assess respiratory response carefully. **Therapeutic levels:** Peak: Life-threatening infections: 25–40 mcg/mL; serious infections: 20–25 mcg/mL; urinary tract infections: 15–20 mcg/mL. **Trough:** Less than 8 mcg/mL. **Toxic levels:** Peak: Greater than 40 mcg/mL; **trough:** Greater than 10 mcg/mL.

PATIENT/FAMILY TEACHING

• Continue antibiotic for full length of treatment. • Space doses evenly. • IM injection may cause discomfort. • Report any hearing, visual, balance, urinary problems, even after therapy is completed. • Do not take other medications without consulting physician.

---

amiodarone ℮

a-mi-**oh**-da-rone
(Nexterone, Pacerone)

■ **BLACK BOX ALERT** ■ Pts should be hospitalized when amiodarone is initiated. Alternative therapies should be tried first before using amiodarone. Only indicated for pts with life-threatening arrhythmias due to risk of toxicity. Pulmonary toxicity may occur without symptoms. Hepatotoxicity is common, usually mild (rarely possible). Can exacerbate arrhythmias. **Do not confuse amiodarone with aMILoride, dronedarone, or Cordarone with Cardura.**

◆CLASSIFICATION

PHARMACOTHERAPEUTIC: Cardiac agent. **CLINICAL:** Antiarrhythmic. Class III.

USES

Management of life-threatening recurrent ventricular fibrillation (VF) or recurrent hemodynamically unstable ventricular tachycardia (VT) unresponsive to other therapy. **OFF-LABEL:** Treatment of atrial fibrillation (e.g., post-operative prevention), primary/secondary prevention of sudden cardiac death due to ventricular arrhythmias, paroxysmal supraventricular tachycardia (SVT). Maintenance of sinus rhythm, rate control, symptomatic nonsustained ventricular tachycardia, or ventricular premature beats.

PRECAUTIONS

Contraindications: Hypersensitivity to amiodarone, iodine. Bradycardia-induced syncope (except in the presence of a pacemaker), second- and third-degree AV block (except in presence of a pacemaker); severe sinus node dysfunction, causing marked sinus bradycardia; cardiogenic shock. **Cautions:** May prolong QT interval. Thyroid disease, electrolyte imbalance, hepatic disease, hypotension, left ventricular dysfunction, pulmonary disease. Pts taking warfarin, surgical pts.

ACTION

Inhibits adrenergic stimulation; affects Na, K, Ca channels; prolongs action potential and refractory period in myocardial tissue. Decreases AV conduction and sinus node function. **Therapeutic Effect:** Suppresses arrhythmias.

PHARMACOKINETICS

Route	Onset	Peak	Duration
PO	3 days–3 wks	1 wk–5 mos	7–50 days after discontinuation

Slowly, variably absorbed from GI tract. Protein binding: 96%. Extensively metabolized in liver. Excreted via bile; not removed by hemodialysis. **Half-life:** 26–107 days; metabolite: 61 days.

LIFESPAN CONSIDERATIONS

Pregnancy/Lactation: Crosses placenta; distributed in breast milk. May adversely affect fetal development. **Children:** Safety and efficacy not established. **Elderly:** May be more sensitive to effects on thyroid function. May experience increased incidence of ataxia, other neurotoxic effects.

INTERACTIONS

DRUG: **QT interval–prolonging medications (e.g., azithromycin, ciprofloxacin, haloperidol, methadone, sotalol)** may increase concentration/effect, risk of QT interval prolongation. My increase concentration/effects of **beta blockers (e.g., atenolol, carvedilol, metoprolol). Calcium channel blockers (e.g., diltiaZEM, verapamil), sofosbuvir** may increase concentration/effect, bradycardic effect. **HERBAL:** Herbals with hypotensive properties (e.g., garlic, ginger, ginkgo biloba) may increase concentration/effects. **FOOD:** Grapefruit products may alter effect. Avoid use during therapy. **LAB VALUES:** May increase serum ALT, AST, alkaline phosphatase, ANA titer. May cause changes in ECG, thyroid function test results. **Therapeutic serum level:** 0.5–2.5 mcg/mL; toxic serum level not established.

AVAILABILITY (Rx)

Infusion (Pre-Mix): Nexterone: 150 mg/100 mL; 360 mg/200 mL. **Injection, Solution:** 150 mg/3 mL, 450 mg/9 mL, 900 mg/18 mL. **Tablets:** *(Pacerone):* 100 mg, 200 mg, 400 mg.

ADMINISTRATION/HANDLING

 IV

Reconstitution • Infusions longer than 2 hrs must be administered/diluted in glass or polyolefin bottles. • Dilute loading dose (150 mg) in 100 mL D$_5$W (1.5 mg/mL). • Dilute maintenance dose (900 mg) in 500 mL D$_5$W (1.8 mg/mL). Concentrations greater than 3 mg/mL cause peripheral vein phlebitis. **Rate of administration** • Does not need protection from light during administration. • Administer through central venous catheter (CVC) if possible, using in-line filter. • Bolus over 10 min (15 mg/min) not to exceed 30 mg/min; then 1 mg/min over 6 hrs; then 0.5 mg/min over 18 hrs. • Infusions longer than 1 hr, concentration not to exceed 2 mg/mL unless CVC used. **Storage** • Store at room temperature. • Stable for 24 hrs when diluted in glass or polyolefin containers; stable for 2 hrs when diluted in PVC containers.

PO

• Give consistently with regard to meals to reduce GI distress. • Do not give with grapefruit products.

IV INCOMPATIBILITIES

Argatroban, heparin, magnesium sulfate.

IV COMPATIBILITIES

Calcium chloride, calcium gluconate, dexmedetomidine, insulin, norepinephrine, potassium chloride, vasopressin.

INDICATIONS/ROUTES/DOSAGE

Ventricular Arrhythmias
PO: **ADULTS, ELDERLY:** Initially, 800–1600 mg/day until initial therapeutic response occurs (usually 1–3 wks), then reduce to 600–800 mg/day for 1 month, then further reduce to maintenance dose of 400 mg/day.
IV infusion: **ADULTS, ELDERLY:** Initially, 150 mg over 10 min, (may repeat if necessary), then 1 mg/min over 6 hrs; then 0.5 mg/min. Continue this rate over at least 18 hrs or until complete transition or oral.

Dosage in Renal Impairment
No dose adjustment.

Dosage in Hepatic Impairment
Use caution.

SIDE EFFECTS

Expected: Corneal microdeposits noted in almost all pts treated for more than 6 mos (can lead to blurry vision). **Occasional (greater than 3%): PO:** Constipation, headache, decreased appetite, nausea, vomiting, paresthesia, photosensitivity, muscular incoordination. **Parenteral:** Hypotension, nausea, fever, bradycardia. **Rare (less than 3%): PO:** Bitter or metallic taste, decreased libido, dizziness, facial flushing, blue-gray coloring of skin (face, arms, and neck), blurred vision, bradycardia, asymptomatic corneal deposits, rash, visual disturbances, halo vision.

ADVERSE EFFECTS/TOXIC REACTIONS

Serious, potentially fatal pulmonary toxicity (alveolitis, pulmonary fibrosis, pneumonitis, acute respiratory distress syndrome) may begin with progressive dyspnea and cough with crackles, decreased breath sounds, pleurisy, HF, or hepatotoxicity. May worsen existing arrhythmias or produce new arrhythmias.

NURSING CONSIDERATIONS

BASELINE ASSESSMENT

Obtain LFT; ECG; CXR in pts with pulmonary disease. Assess B/P, apical pulse immediately before drug is administered (if pulse is 60/min or less or systolic B/P is less than 90 mm Hg, withhold medication, contact physician).

INTERVENTION/EVALUATION

Monitor for symptoms of pulmonary toxicity (progressively worsening dyspnea, cough). Dosage should be discontinued or reduced if toxicity occurs. Assess pulse for quality, rhythm, bradycardia. Monitor ECG for cardiac changes (e.g., widening of QRS interval, prolongation of PR and QT intervals). Assess for nausea, fatigue, paresthesia, tremor. Monitor for signs of hypothyroidism (periorbital edema, lethargy, pudgy hands/feet, cool/pale skin, vertigo, night cramps) and hyperthyroidism (hot/dry skin, bulging eyes [exophthalmos], frequent urination, eyelid edema, weight loss, difficulty breathing). Monitor LFT for hepatotoxicity. If elevated

hepatic enzymes occur, dosage reduction or discontinuation is necessary. Monitor thyroid function test results. Monitor for therapeutic serum level (0.5–2.5 mcg/mL). Toxic serum level not established.

PATIENT/FAMILY TEACHING

• Protect against photosensitivity reaction on skin exposed to sunlight. • Report shortness of breath, cough. • Outpatients should monitor pulse before taking medication. • Do not abruptly discontinue medication. • Compliance with therapy regimen is essential to control arrhythmias. • Restrict salt, alcohol intake. • Avoid grapefruit products. • Recommend ophthalmic exams q6mos. • Report any vision changes, signs/symptoms of cardiac arrhythmias.

amitriptyline

a-mi-**trip**-ti-leen
(Levate ✤)

■ **BLACK BOX ALERT** ■ Increased risk of suicidal thinking and behavior in children, adolescents, young adults 18–24 yrs with major depressive disorder, other psychiatric disorders. **Do not confuse amitriptyline with aminophylline, imipramine, or nortriptyline.**

FIXED-COMBINATION(S)

Limbitrol: amitriptyline/chlordiazePOXIDE (an antianxiety): 12.5 mg/5 mg, 25 mg/10 mg.

◆CLASSIFICATION

PHARMACOTHERAPEUTIC: Tricyclic. **CLINICAL:** Antidepressant.

USES

Treatment of unipolar, major depression. **OFF-LABEL:** Chronic fatigue syndrome, fibromyalgia, functional dyspepsia, chronic tension headache (prevention), irritable bowel syndrome, migraine prevention, neuropathic pain (chronic), postherpetic neuralgia.

✤ Canadian trade name   🦫 Non-Crushable Drug   🔺 High Alert drug

PRECAUTIONS

Contraindications: Hypersensitivity to amitriptyline. Acute recovery period after MI, coadministered with or within 14 days of MAOIs. **Cautions:** Prostatic hypertrophy, history of urinary retention or obstruction, narrow-angle glaucoma, diabetes, seizures, hyperthyroidism, cardiac/hepatic/renal disease, schizophrenia, xerostomia, visual problems, constipation or bowel obstruction, elderly, increased intraocular pressure (IOP), hiatal hernia, suicidal ideation.

ACTION

Blocks reuptake of neurotransmitters (norepinephrine, serotonin) at presynaptic membranes, increasing synaptic concentration in the CNS. **Therapeutic Effect:** Relieves depression; reduces pain associated with chronic pain, migraines.

PHARMACOKINETICS

Widely distributed. Protein binding: 90%. Metabolized in liver. Primarily excreted in urine. Minimal removal by hemodialysis. **Half-life:** 10–26 hrs.

⌛ LIFESPAN CONSIDERATIONS

Pregnancy/Lactation: Crosses placenta; minimally distributed in breast milk. **Children:** More sensitive to increased dosage, toxicity, increased risk of suicidal ideation, worsening of depression. **Elderly:** Increased risk of toxicity. Increased sensitivity to anticholinergic effects. Caution in pts with cardiovascular disease.

INTERACTIONS

DRUG: CNS depressants (e.g., alcohol, morphine, zolpidem) may increase CNS depression. Azelastine, MAOIs (e.g., phenelzine, selegiline) may increase concentration/effect. Aclidinium, ipratropium, tiotropium, umeclidinium may increase concentration/effect, anticholinergic effect. May increase arrhythmogenic effect of dronedarone. **HERBAL:** Herbals with sedative properties (e.g., chamomile, kava kava, valerian) may increase CNS depression.

St. John's wort, Syrian rue may increase concentration/effect. **FOOD:** None known. **LAB VALUES:** May alter ECG readings (flattened T wave), serum glucose (increase or decrease). **Therapeutic serum level:** Peak: 120–250 ng/mL; **toxic serum level:** Greater than 500 ng/mL.

AVAILABILITY (Rx)

Tablets: 10 mg, 25 mg, 50 mg, 75 mg, 100 mg, 150 mg.

ADMINISTRATION/HANDLING

PO

• Give with food or milk if GI distress occurs. Administer higher doses in late afternoon or at bedtime to reduce daytime sedation.

INDICATIONS/ROUTES/DOSAGE

Depression

PO: ADULTS: Initially, 25–50 mg/day as a single dose at bedtime, or in divided doses. May gradually increase in increments of 25–50 mg at 1-wk (or greater) intervals up to 100–300 mg/day. Titrate to lowest effective dosage. **ELDERLY:** Initially, 10–25 mg once daily at bedtime. **ADOLESCENTS:** Initially, 10 mg 3 times/day and 20 mg at bedtime. **Maximum:** 200 mg/day.

Pain Management

PO: ADULTS, ELDERLY: Initially, 10–25 mg once daily at bedtime. May increase gradually in 10–25 mg increments over at least 1 wk up to 150 mg/day.

Migraine Prevention

PO: ADULTS: Initially, 10–25 mg once daily at bedtime. May increase gradually in 10–25 mg increments over at least 1 wk. **Maintenance:** 20–50 mg once daily at bedtime.

Dosage in Renal/Hepatic Impairment

Use with caution.

SIDE EFFECTS

Frequent: Dizziness, drowsiness, dry mouth, orthostatic hypotension, headache, increased appetite, weight gain, nausea, unusual fatigue, unpleasant taste. **Occasional:** Blurred vision, confusion, constipation, hallucinations, delayed micturition, eye pain, arrhythmias, fine muscle tremors, parkinsonian syndrome, anxiety, diarrhea, diaphoresis, heartburn, insomnia. **Rare:** Hypersensitivity, alopecia, tinnitus, breast enlargement, photosensitivity.

ADVERSE EFFECTS/TOXIC REACTIONS

Overdose may produce confusion, seizures, severe drowsiness, changes in cardiac conduction, fever, hallucinations, agitation, dyspnea, vomiting, unusual fatigue, weakness. Abrupt withdrawal after prolonged therapy may produce headache, malaise, nausea, vomiting, vivid dreams. Blood dyscrasias, cholestatic jaundice occur rarely.

NURSING CONSIDERATIONS

BASELINE ASSESSMENT

Observe and record behavior. Assess psychological status, thought content, suicidal ideation, sleep patterns, appearance, interest in environment. For pts on long-term, high-dose therapy, hepatic/renal function tests, blood counts should be performed periodically.

INTERVENTION/EVALUATION

Supervise suicidal-risk pt closely during early therapy (as depression lessens, energy level improves, increasing suicide potential). Assess appearance, behavior, speech pattern, level of interest, mood. Monitor B/P for hypotension, pulse, arrhythmias. **Therapeutic serum level:** Peak: 120–250 ng/mL; **toxic serum level:** Greater than 500 ng/mL. **Maximum:** 200 mg/day.

PATIENT/FAMILY TEACHING

• Go slowly from lying to standing. • Tolerance to postural hypotension, sedative and anticholinergic effects usually develops during early therapy. • Maximum therapeutic effect may be noted in 2–4 wks. • Sensitivity to sun may occur. • Report visual disturbances. • Do not abruptly discontinue medication. • Avoid tasks that require alertness, motor skills until response to drug is established. • Avoid alcohol. • Sips of water may relieve dry mouth.

amivantamab-vmjw

am-ee-van-ti-mab
(Rybrevant)
Do not confuse amivantamab with afatinib, avapritinib, or belantamab.

◆CLASSIFICATION

PHARMACOTHERAPEUTIC: Epidermal growth factor receptor (EGFR) inhibitor, MET inhibitor. **CLINICAL:** Antineoplastic.

USES

First-line treatment of NSCLC with EGFR exon 19 deletions or exon 21 L858R substitution mutations: In combination with lazertinib, for first-line treatment of adults with locally advanced or metastatic NSCLC with EGFR exon 19 deletions or exon 21 L858R substitution mutations. **Previously treated NSCLC with EGFR exon 19 deletions or exon 21 L858 substitution mutations:** In combination with carboplatin and pemetrexed, for treatment of adults with locally advanced or metastatic NSCLC with EGFR exon 19 deletions or exon 21 L858R substitution mutations, whose disease has progressed on or after treatment with an EGFR tyrosine kinase inhibitor.
First-line treatment of NSCLC with EGFR exon 20 insertion mutations: In combination with carboplatin and pemetrexed for the first-line treatment of adults with locally advanced or metastatic non–small-cell lung cancer (NSCLC) with epidermal growth factor receptor (EGFR) exon 20 insertion mutations. **Previously treated NSCLC with EGFR exon 20 insertion mutations:** As a single agent for the treatment of adults with locally advanced or metastatic NSCLC with EGFR exon 20 insertion mutations, whose disease has progressed or after platinum-based chemotherapy.

PRECAUTIONS

Contraindications: Hypersensitivity to amivantamab-vmjw. **Cautions:** Hepatic impairment, pts at risk for interstitial lung disease (e.g., COPD, sarcoidosis, connective disease disease), ocular disease; conditions predisposing to infection (e.g., diabetes, immunocompromised pts, renal failure, open wounds); prior infusion-related reactions.

ACTION

Binds to the EGFR and MET extracellular domains and disrupts EGFR and MET signaling by blocking ligand binding (in exon 20 insertion mutation models, degrading EGFR and MET). The presence of EGFR and MET on tumor cell surfaces also allows for targeted cell destruction by immune effector cells, such as natural killer cells and macrophages, via antibody-dependent cellular cytotoxicity and trogocytosis mechanisms. **Therapeutic Effect:** Inhibits tumor growth.

PHARMACOKINETICS

Widely distributed. Steady-state reached by 9th infusion. Excretion not specified. **Half-life:** 11.3 days.

LIFESPAN CONSIDERATIONS

Pregnancy/Lactation: Avoid pregnancy; may cause fetal harm. Females of reproductive potential must use effective contraception during treatment and for at least 3 mos after discontinuation. Breastfeeding not recommended during treatment and for at least 3 mos after discontinuation. **Children:** Safety and efficacy not established. **Elderly:** No age-related precautions noted.

INTERACTIONS

DRUG: None significant. **HERBAL:** None significant. **FOOD:** None known. **LAB VALUES:** May increase serum alkaline phosphatase, ALT, AST, GGT, glucose. May decrease serum albumin, phosphate, magnesium, sodium, potassium; lymphocytes.

AVAILABILITY (RX)

Injection Solution: 350 mg/7 mL (50 mg/mL).

ADMINISTRATION/HANDLING

 IV

Premedication • Premedicate with an antipyretic (acetaminophen 650–1,000 mg) and an antihistamine (diphenhydramine 25–50 mg [or equivalent]) prior to each dose. A glucocorticoid (dexamethasone 10 mg or methylprednisolone 40 mg [or equivalent]) should be given on days 1 and 2 of first week, then PRN for subsequent doses.

Infusion guidelines • Infusion bag must be made of polyethylene, polypropylene, polyolefin blend, or polyvinyl chloride. • Infuse via dedicated IV line using a sterile, nonpyrogenic, low-protein-binding 0.2 micron in-line filter. • Do not administer as IV push or bolus.

Preparation • Must be prepared by personnel trained in aseptic manipulations and admixing of cytotoxic drugs. • Calculate the number of vials needed for dose based on weight in kg. • Visually inspect for particulate matter or discoloration. Solution should appear colorless to pale yellow. Do not use if solution is cloudy, discolored, or if visible particles are observed. • Remove a volume from a 250 mL NaCl or D_5W infusion bag that is equal to the required volume of vial for dose. • Dilute in 250 mL NaCl or D_5W infusion bag. • Gently invert to mix. Do not shake or agitate.

Rate of administration • *(1,050 mg dose):* **Week 1 (days 1 and 2):** Infuse at 50 mL/hr. May increase to 75 mL/hr if no infusion reactions occur. **Week 2:** Infuse at 85 mL/hr. **Weeks 3, 4, and subsequent wks:** Infuse at 125 mL/hr. • *(1,400 mg dose)* **Week 1 (day 1):** Infuse at 50 mL/hr. May increase to 75 mL/hr if no infusion reactions occur. **Week 1 (day 2):** Infuse at 35 mL/hr. May increase to 50 mL/hr if no infusion reactions occur. **Week 2:** Infuse at 65 mL/hr. **Week 3:** Infuse at 85 mL/hr. **Week 4 and subsequent wks:** Infuse at 125 mL/hr.

Infusion reactions • **Grade 1 or 2 infusion reactions:** Interrupt infusion until symptoms resolve, then resume at 50% of the infusion rate prior to interruption.

If symptoms do not recur after 30 min, may increase infusion rate per guidelines. Premedicate with a corticosteroid prior to subsequent infusions. • **Grade 3 infusion reactions:** Interrupt infusion and treat symptoms until resolved. May resume at 50% of the infusion rate prior to interruption. If symptoms do not recur after 30 min, may increase infusion rate per guidelines. Premedicate with a corticosteroid prior to subsequent infusions. If Grade 4 infusion-related reactions occur, discontinue infusion and treat symptoms. • **Grade 4 infusion reactions or recurrence of Grade 3 reactions:** Permanently discontinue and treat symptoms until resolved.

Storage • Refrigerate unused vials in original carton. • Protect from light. • Diluted solution must be infused within 10 hrs of preparation at room temperature.

🔷 IV INCOMPATABILITIES

Do not mix with other IV solutions or medications.

INDICATIONS/ROUTES/DOSAGE

NSCLC in Combination With Carboplatin and Pemetrexed)

Note: Give initial dose as a split infusion on days 1 (350 mg) and 2 (1,050 mg or 1,400 mg) of first wk. **IV: ADULTS (WEIGHING LESS THAN 80 KG):** 1,400 mg wkly for 4 wks, then 1,750 mg q3wks thereafter starting on wk 7. (**WEIGHING 80 KG OR GREATER:** 1,750 mg wk for 4 wks, then 2,100 mg q3wks thereafter starting on wk 7.

NSCLC (Single Agent in Combination with Lazertinib)

Note: Give initial dose as a split infusion on day 1 (350 mg) and on day 2 (700 mg or 1,050 mg) of first week.
IV: ADULTS (WEIGHING LESS THAN 80 KG): 1,050 mg weekly for 4 wks, then q2wks until disease progression or unacceptable toxicity. (**WEIGHING 80 KG OR GREATER:** 1,400 mg weekly for 4 wks, then q2wks until disease progression or unacceptable toxicity.

Dose Reduction Schedule

(**WEIGHING LESS THAN 80 KG):** First dose reduction: 700 mg. Second dose

reduction: 350 mg. **Unable to tolerate 350-mg dose:** Permanently discontinue. (**WEIGHING 80 KG OR GREATER): First dose reduction:** 1,050 mg. **Second dose reduction:** 700 mg. **Unable to tolerate 700-mg dose:** Permanently discontinue.

Dose Modification

Based on Common Terminology for Adverse Events (CTCAE).

Dermatological Toxicity (Dermatitis, Dry Skin, Pruritus)

Grade 2 toxicity: Start supportive measures. Consider dose reduction if not improved after 2 wks. **Grade 3 toxicity:** Withhold treatment and start supportive measures until improved to Grade 2 or less, then resume at reduced dose. Permanently discontinue if not improved within 2 wks. **Grade 4 toxicity:** Permanently discontinue.

Pulmonary Toxicity

Any grade interstitial lung disease (ILD)/pneumonitis: Withhold treatment if ILD/pneumonitis suspected. Permanently discontinue if ILD/pneumonitis is confirmed.

Other Toxic Reactions

Other Grade 3 toxicities: Withhold treatment until improved to Grade 1 or 0. If symptoms improve within 1 wk, resume at same dose. If symptoms improve in more than 1 wk but within 4 wks, resume at reduced dose. Permanently discontinue if not improved within 4 wks. **Other Grade 4 toxicities:** Withhold treatment until improved to Grade 1 or 0. If symptoms improve within 4 wks, resume at reduced dose. Permanently discontinue if not improved within 4 wks or Grade 4 toxicity recurs.

Dosage in Renal Impairment

Mild to moderate impairment: No dose adjustment. **Severe impairment:** Not specified; use caution.

Dosage in Hepatic Impairment

Mild impairment: No dose adjustment. **Moderate to severe impairment:** Not specified; use caution.

SIDE EFFECTS

Frequent (84%–25%): Rash, skin exfoliation, eczema, arthralgia, musculoskeletal pain, back/neck pain, myalgia, dyspnea, nausea, fatigue, asthenia, edema (facial, lip, periorbital, peripheral), stomatitis, cough. **Occasional (23%–10%):** Constipation, vomiting, pruritus, diarrhea, decreased appetite, dry skin, pyrexia, hypoesthesia, neuralgia, paresthesia, peripheral neuropathy, dizziness, abdominal pain, headache.

ADVERSE EFFECTS/TOXIC REACTIONS

Infusion related-reactions, including chest discomfort, chills, dyspnea, hypotension, nausea, vomiting reported in 66% of pts. ILD/pneumonitis reported in 3% of pts. Dermatological toxicities, including dermatitis, dry skin, pruritus, may occur. Severe cutaneous reactions, including toxic epidermal necrolysis, reported in less than 1% of pts. Ocular toxicities, including blurred vision, conjunctival redness, dry eye, keratitis, uveitis, visual impairment, may occur. Infections, including paronychia (50% of pts), pneumonia (10% of pts), were reported. Hemorrhagic events, including epistaxis, gingival bleeding, hematuria, hemoptysis, mouth/mucosal hemorrhage, reported in 19% of pts.

NURSING CONSIDERATIONS

BASELINE ASSESSMENT

Obtain BMP, LFT; pregnancy test in females of reproductive potential. Confirm compliance of effective contraception. Obtain weight in kilograms. Verify presence of EGFR exon 20 mutations by approved test. Screen for active infection. Administer in an environment equipped to monitor for and manage infusion-related reactions. Question for prior infusion reactions before each infusion. Question history of hepatic impairment, pulmonary/ocular disease. Conduct dermatological exam for baseline status. Offer emotional support.

INTERVENTION/EVALUATION

Obtain BMP, LFT as clinically indicated. Diligently monitor for infusion reactions during each infusion. If infusion reactions occur, interrupt infusion and manage symptoms. Consider ABG, radiologic test if ILD/pneumonitis (excessive cough, dyspnea, fever, hypoxia) is suspected. Consider treatment with corticosteroids if ILD/pneumonitis is confirmed. Assess skin for cutaneous toxicities, sloughing, rash, nail beds for paronychia. Monitor for ocular toxicities, change of vision; oral lesions, mucosal inflammation; bleeding events of any kind. Monitor daily pattern of bowel activity, stool consistency.

PATIENT/FAMILY TEACHING

• Immediately report symptoms of infusion-related reactions such as chills, cough, difficulty breathing, nausea, vomiting. • Pretreatment with acetaminophen, antihistamines, steroidal anti-inflammatories may help reduce infusion reactions. • Due to pretreatment with a corticosteroid, pts with diabetes may experience a transient rise in blood sugar levels. • Report symptoms of lung inflammation (excessive coughing, difficulty breathing, chest pain); toxic skin reactions (itching, peeling, rash, redness, swelling); liver problems (abdominal pain, bruising, clay-colored stool, amber or dark-colored urine, yellowing of the skin or eyes); eye problems (eye dryness/itching/pain/redness, excessive tearing, change of vision, sensitivity to light; infection of the skin around the nailbeds (swelling, redness, pain, pus). • Use effective contraception to avoid pregnancy. Do not breastfeed. • Avoid prolonged sun exposure/tanning beds. Use high-SPF sunscreen, lip balm, clothing to protect against sunburn/skin irritation.

---

amLODIPine

am-**loe**-di-peen
(Katerzia, Norliqva, <u>Norvasc</u>)
Do not confuse amLODIPine with aMILoride, or Norvasc with Navane or Vascor.

FIXED-COMBINATION(S)

Azor: amLODIPine/olmesartan (an angiotensin II receptor antagonist): 5 mg/20 mg, 10 mg/20 mg, 5 mg/40 mg, 10 mg/40 mg. **Caduet:** amLODIPine/atorvastatin (hydroxymethylglutaryl-CoA [HMG-CoA] reductase inhibitor): 2.5 mg/10 mg, 2.5 mg/20 mg, 2.5 mg/40 mg, 5 mg/10 mg, 10 mg/10 mg, 5 mg/20 mg, 10 mg/20 mg, 5 mg/40 mg, 10 mg/40 mg, 5 mg/80 mg, 10 mg/80 mg. **Exforge:** amLODIPine/valsartan (an angiotensin II receptor antagonist): 5 mg/160 mg, 10 mg/160 mg, 5 mg/320 mg, 10 mg/320 mg. **Lotrel:** amLODIPine/benazepril (an angiotensin-converting enzyme [ACE] inhibitor): 2.5 mg/10 mg, 5 mg/10 mg, 5 mg/20 mg, 5 mg/40 mg, 10 mg/20 mg, 10 mg/40 mg. **Tribenzor:** amLODIPine/olmesartan/hydroCHLOROthiazide: 5 mg/20 mg/12.5 mg, 5 mg/40 mg/12.5 mg, 5 mg/40 mg/25 mg, 10 mg/40 mg/12.5 mg, 10 mg/40 mg/25 mg. **Amlodipine/telmisartan:** (an angiotensin II receptor antagonist): 5 mg/40 mg, 5 mg/80 mg, 10 mg/40 mg, 10 mg/80 mg.

◆CLASSIFICATION

PHARMACOTHERAPEUTIC: Calcium channel blocker (dihydropyridine). **CLINICAL:** Antihypertensive, antianginal.

USES

Coronary artery disease: Treatment of symptomatic chronic stable angina. Treatment of confirmed or suspected vasospastic angina (previously referred to as Prinzmetal or variant angina). Treatment of recently documented coronary artery disease (CAD) by angiography and without HF or an ejection fraction less than 40%. **Hypertension:** Management of hypertension in adults and children greater than or equal to 6 yrs of age. **OFF-LABEL:** Raynaud phenomenon.

PRECAUTIONS

Contraindications: Hypersensitivity to amLODIPine. **Cautions:** Hepatic impairment, severe aortic stenosis, hypertrophic cardiomyopathy with outflow tract obstruction.

ACTION

Inhibits calcium movement across cardiac and vascular smooth muscle cell membranes during depolarization. **Therapeutic Effect:** Dilates coronary arteries, peripheral arteries/arterioles. Decreases total peripheral vascular resistance and B/P by vasodilation.

PHARMACOKINETICS

Route	Onset	Peak	Duration
PO	0.5–1 hr	N/A	24 hrs

Widely distributed. Protein binding: 95%–98%. Metabolized in liver. Excreted primarily in urine. Not removed by hemodialysis. **Half-life:** 30–50 hrs (increased in elderly, pts with hepatic cirrhosis).

⌛ LIFESPAN CONSIDERATIONS

Pregnancy/Lactation: Unknown if drug crosses placenta or is distributed in breast milk. **Children:** Safety and efficacy not established in pts younger than 6 yrs. **Elderly:** Half-life may be increased, more sensitive to hypotensive effects.

INTERACTIONS

DRUG: Strong CYP3A4 inhibitors (e.g., **clarithromycin, ketoconazole, ritonavir**) may increase concentration/effect. Strong CYP3A4 inducers (e.g., **carbamazepine, phenytoin, rifampin**) may decrease concentration/effect. May increase concentration/effect of **lomitapide, simvastatin. HERBAL:** Herbals with hypotensive properties (e.g., **garlic, ginger, ginkgo biloba**) may increase risk of hypotension. **FOOD:** None significant. **LAB VALUES:** May increase hepatic enzyme levels.

 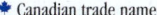

AVAILABILITY (Rx)

Oral Solution: 1 mg/ mL. **Oral Suspension:** 1 mg/mL. **Tablets:** 2.5 mg, 5 mg, 10 mg.

ADMINISTRATION/HANDLING

PO

• May give without regard to food.
• Shake suspension well. Use accurate measuring device (e.g., calibrated oral syringe).

INDICATIONS/ROUTES/DOSAGE

Hypertension

PO: ADULTS: Initially, 2.5–5 once daily. Evaluate after 2–4 wks. Titrate dose. **Maximum:** 10 mg/day. **ELDERLY, ADDITION TO OTHER ANTIHYPERTENSIVES:** Initially, 2.5 mg once daily. Evaluate after 2–4 wks. **Maximum:** 10 mg/day. **CHILDREN 6–17 YRS:** Initially, 2.5 mg once daily. **Usual dose:** 2.5–5 mg once daily.

Angina

PO: ADULTS: 5–10 mg/day as a single dose. **ELDERLY, PTS WITH HEPATIC INSUFFICIENCY:** 5 mg/day as a single dose.

CAD

PO: ADULTS, ELDERLY: 5–10 mg once daily.

Dosage in Renal Impairment

No dose adjustment.

Dosage in Hepatic Impairment

ADULTS, ELDERLY: Hypertension: Initially, 2.5 mg/day. **Angina:** Initially, 5 mg/day. Titrate slowly in pts with severe impairment.

SIDE EFFECTS

Frequent (greater than 5%): Peripheral edema, headache, flushing. **Occasional (5%–1%):** Dizziness, palpitations, nausea, unusual fatigue or weakness (asthenia). **Rare (less than 1%):** Chest pain, bradycardia, orthostatic hypotension.

ADVERSE EFFECTS/ TOXIC REACTIONS

Overdose may produce excessive peripheral vasodilation, marked hypotension with reflex tachycardia, syncope.

NURSING CONSIDERATIONS

BASELINE ASSESSMENT

Assess renal/hepatic function tests, B/P, apical pulse.

INTERVENTION/EVALUATION

Assess B/P (if systolic B/P is less than 90 mm Hg, withhold medication, contact physician). Assess skin for flushing. Question for headache, asthenia.

PATIENT/FAMILY TEACHING

• Do not abruptly discontinue medication. • Compliance with therapy regimen is essential to control hypertension. • Avoid tasks that require alertness, motor skills until response to drug is established. • Do not ingest grapefruit products.

amoxicillin

a-**mox**-i-sil-in
(Novamoxin ✦)
Do not confuse amoxicillin with amoxapine or Atarax.

◆CLASSIFICATION

PHARMACOTHERAPEUTIC: Penicillin. **CLINICAL:** Antibiotic.

USES

Ear, nose, and throat: Infections due to susceptible isolates of *Streptococcus* spp. (alpha- and beta-hemolytic), *Streptococcus pneumoniae, Staphylococcus* spp., or *H. influenzae*. **Genitourinary:** Infections due to isolates of *E. coli, Proteus mirabilis,* or *Enterococcus faecalis*. **Skin and skin structure:** Infections due to susceptible isolates of *Streptococcus* spp. (alpha- and beta-hemolytic), *Staphylococcus* spp., or *E. coli*. **Lower respiratory tract:** Infections due to susceptible isolates of *Streptococcus* spp. (alpha- and beta-hemolytic), *S. pneumoniae, Staphylococcus* spp., or *H. influenzae*. **OFF-LABEL:** Treatment of Lyme disease. Postexposure prophylaxis for anthrax exposure, endocarditis (prophylaxis). Bronchiectasis, prosthetic joint infection.

PRECAUTIONS

Contraindications: Serious hypersensitivity to amoxicillin, other beta-lactams. **Cautions:** History of allergies (esp. cephalosporins), infectious mononucleosis, renal impairment, asthma.

ACTION

Inhibits bacterial cell wall synthesis by binding to PCN-binding proteins. **Therapeutic Effect:** Bactericidal in susceptible microorganisms.

PHARMACOKINETICS

Widely distributed. Protein binding: 20%. Partially metabolized in liver. Primarily excreted in urine. Removed by hemodialysis. **Half-life:** 1–1.3 hrs (increased in renal impairment).

⧗ LIFESPAN CONSIDERATIONS

Pregnancy/Lactation: Crosses placenta, appears in cord blood, amniotic fluid. Distributed in breast milk in low concentrations. May lead to allergic sensitization, diarrhea, candidiasis, skin rash in infant. **Children:** Immature renal function in neonate/young infant may delay renal excretion. **Elderly:** Age-related renal impairment may require dosage adjustment.

INTERACTIONS

DRUG: Allopurinol, probenecid may increase concentration/effect. **HERBAL:** None significant. **FOOD:** None known. **LAB VALUES:** May increase serum ALT, AST, bilirubin, BUN, creatinine, LDH. May cause positive Coombs' test.

AVAILABILITY (Rx)

Capsules: 250 mg, 500 mg. **Powder for Oral Suspension:** 125 mg/5 mL, 200 mg/5 mL, 250 mg/5 mL, 400 mg/5 mL. **Tablets:** 500 mg, 875 mg. **Tablets (Chewable):** 125 mg, 250 mg.

ADMINISTRATION/HANDLING

PO

• Give without regard to food. • Instruct pt to chew/crush chewable tablets thoroughly before swallowing. • Oral suspension dose may be mixed with formula, milk, fruit juice, water, cold drink. • Give immediately after mixing. • After reconstitution, oral suspension is stable for 14 days at either room temperature or refrigerated.

INDICATIONS/ROUTES/DOSAGE

Usual Dosage

PO: ADULTS, ELDERLY: 500–1000 mg q8–12h. **INFANTS, CHILDREN, ADOLESCENTS:** 45–50 mg/kg/day in divided doses q8h. **Maximum Dose:** 500 mg. **NEONATE:** 30 mg/kg/day in divided doses q12h.

Dosage in Renal Impairment

◀**ALERT**▶ Immediate-release 875-mg tablet should not be used in pts with creatinine clearance less than 30 mL/min. Dosage interval is modified based on creatinine clearance. **Creatinine clearance 10–30 mL/min: ADULTS:** 250–500 mg q12h. **CHILDREN:** 8–20 mg/kg/dose q12h. **Creatinine clearance less than 10 mL/min: ADULTS:** 250–500 mg q24h. **CHILDREN:** 8–20 mg/kg/dose q24h.

Dosage in Hepatic Impairment
No dose adjustment.

SIDE EFFECTS

Frequent: GI disturbances (mild diarrhea, nausea, vomiting), headache, oral/vaginal candidiasis. **Occasional:** Generalized rash, urticaria.

ADVERSE EFFECTS/TOXIC REACTIONS

Antibiotic-associated colitis, other superinfections (abdominal cramps, severe watery diarrhea, fever) may result from altered bacterial balance in GI tract. Severe hypersensitivity reactions, including anaphylaxis, acute interstitial nephritis, occur rarely.

NURSING CONSIDERATIONS

BASELINE ASSESSMENT

Question for history of allergies (esp. penicillins, cephalosporins), renal impairment.

INTERVENTION/EVALUATION

Promptly report rash, diarrhea (fever, abdominal pain, mucus and blood in stool may indicate antibiotic-associated colitis). Be alert for superinfection: fever, vomiting, diarrhea, anal/genital pruritus, black "hairy" tongue, oral mucosal changes (ulceration, pain, erythema). Monitor renal/hepatic function tests.

PATIENT/FAMILY TEACHING

• Continue antibiotic for full length of treatment. • Space doses evenly. • Take with meals if GI upset occurs. • Thoroughly crush or chew the chewable tablets before swallowing. • Report rash, diarrhea, other new symptoms.

amoxicillin/clavulanate

a-**mox**-i-sil-in/**klav**-yoo-la-nate
(Augmentin, Augmentin ES 600, Clavulin ✦)
Do not confuse Augmentin with amoxicillin or Azulfidine.

◆ **CLASSIFICATION**

PHARMACOTHERAPEUTIC: Penicillin. **CLINICAL:** Antibiotic.

USES

Lower respiratory tract infections: Caused by beta lactamase–producing isolates of *H. influenzae, M. catarrhalis.* **Acute bacterial otitis media:** Caused by beta lactamase–producing isolates of *H. influenzae, M. catarrhalis.* **Sinusitis:** Caused by beta lactamase–producing isolates of *H. influenzae, M. catarrhalis.* **Skin and skin structure infections:** Caused by beta lactamase–producing isolates of *S. aureus, E. coli,* and *Klebsi-*ella species. **Urinary tract infections:** Caused by beta lactamase–producing isolates of *E. coli, Klebsiella* species, and *Enterobacter* species. **OFF-LABEL:** Diabetic foot infection, intra-abdominal infection, neutropenic fever. Bite wound infection prophylaxis, COPD (acute exacerbation).

PRECAUTIONS

Contraindications: Hypersensitivity to amoxicillin, clavulanate, any penicillins; history of cholestatic jaundice or hepatic impairment with amoxicillin/clavulanate therapy. **Extended-Release:** (additional): Severe renal impairment (creatinine clearance less than 30 mL/min), hemodialysis pt. **Cautions:** History of allergies, esp. cephalosporins; renal impairment, infectious mononucleosis.

ACTION

Amoxicillin inhibits bacterial cell wall synthesis by binding to PCN-binding proteins. Clavulanate inhibits bacterial beta-lactamase protecting amoxicillin from degradation. **Therapeutic Effect:** Amoxicillin is bactericidal in susceptible microorganisms. Clavulanate protects amoxicillin from enzymatic degradation.

PHARMACOKINETICS

Widely distributed. Protein binding: 20%. Partially metabolized in liver. Primarily excreted in urine. Removed by hemodialysis. **Half-life:** 1–1.3 hrs (increased in renal impairment).

⧗ LIFESPAN CONSIDERATIONS

Pregnancy/Lactation: Crosses placenta, appears in cord blood, amniotic fluid. Distributed in breast milk in low concentrations. May lead to allergic sensitization, diarrhea, candidiasis, skin rash in infant. **Children:** Immature renal function in neonate/young infant may delay renal excretion. **Elderly:** Age-related renal impairment may require dosage adjustment.

INTERACTIONS

DRUG: Allopurinol, probenecid may increase concentration/effect. **HERBAL:**

None significant. **FOOD:** None known. **LAB VALUES:** May increase serum ALT, AST. May cause positive Coombs' test.

AVAILABILITY (Rx)

Powder for Oral Suspension: *(Amoclan, Augmentin):* 125 mg–31.25 mg/5 mL, 200 mg–28.5 mg/5 mL, 250 mg–62.5 mg/5 mL, 400 mg–57 mg/5 mL, 600 mg–42.9 mg/5 mL. **Tablets:** *(Augmentin):* 250 mg–125 mg, 500 mg–125 mg, 875 mg–125 mg. **Tablets (Chewable):** *(Augmentin):* 200 mg–28.5 mg, 400 mg–57 mg.

Tablets (Extended-Release): 1,000 mg–62.5 mg.

ADMINISTRATION/HANDLING

PO

• Administer with food. • After reconstitution, oral suspension is stable for 10 days but should be refrigerated. • May mix dose of suspension with milk, formula, or juice and give immediately. • Give without regard to meals. • Give with food to increase absorption, decrease stomach upset. • Instruct pt to chew/crush chewable tablets thoroughly before swallowing. • Do not break, crush, dissolve, or divide extended-release tablets.

INDICATIONS/ROUTES/DOSAGE

Note: Dosage based on amoxicillin component.

Usual Adult Dosage
PO: ADULTS, ELDERLY: 250 mg q8h or 500 mg q8–12h or 875 mg q12h or *(Extended-Release):* 2,000 mg q12h.

Usual Pediatric Dosage
Note: Dosing determined by formulation's amoxicillin/clavulanate ratio.
(Immediate-Release): **INFANTS, CHILDREN, ADOLESCENTS:** (4:1 formulation): 20–40 mg amoxicillin/kg/day in 3 divided doses. **Maximum:** 1500 mg/day. (7:1 formulation): 25–45 mg amoxicillin/kg/day in 2 divided doses. **Maximum:** 1,750 mg/day. (14:1 formulation): 90 mg amoxicillin/kg/day in 2 divided doses; **Maximum:** 4,000 mg/day. **NEONATES:** 30 mg/kg/day (using 125 mg/5 mL suspension) in divided doses q12h.
(Extended-Release): **CHILDREN AND ADOLESCENTS WEIGHING GREATER THAN 40 KG:** 2,000 mg amoxicillin q12h.

Dosage in Renal Impairment
◀**ALERT**▶ Do not use 875-mg tablet or extended-release tablets for creatinine clearance less than 30 mL/min. Dosage and frequency are modified based on creatinine clearance. **Creatinine clearance 10–30 mL/min:** 250–500 mg q12h. **Creatinine clearance less than 10 mL/min:** 250–500 mg q24h. **HD:** 250–500 mg q24h, give dose during and after dialysis. **PD:** 250 mg q12h.

Dosage in Hepatic Impairment
No dose adjustment (see Contraindications).

SIDE EFFECTS

Occasional (9%–4%): Diarrhea, loose stools, nausea, skin rashes, urticaria. **Rare (less than 3%):** Vomiting, vaginitis, abdominal discomfort, flatulence, headache.

ADVERSE EFFECTS/TOXIC REACTIONS

Antibiotic-associated colitis, other superinfections (abdominal cramps, severe watery diarrhea, fever) may result from altered bacterial balance in GI tract. Severe hypersensitivity reactions, including anaphylaxis, acute interstitial nephritis, occur rarely.

NURSING CONSIDERATIONS

BASELINE ASSESSMENT

Question for history of allergies, esp. penicillins, cephalosporins, renal impairment.

INTERVENTION/EVALUATION

Promptly report rash, diarrhea (fever, abdominal pain, mucus and blood in stool may indicate antibiotic-associated colitis). Be alert for signs of superinfection, including fever, vomiting, diarrhea, black "hairy" tongue, ulceration or changes of oral mucosa, anal/genital pruritus. Monitor renal/hepatic tests with prolonged therapy.

PATIENT/FAMILY TEACHING

• Continue antibiotic for full length of treatment. • Space doses evenly. • Take with meals if GI upset occurs. • Thoroughly crush or chew the chewable tablets before swallowing. • Notify physician if rash, diarrhea, other new symptoms occur.

---

amphotericin B

am-foe-**ter**-i-sin

(Abelcet, AmBisome, Fungizone ✦)

◆CLASSIFICATION

PHARMACOTHERAPEUTIC: Polyene antifungal. **CLINICAL:** Antifungal, antiprotozoal.

USES

Abelcet: Treatment of invasive fungal infections refractory or intolerant to Fungizone. **AmBisome:** Empiric treatment of fungal infection in febrile neutropenic pts. *Aspergillus, Candida* species, *Cryptococcus* infections refractory to Fungizone or pt with renal impairment or toxicity with Fungizone. Treatment of cryptococcal meningitis in HIV-infected pts. Treatment of visceral leishmaniasis. **Fungizone:** Treatment of life-threatening fungal infections caused by susceptible fungi, including *Candida* spp., *Histoplasma, Cryptococcus, Aspergillus, Blastomyces.*

PRECAUTIONS

Contraindications: Hypersensitivity to amphotericin B. **Cautions:** Concomitant use with other nephrotoxic drugs; renal impairment.

ACTION

Generally fungistatic but may become fungicidal with high dosages or very susceptible microorganisms. Binds to sterols in fungal cell membrane. **Therapeutic Effect:** Alters fungal cell membrane permeability, allowing loss of potassium, other cellular components, resulting in cell death.

PHARMACOKINETICS

Widely distributed. Protein binding: 90%. Metabolism not specified. Cleared by nonrenal pathways. Minimal removal by hemodialysis. Amphotec and Abelcet are not dialyzable. **Half-life:** Fungizone, 24 hrs (increased in neonates and children); Abelcet, 7.2 days; AmBisome, 100–153 hrs; Amphotec, 26–28 hrs.

⌛ LIFESPAN CONSIDERATIONS

Pregnancy/Lactation: Crosses placenta; unknown if distributed in breast milk. **Children:** Safety and efficacy not established, but use the least amount for therapeutic regimen. **Elderly:** No age-related precautions noted.

INTERACTIONS

DRUG: *(Ambisome):* **Foscarnet** may increase nephrotoxic effect. May decrease therapeutic effect of *Saccharomyces boulardii.* **HERBAL:** None significant. **FOOD:** None known. **LAB VALUES:** May increase serum ALT, AST, alkaline phosphatase, BUN, creatinine. May decrease serum calcium, magnesium, potassium.

AVAILABILITY (Rx)

Injection, Powder for Reconstitution: *(AmBisome, Fungizone):* 50 mg. **Injection, Suspension:** *(Abelcet):* 5 mg/mL (20 mL).

ADMINISTRATION/HANDLING

🔟 IV

• Use strict aseptic technique; no bacteriostatic agent or preservative is present in diluent.

Reconstitution • *(Abelcet):* Shake 20-mL (100-mg) vial gently until contents are dissolved. Withdraw required dose using 5-micron filter needle (supplied by manufacturer). • Dilute with D_5W to 1–2 mg/mL. • *(AmBisome):* Reconstitute each 50-mg vial with 12 mL Sterile Water for Injection to provide concentration of 4 mg/mL. • Shake vial vigorously for 30 sec. Withdraw required dose and inject syringe contents through a 5-micron filter into an infusion of D_5W to provide final concentration of 1–2 mg/mL (0.2–0.5 mg/mL for infants and small children). • *(Fungizone):* Add 10 mL Sterile Water for Injection to each 50-mg vial. • Further dilute with 250–500 mL D₅W. • Final concentration should not exceed 0.1 mg/mL (0.25 mg/mL for central infusion).

Rate of administration • Give by slow IV infusion. Infuse conventional amphotericin over 4–6 hrs; Abelcet over 2 hrs (shake contents if infusion longer than 2 hrs); AmBisome over 1–2 hrs.

Storage • *(Abelcet):* Refrigerate unreconstituted solution. Reconstituted solution is stable for 48 hrs if refrigerated, 6 hrs at room temperature. • *(AmBisome):* Refrigerate unreconstituted solution. Reconstituted vials are stable for 24 hrs when refrigerated. Concentration of 1–2 mg/mL is stable for 6 hrs. • *(Fungizone):* Refrigerate unused vials. • Once reconstituted, vials stable for 24 hrs at room temperature, 7 days if refrigerated. • Diluted solutions stable for 24 hrs at room temperature, 2 days if refrigerated.

🌐 IV INCOMPATIBILITIES

Note: Abelcet, AmBisome, Fungizone: Do not mix with any other drug, diluent, or solution.

🌐 IV COMPATIBILITIES

Note: Abelcet, AmBisome, Fungizone: Do not mix with any other drug, diluent, or solution.

INDICATIONS/ROUTES/DOSAGE

Usual Abelcet Dose
IV infusion: ADULTS, CHILDREN: 5 mg/kg once daily.

Usual AmBisome Dose
IV infusion: ADULTS: 3–6 mg/kg/day. **CHILDREN:** 3–5 mg/kg/day.

Fungizone, Usual Dose
IV infusion: ADULTS, ELDERLY: Dosage based on pt tolerance and severity of infection. Initially, 1-mg test dose is given over 20–30 min (some clinicians believe a test dose is unnecessary). If tolerated, usual dose range is 0.3–1.5 mg/kg/day. Once therapy established, may give q48h at 1–1.5 mg/kg q48h. **Maximum:** 1.5 mg/kg/day. **CHILDREN:** Test dose of 0.1 mg/kg/dose (**maximum:** 1 mg) is infused over 30–60 min. If test dose is tolerated, usual initial dose is 0.25–0.5 mg/kg/day. Gradually increase dose until desired dose achieved. **Maximum:** 1.5 mg/kg/day. Once therapy is established, may give 1–1.5 mg/kg q48h. **NEONATES:** Initially, 1 mg/kg/dose once daily up to 1.5 mg/kg/day for short term. Once therapy established, may give 1–1.5 mg/kg q48h.

Dosage in Renal/Hepatic Impairment
No dose adjustment.

SIDE EFFECTS

Frequent (greater than 10%): Abelcet: Chills, fever, increased serum creatinine, multiple organ failure. **AmBisome:** Hypokalemia, hypomagnesemia, hyperglycemia, hypocalcemia, edema, abdominal pain, back pain, chills, chest pain, hypotension, diarrhea, nausea, vomiting, headache, fever, rigors, insomnia, dyspnea, epistaxis, increased hepatic/renal function test results. **Amphotec:** Chills, fever, hypotension, tachycardia, increased serum creatinine, hypokalemia, bilirubinemia. **Amphocin:** Fever, chills, headache, anemia, hypokalemia, hypomagnesemia, anorexia, malaise, generalized pain, nephrotoxicity.

ADVERSE EFFECTS/TOXIC REACTIONS

Cardiovascular toxicity (hypotension, ventricular fibrillation), anaphylaxis occur rarely. Altered vision/hearing, seizures, hepatic failure, coagulation defects, multiple organ failure, sepsis may occur. Each alternative formulation is less nephrotoxic than conventional amphotericin (Amphocin).

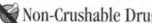
✦ Canadian trade name　　🐾 Non-Crushable Drug　　▣ High Alert drug

NURSING CONSIDERATIONS

BASELINE ASSESSMENT

Obtain BMP, LFT, serum magnesium, ionized calcium. Question for history of allergies, esp. to amphotericin B, sulfite. Avoid, if possible, other nephrotoxic medications. Obtain premedication orders (antipyretics, antihistamines, antiemetics, corticosteroids) to reduce adverse reactions during IV therapy.

INTERVENTION/EVALUATION

Monitor vital signs. Assess for adverse reactions (fever, tremors, chills, anorexia, nausea, vomiting, abdominal pain) q15min twice, then q30min for 4 hrs of initial infusion. If symptoms occur, slow infusion, administer medication for symptomatic relief. For severe reaction, stop infusion and notify physician. Evaluate IV site for phlebitis. Monitor I&O, renal function tests for nephrotoxicity. Monitor CBC, BMP (esp. potassium), LFT, serum magnesium.

PATIENT/FAMILY TEACHING

• Prolonged therapy (wks or mos) is usually necessary. • Fever reaction may decrease with continued therapy. • Muscle weakness may be noted during therapy (due to hypokalemia).

ampicillin

am-pi-sil-in
Do not confuse ampicillin with aminophylline.

◆CLASSIFICATION

PHARMACOTHERAPEUTIC: Penicillin. **CLINICAL:** Antibiotic.

USES

Treatment of infections caused by susceptible strains. **Genitourinary tract including gonorrhea:** *E. coli, P. mirabilis, Enterococcus, Shigella, S. typhosa* and other *Salmonella,* and non–penicillinase-producing *N. gonorrhoeae.* **Respiratory tract:** Non–penicillinase-producing *H. influenzae* and *Staphylococci,* and *Streptococci* including *S. pneumoniae.* **Gastrointestinal tract:** *Shigella, S. typhosa* and other *Salmonella, E. coli, P. mirabilis,* and *Enterococcus.* **Meningitis:** *O. Meningitides.* OFF-LABEL: Endocarditis (prophylaxis); intra-abdominal, pelvic, prosthetic joint infections; osteomyelitis.

PRECAUTIONS

Contraindications: Hypersensitivity to ampicillin or any penicillin. Infections caused by penicillinase-producing organisms. **Cautions:** History of allergies, esp. cephalosporins, renal impairment, asthmatic pts, infectious mononucleosis.

ACTION

Inhibits cell wall synthesis in susceptible microorganisms by binding to PCN binding protein. **Therapeutic Effect:** Bactericidal in susceptible microorganisms.

PHARMACOKINETICS

Widely distributed. Protein binding: 15%–25%. Partially metabolized in liver. Primarily excreted in urine. Removed by hemodialysis. **Half-life:** 1–1.5 hrs (increased in renal impairment).

⧖ LIFESPAN CONSIDERATIONS

Pregnancy/Lactation: Crosses placenta; appears in cord blood, amniotic fluid. Distributed in breast milk in low concentrations. May lead to allergic sensitization, diarrhea, candidiasis, skin rash in infant. **Children:** Immature renal function in neonates/young infants may delay renal excretion. **Elderly:** Age-related renal impairment may require dosage adjustment.

INTERACTIONS

DRUG: Allopurinol, probenecid may increase concentration/effect. **HERBAL:** None significant. **FOOD:** None known. **LAB VALUES:** May increase serum ALT, AST. May cause positive Coombs' test.

AVAILABILITY (Rx)

Capsules: 500 mg. **Injection, Powder for Reconstitution:** 125 mg, 250 mg, 500 mg, 1 g, 2 g.

ADMINISTRATION/HANDLING

 IV

Reconstitution • For IV injection, dilute each vial with 5 mL Sterile Water for Injection or 0.9% NaCl (10 mL for 1- and 2-g vials). **Maximum concentration:** 100 mg/mL for IV push. • For intermittent IV infusion (piggyback), further dilute with 50–100 mL 0.9% NaCl. **Maximum concentration:** 30 mg/mL.

Rate of administration • For IV injection, give over 3–5 min (125–500 mg) or over 10–15 min (1–2 g). For intermittent IV infusion (piggyback), infuse over 15–30 min. • Due to potential for hypersensitivity/anaphylaxis, start initial dose at few drops per min, increase slowly to ordered rate; stay with pt first 10–15 min, then check q10min.

Storage • IV solution, diluted with 0.9% NaCl, is stable for 8 hrs at room temperature or 2 days if refrigerated. • If diluted with D₅W, is stable for 2 hrs at room temperature or 3 hrs if refrigerated. • Discard if precipitate forms.

IM

• Reconstitute each vial with Sterile Water for Injection or Bacteriostatic Water for Injection (consult individual vial for specific volume of diluent). • Stable for 1 hr. • Give deeply in large muscle mass.

PO

• Give orally 1–2 hrs before meals for maximum absorption.

⚛ IV COMPATIBILITIES

Calcium gluconate, dexmedetomidine heparin, insulin, magnesium sulfate, potassium chloride.

INDICATIONS/ROUTES/DOSAGE

Usual Dosage

PO: ADULTS, ELDERLY: 250–500 mg q6h. **ADOLESCENTS, CHILDREN, INFANTS:** 50–100 mg/kg/day in divided doses. **Maximum:** 2 g/day.

IV, IM: ADULTS, ELDERLY: 1–2 g q4–6h or 50–250 mg/kg/day in divided doses. **Maximum:** 12 g/day. **ADOLESCENTS, CHILDREN, INFANTS:** 50–200 mg/kg/day in divided doses q6h. **Maximum:** 8 g/day. **NEONATES:** 50 mg/kg/dose q6–12h or 75 mg/kg/dose q12h.

Dosage in Renal Impairment

Creatinine Clearance	Dosage
10–50 mL/min	Administer q6–12h
Less than 10 mL/min	Administer q12–24h
Hemodialysis	1–2 g q12–24h
Peritoneal dialysis	250 mg q12h
Continuous renal replacement therapy (CRRT)	2g, then 1–2 g q6–8h

Dosage in Hepatic Impairment
No dose adjustment.

SIDE EFFECTS

Frequent: Pain at IM injection site, GI disturbances (mild diarrhea, nausea, vomiting), oral or vaginal candidiasis. **Occasional:** Generalized rash, urticaria, phlebitis, thrombophlebitis (with IV administration), headache. **Rare:** Dizziness, seizures (esp. with IV therapy).

ADVERSE EFFECTS/TOXIC REACTIONS

Antibiotic-associated colitis, other superinfections (abdominal cramps, severe watery diarrhea, fever) may result from altered bacterial balance in GI tract. Severe hypersensitivity reactions, including anaphylaxis, acute interstitial nephritis, occur rarely.

NURSING CONSIDERATIONS

BASELINE ASSESSMENT

Question for history of allergies, esp. penicillins, cephalosporins; renal impairment.

INTERVENTION/EVALUATION

Promptly report rash (although common with ampicillin, may indicate hypersensi-

  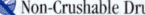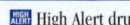

tivity) or diarrhea (fever, abdominal pain, mucus and blood in stool may indicate antibiotic-associated colitis). Evaluate IV site for phlebitis. Check IM injection site for pain, induration. Monitor I&O, urinalysis, renal function tests. Be alert for superinfection: fever, vomiting, diarrhea, anal/genital pruritus, oral mucosal changes (ulceration, pain, erythema).

PATIENT/FAMILY TEACHING

• Continue antibiotic for full length of treatment. • Space doses evenly. • More effective if taken 1 hr before or 2 hrs after food/beverages. • Discomfort may occur with IM injection. • Report rash, diarrhea, or other new symptoms.

ampicillin/ sulbactam

amp-i-**sil**-in/sul-**bak**-tam
(<u>Unasyn</u>)

◆CLASSIFICATION

PHARMACOTHERAPEUTIC: Penicillin. **CLINICAL:** Antibiotic.

USES

Treatment of infections due to susceptible strains. **Skin and skin structure:** Caused by beta lactamase–producing strains of *S. aureus, E. coli, Klebsiella* spp. (including *K. pneumoniae*), *Proteus mirabilis, B. fragilis, Enterobacter* spp., and *Acinetobacter calcoaceticus*. **Intra-abdominal infections:** Caused by beta lactamase–producing strains of *E. coli, Klebsiella* spp. (including *K. pneumoniae*), *Bacteroides* spp. (including *B. fragilis*), and *Enterobacter* spp. **Gynecological infections:** Caused by beta lactamase–producing strains of *E. coli*, and *Bacteroides* spp. (including *B. fragilis*). **OFF-LABEL:** Endocarditis (treatment), community-acquired pneumonia, surgi-

cal prophylaxis, bloodstream, diabetic foot infections.

PRECAUTIONS

Contraindications: Hypersensitivity to ampicillin, any penicillins, or sulbactam. Hx of cholestatic jaundice, hepatic impairment associated with ampicillin/sulbactam. **Cautions:** History of allergies, esp. cephalosporins; renal impairment; infectious mononucleosis; asthmatic pts.

ACTION

Ampicillin inhibits bacterial cell wall synthesis by binding to PCN-binding proteins. Sulbactam inhibits bacterial beta-lactamase, protecting ampicillin from degradation. **Therapeutic Effect:** Bactericidal in susceptible microorganisms.

PHARMACOKINETICS

Widely distributed. Protein binding: 28%–38%. Partially metabolized in liver. Primarily excreted in urine. Removed by hemodialysis. **Half-life:** 1–1.3 hrs (increased in renal impairment).

⧗ LIFESPAN CONSIDERATIONS

Pregnancy/Lactation: Crosses placenta; appears in cord blood, amniotic fluid. Distributed in breast milk in low concentrations. May lead to allergic sensitization, diarrhea, candidiasis, skin rash in infant. **Children:** Safety and efficacy not established in pts younger than 1 yr. **Elderly:** Age-related renal impairment may require dosage adjustment.

INTERACTIONS

DRUG: Allopurinol, probenecid may increase concentration/effect. **Tetracyclines** may decrease therapeutic effect. **HERBAL:** None significant. **FOOD:** None known. **LAB VALUES:** May increase serum ALT, AST, alkaline phosphatase, LDH, creatinine. May cause positive Coombs' test.

AVAILABILITY (Rx)

Injection, Powder for Reconstitution: 1.5 g (ampicillin 1 g/sulbactam 0.5 g), 3 g (ampicillin 2 g/sulbactam 1 g).

ADMINISTRATION/HANDLING

 IV

Reconstitution • For IV injection, dilute with Sterile Water for Injection to provide concentration of 375 mg/mL. • For intermittent IV infusion (piggyback), further dilute with 50–100 mL 0.9% NaCl.

Rate of administration • For IV injection, give slowly over minimum of 10–15 min. • For intermittent IV infusion (piggyback), infuse over 15–30 min. • Due to potential for hypersensitivity/anaphylaxis, start initial dose at few drops per min, increase slowly to ordered rate; stay with pt first 10–15 min, then check q10min.

Storage • IV solution, diluted with 0.9% NaCl, is stable for up to 72 hrs if refrigerated (4 hrs if diluted with D₅W). • Discard if precipitate forms.

IM

• Reconstitute each 1.5-g vial with 3.2 mL Sterile Water for Injection or lidocaine to provide concentration of 250 mg ampicillin/125 mg sulbactam/mL. • Give deeply into large muscle mass within 1 hr after preparation.

☷ IV COMPATIBILITIES

Dexmedetomidine, heparin, insulin.

INDICATIONS/ROUTES/DOSAGE

Usual Dosage Range
IV, IM: ADULTS, ELDERLY, CHILDREN 13 YRS AND OLDER: 1.5–3 g q6h. **Maximum:** 12 g/day. **IV: CHILDREN 12 YRS AND YOUNGER: (Mild to moderate infection):** 100–200 mg ampicillin/kg/day in divided doses q6h. **Maximum dose:** 2,000 mg ampicillin/dose. **(Severe infection):** 200–400 mg ampicillin/kg/day divided q6h. **Maximum dose:** 2,000 mg ampicillin/dose. **NEONATES:** 100 mg (ampicillin)/kg/day in divided doses q8–12h.

Dosage in Renal Impairment
Dosage and frequency are modified based on creatinine clearance and severity of infection.

Creatinine Clearance	Dosage
Greater than 30 mL/min	No dose adjustment
15–30 mL/min	1.5–3 g q12h
5–14 mL/min	1.5–3 g q24h
Hemodialysis	1.5–3 g q12–24h (after HD on dialysis days)
Peritoneal dialysis	1.5–3 g q12–24h
Continuous renal replacement therapy (CRRT)	3 g, then 1.5–3 g q6–12h

Dosage in Hepatic Impairment
No dose adjustment.

SIDE EFFECTS

Frequent: Diarrhea, rash (most common), urticaria, pain at IM injection site, thrombophlebitis with IV administration, oral or vaginal candidiasis. **Occasional:** Nausea, vomiting, headache, malaise, urinary retention.

ADVERSE EFFECTS/TOXIC REACTIONS

Antibiotic-associated colitis, other superinfections (abdominal cramps; severe, watery diarrhea; fever) may result from altered bacterial balance in GI tract. Severe hypersensitivity reactions, including anaphylaxis, acute interstitial nephritis, blood dyscrasias may occur. High dosage may produce seizures.

NURSING CONSIDERATIONS

BASELINE ASSESSMENT

Question for history of allergies, esp. penicillins, cephalosporins; renal impairment.

INTERVENTION/EVALUATION

Promptly report rash (although common with ampicillin, may indicate hypersensitivity) or diarrhea (fever, abdominal pain, mucus and blood in stool may indicate antibiotic-associated colitis). Evaluate IV site for phlebitis. Check IM injection site for pain, induration. Monitor I&O, urinalysis, renal function tests. Be alert for superinfection: fever, vomiting, diarrhea, anal/genital pruritus, oral mucosal changes (ulceration, pain, erythema).

PATIENT/FAMILY TEACHING
• Discomfort may occur with IM injection. • Report rash, diarrhea, or other new symptoms.

anastrozole ℮

an-**as**-troe-zole
(Arimidex)
Do not confuse anastrozole with letrozole, or Arimidex with Imitrex.

◆CLASSIFICATION
PHARMACOTHERAPEUTIC: Aromatase inhibitor. **CLINICAL:** Antineoplastic hormone.

USES
Treatment of advanced breast cancer in postmenopausal women who have developed progressive disease while receiving tamoxifen therapy. First-line therapy in advanced or metastatic breast cancer in postmenopausal women. Adjuvant treatment in early hormone receptor–positive breast cancer in postmenopausal women. **OFF-LABEL:** Treatment of recurrent or metastatic endometrial or uterine cancers; treatment of ovarian cancer. Breast cancer (risk reduction).

PRECAUTIONS
Contraindications: Hypersensitivity to anastrozole. Pregnancy, women who may become pregnant. **Cautions:** Preexisting ischemic cardiac disease, osteopenia (higher risk of developing osteoporosis), hyperlipidemia. May increase fall risk with fractures during therapy in pts with history of osteoporosis.

ACTION
Inhibits aromatase, preventing conversion of androstenedione to estrone, and testosterone to estradiol. **Therapeutic**

Effect: Decreases tumor mass or delays tumor progression.

PHARMACOKINETICS
Widely distributed. Protein binding: 40%. Metabolized in liver. Steady-state plasma levels reached in approximately 7 days. Eliminated by biliary system and, to a lesser extent, kidneys. **Mean Half-life:** 50 hrs in postmenopausal women.

⧗ LIFESPAN CONSIDERATIONS
Pregnancy/Lactation: Crosses placenta; may cause fetal harm. Unknown if distributed in breast milk. **Children:** Safety and efficacy not established. **Elderly:** No age-related precautions noted.

INTERACTIONS
DRUG: Estrogen therapies may reduce concentration/effects. **Tamoxifen** may reduce plasma concentration. **HERBAL:** None significant. **FOOD:** None known. **LAB VALUES:** May elevate serum GGT level in pts with liver metastases. May increase serum ALT, AST, alkaline phosphatase, total cholesterol, LDL.

AVAILABILITY (Rx)
Tablets: 1 mg.

ADMINISTRATION/HANDLING
PO
• Give without regard to food.

INDICATIONS/ROUTES/DOSAGE
Breast Cancer (Advanced or Metastatic)
PO: ADULTS, ELDERLY: 1 mg once daily (continue until tumor progresses).

Breast Cancer (Adjuvant)
PO: ADULTS, ELDERLY: 1 mg once daily (optimal duration of therapy unknown).

Dosage in Renal/Hepatic Impairment
No dose adjustment.

SIDE EFFECTS
Frequent (16%–8%): Asthenia, nausea, headache, hot flashes, back pain, vomiting, cough, diarrhea. **Occasional**

(6%–4%): Constipation, abdominal pain, anorexia, bone pain, pharyngitis, dizziness, rash, dry mouth, peripheral edema, pelvic pain, depression, chest pain, paresthesia. **Rare (2%–1%):** Weight gain, diaphoresis.

ADVERSE EFFECTS/TOXIC REACTIONS

Thrombophlebitis, anemia, leukopenia occur rarely. Vaginal hemorrhage occurs rarely (2% of pts).

NURSING CONSIDERATIONS

BASELINE ASSESSMENT

Obtain bone mineral density, total cholesterol, LDL, mammogram, clinical breast exam.

INTERVENTION/EVALUATION

Monitor for asthenia, dizziness; assist with ambulation if needed. Assess for headache, pain. Offer antiemetic for nausea, vomiting. Monitor for onset of diarrhea; offer antidiarrheal medication.

PATIENT/FAMILY TEACHING

• Notify physician if nausea, asthenia, hot flashes become unmanageable.

anidulafungin

a-**nid**-ue-la-**fun**-jin
(Eraxis)

◆CLASSIFICATION

PHARMACOTHERAPEUTIC: Echinocandin. **CLINICAL:** Antifungal.

USES

Candidemia, *Candida* infections: Intra-abdominal abscess, peritonitis in adults and pts 1 mo of age and older. **Esophageal candidiasis:** Treatment of esophageal candidiasis in adults.

PRECAUTIONS

Contraindications: Hypersensitivity to anidulafungin, other echinocandins. **Cautions:** Hepatic impairment.

ACTION

Inhibits synthesis of the enzyme glucan (vital component of fungal cell formation), preventing fungal cell wall formation. **Therapeutic Effect:** Fungistatic.

PHARMACOKINETICS

Widely distributed. Moderately bound to albumin. Protein binding: 84%–99%. Slow chemical degradation; 30% excreted in feces over 9 days. Not removed by hemodialysis. **Half-life:** 40–50 hrs.

⧗ LIFESPAN CONSIDERATIONS

Pregnancy/Lactation: May cause fetal harm. Crosses placental barrier. Unknown if distributed in breast milk. **Children:** Safety and efficacy not established. **Elderly:** No age-related precautions noted.

INTERACTIONS

DRUG: None significant. **HERBAL:** None significant. **FOOD:** None known. **LAB VALUES:** May increase serum alkaline phosphatase, amylase, ALT, AST, bilirubin, calcium, creatinine, CPK, LDH, lipase. May decrease serum albumin, bicarbonate, magnesium, protein, potassium; Hgb, Hct, WBCs, neutrophils, platelet count. May prolong prothrombin time (PT).

AVAILABILITY (Rx)

Injection, Powder for Reconstitution: 50-mg vial, 100-mg vial.

ADMINISTRATION/HANDLING

 IV

Reconstitution • Reconstitute each 50-mg vial with 15 mL Sterile Water for Injection (100 mg with 30 mL). Swirl, do not shake. • Further dilute 50 mg with 50 mL D₅W or 0.9% NaCl (100 mg with 100 mL, 200 mg with 200 mL).
Rate of administration • Do not exceed infusion rate of 1.1 mg/min. Not for IV bolus injection.
Storage • Refrigerate unused vials. Reconstituted vials are stable for 24 hrs at room temperature. Infusion solution is stable for 48 hrs at room temperature.

🏵 IV COMPATIBILITIES

Heparin, norepinephrine, potassium chloride.

INDICATIONS/ROUTES/DOSAGE

◄ **ALERT** ► Duration of treatment based on pt's clinical response. In general, treatment is continued for at least 14 days after last positive culture.

Candidemia, Other *Candida* Infections
IV: **ADULTS, ELDERLY:** Give single 200-mg loading dose on day 1, followed by 100 mg/day thereafter for at least 14 days after last positive culture.

Esophageal Candidiasis
IV: **ADULTS, ELDERLY:** 200 mg daily for 14–28 days. May transition to fluconazole (oral).

Dosage in Renal/Hepatic Impairment
No dose adjustment.

SIDE EFFECTS

Rare (3%–1%): Diarrhea, nausea, headache, rigors, peripheral edema.

ADVERSE EFFECTS/TOXIC REACTIONS

Hypokalemia occurs in 4% of pts. Hypersensitivity reaction including facial flushing, hypotension, pruritus, urticaria, rash occurs rarely. Hepatitis, elevated LFT, hepatic failure was reported.

NURSING CONSIDERATIONS

BASELINE ASSESSMENT
Obtain CBC, BMP, LFT. Obtain specimens for fungal culture prior to therapy. Treatment may be instituted before results are known.

INTERVENTION/EVALUATION
Monitor for evidence of hepatic dysfunction, hypokalemia. Monitor daily pattern of bowel activity, stool consistency. Assess for rash, urticaria.

PATIENT/FAMILY TEACHING
• For esophageal candidiasis, maintain diligent oral hygiene.

apalutamide

ap-a-**loot**-a-mide
(Erleada)
Do not confuse apalutamide with bicalutamide, enzalutamide, or nilutamide.

◆CLASSIFICATION

PHARMACOTHERAPEUTIC: Anti-androgen. **CLINICAL:** Antineoplastic.

USES

Treatment of nonmetastatic castration-resistant prostate cancer (NM-CRPC), metastatic, castration-sensitive prostate cancer.

PRECAUTIONS

Contraindications: Hypersensitivity to apalutamide. Use in women who are pregnant or may become pregnant. **Cautions:** History of cardiovascular disease (HF, ischemic heart disease), hypothyroidism, conditions predisposing to seizure activity (traumatic brain injury, brain tumor, prior CVA, seizure disorder). Pts at risk for fractures (frequent falls, osteoporosis, chronic corticosteroid therapy), hyperglycemia (e.g., diabetes, recent surgery, chronic use of corticosteroids).

ACTION

Binds directly to ligands of androgen receptor, preventing androgen-receptor translocation, DNA binding, and receptor-mediated transcription. **Therapeutic Effect:** Decreases proliferation of tumor cells, increases apoptosis, resulting in decreased tumor volume.

PHARMACOKINETICS

Widely distributed. Metabolized in liver. Protein binding: 96%. Peak plasma concentration: 2 hrs. Steady-state reached in 4 wks. Excreted in urine (65%), feces (24%). **Half-life:** 3 days.

⧗ LIFESPAN CONSIDERATIONS

Pregnancy/Lactation: Not indicated in female population. Males with female partners of reproductive potential must use effective contraception during treatment and up to 3 mos after discontinuation. May cause fetal harm if administered in pregnant females. May cause decreased fertility in males. **Children:** Safety and efficacy not established. **Elderly:** No age-related precautions noted.

INTERACTIONS

DRUG: Strong **CYP3A4 inhibitors** (e.g., **clarithromycin, ketoconazole, ritonavir**), strong **CYP2C8 inhibitors** (e.g., **gemfibrozil, trimethoprim**), **P-gp inhibitors** (e.g., **amiodarone, azithromycin, captopril, carvedilol, cyclosporine, felodipine, ticagrelor**) may increase concentration/effect. Strong **CYP3A4 inducers** (e.g., **carbamazepine, phenytoin, rifampin**) may decrease concentration/effect. **HERBAL:** None significant. **FOOD:** None known. **LAB VALUES:** May decrease Hgb, Hct, leukocytes, lymphocytes, RBCs. May increase serum cholesterol, glucose, potassium, triglycerides.

AVAILABILITY (Rx)

Tablets: 60 mg, 240 mg.

ADMINISTRATION/HANDLING

PO

• Give without regard to food. • 60-mg tablets may be mixed in applesauce. Mix whole 60-mg tablets in 4 oz of applesauce by stirring. Do not crush or split tablets. • 240-mg tablet can be dispersed in noncarbonated water and given with orange juice, applesauce, or additional water. Place whole 240-mg tablet in a cup. Do not crush or split tablet.

INDICATIONS/ROUTES/DOSAGE

Note: Pts should also receive a gonadotropin-releasing hormone (GnRH) analog concurrently or should have had a bilateral orchiectomy.

Nonmetastatic Castration-Resistant Prostate Cancer, Metastatic Castration-Sensitive Prostate Cancer
PO: ADULTS, ELDERLY: 240 mg once daily (in combination with a gonadotropin-releasing hormone analog agonist or antagonist [if not received orchiectomy]). Continue until disease progression or unacceptable toxicity.

Dose Modification
Based on Common Terminology Criteria for Adverse Effects (CTCAE).

Toxicities or Intolerable Side Effects
Any Grade 3 toxicity or intolerable side effect: Withhold treatment until resolved to Grade 1 or less, then resume at same dose. If applicable, may decrease dose to 180 mg or 120 mg once daily. **Seizures:** Permanently discontinue.

Dosage in Renal/Hepatic Impairment
Mild to moderate impairment: No dose adjustment. **Severe impairment, ESRD:** Not specified; use caution.

SIDE EFFECTS

Frequent (39%–16%): Fatigue, asthenia, hypertension, rash, urticaria, conjunctivitis, stomatitis, diarrhea, nausea, arthralgia, decreased weight. **Occasional (14%–6%):** Hot flush, decreased appetite, early satiety, hypophagia, peripheral edema, penile/scrotal edema, pruritus.

ADVERSE EFFECTS/TOXIC REACTIONS

Anemia, leukopenia, lymphopenia are expected responses to therapy. Increased incidence of falls (16% of pts) and fractures (12% of pts) was reported. Seizures reported in less than 1% of pts. Hypothyroidism reported in 8% of pts. Higher incidence of ischemic heart disease (4% of pts), HF (2% of pts) has occurred.

 Canadian trade name   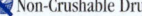 Non-Crushable Drug   **HIGH ALERT** High Alert drug

NURSING CONSIDERATIONS

BASELINE ASSESSMENT

Obtain CBC, BMP, TSH; B/P. Question history of cardiovascular disease (HF, ischemic heart disease), hypothyroidism, seizure disorder. Assess risk for falls and fractures. Receive full medication history and screen for interactions. Offer emotional support.

INTERVENTION/EVALUATION

Monitor CBC, BMP, TSH; B/P periodically. Monitor for symptoms of hypothyroidism (bradycardia, constipation, depression, fatigue, muscle weakness, weight gain), hyperglycemia, seizure activity. Assess skin for rash. Question for any incidence of falls, suspected fractures.

PATIENT/FAMILY TEACHING

• Sexually active men must wear condoms with sexual activity during treatment and for at least 3 mos after last dose. • Women who are pregnant or who plan on becoming pregnant should not handle medication. • Treatment may increase risk of falls and fractures. Go slowly from lying to standing. Use caution during strenuous activity. • Slow heart rate, constipation, depression, fatigue may indicate low thyroid levels. • Immediately report symptoms of seizure activity (confusion, convulsions, loss of consciousness). • Report symptoms of elevated blood sugar levels (blurred vision, headache, increased thirst, frequent urination). • Do not take newly prescribed medications unless approved by the prescriber who originally started treatment.

apixaban

a-**pix**-a-ban
(Eliquis)

■ **BLACK BOX ALERT** ■ Discontinuation in absence of alternative anticoagulation increases risk for thrombotic events. Spinal or epidural hematoma resulting in paralysis may occur with neuraxial anesthesia or spinal/epidural puncture. **Do not confuse apixaban with rivaroxaban, argatroban, or dabigatran.**

◆CLASSIFICATION

PHARMACOTHERAPEUTIC: Factor Xa inhibitor. **CLINICAL:** Anticoagulant.

USES

Reduces risk for stroke, systemic embolism in pts with nonvalvular atrial fibrillation. Prophylaxis of DVT following hip or knee replacement surgery, which may lead to pulmonary embolism (PE). Treatment of DVT and PE and reduces the risk of recurrent DVT/PE following initial therapy. **OFF-LABEL:** Heparin-induced thrombocytopenia. Left ventricular thrombosis (treatment/prevention).

PRECAUTIONS

Contraindications: Severe hypersensitivity to apixaban. Active pathologic bleeding. **Cautions:** Mild to moderate hepatic impairment, severe renal impairment (may increase bleeding risk). Avoid use in pts with severe hepatic impairment, prosthetic heart valve, significant rheumatic heart disease.

ACTION

Selectively, directly, and reversibly inhibits free and clot-bound factor Xa, a key factor in the intrinsic and extrinsic pathway of blood coagulation cascade. **Therapeutic Effect:** Inhibits clot-induced platelet aggregation, fibrin clot formation.

PHARMACOKINETICS

Widely distributed. Peak plasma concentration: 3–4 hrs. Protein binding: 87%. Metabolized in liver. Excreted primarily in urine, feces. **Half-life:** 12 hrs.

⏳ LIFESPAN CONSIDERATIONS

Pregnancy/Lactation: Unknown if distributed in breast milk. **Children:** Safety and efficacy not established. **Elderly:** No age-related precautions noted.

INTERACTIONS

DRUG: Strong CYP3A4 inducers (e.g., **carbamazepine, phenytoin, rifampin**) may decrease level/effect. **Anticoagulants** (e.g., **dabigatran, heparin, warfarin**), **antiplatelets** (e.g., **aspirin, clopidogrel**), **NSAIDs** (e.g., **diclofenac, ibuprofen, naproxen**), **strong CYP3A4 inhibitors** (e.g., **ketoconazole, clarithromycin**) may increase concentration, bleeding risk. **HERBAL:** St. John's wort may decrease concentration/effect. **Herbals with anticoagulant/antiplatelet properties** (e.g., **garlic, ginger, ginkgo biloba**) may increase risk of bleeding. **FOOD:** None known. **LAB VALUES:** May decrease platelet count, Hgb, LFT.

AVAILABILITY (Rx)

Tablets: 2.5 mg, 5 mg.

ADMINISTRATION/HANDLING

◀**ALERT**▶ Discontinuation in absence of alternative anticoagulation increases risk for thrombotic events.

PO

• Give without regard to food. May crush tablets and suspend in 60 mL of water or apple juice, or mixed with applesauce. • If elective surgery or invasive procedures with moderate or high risk for bleeding, discontinue apixaban at least 24–48 hrs prior to procedure.

INDICATIONS/ROUTES/DOSAGE

Nonvalvular Atrial Fibrillation

PO: ADULTS, ELDERLY: 5 mg twice daily. In pts with at least 2 of the following characteristics: age 80 yrs or older, body weight 60 kg or less, serum creatinine 1.5 mg/dL or greater, concurrent use with CYP3A4, or P-gp inhibitors (e.g., ketoconazole, ritonavir), reduce dose to 2.5 mg twice daily.

DVT/PE Treatment

PO: ADULTS, ELDERLY: 10 mg twice daily for 7 days, then 5 mg twice daily.

DVT Prophylaxis (Hip/Knee Replacement)

Note: Begin 12–24 hrs postoperatively. **ADULTS, ELDERLY:** 2.5 mg twice daily (approx. 30 days for hip; 10–14 days for knee).

DVT Prophylaxis, Reduce Risk Recurrent DVT/PE

PO: ADULTS, ELDERLY: 2.5 mg twice daily (after at least 6 mos of treatment).

Dosage in Renal Impairment

DVT/PE/Reduce risk recurrent DVT, postoperative: No adjustment. **Nonvalvular A-fib, HD: SCR LESS THAN 1.5:** No adjustment. **SCR 1.5 OR GREATER, OLDER THAN 80 YRS, WEIGHING 60 KG OR LESS:** 2.5 mg 2 times/day.

Dosage in Hepatic Impairment

Mild impairment: No dose adjustment. **Moderate impairment:** Use caution. **Severe impairment:** Not recommended.

SIDE EFFECTS

Rare (3%–1%): Nausea, ecchymosis.

ADVERSE EFFECTS/TOXIC REACTIONS

Increased risk for bleeding/hemorrhagic events. May cause serious, potentially fatal bleeding, accompanied by one or more of the following: A decrease in Hgb of 2 g/dL or more; a need for 2 or more units of packed RBCs; bleeding occurring at one of the following sites: intracranial, intraspinal, intraocular, pericardial, intra-articular, intramuscular with compartment syndrome, retroperitoneal. Serious reactions include jaundice, cholestasis, cytolytic hepatitis, Stevens-Johnson syndrome, hypersensitivity reaction, anaphylaxis.

NURSING CONSIDERATIONS

BASELINE ASSESSMENT

Obtain CBC. Question history of bleeding disorders, recent surgery, spinal punctures, intracranial hemorrhage, bleeding ulcers, open wounds, anemia, hepatic impairment. Obtain full medication history including herbal products.

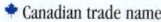 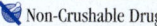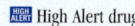

INTERVENTION/EVALUATION

Periodically monitor CBC, stool for occult blood. Be alert for complaints of abdominal/back pain, headache, confusion, weakness, vision change (may indicate hemorrhage). Question for increased menstrual bleeding/discharge. Assess for any sign of bleeding: bleeding at surgical site, hematuria, blood in stool, bleeding from gums, petechiae, ecchymosis.

PATIENT/FAMILY TEACHING

• Do not take/discontinue any medication except on advice from physician. • Avoid alcohol, aspirin, NSAIDs, herbal supplements, grapefruit products. • Consult physician before surgery, dental work. • Use electric razor, soft toothbrush to prevent bleeding. • Report blood-tinged mucus from coughing, heavy menstrual bleeding, headache, vision problems, weakness, abdominal pain, frequent bruising, bloody urine or stool, joint pain or swelling.

---

apremilast

a-**pre**-mi-last
(Otezla)
Do not confuse apremilast with roflumilast.

◆CLASSIFICATION

PHARMACOTHERAPEUTIC: Phosphodiesterase 4 (PDE4) enzyme inhibitor. **CLINICAL:** Antipsoriatic arthritis agent.

USES

Treatment of adults with active psoriatic arthritis. Treatment of adults with plaque psoriasis who are candidates for phototherapy or systemic therapy. Treatment of oral ulcers associated with Behçet's disease.

PRECAUTIONS

Contraindications: Hypersensitivity to apremilast. **Cautions:** History of depression, severe renal impairment, suicidal ideation. Pts with latent infections (e.g., TB, viral hepatitis).

ACTION

Selectively inhibits PDE4, increasing cyclic AMP (cAMP) and regulation of inflammatory mediators. **Therapeutic Effect:** Reduces psoriatic arthritis exacerbations.

PHARMACOKINETICS

Widely distributed. Protein binding: 68%. Peak plasma concentration: 2.5 hrs. Metabolized in liver. Excreted in urine (58%), feces (39%). **Half-life:** 6–9 hrs.

⧗ LIFESPAN CONSIDERATIONS

Pregnancy/Lactation: Unknown if distributed in breast milk. Not recommended for nursing mothers. **Children:** Safety and efficacy not established. **Elderly:** No age-related precautions noted.

INTERACTIONS

DRUG: Strong CYP3A4 inducers (e.g., carbamazepine, phenytoin, rifampin) may decrease concentration/effect. **HERBAL:** None significant. **FOOD:** None significant. **LAB VALUES:** None known.

AVAILABILITY (Rx)

 Tablets: 10 mg, 20 mg, 30 mg.

ADMINISTRATION/HANDLING

PO
• Give without regard to food. Administer whole; do not crush, cut, dissolve, or divide.

INDICATIONS/ROUTES/DOSAGE

Behçet's Disease, Psoriatic Arthritis, Plaque Psoriasis
PO: ADULTS/ELDERLY: Initially, titrate dose from day 1–day 5. **Day 1:** 10 mg in AM only. **Day 2:** 10 mg in AM; 10 mg in PM. **Day 3:** 10 mg in AM; 20 mg in PM. **Day 4:** 20 mg in AM; 20 mg in PM. **Day 5:** 20 mg in AM; 30 mg in PM. **Day 6/maintenance:** 30 mg twice daily.

Dosage in Renal Impairment (Creatinine Clearance less than 30 mL/min)
Days 1–3: 10 mg in AM. **Days 4–5:** 20 mg in AM, using only AM schedule. **Day 6/maintenance:** 30 mg once daily.

Dosage in Hepatic Impairment
No dose adjustment.

SIDE EFFECTS

Occasional (9%–4%): Nausea, diarrhea, headache, upper respiratory tract infection. **Rare (3% or less):** Vomiting, nasopharyngitis, upper abdominal pain.

ADVERSE EFFECTS/TOXIC REACTIONS

Increased risk of depression reported in less than 1% of pts. Weight decrease of 5%–10% of body weight occurred in 10% of pts.

NURSING CONSIDERATIONS

BASELINE ASSESSMENT

Obtain weight, vital signs. Question history of depression, severe renal impairment, suicidal ideations. Screen for prior allergic reactions to drug class. Receive full medication history including herbal products. Assess degree of joint pain, range of motion, mobility.

INTERVENTION/EVALUATION

Monitor for worsening depression, suicidal ideation. Monitor for weight loss. Assess for dehydration if diarrhea occurs. Assess improvement of joint pain, range of motion, mobility.

PATIENT/FAMILY TEACHING

• Report changes in mood or behavior, thoughts of suicide, self-destructive behavior. Report weight loss of any kind. • Increase fluid intake if dehydration suspected. • Immediately notify physician if pregnancy suspected. • Do not chew, crush, dissolve, or divide tablets.

aprepitant/ fosaprepitant

a-**prep**-i-tant/fos-a-**prep**-i-tant
(Cinvanti, Emend)
Do not confuse fosaprepitant with aprepitant, fosamprenavir, or fospropofol.

◆CLASSIFICATION

PHARMACOTHERAPEUTIC: Neurokinin receptor antagonist. **CLINICAL:** Antinausea, antiemetic.

USES

Cinvanti (IV), Emend (PO/IV): Prevention of nausea, vomiting associated with repeat courses of moderately to highly emetogenic cancer chemotherapy. **Emend (PO):** Prevention of postop nausea, vomiting.

PRECAUTIONS

Contraindications: Hypersensitivity to aprepitant or fosaprepitant. Concurrent use with pimozide. **Cautions:** Severe hepatic impairment. Concurrent use of medications metabolized through CYP3A4 (e.g., docetaxel, etoposide, ifosfamide, imatinib, irinotecan, PACLitaxel, vinblastine, vinCRIStine, vinorelbine).

ACTION

Inhibits substance P receptor, augments antiemetic activity of 5-HT$_3$ receptor antagonists. **Therapeutic Effect:** Prevents acute and delayed phases of chemotherapy-induced emesis.

PHARMACOKINETICS

Widely distributed. Crosses blood-brain barrier. Extensively metabolized in liver. Protein binding: greater than 95%. Eliminated primarily by liver metabolism (not excreted renally). **Half-life:** 9–13 hrs.

⌛ LIFESPAN CONSIDERATIONS

Pregnancy/Lactation: Unknown if drug crosses placenta or is distributed in breast milk. **Children:** Safety and efficacy not established. **Elderly:** No age-related precautions noted.

INTERACTIONS

DRUG: Strong CYP3A4 inhibitors (e.g., ketoconazole, clarithromycin) may increase concentration/effect. **Strong CYP3A4 inducers (e.g., carbamaze-**

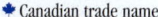 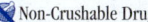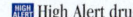

pine, **phenytoin, rifampin**) may decrease concentration/effect. May decrease effectiveness of **hormonal contraceptives, warfarin.** May increase concentration/effects of **bosutinib, budesonide, cobimetinib, neratinib, simeprevir.** **HERBAL:** None significant. **FOOD:** None significant. **LAB VALUES:** May increase serum ALT, AST, alkaline phosphatase, BUN, creatinine, glucose. May produce proteinuria.

AVAILABILITY (Rx)

Capsules: 40 mg, 80 mg, 125 mg.

Injection, Emulsion: *(Cinvanti):* 130 mg/18 mL. *(Aponvie):* **Injection, Powder for Reconstitution:** 150 mg. **Oral Suspension:** 125 mg/5 mL.

ADMINISTRATION/HANDLING
PO

• Give without regard to food. • Administer whole; do not cut, crush, or open capsules. • Suspension (prepared by healthcare provider in oral dispenser). Dispense in pt's mouth along inner cheek. Suspension is stable for 72 hrs if refrigerated or up to 3 hrs at room temperature.

 IV *(Emend)*

Reconstitution • Reconstitute each vial with 5 mL 0.9% NaCl. • Add to 145 mL 0.9% NaCl to provide a final concentration of 1 mg/mL.
Rate of administration • Infuse over 20–30 min 30 min prior to chemotherapy.
Storage • Refrigerate unreconstituted vials. • After reconstitution, solution is stable at room temperature for 24 hrs.
IV Emulsion *(Cinvanti)*
Reconstitution • For 130-mg dose, dilute 18 mL of Cinvanti into 100 mL 0.9% NaCl or D_5W infusion bag. • For 100-mg dose, dilute 14 mL of Cinvanti into 100 mL 0.9% NaCl or D_5W infusion bag. • Mix by gentle inversion (4–5 times). • Do not shake.
Rate of administration • Infuse over 30 minutes. Use only non-DEHP tubing for administration. For IV injection, no further dilution is necessary. Inject over 2 min.

IV INCOMPATIBILITIES
Do not infuse with any solutions containing calcium or magnesium.

INDICATIONS/ROUTES/DOSAGE
Prevention of Nausea/Vomiting Associated With Highly Emetogenic Chemotherapy
IV: ADULTS, ELDERLY: *(Cinvanti):* 130 mg 30 min prior to chemotherapy on day 1 (in combination with a 5-HT_3 antagonist antiemetic on day 1 and oral dexamethasone on days 1-4).
PO: ADULTS, ELDERLY, CHILDREN 12 YRS AND OLDER, CHILDREN LESS THAN 12 YRS WEIGHING 30 KG OR MORE: 125 mg 1 hr prior to chemotherapy on day 1, then 80 mg daily on days 2 and 3 (in combination with a 5-HT3 antagonist antiemetic on day 1 and oral dexamethasone on days 1-4). **CHILDREN 6 MOS TO LESS THAN 12 YRS WEIGHING LESS THAN 30 KG:** 3 mg/kg 1 hr prior to chemotherapy on day 1, then 2 mg/kg daily on days 2 and 3 (in combination with a 5-HT3 antagonist antiemetic on day 1 and oral dexamethasone on days 1-4).

Prevention of Nausea/Vomiting Associated With Moderately Emetogenic Chemotherapy
IV: ADULTS, ELDERLY: *(Cinvanti):* 100 mg 30 min prior to chemotherapy on day 1 (in combination with oral aprepitant 80 mg on days 2 and 3, a 5-HT3 antagonist antiemetic on day 1, and oral dexamethasone on day 1).
PO: ADULTS, ELDERLY, CHILDREN 12 YRS AND OLDER, CHILDREN LESS THAN 12 YRS WEIGHING 30 KG OR MORE: 125 mg 1 hr prior to chemotherapy on day 1, then 80 mg daily on days 2 and 3 (in combination with a 5-HT3 antagonist antiemetic on day 1 and oral dexamethasone on day 1). **CHILDREN 6 MOS TO LESS THAN 12 YRS WEIGHING LESS THAN 30 KG:** 3 mg/kg 1 hr prior to chemotherapy on day 1, then 2 mg/kg daily on days 2 and 3 (in combination with a 5-HT3 antagonist antiemetic on day 1 and oral dexamethasone on day 1).

IV: **ADULTS,   ELDERLY   (SINGLE-DOSE REGIMEN):** *(Emend):* 150 mg over 20–30 min 30 min before chemotherapy. *(Cinvanti):* 130 mg over 30 min or IV injection over 2 min approx. 30 min before chemotherapy.

Prevention of Postop Nausea, Vomiting
PO: **ADULTS, ELDERLY:** 40 mg once within 3 hrs prior to induction of anesthesia.
IV: **ADULTS, ELDERLY:** *(Aponvie):* 32 mg prior to anesthesia induction.

Dosage in Renal/Hepatic Impairment
No dose adjustment. Caution in severe hepatic impairment.

SIDE EFFECTS

Frequent (17%–10%): Fatigue, nausea, hiccups, diarrhea, constipation, anorexia. **Occasional (8%–4%):** Headache, vomiting, dizziness, dehydration, heartburn. **Rare (3% or less):** Abdominal pain, epigastric discomfort, gastritis, tinnitus, insomnia.

ADVERSE EFFECTS/TOXIC REACTIONS

Neutropenia, mucous membrane disorders occur rarely.

NURSING CONSIDERATIONS

BASELINE ASSESSMENT
Assess for dehydration (poor skin turgor, dry mucous membranes, longitudinal furrows in tongue).

INTERVENTION/EVALUATION
Monitor hydration, nutritional status, I&O. Assess bowel sounds for peristalsis. Assist with ambulation if dizziness occurs. Provide supportive measures. Monitor daily pattern of bowel activity, stool consistency.

PATIENT/FAMILY TEACHING
• Relief from nausea/vomiting generally occurs shortly after drug administration. • Report persistent vomiting, headache. • May decrease effectiveness of oral contraceptives

argatroban

ar-**gat**-roe-ban
Do not confuse argatroban with Aggrastat.

◆CLASSIFICATION

PHARMACOTHERAPEUTIC: Direct thrombin inhibitor. **CLINICAL:** Anticoagulant.

USES

Prophylaxis or treatment of thrombosis in heparin-induced thrombocytopenia (HIT) in pts with HIT or at risk of developing HIT undergoing percutaneous coronary procedures.

PRECAUTIONS

Contraindications: Hypersensitivity to argatroban, active major bleeding. **Cautions:** Severe hypertension, immediately following lumbar puncture, spinal anesthesia, major surgery, pts with congenital or acquired bleeding disorders, gastrointestinal ulcerations, hepatic impairment, critically ill pts.

ACTION

Direct thrombin inhibitor that reversibly binds to thrombin-active sites of free and clot-associated thrombin. Inhibits thrombin-catalyzed or thrombin-induced reactions, including fibrin formation, activation of coagulant factors V, VIII, and XIII; inhibits protein C formation, platelet aggregation. **Therapeutic Effect:** Produces anticoagulation.

PHARMACOKINETICS

Distributed primarily in extracellular fluid. Protein binding: 54%. Metabolized in liver. Primarily excreted in the feces, presumably through biliary secretion. **Half-life:** 39–51 min (prolonged in hepatic failure).

⊠ LIFESPAN CONSIDERATIONS

Pregnancy/Lactation: Unknown if excreted in breast milk. **Children:** Safety

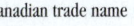 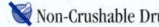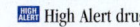

and efficacy not established. **Elderly:** No age-related precautions noted.

INTERACTIONS

DRUG: Anticoagulants (e.g., dabigatran, heparin, rivaroxaban, warfarin), antiplatelets (e.g., aspirin, clopidogrel), NSAIDs (e.g., diclofenac, ibuprofen, naproxen) may increase anticoagulant effect. **HERBAL:** Herbals with anticoagulant/antiplatelet properties (e.g., garlic, ginger, ginkgo biloba) may increase risk of bleeding. **FOOD:** None known. **LAB VALUES:** Prolongs prothrombin time (PT), activated partial thromboplastin time (aPTT), international normalized ratio (INR). May decrease Hgb, Hct.

AVAILABILITY (Rx)

Infusion (Pre-Mix): 50 mg/50 mL. **Injection Solution:** 250 mg/2.5 mL vial.

ADMINISTRATION/HANDLING

 IV

Reconstitution • Dilute each 250-mg vial with 250 mL 0.9% NaCl, D₅W to provide a final concentration of 1 mg/mL.
Rate of administration • Initial rate of administration is based on body weight at 2 mcg/kg/min (e.g., 50-kg pt infuse at 6 mL/hr). Dosage should not exceed 10 mcg/kg/min.
Storage • Discard if solution appears cloudy or an insoluble precipitate is noted. • Following reconstitution, stable for 96 hrs at room temperature or refrigerated. • Avoid direct sunlight.

⬚ IV INCOMPATIBILITIES

Amiodarone.

⬚ IV COMPATIBILITIES

Diltiazem, norepinephrine, vasopressin.

INDICATIONS/ROUTES/DOSAGE

Heparin-Induced Thrombocytopenia (HIT)
IV infusion: ADULTS, ELDERLY: Initially, 2 mcg/kg/min administered as a continuous infusion. After initial infusion, dose may be adjusted until steady-state aPTT is 1.5–3 times initial baseline value, not to exceed 100 sec. Dosage should not exceed 10 mcg/kg/min.

Percutaneous Coronary Intervention
IV infusion: ADULTS, ELDERLY: Initially, administer bolus of 350 mcg/kg over 3–5 min, and begin infusion at 25 mcg/kg/min. Check ACT (activated clotting time) 5–10 min following bolus. If ACT is less than 300 sec, give additional bolus 150 mcg/kg, increase infusion to 30 mcg/kg/min. If ACT is greater than 450 sec, decrease infusion to 15 mcg/kg/min. Recheck ACT in 5–10 min. Once ACT of 300–450 sec achieved, continue dose through duration of procedure.

Dosage in Renal Impairment
No dose adjustment.

Dosage in Hepatic Impairment
Moderate to severe impairment: ADULTS, ELDERLY: Initially, 0.5 mcg/kg/min. **CHILDREN:** Initially, 0.2 mcg/kg/min. Adjust dose in increments of 0.05 mcg/kg/min or less.

SIDE EFFECTS

Frequent (8%–3%): Dyspnea, hypotension, fever, diarrhea, nausea, pain, vomiting, infection, cough.

ADVERSE EFFECTS/TOXIC REACTIONS

Ventricular tachycardia, atrial fibrillation occur occasionally. Major bleeding, sepsis occur rarely.

NURSING CONSIDERATIONS

BASELINE ASSESSMENT

Obtain CBC, PT, aPTT. Determine initial B/P. Minimize need for multiple injection sites, blood draws, catheters.

INTERVENTION/EVALUATION

Assess for any sign of bleeding: bleeding at surgical site, hematuria, melena, bleeding from gums, petechiae, ecchymoses, bleeding from injection sites.

Assess for decreased B/P, increased pulse rate, complaint of abdominal/back pain, severe headache (may indicate hemorrhage). Monitor ACT, PT, aPTT, platelet count, Hgb, Hct. Question for increase in discharge during menses. Assess for hematuria. Observe skin for any occurring ecchymoses, petechiae, hematoma. Use care in removing any dressing, tape.

PATIENT/FAMILY TEACHING
• Use electric razor, soft toothbrush to prevent cuts, gingival trauma. • Report any sign of bleeding, including red/dark urine, black/red stool, coffee-ground vomitus, blood-tinged mucus from cough.

ARIPiprazole

ar-i-**pip**-ra-zole
(Abilify, Abilify Asimtufii, Abilify Maintena, Aristada Initio)
■ **BLACK BOX ALERT** ■ Increased risk of mortality in elderly pts with dementia-related psychosis, mainly due to pneumonia, HF. Increased risk of suicidal thinking and behavior in children, adolescents, young adults 18–24 yrs with major depressive disorder, other psychiatric disorders.
Do not confuse Abilify with Ambien, or ARIPiprazole with esomeprazole, omeprazole, pantoprazole, or RABEprazole (proton pump inhibitors).

◆CLASSIFICATION

PHARMACOTHERAPEUTIC: Quinolinone antipsychotic. **CLINICAL:** Second-generation (atypical) antipsychotic agent.

USES

Bipolar disorder: Acute treatment of bipolar disorder (with acute mania or mixed features) as monotherapy or as adjunct to lithium or valproate in children 10 yrs and older and adults. Maintenance treatment of bipolar disorder in adults.
Schizophrenia: Acute and maintenance treatment of schizophrenia in children 13 yrs and older and adults. **Irritability associated with autism:** Treatment of irritability associated with autistic disorder (symptoms of aggression, deliberate self-injurious behavior, temper tantrums, quick-changing moods) in children 6–17 yrs. **Tourette disorder:** Treatment of Tourette disorder in children 6–18 yrs. **Major depressive disorder (MDD) unipolar:** Adjunctive treatment of MDD in adults with inadequate response to prior antidepressant therapy. **OFF-LABEL:** Treatment of conduct disorders in children/adolescents, agitation/aggression associated with dementia or psychiatric disorders, delusional disorder, Huntington's disease–associated chorea, OCD, Tourette's syndrome.

PRECAUTIONS

Contraindications: Hypersensitivity to ARIPiprazole. **Cautions:** Concurrent use of CNS depressants (including alcohol), disorders in which CNS depression is a feature, cardiovascular or cerebrovascular diseases (may induce hypotension), Parkinson's disease (potential for exacerbation), history of seizures or conditions that may lower seizure threshold (Alzheimer's disease), diabetes mellitus. Pts at risk for pneumonia. Elderly with dementia.

ACTION

Provides partial agonist activity at DOPamine (D2, D3) and serotonin (5-HT$_{1A}$) receptors and antagonist activity at serotonin (5-HT$_{2A}$) receptors. **Therapeutic Effect:** Improves symptoms associated with schizophrenia, bipolar disorder, autism, depression.

PHARMACOKINETICS

Widely distributed. Protein binding: 99%. Reaches steady levels in 2 wks. Metabolized in liver. Excreted in feces (55%), urine (25%). Not removed by hemodialysis. **Half-life:** 75 hrs.

 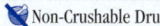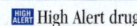

⌛ LIFESPAN CONSIDERATIONS

Pregnancy/Lactation: Unknown if drug crosses placenta. May be distributed in breast milk. Breastfeeding not recommended. **Children:** Safety and efficacy not established. **Elderly:** May increase risk of mortality in pts with dementia-related psychosis.

INTERACTIONS

DRUG: Strong CYP3A4 inducers (e.g., carBAMazepine, rifampin) may decrease concentration/effect. **Strong CYP3A4 inhibitors** (e.g., clarithromycin, ketoconazole, ritonavir), **strong CYP2D6 inhibitors** (e.g., fluoxetine, paroxetine) may increase concentration/effect. **CNS depressants** (e.g., alcohol, morphine, oxycodone, zolpidem) may increase CNS depression. **HERBAL:** Herbals with sedative properties (e.g., chamomile, kava kava, valerian) may increase CNS depression. **FOOD:** None known. **LAB VALUES:** May increase serum glucose. May decrease neutrophils, leukocytes.

AVAILABILITY (Rx)

Injection, Prefilled Syringe: *(Abilify Asimtufii):* 720 mg/2.4 mL, 960 mg/3.2 mL. *(Abilify Maintena):* 300 mg, 400 mg. **Injection, Suspension, Extended-Release, Prefilled Syringe:** *(Aristada Initio):* 675 mg. **Prefilled syringe:** *(Aristada):* 441 mg/1.6 mL, 662 mg/2.4 mL, 882 mg/3.2 mL, 1,064 mg/3.9 mL. **Oral Solution:** 1 mg/mL. **Tablets:** 2 mg, 5 mg, 10 mg, 15 mg, 20 mg, 30 mg. **Orally Disintegrating Tablets:** 10 mg, 15 mg.

ADMINISTRATION/HANDLING

IM *(Abilify Maintena)*

Vial • Reconstitute 400-mg vial with 1.9 mL Sterile Water for Injection (300-mg vial with 1.5 mL) to provide a concentration of 100 mg/0.5 mL. Once reconstituted, administer in gluteal muscle. Do not administer via IV or subcutaneously. **Prefilled Syringe** • Reconstitute at room temperature by rotating syringe plunger to release diluent. Shake until suspension is uniform. • Inject full syringe content immediately following reconstitution.

IM *(Aristada, Aristada Intio)*

• *(Aristada):* Inject into the deltoid (441 mg dose only) or gluteal muscle (441 mg, 662 mg, 882 mg or 1,064 mg). • *(Aristada Initio):* Inject into either the deltoid or gluteal muscle.

PO

• Give without regard to food.

Orally Disintegrating Tablet

• Remove tablet, place entire tablet on tongue. • Do not break, split tablet. • May give without liquid.

INDICATIONS/ROUTES/DOSAGE

Note: May substitute oral solution/tablet mg per mg up to 25 mg. For 30-mg tablets, give 25 mg oral solution. **Strong CYP3A4 inducers:** ARIPiprazole dose should be doubled. **Strong CYP3A4 inhibitors:** ARIPiprazole dose should be reduced by 50%.

Schizophrenia

PO: ADULTS, ELDERLY: Initially, 10–15 mg once daily. May increase dose in 5 mg increments at intervals of 1 wk or more. **Maximum:** 30 mg/day. **CHILDREN 13–17 YRS:** Initially, 2 mg/day for 2 days, then 5 mg/day for 2 days. May further increase to target dose of 10 mg/day. May then increase in increments of 5 mg up to maximum of 30 mg/day. **IM: ADULTS, ELDERLY:** *(Abilify Asimtufii):* 960 mg q2mos (may reduce to 720 mg). When initiated in pts receiving oral aripiprazole, administer the first dose along with oral aripiprazole (10–20 mg) for 14 consecutive days. For pts receiving Abilify Maintena, administer in place of the next scheduled Abilify Maintena injection. *(Abilify Maintena):* **Note:** Overlap oral antipsychotic for 14 days when initiating. Initially, 400 mg monthly (separate doses by at least 26 days). May reduce dose to 300 mg in pts with adverse reactions. *(Aristada Initio):* 675 mg once (single dose) with 30 mg oral aripiprazole with first IM dose of Aristada.

(Aristada): May give Aristada on same day as Aristada Initio or up to 10 days thereafter **OR** administer 21 consecutive days of oral aripiprazole concomitantly with first Aristada injection. Depending on pt needs, treatment with Aristada can be initiated at 441 mg, 662 mg, or 882 mg monthly; 882 mg q6wks; or 1,064 mg q2mos.

Bipolar Disorder
PO: ADULTS, ELDERLY: Monotherapy: Initially, 10–15 mg once daily. May increase in increments of 5–10 mg/day of at least 1-wk intervals to 30 mg/day. **Adjunct to lithium or valproic acid:** Initially, 10–15 mg. May increase to 30 mg/day based on pt tolerance. **CHILDREN 10–17 YRS:** Initially, 2 mg/day for 2 days, then 5 mg/day for 2 days. May further increase to a target of 10 mg/day. Give subsequent dose increases of 5 mg/day. **Maximum:** 30 mg/day.
IM: ADULTS, ELDERLY: *(Abilify Asimtufii):* 960 mg q2mos (may reduce to 720 mg). When initiated in pts receiving oral aripiprazole, administer the first dose along with oral aripiprazole (10–20 mg) for 14 consecutive days. For pts receiving Abilify Maintena, administer in place of the next scheduled Abilify Maintena injection. *(Abilify Maintena):* Initially, 400 mg monthly (separate doses by at least 26 days). May reduce dose to 300 mg in pts with adverse reactions. Tolerability should be established using oral therapy before initiation of parenteral therapy. Continue oral therapy for 14 days during initiation of parenteral therapy.

Major Depressive Disorder (Adjunct to Antidepressants)
PO: ADULTS, ELDERLY: *(Abilify):* Initially, 2–5 mg/day. May increase up to maximum of 15 mg/day. Titrate dose in 5-mg increments of at least 1-wk intervals.

Irritability With Autism
PO: CHILDREN 6–17 YRS: Initially, 2 mg/day for 7 days followed by increase to 5 mg/day. Subsequent increases made in 5-mg increments at intervals of at least 1 wk. **Maximum:** 15 mg/day.

Tourette Disorder
PO: CHILDREN 6–17 YRS WEIGHING 50 KG OR MORE: 2 mg/day for 2 days; then 5 mg/day for 5 days with target dose of 10 mg on day 8. If needed, may further titrate by 5 mg/day at wkly intervals up to 20 mg/day. **Maximum:** 20 mg/day. **LESS THAN 50 KG:** 2 mg/day for 2 days, then 5 mg/day. If needed, may further titrate by 5 mg/day at wkly intervals up to 10 mg/day. **Maximum:** 10 mg/day.

Dosage in Renal/Hepatic Impairment
No dose adjustment.

SIDE EFFECTS
Frequent (11%–5%): Weight gain, headache, insomnia, vomiting. **Occasional (4%–3%):** Light-headedness, nausea, akathisia, drowsiness. **Rare (2% or less):** Blurred vision, constipation, asthenia (loss of strength, energy), anxiety, fever, rash, cough, rhinitis, orthostatic hypotension.

ADVERSE EFFECTS/TOXIC REACTIONS
Extrapyramidal symptoms, neuroleptic malignant syndrome, tardive dyskinesia, hyperglycemia, ketoacidosis, hyperosmolar coma, CVA, TIA occur rarely. Prolonged QT interval occurs rarely. May cause leukopenia, neutropenia, agranulocytosis.

NURSING CONSIDERATIONS

BASELINE ASSESSMENT
Assess behavior, appearance, emotional status, response to environment, speech pattern, thought content. Correct dehydration, hypovolemia. Assess for suicidal tendencies. Question history (or family history) of diabetes. Obtain serum blood glucose level.

INTERVENTION/EVALUATION
Periodically monitor weight. Monitor for extrapyramidal symptoms (abnormal movement), tardive dyskinesia (protrusion of tongue, puffing of cheeks, chewing/puckering of the mouth). Periodically monitor B/P, pulse (particularly in pts with preexisting cardiovascular disease). Monitor serum

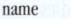 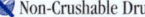

blood glucose levels during therapy. Assess for therapeutic response (greater interest in surroundings, improved self-care, increased ability to concentrate, relaxed facial expression).

PATIENT/FAMILY TEACHING

• Avoid alcohol. • Avoid tasks that require alertness, motor skills until response to drug is established. • Report worsening depression, suicidal ideation, unusual changes in behavior, extrapyramidal effects.

---

asciminib

as-**kim**-i-nib
(Scemblix)
Do not confuse asciminib with abciximab, abemaciclib, afatinib, alectinib, alpelisib, avapritinib, axitinib, bosutinib, dasatinib, imatinib, nilotinib, or ponatinib.

◆CLASSIFICATION

PHARMACOTHERAPEUTIC: BCR-ABL tyrosine kinase inhibitor, STAMP inhibitor. **CLINICAL:** Antineoplastic.

USES

Treatment of adults with Philadelphia chromosome–positive (Ph+) chronic myeloid leukemia (CML) in chronic phase, with *T315I* mutation or previously treated with 2 or more tyrosine kinase inhibitors (TKIs). Newly diagnosed Philadelphia chromosome-positive chronic myeloid leukemia (Ph+ CML) in chronic phase (CP).

PRECAUTIONS

Contraindications: Hypersensitivity to asciminib. **Cautions:** Baseline cytopenias; active infection, conditions predisposing to infection (e.g., diabetes, immunocompromised pts, open wounds), cardiac disease, HF. History of hypertension, pancreatitis.

ACTION

Inhibits viability of cells expressing native or mutant BCR-ABL tyrosine kinase,

including *T315I* mutation, created by the Philadelphia chromosome abnormality. **Therapeutic Effect:** Inhibits tumor cell growth and metastasis.

PHARMACOKINETICS

Widely distributed. Metabolized in liver. Protein binding: 97%. Peak plasma concentration: 2–3 hrs. Excreted in feces (80%), urine (11%). **Half-life:** 5.5–9 hrs.

⧗ LIFESPAN CONSIDERATIONS

Pregnancy/Lactation: Avoid pregnancy; may cause fetal harm. Females of reproductive potential must use effective contraception during treatment and for at least 1 wk after discontinuation. Unknown if distributed in breast milk. Breastfeeding not recommended during treatment and for at least 1 wk after discontinuation. **Children:** Safety and efficacy not established. **Elderly:** No age-related precautions noted.

INTERACTIONS

DRUG: May enhance immunosuppressive effect of **baricitinib, natalizumab, tacrolimus (topical),** and **upadacitinib**. May decrease therapeutic effect of **BCG (intravesical)**. May increase adverse/toxic effects of **vaccines (live)**. **Pimecrolimus** may increase immunosuppressive effect. **Itraconazole** may decrease concentration/effect. **HERBAL:** **Echinacea** may decrease therapeutic effect. **FOOD: Food** may decrease absorption/concentration. **LAB VALUES:** May increase serum amylase, alkaline phosphatase, ALT, AST, bilirubin, cholesterol, creatinine, lipase, potassium, triglycerides, uric acid. May decrease Hgb, Hct, lymphocytes, neutrophils, platelets, RBCs; serum calcium, phosphate.

AVAILABILITY (RX)

 Tablets, Film-Coated: 20 mg, 40 mg.

ADMINISTRATION/HANDLING

PO

• Give without food. Avoid food consumption at least 2 hrs before and 1 hr after dose. • Administer tablets whole; do not break, cut, crush, or divide. Tablets should not be chewed. • If a once-daily-dose regimen is missed by more than 12 hrs, skip dose and give next regularly scheduled time. If a twice-daily-dose regimen is missed by more than 6 hrs, skip dose and give next regularly scheduled time.

INDICATIONS/ROUTES/DOSAGE

CML (Chronic Phase) Newly Diagnosed or Previously Treated With 2 or More TKIs
PO: ADULTS: 80 mg once daily or 40 mg twice daily. Continue until disease progression or unacceptable toxicity.

CML (Chronic Phase) With T315I Mutation
PO: ADULTS: 200 mg twice daily. Continue until disease progression or unacceptable toxicity.

Dose Reduction Schedule for Adverse Events
CML (chronic phase) previously treated with 2 or more TKIs: (First dose reduction): 40 mg once daily or 20 mg twice daily. Permanently discontinue if unable to tolerate reduced dose. CML (chronic phase) with T315I mutation: (First dose reduction): 160 mg twice daily. Permanently discontinue if unable to tolerate reduced dose. Dose Modification Based on Common Terminology Criteria for Adverse Events (CTCAE).

Neutropenia/Thrombocytopenia
ANC less than 1,000 cells/mm³; platelet count less than 50,000 cells/mm³: Withhold treatment until ANC improves to 1,000 cells/mm³ or platelet count improves to 50,000 cells/mm³. If resolved within 2 wks, resume at same dose. If resolved after 2 wks, resume at reduced dose.
Recurrence of neutropenia/thrombocytopenia: Withhold treatment until improved, then resume at reduced dose if not previously done.

Pancreatitis/Elevated Lipase (Asymptomatic)
Serum amylase/lipase elevation greater than 2× upper limit of normal

(ULN): Withhold treatment until serum amylase/lipase improves to less than 1.5× ULN, then resume at reduce dose. If serum amylase/lipase does not improve or recurs at reduced dose, then permanently discontinue.

Other Toxicities
Any Grade 3 or 4 nonhematologic toxicity: Withhold treatment until improved to Grade 1 or 0, then resume at reduced dose. Permanently discontinue if toxicity does not improve.

Dosage in Renal Impairment
Mild to severe impairment: No dose adjustment if not requiring hemodialysis.

Dosage in Hepatic Impairment
No dose adjustment.

SIDE EFFECTS

Note: Frequency and occurrence of side effects may vary based on indicated treatment.
Frequent (42%–21%): Musculoskeletal pain, myalgia, fatigue, asthenia, rash, diarrhea. **Occasional (19% to less than 10%):** Headache, vomiting, abdominal pain, arthralgia, nausea, cough, pruritus, edema, constipation, pyrexia, dizziness, peripheral neuropathy, dyspnea, dry eye, blurry vision, palpitations, decreased appetite, urticaria.

ADVERSE EFFECTS/TOXIC REACTIONS

Myelosuppression (anemia, neutropenia, thrombocytopenia) is an expected response to therapy, but more severe reactions, including febrile neutropenia, may be life threatening. Grade 3 or 4 thrombocytopenia reported in 7% of pts. Grade 3 or 4 neutropenia reported in 8% of pts. Grade 3 anemia reported in 5% of pts. Pancreatitis reported in 3% of pts. Hypertension reported in 19% of pts. Hypersensitivity reactions reported in 32% of pts. Grade 3 or 4 hypersensitivity reaction (bronchospasm, edema, rash) reported in 2% of pts. Arrhythmias, QTc interval prolongation reported in 7% of pts. Cardiovascular toxicities (cardiac ischemia, arterial thrombosis/embolism, HF), infections (upper respiratory tract infections, UTI, pneumonia), hemorrhage (ear, mouth, nose, skin, vaginal) may occur. Plural effusion reported in 2% of pts.

NURSING CONSIDERATIONS

BASELINE ASSESSMENT

Obtain CBC; vital signs; pregnancy test in females of reproductive potential. Confirm compliance of effective contraception. Screen for active infection. Question history of cardiac disease, hypertension, pancreatitis. Receive full medication history and screen for interactions. Offer emotional support.

INTERVENTION/EVALUATION

Monitor CBC for myelosuppression q2wks for 3 mos, then monthly thereafter. Monitor serum amylase/lipase monthly for pancreatitis (severe abdominal pain, nausea, periumbilical ecchymosis [Cullen's sign], flank ecchymosis [Grey Turner's sign]). Monitor ECG for cardiac arrhythmias, ischemia; B/P for hypertension. Obtain echocardiogram if cardiac failure (chest pain, dyspnea, palpitations) is suspected. Diligently screen for infections (cough, dysuria, fatigue, fever, urinary frequency). Monitor for hypersensitivity reactions (bronchospasm, edema, rash), bleeding of any kind. If concomitant use of CYP3A4 substrates, CYP2C9 substrates, P-glycoprotein (P-gp) substrates is unavoidable, monitor for adverse toxic effects.

PATIENT/FAMILY TEACHING

• Treatment may depress your immune system and reduce your ability to fight infection. Report symptoms of infection such as body aches, burning with urination, chills, cough, fatigue, fever. Avoid those with active infection. • Report symptoms of bone marrow depression (e.g., bruising, fatigue, shortness of breath, weight loss; bleeding easily, bloody urine or stool). • Report symptoms of HF (e.g., chest pain, difficulty breathing, palpitations, swelling of extremities); heart arrhythmias (chest pain, dizziness, fainting, palpitations, slow or rapid heart rate, irregular heart rate); allergic reactions (difficulty breathing, rash, swelling). • Persistent, severe abdominal pain that radiates to the back (with or without vomiting) may indicate inflammation of the pancreas. • Use effective contraception to avoid pregnancy. Do not breastfeed. • Report bleeding of any kind.

---

aspirin

as-pir-in
(Ascriptin, Bayer, Bufferin, Durlaza, Ecotrin)
Do not confuse aspirin or Ascriptin with Afrin, Aricept, or Ecotrin with Epogen.

◆CLASSIFICATION

PHARMACOTHERAPEUTIC: Nonsteroidal anti-inflammatory drug (NSAID). **CLINICAL:** Anti-inflammatory, antipyretic, analgesic, anti-platelet.

USES

Analgesic, antipyretic, anti-inflammatory: Temporary relief of headache, pain, and fever causes by colds, muscle aches/pain, menstrual pain, toothache, minor pain of arthritis. **Revascularization procedures:** Adjunctive therapy (e.g., CABG, percutaneous transluminal coronary angioplasty, carotid endarterectomy). **Vascular indications, secondary prevention:** Ischemic stroke, transient ischemic attack, acute coronary syndrome, unstable angina. To reduce risk of death, nonfatal ischemic stroke or TIA; vascular mortality with suspected acute MI; risk of death, nonfatal MI with previous MI, unstable angina; risk of MI, sudden death with stable ischemic heart disease. **OFF-LABEL:** Carotid artery stenting, migraine (acute treatment), polycythemia vera, VTE prevention, adjunctive therapy of Kawasaki disease.

PRECAUTIONS

Contraindications: Hypersensitivity to NSAIDs. Pts with asthma, rhinitis, nasal polyps; use in children (younger than 16 yrs) for viral infections with or without fever. **Cautions:** Platelet/bleeding disorders, severe renal/hepatic impairment, dehydration, erosive gastritis, peptic ulcer disease, sensitivity to tartrazine dyes, elderly (chronic use of doses 325 mg or greater). Avoid use in pregnancy, especially third trimester.

ACTION

Irreversibly inhibits cyclo-oxygenase enzyme, resulting in a decreased formation of prostaglandin precursors. Irreversibly inhibits formation of thromboxane, resulting in inhibiting platelet aggregation. **Therapeutic Effect:** Reduces inflammatory response, intensity of pain; decreases fever; inhibits platelet aggregation.

PHARMACOKINETICS

Route	Onset	Peak	Duration
PO	1 hr	2–4 hrs	4–6 hrs

Rapidly and completely absorbed from GI tract; enteric-coated absorption delayed; rectal absorption delayed and incomplete. Protein binding: High. Widely distributed. Rapidly hydrolyzed to salicylate. **Half-life:** 15–20 min (aspirin); 2–3 hrs (salicylate at low dose); more than 20 hrs (salicylate at high dose).

⌛ LIFESPAN CONSIDERATIONS

Pregnancy/Lactation: Readily crosses placenta; distributed in breast milk. May prolong gestation and labor, decrease fetal birth weight, increase incidence of stillbirths, neonatal mortality, hemor-

rhage. Avoid use during last trimester (may adversely affect fetal cardiovascular system: premature closure of ductus arteriosus). **Children:** Caution in pts with acute febrile illness (Reye's syndrome). **Elderly:** May be more susceptible to toxicity; lower dosages recommended.

INTERACTIONS

DRUG: Alcohol, NSAIDs (e.g., ibuprofen, ketorolac, naproxen) may increase risk of GI effects (e.g., ulceration). **Anticoagulants, (e.g. enoxaparin, warfarin), heparin, thrombolytics, ticagrelor** increase risk of bleeding. **Apixaban, dabigatran, edoxaban, rivaroxaban** may increase anticoagulant effect. **HERBAL: Herbals with anticoagulant/antiplatelet properties (e.g., garlic, ginger, ginkgo biloba)** may increase risk of bleeding. **FOOD:** None known. **LAB VALUES:** May alter serum ALT, AST, alkaline phosphatase, uric acid; prolongs prothrombin time (PT) platelet function assay. May decrease serum cholesterol, potassium, T_3, T_4.

AVAILABILITY (OTC)

Caplets: 325 mg, 500 mg. **Suppositories:** 300 mg. **Tablets:** 325 mg. **Tablets (Chewable):** 81 mg.

🖋 Extended-Release Capsule: **(Durlaza)** 162.5 mg. **Tablets (Enteric-Coated):** 81 mg, 325 mg, 650 mg.

ADMINISTRATION/HANDLING

PO

• Do not break, crush, dissolve, or divide enteric-coated tablets or extended-release capsule. • May give with water, milk, meals if GI distress occurs.

Rectal

• Refrigerate suppositories; do not freeze. • If suppository is too soft, chill for 30 min in refrigerator or run cold water over foil wrapper. • Moisten suppository with cold water before inserting well into rectum.

 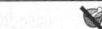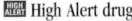

INDICATIONS/ROUTES/DOSAGE

Analgesia, Fever
PO: ADULTS, ELDERLY, CHILDREN 12 YRS AND OLDER AND WEIGHING 50 KG OR MORE: 325–1,000 mg q4–6h prn. **Maximum:** 4 g/day.

Revascularization
PO: ADULTS, ELDERLY: 75–325 mg/day.

MI, Stroke (Risk Reduction)
PO: ADULTS, ELDERLY: 75–100 mg once daily.

Dosage in Renal/Hepatic Impairment
Avoid use in severe impairment.

SIDE EFFECTS

Occasional: GI distress (including abdominal distention, cramping, heartburn, mild nausea); allergic reaction (including bronchospasm, pruritus, urticaria).

ADVERSE EFFECTS/TOXIC REACTIONS

High doses of aspirin may produce GI bleeding and/or gastric mucosal lesions. Dehydrated, febrile children may experience aspirin toxicity quickly. Reye's syndrome, characterized by persistent vomiting, signs of brain dysfunction, may occur in children taking aspirin with recent viral infection (chickenpox, common cold, or flu). Low-grade aspirin toxicity characterized by tinnitus, generalized pruritus (may be severe), headache, dizziness, flushing, tachycardia, hyperventilation, diaphoresis, thirst. Marked toxicity characterized by hyperthermia, restlessness, seizures, abnormal breathing patterns, respiratory failure, coma.

NURSING CONSIDERATIONS

BASELINE ASSESSMENT

Do not give to children or teenagers who have or have recently had viral infections (increases risk of Reye's syndrome). Do not use if vinegar-like odor is noted (indicates chemical breakdown). Assess history of GI bleed, peptic ulcer disease, OTC use of products that may contain aspirin. Assess type, location, duration of pain, inflammation. Inspect appearance of affected joints for immobility, deformities, skin condition. **Therapeutic serum level for antiarthritic effect:** 20–30 mg/dL (toxicity occurs if level is greater than 30 mg/dL).

INTERVENTION/EVALUATION

Monitor urinary pH (sudden acidification, pH from 6.5 to 5.5, may result in toxicity). Assess skin for evidence of ecchymosis. If given as antipyretic, assess temperature directly before and 1 hr after giving medication. Evaluate for therapeutic response: relief of pain, stiffness, swelling; increased joint mobility; reduced joint tenderness; improved grip strength.

PATIENT/FAMILY TEACHING

• Do not, chew, crush, dissolve, or divide enteric-coated tablets. • Avoid alcohol, OTC pain/cold products that may contain aspirin. • Report ringing of the ears or persistent abdominal GI pain, bleeding. • Therapeutic anti-inflammatory effect noted in 1–3 wks. • Behavioral changes, persistent vomiting may be early signs of Reye's syndrome; contact physician.

atezolizumab

a-te-zoe-**liz**-ue-mab
(Tecentriq)
Do not confuse atezolizumab with daclizumab, certolizumab, eculizumab, omalizumab, or tocilizumab.

◆CLASSIFICATION

PHARMACOTHERAPEUTIC: Programmed death-ligand 1 (PD-L1) blocking antibody. Monoclonal antibody. **CLINICAL:** Antineoplastic.

USES

Non-small cell lung cancer (NSCLC):
First-line treatment of metastatic non–small-cell lung cancer (NSCLC) as single-agent therapy in pts whose tumors have high PD-L1 expression, with no EGFR or ALK genomic tumor aberrations, in combination with bevacizumab, paclitaxel, and carboplatin with no EGFR or ALK genomic tumor aberrations or in combination with paclitaxel (protein bound) and carboplatin in pts with no EGFR or ALK genome tumor aberrations. Treatment of metastatic NSCLC as a single agent in pts with disease progression during or following platinum-containing chemotherapy. Pts should have disease progression on approved therapy for EGFR or ALK genomic tumor mutation before receiving atezolizumab. Adjuvant treatment (as a single agent) following resection and platinum-based chemotherapy in adults with stage II to IIIA NSCLC whose tumors have PD-L1 expression on 1% or more of tumor cells. **Small cell lung cancer (SCLC):** First-line treatment of extensive-stage small-cell lung cancer (in combination with carboplatin and etoposide). **Hepatocellular carcinoma (HCC):** Treatment of hepatocellular carcinoma (in combination with bevacizumab). **Melanoma:** Treatment of BRAF V600 mutation-positive unresectable or metastatic melanoma (in combination with cobimetinib and vemurafenib). **Alveolar soft part sarcoma (ASPS):** Treatment of unresectable or metastatic alveolar soft part sarcoma (ASPS) as single agent in adults and pediatric pts 2 yrs of age and older.

PRECAUTIONS

Contraindications: Hypersensitivity to atezolizumab. **Cautions:** Active infection; baseline cytopenias; pts at risk for hyperglycemia (e.g., diabetes, chronic use of corticosteroids); conditions predisposing to infection (e.g., diabetes, renal failure, immunocompromised pts, open wounds); pts at risk for dehydration, electrolyte imbalance; hepatic impairment, peripheral or generalized edema, neuropathy, optic disorders, interstitial lung disease; history of venous thromboembolism, intestinal obstruction, pancreatitis.

ACTION

Binds to PD-L1 to selectively prevent the interaction between PD-L1 and B7.1 receptors. PD-L1 is an immune checkpoint protein expressed on tumor cells. **Therapeutic Effect:** Restores anti-tumor T-cell function. Suppresses tumor growth and improves tumor immunogenicity.

PHARMACOKINETICS

Widely distributed. Metabolism not specified. Steady state reached in 6–9 wks. Elimination not specified. **Half-life:** 27 days.

⧗ LIFESPAN CONSIDERATIONS

Pregnancy/Lactation: Avoid pregnancy; may cause fetal harm. Unknown if distributed in breast milk; however, human immunoglobulin G is present in breast milk. Breastfeeding not recommended during treatment and for at least 5 mos after discontinuation. Females of reproductive potential should use effective contraception during treatment and up to 5 mos after discontinuation. May impair fertility in females. **Children:** Safety and efficacy not established. **Elderly:** No age-related precautions noted.

INTERACTIONS

DRUG: None significant. **HERBAL:** None significant. **FOOD:** None known. **LAB VALUES:** May increase serum alkaline phosphatase, ALT, AST, creatinine, glucose. May decrease serum albumin, sodium; lymphocytes, Hgb, Hct, RBCs.

AVAILABILITY (Rx)

Injection Solution: 840 mg/14 mL, 1,200 mg/20 mL (60 mg/mL).

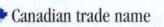 Canadian trade name   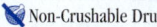 Non-Crushable Drug   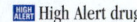 High Alert drug

ADMINISTRATION/HANDLING

IV

Reconstitution • Visually inspect solution for particulate matter or discoloration. Solution should appear clear to slightly yellow. Discard if solution is cloudy or discolored or if visible particles are present. • Do not shake vial. • Withdraw 20 mL of solution from vial and dilute into a 250-mL polyvinyl chloride, polyethylene, or polyolefin infusion bag containing 0.9% NaCl. Dilute with 0.9% NaCl only. • Mix by gentle inversion. • Do not shake. • Discard partially used or empty vials.

Rate of administration • Infuse over 60 min using sterile, nonpyrogenic, low protein-binding, 0.2- to 0.22-micron in-line filter. • If first infusion is tolerated, all subsequent infusions may be delivered over 30 min. • Do not administer as IV bolus.

Storage • Refrigerate diluted solution up to 24 hrs or store at room temperature for no more than 6 hrs (includes time of preparation and infusion). • Do not freeze. • Do not shake.

▓ IV INCOMPATIBILITIES

Do not administer with other medications. Infuse via dedicated line.

INDICATIONS/ROUTES/DOSAGE

NSCLC (Metastatic)

IV: ADULTS, ELDERLY: 840 mg q2wks; or 1,200 mg q3wks; or 1,680 mg q4wks. Administer prior to chemotherapy and bevacizumab when given on the same day. May continue atezolizumab until disease progression or unacceptable toxicity.

NSCLC (Adjuvant Treatment)

IV: ADULTS, ELDERLY: 840 mg q2wks, or 1,200 mg q3wks, or 1,680 mg q4wks (as a single agent). Continue for up to 1 yr unless disease recurrence or unacceptable toxicity occurs.

SCLC

IV: ADULTS, ELDERLY: 840 mg q2wks; or 1,200 mg q3wks; or 1,680 mg q4wks. Administer prior to chemotherapy when given on the same day. May continue atezolizumab until disease progression or unacceptable toxicity.

Hepatocellular Carcinoma

IV: ADULTS, ELDERLY: 840 mg q2 wks; or 1200 mg q3 wks; or 1680 mg q4 wks. Administer prior to bevacizumab when given on the same day. (Bevacizumab is administered at 15 mg/kg q3 wks. May continue atezolizumab until disease progression or unacceptable toxicity.

Melanoma (Unresectable or Metastatic)

Note: Prior to initiating atezolizumab, pts should receive a 28-day treatment cycle of cobimetinib and vemurafenib.

IV: ADULTS, ELDERLY: 840 mg q2 wks; or 1200 mg q3 wks; or 1680 mg q4 wks. (in combination with cobimetinib and vemurafenib). Continue until disease progression or unacceptable toxicity.

ASPS

IV: ADULTS, ELDERLY: 840 mg q2 wks; or 1200 mg q3 wks; or 1680 mg q4 wks. **CHILDREN 2 YRS OF AGE AND OLDER:** 15 mg/kg (up to a maximum 1200 mg) q3 wks. Continue until disease progression or unacceptable toxicity.

Dose Modification

Based on Common Terminology Criteria for Adverse Events (CTCAE). **Withhold treatment for any of the following toxic reactions:** Grade 2 or 3 diarrhea or colitis; Grade 2 pneumonitis; serum AST or ALT elevation 3–5 times upper limit of normal (ULN) or serum bilirubin elevation 1.5–3 times ULN; symptomatic hypophysitis, adrenal insufficiency, hypothyroidism, hyperthyroidism; Grade 3 or 4 hyperglycemia; Grade 3 rash; Grade 2 ocular inflammatory toxicity, Grade 2 or 3 pancreatitis, Grade 3 or 4 infection, Grade 2 infusion-related reactions. **Restarting treatment after interruption of therapy:** Resume treatment when adverse effects return to Grade 0 or 1. **Permanently discontinue** for any of the following toxic reactions: Grade 3 or 4 diarrhea or colitis; Grade 3 or 4 pneumonitis; serum AST or ALT elevation greater than 5 times ULN or serum bilirubin elevation 3 times ULN; Grade 4 hypophysitis; Grade 4 rash; Grade 3 or 4 ocular inflammatory toxicity; Grade 4 or any grade recurrent pancreatitis; Grade 3 or 4 infusion-related reactions; any occurrence of encephalitis, Guillain-Barré, meningitis, meningoencephalitis, myasthenic syndrome/myasthenia gravis.

Dosage in Renal Impairment
No dose adjustment.

Dosage in Hepatic Impairment
Mild impairment: No dose adjustment. **Moderate to severe impairment:** Not specified; use caution.

SIDE EFFECTS

Frequent (52%–18%): Fatigue, decreased appetite, nausea, pyrexia, constipation, diarrhea, peripheral edema. **Occasional (17%–13%):** Abdominal pain, vomiting, dyspnea, back/neck pain, rash, arthralgia, cough, pruritus.

ADVERSE EFFECTS/TOXIC REACTIONS

May cause severe immune-mediated events including adrenal insufficiency (0.4% of pts), interstitial lung disease or pneumonitis (3% of pts), colitis or diarrhea (20% of pts), hepatitis (2%–3% of pts), hypophysitis (0.2% of pts), hyperthyroidism (1% of pts), hypothyroidism (4% of pts), rash (up to 37% of pts), new-onset diabetes with ketoacidosis (0.2% of pts), pancreatitis (0.1% of pts); meningoencephalitis, myasthenic syndrome/myasthenia gravis, Guillain-Barré, ocular inflammatory toxicity (less than 1% of pts). Severe, sometimes fatal infections, including sepsis, herpes encephalitis, mycobacterial infection, occurred in 38% of pts. Urinary tract infections were the most common cause of Grade 3 or higher infection, occurring in 7% of pts. Severe infusion-related reactions reported in less than 1% of pts. Other adverse events, including acute kidney injury, dehydration, dyspnea, encephalitis, hematuria, intestinal obstruction, meningitis, neuropathy, pneumonia, urinary obstruction, venous thromboembolism, were reported.

NURSING CONSIDERATIONS

BASELINE ASSESSMENT
Obtain CBC, BMP, LFT, thyroid panel, pregnancy test in females of reproductive potential. Screen for history of pituitary/pulmonary/thyroid disease, autoimmune disorders, diabetes, hepatic impairment, venous thromboembolism. Conduct full dermatologic/neurologic/ophthalmologic exam. Screen for active infection. Assess hydration status.

INTERVENTION/EVALUATION
Monitor CBC, BMP, LFT, thyroid panel, vital signs. Diligently monitor for immune-mediated adverse events as listed in Adverse Effects/Toxic Reactions. Notify physician if any CTCAE toxicities occur and initiate proper treatment. Obtain chest X-ray if interstitial lung disease, pneumonitis suspected. Due to high risk for dehydration/diarrhea, strictly monitor I&O. Encourage PO intake. If corticosteroid therapy is initiated for immune-mediated events, monitor capillary blood glucose and screen for corticosteroid side effects. Report any changes in neurologic status, including nuchal rigidity with fever, positive Kernig's sign, positive Brudzinski's sign, altered mental status, seizures. Diligently monitor for infection.

PATIENT/FAMILY TEACHING
• Treatment may cause serious or life-threatening inflammatory reactions. Report signs and symptoms of treatment-related inflammatory events in the following body systems: colon (severe abdominal pain or diarrhea); eye (blurry vision, double vision, unequal pupil size, sensitivity to light, eyelid drooping); lung (chest pain, cough, shortness of breath); liver (bruising easily, amber-colored urine, clay-colored/tarry stools, yellowing of skin or eyes); pituitary (persistent or unusual headache, dizziness, extreme weakness, fainting, vision

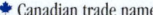 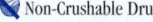

changes); thyroid (trouble sleeping, high blood pressure, fast heart rate [overactive thyroid]), (fatigue, goiter, weight gain [underactive thyroid]), neurologic (confusion, headache, seizures, neck rigidity with fever, severe nerve pain or loss of motor function). • Immediately report allergic reactions, bleeding of any kind, signs of infection. • Treatment may cause severe diarrhea. Drink plenty of fluids. Use effective contraception to avoid pregnancy. Do not breastfeed.

atorvaSTATin

a-**tor**-va-sta-tin
(Atorvaliq, Lipitor)
Do not confuse atorvastatin with atomoxetine, lovastatin, nystatin, pitavastatin, pravastatin, or simvastatin, or Lipitor with labetalol, Levatol, lisinopril, Mevacor, or Zocor.

FIXED-COMBINATION(S)

Caduet: atorvastatin/amLODIPine (calcium channel blocker): 10 mg/2.5 mg, 10 mg/5 mg, 10 mg/10 mg, 20 mg/2.5 mg, 20 mg/5 mg, 20 mg/10 mg, 40 mg/2.5 mg, 40 mg/5 mg, 40 mg/10 mg, 80 mg/5 mg, 80 mg/10 mg.

◆CLASSIFICATION

PHARMACOTHERAPEUTIC: Hydroxymethylglutaryl CoA (HMG-CoA) reductase inhibitor. **CLINICAL:** Antihyperlipidemic.

USES

Heterozygous familial hypercholesterolemia: Reduce elevated cholesterol (total-C), LDL cholesterol (LDL-C), apolipoprotein B (apoB), triglyceride levels, and elevate HDL cholesterol in pts with primary hypercholesterolemia. **Heterozygous familial hypercholesterolemia (pediatric):** Reduce total-C, LDL-C, apoB in pts 10–17 yrs of age with heterozygous familial hypercholesterolemia with LDL-C 190 mg/mL or greater, LDL-C 160 mg/mL or greater with family history of premature cardiovascular disease (CVD), or LDL-C 160 mg/mL or greater with 2 or more other CVD risk factors. **Homozygous familial hypercholesterolemia:** Reduce total-C and LDL-C in pts with homozygous familial hypercholesterolemia as an adjunct to other lipid-lowering treatments. **Prevention of atherosclerotic cardiovascular disease (ASCVD): primary prevention:** Reduce risk of myocardial infarction (MI), stroke, revascularization procedures, and angina in pts without a history of coronary heart disease (CHD) but with multiple CHD risk factors. **Secondary prevention:** Reduce risk of MI, stroke, revascularization procedures, and angina in pts with a history of CHD.

PRECAUTIONS

Contraindications: Hypersensitivity to atorvastatin. Active hepatic disease, breastfeeding, pregnancy or women who may become pregnant, unexplained elevated LFT results. **Cautions:** Anticoagulant therapy; history of hepatic disease; substantial alcohol consumption; pts with prior stroke/TIA; concomitant use of potent CYP3A4 inhibitors; elderly (predisposed to myopathy).

ACTION

Inhibits HMG-CoA reductase, the enzyme that catalyzes the early step in cholesterol synthesis. Results in an increase of expression in LDL receptors on hepatocyte membranes and a stimulation of LDL catabolism. **Therapeutic Effect:** Decreases LDL and VLDL, plasma triglyceride levels; increases HDL concentration.

PHARMACOKINETICS

Widely distributed. Protein binding: greater than 98%. Metabolized in liver. Primarily excreted in feces (biliary). **Half-life:** 14 hrs.

⧖ LIFESPAN CONSIDERATIONS

Pregnancy/Lactation: Distributed in breast milk. Contraindicated during pregnancy. May produce fetal skeletal malformation. **Children:** Safety and efficacy not established. **Elderly:** No age-related precautions noted.

INTERACTIONS

DRUG: Strong CYP3A4 inhibitors (e.g., **clarithromycin, ketoconazole, ritonavir**) may increase concentration/effect. **CycloSPORINE** may increase concentration. **Gemfibrozil, fibrates, niacin, colchicine** may increase concentration/effect. Strong CYP3A4 inducers (e.g., **carbamazepine, phenytoin, rifampin**) may decrease concentration/effect. **HERBAL:** St. John's wort may decrease concentration/effect. **FOOD:** Grapefruit products may increase concentration/effect. **Red yeast rice** may increase concentration/effect. (2.4 mg lovastatin per 600 mg rice). **LAB VALUES:** May increase serum transaminase, creatinine kinase concentrations.

AVAILABILITY (Rx)

🥄 **Oral Suspension:** 20 mg/5 mL.
Tablets: 10 mg, 20 mg, 40 mg, 80 mg.

ADMINISTRATION/HANDLING

PO

• **Tablet:** Give without regard to food or time of day. • **Oral Suspension:** Administer on empty stomach at least 1 hr before or 2 hrs after a meal. May take without regard to time of day.

INDICATIONS/ROUTES/DOSAGE

Prevention of Cardiovascular Disease
PO: ADULTS, ELDERLY: Primary prevention (moderate intensity): 10–20 mg/day; **(high intensity):** 40–80 mg/day. **Secondary prevention (high intensity):** 80 mg/day.

Heterozygous Hypercholesterolemia
PO: ADULTS: Initially, 40–80 mg once daily. **Maximum:** 80 mg/day. **CHILDREN 10–17 YRS:** Initially, 10 mg/day. May increase incrementally by doubling dose at monthly intervals. **Maximum:** 80 mg/day.

Homozygous Familial Hypercholesterolemia
PO: ADULTS, ELDERLY: 80 mg once daily.

Dosage in Renal Impairment
No dose adjustment.

Dosage in Hepatic Impairment
See contraindications.

SIDE EFFECTS

Frequent (16%): Headache. **Occasional (5%–2%):** Myalgia, rash, pruritus, allergy. **Rare (less than 2%–1%):** Flatulence, dyspepsia, depression.

ADVERSE EFFECTS/TOXIC REACTIONS

May cause myopathy (muscle pain, tenderness). Rhabdomyolysis, a life-threatening condition caused by the rapid breakdown of muscle cells, may cause kidney failure and severe disability. Immune-mediated necrotizing myopathy, an autoimmune myopathy, has occurred in pts using statins. May cause hepatotoxicity, jaundice. May cause endocrine dysfunction; increased fasting serum glucose levels. Infections, including nasopharyngitis, UTI, may occur.

NURSING CONSIDERATIONS

BASELINE ASSESSMENT

Obtain cholesterol, triglyceride level, LFT; pregnancy test in females of reproductive potential. Obtain dietary history. Question history of active hepatic disease. Obtain medication history and screen for interactions.

INTERVENTION/EVALUATION

Monitor LFT for hepatoxicity (bruising, jaundice, right upper abdominal pain, nausea, vomiting), serum cholesterol levels. Monitor for muscle weakness/tenderness; rhabdomyolysis (confusion, muscle pain, darkened urine

 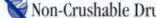

color, vomiting). Obtain CPK level if rhabdomyolysis is suspected.

PATIENT/FAMILY TEACHING

• Follow a low-cholesterol, heart-healthy diet. • Report liver problems (e.g., abdominal pain, bruising, clay-colored stools, amber or dark-colored urine, yellowing of the skin or eyes), muscle tenderness. • Treatment may cause rhabdomyolysis, a life-threatening condition that can cause kidney failure and death. Report muscle pain, fatigue, decreased urine output, or darkened urine color. • There is a high risk of interactions with other medications. Do not take new medication unless approved by prescriber who started treatment. • Avoid excessive alcohol intake; grapefruit products.

avapritinib

a-va-**pri**-ti-nib
(Ayvakit)
Do not confuse avapritinib with acalabrutinib, afatinib, alectinib, axitinib, enasidenib, ibrutinib, or imatinib.

♦**Classification**

PHARMACOTHERAPEUTIC: PDGFR-alpha blocker. Tyrosine kinase inhibitor.
CLINICAL: Antineoplastic.

USES

GI stromal tumor: Treatment of adults with unresectable or metastatic GI stromal tumor (GIST) harboring a platelet-derived growth factor receptor alpha (PDGFRA) exon 18 mutation, including PDGFRA D842V mutations. **ADvSM:** Treatment of adults with advanced systemic mastocytosis (not recommended if platelet count is less than 50,000 cells/mm³). **ISM:** Treatment of adults with indolent systemic mastocytosis (ISM) (not recommended if platelet count is less than 50,000 cells/mm³.

PRECAUTIONS

Contraindications: Hypersensitivity to avapritinib. **Cautions:** Baseline cytopenias, severe hepatic/renal impairment; conditions predisposing to infection (e.g., diabetes, immunocompromised, open wounds). History of intracranial/GI bleeding; anxiety, depression, suicidal ideation/behavior. Avoid concomitant use of strong or moderate CYP3A inhibitors, strong or moderate CYP3A inducers.

ACTION

Blocks PDGFRA targeting PDGFRA, PDGFR, and KIT mutants, which may result in autophosphorylation/activation of these receptors and lead to tumor cell proliferation. Avapritinib inhibits autophosphorylation of PDGFRA, KIT exon mutations. **Therapeutic Effect:** Inhibits tumor growth and survival associated with bowel, esophagus, stomach cancer.

PHARMACOKINETICS

Widely distributed. Metabolized in liver. Protein binding: 99%. Peak plasma concentration: 2–4 hrs. Steady state reached in 15 days. Excreted in feces (70%), urine (18%). **Half-life:** 32–57 hrs.

⌛ LIFESPAN CONSIDERATIONS

Pregnancy/Lactation: Avoid pregnancy; may cause fetal harm. Females and males of reproductive potential must use effective contraception during treatment and for at least 6 wks after discontinuation. Unknown if distributed in breast milk. Breastfeeding not recommended during treatment and for at least 2 wks after discontinuation. May impair fertility in both females and males. **Children:** Safety and efficacy not established. **Elderly:** No age-related precautions noted.

INTERACTIONS

DRUG: Alcohol, other CNS depressants (e.g., lorazepam, oxycodone,

zolpidem) may increase CNS depression. **Strong CYP3A4 inhibitors (e.g., clarithromycin, ketoconazole, ritonavir)** may increase concentration/effect. **Strong CYP3A4 inducers (e.g., carbamazepine, phenytoin, rifampin), moderate CYP3A inducers (e.g., bosentan, nafcillin)** may decrease concentration/effect. **HERBAL: Herbals with sedative properties (e.g., chamomile, kava kava, valerian)** may increase CNS depression. **FOOD:** None significant. **LAB VALUES:** May increase serum alkaline phosphatase, ALT, AST, bilirubin, creatinine. May decrease Hgb, leukocytes, neutrophils, platelets; serum albumin, magnesium, phosphate, potassium, sodium. May increase or decrease serum glucose. May prolong aPTT, PT; increase INR.

AVAILABILITY (Rx)

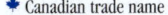 **Tablets:** 25 mg, 50 mg, 100 mg, 200 mg, 300 mg.

ADMINISTRATION/HANDLING

PO
• Give on empty stomach, at least 1 hr before or 2 hrs after meal. • Administer tablets whole; do not break, crush, or divide. Tablet cannot be chewed. • If vomiting occurs after administration, give next dose at regularly scheduled time (do not give additional dose). • If a dose is missed, do not give within 8 hrs of next scheduled dose.

INDICATIONS/ROUTES/DOSAGE

GI Stromal Tumor
PO: **ADULTS, ELDERLY:** 300 mg once daily. Continue until disease progression or unacceptable toxicity. If unable to discontinue moderate CYP3A inhibitor, reduce starting dose to 100 mg once daily.

Advanced Systemic Mastocytosis (AdvSM)
PO: **ADULTS, ELDERLY:** 200 mg once daily. Continue until disease progression or unacceptable toxicity.

Indolent Systemic Mastocytosis (ISM)
PO: **ADULTS, ELDERLY:** 25 mg once daily.

Dose Reduction Schedule for Adverse Events (GI Stromal Tumor)
First dose reduction: 200 mg once daily. **Second dose reduction:** 100 mg once daily. **Unable to tolerate 100 mg dose:** Permanently discontinue.

Dose Reduction Schedule for Adverse Events (Systemic Mastocytosis)
First dose reduction: 100 mg once daily. **Second dose reduction:** 50 mg once daily. **Third dose reduction:** 25 mg once daily. **Unable to tolerate 25-mg dose:** Permanently discontinue.

Dose Modification
Based on Common Terminology Criteria for Adverse Events (CTCAE).

Central Nervous System (CNS) Effects
Grade 1 effects: Continue at same dose or withhold treatment until resolved or improved to baseline, then resume at same dose or reduced dose level. **Grade 2 or 3 effects:** Withhold treatment until resolved, or improved to Grade 1 or baseline, then resume at same dose or reduced dose level. **Grade 4 effects:** Permanently discontinue.

Intracranial Hemorrhage
Grade 1 or 2 intracranial hemorrhage: For first occurrence, withhold treatment until resolved, then resume at reduced dose level. For second occurrence, permanently discontinue. **Grade 3 or 4 intracranial hemorrhage:** Permanently discontinue.

Other Toxicities
Any other Grade 3 or 4 toxicities: Withhold treatment until improved to Grade 2 or less, then resume at same dose or reduced dose level.

Dosage in Renal Impairment
Mild to moderate impairment (CrCl 30–89 mL/min): No dose adjustment. **Severe impairment (CrCl 15–29 mL/min), ESRD:** Not specified; use caution.

Dosage in Hepatic Impairment
Mild to moderate impairment: No dose adjustment. **Severe impairment: (Start-**

 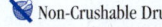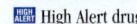

ing dose): GIST: 200 mg once daily. **AdvSM:** 100 mg once daily. **ISM:** 25 mg every other day.

SIDE EFFECTS

Frequent (72%–22%): Edema (conjunctival, face, eye, eyelid, generalized, periorbital, peripheral, localized, orbital, testicular), nausea, fatigue, asthenia, cognitive impairment, vomiting, decreased appetite, diarrhea, increased lacrimation, abdominal pain, constipation, rash, dizziness. **Occasional (17%–8%):** Headache, dyspepsia, sleep disorders, insomnia, somnolence, dysgeusia, ageusia, hair color changes, dyspnea, pyrexia, alopecia, decreased weight, hypertension.

ADVERSE EFFECTS/TOXIC REACTIONS

Myelosuppression (anemia, leukopenia, neutropenia, thrombocytopenia) is an expected response to therapy. Intracranial hemorrhage, subdural hematoma reported in 1%–3% of pts. CNS effects including dizziness, hallucinations, cognitive impairment (e.g., amnesia confusion, dementia, encephalopathy, memory/mental impairment), mood disorders (e.g., agitation, anxiety, depression, dysphoria, personality change, suicidal ideation) reported in 58% of pts. Median onset of CNS effects was 6 wks. Grade 1 or 2 nausea and vomiting has occurred. Other serious reactions including pleural effusion, sepsis (3% of pts); GI hemorrhage, acute kidney injury (2% of pts); pneumonia, tumor hemorrhage (1% of pts) has occurred. Palmar-plantar erythrodysesthesia syndrome (PPES), a chemotherapy-induced skin condition that presents with redness, swelling, numbness, skin sloughing of the hands and feet reported in 1% of pts. Hyperthyroidism, hypothyroidism reported in 3% of pts.

NURSING CONSIDERATIONS

BASELINE ASSESSMENT

Obtain CBC, BMP, LFT; pregnancy test in female pts of reproductive potential. Question history of anxiety, depression, mood disorder, suicidal ideation and behavior; hepatic/renal impairment, intracranial/GI hemorrhage. Assess usual bowel movement patterns, stool characteristics. Assess hydration status. Screen for active infection. Receive full medication history and screen for interactions. Conduct baseline neurologic exam. Offer emotional support.

INTERVENTION/EVALUATION

Obtain CBC, BMP, LFT as clinically appropriate. Conduct regular neurologic exams to assess CNS effects, symptoms of intracranial bleeding (aphasia, blindness, confusion, facial droop, hemiplegia, seizures). Assess skin for dermal toxicities, PPES. Diligently screen for suicidal ideation and behavior; new-onset or worsening of anxiety, depression, mood disorder. Consult mental health professional if mood disorder suspected. Monitor daily pattern of bowel activity, stool consistency; I&Os, hydration status. Monitor for GI bleeding, infections (cough, fatigue, fever); drug toxicities if discontinuation of CYP3A inhibitor is unavoidable.

PATIENT/FAMILY TEACHING

• Treatment may depress your immune system response and reduce your ability to fight infection. Report symptoms of infection such as body aches, chills, cough, fatigue, fever. Avoid those with active infection. • Seek immediate medical attention if thoughts of suicide, new-onset or worsening of anxiety, depression, or changes in mood occur. • Nervous system changes including altered memory, confusion, delirium, difficulty speaking, gait disturbance, numbness, tremors may occur. Avoid tasks that require alertness, motor skills if neurologic effects are occurring. • Report symptoms of liver problems (abdominal pain, bruising, clay-colored stool, amber- or dark-colored urine, yellowing of the skin or eyes); hemorrhagic stroke (confusion, difficulty speaking, one-sided weakness, loss of vision). • Use effective contraception to avoid pregnancy. Do not breastfeed. • Treatment may cause diarrhea, dehydration. Drink plenty of fluids. • There is a high risk of interactions with other medications. Do not take newly prescribed medications unless approved by the prescriber who originally started treatment. • Avoid grapefruit products, herbal supplements (esp. St. John's wort).

avelumab

a-**vel**-ue-mab
(Bavencio)
Do not confuse avelumab with atezolizumab, durvalumab, nivolumab, or olaratumab.

◆CLASSIFICATION

PHARMACOTHERAPEUTIC: Programmed death ligand-1 (PD-L1) blocking antibody. Monoclonal antibody. **CLINICAL:** Antineoplastic.

USES

Merkel cell carcinoma (MCC): Treatment of adults and pediatric pts 12 yrs and older with metastatic Merkel cell carcinoma. **Urothelial carcinoma (UC):** Maintenance treatment of pts with locally advanced or metastatic UC who have not progressed with first-line platinum-containing chemotherapy. Treatment of pts with locally advanced or metastatic UC who have disease progression during or following platinum-containing chemotherapy or have disease progression within 12 mos of neoadjuvant or adjuvant treatment with platinum-containing chemotherapy. **Renal cell carcinoma (RCC):** First-line treatment of advanced renal cell carcinoma (in combination with axitinib). **OFF-LABEL:** Gestational trophoblastic neoplasia.

PRECAUTIONS

Contraindications: Hypersensitivity to avelumab. **Cautions:** Acute infection, conditions predisposing to infection (e.g.,

diabetes, immunocompromised pts, renal failure, open wounds); corticosteroid intolerance, hematologic cytopenias, hepatic impairment, interstitial lung disease, renal insufficiency; history of autoimmune disorders (Crohn's disease, demyelinating polyneuropathy, Guillain-Barré syndrome, Hashimoto's thyroiditis, hyperthyroidism, myasthenia gravis, rheumatoid arthritis, Type I diabetes, vasculitis); CVA, diabetes, intestinal obstruction, pancreatitis.

ACTION

Binds to PD-L1 and blocks interaction with both PD-L1 and B7.1 receptors while still allowing interaction between PD-L2 and PD-L1. PD-L1 is an immune check point protein expressed on tumor cells, down regulating anti-tumor T-cell function. **Therapeutic Effect:** Restores immune responses, including T-cell anti-tumor function.

PHARMACOKINETICS

Widely distributed. Degraded into small peptides and amino acids via proteolytic enzymes. Steady state reached in 4–6 wks. Excretion not specified. **Half-life:** 6.1 days.

▧ LIFESPAN CONSIDERATIONS

Pregnancy/Lactation: Avoid pregnancy; may cause fetal harm. Females of reproductive potential should use effective contraception during treatment and for at least 1 mo after discontinuation. Unknown if distributed in breast milk. However, human immunoglobulin G (IgG) is present in breast milk and is known to cross the placenta. Breastfeeding not recommended during treatment and for at least 1 mo after discontinuation. **Children:** Safety and efficacy not established in pts younger than 12 yrs. **Elderly:** No age-related precautions noted.

INTERACTIONS

DRUG: None significant. **HERBAL:** None significant. **FOOD:** None known. **LAB VALUES:** May decrease Hgb, Hct, lymphocytes, neutrophils, platelets, RBCs. May increase serum alkaline phosphatase,

---

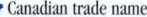 Canadian trade name   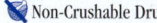 Non-Crushable Drug   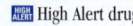 High Alert drug

ALT, AST, amylase, bilirubin, glucose, GGT, lipase.

AVAILABILITY (Rx)

Injection: 200 mg/10 mL (20 mg/mL).

ADMINISTRATION/HANDLING

 IV

Preparation • Visually inspect for particulate matter or discoloration. Solution should appear clear and colorless to slightly yellow in color. • Do not use if solution is cloudy, discolored, or if visible particles are observed. • Withdraw proper volume from vial and inject into a 250-mL bag of 0.9% NaCl or 0.45% NaCl. • Gently invert to mix; avoid foaming. • Do not shake. • Diluted solution should be clear, colorless, and free of particles.

Rate of administration • Infuse over 60 min via dedicated IV line using a sterile, nonpyrogenic, low protein-binding in-line filter.

Storage • Refrigerate unused vials. • May refrigerate diluted solution for no more than 24 hrs or store at room temperature for no more than 4 hrs. If refrigerated, allow diluted solution to warm to room temperature before infusing. • Do not freeze or shake. • Protect from light.

IV INCOMPATIBILITIES

Do not mix or infuse with other medications.

INDICATIONS/ROUTES/DOSAGE

Note: Premedicate with acetaminophen and an antihistamine prior to the first 4 infusions. Consider premedication for subsequent infusions based on prior infusion reactions.

Urothelial Carcinoma

IV: ADULTS, ELDERLY: 800 mg once q2wks. Continue until disease progression or unacceptable toxicity.

Renal Cell Carcinoma (Advanced)

IV: ADULTS, ELDERLY: 800 mg once q2wks. (in combination with axitinib) until disease progression or unacceptable toxicity.

Merkel Cell Carcinoma

IV: ADULTS, ELDERLY, ADOLESCENTS: 800 mg once q2wks. Continue until disease progression or unacceptable toxicity.

Dose Modification

Based on Common Terminology Criteria for Adverse Events (CTCAE).

Infusion-Related Reactions

Grade 1 or 2: Interrupt or decrease rate of infusion. **Grade 3 or 4:** Permanently discontinue.

Endocrine Toxicity

Grade 3 or 4 endocrinopathies: Withhold treatment until resolved to Grade 1 or 0, then resume therapy after corticosteroid taper. Consider hormone replacement therapy if hypothyroidism occurs.

Colitis (Treatment-Induced)

Grade 2 or 3 diarrhea or colitis: Withhold treatment until resolved to Grade 1 or 0, then resume therapy after corticosteroid taper. **Grade 4 diarrhea or colitis; recurrent Grade 3 diarrhea or colitis:** Permanently discontinue.

Hepatic Toxicity

Serum ALT/AST greater than 3 and up to 5 times upper limit normal (ULN) or serum bilirubin greater than 1.5 and up to 3 times ULN): Withhold treatment until resolved to Grade 1 or 0, then resume therapy. **Serum ALT/AST greater than 5 times upper limit normal (ULN) or serum bilirubin greater than 3 times ULN):** Permanently discontinue.

Renal Toxicity

Serum creatinine greater than 1.5 and up to 6 times ULN: Withhold treatment until resolved to Grade 1 or 0, then resume therapy after corticosteroid taper. **Serum creatinine greater than 6 times ULN:** Permanently discontinue.

Other Moderate or Severe Treatment-Induced Reactions

Arthritis, bullous dermatitis, encephalitis, erythema multiform, exfoliative dermatitis, demyelination, Guillain-

Barré syndrome, hemolytic anemia, histiocytic necrotizing lymphadenitis, hypophysitis, hypopituitarism, iritis, myasthenia gravis, myocarditis, myositis, pancreatitis, pemphigoid, psoriasis, Stevens Johnson Syndrome/toxic epidermal necrolysis, rhabdomyolysis, uveitis, vasculitis: Withhold treatment until resolved to Grade 1 or 0, then resume therapy after corticosteroid taper. **Life-threatening adverse effects, recurrent severe immune-mediated reactions; requirement of predniSONE 10 mg/day or greater (or equivalent) for more than 2 wks; persistent Grade 2 or 3 immune-mediated reaction lasting 12 wks or longer:** Permanently discontinue.

Pulmonary Toxicity
Grade 2 pneumonitis: Withhold treatment until resolved to Grade 1 or 0, then resume therapy after corticosteroid taper. **Grade 3 or 4 or recurrent Grade 2 pneumonitis:** Permanently discontinue.

Dosage in Renal/Hepatic Impairment
Not specified; use caution.

SIDE EFFECTS

Note: Percentage of side effects may vary depending on indication of treatment.
Frequent (50%–18%): Fatigue, musculoskeletal pain, diarrhea, rash, infusion reactions (back pain, chills, pyrexia, hypotension), nausea, decreased appetite, peripheral edema, cough. **Occasional (17%–10%):** Constipation, arthralgia, abdominal pain, decreased weight, dizziness, vomiting, hypertension, dyspnea, pruritus, headache.

ADVERSE EFFECTS/TOXIC REACTIONS

Anemia, neutropenia, thrombocytopenia is an expected response to therapy. May cause severe, sometimes fatal cases of immune-mediated reactions such as pneumonitis (1% of pts), hepatitis (1% of pts), colitis (2% of pts), adrenal insufficiency (1% of pts), hypothyroidism, hyperthyroidism (6% of pts), type 1 diabetes mellitus including ketoacidosis (less than 1% of pts), nephritis (less than 1% of pts), other immune-mediated effects (less than 1%). Cellulitis, CVA, dyspnea, ileus, pericardial effusion, small bowel/intestinal obstruction, renal failure, respiratory failure, septic shock, transaminitis, urosepsis may occur.

NURSING CONSIDERATIONS

BASELINE ASSESSMENT
Obtain ANC, CBC, BMP (esp. serum creatinine, creatinine clearance; BUN), TSH, vital signs; pregnancy test in females of reproductive potential. Question history of prior hypersensitivity reaction, infusion-related reactions, allergy to corticosteroids/prednisone. Screen for history of autoimmune disorders, diabetes, pituitary/pulmonary/thyroid disease, renal insufficiency. Obtain nutrition consult. Offer emotional support.

INTERVENTION/EVALUATION
Monitor ANC, CBC, BMP, creatinine clearance, thyroid panel (if applicable); vital signs. Diligently monitor for infusion-related reactions, treatment-related toxicities, esp. during initial infusions. If immune-mediated reactions occur, consider referral to specialist; pt may require treatment with corticosteroids. Screen for allergic reactions, acute infections (cellulitis, sepsis, UTI), hepatitis, pulmonary events (dyspnea, pneumonitis, pneumonia). Monitor strict I&O, hydration status, stool frequency and consistency. Encourage proper calorie intake and nutrition. Assess skin for rash, lesions, dermal toxicities.

PATIENT/FAMILY TEACHING
• Treatment may depress your immune system and reduce your ability to fight infection. Report symptoms of infection such as body aches, burning with urination, chills, cough, fatigue, fever. Avoid those with active infection. • Use effective contraception to avoid pregnancy. Do

 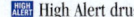

not breastfeed. • Serious adverse reactions may affect lungs, liver, intestines, kidneys, hormonal glands, nervous system, which may require anti-inflammatory medication. • Immediately report any serious or life-threatening inflammatory symptoms in the following body systems: colon (severe abdominal pain/swelling, diarrhea); kidneys (decreased or dark-colored urine, flank pain); lung (chest pain, severe cough, shortness of breath); liver (bruising, dark-colored urine, clay-colored/tarry stools, nausea, yellowing of the skin or eyes); nervous system (paralysis, weakness); pituitary (persistent or unusual headaches, dizziness, extreme weakness, fainting, vision changes); skin (blisters, bubbling, inflammation, rash); thyroid (trouble sleeping, high blood pressure, fast heart rate [overactive thyroid]; fatigue, goiter, weight gain [underactive thyroid]); vascular (low blood pressure, vein/artery pain or irritation). • Do not take any over-the-counter anti-inflammatory medications unless approved by your doctor.

axitinib

ax-**i**-ti-nib
(Inlyta)
Do not confuse axitinib with afatinib, ibrutinib, or imatinib.

◆CLASSIFICATION

PHARMACOTHERAPEUTIC: Vascular endothelial growth factor (VEGF) inhibitor. Tyrosine kinase inhibitor. **CLINICAL:** Antineoplastic.

USES

Renal cell carcinoma (RCC): Indicated in combination with avelumab or pembrolizumab for first-line treatment of pts with advanced RCC. Second-line treatment of advanced RCC as a single agent after failure of one prior systemic therapy. **OFF-LABEL:** Thyroid cancer (differentiated, advanced).

PRECAUTIONS

Contraindications: Hypersensitivity to axitinib. **Cautions:** Pts with increased risk or history of thrombotic events (CVA, MI), GI perforation or fistula formation, renal/hepatic impairment, hypertension, HF. Do not use in pts with untreated brain metastasis or recent active GI bleeding.

ACTION

Inhibits vascular endothelial growth factor receptors. **Therapeutic Effect:** Blocks tumor growth and angiogenesis.

PHARMACOKINETICS

Widely distributed. Metabolized in liver. Protein binding: greater than 99%. Excreted primarily in feces with a lesser amount excreted in urine. **Half-life:** 2.5–6 hrs.

⌛ LIFESPAN CONSIDERATIONS

Pregnancy/Lactation: Avoid pregnancy; may cause fetal harm. Unknown whether distributed in breast milk. **Children:** Safety and efficacy not established. **Elderly:** No age-related precautions noted.

INTERACTIONS

DRUG: **Strong CYP3A4 inhibitors (e.g., erythromycin, ketoconazole, ritonavir)** may significantly increase concentration; do not use concurrently. If used, reduce dose by 50%. Coadministration with **strong CYP3A4 inducers (e.g., carbamazepine, phenytoin, rifampin)** may significantly decrease concentration/effect, do not use concurrently. **HERBAL:** **St. John's wort** may decrease concentration/effect. **FOOD:** **Grapefruit products** may increase concentration/effect. **LAB VALUES:** May decrease Hgb, WBC count, platelets, lymphocytes; serum calcium, alkaline phosphatase, albumin, sodium, phosphate, bicarbonate. May increase serum ALT, AST, bilirubin, BUN, creatinine, serum potassium, lipase, amylase; urine protein. May alter serum glucose.

AVAILABILITY (Rx)

Tablets: 1 mg, 5 mg.

ADMINISTRATION/HANDLING

PO
• Give without regard to food. • Swallow tablets whole with full glass of water.

INDICATIONS/ROUTES/DOSAGE

Renal Cell Carcinoma (Advanced, Second-Line, Single-Agent Therapy)
PO: ADULTS, ELDERLY: Initially, 5 mg twice daily, given approximately 12 hrs apart. If tolerated (for at least 2 consecutive wks with no adverse events above Grade 2, B/P normal, and are not receiving antihypertensive medication), may increase to 7 mg twice daily, then 10 mg twice daily (if BP normal and no antihypertensive use). For adverse effects, may decrease to 3 mg twice daily, then 2 mg twice daily if adverse effects persist.

Renal Cell Carcinoma (Advanced, First-Line Combination Therapy)
With avelumab: Initially, 5 mg q12h. If tolerated for 2 wks or longer, may increase to 7 mg q12h, then 10 mg q12h, or reduce to 3 mg and then 2 mg q12h. *With pembrolizumab:* Initially, 5 mg q12h. If tolerated for 6 wks or longer, may increase to 7 mg q12h, then 10 mg q12h, or reduce to 3 mg and then 2 mg q12h. Continue until disease progression or unacceptable toxicity.

Dose Modification
Dosage with concomitant strong CYP3A4 inhibitors: Reduce dose by 50%. (Avoid concomitant use if possible.)

Dosage in Renal Impairment
Mild to moderate impairment: No dose adjustment. **Severe impairment, ESRD:** Use caution.

Dosage in Hepatic Impairment
Mild impairment: No dose adjustment. **Moderate impairment:** Reduce initial dose by 50%. **Severe impairment:** Not recommended.

SIDE EFFECTS

Frequent (55%–20%): Diarrhea, hypertension, fatigue, decreased appetite, nausea, dysphonia, palmar-plantar erythrodysesthesia (hand-foot) syndrome, weight loss, vomiting, asthenia, constipation. **Occasional (19%–11%):** Hypothyroidism, cough, stomatitis, arthralgia, dyspnea, abdominal pain, headache, peripheral pain, rash, proteinuria, dysgeusia. **Rare (10%–2%):** Dry skin, dyspepsia, dizziness, myalgia, pruritus, epistaxis, alopecia, hemorrhoids, tinnitus, erythema.

ADVERSE EFFECTS/TOXIC REACTIONS

Arterial and venous thrombotic events (MI, CVA), GI perforation, fistula, hemorrhagic events (including cerebral hemorrhage, hematuria, hemoptysis, GI bleeding), hypertensive crisis, cardiac failure have been observed and can be fatal. Hypothyroidism requiring thyroid hormone replacement has been noted. Reversible posterior leukoencephalopathy syndrome (RPLS) has been observed.

NURSING CONSIDERATIONS

BASELINE ASSESSMENT

Obtain BMP, LFT, renal function test, urine protein, serum amylase, lipase, phosphate before initiation of, and periodically throughout, treatment. Offer emotional support. Assess medical history, esp. hepatic function abnormalities. B/P should be well controlled prior to initiating treatment. Stop medication at least 24 hrs prior to scheduled surgery. Monitor thyroid function before and periodically throughout treatment.

INTERVENTION/EVALUATION

Monitor CBC, BMP, LFT, renal function test, urine protein, serum amylase, lipase, phosphate, thyroid tests. Monitor daily pattern of bowel activity, stool consistency. Assess for evidence of bleeding or hemorrhage. Assess for hypertension. For persistent hypertension despite use of antihy-

 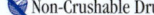

pertensive medications, dose should be reduced. Permanently discontinue if signs or symptoms of RPLS occur (extreme lethargy, increased B/P from pt baseline, pyuria). Contact physician if changes in voice, redness of skin, or rash is noted.

PATIENT/FAMILY TEACHING

• Avoid crowds, those with known infection. • Avoid contact with anyone who recently received live virus vaccine; do not receive vaccinations. • Swallow tablet whole; do not chew, crush, dissolve, or divide. • Avoid grapefruit products. • Report persistent diarrhea, extreme fatigue, abdominal pain, yellowing of skin or eyes, bruising easily; bleeding of any kind, esp. bloody stool or urine; confusion, seizure activity, vision loss, trouble speaking, chest pain; difficulty breathing, leg pain or swelling.

---

azacitidine

ay-za-**sye**-ti-deen
(Onureg, Vidaza)
Do not confuse azacitidine with azathioprine, decitabine, or tizanidine.

◆CLASSIFICATION

PHARMACOTHERAPEUTIC: Antimetabolite, DNA methylation agent.
CLINICAL: Antineoplastic.

USES

Myelodysplastic syndromes (MDSs): Treatment of adults with the following FAB MDS subtypes: Refractory anemia or refractory anemia with ringed sideroblasts (if accompanied by neutropenia or thrombocytopenia or requiring transfusion); refractory anemia with excess blasts; refractory anemia with excess blasts in transformation; chronic myelomonocytic leukemia. **Juvenile myelomonocytic leukemia (JMML):** Treatment of children aged 1 mo and older with newly diagnosed JMML. **Acute myeloid leukemia (AML):** Continued treatment of adults with AML who achieved first complete remission or complete remission with incomplete blood count recovery following intensive induction chemotherapy and are not able to complete intensive curative therapy. **OFF-LABEL:** AML, low intensity therapy.

PRECAUTIONS

Contraindications: Hypersensitivity to azacitidine, mannitol (injection only). Advanced malignant hepatic tumors (injection only). **Cautions:** Baseline cytopenias, conditions predisposing to infection (e.g., diabetes, renal failure, immunocompromised pts, open wounds), hepatic/renal impairment, pts at high risk for tumor lysis syndrome (high tumor burden). Concomitant use of live vaccines is not recommended.

ACTION

Low doses: inhibits DNA methyltransferase, causing hypomethylation of DNA. High doses: direct cytotoxicity to abnormal hematopoietic cells in marrow. **Therapeutic Effect:** Cell death, prevents DNA synthesis, causes cytotoxicity.

PHARMACOKINETICS

Widely distributed. Metabolized hepatic: via hydrolysis and deamination. Protein binding: 6%–12% (oral). Excreted in (IV, SQ) urine (85%), feces (less than 1%); (oral): Urine (less than 2% as unchanged drug). **Half-life:** (IV, SQ): 4 hrs (Oral): 0.5 hrs.

⧗ LIFESPAN CONSIDERATIONS

Pregnancy/Lactation: Avoid pregnancy; may cause fetal harm. Females of reproductive potential must use effective contraception during treatment and for at least 6 mos after discontinuation. Unknown if distributed in breast milk. Breastfeeding not recommended during treatment and for at least 1 wk after discontinuation. May impair fertility. **Males:** Males with female partners of reproductive potential must use effective contraception during treatment and for at least 3 mos after discontinuation. May impair fertility. **Children:** Safety and efficacy not established in pts younger than 1 mo. **Elderly:** May have increased risk of renal toxicity.

INTERACTIONS

DRUG: May increase concentration/effects of **BCG (intravesical), vaccines (live), natalizumab, tacrolimus (topical), tofacitinib.** May decrease concentration/therapeutic effects of **vaccines (live). HERBAL: Echinacea** may decrease therapeutic effect. **FOOD:** None known. **LAB VALUES:** May increase serum alkaline phosphatase, ALT, AST, creatinine. May decrease Hgb, leukocytes, neutrophils, platelets, RBC.

AVAILABILITY (Rx)

Injection, Powder for Reconstitution: 100 mg. **Tablets:** 200 mg, 300 mg.

ADMINISTRATION/HANDLING

◄**ALERT**► Must be prepared by personnel trained in aseptic manipulations and admixing of cytotoxic drugs.

 IV

Reconstitution • Reconstitute each vial with 10 mL Sterile Water for Injection (SWI) to a final concentration of 10 mg/mL. • Vigorously shake vial until contents are fully dissolved. • Visually inspect for particulate matter or discoloration. Solution should appear clear. Do not use if solution is cloudy or discolored.
Adults with MDS • Dilute in a 50–100 mL infusion bag of 0.9% NaCl.
Children With JMML • Dilute in an infusion bag (up to 100 mL) of 0.9% NaCl to a final concentration of 0.9–4 mg/mL.
Rate of administration • Infuse over 10–40 min (must be infused within 1 hr of reconstitution). **Storage •** Store unused vial at room temperature.

SQ

Reconstitution • Reconstitute each vial with 4 mL SWI to a final concentration of 25 mg/mL. • Vigorously shake vial until contents are fully dissolved.

Solution will appear cloudy. Do not filter solution prior to administration. • Use within 1 hr of reconstitution. **Administration •** Doses requiring more than 1 vial should be divided equally into 2 syringes and injected into 2 different sites. • Immediately before administration, contents must be resuspended by inverting the syringe(s) two to three times and rolling the syringe(s) between the palms for 30 sec. • Insert needle subcutaneously into outer thigh, abdomen, or upper arm and inject solution. • Do not inject into areas of active skin disease or injury such as sunburns, skin rashes, inflammation, skin infections, or psoriatic lesions. • Rotate injection sites at least 1 inch away from prior site. • Do not administer IV or intramuscularly.
Storage • When diluted with room-temperature SWI, refrigerate solution up to 8 hrs or store at room temperature for up to 1 hr. When diluted with cold SWI, refrigerate solution for up to 22 hrs. • If refrigerated, allow solution to warm to room temperature for up to 30 mins prior to administration.

PO

• Give without regard to food at the time same each day. • For the first two treatment cycles, give an antiemetic 30 min prior to each dose. Antiemetic prophylaxis may be discontinued after two cycles if nausea or vomiting do not occur. • Administer tablet whole; do not break, cut, or crush. • Tablet cannot be chewed. • If a dose is missed, give as soon as possible that day. Do not double the next dose.

INDICATIONS/ROUTES/DOSAGE

Myelodysplastic Syndrome
◄**ALERT**► Dose adjustment is based on hematologic values. Do not substitute IV form of azacitidine with PO form.
IV, SQ: ADULTS, ELDERLY: 75 mg/m²/day for 7 days repeated q4wks. May increase to 100 mg/m² after two cycles if no benefit is observed and if no toxicities other

than nausea or vomiting have occurred. **Treatment Duration:** Minimum of at least four to six cycles. Additional treatment cycles may be required in pts with complete or partial response. May continue course if pt benefits from further treatment.

Dose Modification
Hematological Laboratory Values
Adults with baseline absolute neutrophil count (ANC) 1,500 cells/mm^3 or greater, platelet count 75,000 cells/mm^3 or greater, and WBC 3,000 cells/mm^3 or greater:

Nadir Count		
Absolute Neutrophil Count	**Platelet Count**	**% Dose in the Next Course**
Less than 500 cells/mm^3:	Less than 25,000 cells/mm^3:	50%
500–1,500 cells/mm^3:	25,000–50,000 cells/mm^3:	67%
Greater than 1,500 cells/mm^3:	Greater than 50,000 cells/mm^3:	100%

Adults with baseline ANC less than 1,500 cells/mm^3, platelet count less than 75,000 cells/mm^3, or WBC less than 3,000 cells/mm^3. Base dose adjustments on nadir counts and bone marrow biopsy cellularity at the time of the nadir as noted below (unless a clear improvement in differentiation is noted at next cycle):

WBC or Platelet Nadir% Decrease in Count (from baseline)	Bone Marrow Biopsy Cellularity at Time of Nadir (%)		
	30–60	15–30	Less than 15
	% Dose in the Next Course		
50–75:	100	50	33
Greater than 75:	75	50	33

If a nadir has occurred, give next course 28 days after the start of preceding course if WBC and platelet count are 25% above

nadir and increasing. If an increase greater than 25% does not occur by day 28, assess count q7days. If a 25% increase does not occur by day 42, reduce dose by 50%.

Renal Toxicity
Decrease in serum bicarbonate level to less than 20 mEq/L: Reduce dose by 50% for the next course. **BUN or serum creatinine elevation:** Delay the next cycle until resolved or improves to baseline, then reduce dose by 50% for the next course.

Acute Myeloid Leukemia (AML)
PO: ADULTS, ELDERLY: 300 mg once daily on days 1–14 of each 28-day cycle. Continue until disease progression or unacceptable toxicity.

Dose Modification
Based on Common Terminology Criteria for Adverse Events (CTCAE).

Gastrointestinal Toxicity, Other Toxic Reactions
Grade 3 or 4 nausea, vomiting, or diarrhea; other toxic reactions: Withhold treatment until improved to Grade 1 or 0, then resume at same dose. If toxicity recurs, withhold treatment until improved to Grade 1 or 0, then reduce dose to 200 mg. If toxicity persists after dose reduction, reduce treatment duration by 7 days. Permanently discontinue if toxicity continues or recurs after dose and schedule reduction.

Neutropenia
Neutrophil count less than 500 cells/mm^3: Withhold treatment until improved to 500 cells/mm^3 or greater, then resume at same dose. **Neutrophil count less than 1,000 cells/mm^3 with fever:** (first occurrence): Withhold treatment until improved to 1,000 cells/mm^3 or greater, then resume at same dose. **(Occurrence in two consecutive cycles):** Withhold treatment until improved to 1,000 cells/mm^3 or greater, then reduce dose to 200 mg. If febrile neutropenia persists after dose reduction, reduce treatment duration by 7 days. Permanently discontinue if

febrile neutropenia recurs after dose and schedule reduction.

Thrombocytopenia

Platelet count less than 50,000 cells/mm³ with bleeding: (First occurrence): Withhold treatment until improved to 50,000 cells/mm³ or greater, then resume at same dose. **(Occurrence in two consecutive cycles):** Withhold treatment until improved to 50,000 cells/mm³ or greater, then reduce dose to 200 mg. If thrombocytopenia with bleeding persists after dose reduction, reduce treatment duration by 7 days. Permanently discontinue if thrombocytopenia with bleeding recurs after dose and schedule reduction.

Juvenile Myelomonocytic Leukemia

Note: Continue treatment up to six cycles if benefit is shown. May consider delaying dose up to 14 days for nonhematologic toxicities. Dose modifications are not recommended for hematological toxicities within the first three cycles. Discontinue treatment if neutrophil count is less 500 cells/mm³ at end of cycle 3 or on day 1 of cycles 5 or 6.
IV: CHILDREN 1 MO TO LESS THAN 1 YR OR WEIGHING LESS THAN 10 KG: 2.5 mg/kg/day for 7 days (in a 28-day cycle) for a minimum of three cycles up to six cycles. **CHILDREN 1 YR AND OLDER AND WEIGHING 10 KG OR GREATER:** 75 mg/m²/day for 7 days (in a 28-day cycle) for a minimum of three cycles up to six cycles.

Dosage in Renal Impairment

No dose adjustment.

Dosage in Hepatic Impairment

IV: No dose adjustment. **PO: Mild impairment:** No dose adjustment. **Moderate to severe impairment:** Not specified; use caution.

SIDE EFFECTS

Note: Frequency and occurrence of side effects may vary based on indicated treatment or drug form.
Frequent (71%–21%): Nausea, vomiting, pyrexia, injection site reactions, constipation, diarrhea, ecchymosis, dyspnea, petechiae, arthralgia, headache, decreased appetite. **Occasional (16%–6%):** Chest pain, myalgia, rash, dizziness, anxiety, abdominal pain, malaise, insomnia, gingival bleeding, hematoma, stomatitis, lethargy, hypotension, anxiety, urticaria. **Rare (5%):** Mouth hemorrhage, dry skin, skin nodule.

ADVERSE EFFECTS/TOXIC REACTIONS

Myelosuppression (anemia, leukopenia, neutropenia, thrombocytopenia) is an expected response to therapy, but more severe reactions including bone marrow depression, febrile neutropenia may be life-threatening. May cause hepatotoxicity in pts with baseline hepatic impairment. Renal toxicities including elevated serum creatinine, renal tubular acidosis, fatal renal failure were reported in pts receiving IV azacitidine. Tumor lysis syndrome may present as acute renal failure, hypocalcemia, hyperuricemia, hyperphosphatemia. Infections including nasopharyngitis, pneumonia, upper respiratory tract infection reported in up to 15% of pts. Other reactions including acute febrile neutrophilic dermatosis, aggravated bone pain, agranulocytosis, anaphylaxis, atrial fibrillation, cardiac failure, cardiorespiratory arrest, catheter site hemorrhage, cerebral hemorrhage, cholecystitis, congestive myopathy, convulsions, dehydration, diverticulitis, eye hemorrhage, general health deterioration, GI bleeding, hemoptysis, interstitial lung disease/pneumonitis, leukemia cutis, loin pain, muscle weakness, necrotizing fasciitis, orthostatic hypotension, pyoderma gangrenosum, splenomegaly, systemic inflammatory response syndrome were reported.

NURSING CONSIDERATIONS

BASELINE ASSESSMENT

Obtain CBC, BMP, LFT, pregnancy test in females of reproductive potential. Confirm compliance of effective contraception. Question history of hepatic/renal impairment. Screen for active infection

---

 Canadian trade name   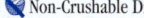 Non-Crushable Drug   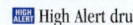 High Alert drug

Due to increased risk of tumor lysis syndrome, assess hydration status prior to each treatment. Offer emotional support.

INTERVENTION/EVALUATION

Obtain CBC, BMP (esp. renal function), LFT prior to each cycle and as clinically indicated. Obtain serum electrolytes, uric acid level if tumor lysis syndrome (acute renal failure, electrolyte imbalance, cardiac arrhythmias, seizures) is suspected. Diligently monitor for infections (cough, fatigue, fever). If serious infection occurs, initiate appropriate antimicrobial therapy. Monitor for myelosuppression (bleeding, bruising, dyspnea, fever, petechiae, weakness), hepatotoxicity (bruising, jaundice, right upper abdominal pain, nausea, vomiting, weight loss). Consider ABG, radiologic test if pneumonitis (excessive cough, dyspnea, fever, hypoxia) is suspected. Consider treatment with corticosteroids if pneumonitis is confirmed. Conduct routine head-to-toe assessments to evaluate for general health deterioration. Monitor daily pattern of bowel activity, stool consistency.

PATIENT/FAMILY TEACHING

• Treatment may depress your immune system response and reduce your ability to fight infection. Report symptoms of infection such as body aches, chills, cough, fatigue, fever. Avoid those with active infection. • Report symptoms of bone marrow depression such as bruising, fatigue, fever, shortness of breath, weight loss; bleeding easily, bloody urine or stool. • Report liver problems (abdominal pain, bruising, clay-colored stool, amber or dark-colored urine, yellowing of the skin or eyes), inflammation of the lung (excessive cough, difficulty breathing, chest pain), bleeding of any kind. • Therapy may cause tumor lysis syndrome (a condition caused by the rapid breakdown of cancer cells), which can cause kidney failure and can be fatal. Report decreased urination, amber-colored urine; confusion, difficulty breathing, fatigue, fever, muscle or joint pain, palpitations, seizures, vomiting. • Severe diarrhea or vomiting may cause dehydration, electrolyte imbalance. Report diarrhea or vomiting that does not improve with medical management. Drink plenty of fluids. • Use effective contraception to avoid pregnancy. Do not breastfeed.

azithromycin

a-**zith**-roe-**mye**-sin
(AzaSite, Zithromax)
Do not confuse azithromycin with azaTHIOprine or erythromycin, or Zithromax with Fosamax or Zovirax.

◆**CLASSIFICATION**

PHARMACOTHERAPEUTIC: Macrolide.
CLINICAL: Antibiotic.

USES

Acute bacterial exacerbations of chronic bronchitis, acute bacterial sinusitis due to *H. influenzae, M. catarrhalis,* or *S. pneumoniae.* **Community-acquired pneumonia** due to *C. pneumoniae, H. influenzae, M. pneumoniae,* or *S. pneumoniae.* **Pharyngitis/tonsillitis** caused by *S. pyogenes* as an alternative to first-line therapy. **Uncomplicated skin and skin structure infections** due to *S. aureus, S. pyogenes, S. agalactiae.* **Urethritis and cervicitis** due to *C. trachomatis* or *N. gonorrhoeae.* **Genital ulcer disease in males** due to *H. ducreyi* (chancroid). **Acute otitis media** caused by *H. influenzae, M. catarrhalis, S. pneumoniae.* **OFF-LABEL:** Prophylaxis of endocarditis. Prevention of pulmonary exacerbations in pts with cystic fibrosis. Infectious diarrhea, Lyme disease, pertussis, surgical prophylaxis (uterine evacuation). **Ophthalmic:** Treatment of bacterial conjunctivitis caused by susceptible infections due to *H. influenzae, S. aureus, S. mitis, S. pneumoniae.*

PRECAUTIONS

Contraindications: Hypersensitivity to azithromycin, erythromycin, or other macrolide antibiotics. History of cholestatic jaundice/hepatic impairment associated with prior azithromycin therapy. **Cautions:** Hepatic/renal impairment, myasthenia gravis, hepatocellular and/or cholestatic hepatitis (with or without jaundice), hepatic necrosis. May prolong QT interval.

ACTION

Binds to ribosomal receptor sites of susceptible organisms, inhibiting RNA-dependent protein synthesis. **Therapeutic Effect:** Bacteriostatic or bactericidal, depending on drug dosage.

PHARMACOKINETICS

Widely distributed. Protein binding: 7%–50%. Metabolized in liver. Excreted primarily by biliary excretion. **Half-life:** 68 hrs.

LIFESPAN CONSIDERATIONS

Pregnancy/Lactation: Unknown if distributed in breast milk. **Children:** Safety and efficacy not established in pts younger than 16 yrs for IV use and younger than 6 mos for oral use. **Elderly:** No age-related precautions in those with normal renal function.

INTERACTIONS

DRUG: QT interval–prolonging medications (e.g., **amiodarone, certinib, haloperidol, moxifloxacin**) may increase risk of QT interval prolongation, cardiac arrhythmias. May increase concentration/effect of **colchicine, cycloSPORINE, dabigatran, edoxaban, pazopanib, topotecan, HERBAL:** None significant. **FOOD:** None known. **LAB VALUES:** May increase serum creatine phosphokinase (CPK), ALT, AST, bilirubin, LDH, potassium.

AVAILABILITY (Rx)

Injection, Powder for Reconstitution: 500 mg. **Ophthalmic Solution:** 1%. **Oral Packet:** 1g. **Oral Suspension:** 100 mg/5 mL, 200 mg/5 mL. **Tablets:** 250 mg, 500 mg, 600 mg.

ADMINISTRATION/HANDLING

IV

Reconstitution • Reconstitute each 500-mg vial with 4.8 mL Sterile Water for Injection to provide concentration of 100 mg/mL. • Shake well to ensure dissolution. • Further dilute with 250 or 500 mL 0.9% NaCl or D₅W to provide final concentration of 2 mg/mL with 250 mL diluent or 1 mg/mL with 500 mL diluent.

Rate of administration • Infuse over 60 min (2 mg/mL). Infuse over 3 hrs (1 mg/mL).

Storage • Store vials at room temperature. • Following reconstitution, diluted solution is stable for 24 hrs at room temperature or 7 days if refrigerated.

PO

• Give without regard to food. • May store suspension at room temperature. Stable for 10 days after reconstitution.

Ophthalmic

• Place gloved finger on lower eyelid and pull out until a pocket is formed between eye and lower lid. • Place prescribed number of drops into pocket. • Instruct pt to close eye gently for 1 to 2 min (so that medication will not be squeezed out of sac) and to apply digital pressure to lacrimal sac at inner canthus for 1 min to minimize systemic absorption.

IV INCOMPATIBILITIES

Potassium chloride.

IV COMPATIBILITIES

Dexmedetomidine.

INDICATIONS/ROUTES/DOSAGE

Usual Dosage Range

PO: ADULTS, ELDERLY: 500 mg once, then 250 mg daily for 4 days or 500 mg daily for 3 days. **ADOLESCENTS, CHILDREN, INFANTS:** 5–12 mg/kg/dose

(usually 10–12 mg/kg on day 1, then 5–6 mg/kg thereafter). **Usual maximum total course:** 1,500–2,000 mg. **NEONATES:** 10 mg/kg once daily.
IV: ADULTS, ELDERLY: 250–500 mg once daily **ADOLESCENTS, CHILDREN, INFANTS, NEONATES:** 10 mg/kg once daily. **Maximum:** 500 mg/dose.

Bacterial Conjunctivitis
Ophthalmic: ADULTS, ELDERLY: 1 drop in affected eye twice daily for 2 days, then 1 drop once daily for 5 days.

Dosage in Renal/Hepatic Impairment
Use caution.

SIDE EFFECTS

Occasional: Systemic: Nausea, vomiting, diarrhea, abdominal pain. **Ophthalmic:** Eye irritation. **Rare: Systemic:** Headache, dizziness, allergic reaction.

ADVERSE EFFECTS/TOXIC REACTIONS

Antibiotic-associated colitis, other super-infections may result from altered bacterial balance in GI tract. Acute interstitial nephritis, hepatotoxicity occur rarely.

NURSING CONSIDERATIONS

BASELINE ASSESSMENT
Question for history of hepatitis, allergies to azithromycin, erythromycins. Assess for infection (WBC count, appearance of wound, evidence of fever).

INTERVENTION/EVALUATION
Check for GI discomfort, nausea, vomiting. Monitor daily pattern of bowel activity and stool consistency. Monitor LFT, CBC. Assess for hepatotoxicity: malaise, fever, abdominal pain, GI disturbances. Be alert for superinfection: Fever, vomiting, diarrhea, anal/genital pruritus, oral mucosal changes (ulceration, pain, erythema).

PATIENT/FAMILY TEACHING
• Continue therapy for full length of treatment. • Avoid concurrent adminis-

tration of aluminum- or magnesium-containing antacids. • Bacterial conjunctivitis: Do not wear contact lenses.

aztreonam

az-**tree**-o-nam
(Azactam, Cayston)

◆CLASSIFICATION

PHARMACOTHERAPEUTIC: Monobactam. **CLINICAL:** Antibiotic.

USES

Urinary tract infections (complicated and uncomplicated) (including pyelonephritis and cystitis [initial and recurrent]): Caused by *E. coli, K. pneumoniae, P. mirabilis, P. aeruginosa, E. cloacae, K. oxytoca, Citrobacter* species and *S. marcescens.* **Lower respiratory tract infections (including pneumonia and bronchitis):** Caused by *E. coli, K. pneumoniae, P. aeruginosa, H. influenzae, P. mirabilis, Enterobacter* species, and *S. marcescens.* Septicemia caused by *E. coli, K. pneumoniae, P. aeruginosa, P. mirabilis, S. marcescens* and *Enterobacter* species. **Skin and skin-structure infections (including those associated with postoperative wounds, ulcers, and burns):** Caused by *E. coli, P. mirabilis, S. marcescens, Enterobacter* species, *P. aeruginosa, K. pneumoniae,* and *Citrobacter* species. **Intra-abdominal infections (including peritonitis):** Caused by *E. coli, Klebsiella* species including *K. pneumoniae, Enterobacter* species including *E. cloacae, P. aeruginosa, Citrobacter* species including *C. freundii,* and *Serratia* species including *S. marcescens.* **Gynecologic infections (including endometritis and pelvic cellulitis):** Caused by *E. coli, K. pneumoniae, Enterobacter* species including *E. cloacae,* and *P. mirabilis.* **Oral inhalation: (Cayston):** Improve respiratory symptoms in cystic fibrosis pts with

P. aeruginosa. **OFF-LABEL:** Surgical prophylaxis. Bacterial meningitis, osteomyelitis.

PRECAUTIONS

Contraindications: Hypersensitivity to aztreonam. **Cautions:** History of allergy, esp. cephalosporins, penicillins; renal impairment; bone marrow transplant pts with risk factors for toxic epidermal necrolysis (TEN).

ACTION

Binds to penicillin-binding proteins, which inhibits bacterial cell wall synthesis. **Therapeutic Effect:** Bactericidal.

PHARMACOKINETICS

Widely distributed. Protein binding: 56%–60%. Partially metabolized by hydrolysis. Primarily excreted in urine. Removed by hemodialysis. **Half-life:** 1.4–2.2 hrs (increased in renal/hepatic impairment).

⧗ LIFESPAN CONSIDERATIONS

Pregnancy/Lactation: Crosses placenta, distributed in amniotic fluid; low concentration in breast milk. **Children:** Safety and efficacy not established in pts younger than 9 mos. **Elderly:** Age-related renal impairment may require dosage adjustment.

INTERACTIONS

DRUG: None significant. **HERBAL:** None significant. **FOOD:** None known. **LAB VALUES:** May increase serum alkaline phosphatase, creatinine, LDH, ALT, AST levels. Produces a positive Coombs' test. May prolong partial thromboplastin time (PTT), prothrombin time (PT).

AVAILABILITY (Rx)

Injection, Powder for Reconstitution: *(Azactam):* 1 g, 2 g. **Oral Inhalation, Powder for Reconstitution:** *(Cayston):* 75 mg.

ADMINISTRATION/HANDLING

 IV

Reconstitution • For IV push, dilute each gram with 6–10 mL Sterile Water for Injection. • For intermittent IV infusion, further dilute with 50–100 mL D₅W or 0.9% NaCl. Final concentration not to exceed 20 mg/mL.

Rate of administration • For IV push, give over 3–5 min. • For IV infusion, administer over 20–60 min.

Storage • Store vials at room temperature. • Solution appears colorless to light yellow. • Following reconstitution, solution is stable for 48 hrs at room temperature or 7 days if refrigerated. • Discard if precipitate forms. Discard unused portions.

IM

• Reconstitute with at least 3 mL diluent per gram of aztreonam. • Shake immediately, vigorously after adding diluent. • Inject deeply into large muscle mass. • Following reconstitution, solution is stable for 48 hrs at room temperature or 7 days if refrigerated.

Inhalation

• Administer only with an Altera nebulizer system. • Nebulize over 2–3 min. • Give bronchodilator 15 min–4 hrs (short-acting) or 30 min–12 hrs (long-acting) before administration. • Reconstituted solution must be used immediately.

⊞ IV COMPATIBILITIES

Calcium gluconate, dexmedetomidine, heparin, insulin, magnesium sulfate, potassium chloride, propofol.

INDICATIONS/ROUTES/DOSAGE

Note: Doses greater than 1 gram should be given IV.

Usual Dosage

IM/IV: ADULTS, ELDERLY: 1–2 g q6–12h. **CHILDREN:** 90–120 mg/kg/day in divided doses q6–8h. **NEONATES:** 30 mg/kg/dose q6–12h.

Cystic Fibrosis

Note: Pretreatment with a bronchodilator is recommended.

Inhalation (nebulizer): ADULTS, CHILDREN 7 YRS OR OLDER: 75 mg 3 times/day (at least 4 hrs apart) for 28 days, followed by 28 days off therapy.

Dosage in Renal Impairment

Dosage and frequency are modified based on creatinine clearance and severity of infection:

Creatinine Clearance	Dosage
10–30 mL/min	50% usual dose at usual intervals
Less than 10 mL/min	25% usual dose at usual intervals
Hemodialysis	500 mg–2 g, then 25% of initial dose at usual interval
Continuous renal replacement therapy (CRRT)	2 g, then 1 g q8–12h or 2g q12h

Dosage in Hepatic Impairment

Use with caution.

SIDE EFFECTS

Frequent (greater than 5%): Cayston: Cough, nasal congestion, wheezing, pharyngolaryngeal pain, pyrexia, chest discomfort, abdominal pain, vomiting. **Occasional (less than 3%):** Discomfort and swelling at IM injection site, nausea, vomiting, diarrhea, rash. **Rare (less than 1%):** Phlebitis or thrombophlebitis at IV injection site, abdominal cramps, headache, hypotension.

ADVERSE EFFECTS/TOXIC REACTIONS

Antibiotic-associated colitis, other superinfections may result from altered bacterial balance in GI tract. Severe hypersensitivity reactions, including anaphylaxis, occur rarely.

NURSING CONSIDERATIONS

BASELINE ASSESSMENT

Question for history of allergies, esp. to aztreonam, other antibiotics.

INTERVENTION/EVALUATION

Evaluate for phlebitis, pain at IM injection site. Assess for GI discomfort, nausea, vomiting. Monitor daily pattern of bowel activity, stool consistency. Assess skin for rash. Be alert for superinfection: fever, vomiting, diarrhea, anal/genital pruritus, oral mucosal changes (ulceration, pain, erythema). Monitor renal/hepatic function.

PATIENT/FAMILY TEACHING

• Report nausea, vomiting, diarrhea, rash.

baclofen

bak-loe-fen
(Fleqsuvy, Gablofen, Lioresal, Lyvispah, Ozobax)

■ BLACK BOX ALERT ■ Abrupt withdrawal of intrathecal form has resulted in severe hyperpyrexia, obtundation, rebound or exaggerated spasticity, muscle rigidity, leading to organ failure, death.
Do not confuse baclofen with Bactroban or Beclovent, or Lioresal with lisinopril or Lotensin.

◆CLASSIFICATION

PHARMACOTHERAPEUTIC: Skeletal muscle relaxant. **CLINICAL:** Antispastic, analgesic in trigeminal neuralgia.

USES

Oral: Treatment of spasticity resulting from multiple sclerosis, particularly for the relief of flexor spasms and concomitant pain, clonus, and muscular rigidity. **Intrathecal:** Management of severe spasticity of spinal cord or cerebral origin in pts 4 yrs of age and older. **OFF-LABEL:** Treatment of intractable hiccups or pain, muscle spasm, and/or musculoskeletal pain.

PRECAUTIONS

Contraindications: Hypersensitivity to baclofen. **Intrathecal:** IV, IM, SQ, or epidural administration in addition to intrathecal use. **Cautions:** Renal impairment, seizure disorder, elderly, autonomic dysreflexia, reduced GI motility, GI or urinary obstruction; respiratory, pulmonary, peptic ulcer disease.

ACTION

Inhibits transmission of monosynaptic or polysynaptic reflexes at spinal cord level possibly by hyperpolarization of primary afferent fiber terminals. **Therapeutic Effect:** Relieves muscle spasticity.

PHARMACOKINETICS

Widely distributed. Protein binding: 30%. Partially metabolized in liver. Primarily excreted in urine. **Half-life:** 2.5–4 hrs.

⌛ LIFESPAN CONSIDERATIONS

Pregnancy/Lactation: Unknown if crosses placenta or distributed in breast milk. **Children:** Safety and efficacy not established in pts younger than 12 yrs. Limited published data in children. **Elderly:** Increased risk of CNS toxicity (hallucinations, sedation, confusion, mental depression); age-related renal impairment may require decreased dosage.

INTERACTIONS

DRUG: CNS depressants (e.g., alcohol, morphine, oxyCODONE, zolpidem) may increase CNS depressant effect. **HERBAL: Herbals with sedative properties (e.g., chamomile, kava kava, valerian)** may increase CNS depression. **FOOD:** None known. **LAB VALUES:** May increase serum ALT, AST, alkaline phosphatase, glucose.

AVAILABILITY (Rx)

Intrathecal Injection Solution: 500 mcg/mL, 1,000 mcg/mL, 2,000 mcg/mL. **Oral packet:** 5 mg, 10 mg, 20 mg. **Oral Solution:** 5 mg/5 mL. **Oral Suspension:** 25 mg/5 mL (5 mg/mL). **Tablets:** 5 mg, 10 mg, 20 mg.

ADMINISTRATION/HANDLING

PO
• Administer without regard to food (give with food to reduce nausea). **Oral Suspension:** Shake well before administration. • Discard unused portion 2 mos after first opening. • A calibrated measuring device is recommended to measure/deliver prescribed dose. **Oral Granules:** Empty entire contents of packet into the mouth. Granules will dissolve in the mouth or can be swallowed. May give with liquids or soft foods. • Contents of each packet can be emptied and mixed with up to 15 mL of liquid or soft food and administered within 2 hrs of mixing. **Oral Solution** • Store refrigerated. A calibrated measuring device is recommended when administering.

Intrathecal

• For screening, a 50 mcg/mL concentration should be used for injection. • For maintenance therapy, solution should be diluted for pts who require concentrations other than 500 mcg/mL or 2,000 mcg/mL.

INDICATIONS/ROUTES/DOSAGE

◄ **ALERT** ► Avoid abrupt withdrawal.

Spasticity

PO: ADULTS, CHILDREN 12 YRS AND OLDER: Initially, 5 mg 1–3 times daily. May increase by 5 mg/dose at 3-day intervals until optimal response achieved. Range: 40–80 mg/day. **Maximum:** 80 mg/day. **ELDERLY:** Initially, 5 mg 2–3 times daily. May gradually increase dosage.

Intrathecal Dose

ADULTS, ELDERLY, CHILDREN 4 YRS AND OLDER: Initially, 50 mcg as screening dose (25 mcg in very small pediatric pts) for 1 dose; observe pt for 4–8 hrs for positive response (decrease in muscle tone and/or frequency and/or severity of spasm). If response is inadequate, give 75 mcg 24h after 1st dose. If response is still inadequate, give 100 mcg 24h after 2nd dose. **Initial pump dose:** Give double screening dose (unless efficacy of bolus maintained greater than 8 hrs, then screening dose). After 24h, dose may be increased/decreased only once q24h until satisfactory response.

Dosage in Renal Impairment

Use caution.

Dosage in Hepatic Impairment

No dose adjustment.

SIDE EFFECTS

Frequent (greater than 10%): Transient drowsiness, asthenia, dizziness, nausea, vomiting. **Occasional (10%–2%):** Headache, paresthesia, constipation, anorexia, hypotension, confusion, nasal congestion. **Rare (less than 1%):** Paradoxical CNS excitement or restlessness, slurred speech, tremor, dry mouth, diarrhea, nocturia, impotence.

ADVERSE EFFECTS/TOXIC REACTIONS

Abrupt discontinuation may produce hallucinations, seizures. Overdose results in blurred vision, seizures, myosis, mydriasis, severe muscle weakness, strabismus, respiratory depression, vomiting.

NURSING CONSIDERATIONS

BASELINE ASSESSMENT

Record onset, type, location, duration of muscular spasm, pain. Check for immobility, stiffness, swelling.

INTERVENTION/EVALUATION

For pts on long-term therapy, BMP, LFT, CBC should be performed periodically. Assess for paradoxical reaction. Observe for drowsiness, dizziness, ataxia. Assist with ambulation at all times. Evaluate for therapeutic response: Decreased intensity of skeletal muscle spasm, pain.

PATIENT/FAMILY TEACHING

• Drowsiness usually decreases with continued therapy. • Avoid tasks that require alertness, motor skills until response to drug is established. • Do not abruptly withdraw medication after long-term therapy (may result in muscle rigidity, rebound spasticity, high fever, altered mental status). • Avoid alcohol, CNS depressants.

baricitinib

bar-i-**sye**-ti-nib
(Olumiant)

■ **BLACK BOX ALERT** ■ Increased risk for developing bacterial, viral, invasive fungal infections including tuberculosis, cryptococcosis, pneumocystosis, that may lead to hospitalization or death. Infections often occurred in combination with immunosuppressants (methotrexate, other disease-modifying antirheumatic drugs). Closely monitor for development of infection. Test for latent tuberculosis prior to treatment and during treatment, regardless of initial result. Treatment of latent TB should be initiated before initiation. Lymphomas, other malignancies were reported. Thromboembolic events including DVT, pulmonary embolism, arterial thrombosis have occurred.

Do not confuse baricitinib with ceritinib, gefitinib, tofacitinib, or sunitinib.

◆CLASSIFICATION

PHARMACOTHERAPEUTIC: Janus-associated kinase inhibitor. **CLINICAL:** Antirheumatic agent. Disease modifying.

USES

Rheumatoid arthritis (RA): Treatment of adults with moderately to severely active rheumatoid arthritis who have had an inadequate response to one or more TNF antagonist therapies. May be used alone or in combination with methotrexate or other nonbiologic disease-modifying antirheumatic drugs (DMARDs). **COVID-19:** Treatment of COVID-19 in hospitalized adults requiring supplemental oxygen, noninvasive or invasive mechanical ventilation, or extracorporeal membrane oxygenation (ECMO). **Alopecia areata:** Treatment of adults with severe alopecia areata.

PRECAUTIONS

Hypersensitivity to baricitinib. **Cautions:** Baseline cytopenias; hepatic/renal impairment, elderly, hypercholesterolemia; history of arterial or venous thromboembolic events (CVA, DVT, MI, PE), pts at risk for thrombosis (immobility, indwelling venous catheter/access device, morbid obesity, underlying atherosclerosis, genetic hypercoagulable conditions); recent travel or residence in TB or mycosis endemic areas; history of chronic opportunistic infections (esp. bacterial, invasive fungal, mycobacterial, protozoal, viral, TB); history of HIV, herpes zoster, hepatitis B or C virus infection; conditions predisposing to infection (e.g., diabetes, renal failure, immunocompro-

mised pts, open wounds), pts at risk for GI perforation (e.g., Crohn's disease, diverticulitis, GI tract malignancies, peptic ulcers, peritoneal malignancies), pts who reside or travel to where TB is endemic. Concomitant use of strong organic anion transporter 2 (OAT3) inhibitors (e.g., probenecid), JAK inhibitors, biologic DMARDs, potent immunosuppressants (e.g., azathioprine or cyclosporine) not recommended.

ACTION

Inhibits JAK enzymes, which are intracellular enzymes involved in stimulating hematopoiesis and immune cell function via a signaling pathway. **Therapeutic Effect:** Reduces inflammation, tenderness, swelling of joints; slows or prevents progressive joint destruction in rheumatoid arthritis (RA).

PHARMACOKINETICS

Widely distributed. Metabolized in liver. Protein binding: 50%. Peak plasma concentration: 1 hr. Excreted in urine (75%), feces (20%). **Half-life:** 12 hrs.

⏳ LIFESPAN CONSIDERATIONS

Pregnancy/Lactation: Unknown if distributed in breast milk. Breastfeeding not recommended. **Children:** Safety and efficacy not established. **Elderly:** Increased risk for serious infections, malignancy.

INTERACTIONS

DRUG: May decrease therapeutic effects of **live vaccines, BCG (intravesical). Immunosuppressants (e.g., azathioprine, cyclosporine)** may increase risk for immunosuppression, infection. May increase adverse/toxic effects of **natalizumab, tacrolimus, tofacitinib, vaccines (live). Probenecid** may increase concentration/effect. **HERBAL:** None significant. **FOOD:** None known. **LAB VALUES:** May increase serum ALT, AST, CPK, cholesterol (HDL, LDL, total), triglycerides; platelets. May decrease ANC, Hgb, absolute lymphocyte count.

AVAILABILITY (Rx)

Tablets: 1 mg, 2 mg, 4 mg.

ADMINISTRATION/HANDLING

PO

• Give without regard to food. • For pts unable to swallow, tablets may be dispersed in 5–10 mL water (tablets may be crushed to facilitate dispersion). Administer immediately.

INDICATIONS/ROUTES/DOSAGE

◄**ALERT**► Rheumatoid Arthritis, Alopecia Areata: Avoid initiation or interrupt treatment in pts with severe, active infection (systemic/localized), absolute lymphocyte count less than 500 cells/mm3, ANC less than 1000 cells/mm3, Hgb less than 8 g/dL. Do not use in combination with biologic DMARDs or with strong immunosuppressants (e.g., azathioprine or cyclosporine). COVID-19: Avoid initiation or interrupt treatment in pts with lymphopenia (ALC less than 200 cells/mm3) or neutropenia (ANC less than 500 cells/mm3).

Rheumatoid Arthritis

PO: ADULTS, ELDERLY: 2 mg once daily.

COVID-19

PO: ADULTS, ELDERLY: 4 mg once daily for 14 days or until hospital discharge, whichever occurs first.

Alopecia Areata

PO: ADULTS, ELDERLY: 2 mg once daily. May increase to 4 mg once daily.

Dose Modification

Anemia

Hgb less than 8 g/dL: Withhold treatment until Hgb is greater than or equal to 8 gm/dL.

Lymphopenia

Absolute lymphocyte count (ALC) less than 500 cells/mm³: Withhold treatment until ALC is greater than or equal to 500 cells/mm³.

Neutropenia

ANC less than 1,000 cells/mm³: Withhold treatment until ANC is greater than or equal to 1,000 cells/mm³.

Serious Infection

Withhold treatment until serious infection is resolved, then resume as clinically indicated.

Dosage in Renal Impairment

Rheumatoid Arthritis: eGFR 30–59 mL/min: 1 mg daily. **Less than 30 mL/min:** Not recommended. **Alopecia Areata: eGFR 30–59 mL/min:** Reduce to 2 mg or 1 mg based on dose. **Less than 30 mL/min:** Not recommended. **COVID-19: eGFR 30–59 mL/min:** 2 mg once daily. **eGFR 15–29 mL/min:** 1 mg daily. **Less than 15 mL/min:** Not recommended.

Dosage in Hepatic Impairment

Mild to moderate impairment: No dose adjustment. **Severe impairment:** Not recommended.

SIDE EFFECTS

Rare (2%–1%): Nausea, acne, fatigue, genital *Candida* infections, abdominal pain, weight increase.

ADVERSE EFFECTS/TOXIC REACTIONS

Neutropenia, lymphopenia may increase risk of infection. Serious and sometimes fatal infections (bacterial, mycobacterial, viral, invasive fungal, other opportunistic infection) may occur. Serious infections may include aspergillosis, BK virus, cellulitis, cryptococcosis, cytomegalovirus, esophageal candidiasis, herpes zoster histoplasmosis, listeriosis, pneumocystosis, pneumonia, tuberculosis, UTI, sepsis. Upper respiratory tract infections including epiglottitis, laryngitis, nasopharyngitis, pharyngitis, pharyngotonsillitis, sinusitis, tracheitis, tonsillitis reported in 16% of pts. May increase risk of new malignancies. May induce viral reactivation of hepatitis B or C virus infection, herpes zoster, HIV. Thrombosis including DVT, pulmonary embolism, arterial thrombosis have occurred. May increase risk of GI perforation. Platelet count greater than 600,000 cells/mm³ occurred in 1% of pts.

NURSING CONSIDERATIONS

BASELINE ASSESSMENT

Obtain CBC, BMP, LFT, lipid panel; pregnancy test in females of reproductive potential. Assess onset, location, duration of pain, inflammation. Inspect appearance of affected joints for immobility, deformities. Evaluate for active TB and test for latent infection prior to and during treatment. Induration of 5 mm or greater with purified protein derivative (PPD) is considered a positive result when assessing for latent TB. Consider treatment with antimycobacterial therapy in pts with latent TB. Question history of arterial/venous thrombosis, hepatic/renal impairment, HIV infection, hepatitis B or C virus infection, diverticulitis, malignancies. Screen for active infection. Assess skin for open wounds. Receive full medication history and screen for interactions.

INTERVENTION/EVALUATION

Assess for therapeutic response: Relief of pain, stiffness, swelling; increased joint mobility; reduced joint tenderness; improved grip strength. Monitor CBC, LFT periodically. Monitor for TB regardless of baseline PPD. Consider discontinuation if acute infection, opportunistic infection, sepsis occurs; initiate appropriate antimicrobial therapy. Immediately report any hemorrhaging, melena, abdominal pain, hemoptysis (may indicate GI perforation). Monitor for symptoms of DVT (leg or arm pain/swelling), CVA (aphasia, altered mental status, headache, hemiplegia, vision loss), MI (chest pain, dyspnea, syncope, diaphoresis, arm/jaw pain), PE (chest pain, dyspnea, tachycardia).

PATIENT/FAMILY TEACHING

• Treatment may depress your immune response and reduce your ability to fight infection. Report symptoms of infection such as body aches, chills, cough, fatigue, fever. Avoid those with active infection. • Expect routine tuberculosis screening. Report any travel plans to possible endemic areas. • Do not receive live vaccines. • Report symptoms of DVT (swelling, pain, hot feeling in the arms or legs; discoloration of extremity), lung embolism (difficulty breathing, chest pain, rapid heart rate), stroke (confusion, one-sided weakness or paralysis, difficulty

speaking). • Treatment may cause life-threatening arterial blood clots; report symptoms of heart attack (chest pain, difficulty breathing, jaw pain, nausea, pain that radiates to the arm or jaw, sweating), stroke (blindness, confusion, one-sided weakness, loss of consciousness, trouble speaking, seizures). • Report symptoms of liver problems such as bruising, confusion, dark or amber-colored urine, right upper abdominal pain, or yellowing of the skin or eyes. • Immediately report severe or persistent abdominal pain, bloody stool, fever; may indicate tear in GI tract. • Treatment may cause reactivation of chronic viral infections, new cancers.

beclomethasone

be-kloe-**meth**-a-sone
(Beconase AQ, QNASL, QVAR RediHaler)
Do not confuse beclomethasone with betamethasone or dexamethasone, or Beconase with baclofen.

◆**CLASSIFICATION**

PHARMACOTHERAPEUTIC: Adrenocorticosteroid. **CLINICAL:** Anti-inflammatory, immunosuppressant.

USES

Inhalation: (QVAR RediHaler): Maintenance and prophylactic treatment of asthma in pts 4 yrs and older. **Intranasal: Beconase AQ:** Relief of symptoms of seasonal/perennial allergic and nonallergic rhinitis in adults and children 6 yrs and older; prevention of nasal polyp recurrence after surgical removal in pts 6 yrs and older. **QNASL:** Treatment of seasonal and perennial allergic rhinitis in adults and children 4 yrs and older.

PRECAUTIONS

Contraindications: Hypersensitivity to beclomethasone. **Oral Inhalation:** Acute exacerbation of asthma, status asthmaticus. **Cautions:** Cardiovascular disease, cataracts, diabetes, elderly, glaucoma, hepatic/renal impairment, myasthenia gravis, risk for osteoporosis, peptic ulcer disease, seizure disorder, thyroid disease, ulcerative colitis; following acute MI. Avoid use in pts with untreated viral, fungal, or bacterial systemic infections.

ACTION

Controls or prevents inflammation by altering rate of protein synthesis; depresses migration of polymorphonuclear leukocytes, fibroblasts; reverses capillary permeability. **Therapeutic Effect: Inhalation:** Inhibits bronchoconstriction, produces smooth muscle relaxation, decreases mucus secretion. **Intranasal:** Decreases response to seasonal, perennial rhinitis.

PHARMACOKINETICS

Rapidly absorbed from pulmonary, nasal, GI tissue. Metabolized in liver. Protein binding: 87%. Excreted in feces (60%), urine (12%). **Half-life:** 2–4.5 hrs.

⌛ LIFESPAN CONSIDERATIONS

Pregnancy/Lactation: Unknown if crosses placenta or distributed in breast milk. **Children:** Prolonged treatment/high dosages may decrease short-term growth rate, cortisol secretion. **Elderly:** No age-related precautions noted.

INTERACTIONS

DRUG: May increase concentration/effect of **desmopressin, loxapine.** May decrease effect of **aldesleukin. HERBAL:** None significant. **FOOD:** None known. **LAB VALUES:** None significant.

AVAILABILITY (Rx)

Oral Inhalation: *(QVAR RediHaler):* 40 mcg/inhalation, 80 mcg/inhalation. **Nasal Inhalation:** *(Beconase AQ):* 42 mcg/

inhalation. *(QNASL):* 40 mcg/actuation, 80 mcg/actuation.

ADMINISTRATION/HANDLING

Inhalation
• Shake container well. • Instruct pt to exhale completely, place mouthpiece between lips, inhale, hold breath as long as possible before exhaling. • Allow at least 1 min between inhalations. • Rinse mouth after each use (decreases dry mouth, hoarseness, thrush).

Intranasal
• Instruct pt to clear nasal passages as much as possible before use. • Tilt pt's head slightly forward. • Insert spray tip into nostril, pointing toward nasal passages, away from nasal septum. • Spray into one nostril while pt holds the other nostril closed, concurrently inhaling through nose to permit medication as high into nasal passages as possible.

INDICATIONS/ROUTES/DOSAGE

Asthma
Oral inhalation: *(QVAR RediHaler):* **ADULTS, ELDERLY, CHILDREN 12 YRS AND OLDER:** (Pts not on inhaled corticosteroids): Initially 40–80 mcg twice daily. (Previously on inhaled corticosteroids): Initially, 40–320 mcg twice daily. **Maximum:** 320 mcg twice daily. **CHILDREN 4–11 YRS:** Initially, 40 mcg twice daily. **Maximum:** 80 mcg twice daily.

Allergic/Nonallergic Rhinitis, Prevention of Recurrence of Nasal Polyps
Nasal inhalation: *(Beconase AQ):* **ADULTS, ELDERLY, CHILDREN 12 YRS AND OLDER:** 1–2 sprays (42 or 84 mcg) in each nostril twice daily. **Maximum:** 336 mcg/day. **CHILDREN 6–11 YRS:** 1 spray (42 mcg) in each nostril twice daily (total dose: 168 mcg daily). May increase to 2 sprays (84 mcg) 2 times/day (total dose: 336 mcg daily). Once adequate control achieved, decrease to 1 spray (42 mcg)

in each nostril twice daily (total dose: 168 mcg daily).

Allergic Rhinitis
Nasal inhalation: *(QNASL):* **ADULTS, ELDERLY, CHILDREN 12 YRS AND OLDER:** 80 mcg/spray: 2 sprays in each nostril daily. **Maximum:** 320 mcg (4 sprays/day). **CHILDREN 4–11 YRS:** 40 mcg/spray: 1 spray each nostril once daily. **Maximum:** 80 mcg/day.

Dosage in Renal/Hepatic Impairment
No dose adjustment.

SIDE EFFECTS

Frequent: Inhalation (14%–4%): Throat irritation, dry mouth, hoarseness, cough. **Intranasal:** Nasal burning, mucosal dryness. **Occasional: Inhalation (3%–2%):** Localized fungal infection (thrush). **Intranasal:** Nasal-crusting epistaxis, sore throat, ulceration of nasal mucosa. **Rare: Inhalation:** Transient bronchospasm, esophageal candidiasis. **Intranasal:** Nasal and pharyngeal candidiasis, eye pain.

ADVERSE EFFECTS/TOXIC REACTIONS

Acute hypersensitivity reaction (urticaria, angioedema, severe bronchospasm) occurs rarely. Change from systemic to local steroid therapy may unmask previously suppressed bronchial asthma condition.

NURSING CONSIDERATIONS

BASELINE ASSESSMENT

Question for history of asthma, rhinitis. Question for hypersensitivity to corticosteroids.

INTERVENTION/EVALUATION

Monitor respiratory status. Auscultate lung sounds. Observe for signs of oral candidiasis. In pts receiving bronchodilators by inhalation concomitantly with inhaled steroid therapy, advise use of bronchodilator several minutes before corticosteroid aerosol (enhances penetration of steroid into bronchial tree).

PATIENT/FAMILY TEACHING

• Do not change dose schedule or stop taking drug; must taper off gradually under medical supervision. • **Inhalation:** Maintain diligent oral hygiene. • Rinse mouth with water immediately after inhalation (prevents mouth/throat dryness, fungal infection of mouth). • Report sore throat or mouth. • **Intranasal:** Report symptoms that do not improve; or if sneezing, nasal irritation occurs. • Clear nasal passages prior to use. • Improvement may take days to several weeks.

benazepril

ben-**ay**-ze-pril
(Lotensin)

■ BLACK BOX ALERT ■ May cause fetal injury, mortality. Discontinue as soon as possible once pregnancy is detected.
Do not confuse benazepril with enalapril, lisinopril, or Benadryl, or Lotensin with Lioresal.

FIXED-COMBINATION(S)

Lotensin HCT: benazepril/hydrochlorothiazide (a diuretic): 5 mg/6.25 mg, 10 mg/12.5 mg, 20 mg/12.5 mg, 20 mg/25 mg. **Lotrel:** benazepril/amLODIPine (a calcium blocker): 2.5 mg/10 mg, 5 mg/10 mg, 5 mg/20 mg, 5 mg/40 mg, 10 mg/20 mg, 10 mg/40 mg.

◆CLASSIFICATION

PHARMACOTHERAPEUTIC: Angiotensin-converting enzyme (ACE) inhibitor. **CLINICAL:** Antihypertensive.

USES

Treatment of hypertension in adults and children 6 yrs and older. Used alone or in combination with other antihypertensives.

PRECAUTIONS

Contraindications: Hypersensitivity to benazepril. History of angioedema with or without previous treatment with ACE inhibitors. Use with aliskiren in pts with diabetes. Coadministration with or within 36 hrs of switching to or from a neprilysin inhibitor (e.g., sacubitril). **Cautions:** Renal impairment; hypertrophic cardiomyopathy without flow tract obstruction; severe aortic stenosis; before, during, or immediately following major surgery; unstented renal artery stenosis; diabetes mellitus, pregnancy, breastfeeding. Concomitant use of potassium-sparing diuretics, potassium supplements.

ACTION

Decreases rate of conversion of angiotensin I to angiotensin II, a potent vasoconstrictor. Results in lower levels of angiotensin II, causing an increase in plasma renin activity and decreased aldosterone secretion. **Therapeutic Effect:** Lowers B/P.

PHARMACOKINETICS

Widely distributed. Metabolized in liver. Protein binding: 97%. Peak plasma concentration: 2–4 hrs. Minimal removal by hemodialysis. **Half-life:** 35 min; metabolite, 10–11 hrs.

⏳ LIFESPAN CONSIDERATIONS

Pregnancy/Lactation: Crosses placenta. Unknown if distributed in breast milk. May cause fetal, neonatal mortality or morbidity. **Children:** Safety and efficacy not established. **Elderly:** May be more sensitive to hypotensive effects.

INTERACTIONS

DRUG: Aliskiren may increase hyperkalemic effect. May increase potential for allergic reactions to **allopurinol. Angiotensin II receptor blockers (ARB)** (e.g., **losartan, valsartan**) may increase adverse effects. May increase adverse effects of **lithium, sacubitril. HERBAL: Herbals with hypertensive properties** (e.g., **licorice, yohimbe**) or **hypotensive properties** (e.g., **garlic, ginger, ginkgo biloba**) may alter effects. **FOOD:** None known. **LAB VALUES:** May increase serum potassium, ALT, AST, alkaline phosphatase, bilirubin, BUN, creatinine, glucose. May decrease serum sodium; Hgb, Hct. May cause positive ANA titer.

AVAILABILITY (Rx)

Tablets: 5 mg, 10 mg, 20 mg, 40 mg.

ADMINISTRATION/HANDLING

• Give without regard to food.

INDICATIONS/ROUTES/DOSAGE

Hypertension
PO: ADULTS, ELDERLY: Initially, 10 mg once daily. Evaluate response after 2–4 wks. May titrate dose as needed up to 40 mg/day in 1 or 2 divided doses. **CHILDREN 6 YRS AND OLDER:** Initially, 0.2 mg/kg/day (up to 10 mg/day). Maintenance: 0.1–0.6 mg/kg/day. **Maximum:** 40 mg/day.

Dosage in Renal Impairment
CrCl less than 30 mL/min: ADULTS: Initially, 5 mg/day titrated up to maximum of 40 mg/day. **CHILDREN:** Not recommended. **HD, PD:** 25%–50% of usual dose; supplement dose not necessary.

Dosage in Hepatic Impairment
Use caution.

SIDE EFFECTS

Frequent (6%–3%): Cough, headache, dizziness. **Occasional (2%):** Fatigue, drowsiness, nausea. **Rare (less than 1%):** Rash, fever, myalgia, diarrhea, loss of taste.

ADVERSE EFFECTS/TOXIC REACTIONS

Excessive hypotension ("first-dose syncope") may occur in pts with HF, severe salt or volume depletion. Angioedema, hyperkalemia occur rarely. Agranulocytosis, neutropenia may be noted in pts with renal impairment, collagen vascular disease (scleroderma, systemic lupus erythematosus). Nephrotic syndrome may occur in pts with history of renal disease.

NURSING CONSIDERATIONS

BASELINE ASSESSMENT

Obtain CBC before therapy begins and q2wks for 3 mos, then periodically thereafter. Obtain B/P immediately before each dose, in addition to regular monitoring (be alert to fluctuations).

INTERVENTION/EVALUATION

Assist with ambulation if dizziness occurs. Monitor B/P, renal function, urinary protein, serum potassium. Monitor CBC with differential if pt has collagen vascular disease or renal impairment. If excessive reduction in B/P occurs, place pt in supine position with legs elevated. Increased surveillance is recommended in pts with renal impairment, autoimmune disease, or taking drugs that affect leukocytes or immune response.

PATIENT/FAMILY TEACHING

• To reduce hypotensive effect, go from lying to standing slowly. • Full therapeutic effect may take 2–4 wks. • Skipping doses or noncompliance with drug therapy may produce severe rebound hypertension. • Report dizziness, persistent cough.

bendamustine

ben-da-**mus**-teen
(Belrapzo, Bendeka, Treanda)
Do not confuse bendamustine with carmustine or lomustine.

◆CLASSIFICATION

PHARMACOTHERAPEUTIC: Alkylating agent. **CLINICAL:** Antineoplastic.

USES

Chronic lymphocytic leukemia (CLL): Treatment of CLL. **Non-Hodgkin's lymphoma (NHL):** Treatment of indolent B-cell NHL that has progressed during or within 6 mos of treatment with riTUXimab or a riTUXimab-containing regimen. **OFF-LABEL:** Hodgkin's lymphoma (relapsed/refractory), multiple myeloma (salvage therapy), Waldenström marcoglobulinemia (refractory).

PRECAUTIONS

Contraindications: Hypersensitivity to bendamustine. (Bendeka only): polyethylene glycol 400, or propylene glycol mono-thioglycerol. **Cautions:** Baseline cytopenias, hepatic/renal impairment, conditions predisposing to infection (e.g., diabetes, renal failure, immunocompromised pts, open wounds); dermatologic disease, HF, dehydration; pts at high risk for tumor lysis syndrome (high tumor burden); history of hepatitis B virus infection, herpes zoster infection.

ACTION

Alkylates and cross-links double-stranded DNA. **Therapeutic Effect:** Inhibits tumor cell growth, causes cell death.

PHARMACOKINETICS

Widely distributed. Metabolized in liver and via hydrolysis to metabolites. Protein binding: 94%–96%. Excreted in urine (50%), feces (25%). **Half-life:** 40 min.

⧗ LIFESPAN CONSIDERATIONS

Pregnancy/Lactation: May cause fetal harm. Unknown if distributed in breast milk. Impaired spermatogenesis, azoospermia have been reported in male pts. **Children:** Safety and efficacy not established. **Elderly:** No age-related precautions noted.

INTERACTIONS

DRUG: CYP1A2 inducers (e.g., **carbamazepine, rifampicin**) may decrease

---

concentration/effect. **CYP1A2 inhibitors (e.g., ciprofloxacin, fluvoxamine)** may increase concentration/effect. May decrease therapeutic effect of **BCG (intravesical).** **HERBAL:** None significant. **FOOD:** None known. **LAB VALUES:** May increase serum AST, bilirubin, creatinine, glucose, uric acid. May decrease WBCs, neutrophils, Hgb, platelets; serum potassium, sodium, calcium.

AVAILABILITY (Rx)

Injection Powder for Reconstitution: *(Treanda):* 25 mg, 100 mg. Single dose vial: 45 mg/0.5 mL, 180 mg/2 mL. **Injection Solution:** *(Belrapzo, Bendeka):* Multidose vial: 100 mg/4 mL.

ADMINISTRATION/HANDLING

 IV

Trenanda
Reconstitution • Reconstitute each 100-mg vial with 20 mL Sterile Water for Injection (25-mg vial with 5 mL) for final concentration of 5 mg/mL. • Powder should completely dissolve in 5 min. • Discard if particulate matter is observed. • Withdraw volume needed for required dose (based on 5 mg/mL concentration) and immediately transfer to 500-mL infusion bag of 0.9% NaCl for final concentration of 0.2–0.6 mg/mL. • Reconstituted solution must be transferred to infusion bag within 30 min of reconstitution. • After transferring, thoroughly mix contents of infusion bag.
Rate of administration • Infuse over 30 min for CLL or 60 min for NHL.
Storage • Reconstituted solution should appear clear and colorless to pale yellow. • Final solution is stable for 24 hrs if refrigerated or 3 hrs at room temperature. • Administration must be completed within these stability time frames.

Belrapzo
Dilution • Allow vial to warm to room temperature. • Withdraw the volume needed for required dose and transfer into

a 500 mL infusion bag of 0.9% NaCl for a final concentration of 0.05-0.7 mg/mL.
Rate of administration • Infuse over 30 mon for CLL or 60 min for NHL.
Storage • Refrigerate diluted solution for up to 24 hrs or store at room temperature for up to 3 hrs. • Refrigerate multidose vials. • Partially used vials are stable for up to 28 days when refrigerated in original carton. • Each vial is not recommended for more than a total of 6 dose withdrawals.

Bendeka
Dilution • Allow vial to warm to room temperature. • Withdraw the volume needed for required dose and transfer into a 50 mL infusion bag 0.9% NaCl to a final concentration of 0.49-5.6 mg/mL.
Rate of administration • Infuse over 10 min.
Storage • Refrigerate diluted solution for up to 24 hrs or store at room temperature for up to 6 hrs. • Refrigerate multidose vials. • Partially used vials are stable for up to 28 days when refrigerated in original carton. • Each vial is not recommended for more than a total of 6 dose withdrawals.

INDICATIONS/ROUTES/DOSAGE

◄ALERT► Antiemetics are recommended to prevent nausea and vomiting.
Chronic Lymphocytic Leukemia
IV: ADULTS/ELDERLY: 100 mg/m^2 given over 30 min daily on days 1 and 2 of a 28-day cycle as a single agent, up to 6 cycles.

Non-Hodgkin's Lymphoma
IV: ADULTS/ELDERLY: 120 mg/m^2 on days 1 and 2 of a 21-day cycle as a single agent, up to 8 cycles.

Dose Modification
Hematologic toxicity Grade 4 or greater: Withhold until ANC 1,000 cells/mm^3 or greater, platelet 75,000 cells/mm^3 or greater. **CLL: toxicity Grade 3 or greater:** Reduce dose to 50 mg/m^2 on days 1 and 2 of each treatment cycle. **Recurrence:** Reduce dose to 25 mg/^{2} on days 1 and 2 of each cycle. **NHL: hematologic toxicity Grade 4 or nonhematologic**

toxicity Grade 3 or greater: Reduce dose to 90 mg/m² on days 1 and 2 of each cycle. **Recurrence:** Reduce dose to 60 mg/m² on days 1 and 2 of each treatment cycle.

Dosage in Renal Impairment

Not recommended in pts with CrCl less than 30 mL/min.

Dosage in Hepatic Impairment

Not recommended in pts with serum ALT/AST 2.5–10 times ULN and total bilirubin 1.5–3 times ULN, or total bilirubin greater than 3 times ULN.

SIDE EFFECTS

Note: Frequency and occurrence of side effects may vary depending on indication of treatment.

Frequent (75%–21%): Nausea, fatigue, vomiting, anorexia, diarrhea, pyrexia, constipation, decreased appetite, cough, headache. **Occasional (18%–6%):** Decreased weight, rash, dyspnea, stomatitis, dehydration, back pain, dizziness, chills, peripheral edema, abdominal pain, insomnia, dyspepsia, asthenia, pharyngeal pain, anxiety, dysgeusia, tachycardia, depression, chest pain, infusion site pain, catheter site pain, arthralgia, pruritus, hypotension. **Rare (5%):** Extremity pain, bone pain, abdominal distension, wheezing, nasal congestion, dry skin, night sweats, hyperhidrosis.

ADVERSE EFFECTS/TOXIC REACTIONS

Grade 3–4 myelosuppression reported in 98% of pts. Infections including sepsis, septic shock, herpes zoster, upper respiratory tract infection, UTI, sinusitis, pneumonia, febrile neutropenia, oral candidiasis, nasopharyngitis were reported. Reactivation of cytomegalovirus, hepatitis B virus, mycobacterium tuberculosis, herpes zoster was reported. Tumor lysis syndrome may present as acute renal failure, hypocalcemia, hyperuricemia, hyperphosphatemia. Infusion reactions (e.g., chills, fever, pruritus, rash), anaphylaxis were reported. Fatal skin reactions including Stevens-Johnson syndrome, toxic epidermal necrolysis, DRESS syndrome (drug reaction with eosinophilia and systemic symptoms, also known as multiorgan hypersensitivity) have been reported. DRESS may present with facial swelling, eosinophilia, fever, lymphadenopathy, rash, which may be associated with other organ systems, such as hepatitis, hematologic abnormalities, myocarditis, nephritis. Serious, sometimes fatal, hepatotoxicity may occur. Premalignant and malignant disease including myelodysplastic syndrome, myeloproliferative disorders, acute myeloid leukemia, bronchial carcinoma were reported. Skin and soft tissue infusion site extravasation with secondary cellulitis, exfoliation may occur. Other reactions may include acute renal failure, cardiac failure, pulmonary fibrosis, hemolysis, dermatitis, skin necrosis, atrial fibrillation, myocardial infarction, pneumonitis.

NURSING CONSIDERATIONS

BASELINE ASSESSMENT

Obtain CBC, BMP, LFT; pregnancy test in females of reproductive potential. Screen for active infection. Assess usual bowel movement patterns, stool characteristics. Ensure adequate hydration in pts at risk for tumor lysis syndrome. Question history of hepatic/renal impairment; history of hepatitis B virus infection, herpes zoster infection. Conduct baseline dermatologic exam. Receive full medication history and screen for interactions. Ensure patency of IV access. Offer emotional support.

INTERVENTION/EVALUATION

Monitor CBC for myelosuppression; BMP; LFT for hepatotoxicity; renal function (CrCl, GFR). Hematologic nadirs usually occur in 3rd wk of therapy. An increase of serum creatinine greater than 0.4 mg/dL from baseline may indicate renal injury. Obtain serum calcium, phosphate, uric acid if tumor lysis syndrome is suspected (presents as acute renal failure, electrolyte imbalance, cardiac arrhythmias, seizures). Monitor for infusion-related reactions, hypersensitivity reactions (anaphylaxis, chills, fever, rash), renal toxicity (anuria, hypertension, generalized edema, flank pain), extravasation injuries (redness, swelling, pain, necrosis of injection site), secondary malignancies, HBV reactivation (amber- to orange-colored urine, fatigue, jaundice, nausea, vomiting). Assess skin for dermal toxicities, DRESS. Monitor daily pattern of bowel activity, stool consistency; I&Os. Ensure adequate hydration, nutrition. Monitor for infections (cough, fatigue, fever). If serious infection, sepsis occurs, initiate appropriate antimicrobial therapy.

PATIENT/FAMILY TEACHING

• Treatment may depress your immune system response and reduce your ability to fight infection. Report symptoms of infection such as body aches, chills, cough, fatigue, fever. Avoid those with active infection. • Report symptoms of bone marrow depression such as bruising, fatigue, fever, shortness of breath, weight loss; bleeding easily, bloody urine or stool. • Therapy may cause life-threatening tumor lysis syndrome (a condition caused by the rapid breakdown of cancer cells), which can cause kidney failure. Report decreased urination, amber-colored urine; confusion, difficulty breathing, fatigue, fever, muscle or joint pain, palpitations, seizures, vomiting. • Treatment may cause diarrhea, dehydration. Drink plenty of fluids. • Use effective contraception. Do not breastfeed. • Report liver problems (abdominal pain, bruising, clay-colored stool, amber- or dark-colored urine, yellowing of the skin or eyes), kidney problems (decreased urine output, flank pain, darkened urine), skin reactions (rash, skin eruptions); UTI (fever, urinary frequency, burning during urination, foul-smelling urine), skin problems (rash, sloughing, necrotic tissue, dermal toxicity). • Report symptoms of drug-induced hypersensitivity syndrome (fever, swollen face/lymph nodes, skin rash/peeling/inflammation). • Allergic reactions such as chills, fever, rash may occur during infusion. Anaphylaxis (difficulty breathing, low blood pressure, severe rash, swelling of lips

and tongue, rapid heart rate, can be life threatening. If allergic reaction occurs, seek immediate medical attention. • Treatment may cause reactivation of chronic viral infections, new cancers.

benralizumab

ben-ra-**liz**-ue-mab
(Fasenra, Fasenra Pen)
Do not confuse benralizumab with certolizumab, daclizumab, eculizumab, efalizumab, mepolizumab, natalizumab, omalizumab, pembrolizumab, reslizumab, tocilizumab, or vedolizumab.

◆**CLASSIFICATION**

PHARMACOTHERAPEUTIC: Interleukin-5 receptor alpha-directed cytolytic. Monoclonal antibody. **CLINICAL:** Antiasthmatic.

USES

Add-on maintenance treatment of pts with severe asthma, aged 6 yrs and older, and with an eosinophilic phenotype. Treatment of adults with eosinophilic granulomatosis with polyangiitis (EGPA).

PRECAUTIONS

Contraindications: Hypersensitivity to benralizumab. **Cautions:** History of helminth (parasite) infection; long-term use of corticosteroids. Not indicated for treatment of other eosinophilic conditions; relief of acute bronchospasm or status asthmaticus.

ACTION

Inhibits signaling of interleukin-5 cytokine, reducing production and survival of eosinophils responsible for asthmatic inflammation and pathogenesis. **Therapeutic Effect:** Prevents inflammatory process; relieves signs/symptoms of asthma.

PHARMACOKINETICS

Widely distributed. Degraded into small peptides and amino acids via proteolytic enzymes. **Half-life:** 15 days.

⧖ LIFESPAN CONSIDERATIONS

Pregnancy/Lactation: Unknown if distributed in breast milk. However, human immunoglobulin G is present in breast milk and is known to cross placenta. **Children:** Safety and efficacy not established in pts younger than 6 yrs. **Elderly:** No age-related precautions noted.

INTERACTIONS

DRUG: None significant. **HERBAL:** None significant. **FOOD:** None known. **LAB VALUES:** None known.

AVAILABILITY (Rx)

Injection Solution, Prefilled Syringe: 30 mg/mL, 10 mg/0.5 mL. **Auto-Injector:** 30 mg/mL.

ADMINISTRATION/HANDLING

SQ

Preparation • Remove prefilled syringe from refrigerator and allow solution to warm to room temperature (approx. 30 min) with needle cap intact. • Visually inspect for particulate matter or discoloration. Solution should appear clear, colorless to slightly yellow in color. Do not use if solution is cloudy, discolored, or visible particles are observed.
Administration • Follow manufacturer guidelines regarding use of plunger. • Insert needle subcutaneously into upper arm, outer thigh, or abdomen and inject solution. • Do not inject into areas of active skin disease or injury such as sunburns, skin rashes, inflammation, skin infections, or active psoriasis. • Do not administer IV or intramuscularly. • Rotate injection sites.
Storage • Refrigerate prefilled syringes in original carton until time of use. Once warmed to room temperature, do not place back into refrigerator. • Do not freeze or expose to heating sources. • Do not shake. • Protect from light.

INDICATIONS/ROUTES/DOSAGE

Asthma (Severe)

SQ: ADULTS, ELDERLY; CHILDREN 12 YRS OF AGE, 6–11 YRS OF AGE WEIGHING 35 KG OR MORE: 30 mg once q4wks for the first 3 doses, then once q8wks thereafter. **CHILDREN 6–11 YRS OF AGE WEIGHING LESS THAN 35 KG:** 10 mg q4wks for first 3 doses, then once q8wks thereafter. Continue for minimum of 4 mos to determine efficacy.

EGPA

SQ: ADULTS, ELDERLY: 30 mg q4wks.

Dosage in Renal/Hepatic Impairment
Not specified; use caution.

SIDE EFFECTS

Occasional (8%–3%): Headache, pyrexia.

ADVERSE EFFECTS/TOXIC REACTIONS

Hypersensitivity reactions including anaphylaxis, angioedema, bronchospasm, hypotension, urticaria, rash were reported. Hypersensitivity reactions typically occurred hrs to days after administration. Infections including bacterial/viral pharyngitis may occur. Unknown if treatment will influence the immunological response to helminth (parasite) infection.

NURSING CONSIDERATIONS

BASELINE ASSESSMENT

Obtain apical pulse, oxygen saturation. Auscultate lung fields. Question history of parasitic infection, hypersensitivity reaction. Pts with preexisting helminth (parasite) infection should be treated prior to initiation. Inhaled or systemic corticosteroids should not be suddenly discontinued upon initiation. Corticosteroids that are not gradually reduced may cause withdraw symptoms or unmask conditions that were originally suppressed with corticosteroid therapy.

INTERVENTION/EVALUATION

Monitor rate, depth, rhythm of respirations. Assess lungs for wheezing, rales. Monitor oxygen saturation. Interrupt or discontinue treatment if hypersensitivity reaction, opportunistic infection (esp. parasite infection, herpes zoster infection); worsening of asthma-related symptoms (esp. in pts tapering off corticosteroids) occurs. Obtain pulmonary function test to assess disease improvement. Monitor for increased use of rescue inhalers; may indicate deterioration of asthma.

PATIENT/FAMILY TEACHING

• Treatment not indicated for relief of acute asthmatic episodes. • Have a rescue inhaler readily available. • Increased use of rescue inhaler may indicate worsening of asthma. • Seek medical attention if asthma symptoms worsen or remain uncontrolled after starting therapy. • Immediately report allergic reactions such as difficulty breathing, itching, hives, rash, swelling of the face or tongue. • Report infections of any kind. • Do not stop corticosteroid therapy unless directed by prescriber.

bethanechol

be-**than**-e-kole
(Duvoid ✦)
Do not confuse bethanechol with betaxolol.

◆CLASSIFICATION

PHARMACOTHERAPEUTIC: Parasympathomimetic choline ester. **CLINICAL:** Cholinergic.

USES

Treatment of acute postoperative and postpartum nonobstructive urinary retention, neurogenic atony of urinary bladder with retention.

PRECAUTIONS

Contraindications: Hypersensitivity to bethanechol. Mechanical obstruction of GI/GU tract, GI or bladder wall instability, hyperthyroidism, asthma, peptic ulcer disease, epilepsy, pronounced bradycardia or hypotension, parkinsonism, CAD, vasomotor instability, bladder neck obstruction, spastic GI disturbances, acute inflammatory lesions of the GI tract, peritonitis, marked vagotonia. **Cautions:** Bladder reflux infection.

ACTION

Stimulates parasympathetic nervous system, increasing bladder muscle tone and causing contractions, which initiates urination. Also stimulates gastric motility, increasing gastric tone, and may restore peristalsis. **Therapeutic Effect:** May initiate urination, bladder emptying. Stimulates gastric, intestinal motility.

PHARMACOKINETICS

Route	Onset	Peak	Duration
PO	30–90 min	60 min	6 hrs

Poorly absorbed following PO administration. Does not cross blood-brain barrier. **Half-life:** Unknown.

⧗ LIFESPAN CONSIDERATIONS

Pregnancy/Lactation: Unknown if crosses placenta or distributed in breast milk. **Children/Elderly:** No age-related precautions noted.

INTERACTIONS

DRUG: None Significant. **HERBAL:** None significant. **FOOD:** None known. **LAB VALUES:** May increase serum amylase, lipase, ALT, AST.

AVAILABILITY (Rx)

Tablets: 5 mg, 10 mg, 25 mg, 50 mg.

ADMINISTRATION/HANDLING

PO

• Administer 1 hr before or 2 hrs after meals to reduce nausea/vomiting.

INDICATIONS/ROUTES/DOSAGE

Nonobstructive Urinary Retention, Neurogenic Bladder
PO: ADULTS, ELDERLY: Usual dose: 10–50 mg 3–4 times/day. Minimum effective dose determined by giving 5–10 mg initially, repeating same amount at 1-hr intervals until desired response is achieved or a maximum of 50 mg is reached.

Dosage in Renal/Hepatic Impairment
No dose adjustment.

SIDE EFFECTS

Occasional: Belching, changes in vision, blurred vision, diarrhea, urinary urgency or frequency. **Rare:** Dyspnea, chest tightness, bronchospasm.

ADVERSE EFFECTS/TOXIC REACTIONS

Overdose produces CNS stimulation (insomnia, anxiety, orthostatic hypotension), cholinergic stimulation (headache, increased salivation/diaphoresis, nausea, vomiting, flushed skin, abdominal pain, seizures).

NURSING CONSIDERATIONS

BASELINE ASSESSMENT

Ensure pt has emptied bladder prior to procedure.

INTERVENTION/EVALUATION

Monitor urine output. Palpate bladder for evidence of urinary retention. Obtain bladder scan to assess urinary volume.

PATIENT/FAMILY TEACHING.

• Report nausea, vomiting, diarrhea, diaphoresis, increased salivary secretions, irregular heartbeat, muscle weakness, severe abdominal pain, difficulty breathing.

---

bevacizumab

be-va-**siz**-ue-mab
(Alymsys, Avastin, Mvasi, Vegzelma, Zirabev)
Do not confuse Avastin with Astelin, or bevacizumab with cetuximab or riTUXimab.

◆CLASSIFICATION

PHARMACOTHERAPEUTIC: Vascular endothelial growth factor (VEGF) inhibitor. Monoclonal antibody. **CLINICAL:** Antineoplastic.

USES

Cervical cancer: Persistent, recurrent, or metastatic cervical cancer (in com-

bination with paclitaxel and cisplatin or paclitaxel and topotecan). **Colorectal cancer:** Metastatic colorectal cancer in combination with fluorouracil-based therapy for first- or second-line treatment. Metastatic colorectal cancer in combination with fluoropyrimidine-irinotecan– or fluoropyrimidine-oxaliplatin–based therapy for pts having progressed on a first-line bevacizumab regimen. **Epithelial ovarian, fallopian tube, or primary peritoneal cancer:** In combination with carboplatin and paclitaxel followed by bevacizumab as a single agent for stage III or IV disease following initial surgical resection; in combination with paclitaxel, liposomal doxorubicin, or topotecan for platinum-resistant recurrent disease in pts who received no more than two prior therapy regimens; in combination with carboplatin and paclitaxel or carboplatin and gemcitabine followed by bevacizumab as a single agent for platinum-sensitive recurrent disease. **Glioblastoma:** Recurrent glioblastoma in adults. **Hepatocellular carcinoma (HCC):** In combination with atezolizumab in pts with unresectable or metastatic HCC who have not received prior systemic therapy. **Non-Squamous non–small-cell lung cancer (NSCLC):** First-line treatment for unresectable, locally advanced, recurrent or metastatic non-squamous NSCLC in combination with carboplatin and paclitaxel. **Renal cell carcinoma (RCC):** Metastatic RCC in combination with interferon alfa. **OFF-LABEL:** Age-related macular degeneration, breast cancer, endometrial cancer, malignant pleural mesothelioma, soft tissue sarcoma.

PRECAUTIONS

Contraindications: Hypersensitivity to bevacizumab. **Cautions:** Cardiovascular disease, acquired coagulopathy, preexisting hypertension, pts at risk of thrombocytopenia. Pts with CNS metastasis. Do not administer within 28 days of major surgery or active bleeding. Pts at risk for hemorrhage (e.g., history of GI bleeding, fistulas, coagulation disorders, recent

---

trauma; concomitant use of anticoagulants, NSAIDS, antiplatelets), history of thromboembolism (CVA, DVT, MI), transient ischemic attack [TIA]), GI perforation or hemorrhage; pts at risk for thrombosis (immobility, indwelling venous catheter/access device, morbid obesity, genetic hypercoagulable conditions).

ACTION

Binds to and neutralizes vascular endothelial growth factor, preventing association with endothelial receptors. **Therapeutic Effect:** Inhibition of microvascular growth retards growth of all tissue, including metastatic tissue.

PHARMACOKINETICS

Clearance varies by body weight, gender, tumor burden. **Half-life:** 20 days (range: 11–50 days).

⌛ LIFESPAN CONSIDERATIONS

Pregnancy/Lactation: May possess teratogenic effects. Potential for fertility impairment. May decrease maternal and fetal body weight, increase risk of skeletal fetal abnormalities. Breastfeeding not recommended. **Children:** Safety and efficacy not established. **Elderly:** Higher incidence of severe adverse reactions in pts older than 65 yrs.

INTERACTIONS

DRUG: May increase cardiotoxic effect of **anthracyclines.** May decrease therapeutic effect of **BCG (intravesical). Sunitinib** may increase adverse effects. **HERBAL:** None significant. **FOOD:** None known. **LAB VALUES:** May decrease Hgb, Hct, platelet count, WBC; serum potassium, sodium. May increase urine protein.

AVAILABILITY (Rx)

Injection Solution: 100 mg/4 mL, 400 mg/16 mL vials.

ADMINISTRATION/HANDLING

 IV

◀ALERT▶ Do not give by IV push or bolus.

Reconstitution • Dilute prescribed dose in 100 mL 0.9% NaCl. • Avoid dextrose-containing solutions. • Discard any unused portion.
Rate of administration • Usually given following other chemotherapy. Infuse initial dose over 90 min. • If first infusion is well tolerated, second infusion may be administered over 60 min. • If 60-min infusion is well tolerated, all subsequent infusions may be administered over 30 min.
Storage • Diluted solution may be stored for up to 8 hrs if refrigerated.

⚙ IV INCOMPATIBILITIES

Do not mix with dextrose solutions.

INDICATIONS/ROUTES/DOSAGE

Colorectal Cancer (In Combination With Fluorouracil-Based Chemotherapy)
IV: **ADULTS, ELDERLY:** 5 mg/kg q2wks (in combination with bolus-IFL) or 10 mg/kg q2wks in combination with FOLFOX4).

Colorectal Cancer Progression (Following First-Line Therapy Containing Bevacizumab)
IV: **ADULTS, ELDERLY:** 5 mg/kg q2wks or 7.5 mg/kg q3wks (in combination with fluoropyrimidine-irinotecan– or fluoropyrimidine-oxaliplatin–based regimen).

Non-Squamous Non–Small-Cell Lung Cancer (NSCLC)
IV: **ADULTS, ELDERLY:** 15 mg/kg q3wks (in combination with CARBOplatin and PACLitaxel) for 6 cycles.

Metastatic Renal Cell Carcinoma
IV: **ADULTS, ELDERLY:** 10 mg/kg once q2wks (with interferon alfa).

Glioblastoma
IV: **ADULTS, ELDERLY:** 10 mg/kg q2wks (as monotherapy).

Ovarian Cancer (Platinum-Resistant)
IV: **ADULTS, ELDERLY:** 10 mg/kg q2wks with PACLitaxel, DOXOrubicin (liposomal), or wkly topotecan or 15 mg/kg q3wks (with topotecan q3wks).

Ovarian Cancer (Platinum-Sensitive)
IV: **ADULTS, ELDERLY:** 15 mg/kg q3wks with CARBOplatin/PACLitaxel for 6–8 cycles, then 15 mg/kg q3wks as a single agent or 15 mg/kg with CARBOplatin/gemcitabine for 6–10 cycles, then continue 15 mg/kg q3wks as a single agent. Continue until disease progression or unacceptable toxicity.

Ovarian Cancer (Following Initial Surgery)
IV: **ADULTS, ELDERLY:** 15 mg/kg q3wks with CARBOplatin/PACLitaxel for 6 cycles, then 15 mg/kg q3wks as a single agent for total of up to 22 cycles. Continue until disease progression.

Cervical Cancer
IV: **ADULTS, ELDERLY:** 15 mg/kg q3wks (in combination with PACLitaxel and either CISplatin or topotecan). Continue until disease progression or unacceptable toxicity.

Hepatocellular Carcinoma (HCC)
IV: **ADULTS, ELDERLY:** 15 mg/kg q3wks (after administration of 1,200 mg of atezolizumab on same day). If atezolizumab is discontinued, may continue as monotherapy until disease progression or unacceptable toxicity.

Dose Adjustment for Toxicity
Temporary suspension: Mild to moderate proteinuria, severe hypertension not controlled with medical management. **Permanent discontinuation:** Wound dehiscence requiring intervention, GI perforation, tracheoesophageal fistula, Grade 4 fistula, fistula formation involving any internal organ, hypertensive crisis, serious bleeding, nephrotic syndrome, arterial or venous thromboembolism, hypertensive encephalopathy, posterior reversible encephalopathy syndrome, severe infusion reaction, HF.

Dosage in Renal/Hepatic Impairment
No dose adjustment.

SIDE EFFECTS
Frequent (73%–25%): Asthenia, vomiting, anorexia, hypertension, epistaxis, stoma-titis, constipation, headache, dyspnea. **Occasional (21%–15%):** Altered taste, dry skin, exfoliative dermatitis, dizziness, flatulence, excessive lacrimation, skin discoloration, weight loss, myalgia. **Rare (8%–6%):** Nail disorder, skin ulcer, alopecia, confusion, abnormal gait, dry mouth.

ADVERSE EFFECTS/TOXIC REACTIONS
Fatal GI perforations reported in up to 3% of pts. Serious fistula formations in bladder, biliary, bronchopleural, tracheoesophageal, renal, vaginal sites may occur. Necrotizing fasciitis due to poor wound healing complications, GI perforation may occur. Severe bleeding events including CNS hemorrhage, GI bleeding, epistaxis, hemoptysis, hematemesis, pulmonary hemorrhage, vaginal bleeding were reported. Thromboembolic events including CVA, DVT, MI, TIA. Posterior reversible encephalopathy syndrome (PRES) reported in less than 1% of pts. Renal injury, proteinuria, nephrotic syndrome may occur. Infusion-related reactions including altered mental status, chest pain, diaphoresis, hypertension crisis, hypoxia, rigors, wheezing may occur. Palmar-plantar erythrodysesthesia (redness, swelling, numbness, skin sloughing of the hands and feet) reported in 5% of pts. Other reactions may include ovarian failure, HF.

NURSING CONSIDERATIONS
BASELINE ASSESSMENT
Obtain CBC, serum potassium, sodium levels at regular intervals during therapy. Assess for proteinuria with urinalysis. For pts with 2+ or greater urine dipstick reading, a 24-hr urine collection is advised. Question history as listed in Precautions. Screen for active infection. Offer emotional support.

INTERVENTION/EVALUATION
Monitor CBC for myclosuppression; renal function (CrCl, GFR). Monitor

for GI perforation, GI bleeding, bloody stool; symptoms of intracranial bleeding (aphasia, blindness, confusion, facial droop, hemiplegia, seizures); symptoms of MI (chest pain, diaphoresis, left arm/jaw pain, increased serum troponin, ST segment elevation), CVA (aphasia, altered mental status, facial droop, hemiplegia, vision loss), DVT (leg or arm pain/swelling), PE (chest pain, dyspnea, tachycardia), HF (dyspnea, peripheral edema, palpitations, exercise intolerance). Monitor B/P for hypertension. Persistent hypertension despite medical management may indicate hypertensive crisis. Reversible posterior leukoencephalopathy syndrome should be considered in pts with seizure, headache, visual disturbances, confusion, altered mental status. An increase of serum creatinine greater than 0.4 mg/dL from baseline may indicate renal injury. Monitor for infusion-related reactions. Assess proteinuria with urinalysis. Monitor daily pattern of bowel activity, stool consistency.

PATIENT/FAMILY TEACHING

• Treatment may depress your immune system and reduce your ability to fight infection. Report symptoms of infection such as body aches, burning with urination, chills, cough, fatigue, fever. Avoid those with active infection. • Treatment may worsen high blood pressure. • Therapy may cause life-threatening blood clots or bleeding; report symptoms of heart attack (chest pain, difficulty breathing, jaw pain, nausea, pain that radiates to the left arm, sweating), DVT (swelling, pain, hot feeling in the arms or legs; discoloration of extremity), stroke (confusion, difficulty speaking, one-sided weakness or paralysis, loss of vision). • Stomach/pelvic pain, vomiting, fever may indicate GI perforation (tear). • Neurologic changes including altered mental status, seizures, headache, blurry vision, trouble speaking, one-sided weakness may indicate stroke, high blood pressure crisis, or life-threatening brain swelling. • Report abdominal pain, vomiting, constipation, headache. • Do not receive immunizations without physician's approval (lowers body's resistance). • Avoid pregnancy.

bexagliflozin

bex-a-gli-**floe**-zin
(Brenzavvy)
Do not confuse bexagliflozin with canagliflozin, dapagliflozin, empagliflozin, ertugliflozin.

◆CLASSIFICATION

PHARMACOTHERAPEUTIC: Sodium-glucose cotransporter 2 (SGLT2) inhibitor. **CLINICAL:** Antidiabetic.

USES

Adjunct treatment to diet and exercise to improve glycemic control in pts with type 2 diabetes mellitus.

PRECAUTIONS

Contraindications: Hypersensitivity to bexagliflozin; other SGLT2 inhibitors; pts on dialysis. **Cautions:** Mild to moderate renal impairment (CrCl greater 30 mL/min), hypovolemia/dehydration, elderly; pts at risk for lower leg amputation (diabetic foot ulcers, peripheral vascular disease); recent genital mycotic infection; pts at risk for diabetic ketoacidosis (insulin dose reduction, acute febrile illness, reduced calorie intake, surgery, alcohol abuse). Concomitant use of loop diuretics, other hypoglycemic agents (e.g., insulin, insulin secretagogues). Not recommended in pts with diabetic ketoacidosis, type 1 diabetes mellitus; severe renal impairment (eGFR less than 30 mL/min), severe hepatic impairment.

ACTION

Inhibits SGLT2, the transporter responsible for reabsorption of the majority of glucose from the renal glomerular filtrate in the proximal renal tubule, reducing reabsorption of filtered glucose and lowering the renal threshold for glucose. **Therapeutic Effect:** Increases urinary excretion of glucose; lowers serum glucose levels.

PHARMACOKINETICS

Widely distributed. Metabolized in liver by glucuronidation. Protein binding: 93%. Peak plasma concentration: 2–4 hrs. Excreted in feces (51%), urine (41%). **Half-life:** 12 hrs.

⧗ LIFESPAN CONSIDERATIONS

Pregnancy/Lactation: Not recommended during second or third trimester. Unknown if distributed in breast milk. Breastfeeding not recommended. **Children:** Safety and efficacy not established in pts younger than 18 yrs. **Elderly:** May have increased risk for adverse effects (dehydration, hypotension, syncope).

INTERACTIONS

DRUG: **Insulin, insulin secretagogues (e.g., glyBURIDE)** may increase risk of hypoglycemia. **UGT enzyme inducers (e.g., carBAMazepine, phenytoin, rifampicin)** may decrease concentration/effect. May decrease concentration/effect of **lithium.** **HERBAL:** **Herbals with hypoglycemic properties (e.g., fenugreek, flaxseed, ginseng, gotu kola)** may increase risk of hypoglycemia. **FOOD:** None known. **LAB VALUES:** May increase low-density lipoprotein cholesterol (LDL-C), serum creatinine. May decrease eGFR. May interfere with 1,5-anhydroglucitol (1,5-AG) assay.

AVAILABILITY (Rx)

Tablets: 20 mg.

ADMINISTRATION/HANDLING

PO
• Give without regard to food. • Administer tablet whole; do not cut or crush. • Tablet cannot be chewed. • If a dose is missed, give as soon as possible that day. Do not double the next dose.

INDICATIONS/ROUTES/DOSAGE

Type 2 Diabetes Mellitus
PO: **ADULTS, ELDERLY:** 20 mg once daily in the morning.

Dosage in Renal Impairment
eGFR 30 mL/min or greater: No dose adjustment. **eGFR less than 30mL/min:** Not recommended. **Pts on dialysis:** Contraindicated.

Dosage in Hepatic Impairment
Mild to moderate impairment: No dose adjustment. **Severe impairment:** Not recommended.

SIDE EFFECTS

Occasional (7%): Increased urination. **Rare (3%–2%):** Thirst, vaginal pruritus.

ADVERSE EFFECTS/TOXIC REACTIONS

Symptomatic hypotension (orthostatic hypotension, postural dizziness, syncope) may occur, esp. in pts who are elderly, use concomitant loop diuretics, or have baseline systolic hypotension. Intravascular volume depletion may cause acute kidney injury requiring dialysis. Hypoglycemic events were reported, esp. in pts using concomitant hypoglycemic medications. Fatal cases of ketoacidosis were reported. Infections including urosepsis, pyelonephritis, UTI, genital mycotic infections (male and female), upper respiratory tract infection may occur. May increase risk of lower limb amputations. Necrotizing fasciitis of the perineum (Fournier's gangrene), a life-threatening necrotizing infection of the genital and perineum region that requires urgent surgical intervention, has been reported. May increase risk of fractures.

NURSING CONSIDERATIONS

BASELINE ASSESSMENT

Obtain BUN, serum creatinine, eGFR, CrCl, blood glucose level, Hgb A1c; B/P. Assess hydration status. Correct volume depletion prior to initiation. Assess pt's understanding of diabetes management, routine home glucose monitoring. Obtain dietary consult for nutritional education. Question history of hepatic/renal impairment, type 1 diabetes, ketoacidosis. Receive full medication history and screen

  Canadian trade name   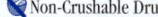 Non-Crushable Drug   🄷🄸 High Alert drug

for interactions. Screen for risks of lower limb amputation (e.g., peripheral vascular disease, diabetic foot ulcers).

INTERVENTION/EVALUATION

Monitor BUN, serum creatinine, eGFR, CrCl, blood glucose level, Hgb A1c; B/P periodically. Monitor for hypoglycemia (anxiety, confusion, diaphoresis, diplopia, dizziness, headache, hunger, perioral numbness, tachycardia, tremors), hyperglycemia (fatigue, Kussmaul respirations, polyphagia, polyuria, polydipsia, nausea, vomiting), ketoacidosis (e.g., dehydration, confusion, extreme thirst, sweet-smelling breath, Kussmaul respirations, nausea). Pts presenting with metabolic acidosis should be screened for ketoacidosis, regardless of serum glucose levels. Concomitant use of beta blockers (e.g., carvedilol, metoprolol) may mask symptoms of hypoglycemia. Monitor for acute kidney injury (dark-colored urine, flank pain, decreased urine output, muscle aches), infections (cough, fatigue, fever), urinary tract infection (dysuria, fever, flank pain, malaise), mycotic infections, Fournier's gangrene (perineal necrosis). Screen for glucose-altering conditions: fever, stress, surgical procedures, trauma. Encourage fluid intake. Monitor I&Os.

PATIENT/FAMILY TEACHING

• Diabetes mellitus requires lifelong control. Diet and exercise are principal parts of treatment; do not skip or delay meals. Test blood sugar regularly. Monitor daily calorie intake. • When taking combination drug therapy or when glucose conditions are altered (excessive alcohol ingestion, insufficient carbohydrate intake, hormone deficiencies, critical illness), have a low blood sugar treatment available (e.g., glucagon, oral dextrose). • Therapy may increase risk for dehydration and low blood pressure, which may cause kidney failure. Report decreased urination, amber-colored urine, flank pain, fatigue, swelling of the hands or feet. Drink enough fluids to maintain adequate hydration. • Genital itching or discharge may indicate yeast in-

fection. • Report symptoms of perineal necrosis (e.g., discoloration, pain, swelling of the scrotum, penis, or perineum). • Report symptoms of UTI, kidney infection (back pain, pelvic pain, burning while urinating, cloudy or foul-smelling urine). • Go slowly from lying to standing. • Do not breastfeed.

bictegravir/emtricitabine/tenofovir

bik-**teg**-ra-vir/**em**-trye-**sye**-ta-been/ ten-**oh**-foe-veer
(Biktarvy)

■ **BLACK BOX ALERT** ■ Serious, sometimes fatal lactic acidosis and severe hepatomegaly with steatosis (fatty liver) have been reported. Severe exacerbations of hepatitis B virus (HBV) reported in pts co-infected with HIV-1 and HBV following discontinuation. If discontinuation occurs, monitor hepatic function for at least several months. Initiate anti-HBV therapy if warranted.

Do not confuse bictegravir/ emtricitabine/tenofovir (Biktarvy) with elvitegravir/cobicistat/ emtricitabine/tenofovir (Stribild), emtricitabine/rilpivirine/tenofovir (Complera), efavirenz/ emtricitabine/tenofovir (Atripla), or emtricitabine/ tenofovir (Truvada).

FIXED-COMBINATION(S)

Biktarvy: bictegravir/emtricitabine/ tenofovir: 50 mg/200 mg/25 mg.

◆**CLASSIFICATION**

PHARMACOTHERAPEUTIC: Integrase inhibitor, nucleoside reverse transcriptase inhibitor, nucleotide reverse transcriptase inhibitor. **CLINICAL:** Antiretroviral.

USES

Indicated as complete regimen for treatment of HIV-1 infection in adults and pediatric pts weighing 14 kg or more who are antiretroviral naive or to replace the current antiretroviral regimen in pts who are virologically suppressed (HIV-1 RNA less than 50 copies/mL) on a stable antiretroviral regimen with no history of treatment failure and no known substitutions associated with resistance to the individual components of bictegravir/emtricitabine/tenofovir.

PRECAUTIONS

Contraindications: Hypersensitivity to bictegravir/emtricitabine/tenofovir. Concomitant use of dofetilide, rifampin. **Cautions:** Mild to moderate hepatic/renal impairment. History of depression, suicidal ideation; hepatitis B or C virus infection. Concomitant use of nephrotoxic medications. Not recommended in pts with creatinine clearance less than 30 mL/min; severe hepatic impairment.

ACTION

Bictegravir inhibits strand transfer activity of HIV-1 integrase, essential for viral replication. Emtricitabine inhibits HIV-1 reverse transcriptase by competing with natural substrates, resulting in chain termination. Tenofovir inhibits HIV reverse transcriptase by interfering with HIV viral RNA-dependent DNA polymerase. **Therapeutic Effect:** Interferes with HIV replication, slowing progression of HIV infection.

PHARMACOKINETICS

Widely distributed. Bictegravir metabolized in liver. Emtricitabine phosphorylated by cellular enzymes. Tenofovir metabolized by enzymatic hydrolysis, mediated by macrophages and hepatocytes. Protein binding: (bictegravir): Greater than 99%; (emtricitabine): Less than 4%; (tenofovir): 80%. Peak plasma concentration: (bictegravir): 2–4 hrs; (emtricitabine): 1.5–2 hrs; (tenofovir): 0.5–2 hrs. Bictegravir excreted in feces (60%), urine (35%). Emtricitabine excreted in urine (70%), feces (14%). Tenofovir excreted in urine, feces (32%), (less than 1%). **Half-life:** (bictegravir): 17 hrs; (emtricitabine): 10 hrs; (tenofovir): 0.5 hrs.

⌛ LIFESPAN CONSIDERATIONS

Pregnancy/Lactation: Breastfeeding not recommended due to risk of postnatal HIV transmission. Distributed in breast milk. **Children:** Safety and efficacy not established in children weighing less than 14 kg. **Elderly:** Not specified; use caution.

INTERACTIONS

DRUG: May significantly increase concentration/effect of **dofetilide** (contraindicated). **Rifampin** may significantly decrease concentration/effect (contraindicated). **Carbamazepine, oxcarbazepine, phenobarbital, primidone** may decrease concentration of tenofovir. **Adefovir, fosphenytoin, phenytoin** may decrease therapeutic effect of tenofovir. **HERBAL:** St. John's wort may decrease concentration/effect of bictegravir, tenofovir. **FOOD:** None known. **LAB VALUES:** May increase serum amylase, ALT, AST, cholesterol, creatine kinase, creatinine. May decrease neutrophils.

AVAILABILITY (Rx)

Fixed-Dose Combination Tablets: bictegravir 50 mg/emtricitabine 200 mg/tenofovir 25 mg, bictegravir 30 mg/emtricitabine 120 mg/tenofovir 15 mg.

ADMINISTRATION/HANDLING

PO

• Give without regard to food. • Administer at least 2 hrs before medications containing aluminum, calcium, iron, magnesium (supplements, antacids, laxatives).

INDICATIONS/ROUTES/DOSAGE

HIV Infection

PO: ADULTS, ELDERLY, CHILDREN WEIGHING AT LEAST 25 KG: 1 tablet (bictegravir 50 mg/emtricitabine 200 mg/tenofovir 25 mg) once daily. **CHILDREN WEIGHING 14–24 KG:** 1 tablet (bictegravir 30 mg/emtricitabine120 mg/tenofovir 15 mg) once daily.

Dosage in Renal Impairment

CrCl greater than or equal to 30 mL/min: No dose adjustment. **CrCl less than or equal to 30 mL/min:** Not recommended.

Dosage in Hepatic Impairment

Mild to moderate impairment: No dose adjustment. **Severe impairment:** Not recommended.

SIDE EFFECTS

Occasional (6%–2%): Diarrhea, nausea, headache, fatigue, abnormal dreams, dizziness, insomnia, vomiting, flatulence, dyspepsia, abdominal pain, rash.

ADVERSE EFFECTS/TOXIC REACTIONS

If therapy is discontinued, pts coinfected with hepatitis B virus have an increased risk for viral replication, worsening of hepatic function, and may experience hepatic decompensation and/or failure. May induce immune reconstitution syndrome (inflammatory response to dormant opportunistic infections, such as *Mycobacterium avium*, cytomegalovirus, PCP, tuberculosis, or acceleration of autoimmune disorders such as Graves' disease, polymyositis, Guillain-Barré). Acute renal failure, Fanconi syndrome (renal tubular injury with severe hypophosphatemia) were reported. Fatal cases of lactic acidosis, severe hepatomegaly with steatosis have occurred. Suicidal ideation, depression, suicide attempt reported in less than 1% of pts (primarily occurred in pts with prior psychiatric illness).

NURSING CONSIDERATIONS

BASELINE ASSESSMENT

Obtain BUN, serum creatinine, creatinine clearance, GFR; CD4+ count, viral load, HIV-1 RNA level; urine glucose, urine protein. Obtain serum phosphate level in pts with chronic kidney disease. Test all pts for hepatitis B virus infection. Question history of depression, suicidal ideation. Receive full medication history (including herbal products); screen for contraindications/interactions. Offer emotional support.

INTERVENTION/EVALUATION

Monitor CD4+ count, viral load, HIV-1 RNA level for treatment effectiveness. Monitor renal function as clinically indicated. An increase in serum creatinine greater than 0.4 mg/dL from baseline may indicate renal impairment. If discontinuation of drug regimen occurs, monitor hepatic function for at least several months. Initiate anti-HBV therapy if warranted. Cough, dyspnea, fever, excess of band cells on CBC may indicate acute infection (WBC count may be unreliable in pts with uncontrolled HIV infection). Screen for immune reconstitution syndrome. Monitor daily pattern of bowel activity, stool consistency; I&Os.

PATIENT/FAMILY TEACHING

• Drug resistance can form if therapy is interrupted; do not run out of supply. • As immune system strengthens, it may respond to dormant infections hidden within the body. Report body aches, chills, cough, fever, night sweats, shortness of breath. • Treatment may cause kidney failure. Report flank pain, darkened urine, decreased urine output. • Practice safe sex with barrier methods or abstinence. • Do not breastfeed.

bimekizumab-bkzx

bye-me-**kiz**-ue-mab
(Bimzelx)
Do not confuse bimekizumab with ixekizumab, mirikizumab, risankizumab, or tildrakizumab.

◆CLASSIFICATION

PHARMACOTHERAPEUTIC: Interleukin-17A and F antagonist. Monoclonal antibody. **CLINICAL:** Antipsoriatic agent.

USES

Treatment of moderate to severe plaque psoriasis in adults who are candidates for systemic therapy or phototherapy.

PRECAUTIONS

Contraindications: Hypersensitivity to bimekizumab-bkzx. **Cautions:** Hepatic impairment; pts at risk for suicide ideation and behavior; history of inflammatory bowel disease (e.g., ulcerative colitis, Crohn's disease); conditions predisposing to infection (e.g., diabetes, immunocompromised pts, renal failure, open wounds), chronic opportunistic infections (e.g., herpes virus infection, fungal infections); prior exposure to tuberculosis (TB) or use in pts who reside or travel to areas where TB is endemic. Avoid use during active infection or active TB infection. Concomitant use of live vaccines is not recommended.

ACTION

Selectively binds to interleukin-17A (IL-17A), IL-17F, 17-AF cytokines and inhibits interaction with IL-17 receptor. IL-17 is a cytokine that is involved in inflammatory and immune response. **Therapeutic Effect:** Alters biologic immune response; reduces inflammation of psoriatic lesions.

PHARMACOKINETICS

Widely distributed. Degraded into small peptides via catabolic pathway. Peak plasma concentration: 3–4 days. **Half-life:** 23 days.

⏳ LIFESPAN CONSIDERATIONS

Pregnancy/Lactation: Unknown if distributed in breastmilk. However, human immunoglobulin G (IgG) is present in breastmilk and is known to cross the placenta. **Children:** Safety and efficacy not established. **Elderly:** No age-related precautions noted.

INTERACTIONS

DRUG: May decrease levels/therapeutic effects of **vaccines (live).** May increase levels/adverse effects of **BCG** (intravesical)**, vaccines (live).** May alter **CYP450 substrates with a narrow therapeutic index (e.g., cyclosporine, warfarin). HERBAL:** None significant. **FOOD:** None known. **LAB VALUES:** May increase serum alkaline phosphatase, ALT, AST, bilirubin.

AVAILABILITY (Rx)

Injection Solution, Prefilled Syringe or Auto-Injector: 160 mg/mL.

ADMINISTRATION/HANDLING

SQ

Preparation • Remove carton from refrigerator and allow solution to warm to room temperature (approx. 30–45 min) without removing prefilled syringes or auto-injectors (protects solution from light). • Visually inspect for particulate matter or discoloration. Solution should appear clear to slightly opalescent, colorless to pale brownish-yellow. Do not use if solution is cloudy, discolored, or visible particles are observed.

Administration • Dose requires 2 separate injections at different sites. Insert needle subcutaneously into outer thigh, abdomen, or back of upper arm and inject solution. • Do not inject within 2 inches (5 cm) of navel or into areas of active skin disease or injury such as sunburns, skin rashes, inflammation, skin infections, or psoriatic lesions. • Rotate injection sites. • Do not administer IV or intramuscularly. • If a dose is missed, administer as soon as possible, then give next dose at regularly scheduled time.

Storage • Refrigerate prefilled syringes/auto-injectors in original carton until time of use. • Protect from light. • Do not shake. • Do not freeze or expose to heating sources.

INDICATIONS/ROUTES/DOSAGE

Plaque Psoriasis (Severe)

SQ: ADULTS: 320 mg (given as two injections of 160 mg at different sites) once at wk 0, 4, 8, 12, and 16, then q8wks thereafter. **PTS WEIGHING GREATER THAN 120 KG:** Consider dose of 320 mg q4wks after wk 16.

Dosage in Hepatic/Renal Impairment
Not specified; use caution.

SIDE EFFECTS

Rare (3%–1%): Headache, injection site reactions (bruising, edema/swelling erythema, pain), acne, folliculitis, fatigue.

ADVERSE EFFECTS/TOXIC REACTIONS

May increase risk of suicidal ideation and behavior. Infections occurred in 36% of pts. Upper respiratory tract infections, *Candida* infections, tinea infections, gastroenteritis, and herpes simplex infections were reported. May cause elevation of hepatic enzymes greater than 3 times upper limit of normal. Inflammatory bowel disease, including ulcerative colitis and Crohn's disease, may occur. Neutropenia reported in less than 1% of pts.

NURSING CONSIDERATIONS

BASELINE ASSESSMENT

Obtain LFT. Consider completion of age-appropriate immunizations prior to initiation. Evaluate for active TB and test for latent infection prior to initiation and periodically during therapy. An induration of 5 mm or greater with tuberculin skin testing should be considered a positive test result when assessing if treatment for latent tuberculosis is necessary. Screen for active or chronic infection. Question history of inflammatory bowel disease; mood disorder, suicidal ideation and behavior. Conduct dermatological exam; record characteristics of psoriatic lesions. Assess pt's willingness to self-inject medication. Teach proper injection techniques.

INTERVENTION/EVALUATION

Monitor LFT periodically. Monitor for symptoms of tuberculosis (cough, fatigue, hemoptysis, nocturnal sweating, weight loss), including those who tested negative for latent TB infection prior to initiating therapy. Interrupt or discontinue treatment if serious infection, opportunistic infection, or sepsis occurs. Diligently monitor for suicidal ideation and behavior; new-onset or worsening of anxiety, depression, mood disorder. Consult mental health professional if mood disorder is suspected. Monitor for symptoms of inflammatory bowel disease (abdominal cramping/pain, diarrhea, fatigue, melena, reduced appetite, weight loss). Assess skin for improvement of psoriatic lesions.

PATIENT/FAMILY TEACHING

• Treatment may depress your immune system and reduce your ability to fight infection. Report symptoms of infection such as body aches, burning with urination, chills, cough, fatigue, fever; fungal infections. Avoid those with active infection. • Do not receive live vaccines. • Expect routine tuberculosis screening. Report symptoms of tuberculosis such as cough, fatigue, night sweats, weight loss, or coughing up blood. • Report travel plans to possible endemic areas. • Seek immediate medical attention if thoughts of suicide, new-onset or worsening of anxiety, depression, or changes in mood occurs. • Report liver problems (abdominal pain, bruising, clay-colored stool, amber or dark colored urine, yellowing of the skin or eyes); symptoms of bowel inflammation (abdominal cramping/pain, bloody stool, diarrhea, fatigue, reduced appetite, weight loss).

binimetinib

bin-i-**me**-ti-nib
(Mektovi)
Do not confuse binimetinib with alectinib, bosutinib, brigatinib, cobimetinib, neratinib or trametinib, or Mektovi with Mekinist.

◆CLASSIFICATION

PHARMACOTHERAPEUTIC: Mitogen-activated extracellular (MEK) kinase inhibitor. **CLINICAL:** Antineoplastic.

USES

Metastatic melanoma: Treatment of pts with unresectable or metastatic melanoma with a BRAF V600E or V600K mutation

---

(in combination with encorafenib). **Non–small-cell lung cancer (NSCLC):** In combination with encorafenib, for the treatment of adults with metastatic NSCLC with a BRAF V600E mutation.

PRECAUTIONS

Contraindications: Hypersensitivity to binimetinib. **Cautions:** Baseline cytopenias; pts at risk for hemorrhage (e.g., history of GI bleeding, coagulation disorders, recent trauma; concomitant use of anticoagulants, NSAIDs, antiplatelets), hepatic/renal impairment, pulmonary disease, cardiovascular disease, HF. History of thromboembolism (deep vein thrombosis [DVT], pulmonary embolism [PE]); pts at risk for thrombosis (immobility, indwelling venous catheter/access device, morbid obesity, genetic hypercoagulable conditions).

ACTION

Potent and selective inhibitor of mitogen-activated extracellular kinase (MEK) pathway. Reversibly inhibits MEK1 and MEK2, which are upstream regulators of the ERK pathway. The ERK pathway promotes cellular proliferation. MEK1 and MEK2 are part of the BRAF pathway. **Therapeutic Effect:** Increases apoptosis and reduces tumor growth.

PHARMACOKINETICS

Widely distributed. Metabolized in liver. Protein binding: 97%. Peak plasma concentration: 1.6 hrs. Excreted in feces (62%), urine (31%). **Half-life:** 3.5 hrs.

⧗ LIFESPAN CONSIDERATIONS

Pregnancy/Lactation: Avoid pregnancy; may cause fetal harm. Females of reproductive potential should use effective contraception during treatment and for up to 4 wks after discontinuation. Unknown if distributed in breast milk. Breastfeeding not recommended during treatment and up to 3 days after discontinuation. **Children:** Safety and efficacy not established. **Elderly:** No age-related precautions noted.

INTERACTIONS

DRUG: None significant. **HERBAL:** None significant. **FOOD:** None known. **LAB VALUES:** May increase serum alkaline phosphatase, ALT, AST, creatine phosphokinase, creatinine, GGT. May decrease Hct, Hgb, leukocytes, lymphocytes, neutrophils, RBCs; serum sodium.

AVAILABILITY (Rx)

Tablets: 15 mg.

ADMINISTRATION/HANDLING

PO
• Give without regard to food. • If a dose is missed or vomiting occurs after administration, give next dose at regularly scheduled time. • Do not give a missed dose within 6 hrs of next dose.

INDICATIONS/ROUTES/DOSAGE

Metastatic Melanoma
PO: ADULTS, ELDERLY: 45 mg twice daily (in combination with encorafenib). Continue until disease progression or unacceptable toxicity.

NSCLC
PO: ADULTS, ELDERLY: 45 mg twice daily (in combination with encorafenib). Continue until disease progression or unacceptable toxicity.

Dose Reduction for Adverse Reactions
First dose reduction: 30 mg twice daily. **Unable to tolerate 30 mg dose:** Permanently discontinue.

Dose Modification
Based on Common Terminology Criteria for Adverse Events (CTCAE). See prescribing information for encorafenib for recommended dose modification. If encorafenib is discontinued, binimetinib must also be discontinued.

Cardiomyopathy
Asymptomatic, absolute decrease in left ventricular ejection fraction (LVEF) greater than 10% from baseline and below lower limit of normal (LLN):

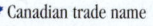 ♣ Canadian trade name   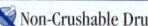 Non-Crushable Drug   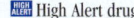 High Alert drug

Withhold treatment for up to 4 wks. If LVEF is at or above LLN, and the decrease from baseline is 10% or less, and pt is asymptomatic, then resume at reduced dose. If LVEF does not recover within 4 wks, permanently discontinue. **Symptomatic HF or absolute decrease in LVEF of greater than 20% from baseline that is also below LLN:** Permanently discontinue.

Dermatologic Reactions

Grade 2 skin reaction: If not improved within 2 wks, withhold treatment until improved to Grade 1 or 0. Resume at same dose for first occurrence or reduce dose if reaction is recurrent. **Grade 3 skin reaction:** Withhold treatment until improved to Grade 1 or 0. Resume at same dose for first occurrence or reduce dose if reaction is recurrent. **Grade 4 skin reaction:** Permanently discontinue.

Hepatotoxicity

Grade 2 serum ALT, AST elevation: Maintain dose. If not improved within 2 wks, withhold treatment until improved to Grade 1 or 0 (or to pretreatment baseline), then resume at same dose. **Grade 3 or 4 serum ALT, AST elevation:** See Other Adverse Reactions.

Ocular Toxicities

Symptomatic serious retinopathy; retinal pigment epithelial detachment: Withhold treatment for up to 10 days. If symptoms improve and become asymptomatic, resume at same dose. If not improved, resume at reduced dose or permanently discontinue. **Retinal vein occlusion:** Permanently discontinue.

Pulmonary Toxicity

Grade 2 interstitial lung disease: Withhold treatment for up to 4 wks. If improved to Grade 1 or 0, resume at reduced dose. If not resolved within 4 wks, permanently discontinue. **Grade 3 or 4 interstitial lung disease:** Permanently discontinue.

Rhabdomyolysis, Elevated Serum CPK

Grade 4 asymptomatic CPK elevation; any CPK elevation with symp- **toms or with renal impairment:** Withhold treatment for up to 4 wks. If improved to Grade 1 or 0, resume at reduced dose. If not resolved within 4 wks, permanently discontinue.

Uveitis

Grade 1–3 uveitis: Withhold treatment for up to 6 wks if Grade 1 or 2 uveitis does not respond to medical therapy or if Grade 3 uveitis occurs. If improved, resume at same dose or reduced dose. If not improved, permanently discontinue. **Grade 4 uveitis:** Permanently discontinue.

Other Adverse Reactions (Including Hemorrhage)

Any recurrent Grade 2 reaction; first occurrence of any Grade 3 reaction: Withhold treatment for up to 4 wks. If improved to Grade 1 or 0 (or to pretreatment baseline), resume at reduced dose. If not improved, permanently discontinue. **First occurrence of any Grade 4 reaction:** Permanently discontinue or withhold treatment for up to 4 wks. If improved to Grade 1 or 0 (or to pretreatment baseline), resume at reduced dose. If not improved, permanently discontinue. **Recurrent Grade 3 reaction:** Consider permanent discontinuation. **Recurrent Grade 4 reaction:** Permanently discontinue.

Thromboembolism

Uncomplicated deep vein thrombosis (DVT); pulmonary embolism (PE): Withhold treatment until improved to Grade 1 or 0, then resume at reduced dose. **Life-threatening PE:** Permanently discontinue.

Dosage in Renal Impairment

Mild to severe impairment: Not specified; use caution.

Dosage in Hepatic Impairment

Mild impairment: No dose adjustment. **Moderate to severe impairment:** 30 mg twice daily.

SIDE EFFECTS

Frequent (43%–20%): Fatigue, nausea, diarrhea, vomiting, abdominal pain, constipation, rash, visual impairment.

Occasional (18%–13%): Pyrexia, dizziness, peripheral edema.

ADVERSE EFFECTS/TOXIC REACTIONS

Myelosuppression (anemia, leukopenia, lymphopenia, neutropenia) is an expected response to therapy. Cardiomyopathy reported in 7% of pts. DVT reported in 6% of pts. PE reported in 3% of pts. Ocular toxicities including serious retinopathy, retinal detachment, macular edema, retinal vein occlusion may occur. Uveitis, including iritis and iridocyclitis, occurred in 4% of pts. Interstitial lung disease, pneumonitis reported in less than 1% of pts. Grade 3 or 4 hepatotoxicity reported in 3%–6% of pts. Rhabdomyolysis occurs rarely. Serious hemorrhagic events including GI bleeding, rectal bleeding (4% of pts), hematochezia (3% of pts) may occur. Fatal intracranial hemorrhage reported in 2% of pts in the setting of new or progressive brain metastases. Colitis, panniculitis reported in less than 10% of pts.

NURSING CONSIDERATIONS

BASELINE ASSESSMENT

Confirm presence of BRAF V600E or V600K mutation in tumor specimen before initiation. Obtain baseline CBC, BMP, LFT, CPK; pregnancy test in females of reproductive potential. Question history of cardiovascular disease, genetic hypercoagulable conditions, hypersensitivity reactions, HF, pulmonary disease, thrombosis. Obtain echocardiogram for LVEF. Screen for active infection. Verify use of effective contraception in females of reproductive potential. Offer emotional support.

INTERVENTION/EVALUATION

Monitor CBC for cytopenias; LFT for hepatotoxicity (bruising, hematuria, jaundice, right upper abdominal pain, nausea, vomiting, weight loss); CPK for rhabdomyolysis (amber-colored urine, flank pain, decreased urine output, muscle aches). Assess skin for dermal toxicities. Assess for eye pain/redness, visual changes at each office visit. Assess LVEF by echocardiogram 1 mo after initiation, then q2–3mos thereafter during treatment. If treatment withheld due to change in LVEF, monitor LVEF q2wks. Monitor for symptoms of DVT (leg or arm pain/swelling), PE (chest pain, dyspnea, tachycardia), HF (dyspnea, peripheral edema, palpitations, exercise intolerance). Monitor for GI bleeding, bloody stool; symptoms of intracranial bleeding (aphasia, blindness, confusion, facial droop, hemiplegia, seizures). Obtain ABG, radiologic test if interstitial lung disease or pneumonitis suspected. Diligently screen for infections.

PATIENT/FAMILY TEACHING

• Treatment may depress your immune system and reduce your ability to fight infection. Report symptoms of infection such as body aches, chills, cough, fatigue, fever. Avoid those with active infection. • Expect frequent cardiac function tests, eye exams, skin exams. • Therapy may cause toxic skin reactions, vision changes, or decrease the heart's ability to pump blood. • Report GI bleeding such as bloody stools or rectal bleeding. • Report symptoms of liver problems (bruising, confusion; amber, dark, orange-colored urine; right upper abdominal pain, yellowing of the skin or eyes); lung problems (severe cough, difficulty breathing, lung pain, shortness of breath), DVT (swelling, pain, hot feeling in the arms or legs; discoloration of extremity), lung embolism (difficulty breathing, chest pain, rapid heart rate), hemorrhagic stroke (confusion, difficulty speaking, one-sided weakness or paralysis, loss of vision), HF (shortness of breath, palpitations; swelling of legs, ankle, feet); rhabdomyolysis (dark-colored urine, decreased urinary output, fatigue, muscle aches). • Report any vision changes, eye redness. • Use effective contraception to avoid pregnancy. Do not breastfeed.

B

bisoprolol

bi-**soe**-proe-lol
(Apo-Bisoprolol ✦)
Do not confuse bisoprolol with metoprolol.

FIXED-COMBINATION(S)

Ziac: bisoprolol/hydroCHLOROthiazide (a diuretic): 2.5 mg/6.25 mg, 5 mg/6.25 mg, 10 mg/6.25 mg.

◆CLASSIFICATION

PHARMACOTHERAPEUTIC: Beta₁ selective adrenergic blocker. **CLINICAL:** Antihypertensive.

USES

Management of hypertension, alone or in combination with other medications. **OFF-LABEL:** Angina, atrial fibrillation/flutter, maintenance of ventricular control, HF with reduced ejection fraction, ventricular arrhythmias.

PRECAUTIONS

Contraindications: Hypersensitivity to bisoprolol. Cardiogenic shock, marked sinus bradycardia, overt HF, second- or third-degree heart block (except in pts with pacemaker). **Cautions:** Concurrent use of digoxin, verapamil, diltiaZEM. History of HF, severe anaphylaxis to allergens, renal/hepatic impairment, hyperthyroidism, diabetes, bronchospastic disease, myasthenia gravis, psychiatric disease, peripheral vascular disease, Raynaud's disease.

ACTION

Selectively blocks beta₁-adrenergic receptors. **Therapeutic Effect:** Slows sinus heart rate, decreases B/P.

PHARMACOKINETICS

Widely distributed. Protein binding: 26%–33%. Metabolized in liver. Primarily excreted in urine. Not removed by hemodialysis. **Half-life:** 9–12 hrs (increased in renal impairment).

⧗ LIFESPAN CONSIDERATIONS

Pregnancy/Lactation: Readily crosses placenta; distributed in breast milk. Avoid use during first trimester. May cause bradycardia, apnea, hypoglycemia, hypothermia during delivery, low-birth-weight infants. **Children:** Safety and efficacy not established. **Elderly:** Age-related peripheral vascular disease may increase risk of decreased peripheral circulation.

INTERACTIONS

DRUG: Alpha₂ agonists (e.g., cloNIDine) may increase AV-blocking effect. **Strong CYP3A4 inducers (e.g., carBAMazepine, phenytoin, rifAMPin)** may decrease concentration/effect. **Dronedarone, rivastigmine** may increase bradycardic effect. May increase vasoconstriction of **ergot derivatives (e.g., dihydroergotamine, ergotamine). HERBAL:** Herbals with hypertensive properties (e.g., licorice, yohimbe) or hypotensive properties (e.g., garlic, ginger, ginkgo biloba) may alter effects. **FOOD:** None known. **LAB VALUES:** May increase ANA titer, serum BUN, creatinine, potassium, uric acid, lipoproteins, triglycerides.

AVAILABILITY (Rx)

Tablets: 5 mg, 10 mg.

ADMINISTRATION/HANDLING

PO
• Give without regard to food.

INDICATIONS/ROUTES/DOSAGE

Hypertension
PO: ADULTS, ELDERLY: Initially, 2.5–5 mg once daily. Titrate at wkly or longer intervals. Usual dose: 2.5–10 mg once daily. **Maximum:** 20 mg/day.

Dosage in Renal Impairment
CrCl less than 40 mL/min: ADULTS, ELDERLY: Initially, give 2.5 mg.

Dosage in Hepatic Impairment
Cirrhosis, hepatitis: Initially, 2.5 mg.

SIDE EFFECTS

Frequent (11%–8%): Fatigue, headache. **Occasional (4%–2%):** Dizziness, arthralgia, peripheral edema, URI, rhinitis, pharyngitis, diarrhea, nausea, insomnia. **Rare (less than 2%):** Chest pain, asthenia, dyspnea, vomiting, bradycardia, dry mouth, diaphoresis, decreased libido, impotence.

ADVERSE EFFECTS/ TOXIC REACTIONS

Overdose may produce profound bradycardia, hypotension. Abrupt withdrawal may result in diaphoresis, palpitations, headache, tremors. May precipitate HF, MI in pts with cardiac disease, thyroid storm in pts with thyrotoxicosis, peripheral ischemia in those with existing peripheral vascular disease. Hypoglycemia may occur in previously controlled diabetes. Thrombocytopenia, unusual bruising/bleeding occur rarely.

NURSING CONSIDERATIONS

BASELINE ASSESSMENT

Assess BUN, serum creatinine; GFR. Assess B/P, apical pulse immediately before drug is administered (if pulse is 60/min or less or systolic B/P is less than 90 mm Hg, withhold medication, contact physician).

INTERVENTION/EVALUATION

Monitor B/P, pulse for quality, irregular rate, bradycardia. Assist with ambulation if dizziness occurs. Assess for peripheral edema. Monitor daily pattern of bowel activity, stool consistency. Assess neurologic status.

PATIENT/FAMILY TEACHING

• Do not abruptly discontinue medication. • Compliance with therapy regimen is essential to control hypertension. • If dizziness occurs, sit or lie down immediately. • Avoid tasks that require alertness, motor skills until response to drug is established. • Take pulse properly before each dose and report excessively slow pulse rate (less than 60 beats/min). Report numbness of extremities, dizziness. • Do not use nasal decongestants, OTC cold preparations (stimulants) without physician's approval. • Restrict salt, alcohol intake.

blinatumomab

blin-a-**toom**-oh-mab
(Blincyto)

■ **BLACK BOX ALERT** ■ Cytokine release syndrome (CRS) or neurologic toxicities, which may be life threatening or fatal, have occurred. Interrupt or discontinue treatment as recommended.
Do not confuse blinatumomab with ibritumomab or tositumomab.

◆CLASSIFICATION

PHARMACOTHERAPEUTIC: Anti-CD19/CD3 bispecific T-cell engager. Monoclonal antibody. **CLINICAL:** Antineoplastic.

USES

Treatment of adults and pediatric pts 1 mo and older with CD19-positive B-cell precursor acute lymphoblastic leukemia (ALL) in first or second complete remission with minimal residual disease (MRD) greater than or equal to 0.1%. Treatment of relapsed or refractory CD19-positive B-cell precursor acute lymphoblastic leukemia (ALL). Treatment of CD19-positive Philadelphia chromosome–negative B-cell precursor ALL in the consolidation phase of multiphase chemotherapy.

PRECAUTIONS

Contraindications: Hypersensitivity to blinatumomab. **Cautions:** Baseline cytopenias; active infection or pts at increased risk of infection (diabetes, indwelling catheters), hepatic/renal impairment, high tumor burden, history of cognitive or seizure disorders, syncope, elderly.

ACTION

Binds to CD19 expressed on B cells and CD3 expressed on T cells. Activates endogenous T cells, forming a cytolytic synapse between a cytotoxic T cell and the cancer target B cell. **Therapeutic Effect:** Inhibits tumor cell growth and metastasis in ALL.

PHARMACOKINETICS

Widely distributed. Metabolized into small peptides and amino acids via catabolic pathway. Protein binding: Not specified. Steady state reached within 24 hrs. Excretion not specified; negligible amounts excreted in urine. **Half-life:** 2.1 hrs.

⧗ LIFESPAN CONSIDERATIONS

Pregnancy/Lactation: May cause fetal harm. Avoid pregnancy. Unknown if distributed in breast milk. Must either discontinue drug or discontinue breastfeeding. **Children:** Safety and efficacy not established. **Elderly:** May have increased risk of neurologic toxicities, including cognitive disorder, encephalopathy, confusion, seizure; serious infections, hepatic impairment.

INTERACTIONS

DRUG: May decrease therapeutic effect of **BCG (intravesical), vaccines (live).** May increase adverse effects of **natalizumab, vaccines (live). HERBAL:** Echinacea may decrease therapeutic effect. **FOOD:** None known. **LAB VALUES:** May decrease immunoglobulins, Hgb, Hct, neutrophils, leukocytes, platelets; serum albumin, magnesium, phosphate, potassium. May increase serum ALT, AST, bilirubin, GGT, glucose; body weight.

AVAILABILITY (Rx)

Injection, Lyophilized Powder for Reconstitution: 35 mcg/vial.

ADMINISTRATION/HANDLING

 IV

• Do not flush infusion line after administration, esp. when changing infusion bags. Flushing of infusion line can result in excess dosage and complications. • At end of infusion, any used solution in IV bag and IV lines should be disposed of in accordance with local requirements.

Premedication • Premedicate with dexamethasone 20 mg IV 1 hr prior to the first dose of each cycle, prior to step dose (such as cycle 1 on day 8), or when restarting an infusion after an interruption of 4 or more hrs.

Reconstitution • Reconstitution guidelines are highly specific. Infusion bags must be prepared by personnel trained in aseptic preparations and admixing of oncologic drugs following strict environmental specifications at a USP 797 compliant facility using ISO Class 5 laminar flow hood or better. • See manufacturer guidelines for details.

Rate of administration • Administer as continuous IV infusion at a constant flow rate using an infusion pump. The pump should be programmable, lockable, nonelastomeric, and have an alarm. • Infusion bags should be infused over 24–48 hrs. Infuse the total 240-mL solution according to the instructions on the pharmacy label of the bag at one of the following constant rates: 10 mL/hr over 24 hrs, or 5 mL/hr over 48 hrs. • Infuse via dedicated line. • Use sterile, nonpyrogenic, low protein-binding, 0.2-micron in-line filter.

Storage • Refrigerate unused vials and IV solution stabilizer until time of use. • Protect from light. • Do not freeze. • Reconstituted vials may be stored at room temperature up to 4 hrs or refrigerated up to 24 hrs. • Prepared IV bag solutions may be stored at room temperature up to 48 hrs or refrigerated up to 8 days. • If prepared IV bag solution is not administered within the infusion time frame and temperature indicated, it must be discarded; do not refrigerate again.

INDICATIONS/ROUTES/DOSAGE

Note: Hospitalization is recommended for the first 9 days of the first cycle and the first 2 days of the second cycle. For all subsequent cycle starts and reinitiation (e.g., if treatment is interrupted for 4 or more hrs), supervision by a healthcare professional or hospitalization is recommended.

Relapsed or Refractory B-Cell Precursor ALL
IV: ADULTS, ELDERLY, CHILDREN: A treatment course consists of up to 2 cycles for induction followed by 3 additional cycles for consolidation and up to 4 additional cycles of continued therapy. Cycles 1–5 consist of 4 wks of continuous IV infusion followed by a 2-wk treatment-free interval. Cycles 6–9 consist of 4 wks of continuous IV infusion followed by an 8-wk treatment-free interval. **PTS WEIGHING 45 KG OR MORE:** (Induction cycle 1): Administer 9 mcg/day on days 1–7, then at 28 mcg/day on days 8–28 as continuous infusion. (Induction cycle 2, consolidation cycles 3–5, continued therapy cycles 6–9): Administer 28 mcg/day on days 1–28. **PTS WEIGHING LESS THAN 45 KG:** (Cycle 1): 5 mcg/m²/day (not to exceed 9 mcg/day) on days 1–7 and 15 mcg/m²/day (**Maximum:** 28 mcg/day) on days 8–28 as continuous infusion. (Induction cycle 2, consolidation cycles 3–5, continued therapy cycles 6–9): Administer 15 mcg/m²/day (**Maximum:** 28 mcg/day) on days 1–28.

MRD-Positive B-Cell Precursor ALL
Note: Hospitalization is recommended for the first 3 days of the first cycle and the first 2 days of the second cycle. For all subsequent cycle starts and reinitiations (e.g., if treatment is interrupted for 4 or more hrs), supervision by a healthcare professional or hospitalization is recommended.
IV: ADULTS, ELDERLY, CHILDREN: A treatment course consists of 1 induction cycle followed by up to 3 additional cycles for consolidation. Each cycle consists of 4 wks of continuous infusion followed by a 2-wk treatment-free interval. **PTS WEIGHING 45 KG OR MORE:** Administer 28 mcg/day on days 1–28. **PTS WEIGHING LESS THAN 45**

KG: Administer 15 mcg/m²/day (**Maximum:** 28 mcg/day) on days 1–28.

B-cell Precursor ALL (Consolidation Phase)
IV: ADULTS, ELDERLY, CHILDREN: A single cycle of monotherapy in consolidation is 28 days of continuous infusion followed by a 14-day treatment-free interval (total 42 days). **PTS WEIGHING 45 KG OR MORE:** Administer 28 mcg/day on days 1–28. **PTS WEIGHING LESS THAN 45 KG:** Administer 15 mcg/m²/day. **Maximum:** 28 mcg/day on days 1–28.

Dose Modification
Based on Common Terminology Criteria for Adverse Events (CTCAE). **Note:** If interruption after an adverse event is no longer than 7 days, continue the same cycle to a total of 28 days of infusion inclusive of the days before and after the interruption in that cycle. If interruption due to an adverse event is longer than 7 days, start new cycle.

Cytokine Release Syndrome
Grade 3: Withhold until resolved, then restart at 9 mcg/day. Increase dose to 28 mcg/day after 7 days if toxicity does not occur. **Grade 4:** Permanently discontinue.

Neurological Toxicity
Grade 3: Withhold until no more than Grade 1 for at least 3 days, then restart at 9 mcg/day. Increase dose to 28 mcg/day after 7 days if toxicity does not recur. If toxicity occurred at 9 mcg/day, or if toxicity takes more than 7 days to resolve, permanently discontinue. **Grade 4:** Permanently discontinue.

Seizure
Permanently discontinue if more than one seizure occurs.

Other Clinically Relevant Adverse Reactions
Grade 3: Withhold until no more than Grade 1, then restart at 9 mcg/day. Increase dose to 28 mcg/day after 7 days if toxicity does not recur. If toxicity takes more than 14 days to resolve, perma-

nently discontinue. **Grade 4:** Consider permanent discontinuation.

Elevated Hepatic Enzymes

Interrupt treatment if ALT/AST rise to greater than 5 times upper limit of normal (ULN) or bilirubin rises to more than 3 times ULN. Consider dose recommendation as listed in other clinically relevant adverse reactions or as ordered by prescriber.

Dosage in Renal Impairment

CrCl equal to or greater than 30 mL/min: No dose adjustment. **CrCl less than 30 mL/min or hemodialysis:** Not specified; use caution.

Dosage in Hepatic Impairment

Not specified; use caution.

SIDE EFFECTS

Frequent (62%–36%): Pyrexia, headache. **Occasional (25%–5%):** Peripheral edema, nausea, tremor, constipation, diarrhea, cough, fatigue, dyspnea, insomnia, chills, abdominal pain, dizziness, back pain, extremity pain, vomiting, bone pain, chest pain, decreased appetite, arthralgia, hypotension, hypertension, tachycardia, confusion, paresthesia. **Rare (4%–2%):** Aphasia, memory impairment.

ADVERSE EFFECTS/TOXIC REACTIONS

Myelosuppression (anemia, leukopenia, neutropenia, thrombocytopenia) is an expected outcome of treatment. Cytokine release syndrome (CRS) may be life threatening or fatal. Symptoms of CRS may include asthenia, hypotension, nausea, pyrexia; elevated ALT/AST, bilirubin; disseminated intravascular coagulation (DIC), capillary leak syndrome, hemophagocytic lymphohistiocytosis/macrophage activation syndrome (HLH/MAS). Infusion reactions have occurred and may be clinically indistinguishable from CRS. Neurologic toxicities such as altered level of consciousness, balance disorders, confusion, disorientation encephalopathy, seizures, speech disorders, syncope occurred in approx. 50%

of pts and may affect ability to drive or operate machinery. Median time to onset of neurologic toxicity was 7 days. CTCAE Grade 3 toxicities or higher occurred in 15% of pts. Serious infections such as opportunistic infections, bacterial/viral/fungal infections, sepsis, pneumonia, catheter-site infections occurred in 25% of pts. Other life-threatening or fatal events may include tumor lysis syndrome, neutropenia/febrile neutropenia, leukoencephalopathy. Medication preparation and administration errors have occurred, resulting in underdose or overdose.

NURSING CONSIDERATIONS

BASELINE ASSESSMENT

Obtain CBC, BMP, LFT, serum magnesium, phosphate, ionized calcium, vital signs. Consider electrolyte correction before starting treatment. Screen for home medications requiring narrow therapeutic index. Screen for active infection, history of seizures, hepatic/renal impairment, cognitive disorders. Verify pregnancy status in women of childbearing potential. Assess plans of breastfeeding. Conduct full neurologic assessment. Offer emotional support.

INTERVENTION/EVALUATION

Monitor CBC, LFT, serum electrolytes (correct as indicated), vital signs. Monitor closely for cytokine release syndrome, neurologic toxicities, serious infection, tumor lysis syndrome, hepatic impairment. Keep area around IV site clean to reduce risk of infection. Do not adjust setting of infusion pump. Pump changes may result in dosing errors. Do not flush IV line after infusion completion. Initiate fall precautions. Monitor I&O.

PATIENT/FAMILY TEACHING

• Treatment may cause life-threatening side effects that must be immediately treated by medical personnel. • Report symptoms of cytokine release syndrome, such as chills, facial swelling, fever, low blood pressure, nausea, vomiting, weakness; any infusion-related reactions, such as difficulty breathing or skin rash.

• Report any neurologic problems, such as confusion, difficulty speaking or slurred speech, loss of consciousness, loss of balance, or seizures. • Treatment may lower your white blood cell count and increase your risk of infection. Report any signs of infection, such as fever, cough, fatigue, or burning with urination. Keep area around IV catheter clean at all times to reduce risk of infection. • Do not change or alter settings on infusion pump, even if the pump alarm sounds. Any changes made to the infusion pump by anyone other than trained medical personnel can result in a dose that is too high or too low and may be life threatening. • Report symptoms of liver problems, such as bruising, confusion, dark or amber-colored urine, right upper abdominal pain, or yellowing of the skin or eyes. • Avoid tasks that require alertness, motor skills until response to drug is established. Do not drive or operate machinery. • Hospitalization is required when starting therapy.

---

bortezomib

bor-**tez**-oh-mib
(Velcade)

◆CLASSIFICATION

PHARMACOTHERAPEUTIC: Proteasome inhibitor. **CLINICAL:** Antineoplastic.

USES

Treatment of relapsed or refractory mantle cell lymphoma. Treatment of multiple myeloma. **OFF-LABEL:** Treatment of Waldenström's macroglobulinemia; peripheral or cutaneous T-cell lymphoma; systemic light-chain amyloidosis. Antibody-mediated rejection in cardiac transplantation, relapsed/refractory follicular lymphoma.

PRECAUTIONS

Contraindications: Hypersensitivity to bortezomib, boron, or mannitol; intra-

thecal administration. **Cautions:** Concomitant use of CYP3A4 inhibitors, history of syncope, concomitant use of antihypertensives; dehydration, diabetes, hepatic impairment, preexisting cardiac disease, neuropathy.

ACTION

Inhibits proteasomes (enzyme complexes regulating protein homeostasis within the cell). **Therapeutic Effect:** Produces cell-cycle arrest, apoptosis.

PHARMACOKINETICS

Widely distributed. Protein binding: 83%. Primarily metabolized by enzymatic action. Significant biliary excretion, with lesser amount excreted in urine. **Half-life:** 9–15 hrs.

⏳ LIFESPAN CONSIDERATIONS

Pregnancy/Lactation: May cause degenerative effects in ovary, degenerative changes in testes. May affect male/female fertility. Breastfeeding not recommended. **Children:** Safety and efficacy not established. **Elderly:** Increased incidence of Grade 3 or 4 thrombocytopenia.

INTERACTIONS

DRUG: CYP3A4 inhibitors (e.g., itraconazole, ketoconazole) may increase concentration/toxicity. CYP3A4 inducers (e.g., carbamazepine, phenytoin, rifampin) may decrease concentration/effect (avoid use). **HERBAL:** Green tea, green tea extracts may decrease effect. Herbals with hypotensive effects (e.g., garlic, ginkgo biloba, ginger) may enhance the hypotensive effect. **FOOD:** None significant. **LAB VALUES:** May significantly decrease WBC, Hgb, Hct, platelet count, neutrophils.

AVAILABILITY (Rx)

Injection, Powder for Reconstitution: 3.5 mg.

ADMINISTRATION/HANDLING

 IV

Reconstitution • Reconstitute vial with 3.5 mL 0.9% NaCl to provide a concentration of 1 mg/mL.

Rate of administration • Give as bolus IV injection over 3–5 sec.

Storage • Store unopened vials at room temperature. • Once reconstituted, solution may be stored at room temperature for up to 3 days or for 5 days if refrigerated.

SQ

Reconstitution • Reconstitute vial with 1.4 mL 0.9% NaCl to provide a concentration of 2.5 mg/mL.

INDICATIONS/ROUTES/DOSAGE

Mantle Cell Lymphoma (Initial Treatment)
IV: ADULTS, ELDERLY: 1.3 mg/m^2 days 1, 4, 8, 11 of a 21-day cycle for 6 cycles (in combination with riTUXimab, cyclophosphamide, DOXOrubicin, and predniSONE). If response is seen at cycle 6, may continue for 2 additional cycles.

Multiple Myeloma (Initial Treatment)
IV, SQ: ADULTS, ELDERLY: (with melphalan and predniSONE): 1.3 mg/m^2 on days 1, 4, 8, 11, 22, 25, 29, 32 of a 42-day cycle for 4 cycles, then 1.3 mg/m^2 once wkly on days 1, 8, 22, 29 of a 42-day cycle for 5 cycles.

Relapsed Multiple Myeloma, Relapsed Mantle Cell Lymphoma
IV, SQ: ADULTS, ELDERLY: 1.3 mg/m^2 twice wkly for 2 wks (days 1, 4, 8, and 11), followed by a 10-day rest period (days 12–21). For extended therapy of more than eight cycles, may give on standard schedule or, for relapsed multiple myeloma, on a maintenance schedule of once wkly for 4 wks (days 1, 8, 15, and 22), followed by a 13-day rest period (days 23–35).

Dosage Adjustment Guidelines
Withhold therapy at onset of CTCAE Grade 3 nonhematologic or Grade 4 hematologic toxicities, excluding neuropathy. When symptoms resolve, resume therapy at a 25% reduced dosage.

Dosage Adjustment Guidelines With Neuropathic Pain, Peripheral Sensory Neuropathy
For CTCAE Grade 1 toxicity with pain or Grade 2 (interfering with function but not activities of daily living [ADL]), 1 mg/m^2. For Grade 2 toxicity with pain or Grade 3 (interfering with ADL), withhold drug until toxicity is resolved, then reinitiate with 0.7 mg/m^2. For Grade 4 toxicity (permanent sensory loss that interferes with function), discontinue bortezomib.

Dosage in Renal Impairment
No dose adjustment.

Dosage in Hepatic Impairment
Mild impairment: No dose adjustment. **Moderate (bilirubin greater than 1.5–3 times upper limit of normal [ULN]) to severe (bilirubin greater than 3 times ULN) impairment:** Decrease initial dose to 0.7 mg/m^2 (based on tolerance may increase to 1 mg/m^2 or decrease to 0.5 mg/m^2).

SIDE EFFECTS

Expected (65%–36%): Fatigue, malaise, asthenia, nausea, diarrhea, anorexia, constipation, fever, vomiting. **Frequent (28%–21%):** Headache, insomnia, arthralgia, limb pain, edema, paresthesia, dizziness, rash. **Occasional (18%–11%):** Dehydration, cough, anxiety, bone pain, muscle cramps, myalgia, back pain, abdominal pain, taste alteration, dyspepsia, pruritus, hypotension (including orthostatic hypotension), rigors, blurred vision.

ADVERSE EFFECTS/TOXIC REACTIONS

Thrombocytopenia reported in 40% of pts. GI, intracerebral hemorrhage are associated with drug-induced thrombocytopenia. Anemia occurs in 32% of pts. New onset or worsening of existing neuropathy occurs in 37% of pts. Symptoms may improve in some pts upon drug discontinuation. Pneumonia occurs occasionally.

NURSING CONSIDERATIONS

BASELINE ASSESSMENT
Obtain CBC. Ensure adequate hydration prior to initiation of therapy. Antiemetics, antidiarrheals may be effective in

preventing, treating nausea, vomiting, diarrhea. Offer emotional support.

INTERVENTION/EVALUATION

Routinely assess B/P; monitor pt for orthostatic hypotension. Maintain strict I&O. Monitor CBC, esp. platelet count, throughout treatment. Monitor renal, hepatic, pulmonary function throughout therapy. Encourage adequate fluid intake to prevent dehydration. Monitor temperature and be alert to high potential for fever. Monitor for peripheral neuropathy (burning sensation, neuropathic pain, paresthesia, hyperesthesia). Avoid IM injections, rectal temperatures, other traumas that may induce bleeding.

PATIENT/FAMILY TEACHING

• Report new/worsening vomiting, bruising/bleeding, breathing difficulties. • Discuss importance of pregnancy testing, avoidance of pregnancy, measures to prevent pregnancy. • Increase fluid intake. • Avoid tasks that require mental alertness, motor skills until response to drug is established.

---

bosutinib

boe-**sue**-ti-nib
(Bosulif)

◆CLASSIFICATION

PHARMACOTHERAPEUTIC: BCR-ABL tyrosine kinase inhibitor. **CLINICAL:** Antineoplastic.

USES

Treatment of adults and pts 1 yr of age and older with chronic phase Ph+ chronic myelogenous leukemia (CML), newly-diagnosed or resistant or intolerant to prior therapy; adults with accelerated or blast phase Ph+ CML with resistance or intolerance to prior therapy.

PRECAUTIONS

Contraindications: Hypersensitivity to bosutinib. **Cautions:** Baseline cytopenias; hepatic impairment, recent diarrhea, pulmonary edema, HF, fluid retention. History of pancreatitis, moderate to severe renal impairment. Avoid concurrent use of CYP3A4 inducers/inhibitors.

ACTION

Inhibits Bcr-Abl tyrosine kinase, a translocation-created enzyme, created by the Philadelphia chromosome abnormality noted in chronic myelogenous leukemia (CML). Inhibits Src-family kinase, including Src, Lyn, and Hck. **Therapeutic Effect:** Inhibits cancer cell growth and proliferation in chronic, accelerated, or blast phase CML.

PHARMACOKINETICS

Widely distributed. Protein binding: 94%. Metabolized in liver. Excreted in feces (91%), urine (3%). **Half-life:** 22.5 hrs.

⧗ LIFESPAN CONSIDERATIONS

Pregnancy/Lactation: Avoid pregnancy; may cause fetal harm. Females of reproductive potential must use effective contraception during treatment and for at least 2 wks after discontinuation. Unknown if distributed in breast milk. Breastfeeding not recommended during treatment and for at least 2 wks after discontinuation. **Children:** Safety and efficacy not established. **Elderly:** No age-related precautions noted.

INTERACTIONS

DRUG: Strong CYP3A inhibitors and/or P-glycoprotein (P-gp) inhibitors (e.g., clarithromycin, ketoconazole, ritonavir, miSOPROStol, nafcillin), moderate CYP3A4 inhibitors (e.g., ciprofloxacin, diltiaZEM, erythromycin, verapamil) may increase concentration/effect. Strong CYP3A4 inducers (e.g., rifAMPin, phenytoin, PHENobarbital), moderate CYP3A4 inducers (e.g., dexamethasone, modafinil, nafcillin) may decrease concentration/effect. **HERBAL:** St. John's wort may decrease effectiveness. **Bitter orange, pomegran-**

ate, star fruit may increase concentration/ effect. **FOOD: Grapefruit products** may decrease concentration/effect. **LAB VALUES:** May decrease Hgb, platelets, WBCs, serum phosphate. May increase serum ALT, AST, bilirubin, lipase.

AVAILABILITY (Rx)

Capsules: 50 mg, 100 mg.

Tablets: 100 mg, 400 mg, 500 mg.

ADMINISTRATION/HANDLING

PO
• Give with food. Do not break, crush, dissolve, or divide tablets. • Give capsules whole (may open and mix with applesauce or yogurt). • Ensure mixture is swallowed immediately without chewing. • If a dose is missed beyond 12 hrs, skip the dose and resume usual dose the following day.

INDICATIONS/ROUTES/DOSAGE

AP or BP Ph+CML (Resistant or Intolerant to Prior Therapy)

PO: ADULTS, ELDERLY: 500 mg once daily. Continue until disease progression or unacceptable toxicity. May increase to a maximum of 600 mg daily in pts not reaching complete hematologic, cytogenetic, or molecular response and do not have Grade 3 or greater adverse reactions.

Newly-Diagnosed CP PH+ CML

PO: ADULTS, ELDERLY: 400 mg once daily. **CHILDREN:** 300 mg/^{2} once daily. **(CP Ph+ CML w/ resistance or intolerance to prior therapy):** 400 mg/m² orally once daily. Continue until disease progression or unacceptable toxicity.

CML With Baseline Renal Impairment

Ph+CML (intolerant): CrCl less than 30 mL/min: 300 mg once daily. CrCl 30–50 mL/min: 400 mg once daily. **Ph+CML (newly diagnosed):** CrCl less than 30 mL/min: 200 mg once daily. CrCl 30–50 mL/min: 300 mg once daily.

CML With Baseline Hepatic Impairment

PO: ADULTS: 200 mg once daily with food.

Dosage Modification
Hepatotoxicity: Withhold treatment until serum ALT, AST less than or equal to 2.5 times ULN. Then, resume at 400 mg once daily with food. Discontinue if recovery lasts longer than 4 wks or hepatotoxicity, including elevated serum bilirubin levels greater than 2 times ULN. **Severe diarrhea:** Withhold until recovery to low-grade diarrhea. Then, resume at 400 mg once daily with food. **Myelosuppression:** Withhold until absolute neutrophil count greater than 1,000 cells/mm³ and platelet count greater than 50,000 cells/mm³. Then, resume at same dose if recovery occurs within 2 wks. May reduce dose to 400 mg for recovery lasting greater than 2 wks.

SIDE EFFECTS

Frequent (82%–35%): Diarrhea, nausea, vomiting, abdominal pain, rash. **Occasional (26%–10%):** Pyrexia, fatigue, headache, cough, peripheral edema, arthralgia, anorexia, upper respiratory infection, asthenia, back pain, nasopharyngitis, dizziness, pruritus.

ADVERSE EFFECTS/TOXIC REACTIONS

Severe fluid retention may result in pleural effusion, pericardial effusion, pulmonary edema, ascites. Neutropenia, thrombocytopenia, anemia is an expected response of drug therapy. Severe diarrhea may result in fluid loss, electrolyte imbalance, hypotension. Hepatotoxicity occurred in 7%–9% of pts.

NURSING CONSIDERATIONS

BASELINE ASSESSMENT

Obtain CBC, BMP, LFT; pregnancy test in females of reproductive potential, baseline weight. Obtain full medication history, including vitamins, herbal products. Screen for peripheral edema, signs/symptoms of HF, anemia. Offer emotional support.

INTERVENTION/EVALUATION

Weigh daily and monitor for unexpected rapid weight gain, edema. Monitor for changes in serum electrolytes, LFT during treatment. Offer antiemetics for nausea, vomiting. Monitor daily pattern of bowel activity, stool consistency. Monitor CBC for neutropenia, thrombocytopenia, anemia. Assess for bruising, hematuria, jaundice, right upper abdominal pain, weight loss, or acute infection (fever, diaphoresis, lethargy, productive cough).

PATIENT/FAMILY TEACHING

• Take with meals. • Drink plenty of fluids (diarrhea may result in dehydration). • Swallow whole; do not break, chew, crush, dissolve, or divide tablets. • Use effective contraception to avoid pregnancy. Do not breastfeed. • Report urine changes, bloody or clay-colored stools, upper abdominal pain, nausea, vomiting, bruising, persistent diarrhea, fever, cough, difficulty breathing, chest pain. • Immediately report any newly prescribed medications. • Avoid alcohol, grapefruit products. • Discuss using antacids for indigestion, heartburn, upset stomach (omeprazole, lansoprazole, pantoprazole may reduce absorption, concentration of bosutinib). • Separate antacid dosing by more than 2 hrs before and after medication.

---

brentuximab vedotin

bren-**tux**-i-mab ve-**doe**-tin
(Adcetris)
■ **BLACK BOX ALERT** ■ JC virus infection resulting in progressive multifocal leukoencephalopathy and death can occur.

◆CLASSIFICATION

PHARMACOTHERAPEUTIC: Monoclonal antibody, anti-CD30. **CLINICAL:** Antineoplastic.

USES

Classical Hodgkin's lymphoma (cHL): Treatment of adults with relapsed or refractory classical Hodgkin's lymphoma after failure of autologous hematopoietic stem cell transplant (HSCT) or after failure of at least two prior multiagent chemotherapy regimens or in pts who are not transplant candidates. Treatment of classical Hodgkin's lymphoma, previously untreated stage III or IV in combination with doxorubicin, vinblastine, and dacarbazine. Treatment of adults with classical Hodgkin's lymphoma in adults at high risk of relapse or progression as post autologous HSCT consolidation. Treatment of pts 2 yrs and older with previously untreated high-risk classical Hodgkin's lymphoma (cHL), in combination with doxorubicin, vincristine, etoposide, prednisone, and cyclophosphamide. **Systemic anaplastic large cell lymphoma (sALCL):** Treatment adults with of systemic anaplastic large-cell lymphoma (sALCL) after failure of at least one prior multiagent chemotherapy regimen. Treatment of adults with previously untreated systemic ALCL, peripheral T-cell lymphoma (CD30-expressing) in combination with cyclophosphamide, DOXOrubicin, and predniSONE. **Cutaneous anaplastic large cell lymphoma (pcALCL)/CD30-expressing mycosis fungoides (MF):** Treatment of primary cutaneous ALCL or CD30-expressing mycosis fungoides. in adults receiving prior systemic therapy.

PRECAUTIONS

Contraindications: Hypersensitivity to brentuximab. Avoid use with bleomycin (increased risk for pulmonary toxicity). **Cautions:** Renal/hepatic impairment, peripheral neuropathy, infusion reactions, neutropenia, tumor lysis syndrome, Stevens-Johnson syndrome, pregnancy.

ACTION

Binds to CD30-expressing cells, allowing the antibody to direct the drug to a target on lymphoma cells, disrupting the microtubule network within the cell. **Therapeutic Effect:** Induces cell cycle arrest, cell death.

PHARMACOKINETICS

Widely distributed. Minimally metabolized Protein binding: 68%–82%. Excreted primarily in feces (72%). **Half-life:** 4–6 days.

⌛ LIFESPAN CONSIDERATIONS

Pregnancy/Lactation: May cause fetal harm (embryo-fetal toxicities). Unknown if distributed in breast milk. **Children/ Elderly:** Safety and efficacy not established.

INTERACTIONS

DRUG: Strong CYP3A4 inhibitors (e.g., atazanavir, clarithromycin, ketoconazole) may increase concentration/effect. **CYP3A4 inducers (e.g., carbamazepine, phenytoin, rifampin)** may decrease concentration/effect. May decrease therapeutic effect of **BCG (intravesical), vaccines (live).** May increase adverse effects of **bleomycin, natalizumab, vaccines (live). HERBAL:** Echinacea may decrease effect. **FOOD:** None known. **LAB VALUES:** May decrease Hgb, Hct, WBC, RBC, platelets. May increase serum bicarbonate, lactate dehydrogenase, glucose, albumin, magnesium, sodium.

AVAILABILITY (Rx)

Injection, Powder for Reconstitution: 50-mg single-use vial.

ADMINISTRATION/HANDLING

 IV

Reconstitution • Reconstitute each 50-mg vial with 10.5 mL Sterile Water for Injection, directing the stream toward wall of vial and not at powder. • Gently swirl (do not shake). • This will yield a concentration of 5 mg/mL. • The dose for pts weighing over 100 kg should be calculated for 100 kg. • Reconstituted solution must be transferred to infusion bag with a minimum 100 mL diluent, yielding a final concentration of 0.4–1.8 mg/mL brentuximab. • Gently invert bag to mix solution.
Rate of administration • Infuse over 30 min.
Storage • Discard if solution contains particulate or is discolored; solution should appear clear to slightly opalescent, colorless. • May store solution at 36°–46°F. • Use within 24 hrs after reconstitution.

▓ IV COMPATIBILITIES

0.9% NaCl, D_5W, lactated Ringer's.

INDICATIONS/ROUTES/DOSAGE

◄**ALERT**► Do not give by IV bolus or IV push.

cHL (Relapsed)

IV infusion: ADULTS, ELDERLY: 1.8 mg/kg (**Maximum:** 180 mg) q3wks. Continue treatment until disease progression or unacceptable toxicity.

cHL Consolidation

IV infusion: ADULTS/ELDERLY: 1.8 mg/kg (**Maximum:** 180 mg) q3wks. Continue treatment until a maximum of 16 cycles, disease progression, or unacceptable toxicity occurs. Begin within 4–6 wks post HSCT or upon recovery from HSCT.

cHL (Previously Untreated)

IV infusion: ADULTS, ELDERLY: 1.2 mg/kg (**Maximum:** 120 mg) q2wks (in combination with doxorubicin, vinblastine, and dacarbazine [AVD]). Begin within 1 hr after completion of AVD until a maximum of 12 doses, disease progression, or unacceptable toxicity occurs. CHILDREN 2 YRS AND OLDER: 1.8 mg/kg (**Maximum:** 180 mg) q3wks for a maximum of 5 doses (in combination with doxorubicin, vincristine, etoposide, prednisone, and cyclophosphamide).

sALCL (Relapsed)

IV infusion: ADULTS/ELDERLY: 1.8 mg/kg (**Maximum:** 180 mg) infused over 30 min q3wks. Continue treatment until disease progression or unacceptable toxicity occurs.

sALCL, Peripheral T-Cell Lymphoma (CD30-Expressing), Previously Untreated

IV infusion: ADULTS/ELDERLY: 1.8 mg/kg (**Maximum:** 180 mg) q3wks for 6–8 doses (in combination with cyclophosphamide, DOXOrubicin, and predniSONE).

pcALCL or CD30-Expressing MF
IV infusion: ADULTS/ELDERLY: 1.8 mg/kg (**Maximum:** 180 mg) q3wks for up to 16 cycles until disease progression or unacceptable toxicity.

Dosage in Renal Impairment
CrCl less than 30 mL/min: Avoid use.

Dosage in Hepatic Impairment
Mild impairment: Initial dose 1.2 mg/kg (**Maximum:** 120 mg) q3wks. **Moderate to severe impairment:** Avoid use.

SIDE EFFECTS
◄**ALERT**► Effects present as mild, manageable.
Frequent (52%–22%): Peripheral neuropathy, fatigue, respiratory tract infection, nausea, diarrhea, fever, rash, abdominal pain, cough, vomiting. **Occasional (19%–11%):** Headache, dizziness, constipation, chills, bone/muscle pain, insomnia, peripheral edema, alopecia. **Rare (10%–5%):** Anxiety, muscle spasm, decreased appetite, dry skin.

ADVERSE EFFECTS/TOXIC REACTIONS
Myelosuppression characterized as neutropenia (54% of pts), peripheral neuropathy (52% of pts), thrombocytopenia (28% of pts), anemia (19% of pts) have occurred. Infusion reactions (including anaphylaxis), Stevens-Johnson syndrome have been reported. Tumor lysis syndrome may lead to acute renal failure. Progressive multifocal leukoencephalopathy (changes in mood, confusion, loss of memory, decreased strength or weakness on one side of body, changes in speech, walking, and vision) has been reported.

NURSING CONSIDERATIONS

BASELINE ASSESSMENT
Obtain CBC prior to initiation and before each dosing cycle. Question for evidence of peripheral neuropathy (hypoesthesia, hyperesthesia, paresthesia, burning sensation, neuropathic pain or weakness). Offer emotional support.

INTERVENTION/EVALUATION
Monitor CBC as clinically indicated. Offer antiemetics to control nausea, vomiting. Monitor for hematologic toxicity (fever, sore throat, signs of local infection, bruising, unusual bleeding), symptoms of anemia (excessive fatigue, weakness). Monitor and report nausea, vomiting, diarrhea. Monitor daily pattern of bowel activity, stool consistency. Assess skin for evidence of rash. Pts experiencing new or worsening neuropathy may require a delay, dose change, or discontinuation of treatment.

PATIENT/FAMILY TEACHING
• Treatment may depress immune system response and reduce ability to fight infection. Report symptoms of infection such as body aches, chills, cough, fatigue, fever. Avoid those with active infection. • Report symptoms of bone marrow depression (e.g., bruising, fatigue, fever, shortness of breath, weight loss; bleeding easily, bloody urine or stool). • Do not receive immunizations without physician's approval (drug lowers body resistance). • Report neurologic changes, neuropathy, or stroke-like symptoms (confusion, difficulty speaking, altered gait).

brexpiprazole

brex-**pip**-ra-zole
(Rexulti)

■ **BLACK BOX ALERT** ■ Elderly pts with dementia-related psychosis are at increased risk of death, mainly due to HF, pneumonia. Increased risk of suicidal thoughts and behaviors in pts aged 24 yrs and younger with major depression, other psychiatric disorders.

Do not confuse brexpiprazole with ARIPiprazole, esomeprazole, omeprazole, or pantoprazole, or RABEprazole.

◆**CLASSIFICATION**

PHARMACOTHERAPEUTIC: DOPamine agonist. **CLINICAL:** Second-generation (atypical) antipsychotic agent.

 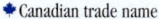

USES

Adjunctive therapy to antidepressants for the treatment of major depressive disorder in adults. Treatment of schizophrenia in adults and pts 13 yrs and older. Treatment of agitation associated with dementia due to Alzheimer's disease. **OFF-LABEL:** Psychosis/agitation associated with dementia (other than Alzheimer's disease).

PRECAUTIONS

Contraindications: Hypersensitivity to brexpiprazole. **Cautions:** Concurrent use of CNS depressants (including alcohol), antihypertensives; disorders in which CNS depression is a feature; cardiovascular or cerebrovascular disease (may induce hypotension), Parkinson's disease, Parkinson's disease dementia, Lewy body dementia, history of seizures or conditions that may lower seizure threshold (Alzheimer's disease). Pts at risk for aspiration pneumonia, elderly, HF, diabetes. Pts at high risk for suicide. Preexisting low WBC/ANC, history of drug-induced leukopenia/neutropenia, dehydration. Potential for cognitive and motor impairment (caution when driving or operating machinery).

ACTION

Provides partial agonist activity at DOPamine and serotonin (5-HT$_1$A) receptors and antagonist activity at serotonin (5-HT$_2$A) receptors. **Therapeutic Effect:** Diminishes schizophrenic, depressive behavior.

PHARMACOKINETICS

Widely distributed. Metabolized in liver. Protein binding: greater than 99%. Peak plasma concentration: 4 hrs. Steady state reached in 10–12 days. Excreted in urine (25%), feces (46%). **Half-life:** 86–91 hrs.

⌛ LIFESPAN CONSIDERATIONS

Pregnancy/Lactation: Unknown if distributed in breast milk. May cause extrapyramidal and/or withdrawal symptoms in neonates if given in third trimester. **Children:** Safety and efficacy not established. **Elderly:** May have increased risk for adverse effects due to age-related hepatic, renal, cardiac disease. May increase risk of death in elderly pts with dementia-related psychosis.

INTERACTIONS

DRUG: **Alcohol** may potentiate cognitive and motor effects. **Strong CYP3A4 inducers (e.g., carBAMazepine, phenytoin, rifAMPin)** may decrease concentration/effect. **Strong CYP3A4 inhibitors (e.g., itraconazole, ketoconazole), strong CYP2D6 inhibitors (e.g., FLUoxetine, PARoxetine)** may increase concentration/effect. **Metoclopramide** may increase adverse effects. **HERBAL:** St John's wort may decrease concentration. **Kava kava, valerian** may increase CNS depression. **FOOD:** None known. **LAB VALUES:** May decrease leukocytes, neutrophils. May increase serum blood glucose, lipid levels.

AVAILABILITY (Rx)

Tablets: 0.25 mg, 0.5 mg, 1 mg, 2 mg, 3 mg, 4 mg.

ADMINISTRATION/HANDLING

PO
• Give without regard to food.

INDICATIONS/ROUTES/DOSAGE

Major Depressive Disorder (MDD)
PO: **ADULTS, ELDERLY:** Initially, 0.5–1 mg once daily. May increase at weekly intervals up to 1 mg (if initial dose is 0.5 mg) once daily, then up to target dose of 2 mg once daily. **Maximum:** 3 mg once daily.

Schizophrenia
PO: **ADULTS, ELDERLY:** Initially, 1 mg once daily on days 1–4. May increase to 2 mg once daily on days 5–7, then to 4 mg once daily on day 8 based on clinical response and tolerability. **Maximum:** 4 mg once daily. **CHILDREN 13 YRS AND OLDER:** Initially, 0.5 mg once daily on days 1–4. On days 5–7, titrate to 1 mg once daily. On day 8, titrate to 2 mg based on clinical response and tolerability. Wkly dose increases can

be made in 1-mg increments to a recommended target dose of 2–4 mg once daily. **Maximum:** 4 mg once daily.

Agitation-Associated Dementia Due to Alzheimer's Disease
PO: ADULTS, ELDERLY: Initially, 0.5 mg once daily on days 1–7. On days 8–14, increase dose to 1 mg once daily, then to 2 mg once daily on day 15. **Maximum:** 3 mg once daily after at least 14 days.

Dosage in Renal Impairment
CrCl less than 60 mL/min: Maximum: 2 mg once daily for MDD, or 3 mg once daily for schizophrenia.

Dosage in Hepatic Impairment
Maximum: 2 mg once daily for MDD, or 3 mg once daily for schizophrenia. **CYP2D6 poor metabolizers or pts taking strong CYP2D6 inhibitors or strong CYP3A4 inhibitors:** Administer half of the usual dose. **CYP2D6 poor metabolizers taking strong/moderate CYP3A4 inhibitors or pts taking strong/moderate CYP2D6 inhibitors with strong/moderate CYP3A4 inhibitors:** Administer a quarter of the usual dose. **Pts taking strong CYP3A4 inducers:** Double the usual dose over 1–2 wks.

SIDE EFFECTS
Occasional (9%–4%): Headache, nasopharyngitis, dyspepsia, akathisia, somnolence, tremor. **Rare (3%–1%):** Constipation, fatigue, increased appetite, weight gain, anxiety, restlessness, dizziness, diarrhea, blurry vision, dry mouth, salivary hypersecretion, abdominal pain, flatulence, myalgia, abnormal dreams, insomnia, hyperhidrosis.

ADVERSE EFFECTS/TOXIC REACTIONS
May increase risk of death in elderly pts with dementia-related psychosis. Most deaths appeared to be cardiovascular (e.g., HF, sudden death) or infectious (e.g., pneumonia) in nature. Increased incidence of suicidal thoughts and behaviors in pts 24 yrs and younger was reported. May increase risk of neuroleptic malignant

syndrome (NMS). Symptoms of NMS may include hyperpyrexia, muscle rigidity, altered mental status, autonomic instability (irregular pulse or blood pressure, tachycardia, diaphoresis, and cardiac dysrhythmia), elevated creatinine, phosphokinase, myoglobinuria (rhabdomyolysis), acute renal failure. Metabolic changes such as hyperglycemia, ketoacidosis, hyperosmolar coma, diabetes, dyslipidemia, dystonia, and weight gain may occur. Other adverse effects may include leukopenia, neutropenia, agranulocytosis, orthostatic hypotension, syncope, cerebrovascular events (e.g., CVA, transient ischemic attack), seizures, hyperthermia, dysphagia, cognitive or motor impairment, tardive dyskinesia.

NURSING CONSIDERATIONS

BASELINE ASSESSMENT
Obtain BMP, capillary blood glucose, vital signs; CBC in pts with preexisting low WBC or history of leukopenia or neutropenia. Receive full medication history and screen for drug interactions. Assess behavior, appearance, emotional state, response to environment, speech pattern, thought content. Correct dehydration, hypovolemia. Assess for suicidal tendencies, history of dementia-related psychosis, HF, CVA, NMS, diabetes.

INTERVENTION/EVALUATION
Monitor weight, BMP, capillary blood glucose, vital signs. Diligently monitor for extrapyramidal symptoms, tardive dyskinesia, hypotension, syncope, cerebrovascular or cardiovascular dysfunction, NMS. Assess for therapeutic response (greater interest in surroundings, improved self-care, increased ability to concentrate, relaxed facial expression).

PATIENT/FAMILY TEACHING
• Avoid alcohol. • Avoid tasks that require alertness, motor skills until response to drug is established. • Report worsening depression, suicidal ideation, abnormal changes in behavior. • Treatment may cause life-threatening conditions such as involuntary, uncontrollable

movements, elevated body temperature, altered mental status, high or low blood pressure, seizures. • Pts with HF or active pneumonia are at increased risk of sudden death. • Immediately report fever, cough, increased sputum production, palpitations, fainting, or signs of HF.

brigatinib

bri-**ga**-ti-nib
(Alunbrig)
Do not confuse brigatinib with axitinib, cabozantinib, ceritinib, crizotinib, erlotinib, imatinib.

◆CLASSIFICATION

PHARMACOTHERAPEUTIC: Anaplastic lymphoma tyrosine kinase inhibitor. **CLINICAL:** Antineoplastic.

USES

First-line treatment of pts with anaplastic lymphoma kinase (ALK)–positive metastatic non–small-cell lung cancer (NSCLC).

PRECAUTIONS

Contraindications: Hypersensitivity to brigatinib. **Cautions:** Baseline cytopenias. History of symptomatic bradycardia, bradyarrhythmias, diabetes, hepatic/renal impairment, hypertension, ocular disease, pancreatitis, pulmonary disease. Concomitant use of strong CYP3A inhibitors, beta blockers, calcium channel blockers (see Interactions).

ACTION

A broad-spectrum kinase inhibitor (activity against EGFR, ALK, ROSI, IGF-1R and FLT-3). Inhibits ALK downstream signaling proteins. Has activity against cells expressing EML4-ALK. **Therapeutic Effect:** Expresses anti-tumor activity against EML-ALK mutant forms shown in NSCLC in pts progressed with crizotinib.

PHARMACOKINETICS

Widely distributed. Metabolized in liver. Protein binding: 66%. Peak plasma concentration: 1–4 hrs. Excreted in feces (65%), urine (25%). **Half-life:** 25 hrs.

⧗ LIFESPAN CONSIDERATIONS

Pregnancy/Lactation: Avoid pregnancy; may cause fetal harm. Females of reproductive potential should use effective nonhormonal contraception during treatment and for at least 4 mos after discontinuation. Unknown if distributed in breast milk. Breastfeeding not recommended during treatment and for at least 1 wk after discontinuation. **Males:** Males with female partners of reproductive potential should use barrier methods during sexual activity during treatment for at least 3 mos after discontinuation. **Children:** Safety and efficacy not established. **Elderly:** No age-related precautions noted.

INTERACTIONS

DRUG: Strong **CYP3A4 inhibitors** (e.g., **clarithromycin, itraconazole, ritonavir**) may increase concentration/effect. Strong **CYP3A4 inducers** (e.g., **carbamazepine, phenytoin, rifampin**) may decrease concentration/effect. **HERBAL:** **St. John's wort** may decrease concentration/effect. **FOOD:** **Grapefruit products** may increase concentration/effect. **LAB VALUES:** May increase serum alkaline phosphatase, ALT, AST, amylase, bilirubin, CPK, glucose, lipase. May decrease Hct, Hgb, lymphocytes, RBCs; serum phosphate. May prolong aPTT.

AVAILABILITY (Rx)

Tablets: 30 mg, 90 mg, 180 mg.

ADMINISTRATION/HANDLING

PO
• Give with or without food. • Administer tablets whole; do not break, crush, cut, or divide. • If a dose is missed or vomiting occurs after administration, do

not give extra dose. Administer next dose at regularly scheduled time.

INDICATIONS/ROUTES/DOSAGE

Non–Small-Cell Lung Cancer (Metastatic, ALK-Positive)

PO: ADULTS, ELDERLY: 90 mg once daily for 7 days. If 90-mg dose is tolerated, then increase to 180 mg once daily. Continue until disease progression or unacceptable toxicity. **Note:** If treatment is interrupted for 14 days (or more) for reasons other than toxic reactions, restart at 90 mg once daily for 7 days before increasing to the dose that was previously tolerated.

Dose Reduction Schedule

First dose reduction: 90 MG ONCE DAILY: Reduce to 60 mg once daily. **180 MG ONCE DAILY:** Reduce to 120 mg once daily. **Second dose reduction: 90 MG ONCE DAILY:** Permanently discontinue. **180 MG ONCE DAILY:** Reduce to 90 mg once daily. **Third dose reduction: 90 MG ONCE DAILY:** N/A. **180 MG ONCE DAILY:** Reduce to 60 mg once daily. **Note:** Once dose has been reduced, do not subsequently increase dose. If pt is unable to tolerate 60-mg dose, permanently discontinue.

Dose Modification

Based on Common Terminology Criteria for Adverse Events (CTCAE).

Symptomatic Bradycardia

Withhold treatment until recovery to asymptomatic bradycardia or to a heart rate of 60 bpm or greater, then resume at reduced dose level (if pt not taking concomitant medications known to cause bradycardia). **Symptomatic bradycardia in pts taking concomitant medications known to cause bradycardia:** Withhold treatment until recovery to asymptomatic bradycardia or heart rate of 60 bpm or greater. If concomitant medication can be adjusted or discontinued, then resume at same dose. If concomitant medication cannot be ad-

justed or discontinued, then resume at reduced dose level. **Life-threatening bradycardia in pts who are not taking concomitant medications known to cause bradycardia:** Permanently discontinue. **Life-threatening bradycardia in pts who are taking concomitant medications known to cause bradycardia:** Withhold treatment until recovery to asymptomatic bradycardia or heart rate of 60 bpm or greater. If concomitant medication can be adjusted or discontinued, then resume at reduced dose level with frequent monitoring. Permanently discontinue if symptomatic bradycardia recurs despite dose reduction.

CPK Elevation

Grade 3 CPK elevation (greater than 5 times upper limit of normal [ULN]): Withhold treatment until recovery to baseline or less than or equal to 2.5 times ULN, then resume at same dose. **Grade 4 CPK elevation (greater than 10 times ULN) or recurrence of Grade 3 CPK elevation:** Withhold treatment until recovery to baseline or less than or equal to 2.5 times ULN, then resume at reduced dose level.

Hyperglycemia

Grade 3 serum glucose elevation (greater than 250 mg/dL or 13.9 mmol/L): If adequate medical management of hyperglycemia cannot be achieved, withhold treatment until adequately controlled. Consider dose reduction or permanent discontinuation.

Hypertension

Grade 3 hypertension (systolic B/P greater than or equal to 160 mm Hg or diastolic B/P greater than or equal to 100 mm Hg); concomitant use of more than one antihypertensive drug; required medical intervention; requirement of aggressive hypertensive therapy: Withhold treatment until recovery to Grade 1 or 0, then resume at reduced dose level. **Grade 4 hypertension (first occur**

✦ Canadian trade name   ◆ Non-Crushable Drug   ▦ High Alert drug

rence) or recurrence of Grade 3 hypertension: Withhold treatment until recovery to Grade 1 or 0, then either resume at reduced dose level or permanently discontinue. **Recurrence of Grade 4 hypertension:** Permanently discontinue.

Lipase/Amylase Elevation
Grade 3 serum amylase or lipase elevation (greater than 2 times upper limit of normal [ULN]): Withhold treatment until recovery to Grade 1 or 0 (or baseline), then resume at same dose. **Grade 4 serum amylase or lipase elevation (greater than 5 times ULN) or recurrence of Grade 3 serum lipase or amylase elevation:** Withhold treatment until recovery to Grade 1 or 0, then resume at reduced dose level.

Pulmonary Toxicity
Grade 1 pulmonary symptoms during the first 7 days of therapy: Withhold treatment until recovery to baseline, then resume at same dose level. Do not increase dose if interstitial lung disease (ILD)/pneumonitis suspected. **Grade 1 pulmonary symptoms after the first 7 days of therapy:** Withhold treatment until recovery to baseline, then resume at same dose level. **Grade 2 pulmonary symptoms during the first 7 days of therapy:** Withhold treatment until recovery to baseline, then resume at reduced dose level. Do not increase dose if ILD/pneumonitis suspected. **Grade 2 pulmonary symptoms after the first 7 days of therapy:** Withhold treatment until recovery to baseline, then resume at same dose level. If ILD/pneumonitis is suspected, resume at reduced dose level. With any recurrence of ILD/pneumonitis or any Grade 3 or 4 pulmonary symptoms, permanently discontinue.

Visual Disturbance
Grade 2 or 3 visual disturbance: Withhold treatment until recovery to baseline, then resume at reduced dose level. **Grade 4 visual disturbance:** Permanently discontinue.

Other Toxicities
Any other Grade 3 toxicity: Withhold treatment until recovery to baseline, then resume at same dose level. **Recurrence of any other Grade 3 toxicity:** Withhold treatment until recovery to baseline, then either resume at reduced dose level or permanently discontinue. **First occurrence of any other Grade 4 toxicity:** Withhold treatment until recovery to baseline, then either resume at reduced dose level or permanently discontinue. **Recurrence of any other Grade 4 toxicity:** Permanently discontinue. **Concomitant use of strong CYP3A inhibitors:** Reduce daily dose by 50% if strong CYP3A inhibitor cannot be discontinued. If strong CYP3A inhibitor is discontinued, then resume the dose that was previously tolerated before starting CYP3A inhibitor.

Dosage in Renal Impairment
Mild to moderate impairment: No dose adjustment. **Severe impairment:** Not specified; use caution.

Dosage in Hepatic Impairment
Mild impairment: No dose adjustment. **Moderate to severe impairment:** Not specified; use caution.

SIDE EFFECTS

Frequent (33%–19%): Nausea, fatigue, headache, dyspnea, vomiting, decreased appetite, diarrhea, constipation. **Occasional (18%–9%):** Cough, abdominal pain, rash (acneiform dermatitis, exfoliative rash, pruritic rash, pustular rash), pyrexia, arthralgia, peripheral neuropathy, muscle spasm, extremity pain, hypertension, back pain, myalgia.

ADVERSE EFFECTS/TOXIC REACTIONS

Anemia, leukopenia are expected responses to therapy. Serious events, such as ILD/pneumonitis (3%–9% of pts), hypertension (6%–21% of pts), symptomatic bradycardia (6%–7% of pts), visual disturbance (blurred vision, diplopia, reduced visual acuity, macular edema, vitreous floaters, visual field defect, vitreous detachment, cataract [7%–10% of pts]), CPK elevation (27%–48% of pts), pancreatic enzyme elevation (27%–39%), hyperglycemia (43% of pts), may occur.

NURSING CONSIDERATIONS

BASELINE ASSESSMENT

Obtain CBC, BMP, LFT; pregnancy test in females of reproductive potential. Obtain baseline ECG in pts with history of arrhythmia, HF. Question plans for breastfeeding. Question history of hepatic/renal impairment, diabetes, cardiac/pulmonary disease, hypertension, pancreatitis. Receive full medication history and screen for interactions. Assess visual acuity. Verify ALK-positive NSCLC test prior to initiation. Obtain nutritional consult. Offer emotional support.

INTERVENTION/EVALUATION

Monitor CBC, CPK, BMP, LFT; vital signs (esp. heart rate) periodically. Obtain serum amylase, lipase in pts with severe abdominal pain, nausea, periumbilical ecchymosis (Cullen's sign), flank ecchymosis (Grey Turner's sign). Monitor for hepatotoxicity, hyperglycemia, vision changes, myalgia, musculoskeletal pain, interstitial lung disease/pneumonitis. If treatment-related toxicities occur, consider referral to specialist; pt may require treatment with corticosteroids. Screen for acute infections. Monitor I&O, hydration status, stool frequency and consistency. Encourage proper calorie intake and nutrition. Assess skin for rash, lesions.

PATIENT/FAMILY TEACHING

• Treatment may depress your immune system and reduce your ability to fight infection. Report symptoms of infection, such as body aches, burning with urination, chills, cough, fatigue, fever. Avoid those with active infection. • Therapy may decrease your heart rate, which may be life threatening; report dizziness, chest pain, palpitations, or fainting. • Worsening cough, fever, or shortness of breath may indicate severe lung inflammation. • Use effective contraception to avoid pregnancy. Do not breastfeed. • Blurry vision, confusion, frequent urination, increased thirst, fruity breath may indicate high blood sugar levels. • Report abdominal pain, bruising around belly button or flank bruising, black/tarry stools, dark-colored urine, decreased urine output, severe muscle aches, yellowing of the skin or eyes. • Do not take newly prescribed medication unless approved by the doctor who originally started treatment. • Do not ingest grapefruit products.

budesonide

bue-**des**-oh-nide
(Eohilia, Ortikos, Pulmicort Flexhaler, Pulmicort, Tarpeyo, Uceris)
Do not confuse budesonide with Budeprion.

FIXED-COMBINATION(S)

Airsupra: budesonide/albuterol (bronchodilator): 80 mcg/90 mcg. **Symbicort:** budesonide/formoterol (bronchodilator): 80 mcg/4.5 mcg, 160 mcg/4.5 mcg. **Symbicort Aerosphere:** budesonide/formoterol: 160 mcg/4.8 mcg.

◆CLASSIFICATION

PHARMACOTHERAPEUTIC: Glucocorticosteroid. **CLINICAL:** Anti-inflammatory, antiallergy.

USES

Nasal: (OTC): Relief of hay fever, other upper respiratory allergies in adults and children 6 yrs and older. **Nebulization, oral inhalation:** Maintenance or prophylaxis therapy for asthma in pts 6 yrs and older (dry powder inhaler) or 12 mos to

---

8 yrs (nebulization). **PO:** Treatment of mild to moderate active Crohn's disease. Maintenance of clinical remission of mild to moderate Crohn's disease. Induction of remission in active, mild to moderate ulcerative colitis. **Eohilia:** Treatment in adults and children 11 yrs and older with eosinophilic esophagitis (EoE). **Tarpeyo:** Reduce proteinuria in adults with primary immunoglobulin A nephropathy (IgAN) at risk of rapid disease progression, generally a urine protein-to-creatinine ratio (UPCR) greater than or equal to 1.5 g/g. **OFF-LA-BEL: PO:** Treatment of eosinophilic esophagitis, autoimmune hepatitis, microscopic colitis. **Nebulization/inhalation:** Treatment of COPD (maintenance), eosinophilic esophagitis.

PRECAUTIONS

Contraindications: Hypersensitivity to budesonide (nebulization/inhalation), primary treatment of status asthmaticus, acute episodes of asthma. Not for relief of acute bronchospasms. **Nasal:** Use in children younger than 6 yrs of age. **Cautions:** Thyroid disease, hepatic impairment, renal impairment, cardiovascular disease, diabetes, glaucoma, cataracts, myasthenia gravis, pts at risk for osteoporosis, seizures, GI disease, post acute MI, elderly.

ACTION

Inhibits accumulation of inflammatory cells; controls rate of protein synthesis; decreases migration of polymorphonuclear leukocytes (reverses capillary permeability and lysosomal stabilization at cellular level). **Therapeutic Effect:** Relieves symptoms of allergic rhinitis, asthma, Crohn's disease.

PHARMACOKINETICS

Form	Onset	Peak	Duration
Pulmicort Respules	2–8 days	4–6 wks	—
Rhinocort Aqua	10 hrs	2 wks	—

Minimally absorbed from nasal tissue; moderately absorbed from inhalation.

Protein binding: 88%. Primarily metabolized in liver. **Half-life:** 2–3 hrs.

⧗ LIFESPAN CONSIDERATIONS

Pregnancy/Lactation: Unknown if drug crosses placenta or is distributed in breast milk. **Children:** Prolonged treatment or high dosages may decrease short-term growth rate, cortisol secretion. **Elderly:** No age-related precautions noted.

INTERACTIONS

DRUG: **Strong CYP3A4 inhibitors (e.g., clarithromycin, ketoconazole, ritonavir)** may increase concentration/effect. **Strong CYP3A4 inducers (e.g., carbamazepine, phenytoin, rifampin)** may decrease concentration/effect. May decrease effect of **aldesleukin.** **HERBAL:** None significant. **FOOD: Grapefruit products** may increase concentration/effect. **LAB VALUES:** May decrease serum potassium.

AVAILABILITY (Rx)

Oral Inhalation Powder: *(Pulmicort Flexhaler):* 90 mcg per inhalation; 180 mcg per inhalation. **Inhalation Suspension for Nebulization:** *(Pulmicort):* 0.25 mg/2 mL; 0.5 mg/2 mL; 1 mg/2 mL. **Nasal Spray:** 32 mcg/spray. **Oral suspension:** 2 mg/10 mL single-dose stick packs.

🦫 **Delayed-Release Capsules:** 3 mg. *(Tarpeyo):* 4 mg. **Extended-Release Capsules:** *(Uceris):* 9 mg. *(Ortikos):* 6 mg, 9 mg.

ADMINISTRATION/HANDLING

Inhalation
• Hold inhaler in upright position to load dose. Do not shake prior to use. Prime prior to first use only. • Place mouthpiece between lips and inhale forcefully and deeply. Do not exhale through inhaler; do not use a spacer. • Rinsing mouth after each use decreases incidence of candidiasis.

Intranasal
• Instruct pt to clear nasal passages before use. • Tilt pt's head slightly for-

ward. • Insert spray tip into nostril, pointing toward nasal passages, away from nasal septum. • Spray into one nostril while pt holds other nostril closed and concurrently inspires through nostril to allow medication as high into nasal passages as possible.

Nebulization
• Shake well before use. • Administer with mouthpiece or face mask. • Rinse mouth following treatment.

PO
• *(Eohilia)* Do NOT mix with food or liquid. • Shake stick pack for at least 10 sec prior to opening. • Administer all of the suspension. Do not allow eating or drinking for 30 min after dose. • Avoid consumption of grapefruit juice for the duration of therapy.
• *(Tarpeyo)* Administer in morning at least 1 hr before a meal. • Administer whole; do not open, crush, or allow chewing. **Capsule, delayed-release particles** • Administer in morning without regard to food. • Administer whole; do not crush or allow chewing (may open and mix with applesauce).
• *(Ortikos)* Administer in morning without regard to food. • Administer whole; do not crush or allow chewing.
• *(Uceris)* Administer in morning without regard to food. • Administer whole; do not crush, break, or allow chewing.

INDICATIONS/ROUTES/DOSAGE

Rhinitis
Intranasal: (Rx): ADULTS, ELDERLY, CHILDREN 6 YRS AND OLDER: 1 spray (32 mcg) in each nostril once daily. **Maximum:** 4 sprays in each nostril once daily for adults and children 12 yrs and older; 2 sprays in each nostril once daily for children 6–11 yrs.

Upper Respiratory Symptoms
Intranasal: (OTC): ADULTS, ELDERLY, CHILDREN 6 YRS AND OLDER: 2 sprays in each nostril once daily. May decrease to 1 spray in each nostril once daily.

Bronchial Asthma
Nebulization: CHILDREN 12 MOS–8 YRS: (Previous therapy with bronchodilators alone): 0.5 mg/day as single dose or 2 divided doses. **Maximum:** 0.5 mg/day. **(Previous therapy with inhaled corticosteroids):** 0.5 mg/day as single dose or 2 divided doses. **Maximum:** 1 mg/day. **(Previous therapy of oral corticosteroids):** 1 mg/day as single dose or 2 divided doses. **Maximum:** 1 mg/day.
Oral inhalation: (Pulmicort Flexhaler): **ADULTS, ELDERLY:** 90–360 mcg 2 times/day. **Maximum:** 720 mcg 2 times/day. **CHILDREN 6 YRS AND OLDER:** 180 mcg 2 times/day. **Maximum:** 360 mcg 2 times/day.

Crohn's Disease
PO (capsule): ADULTS, ELDERLY: 9 mg once daily for up to 8 wks. Recurring episodes may be treated with a repeat 8-wk course of treatment. **Maintenance of remission:** 6 mg once daily for up to 3 mos.

Ulcerative Colitis
PO (tablet): ADULTS, ELDERLY: 9 mg once daily in morning for up to 8 wks.

Reduce Proteinuria
PO: ADULTS, ELDERLY: 16 mg once daily for 9 mos. When discontinuing therapy, reduce dose to 8 mg once daily for the last 2 wks of therapy.

Eosinophilic Esophagitis (EoE)
PO: ADULTS, CHILDREN 11 YRS AND OLDER: 2 mg orally twice daily for 12 wks.

Dosage in Renal/Hepatic Impairment
No dose adjustment.

SIDE EFFECTS

Frequent (greater than 3%): Nasal: Mild nasopharyngeal irritation, burning, stinging, dryness; headache, cough. **Inhalation:** Flu-like symptoms, headache, pharyngitis. **Occasional (3%–1%): Nasal:** Dry mouth, dyspepsia, rebound congestion, rhinorrhea, loss of taste. **Inhalation:** Back pain, vomiting, altered taste, voice changes, abdominal pain, nausea, dyspepsia.

ADVERSE EFFECTS/TOXIC REACTIONS

Acute hypersensitivity reaction (urticaria, angioedema, severe bronchospasm) occurs rarely.

 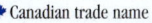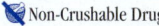

NURSING CONSIDERATIONS

BASELINE ASSESSMENT

Question for hypersensitivity to any corticosteroids, components. Auscultate lung sounds.

INTERVENTION/EVALUATION

Monitor for relief of symptoms. Auscultate lung sounds. Observe proper use of medication delivery device to ensure correct technique.

PATIENT/FAMILY TEACHING

• Improvement noted in 24 hrs, but full effect may take 3–7 days. • Report if no improvement in symptoms or if sneezing, nasal irritation occurs.

bumetanide

bue-**met**-a-nide
(Bumex, Burinex)

■ **BLACK BOX ALERT** ■ Excess dosage can lead to profound diuresis with fluid and electrolyte loss.
Do not confuse bumetanide with Buminate.

◆CLASSIFICATION

PHARMACOTHERAPEUTIC: Loop diuretic. **CLINICAL:** Diuretic.

USES

Management of edema secondary to HF, renal disease, (including nephrotic syndrome), or hepatic disease.

PRECAUTIONS

Contraindications: Hypersensitivity to bumetanide. Anuria, hepatic coma, severe electrolyte depletion (until condition improves or is corrected). **Cautions:** Severe hypersensitivity to sulfonamides; hypotension.

ACTION

Enhances excretion of sodium, chloride, and, to lesser degree, potassium by direct action at ascending limb of loop of Henle and in proximal tubule. **Therapeutic Effect:** Produces diuresis.

PHARMACOKINETICS

Route	Onset	Peak	Duration
PO	30–60 min	60–120 min	4–6 hrs
IV	Rapid	15–30 min	2–3 hrs

Completely absorbed from GI tract (absorption decreased in HF, nephrotic syndrome). Protein binding: 94%–96%. Partially metabolized in liver. Primarily excreted in urine. Not removed by hemodialysis. **Half-life:** 1–1.5 hrs.

⧗ LIFESPAN CONSIDERATIONS

Pregnancy/Lactation: Unknown if drug is distributed in breast milk. **Children:** Safety and efficacy not established. **Elderly:** May be more sensitive to hypotension/electrolyte effects. Increased risk for circulatory collapse or thrombolytic episode. Age-related renal impairment may require reduced or extended dosage interval.

INTERACTIONS

DRUG: Agents inducing hypokalemia (e.g., metOLazone, hydroCHLOROthiazide) may increase risk of hypokalemia. **NSAIDs (e.g., diclofenac, naproxen)** may decrease effect. May increase hyponatremic effect of **desmopressin. HERBAL: Herbals with hypertensive properties (e.g., licorice, yohimbe)** or **hypotensive properties (e.g., garlic, ginger, ginkgo biloba)** may alter effects. **FOOD:** None known. **LAB VALUES:** May increase serum glucose, BUN, uric acid; urinary phosphate. May decrease serum calcium, chloride, magnesium, potassium, sodium.

AVAILABILITY (Rx)

Injection Solution: 0.25 mg/mL. **Tablets:** 0.5 mg, 1 mg, 2 mg.

ADMINISTRATION/HANDLING

💊 IV

Rate of administration • May give undiluted but is compatible with D_5W, 0.9%

NaCl, or lactated Ringer's solution. • Administer IV push over 1–2 min. • May give through Y tube or 3-way stopcock. • May give as continuous infusion. **Storage** • Store at room temperature. • Stable for 24 hrs if diluted.

PO
• Give without regard to food.

▨ IV COMPATIBILITIES

Dexmedetomidine, diltiazem, propofol.

INDICATIONS/ROUTES/DOSAGE

Edema, HF
Note: Maximum recommended dose is 10 mg/day to avoid toxicity.
PO, IV: ADULTS, ELDERLY: Initially, 0.5–1 mg once, then titrate PRN to an effective dose. **Refractory edema; acute decompensation in pts taking PO loop diuretics: IV:** (Bolus/intermittent dosing): Initially, administer 1–2.5 times the total daily oral effective dose, then titrate PRN to an effective dose. **Continuous infusion:** Initially, 0.5–1 mg/hr; if diuretic response is not adequate, repeat IV bolus dose and increase continuous infusion up to 2 mg/hr.

Usual Pediatric Dosage
IV, IM, PO: CHILDREN: 0.01–0.1 mg/kg/dose q6–24h. **Maximum:** 10 mg/day. **NEONATES:** 0.01–0.05 mg/kg/dose q12–48h.

Dosage in Renal/Hepatic Impairment
Use caution; contraindicated in anuria, hepatic coma.

SIDE EFFECTS

Expected: Increased urinary frequency and urine volume. **Frequent (5%):** Muscle cramps, dizziness, hypotension, headache, nausea. **Occasional (3%–1%):** Impaired hearing, pruritus, ECG changes, weakness, hives, abdominal pain, dyspepsia, musculoskeletal pain, rash, nausea, vomiting. **Rare (less than 1%):** Chest pain, ear pain, fatigue, dry mouth, premature ejaculation, impotence, nipple tenderness.

ADVERSE EFFECTS/TOXIC REACTIONS

Vigorous diuresis may lead to profound water and electrolyte depletion, resulting in hypokalemia, hyponatremia, dehydration, coma, circulatory collapse. Ototoxicity manifested as deafness, vertigo, tinnitus may occur, esp. in pts with severe renal impairment or those taking other ototoxic drugs. Blood dyscrasias, acute hypotensive episodes have been reported.

NURSING CONSIDERATIONS

BASELINE ASSESSMENT
Obtain vital signs, esp. B/P for hypotension, before administration. Assess for edema. Observe skin turgor, mucous membranes for hydration status. Initiate I&O, obtain baseline weight.

INTERVENTION/EVALUATION
Continue to monitor B/P, vital signs, electrolytes, I&O, weight. Note extent of diuresis. Watch for changes from initial assessment (hypokalemia may result in muscle weakness, tremor, muscle cramps, altered mental status, cardiac arrhythmias; hyponatremia may result in confusion, thirst, cold/clammy skin).

PATIENT/FAMILY TEACHING
• Expect increased urinary frequency/volume. • Report auditory abnormalities (e.g., sense of fullness in ears, tinnitus). • Eat foods high in potassium such as whole grains (cereals), legumes, meat, bananas, apricots, orange juice, potatoes (white, sweet), raisins. • Rise slowly from sitting/lying position.

buPROPion

bue-**proe**-pee-on
(Aplenzin, Forfivo XL, Wellbutrin SR, Wellbutrin XL)

■ **BLACK BOX ALERT** ■ Increased risk of suicidal thinking and behavior in children, adolescents, young adults 18–24 yrs with major depressive disorder, other psychiatric disorders. Agitation, hostility, depressed mood also reported. Use in smoking cessation may cause serious neuropsychiatric events.

Do not confuse Aplenzin with Relenza, buPROPion with busPIRone, Wellbutrin SR with Wellbutrin XL.

FIXED-COMBINATION(S)

Auvelity: bupropion/dextromethorphan (an NMDA receptor antagonist): 105 mg/45 mg.

◆CLASSIFICATION

PHARMACOTHERAPEUTIC: Dopamine/norepinephrine reuptake inhibitor. **CLINICAL:** Antidepressant, smoking cessation aid.

USES

Treatment of unipolar major depressive disorder (MDD) in adults. Prevention of seasonal MDD in pts with seasonal affective disorder (SAD). Aid to smoking cessation treatment. **OFF-LABEL:** Treatment of ADHD in adults, children. Depression associated with bipolar disorder. SSRI-induced sexual dysfunction.

PRECAUTIONS

Contraindications: Hypersensitivity to buPROPion. Current or prior diagnosis of anorexia nervosa or bulimia, seizure disorder, use of MAO inhibitors (concurrently or within 14 days of discontinuing either bupropion or the MAOI); pts undergoing abrupt discontinuation of alcohol or sedatives. Initiation of buPROPion in pts receiving linezolid or IV methylene blue. **Aplenzin, Forfivo XL, Wellbutrin XL (additional):** Conditions increasing seizure risk, severe head injury, stroke, CNS tumor/infection. **Forfivo XL (additional):** Pts receiving other dosage forms of bupropion. **Cautions:** History of seizure, cranial or head trauma, cardiovascular disease, history of hypertension or coronary artery disease, elderly, pts at high risk for suicide, renal/hepatic impairment. Concurrent

use of antipsychotics, antidepressants, theophylline, steroids, stimulants, hypoglycemic agents, excessive use of alcohol, sedatives/hypnotics, opioids.

ACTION

Blocks reuptake of neurotransmitters, (DOPamine, norepinephrine) at CNS presynaptic membranes. **Therapeutic Effect:** Relieves depression. Eliminates nicotine withdrawal symptoms.

PHARMACOKINETICS

Widely distributed. Protein binding: 84%. Crosses the blood-brain barrier. Metabolized in liver. Primarily excreted in urine. **Half-life:** 14 hrs.

⧗ LIFESPAN CONSIDERATIONS

Pregnancy/Lactation: Unknown if drug crosses placenta or is distributed in breast milk. **Children:** More sensitive to increased dosage, toxicity; increased risk of suicidal ideation, worsening of depression. Safety and efficacy not established. **Elderly:** More sensitive to anticholinergic, sedative, cardiovascular effects. Age-related renal impairment may require dosage adjustment.

INTERACTIONS

DRUG: MAOIs (e.g., **phenelzine, selegiline**) may increase hypertensive effect. May decrease concentration of **tamoxifen.** May increase concentration of **aripiprazole, brexpiprazole, iloperidone, metoclopramide, thioridazine.** May increase adverse effects of **citalopram, vortioxetine. HERBAL: FOOD:** None known. **LAB VALUES:** May decrease WBC.

AVAILABILITY (Rx)

Tablets: 75 mg, 100 mg.

⧗ **Extended-Release Tablets: (24 hr): (Aplenzin):** 174 mg, 348 mg, 522 mg **(Forfivo XL):** 450 mg **(Wellbutrin XL):** 150 mg, 300 mg. **Generic:** 150 mg, 300 mg, 450 mg. **Sustained-Release Tablets: (12 hr): (Wellbutrin SR):** 100 mg, 150 mg, 200 mg.

ADMINISTRATION/HANDLING

PO

• Give without regard to food (give with food if GI irritation occurs). • Tablets should be administered whole; do not crush, divide, or allow chewing. *(Immediate-Release):* Administer 3–4 times daily. Maximum single dose: 150 mg. *(12 hr Extended-Release):* Administer 2 times/day with at least 8 hr between doses. Maximum single dose: 200 mg. *(24 hr Extended-Release):* Administer once daily with at least 24 hr between doses.

INDICATIONS/ROUTES/DOSAGE

MDD

PO: *(Immediate-Release):* **ADULTS, ELDERLY:** Initially, 100 mg twice daily. May increase to 100 mg 3 times/day no sooner than 3 days after beginning therapy. **Maximum:** 150 mg 3 times/day. **PO:** *(Sustained-Release):* **ADULTS, ELDERLY:** Initially, 150 mg/day as a single dose in the morning. May increase to 150 mg twice daily as early as day 4 after beginning therapy. **Maximum:** 400 mg/day in 2 divided doses. Do not exceed 200 mg in a single dose. **PO:** *(Extended-Release):* **ADULTS, ELDERLY:** 150 mg once daily in the morning. May increase to 300 mg once daily as early as day 4. If no clinical improvement after 2 wks, may increase to 450 mg once daily. **Maximum:** 450 mg/day. *(Aplenzin):* Initially, 174 mg once daily in morning; may increase as soon as 4 days to 348 mg/day.

Smoking Cessation

NOTE: Treatment should be initiated before the pt's planned quit day (within the first 2 wks of treatment), while pt is still smoking.
PO: ADULTS, ELDERLY: Initially, 150 mg/day for 3 days, then 150 mg twice daily for 7–12 wks.

SAD

Note: Initiate treatment in autumn before symptom onset; discontinue in early spring with dose tapering.

PO: ADULTS, ELDERLY: *(Wellbutrin XL):* 150 mg/day for 1 wk, then 300 mg/day. *(Aplenzin):* 174 mg once daily. May increase after 1 wk to 348 mg once daily.

Dosage in Renal Impairment

Use caution.

Dosage in Hepatic Impairment

Mild to moderate impairment: Use caution, reduce dosage. **Severe impairment:** Use extreme caution. **Maximum:** *(Aplenzin):* 174 mg every other day. *(Wellbutrin):* 75 mg/day. *(Wellbutrin SR):* 100 mg/day or 150 mg every other day. *(Wellbutrin XL):* 150 mg every other day. *(Zyban):* 150 mg every other day.

SIDE EFFECTS

Frequent (32%–18%): Constipation, weight gain or loss, nausea, vomiting, anorexia, dry mouth, headache, diaphoresis, tremor, sedation, insomnia, dizziness, agitation. **Occasional (10%–5%):** Diarrhea, akinesia, blurred vision, tachycardia, confusion, hostility, fatigue.

ADVERSE EFFECTS/TOXIC REACTIONS

Risk of seizures increases in pts taking more than 150 mg/dose; in pts with history of bulimia, seizure disorders, discontinuing drugs that may lower seizure threshold.

NURSING CONSIDERATIONS

BASELINE ASSESSMENT

Assess psychological status, thought content, suicidal tendencies, appearance. For pts on long-term therapy, hepatic/renal function tests should be performed periodically.

INTERVENTION/EVALUATION

Supervise suicidal-risk pt closely during early therapy and dose changes (as depression lessens, energy level improves, increasing suicide potential). Assess appearance, behavior, speech pattern, level of interest, mood changes.

PATIENT/FAMILY TEACHING

• Full therapeutic effect may be noted in approx. 4 wks. • Avoid tasks that

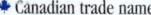

require alertness, motor skills until response to drug is established. • Report signs/symptoms of seizure, worsening depression, suicidal ideation, unusual behavioral changes. • Avoid alcohol. • Do not chew, crush, dissolve, or divide sustained-, extended-release tablets.

busPIRone

bue-**spye**-rone
Do not confuse busPIRone with buPROPion.

◆CLASSIFICATION

PHARMACOTHERAPEUTIC: Nonbarbiturate. **CLINICAL:** Antianxiety.

USES

Management of generalized anxiety disorders. Short-term relief of symptoms of anxiety. **OFF-LABEL:** Shivering (targeted temperature management), unipolar depression (augmentation).

PRECAUTIONS

Contraindications: Hypersensitivity to busPIRone. Concomitant use of MAOIs intended to treat depression or within 14 days of discontinuing MAOIs intended to treat depression. Concomitant use of MAOIs within 14 days of discontinuing buspirone. Initiation of buspirone in pts receiving IV methylene blue or linezolid. **Cautions:** Concurrent use of MAOIs, severe hepatic/renal impairment (not recommended).

ACTION

Binds to serotonin, DOPamine at presynaptic neurotransmitter receptors in CNS. **Therapeutic Effect:** Produces anxiolytic effect.

PHARMACOKINETICS

Widely distributed. Protein binding: 95%. Metabolized in liver. Primarily excreted in urine. Not removed by hemodialysis. **Half-life:** 2–3 hrs.

⏳ LIFESPAN CONSIDERATIONS

Pregnancy/Lactation: Unknown if drug crosses placenta or is distributed in breast milk. **Children:** Safety and efficacy not established. **Elderly:** No age-related precautions noted.

INTERACTIONS

DRUG: CNS depressants (e.g., alcohol, morphine, oxyCODONE, zolpidem) may increase CNS depressant effect. May increase adverse effects of **MAOIs (e.g., phenelzine, selegiline).** May increase serotonergic effects of **SSRIs (e.g., citalopram, FLUoxetine, sertraline). CYP3A4 inhibitors (e.g., erythromycin, ketoconazole)** may increase concentration/effect. **CYP3A4 inducers (e.g., rifAMPin)** may decrease concentration/effect. **HERBAL: Herbals with sedative properties (e.g., chamomile, kava kava, valerian)** may increase CNS depression. **St. John's wort, Yohimbe** may decrease concentration/effect. **FOOD: Grapefruit products** may increase concentration, risk of toxicity. **LAB VALUES:** May produce false-positive urine metanephrine/catecholamine assay test.

AVAILABILITY (Rx)

Tablets: 5 mg, 7.5 mg, 10 mg, 15 mg, 30 mg.

ADMINISTRATION/HANDLING

PO
• Administer in consistent manner regarding food (always with food or always without food).

INDICATIONS/ROUTES/DOSAGE

Anxiety Disorders
PO: ADULTS, ELDERLY: Initially, 10–15 mg/day in 2–3 divided doses. May increase every 2–3 days in increments of 5 mg/day up to a maximum of 60 mg/day. **Usual dose:** 20–30 mg/day in 2–3 divided doses.

Dosage in Renal/Hepatic Impairment
Not recommended in pts with severe hepatic or renal impairment.

B

SIDE EFFECTS

Frequent (12%–6%): Dizziness, drowsiness, nausea, headache. **Occasional (5%–2%):** Nervousness, fatigue, insomnia, dry mouth, light-headedness, mood swings, blurred vision, poor concentration, diarrhea, paresthesia. **Rare:** Muscle pain/stiffness, nightmares, chest pain, involuntary movements.

ADVERSE EFFECTS/TOXIC REACTIONS

No evidence of drug tolerance, psychological or physical dependence, withdrawal syndrome. Overdose may produce severe nausea, vomiting, dizziness, drowsiness, abdominal distention, excessive pupil constriction.

NURSING CONSIDERATIONS

BASELINE ASSESSMENT

Assess degree/manifestations of anxiety. Offer emotional support. Assess motor responses (agitation, trembling, tension), autonomic responses (cold, clammy hands; diaphoresis).

INTERVENTION/EVALUATION

For pts on long-term therapy, CBC, LFT, renal function tests should be performed periodically. Assist with ambulation if drowsiness, dizziness occur. Evaluate for therapeutic response: calm facial expression, decreased restlessness, lessened insomnia, mental status.

PATIENT/FAMILY TEACHING

• Improvement may be noted in 7–10 days, but optimum therapeutic effect generally takes 3–4 wks. • Drowsiness usually disappears during continued therapy. • If dizziness occurs, slowly go from lying to standing. • Avoid tasks that require alertness, motor skills until response to drug is established. • Avoid alcohol, grapefruit products. • Be consistent in taking with regard to food.

C

cabazitaxel

ka-**baz**-i-**tax**-el
(Jevtana)

■ BLACK BOX ALERT ■ All pts should be premedicated with a corticosteroid, an antihistamine, and an H₂ serum antagonist prior to infusion. Severe hypersensitivity reactions have occurred. Immediately discontinue infusion and give appropriate treatment if hypersensitivity reaction occurs. Neutropenic deaths reported. CBC, particularly ANC, should be obtained prior to and during treatment. Do not administer with neutrophil count 1,500 cells/mm³ or less.

Do not confuse cabazitaxel with PACLitaxel or Paxil, or Jevtana with Januvia, Levitra, or Sentra.

◆CLASSIFICATION

PHARMACOTHERAPEUTIC: Microtubule inhibitor. **CLINICAL:** Antineoplastic.

USES

Used in combination with predniSONE for treatment of castration-resistant metastatic prostate cancer previously treated with a DOCEtaxel-containing regimen.

PRECAUTIONS

Contraindications: Hypersensitivity to cabazitaxel. Severe hepatic impairment (total serum bilirubin greater than 3 times upper limit of normal [ULN]). Neutrophil count of 1,500 cells/mm³ or less, history of hypersensitivity to polysorbate 80. **Cautions:** Mild to moderate hepatic impairment (bilirubin equal to or less than 3 times ULN), elderly, pregnancy, renal impairment (CrCl less than 30 mL/min). Pts at risk for developing GI complications (e.g., GI ulceration, concomitant use of NSAIDs).

ACTION

Binds to tubulin to promote assembly into microtubules and inhibits disassembly, which stabilizes microtubules. Inhibits microtubule depolymerization/cell division. **Therapeutic Effect:** Arrests the cell cycle, inhibiting tumor proliferation.

PHARMACOKINETICS

Widely distributed. Metabolized in liver. Protein binding: 89%–92%. Excreted in feces (76%), urine (3.7%). **Half-life:** 95 hrs.

⧗ LIFESPAN CONSIDERATIONS

Pregnancy/Lactation: May cause fetal harm. Crosses placental barrier. Breastfeeding not recommended. **Children:** Safety and efficacy not established. **Elderly:** Pts 65 yrs and older have 5% greater risk of developing neutropenia, fatigue, dizziness, fever, urinary tract infection, dehydration.

INTERACTIONS

DRUG: Strong CYP3A4 inhibitors (e.g., atazanavir, clarithromycin, ketoconazole, ritonavir) may increase concentration/effect; avoid use. Strong CYP3A4 inducers (e.g., carBAMazepine, phenytoin, rifAMPin) may decrease cabazitaxel concentration effects. May decrease concentration/therapeutic effects of **vaccines (live).** May increase concentration/effects of **BCG (intravesical), vaccines (live). HERBAL:** Echinacea may decrease therapeutic effect. **FOOD:** Grapefruit products may increase concentration/effect. **LAB VALUES:** May increase serum bilirubin. May decrease Hgb, Hct, neutrophils, platelets.

AVAILABILITY (Rx)

Injection: 60 mg/1.5 mL.

ADMINISTRATION/HANDLING

◄ ALERT ► Wear gloves during preparation, handling. Two-step dilution process must be performed under aseptic conditions to prepare second (final) infusion solution. Medication undergoes two dilutions. After second dilution, administration should be initiated within 30 min.

Reconstitution • Step 1, first dilution: Each vial of cabazitaxel contains 60 mg/1.5 mL.; must first be mixed with entire contents of supplied diluent. • Once reconstituted, solution contains 10 mg/mL of cabazitaxel. • When transferring diluent, direct needle onto inside vial wall and inject slowly to limit foaming. • Remove syringe and needle, then gently mix initial diluted solution by repeated inversions for at least 45 sec to ensure full mixing of drug and diluent. • Do not shake. • Allow any foam to dissipate. • **Step 2, final dilution:** Withdraw recommended dose and further dilute with 250 mL 0.9% NaCl or D_5W. • If dose greater than 65 mg is required, use larger volume of 0.9% NaCl or D_5W so that concentration of 0.26 mg/mL is not exceeded. • Concentration of final diluted solution should be between 0.10 and 0.26 mg/mL.

Rate of administration • Infuse over 1 hr using in-line 0.22-micron filter.

Storage • Store vials at room temperature. • First dilution solution stable for 30 min. • Final diluted solution stable for 8 hrs at room temperature or 24 hrs if refrigerated.

INDICATIONS/ROUTES/DOSAGE

◀ALERT▶ Antihistamine (dexchlorpheniramine 5 mg, diphenhydrAMINE 25 mg, or equivalent antihistamine), corticosteroid (dexAMETHasone 8 mg or equivalent), and H_2 antagonist (e.g., famotidine) should be given at least 30 min prior to each dose to reduce risk/severity of hypersensitivity.

Metastatic Prostate Cancer
◀ALERT▶ Monitoring of CBC is essential on wkly basis during cycle 1 and before each treatment cycle thereafter so that the dose can be adjusted.
IV infusion: ADULTS, ELDERLY: 20–25 mg/m² given as 1-hr infusion q3wks in combination with predniSONE.

Dose Modification
Grade 3 neutropenia, febrile neutropenia, Grade 3 or persistent diarrhea, neuropathy: Reduce dosage to 20 mg/m² after treatment interruption.

Dosage With Strong CYP3A Inhibitors
Consider dose reduction by 25%.

Dosage in Renal Impairment
CrCl less than 15 mL/min: Use caution.

Dosage in Hepatic Impairment
Mild impairment: 20 mg/m². **Moderate impairment:** 15 mg/m². **Severe impairment:** Contraindicated.

SIDE EFFECTS

Frequent (47%–16%): Diarrhea, fatigue, nausea, vomiting, constipation, esthesia, abdominal pain, anorexia, back pain. **Occasional (13%–5%):** Peripheral neuropathy, fever, dyspnea, cough, arthralgia, dysgeusia, dyspepsia, alopecia, peripheral edema, weight decrease, urinary tract infection, dizziness, headache, muscle spasm, dysuria, hematuria, mucosal inflammation, dehydration.

ADVERSE EFFECTS/TOXIC REACTIONS

Myelosuppression (anemia, neutropenia, thrombocytopenia) is an expected response to therapy, but more severe reactions including severe neutropenia, febrile neutropenia may be life threatening. Hypersensitivity reaction may include generalized rash, erythema, hypotension, bronchospasm. 94% of pts develop Grade 1–4 neutropenia and associated complications including anemia, thrombocytopenia, sepsis. GI abnormalities, hypertension, arrhythmias, renal failure may occur.

NURSING CONSIDERATIONS

BASELINE ASSESSMENT
Obtain ANC, CBC, BMP, LFT, serum testosterone. Assess ANC, CBC prior to each infusion. Question history of hypersensitivity reaction; renal/hepatic impairment; intolerance to corticosteroids. Receive full medication history and screen for interactions.

INTERVENTION/EVALUATION
Monitor CBC, ANC on wkly basis during cycle 1 and before each treatment cycle thereafter; do not administer if ANC less than 1,500 cells/mm³. Monitor serum ALT, AST, renal function. Monitor for hypersensitivity reaction (rash, erythema, dyspnea). Encourage adequate fluid intake. Monitor daily pattern of bowel activity, stool consistency. Offer antiemetics if nausea, vomiting occur. Closely monitor for signs/symptoms of neutropenia.

C

PATIENT/FAMILY TEACHING

• Treatment may depress your immune system and reduce your ability to fight infection. Report symptoms of infection such as body aches, burning with urination, chills, cough, fatigue, fever. Avoid those with active infection. • Report symptoms of bone marrow depression (e.g., bruising, fatigue, fever, shortness of breath, weight loss; bleeding easily, bloody urine or stool). • Report fever, chills, persistent sore throat, unusual bruising/bleeding, pale skin, fatigue. • Avoid tasks that require alertness, motor skills until response to drug is established. • Maintain strict oral hygiene. • Do not have immunizations without physician approval (drug lowers body's resistance). • Avoid those who have received a live virus vaccine. • Avoid grapefruit products. • Diarrhea may cause dehydration; drink plenty of fluids.

cabotegravir/ rilpivirine

ka-boe-**teg**-ra-vir/ril-pi-**vir**-een
(Cabenuva)
Do not confuse cabotegravir with cabozantinib, dolutegravir, elvitegravir, or raltegravir; or rilpivirine with etravirine.

◆ CLASSIFICATION

PHARMACOTHERAPEUTIC: Integrase strand transfer inhibitor (INSTI), non-nucleoside reverse transcriptase inhibitor (NNRTI). **CLINICAL:** Antiretroviral agent (anti-HIV).

USES

Treatment of HIV-1 infection in adults and adolescents 12 yrs of age and older and weighing at least 35 kg to replace the current antiretroviral regimen in pts who are virologically suppressed (HIV-1 RNA less than 50 copies/mL) on a stable antiretroviral regimen with no history of treatment failure and with no known or suspected resistance to either cabotegravir or rilpivirine.

PRECAUTIONS

Contraindications: Hypersensitivity to cabotegravir or rilpivirine. Concomitant use of carBAMazepine, oxcarbazepine, PHENobarbital, phenytoin; rifabutin, rifAMPin; rifapentine; dexAMETHasone, St. John's wort. **Cautions:** Hepatic/renal impairment, psychiatric disorders (e.g., depression, psychosis, suicidal ideation). Concomitant use of other antiretrovirals is not recommended.

ACTION

Cabotegravir inhibits HIV integrase by blocking strand transfer of retroviral DNA integration (essential for HIV replication cycle). Rilpivirine blocks noncompetitive HIV-1 reverse transcriptase (does not inhibit DNA polymerases). **Therapeutic Effect:** Interferes with HIV replication, slowing progression of HIV infection.

PHARMACOKINETICS

Widely distributed. Cabotegravir metabolized by enzymatic activity via glucuronidation. Rilpivirine metabolized in liver. Protein binding: 99% (or greater). Peak plasma concentration: (cabotegravir): 7 days; (rilpivirine): 3–4 days. Cabotegravir excreted in feces (59%), urine (27%). Rilpivirine excreted in feces (85%), urine (6%). **Half-life:** (cabotegravir): 5.6–11.5 wks; (rilpivirine): 13–28 wks. Cabotegravir and rilpivirine can remain in systemic circulation for up to 12 mos after discontinuation.

⧗ LIFESPAN CONSIDERATIONS

Pregnancy/Lactation: Unknown if distributed in breast milk. Breastfeeding not recommended due to risk of postnatal HIV transmission. **Children:** Safety and efficacy not established in pts younger than 12 yrs or weighing less than 35 kg. **Elderly:** Safety and efficacy not established.

INTERACTIONS

DRUG: Strong CYP3A4 inducers (e.g., **carBAMazepine, phenytoin, rifAMPin)**

may decrease concentration/effect; use contraindicated. **DexAMETHasone** (more than 1 dose) may decrease concentration/effect of rilpivirine. **Macrolide antibiotics (e.g., azithromycin, clarithromycin)** may increase concentration/effect of rilpivirine; may increase risk of torsade de pointes. **HERBAL:** St. John's wort may decrease concentration/effect. **FOOD:** None known. **LAB VALUES:** May increase serum ALT, AST, bilirubin, creatine phosphokinase, lipase.

AVAILABILITY (Rx)

Injection Suspension, Long-Acting (Co-Packaged Kit): cabotegravir 400 mg/2 mL (200 mg/mL) with rilpivirine 600 mg/2 mL (300 mg/mL), cabotegravir 600mg/3 mL (200 mg/mL) with rilpivirine 900 mg/3 mL (300 mg/mL).

ADMINISTRATION/HANDLING

Intramuscular

Note: Initiate treatment on the last day of current antiretroviral therapy (with or without an oral lead-in of cabotegravir and rilpivirine according to manufacturer guidelines). Cabotegravir and rilpivirine must be given at the same appointment by a healthcare professional. May give up to 7 days before or after scheduled injections. If a dose is missed, see manufacturer guidelines for recommendations.

Preparation • Remove vials from refrigerator and allow suspension to warm to room temperature (approx. 15 min). • Visually inspect for particulate matter or discoloration (brown tinted glass may impair inspection). Cabotegravir suspension should appear white to light pink. Rilpivirine suspension should appear white to off-white. • Shake vials well until suspension is uniform. Small air bubbles may be present. • Transfer suspension into supplied syringes (see manufacturer guidelines).

Administration • Insert each needle intramuscularly into separate gluteal sites at least 2 cm apart or on opposite sides and inject suspension(s). Do not give IV or SQ. • Do not inject into areas of active skin disease or injury such as sunburns,

skin rashes, inflammation, skin infections, or active psoriasis.

Storage • Refrigerate vials in original carton until time of use. Do not freeze. • Vials warmed to room temperature may remain in carton for up to 6 hrs. Do not return to refrigerator. • Suspension-filled syringes may be stored at room temperature for up to 2 hrs. Do not refrigerate.

INDICATIONS/ROUTES/DOSAGE

Note: For gluteal IM administration only.
HIV-1 Infection

IM: ADULTS, CHILDREN 12 YRS AND OLDER WEIGHING AT LEAST 35 KG: Monthly regimen: Initially, 600 mg (cabotegravir) and 900 mg (rilpivirine) once on the last day of current antiretroviral therapy, then continue with injections of 400 mg (cabotegravir) and 600 mg (rilpivirine) monthly thereafter. **Every 2-mo regimen:** Initially, (on the last day of current antiretroviral therapy), 600 mg (cabotegravir) and 900 mg (rilpivirine) once monthly for 2 consecutive mos, then 600 mg (cabotegravir) and 900 mg (rilpivirine) q2 mos thereafter (begin 2 mos after last initiation injection).

Dose Modification

Switching Regimen from Monthly to Every 2 mos: Give 600 mg (cabotegravir) and 900 mg (rilpivirine) once 1 mo after last maintenance dose, then continue same dose q2mos. **Switching Regimen from Every 2 mos to Monthly:** Give 400 mg (cabotegravir) and 600 mg (rilpivirine) once 2 mos after last maintenance dose, then continue same dose monthly.

Dosage in Renal Impairment

Mild to moderate impairment: No dose adjustment. **Severe impairment:** Recommend increased monitoring for adverse effects/toxic reactions. Recommend increased monitoring for adverse effects/toxic reactions. **ESRD:** Not specified; use caution.

Dosage in Hepatic Impairment

Mild to moderate impairment: No dose adjustment. **Severe impairment:** Not specified; use caution.

C

SIDE EFFECTS

Frequent (83%): Injection site reactions (pain/discomfort, nodules, induration, swelling, erythema, pruritus, bruising/discoloration, warmth, hematoma). **Occasional (8%–5%):** Pyrexia, fatigue, malaise, asthenia. **Rare (4% to less than 2%):** Headache, musculoskeletal pain, myalgia, nausea, insomnia, somnolence, rash, abdominal pain, weight gain, anxiety, abnormal dreams.

ADVERSE EFFECTS/TOXIC REACTIONS

Hypersensitivity reactions, including angioedema, dyspnea, hepatitis; severe rash that is accompanied by blisters, fatigue, fever, muscle and joint pain, oral lesions may occur. Serious postinjection reactions (abdominal cramping, agitation, bronchospasm, chest or back pain, dizziness, flushing, oral numbness, sweating) reported in less than 1% of pts. Hepatotoxicity may occur in pts with or without prior hepatic impairment. Drug reaction with eosinophilia and systemic symptoms (DRESS), also known as multiorgan hypersensitivity, has been reported. DRESS may present as facial swelling, eosinophilia, fever, lymphadenopathy, rash, which may involve other organ systems, such as hepatitis, hematologic abnormalities, myocarditis, nephritis. May increase risk of suicidal behavior and ideation. Other psychological disorders may include depression, dysphoria, irritability, mood swings.

NURSING CONSIDERATIONS

BASELINE ASSESSMENT

Obtain LFT, CD4+ count, viral load, HIV-1 RNA level; pregnancy test in females of reproductive potential. Pts should be carefully selected for treatment and must agree to comply with the required dosing schedule. Advise pts that noncompliance may cause drug resistance and viral rebound. Question history of hepatic/renal impairment; psychiatric disorder, suicidal ideation and behavior. Receive full medication history (including herbal products) and screen for contraindications/interactions. Concomitant use of other medications may need to be adjusted or discontinued.

INTERVENTION/EVALUATION

Monitor CD4+ count, viral load, HIV-1 RNA level for treatment effectiveness. Monitor LFT for hepatic injury (bruising, jaundice, right upper abdominal pain, nausea, vomiting, weight loss). Cough, dyspnea, fever, excess band cells on CBC may indicate acute infection (WBC may be unreliable in pts with uncontrolled HIV infection). Diligently assess for suicidal ideation and behavior; new-onset or worsening of anxiety, depression, mood disorder. Consult mental health professional if mood disorder is suspected. Monitor for hypersensitive reactions, serious injection reactions, symptoms of DRESS.

PATIENT/FAMILY TEACHING

• Treatment does not cure HIV infection or reduce risk of transmission. Practice safe sex with barrier methods or abstinence. • Drug resistance or viral rebound can form if treatment is interrupted; do not miss scheduled injection appointments. • As immune system strengthens, it may respond to dormant infections hidden within the body. Report any new fever, chills, body aches, cough, night sweats, shortness of breath. • Report symptoms of drug-induced hypersensitivity syndrome (e.g., fever, swollen face/lymph nodes, skin rash/peeling/inflammation). • Seek immediate medical attention if thoughts of suicide, new-onset or worsening of anxiety, depression, or changes in mood occurs. • There is a high risk of interactions with other medications. Do not take newly prescribed medications unless approved by prescriber who originally started therapy. Do not take herbal products, esp. St John's wort. • Breastfeeding not recommended. • Report liver problems (abdominal pain, bruising, clay-colored stool, amber or dark-colored urine, yellowing of the skin or eyes), rash. • Severe allergic reactions may occur. Seek immediate medical attention if difficulty breathing, dizziness, fast heart rate, itching, hives, rash; swelling of the face, lips, or tongue occurs.

cabozantinib

ka-boe-**zan**-ti-nib
(Cabometyx, Cometriq)

◆ CLASSIFICATION

PHARMACOTHERAPEUTIC: Tyrosine kinase inhibitor. **CLINICAL:** Antineoplastic.

USES

Renal cell carcinoma (RCC): Treatment of advanced RCC as monotherapy. Treatment of advanced RCC as a first-line treatment in combination with nivolumab. **Hepatocellular carcinoma (HCC):** Treatment of HCC in adults previously treated with sorafenib. **Differentiated thyroid cancer (DTC):** Treatment of adults and children 12 yrs of age and older with locally advanced or metastatic DTC that has progressed following prior VEGFR-targeted therapy and who are radioactive iodine refractory or ineligible. **Medullary thyroid cancer (MTC):** Treatment of progressive, metastatic MTC.

PRECAUTIONS

Contraindications: Hypersensitivity to cabozantinib. **Cautions:** Baseline cytopenias, hepatic impairment, thyroid dysfunction; recent surgery or dental procedures, open wounds, chronic electrolyte imbalance, dehydration, hypertension; recent history of hemorrhagic events, hemoptysis.

ACTION

Inhibits tyrosine kinase activity in tumor cells. Inhibits cell migration, proliferation, survival, and angiogenesis (new blood vessel formation). **Therapeutic Effect:** Inhibits tumor cell growth and metastasis.

PHARMACOKINETICS

Widely distributed. Metabolized in liver. Protein binding: 99%. Peak plasma concentration: 3–4 hrs. Excreted in feces (54%), urine (27%). **Half-life:** 99 hrs.

⏳ LIFESPAN CONSIDERATIONS

Pregnancy/Lactation: Avoid pregnancy; may cause fetal harm. Females of reproductive potential must use effective contraception during treatment and for at least 4 months after discontinuation. Unknown if distributed in breast milk. Breastfeeding not recommended during treatment and for at least 4 months after discontinuation. May impair fertility in both females and males. **Children:** Safety and efficacy not established in pts younger than 12 yrs. **Elderly:** No age-related precautions noted.

INTERACTIONS

DRUG: Strong **CYP3A4 inhibitors (e.g., clarithromycin, ketoconazole, ritonavir)** may increase concentration/effect. Strong **CYP3A4 inducers (e.g., carBAMazepine, phenytoin, rifAMPin)** may decrease concentration/effect. **HERBAL:** St John's wort may decrease effect. **FOOD:** Grapefruit products may increase concentration/effect. **High-fat meals** may increase absorption/exposure. **LAB VALUES:** May decrease lymphocytes, neutrophils, platelets; serum albumin, calcium, magnesium, phosphorus, potassium, sodium. May increase serum alkaline phosphatase, ALT, AST, bilirubin, lipase, TSH, urine protein.

AVAILABILITY (Rx)

Cabometyx (Tablets): 20 mg, 40 mg, 60 mg.
Cometriq (Capsules): 20 mg, 80 mg.

ADMINISTRATION/HANDLING

PO
• Give on empty stomach only; do not eat for at least 2 hrs before and at least 1 hr after taking. • Give with water. • Administer capsules whole; do not break, cut, dissolve, or divide. Do not crush tablets.

 Canadian trade name   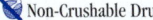 Non-Crushable Drug   🔴 High Alert drug

C

INDICATIONS/ROUTES/ DOSAGES

Note: Do not substitute capsules with tablets.

Metastatic Medullary Thyroid Cancer (Progressive)
PO: *(Cometriq):* ADULTS, ELDERLY: 140 mg once daily.

Dose Reduction Schedule (Cometriq)
Previously Taking 140 mg Daily Dose: Reduce to 100 mg daily. **Previously Taking 100 mg Daily Dose:** Reduce to 60 mg daily. **Previously Taking 60 mg Daily Dose:** If tolerated, resume at same dose. If not tolerated, permanently discontinue.

Dose Modification (Cometriq)
Based on Common Terminology Criteria for Adverse Events (CTCAE).

Hematological/Non-hematological Reactions
Grade 4 Hematological Reactions; Grade 3 or 4 Nonhematological Reactions; Intolerable Grade 2 Reactions; Osteonecrosis of the Jaw: Withhold treatment until improved to Grade 1 or 0 (or baseline), then resume at reduced dose per dose reduce schedule.

Concomitant Use of Strong CYP3A4 Inhibitors
If use of strong CYP3A4 inhibitor is unavoidable, reduce daily dose by 40 mg. If strong CYP3A inhibitor is discontinued for 2–3 days, may resume previous cabozantinib dose taken before use of strong CYP3A inhibitor.

Concomitant Use of Strong CYP3A4 Inducer
If use of strong CYP3A4 inducer is unavoidable, increase daily dose by 40 mg. If strong CYP3A inducer is discontinued for 2–3 days, may resume previous cabozantinib dose taken before use of strong CYP3A inducer. Do not exceed 180 mg daily.

Hepatocellular Carcinoma
PO: *(Cabometyx):* ADULTS, ELDERLY: 60 mg once daily. Continue until disease progression or unacceptable toxicity.

Renal Cell Carcinoma
PO: *(Cabometyx):* ADULTS, ELDERLY: 60 mg once daily. Continue until disease progression or unacceptable toxicity. **In combination with nivolumab:** 40 mg daily with nivolumab 240 mg q2wks or 480 mg q4wks. Continue until disease progression or unacceptable toxicity.

Differentiated Thyroid Cancer
PO: *(Cabometyx):* ADULTS, CHILDREN 12 YRS AND OLDER WITH BSA GREATER THAN OR EQUAL TO 1.2 m²: 60 mg once daily until disease progression or unacceptable toxicity. BSA LESS THAN 1.2 m²: 40 mg once daily until disease progression or unacceptable toxicity.

Dose Reduction Schedule (Cabometyx)
Previously Taking 60 mg Daily Dose: Reduce to 40 mg daily. **Previously Taking 40 mg Daily Dose:** Reduce to 20 mg daily. **Previously Taking 20 mg Daily Dose:** Reduce to 20 mg every other day. **Previously Taking Lowest Dose:** If tolerated, resume at same dose. If lowest dose is not tolerated, permanently discontinue.

Dose Modification (Cabometyx)
Based on Common Terminology Criteria for Adverse Events (CTCAE).

Diarrhea
Grade 2–4 Diarrhea: Withhold treatment until improved to Grade 1 or 0, then resume at reduced dose.

Hepatotoxicity (in Combination with Nivolumab)
Note: Consider treating hepatotoxicity with corticosteroid therapy.
Serum Alt or Ast 3–10 Times Upper Limit of Normal (Uln) with Total Bilirubin Less Than 2 Times Uln: Withhold cabozantinib and nivolumab until improved to Grade 1 or 0, then rechallenge with cabozantinib and/or nivolumab. **Serum Alt or Ast Greater Than 10 Times Uln; Serum Alt or Ast Greater Than 3 Times Uln with Total Bilirubin 2 Times Uln or Greater:** Permanently discontinue cabozantinib and nivolumab.

Hypertension, Hypertensive Crisis
Grade 3 Hypertension: Withhold treatment until improved to Grade 2 or less, then resume at reduced dose. **Grade 4 Hypertension; Uncontrolled Hypertension:** Permanently discontinue.

Osteonecrosis of the Jaw (ONJ)
Any Grade ONJ: Withhold treatment until completely resolved, then resume at reduced dose.

Palmar-Plantar Erythrodysesthesia (PPES)
Intolerable Grade 2 or 3 Ppes: Withhold treatment until improved to grade 1 or 0, then resume at reduced dose.

Proteinuria
Grade 2 or 3 Proteinuria: Withhold treatment until improved to Grade 1 or 0, then resume at reduced dose. Permanently discontinue if nephrotic syndrome occurs.

Any Other Adverse Reactions
Intolerable Grade 2 Adverse Reaction; Grade 3 or 4 Adverse Reaction: Withhold treatment until improved to Grade 1 or 0 (or baseline), then resume at reduced dose.

Concomitant Use of Strong CYP3A4 Inhibitors
If use of strong CYP3A4 inhibitor is unavoidable, reduce daily dose by 20 mg. If strong CYP3A inhibitor is discontinued for 2–3 days, may resume previous cabozantinib dose taken before use of strong CYP3A inhibitor.

Concomitant Use of Strong CYP3A4 Inducer
If use of strong CYP3A4 inducer is unavoidable, increase daily dose by 20 mg. If strong CYP3A inducer is discontinued for 2–3 days, may resume previous cabozantinib dose taken before use of strong CYP3A inducer.

Discontinuation of Treatment
Permanently discontinue treatment for Grade 3 or 4 hemorrhage, GI perforation (any grade), Grade 4 fistula, acute myocardial infarction (any grade), Grade 2–4 cerebral infarction, Grade 3 or 4 arterial thromboembolic events, Grade 4 venous thromboembolic events, reversible posterior leukoencephalopathy syndrome.

Dosage in Renal Impairment
Mild to moderate impairment: No dose adjustment. **Severe impairment:** Use caution.

Dosage in Hepatic Impairment
(Cabometyx): **Mild impairment:** No dose adjustment. **Moderate impairment:** For children with BSA less than 1.2 m^2, reduce starting dose of 60 mg once daily to 40 mg once daily or 40 mg once daily to 20 mg once daily. **Severe impairment:** Not recommended. **(Cometriq):** **Mild to moderate impairment:** Reduce to 80 mg once daily. **Severe impairment:** Not recommended.

SIDE EFFECTS

Frequent (63%–34%): Diarrhea, stomatitis, weight loss, decreased appetite, nausea, fatigue, oral pain, dysgeusia. **Occasional (27%–7%):** Constipation, abdominal pain, vomiting, asthenia, dysphonia, dry skin, headache, alopecia, dizziness, arthralgia, dysphagia, muscle spasms, erythema, dyspepsia, anxiety, musculoskeletal pain, paresthesia, peripheral neuropathy, hyperkeratosis.

ADVERSE EFFECTS/TOXIC REACTIONS

Myelosuppression (anemia, leukopenia, lymphopenia, neutropenia, thrombocytopenia) is an expected response to therapy. Thyroid dysfunction, mainly hypothyroidism, reported in 19% of pts. GI perforation reported in 1% of pts. Hemorrhagic events reported in 5% of pts. Hepatotoxicity, adrenal insufficiency reported in pts receiving concomitant nivolumab therapy. Malignant hypertension may occur despite continued medical management. Thromboembolic events including venous/arterial thromboembolism, cerebral infarction, MI have been reported. May cause ineffective wound healing or wound dehiscence requiring medical intervention. Osteonecrosis of the

---

✦ Canadian trade name   🦋 Non-Crushable Drug   🔲 High Alert drug

jaw may present as mandibular pain, jaw bone erosion, periodontal/gingival infection or ulceration, osteomyelitis, slow healing of the mouth after dental procedures. Palmar-plantar erythrodysesthesia syndrome (PPES), a chemotherapy-induced skin condition that presents as redness, swelling, numbness, skin sloughing of the hands and feet, may occur. Reversible posterior leukoencephalopathy syndrome (RPLS) reported in less than 1% of pts. Proteinuria may indicate nephrotic syndrome.

NURSING CONSIDERATIONS

BASELINE ASSESSMENT

Obtain CBC with differential, BMP, LFT, pregnancy test in females of reproductive potential; vital signs. Assess for recent surgeries, dental procedures. Obtain negative urine pregnancy before initiating treatment. Receive full medication history, including herbal products. Question history of hypertension, hepatic impairment, thyroid dysfunction, hemorrhagic events, thromboembolic events such as CVA, DVT, MI, pulmonary embolism. Assess for open wounds, skin lesions.

INTERVENTION/EVALUATION

Monitor CBC, serum electrolytes, urinalysis. Routinely assess vital signs and report any change in B/P. Persistent diastolic hypertension may indicate hypertensive crisis. Obtain ECG for palpitations, chest pain. RPLS should be considered in pt with seizure, headache, visual disturbances, confusion, altered mental status. Assess hydration status. Encourage fluid intake. Immediately report melena, abdominal pain, hematemesis (may indicate GI perforation), bleeding of any kind. Monitor for symptoms of DVT (leg or arm pain/swelling), CVA (aphasia, altered mental status, headache, hemiplegia, vision loss); MI (chest pain, dyspnea, syncope, diaphoresis, arm/jaw pain), pulmonary embolism (chest pain, dyspnea, tachycardia). Monitor skin for poor healing of chronic wounds, new skin lesions. Monitor for osteonecrosis of the jaw. Monitor daily bowel activity and stool consistency.

PATIENT/FAMILY TEACHING

• Treatment may depress the immune system and reduce the ability to fight infection. Report symptoms of infection such as body aches, burning with urination, chills, cough, fatigue, fever. Avoid those with active infection. • There is a high risk of interactions with other medications. Do not take newly prescribed medications unless approved by prescriber who originally started therapy. • Report liver problems (abdominal pain, bruising, clay-colored stool, amber or dark colored urine, yellowing of the skin or eyes), toxic skin reactions (sloughing, rash, poor healing of wounds), thyroid dysfunction (fatigue, goiter, weight gain), toxic skin reactions (sloughing, rash, poor healing of wounds), jaw pain or oral lesions; bleeding of any kind. • Neurologic changes, including blurry vision, confusion, headache, one-sided weakness, seizures, trouble speaking, may indicate high blood pressure crisis or stroke. • Posterior reversible encephalopathy syndrome, a dysfunction of the brain that may cause a stroke or bleeding in the brain, may occur. • Use effective contraception to avoid pregnancy. Do not breastfeed. Fertility may be impaired. • Treatment may cause life-threatening arterial blood clots; report symptoms of heart attack (chest pain, difficulty breathing, jaw pain, nausea, pain that radiates to the arm or jaw, sweating), stroke (blindness, confusion, one-sided weakness, loss of consciousness, trouble speaking, seizures), lung embolism (difficulty breathing, chest pain, rapid heart rate). • Immediately report severe or persistent abdominal pain, bloody stool, fever; may indicate tear in GI tract. • Notify physician before any planned surgeries or dental procedures. • Do not ingest grapefruit products. • Do not take with food. Do not eat at least 2 hrs before or 1 hr after any dose. • Severe diarrhea may lead to dehydration; drink plenty of fluids.

calcium acetate

(Eliphos, PhosLo)

calcium carbonate

(Apo-Cal ✿, Caltrate 600 ✿, OsCal ✿, Titralac, Tums)

calcium chloride

(Cal-Citrate, Citracal, Osteocit ✿)

calcium glubionate

calcium gluconate

kal-si-um
Do not confuse Citracal with Citrucel, OsCal with Asacol, or PhosLo with Prosom.

◆CLASSIFICATION

PHARMACOTHERAPEUTIC: Electrolyte replenisher. **CLINICAL:** Antacid, antihypocalcemic, antihyperkalemic, antihypermagnesemic, antihyperphosphatemic.

USES

Parenteral (calcium chloride): Treatment of hypocalcemia and conditions secondary to hypocalcemia (e.g., seizures, arrhythmias), emergency treatment of severe hypermagnesemia; **(calcium gluconate):** Treatment of hypocalcemia and conditions secondary to hypocalcemia (e.g., seizures, arrhythmias). **Calcium carbonate:** Antacid, dietary supplement. **Calcium acetate:** Controls hyperphosphatemia in end-stage renal disease. **OFF-LABEL Calcium chloride:** Calcium channel blocker overdose, severe hyperkalemia, malignant arrhythmias associated with hypermagnesemia.

PRECAUTIONS

Contraindications: Hypersensitivity to calcium formulation. **All preparations:** Cal-

cium-based renal calculi, hypercalcemia, ventricular fibrillation. **Calcium chloride:** Digoxin toxicity. **Calcium gluconate: Neonates:** Concurrent IV use with cefTRIAXone. **Cautions:** Chronic renal impairment, hypokalemia, concurrent use with digoxin.

ACTION

Essential for function, integrity of nervous, muscular, skeletal systems. Plays an important role in normal cardiac/renal function, respiration, blood coagulation, cell membrane and capillary permeability. Assists in regulating release/storage of hormones/neurotransmitters. Neutralizes/reduces gastric acid (increases pH). **Calcium acetate:** Binds with dietary phosphate, forming insoluble calcium phosphate. **Calcium chloride, calcium gluconate:** Moderates nerve and muscle performance by regulating action potential excitation threshold. **Therapeutic Effect:** Replaces calcium in deficiency states; controls hyperphosphatemia in end-stage renal disease; relieves heartburn, indigestion.

PHARMACOKINETICS

Moderately absorbed from small intestine (absorption depends on presence of vitamin D metabolites, pH). Primarily eliminated in feces.

⧖ LIFESPAN CONSIDERATIONS

Pregnancy/Lactation: Distributed in breast milk. Unknown whether calcium chloride or calcium gluconate is distributed in breast milk. **Children:** Risk of extreme irritation, possible tissue necrosis or sloughing with IV calcium preparations. Restrict IV use due to small vasculature. **Elderly:** Oral absorption may be decreased.

INTERACTIONS

DRUG: Hypercalcemia may increase **digoxin** toxicity. Oral form may decrease absorption of **bisphosphonates (e.g., risedronate), calcium channel blockers (e.g., amLODIPine, dilTIAZem, verapamil), tetracycline derivatives, thyroid products. HERBAL:** None signifi-

---

✿ Canadian trade name   ▼ Non-Crushable Drug   🄷🄰 High Alert drug

cant. **FOOD:** **Food** may increase calcium absorption. **LAB VALUES:** May increase serum pH, calcium, gastrin. May decrease serum phosphate, potassium.

AVAILABILITY (Rx)

Calcium Acetate (667 mg = 169 mg calcium)
Capsules: 667 mg. **Tablets:** *(Eliphos):* 667 mg.

Calcium Carbonate (1 g = 400 mg calcium)
Tablets: 500 mg, 600 mg, 1,250 mg, 1,500 mg. **Tablets (Chewable):** 500 mg, 750 mg, 1,000 mg.

Calcium Chloride
Injection Solution: 10% (100 mg/mL) equivalent to 27.2 mg elemental calcium per mL.

Calcium Gluconate (1 g = 93 mg calcium)
Injection Solution: 10%.

ADMINISTRATION/HANDLING

 IV

Dilution: *(Calcium Chloride):* May give undiluted (in emergency situations) or dilute 1 g with 100 mL 0.9% NaCl. *(Calcium Gluconate):* May give undiluted or may dilute 1–2 g with 100 mL 0.9% NaCl or D5W.
Rate of administration: *(Calcium Chloride):* **Note:** Rapid administration may produce bradycardia, metallic/chalky taste, hypotension, sensation of heart, peripheral vasodilation. • **IV push:** Infuse slowly at maximum rate of 100 mg/min (in cardiac arrest, may administer over 10–20 sec). • **IV infusion:** Dilute to maximum final concentration of 20 mg/mL and infuse over 1 hr or no faster than 45–90 mg/kg/hr. Give via a central line. Do **NOT** use scalp, small hand or foot veins. Stop infusion if pt complains of pain or discomfort. *(Calcium Gluconate):* **Note:** Rapid administration may produce vasodilation, hy-

potension, arrhythmias, syncope, cardiac arrest. • **IV push:** Infuse slowly over 3–5 min or at maximum rate of 200 mg/min (in cardiac arrest, may administer over 10–20 sec). • **IV infusion:** Dilute 1–2 g in 100 mL 0.9% NaCl or D5W and infuse over 1 hr.
Storage • Store at room temperature. • Once diluted, stable for 24 hrs at room temperature.

PO
(Calcium Acetate): Administer with meals. *(Calcium Carbonate):* Administer with meals. Instruct pt to thoroughly chew chewable tablets before swallowing.

🔳 IV INCOMPATIBILITIES
Calcium chloride: propofol.

🔳 IV COMPATIBILITIES
Calcium chloride: Amiodarone, dobutamine, milrinone. **Calcium gluconate:** Amiodarone, clevidipine, heparin, potassium chloride, propofol.

INDICATIONS/ROUTES/DOSAGE

Hyperphosphatemia
PO: *(Calcium Acetate):* **ADULTS, ELDERLY:** Initially, 1,334 mg 3 times/day with meals. May increase gradually (q2–3wks) to decrease serum phosphate level to less than 6 mg/dL as long as hypercalcemia does not develop. **Usual dose:** 1,334–2,001 mg with each meal.

Hypocalcemia
IV: *(Calcium Chloride):* **ADULTS, ELDERLY:** 1 g diluted in 100 mL D5W or 0.9% NaCl. Infuse via central line over 10–20 min. Do not exceed 100 mg/min except in emergency situations. **CHILDREN, NEONATES:** 10–20 mg/kg/dose, repeat q4–6h, if needed. **IV:** *(Calcium Gluconate):* **ADULTS, ELDERLY:** **(Mild):** 1–2 g over 60 min. May repeat after 10–60 min.

Antacid

PO: *(Calcium Carbonate):* ADULTS, ELDERLY: 1–4 tabs as needed. **Maximum:** 8,000 mg/day. CHILDREN 12 YRS AND OLDER: 1,000–3,000 mg for up to 2 wks. **Maximum:** 7,500 mg/day. CHILDREN 6–11 YRS: 800 mg/day for up to 2 wks. **Maximum:** 2,400 mg/day. CHILDREN 2–5 YRS: 400 mg/day for up to 2 wks. **Maximum:** 1,200 mg/day.

Supplement

PO: *(Calcium Carbonate):* ADULTS, ELDERLY: 500 mg–4 g/day in 1–3 divided doses. CHILDREN OLDER THAN 4 YRS: 750 mg 3 times/day. CHILDREN 2–4 YRS: 750 mg 2 times/day. *(Calcium Citrate):* ADULTS, ELDERLY: 0.5–2 g 2–4 times/day. CHILDREN: 45–65 mg/kg/day in 4 divided doses.

Dosage in Renal/Hepatic Impairment
No dose adjustment.

SIDE EFFECTS

Frequent: PO: Chalky taste. **Parenteral:** Pain, rash, redness, burning at injection site; flushing, nausea, vomiting, diaphoresis, hypotension. **Occasional: PO:** Mild constipation, fecal impaction, peripheral edema, metabolic alkalosis (muscle pain, restlessness, slow respirations, altered taste). **Calcium carbonate:** Milk-alkali syndrome (headache, decreased appetite, nausea, vomiting, unusual fatigue). **Rare:** Urinary urgency, painful urination.

ADVERSE EFFECTS/TOXIC REACTIONS

Hypercalcemia: Early signs: Constipation, headache, dry mouth, increased thirst, irritability, decreased appetite, metallic taste, fatigue, weakness, depression. **Later signs:** Confusion, drowsiness, hypertension, photosensitivity, arrhythmias, nausea, vomiting, painful urination.

NURSING CONSIDERATIONS

BASELINE ASSESSMENT

Assess B/P, ECG and cardiac rhythm, renal function, serum magnesium, phosphate, calcium, ionized calcium.

INTERVENTION/EVALUATION

Monitor BMP, serum ionized calcium, magnesium, phosphate; B/P, cardiac rhythm, renal function. Monitor for signs of hypercalcemia.

PATIENT/FAMILY TEACHING
• Do not take within 1–2 hrs of other oral medications, fiber-containing foods. • Avoid excessive use of alcohol, tobacco, caffeine.

canagliflozin

kan-a-gli-**floe**-zin
(Invokana)
Do not confuse canagliflozin with bexagliflozin, dapagliflozin, empagliflozin, or ertugliflozin.

FIXED-COMBINATION(S)

Invokamet: canagliflozin/metFORMIN (an antidiabetic): 50 mg/500 mg, 50 mg/1,000 mg, 150 mg/500 mg, 150 mg/1,000 mg.

◆CLASSIFICATION

PHARMACOTHERAPEUTIC: Sodium-glucose cotransporter 2 (SGLT2) inhibitor. **CLINICAL:** Antidiabetic.

USES

Adjunctive treatment to diet and exercise to improve glycemic control in pts with type 2 diabetes mellitus; risk reduction of major cardiovascular events (cardiovascular death, nonfatal MI, and nonfatal stroke) in adults with type 2 diabetes and established CV disease; reduce risk of end-stage kidney disease, doubling of serum creatinine, cardiovascular death,

---

and hospitalization for HF in pts with type 2 diabetes mellitus and diabetic nephropathy with albuminuria.

PRECAUTIONS

Contraindications: Hypersensitivity to canagliflozin; pts on dialysis. **Cautions:** Concomitant use of loop diuretics, other hypoglycemic agents (e.g., insulin, insulin secretagogues), baseline systolic hypotension, renal impairment, hypovolemia/dehydration, pts at risk for lower leg amputation (diabetic foot ulcers, peripheral vascular disease); recent genital mycotic infection; pts at risk for diabetic ketoacidosis (insulin dose reduction, acute febrile illness, reduced calorie intake, surgery, alcohol abuse, history of pancreatitis). Not recommended in pts with active bladder cancer, diabetic ketoacidosis, type 1 diabetes mellitus, mild to moderate renal impairment when used for glycemic control.

ACTION

Inhibits SGLT2 in proximal renal tubule, reducing reabsorption of filtered glucose from tubular lumen and lowering renal threshold for glucose. Reduces reabsorption of sodium and increases delivery of sodium to the distal tubule. **Therapeutic Effect:** Increases urinary excretion of glucose; lowers serum glucose levels. Reduces cardiac preload and afterload; downregulates sympathetic activity.

PHARMACOKINETICS

Widely distributed. Metabolized in liver. Peak plasma concentration: 1–2 hrs. Protein binding: 99%. Excreted in feces (42%), urine (33%). **Half-life:** 11–13 hrs.

⌛ LIFESPAN CONSIDERATIONS

Pregnancy/Lactation: Not recommended during second or third trimester. Unknown if distributed in breast milk. Breastfeeding not recommended. **Children:** Safety and efficacy not established. **Elderly:** May have increased risk for adverse reactions (e.g., hypotension, syncope, dehydration).

INTERACTIONS

DRUG: May increase concentration effects of **digoxin, hypoglycemic-associated agents (e.g., glyBURIDE), insulins, loop diuretics (e.g., furosemide).** May decrease concentration of **lithium.** **HERBAL:** Herbals with hypoglycemic properties (e.g., fenugreek, flaxseed, ginseng, gotu kola) may increase risk of hypoglycemia. **FOOD:** None known. **LAB VALUES:** May increase serum low-density lipoprotein-cholesterol (LDL-C), Hgb, creatinine, magnesium, phosphate, potassium. May decrease glomerular filtration rate. Expected to result in positive urine glucose test. May interfere with 1,5-anhydrogluitol (1,5-AG) assay.

AVAILABILITY (Rx)

Tablets: 100 mg, 300 mg.

ADMINISTRATION/HANDLING

PO

• May give without regard to food. Recommended before the first meal of the day.

INDICATIONS/ROUTES/DOSAGE

Type 2 Diabetes Mellitus
PO: ADULTS/ELDERLY: 100 mg daily before first meal. May increase to 300 mg daily after 4–12 wks if further treatment needed to achieve glycemic goals.

Atherosclerotic Cardiovascular Disease
PO: ADULTS, ELDERLY: 100–300 mg once daily.

Diabetic Kidney Disease
PO: ADULTS, ELDERLY: 100 mg once daily prior to the first meal of day in pts with urinary albumin excretion greater than 300 mg/day. No further dose titration is necessary.

Dose Modification
Concomitant use of insulin, insulin secretagogue Consider lowering dose of insulin or insulin secretagogue to reduce hypoglycemic events.
Concomitant Use of UGT Inducers (e.g., Rifampin, Phenytoin, Ritonavir)
eGFR 60 mL/min or greater: Increase dose to 200 mg once daily in pts

taking concurrent 100-mg dose. May increase dose to 300 mg once daily in pts tolerating 200-mg dose who require additional glycemic control. **eGFR less than 60 mL/min:** Increase dose to 200 mg once daily in pts taking concurrent 100 mg dose. Consider additional anti-hyperglycemic agents who require additional glycemic control.

Dosage in Renal Impairment
GFR 30–59 mL/min: 100 mg daily (maximum). **GFR less than 30 mL/min:** Initiation of therapy not recommended. (Pts established on canagliflozin may continue 100 mg once daily).

Dosage in Hepatic Impairment
No dose adjustment.

SIDE EFFECTS
Occasional (5%): Increased urination. **Rare (3%–2%):** Thirst, nausea, constipation.

ADVERSE EFFECTS/TOXIC REACTIONS
May increase risk of lower limb amputations. Symptomatic hypotension (orthostatic hypotension, postural dizziness, syncope) may occur, esp. in pts who are elderly, use concomitant loop diuretics, or have baseline systolic hypotension. Intravascular volume depletion/contraction may cause acute kidney injury requiring dialysis. Fatal cases of ketoacidosis were reported. Hypoglycemic events were reported in pts using concomitant insulin, insulin secretagogues. Infections including influenza, nasopharyngitis, pyelonephritis, urosepsis, UTI, genital mycotic infections (male and female), upper respiratory tract infection may occur. Necrotizing fasciitis of the perineum (Fournier's gangrene), a life-threatening necrotizing infection of the genital and perineum region that requires urgent surgical intervention, has been reported. An increased risk of bone fracture was reported. Hypersensitivity reactions including anaphylaxis, angioedema, urticaria have occurred.

NURSING CONSIDERATIONS

BASELINE ASSESSMENT
Obtain BUN, serum creatinine, eGFR, CrCl, blood glucose level, Hgb A1c; B/P. Assess hydration status. Correct volume depletion before initiation. Assess pt's understanding of diabetes management, routine home glucose monitoring. Obtain dietary consult for nutritional education. Question history of renal impairment, type 1 diabetes, ketoacidosis. Screen for risks of lower limb amputation (e.g., peripheral vascular disease, diabetic foot ulcers). In pts requiring surgery, consider suspending treatment at least 3 days before surgery.

INTERVENTION/EVALUATION
Monitor BUN, serum creatinine, eGFR, CrCl, blood glucose level, Hgb A1c; B/P periodically. Monitor for ketoacidosis (e.g., dehydration, confusion, extreme thirst, sweet-smelling breath, Kussmaul respirations, nausea), hypoglycemia (anxiety, confusion, diaphoresis, diplopia, dizziness, headache, hunger, perioral numbness, tachycardia, tremors), hyperglycemia (fatigue, Kussmaul respirations, polyphagia, polyuria, polydipsia, nausea, vomiting). Pts presenting with metabolic acidosis should be screened for ketoacidosis, regardless of serum glucose levels. Concomitant use of beta blockers (e.g., carvedilol, metoprolol) may mask symptoms of hypoglycemia. Monitor for acute kidney injury (dark-colored urine, flank pain, decreased urine output, muscle aches), infections (cough, fatigue, fever), urinary tract infections (dysuria, fever, flank pain, malaise), mycotic infections, Fournier's gangrene (perineal necrosis). Screen for glucose-altering conditions (fever, increased activity or stress, surgical procedures). Monitor weight, I&Os. Monitor for hypersensitivity reactions (anaphylaxis, angioedema, urticaria). Diligently monitor for new leg ulcers, sores, pain; wound may lead to amputation.

PATIENT/FAMILY TEACHING

• Diabetes mellitus requires lifelong control. Diet and exercise are principal parts of treatment; do not skip or delay meals. Test blood sugar regularly. Monitor daily calorie intake. • When taking combination drug therapy or when glucose conditions are altered (excessive alcohol ingestion, insufficient carbohydrate intake, hormone deficiencies, critical illness), have a low blood sugar treatment available (e.g., glucagon, oral dextrose). • Genital itching or discharge may indicate yeast infection. • Report symptoms of perineal necrosis (e.g., discoloration, pain, swelling of the scrotum, penis, or perineum). • Therapy may increase risk for dehydration, low blood pressure, which may cause kidney failure. Report decreased urination, amber-colored urine, flank pain, fatigue, swelling of the hands or feet. Drink enough fluids to maintain adequate hydration. Pts with HF should be cautious of overhydration. • Report symptoms of UTI, kidney infection (back pain, pelvic pain, burning while urinating, cloudy or foul-smelling urine), allergic reactions (difficulty breathing, rash, wheezing; swelling of the face or tongue). • Go slowly from lying to standing. • Do not breastfeed. • Treatment may cause loss of limbs; immediately report new leg ulcers, pain, tenderness.

---

capecitabine `TOP 100` `HIGH ALERT`

kap-e-**sye**-ta-bine
(Xeloda)

■ **BLACK BOX ALERT** ■ May increase anticoagulant effect of warfarin. Fatal hemorrhagic events have occurred.

Do not confuse capecitabine with decitabine or emtricitabine, or Xeloda with Xenical.

◆CLASSIFICATION

PHARMACOTHERAPEUTIC: Antimetabolite. **CLINICAL:** Antineoplastic.

USES

Colorectal cancer: Adjuvant treatment of Stage III colon cancer as a single agent or as a component of a combination chemotherapy regimen. Perioperative treatment of locally advanced rectal cancer as a component of chemo-radiotherapy. Treatment of unresectable or metastatic colorectal cancer as a single agent or as a component of a combination chemotherapy. **Breast cancer:** Treatment of advanced or metastatic breast cancer as a single agent if an anthracycline- or taxane-containing chemotherapy is not indicated. Treatment of advanced or metastatic breast cancer in combination with DOCEtaxel after disease progression on prior anthracycline-containing chemotherapy. **Gastric, esophageal, or gastroesophageal junction cancer:** Treatment of unresectable or metastatic gastric, esophageal, or gastroesophageal junction cancer as a component of combination chemotherapy. Treatment of HER2-overexpressing metastatic gastric or gastroesophageal junction adenocarcinoma in pts who have not received prior treatment for metastatic disease. **Pancreatic cancer:** Adjuvant treatment of pancreatic adenocarcinoma as a component of a combination chemotherapy. **OFF-LABEL:** Anal carcinoma, biliary tract cancer (advanced/adjuvant), breast cancer (adjuvant, triple egative), gastric cancer (adjuvant), head/neck cancer, neuroendocrine tumors, ovarian cancer, pancreatic cancer (locally advanced or metastatic), small bowel adenocarcinoma.

PRECAUTIONS

Contraindications: Severe renal impairment (CrCl less than 30 mL/min), dihydropyrimidine dehydrogenase (DPD) deficiency, hypersensitivity to capecitabine, 5-fluorouracil (5-FU). **Cautions:** Existing bone marrow depression, hepatic impairment, mild to moderate renal impairment, previous cytotoxic therapy/radiation therapy, elderly (60 yrs of age or older).

ACTION

Enzymatically converted to 5-fluorouracil (5-FU). Inhibits enzymes necessary for synthesis of essential cellular components. **Therapeutic Effect:** Inhibits thymidylate synthetase; blocks methylation of deoxyuridylic acid to thymidylic acid, interfering with DNA, RNA synthesis. Specific for the G_1 and S phases of the cell cycle.

PHARMACOKINETICS

Widely distributed. Protein binding: less than 60%. Metabolized in liver. Primarily excreted in urine. **Half-life:** 45 min.

⧖ LIFESPAN CONSIDERATIONS

Pregnancy/Lactation: May cause fetal harm. Unknown if distributed in breast milk. **Children:** Safety and efficacy not established. **Elderly:** May be more sensitive to GI side effects.

INTERACTIONS

DRUG: May increase concentration, toxicity of **warfarin. Bone marrow depressants** may increase myelosuppressive effect. May decrease concentration/therapeutic effects of **vaccines (live).** May increase levels/effects of **BCG (intravesical), vaccines (live). Allopurinol** may decrease concentration/effect. **HERBAL: Echinacea** may decrease therapeutic effect. **FOOD:** None known. **LAB VALUES:** May increase serum alkaline phosphatase, bilirubin, ALT, AST. May decrease Hgb, Hct, WBC. May increase PT/INR.

AVAILABILITY (Rx)

Tablets: 150 mg, 500 mg.

ADMINISTRATION/HANDLING

• Give within 30 min after meals with water. • Administer at approximately the same time each day (12 hrs apart). Administer whole (do not cut, crush or allow chewing).

INDICATIONS/ROUTES/DOSAGE

Colon Cancer
PO: ADULTS, ELDERLY: Adjuvant treatment: (single agent): 1,250 mg/m² twice daily for the first 14 days of each 21-day cycle for a maximum of eight cycles. **(In combination with oxaliplatin-containing regimens):** 1,000 mg/m² twice daily for the first 14 days of each 21-

day cycle for a maximum of eight cycles. **Perioperative treatment: (with radiation therapy):** 825 mg/m² twice daily. **(Without radiation therapy):** 1,250 mg/m² twice daily. **Unresectable or metastatic: (single agent):** 1,250 mg/m² twice daily for the first 14 days of each 21-day cycle until disease progression or unacceptable toxicity. **(In combination with oxaliplatin):** 1,000 mg/m² twice daily for the first 14 days of each 21-day cycle until disease progression or unacceptable toxicity.

Breast Cancer, Advanced or Metastatic
PO: ADULTS, ELDERLY: (Single agent): 1,000 mg/m² or 1,250 mg/m² twice daily for the first 14 days of each 21-day cycle until disease progression or unacceptable toxicity. **(In combination with DOCETaxel):** 1,000 mg/m² or 1,250 mg/m² twice daily for the first 14 days of a 21-day cycle until disease progression or unacceptable toxicity.

Gastric, Esophageal, or Gastroesophageal Junction Cancer
PO: ADULTS, ELDERLY: Unresectable or metastatic: 625 mg/m² twice daily on days 1–21 of each 21-day cycle for a maximum of eight cycles (in combination with platinum-containing chemotherapy) **OR** 850 mg/m² or 1,000 mg/m² twice daily for the first 14 days of each 21-day cycle until disease progression or unacceptable toxicity (in combination with oxaliplatin). **HER2-overexpressing metastatic adenocarcinoma of the gastroesophageal junction or stomach:** 1,000 mg/m² twice daily for the first 14 days of each 21-day cycle until disease progression or unacceptable toxicity (in combination with CISplatin and trastuzumab).

Pancreatic Cancer
PO: ADULTS, ELDERLY: 830 mg/m² twice daily for the first 21 days of each 28-day cycle for maximum of six cycles (in combination with gemcitabine).

Dosage in Renal Impairment
CrCl 51–80 mL/min: No adjustment. **CrCl 30–50 mL/min:** 75% of normal dose. **CrCl less than 30 mL/min:** Contraindicated.

Dosage in Hepatic Impairment

No dose adjustment at start of therapy; interrupt therapy for Grade 3 or 4 hyperbilirubinemia until bilirubin is 3 times ULN or less.

SIDE EFFECTS

Frequent (55%–25%): Diarrhea, nausea, vomiting, stomatitis, fatigue, anorexia, dermatitis. **Occasional (24%–10%):** Constipation, dyspepsia, headache, dizziness, insomnia, edema, myalgia, pyrexia, dehydration, dyspnea, back pain. **Rare (less than 10%):** Mood changes, depression, sore throat, epistaxis, cough, visual abnormalities.

ADVERSE EFFECTS/TOXIC REACTIONS

Serious reactions include myelosuppression (neutropenia, thrombocytopenia, anemia), cardiovascular toxicity (angina, cardiomyopathy, DVT), respiratory toxicity (dyspnea, epistaxis, pneumonia), lymphedema. Palmar-plantar erythrodysesthesia syndrome (PPES), presenting as redness, swelling, numbness, skin sloughing of hands and feet, may occur.

NURSING CONSIDERATIONS

BASELINE ASSESSMENT

Assess sensitivity to capecitabine or 5-fluorouracil. Obtain baseline Hgb, Hct, serum chemistries, renal function. Offer emotional support.

INTERVENTION/EVALUATION

Monitor for severe diarrhea, nausea, vomiting; if dehydration occurs, fluid and electrolyte replacement therapy should be initiated. Assess hands/feet for PPES. Monitor CBC for evidence of bone marrow depression. Monitor renal/hepatic function. Monitor for blood dyscrasias (fever, sore throat, signs of local infection, unusual bruising/bleeding from any site), symptoms of anemia (excessive fatigue, weakness).

PATIENT/FAMILY TEACHING

• Report nausea, vomiting, diarrhea, hand-and-foot syndrome, stomatitis. • Do not have immunizations without physician's approval (drug lowers body's resistance).

• Avoid contact with those who have recently received live virus vaccine. • Promptly report fever higher than 100.5°F, sore throat, signs of local infection, unusual bruising/bleeding from any site.

capivasertib

cap-**eye**-va-**ser**-tib
(Truqap)
Do not confuse capivasertib with baricitinib, cabozantinib, or certinib.

◆CLASSIFICATION

PHARMACOTHERAPEUTIC: Kinase inhibitor. **CLINICAL:** Antineoplastic.

USES

In combination with fulvestrant, for treatment of adults with hormone receptor (HR)-positive, human epidermal growth factor receptor 2 (HER2)-negative, locally advanced or metastatic breast cancer with one or more *PIK3CA/AKT1/PTEN* alterations following progression on at least one endocrine-based regimen in the metastatic setting or recurrence on or within 12 mos of completing adjuvant therapy.

PRECAUTIONS

Contraindications: Hypersensitivity to capivasertib. **Cautions:** Baseline cytopenias, renal impairment, pts at risk for hyperglycemia (e.g., diabetes, chronic use of corticosteroids), diabetic ketoacidosis (insulin dose reduction, acute febrile illness, surgery, alcohol abuse). Avoid concomitant use of strong or moderate CYP3A inhibitors or inducers.

ACTION

Inhibits phosphorylation/activation of downstream serine/threonine-protein (AKT) kinase substrates, blocking upstream signaling pathways of ATK1 and PIK3CA mutations, and PTEN alterations. **Therapeutic Effect:** Inhibits tumor growth.

PHARMACOKINETICS

Widely distributed. Metabolized in liver. Protein binding: 22%. Peak plasma concentration: 1–2 hrs. Steady-state reached by third and fourth dose of each week, starting week 2. Excreted in feces (50%), urine (45%). **Half-life:** 8.3 hrs.

⧗ LIFESPAN CONSIDERATIONS

Pregnancy/Lactation: Avoid pregnancy; may cause fetal harm. Females of reproductive potential should use effective contraception during treatment and for at least 1 mo after discontinuation. Unknown if distributed in breast milk. Breastfeeding not recommended. **Males:** Males with female partners of reproductive potential should use effective contraception during treatment and for at least 4 mos after discontinuation. **Children:** Safety and efficacy not established. **Elderly:** May have increased risk of grade 3–5 reactions, dose reductions, or permanent discontinuation.

INTERACTIONS

DRUG: **Strong CYP3A4 inhibitors (e.g., clarithromycin, ketoconazole, ritonavir), moderate CYP3A4 inhibitors (e.g., dilTIAZem, fluconazole, verapamil)** may increase concentration/effect. **Strong CYP3A4 inducers (e.g., carBAMazepine, phenytoin, riFAMPin), moderate CYP3A4 inducers (e.g., dexamethasone, modafinil, nafcillin)** may decrease concentration/effect. **HERBAL:** **St. John's wort** may decrease concentration/effect. **FOOD:** None known. **LAB VALUES:** May increase serum ALT, creatinine, glucose, triglycerides; urine protein. May decrease Hgb, leukocytes, lymphocytes, neutrophils, platelets; serum calcium, potassium. May decrease eGFR.

AVAILABILITY (Rx)

Tablets: 160 mg, 200 mg.

ADMINISTRATION/HANDLING

PO
• Give without regard to food. • Administer tablet whole; do not break, crush, or divide. Tablet cannot be chewed. Do not give if tablet is broken, cracked, or not intact. • If vomiting occurs after administration, give next dose at the regularly scheduled time (do not give additional dose). • If a dose is missed by more than 4 hrs, skip the dose and resume at the next regularly scheduled time.

INDICATIONS/ROUTES/DOSAGE

Note: Administer a luteinizing hormone-releasing hormone agonist (e.g., leuprolide) for males or for premenopausal and perimenopausal females per clinical guidelines.

Breast Cancer (HR-Positive, HER2-Negative, Locally Advanced or Metastatic)

PO: **ADULTS, ELDERLY:** 400 mg twice daily (in combination with fulvestrant) for 4 days, followed by 3 days off each week. Continue until disease progression or unacceptable toxicity.

Dose Reduction Schedule for Adverse Events

First dose reduction: 320 mg twice daily for 4 days, followed by 3 days off each week. **Second dose reduction:** 200 mg twice daily for 4 days, followed by 3 days off each week. **Unable to tolerate 200 mg dose:** Permanently discontinue.

Dose Modification

Based on Common Terminology Criteria for Adverse Events (CTCAE).

Diarrhea

Grade 2: Withhold treatment until improved to grade 1 or 0. If recovery occurs in 28 days or less, resume at same dose or reduced dose. If recovery occurs in 29 days or more, resume at reduced dose. If grade 2 diarrhea recurs, reduce dose. **Grade 3:** Withhold treatment until improved to grade 1 or 0. If recovery occurs in 28 days or less, resume at same dose or reduced dose. If recovery occurs in 29 days or more, permanently discontinue. **Grade 4:** Permanently discontinue.

Hyperglycemia

Fasting glucose level greater than upper limit of normal (ULN) to 160

mg/dL (or greater than ULN to 8.9 mmol/L); Hgb A1c greater than 7%: Consider starting or increasing oral antidiabetic treatment. **Fasting glucose level 161–250 mg/dL (or 9–13.9 mmol/L):** Withhold treatment until fasting glucose level improves to 160 mg/dL (or 8.9 mmol/L) or less. If recovery occurs in 28 days or less, resume at same dose. If recovery occurs in 29 days or more, resume at reduced dose. **Fasting glucose level 251–500 mg/dL (or 14–27.8 mmol/L):** Withhold treatment until fasting glucose level improves to 160 mg/dL (or 8.9 mmol/L) or less. If recovery occurs in 28 days or less, resume at reduced dose. If recovery does not occur within 28 days, permanently discontinue. **Fasting glucose level greater than 500 mg/dL (or greater than 27.8 mmol/L); life-threatening sequela of hyperglycemia at any fasting glucose level:** Permanently discontinue treatment if persists greater than 24 hrs. If fasting glucose level is less than 500 mg/dL (or greater than 87.8 mmol/L) within 24 hrs, follow guidance according to relevant grade.

Other Adverse Reactions
Other grade 2 reactions: Withhold treatment until improves to grade 1 or 0, then resume at same dose. **Other grade 3 reactions:** Withhold treatment until improved to grade 1 or 0. If recovery occurs in 28 days or less, resume at same dose. If recovery occurs in 29 days or more, resume at reduced dose. **Other grade 4 reactions:** Permanently discontinue.

Skin Toxicity
Grade 2 cutaneous reactions: Withhold treatment until improves to grade 1 or 0, then resume at same dose. If grade 2 cutaneous reactions persist or recur, reduce dose. **Grade 3:** Withhold treatment until improves to grade 1 or 0. If recovery occurs in 28 days or less, resume at same dose. If recovery occurs in 29 days or more, resume at reduced dose. If grade 3 cutaneous reactions recur, permanently discontinue. **Grade 4:** Permanently discontinue.

Concomitant Use of CYP3A4 Inhibitor
If strong or moderate CYP3A inhibitor cannot be avoided, reduce capivasertib dose to 320 mg twice daily for 4 days, followed by 3 days off each week. If strong or moderate CYP3A inhibitor is discontinued for 3–5 half-lives, resume capivasertib dose prior to use of CYP3A inhibitor.

Dosage in Renal Impairment
Mild to moderate impairment: No dose adjustment. **Severe impairment:** Not specified; use caution.

Dosage in Hepatic Impairment
Mild impairment: No dose adjustment. **Moderate impairment:** No dose adjustment. However, an increase of clinical monitoring is recommended. **Severe impairment:** Not specified; use caution.

SIDE EFFECTS

Frequent (77%–38%): Diarrhea, nausea, stomatitis, vomiting, fatigue. **Occasional (19%–17%):** Hyperglycemia, decreased appetite, headache.

ADVERSE EFFECTS/TOXIC REACTIONS

Severe hyperglycemia, including ketoacidosis, may occur. Severe diarrhea may cause dehydration, electrolyte imbalance, renal injury. Grade 3 or 4 diarrhea reported in 9% of pts. Cutaneous reactions, including erythema multiform, palmar-plantar erythrodysesthesia, may occur. Drug reaction with eosinophilia and systemic symptoms (DRESS), also known as multiorgan hypersensitivity, has been reported. DRESS may present with facial swelling, eosinophilia, fever, lymphadenopathy, and rash, which may be associated with other organ systems, such as hepatitis, hematological abnormalities, myocarditis, nephritis. Renal injuries, including acute kidney injury, renal failure, renal impairment, may occur. Urinary tract infections (UTI) reported in 14 % of pts.

NURSING CONSIDERATIONS

BASELINE ASSESSMENT

Obtain CBC, BMP, fasting glucose level, Hgb A1c; pregnancy test in females of reproductive potential. Verify use of effective contraception. Confirm presence of *PIK3CA/AKT1/PTEN* alterations in tumor specimen. Question history of diabetes, ketoacidosis. Recommend adequate glycemic control prior to initiation. Screen for active infection. Assess usual bowel movement patterns, stool characteristics. Assess hydration status. Receive full medication history and screen for interactions. Offer emotional support.

INTERVENTION/EVALUATION

Monitor CBC, renal function as clinically indicated. Obtain fasting glucose level q2wks for 4 wks, then monthly. Monitor Hbg A1c q3mos. Monitor for hyperglycemia (fatigue, polyuria, nausea, vomiting), ketoacidosis (e.g., dehydration, confusion, Kussmaul respirations, nausea, polydipsia, sweet-smelling breath), acute kidney injury (dark-colored urine, flank pain, decreased urine output, muscle aches), infections (cough, fatigue, fever), UTI (dysuria, fever, flank pain, malaise); skin toxicities, cutaneous reactions, symptoms of DRESS. If treatment-related toxicities occur, consider referral to specialist. Monitor daily pattern of bowel activity, stool consistency, I&Os. Recommend antidiarrheal agents (e.g., loperamide) at first sign of loose stool. Encourage adequate hydration.

PATIENT/FAMILY TEACHING

• Treatment may depress your immune system and reduce your ability to fight infection. Report symptoms of infection such as body aches, burning with urination, chills, cough, fatigue, fever. Avoid those with active infection. • Treatment may cause severe rashes, peeling, or blistering of the skin. • Severe diarrhea may cause dehydration, kidney injuries. Drink plenty of fluids. Report diarrhea that does not improve with medical management. • Decreased urination, amber-colored urine, flank pain, fatigue, swelling of the hands or feet may indicate kidney impairment. • Report symptoms of high blood sugar levels (blurred vision, confusion, excessive thirst/hunger, headache, frequent urination); toxic skin reactions (itching, peeling, rash, redness, swelling); UTI (fever, urinary frequency, burning during urination, foul smelling urine). • Use effective contraception to avoid pregnancy. Do not breastfeed. • There is a high risk of interactions with other medications. Do not take any newly prescribed medications unless approved by prescriber who originally started treatment. Avoid herbal supplements.

capmatinib

kap-**ma**-ti-nib
(Tabrecta)
Do not confuse capmatinib with cabozantinib, capecitabine, ceritinib, cobimetinib, crizotinib, or imatinib.

◆CLASSIFICATION

PHARMACOTHERAPEUTIC: Mesenchymal-epithelial transition (MET) tyrosine kinase inhibitor. **CLINICAL:** Antineoplastic.

USES

Treatment of adults with metastatic non–small-cell lung cancer (NSCLC) whose tumors have a mutation that leads to MET exon 14 skipping.

PRECAUTIONS

Contraindications: Hypersensitivity to capmatinib. **Cautions:** Baseline cytopenias; hepatic impairment, pulmonary disease; concomitant use of CYP3A inhibitors, CYP1A2 substrates, P-glycoprotein substrates, breast cancer resistance protein (BCRP) substrates. Avoid concomitant use of strong or moderate CYP3A inducers.

ACTION

Inhibits MET phosphorylation (including the mutant variant produced by exon 14 skipping), which increases downstream MET signaling. **Therapeutic Effect:** Decreases tumor cell growth.

PHARMACOKINETICS

Widely distributed. Metabolized in liver and by aldehyde oxidase. Protein binding: 96%. Peak plasma concentration: 1–2 hrs. Steady state reached in 3 days. Excreted in feces (78%), urine (22%). **Half-life:** 6.5 hrs.

⧗ LIFESPAN CONSIDERATIONS

Pregnancy/Lactation: Avoid pregnancy; may cause fetal harm. Female and male pts of reproductive potential must use effective contraception during treatment and for at least 7 days after discontinuation. Unknown if distributed in breast milk. Breastfeeding not recommended during treatment and for at least 7 days after discontinuation. **Children:** Safety and efficacy not established. **Elderly:** No age-related precautions noted.

INTERACTIONS

DRUG: Strong CYP3A4 inducers (e.g., carBAMazepine, phenytoin, rifAMPin), moderate CYP3A4 inducers (e.g., bosentan, nafcillin) may decrease concentration/effect. **HERBAL:** None significant. **FOOD:** None known. **LAB VALUES:** May increase serum alkaline phosphatase, ALT, AST, amylase, creatinine, GGT, lipase, potassium. May decrease serum albumin, glucose, phosphate, sodium, magnesium; Hgb, leukocytes, lymphocytes.

AVAILABILITY (Rx)

Tablets: 150 mg, 200 mg.

ADMINISTRATION/HANDLING

PO
• Give with or without regard to food. • Administer tablets whole; do not break, crush, or divide. Tablet cannot be chewed. • If vomiting occurs after administration, give next dose at regularly scheduled time (do not give additional dose).

INDICATIONS/ROUTES/DOSAGE

Non–Small-Cell Lung Cancer
PO: ADULTS, ELDERLY: 400 mg twice daily. Continue until disease progression or unacceptable toxicity.

Dose Reduction Schedule for Adverse Events
First dose reduction: 300 mg twice daily. **Second dose reduction:** 200 mg twice daily. **Unable to tolerate 200 mg dose:** Permanently discontinue.

Dose Modification
Based on Common Terminology Criteria for Adverse Events (CTCAE).

Serum ALT/AST Elevation
Grade 3 serum ALT/AST elevation (without total bilirubin elevation): Withhold treatment until improved to baseline. If improved within 7 days, resume at same dose. If not improved within 7 days, resume at reduced dose level. **Grade 4 serum ALT/AST elevation (without total bilirubin elevation):** Permanently discontinue. **Serum ALT/AST elevation greater than 3 times ULN (with total bilirubin elevation greater than 2 times ULN):** Permanently discontinue.

Hyperbilirubinemia
Grade 2 increased total bilirubin (without ALT/AST elevation): Withhold treatment until improved to baseline. If improved within 7 days, resume at same dose. If not improved within 7 days, resume at reduced dose level. **Grade 3 increased total bilirubin (without ALT/AST elevation):** Withhold treatment until improved to baseline. If improved within 7 days, resume at reduced dose level. If not improved within 7 days, permanently discontinue. **Grade 4 increased total bilirubin (without ALT/AST elevation):** Permanently discontinue.

Interstitial Lung Disease (ILD)
Any grade treatment-related ILD: Permanently discontinue.

Other Toxicities
Any Grade 2 toxicities: No dose adjustment. If intolerable, consider with-

holding treatment until resolved, then resume at reduced dose level. **Any Grade 3 toxicity:** Withhold treatment until resolved, then resume at reduced dose level. **Any Grade 4 toxicities:** Permanently discontinue.

Dosage in Renal Impairment
Mild to moderate impairment: No dose adjustment. **Severe impairment:** Not specified; use caution.

Dosage in Hepatic Impairment
Mild to severe impairment: Not specified; use caution.

SIDE EFFECTS
Frequent (52%–18%): Peripheral edema, fatigue, asthenia, nausea, vomiting, dyspnea, decreased appetite, constipation, diarrhea, cough. **Occasional (15%–less than 10%):** Noncardiac chest pain, back pain, pyrexia, decreased weight, pruritus, urticaria.

ADVERSE EFFECTS/TOXIC REACTIONS
Myelosuppression (anemia, leukopenia, lymphopenia) is an expected response to therapy. Pneumonitis, ILD reported in 5% of pts. Hepatotoxicity reported in 13% of pts. Photosensitivity reactions from UV exposure may increase risk of sunburn, skin erythema. Acute kidney injury, cellulitis reported in less than 10% of pts.

NURSING CONSIDERATIONS

BASELINE ASSESSMENT
Obtain CBC, BMP, LFTs; pregnancy test in females of reproductive potential. Confirm compliance of effective contraception. Confirm presence of mutation that leads to MET exon 14 skipping in tumor expression. Question history of hepatic impairment, pulmonary disease. Screen for active infection. Receive full medication history and screen for interactions. Offer emotional support.

INTERVENTION/EVALUATION
Monitor LFT q2wks for 3 mos, then monthly thereafter (or more frequently in pts with

hepatotoxicity). Monitor BUN, CrCl, serum creatinine periodically for acute kidney injury. An increase of serum creatinine greater than 0.4 mg/dL from baseline may indicate renal impairment. Consider ABG, radiologic test if ILD/pneumonitis (excessive cough, dyspnea, fever, hypoxia) is suspected. Monitor for drug toxicities if discontinuation or dose reduction of concomitant CYP3A inhibitor, P-glycoprotein inhibitor, CYP1A2 inhibitor is unavoidable.

PATIENT/FAMILY TEACHING
• Treatment may depress your immune system response and reduce your ability to fight infection. Report symptoms of infection such as body aches, chills, cough, fatigue, fever. Avoid those with active infection. • Report symptoms of lung inflammation (excessive coughing, difficulty breathing, chest pain); toxic skin reactions (itching, peeling, rash, redness, swelling); liver problems (abdominal pain, bruising, clay-colored stool, amber- or dark-colored urine, yellowing of the skin or eyes), kidney problems (decreased urine output, flank pain, darkened urine). • Use effective contraception to avoid pregnancy. Do not breastfeed. • Avoid prolonged sun exposure/tanning beds. Use high SPF sunscreen, lip balm, clothing to protect against sunburn. • There is a high risk of interactions with other medications. Do not take newly prescribed medications unless approved by prescriber who originally started therapy. • Avoid grapefruit products, herbal supplements (esp. St. John's wort).

carBAMazepine

kar-ba-**maz**-e-peen
(Carbatrol, Epitol, Equetro, Tegretol, Tegretol XR)

■ **BLACK BOX ALERT** ■ Potentially fatal aplastic anemia, agranulocytosis reported. Potentially fatal, severe dermatologic reactions (e.g., Stevens-Johnson syndrome, toxic epidermal necrolysis) may occur. Risk increased in pts with the variant HLA-β* 1502 allele, almost exclusively in pts of Asian ancestry. **Do not confuse carBAMazepine with oxcarbazepine, eslicarbazepine, or Tegretol with Mebaral, Toprol XL, Toradol, or Trental.**

◆**CLASSIFICATION**

PHARMACOTHERAPEUTIC: Iminostilbene derivative. **CLINICAL:** Anticonvulsant.

USES

Bipolar disorder: Acute treatment of hypomania and mild to moderate mania episode with mixed features associated with bipolar disorder. **Seizures:** Monotherapy and adjunctive therapy in pts with focal (partial) onset, generalized onset seizures. **Neuropathic pain:** Treatment of trigeminal or glossopharyngeal neuralgia.

PRECAUTIONS

Contraindications: Concomitant use or within 14 days of use of MAOIs, myelosuppression. Concomitant use of delavirdine or other NNRT inhibitors that are substrates of CYP3A4. Hypersensitivity to carBAMazepine, tricyclic antidepressants. **Cautions:** High risk of suicide, increased IOP, hepatic or renal impairment, history of cardiac impairment, ECG abnormalities, elderly.

ACTION

Decreases sodium ion influx into neuronal membranes (may depress activity in thalamus, decreasing synaptic transmission or decreasing temporal stimulation, leading to neural discharge). **Therapeutic Effect:** Produces anticonvulsant effect.

PHARMACOKINETICS

Widely distributed. Protein binding: 75%–90%. Metabolized in liver. Primarily excreted in urine. Not removed by hemodialysis. **Half-life:** 25–65 hrs (decreased with chronic use).

⌛ LIFESPAN CONSIDERATIONS

Pregnancy/Lactation: Crosses placenta; distributed in breast milk. Accumulates in fetal tissue. **Children:** Behavioral changes more likely to occur. **Elderly:** More susceptible to confusion, agitation, AV block, bradycardia, syndrome of inappropriate antidiuretic hormone (SIADH).

INTERACTIONS

DRUG: **CYP3A4 inhibitors (e.g., cimetidine, clarithromycin, azole antifungals, protease inhibitors)** may increase concentration/effect. **CYP3A4 inducers (e.g., rifAMPin, phenytoin)** may decrease concentration/effects. May decrease concentration/effects of **abemaciclib, apixaban, axitinib, BCG (intravesical), bosutinib, brigatinib, dronedarone, hormonal contraceptives, NIFEdipinee, ranolazine, regorafenib, traZODone, vorapaxar, voriconazole, warfarin.** **HERBAL:** **Gotu kola, kava kava, valerian** may increase CNS depression. **FOOD:** **Grapefruit products** may increase concentration/effect. **LAB VALUES:** May increase serum BUN, glucose, alkaline phosphatase, bilirubin, ALT, AST, cholesterol, HDL, triglycerides. May decrease serum calcium, thyroid hormone (T_3, T_4 index) levels. **Therapeutic serum level:** 4–12 mcg/mL; **toxic serum level:** Greater than 12 mcg/mL.

AVAILABILITY (Rx)

Oral Suspension: 100 mg/5 mL. **Tablets:** 200 mg. **Tablets:** *(Chewable):* 100 mg.

🔖 **Capsules:** *(Extended-Release):* 100 mg, 200 mg, 300 mg. **Tablets:** *(Extended-Release):* 100 mg, 200 mg, 400 mg.

ADMINISTRATION/HANDLING

PO

• Store oral suspension, tablets at room temperature. • To reduce GI distress, give tablets or extended-release tablets with food. May give extended-release capsules without regard to food. Give extended-release capsules whole; do not cut or crush. Capsules may be opened and beads sprinkled on food (e.g., applesauce). • Give extended-release tablets whole; do not break, cut, or crush. Extended-release formulations cannot be chewed. • Shake oral suspension well. Do not administer simultaneously with other liquid medicine.

INDICATIONS/ROUTES/DOSAGE

◄**ALERT**► Suspension must be given on a 3–4 times/day schedule; tablets on a 2–4 times/day schedule; extended-release capsules 2 times/day. **(Carnexiv):** 70% of total oral dose given as four 30-min infusions separated by 6 hrs.

Seizure Control
PO: ADULTS, ELDERLY: Initially, 2–3 mg/kg/day (100–200 mg/day) in 2–4 divided doses (based on formulation chosen). May increase dose by 200 mg or less per day in time increments of at least q5days. **Usual dose:** 800–1,200 mg/day in 2–4 divided doses. **Maximum: ADULTS, ELDERLY:** 1,600 mg/day; **ADOLESCENTS (Immediate-Release):** Initially, 200 mg twice daily. Titrate up to 200 mg/day at wkly intervals. **Maintenance:** 800–1,200 mg/day in 3–4 divided doses. **Oral suspension:** 100 mg 4 times/day. Titrate up to 200 mg/day at wkly intervals. **Maintenance:** 800–1,200 mg/day in 3–4 divided doses. **(Extended-Release):** Initially, 200 mg 2 times/day. May increase by 200 mg/day at wkly intervals. Maintenance: 800–1,200 mg/day in 2 divided doses. **CHILDREN 6–12 YRS: (Immediate-Release):** Initially, 100 mg twice daily (tablets) or 50 mg 4 times/day (oral suspension). May increase by 100 mg/day at wkly intervals. **Usual dose:** 400–800 mg/day. **Maximum:** 1,000 mg/day. **(Extended-Release):** Initially, 100 mg 2 times/day. May increase by 100 mg/day at wkly intervals. **(Usual Range):** 400–800 mg/day in 2 divided doses. **Maximum:** 1,000 mg/day. **CHILDREN YOUNGER THAN 6 YRS: (Immediate-Release):** Initially, 10–20 mg/kg/day 2–3 times/day (tablets) or 4 times/day (suspension). May increase at wkly intervals until optimal response and therapeutic levels are achieved. **Maximum:** 35 mg/kg/day in 3–4 divided doses.

Neuropathic Pain
PO: ADULTS, ELDERLY: Initially, 200–400 mg/day in 2–4 divided doses, gradually increasing (e.g., over several weeks) in increments of 200 mg/day as needed. **Usual dose:** 600–800 mg daily. **Maximum:** 1,200 mg/day.

Bipolar Disorder
PO: ADULTS, ELDERLY: Initially, 100–400 mg/day in 2–4 divided doses. May adjust dose in 200-mg increments q1–4 days. **Usual range:** 600–1,200 mg/day. **Maximum:** 1,600 mg/day in divided doses.

Dosage in Renal Impairment
CrCl less than 10 mL/min: 75% of normal dose. **HD:** 75% of normal dose. **CRRT:** 75% of normal dose.

Dosage in Hepatic Impairment
Use caution.

SIDE EFFECTS

Frequent (greater than 10%): Vertigo, somnolence, ataxia, fatigue, leukopenia, rash, urticaria, nausea, vomiting. **Occasional (10%–1%):** Headache, diplopia, blurred vision, thrombocytopenia, dry mouth, edema, fluid retention, increased weight. **Rare (less than 1%):** Tremors, visual disturbances, lymphadenopathy, jaundice, involuntary muscle movements, nystagmus, dermatitis.

ADVERSE EFFECTS/TOXIC REACTIONS

Toxic reactions appear as blood dyscrasias (aplastic anemia, agranulocytosis, thrombocytopenia, leukopenia, leukocytosis, eosinophilia), cardiovascular disturbances (HF, hypotension/hypertension, thrombophlebitis, arrhythmias), dermatologic effects (rash, urticaria, pruritus, photosensitivity). Abrupt withdrawal may precipitate status epilepticus.

NURSING CONSIDERATIONS

BASELINE ASSESSMENT
CBC, serum iron determination, urinalysis, BUN should be performed before therapy

begins and periodically during therapy. **Seizures:** Review history of seizure disorder (intensity, frequency, duration, level of consciousness [LOC]). Initiate seizure precautions. **Neuralgia:** Assess facial pain, stimuli that may cause facial pain. **Bipolar:** Assess mental status, cognitive abilities.

INTERVENTION/EVALUATION

Seizures: Observe frequently for recurrence of seizure activity. Monitor therapeutic levels. Assess for clinical improvement (decrease in intensity, frequency of seizures). Assess for clinical evidence of early toxicity (fever, sore throat, mouth ulcerations, unusual bruising/bleeding, joint pain). **Neuralgia:** Avoid triggering tic douloureux (draft, talking, washing face, jarring bed, hot/warm/cold food or liquids). **Bipolar:** Monitor for suicidal ideation, behavioral changes. Observe for excessive sedation. **Therapeutic serum level:** 4–12 mcg/mL; **toxic serum level:** Greater than 12 mcg/mL.

PATIENT/FAMILY TEACHING

• Do not abruptly discontinue medication after long-term use (may precipitate seizures). • Strict maintenance of therapy is essential for seizure control. • Avoid tasks that require alertness, motor skills until response to drug is established. • Report visual disturbances. • Blood tests should be repeated frequently during first 3 mos of therapy and at monthly intervals thereafter for 2–3 yrs. • Do not take oral suspension simultaneously with other liquid medicine. • Do not ingest grapefruit products. • Report serious skin reactions.

carbidopa/levodopa

kar-bi-doe-pa/**lee**-voe-doe-pa
(Apo-Levocarb ✦, Dhivy, Duopa, Rytary, Sinemet)
Do not confuse Sinemet with Serevent.

FIXED-COMBINATION(S)

Stalevo: carbidopa/levodopa/entacapone (antiparkinson agent): 12.5 mg/50 mg/200 mg, 18.75 mg/75 mg/200 mg, 25 mg/100 mg/200 mg, 31.25 mg/125 mg/200 mg, 37.5 mg/150 mg/200 mg, 50 mg/200 mg/200 mg.

◆CLASSIFICATION

PHARMACOTHERAPEUTIC: DOPamine precursor. Decarboxylase inhibitor. **CLINICAL:** Antiparkinson agent.

USES

Parkinson's disease: Treatment of Parkinson's disease, postencephalitic parkinsonism, symptomatic parkinsonism following CNS injury by carbon monoxide poisoning, manganese intoxication. **Duopa:** Treatment of motor fluctuations in advanced Parkinson's disease. **OFF-LABEL:** Restless legs syndrome.

PRECAUTIONS

Contraindications: Hypersensitivity to carbidopa/levodopa. Concurrent use with MAOIs or use within 14 days. (Tablets only): Narrow-angle glaucoma. **Cautions:** History of MI, arrhythmias, bronchial asthma, emphysema, severe cardiac, pulmonary, renal/hepatic impairment; active peptic ulcer, treated open-angle glaucoma, seizure disorder, pts at risk for hypotension; elderly.

ACTION

Levodopa is converted to DOPamine in basal ganglia, increasing DOPamine concentration in brain, inhibiting hyperactive cholinergic activity. Carbidopa prevents peripheral breakdown of levodopa, making more levodopa available for transport into brain. **Therapeutic Effect:** Treats symptoms (e.g., stiffness, tremors) associated with Parkinson's disease.

PHARMACOKINETICS

Widely distributed. Excreted primarily in urine. Levodopa is converted to DOPamine. Excreted primarily in urine. **Half-life:** 1–2 hrs (carbidopa); 1–3 hrs (levodopa).

⧗ LIFESPAN CONSIDERATIONS

Pregnancy/Lactation: Unknown if drug crosses placenta or is distributed in breast milk. May inhibit lactation. Breastfeeding not recommended. **Children:** Safety and efficacy not established. **Elderly:** More sensitive to effects of levodopa. Anxiety, confusion, nervousness more common when receiving anticholinergics.

INTERACTIONS

DRUG: **Antipsychotics, pyridoxine** may decrease therapeutic effect. May increase adverse effects of **MAOIs (e.g., phenelzine, selegiline).** **HERBAL:** None significant. **FOOD:** **High-protein** diets may cause decreased or erratic response to levodopa. **LAB VALUES:** May increase serum BUN, LDH, alkaline phosphatase, bilirubin, ALT, AST. May decrease Hgb, Hct, WBC.

AVAILABILITY (Rx)

Enteral Suspension: *(Duopa):* 100-mL cassette containing 4.63 mg carbidopa and 20 mg levodopa per mL. **Tablets:** *(Immediate-Release [Sinemet]):* 10 mg carbidopa/100 mg levodopa, 25 mg carbidopa/100 mg levodopa, 25 mg carbidopa/250 mg levodopa. *[Dhivy]:* 25 mg/100 mg (each tablet with 3 functional scores with each segment 6.25 mg/25 mg. **Tablets:** *(Orally Disintegrating Immediate-Release):* 10 mg carbidopa/100 mg levodopa, 25 mg carbidopa/100 mg levodopa, 25 mg carbidopa/250 mg levodopa.

🦢 **Capsules:** *(Extended-Release [Rytary]):* carbidopa/levodopa: 23.75 mg/95 mg, 36.25 mg/145 mg, 48.75 mg/195 mg, 61.25 mg/245 mg. **Tablets:** *(Extended-Release):* 25 mg carbidopa/100 mg levodopa, 50 mg carbidopa/200 mg levodopa.

ADMINISTRATION/HANDLING

Note: Space doses evenly over waking hours.
Enteral Suspension
• Refrigerate. Remove 20 min prior to administration.
PO
• Scored tablets may be crushed. • Give **Extended-release capsule:** May give without regard to food. Administer whole (do not crush, divide, or allowing chewing). • May be opened, sprinkled on applesauce, and

given immediately. **Oral tablets:** Administer with meals to decrease GI upset. • Controlled-release tablet should not be chewed, crushed. *Dhivy* tablets may be broken at score lines. • *(Orally Disintegrating Tablet):* Place orally disintegrating tablet on top of tongue. Tablet will dissolve in seconds; pt to swallow with saliva. Not necessary to administer with liquid.

INDICATIONS/ROUTES/DOSAGE
Parkinsonism

PO: ADULTS, ELDERLY: *(Immediate-Release Orally Disintegrating Tablet):* Initially, 10 mg carbidopa/100 mg levodopa PO 3–4 times daily or 25/100 mg 3 times/day. May increase daily or every other day by 1 tablet (25/100 mg) up to 200/2,000 mg daily divided in 4 or more doses/day. *(Extended-Release):* Initially, 50/200 mg 2 times/day at least 6 hrs apart. May adjust dose no faster than 3 days up to a maximum of 2,400 mg levodopa/day. *(Rytary):* Initially, 23.75/95 mg 3 times/day for 3 days, then to 36.25/145 mg 3 times/day. Frequency may be increased to maximum of 5 times/day if needed and tolerated. **Maximum daily dose:** 612.5/2,450 mg/day. *(Enteral Suspension):* **Maximum:** 2,000 mg (1 container) over 16 hrs through NJ or PEG tube via infusion pump. Also take oral immediate-release in evening after disconnecting pump. Refer to manufacturer's guidelines for morning dose, continuous dose escalation, titration instructions.

Dosage in Renal/Hepatic Impairment
Use caution.

SIDE EFFECTS

Frequent (80%–50%): Involuntary movements of face, tongue, arms, upper body; nausea/vomiting; anorexia. **Occasional:** Depression, anxiety, confusion, nervousness, urinary retention, palpitations, dizziness, light-headedness, decreased appetite, blurred vision, constipation, dry mouth, flushed skin, headache, insomnia, diarrhea, unusual fatigue, darkening of urine and sweat. **Rare:** Hypertension, ulcer, hemolytic anemia (marked by fatigue).

━ Canadian trade name ━ Non-Crushable Drug ━ High Alert drug

C

ADVERSE EFFECTS/TOXIC REACTIONS

High incidence of involuntary choreiform, dystonic, dyskinetic movements may occur in pts on long-term therapy. Numerous mild to severe CNS and psychiatric disturbances may occur (reduced attention span, anxiety, nightmares, daytime drowsiness, euphoria, fatigue, paranoia, psychotic episodes, depression, hallucinations).

NURSING CONSIDERATIONS

BASELINE ASSESSMENT

Assess symptoms of Parkinson's disease (e.g., muscular rigidity, pen rolling motion, gait disturbance, tremors), emotional state. Receive full medication history and screen for interactions.

INTERVENTION/EVALUATION

Be alert to neurologic effects (headache, lethargy, mental confusion, agitation). Monitor for evidence of dyskinesia (difficulty with movement). Assess for clinical reversal of symptoms (improvement of tremor of head and hands at rest, mask-like facial expression, shuffling gait, muscular rigidity). Monitor B/P (standing, sitting, supine).

PATIENT/FAMILY TEACHING

• Avoid tasks that require alertness, motor skills until response to drug is established. • Take with food to minimize GI upset. • Effects may be delayed from several wks to mos. • May cause darkening of urine or sweat (not harmful). • Report any uncontrolled movement of face, eyelids, mouth, tongue, arms, hands, legs; mental changes; palpitations; severe or persistent nausea/vomiting; difficulty urinating. • Report exacerbations of asthma, underlying depression, psychosis.

CARBOplatin **HIGH ALERT**

kar-boe-**plat**-in
(Paraplatin)

■ **BLACK BOX ALERT** ■ Must be administered by personnel trained in administration/handling of chemotherapeutic agents (high potential for severe reactions, including anaphylaxis [may occur within minutes of administration] and sudden death). Profound myelosuppression (anemia, thrombocytopenia) has occurred. Vomiting may occur.
Do not confuse CARBOplatin with CISplatin or oxaliplatin, or with Platinol.

◆CLASSIFICATION

PHARMACOTHERAPEUTIC: Alkylating agent. Platinum analog. **CLINICAL:** Antineoplastic.

USES

Ovarian cancer: Treatment of advanced ovarian carcinoma. Palliative treatment of recurrent ovarian cancer. **OFF-LABEL:** Hodgkin's and non-Hodgkin's lymphomas, malignant melanoma, treatment of breast, bladder, cervical, endometrial, esophageal, small-cell lung, non–small-cell lung, head and neck, testicular carcinomas; germ cell tumors, osteogenic sarcoma. Anal cancer (advanced), gastric cancer, gestational trophoblastic neoplasia, malignant pleural mesothelioma, Merkel cell carcinoma, neuroendocrine tumors, prostate cancer (castraton resistant, metastatic) thyroid carcinoma.

PRECAUTIONS

Contraindications: Hypersensitivity to CARBOplatin. History of severe allergic reaction to CISplatin, platinum compounds, mannitol; severe bleeding, severe myelosuppression. **Cautions:** Moderate bone marrow depression, renal impairment, elderly.

ACTION

Inhibits DNA synthesis by cross-linking with DNA strands, preventing cell division. **Therapeutic Effect:** Interferes with DNA function.

PHARMACOKINETICS

Protein binding: Low. Hydrolyzed in solution to active form. Primarily excreted in urine. **Half-life:** 2.6–5.9 hrs.

LIFESPAN CONSIDERATIONS

Pregnancy/Lactation: If possible, avoid use during pregnancy, esp. first trimester. May cause fetal harm. Unknown if distributed in breast milk. Breastfeeding not recommended. **Children:** Safety and efficacy not established. **Elderly:** Peripheral neurotoxicity increased, myelotoxicity may be more severe. Age-related renal impairment may require decreased dosage, careful monitoring of blood counts.

INTERACTIONS

DRUG: Bone marrow depressants (e.g., cladribine) may increase myelosuppression. May increase adverse effects of **cloZAPine, natalizumab, leflunomide.** May increase immunosuppressive effect of **baricitinib.** May increase concentration/effect of **bexarotene.** May decrease therapeutic effect of **BCG (intravesical), vaccines (live).** May increase adverse effects of **vaccines (live). HERBAL: Echinacea** may decrease therapeutic effect. **FOOD:** None known. **LAB VALUES:** May decrease serum calcium, magnesium, potassium, sodium. May increase serum BUN, alkaline phosphatase, bilirubin, creatinine, AST.

AVAILABILITY (Rx)

Injection Solution: 10 mg/mL (5 mL, 15 mL, 45 mL, 60 mL, 100 mL).

ADMINISTRATION/HANDLING

◄ ALERT ► May be carcinogenic, mutagenic, teratogenic. Handle with extreme care during preparation/administration.

 IV

Reconstitution • Dilute with D_5W or 0.9% NaCl to a final concentration as low as 0.5 mg/mL.
Rate of administration • Infuse over 15–60 min. • Rarely, anaphylactic reaction occurs minutes after administration. Use of epinephrine, corticosteroids alleviates symptoms.

Storage • Store vials at room temperature. • After dilution, solution is stable for 8 hrs.

IV COMPATIBILITIES

D5W, 0.9% NaCl.

INDICATIONS/ROUTES/DOSAGE

Note: Doses commonly calculated by target AUC.
Ovarian Carcinoma
IV: ADULTS: 300 mg/m$_2$ on day 1 in combination with cyclophosphamide (600 mg/m$_2$ IV on day 1), repeated q4wk 6 cycles. **Recurrent ovarian cancer:** 360 mg/m$_2$ on day 1, repeated q4wks as a single agent.

Dose Modification
Platelets less than 50,000 cells/ mm³ or ANC less than 500 cells/ mm³: Give 75% of dose.

Dosage in Renal Impairment
Initial dosage is based on creatinine clearance; subsequent dosages are based on pt's tolerance, degree of myelosuppression.

Creatinine Clearance	Dosage Day 1
60 mL/min or greater	360 mg/m²
41–59 mL/min	250 mg/m²
16–40 mL/min	200 mg/m²

Dosage in Hepatic Impairment
No dose adjustment.

SIDE EFFECTS

Frequent (80%–65%): Nausea, vomiting. **Occasional (17%–4%):** Generalized pain, diarrhea/constipation, peripheral neuropathy. **Rare (3%–2%):** Alopecia, asthenia, hypersensitivity reaction (erythema, pruritus, rash, urticaria).

ADVERSE EFFECTS/TOXIC REACTIONS

Myelosuppression may be severe, resulting in anemia, infection (sepsis, pneumonia), major bleeding. Prolonged treatment may result in peripheral neuropathy. Ototoxicity, vision loss were reported. Hypersensitivity reactions, including anaphylaxis, may occur.

NURSING CONSIDERATIONS

BASELINE ASSESSMENT

Obtain ECG, CBC, BMP, LFT. Do not repeat treatment until WBC recovers from previous therapy. Transfusions may be needed in pts receiving prolonged therapy (myelosuppression increased in those with previous therapy, renal impairment). Offer emotional support.

INTERVENTION/EVALUATION

Monitor CBC, BMP, LFT; pulmonary function. Monitor for fever, sore throat, signs of local infection, unusual bruising/bleeding from any site, symptoms of anemia (excessive fatigue, weakness).

PATIENT/FAMILY TEACHING

• Nausea and vomiting are common side effects that may require anti-nausea medication. • Do not have immunizations without physician's approval (drug lowers body's resistance). • Avoid contact with those who have recently received live virus vaccine.

---

carfilzomib

kar-**fil**-zoh-mib
(Kyprolis)
Do not confuse carfilzomib with crizotinib, ixazomib, PAZOpanib.

◆CLASSIFICATION

PHARMACOTHERAPEUTIC: Proteasome inhibitor. **CLINICAL:** Antineoplastic.

USES

Multiple myeloma: Treatment (monotherapy) of relapsed or refractory multiple myeloma in adults who have received 1 or more lines of therapy. Treatment of relapsed or refractory multiple myeloma (in combination with dexAMETHasone, or with lenalidomide and dexAMETHa-sone, or with daratumumab and dexAMETHasone) in adults who have received 1–3 prior lines of therapy. **OFF-LABEL:** Waldenstrom macroglobulinemia, multiple myeloma (newly diagnosed).

PRECAUTIONS

Contraindications: Hypersensitivity to carfilzomib. **Cautions:** Preexisting HF, decreased left ventricular ejection fraction, myocardial abnormalities, complications of pulmonary hypertension (e.g., dyspnea), hepatic impairment, thrombocytopenia.

ACTION

Blocks action of proteasomes (responsible for intracellular protein homeostasis). **Therapeutic Effect:** Causes cell cycle arrest and apoptosis of cancer cells.

PHARMACOKINETICS

Widely distributed. Metabolized via hydrolysis and peptidase cleavage. Protein binding: 97%–98%. Excreted primarily extrahepatically. Minimal removal by hemodialysis. **Half-life:** Equal to or less than 1 hr on day 1 of cycle 1. Proteasome inhibition was maintained for 48 hrs or longer following first dose of carfilzomib for each week of dosing.

⧗ LIFESPAN CONSIDERATIONS

Pregnancy/Lactation: Avoid pregnancy. May cause fetal harm. Unknown if excreted in breast milk. **Children:** Safety and efficacy not established. **Elderly:** No age-related precautions noted.

INTERACTIONS

DRUG: May decrease levels/effect of **BCG (intravesical), vaccines (live)**. May increase myelosuppressive effect of **myelosuppressants (e.g., cladribine). Hormonal contraceptives** may increase concentration/effect. **HERBAL:** None significant. **FOOD:** None known. **LAB VALUES:** May increase serum creatinine, glucose, creatinine, ALT, AST, bilirubin, calcium. May decrease RBC, Hgb, Hct, absolute neutrophil count

(ANC), platelet count; serum magnesium, phosphate, potassium, sodium.

AVAILABILITY (Rx)

Injection Powder for Reconstitution (Single-Use Vial): 10 mg, 30 mg, 60 mg.

ADMINISTRATION/HANDLING

 IV

Reconstitution • Reconstitute 60-mg vial with 29 mL Sterile Water for Injection (30-mg vial with 15 mL, 10 mg with 5 mL), directing solution to inside wall of vial (minimizes foaming). • Swirl and invert vial slowly for 1 min or until completely dissolved. • Do not shake. • If foaming occurs, rest vial for 2–5 min until subsided. • Withdraw calculated dose from vial and dilute into 50–100 mL D_5W (depending on dose and infusion duration). • Final concentration of reconstituted solution: 2 mg/mL.

Rate of administration • Infuse over 10–30 min (depending on the dose regimen) via dedicated IV line. Flush line before and after with NaCl or D_5W. • Do not administer as a bolus.

Storage • Refrigerate unused vials. • Reconstituted solution may be refrigerated up to 24 hrs. • At room temperature, use diluted solution within 4 hrs.

⬡ IV INCOMPATIBILITIES

Do not mix with other IV medications or additives. Flush IV administration line with NaCl or D_5W immediately before and after carfilzomib administration.

INDICATIONS/ROUTES/DOSAGE

◀**ALERT**▶ Dose is calculated using pt's actual body surface area at baseline. Pts with a body surface area greater than 2.2 m^2 should receive dose based on a body surface area of 2.2 m^2. No dose adjustment needed for weight changes of less than or equal to 20%.

◀**ALERT**▶ Prior to each dose in cycle 1, give 250 mL to 500 mL NaCl bolus. Give an additional 250 mL to 500 mL IV fluid following administration. Continue IV hydra-

tion in subsequent cycles (reduces risk of renal toxicity, tumor lysis syndrome). Premedicate with dexAMETHasone 4 mg PO or IV prior to all doses during cycle 1 and prior to all doses during first cycle of dose escalation to 27 mg/m^2 (reduces incidence, severity of infusion reactions). Reinstate dexAMETHasone premedication (4 mg PO or IV) if symptoms develop or reappear during subsequent cycles.

Multiple Myeloma, Relapsed/Refractory (Single-Agent 20/27 mg/m^2 Regimen)
IV: ADULTS, ELDERLY: Cycle 1: 20 mg/m^2 over 10 min on days 1 and 2. If tolerated, increase to 27 mg/m^2 over 10 min on days 8, 9, 15, and 16 of a 28-day cycle. **Cycles 2–12:** 27 mg/m^2 over 10 min on days 1, 2, 8, 9, 15, and 16 of a 28-day cycle. **Cycles 13 and beyond:** 27 mg/m^2 over 10 min on days 1, 2, 15, and 16 of a 28-day cycle. Continue until disease progression or unacceptable toxicity.

Multiple Myeloma, Relapsed/Refractory (Single-Agent 20/56 mg/m^2 Regimen)
IV: ADULTS, ELDERLY: Cycle 1: 20 mg/m^2 over 30 min on days 1 and 2. If tolerated, increase to 56 mg/m^2 over 30 min on days 8, 9, 15, and 16 of a 28-day cycle. **Cycles 2–12:** 56 mg/m^2 over 30 min on days 1, 2, 8, 9, 15, and 16 of a 28-day cycle. **Cycles 13 and beyond:** 56 mg/m^2 over 30 min on days 1, 2, 15, and 16 of a 28-day cycle. Continue until disease progression or unacceptable toxicity.

Multiple Myeloma, Relapsed/Refractory (in Combination With Lenalidomide and DexAMETHasone)
IV: ADULTS, ELDERLY: Cycle 1: 20 mg/m^2 over 10 min on days 1 and 2. If tolerated, increase to 27 mg/m^2 over 10 min on days 8, 9, 15, and 16 of a 28-day cycle. **Cycles 2–12:** 27 mg/m^2 over 10 min on days 1, 2, 8, 9, 15, and 16 of a 28-day cycle. **Cycles 13–18:** 27 mg/m^2 over 10 min on days 1, 2, 15, and 16 of a 28-day cycle. Beginning with cycle 19, lenalidomide and dexAMETHasone may be continued (until disease progression or unacceptable toxicity) without carfilzomib.

 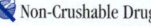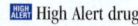

Multiple Myeloma, Relapsed/Refractory (in Combination With DexAMETHasone)

IV: ADULTS, ELDERLY: Cycle 1: 20 mg/m^2 over 30 min on days 1 and 2. If tolerated, increase to 56 mg/m^2 over 30 min on days 8, 9, 15, and 16 of a 28-day cycle. **Cycle 2 and beyond:** 56 mg/m^2 over 30 min on days 1, 2, 8, 9, 15, and 16 of a 28-day cycle. Continue until disease progression or unacceptable toxicity.

Multiple Myeloma, Relapsed/Refractory (in Combination With DexAMETHasone; 20/70 mg/m^2 Regimen [once-wkly dosing])

IV: ADULTS, ELDERLY: Cycle 1: 20 mg/m^2 over 30 min on day 1. Increase dose to 70 mg/m^2 over 30 min on days 8 and 15 of a 28-day treatment cycle. **Cycle 2 and beyond:** 70 mg/m^2 over 30 min on days 1, 8, and 15 of a 28-day treatment cycle. Continue until disease progression or unacceptable toxicity.

Multiple Myeloma, Relapsed/Refractory (in Combination With Daratumumab and DexAMETHasone; 20/56 mg/m^2 Regimen [twice-wkly dosing])

IV: ADULTS, ELDERLY: Cycle 1: 20 mg/m^2 on days 1 and 2; if tolerated, increase to 56 mg/m^2 on days 8, 9, 15, and 16 of a 28-day cycle. **Cycles 2 and thereafter:** 56 mg/m^2 on days 1, 2, 8, 9, 15, and 16 of a 28-day cycle; continue until disease progression or unacceptable toxicity.

Multiple Myeloma, Relapsed/Refractory (in Combination With Daratumumab and DexAMETHasone; 20/70 mg/m^2 Regimen [once-wkly dosing])

IV: Cycle 1: 20 mg/m^2 on day 1; if tolerated, increase dose to 70 mg/m^2 on days 8 and 15 of a 28-day cycle. **Cycles 2 and thereafter:** 70 mg/m^2 over on days 1, 8, and 15 of a 28-day cycle; continue until disease progression or unacceptable toxicity.

Dose Modification

Hematologic Toxicity

Grade 3 or 4 neutropenia: Withhold dose. Continue at same dose if fully recovered prior to next scheduled dose. If recovered to Grade 2, reduce dose by one dose level. If dose tolerated, may escalate to previous dose. **Grade 4 thrombo-**

cytopenia: Withhold dose. Continue at same dose if fully recovered prior to next scheduled dose. If recovered to Grade 3, reduce dose by one dose level. If dose tolerated, may escalate to previous dose.

Cardiotoxicity

Grade 3 or 4, new onset or worsening of HF, decreased LVF, myocardial ischemia: Withhold dose until resolved or at baseline. After resolution, restart at reduced dose level. If dose tolerated, may escalate to previous dose.

Hepatotoxicity

Grade 3 or 4 elevation of bilirubin, transaminases: Withhold dose until resolved or at baseline. After resolution, restart at reduced dose level. If dose tolerated, may escalate to previous dose.

Peripheral Neuropathy

Grade 3 or 4: Withhold dose until resolved or at baseline. After resolution, restart at reduced dose level. If dose tolerated, may escalate to previous dose.

Pulmonary Toxicity

Pulmonary hypertension: Withhold dose until resolved or at baseline. After resolution, restart at reduced dose level. If dose tolerated, may escalate to previous dose. **Grade 3 or 4 pulmonary complications:** Withhold dose until resolved or at baseline. After resolution, restart at reduced dose level. If dose tolerated, may escalate to previous dose.

Renal Toxicity

Serum creatinine 2 times or greater from baseline: Withhold dose until renal function improves to Grade 1 or baseline. After resolution, restart at reduced dose level. If dose tolerated, may escalate to previous dose.

Dosage in Renal/Hepatic Impairment

No dose adjustment.

SIDE EFFECTS

Frequent (56%–20%): Fatigue, anemia, nausea, exertional dyspnea, diarrhea, fever, headache, cough, peripheral edema, vomiting, constipation, back pain. **Occasional**

(18%–14%): Insomnia, chills, arthralgia, muscle spasms, hypertension, asthenia, extremity pain, dizziness, hypoesthesia (decreased sensitivity to touch), anorexia.

ADVERSE EFFECTS/TOXIC REACTIONS

Pneumonia (10% of pts), acute renal failure (4% of pts), pyrexia (3% of pts), and HF (3% of pts) were reported. Adverse reactions leading to discontinuation occurred in 15% of pts. Upper respiratory tract infection reported in 28% of pts. HF, pulmonary edema, decrease in ejection fraction were reported in 7% of pts. Infusion reaction characterized by chills, fever, wheezing, facial flushing, dyspnea, vomiting, chest tightness can occur immediately following or up to 24 hrs after administration. Tumor lysis syndrome occurs rarely.

NURSING CONSIDERATIONS

BASELINE ASSESSMENT

Obtain accurate height and weight. Obtain full history of home medications including vitamins, herbal products. Ensure hydration status and maintain throughout treatment. Obtain CBC, BMP, LFT. Assess vital signs, O_2 saturation. Platelet nadirs occur around day 8 of each 28-day cycle and recover to baseline by start of the next 28-day cycle. Offer emotional support.

INTERVENTION/EVALUATION

Monitor for fluid overload. Monitor platelet count frequently; adjust dose according to grade of thrombocytopenia. Obtain serum ALT, AST, bilirubin for evidence of hepatotoxicity. Monitor vital signs, O_2 saturation routinely. Monitor cardiac function and manage as needed. Assess for palpitations, tachycardia. Assess for anemia-related dizziness, exertional dyspnea, fatigue, weakness, syncope. Monitor for acute infection (fever, diaphoresis, lethargy, oral mucosal changes, productive cough), bloody stools, bruising, hematuria, DVT, pulmonary embolism. Encourage nutritional intake and assess anorexia, weight loss. Monitor daily pattern of bowel activity, stool consistency. Offer antiemetics if nausea, vomiting occur. Monitor for symptoms of neutropenia.

PATIENT/FAMILY TEACHING

• Immediately report any newly prescribed medications. • May alter taste of food or decrease appetite. • Report bloody stool/urine, increased bruising, difficulty breathing, weakness, dizziness, palpitations, weight loss. • Maintain strict oral hygiene. • Do not have immunizations without physician approval (drug lowers body's resistance). • Avoid those who have recently taken live virus vaccine. • Avoid crowds, those with symptoms of viral illness.

◆CLASSIFICATION

PHARMACOTHERAPEUTIC: Serotonin receptor antagonist. **CLINICAL:** Second-generation (atypical) antipsychotic.

USES

Treatment of schizophrenia. **Bipolar disorder:** Acute treatment of mania or mixed episodes associated with bipolar disorder in adults. Treatment of depressive episodes associated with bipolar I disorder (bipolar depression) in adults. **Major depressive disorder (unipolar) (MDD):** Adjunctive therapy to antidepressants for the treatment of major depressive disorder (MDD) in adults with inadequate response to antidepressants.

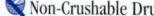

PRECAUTIONS

Contraindications: Hypersensitivity to cariprazine. **Cautions:** Baseline cytopenias; debilitation, diabetes, dyslipidemia, elderly, hepatic impairment, Parkinson's disease, pts at risk for hypotension (dehydration, hypovolemia, concomitant use of antihypertensives), pts at risk for aspiration, dysphagia; history of cardiovascular disease (e.g., ischemic heart disease, HF, cardiac arrhythmias); pts at risk for CVA, TIA; hx of seizures. Concomitant use of medications that lower seizure threshold. Avoid concomitant use of CYP3A inducers.

ACTION

Partial agonist of central DOPamine D_2 and serotonin 5-HT$_{1A}$ receptors and antagonist of serotonin 5-HT$_{2A}$ receptors. **Therapeutic Effect:** Diminishes symptoms of psychotic behavior.

PHARMACOKINETICS

Widely distributed. Metabolized in liver. Protein binding: 91%–97%. Peak plasma concentration: 3–6 hrs. Mean plasma concentrations decrease approx. 50% after 1 wk from last dose. Excreted primarily in urine (21%). **Half-life:** 2–4 days.

⧗ LIFESPAN CONSIDERATIONS

Pregnancy/Lactation: Avoid pregnancy; may cause fetal harm. May increase risk of extrapyramidal symptoms and/or withdrawal syndrome in neonates. Unknown if distributed in breast milk. Must either discontinue drug or discontinue breastfeeding. **Children:** Safety and efficacy not established. **Elderly:** May increase risk of adverse effects due to age-related cardiac/hepatic/renal impairment.

INTERACTIONS

DRUG: Strong CYP3A inhibitors (e.g., clarithromycin, ketoconazole, ritonavir) may increase concentration/effect. **Strong CYP3A inducers (e.g., carBAMazepine, rifAMPin), moderate CYP3A inducers (e.g., nafcillin)** may decrease concentration/effect; avoid use. **Alcohol, antidepressants (e.g., sertraline, nortriptyline), benzodiazepines (e.g., diazePAM, LORazepam), opioids (e.g., morphine), phenothiazines (e.g., thioridazine), sedative/hypnotics (e.g., zolpidem)** may increase CNS depression. **Metoclopramide** may increase adverse effects. **HERBAL: Herbs with sedative properties (e.g., chamomile, kava kava, valerian)** may increase CNS depression. **FOOD:** None significant. **LAB VALUES:** May increase serum ALT, AST, CPK. May decrease serum sodium.

AVAILABILITY (Rx)

💊 Capsules: 1.5 mg, 3 mg, 4.5 mg, 6 mg.

ADMINISTRATION/HANDLING

PO

Give without regard to food. Administer whole; do not break, crush, cut, or open capsule.

INDICATIONS/ROUTES/DOSAGE

Note: Due to the long half-life of cariprazine and its active metabolites, changes in dose will not fully reflect in the plasma for several wks.

Schizophrenia
PO: ADULTS, ELDERLY: Initially, 1.5 mg once daily. May increase to 3 mg on day 2 if tolerated. May further increase in increments of 1.5–3 mg based on clinical response and tolerability. **Range:** 1.5–6 mg once daily.

Bipolar I Disorder (Manic or Mixed Episodes)
PO: ADULTS, ELDERLY: 1.5 mg once on day 1, then increase to 3 mg once daily on day 2. May further increase in increments of 1.5–3 mg based on clinical response and tolerability. **Range:** 3–6 mg once daily.

Depressive Episodes Associated With Bipolar I Disorder (Bipolar Depression)
PO: ADULTS, ELDERLY: Initially, 1.5 mg once daily. Based on clinical response and tolerability, dose may be increased to

3 mg once daily on day 15. **Maximum:** 3 mg once daily.

Adjunctive Therapy to Antidepressants in MDD

PO: ADULTS, ELDERLY: Initially, 1.5 mg once daily. May increase to 3 mg once daily on day 15. **Maximum:** 3 mg once daily.

Concomitant Use of Strong CYP3A Inhibitors

Pts starting strong CYP3A inhibitor while on stable dose of cariprazine: Reduce maintenance cariprazine dose by 50%. Pts taking cariprazine 4.5 mg/day should reduce dosage to 1.5 mg/day or 3 mg/day. Pts taking 1.5 mg/day, adjust dosing to every other day. If the strong CYP3A inhibitor is discontinued, cariprazine may need to be increased. **Pts starting cariprazine while on CYP3A inhibitor:** 1.5 mg once on day 1; no dose on day 2; 1.5 mg once on day 3. After day 3, increase dose to 3 mg once daily as tolerated. If strong CYP3A inhibitor is discontinued, cariprazine may need to be increased.

Dosage in Renal/Hepatic Impairment

Mild to moderate impairment: No dose adjustment. **Severe impairment:** Treatment not recommended.

SIDE EFFECTS

Frequent (26%–11%): Bradykinesia, cogwheel rigidity, drooling, dyskinesia, masked faces, muscle rigidity, dystonia, tremor, salivary hypersecretion, torticollis, trismus, insomnia, akathisia, headache. **Occasional (5%–3%):** Nausea, constipation, restlessness, vomiting, dizziness, agitation, anxiety, dyspepsia, abdominal pain, diarrhea, fatigue, asthenia, back pain, toothache, hypertension, decreased appetite. **Rare (2%–1%):** Dry mouth, weight gain, extremity pain, somnolence, sedation, cough, tachycardia, arthralgia.

ADVERSE EFFECTS/TOXIC REACTIONS

May increase risk of hypotension, orthostatic hypotension, syncope; diabetes mellitus, DKA, hyperglycemia, hyperglycemic hyperosmolar nonketotic coma; leukopenia, neutropenia, febrile neutropenia; aspiration, dysphagia, gastritis, gastric reflux; extrapyramidal symptoms including akathisia, dystonia, parkinsonism, tardive dyskinesia; suicidal ideation. May cause neuroleptic malignant syndrome (NMS), manifested by altered mental status, cardiac arrhythmias, diaphoresis, labile blood pressure, malignant hyperthermia, muscle rigidity, rhabdomyolysis, renal failure. May increase risk of death in pts with dementia-related psychosis. Cognitive and motor impairment reported in 7% of pts. May increase seizure-like activity related to decrease in seizure threshold. Infectious processes including nasopharyngitis, urinary tract infection reported in 1% of pts. Hypersensitivity reactions including angioedema, rash, pruritus have occurred.

NURSING CONSIDERATIONS

BASELINE ASSESSMENT

Obtain Hgb A1c in pts with diabetes; ANC, CBC in pts with baseline leukopenia, neutropenia. Receive full medication history, including herbal products, and screen for interactions. Assess appearance, behavior, speech pattern, levels of interest. Verify pregnancy status. Question history of diabetes, cardiovascular disease, CVA, dysphagia, hepatic impairment, hypersensitivity reaction, TIA, seizures.

INTERVENTION/EVALUATION

Monitor ANC, CBC, fasting lipid profile, fasting plasma glucose levels if clinically indicated. Assess mental status for anxiety, depression, suicidal ideation (esp. at initiation and with change in dosage), social function. Due to long half-life, any change in dosage will not be fully reflected for several wks; monitor closely for adverse effects during the following wks. Monitor for hypersensitivity reaction, dysphagia, tardive dyskinesia, extrapyramidal symptoms, metabolic changes including hyperglycemia. Screen for infection. Monitor for neuroleptic malignant syndrome.

PATIENT/FAMILY TEACHING

• Immediately report thoughts of suicide or plans to commit suicide. • Avoid tasks that require alertness until response to drug is established. • Therapy may increase blood sugar levels. Monitor for blurry vision, confusion, frequent urination, fruity-smelling breath, thirst, weakness. • Treatment may cause fetal harm. Avoid pregnancy. Do not breastfeed. • Treatment may lower ability to fight infection. • Do not ingest grapefruit products or herbal products. • Report drooling, muscle rigidity, lockjaw, tremors, or inability to control muscle movements. • Treatment may increase risk of seizures. • Report confusion, palpitations, profuse sweating, fluctuating blood pressure, unusually high core body temperature, muscle rigidity, dark-colored urine or decreased urine output; may indicate life-threatening neurologic event called neuroleptic malignant syndrome (NMS).

---

carvedilol   `TOP 100` `HIGH ALERT`

kar-**ve**-dil-ole
(Apo-Carvedilol 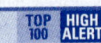, Coreg, Coreg CR)
Do not confuse carvedilol with atenolol or carteolol, or Coreg with Corgard, Cortef, or Cozaar.

◆CLASSIFICATION

PHARMACOTHERAPEUTIC: Beta-adrenergic blocker. **CLINICAL:** Antihypertensive.

USES

Heart failure with reduced ejection fraction: Treatment of mild to severe HF of ischemic or cardiomyopathic origin or to reduce cardiovascular mortality in clinically stable pts who have survived the acute phase of a myocardial infarction (MI) and have a left ventricular ejection fraction of less than or equal to 40% (with or without symptomatic HF). **Hypertension:** Management of hypertension (used alone or in combination with other antihypertensive agents). **OFF-LABEL:** Treatment of angina pectoris atrial fibrillation/flutter. Nonsustained ventricular tachycardia or PVCs (symptomatic), variceal hemorrhage.

PRECAUTIONS

Contraindications: Prior hypersensitivity reactions (e.g., anaphylaxis, angioedema Stevens-Johnson syndrome), bronchial asthma or related bronchospastic conditions, cardiogenic shock, decompensated HF requiring intravenous inotropic therapy, severe hepatic impairment, second- or third-degree AV block, severe bradycardia, or sick sinus syndrome (except in pts with pacemaker). **Cautions:** Diabetes, myasthenia gravis, mild to moderate hepatic impairment. Withdraw gradually to avoid acute tachycardia, hypertension, and/or ischemia. Pts suspected of having Prinzmetal's angina, pheochromocytoma.

ACTION

Possesses nonselective beta-blocking and alpha-adrenergic blocking activity. Causes vasodilation. **Therapeutic Effect: Hypertension:** Reduces cardiac output, exercise-induced tachycardia, reflex orthostatic tachycardia; reduces peripheral vascular resistance. **HF:** Decreases pulmonary capillary wedge pressure, heart rate, systemic vascular resistance; increases stroke volume index.

PHARMACOKINETICS

Route	Onset	Peak	Duration
PO	30 min	1–2 hrs	24 hrs

Widely distributed. Protein binding: 98%. Metabolized in liver. Excreted primarily via bile into feces. Minimally removed by hemodialysis. **Half-life:** 7–10 hrs. Food delays rate of absorption.

⌛ LIFESPAN CONSIDERATIONS

Pregnancy/Lactation: Unknown if drug crosses placenta or is distributed in breast milk. May cause bradycardia, apnea, hypoglycemia, hypothermia during delivery; may contribute to low birth-weight infants. **Children:** Safety and efficacy not established. **Elderly:** Incidence of dizziness may be increased.

INTERACTIONS

DRUG: CYP2C9 inhibitors (e.g., amiodarone, fluoxetine, paroxetine), digoxin may increase concentration/effect. May decrease bronchodilation effect of **beta$_2$ agonists (e.g., albuterol, salmeterol).** May increase concentration/effects of **PAZOpanib, topotecan. Rivastigmine** may increase risk of bradycardia. **HERBAL: Herbals with hypertensive properties (e.g., licorice, yohimbe)** or **hypotensive properties (e.g., garlic, ginger, ginkgo biloba)** may alter effects. **FOOD:** None known. **LAB VALUES:** May increase serum creatinine, bilirubin, ALT, AST, PT.

AVAILABILITY (Rx)

Tablets *(Immediate-Release):* 3.125 mg, 6.25 mg, 12.5 mg, 25 mg.

Capsules: *(Extended-Release):* 10 mg, 20 mg, 40 mg, 80 mg.

ADMINISTRATION/HANDLING

PO

• Give with food to minimize risk of orthostatic hypotension. • Do not crush or cut extended-release capsules. • Capsules may be opened and sprinkled on applesauce for immediate use.

INDICATIONS/ROUTES/DOSAGE

Hypertension

PO: *(Immediate-Release):* **ADULTS, ELDERLY:** Initially, 6.25 mg twice daily. Titrate as needed at 1 wk or greater intervals. **Usual dose:** 6.25–25 mg twice daily. *(Extended-Release):* Initially, 20 mg once daily. Titrate as needed at 1 wk or greater intervals. **Usual dose:** 20–80 mg/day..

HF

PO: *(Immediate-Release):* **ADULTS, ELDERLY:** Initially, 3.125 mg twice daily. May double at 2-wk intervals to target dose. **Maximum: WEIGHING MORE THAN 85 KG:** 50 mg twice daily; **LESS THAN 85 KG:** 25 mg twice daily. *(Extended-Release):* Initially, 10 mg once daily for 2 wks. May increase to 20 mg, 40 mg, and 80 mg over successive intervals of at least 2 wks. **Maximum:** 80 mg/day.

Left Ventricular Dysfunction Following MI

PO: ADULTS, ELDERLY: *(Immediate-Release):* Initially, 6.25 mg twice daily. May increase after 3-10 days to 12.5 mg twice daily, then to a target dose of 25 mg twice daily. *(Extended-Release):* Initially, 10-20 mg once daily. May increase after 3-10 days, to 40 mg once daily, then to a target dose of 80 mg once daily.

Dosage in Renal Impairment

No dose adjustment.

Dosage in Hepatic Impairment

Contraindicated in severe impairment.

SIDE EFFECTS

Frequent (6%–4%): Fatigue, dizziness. **Occasional (2%):** Diarrhea, bradycardia, rhinitis, back pain. **Rare (less than 2%):** Orthostatic hypotension, drowsiness, UTI, viral infection.

ADVERSE EFFECTS/TOXIC REACTIONS

Overdose may cause profound bradycardia, hypotension, bronchospasm, cardiac insufficiency, cardiogenic shock, cardiac arrest. Abrupt withdrawal may result in diaphoresis, palpitations, headache, tremors. May precipitate HF, MI in pts with cardiac disease; thyroid storm in pts with thyrotoxicosis; peripheral ischemia in pts with existing peripheral vascular disease. Hypoglycemia may occur in pts with previously controlled diabetes. May mask symptoms of hypoglycemia (anxiety, confusion, diaphoresis, diplopia, dizziness, headache, hunger, perioral numbness, tachycardia, tremors).

NURSING CONSIDERATIONS

BASELINE ASSESSMENT
Assess B/P, apical pulse immediately before drug is administered (if pulse is 60 beats/min or less or systolic B/P is less than 90 mm Hg, withhold medication, contact physician). Receive full medication history and screen for interactions.

INTERVENTION/EVALUATION
Monitor B/P for hypotension, respirations for dyspnea. Take standing systolic B/P 1 hr after dosing as guide for tolerance. Assess pulse for quality, regularity, rate; monitor for bradycardia. Monitor ECG for cardiac arrhythmias. Assist with ambulation if dizziness occurs. Assess for evidence of HF: Dyspnea (particularly on exertion or lying down), night cough, peripheral edema, distended neck veins. Monitor I&O (increase in weight, decrease in urine output may indicate HF).

PATIENT/FAMILY TEACHING
• Full therapeutic effect of B/P may take 1–2 wks. • Take with food. • Abruptly stopping treatment or missing multiple doses may cause beta-blocker withdrawal symptoms (fast heart rate, high blood pressure, palpitations, sweating, tremors). • Compliance with therapy regimen is essential to control hypertension. • Report excessive fatigue, prolonged dizziness. • Do not use nasal decongestants, OTC cold preparations (stimulants) without physician's approval. • Monitor B/P, pulse before taking medication. • Restrict salt, alcohol intake.

caspofungin

kas-poe-**fun**-jin
(<u>Cancidas</u>)

◆CLASSIFICATION
PHARMACOTHERAPEUTIC: Echinocandin antifungal. **CLINICAL:** Antifungal.

USES
Treatment of invasive aspergillosis, in pts refractory to or intolerant of other therapies. Treatment of candidemia and *Candida* infections (intra-abdominal abscess, peritonitis, pleural space infections). Treatment of esophageal candidiasis. Empiric therapy for presumed fungal infections in febrile neutropenia. **OFF-LABEL:** Oropharyngeal refractory disease. Prophylaxis in invasive fungal infections.

PRECAUTIONS
Contraindications: Hypersensitivity to caspofungin. **Cautions:** Concurrent use of cycloSPORINE; hepatic impairment.

ACTION
Inhibits synthesis of glucan, a vital component of fungal cell wall formation, damaging fungal cell membrane. **Therapeutic Effect:** Inhibits growth and reproduction of fungi.

PHARMACOKINETICS
Widely distributed. Protein binding: 97%. Metabolized in liver. Excreted in urine (50%), feces (30%). Not removed by hemodialysis. **Half-life:** 40–50 hrs.

⊠ LIFESPAN CONSIDERATIONS

Pregnancy/Lactation: May cause fetal harm. Crosses placental barrier. Distributed in breast milk. **Children:** Safety and efficacy not established in pts younger than 3 mos. **Elderly:** Age-related moderate renal impairment may require dosage adjustment.

INTERACTIONS

DRUG: CycloSPORINE may increase concentration/effect. **RifAMPin** may decrease concentration/effect. May decrease therapeutic effect of *Saccharomyces boulardii*. **HERBAL:** None significant. **FOOD:** None known. **LAB VALUES:** May increase serum alkaline phosphatase, bilirubin, creatinine, ALT, AST, urine protein. May decrease serum albumin, bicarbonate, potassium, magnesium; Hgb, Hct.

AVAILABILITY (Rx)

Injection Powder for Reconstitution: 50-mg, 70-mg vials.

ADMINISTRATION/HANDLING

 IV

Reconstitution • Allow vial to warm to room temperature • Reconstitute 50-mg or 70-mg vial with 0.9% NaCl, Sterile Water for Injection, or Bacteriostatic Water for Injection. Further dilute in 0.9% NaCl or D_5W to maximum concentration of 0.5 mg/mL.
Rate of administration • Infuse over 60 min.
Storage • Refrigerate unused vials. • Reconstituted vial may be stored at room temperature for up to 1 hr. • Diluted solution may be stored at room temperature for 24 hrs or 48 hrs if refrigerated. • Discard if solution contains particulate or is discolored.

⊞ IV INCOMPATIBILITIES

Potassium phosphates.

⊞ IV COMPATIBILITIES

Heparin, insulin, magnesium sulfate, norepinephrine, potassium chloride.

INDICATIONS/ROUTES/DOSAGE

Note: Maximum loading dose and daily maintenance dose in children should not exceed 70 mg, regardless of the pt's calculated dose.

Aspergillosis (Refractory or Intolerant to Other Therapies), *Candida* Infections
IV: ADULTS: Initially, 70 mg on day 1, then 50 mg once daily. **CHILDREN 3 MOS TO 17 YRS:** Dosage based on the pt's body surface area. For all indications, administer a single 70-mg/m^2 loading dose on day 1, then 50 mg/m^2 once daily thereafter.

Esophageal Candidiasis
IV: ADULTS: Initially, 70 mg on day 1, then 50 mg once 14–21 days. **CHILDREN 3 MOS TO 17 YRS:** Dosage based on the pt's body surface area, administer a single 70-mg/m^2 loading dose on day 1, then 50 mg/m^2 once daily thereafter.

Dosage in Renal Impairment
No dose adjustment.

Dosage in Hepatic Impairment
Mild impairment: No dose adjustment. **Moderate impairment:** Decrease dose to 35 mg/day. **Severe impairment; children with any degree of hepatic impairment:** Not studied.

SIDE EFFECTS

Frequent (26%): Fever. **Occasional (11%–4%):** Headache, nausea, phlebitis. **Rare (3% or less):** Paresthesia, vomiting, diarrhea, abdominal pain, myalgia, chills, tremor, insomnia.

ADVERSE EFFECTS/TOXIC REACTIONS

Hypersensitivity reaction (rash, facial edema, pruritus, sensation of warmth), including anaphylaxis, may occur. May

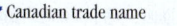 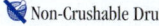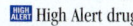

cause hepatic dysfunction, hepatitis (drug-induced), or hepatic failure.

NURSING CONSIDERATIONS

BASELINE ASSESSMENT
Obtain CBC, BMP, LFT. Determine baseline temperature. Question history of prior hypersensitivity reaction.

INTERVENTION/EVALUATION
Assess for signs/symptoms of hepatic dysfunction. Monitor LFT in pts with preexisting hepatic impairment. Monitor CBC, serum potassium. Monitor for fever, hypersensitivity reaction.

PATIENT/FAMILY TEACHING
• Report rash, facial swelling, itching, difficulty breathing, abdominal pain, yellowing of skin or eyes, dark-colored urine, nausea.

ceFAZolin

sef-a-**zoe**-lin
Do not confuse ceFAZolin with cefOXitin, cefprozil, cefTRIAXone, or cephalexin.

◆CLASSIFICATION
PHARMACOTHERAPEUTIC: First-generation cephalosporin. **CLINICAL:** Antibiotic.

USES
Treatment of the following infections when caused by susceptible bacteria: **Respiratory tract infections** due to *S. pneumoniae, S. aureus,* and *S. pyogenes.* **Urinary tract infections** due to *Escherichia coli* and *Proteus mirabilis.* Skin and skin structure infections due to *S. aureus, S. pyogenes,* and *S. agalactiae.* **Biliary infections** due to *E. coli,* various isolates of *Streptococci, P. mirabilis,* and *S. aureus.* **Bone and joint infections** due to *S. aureus.* **Genital infections** due to *E. coli,* and *P. mirabilis.* **Septicemia** due to

S. pneumoniae, S. aureus, P. mirabilis, and *E. coli.* **Endocarditis** due to *S. aureus* and *S. pyogenes.* **OFF-LABEL:** Prophylaxis against infective endocarditis. Treatment of peritonitis, toxic shock syndrome.

PRECAUTIONS
Contraindications: History of hypersensitivity/anaphylactic reaction to ceFAZolin, cephalosporins. **Cautions:** Severe renal impairment, history of penicillin allergy, history of seizures.

ACTION
Binds to bacterial cell membranes, inhibits cell wall synthesis. **Therapeutic Effect:** Bactericidal.

PHARMACOKINETICS
Widely distributed. Protein binding: 85%. Primarily excreted unchanged in urine. Moderately removed by hemodialysis. **Half-life:** 1.4–1.8 hrs (increased in renal impairment).

⧖ LIFESPAN CONSIDERATIONS
Pregnancy/Lactation: Readily crosses placenta; distributed in breast milk. **Children:** No age-related precautions noted. **Elderly:** Age-related renal impairment may require reduced dosage.

INTERACTIONS
DRUG: **Probenecid** may increase concentration/effect. **HERBAL:** None significant. **FOOD:** None known. **LAB VALUES:** May increase serum BUN, alkaline phosphatase, bilirubin, creatinine, LDH, ALT, AST. May cause positive direct/indirect Coombs' test.

AVAILABILITY (Rx)
Injection, Powder for Reconstitution: 500 mg, 1 g. **Ready-to-Hang Infusion:** 1 g/50 mL, 2 g/100 mL.

ADMINISTRATION/HANDLING
 IV

Reconstitution • Reconstitute each 1 g with at least 10 mL Sterile Water for Injection or 0.9% NaCl. • May further dilute in 50–100 mL D$_5$W or 0.9% NaCl (decreases incidence of thrombophlebitis).

Rate of administration • For IV push, administer over 3–5 min (**maximum concentration:** 100 mg/mL). • For intermittent IV infusion (piggyback), infuse over 30–60 min (**maximum concentration:** 20 mg/mL).

Storage • Solution appears light yellow to yellow in color. • Reconstituted solution stable for 24 hrs at room temperature or for 10 days if refrigerated. • IV infusion (piggyback) stable for 48 hrs at room temperature or for 14 days if refrigerated.

IM

• To minimize discomfort, inject deep IM slowly. • Less painful if injected into gluteus maximus rather than lateral aspect of thigh.

▨ IV COMPATIBILITIES

Calcium gluconate, dexmedetomidine, diltiazem, heparin, insulin, magnesium sulfate.

INDICATIONS/ROUTES/DOSAGE

Usual Dosage Range

IV, IM: ADULTS: 1–1.5 g q6–12h (usually q8h). **Maximum:** 12 g/day. **CHILDREN OLDER THAN 1 MO (Mild to Moderate Infection):** 25–100 mg/kg/day divided q6–8h. **Maximum:** 6 g/day. **(Severe Infection):** 100–150 mg/kg/day divided q6–8h. **Maximum:** 12 g/day. **NEONATES:** 50–150 mg/kg/day in 2–4 divided doses.

Dosage in Renal Impairment

Dosing frequency is modified based on creatinine clearance.

Creatinine Clearance	Dosage
11–34 mL/min	50% usual dose q12h
10 mL/min or less	50% usual dose q18–24h
HD	500 mg–1 g q24h
PD	500 mg q12h
CRRT	
CVVH	Loading dose 2 g, then 1–2 g q12h
CVVHD/CVVHDF	Loading dose 2 g, then 1 g q8h or 2 g q12h

Dosage in Hepatic Impairment

No dose adjustment.

SIDE EFFECTS

Frequent: Discomfort with IM administration, oral candidiasis (thrush), mild diarrhea, mild abdominal cramping, vaginal candidiasis. **Occasional:** Nausea, serum sickness–like reaction (fever, joint pain; usually occurs after second course of therapy and resolves after drug is discontinued). **Rare:** Allergic reaction (rash, pruritus, urticaria), thrombophlebitis (pain, redness, swelling at injection site).

ADVERSE EFFECTS/TOXIC REACTIONS

Antibiotic-associated colitis, other superinfections (abdominal cramps, severe watery diarrhea, fever) may result from altered bacterial balance in GI tract. Nephrotoxicity may occur, esp. in pts with preexisting renal disease. Pts with history of penicillin allergy are at increased risk for developing severe hypersensitivity reaction (severe pruritus, angioedema, bronchospasm, anaphylaxis).

NURSING CONSIDERATIONS

BASELINE ASSESSMENT

Obtain CBC, renal function test. Question for history of allergies, particularly cephalosporins, penicillins.

INTERVENTION/EVALUATION

Evaluate IM site for induration and tenderness. Assess oral cavity for white patches on mucous membranes, tongue (thrush). Monitor daily pattern of bowel activity, stool consistency. Mild GI effects may be tolerable (increasing severity may indicate onset of antibiotic-associated colitis). Monitor I&O, renal function tests for nephrotoxicity. Be alert for superinfection: fever, vomiting, diarrhea, anal/genital pruritus, oral mucosal changes (ulceration, pain, erythema).

PATIENT/FAMILY TEACHING

• Discomfort may occur with IM injection.

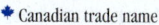 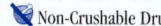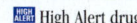

C

cefdinir

sef-di-neer
(Omnicef ✦)

◆CLASSIFICATION

PHARMACOTHERAPEUTIC: Third-generation cephalosporin. **CLINICAL:** Antibiotic.

USES

Community-acquired pneumonia, acute exacerbations of chronic bronchitis, acute maxillary sinusitis, acute bacterial otitis media caused by *H. influenzae* (including β-lactamase producing strains), *S. pneumoniae* (penicillin-susceptible strains only), and *M. catarrhalis* (including β-lactamase producing strains) **Pharyngitis/tonsillitis** caused by *S. pyogenes.* **Uncomplicated skin and skin structure infections** caused by *S. aureus* (including β-lactamase producing strains) and *S. pyogenes.* **OFF-LABEL:** Urinary tract infections.

PRECAUTIONS

Contraindications: Hypersensitivity to cefdinir. History of anaphylactic reaction to cephalosporins. **Cautions:** Hypersensitivity to penicillins; renal impairment.

ACTION

Binds to bacterial cell membranes, inhibits cell wall synthesis. **Therapeutic Effect:** Bactericidal.

PHARMACOKINETICS

Widely distributed. Protein binding: 60%–70%. Not appreciably metabolized. Primarily excreted in urine. Minimally removed by hemodialysis. **Half-life:** 1–2 hrs (increased in renal impairment).

⧗ LIFESPAN CONSIDERATIONS

Pregnancy/Lactation: Crosses placenta. Not detected in breast milk. **Children:** Newborns, infants may have lower renal clearance. **Elderly:** Age-related renal impairment may require decreased dosage or increased dosing interval.

INTERACTIONS

DRUG: Antacids, iron preparations may interfere with absorption. **Probenecid** increases concentration/effect. **HERBAL:** None significant. **FOOD:** None known. **LAB VALUES:** May produce false-positive reaction for urine ketones. May increase serum alkaline phosphatase, bilirubin, LDH, ALT, AST.

AVAILABILITY (Rx)

🐾 **Capsules:** 300 mg. **Powder for Oral Suspension:** 125 mg/5 mL, 250 mg/5 mL.

ADMINISTRATION/HANDLING

PO
• Give without regard to food. Give at least 2 hrs before or after antacids or iron supplements. • Twice-daily doses should be given 12 hrs apart. • Shake oral suspension well before administering. • Store mixed suspension at room temperature for 10 days.

INDICATIONS/ROUTES/DOSAGE

Usual Dosage Range
PO: ADULTS, ELDERLY: 300 mg q12h or 600 mg once daily. **CHILDREN 6 MOS–12 YRS:** 7 mg/kg q12h or 14 mg/kg once daily. **Maximum:** 600 mg/day.

Dosage in Renal Impairment
CrCl less than 30 mL/min: 300 mg/day or 7 mg/kg as single daily dose. **Maximum:** 300 mg. **Hemodialysis pts:** 300 mg or 7 mg/kg/dose every other day. **Maximum:** 300 mg.

Dosage in Hepatic Impairment
No dose adjustment.

SIDE EFFECTS

Frequent: Oral candidiasis, mild diarrhea, mild abdominal cramping, vaginal candidiasis. **Occasional**: Nausea, serum sickness–like reaction (fever, joint pain; usually occurs after second course of therapy and resolves after drug is discontinued). **Rare**: Allergic reaction (rash, pruritus, urticaria).

ADVERSE EFFECTS/TOXIC REACTIONS

Antibiotic-associated colitis, other superinfections (abdominal cramps, severe watery diarrhea, fever) may result from altered bacterial balance in GI tract. Nephrotoxicity may occur, esp. in pts with preexisting renal disease. Pts with history of penicillin allergy are at increased risk for developing a severe hypersensitivity reaction (severe pruritus, angioedema, bronchospasm, anaphylaxis).

NURSING CONSIDERATIONS

BASELINE ASSESSMENT

Obtain CBC, renal function test. Question for hypersensitivity to cefdinir or other cephalosporins, penicillins.

INTERVENTION/EVALUATION

Observe for rash. Monitor daily pattern of bowel activity, stool consistency. Mild GI effects may be tolerable (increasing severity may indicate onset of antibiotic-associated colitis). Be alert for superinfection: Fever, vomiting, diarrhea, anal/genital pruritus, oral mucosal changes (ulceration, pain, erythema). Monitor hematology reports.

PATIENT/FAMILY TEACHING

• Take antacids 2 hrs before or following medication. • Continue medication for full length of treatment; do not skip doses. • Doses should be evenly spaced. • Report persistent severe diarrhea, rash, muscle aches, fever, enlarged lymph nodes, joint pain.

cefepime

sef-e-**peem**
Do not confuse cefepime with cefixime or cefTAZidime.

◆CLASSIFICATION

PHARMACOTHERAPEUTIC: Fourth-generation cephalosporin. **CLINICAL:** Antibiotic.

USES

Pneumonia caused by susceptible strains of *S. pneumoniae, P. aeruginosa, K. pneumoniae,* or *Enterobacter* species. **Empiric therapy for febrile neutropenic pts** at high risk for severe infection. **Uncomplicated/complicated UTIs (including pyelonephritis)** caused by susceptible isolates of *E. coli, K. pneumoniae,* or *P. mirabilis.* **Uncomplicated skin and skin structure infections** caused by *S. aureus* (methicillin-susceptible isolates only) or *S. pyogenes.* **Complicated intra-abdominal infections (used in combination With metronidazole)** caused by susceptible isolates of *E. coli,* viridans group Streptococci, *P. aeruginosa, K. pneumoniae, Enterobacter* species, or *B. fragilis.* **OFF-LABEL:** Gram-negative bacteremia, acute pulmonary exacerbations in cystic fibrosis; diabetic foot infection, neutropenic fever (high-risk cancer pts), osteomyelitis, peritonitis, prosthetic joint infection, sepsis/septic shock, septic arthritis.

PRECAUTIONS

Contraindications: History of anaphylactic reaction to penicillins, hypersensitivity to cefepime, cephalosporins. **Cautions:** Renal impairment, history of seizure disorder, GI disease (colitis), elderly.

ACTION

Binds to bacterial cell wall membranes, inhibits cell wall synthesis. **Therapeutic Effect:** Bactericidal.

 ✜ Canadian trade name 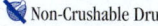 Non-Crushable Drug 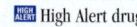 High Alert drug

C

PHARMACOKINETICS

Widely distributed. Protein binding: 20%. Primarily excreted in urine. Removed by hemodialysis. **Half-life:** 2–2.3 hrs (increased in renal impairment, elderly pts).

⏳ LIFESPAN CONSIDERATIONS

Pregnancy/Lactation: Unknown if distributed in breast milk. **Children:** No age-related precautions noted in pts older than 2 mos. **Elderly:** Age-related renal impairment may require reduced dosage or increased dosing interval. Elderly pts with renal insufficiency may have an increased risk of encephalopathy, seizures.

INTERACTIONS

DRUG: Probenecid may increase concentration/effect. May increase concentration/effect of **aminoglycosides**. **HERBAL:** None significant. **FOOD:** None known. **LAB VALUES:** May increase serum BUN, alkaline phosphatase, bilirubin, LDH, ALT, AST. May cause positive direct/indirect Coombs' test.

AVAILABILITY (Rx)

Injection, Powder for Reconstitution: 1 g, 2 g. **Injection, Premix:** 1 g (50 mL), 2 g (100 mL).

ADMINISTRATION/HANDLING

 IV

Reconstitution • Add 10 mL of diluent for 1-g and 2-g vials. • Further dilute with 50–100 mL 0.9% NaCl or D₅W. **Rate of administration** • For intermittent IV infusion (piggyback), infuse over 30 min. For IV push, administer over 5 min.
Storage • Solution is stable for 24 hrs at room temperature, 7 days if refrigerated.

IM
• Add 2.4 mL Sterile Water for Injection, 0.9% NaCl, or D₅W to 1-g and 2-g vials. • Inject into a large muscle mass (e.g., upper gluteus maximus).

🕸 IV INCOMPATIBILITIES

Nicardipine, propofol.

🕸 IV COMPATIBILITIES

Dexmedetomidine, insulin.

INDICATIONS/ROUTES/DOSAGE

Usual Dosage Range

IV: ADULTS, ELDERLY: 1–2 g q8–12h. **CHILDREN:** 50 mg/kg q8–12h. **Maximum:** 2,000 mg/dose. **NEONATES:** 30 mg/kg q12h up to 50 mg/kg q8–12h.

Dosage in Renal Impairment

Dosage and frequency are modified based on creatinine clearance and severity of infection.

Creatinine Clearance Dosage

Creatinine Clearance	Dosage
30–60 mL/min	500 mg q24h–2 g q12h
11–29 mL/min	500 mg–2 g q24h
10 mL/min or less	250 mg–1 g q24h
Hemodialysis	Initially, 1 g, then 0.5–1 g q24h or 1–2 g q48–72h
Peritoneal dialysis	Normal dose q48h
Continuous renal replacement therapy	Initially, 2 g, then 1 g q8h or 2 g q12h

Dosage in Hepatic Impairment

No dose adjustment.

SIDE EFFECTS

Frequent: Discomfort with IM administration, oral candidiasis (thrush), mild diarrhea, mild abdominal cramping, vaginal candidiasis. **Occasional:** Nausea, serum sickness–like reaction (fever, joint pain; usually occurs after second course of therapy and resolves after drug is discontinued). **Rare:** Allergic reaction (rash, pruritus, urticaria), thrombophlebitis (pain, redness, swelling at injection site).

ADVERSE EFFECTS/TOXIC REACTIONS

Antibiotic-associated colitis, other superinfections (abdominal cramps, severe watery diarrhea, fever) may result from altered bacterial balance in GI tract. Nephrotoxicity may occur, esp. in pts with preexisting renal disease. Pts with history of penicillin allergy are at increased risk for developing a severe hypersensitivity reaction (severe pruritus, angioedema, bronchospasm, anaphylaxis).

NURSING CONSIDERATIONS

BASELINE ASSESSMENT
Obtain CBC, renal function test. Question for history of allergies, particularly cephalosporins, penicillins.

INTERVENTION/EVALUATION
Evaluate IM site for induration and tenderness. Assess oral cavity for white patches on mucous membranes, tongue (thrush). Monitor daily pattern of bowel activity, stool consistency. Mild GI effects may be tolerable (increasing severity may indicate onset of antibiotic-associated colitis). Monitor I&O, CBC, renal function tests for nephrotoxicity. Be alert for superinfection: Fever, vomiting, diarrhea, anal/genital pruritus, oral mucosal changes (ulceration, pain, erythema).

PATIENT/FAMILY TEACHING
• Discomfort may occur with IM injection. • Continue therapy for full length of treatment. • Doses should be evenly spaced. • Report persistent diarrhea.

---

cefotaxime

sef-oh-**tax**-eem
Do not confuse cefotaxime with cefOXitin, ceftizoxime, or cefuroxime.

◆CLASSIFICATION
PHARMACOTHERAPEUTIC: Third-generation cephalosporin. **CLINICAL:** Antibiotic.

USES
Treatment of bacteremia/septicemia, bone and joint infections, CNS infections (e.g., meningitis), genitourinary infections, gynecologic infections, intra-abdominal infections, lower respiratory tract infections (e.g., pneumonia), skin and skin structure infections caused by susceptible strains of microorganisms including *S. pneumoniae, S. pyogenes* (Group A Streptococci) *S. aureus* (penicillinase and non-penicillinase producing), *E. coli, Klebsiella* species, *H. influenzae, P. mirabilis, S. marcescens, Enterobacter* species, indole-positive *Proteus* and *Pseudomonas* species (including *P. aeruginosa*). **OFF-LABEL:** Surgical prophylaxis, bite wound, COPD (acute exacerbation), gonococcal infection, Lyme disease, *Salmonella* species infection, skin/soft tissue necrotizing infections.

PRECAUTIONS
Contraindications: History of hypersensitivity/anaphylactic reaction to cefotaxime, cephalosporins. **Cautions:** History of penicillin allergy, colitis, renal impairment with CrCl less than 30 mL/min.

ACTION
Binds to bacterial cell membranes, inhibits cell wall synthesis. **Therapeutic Effect:** Bactericidal.

PHARMACOKINETICS
Widely distributed to CSF. Protein binding: 30%–50%. Partially metabolized in liver. Primarily excreted in urine. Moderately removed by hemodialysis. **Half-life:** 1 hr (increased in renal impairment).

⧖ LIFESPAN CONSIDERATIONS
Pregnancy/Lactation: Readily crosses placenta. Distributed in breast milk. **Children:** No age-related precautions noted. **Elderly:** Age-related renal impairment may require dosage adjustment.

INTERACTIONS
DRUG: Probenecid may increase concentration/effect. **HERBAL:** None significant. **FOOD:** None known. **LAB VALUES:** May cause positive direct/indirect Coombs' test. May increase serum BUN, creatinine, ALT, AST, alkaline phosphatase.

C

AVAILABILITY (Rx)

Injection, Powder for Reconstitution: 1 g, 2 g.

ADMINISTRATION/HANDLING

 IV

Reconstitution • Reconstitute with 10 mL Sterile Water for Injection or 0.9% NaCl to provide a maximum concentration of 100 mg/mL. • May further dilute with 50–100 mL 0.9% NaCl or D₅W.

Rate of administration • For IV push, administer over 3–5 min. • For intermittent IV infusion (piggyback), infuse over 15–30 min.

Storage • Solution appears light yellow to amber. • IV infusion (piggyback) is stable for 24 hrs at room temperature, 5 days if refrigerated. • Discard if precipitate forms.

IM

• Reconstitute with Sterile Water for Injection or Bacteriostatic Water for Injection to provide a concentration of 230–330 mg/mL. • To minimize discomfort, inject deep IM slowly. Less painful if injected into gluteus maximus than lateral aspect of thigh. For 2-g IM dose, give at 2 separate sites.

IV COMPATIBILITIES

Dexmedetomidine, diltiazem, magnesium sulfate, propofol.

INDICATIONS/ROUTES/DOSAGE

Usual Dosage Range

IV, IM: ADULTS, ELDERLY: Uncomplicated infection: 1 g q12h. **Moderate to severe infection:** 1–2 g q8h. **Life-threatening infection:** 2 g q4h. **INFANTS, CHILDREN, ADOLESCENTS:** 150–180 mg/kg/day in divided doses q8h. **Maximum:** 8 g/day. **NEONATES:** 50 mg/kg/dose q6–12h.

Dosage in Renal Impairment

Creatinine Clearance	Dosage Interval
10–50 mL/min	6–12 hrs
Less than 10 mL/min	24 hrs
Hemodialysis	1–2 g q24h
Peritoneal dialysis	1g q24h
CVVH	1–2 g q8–12h
CVVHD	1–2g q8h
CVVHDF	1–2g q6–8h

Dosage in Hepatic Impairment

No dose adjustment.

SIDE EFFECTS

Frequent: Discomfort with IM administration, oral candidiasis (thrush), mild diarrhea, mild abdominal cramping, vaginal candidiasis. **Occasional:** Nausea, serum sickness–like reaction (fever, joint pain; usually occurs after second course of therapy and resolves after drug is discontinued). **Rare:** Allergic reaction (rash, pruritus, urticaria), thrombophlebitis (pain, redness, swelling at injection site).

ADVERSE EFFECTS/TOXIC REACTIONS

Antibiotic-associated colitis, other superinfections (abdominal cramps, severe watery diarrhea, fever) may result from altered bacterial balance in GI tract. Nephrotoxicity may occur, esp. in pts with preexisting renal disease. Pts with history of penicillin allergy are at increased risk for developing a severe hypersensitivity reaction (severe pruritus, angioedema, bronchospasm, anaphylaxis).

NURSING CONSIDERATIONS

BASELINE ASSESSMENT

Question for history of allergies, particularly cephalosporins, penicillins.

INTERVENTION/EVALUATION

Check IM injection sites for induration, tenderness. Assess oral cavity for white patches on mucous membranes, tongue (thrush). Monitor daily pattern of bowel activity, stool consistency. Mild GI effects may be tolerable (increasing severity may indicate onset of antibiotic-associated colitis). Monitor I&O, renal function tests for nephrotoxicity. Be alert for superinfection: Fever, vomiting, diarrhea, anal/genital pruritus, oral mucosal changes (ulceration, pain, erythema).

PATIENT/FAMILY TEACHING

• Discomfort may occur with IM injection. • Doses should be evenly spaced. • Continue antibiotic therapy for full length of treatment.

---

ceftaroline

sef-**tar**-o-leen
(Teflaro)

◆CLASSIFICATION

PHARMACOTHERAPEUTIC: Fifth-generation cephalosporin. **CLINICAL:** Antibiotic.

USES

Treatment of susceptible infections due to gram-positive and gram-negative organisms, including *S. pneumoniae, S. aureus* (methicillin-susceptible only), *H. influenzae, Klebsiella pneumoniae, E. coli,* including acute bacterial skin and skin structure infections in adults and pts at least 34 wks gestational age and 12 days postnatal age, community-acquired bacterial pneumonia in adults and pts 2 mos of age and older. **OFF-LABEL:** Bloodstream infections. Hospital-acquired or ventilator-associated pneumonia.

PRECAUTIONS

Contraindications: History of hypersensitivity/anaphylactic reaction to ceftaroline, cephalosporins. **Cautions:** History of allergy to penicillin, severe renal impairment with CrCl less than 50 mL/min, elderly.

ACTION

Binds to bacterial cell membranes, inhibits cell wall synthesis. **Therapeutic Effect:** Bactericidal.

PHARMACOKINETICS

Widely distributed. Protein binding: 20%. Not metabolized. Primarily excreted in urine. Hemodialyzable. **Half-life:** 1.6 hrs (increased in renal impairment).

⌛ LIFESPAN CONSIDERATIONS

Pregnancy/Lactation: Unknown if distributed in breast milk. **Children:** No age-related precautions noted. **Elderly:** Age-related renal impairment may require dose adjustment.

INTERACTIONS

DRUG: Probenecid may increase concentration /effect. May alter concentration/effect of **aminoglycosides (e.g., gentamicin). HERBAL:** None significant. **FOOD:** None known. **LAB VALUES:** May cause positive direct/indirect Coombs' test. May increase serum BUN, creatinine. May decrease serum potassium.

AVAILABILITY (Rx)

Injection, Powder for Reconstitution: 400-mg, 600-mg single-use vial.

ADMINISTRATION/HANDLING

◀**ALERT**▶ Give by intermittent IV infusion (piggyback). Do not give IV push.
Reconstitution • Reconstitute either 400-mg or 600-mg vial with 20 mL Sterile Water for Injection. • Mix gently to dissolve powder. • Further dilute with 50–250 mL D$_5$W, 0.9% NaCl.
Rate of administration • Infuse over 5–60 min.
Storage • Discard if particulate is present. • Following reconstitution, solution should appear clear, light to dark yellow. • Solution is stable for 6 hrs at room temperature or 24 hrs if refrigerated.

C

 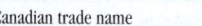

✲ IV INCOMPATIBILITIES

Potassium phosphate, sodium phosphate.

✲ IV COMPATIBILITIES

Calcium gluconate, diltiazem, heparin, insulin, magnesium sulfate, norepinephrine, potassium chloride, propofol, vasopressin.

INDICATIONS/ROUTES/DOSAGE

Usual Dosage

IV: ADULTS, ELDERLY: 600 mg q12h. **CHILDREN 2–18 YRS (WEIGHING MORE THAN 33 KG):** 400 mg q8h or 600 mg q12h. **(WEIGHING 33 KG OR LESS):** 12 mg/kg q8h. **CHILDREN 2 MOS TO LESS THAN 2 YRS:** 8 mg/kg q8h. **GESTATIONAL AGE 34 WKS AND OLDER AND POSTNATAL AGE 12 DAYS AND OLDER:** 6 mg/kg q8h.

Dosage in Renal Impairment

Creatinine Clearance	Dosage
30–50 mL/min	400 mg q12h
15–29 mL/min	300 mg q12h
End-stage renal disease, hemodialysis	200 mg every 12 hrs (give after dialysis)

Dosage in Hepatic Impairment

No dose adjustment.

SIDE EFFECTS

Occasional (5%–4%): Diarrhea, nausea. **Rare (3%–2%):** Allergic reaction (rash, pruritus, urticaria), phlebitis.

ADVERSE EFFECTS/TOXIC REACTIONS

Antibiotic-associated colitis, other superinfections (abdominal cramps, severe watery diarrhea, fever) may result from altered bacterial balance in GI tract. Nephrotoxicity may occur, esp. with preexisting renal disease. Pts with history of penicillin allergy are at increased risk for developing a severe hypersensitivity reaction (severe pruritus, angioedema, bronchospasm, anaphylaxis).

NURSING CONSIDERATIONS

BASELINE ASSESSMENT

Obtain CBC, renal function test. Question for hypersensitivity to other cephalosporins, penicillins. For pts on hemodialysis, administer medication after dialysis.

INTERVENTION/EVALUATION

Assess oral cavity for white patches on mucous membranes, tongue (thrush). Monitor daily pattern of bowel activity, stool consistency. Mild GI effects may be tolerable, but increasing severity may indicate onset of antibiotic-associated colitis. Monitor I&O, renal function tests for evidence of nephrotoxicity. Be alert for superinfection: Fever, vomiting, severe genital/anal pruritus, moderate to severe diarrhea, oral mucosal changes (ulceration, pain, erythema).

PATIENT/FAMILY TEACHING

• Continue medication for full length of treatment. • Doses should be evenly spaced.

cefTAZidime

sef-**taz**-i-deem
(Tazicef)
Do not confuse cefTAZidime with ceFAZolin, cefepime, or cefTRIAXone.

◆CLASSIFICATION

PHARMACOTHERAPEUTIC: Third-generation cephalosporin. **CLINICAL:** Antibiotic.

USES

Treatment of lower respiratory tract infections (e.g., pneumonia), skin and skin structure infections, UTIs, bacterial septicemia, bone and joint infections, gynecologic infections, intra-abdominal Infections, CNS infections (e.g., meningitis) caused by susceptible strain of microorganisms including *P. aeruginosa* and other *Pseudomonas* spp.; *H. influenzae, Klebsiella* spp.; *Enterobacter* spp.; *P. mirabilis; E. coli; Serratia* spp.; *Citrobacter* spp.; *S. pneumoniae;* and *S. aureus* (methicillin-susceptible strains). **OFF-LABEL:** Bacterial endophthalmitis; acute pulmonary exacerbation in cystic fibrosis, diabetic foot infection, peritonitis.

PRECAUTIONS

Contraindications: History of hypersensitivity/anaphylactic reaction to cefTAZidime, cephalosporins. **Cautions:** Severe renal impairment, history of penicillin allergy, seizure disorder.

ACTION

Binds to bacterial cell membranes, inhibits cell wall synthesis. **Therapeutic Effect:** Bactericidal.

PHARMACOKINETICS

Widely distributed, including to CSF. Protein binding: 5%–17%. Primarily excreted in urine. Removed by hemodialysis. **Half-life:** 2 hrs (increased in renal impairment).

⧗ LIFESPAN CONSIDERATIONS

Pregnancy/Lactation: Readily crosses placenta. Distributed in breast milk. **Children:** No age-related precautions noted. **Elderly:** Age-related renal impairment may require dosage adjustment.

INTERACTIONS

DRUG: Probenecid may increase concentration/effect. May alter concentration/effect of **aminoglycosides (e.g., gentamicin). HERBAL:** None significant. **FOOD:** None known. **LAB VALUES:** May increase serum BUN, alkaline phosphatase, creatinine, LDH, ALT, AST. May cause positive direct/indirect Coombs' test.

AVAILABILITY (Rx)

Injection Powder for Reconstitution: 1 g, 2 g. **Injection Premix:** 1 g/50 mL.

ADMINISTRATION/HANDLING

◀**ALERT**▶ Give by IM injection, direct IV injection (IV push), or intermittent IV infusion (piggyback).

 IV

Reconstitution • Add 10 mL Sterile Water for Injection to each 1 g to provide concentration of 90 mg/mL. • May further dilute with 50–100 mL 0.9% NaCl, D5W, or other compatible diluent.
Rate of administration • For IV push, administer over 3–5 min (**maximum concentration:** 180 mg/mL). • For intermittent IV infusion (piggyback), infuse over 15–30 min.
Storage • Solution appears light yellow to amber, tends to darken (color change does not indicate loss of potency). • IV infusion (piggyback) stable for 12 hrs at room temperature or 3 days if refrigerated. • Discard if precipitate forms.

IM

Reconstitution • Add 1.5 mL Sterile Water for Injection or lidocaine 1% to 500-mg vial or 3 mL to 1-g vial to provide a concentration of 280 mg/mL. • To minimize discomfort, inject deep IM slowly. Less painful if injected into gluteus maximus than lateral aspect of thigh.

▦ IV INCOMPATIBILITIES

Amiodarone, ibuprofen.

▦ IV COMPATIBILITIES

Dexmedetomidine, diltiazem, heparin, insulin.

INDICATIONS/ROUTES/DOSAGE
Usual Dosage Range
IV, IM: ADULTS, ELDERLY: 1–2 g q8–12h. **IV: CHILDREN 1 MO–12 YRS: Mild to moderate infection:** 90–150 mg/kg/day in divided doses q8h. **Maximum:** 6 g/day. **Severe infection:** 200–300 mg/kg/day in divided doses q8h. **Maxi**

C

mum: 6 g/day. **NEONATES 0–4 WKS:** 50 mg/kg/dose q8–12h.

Dosage in Renal Impairment
Dosage and frequency are modified based on creatinine clearance and severity of infection.

Creatinine Clearance	Dosage
31–50 mL/min	1g q12h
16–30 mL/min	1g q24h
6–15 mL/min	500 mg q24h
Less than 6 mL/min	500 mg q48h
Hemodialysis	0.5–1 g q24h or 1–2 g q48–72h (give post hemodialysis on dialysis days)
Peritoneal dialysis	Initially, 1 g, then 0.5 g q24h
Continuous renal replacement therapy	Initially, 2 g, then 1 g q8h or 2 g q12h

Dosage in Hepatic Impairment
No dose adjustment.

SIDE EFFECTS

Frequent: Discomfort with IM administration, oral candidiasis (thrush), mild diarrhea, mild abdominal cramping, vaginal candidiasis. **Occasional:** Nausea, serum sickness–like reaction (fever, joint pain; usually occurs after second course of therapy and resolves after drug is discontinued). **Rare:** Allergic reaction (pruritus, rash, urticaria), thrombophlebitis (pain, redness, swelling at injection site).

ADVERSE EFFECTS/TOXIC REACTIONS

Antibiotic-associated colitis, other superinfections (abdominal cramps, severe watery diarrhea, fever) may result from altered bacterial balance in GI tract. Nephrotoxicity may occur, esp. in pts with preexisting renal disease. Pts with history of penicillin allergy are at increased risk for developing a severe hypersensitivity reaction (severe pruritus, angioedema, bronchospasm, anaphylaxis).

NURSING CONSIDERATIONS

BASELINE ASSESSMENT
Obtain CBC, renal function test. Question for history of allergies, particularly cephalosporins, penicillins.

INTERVENTION/EVALUATION
Evaluate IV site for phlebitis (heat, pain, red streaking over vein). Assess IM injection sites for induration, tenderness. Check oral cavity for white patches on mucous membranes, tongue (thrush). Monitor daily pattern of bowel activity, stool consistency. Mild GI effects may be tolerable (increasing severity may indicate onset of antibiotic-associated colitis). Monitor I&O, renal function tests for nephrotoxicity. Be alert for superinfection: fever, vomiting, diarrhea, anal/genital pruritus, oral mucosal changes (ulceration, pain, erythema).

PATIENT/FAMILY TEACHING
• Discomfort may occur with IM injection. • Doses should be evenly spaced. • Continue antibiotic therapy for full length of treatment.

cefTAZidime/avibactam

sef-**taz**-i-deem/**a**-vi-**bak**-tam
(Avycaz)
Do not confuse cefTAZidime with ceFAZolin or cefepime, or avibactam with sulbactam or tazobactam.

◆CLASSIFICATION

PHARMACOTHERAPEUTIC: Cephalosporin/beta-lactamase inhibitor. **CLINICAL:** Antibacterial.

USES

Used in combination with metroNIDAZOLE for treatment of complicated intra-abdominal infections caused by the following susceptible microorganisms:

E. cloacae, E. coli, K. pneumoniae, K. oxytoca, P. mirabilis, P. stuartii, and P. aeruginosa in adults and pediatric pts 3 mos and older. Treatment of complicated urinary tract infections, including pyelonephritis, caused by the following susceptible microorganisms: C. freundii, C. koseri, E. aerogenes, E. cloacae, E. coli, K. pneumoniae, Proteus spp., and P. aeruginosa in adults and pediatric pts 3 mos and older. Treatment of hospital-acquired bacterial pneumonia and ventilator-associated bacterial pneumonia (HAP/VAP) caused by the following susceptible microorganisms: K. pneumoniae, E. cloacae, E. coli, Serratia marcescens, P. mirabilis, P. aeruginosa, and Haemophilus influenzae.

PRECAUTIONS

Contraindications: Hypersensitivity to avibactam-containing products, cefTAZidime, cephalosporins. **Cautions:** History of renal impairment, seizure disorder, encephalopathy, recent C. difficile infection or antibiotic-associated colitis. Hypersensitivity to penicillins, other beta-lactams.

ACTION

Inhibits cell wall synthesis by binding to bacterial cell membrane. Bacterial action of cefTAZidime is mediated through binding to essential penicillin-binding proteins. Avibactam inactivates some beta-lactamases and protects cefTAZidime from degradation by certain beta-lactamases. **Therapeutic Effect:** Bactericidal.

PHARMACOKINETICS

Widely distributed. Excreted unchanged as parent drug; not significantly metabolized in liver. Protein binding: less than 10%. Removed extensively by hemodialysis (55% of dose). Eliminated in urine (80%–90% unchanged). **Half-life:** 2.7 hrs (dependent on dose and severity of renal impairment).

⧗ LIFESPAN CONSIDERATIONS

Pregnancy/Lactation: CefTAZidime is excreted in breast milk in low concentrations. Unknown if avibactam is excreted in breast milk. **Children:** Safety and efficacy not established. **Elderly:** May have increased risk of adverse effects (due to renal impairment).

INTERACTIONS

DRUG: May decrease therapeutic effect of **BCG (intravesical). Probenecid** may increase concentration/effect of avibactam. May alter concentration/effect of **aminoglycosides (e.g., gentamicin).** **HERBAL:** None significant. **FOOD:** None known. **LAB VALUES:** May increase serum alkaline phosphatase, ALT, GGT, LDH. May decrease platelets, eosinophils, leukocytes, lymphocytes, serum potassium. May result in positive Coombs' test or false-positive elevated urine glucose.

AVAILABILITY (Rx)

◀**ALERT**▶ CefTAZidime/avibactam is a combination product.
Injection, Powder for Reconstitution: 2 gm cefTAZidime/0.5 gm avibactam.

ADMINISTRATION/HANDLING
 IV

Reconstitution • Reconstitute vial with 10 mL of one of the following solutions: 0.9% NaCl, Sterile Water for Injection, or 5% Dextrose Injection. • Shake gently until powder is completely dissolved. • Visually inspect for particulate matter or discoloration. Solution should appear clear to slightly yellow in color. • Final concentration of vial will equal approx. 0.167 g/mL of cefTAZidime and 0.042 g/mL of avibactam. • Further dilute with 50 mL to 250 mL 0.9% NaCl or 5% Dextrose Injection. **Rate of administration** • Infuse over 2 hrs.
Storage • Diluted solution may be stored at room temperature up to 12 hrs or refrigerated up to 24 hrs. • Infuse within 12 hrs once removed from refrigerator. • Do not freeze.

▦ IV COMPATABILITIES

Dexmedetomidine, heparin, magnesium sulfate, norepinephrine, potassium chloride, potassium phosphates.

INDICATIONS/ROUTES/DOSAGE

Complicated Intra-Abdominal Infections
IV: ADULTS, ELDERLY: 2.5 g (cefTAZidime 2 g/avibactam 0.5 g) q8h for 5–14 days (in combination with metroNIDAZOLE). **INFANTS 6 MOS AND OLDER, CHILDREN, ADOLESCENTS YOUNGER THAN 18 YRS:** 50 mg cefTAZidime/kg/dose q8h; **Maximum:** 2g cefTAZidime/dose. **INFANTS 3 MOS TO LESS THAN 6 MOS:** 40 mg cefTAZidime/kg/dose q8h.

Complicated Urinary Tract Infections Including Pyelonephritis
IV: ADULTS, ELDERLY: 2.5 g (2 g cefTAZidime/0.5 g avibactam) q8h for 7–14 days. **INFANTS 6 MOS AND OLDER, CHILDREN, ADOLESCENTS YOUNGER THAN 18 YRS:** 50 mg cefTAZidime/kg/dose q8h. **Maximum:** 2 g cefTAZidime/dose. **INFANTS 3 MOS TO LESS THAN 6 MOS:** 40 mg cefTAZidime/kg/dose q8h.

HAP/VAP
IV: ADULTS, ELDERLY: 2.5 g (2 g cefTAZidime/0.5 g avibactam) q8h for 7–14 days.

Dosage in Renal Impairment
Note: Infuse after hemodialysis on hemodialysis days. Dosage is modified based on creatinine clearance.

Creatinine Clearance	Dosage
Greater than 50 mL/min	2.5 g (2 g/0.5 g) q8h
31–50 mL/min	1.25 g (1 g/0.25 g) q8h
16–30 mL/min	0.94 g (0.75 g/0.19 g) q12h
6–15 mL/min	0.94 g (0.75 g/0.19 g) q24h
Less than or equal to 5 mL/min	0.94 g (0.75 g/0.19 g) q48h

Dosage in Hepatic Impairment
No dose adjustment.

SIDE EFFECTS

Occasional (14%–5%): Vomiting, nausea, abdominal pain, anxiety, rash. **Rare (4%–2%):** Constipation, dizziness.

ADVERSE EFFECTS/TOXIC REACTIONS

May cause worsening of renal function or acute renal failure in pts with renal impairment. Clinical cure rates were lower in pts with CrCl 30–50 mL/min compared with those with CrCl greater than 50 mL/min, and in pts receiving metroNIDAZOLE combination therapy. Blood and lymphatic disorders such as agranulocytosis, hemolytic anemia, leukopenia, lymphocytosis, neutropenia, thrombocytopenia were reported. Hypersensitivity reactions, including anaphylaxis or severe skin reactions, have been reported in pts treated with beta-lactam antibacterial drugs. *C. difficile*–associated diarrhea, with severity ranging from mild diarrhea to fatal colitis, may occur more than 2 mos after treatment completion. CNS reactions including asterixis, coma, encephalopathy, neuromuscular excitability, myoclonus, nonconvulsive status epilepticus, seizures have been reported in pts receiving cefTAZidime, esp. in pts with renal impairment. May increase risk of development of drug-resistant bacteria when used in the absence of a proven or strongly suspected bacterial infection. Skin and subcutaneous tissue disorders such as angioedema, erythema multiforme, pruritus, Stevens-Johnson syndrome, toxic epidermal necrolysis were reported in pts receiving cefTAZidime. Other reported adverse effects, including infusion site inflammation/hematoma/thrombosis, jaundice, candidiasis, dysgeusia, paresthesia, tubulointerstitial nephritis, vaginal inflammation, occur rarely.

NURSING CONSIDERATIONS

BASELINE ASSESSMENT

Obtain CBC, BUN, serum creatinine, potassium; CrCl, eGFR, LFT; bacterial culture and sensitivity; vital signs. Question history of recent *C. difficile* infection, renal impairment, seizure disorder; hypersensitivity reaction to beta-lactams, carbapenem, cephalosporins, PCN. Assess skin for wounds; assess hydration status. Question pt's usual stool characteristics (color, frequency, consistency).

INTERVENTION/EVALUATION

Monitor CBC, BMP, renal function periodically. For pts with changing renal function, monitor renal function test daily and adjust dose accordingly. Diligently monitor I&Os. Observe daily pattern of bowel activity, stool consistency (increased severity may indicate antibiotic-associated colitis). If frequent diarrhea occurs, obtain *C. difficile* toxin screen and initiate isolation precautions until test result confirmed; manage proper fluids levels/PO intake, electrolyte levels, protein intake. Antibacterial drugs that are not directed against *C. difficile* infection may need to be discontinued. Report any sign of hypersensitivity reaction.

PATIENT/FAMILY TEACHING

• It is essential to complete drug therapy despite symptom improvement. Early discontinuation may result in antibacterial resistance or increased risk of recurrent infection. • Report any episodes of diarrhea, esp. in the mos following treatment completion. Frequent diarrhea, fever, abdominal pain, blood-streaked stool may indicate infectious diarrhea and may be contagious to others. • Report abdominal pain, black/tarry stools, bruising, yellowing of skin or eyes; dark urine, decreased urine output; skin problems such as development of sores, rash, skin bubbling/necrosis. • Drink plenty of fluids. • Report any nervous system changes such as anxiety, confusion, hallucinations, muscle jerking, or seizure-like activity. • Severe allergic reactions such as hives, palpitations, shortness of breath, rash, tongue-swelling may occur.

ceftobiprole medocaril

sef-**toe**-bye-prole me-**dok**-a-ril
(Zevtera)
Do not confuse ceftobiprole with cefazolin, ceftaroline, ceftazidime, or ceftriaxone.

◆CLASSIFICATION

PHARMACOTHERAPEUTIC: Cephalosporin. **CLINICAL:** Antibiotic.

USES

Staphylococcus aureus **Bloodstream (SAB) Infections:** Treatment of adults with SAB (bacteremia), including those with right-sided infective endocarditis caused by methicillin-susceptible and methicillin-resistant isolates. **Acute Bacterial Skin and Skin Structure Infections (ABSSSI):** Treatment of adults with ABSSSI caused by susceptible isolates of the following gram-positive and gram-negative microorganisms: *Staphylococcus aureus* (methicillin-susceptible and methicillin-resistant isolates), *Streptococcus pyogenes*, and *Klebsiella pneumoniae*. **Community-Acquired Bacterial Pneumonia (CABP):** Treatment of adult and pediatric pts aged 3 mos to less than 18 yrs) with CABP caused by susceptible isolates of the following gram-positive and gram-negative microorganisms: *Staphylococcus aureus* (methicillin-susceptible isolates), *S. pneumoniae*, *H. influenzae*, *H. parainfluenzae*, *E. coli*, and *Klebsiella pneumoniae*.

PRECAUTIONS

Contraindications: Hypersensitivity to ceftobiprole, cephalosporins. **Cautions:** History of seizure disorder, renal impairment, hypersensitivity reaction to penicillin. Avoid concomitant use of OATP1B1 and OATP1B3 substrates.

ACTION

Binds to bacterial cell membranes, inhibiting cell wall synthesis. **Therapeutic Effect:** Bactericidal.

PHARMACOKINETICS

Widely distributed. Minimally metabolized. Protein binding: 16%. Excreted in urine (83%). **Half-life:** 3.3 hrs.

LIFESPAN CONSIDERATIONS

Pregnancy/Lactation: Unknown if distributed in breast milk. **Children:** Safety and efficacy not established in pts younger than 3 mos. **Elderly:** No age-related precautions noted.

C

INTERACTIONS

DRUG: May increase concentration/effects of **OATP1B1 and OATP1B3 substrates (e.g., atorvastatin, losartan, simvastatin, valsartan). HERBAL:** None significant. **FOOD:** None known. **LAB VALUES:** May increase serum alkaline phosphatase, ALT, AST, bilirubin, GGT, lactate dehydrogenase. May decrease leukocytes, platelets; serum potassium. May cause false positive dipstick test results (e.g., urine glucose, ketones, proteins; occult blood). May cause positive direct/indirect Coombs test.

AVAILABILITY (Rx)

Injection, Powder for Reconstitution: 667 mg.

ADMINISTRATION/HANDLING

IV

Reconstitution • For adults and children 12 yrs and older, reconstitute vial with 10 mL of sterile water or D5W. For children aged 3 mos to less than 12 yrs, reconstitute only with 10 mL of D5W. • Shake vial vigorously until powder is completely dissolved (may take up to 10 min). Allow foam to dissipate. • Visually inspect for particulate matter or discoloration. Solution should appear clear to slightly opalescent and yellowish. Do not use if solution is cloudy, discolored, or if visible particles are observed.

Dilution • **Adults:** Transfer 10 mL from reconstituted vial into 250 mL infusion bag containing 0.9% NaCl or D5W for a final concentration of 2.67 mg/mL (667 mg/250 mL). • **Adults with creatinine clearance less than 30mL/min:** Transfer 5 mL from reconstituted vial into 125 mL infusion bag containing 0.9% NaCl or D5W for a final concentration of 2.67 mg/mL (333 mg/125 mL). • **Children 12 yrs to less than 18 yrs (with or without renal impairment):** Transfer the volume required for weight-based dose from reconstituted vial into an infusion bag containing 0.9% NaCl or D5W. Do not exceed a diluted volume greater than 250 mL or a final concentration greater than 667 mg/250 mL (2.67 mg/mL). • **Children 3 mos to less than 12 yrs; children 2 yrs to less than 12 yrs with renal impairment:** Transfer the volume required for weight-based dose from reconstituted vial into an infusion bag containing D5W. Do not exceed a diluted volume greater than 125 mL or a final concentration greater than 667 mg/125 mL (5.33 mg/mL).

Rate of Administration • Infuse over 2 hrs.

Storage • Refrigerate unused vial in original carton. Protect from light. • Reconstituted vial may be refrigerated up to 24 hrs or stored at room temperature for up to 1 hr. • Allow refrigerated solutions to warm to room temperature prior to infusion. • Do not freeze vials or diluted solution. **Diluted solutions for adults and children 12 to less than 18 yrs:** Solutions diluted in D5W infusion bag may be refrigerated (protected from light) for up to 94 hrs or stored at room temperature (not protected from light) for up to 6 hrs. Solutions diluted in 0.9% NaCl infusion bag may be refrigerated (protected from light) for up to 24 hrs or stored at room temperature (not protected from light) for up to 4 hrs. **Diluted solutions for children less than 12 yrs:** Solutions diluted in D5W infusion bag may be refrigerated (protected from light) for up to 24 hrs or stored at room temperature (not protected from light) for up to 6 hrs.

IV COMPATABILITIES

5% Dextrose injection, 0.9% NaCl.

INDICATIONS/ROUTES/DOSAGE

Note: In adult pts with creatinine clearance *greater* than 150 mL/min, increase frequency of 667 mg dose to q6h.

SAB

IV: ADULTS: 667 mg q6h on days 1–8, then q8h on day 9 and thereafter. **Duration of treatment:** Up to 42 days.

ABSSSI

IV: ADULTS: 667 mg q8h for 5–14 days.

CABP

IV: ADULTS: 667 mg q8h for 5–14 days.
CHILDREN 12 YRS TO LESS THAN 18 YRS: 13.3 mg/kg q8h for 7–14 days. **Maximum:** 667 mg/dose.
CHILDREN 3 MOS TO LESS THAN 12 YRS: 20 mg/kg q8h for 7–14 days. **Maximum:** 667 mg/dose.

Dosage in Renal Impairment
Adults With SAB, ABSSSI, CABP

Indication	Creatinine Clearance	Dose	Frequency*
SAB	30–49 mL/min	667 mg	q8h on days 1–8, then q12h starting day 9
	15–29 mL/min	333 mg	q8h on days 1–8, then q12h starting day 9
	Less than 15 mL/min including Hemodialysis	333 mg	q24h
ABSSSI, CABP	30–49 mL/min	667 mg	q12h
	15–29 mL/min	333 mg	q12h
	Less than 15 mL/min including Hemodialysis	333 mg	q24h

*Duration of treatment is up to 42 days for SAB; 5–14 days for ABSSSI, CABP.

Children With CABP

Pediatric Age Group	Estimated Glomerular Filtration Rate (eGFR)	Dosage Regimen*
12 yrs to less than 18 yrs	30–49 mL/min/1.73 m²	10 mg/kg (up to 667 mg) q12h
	15–29 mL/min/1.73 m²	10 mg/kg (up to 333 mg) q12h
6 yrs to less than 12 yrs	30–49 mL/min/1.73 m²	10 mg/kg (up to 667 mg) q12h
	15–29 mL/min/1.73 m²	10 mg/kg (up to 333 mg) q24h
2 yrs to less than 6 yrs	30–49 mL/min/1.73 m²	13.3 mg/kg q12h (up to 667 mg)
	15–29 mL/min/1.73 m²	13.3 mg/kg q24h (up to 333 mg)

*Duration of treatment is 7–14 days.

Dosage in Hepatic Impairment
Not specified; use caution.

SIDE EFFECTS

Note: Side effects may vary depending on indication of treatment.
Occasional (10%–5%): Nausea, vomiting, diarrhea, hypertension, insomnia. **Rare (4%–2%):** Pyrexia, phlebitis, abdominal pain, headache, dizziness, dyspnea, dysgeusia, rash, anxiety.

ADVERSE EFFECTS/TOXIC REACTIONS

An increase in mortality was reported with unapproved use in ventilator-associated bacterial pneumonia. Hypersensitivity reactions, including angioedema, anaphylaxis, bronchospasm, pruritus, wheezing may occur. Central nervous system (CNS) reactions including asterixis, coma, encephalopathy, myoclonus, neuromuscular excitability, nonconvulsive status epilepticus (NCSE); seizures may occur, especially in pts with history of seizures, CNS disorders.
Clostridium difficile–associated diarrhea, with severity ranging from mild diarrhea to fatal colitis, was reported. *C. difficile* infection may occur more than 2 mos after completion of treatment. May increase risk of development of drug-resistant bacteria when used in the absence of a proven or strongly suspected bacterial infection. Fungal infections including *Candida* infection, oral candidiasis, vulvovaginal candidiasis, tinea pedis was reported.

NURSING CONSIDERATIONS

BASELINE ASSESSMENT

Obtain BUN, serum creatinine, CrCl, GFR in pts with renal impairment. Question history of renal impairment, seizure disorder, recent *C. difficile* infection; hypersensitivity reaction to cephalosporins, penicillin. Obtain bacterial culture and sensitivity prior to initiation. Question pt's usual stool characteristics (color, frequency, consistency).

INTERVENTION/EVALUATION

Monitor BUN, serum creatinine, CrCl, eGFR, in pts with renal impairment. Observe daily pattern of bowel activity, stool consistency (increased severity may indicate antibiotic-associated colitis). If frequent diarrhea occurs, obtain *C. difficile* toxin screen and initiate isolation precautions until test result is confirmed; manage hydration, electrolyte levels, protein intake. Antibacterial drugs that are not directed against *C. difficile* infection may need to be discontinued. Monitor for CNS reactions (agitation, anxiety, confusion, insomnia, myoclonus, seizures); hypersensitivity reactions (angioedema, dyspnea, hemodynamic instability, itching, urticaria).

PATIENT/FAMILY TEACHING

• It is essential to complete drug therapy despite improvement of symptoms. Early discontinuation may result in antibacterial resistance or may increase risk of recurrent infection. • Report any episodes of diarrhea, especially in the following months after last dose. Frequent, loose, foul-smelling stool; abdominal pain, dehydration, fever may indicate infectious diarrhea and may be contagious to others. • Report abdominal pain, black/tarry stools, bruising, yellowing of skin or eyes; dark urine, decreased urine output. • Report nervous system changes such as anxiety, confusion, hallucinations, muscle jerking, or seizure-like activity. • Severe allergic reactions such as hives, palpitations, shortness of breath, rash, tongue/facial swelling may occur.

ceftolozane/ tazobactam

cef-**tol**-oh-zane/tay-zoe-**bak**-tam (Zerbaxa)

Do not confuse ceftolozane with cefTAZidime, or tazobactam with avibactam or sulbactam.

◆CLASSIFICATION

PHARMACOTHERAPEUTIC: Cephalosporin/beta-lactamase inhibitor. **CLINICAL:** Antibacterial.

USES

Used in combination with metronidazole for treatment of complicated intra-abdominal infections caused by the following susceptible gram-negative and gram-positive microorganisms: *B. fragilis, E. cloacae, E. coli, K. oxytoca, K. pneumoniae, P. mirabilis, P. aeruginosa, S. anginosus, S. constellatus,* and *S. salivarius* in pts 18 yrs or older and pts ranging from birth to less than 18 yrs old. Treatment of complicated urinary tract infections, including pyelonephritis, caused by the following susceptible gram-negative microorganisms: *E. coli, K. pneumoniae, P. mirabilis,* and *P. aeruginosa* in pts 18 yrs or older and pts ranging from birth to less than 18 yrs old. Treatment of hospital-acquired pneumonia and ventilator-associated bacterial pneumonia in pts 18 yrs and older caused by *E. cloacae, E. coli, Haemophilus influenzae, K. oxytoca, K. pneumoniae, P. mirabilis, P. aeruginosa,* and *Serratia marcescens.* **OFF-LABEL:** Serious infections due to multidrug-resistant *P. aeruginosa.*

PRECAUTIONS

Contraindications: Hypersensitivity to ceftolozane/tazobactam, piperacillin/ tazobactam, or other beta-lactams. **Cautions:** History of atrial fibrillation, electrolyte imbalance–associated arrhythmias, recent *C. difficile* infection or antibiotic-associated colitis, renal/hepatic impairment, seizure disorder; prior hypersensitivity to penicillins, other cephalosporins.

ACTION

Inhibits cell wall synthesis by binding to bacterial cell membrane. Bacterial action of ceftolozane is mediated through binding to essential penicillin-binding proteins. Tazobactam inactivates certain beta-lactamases and binds to certain chromosomal and plasmid-mediated bacterial beta-lactamases. **Therapeutic Effect:** Bactericidal.

PHARMACOKINETICS

Widely distributed. Excreted unchanged as parent drug; not significantly metabolized in liver. Protein binding: 16%–30%. Eliminated in urine (95% unchanged). Removed extensively by hemodialysis. **Half-life:** 2.7 hrs (dependent on dose and severity of renal impairment).

⧖ LIFESPAN CONSIDERATIONS

Pregnancy/Lactation: Unknown if distributed in breast milk. **Children:** No age-related precautions noted. **Elderly:** May have increased risk of adverse effects (due to renal impairment).

INTERACTIONS

DRUG: Probenecid may increase concentration/effect. **HERBAL:** None significant. **FOOD:** None known. **LAB VALUES:** May increase serum alkaline phosphatase, ALT, AST, GGT. May decrease Hgb, Hct, platelets; serum potassium, magnesium, phosphate. May result in positive Coombs' test.

AVAILABILITY (Rx)

◀ **ALERT** ▶ Ceftolozane/tazobactam is a combination product.
Injection Powder for Reconstitution: 1 g ceftolozane/0.5 g tazobactam.

ADMINISTRATION/HANDLING

 IV

Reconstitution • Reconstitute vial with 10 mL of Sterile Water for Injection or 0.9% NaCl. • Shake gently until powder is completely dissolved. • Fi-

nal volume of vial will equal approx. 11.4 mL. • Visually inspect for particulate matter or discoloration. Solution should appear clear, colorless to slightly yellow in color. • Withdraw required volume from reconstituted vial and inject into diluent bag containing 100 mL 0.9% NaCl or 5% dextrose injection as follows:

Ceftolozane/ Tazobactam	Volume to Withdraw From Reconstituted Vial
1.5 g (1 g/0.5 g)	11.4 mL
750 mg (500 mg/250 mg)	5.7 mL
375 mg (250 mg/125 mg)	2.9 mL
150 mg (100 mg/50 mg)	1.2 mL

Rate of administration • Infuse over 60 min.
Storage • Refrigerate intact vials. • Reconstituted vial may be held for 1 hr prior to transfer to diluent bag. • May refrigerate diluted solution up to 7 days or store at room temperature up to 24 hrs. • Do not freeze.

⊞ IV INCOMPATIBILIES

Nicardipine.

⊞ IV COMPATIBILITIES

Amiodarone, calcium gluconate, dexmedetomidine, diltiazem, heparin, insulin, magnesium sulfate, potassium chloride, potassium phosphates, sodium phosphates, vasopressin.

INDICATIONS/ROUTES/DOSAGE

Complicated Intra-Abdominal Infections
IV: ADULTS, ELDERLY: 1.5 g (ceftolozane 1 g/tazobactam 0.5 g) q8h for 4–14 days (in combination with metroNIDAZOLE).

Complicated Urinary Tract Infections Including Pyelonephritis, Complicated Intra-Abdominal Infections
IV: ADULTS, ELDERLY: 1.5 g (ceftolozane 1 g/tazobactam 0.5 g) q8h for 7 days. **BIRTH TO LESS THAN 18 YRS:** 30 mg/kg q8h up to a maximum dose of 1.5 g q8h for 7–14 days.

Hospital-Acquired or Ventilator-Associated

IV: ADULTS, ELDERLY: 3 g (ceftolozane) q8h for 7 days (longer course may be required).

Dosage in Renal Impairment

CrCl 30–50 mL/min: 750 mg (500 mg/250 mg) q8h. **CrCl 15–29 mL/min:** 375 mg (250 mg/125 mg) q8h. **End-stage renal disease or on hemodialysis:** 750 mg (500 mg/250 mg) loading dose, then 150 mg (100 mg/50 mg) maintenance dose q8h for the remainder of the treatment period. **Note:** Administer after hemodialysis on hemodialysis days.

Dosage in Hepatic Impairment

No dose adjustment.

SIDE EFFECTS

Occasional (6%–3%): Nausea, diarrhea, pyrexia, insomnia, headache, vomiting. **Rare (2%–1%):** Constipation, anxiety, hypotension, rash, abdominal pain, dizziness, tachycardia, dyspnea, urticaria, gastritis, abdominal distention, dyspepsia, flatulence.

ADVERSE EFFECTS/TOXIC REACTIONS

Clinical cure rates were lower in pts with CrCl 30–50 mL/min compared with those with CrCl greater than 50 mL/min, and in pts receiving metroNIDAZOLE combination therapy. Hypersensitivity reactions including anaphylaxis or severe skin reactions have been reported with use of beta-lactam antibacterial drugs. *Clostridium difficile*–associated diarrhea, with severity ranging from mild diarrhea to fatal colitis, may occur more than 2 mos after treatment completion. May increase risk of development of drug-resistant bacteria when used in the absence of a proven or strongly suspected bacterial infection. Atrial fibrillation reported in 1.2% of pts. Other reported adverse events such as angina pectoris, infections (candidiasis, oropharyngeal infection, fungal urinary tract infection), paralytic ileus, venous thrombosis occur rarely.

NURSING CONSIDERATIONS

BASELINE ASSESSMENT

Obtain CBC, serum BUN, creatinine; CrCl, eGFR, LFT; bacterial culture and sensitivity; vital signs. Question history of atrial fibrillation, recent *C. difficile* infection, hepatic/renal impairment, hypersensitivity reaction to beta-lactams, cephalosporins, penicillins, carbapenem. Assess skin for wounds; assess hydration status. Question pt's usual stool characteristics (color, frequency, consistency).

INTERVENTION/EVALUATION

Monitor CBC, BMP, renal function test periodically; serum magnesium, ionized calcium in pts at risk for arrhythmias. For pts with changing renal function, monitor renal function test daily and adjust dose accordingly. Diligently monitor I&Os. Observe daily pattern of bowel activity, stool consistency (increased severity may indicate antibiotic-associated colitis). If frequent diarrhea occurs, obtain *C. difficile* toxin screen and initiate isolation precautions until test result confirmed; manage proper fluids levels/PO intake, electrolyte levels, protein intake. Antibacterial drugs that are not directed against *C. diffcile* infection may need to be discontinued. Report any signs of hypersensitivity reaction.

PATIENT/FAMILY TEACHING

• It is essential to complete drug therapy despite symptom improvement. Early discontinuation may result in antibacterial resistance or increased risk of recurrent infection. • Report any episodes of diarrhea, esp. the following mos after treatment completion. Frequent diarrhea, fever, abdominal pain, blood-streaked stool may indicate infectious diarrhea and may be contagious to others. • Report abdominal pain, black/tarry stools, bruising, yellowing of skin or eyes; dark urine, decreased urine output. • Drink plenty of fluids. • Severe allergic reactions such as hives, palpitations, rash, shortness of breath, tongue swelling may occur.

C

cefTRIAXone

sef-trye-**ax**-own
**Do not confuse cefTRIAXone
with ceFAZolin, cefOXitin, or
ceftazidime.**

◆CLASSIFICATION

PHARMACOTHERAPEUTIC: Third-
generation cephalosporin. **CLINI-
CAL:** Antibiotic.

USES

Treatment of bloodstream infections, bone
and joint infections (e.g., osteomyelitis),
gonococcal infection, intra-abdominal
infection, lower respiratory tract infection (e.g., community-acquired pneumonia), bacterial meningitis, otitis media,
pelvic inflammatory disease, skin/soft
tissue infections, surgical prophylaxis,
complicated UTI caused by susceptible
strains of microorganisms including *S.
pneumoniae*, *S. aureus*, *H. influenzae*,
K. pneumoniae, *E. coli*, *E. erogenes*, *P.
mirabilis*, *S. marcescens*, and *P. aeruginosa*. **OFF-LABEL:** Bite wound infection,
COPD (acute exacerbation), diabetic
wound infection, endocarditis, Lyme disease, toxic shock syndrome, *Salmonella*
infection.

PRECAUTIONS

Contraindications: History of hypersensitiv-
ity/anaphylactic reaction to cefTRIAXone,
cephalosporins. Hyperbilirubinemic neonates, esp. premature infants, should not
be treated with cefTRIAXone (can displace
bilirubin from its binding to serum albumin, causing bilirubin encephalopathy). Do
not administer with calcium-containing IV
solutions, including continuous calcium-
containing infusion such as parenteral
nutrition (in neonates) due to the risk of
precipitation of cefTRIAXone-calcium salt.
Cautions: Hepatic impairment, history of
GI disease (esp. ulcerative colitis, antibiotic-associated colitis). History of penicillin
allergy.

ACTION

Binds to bacterial cell membranes, inhibits cell wall synthesis. **Therapeutic
Effect:** Bactericidal.

PHARMACOKINETICS

Widely distributed, including to CSF. Protein
binding: 83%–96%. Primarily excreted in
urine. Not removed by hemodialysis. **Half-
life: IV:** 4.3–4.6 hrs; **IM:** 5.8–8.7 hrs (increased in renal impairment).

⧗ LIFESPAN CONSIDERATIONS

Pregnancy/Lactation: Readily crosses
placenta. Distributed in breast milk. **Children:** May displace bilirubin from serum
albumin. Contraindicated in hyperbilirubinemic neonates. **Elderly:** Age-related
renal impairment may require dosage
adjustment.

INTERACTIONS

DRUG: Probenecid may increase concen-
tration/effect. **Calcium salts** may increase
adverse/toxic effects. **HERBAL:** None significant. **FOOD:** None known. **LAB VALUES:** May
increase serum BUN, alkaline phosphatase,
bilirubin, creatinine, LDH, ALT, AST. May cause
positive direct/indirect Coombs' test.

AVAILABILITY (Rx)

Injection, Powder for Reconstitution: 250
mg, 500 mg, 1 g, 2 g. **Intravenous Solution:** 1 g/50 mL, 2 g/50 mL.

ADMINISTRATION/HANDLING

 IV

Reconstitution • Add 2.4 mL Sterile
Water for Injection to each 250 mg to
provide concentration of 100 mg/
mL. • May further dilute with 50–100
mL 0.9% NaCl, D₅W.
Rate of administration • For IV push,
administer over 1–4 min (**maximum
concentration:** 40 mg/mL). • For
intermittent IV infusion (piggyback), infuse over 30 min.
Storage • Solution appears light yellow to amber. • IV infusion (piggyback)
is stable for 2 days at room temperature,

10 days if refrigerated. • Discard if precipitate forms.

IM

• Add 0.9 mL Sterile Water for Injection, 0.9% NaCl, D_5W, or lidocaine to each 250 mg to provide concentration of 250 mg/mL. • To minimize discomfort, inject deep IM slowly. Less painful if injected into gluteus maximus than lateral aspect of thigh.

▓ IV COMPATIBILITIES

Acetaminophen, dexmedetomidine, diltiazem, heparin, propofol.

INDICATIONS/ROUTES/DOSAGE

Usual Dosage Range

IM/IV: ADULTS, ELDERLY: 1–2 g q12–24h. **INFANTS, CHILDREN, ADOLESCENTS:** 50–75 mg/kg/dose q24h. **NEONATES:** 50 mg/kg/dose given once daily.

Dosage in Renal/Hepatic Impairment

Dosage modification is usually unnecessary, but hepatic/renal function test results should be monitored in pts with renal and hepatic impairment or severe renal impairment.

SIDE EFFECTS

Frequent: Discomfort with IM administration, oral candidiasis (thrush), mild diarrhea, mild abdominal cramping, vaginal candidiasis. **Occasional:** Nausea, serum sickness–like reaction (fever, joint pain; usually occurs after second course of therapy and resolves after drug is discontinued). **Rare:** Allergic reaction (rash, pruritus, urticaria), thrombophlebitis (pain, redness, swelling at injection site).

ADVERSE EFFECTS/TOXIC REACTIONS

Antibiotic-associated colitis, other superinfections (abdominal cramps, severe watery diarrhea, fever) may result from altered bacterial balance in GI tract. Nephrotoxicity may occur, esp. in pts with preexisting renal disease. Pts with history of penicillin allergy are at increased risk for developing a severe hypersensitivity reaction (severe pruritus, angioedema, bronchospasm, anaphylaxis).

NURSING CONSIDERATIONS

BASELINE ASSESSMENT

Obtain CBC, renal function test. Question for history of allergies, particularly cephalosporins, penicillins.

INTERVENTION/EVALUATION

Assess oral cavity for white patches on mucous membranes, tongue (thrush). Monitor daily pattern of bowel activity, stool consistency. Mild GI effects may be tolerable (increasing severity may indicate onset of antibiotic-associated colitis). Monitor I&O, renal function tests for nephrotoxicity, CBC. Be alert for superinfection: Fever, vomiting, diarrhea, anal/genital pruritus, oral mucosal changes (ulceration, pain, erythema).

PATIENT/FAMILY TEACHING

• Discomfort may occur with IM injection. • Doses should be evenly spaced. • Continue antibiotic therapy for full length of treatment.

cefuroxime

sef-ue-**rox**-eem
Do not confuse cefuroxime with cefotaxime, cefprozil, or deferoxamine.

◆CLASSIFICATION

PHARMACOTHERAPEUTIC: Second-generation cephalosporin. **CLINICAL:** Antibiotic.

USES

Treatment of bone and joint infections, COPD (acute exacerbation), lower respiratory tract infections, Lyme disease, otitis media, septicemia, bacterial sinusitis, skin and skin structure infections, *Streptococcal* pharyngitis, surgical prophylaxis, UTI caused by susceptible strains of microorganisms including *S. pneumoniae, H. influenzae* (including ampicillin-resistant strains), *Enterobacter* spp., *Klebsiella* spp., *S. aureus* (penicillinase- and non-penicillinase-producing strains), *S. pyogenes*, *E. coli*. **OFF-LABEL:** Bite wound infection, intra-abdominal infection. Otitis media (acute).

PRECAUTIONS

Contraindications: History of hypersensitivity/anaphylactic reaction to cefuroxime, cephalosporins. **Cautions:** Severe renal impairment, history of penicillin allergy. Pts with hx of colitis, GI malabsorption, seizures.

ACTION

Binds to bacterial cell membranes, inhibits cell wall synthesis. **Therapeutic Effect:** Bactericidal.

PHARMACOKINETICS

Rapidly absorbed from GI tract. Protein binding: 33%–50%. Widely distributed, including to CSF. Primarily excreted unchanged in urine. Moderately removed by hemodialysis. **Half-life:** 1.3 hrs (increased in renal impairment).

LIFESPAN CONSIDERATIONS

Pregnancy/Lactation: Readily crosses placenta. Distributed in breast milk. **Children:** No age-related precautions noted. **Elderly:** Age-related renal impairment may require dosage adjustment.

INTERACTIONS

DRUG: Probenecid may increase concentration/effect. **Antacids, H_2-receptor antagonists (e.g., famotidine), proton pump inhibitors (e.g., pantoprazole)** may decrease absorption. May decrease therapeutic effect of **BCG (intravesical)**. **HERBAL:** None significant. **FOOD:** None known. **LAB VALUES:** May increase serum BUN, creatinine, alkaline phosphatase, bilirubin, LDH, ALT, AST. May cause positive direct/indirect Coombs' test.

AVAILABILITY (Rx)

Injection Powder for Reconstitution: 750 mg, 1.5 g. **Tablets:** 250 mg, 500 mg.

ADMINISTRATION/HANDLING

IV

Reconstitution • Reconstitute 750 mg in 8 mL (1.5 g in 14 mL) Sterile Water for Injection to provide a concentration of 100 mg/mL. • For intermittent IV infusion (piggyback), further dilute with 50–100 mL 0.9% NaCl or D₅W.
Rate of administration • For IV push, administer over 3–5 min. • For intermittent IV infusion (piggyback), infuse over 15–30 min.
Storage • Solution appears light yellow to amber (may darken, but color change does not indicate loss of potency). • IV infusion (piggyback) is stable for 24 hrs at room temperature, 7 days if refrigerated. • Discard if precipitate forms.

IM
• To minimize discomfort, inject deep IM slowly in large muscle mass.

PO
• Give tablets without regard to food. • if GI upset occurs, give with food, milk. • Avoid crushing tablets due to bitter taste.

IV COMPATIBILITIES

Dexmedetomidine, diltiazem, propofol.

INDICATIONS/ROUTES/DOSAGE

Usual Dosage
IV, IM: ADULTS, ELDERLY: 750 mg–1.5 g q8h up to 1.5 g q6h for severe infections. **INFANTS, CHILDREN, ADOLESCENTS:** 100–150 mg/kg/day in divided doses q8h. **Maximum:** 6,000 mg/day. **NEONATES:** 50 mg/kg/dose q8–12h.
PO: ADULTS, ELDERLY: 250–500 mg twice daily **INFANTS, CHILDREN, ADOLESCENTS:** 20–30 mg/kg/day in 2 divided doses. **Maximum:** 1 g/day (500 mg/dose).

Dosage in Renal Impairment
Adult dosage frequency is modified based on creatinine clearance and severity of infection.

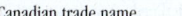

C

Creatinine Clearance	Dosage
IV	
Greater than 20 mL/min	q8h
10–20 mL/min	q12h
Less than 10 mL/min	q24h
Peritoneal dialysis	Dose q24h
Continuous renal re-placement therapy	1 g q12h
PO	
Greater than 30 mL/min	No adjustment
10–29 mL/min	q24h
Less than 10 mL/min	q48h

Dosage in Hepatic Impairment
No dose adjustment.

SIDE EFFECTS

Frequent: Discomfort with IM administration, oral candidiasis (thrush), mild diarrhea, mild abdominal cramping, vaginal candidiasis. **Occasional:** Nausea, serum sickness–like reaction (fever, joint pain; usually occurs after second course of therapy and resolves after drug is discontinued). **Rare:** Allergic reaction (rash, pruritus, urticaria), thrombophlebitis (pain, redness, swelling at injection site).

ADVERSE EFFECTS/TOXIC REACTIONS

Antibiotic-associated colitis, other superinfections (abdominal cramps, severe watery diarrhea, fever) may result from altered bacterial balance in GI tract. Nephrotoxicity may occur, esp. in pts with preexisting renal disease. Pts with history of penicillin allergy are at increased risk for developing a severe hypersensitivity reaction (severe pruritus, angioedema, bronchospasm anaphylaxis).

NURSING CONSIDERATIONS

BASELINE ASSESSMENT

Obtain CBC, renal function test. Question for history of allergies, particularly cephalosporins, penicillins.

INTERVENTION/EVALUATION

Assess oral cavity for white patches on mucous membranes, tongue (thrush).

Monitor daily pattern of bowel activity, stool consistency. Mild GI effects may be tolerable (increasing severity may indicate onset of antibiotic-associated colitis). Monitor I&O, renal function tests for nephrotoxicity. Be alert for superinfection: Fever, vomiting, diarrhea, anal/genital pruritus, oral mucosal changes (ulceration, pain, erythema).

PATIENT/FAMILY TEACHING

• Discomfort may occur with IM injection. • Doses should be evenly spaced. • Continue antibiotic therapy for full length of treatment. • May cause GI upset (may take with food, milk).

celecoxib
TOP 100

sel-e-**kox**-ib
(CeleBREX, Elyxyb)

■ **BLACK BOX ALERT** ■ Increased risk of serious cardiovascular thrombotic events, including MI, CVA. Contraindicated in the setting of coronary artery bypass graft (CABG) surgery. Increased risk of severe GI reactions, including ulceration, bleeding, perforation of stomach, intestines.
Do not confuse CeleBREX with CeleXA, Cerebyx, or Clarinex.

FIXED-COMBINATION(S)

Seglentis: celecoxib/traMADol (an analgesic): 56 mg/44 mg.

◆CLASSIFICATION

PHARMACOTHERAPEUTIC: NSAID, COX-2 selective. **CLINICAL:** Anti-inflammatory.

USES

Anti-inflammatory: Relief of signs/symptoms of ankylosing spondylitis or rheumatoid arthritis. **Dysmenorrhea:** Management of primary dysmenorrhea. **Juvenile idiopathic arthritis (JIA):** Management of signs/symptoms of JIA in pts 2 yrs and older and weighing 10 kg or more. **Migraine:** Acute treatment of migraine with or without aura. **Osteoarthritis (OA):** Management of the signs and symptoms of OA. **Pain (acute):** Management of acute pain in adults. **OFF-LABEL:** Treatment of gout (acute flares).

PRECAUTIONS

◄ALERT► May increase cardiovascular risk when high doses are given to prevent colon cancer.

Contraindications: Hypersensitivity to celecoxib, sulfonamides, aspirin, other NSAIDs. Active GI bleeding. Pts experiencing asthma, urticaria, or allergic reactions to aspirin, other NSAIDs. Treatment of perioperative pain in coronary artery bypass graft (CABG) surgery. **Cautions:** History of GI disease (bleeding/ulcers); concurrent use with aspirin, anticoagulants, smoking; alcohol, elderly, debilitated pts, hypertension, asthma, renal/hepatic impairment. Pts with edema, cerebrovascular disease, ischemic heart disease, HF, known or suspected deficiency of cytochrome P450 isoenzyme 2C9. Pediatric pts with systemic-onset juvenile idiopathic arthritis.

ACTION

Inhibits cyclooxygenase-2, the enzyme responsible for prostaglandin synthesis. **Therapeutic Effect:** Reduces inflammation, relieves pain.

PHARMACOKINETICS

Widely distributed. Protein binding: 97%. Metabolized in liver. Primarily eliminated in feces. **Half-life:** 11.2 hrs.

⏳ LIFESPAN CONSIDERATIONS

Pregnancy/Lactation: Unknown if drug crosses placenta or is distributed in breast milk. Avoid use during third trimester (may adversely affect fetal cardiovascular system: premature closure of ductus arteriosus). **Children:** Safety and efficacy not established. **Elderly:** No age-related precautions noted.

INTERACTIONS

DRUG: May increase concentration/effects of **lithium, methotrexate. Aspirin** may increase adverse effects. May increase nephrotoxic effects of **cycloSPORINE, tenofovir. HERBAL: Herbals with anticoagulant/antiplatelet properties (e.g., garlic, ginger, ginkgo biloba)** may increase adverse effects. **FOOD:** None known. **LAB VALUES:** May increase serum ALT, AST, alkaline phosphatase, creatinine, BUN. May decrease serum phosphate.

AVAILABILITY (Rx)

Solution, Oral: *(Elyxyb):* 120 mg/4.8 mL.

Capsules: 50 mg, 100 mg, 200 mg, 400 mg.

ADMINISTRATION/HANDLING

PO
• May give without regard to food.
• Capsules may be swallowed whole or opened and mixed with applesauce. Administer immediately with water. **Oral solution** • Give without regard to food. • Administer full dose directly from bottle. Use calibrated measuring device for partial doses.

INDICATIONS/ROUTES/DOSAGE

Note: Consider reduced initial dose of 50% in poor CYP2C9 metabolizers.

Osteoarthritis
PO: ADULTS, ELDERLY: 200 mg/day as a single dose or 100 mg twice daily.

Rheumatoid Arthritis (RA)
PO: ADULTS, ELDERLY: 100–200 mg twice daily.

Juvenile Rheumatoid Arthritis (JRA)
PO: CHILDREN 2 YRS AND OLDER, WEIGHING MORE THAN 25 KG: 100 mg twice daily. **WEIGHING 10–25 KG:** 50 mg twice daily.

Acute Pain, Primary Dysmenorrhea
PO: ADULTS, ELDERLY: Initially, 400 mg with additional 200 mg on day 1, if needed. **Maintenance:** 200 mg twice daily as needed.

Ankylosing Spondylitis
PO: ADULTS, ELDERLY: 200 mg/day as a single dose or in 2 divided doses. May in-

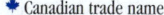 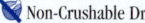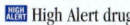

crease to 400 mg/day if no effect is seen after 6 wks.

Acute Migraine
PO: ADULTS: 120 mg once. Maximum: 120 mg/24 hr period.

Dosage in Renal Impairment
Mild to moderate impairment: No dose adjustment. Use caution in pts requiring long-term therapy. **Severe impairment:** Not recommended.

Dosage in Hepatic Impairment
Mild impairment: No dose adjustment. **Moderate impairment:** Reduce dose by 50%. **Severe impairment:** Not recommended. Not recommended in severe hepatic impairment.

SIDE EFFECTS

Frequent (16%–5%): Diarrhea, dyspepsia, headache, upper respiratory tract infection. **Occasional (less than 5%):** Abdominal pain, flatulence, nausea, back pain, peripheral edema, dizziness, insomnia, rash.

ADVERSE EFFECTS/TOXIC REACTIONS

May increase risk of cardiovascular thrombotic events, including MI, stroke. Severe, sometimes fatal, GI events, including GI bleeding; perforation of esophagus, small intestine, colon may occur. Severe hepatic injury, including fulminant hepatitis, hepatic necrosis/failure, was reported. Elevated serum ALT/AST reported in 15% of pts. May increase risk of HF, edema. Long-term use may cause renal papillary necrosis, renal toxicity. Dermatological toxicities, including Stevens-Johnson syndrome, erythema multiforme, toxic and epidermal necrolysis, was reported. Drug reaction with eosinophilia and systemic symptoms (DRESS), also known as multiorgan hypersensitivity, has been reported. DRESS may present with facial swelling, eosinophilia, fever, lymphadenopathy, and rash, which may be associated with other organ systems, such as hepatitis, hematological abnormalities, myocarditis, and nephritis.

BASELINE ASSESSMENT
Assess onset, type, location, duration of pain/inflammation. Inspect appearance of affected joints for immobility, deformity, skin condition. Assess for allergy to sulfa, aspirin, or NSAIDs (contraindicated).

INTERVENTION/EVALUATION
Assess for therapeutic response: pain relief; decreased stiffness, swelling; increased joint mobility; reduced joint tenderness; improved grip strength. Observe for bleeding, bruising, weight gain.

PATIENT/FAMILY TEACHING
• If GI upset occurs, take with food. • Avoid aspirin, alcohol (increases risk of GI bleeding). • Immediately report chest pain, jaw pain, sweating, confusion, difficulty speaking, one-sided weakness (may indicate heart attack or stroke).

cemiplimab-rwic

se-**mip**-li-mab
(Libtayo)
Do not confuse cemiplimab with cosibelimab.

◆CLASSIFICATION

PHARMACOTHERAPEUTIC: Programmed death receptor-1 (PD-1) blocking antibody. **CLINICAL:** Antineoplastic.

USES

Cutaneous squamous cell carcinoma (CSCC): Treatment of adults with metastatic or locally advanced CSCC who are not candidates for curative surgery or curative radiation. **Basal cell carcinoma (BCC):** Treatment of adults with locally advanced or metastatic BCC who have been previously treated with a hedgehog pathway inhibitor or for whom a hedgehog pathway inhibitor is not appropriate. **Non–small-cell lung cancer (NSCLC):** In combination with platinum-based chemotherapy for first-line treatment of adults with

NSCLC with no EGFR, ALK, or ROS1 aberrations, and is metastatic or locally advanced where pts are not candidates for surgical resection or definitive chemoradiation. As single agent for first-line treatment of adults with NSCLC whose tumors have high PD-L1 expression (Tumor Proportion Score greater than or equal to 50%) with no EGFR, ALK, or ROS1 aberrations, and is metastatic or locally advanced where pts are not candidates for surgical resection or definitive chemoradiation.

PRECAUTIONS

Contraindications: Hypersensitivity to cemiplimab-rwic. **Cautions:** Baseline cytopenias, pts at risk for interstitial lung disease (e.g., COPD, sarcoidosis, connective disease disease); history of autoimmune disorders (Crohn's disease, demyelinating polyneuropathy, Guillain-Barré syndrome, Hashimoto's thyroiditis, hyperthyroidism, myasthenia gravis, rheumatoid arthritis, type 1 diabetes, vasculitis); hypothyroidism, pancreatitis; solid organ transplant, allogeneic hematopoietic stem cell transplantation.

ACTION

Binds to PD-1 ligands, blocking interaction with PD-L1 and PD-L2. PD-L1 is an immune checkpoint protein expressed on tumor cells that downregulates antitumor T-cell function. **Therapeutic Effect:** Restores immune responses (including T-cell antitumor function), decreasing tumor growth and proliferation.

PHARMACOKINETICS

Widely distributed. Metabolism not specified. Steady state reached in 4 mos. Excretion not specified. **Half-life:** 22 days.

⌛ LIFESPAN CONSIDERATIONS

Pregnancy/Lactation: Avoid pregnancy; may cause fetal harm. Females of reproductive potential must use effective contraception during treatment and for at least 4 mos after discontinuation. Breastfeeding not recommended during

treatment and for at least 4 mos after discontinuation. Human immunoglobulin G (IgG) is present in breast milk and known to cross the placenta. **Children:** Safety and efficacy not established. **Elderly:** No age-related precautions noted.

INTERACTIONS

DRUG: None known. **HERBAL:** None significant. **FOOD:** None known. **LAB VALUES:** May increase serum alkaline phosphatase, ALT, AST, bilirubin, calcium, creatinine. May decrease serum albumin, magnesium, potassium, sodium; Hgb, leukocytes, lymphocytes, RBCs.

AVAILABILITY (Rx)

Injection Solution: 350 mg/7 mL (50 mg/mL).

ADMINISTRATION/HANDLING
 IV

Infusion Guidelines • Infuse via dedicated IV line using a sterile, nonpyrogenic, low-protein-binding 0.2- to 5-micron, in-line filter. • Do not administer as IV push or bolus.

Preparation • Must be prepared by personnel trained in aseptic manipulations and admixing of cytotoxic drugs. • Visually inspect for particulate matter or discoloration. Solution should appear clear to slightly opalescent, colorless to pale yellow. Do not use if solution is cloudy or discolored. Trace amounts of translucent to white particles may be present. • Dilute into an infusion bag containing D5W or 0.9% NaCl to a final concentration of 1–20 mg/mL. • Mix by gentle inversion. Do not shake or agitate.

Rate of Administration • Infuse over 30 min.

Infusion Reactions • Grade 1 or 2 infusion reactions: Interrupt or slow infusion rate. **Grade 3 or 4 infusion reactions:** Permanently discontinue.

Storage • Refrigerate unused vials in original carton. Protect from light. • May refrigerate diluted solution for up to 24 hrs or store at room temperature up to 8 hrs (includes infusion time). • Do not shake, agitate, or freeze. • If refrigerated, allow diluted solution to warm to room temperature.

INDICATIONS/ROUTES/DOSAGE

CSCC, BCC (Metastatic or Locally Advanced)
IV: ADULTS: 350 mg q3wks for up to 24 mos. Continue until disease progression or unacceptable toxicity.

NSCLC (Metastatic or Locally Advanced)
IV: ADULTS: 350 mg q3wks until disease progression or unacceptable toxicity.

Dose Modification
Based on Common Terminology Criteria for Adverse Events (CTCAE). No dose reduction is required. Based on severity of adverse reactions, withhold treatment and consider starting corticosteroid therapy. Resume treatment if symptoms improve to Grade 1 or 0 after corticosteroid taper.

Immune-Mediated Adverse Reactions
Withhold Treatment for the Following Adverse Reactions: Grade 2 pneumonitis; Grade 2 or 3 colitis; clinically unstable Grade 3 or 4 endocrinopathies; Grade 2 or 3 nephritis with renal dysfunction; Grade 2 neurological toxicities; *suspected* Stevens-Johnson syndrome, toxic epidermal necrolysis, or drug reaction with eosinophilia and systemic symptoms (DRESS); serum ALT/AST greater than 3–8 times ULN or total serum bilirubin greater than 1.5–3 times ULN (hepatitis with no tumor involvement of the liver); baseline serum ALT/AST greater than 1–3 times ULN that increases to greater than 5–10 times ULN, or baseline serum ALT/AST greater than 3–5 times ULN that increases to greater than 8–10 times ULN (hepatitis with tumor involvement of the liver). **Permanently Discontinue for the Following Adverse Reactions:** Grade 3 or 4 pneumonitis; Grade 4 colitis; clinically unstable Grade 3 or 4 endocrinopathies

depending on severity; Grade 4 nephritis with renal dysfunction; Grade 2–4 myocarditis; Grade 3 or 4 neurological toxicities; *confirmed* Stevens-Johnson syndrome, toxic epidermal necrolysis, or DRESS; serum ALT/AST greater than 8 times ULN or total serum bilirubin greater than 3 times ULN (hepatitis with no tumor involvement of the liver); serum ALT/AST greater than 10 times ULN or total serum bilirubin greater than 3 times ULN (hepatitis with tumor involvement of the liver); Grade 3 or 4 infusion-related reactions; recurrent, severe, immune-mediated reaction requiring immunosuppressive therapy; symptoms that do not improve to Grade 1 or 0 within 12 wks of starting corticosteroid therapy or unable to tolerate corticosteroid reduction to less than 10 mg prednisone (or equivalent)/day.

Other Immune-Mediated Adverse Reactions
Unless specified, withhold treatment for other Grade 3 immune-mediated adverse reactions until improved to Grade 1 or 0. Permanently discontinue for other Grade 4 immune-mediated adverse reactions, recurrent Grade 3 immune-mediated adverse reactions requiring an immunosuppressant, or unable to tolerate corticosteroid reduction to less than 10 mg prednisone (or equivalent)/day.

Dosage in Hepatic/Renal Impairment
No dose adjustment.

SIDE EFFECTS

Frequent (38%–21%): Fatigue, asthenia, rash, musculoskeletal pain, diarrhea, pruritus, nausea. **Occasional (17%–10%):** Hypertension, constipation, cough, vomiting, decreased appetite, headache, dizziness, actinic keratosis.

ADVERSE EFFECTS/TOXIC REACTIONS

Anemia, lymphopenia are expected responses to therapy. May cause severe and/or fatal immune-mediated adverse reactions including acute kidney injury, nephritis; colitis, hepatitis, pancreatitis, pneumonitis; adrenal insufficiency, hypoparathyroidism, hyperthyroidism, hypophysitis, thyroiditis, type 1 diabetes mellitus including ketoacidosis; autoimmune neuropathy, encephalitis, Guillain-Barre syndrome, meningitis, myasthenia gravis, myelitis, nerve paresis; myocarditis, pericarditis, vasculitis; iritis, uveitis; myositis, polymyositis, rhabdomyolysis; aplastic anemia, hemolytic anemia, hemophagocytic lymphohistiocytosis, histiocytic necrotizing lymphadenitis, immune thrombocytopenia; sarcoidosis, systemic inflammatory response syndrome. Immune-mediated adverse reactions can affect any organ at any time. Solid organ transplant rejection, allogeneic hematopoietic stem cell transplantation complications were reported. May cause cytomegalovirus infection/reactivation in pts with corticosteroid-refractory immune-related colitis. Dermatologic toxicities including Stevens-Johnson syndrome, toxic epidermal necrolysis may occur. DRESS, also known as multiorgan hypersensitivity, has been reported. DRESS may present with facial swelling, eosinophilia, fever, lymphadenopathy, and rash, which may be associated with other organ systems, such as hepatitis, hematological abnormalities, myocarditis, nephritis. Life-threatening infusion reactions may occur. Upper respiratory tract infections reported in 14% of pts.

NURSING CONSIDERATIONS

BASELINE ASSESSMENT

Obtain CBC, BMP, LFT, thyroid panel; pregnancy test in females of reproductive potential; vital signs. Confirm compliance with effective contraception. Screen for history of autoimmune disorders, diabetes, pituitary/pulmonary/thyroid disease. Perform full dermatological exam if treated for squamous or basal cell carcinoma; assess skin for moles, lesions, papillomas. Administer in an environment equipped to monitor for and manage infusion-related reactions. Question for prior infusion-related reactions before each infusion. Screen for active infection. Offer emotional support.

INTERVENTION/EVALUATION

Monitor CBC, LFT, renal function, thyroid panel as clinically indicated. Assess for infusion reactions during each infusion. If reactions occur, interrupt or decrease the infusion rate. Immune-mediated reactions can affect any organ. Early detection and management are vital. Conduct a complete head-to-toe assessment frequently. Radiological examination, blood sampling, and/or treatment with corticosteroids should be considered if an immune-mediated reaction is suspected. Assess for eye pain/redness, visual changes at each office visit and at regular intervals. Monitor daily pattern of bowel activity, stool consistency. Assess skin for rash, lesions, dermatological toxicities; symptoms of DRESS. Monitor blood glucose levels in pts treated with corticosteroids.

PATIENT/FAMILY TEACHING

• Immediately report symptoms of infusion-related reactions such as chills, cough, difficulty breathing, nausea, vomiting. • Report symptoms of drug-induced hypersensitivity syndrome (e.g., fever, swollen face/lymph nodes, skin rash/peeling/inflammation). • Serious adverse reactions may affect lungs, liver, intestines, kidneys, hormonal glands, nervous system (or any organ), which may require anti-inflammatory medication. Immediately report any symptoms in the following body systems: Colon (severe abdominal pain/swelling, diarrhea); eyes (pain, redness, vision problems), heart (chest pain, difficulty breathing), kidneys (decreased or dark-colored urine, flank pain); lung (chest pain, severe cough, shortness of breath); liver (bruising, dark-colored urine, clay-colored/tarry stools, nausea, yellowing of the skin or eyes); nervous system (confusion, difficulty breathing or swallowing; paralysis, weakness), pituitary (persistent or unusual headaches, dizziness, extreme weakness, fainting, vision changes); skin (blisters, bubbling, inflammation, rash); thyroid (trouble sleeping, high blood pressure, fast heart rate [overactive thyroid]; fatigue, goiter, weight gain [underactive thyroid]); vascular (low blood pressure, vein/artery pain or irritation). • Use effective contraception to avoid pregnancy. Do not breastfeed.

cephalexin

sef-a-**lex**-in
Do not confuse cephalexin with ce-faclor, ceFAZolin, or ciprofloxacin.

◆CLASSIFICATION
PHARMACOTHERAPEUTIC: First-generation cephalosporin. **CLINICAL:** Antibiotic.

USES
Respiratory tract infections caused by *S. pneumoniae, S. pyogenes.* **Otitis media** caused by *S. pneumoniae, H. influenzae, S. aureus, S. pyogenes,* and *M. catarrhalis.* **Skin and skin structure infections** caused by *S. pneumoniae, S. pyogenes.* **Bone infections** caused by *S. aureus, P. mirabilis.* **Genitourinary tract infections** (including acute prostatitis). **OFF-LABEL:** Suppression of prosthetic joint infection. Endocarditis (prophylaxis) caused by *E. coli, P. mirabilis,* and *K. pneumoniae.*

PRECAUTIONS
Contraindications: History of hypersensitivity/anaphylactic reaction to cephalexin, cephalosporins. **Cautions:** Renal impairment, history of GI disease (esp. ulcerative colitis, antibiotic-associated colitis), history of penicillin allergy.

ACTION
Binds to bacterial cell membranes, inhibits cell wall synthesis. **Therapeutic Effect:** Bactericidal.

PHARMACOKINETICS
Widely distributed. Protein binding: 10%–15%. Primarily excreted unchanged in urine. Moderately removed by hemodialysis. **Half-life:** 0.9–1.2 hrs (increased in renal impairment).

⧗ LIFESPAN CONSIDERATIONS
Pregnancy/Lactation: Readily crosses placenta. Distributed in breast milk. **Children:** No age-related precautions noted. **Elderly:** Age-related renal impairment may require dosage adjustment.

INTERACTIONS
DRUG: Probenecid may increase concentration/effect. **HERBAL:** None significant. **FOOD:** None known. **LAB VALUES:** May increase serum BUN, creatinine, alkaline phosphatase, bilirubin, LDH, ALT, AST. May cause positive direct/indirect Coombs' test.

AVAILABILITY (Rx)
Capsules: 250 mg, 500 mg, 750 mg. **Powder for Oral Suspension:** 125 mg/5 mL, 250 mg/5 mL. **Tablets:** 250 mg, 500 mg.

ADMINISTRATION/HANDLING
PO
Oral • Give without regard to food. If GI upset occurs, give with food, milk. **Oral Suspension** • After reconstitution, oral suspension is stable for 14 days if refrigerated. • Shake oral suspension well before using. Give with accurate measuring device.

INDICATIONS/ROUTES/DOSAGE
Usual Dosage Range
PO: ADULTS, ELDERLY: 250–1,000 mg q6h or 500 mg q12h. **Maximum:** 4 g/day. **INFANTS, CHILDREN, ADOLESCENTS: (Mild to moderate infections):** 25–50 mg/kg/day divided q6–12h. **Maximum:** 2 g/day. **(Severe infections):** 75–100 mg/kg/day divided q6–8h. **Maximum:** 4 g/day.

Dosage in Renal Impairment
After usual initial dose, dosing frequency is modified based on creatinine clearance and severity of infection.

Creatinine Clearance	Dosage
60 mL/min or greater	No adjustment
30–59 mL/min	Maximum: 1,000 mg/day
15–29 mL/min	250 mg q8-12h
5–14 mL/min	250 mg q24h
1–4 mL/min	250 mg q48-60h
Hemodialysis	250–500 mg q12–24h (administer after dialysis session)

Dosage in Hepatic Impairment
No dose adjustment.

SIDE EFFECTS

Frequent: Oral candidiasis, mild diarrhea, mild abdominal cramping, vaginal candidiasis. **Occasional:** Nausea, serum sickness–like reaction (fever, joint pain; usually occurs after second course of therapy and resolves after drug is discontinued). **Rare:** Allergic reaction (rash, pruritus, urticaria).

ADVERSE EFFECTS/TOXIC REACTIONS

Antibiotic-associated colitis, other superinfections (abdominal cramps, severe watery diarrhea, fever) may result from altered bacterial balance in GI tract. Nephrotoxicity may occur, esp. in pts with preexisting renal disease. Pts with history of penicillin allergy are at increased risk for developing a severe hypersensitivity reaction (severe pruritus, angioedema, bronchospasm, anaphylaxis).

NURSING CONSIDERATIONS

BASELINE ASSESSMENT

Obtain CBC, renal function test. Question for history of allergies, particularly cephalosporins, penicillins.

INTERVENTION/EVALUATION

Assess oral cavity for white patches on mucous membranes, tongue (thrush). Monitor daily pattern of bowel activity, stool consistency. Mild GI effects may be tolerable (increasing severity may indicate onset of antibiotic-associated coli-

tis). Monitor I&O, renal function tests for nephrotoxicity. Be alert for superinfection: fever, vomiting, diarrhea, anal/genital pruritus, oral mucosal changes (ulceration, pain, erythema). With prolonged therapy, monitor renal/hepatic function tests.

PATIENT/FAMILY TEACHING

• Doses should be evenly spaced. • Continue therapy for full length of treatment. • May cause GI upset (may take with food, milk). • Refrigerate oral suspension. • Report persistent diarrhea.

ceritinib

se-**ri**-ti-nib
(Zykadia)
Do not confuse ceritinib with crizotinib, gefitinib, imatinib, or lapatinib.

◆CLASSIFICATION

PHARMACOTHERAPEUTIC: Anaplastic lymphoma kinase inhibitor. **CLINICAL:** Antineoplastic.

USES

Treatment of pts with anaplastic lymphoma kinase (ALK)–positive metastatic non–small-cell lung cancer (NSCLC).

PRECAUTIONS

Contraindications: Hypersensitivity to ceritinib. **Cautions:** Bradyarrhythmias/ventricular arrhythmias, diabetes, dehydration, electrolyte imbalance (e.g., hypomagnesemia, hypokalemia), hepatic impairment, HF, ocular disease, pulmonary disease. Concomitant use of QT-interval-prolonging medications. Not recommended in pts with congenital long QT syndrome. Avoid use of medications that cause bradycardia.

ACTION

Potent inhibitor of ALK involved in the pathogenesis of NSCLC. ALK gene abnormalities may result in expression of oncogenic fusion proteins, resulting in increased cell proliferation/survival in tumor cells. **Therapeutic Effect:** Reduces proliferation of tumor cells expressing the genetic abnormality.

PHARMACOKINETICS

Widely distributed. Metabolized in liver. Peak plasma concentration: 4–6 hrs. Protein binding: 97%. Eliminated in feces (92%), urine (1.3%). **Half-life:** 41 hrs.

⧗ LIFESPAN CONSIDERATIONS

Pregnancy/Lactation: Avoid pregnancy; may cause fetal harm. Contraception recommended during treatment and for at least 2 wks after discontinuation. Unknown if distributed in breast milk. **Children:** Safety and efficacy not established. **Elderly:** No age-related precautions noted.

INTERACTIONS

DRUG: Strong CYP3A4 inhibitors (e.g., clarithromycin, ketoconazole, ritonavir) may increase concentration/effect; avoid use. **Strong CYP3A4 inducers (e.g., carBAMazepine, phenytoin, rifAMPin)** may decrease concentration/effect; avoid use. **QT interval-prolonging medications (e.g., amiodarone, azithromycin, haloperidol, moxifloxacin)** may increase risk of QT interval prolongation, cardiac arrhythmias. **Dronedarone** may increase risk of bradycardia. May increase concentration/effects of **aprepitant, bosutinib, budesonide, cobimetinib, eletriptan, ivabradine.** **HERBAL:** None significant. **FOOD: Grapefruit products** may increase concentration/effect; avoid use. **LAB VALUES:** May decrease Hgb, phosphate. May increase serum ALT, AST, bilirubin, creatinine, glucose, lipase.

AVAILABILITY (Rx)

 Tablets: 150 mg.

ADMINISTRATION/HANDLING

PO
• Give with food. • Administer whole; do not break, cut, or open. • If a dose is missed, take dose unless next dose due

within 12 hrs. If vomiting occurs, do not administer an additional dose.

INDICATIONS/ROUTES/DOSAGE

Non–Small-Cell Lung Cancer
PO: **ADULTS/ELDERLY:** 450 mg once daily until disease progression or unacceptable toxicity.

Dose Modification
Cardiotoxicity
QTc interval greater than 500 msec on at least 2 separate ECGs: Withhold until QTc interval is less than 481 msec, or recovery to baseline (if baseline QTc interval is greater than or equal to 481 msec), then resume with a 150-mg dose reduction. **QTc prolongation in combination with torsades de pointes or polymorphic ventricular tachycardia or serious arrhythmia:** Permanently discontinue. **Symptomatic, non-life-threatening bradycardia:** Withhold until recovery to asymptomatic bradycardia or heart rate of 60 beats/min or greater. Evaluate concomitant medications known to cause bradycardia and adjust dose as tolerated (reduction not specified). **Clinically significant, life-threatening bradycardia requiring intervention or life-threatening bradycardia in pts taking concomitant medications known to cause bradycardia or hypotension:** Withhold until recovery to asymptomatic bradycardia or heart rate of 60 beats/min or greater. If concomitant medication can be adjusted or discontinued, then resume with a 150-mg dose reduction. **Life-threatening bradycardia in pts who are not taking concomitant medications known to cause bradycardia or hypotension:** Permanently discontinue.

Concomitant Use of Strong CYP3A Inhibitors
If concomitant use unavoidable, reduce ceritinib dose by one third, rounded to the nearest 150-mg dose strength. After discontinuation of a strong CYP3A inhibitor, resume ceritinib dose that was taken prior to initiating strong CYP3A inhibitor.

Gastrointestinal Toxicity
Severe or intolerable diarrhea, nausea, vomiting despite optimal antiemetic or antidiarrheal therapy: Withhold until improved, then resume with a 150-mg dose reduction.

Hepatotoxicity
ALT, AST greater than 5 times upper limit of normal (ULN) with total bilirubin elevation less than or equal to 2 times ULN: Withhold until recovery to baseline or less than or equal to 2 times ULN, then resume with a 150-mg dose reduction.
ALT, AST greater than 3 times ULN with total bilirubin elevation greater than or equal to 2 times ULN in the absence of cholestasis or hemolysis: Permanently discontinue.

Hyperglycemia
Persistent hyperglycemia greater than 250 mL/dL despite optimal antihyperglycemic therapy: Withhold until hyperglycemia is adequately controlled, then resume with a 150-mg dose reduction. If adequate control cannot be achieved with optimal medical management, then permanently discontinue.

Pulmonary Toxicity
Any grade treatment related to interstitial lung disease/pneumonitis: Permanently discontinue.

Intolerability/Toxicity
If unable to tolerate 300-mg dose: Permanently discontinue.

Dosage in Renal Impairment
Mild to moderate impairment: CrCl 30–90 mL/min: No dose adjustment. **Severe impairment:** Not specified; use caution.

Dosage in Hepatic Impairment
Mild to moderate impairment: No dose adjustment. **Severe impairment:** Decrease dose by 1/3 (round to nearest 150 mg).

SIDE EFFECTS

Frequent (86%–52%): Diarrhea, nausea, vomiting, abdominal pain, fatigue, asthenia. **Occasional (34%–9%):** Decreased appetite, constipation, paresthesia, muscular weakness, gait disturbance, peripheral motor/sensory neuropathy, hypotonia, polyneuropathy, dyspepsia, gastric reflux disease, dysphagia, rash, maculopapular rash, acneiform dermatitis, vision impairment, blurred vision, photopsia, presbyopia, reduced visual acuity.

ADVERSE EFFECTS/TOXIC REACTIONS

Approximately 60% of pts required at least one dose reduction. Median time to first dose reduction was approximately 7 wks. Decreased Hgb levels reported in 84% of pts. Severe or persistent GI toxicity including nausea, vomiting, diarrhea occurred in 96% of pts; severe cases reported in 14% of pts. Drug-induced hepatotoxicity with elevation of serum ALT 5 times ULN occurred in 27% of pts. Bradycardia, severe interstitial lung disease (ILD), QT interval prolongation, ILD reported in 3% of pts. Grade 3–4 hyperglycemia reported in 13% of pts; diabetics have a sixfold increase in risk; pts receiving corticosteroids have twofold increase in risk. Fatal adverse reactions including pneumonia, respiratory failure, ILD/pneumonitis, pneumothorax, gastric hemorrhage, general physical health deterioration, tuberculosis, cardiac tamponade, sepsis occurred in 5% of pts.

NURSING CONSIDERATIONS

BASELINE ASSESSMENT
Obtain CBC, BMP, LFT; pregnancy test in females of reproductive potential. Obtain baseline ECG in pts with history of arrhythmias, HF, electrolyte imbalance, or concurrent use of medications known to prolong QTc interval. Question possibility of pregnancy or plans of breastfeeding. Assess hydration status. Screen for history/comorbidities. Receive full medication history including herbal products, esp. CYP3A in-

hibitors or inducers, medications that prolong QT interval. Assess visual acuity. Verify ALK-positive NSCLC test prior to initiation.

INTERVENTION/EVALUATION

Monitor CBC routinely; LFT monthly (or more frequently in pts with elevated hepatic enzymes). Obtain BMP, serum ionized calcium, magnesium if arrhythmia or dehydration occurs. Monitor vital signs (esp. heart rate). Obtain ECG for bradycardia, chest pain, dyspnea; chest X-ray if ILD, pneumonitis, pneumothorax suspected. Worsening cough, fever, or shortness of breath may indicate pneumonitis. Monitor for hepatic dysfunction, hyperglycemia, sepsis, vision changes. Assess hydration status. Encourage PO intake. Offer antidiarrheal medication for loose stool, antiemetic for nausea, vomiting.

PATIENT/FAMILY TEACHING

• Most pts experience diarrhea, nausea, vomiting, which may lead to dehydration; drink plenty of fluids. • Report history of heart problems, including extremity swelling, HF, congenital long QT syndrome, palpitations, syncope. Therapy may decrease your heart rate; report dizziness, chest pain, palpitations, or fainting. • Worsening cough, fever, or shortness of breath may indicate severe lung inflammation. • Avoid pregnancy; contraception recommended during treatment and up to 2 wks after final dose. Do not breastfeed. • Blurry vision, confusion, frequent urination, increased thirst, fruity breath may indicate high blood sugar levels. • Report any yellowing of skin or eyes, upper abdominal pain, bruising, black/tarry stools, dark urine. • Immediately report any newly prescribed medications. • Take on empty stomach only; do not eat 2 hrs before or 2 hrs after any dose. • Avoid alcohol. Do not consume grapefruit products.

---

certolizumab pegol

ser-toe-**liz**-ue-mab
(Cimzia)

■**BLACK BOX ALERT**■ Serious, sometimes fatal cases of tuberculosis, invasive fungal infections, or other opportunistic infections, including viral and bacterial infection, have been reported in children/adolescents receiving other TNF-blocking medications. Lymphoma reported in children/adolescents receiving other TNF-blocking medications.

◆**CLASSIFICATION**

PHARMACOTHERAPEUTIC: Antirheumatic, disease modifying, GI agent. Tumor necrosis factor (TNF) blocker. **CLINICAL:** Anti-inflammatory agent.

USES

Ankylosing spondylitis (AS): Treatment of adults with active AS. **Non-radiographic axial spondyloarthritis (nr-axSpA):** Treatment of adults with nr-axSpA with objective signs of inflammation. **Crohn's disease:** Reduces signs and symptoms of Crohn's disease and maintains clinical response in adults with moderately to severely active disease who have had an inadequate response to conventional therapy. **Plaque psoriasis (PsO):** Treatment of adults with moderate-to-severe PsO who are candidates for systemic therapy or phototherapy. **Psoriatic arthritis (PsA):** Treatment of adults with active PsA. **Rheumatoid arthritis (RA):** Treatment of adults with moderately to severely active RA.

PRECAUTIONS

Contraindications: Hypersensitivity to certolizumab. **Cautions:** Chronic, latent, or localized infection; preexisting or recent-onset CNS demyelinating disorders, moderate to severe HF, underlying hematologic disorders, elderly. Pts who have resided in regions where TB is endemic, pts who are hepatitis B virus carriers. Use of live vaccines.

ACTION

Binds to and neutralizes human TNF-alpha activity. Elevated levels of TNF-alpha play a role in inflammation (Crohn's disease) and joint destruction (RA). **Therapeutic Effect:** Reduces symptoms of Crohn's disease and joint destruction associated with rheumatoid arthritis.

PHARMACOKINETICS

Higher clearance with increasing body weight. Peak plasma concentrations: 54–171 hrs. **Half-life:** 14 days.

⧗ LIFESPAN CONSIDERATIONS

Pregnancy/Lactation: Unknown if distributed in breast milk. **Children:** Safety and efficacy not established. **Elderly:** Use cautiously due to higher risk of infection.

INTERACTIONS

DRUG: May increase adverse effects of **abatacept, anakinra, canakinumab, natalizumab, vaccines (live), vedolizumab.** May decrease therapeutic effects of **BCG (intravesical), vaccines (live). HERBAL: Echinacea** may decrease therapeutic effect. **FOOD:** None known. **LAB VALUES:** May increase serum alkaline phosphatase, ALT, AST, bilirubin; aPTT.

AVAILABILITY (Rx)

Injection, Powder for Reconstitution: 200 mg. **Injection, Solution:** 200 mg/mL in a single-use prefilled syringe.

ADMINISTRATION/HANDLING

SQ

Reconstitution • Bring to room temperature before reconstitution. • Reconstitute with 1 mL Sterile Water for Injection. • Gently swirl without shaking, using syringe with 20-gauge needle. • Leave undisturbed to fully reconstitute (may take as long as 30 min). • Using a new 20-gauge needle, withdraw reconstituted solution into syringe for final concentration of 1 mL (200 mg). Use separate syringes for multiple vials. • Switch each 20-gauge needle to a 23-gauge needle and inject full contents of each syringe subcutaneously into separate sites on the abdomen or thigh. **Storage** • Store vial in refrigerator. • Once powder reconstituted, solution should appear clear to opalescent, colorless to pale yellow. • Discard if solution is discolored or contains precipitate. • Reconstituted solution is stable for up to 2 hrs at room temperature or 24 hrs if refrigerated.

INDICATIONS/ROUTES/DOSAGE

Note: Each 400-mg dose is given as two injections of 200 mg each.

Crohn's Disease
SQ: Initially, 400 mg (given as two subcutaneous injections of 200 mg) and at weeks 2 and 4. **Maintenance:** In pts who obtain a therapeutic response, 400 mg q4wks.

Rheumatoid Arthritis, Ankylosing Spondylitis, Psoriatic Arthritis
SQ: ADULTS, ELDERLY: Initially, 400 mg and at weeks 2 and 4. **Maintenance:** 200 mg q2wks or 400 mg q4wks.

Plaque Psoriasis
SQ: ADULTS, ELDERLY: 400 mg every other week. **PTS WEIGHING 90 KG OR LESS:** 400 mg at wks 0, 2, and 4, then 200 mg every other wk may be used.

Axial Spondyloarthritis, Nonradiographic
SQ: ADULTS, ELDERLY: Initially, 400 mg, repeat dose 2 and 4 wks after initial dose. **Maintenance:** 200 mg q2wks or 400 mg q4wks.

Dosage Modification
Discontinue for hypersensitivity reaction, lupus-like syndrome, serious infection, sepsis, hepatitis B virus reactivation.

Dosage in Renal/Hepatic Impairment
No dose adjustment.

SIDE EFFECTS

Occasional (6%): Arthralgia. **Rare (less than 1%):** Abdominal pain, diarrhea.

ADVERSE EFFECTS/TOXIC REACTIONS

Upper respiratory tract infection occurs in 20% of pts. UTI occurs in 7% of pts. Serious infections such as pneumonia, pyelonephritis occur in 3% of pts. Hypersensitivity reaction (rash, urticaria, hypotension, dyspnea) occurs rarely. May increase risk of malignancies (e.g., lymphoma).

NURSING CONSIDERATIONS

BASELINE ASSESSMENT
Obtain baseline CBC, urinalysis, C-reactive protein. Do not initiate treatment in pts with active infections, including chronic or localized infection. TB test should be obtained before initiation.

INTERVENTION/EVALUATION
Monitor pts for infection during and after treatment. If pt develops an infection, treatment should be discontinued. Monitor lab results, especially WBC count, urinalysis, C-reactive protein for evidence of infection.

PATIENT/FAMILY TEACHING
• Report cough, fever, flu-like symptoms. • Do not receive live virus vaccine during treatment or within 3 mos after last dose.

---

cetirizine

se-**teer**-i-zeen
(Apo-Cetirizine ✱, Quzyttir, Reactine ✱, Zerviate, ZyrTEC ALLERGY)
Do not confuse cetirizine with levocetirizine, or ZyrTEC with Xanax, Zantac, Zocor, or ZyPREXA.

FIXED-COMBINATION(S)

ZyrTEC D 12 Hour Tablets: cetirizine/pseudoephedrine: 5 mg/120 mg.

◆CLASSIFICATION

PHARMACOTHERAPEUTIC: Histamine H_1 antagonist (second generation). **CLINICAL:** Antihistamine.

USES

PO: Relief of symptoms associated with allergic rhinitis. Treatment of uncomplicated skin manifestations of chronic spontaneous urticaria. **Quzyttir:** Treatment of new-onset acute urticaria. **Zerviate:** Treatment of ocular itching associated with allergic conjunctivitis. **OFF-LABEL:** Anaphylaxis (adjunct), angioedema, infusion reaction (premedication).

PRECAUTIONS

Contraindications: Hypersensitivity to cetirizine, hydrOXYzine. **Cautions:** Elderly, hepatic/renal impairment.

ACTION

Competes with histamine for H_1-receptor sites on effector cells in GI tract, blood vessels, respiratory tract. **Therapeutic Effect:** Prevents allergic response; produces mild bronchodilation; blocks histamine-induced bronchitis.

PHARMACOKINETICS

Route	Onset	Peak	Duration
PO	Less than 1 hr	4–8 hrs	Less than 24 hrs

Widely distributed. Minimally metabolized in liver. Protein binding: 93%. Primarily excreted in urine. **Half-life:** 6.5–10 hrs.

⧗ LIFESPAN CONSIDERATIONS

Pregnancy/Lactation: Not recommended during first trimester of pregnancy. Distributed in breast milk. Breastfeeding not recommended. **Children:** Less likely to cause anticholinergic effects. **Elderly:** More sensitive to anticholinergic effects (e.g., dry mouth, urinary retention). Dizziness, sedation, confusion may occur.

INTERACTIONS

DRUG: Alcohol, CNS depressants (e.g., LORazepam, morphine, zolpidem) may increase CNS depression. Anticholinergics (e.g., aclidinium, ipratropium, umeclidinium) may increase anticholinergic effect. **HERBAL:** Herbs with sedative properties (e.g., chamomile, kava kava, valerian) may increase CNS depression. **FOOD:** None known. **LAB VALUES:** May suppress wheal and flare reactions to antigen skin testing unless drug is discontinued 4 days before testing.

AVAILABILITY (Rx)

Capsules: 10 mg. **Injection:** 10 mg/mL. **Ophthalmic:** 0.24%. **Oral Solution:** 5 mg/5 mL. **Tablets:** 5 mg, 10 mg. **Tablets (Chewable):** 5 mg, 10 mg. **Tablets (Dispersible):** 10 mg.

ADMINISTRATION/HANDLING

PO
• Give without regard to food. **Chewable tablet** • Must be chewed before swallowing. May give with or without water.
IV
• Administer IV push over 1–2 min.
Ophthalmic
• Remove contact lenses before administration (wait at least 10 min before inserting contact lenses). • Use immediately after opening. Wash hands; do not touch dropper tip to eyelids.

INDICATIONS/ROUTES/DOSAGE

◄**ALERT**► May cause drowsiness at dosage greater than 10 mg/day.

Allergic Rhinitis, Urticaria
PO: ADULTS, CHILDREN OLDER THAN 5 YRS: Initially, 5–10 mg/day as single dose. **Maximum:** 10 mg/day. **ELDERLY:** 5 mg once daily. **Maximum:** 5 mg/day. **CHILDREN 2–5 YRS:** 2.5 mg/day. May increase up to 5 mg/day as a single dose or in 2 divided doses. **CHILDREN 12–23 MOS:** Initially, 2.5 mg/day. May increase up to 5 mg/day in 2 divided doses. **CHILDREN 6–11 MOS:** 2.5 mg once daily.

Acute Urticaria
IV: ADULTS, ELDERLY: Initially, 10 mg once daily. **CHILDREN 12 YRS AND OLDER, ADOLESCENTS:** 10 mg q24h. **CHILDREN 6–11 YRS:** 5–10 mg q24h. **CHILDREN 6 MOS TO 5 YRS:** 2.5 mg q24h.

Allergic Conjunctivitis
OPHTH: ADULTS, ELDERLY, ADOLESCENTS, CHILDREN 2 YRS AND OLDER: Instill 1 drop in affected eye twice daily (about 8 hrs apart).

Dosage in Renal Impairment
Adults: GFR 50 mL/min or less: 5 mg once daily. **Children:** GFR 10 29 mL/min: reduce dose by 50 %. GFR <10 mL/min: Not recommended.

Dosage in Hepatic Impairment
No dose adjustment.

SIDE EFFECTS

Occasional (10%–2%): Pharyngitis, dry mucous membranes, nausea, vomiting, abdominal pain, headache, dizziness, fatigue, thickening of mucus, drowsiness, photosensitivity, urinary retention.

ADVERSE EFFECTS/TOXIC REACTIONS

Children may experience paradoxical reaction (restlessness, insomnia, euphoria, nervousness, tremor). Dizziness, sedation, confusion more likely to occur in elderly.

NURSING CONSIDERATIONS

BASELINE ASSESSMENT
Assess lung sounds. Assess severity of rhinitis, urticaria, other symptoms.

INTERVENTION/EVALUATION
For upper respiratory allergies, increase fluids to maintain thin secretions and offset thirst. Monitor symptoms for therapeutic response.

PATIENT/FAMILY TEACHING
• Avoid tasks that require alertness, motor skills until response to drug is established. • Avoid alcohol.

---

cetuximab

se-**tux**-i-mab
(Erbitux)

■ **BLACK BOX ALERT** ■ Severe infusion reactions (bronchospasm, stridor, urticaria, hypotension, cardiac arrest) have occurred, especially with first infusion in pts with head and neck cancer. Cardiopulmonary arrest reported in pts receiving radiation in combination with cetuximab. **Do not confuse cetuximab with bevacizumab.**

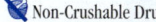

◆CLASSIFICATION

PHARMACOTHERAPEUTIC: Epidermal growth factor receptor (EGFR) inhibitor, monoclonal antibody. **CLINICAL:** Antineoplastic.

USES

Colorectal cancer, metastatic: In combination with FOLFIRI (irinotecan, fluorouracil, leucovorin) for first-line treatment. In combination with irinotecan in pts who are refractory to irinotecan-based chemotherapy. As a single-agent in pts who have not responded to oxaliplatin- and irinotecan-based chemotherapy or who are intolerant to irinotecan. In combination with encorafenib, for the treatment of adults with metastatic colorectal cancer (CRC) with a BRAF V600E mutation. **Head and neck cancer, squamous cell:** In combination with radiation therapy for the initial treatment of locally or regionally advanced squamous cell carcinoma of the head and neck (SCCHN). In combination with platinum-based therapy with fluorouracil for the first-line treatment of pts with recurrent locoregional disease or metastatic SCCHN. As a single-agent for the treatment of pts with recurrent or metastatic SCCHN for whom prior platinum-based therapy has failed. **OFF-LABEL:** Penile cancer (skin cancer advanced or metastatic), squamous cell skin cancer (unresectable).

PRECAUTIONS

Contraindications: Hypersensitivity to cetuximab. **Cautions:** Preexisting IgE antibodies to cetuximab, coronary artery disease, HF, arrhythmias, pulmonary disease.

ACTION

Specifically binds to and inhibits epidermal growth factor receptor (EGFR), blocking phosphorylation/activation of receptor-associated kinases. **Therapeutic Effect:** Inhibits tumor cell growth, inducing apoptosis (cell death).

PHARMACOKINETICS

Reaches steady-state levels by the third wkly infusion. Clearance decreases as dose increases. **Half-life:** 114 hrs (range: 75–188 hrs).

⏳ LIFESPAN CONSIDERATIONS

Pregnancy/Lactation: Crosses placental barrier; may cause fetal harm; abortifacient. Breastfeeding not recommended. **Children:** Safety and efficacy not established. **Elderly:** No age-related precautions noted.

INTERACTIONS

DRUG: None significant. **HERBAL:** None significant. **FOOD:** None known. **LAB VALUES:** May decrease WBCs; serum calcium, magnesium, potassium.

AVAILABILITY (Rx)

Injection Solution: 2 mg/mL (50 mL, 100 mL).

ADMINISTRATION/HANDLING

🖐 IV

◄**ALERT►** Do not give by IV push or bolus.

Reconstitution • Does not require reconstitution. **•** Solution should appear clear, colorless; may contain a small amount of visible, white particulates. **•** Do not shake or dilute. **•** Infuse with a low protein-binding 0.22-micron in-line filter.

Rate of administration • First dose should be given as a 120-min infusion. **•** Maintenance infusion should be infused over 60 min. **•** Maximum infusion rate should not exceed 5 mL/min (10 mg/min).

Storage • Refrigerate vials. **•** Infusion containers are stable for up to 12 hrs if refrigerated, up to 8 hrs at room temperature. **•** Discard unused portions.

▦ IV COMPATIBILITIES

Irinotecan (Camptosar).

INDICATIONS/ROUTES/DOSAGE

Metastatic Colorectal Cancer

Cetuximab single-agent therapy or in combination with irinotecan or FOLFIRI (irinotecan, fluorouracil, and leucovorin): **Note:** When given in combination with irinotecan or FOLFIRI, complete cetuximab dose 1 hr prior to chemotherapy.
IV: ADULTS, ELDERLY: Initially, 400 mg/m^2 as a loading dose. **Maintenance:** 250 mg/m^2 infused over 60 min wkly or 500 mg/m^2 infused over 120 min q2wks. Continue until disease progression or unacceptable toxicity. In combination with encorafenib: Initially, 400 mg/m^2 a loading dose. Maintenance: 250 mg/m^2 infused over 60 min wkly. Continue until disease progression or unacceptable toxicity.

Head and Neck Cancer (Squamous Cell)

Note: When given in combination with platinum/fluorouracil chemotherapy, complete cetuximab dose 1 hr prior to chemotherapy.
IV: ADULTS, ELDERLY: With radiation therapy: Initially, 400 mg/m^2 1 wk prior to initiation of radiation therapy course. Then 250 mg/m2 once wkly for duration of radiation therapy (6–7 weeks). Complete cetuximab 1 hr prior to radiation therapy. **Single-agent cetuximab or in combination with a platinum-based therapy with fluorouracil:** *Weekly dosing:* Initially, 400 mg/m^2, then 250 mg/m^2 wkly. *Biweekly dosing:* (Initial and subsequent doses): 500 mg/m^2 once q2wks. Continue until disease progression or unacceptable toxicity.

Dosage in Renal/Hepatic Impairment

No dose adjustment.

SIDE EFFECTS

Frequent (90%–25%): Acneiform rash, malaise, fever, nausea, diarrhea, constipation, headache, abdominal pain, anorexia, vomiting. **Occasional (16%–10%):** Nail disorder, back pain, stomatitis, peripheral edema, pruritus, cough, insomnia. **Rare (9%–5%):** Weight loss, depression, dyspepsia, conjunctivitis, alopecia.

ADVERSE EFFECTS/TOXIC REACTIONS

Anemia occurs in 10% of pts. Severe infusion reaction (rapid onset of airway obstruction, hypotension, severe urticaria) occurs rarely. Dermatologic toxicity, pulmonary embolus, leukopenia, renal failure occur rarely.

NURSING CONSIDERATIONS

BASELINE ASSESSMENT

Obtain CBC, BMP, pregnancy test in females of reproductive potential. Question history of hypersensitivity reaction. Offer emotional support.

INTERVENTION/EVALUATION

Monitor for evidence of infusion reaction (rapid onset of bronchospasm, stridor, hoarseness, urticaria, hypotension) during infusion and for at least 1 hr postinfusion. Pts may experience first severe infusion reaction during later infusions. Assess skin for evidence of dermatologic toxicity (development of inflammatory sequelae, dry skin, exfoliative dermatitis, rash). Monitor CBC, serum electrolytes, acute onset or worsening pulmonary symptoms.

PATIENT/FAMILY TEACHING

• Do not have immunizations without physician's approval (drug lowers resistance). • Avoid contact with anyone who recently received a live virus vaccine. • Avoid crowds, those with infection. • Wear sunscreen, limit sun exposure (sunlight can exacerbate skin reactions). • Avoid pregnancy. • Report cardiac or lung symptoms, severe rash.

---

chlorambucil 🟥HIGH ALERT

klor-**am**-bue-sil
(Leukeran)
■ **BLACK BOX ALERT** ■ May cause myelosuppression. Affects fertility; potential for carcinogenic, mutagenic, teratogenic effects. May cause azoospermia.

Do not confuse Leukeran with Alkeran, Leukine, or Myleran.

◆CLASSIFICATION

PHARMACOTHERAPEUTIC: Alkylating agent, nitrogen mustard. CLINICAL: Antineoplastic.

USES

Treatment of chronic lymphocytic leukemia (CLL), Hodgkin's and non-Hodgkin's lymphomas (NHL). OFF-LABEL: Nephrotic syndrome in children, Waldenström's macroglobulinemia.

PRECAUTIONS

Contraindications: Hypersensitivity to chlorambucil. Previous allergic reaction to other alkylating agents, prior resistance to chlorambucil, pregnancy. Extreme Cautions: Treatment within 4 wks after full-course radiation therapy or myelosuppressive drug regimen. Cautions: History of bone marrow suppression, head trauma, hepatic impairment, nephrotic syndrome, seizure disorder; administration of live vaccines to immunocompromised pts.

ACTION

Inhibits DNA, RNA synthesis by crosslinking with DNA strands. Therapeutic Effect: Interferes with DNA replication and RNA transcription.

PHARMACOKINETICS

Widely distributed. Protein binding: 99%. Metabolized in liver. Not removed by hemodialysis. Half-life: 1.5 hrs; metabolite, 2.5 hrs.

⊠ LIFESPAN CONSIDERATIONS

Pregnancy/Lactation: If possible, avoid use during pregnancy, esp. first trimester. Breastfeeding not recommended. Children: No age-related precautions noted. When taken for nephrotic syndrome, may increase risk of seizures. Elderly: No age-related precautions noted.

INTERACTIONS

DRUG: May decrease therapeutic effect of BCG (intravesical), vaccines (live). May increase adverse effects of vaccines (live). May increase myelosuppressive effect of myelosuppressants (e.g., cladribine). HERBAL: Echinacea may decrease therapeutic effect. FOOD: Acidic foods, spicy foods may delay absorption. LAB VALUES: May increase serum alkaline phosphatase, AST, uric acid.

AVAILABILITY (Rx)

Tablets: 2 mg.

ADMINISTRATION/HANDLING

PO
• May administer as a single daily dose (preferably on an empty stomach).

INDICATIONS/ROUTES/DOSAGE

Usual Dosage
PO: ADULTS, ELDERLY: 0.1–0.2 mg/kg daily for 3–6 wks as required (usually 4–10 mg/day for the average pt).

Dosage in Renal Impairment
CrCl 10–50 mL/min: 75% of dose. CrCl less than 10 mL/min: 50% of dose.

Dosage in Hepatic Impairment
Use caution.

SIDE EFFECTS

Expected: GI effects (nausea, vomiting, anorexia, diarrhea, abdominal distress), generally mild, last less than 24 hrs, occur only if single dose exceeds 20 mg. Occasional: Rash, dermatitis, pruritus, oral ulcerations. Rare: Alopecia, urticaria, erythema, hyperuricemia.

ADVERSE EFFECTS/TOXIC REACTIONS

Hematologic toxicity due to severe myelosuppression occurs frequently, manifested as neutropenia, anemia, thrombocytopenia. After discontinuation of therapy, thrombocytopenia, neutropenia usually last for 1–2 wks but may persist for 3–4 wks. Neutrophil count may continue to decrease for up to 10 days after last dose. Toxicity appears to be less severe with intermittent drug administration. Overdosage may produce seizures in children. Excessive serum uric acid level, hepatotoxicity occur rarely.

NURSING CONSIDERATIONS

BASELINE ASSESSMENT

Obtain CBC before therapy and wkly during therapy, WBC count 3–4 days following each wkly, CBC during first 3–6 wks of therapy (4–6 wks if pt on intermittent dosing schedule).

INTERVENTION/EVALUATION

Monitor CBC, serum uric acid, LFT. Monitor for hematologic toxicity (fever, sore throat, signs of local infection, unusual bruising/bleeding from any site), symptoms of anemia (excessive fatigue, weakness). Assess skin for rash, pruritus, urticaria.

PATIENT/FAMILY TEACHING

• Treatment may depress your immune system and reduce your ability to fight infection. Report symptoms of infection such as body aches, burning with urination, chills, cough, fatigue, fever. Avoid those with active infection. • Report symptoms of bone marrow depression (e.g., bruising, fatigue, fever, shortness of breath, weight loss; bleeding easily, bloody urine or stool). • Increase fluid intake (may protect against hyperuricemia). • Avoid acidic or spicy foods; may delay absorption of medication. • Do not have immunizations without physician's approval (drug lowers resistance). • Avoid contact with those who have recently received live virus vaccine.

ciprofloxacin

sip-roe-**flox**-a-sin
(Cetraxal, Ciloxan, Cipro, Otiprio)
■ **BLACK BOX ALERT** ■ May increase risk of tendonitis, tendon rupture. May exacerbate myasthenia gravis.

Do not confuse Ciloxan with Cytoxan, or Cipro with Ceftin, or ciprofloxacin with cephalexin.

FIXED-COMBINATION(S)

Cipro HC Otic: ciprofloxacin/hydrocortisone (a steroid): 0.2%/1%. **CiproDex Otic:** ciprofloxacin/dexAMETHasone (a corticosteroid): 0.3%/0.1%.

◆CLASSIFICATION

PHARMACOTHERAPEUTIC: Fluoroquinolone. **CLINICAL:** Antibiotic.

USES

Treatment of susceptible infections including UTI; acute, uncomplicated cystitis in females; chronic bacterial prostatitis, bone/joint infections, intra-abdominal infections (in combination with metronidazole), skin and skin structure infections; lower respiratory tract infections caused by susceptible microorganisms including *E. coli, K. pneumoniae, E. cloacae, P. mirabilis, P. vulgaris, P. stuartii, M. morganii, C. freundii, P. aeruginosa,* methicillin-susceptible *S. aureus,* methicillin-susceptible *S. epidermidis,* or *S. pyogenes* **Ophthalmic:** Treatment of bacterial conjunctivitis, corneal ulcers. **Otic:** Treatment of acute otitis externa due to susceptible strains of *P. aeruginosa* or *S. aureus.* **OFF-LABEL:** Bite wound, chancroid, COPD (acute exacerbation), Crohn's disease (adjunct perianal fistulas), diabetic foot infection, endocarditis, bacterial meningitis, neutropenia, prosthetic joint infection, *Shigella* GI infection, surgical prophylaxis..

PRECAUTIONS

Contraindications: Hypersensitivity to ciprofloxacin, other quinolones. Concurrent use of tiZANidine. **Cautions:** Renal impairment, CNS disorders, seizures, rheumatoid arthritis, history of QT prolongation, uncorrected hypokalemia, hypomagnesemia, myasthenia gravis. Suspension not used through feeding or gastric tubes. Use in children (due to adverse events to joints/surrounding tissue).

ACTION

Inhibits enzyme, DNA gyrase, in susceptible bacteria, interfering with bacterial cell replication. **Therapeutic Effect:** Bactericidal.

PHARMACOKINETICS

Widely distributed, including to CSF. Protein binding: 20%–40%. Metabolized in liver. Primarily excreted in urine. Minimal removal by hemodialysis. **Half-life:** 3–5 hrs (increased in renal impairment, elderly).

⧖ LIFESPAN CONSIDERATIONS

Pregnancy/Lactation: Unknown if distributed in breast milk. If possible, do not use during pregnancy/lactation (risk of arthropathy to fetus/infant). **Children:** Arthropathy may occur. **Elderly:** Age-related renal impairment may require dosage adjustment.

INTERACTIONS

DRUG: **Antacids, calcium, magnesium, zinc, iron preparations, sucralfate** may decrease absorption. May increase effects of **caffeine, oral anticoagulants (e.g., warfarin).** May increase concentration/effect of **pimozide, TIZanidine.** May increase concentration, toxicity of **theophylline. HERBAL:** None significant. **FOOD:** None known. **LAB VALUES:** May increase serum alkaline phosphatase, creatine kinase (CK), LDH, ALT, AST.

AVAILABILITY (Rx)

Infusion Solution: 200 mg/100 mL, 400 mg/200 mL. **Ophthalmic Ointment:** *(Ciloxan):* 0.3%. **Ophthalmic Solution:** *(Ciloxan):* 0.3%. **Otic Solution:** *(Cetraxal):* 0.2% (single-dose container: 0.25 mL). *(Otiprio):* 6%. **Suspension, Oral:** 250 mg/5 mL, 500 mg/5 mL. **Tablets:** 100 mg, 250 mg, 500 mg, 750 mg.

ADMINISTRATION/HANDLING

 IV

Reconstitution • Available prediluted in infusion container ready for use. Final concentration not to exceed 2 mg/mL.

Rate of administration • Infuse over 60 min (reduces risk of venous irritation). **Storage** • Store at room temperature. • Solution appears clear, colorless to slightly yellow.

PO

• May be given with food to minimize GI upset. • Give at least 2 hrs before or 6 hrs after antacids, calcium, iron, zinc-containing products. • Do not administer suspension through feeding or gastric tubes. • **NG tube:** Crush immediate-release tablet and mix with water. Flush tube before/after administration.

Ophthalmic

• Place gloved finger on lower eyelid and pull out until a pocket is formed between eye and lower lid. • Place ointment or drops into pocket. • Instruct pt to close eye gently for 1–2 min (so that medication will not be squeezed out of the sac). • Instruct pt using ointment to roll eyeball to increase contact area of drug to eye. • Instruct pt using solution to apply digital pressure to lacrimal sac at inner canthus for 1 min to minimize systemic absorption. • Do not use ophthalmic solution for injection.

▩ IV INCOMPATIBILITIES

Furosemide, heparin.

▩ IV COMPATIBILITIES

Calcium gluconate, dexmedetomidine, diltiazem, potassium chloride.

INDICATIONS/ROUTES/DOSAGE

Note: Not recommended as first choice in pregnancy/lactation or in children younger than 18 yrs due to adverse events related to joints/surrounding tissue.

Usual Dosage Range

PO: ADULTS, ELDERLY: 250–750 mg q12h. **CHILDREN:** 10–20 mg/kg/dose q12h. **Maximum:** 750 mg/dose.
IV: ADULTS, ELDERLY: 200–400 mg q12h. **CHILDREN:** 10 mg/kg q8–12h. **Maximum:** 400 mg/dose.

Usual Ophthalmic Dosage

Adults, Elderly, Children: *(Solution):* 1–2 drops q2h while awake for 2 days, then 1–2 drops q4h while awake for 5 days. *(Ointment):* Apply 3 times/day for 2 days, then 2 times/day for 5 days.

Usual Otic Dosage

Adults, Elderly, Children: Otic solution 0.2%: Instill 0.25 mL (0.5 mg) 2 times/day for 7 days. **Otic suspension 6%:** Instill 0.2 mL as a single dose.

Dosage in Renal Impairment

Dosage and frequency are modified based on creatinine clearance and the severity of the infection.

Creatinine Clearance	Dosage
Immediate-Release	
30–50 mL/min	PO: 250–500 mg q12h
5–29 mL/min	250–500 mg q18h
ESRD, HD, PD	250–500 mg q24h
Extended-Release	
< 30 mL/min	500 mg q24h
ESRD, HD, PD	500 mg q24h
IV 5–29 mL/min	200–400 mg q18–24h

Dosage in Hepatic Impairment

No dose adjustment.

SIDE EFFECTS

Frequent (5%–2%): Nausea, diarrhea, dyspepsia, vomiting, constipation, flatulence, confusion, crystalluria. **Ophthalmic:** Burning, crusting in corner of eye. **Occasional (less than 2%):** Abdominal pain/discomfort, headache, rash. **Ophthalmic:** Altered taste, sensation of foreign body in eye, eyelid redness, itching. **Rare (less than 1%):** Dizziness, confusion, tremors, hallucinations, hypersensitivity reaction, insomnia, dry mouth, paresthesia.

ADVERSE EFFECTS/TOXIC REACTIONS

Superinfection (esp. enterococcal, fungal), nephropathy, cardiopulmo-

nary arrest, cerebral thrombosis may occur. Hypersensitivity reaction (rash, pruritus, blisters, edema, burning skin), photosensitivity have occurred. Sensitization to ophthalmic form may contraindicate later systemic use of ciprofloxacin. May exacerbate muscle weakness in pts with myasthenia gravis. Dermatologic conditions such as toxic epidermal necrolysis, Stevens-Johnson syndrome have been reported. Cases of severe hepatotoxicity have occurred. May increase risk of tendonitis, tendon rupture.

NURSING CONSIDERATIONS

BASELINE ASSESSMENT

Question for history of hypersensitivity to ciprofloxacin, quinolones; myasthenia gravis, renal/hepatic impairment.

INTERVENTION/EVALUATION

Obtain urinalysis for microscopic analysis for crystalluria prior to and during treatment. Evaluate food tolerance. Monitor daily pattern of bowel activity, stool consistency. Encourage hydration (reduces risk of crystalluria). Monitor for dizziness, headache, visual changes, tremors. Assess for chest, joint pain. **Ophthalmic:** Observe therapeutic response.

PATIENT/FAMILY TEACHING

• It is essential to complete drug therapy despite improvement of symptoms. Early discontinuation may result in antibacterial resistance or increase the risk of recurrent infection. • Frequent diarrhea, fever, abdominal pain, blood-streaked stool may indicate infectious diarrhea and may be contagious to others. • Maintain adequate hydration. • Do not take antacids within 2 hrs of ciprofloxacin (reduces/destroys effectiveness). • Shake suspension well before using; do not chew microcapsules in suspension. • Report tendon pain or swelling. • Avoid exposure to sunlight/artificial light (may cause photosensitivity reaction).

C

CISplatin

HIGH ALERT

sis-**pla**-tin

■ **BLACK BOX ALERT** ■ Cumulative renal toxicity may be severe. Dose-related toxicities include myelosuppression, nausea, vomiting. Ototoxicity, especially pronounced in children, noted by tinnitus, loss of high-frequency hearing, deafness. Must be administered by personnel trained in administration/handling of chemotherapeutic agents. Anaphylactic reaction can occur within minutes of administration. Avoid confusion between CISplatin and CARBOplatin.

Do not confuse CISplatin with CARBOplatin or oxaliplatin.

◆CLASSIFICATION

PHARMACOTHERAPEUTIC: Alkylating agent. **CLINICAL:** Antineoplastic.

USES

Treatment of advanced testicular cancers, advanced ovarian cancers, advanced bladder cancer. **OFF-LABEL:** Breast, cervical, endometrial, esophageal, gastric, head and neck, lung (small-cell, non-small-cell) carcinomas; Hodgkin's and non-Hodgkin's lymphomas; malignant melanoma, neuroblastoma, osteosarcoma, pancreatic cancer, soft tissue sarcoma.

PRECAUTIONS

Contraindications: Hypersensitivity to CISplatin. **Cautions:** Baseline cytopenias, renal impairment, hearing impairment, elderly.

ACTION

Inhibits DNA synthesis by cross-linking with DNA strands. Cell cycle–phase nonspecific. **Therapeutic Effect:** Prevents cellular division.

PHARMACOKINETICS

Widely distributed. Protein binding: greater than 90%. Undergoes rapid nonenzymatic conversion to inactive metabolite. Excreted in urine. Removed by hemodialysis. **Half-life:** 58–73 hrs (increased in renal impairment).

☒ LIFESPAN CONSIDERATIONS

Pregnancy/Lactation: If possible, avoid use during pregnancy, esp. first trimester. Breastfeeding not recommended. **Children:** Ototoxic effects may be more severe. **Elderly:** Age-related renal impairment may require dosage adjustment.

INTERACTIONS

DRUG: Bone marrow depressants (e.g., cladribine) may increase myelosuppression. **Live virus vaccines** may decrease concentration/effect. May increase concentration/effects of **vaccines (live). HERBAL:** Echinacea may decrease therapeutic effect. **FOOD:** None known. **LAB VALUES:** May increase serum BUN, creatinine, uric acid, AST. May decrease CrCl, serum calcium, magnesium, phosphate, potassium, sodium. May cause positive Coombs' test.

AVAILABILITY (Rx)

Injection Solution: 1 mg/mL (50 mL, 100 mL, 200 mL).

ADMINISTRATION/HANDLING

◄**ALERT**► Wear protective gloves during handling. May be carcinogenic, mutagenic, teratogenic. Handle with extreme care during preparation/administration.

 IV

Dilution • Dilute desired dose in 250–1,000 mL 0.9% NaCl, D₅/0.45% NaCl, or D₅/0.9% NaCl to concentration of 0.05–2 mg/mL. Solution should have final NaCl concentration of 0.2% or greater.
Rate of administration • Infuse over 30 min to 4 hrs at a rate of 1 mg/min (rate varies by protocol). • Monitor for anaphylactic reaction during first few minutes of infusion.

Storage • Protect from sunlight. • Do not refrigerate (may precipitate). Discard if precipitate forms. IV infusion: Stable for 72 hrs at 39°F–77°F.

⚙ IV INCOMPATIBILITIES

Do no dilute in **D5W.**

⚙ IV COMPATIBILITIES

Granisetron, mannitol, ondansetron, palonosetron.

INDICATIONS/ROUTES/DOSAGE

Note: Pretreatment hydration with 1–2 liters of fluid recommended. Adequate hydration, urine output greater than 100 mL/hr should be maintained for 24 hrs after administration. Verify any CISplatin dose exceeding 100 mg/m^2/course.

Bladder Cancer
IV: ADULTS, ELDERLY: 50–70 mg/m^2 q3–4wks.

Ovarian Cancer
IV: ADULTS, ELDERLY: 75–100 mg/m^2 q3–4wks.

Testicular Cancer
IV: ADULTS, ELDERLY: 20 mg/m^2 daily for 5 days repeated q3wks (in combination with bleomycin and etoposide).

Dosage in Renal Impairment
Dosage is modified based on CrCl, BUN.
◄ALERT► Repeated courses of CISplatin should not be given until serum creatinine is less than 1.5 mg/100 mL and/or BUN is less than 25 mg/100 mL.

Creatinine Clearance	Dosage
10–50 mL/min	75% of normal dose
Less than 10 mL/min	50% of normal dose
Hemodialysis	50% of dose post dialysis
Peritoneal dialysis	50% of dose
Continuous renal replacement therapy	75% of dose

Dosage in Hepatic Impairment
No dose adjustment.

SIDE EFFECTS

Frequent: Nausea, vomiting (occurs in more than 90% of pts, generally beginning 1–4 hrs after administration and lasting up to 24 hrs); myelosuppression (affecting 25%–30% of pts, with recovery generally occurring in 18–23 days). **Occasional:** Peripheral neuropathy (with prolonged therapy [4–7 mos]). Pain/redness at injection site, loss of taste, appetite. **Rare:** Hemolytic anemia, blurred vision, stomatitis.

ADVERSE EFFECTS/TOXIC REACTIONS

Anaphylactic reaction (angioedema, wheezing, tachycardia, hypotension) may occur in first few minutes of administration in pt previously exposed to CISplatin. Nephrotoxicity occurs in 28%–36% of pts treated with a single dose, usually during second wk of therapy. Ototoxicity (tinnitus, hearing loss) occurs in 31% of pts treated with a single dose (more severe in children). Symptoms may become more frequent, severe with repeated doses.

NURSING CONSIDERATIONS

BASELINE ASSESSMENT

Obtain CBC, BMP, LFT. Pts should be well hydrated before and 24 hrs after medication to ensure adequate urinary output (100 mL/hr), decrease risk of nephrotoxicity.

INTERVENTION/EVALUATION

Measure all emesis, urine output (general guideline requiring immediate notification of physician: 750 mL/8 hrs, urinary output less than 100 mL/hr). Monitor I&O q1–2h beginning with pretreatment hydration, continue for 48 hrs after dose. Assess vital signs q1–2h during infusion. Monitor urinalysis, serum electrolytes, LFT, renal function tests, CBC, platelet count for changes from baseline.

✦ Canadian trade name   🥄 Non-Crushable Drug   High Alert drug

C

PATIENT/FAMILY TEACHING
• Report signs of ototoxicity (tinnitus, hearing loss). • Do not have immunizations without physician's approval (lowers body's resistance). • Avoid contact with those who have recently taken oral polio vaccine. • Report if nausea/vomiting continues at home. • Report signs of peripheral neuropathy.

---

citalopram

sye-**tal**-o-pram
(CeleXA)

■ **BLACK BOX ALERT** ■ Increased risk of suicidal thinking and behavior in children, adolescents, young adults 18–24 yrs with major depressive disorder, other psychiatric disorders.
Do not confuse CeleXA with CeleBREX, Cerebyx, Ranexa, or ZyPREXA.

◆CLASSIFICATION

PHARMACOTHERAPEUTIC: Selective serotonin reuptake inhibitor. **CLINICAL:** Antidepressant.

USES

Treatment of unipolar major depression in adults. **OFF-LABEL:** Obsessive compulsive disorder (OCD), social anxiety disorder (SAD), generalized anxiety disorder (GAD), panic disorder, aggressive/agitated behavior associated with dementia, binge eating disorder, posttraumatic stress disorder, premenstrual dysphoric disorder (PMDD), vasomotor symptoms associated with menopause.

PRECAUTIONS

Contraindications: Hypersensitivity to citalopram, use of MAOIs intended to treat psychiatric disorders (concurrently or within 14 days of discontinuing either citalopram or MAOI), initiation in pts receiving linezolid or methylene blue. Concurrent use with pimozide. **Cautions:** El-

derly, hepatic/renal impairment, seizure disorder. Not recommended in pts with congenital long QT syndrome, bradycardia, recent MI, uncompensated HF, hypokalemia, or hypomagnesemia; pts at high risk of suicide.

ACTION

Blocks uptake of the neurotransmitter serotonin at CNS presynaptic neuronal membranes, increasing its availability at postsynaptic receptor sites. **Therapeutic Effect:** Relieves symptoms of depression.

PHARMACOKINETICS

Widely distributed. Protein binding: 80%. Extensively metabolized in liver. Excreted in urine. **Half-life:** 35 hrs.

⏳ LIFESPAN CONSIDERATIONS

Pregnancy/Lactation: Distributed in breast milk. **Children:** May cause increased anticholinergic effects, hyperexcitability. **Elderly:** More sensitive to anticholinergic effects (e.g., dry mouth), more likely to experience dizziness, sedation, confusion, hypotension, hyperexcitability.

INTERACTIONS

DRUG: CYP2C19 inhibitors (e.g., fluconazole), QT-interval-prolonging medications (e.g., amiodarone, azithromycin, ciprofloxacin, haloperidol) may increase risk of QT prolongation. **Linezolid, MAOIs (e.g., phenelzine, selegiline), triptans** may cause serotonin syndrome (excitement, diaphoresis, rigidity, hyperthermia, autonomic hyperactivity, coma). **Strong CYP3A4 inducers (e.g., carBAMazepine, phenytoin, rifAMPin)** may decrease concentration/effect. **HERBAL:** St. John's wort may decrease concentration/effect. **FOOD:** None known. **LAB VALUES:** May decrease serum sodium.

AVAILABILITY (Rx)

Capsule: 30 mg. **Oral Solution:** 10 mg/5 mL. **Tablets:** 10 mg, 20 mg, 40 mg.

ADMINISTRATION/HANDLING

PO
• Give without regard to food.

INDICATIONS/ROUTES/DOSAGE

Note: Doses greater than 40 mg not recommended.

Depression
PO: ADULTS YOUNGER THAN 60 YRS: Initially, 20 mg once daily in the morning or evening. May increase in 20-mg increments at intervals of no less than 1 wk. **Maximum:** 40 mg/day. **ELDERLY 60 YRS OR OLDER:** 10–20 mg once daily. **Maximum:** 20 mg/day.

Dose Modification
Hepatic impairment; poor metabolizers of CYP2C19; concomitant use of CYP2C19 inhibitors: 20 mg once daily. **Maximum:** 20 mg/day.

Dosage in Renal Impairment
Mild to moderate impairment: No dose adjustment. **Severe impairment:** Use caution.

SIDE EFFECTS

Frequent (21%–11%): Nausea, dry mouth, drowsiness, insomnia, diaphoresis. **Occasional (8%–4%):** Tremor, diarrhea, abnormal ejaculation, dyspepsia, fatigue, anxiety, vomiting, anorexia. **Rare (3%–2%):** Sinusitis, sexual dysfunction, menstrual disorder, abdominal pain, agitation, decreased libido.

ADVERSE EFFECTS/TOXIC REACTIONS

Overdose manifested as dizziness, drowsiness, tachycardia, confusion, seizures, torsades de pointes, ventricular tachycardia, sudden death. Serotonin syndrome or neuroleptic malignant syndrome (NMS)–like reactions have been reported.

NURSING CONSIDERATIONS

BASELINE ASSESSMENT
Obtain CBC, LFT in pts on long-term therapy. Observe, record behavior. Assess psychological status, thought content, sleep pattern, appearance, interest in environment. Screen for bipolar disorder.

INTERVENTION/EVALUATION
Supervise suicidal-risk pt closely during early therapy (as depression lessens, energy level improves, increasing suicide potential). Assess appearance, behavior, speech pattern, level of interest, mood.

PATIENT/FAMILY TEACHING
• Do not stop taking medication or increase dosage. • Avoid alcohol. • Avoid tasks that require alertness, motor skills until response to drug is established. • Report worsening depression, suicidal ideation, unusual changes in behavior.

---

clarithromycin

kla-**rith**-roe-**mye**-sin
(Apo-Clarithromycin ♣, PMS-Clarithromycin ♣)
Do not confuse clarithromycin with Claritin, clindamycin, or erythromycin.

◆CLASSIFICATION

PHARMACOTHERAPEUTIC: Macrolide. **CLINICAL:** Antibiotic.

USES

Treatment of acute bacterial exacerbation of chronic bronchitis, otitis media, acute maxillary sinusitis, *Mycobacterium avium* complex (MAC), pharyngitis, tonsillitis, *H. pylori* duodenal ulcer, community-acquired pneumonia, skin and soft tissue infections. Prevention of MAC disease caused by susceptible microorganisms including *H. influenzae, H. parainfluenzae, M. catarrhalis, S. pneumoniae, S. aureus, H. pylori*, and *S. pyogenes*. **OFF-LABEL:** Prophylaxis of infective endocarditis (before invasive dental procedures), pertussis, Lyme disease.

PRECAUTIONS

Contraindications: Hypersensitivity to clarithromycin, other macrolide antibiotics. History of QT prolongation or ventricular arrhythmias, including torsades de pointes. History of cholestatic jaundice or hepatic impairment with prior use of clarithromycin. Concomitant use with colchicine (in pts with renal/hepatic impairment), statins, pimozide, ergotamine, dihydroergotamine. **Cautions:** Hepatic/renal impairment, elderly with severe renal impairment, myasthenia gravis, coronary artery disease. Pts at risk of prolonged cardiac repolarization. Avoid use with uncorrected electrolytes (e.g., hypokalemia, hypomagnesemia), clinically significant bradycardia, class IA or III antiarrhythmics (see Classification).

ACTION

Binds to ribosomal receptor sites of susceptible organisms, inhibiting protein synthesis of bacterial cell wall. **Therapeutic Effect:** Bacteriostatic; may be bactericidal with high dosages or very susceptible microorganisms.

PHARMACOKINETICS

Widely distributed (except CNS). Protein binding: 65%–75%. Metabolized in liver. Primarily excreted in urine. Not removed by hemodialysis. **Half-life:** 3–7 hrs; metabolite, 5–9 hrs (increased in renal impairment).

☒ LIFESPAN CONSIDERATIONS

Pregnancy/Lactation: Unknown if distributed in breast milk. **Children:** Safety and efficacy not established in pts younger than 6 mos. **Elderly:** Age-related renal impairment may require dosage adjustment.

INTERACTIONS

DRUG: May increase concentration/effects of **acalabrutinib, ado-trastuzumab, axitinib, bosutinib, budesonide, eletriptan, lovastatin.** May increase QT-prolonging effects of **dronedarone.** **HERBAL:** None significant. **FOOD:** None known. **LAB VALUES:** May increase serum BUN, ALT, AST, alkaline phosphatase, LDH, creatinine, PT. May decrease WBC.

AVAILABILITY (Rx)

Oral Suspension: 125 mg/5 mL, 250 mg/5 mL. **Tablets:** 250 mg, 500 mg.

Tablets (Extended-Release): 500 mg.

ADMINISTRATION/HANDLING

PO
• Give immediate-release tablets, oral suspension without regard to food. • Give q12h (rather than twice daily). • Shake suspension well before each use. • Extended-release tablets should be given with food. • Do not break, crush, dissolve, or divide extended-release tablets.

INDICATIONS/ROUTES/DOSAGE

Usual Dosage Range
PO: ADULTS, ELDERLY: 250–500 mg q12h or 1,000 mg once daily (2 × 500-mg extended-release tablets). **CHILDREN 6 MOS AND OLDER:** *(Immediate-Release):* 7.5 mg/kg q12h. **Maximum:** 500 mg/dose.

Dosage in Renal Impairment
CrCl less than 30 mL/min: Reduce dose by 50% and administer once or twice daily. **HD:** Administer dose after dialysis complete.

Combination With Atazanavir or Ritonavir

CrCl 30–60 mL/min	Decrease dose by 50%
CrCl less than 30 mL/min	Decrease dose by 75%

Dosage in Hepatic Impairment
No dose adjustment.

SIDE EFFECTS

Occasional (6%–3%): Diarrhea, nausea, altered taste, abdominal pain. **Rare (2%–1%):** Headache, dyspepsia.

ADVERSE EFFECTS/TOXIC REACTIONS

Antibiotic-associated colitis, other superinfections (abdominal cramps, severe watery diarrhea, fever) may result from altered bacterial balance in GI tract. Hepatotoxicity, thrombocytopenia occur rarely.

NURSING CONSIDERATIONS

BASELINE ASSESSMENT
Question for allergies to clarithromycin, erythromycins.

INTERVENTION/EVALUATION
Monitor daily pattern of bowel activity, stool consistency. Mild GI effects may be tolerable, but increasing severity may indicate onset of antibiotic-associated colitis. Be alert for superinfection: Fever, vomiting, diarrhea, anal/genital pruritus, oral mucosal changes (ulceration, pain, erythema).

PATIENT/FAMILY TEACHING
• It is essential to complete drug therapy despite improvement of symptoms. Early discontinuation may result in antibacterial resistance or increase the risk of recurrent infection. • Frequent diarrhea, fever, abdominal pain, blood-streaked stool may indicate infectious diarrhea and may be contagious to others. • Biaxin may be taken without regard to food. Take Biaxin XL with food.

---

clevidipine

clev-eye-di-peen
(Cleviprex)
Do not confuse clevidipine with amlodipine, cladribine, clofarabine, clozapine, or Cleviprex with Claravis.

◆**CLASSIFICATION**

PHARMACOTHERAPEUTIC: Dihydropyridine calcium channel blocker. **CLINICAL:** Antihypertensive.

USES
Management of hypertension when oral therapy is not feasible or not desirable. **OFF-LABEL:** Acute ischemic stroke (B/P management).

PRECAUTIONS
Contraindications: Hypersensitivity to clevidipine. Allergy to soy or egg products; abnormal lipid metabolism (e.g., acute pancreatitis, lipoid nephrosis, pathologic hyperlipidemia if accompanied by hyperlipidemia), severe aortic stenosis. **Cautions:** HF; lipid metabolism dysfunction.

ACTION
Causes potent arterial vasodilation by inhibiting the influx of calcium during depolarization in arterial smooth muscle. **Therapeutic Effect:** Decreases mean arterial pressure (MAP) by reducing systemic vascular resistance.

PHARMACOKINETICS
Widely and rapidly distributed. Full recovery of therapeutic B/P occurs 5–15 min. after discontinuation. Onset of effects: 2–4 min. Metabolized via hydrolysis by esterases in blood and extravascular tissue. Protein binding: 99.5%. Excreted in urine (74%), feces (22%). **Half-life:** 15 min.

⧗ LIFESPAN CONSIDERATIONS
Pregnancy/Lactation: Unknown if distributed in breast milk. May depress uterine contractions during labor and delivery. **Children:** Safety and efficacy not established. **Elderly:** Start at low end of dosing range. May experience greater hypotensive effect.

INTERACTIONS
DRUG: None significant. **HERBAL:** **Herbals with hypotensive properties (e.g., garlic, ginger, hawthorn)** may enhance effect. **Yohimbe** may decrease effect. **FOOD:** None known. **LAB VALUES:** May increase serum BUN, potassium, triglycerides, uric acid.

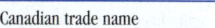

C

AVAILABILITY (Rx)

Injection, Emulsion: 50 mL (0.5 mg/mL), 100 mL (0.5 mg/mL).

ADMINISTRATION/HANDLING

 IV

Preparation • Do not dilute. • To ensure uniformity of emulsion, gently invert vial several times before use. • Visually inspect for particulate matter or discoloration. Emulsion should appear milky white. Discard if discoloration or particulate matter is observed.
Rate of administration • Titrate to desired effect using infusion pump via peripheral or central line.
Storage • Refrigerate unused vial in original carton. • May store at controlled room temperature (77°F) for up to 2 mos. • Do not freeze. • Do not return to refrigerator once warmed to room temperature. Once the stopper is punctured, use within 12 hrs. • Discard unused portions.

⊞ IV INCOMPATIBILITIES

May be administered with, but not diluted in, solutions including Sterile Water for Injection, 0.9% NaCl, dextrose-containing solutions, lactated Ringer's, 10% amino acid. Do not administer with other medications.

INDICATIONS/ROUTES/DOSAGE

Note: Individualize dosage depending on desired B/P and pt response. See manufacturer guidelines for dose conversion.
Hypertension
IV: ADULTS, ELDERLY: Initiate infusion at 1–2 mg/hr. **Titration:** Initially, dosage may be doubled at short (90-sec) intervals. As B/P approaches goal, an increase in dosage should be less than double, and time intervals between dose adjustments should be lengthened to q5–10 min. **Maintenance:** Desired therapeutic effect generally occurs at a rate of 4–6 mg/hr (pts with severe hypertension may

require limited doses up to 32 mg/hr).
Maximum: 16 mg/hr (no more than 21 mg/hr or 1000 mL is recommended per 24 hrs due to lipid load).

Dosage in Renal Impairment
No dose adjustment.

Dosage in Hepatic Impairment
Not specified; use caution.

SIDE EFFECTS

Occasional (6%–3%): Headache, insomnia, nausea, vomiting. **Rare (less than 1%):** Syncope, dyspnea.

ADVERSE EFFECTS/TOXIC REACTIONS

May cause atrial fibrillation, hypotension, reflex tachycardia. Rebound hypertension may occur in pts who are not transitioned to oral antihypertensives after discontinuation. Dihydropyridine calcium channel blockers are known to have negative inotropic effects, which may exacerbate HF. Rebound hypertension may cause emergent hypertensive crisis, which may cause CVA, myocardial infarction, renal failure, HF, seizures.

NURSING CONSIDERATIONS

BASELINE ASSESSMENT

Screen for history of defective lipid metabolism, pancreatitis, hypertriglyceridemia, severe aortic stenosis; allergy to soy products, eggs products. Assess B/P, apical pulse immediately before initiation.

INTERVENTION/EVALUATION

Monitor B/P, pulse rate. Generally, an increase of 1–2 mg/hour will produce an additional 2–4 mm Hg decrease in systolic B/P. If an oral antihypertensive is required to wean off infusion, consider the delay of onset of oral medication's effect. Pts who receive prolonged IV infusions and are not changed to other antihypertensives should be monitored for rebound hypertension for at least 8 hrs after discontinuation. Obtain serum triglyceride level in pts receiving prolonged infusions. Monitor for atrial fibrillation, hypotension, reflex tachycardia; exacerbation of HF in pts with history of HF. Beta blockers should be discontinued only after a gradual reduction in dose.

PATIENT/FAMILY TEACHING

• In some pts, an oral blood pressure medication may need to be started; compliance is essential to control high blood pressure. • Life-threatening high blood pressure crisis may occur up to 8 hrs after stopping infusion; report severe anxiety, chest pain, difficulty breathing, headache, stroke-like symptoms (confusion, difficulty speaking, paralysis, one-sided weakness, vision loss).

clindamycin

klin-da-**mye**-sin
(Cleocin, Cleocin T, Clindagel, Clindesse)

■ **BLACK BOX ALERT** ■ May cause severe, potentially fatal colitis characterized by severe, persistent diarrhea, severe abdominal cramps, passage of blood and mucus.
Do not confuse Cleocin with Clinoril or Cubicin, or clindamycin with clarithromycin, Claritin, or vancomycin.

◆**CLASSIFICATION**

PHARMACOTHERAPEUTIC: Lincosamide. **CLINICAL:** Antibiotic.

USES

Systemic: Treatment of bone/joint, gynecological, intra-abdominal, lower respiratory tract, septicemia, skin/soft tissue infections caused by susceptible microorganisms including *S. aureus* (methicillin-susceptible strains), *S. pneumoniae* (penicillin-susceptible strains), *S. pyogenes*, and anaerobes (e.g., *Clostridium perfringens, Fusobacterium necrophorum, Fusobacterium nucleatuum, Peptostreptococcus*

anaerobius, Prevotella melaninogenica). **Topical:** Treatment of acne vulgaris. **Intravaginal:** Treatment of bacterial vaginosis. **OFF-LABEL:** Treatment of babesiosis, bacterial vaginosis, bite wound infection, diabetic foot infection, neutropenic fever (empiric therapy), prosthetic joint infection, surgical prophylaxis, *Pneumocystis jiroveci* pneumonia (PCP), sinusitis, toxoplasmosis.

PRECAUTIONS

Contraindications: Hypersensitivity to clindamycin. **Cautions:** Severe hepatic dysfunction; history of GI disease (especially colitis).

ACTION

Inhibits protein synthesis of bacterial cell wall by binding to bacterial ribosomal receptor sites. Topically, decreases fatty acid concentration on skin. **Therapeutic Effect:** Bacteriostatic or bactericidal.

PHARMACOKINETICS

Widely distributed. Protein binding: 92%–94%. Metabolized in liver. Primarily excreted in urine. Not removed by hemodialysis. **Half-life:** 1.6–5.3 hrs (increased in renal/hepatic impairment, premature infants).

⧖ LIFESPAN CONSIDERATIONS

Pregnancy/Lactation: Readily crosses placenta. Distributed in breast milk. **Topical/Vaginal:** Unknown if distributed in breast milk. **Children:** Caution in pts younger than 1 mo. **Elderly:** No age-related precautions noted.

INTERACTIONS

DRUG: Strong CYP34A inhibitors (e.g., clarithromycin, ketoconazole, ritonavir), moderate CYP3A4 inhibitors (e.g., diltiazem, verapamil) may increase concentration/effect. **HERBAL:** None significant. **FOOD:** None known. **LAB VALUES:** May increase serum alkaline phosphatase, ALT, AST.

C

AVAILABILITY (Rx)

 Capsules: 75 mg, 150 mg, 300 mg. **Vaginal Cream:** 2%. **Topical Gel:** 1%. **Infusion, Premix:** 300 mg/50 mL, 600 mg/50 mL, 900 mg/50 mL. **Injection Solution:** 150 mg/mL. **Lotion:** 1%. **Oral Solution:** 75 mg/5 mL. **Vaginal Suppositories:** 100 mg. **Topical Swabs:** 1%.

ADMINISTRATION/HANDLING

IV

Reconstitution • Dilute 300–600 mg with 50 mL D$_5$W or 0.9% NaCl (900–1,200 mg with 100 mL).
Rate of administration • Infuse over at least 10–60 min at rate not exceeding 30 mg/min. Severe hypotension, cardiac arrest can occur with rapid administration. • No more than 1.2 g should be given in a single infusion.
Storage • Reconstituted IV infusion (piggyback) is stable for 16 days at room temperature, 32 days if refrigerated.

PO

• After reconstitution, oral solution is stable for 2 wks at room temperature. • Do not refrigerate oral solution (avoids thickening). • Give with at least 8 oz water (minimizes esophageal ulceration). • Give without regard to food.

Topical

• Wash skin; allow to dry completely before application. • Shake topical lotion well before each use. • Apply liquid, solution, or gel in thin film to affected area. • Avoid contact with eyes or abraded areas.

Vaginal, Cream or Suppository

• Use one applicatorful or suppository at bedtime. • Fill applicator that comes with cream or suppository to indicated level. • Instruct pt to lie on back with knees drawn upward and spread apart. • Insert applicator into vagina and push plunger to release medication. • Withdraw, wash applicator with soap and warm water. • Wash hands promptly to avoid spreading infection.

IV COMPATIBILITIES

Heparin, potassium chloride.

INDICATIONS/ROUTES/DOSAGE

Usual Dosage

IV, IM: ADULTS, ELDERLY: 600–2,700 mg/day in 2–4 divided doses. **Maximum:** 4,800 mg/day IV for severe infections. **INFANTS, CHILDREN, ADOLESCENTS:** 20–40 mg/kg/day divided q6–8h. **Maximum:** 2,700 mg/day. **NEONATES:** 5–9 mg/kg/dose q8h.
PO: ADULTS, ELDERLY: 150–450 mg q6h. **Maximum:** 1,800 mg/day. **INFANTS, CHILDREN, ADOLESCENTS:** 10–25 mg/kg/day in divided doses q8h. **Maximum:** 1,800 mg/day. **NEONATES:** 5–9 mg/kg/dose q8h.

Bacterial Vaginosis

Intravaginal: *(Cream):* **ADULTS:** One applicatorful at bedtime for 3 days in nonpregnant pts or for 7 days in pregnant pts. *(Clindesse):* **ADULTS:** One applicatorful once daily as single dose in nonpregnant pts. **Suppository: ADULTS:** Once daily into vagina at bedtime for 3 days.

Acne Vulgaris

Topical: ADULTS: Apply thin layer to affected area twice daily (pledget, lotion, solution); once daily (gel, foam).

Dosage in Renal/Hepatic Impairment

No dose adjustment.

SIDE EFFECTS

Frequent: Systemic: Abdominal pain, nausea, vomiting, diarrhea. **Topical:** Dry, scaly skin. **Vaginal:** Vaginitis, pruritus. **Occasional: Systemic:** Phlebitis; pain, induration at IM injection site; allergic reaction, urticaria, pruritus. **Topical:** Contact dermatitis, abdominal pain, mild diarrhea, burning, stinging. **Vaginal:** Headache, dizziness, nausea, vomiting, abdominal pain. **Rare: Vaginal:** Hypersensitivity reaction.

ADVERSE EFFECTS/TOXIC REACTIONS

Antibiotic-associated colitis, other superinfections (abdominal cramps, severe watery diarrhea, fever) may occur during and several wks after clindamycin therapy (including topical form). Blood dyscrasias (leukopenia, thrombocytopenia), nephrotoxicity (proteinuria, azotemia, oliguria) occur rarely. Thrombophlebitis with IV administration.

NURSING CONSIDERATIONS

BASELINE ASSESSMENT

Obtain WBC. Question pt for history of allergies. Avoid, if possible, concurrent use of neuromuscular blocking agents.

INTERVENTION/EVALUATION

Monitor daily pattern of bowel activity, stool consistency. Report diarrhea promptly due to potential for serious colitis (even with topical or vaginal administration). Assess skin for rash (dryness, irritation) with topical application. With all routes of administration, be alert for superinfection: fever, vomiting, diarrhea, anal/genital pruritus, oral mucosal changes (ulceration, pain, erythema).

PATIENT/FAMILY TEACHING

• It is essential to complete drug therapy despite improvement of symptoms. Early discontinuation may result in antibacterial resistance or increase the risk of recurrent infection. • Frequent diarrhea, fever, abdominal pain, blood-streaked stool may indicate infectious diarrhea and may be contagious to others. • Take oral doses with at least 8 oz water. • Use caution when applying topical clindamycin concurrently with peeling or abrasive acne agents, soaps, alcohol-containing cosmetics to avoid cumulative effect. • Do not apply topical preparations near eyes, abraded areas. • **Vaginal:** In event of accidental contact with eyes, rinse with large amounts of cool tap water. • Do not engage in sexual intercourse during treatment. • Wear sanitary pad to protect clothes against stains. Tampons should not be used.

clofarabine

kloe-**far**-a-bine
(Clolar)
Do not confuse clofarabine with cladribine or clevidipine.

◆CLASSIFICATION

PHARMACOTHERAPEUTIC: Antimetabolite (purine analog). **CLINICAL:** Antineoplastic.

USES

Treatment of pediatric pts (1–21 yrs) with relapsed or refractory acute lymphoblastic leukemia (ALL) (after at least 2 prior regimens). **OFF-LABEL:** Treatment of acute myelogenous leukemia (AML), refractory Langerhans cell histiocytosis.

PRECAUTIONS

Contraindications: Hypersensitivity to clofarabine. **Cautions:** Dehydration, hypotension, concomitant nephrotoxic or hepatotoxic medications, renal/hepatic impairment.

ACTION

Metabolized intracellularly to clofarabine triphosphate. Inhibits ribonucleoside reductase, which inhibits DNA synthesis. Competes with DNA polymers, decreasing cell replication. **Therapeutic Effect:** Decreases cell replication, inhibits cell repair. Produces cell death.

PHARMACOKINETICS

Protein binding: 47%. Metabolized intracellularly. Primarily excreted in urine (40%–60% unchanged). **Half-life:** 5.2 hrs.

C

⧗ LIFESPAN CONSIDERATIONS

Pregnancy/Lactation: May cause fetal harm. Breastfeeding not recommended. **Children:** Safety and efficacy not established in pts younger than 1 yr. **Elderly:** No age-related precautions noted.

INTERACTIONS

DRUG: May decrease therapeutic effect of **BCG (intravesical), vaccines (live).** May increase adverse effects of **vaccines (live). HERBAL:** Echinacea may decrease therapeutic effect. **Herbals with hypertensive properties (e.g., licorice, yohimbe)** or **hypotensive properties (e.g., garlic, ginger, ginkgo biloba)** may alter effects. **FOOD:** None known. **LAB VALUES:** May increase serum creatinine, uric acid, ALT, AST, bilirubin.

AVAILABILITY (Rx)

Injection Solution: 1 mg/mL (20-mL vial).

ADMINISTRATION/HANDLING

 IV

Reconstitution • Filter clofarabine through sterile, 0.2-micrometer syringe filter prior to dilution with D_5W or 0.9% NaCl to final concentration of 0.15–0.4 mg/mL. **Rate of administration** • Administer over 2 hrs. • Continuously infuse IV fluids to decrease risk of tumor lysis syndrome, other adverse events. **Storage** • Store at room temperature. • Use diluted solution within 24 hrs.

▩ IV INCOMPATIBILITIES

Do not administer any other medication through same IV line.

INDICATIONS/ROUTES/DOSAGE

Acute Lymphoblastic Leukemia (ALL)
IV: CHILDREN 1–21 YRS: 52 mg/m² over 2 hrs once daily for 5 consecutive days; repeat q2–6wks following recovery or return to baseline organ function. (Subsequent cycles should begin no sooner than 14 days from day 1 of previous cycle and when ANC is 750 cells/mm³ or greater.)

Dosage in Renal Impairment
Dosage is modified based on creatinine clearance.

Creatinine Clearance	Dosage
30–60 mL/min	Decrease dose by 50%
Less than 30 mL/min	Use with caution

Dosage in Hepatic Impairment
Baseline impairment: No dose adjustment. **Hepatotoxicity during treatment; Grade 3 or higher increase in bilirubin:** Discontinue treatment. May restart at 25% dose reduction following recovery to baseline.

SIDE EFFECTS

Frequent (83%–20%): Vomiting, nausea, diarrhea, pruritus, headache, fever, dermatitis, rigors, abdominal pain, fatigue, tachycardia, epistaxis, anorexia, petechiae, limb pain, hypotension, anxiety, constipation, edema. **Occasional (19%–11%):** Cough, mucosal inflammation, erythema, flushing, hematuria, dizziness, gingival bleeding, injection site pain, respiratory distress, pharyngitis, back pain, palmar-plantar erythrodysesthesia syndrome, myalgia, oral candidiasis, hypertension, depression, irritability, arthralgia, anorexia. **Rare (10%):** Tremor, weight gain, drowsiness.

ADVERSE EFFECTS/TOXIC REACTIONS

Neutropenia occurred in 57% of pts; pericardial effusion in 35%; left ventricular systolic dysfunction in 27%; hepatomegaly, jaundice in 15%; pleural effusion, pneumonia, bacteremia in 10%; capillary leak syndrome in less than 10%.

NURSING CONSIDERATIONS

BASELINE ASSESSMENT

Obtain, BMP, LFT; pregnancy test in females of reproductive potential. Question history of hepatic/renal impairment. Offer emotional support.

C

INTERVENTION/EVALUATION

Monitor CBC, renal function test, LFT, serum uric acid. Monitor respiratory status, cardiac function. Monitor daily pattern of bowel activity, stool consistency. Assess for GI disturbances. Assess skin for pruritus, dermatitis, petechiae, erythema on palms of hands and soles of feet. Assess for fever, sore throat; obtain blood cultures to detect evidence of infection. Ensure adequate hydration.

PATIENT/FAMILY TEACHING

• Do not have immunizations without physician's approval (drug lowers resistance). • Avoid contact with anyone who recently received a live virus vaccine. • Avoid crowds, those with infection. • Avoid pregnancy; pts of childbearing potential should use effective contraception. • Maintain strict oral hygiene and frequent handwashing. • Report fever, respiratory distress, prolonged nausea, vomiting, diarrhea, easy bruising.

clonazePAM

kloe-**naz**-e-pam
(KlonoPIN, Rivotril ✦)

■ **BLACK BOX ALERT** ■ Concomitant use with opioids may result in profound sedation, respiratory depression, coma, and death. The use of clonazePAM exposes users to risks of abuse, misuse, and addiction. Continued use may lead to significant physical dependence.
Do not confuse clonazePAM or KlonoPIN with cloBAZam, cloNIDine, cloZAPine, or LORazepam.

◆CLASSIFICATION

PHARMACOTHERAPEUTIC: Benzodiazepine (Schedule IV). **CLINICAL:** Anticonvulsant, antianxiety.

USES

Seizures: Monotherapy or adjunctive therapy in treatment of Lennox-Gastaut syndrome (petit mal variant epilepsy); akinetic, myoclonic seizures; absence seizures (petit mal) unresponsive to succinimides. **Panic disorder:** Treatment of panic disorder with or without agoraphobia. **OFF-LABEL:** Anxiety, agitation, myoclonus, REM sleep behavior disorder, tardive dyskinesia, vertigo (acute episodes).

PRECAUTIONS

Contraindications: Hypersensitivity to clonazePAM. Active narrow-angle glaucoma, severe hepatic disease. **Cautions:** Renal/hepatic impairment, impaired gag reflex, chronic respiratory disease, elderly, debilitated pts, depression, pts at risk of suicide or drug dependence, concomitant use of other CNS depressants.

ACTION

Enhances activity of GABA; depresses nerve impulse transmission in motor cortex. **Therapeutic Effect:** Produces anxiolytic, anticonvulsant effects.

PHARMACOKINETICS

Route	Onset	Peak	Duration
PO	20–60 min	—	12 hrs or less

Widely distributed. Protein binding: 85%. Metabolized in liver. Excreted in urine. Not removed by hemodialysis. **Half-life:** 18–50 hrs.

⧖ LIFESPAN CONSIDERATIONS

Pregnancy/Lactation: Crosses placenta. May be distributed in breast milk. Chronic ingestion during pregnancy may produce withdrawal symptoms, CNS depression in neonates. **Children:** Long-term use may adversely affect physical/mental development. **Elderly:** Not recommended in elderly due to anticholinergic effects, potential for sedation, orthostatic hypotension.

INTERACTIONS

DRUG: Alcohol, other CNS depressants (e.g., **lorazePAM, morphine, zolpidem**) may increase CNS depressant effect. **Strong CYP3A4 inhibitors (e.g., clarithromycin, ketoconazole, rito-**

navir) may increase concentration/effect. **Strong CYP3A4 inducers (e.g., carBAMazepine, phenytoin, rifAMPin)** may decrease concentration/effect. **HERBAL:** Herbs with sedative properties (e.g., chamomile, kava kava, valerian) may increase CNS depression. **Yohimbine** may diminish the therapeutic effect. **FOOD:** None known. **LAB VALUES:** None significant.

AVAILABILITY (Rx)

Tablets: 0.5 mg, 1 mg, 2 mg. **Tablets (Orally Disintegrating):** 0.125 mg, 0.25 mg, 0.5 mg, 1 mg, 2 mg.

ADMINISTRATION/HANDLING

PO
• Give without regard to food. • Swallow whole with water.

Orally Disintegrating Tablet
• Open pouch, peel back foil; do not push tablet through foil. • Remove tablet with dry hands, place in mouth. • Swallow with or without water. • Use immediately after removing from package.

INDICATIONS/ROUTES/DOSAGE

Seizures
PO: ADULTS, ELDERLY: (Monotherapy): Initially, 0.5–1.5 mg/day in 1–3 divided doses. **(Adjunctive therapy):** Initially, 0.5–1 mg/day in 1–3 divided doses. May increase in 0.5- to 1-mg increments every 3–7 days until seizures are controlled or adverse effects occur. **Maintenance:** 2–8 mg/day in 1–2 divided doses. **Maximum:** 20 mg/day. **CHILDREN 10 YRS AND OLDER OR WEIGHING 30 KG OR MORE:** Initially, 0.01–0.05 mg/kg/day in 2 or 3 doses **(maximum initial dose:** 0.05 mg 3 times/day). May increase in increments of 25% or 0.5–1 mg q3–7 days. **Maintenance:** 0.05–0.2 mg/kg/day in 2–3 divided doses. **Maximum:** 20 mg/day. **INFANTS, CHILDREN YOUNGER THAN 10 YRS OR WEIGHING LESS THAN 30 KG:** 0.01–0.03 mg/kg/day **(maximum initial dose:** 0.05 mg/kg/day) in 2–3 divided doses; may be increased by no more than 0.25–0.5

mg every 3 days until seizures are controlled or adverse effects occur. **Maintenance:** 0.1–0.2 mg/kg/day in 3 divided doses. **Maximum:** 0.2 mg/kg/day.

Panic Disorder
PO: ADULTS, ELDERLY: Initially, 0.25–1 mg/day in 1 or 2 divided doses. May increase in increments of 0.25–0.5 mg q3days or longer. **Usual dose:** 1–3 mg/day in 1–4 divided doses. **Maximum:** 4 mg/day. **Note:** Discontinue gradually by 0.125 mg twice daily q3days until completely withdrawn.

Dosage in Renal Impairment
Use caution.

Dosage in Hepatic Impairment
Mild to moderate impairment: Use with caution. **Severe impairment:** Contraindicated.

SIDE EFFECTS

Frequent (37%–11%): Mild, transient drowsiness; ataxia, behavioral disturbances (aggression, irritability, agitation), esp. in children. **Occasional (10%–5%):** Dizziness, ataxia, URI, fatigue. **Rare (4% or less):** Impaired memory, dysarthria, nervousness, sinusitis, rhinitis, constipation, allergic reaction.

ADVERSE EFFECTS/TOXIC REACTIONS

Abrupt withdrawal may result in pronounced restlessness, irritability, insomnia, hand tremors, abdominal/muscle cramps, diaphoresis, vomiting, status epilepticus. Overdose results in drowsiness, confusion, diminished reflexes, coma. **Antidote:** Flumazenil (see Appendix H for dosage).

NURSING CONSIDERATIONS

BASELINE ASSESSMENT
Review history of seizure disorder (frequency, duration, intensity, level of consciousness [LOC]). For panic attack, assess motor responses (agitation, trembling, tension), autonomic responses (cold/clammy hands, diaphoresis).

C

INTERVENTION/EVALUATION

Observe for excess sedation, respiratory depression, suicidal ideation. Assess children, elderly for paradoxical reaction, particularly during early therapy. Initiate seizure precautions, observe frequently for recurrence of seizure activity. Assist with ambulation if drowsiness, ataxia occur. For pts on long-term therapy, CBC, BMP, LFT should be performed periodically. Evaluate for therapeutic response: Decreased intensity and frequency of seizures or, if used in panic attack, calm facial expression, decreased restlessness.

PATIENT/FAMILY TEACHING

• Avoid tasks that require alertness, motor skills until response to drug is established. • Do not abruptly discontinue medication after long-term therapy. • Strict maintenance of drug therapy is essential for seizure control. • Avoid alcohol. • Report depression, thoughts of suicide/self-harm, excessive drowsiness, GI symptoms, worsening or loss of seizure control.

cloNIDine

klon-i-deen
(Catapres-TTS, Duraclon, Kapvay, Nexixclon XR)

■**BLACK BOX ALERT** ■ Epidural: Not to be used for perioperative, obstetric, or postpartum pain. Must dilute concentrated epidural injectable (500 mcg/mL) prior to use.
Do not confuse Catapres with Cataflam, or cloNIDine with clomiPHENE, clonazePAM, KlonoPIN, or quiNIDine.

◆CLASSIFICATION

PHARMACOTHERAPEUTIC: Alpha₂-adrenergic agonist. **CLINICAL:** Antihypertensive.

USES

Immediate-release, extended-release (Nexiclon), transdermal patch: Treatment of hypertension alone or in combination with other antihypertensive agents.

Kapvay: Treatment of attention-deficit hyperactivity disorder (ADHD). Monotherapy or adjuvant therapy in children ages 6–12 years yrs, adolescents, and adults. **Epidural: (additional):** Combined with opiates for relief of severe cancer pain. **OFF-LABEL:** Opioid withdrawal, vasomotor symptoms associated with menopause, ICU sedation (transition from dexmedeTOMIDine). Tourette's syndrome, insomnia in children.

PRECAUTIONS

Contraindications: Hypersensitivity to cloNIDine. **Epidural:** Contraindicated in pts with bleeding diathesis or infection at the injection site; pts receiving anticoagulation therapy. **Cautions:** Depression, elderly. Severe coronary insufficiency, recent MI, cerebrovascular disease, chronic renal impairment, preexisting bradycardia, sinus node dysfunction, conduction disturbances; concurrent use with digoxin, dilTIAZem, metoprolol, verapamil.

ACTION

Stimulates alpha₂-adrenergic receptors in the brainstem, reducing sympathetic outflow from the CNS. **Epidural:** Prevents pain signal transmission to brain and produces analgesia at pre- and post-alpha-adrenergic receptors in spinal cord. **ADHD:** Mechanism of action unknown. **Therapeutic Effect:** Reduces peripheral resistance; decreases B/P, heart rate. Produces analgesia.

PHARMACOKINETICS

Route	Onset	Peak	Duration
PO	0.5–1 hr	2–4 hrs	6–10 hrs

Widely distributed. Transdermal best absorbed from chest and upper arm; least absorbed from thigh. Protein binding: 20%–40%. Metabolized in liver. Primarily excreted in urine. Minimally removed by hemodialysis. **Half-life:** 6–20 hrs (increased in renal impairment).

⧖ LIFESPAN CONSIDERATIONS

Pregnancy/Lactation: Crosses placenta. Distributed in breast milk. **Chil-**

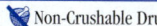

C

dren:** More sensitive to effects; use caution. **Elderly:** Not recommended in elderly due to high risk of CNS adverse effects, orthostatic hypotension. Avoid as first-line antihypertensive.

INTERACTIONS

DRUG: CNS depressants (e.g., alcohol, morphine, oxyCODONE, zolpidem) may increase CNS depression. May increase AV blocking effect of **beta blockers (e.g., atenolol, carvedilol, metoprolol).** Tricyclic antidepressants **(e.g., amitriptyline, doxepin, nortriptyline)** may decrease effect (may require increased dose of cloNIDine). **Digoxin, dilTIAZem, metoprolol, verapamil** may increase risk of serious bradycardia. **HERBAL: Herbs with sedative properties (e.g., chamomile, kava kava, valerian)** may increase CNS depression. **Herbals with hypertensive properties (e.g., licorice, yohimbe)** or **hypotensive properties (e.g., garlic, ginger, ginkgo biloba)** may alter effects. **FOOD:** None known. **LAB VALUES:** None significant.

AVAILABILITY (Rx)

Injection Solution: 100 mcg/mL, 500 mcg/mL. **Tablets:** 0.1 mg, 0.2 mg, 0.3 mg. **Transdermal Patch:** 2.5 mg (release at 0.1 mg/24 hrs), 5 mg (release at 0.2 mg/24 hrs), 7.5 mg (release at 0.3 mg/24 hrs).

Extended-Release Tablets: *(Kapvay):* 0.1 mg. *(Nexiclon XR):* 0.17 mg (scored).

ADMINISTRATION/HANDLING

PO
• Give without regard to food. *(Kapvay):*
• Swallow whole (do not crush, chew, or split). *(Nexiclon):* • May split in half. Take preferably at bedtime.

Transdermal
• Apply transdermal system to dry, hairless area of intact skin on upper arm or chest. • Rotate sites (prevents skin irritation). • Do not trim patch to adjust dose.

Epidural
• Must be administered only by medical personnel trained in epidural management.

⊞ IV INCOMPATIBILITIES
None known.

⊞ IV COMPATIBILITIES
Bupivacaine, lidocaine, ropivacaine.

INDICATIONS/ROUTES/DOSAGE

Hypertension
PO: ADULTS: *(Immediate-Release):* Initially, 0.1 mg twice a day. Increase by 0.1 mg/day at wkly intervals. **Dosage range:** 0.2–0.6 mg/day in 2 divided doses. **ELDERLY:** Initially, 0.1 mg at bedtime. May increase gradually. *Extended-Release Tablet (Nexiclon XR):* Initially, 0.17 mg once daily at bedtime. May increase by 0.09 mg/day. **Usual range:** 0.17–0.52 mg once daily. **Maximum:** 0.52 mg/day.
Transdermal: ADULTS, ELDERLY: Initially, system delivering 0.1 mg/24 hrs applied once q7days. May increase by 0.1 mg at 1- to 2-wk intervals. **Usual dosage range:** 0.1–0.3 mg once wkly.

Attention-Deficit Hyperactivity Disorder (ADHD)
Note: When discontinuing, taper gradually over 1–2 wks. *(Extended-Release Tablets):* Taper by 0.1 mg or less q3–7 days.
PO: CHILDREN WEIGHING 45 KG OR LESS: *(Immediate-Release):* Initially 0.05 mg/day at bedtime. May increase in increments of 0.05 mg/day q3–7days up to a maximum of 0.2 mg/day (27–40.5 kg), 0.3 mg/day (40.5–45 kg). **MORE THAN 45 KG:** *(Immediate-Release):* 0.1 mg at bedtime. May increase 0.1 mg/day q3–7 days. **Maximum:** 0.4 mg/day. *(Extended-Release Tablet [Kapvay]):* **CHILDREN 6 YRS AND OLDER:** Initially, 0.1 mg daily at bedtime. May increase in increments of 0.1 mg/day at wkly intervals (**maximum:** 0.4 mg/day).

Doses should be taken twice daily with higher split dose given at bedtime.

Severe Pain
Epidural: ADULTS, ELDERLY: 30–40 mcg/hr. **CHILDREN:** Range: 0.5–2 mcg/kg/hr, not to exceed adult dose.

Dosage in Renal/Hepatic Impairment
No dose adjustment.

SIDE EFFECTS

Frequent (40%–10%): Dry mouth, drowsiness, dizziness, sedation, constipation. **Occasional (5%–1%): Tablets, injection:** Depression, pedal edema, loss of appetite, decreased sexual function, itching eyes, dizziness, nausea, vomiting, nervousness. **Transdermal:** Pruritus, redness, or darkening of skin. **Rare (less than 1%):** Nightmares, vivid dreams, feeling of coldness in distal extremities (esp. the digits).

ADVERSE EFFECTS/TOXIC REACTIONS

Overdose produces profound hypotension, irritability, bradycardia, respiratory depression, hypothermia, miosis (pupillary constriction), arrhythmias, apnea. Abrupt withdrawal may result in rebound hypertension associated with nervousness, agitation, anxiety, insomnia, paresthesia, tremor, flushing, diaphoresis. May produce sedation in pts with acute CVA.

NURSING CONSIDERATIONS

BASELINE ASSESSMENT
Obtain B/P prior to each dose.

INTERVENTION/EVALUATION
Monitor B/P, pulse, mental status. Monitor daily pattern of bowel activity, stool consistency. If cloNIDine is to be withdrawn, discontinue concurrent betablocker therapy several days before discontinuing cloNIDine (prevents cloNIDine withdrawal hypertensive crisis). Slowly reduce cloNIDine dosage over 2–4 days

PATIENT/FAMILY TEACHING
• Avoid tasks that require alertness, motor skills until response to drug is established. • To reduce hypotensive effect, rise slowly from lying to standing. • Skipping doses or voluntarily discontinuing drug may produce severe rebound hypertension. • Avoid alcohol. • If patch loosens during 7-day application period, secure with adhesive cover.

clopidogrel

kloe-**pid**-oh-grel
(Plavix)

■ BLACK BOX ALERT ■ Diminished effectiveness in CYP2C19 metabolizers increases risk for cardiovascular events. Pts with CYP2C19*2 and/or CYP2C19*3 alleles may have reduced platelet inhibition.
Do not confuse Plavix with Elavil or Paxil.

◆CLASSIFICATION

PHARMACOTHERAPEUTIC: Thienopyridine derivative. **CLINICAL:** Antiplatelet.

USES

Acute coronary syndrome (ACS): Reduce rate of myocardial infarction (MI) and stroke in pts with non-ST-segment elevation acute coronary syndrome (unstable angina/non-ST-elevation MI [NSTEMI]), including pts who are managed medically and those managed with coronary revascularization (administer with aspirin). Reduce the rate of MI and stroke in pts with acute ST-elevation myocardial infarction (STEMI) who are to be managed medically (administer with aspirin). **MI, ischemic stroke, peripheral atherosclerotic disease:** Reduce the rate of MI and stroke in pts with established peripheral arterial disease or history of recent (MI) or stroke. **OFF-LABEL:** Percutaneous coronary intervention for stable ischemic heart disease, symptomatic carotid artery atherosclerosis, carotid artery stenting, CABG surgery, stable ischemic heart disease, TAVR/transcatheter mitral valve repair (thromboprophylaxis).

PRECAUTIONS

Contraindications: Hypersensitivity to clopidogrel. Active bleeding (e.g., peptic ulcer, intracranial hemorrhage). **Cautions:** Severe hepatic/renal impairment, pts at risk of increased bleeding (e.g., trauma), concurrent use of anticoagulants. Avoid concurrent use of CYP2C19 inhibitors (e.g., omeprazole).

ACTION

Active metabolite irreversibly blocks $P2Y_{12}$ component of ADP receptors on platelet surface, preventing activation of GPIIb/IIIa receptor complex. **Therapeutic Effect:** Inhibits platelet aggregation.

PHARMACOKINETICS

Route	Onset	Peak	Duration
PO	2 hrs	5–7 days (with repeated doses of 75 mg/day)	5 days after last dose

Widely distributed. Protein binding: 98%. Metabolized in liver. Eliminated equally in the urine and feces. **Half-life:** 8 hrs.

⏳ LIFESPAN CONSIDERATIONS

Pregnancy/Lactation: Unknown if drug crosses placenta or is distributed in breast milk. **Children:** Safety and efficacy not established. **Elderly:** No age-related precautions noted.

INTERACTIONS

DRUG: May increase adverse effects of **apixaban, dabigatran, edoxaban, warfarin. Strong CYP2C19 inhibitors (e.g., fluvoxaMINE, FLUoxetine)** may decrease concentration/effect. **Chronic use of NSAIDs (e.g., diclofenac, meloxicam, naproxen)** may increase risk of GI bleeding. **HERBAL: Herbals with anticoagulant/antiplatelet properties (e.g., garlic, ginger, ginkgo biloba), glucosamine** may increase risk of bleeding. **FOOD: Grapefruit products** may decrease therapeutic effect. **LAB VALUES:** May increase serum bilirubin, ALT, AST, cholesterol, uric acid. May decrease neutrophil count, platelet count.

AVAILABILITY (Rx)

Tablets: 75 mg, 300 mg.

ADMINISTRATION/HANDLING

PO
• Give without regard to food. Tablets cannot be crushed, cut, or chewed. • Avoid grapefruit products.

INDICATIONS/ROUTES/DOSAGE

Recent MI, Stroke, PAD
PO: ADULTS, ELDERLY: 75 mg once daily without a loading dose.

ACS
PO: ADULTS, ELDERLY: 300 mg loading dose (pts needing antiplatelet effect within hrs), then 75 mg once daily.

Dosage in Renal Impairment
No dose adjustment.

Dosage in Hepatic Impairment
Use caution.

SIDE EFFECTS

Frequent (15%): Skin disorders. **Occasional (8%–6%):** Upper respiratory tract infection, chest pain, flu-like symptoms, headache, dizziness, arthralgia. **Rare (5%–3%):** Fatigue, edema, hypertension, abdominal pain, dyspepsia, diarrhea, nausea, epistaxis, dyspnea, rhinitis.

ADVERSE EFFECTS/TOXIC REACTIONS

Agranulocytosis, aplastic anemia/pancytopenia, thrombotic thrombocytopenic purpura (TTP) occur rarely. Hepatitis, hypersensitivity reaction, anaphylactoid reaction have been reported. Discontinuation may increase risk of cardiovascular events.

NURSING CONSIDERATIONS

BASELINE ASSESSMENT

Obtain platelet count. Question history of hemorrhagic events, traumatic bleeding. Obtain medication history and screen for interactions.

INTERVENTION/EVALUATION

Monitor platelet count for evidence of thrombocytopenia. Assess Hgb, Hct, for evidence of bleeding; serum ALT, AST, bilirubin, BUN, creatinine; signs/symptoms of hepatic insufficiency during therapy.

PATIENT/FAMILY TEACHING

• It may take longer to stop bleeding during drug therapy. • Report any unusual bleeding. • Inform physicians, dentists if clopidogrel is being taken, esp. before surgery is scheduled or before taking any new drug.

cobimetinib

koe-bi-**me**-ti-nib
(Cotellic)
Do not confuse cobimetinib with cabozantinib, imatinib, or trametinib.

◆CLASSIFICATION

PHARMACOTHERAPEUTIC: MEK inhibitor. **CLINICAL:** Antineoplastic.

USES

Metastatic melanoma: Treatment of pts with unresectable or metastatic melanoma with a BRAF V600E or V600K mutation, in combination with vemurafenib. **Histiocytic neoplasms:** As a single agent for the treatment of adults with histiocytic neoplasms.

PRECAUTIONS

Contraindications: Hypersensitivity to cobimetinib. **Cautions:** Baseline anemia, lymphopenia, thrombocytopenia;

cardiomyopathy, hepatic/renal impairment, HF, hypertension, ocular disorders; pts at risk for bleeding (history of gastrointestinal, genitourinary, intracranial, reproductive system bleeding), electrolyte imbalance. Not recommended in pts taking moderate or strong CYP3A inhibitors.

ACTION

Potent and selective inhibitor of mitogen-activated extracellular kinase (MEK) pathway. Reversibly inhibits MEK1 and MEK2, which are upstream regulators of the ERK pathway. The ERK pathway promotes cellular proliferation. MEK1 and MEK2 are part of the BRAF pathway. **Therapeutic Effect:** Causes apoptosis and reduces tumor growth.

PHARMACOKINETICS

Widely distributed. Metabolized in liver. Protein binding: 95%. Peak plasma concentration: 2.4 hrs. Steady state reached in 9 days. Eliminated in feces (76%), urine (18%). **Half-life:** 44 hrs.

⧖ LIFESPAN CONSIDERATIONS

Pregnancy/Lactation: Avoid pregnancy; may cause fetal harm/malformations. Females of reproductive potential should use effective contraception during treatment and up to 2 wks after discontinuation. Unknown if distributed in breast milk. Breastfeeding not recommended. May reduce fertility in females and males. **Children/Elderly:** Safety and efficacy not established.

INTERACTIONS

DRUG: **Strong CYP3A4 inhibitors** (e.g., **clarithromycin, ketoconazole, ritonavir**), **moderate CYP3A4 inhibitors** (e.g., **atazanavir, ciprofloxacin**) may increase concentration/effect. **Strong CYP3A4 inducers** (e.g., **car-BAMazepine, phenytoin, rifAMPin**), **moderate CYP3A4 inducers** (e.g., **bosentan, nafcillin**) may decrease concentration/effect. **HERBAL:** None significant. **FOOD: Grapefruit products** may increase serum concentration/effect. **LAB VALUES:** Many increase serum alkaline phosphatase, ALT, AST, creatine phosphokinase, creatinine, GGT. May decrease Hct, Hgb, lymphocytes, platelets, RBCs; serum albumin, calcium, sodium. May increase or decrease serum potassium.

AVAILABILITY (Rx)

Tablets: 20 mg.

ADMINISTRATION/HANDLING

PO
• Give without regard to food. Tablets should not be crushed, chewed, or cut. • If dose is missed or vomiting occurs during administration, give next dose at regularly scheduled time.

INDICATIONS/ROUTES/DOSAGE

Metastatic Melanoma
PO: ADULTS, ELDERLY: 60 mg (three 20-mg tablets) once daily for first 21 days of 28-day cycle (in combination with vemurafenib). Continue until disease progression or unacceptable toxicity.

Histiocytic Neoplasms
PO: ADULTS, ELDERLY: **(Single agent):** 60 mg once daily for 21 days of 28-day cycle.

Concomitant Use of CYP3A Inhibitors
Reduce dose to 20 mg once daily if short-term (14 days or less) use of moderate CYP3A inhibitors is unavoidable. May resume 60-mg once-daily dose once the short-term CYP3A inhibitor is discontinued. Use an alternative strong or moderate CYP3A inhibitor in pts already taking reduced dose of 20 mg or 40 mg daily.

Dose Modification
Based on Common Terminology Criteria for Adverse Events (CTCAE) grading 1–4. See prescribing information for vemurafenib for recommended dose modification.

Dose Reduction Schedule
First dose reduction: 40 mg once daily. **Second dose reduction:** 20 mg once daily. Permanently discontinue if unable to tolerate 20 mg once daily.

Cardiomyopathy
Asymptomatic decrease in left ventricular ejection fraction (LVEF) greater than 10% from baseline and less than institutional lower limit of normal (LLN): Withhold treatment for 2 wks, then reassess LVEF. Resume at next lower dose level if LVEF is at or above LLN and the decrease from baseline is 10% or less. Permanently discontinue if LVEF is less than LLN or the decrease from baseline LVEF is more than 10%. **Symptomatic decrease of LVEF from baseline:** Withhold treatment for up to 4 wks, then reassess LVEF. Resume at next lower dose level if symptoms resolve, LVEF is at or above LLN, and the decrease from baseline LVEF is 10% or less. Permanently discontinue if symptoms persist, LVEF is less than LLN, or the decrease from baseline LVEF is more than 10%.

Dermatologic Reactions
Grade 2 (intolerable); Grade 3 or 4: Withhold or reduce dose.

Hepatotoxicity or Hepatic Laboratory Abnormalities
First occurrence, Grade 4: Withhold treatment for up to 4 wks. If improved to Grade 0 or 1, resume at next lower dose level. If not improved to Grade 0 or 1 within 4 wks, permanently discontinue. **Recurrent Grade 4:** Permanently discontinue.

Hemorrhage
Grade 3: Withhold treatment for up to 4 wks. If not improved to Grade 0 or 1, resume at next lower dose level. If not improved within 4 wks, permanently discontinue. **Grade 4:** Permanently discontinue.

New Primary Malignancies (Cutaneous or Noncutaneous)
No dose adjustment.

Nonspecific Adverse Effects
Any intolerable Grade 2; any Grade 3: Withhold for up to 4 wks. If improved to Grade 0 or 1, resume at next lower dose level. If not improved within 4 wks, permanently discontinue. **First occurrence of any Grade 4:** Permanently discontinue.

Ocular Toxicities

Serious retinopathy: Withhold treatment for up to 4 wks. If signs and symptoms improve, resume at next lower dose level. If not improved or symptoms recur at the lower dose within 4 wks, permanently discontinue. **Retinal vein occlusion:** Permanently discontinue.

Photosensitivity

Grade 2 (intolerable); Grade 3 or 4: Withhold treatment for up to 4 wks. If improved to Grade 0 or 1, resume at next lower dose level. If not improved within 4 wks, permanently discontinue.

Rhabdomyolysis, CPK Level Elevations

Grade 4 CPK elevation or any CPK elevation with myalgia: Withhold treatment for up to 4 wks. If improved to Grade 3 or lower, resume at next lower dose level. If not improved within 4 wks, permanently discontinue.

Severe Hypersensitivity Reaction

Permanently discontinue.

Dosage in Renal Impairment

Mild to moderate impairment: No dose adjustment. **Severe impairment:** Not specified; use caution.

Dosage in Hepatic Impairment

Mild impairment: No dose adjustment. **Moderate to severe impairment:** Not specified; use caution.

SIDE EFFECTS

Frequent (60%–24%): Diarrhea, photosensitivity, sunburn, solar dermatitis, nausea, pyrexia, vomiting. **Occasional (16%–10%):** Acneiform dermatitis, stomatitis, aphthous stomatitis, mouth ulceration, mucosal inflammation, alopecia, hypertension, vision impairment, blurred vision, reduced visual acuity, hyperkeratosis, erythema, chills.

ADVERSE EFFECTS/TOXIC REACTIONS

Myelosuppression (anemia lymphopenia, thrombocytopenia) is an expected response to therapy. New primary malignancies, including squamous cell carcinoma, keratoacanthoma, secondary-primary melanomas, were reported. Serious, sometimes fatal hemorrhagic events, including GI bleeding (4% of pts), intracranial bleeding (1% of pts), hematuria (2% of pts), reproductive system hemorrhage (2% of pts), have occurred. Other hemorrhagic events may include cerebral/conjunctival/intracranial/gingival/hemorrhoidal/ovarian/pulmonary/rectal/uterine/vaginal bleeding; ecchymosis, epistaxis. Grade 3 or 4 cardiomyopathy reported in 26% of pts. Grade 3 or 4 skin reactions including severe rash occurred in 16% of pts. Ocular toxicities, including retinopathy, chorioretinopathy, retinal detachment, reported in 26% of pts. Grade 3 or 4 CPK level elevations occurred in 14% of pts and may lead to rhabdomyolysis. Hepatotoxicity reported in 7%–11% of pts. Severe photosensitivity reported in 47% of pts.

NURSING CONSIDERATIONS

BASELINE ASSESSMENT

Confirm presence of BRAF V600E or V600K mutation in tumor specimen prior to initiation. Obtain baseline CBC, BMP, LFT, CPK; serum albumin, magnesium, phosphate, ionized calcium; urine pregnancy; vital signs. Obtain ophthalmologic exam with visual acuity; ECG, echocardiogram for LVEF. Assess skin for moles, lesions, papillomas. Verify use of effective contraception in females of reproductive potential. Receive full medication history, including herbal products. Question history as listed in Precautions. Assess hydration status.

INTERVENTION/EVALUATION

Monitor CBC, BMP, LFT, CPK; serum albumin, magnesium, phosphate, ionized calcium; vital signs. Assess skin for new lesions, dermal toxicities at least q2mos during treatment and for least 6 mos after discontinuation. Assess LVEF by echocardiogram 1 mo after initiation, then q3mos thereafter until discontinuation. If treatment

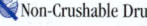

interrupted due to change in LVEF, monitor LVEF at 2 wks, 4 wks, 10 wks, and 16 wks, and then as indicated. Conduct ophthalmologic examinations regularly, esp. with any new or worsening visual disturbances. Assess for eye pain, visual changes. Immediately report GI bleeding, hematuria, unusual reproductive system hemorrhage; symptoms of intracranial bleeding (aphasia, blindness, confusion, facial droop, hemiplegia, seizures). Monitor for hepatotoxicity; monitor for signs of rhabdomyolysis, such as dark-colored urine, flank pain, decreased urine output, muscle aches. Due to high risk of diarrhea, strictly monitor I&O.

PATIENT/FAMILY TEACHING

• Blood levels monitoring, cardiac function tests, eye exams, skin exams will be conducted frequently. • Treatment may lead to severe anemia, HF, kidney failure, new cancers, severe light sensitivity, liver dysfunction, skin toxicities (such as severe rash, peeling), vision changes. • Report bloody stools, bloody urine, unusual reproductive system bleeding, nosebleeds, coughing up blood; abdominal or flank pain, dark-colored urine, decreased urinary output; stroke-like symptoms; new skin moles or lesions, rash; eye pain, vision changes; heart problems such as shortness of breath, dizziness, fainting, palpitations. • Report any newly prescribed medications. • Avoid sunlight, tanning beds. Wear protective clothing, high-SPF sunscreen, and lip balm when outdoors. • Use contraception to avoid pregnancy. Do not breastfeed. Treatment may reduce fertility.

---

colchicine

kol-chi-seen
(Colcrys, Lodoco, Mitigare)
Do not confuse colchicine with Cortrosyn.

◆CLASSIFICATION

PHARMACOTHERAPEUTIC: Alkaloid.
CLINICAL: Antigout.

USES

Prevention, treatment of acute gouty arthritis. Used to reduce frequency of recurrence of familial Mediterranean fever (FMF) in adults and children 4 yrs and older. **Lodoco:** Reduce risk of myocardial infarction (MI), stroke, coronary revascularization, cardiovascular death in adults with established atherosclerotic disease or multiple risk factors for cardiovascular disease. **OFF-LABEL:** Treatment of Behcet's disease, pericarditis (recurrent or acute), stable ischemic heart disease (prevention of CV events), vasculitis.

PRECAUTIONS

Contraindications: Hypersensitivity to colchicine. Concomitant use of a P-glycoprotein (e.g., cycloSPORINE) or strong CYP3A4 inhibitor (e.g., clarithromycin) in presence of renal or hepatic impairment. **Mitigare:** Pts with both renal/hepatic impairment. **Cautions:** Hepatic impairment, elderly, debilitated pts, renal impairment. Concomitant use of cycloSPORINE, dilTIAZem, verapamil, fibrates, statins may increase risk of myopathy.

ACTION

Disrupts cytoskeletal functions by preventing activation, degranulation, and migration of neutrophils associated with gout symptoms. In FMF, may interfere with intracellular assembly of inflammasome complex present in neutrophils and monocytes. **Therapeutic Effect:** Reduces inflammatory process.

PHARMACOKINETICS

Widely distributed. Oral bioavailability: 45%. Highest concentration is in liver, spleen, kidney. Protein binding: 30%–50%. Re-enters intestinal tract by biliary secretion and is reabsorbed from intestines. Partially metabolized in liver via CYP3A4. Eliminated primarily in feces. **Half-life:** 27–31 hrs.

⧗ LIFESPAN CONSIDERATIONS

Pregnancy/Lactation: Drug crosses placenta and is distributed in breast milk.

Children: Safety and efficacy not established. **Elderly:** May be more susceptible to cumulative toxicity. Age-related renal impairment may increase risk of myopathy.

INTERACTIONS

DRUG: CYP3A4 inhibitors (e.g., **clarithromycin, ketoconazole, ritonavir**), **P-glycoprotein/ABCB1 inhibitors** (**e.g., amiodarone**) may increase concentration/effect. May increase concentration/effect; risk of adverse effects (myopathy) of **HMG-CoA inhibitors (statins)** (**e.g., atorvastatin**). **HERBAL:** None significant. **FOOD: Grapefruit products** may increase concentration/toxicity. **LAB VALUES:** May increase serum alkaline phosphatase, AST. May decrease platelet count.

AVAILABILITY (Rx)

Tablets: *(Colcrys):* 0.6 mg. *(Lodoco):* 0.5 mg. **Capsule:** *(Mitigare):* 0.6 mg.

ADMINISTRATION/HANDLING

PO
• Give without regard to food. • Give with adequate water and maintain fluid intake.

INDICATIONS/ROUTES/DOSAGE

Acute Gouty Arthritis (Colcrys)
PO: ADULTS, ELDERLY: Initially, 1.2 mg at first sign of gout flare, then 0.6 mg 1 hr later. **Maximum:** 1.8 mg/day on day 1. **Day 2 and thereafter:** 0.6 mg 1–2 times daily until flare resolves.

Gout Prophylaxis (Colcrys, Mitigare)
Note: Duration of prophylaxis is 6 mos or 3 mos (pts without tophi) to 6 mos (pts with 1 or more tophi)
PO: ADULTS, ELDERLY: 0.6 mg 1–2 times/day. **Maximum:** 1.2 mg/day.

FMF (Colcrys)
PO: ADULTS, ELDERLY: 1.2–2.4 mg/day in 1–2 divided doses. Titrate dose in 0.6-mg increments. **Maximum:** 3 mg/day. **CHILDREN 12 YRS AND OLDER:** 1.2–2.4 mg/day in 1–2 divided doses. **CHILDREN 7–11 YRS:** 0.9–1.8 mg/day in 1–2 divided doses. **CHILDREN 4–6 YRS:** 0.3–1.8 mg/day

in 1–2 divided doses. **Note:** Increase or decrease dose by 0.3 mg/day, not to exceed maximum dose of 2.4 mg/day.

Pericarditis
PO: ADULTS TO AGE 70 YRS WEIGHING 70 KG OR MORE: 0.5–0.6 mg BID. **WEIGHING LESS THAN 70 KG:** 0.5–0.6 mg/day 3 mos. **ADULTS OLDER THAN 70 YRS WEIGHING 70 KG OR MORE:** 0.25–0.3 mg BID. **WEIGHING <70 KG:** 0.25–0.3 mg/day 3 mos.

Risk Reduction for Prevention of CV Events
PO: *(Lodoco):* **ADULTS, ELDERLY:** 0.5 mg once daily.

Dosage in Renal Impairment

Creatinine Clearance	Dosage
Less than 30 mL/min	
FMF	0.3 mg initially
Gout prophylaxis	0.3 mg/day
Gout flare	No reduction
HD	
FMF	0.3 mg as single dose
Gout prophylaxis	0.3 mg 2–4 times/wk

Dosage in Hepatic Impairment
Use caution.

SIDE EFFECTS

Frequent: Nausea, vomiting, abdominal discomfort. **Occasional:** Anorexia. **Rare:** Hypersensitivity reaction, including angioedema.

ADVERSE EFFECTS/TOXIC REACTIONS

Bone marrow depression (aplastic anemia, agranulocytosis, thrombocytopenia) may occur with long-term therapy. Overdose initially causes burning feeling in skin/throat; severe diarrhea, abdominal pain. Second stage manifests as fever, seizures, delirium, renal impairment (hematuria, oliguria). Third stage causes hair loss, leukocytosis, stomatitis.

NURSING CONSIDERATIONS

BASELINE ASSESSMENT

Obtain baseline laboratory studies. **Gout:** Assess involved joints for pain, mobility, edema. **Mediterranean fever:** Assess abdominal pain, fever, chills, erythema, swollen skin lesions.

INTERVENTION/EVALUATION

Discontinue medication immediately if GI symptoms occur. Encourage high fluid intake (3,000 mL/day). Monitor I&O (output should be at least 2,000 mL/day), CBC, hepatic/renal function tests. Monitor serum uric acid. Assess for therapeutic response: Relief of pain, stiffness, swelling; increased joint mobility; reduced joint tenderness; improved grip strength.

PATIENT/FAMILY TEACHING

• Drink 8–10 (8-oz) glasses of fluid daily while taking medication. • Report skin rash, sore throat, fever, unusual bruising/bleeding, weakness, fatigue, numbness. • Stop medication as soon as gout pain is relieved or at first sign of nausea, vomiting, diarrhea. • Avoid grapefruit products.

crizotinib

kriz-**o**-ti-nib
(Xalkori)

♦CLASSIFICATION

PHARMACOTHERAPEUTIC: Tyrosine kinase inhibitor. Anaplastic lymphoma kinase inhibitor. **CLINICAL:** Antineoplastic.

USES

Non–small-cell lung cancer (NSCLC): Treatment of metastatic NSCLC that is anaplastic lymphoma kinase (ALK) positive or is ROS-1 positive in adults. **Anaplastic large cell lymphoma (ALCL):** Treatment of ALCL systemic ALK-positive, relapsed or refractory in young adults and children 1 yr of age and older. **Inflammatory myofibroblastic tumor (IMT):** Treatment of adult and pediatric pts 1 yr of age and older with unresectable, recurrent, or refractory IMT that is ALK-positive.

PRECAUTIONS

Contraindications: Hypersensitivity to crizotinib. **Cautions:** Baseline hepatic impairment, congenital long QT interval syndrome. Pregnancy (avoid use). Concomitant use of CYP3A4 inducers/inhibitors, medications known to cause bradycardia, renal impairment.

ACTION

Inhibits receptor tyrosine kinases, including anaplastic lymphoma kinase (ALK), hepatocyte growth factor receptors (HGFR, c-Met), recepteur d'origine nantais (RON). ALK gene abnormalities due to mutation may result in expression of oncogenic fusion proteins. **Therapeutic Effect:** Inhibits tumor cell proliferation of cells expressing genetic alteration.

PHARMACOKINETICS

Widely distributed. Metabolized in liver. Peak plasma concentration: 4–6 hrs. Protein binding: 91%. Excreted in feces (63%) and urine (22%). **Half-life:** 42 hrs.

⧖ LIFESPAN CONSIDERATIONS

Pregnancy/Lactation: Avoid pregnancy. May cause fetal harm. Contraception should be considered during therapy and for at least 12 wks after discontinuation. Do not initiate therapy until pregnancy status confirmed. Unknown if crosses placenta or distributed in breast milk. Nursing mothers must discontinue either nursing or drug therapy. **Children:** Safety and efficacy not established. **Elderly:** No age-related precautions noted.

INTERACTIONS

DRUG: Strong CYP3A4 inhibitors (e.g., clarithromycin, ketoconazole, ritonavir) may increase concentration/effect. **Strong CYP3A4 inducers (e.g., carBAMazepine, phenytoin, rifAMPin)** may decrease concentration/effect. May increase concentration/effect of **aprepitant, bosutinib, budesonide, cobimetinib, cycloSPORINE, ivabradine, neratinib, sirolimus, tacrolimus.** **HERBAL:** St. John's wort may decrease concentration/effect. **FOOD: Grapefruit products** may increase concentration/toxicity (potential for torsades, myelotoxicity). **LAB VALUES:** May increase serum ALT, AST, alkaline phosphatase, bilirubin. May decrease neutrophils, platelets, lymphocytes.

AVAILABILITY (Rx)

Oral pellets: 20 mg, 50 mg, 150 mg.

Capsules: 200 mg, 250 mg.

ADMINISTRATION/HANDLING

Capsules

• May give without regard to food. • Avoid grapefruit products. • Administer capsules whole. Do not break, crush, dissolve, or divide capsules. **Oral pellets:** Supplied encapsulated in shells (cannot be swallowed.) • Pellets can not be chewed or crushed. • Open shell(s) and empty contents directly into the pt's mouth or into a consumer-supplied oral dosing aid. Immediately after administration, give a sufficient amount of water to ensure all medication is swallowed.

INDICATIONS/ROUTES/DOSAGE

NSCLC

PO: ADULTS: 250 mg twice daily. Continue until disease progression or unacceptable toxicity.

ALCL

PO: ADULTS, CHILDREN 1-18 YRS: 280 mg/m² twice daily based on body surface area (BSA). Continue until disease progression or unacceptable toxicity.

IMT

PO: ADULTS, ELDERLY: 250 mg twice daily. **CHILDREN:** 280 mg/m² twice daily based on BSA. Continue until disease progression or unacceptable toxicity.

Body Surface Area	Recommended Dose
0.38 to 0.46 m²	120 mg twice daily
0.47 to 0.51 m²	140 mg twice daily
0.52 to 0.61 m²	150 mg twice daily
0.62 to 0.80 m²	200 mg twice daily
0.81 to 0.97 m²	250 mg twice daily
0.98 to 1.16 m²	300 mg twice daily
1.17 to 1.33 m²	350 mg twice daily
1.34 to 1.51 m²	400 mg twice daily
1.52 to 1.69 m²	450 mg twice daily
1.70 m² or greater	500 mg twice daily

Dosage Modification

Interrupt and/or reduce to 200 mg twice daily based on graded protocol, including hematologic toxicity (Grade 4), elevated LFT with bilirubin elevation (Grade 1), QT prolongation (Grade 3). May reduce to 250 mg once daily if indicated. Discontinue treatment for QT prolongation (Grade 4), elevated LFT with bilirubin elevation (Grades 2, 3, 4), pneumonitis of any grade.

Hematologic Toxicity

Grade 3 toxicity (WBC 1,000–2,000 cells/mm³, ANC 500–1,000 cells/mm³, platelets 25,000–50,000 cells/mm³), Grade 3 anemia: Withhold treatment until recovery to Grade 2 or less, then resume at same dosage. **Grade 4 toxicity (WBC less than 1,000 cells/mm³, ANC less than 500 cells/mm³, platelets less than 25,000 cells/mm³), Grade 4 anemia:** Withhold treatment until recovery to Grade 2 or less, then resume at 200 mg twice daily. **Grade 4 toxicity on 200 mg twice daily:** Withhold treatment until recovery to Grade 2 or less, then resume at 250 mg once daily. **Recurrent Grade 4 toxicity on 250 mg once daily:** Permanently discontinue.

Cardiotoxicity

Grade 3 QTc prolongation on at least 2 separate ECGs: Withhold treatment until recovery to baseline or Grade 1 or less. Resume at 200 mg twice daily. **Recurrent Grade 3 QTc prolongation on 200 mg twice daily:** Withhold treatment until recovery to baseline or Grade 1 or less. Resume at 250 mg once daily. **Recurrent Grade 3 QTc prolongation on 250 mg once daily:** Permanently discontinue.

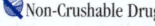

Bradycardia
Grades 2 or 3: Withhold until recovery to asymptomatic bradycardia or heart rate 60 or more beats/min, evaluate concomitant medications, then resume at 200 mg twice daily. **Grade 4 due to crizotinib:** Permanently discontinue. **Grade 4 associated with concurrent medications known to cause bradycardia/hypotension:** Withhold until recovery to asymptomatic bradycardia or heart rate 60 or more beats/min, and if concurrent medications can be stopped, resume at 250 mg once daily.

Pulmonary Toxicity
Permanently discontinue.

Dosage in Renal Impairment
CrCl less than 30 mL/min: 250 mg once daily.

Dosage in Hepatic Impairment
No dose adjustment (see dose for hepatotoxicity during treatment).

SIDE EFFECTS

Frequent (62%–27%): Diplopia, photopsia, photophobia, blurry vision, visual field defect, vitreous floaters, reduced visual acuity, nausea, diarrhea, vomiting, peripheral/localized edema, constipation. **Occasional (20%–4%):** Fatigue, decreased appetite, dizziness, neuropathy, paresthesia, dysgeusia, dyspepsia, dysphagia, esophageal obstruction/pain/spasm/ulcer, odynophagia, reflux esophagitis, rash, abdominal pain/tenderness, stomatitis, glossodynia, glossitis, cheilitis, mucosal inflammation, oropharyngeal pain/discomfort, bradycardia, headache, cough. **Rare (3%–1%):** Musculoskeletal chest pain, insomnia, dyspnea, arthralgia, nasopharyngitis, rhinitis, pharyngitis, URI, back pain, complex renal cysts, chest pain/tightness.

ADVERSE EFFECTS/TOXIC REACTIONS

Severe, sometimes fatal treatment-related pneumonitis, pneumonia, dyspnea, pulmonary embolism in less than 2% of pts was noted. Grade 3–4 elevation of hepatic enzymes, increased QT prolongation may require discontinuation. May cause thrombocytopenia, neutropenia, lymphopenia. Severe/worsening vitreous floaters, photopsia may indicate retinal hole, retinal detachment.

BASELINE ASSESSMENT

Assess vital signs, O_2 saturation. Obtain baseline CBC with differential, serum chemistries, LFT, PT/INR, ECG; pregnancy test in females of reproductive potential. Obtain full medication history including vitamins, herbal products. Detection of ALK-positive NSCLC test needed prior to treatment. Assess history of tuberculosis, HIV, HF, bradyarrhythmias, electrolyte imbalance, medications that prolong QT interval. Assess visual acuity, history of vitreous floaters. Offer emotional support.

INTERVENTION/EVALUATION

Assess vital signs, O_2 saturation routinely. Monitor CBC with differential monthly, LFT, monthly; increase testing for Grades 2, 3, 4 adverse effects. Obtain ECG for bradycardia, electrolyte imbalance, chest pain, difficulty breathing. Monitor for bruising, hematuria, jaundice, right upper abdominal pain, weight loss, or acute infection (fever, diaphoresis, lethargy, oral mucosal changes, productive cough). Worsening cough, fever, or shortness of breath may indicate pneumonitis. Consider ophthalmological evaluation for vision changes. Reinforce birth control compliance.

PATIENT/FAMILY TEACHING

• Report urine changes, bloody or clay-colored stools, upper abdominal pain, nausea, vomiting, bruising, fever, cough, difficulty breathing. • Report history of liver abnormalities or heart problems, including long QT syndrome, syncope, palpitations, extremity swelling. • Immediately report any newly prescribed medications, suspected pregnancy, or vision changes, including light flashes, blurred vision, photophobia, or new or increased floaters. • Use contraception to avoid pregnancy. Do not breastfeed. • Avoid alcohol, grapefruit products.

cyclobenzaprine

sye-kloe-**ben**-za-preen
(Amrix, Fexmid)
Do not confuse cyclobenzaprine with cycloSERINE or cyproheptadine.

◆CLASSIFICATION

PHARMACOTHERAPEUTIC: Centrally acting muscle relaxant. **CLINICAL:** Skeletal muscle relaxant.

USES

Short term (2–3 wks) treatment of muscle spasm associated with acute, painful musculoskeletal conditions. **OFF-LABEL:** Treatment of muscle spasms associated with temporomandibular joint pain (TMJ), fibromyalgia.

PRECAUTIONS

Contraindications: Hypersensitivity to cyclobenzaprine. Acute recovery phase of MI, arrhythmias, HF, heart block, conduction disturbances, hyperthyroidism, use within 14 days of MAOIs. **Cautions:** Hepatic impairment, history of urinary hesitancy or retention, angle-closure glaucoma, increased intraocular pressure (IOP), elderly.

ACTION

Centrally acting skeletal muscle relaxant that reduces tonic somatic muscle activity at level of brainstem. Influences both alpha and gamma motor neurons. **Therapeutic Effect:** Relieves local skeletal muscle spasm.

PHARMACOKINETICS

Route	Onset	Peak	Duration
PO	1 hr	3–4 hrs	12–24 hrs

Widely distributed. Protein binding: 93%. Metabolized in GI tract and liver. Primarily excreted in urine. **Half-life:** 8–37 hrs.

⌛ LIFESPAN CONSIDERATIONS

Pregnancy/Lactation: Unknown if drug crosses placenta or is distributed in breast milk. **Children:** Safety and efficacy not established. **Elderly:** Increased sensitivity to anticholinergic effects (e.g., confusion, urinary retention). Increased risk of falls, fractures. Not recommended.

INTERACTIONS

DRUG: Alcohol, other CNS depressant medications (e.g., LORazepam, morphine, zolpidem) may increase CNS depression. **MAOIs** (e.g., phenelzine, selegiline) may increase risk of hypertensive crisis, seizures. **Anticholinergics** (e.g., aclidinium, ipratropium, umeclidinium) may increase anticholinergic effect. **HERBAL:** Herbals with sedative properties (e.g., chamomile, kava kava, valerian) may increase CNS depression. **FOOD:** None known. **LAB VALUES:** None significant.

AVAILABILITY (Rx)

Tablets: 5 mg, 7.5 mg, 10 mg.
Capsules: *(Extended-Release [Amrix]):* 15 mg, 30 mg.

ADMINISTRATION/HANDLING

PO
• Give without regard to food. • Do not break, crush, dissolve, or divide extended-release capsule (may sprinkle capsule contents on applesauce and give immediately. Do not allow chewing). • Give extended-release capsule at same time each day.

INDICATIONS/ROUTES/DOSAGE

◄**ALERT**► Do not use longer than 2–3 wks.

Acute, Painful Musculoskeletal Conditions

PO: ADULTS, ELDERLY, CHILDREN 15 YRS AND OLDER: Initially, 5 mg 3 times/day. May increase to 10 mg 3 times/day.

PO: *(Extended-Release)*, ADULTS: 15–30 mg once daily. Not recommended in elderly.

Dosage in Renal Impairment
No dose adjustment.

Dosage in Hepatic Impairment
Note: Extended-release capsule not recommended in pts with hepatic impairment. **Mild impairment:** 5 mg 3 times/day. **Moderate to severe impairment:** Not recommended.

SIDE EFFECTS

Frequent (39%–11%): Drowsiness, dry mouth, dizziness. **Rare (3%–1%):** Fatigue, asthenia, blurred vision, headache, anxiety, confusion, nausea, constipation, dyspepsia, unpleasant taste.

ADVERSE EFFECTS/TOXIC REACTIONS

Overdose may cause visual hallucinations, hyperactive reflexes, muscle rigidity, vomiting, hyperpyrexia.

NURSING CONSIDERATIONS

BASELINE ASSESSMENT

Record onset, type, location, duration of muscular spasm. Check for immobility, stiffness, swelling.

INTERVENTION/EVALUATION

Assist with ambulation. Assess for therapeutic response: Relief of pain; decreased stiffness, swelling; increased joint mobility; reduced joint tenderness; improved grip strength.

PATIENT/FAMILY TEACHING

• Avoid tasks that require alertness, motor skills until response to drug is established. • Drowsiness usually diminishes with continued therapy. • Avoid alcohol, other depressants while taking medication. • Avoid sudden changes in posture. • Sugarless gum, sips of water may relieve dry mouth.

cycloPHOSphamide HIGH ALERT

sye-kloe-**foss**-fa-mide
(Procytox ✦)
Do not confuse cycloPHOSphamide with cycloSPORINE or ifosfamide.

◆CLASSIFICATION

PHARMACOTHERAPEUTIC: Alkylating agent. **CLINICAL:** Antineoplastic.

USES

Treatment of acute lymphocytic, acute non-lymphocytic, chronic myelocytic, chronic lymphocytic leukemias; ovarian, breast carcinomas; neuroblastoma; retinoblastoma; Hodgkin's, non-Hodgkin's lymphomas; multiple myeloma; mycosis fungoides; nephrotic syndrome in children. **OFF-LABEL:** Castleman's disease, dermatomyositis, Ewing sarcoma, graft versus host disease, hematopoietic stem cell/marrow transplant, interstitial pneumonia, lupus nephritis, osteocarcoma, ovarian germ cell tumors, pheochromocytoma (malignant), systemic light chain amyloidosis, Waldenstrom macroglobulinemia.

PRECAUTIONS

Contraindications: Hypersensitivity to cycloPHOSphamide. Urinary outflow obstruction. **Cautions:** Severe leukopenia, thrombocytopenia, tumor infiltration of bone marrow, previous therapy with other antineoplastic agents, radiation, renal/hepatic/cardiac impairment, active UTI.

ACTION

Inhibits DNA, RNA protein synthesis by cross-linking with DNA, RNA strands. Cell cycle–phase nonspecific. **Therapeutic Effect:** Prevents cell growth. Potent immunosuppressant.

PHARMACOKINETICS

Widely distributed. Protein binding: 10%–60%. Crosses blood-brain barrier.

Metabolized in liver. Primarily excreted in urine. Removed by hemodialysis. **Half-life:** 3–12 hrs.

⌛ LIFESPAN CONSIDERATIONS

Pregnancy/Lactation: If possible, avoid use during pregnancy. Use of effective contraception during therapy and up to 1 yr after completion of therapy is recommended. May cause fetal malformations (limb abnormalities, cardiac anomalies, hernias). Distributed in breast milk. Breastfeeding not recommended. **Children:** No age-related precautions noted. **Elderly:** Age-related renal impairment may require dosage adjustment.

INTERACTIONS

DRUG: CYP2B6 inducers (e.g., carBAMazepine, PHENobarbital, phenytoin) may decrease concentration/effect. **Anthracycline agents (e.g., DOXOrubicin, epiRUBicin)** may increase risk of cardiomyopathy. **Live virus vaccines** may potentiate virus replication, increase vaccine side effects, decrease pt's antibody response to vaccine. **HERBAL:** Pts with an estrogen-dependent tumor should avoid **black cohosh, dong quai. Echinacea** may decrease concentration/effect. **FOOD:** None known. **LAB VALUES:** May increase serum uric acid.

AVAILABILITY (Rx)

Capsules: 25 mg, 50 mg.

Injection, Powder for Reconstitution: 500 mg, 1 g, 2 g. **Injection, Solution:** 500mg/2.5 mL, 1 g/5 mL, 2 g/10mL.

ADMINISTRATION/HANDLING

◀**ALERT**▶ May be carcinogenic, mutagenic, teratogenic. Handle with extreme care during preparation/administration.

🖐 **IV**

Reconstitution • Reconstitute each 100 mg with 5 mL Sterile Water for Injection, 0.9% NaCl, or D$_5$W to provide concentration of 20 mg/mL. • Shake to dissolve. • Allow to stand until clear.

Rate of administration • Infusion rates vary based on protocol. May give by direct IV injection, IV piggyback, or continuous IV infusion.

Storage • Reconstituted solution in 0.9% NaCl is stable for 24 hrs at room temperature or up to 6 days if refrigerated.

PO

• Give on an empty stomach. If GI upset occurs, give with food. • Do not cut or crush. • To minimize risk of bladder irritation, do not give at bedtime.

🔲 IV COMPATIBILITIES

Granisetron, ondansetron, palonosetron, propofol.

INDICATIONS/ROUTES/DOSAGE

Note: Hematologic toxicity may require dose reduction.

Usual Dosage (Refer to Individual Protocols)

IV: ADULTS, ELDERLY, CHILDREN: (Single agent): 40–50 mg/kg in divided doses over 2–5 days or 10–15 mg/kg q7–10 days or 3–5 mg/kg twice wkly.
PO: ADULTS, ELDERLY, CHILDREN: 1–5 mg/kg/day.

Nephrotic Syndrome

PO: ADULTS, CHILDREN: 2 mg/kg/day for 8–12 wks. **Maximum cumulative dose:** 168 mg/kg.

Dosage in Renal/Hepatic Impairment
No dose adjustment. Use caution.

SIDE EFFECTS

Expected: Marked leukopenia 8–15 days after initiation. **Frequent:** Nausea, vomiting (beginning about 6 hrs after administration and lasting about 4 hrs); alopecia (33%). **Occasional:** Diarrhea, darkening of skin/fingernails, stomatitis, headache, diaphoresis. **Rare:** Pain/redness at injection site.

ADVERSE EFFECTS/TOXIC REACTIONS

Myelosuppression (leukopenia, anemia, thrombocytopenia, hypoprothrombinemia) is an expected response to therapy. Expect leukopenia to resolve in 17–28 days. Anemia generally occurs after large doses or prolonged therapy. Thrombocytopenia may occur 10–15 days after drug initiation. Hemorrhagic cystitis occurs commonly in long-term therapy (esp. in children). Pulmonary fibrosis, cardiotoxicity noted with high doses. Amenorrhea, azoospermia, hyperkalemia may occur.

NURSING CONSIDERATIONS

BASELINE ASSESSMENT

Obtain CBC wkly during therapy or until maintenance dose is established, then at 2- to 3-wk intervals. Question history of urinary outlet flow obstruction, hepatic/renal impairment, active infections. Obtain pregnancy test in females of reproductive potential.

INTERVENTION/EVALUATION

Monitor CBC, serum BUN, creatinine, electrolytes, urine output. Monitor WBC counts closely during initial therapy. Monitor for hematologic toxicity (fever, sore throat, signs of local infection, unusual bruising/bleeding from any site), symptoms of anemia (excessive fatigue, weakness). Recovery from marked leukopenia due to myelosuppression can be expected in 17–28 days.

PATIENT/FAMILY TEACHING

• Drink plenty of fluids to hydrate and promote urination (assists in preventing cystitis) at least 24 hrs before, during, after therapy. • Do not have immunizations without physician's approval (drug lowers resistance). • Avoid contact with those who have recently received live virus vaccine. • Promptly report fever, sore throat, signs of local infection, difficulty or pain with urination, unusual bruising/bleeding from any site. • Hair loss is reversible, but new hair growth may have different color, texture. • Avoid pregnancy for up to 1 yr after completion of treatment.

cycloSPORINE

sye-kloe-**spor**-in
(Cequa, Gengraf, Neoral, Restasis, SandIMMUNE, Verkazia, Vevye)
■ **BLACK BOX ALERT** ■ Only physicians experienced in management of immunosuppressive therapy and organ transplant pts should prescribe. Renal impairment may occur with high dosage. Increased risk of neoplasia, susceptibility to infections. May cause hypertension, nephrotoxicity. Psoriasis pts: Increased risk of developing skin malignancies. The modified/nonmodified formulations are not bioequivalent and cannot be used interchangeably without close monitoring.
Do not confuse cycloSPORINE with cycloSERINE or cycloPHOS-phamide, Gengraf with ProGraf, Neoral with Neurontin or Nizoral, or SandIMMUNE with SandoSTATIN.

◆CLASSIFICATION

PHARMACOTHERAPEUTIC: Calcineurin inhibitor. **CLINICAL:** Immunosuppressant.

USES

Nonmodified: Prevents organ rejection of kidney, liver, heart in combination with steroid therapy and an antiproliferative immunosuppressive agent. Treatment of chronic allograft rejection in those previously treated with other immunosuppressives. **Modified:** Prophylaxis of organ rejection in kidney, liver, and heart allogeneic transplants (in combination with azathioprine and corticosteroids). Treatment of pts with severe active, rheumatoid arthritis not adequately responding to methotrexate. Treatment of adult, nonimmunocompromised pts with severe, recalcitrant, plaque psoriasis who have not responded to at least one systemic therapy or in pts for whom other systemic therapies are contraindicated, or cannot be tolerated. **Ophthalmic:** Dry eye. Keratoconjunctivitis sicca, vernal keratoconjunctivitis. **OFF-LABEL:** Allogenic stem cell transplants for prevention/treatment of graft-vs-host disease; focal segmental glomerulosclerosis, lupus nephritis, severe ulcerative colitis, aplastic anemia, immune thrombocytopenia, myasthenia gravis, uveitis.

PRECAUTIONS

Contraindications: History of hypersensitivity to cycloSPORINE, polyoxyethylated castor oil; rheumatoid arthritis and psoriasis, renal dysfunction, uncontrolled hypertension, renal impairment, or malignancies in treatment of psoriasis or rheumatoid arthritis. **Cautions:** Hepatic/renal impairment. History of seizures. Avoid live vaccines.

ACTION

Inhibits cellular, humoral immune responses by inhibiting interleukin-2, a proliferative factor needed for T-cell activity. **Therapeutic Effect:** Prevents organ rejection, relieves symptoms of psoriasis, arthritis.

PHARMACOKINETICS

Widely distributed. Protein binding: 90%. Metabolized in liver. Eliminated primarily by biliary or fecal excretion. Not removed by hemodialysis. **Half-life:** Adults, 10–27 hrs; children, 7–19 hrs.

⌛ LIFESPAN CONSIDERATIONS

Pregnancy/Lactation: Readily crosses placenta. Distributed in breast milk. Breastfeeding not recommended. **Children:** No age-related precautions noted in transplant pts. **Elderly:** Increased risk of hypertension, increased serum creatinine.

INTERACTIONS

DRUG: May increase concentration/effects of **aliskiren, atorvastatin, dronedarone, lovastatin, pazopanib, simvastatin. Strong CYP3A4 inhibitors (e.g., clarithromycin, ketoconazole, ritonavir)** may increase concentration/effect. **Strong CYP3A4 inducers (e.g., carBAMazepine, phenytoin, rifAMPin)** may decrease concentration/effect. **Vaccines (live)** may alter concentration/effects. **HERBAL:** Echinacea may decrease therapeutic effect. **FOOD:** Grapefruit products may increase absorption/immunosuppression, risk of toxicity. **LAB VALUES:** May increase serum BUN, alkaline phosphatase, amylase, bilirubin, creatinine, potassium, uric acid, ALT, AST. May decrease serum magnesium. **Therapeutic peak serum level:** 50–400 ng/mL; **toxic serum level:** Greater than 400 ng/mL.

AVAILABILITY (Rx)

🖋 **Capsules:** *(Gengraf, Neoral [Modified], SandIMMUNE [Nonmodified]):* 25 mg, 50 mg, 100 mg. **Injection, Solution:** *(SandIMMUNE):* 50 mg/mL. **Ophthalmic Emulsion:** *(Restasis):* 0.05%. *(Verkazia):* 0.1%. **Ophthalmic Solution *(Cequa):*** 0.09%. *(Vevye):* 0.1%. **Oral Solution:** *(Gengraf, Neoral [Modified], SandIMMUNE [Nonmodified]):* 100 mg/mL.

ADMINISTRATION/HANDLING

◀**ALERT**▶ Oral solution available in bottle form with calibrated liquid measuring device. Oral form should replace IV administration as soon as possible.

 IV

Reconstitution • Dilute each mL (50 mg) concentrate with 20–100 mL 0.9% NaCl or D_5W (**maximum concentration:** 2.5 mg/mL).
Rate of administration • Infuse over 2–6 hrs. • Monitor pt continuously for hypersensitivity reaction (facial flushing, dyspnea).

Storage • Store parenteral form at room temperature. • Protect IV solution from light. • After diluted, stable for 6 hrs in PVC; 24 hrs in non-PVC or glass.

PO

• Administer consistently with relation to time of day and meals. • Oral solution may be mixed in glass container with milk, chocolate milk, orange juice, or apple juice (preferably at room temperature). Stir well. • Drink immediately. • Add more diluent to glass container. Mix with remaining solution to ensure total amount is given. • Dry outside of calibrated liquid measuring device before replacing cover. • Do not rinse with water. • Avoid refrigeration of oral solution (solution may separate). • Discard oral solution after 2 mos once bottle is opened.

Ophthalmic

• Invert vial several times to obtain uniform suspension. • Instruct pt to remove contact lenses before administration (may reinsert 15 min after administration). • May use with artificial tears.

🔲 IV COMPATIBILITIES

Propofol.

INDICATIONS/ROUTES/DOSAGE

Note: The modified/nonmodified formulations are not bioequivalent and cannot be used interchangeably without close monitoring. Refer to institutional protocols. Dosing in clinical practice may differ greatly compared to manufacturer's labeling.

Transplantation, Prevention of Organ Rejection

Note: Initial dose given 4–12 hrs prior to transplant or postoperatively.
PO: ADULTS, ELDERLY, CHILDREN: Nonmodified: Refer to institutional protocol for specific dosing. **Modified:** (dose dependent upon type of transplant): **Renal:** 6–12 mg/kg/day in 2 divided doses. **Hepatic:** 4–12

mg/kg/day in 2 divided doses. **Heart:** 4–10 mg/kg/day in 2 divided doses.
IV: ADULTS, ELDERLY, CHILDREN: Nonmodified: Initially, 5–6 mg/kg/dose daily. Switch to oral as soon as possible.

Rheumatoid Arthritis

PO: ADULTS, ELDERLY: Modified: Initially, 2.5 mg/kg a day in 2 divided doses. May increase by 0.5–0.75 mg/kg/day after 8 wks with additional increases made at 12 wks. **Maximum:** 4 mg/kg/day.

Psoriasis

PO: ADULTS, ELDERLY: Modified: Initially, 1–3 mg/kg/day in 2 divided doses. May increase by 0.5 mg/kg/day after 4 wks; additional increases may be made q2wks. **Maximum:** 4 mg/kg/day.

Dry Eye

Ophthalmic: ADULTS, ELDERLY: *(Vevye):* Instill 1 drop in each affected eye q12h.

Keratoconjuntivitis Sicca

Ophthalmic: ADULTS, ELDERLY: *(Cequa, Restasis):* 1 drop in each eye twice daily (12 hrs apart).

Vernal Keratoconjunctivitis

Ophthalmic: ADULTS, ELDERLY: *(Verkazia):* 1 drop in each affected eye 4 times/day until symptoms resolve.

Dosage in Renal Impairment

Modify dose if serum creatinine levels 25% or above pretreatment levels.

Dosage in Hepatic Impairment

Mild to moderate impairment: No dose adjustment. **Severe impairment:** Use caution.

SIDE EFFECTS

Frequent (26%–12%): Mild to moderate hypertension, hirsutism, tremor. **Occasional (4%–2%):** Acne, leg cramps, gingival hyperplasia (red, bleeding, tender gums), paresthesia, diarrhea, nausea, vomiting, headache. **Rare (less than 1%):** Hypersensitivity reaction, abdominal discomfort, gynecomastia, sinusitis.

ADVERSE EFFECTS/TOXIC REACTIONS

Mild nephrotoxicity occurs in 25% of renal transplants, 38% of cardiac transplants, 37% of liver transplants, generally 2–3 mos after transplantation (more severe toxicity may occur soon after transplantation). Hepatotoxicity occurs in 4% of renal, 7% of cardiac, and 4% of liver transplants, generally within first mo after transplantation. Both toxicities usually respond to dosage reduction. Severe hyperkalemia, hyperuricemia occur occasionally.

NURSING CONSIDERATIONS

BASELINE ASSESSMENT

Obtain BMP, LFT. If nephrotoxicity occurs, mild toxicity is generally noted 2–3 mos after transplantation; more severe toxicity noted early after transplantation; hepatotoxicity may be noted during first mo after transplantation.

INTERVENTION/EVALUATION

Diligently monitor serum BUN, creatinine, bilirubin, ALT, AST, LDH levels for evidence of hepatotoxicity/nephrotoxicity (mild toxicity noted by slow rise in serum levels; more overt toxicity noted by rapid rise in levels; hematuria also noted in nephrotoxicity). Monitor serum potassium for hyperkalemia. Encourage diligent oral hygiene (gingival hyperplasia). Monitor B/P for evidence of hypertension. **Note:** Reference ranges dependent on organ transplanted, organ function, cycloSPORINE toxicity. Trough levels should be obtained immediately prior to next dose. **Therapeutic serum level:** 50–400 ng/mL; **toxic serum level:** Greater than 400 ng/mL.

PATIENT/FAMILY TEACHING

• Report severe headache, persistent nausea/vomiting, unusual swelling of extremities, chest pain. • Avoid grapefruit products (increases concentration/effects), St. John's wort (decreases concentration). • Do not take any newly prescribed or OTC medications unless approved by the prescriber who originally started treatment.

cytarabine ■HIGH ALERT

sye-**tar**-a-bine
(Cytosar-U ✦)

■ **BLACK BOX ALERT** ■ Must be administered by personnel trained in administration/handling of chemotherapeutic agents. **Conventional:** Potent myelosuppressant. High risk of multiple toxicities (GI, CNS, pulmonary, cardiac). **Liposomal:** Chemical arachnoiditis, manifested by profound nausea, vomiting, fever, may be fatal if untreated. **Do not confuse cytarabine with cladribine, clofarabine, Cytosar, Cytoxan, DAUNOrubicin, vidarabine, or vinorelbine, or Cytosar with cytarabine, Cytovene, Cytoxan, or Neosar.**

FIXED COMBINATION(S)

Vyxeos: cytarabine/DAUNOrubicin (a nucleoside metabolic inhibitor): 100 mg/44 mg.

◆CLASSIFICATION

PHARMACOTHERAPEUTIC: Antimetabolite. **CLINICAL:** Antineoplastic.

USES

Conventional: Remission induction (in combination with other chemotherapeutic agents) in acute myeloid leukemia (AML), treatment of acute lymphoblastic leukemia (ALL) and chronic myeloid leukemia (CML) in blast phase, prophylaxis and treatment of meningeal leukemia. **OFF-LABEL:** Acute promyelocytic leukemia, chronic lymphocytic leukemia, Hodgkin's lymphoma (relapsed/refractory), non-Hodgkin's lymphomas, primary CNS lymphoma.

PRECAUTIONS

Contraindications: Hypersensitivity to cytarabine. **Liposomal:** Active meningeal infection. **Cautions:** Renal/hepatic impairment, prior drug-induced bone marrow suppression.

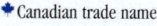 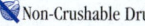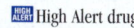

ACTION

Inhibits DNA polymerase. Cell cycle–specific for S phase of cell division. **Therapeutic Effect:** Inhibits DNA synthesis. Potent immunosuppressive activity.

PHARMACOKINETICS

Widely distributed; moderate amount crosses blood-brain barrier. Protein binding: 15%. Primarily excreted in urine. **Half-life:** 1–3 hrs.

⧗ LIFESPAN CONSIDERATIONS

Pregnancy/Lactation: If possible, avoid use during pregnancy. May cause fetal malformations. Unknown if distributed in breast milk. Breastfeeding not recommended. **Children:** No age-related precautions noted. **Elderly:** Age-related renal impairment may require dosage adjustment.

INTERACTIONS

DRUG: May decrease therapeutic effect of **BCG (intravesical)**, **vaccines (live)**. May increase adverse effects of **vaccines (live)**. May increase adverse effects of **natalizumab**. **HERBAL: Echinacea** may decrease therapeutic effect. **FOOD:** None known. **LAB VALUES:** May increase serum alkaline phosphatase, bilirubin, uric acid, AST.

AVAILABILITY (Rx)

Injection, Solution: 20 mg/mL, 100 mg/mL.

ADMINISTRATION/HANDLING

◄**ALERT**► May give by subcutaneous, IV push, IV infusion, intrathecal routes at concentration not to exceed 100 mg/mL. May be carcinogenic, mutagenic, teratogenic (embryonic deformity). Handle with extreme care during preparation/administration.

 IV, Intrathecal

Reconstitution • Dilute with 250–1,000 mL D$_5$W or 0.9% NaCl for IV infusion. • **Intrathecal:** Reconstitute vial with preservative-free 0.9% NaCl or pt's spinal fluid. Dose usually administered in 5–15 mL of solution, after equivalent volume of CSF removed.

Rate of administration • Conventional: For IV infusion, give over 1–3 hrs or as continuous infusion.
Storage • Conventional: Store at room temperature. • Reconstituted solution is stable for 48 hrs at room temperature. • Use diluted solution within 24 hrs. • Discard if slight haze develops.

▦ IV COMPATIBILITIES

Granisetron, ondansetron, propofol.

INDICATIONS/ROUTES/DOSAGE

Usual Dosage for Induction (Conventional) (Refer to Individual Protocols)
IV: ADULTS, ELDERLY, CHILDREN: (Induction): Usual dose (in combination with other anticancer drugs): 100 mg/m2/day by continuous IV infusion (days 1-7) or 100 mg/m2 IV q12h (days 1-7).

Dosage in Renal/Hepatic Impairment
No dose adjustment.

SIDE EFFECTS

Frequent (33%–16%): Asthenia, fever, pain, altered taste/smell, nausea, vomiting (risk greater with IV push than with continuous IV infusion). **Intrathecal (28%–11%):** Headache, asthenia, altered taste/smell, confusion, drowsiness, nausea, vomiting. **Occasional: IV (11%–7%):** Abnormal gait, drowsiness, constipation, back pain, urinary incontinence, peripheral edema, headache, confusion. **Intrathecal (7%–3%):** Peripheral edema, back pain, constipation, abnormal gait, urinary incontinence.

ADVERSE EFFECTS/TOXIC REACTIONS

Myelosuppression (leukopenia, anemia, thrombocytopenia, megaloblastosis, reticulocytopenia), occurring minimally after single IV dose. Leukopenia, anemia, thrombocytopenia should be expected with daily or continuous IV therapy. Cytarabine syndrome (fever, myalgia, rash, conjunctivitis, malaise, chest pain), hyperuricemia may occur. High-dose therapy may produce severe CNS, GI, pulmonary toxicity.

NURSING CONSIDERATIONS

BASELINE ASSESSMENT

Obtain baseline CBC, renal function, LFT. Leukocyte count decreases within 24 hrs after initial dose, continues to decrease for 7–9 days followed by brief rise at 12 days, decreases again at 15–24 days, then rises rapidly for next 10 days. Platelet count decreases 5 days after drug initiation to its lowest count at 12–15 days, then rises rapidly for next 10 days. Offer emotional support.

INTERVENTION/EVALUATION

Monitor BMP, LFT; serum uric acid. Monitor CBC for myelosuppression. Monitor for blood dyscrasias (fever, sore throat, signs of local infection, unusual bruising/bleeding from any site), symptoms of anemia (excessive fatigue, weakness). Monitor for signs of neuropathy (gait disturbances, handwriting difficulties, paresthesia).

PATIENT/FAMILY TEACHING

• Increase fluid intake (may protect against hyperuricemia). • Do not have immunizations without physician's approval (drug lowers resistance). • Avoid contact with those who have recently received live virus vaccine. • Promptly report fever, sore throat, signs of local infection, unusual bruising/bleeding from any site.

dabigatran

dab-i-**gah**-tran
(Pradaxa)

■ **BLACK BOX ALERT** ■ Risk of thrombotic events (e.g., stroke) is increased if discontinued for a reason other than pathological bleeding. Spinal or epidural hematoma may occur with neuraxial anesthesia.

◆CLASSIFICATION

PHARMACOTHERAPEUTIC: Direct thrombin inhibitor. **CLINICAL:** Anticoagulant.

USES

Nonvalvular atrial fibrillation: Indicated to reduce risk of stroke, systemic embolism in pts with nonvalvular atrial fibrillation. **Deep venous thrombosis (DVT and pulmonary embolism [PE]) treatment and prevention:** Treatment of deep vein thrombosis (DVT) and pulmonary embolism (PE) in pts who have been treated with a parenteral anticoagulant for at least 5 days and to reduce risk of recurrence of DVT and PE in previously treated pediatric pts aged 3 mos to 11 yrs (oral pellets), pediatric pts aged 8–17 yrs (capsules), and adults. **Venous thromboembolism prophylaxis:** Prophylaxis of DVT and PE in pts who have undergone hip replacement surgery.

PRECAUTIONS

Contraindications: Severe hypersensitivity to dabigatran. Active major bleeding, pts with mechanical prosthetic heart valves. **Cautions:** Renal impairment (CrCl 15–30 mL/min), moderate hepatic impairment, invasive procedures, spinal anesthesia, major surgery, pts with congenital or acquired bleeding disorders, elderly, concurrent use of medications that increase risk of bleeding, valvular heart disease.

ACTION

Reversible direct thrombin inhibitor that inhibits both free and fibrin-bound thrombin. **Therapeutic Effect:** Inhibits coagulation. Prevents thrombin-mediated effects, including cleavage of fibrinogen to fibrin; activation of factors V, VIII, XI, and XIII; and inhibition of thrombin-induced platelet aggregation.

PHARMACOKINETICS

Metabolized in liver. Protein binding: 35%. Eliminated primarily in urine. **Half-life:** 12–17 hrs.

⧗ LIFESPAN CONSIDERATIONS

Pregnancy/Lactation: Unknown if distributed in breast milk. **Children:** Safety and efficacy not established in pts younger than 3 mos. **Elderly:** Severe renal impairment may require dosage adjustment.

INTERACTIONS

DRUG: **Dronedarone, P-glycoprotein/ABCB1 inhibitors (e.g., amiodarone, colchicine, omeprazole)** may increase concentration/effect. **Antacids, P-glycoprotein (P-gp)/ABCB1 inducers (e.g., carBAMazepine, phenytoin)** may decrease concentration/effect. **Apixaban, edoxaban** may increase anticoagulant effect. **Aspirin, vorapaxar** may increase adverse effects. **HERBAL:** **Herbals with anticoagulant/antiplatelet properties (e.g., garlic, ginger, ginkgo biloba)** may increase effect. **FOOD:** **High-fat meal** delays absorption approx. 2 hrs. **LAB VALUES:** May increase aPTT, PT, INR.

AVAILABILITY (Rx)

Oral Pellets: 20 mg, 30 mg, 40 mg, 50 mg, 110 mg, 150 mg per packet.

Capsules: 75 mg, 110 mg, 150 mg.

ADMINISTRATION/HANDLING

PO

Capsules • May be given without regard to food. Administer with water. • Do not break, cut, open, or allow chewing of capsules. ***Oral pellets*** • May mix with 2 tsp of mashed carrots, applesauce, or mashed banana. • May administer with apple juice (spooned directly into the pt's mouth and swallowed with apple juice or added to 1–2 oz of apple juice). Do not administer via syringe or feeding tube or with milk, milk products, or soft foods containing milk products.

INDICATIONS/ROUTES/DOSAGE

◄ALERT► Medication should be discontinued prior to invasive or surgical procedures. Note: Oral pellets are NOT substitutable on a milligram-to-milligram basis with other dabigatran dosage forms.

Treatment/Prevention of DVT/PE
PO: *(Capsules):* **ADULTS, ELDERLY:** 150 mg twice daily (after at least 5 days of treatment with parenteral anticoagulants). **PEDIATRIC PTS 8–17 YRS: (11–15 KG):** 75 mg twice daily. **(16–25 KG):** 110 mg twice daily. **(26–40 KG):** 150 mg twice daily. **(41–60 KG):** 185 mg twice daily. **(61–80 KG):** 220 mg twice daily. **(81 KG or greater):** 260 mg twice daily. *(Oral Pellets):* Can be used for pts 3 mos to less than 12 yrs (as soon as able to swallow soft food). Refer to manufacturer's prescribing information for dosage.

Nonvalvular Atrial Fibrillation
PO: ADULTS, ELDERLY: 150 mg twice daily (to reduce risk of stroke/systemic embolism).

Prophylaxis Following Hip Surgery
PO: ADULTS, ELDERLY: 110 mg on day one (1–4 hr postoperative and established hemostasis), then 220 mg daily for a minimum of 10–14 days up to 35 days.

Dosage in Renal Impairment
Nonvalvular atrial fibrillation: CrCl 15–30 mL/min: Reduce dose to 75 mg twice daily. **CrCl less than 15 mL/min, or HD:** Not recommended (HD removes ~60% over 2–3 hrs). **CrCl 30–50 mL/min with concomitant use of P-gp inhibitors:** Reduce dose to 75 mg twice daily if given with P-gp inhibitors dronedarone or ketoconazole (systemic). **CrCl less than 30 mL/min with concomitant use of P-gp inhibitors:** Avoid coadministration. **Treatment/Prevention of DVT/PE: CrCl less than or equal to 30 mL/min:** Not specified. **CrCl less than 50 mL/min with concomitant use of P-gp inhibitors:** Avoid coadministration. **Prophylaxis following hip surgery: CrCl less than or equal to 30 mL/min:** Not specified. **CrCl less than 50 mL/min with concomitant use of P-gp inhibitors:** Avoid coadministration.

Dosage in Hepatic Impairment
No dosage adjustment.

SIDE EFFECTS
Frequent (less than 16%): Dyspepsia (heartburn, nausea, indigestion), diarrhea, upper abdominal pain.

ADVERSE EFFECTS/TOXIC REACTIONS
Severe, sometimes fatal, hemorrhagic events, including intracranial hemorrhage, hemorrhagic stroke, GI bleeding, may occur. Hypersensitivity reactions, including anaphylaxis, reported in less than 1% of pts.

NURSING CONSIDERATIONS

BASELINE ASSESSMENT
Obtain CBC. Question history of mechanical heart valve, recent surgery; hepatic, renal impairment; recent spinal, epidural procedures; recent hemorrhagic events (intracranial hemorrhage, hemorrhagic stroke, GI/GU bleeding). Receive full medication history and screen for interactions. Screen for active bleeding.

INTERVENTION/EVALUATION
Obtain aPTT, platelet count if bleeding occurs. Assess for any signs of bleeding (hematuria, melena, bleeding from gums, petechiae, bruising), hematoma, hypotension, tachycardia, abdominal pain. Question for increase in discharge during menses. Use care when removing adhesives, tape. Monitor for symptoms

D

of intracranial hemorrhage (altered mental status, aphasia, lethargy, hemiparesis, hemiplegia, seizures, vision changes).

PATIENT/FAMILY TEACHING

• Treatment may increase risk of bleeding. • Report dark or bloody urine, black or bloody stool, coffee-ground vomitus, bloody sputum, nosebleeds. • Stroke-like symptoms may indicate bleeding into the brain; report difficulty speaking, headache, numbness, paralysis, vision changes, seizures. • Use electric razor, soft toothbrush to prevent bleeding. • Do not take newly prescribed medications, including OTC medications such as ibuprofen or naproxen, unless approved by physician who originally started treatment. • Stopping therapy may increase the risk of blood clots or stroke.

dabrafenib

da-**braf**-e-nib
(Tafinlar)
Do not confuse dabrafenib with dasatinib.

◆CLASSIFICATION

PHARMACOTHERAPEUTIC: BRAF kinase inhibitor. **CLINICAL:** Antineoplastic.

USES

Melanoma (unresectable or metastatic): Treatment of unresectable or metastatic melanoma with BRAF V600E mutation (single-agent therapy) or in pts with BRAF V600E or V600K mutations (in combination with trametinib). **Melanoma: (Adjuvant):** Adjuvant treatment of melanoma (in combination with trametinib) in pts with a BRAF V600E or BRAF V600K mutation, and lymph node involvement. **Non–small-cell lung cancer (NSCLC):** Treatment

of metastatic (NSCLC) in combination with trametinib in pts with BRAF V600E mutation. **Anaplastic thyroid cancer (ATC):** Treatment of locally advanced or metastatic ATC (in combination with trametinib) in pts with BRAF V600E mutation and with no satisfactory locoregional treatment options. **Solid tumors:** Treatment of adult and pediatric pts 6 yrs of age and older with unresectable or metastatic solid tumors with *BRAF* V600E mutation who have progressed following prior treatment and have no satisfactory alternative treatment options. **Low-grade glioma (LGG):** Treatment of pts 1 yr of age and older (in combination with trametinib) with LGG with a BRAF V600E mutation who require systemic therapy. ◄**ALERT**► Not indicated for treatment of wild-type BRAF melanomas, wild-type BRAF NSCLC, or wild-type BRAF anaplastic thyroid cancer.

PRECAUTIONS

Contraindications: Hypersensitivity to dabrafenib. **Cautions:** Diabetes, hepatic/renal impairment, dehydration, glucose-6-phosphate dehydrogenase (G6PD) deficiency, pts at increased risk for arrhythmias, HF.

ACTION

Selectively inhibits some mutant forms of protein kinase B-raf (BRAF). **Therapeutic Effect:** Inhibits tumor cell growth and survival.

PHARMACOKINETICS

Widely distributed. Metabolized in liver. Protein binding: 99.7%. Peak plasma concentration: 2 hrs. Excreted in feces (71%), urine (23%). **Half-life:** 8 hrs.

⧗ LIFESPAN CONSIDERATIONS

Pregnancy/Lactation: Avoid pregnancy; may cause fetal harm. Must use effective nonhormonal contraception during treatment and for at least 2 wks after discontinuation (intrauterine device, barrier methods). Unknown if distributed in breast milk. May impair fertility in females and males. **Children:** Safety and efficacy not established. **Elderly:** May have increased risk of adverse effects, skin lesions.

INTERACTIONS

DRUG: Strong **CYP2C8 inhibitors** (e.g., gemfibrozil), strong **CYP3A4 inhibitors** (e.g., clarithromycin, ketoconazole, ritonavir) may increase concentration/effect. Strong **CYP3A4 inducers** (e.g., carBAMazepine, phenytoin, rifAMPin) may decrease concentration/effect. May increase concentration/effects of **pazopanib, topotecan, voxilaprevir.** May decrease concentration/effect of **abemaciclib, axitinib, neratinib, olaparib, ranolazine.** May decrease effectiveness of **hormonal contraceptives. HERBAL:** None significant. **FOOD: High-fat meals** may decrease absorption/effect. **LAB VALUES:** May increase serum glucose, alkaline phosphatase. May decrease serum phosphate, sodium.

AVAILABILITY (Rx)

Tablets (for Oral Suspension): 10 mg.

Capsules: 50 mg, 75 mg.

ADMINISTRATION/HANDLING

PO

Capsules: Give at least 1 hr before or at least 2 hrs after meal. • Do not break, crush, open, or divide capsule. • Missed dose may be given up to 6 hrs before next dose.
Tablets for oral suspension: Tablets should not be swallowed whole, chewed or crushed. Gently stir the water and prescribed number of tablets until fully dissolved. Use immediately.

INDICATIONS/ROUTES/DOSAGE

Melanoma (Metastatic/unresectable) (with BRAF V600E mutation) (single agent)
PO: ADULTS, ELDERLY: 150 mg twice daily (about 12 hrs apart). Continue until disease progression or unacceptable toxicity.

Melanoma, NSCLC, Anaplastic Thyroid Cancer (in combination with trametinib)
PO: ADULTS, ELDERLY: 150 mg twice daily. Continue until disease progression or unacceptable toxicity.

Melanoma (Adjuvant) (in combination with trametinib)
PO: ADULTS, ELDERLY: 150 mg twice daily until disease recurrence or unacceptable toxicity for up to 1 yr.

Solid Tumors (in combination with trametinib)
PO: ADULTS, ELDERLY: 150 mg twice daily. **CHILDREN 6–17 YRS OF AGE: (51 KG OR GREATER):** 150 mg twice daily. **(38–50 KG):** 100 mg twice daily. **(26–37 KG):** 75 mg twice daily until disease progression or unacceptable toxicity. *(Oral suspension):* 51 KG OR GREATER: 150 mg twice daily. 46–50 KG: 130 mg twice daily. 42–46 KG: 110 mg twice daily. 38–41 KG: 100 mg twice daily. 34–37 KG: 90 mg twice daily. 30–33 KG: 80 mg twice daily. 26–29 KG: 70 mg twice daily. 22–25 KG: 60 mg twice daily. 18–21 KG: 50 mg twice daily. 14–17 KG: 40 mg twice daily. 10–13 KG: 30 mg twice daily. 8–9 KG: 20 mg twice daily.

LGG
PO: CHILDREN 51 KG OR GREATER: 150 mg twice daily. **CHILDREN 1 YR OF AGE AND OLDER:** *(Oral Suspension):* 51 KG or greater: 150 mg twice daily; 46–50 KG: 130 mg twice daily; 42–46 KG: 110 mg twice daily; 38–41 KG: 100 mg twice daily; 34–37 KG: 90 mg twice daily; 30–33 KG: 80 mg twice daily; 26–29 KG: 70 mg twice daily; 22–25 KG: 60 mg twice daily; 18–21 KG: 50 mg twice daily; 14–17 KG: 40 mg twice daily; 10–13 KG: 30 mg twice daily; 8–9 KG: 20 mg twice daily.

Dose Modification
Based on Common Terminology Criteria for Adverse Events (CTCAE).

DABRAFENIB (TAFINLAR)

Dosage Reductions for Capsules

Dosage	First Dose Reduction	Second Dose Reduction	Third Dose Reduction
150 mg twice daily	100 mg	75 mg	50 mg
100 mg twice daily	75 mg	50 mg	N/A
75 mg twice daily	50 mg	N/A	N/A

Dosage Reductions for Oral Suspension

Body Weight	First Dose Reduction	Second Dose Reduction	Third Dose Reduction
≥51 kg (150 mg twice daily)	100 mg twice daily	80 mg twice daily	50 mg twice daily
46–50 kg (130 mg twice daily)	90 mg twice daily	70 mg twice daily	40 mg twice daily
42–45 kg (110 mg twice daily)	70 mg twice daily	60 mg twice daily	40 mg twice daily
38–41 kg (100 mg twice daily)	70 mg twice daily	50 mg twice daily	30 mg twice daily
34–37 kg (90 mg twice daily)	60 mg twice daily	50 mg twice daily	30 mg twice daily
30–33 kg (80 mg twice daily)	50 mg twice daily	40 mg twice daily	30 mg twice daily
26–29 kg (70 mg twice daily)	50 mg twice daily	40 mg twice daily	20 mg twice daily
22–25 kg (60 mg twice daily)	40 mg twice daily	30 mg twice daily	20 mg twice daily
18–21 kg (50 mg twice daily)	30 mg twice daily	20 mg twice daily	10 mg twice daily
14–17 kg (40 mg twice daily)	30 mg twice daily	20 mg twice daily	10 mg twice daily
10–13 kg (30 mg twice daily)	20 mg twice daily	10 mg twice daily	N/A
8–9 kg (20 mg twice daily)	10 mg twice daily	N/A	N/A

Cardiac
Symptomatic HF; absolute decrease in LVEF greater than 20% from baseline that is below the lower limit of normal: Withhold treatment until cardiac function improves, then resume at same dose.

Febrile Drug Reaction
Fever 101.3°F–104°F: Withhold treatment until resolved. Then resume at same dose (or at reduced dose level). **Fever greater than 104°F; fever associated with dehydration, hypotension, renal failure:** Withhold treatment until resolved, then resume at reduced dose level (or permanently discontinue).

Dermatologic Toxicity
Intolerable Grade 2 or any Grade 3 or 4 dermatologic toxicity: Withhold treatment for up to 3 wks. If improved, resume at reduced dose level. If not improved, permanently discontinue.

New Primary Malignancies
Noncutaneous RAS mutation-positive malignancies: Permanently discontinue.

Uveitis
Uveitis (including iritis and iridocyclitis): If mild to moderate uveitis does not improve with ocular therapy or if severe uveitis occurs, withhold treatment for up to 6 wks. If improved to Grade 1 or 0, resume at same dose (or at reduced dose level). If not improved, permanently discontinue.

Any Other Toxicity

Intolerable Grade 2 or any Grade 3 toxicity: Withhold treatment until improved to Grade 1 or 0, then resume at reduced dose level. If not improved, permanently discontinue. **First occurrence of any Grade 4 toxicity:** Withhold treatment until improved to Grade 1 or 0, then resume at reduced dose level (or permanently discontinue). **Recurrence of any Grade 4 toxicity:** Permanently discontinue.

Dosage in Renal Impairment

Mild to moderate impairment: No dosage adjustment. **Severe impairment:** Not specified; use caution.

Dosage in Hepatic Impairment

Mild impairment: No dosage adjustment. **Moderate to severe impairment:** Not specified; use caution.

SIDE EFFECTS

Frequent (37%–17%): Hyperkeratosis, headache, pyrexia, arthralgia, alopecia, rash. **Occasional (12%–10%):** Back pain, cough, myalgia, constipation, nasopharyngitis, fatigue.

ADVERSE EFFECTS/TOXIC REACTIONS

Cutaneous squamous cell carcinoma (cuSCC) and keratoacanthomas reported in 7% of pts (esp. elderly, prior skin cancer, chronic sun exposure). Skin reactions including palmar-plantar erythrodysesthesia syndrome (PPES), papilloma have occurred. May increase cell proliferation of wild-type BRAF melanoma or new malignant melanomas. Eye conditions including uveitis, iritis reported. Hyperglycemia reported in 6% of pts. Serious febrile drug reactions including hypotension, rigors, dehydration reported in 4% of pts. Pts with G6PD deficiency have increased risk of hemolytic anemia. Pancreatitis, interstitial nephritis, bullous rash reported in less than 10% of pts. Hemorrhagic events including GI bleeding, major organ bleeding may occur in pts receiving concomitant trametinib therapy. Cardiomyopathy with an absolute decrease in LVEF greater than 10% was reported.

NURSING CONSIDERATIONS

BASELINE ASSESSMENT

Obtain BMP, blood glucose level; pregnancy test in females of reproductive potential. Confirm BRAF V600 mutation status. Make note of current moles, lesions for future comparison. Conduct ophthalmologic exam, visual acuity. Receive full medication history (including herbal products) and screen for interactions. Offer emotional support.

INTERVENTION/EVALUATION

Monitor serum electrolytes; serum blood glucose periodically (esp. in pts with diabetes). Obtain CBC if hemolytic anemia suspected in pts with G6PD deficiency. Monitor for signs of hyperglycemia. Assess skin for new moles, lesions q2 mos during treatment and at least 6 mos after discontinuation. Immediately report any vision changes, eye pain/swelling, febrile drug reactions, worsening renal function. Monitor I&Os. Consider echocardiogram in pts suspected of cardiomyopathy, decreased LVEF (chest pain, edema, dyspnea, palpitations).

PATIENT/FAMILY TEACHING

• Treatment may increase risk of new cancers. • Use effective contraception to avoid pregnancy. Do not breastfeed. • Report symptoms of high blood sugar levels (confusion, excessive thirst/hunger, headache, frequent urination); toxic skin reactions (itching, peeling, rash, redness, swelling); eye pain/swelling, vision changes; new moles or lesions of the skin. • Fevers may be complicated by low blood pressure, dehydration, or kidney failure. • Minimize exposure to sunlight. • Report bleeding of any kind. • Therapy may reduce your heart's ability to pump effectively; report difficulty breathing, chest pain, dizziness, palpitations, swelling of the legs or feet. • Do not take newly prescribed medications unless approved by the prescriber who originally started treatment.

 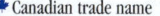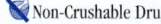

dacomitinib

dak-oh-**mi**-ti-nib
(Vizimpro)

Do not confuse dacomitinib with afatinib, dabrafenib, dasatinib, erlotinib, gefitinib, or osimertinib.

◆CLASSIFICATION

PHARMACOTHERAPEUTIC: Tyrosine kinase inhibitor. Epidermal growth factor receptor (EGFR) inhibitor. **CLINICAL:** Antineoplastic.

USES

First-line treatment of metastatic non–small-cell lung cancer (NSCLC) with EGFR exon 19 deletion or exon 21 L858R substitution mutations.

PRECAUTIONS

Contraindications: Hypersensitivity to dacomitinib. **Cautions:** Baseline cytopenias; dehydration, diabetes, hepatic impairment; history of pulmonary disease.

ACTION

Irreversibly inhibits kinase activity of human EGFR family and certain EGFR mutations. **Therapeutic Effect:** Inhibits tumor cell growth and metastasis.

PHARMACOKINETICS

Widely distributed. Metabolized in liver. Protein binding: 98%. Peak plasma concentration: 6 hrs. Excreted in feces (79%), urine (3%). **Half-life:** 70 hrs.

⧗ LIFESPAN CONSIDERATIONS

Pregnancy/Lactation: Avoid pregnancy; may cause fetal harm. Females of reproductive potential should use effective contraception during treatment and for at least 17 days after discontinuation. Unknown if distributed in breast milk. Breastfeeding not recommended during treatment and for at least 17 days after discontinuation. **Children:** Safety and efficacy not established. **Elderly:** May have higher risk of Grade 3 and 4 toxic reactions; higher frequency of treatment interruptions or discontinuation.

INTERACTIONS

DRUG: Histamine H_2 receptor antagonists (e.g., famotidine), proton pump inhibitors (e.g., omeprazole, pantoprazole) may decrease concentration/effect. May increase concentration/effects of **CYP2D6 substrates** (e.g., amitriptyline, carvedilol, FLUoxetine, tamoxifen). **HERBAL:** None significant. **FOOD:** None known. **LAB VALUES:** May increase serum alkaline phosphatase, ALT, AST, bilirubin, creatinine, glucose. May decrease serum albumin, calcium, potassium, sodium, magnesium; Hgb, Hct, lymphocytes, RBC count.

AVAILABILITY (Rx)

Tablets: 15 mg, 30 mg, 45 mg.

ADMINISTRATION/HANDLING

PO
• Give without regard to food. • If a dose is missed or vomiting occurs after administration, skip dose and give at next regularly scheduled time. • Give at least 6 hrs before or at least 10 hrs after antacid or H_2 receptor antagonists (e.g., famotidine). Avoid concomitant use proton pump inhibitor (PPIs).

INDICATIONS/ROUTES/DOSAGE

Non–Small-Cell Lung Cancer
PO: ADULTS, ELDERLY: 45 mg once daily. Continue until disease progression or unacceptable toxicity.

Reduction Schedule for Adverse Reactions
First dose reduction: 30 mg. **Second dose reduction:** 15 mg.

Dose Modification
Based on Common Terminology Criteria for Adverse Events (CTCAE).

Dermatologic Toxicity
Grade 2 skin reaction: Withhold treatment until improved to Grade 1 or 0, then

resume at same dose level. **Recurrent or persistent Grade 2 skin reaction, Grade 3 or 4 skin reaction:** Withhold treatment until improved to Grade 1 or 0, then resume at reduced dose level.

GI Toxicity
Grade 2 diarrhea: Withhold treatment until improved to Grade 1 or 0, then resume at same dose level. **Recurrent Grade 2 diarrhea, Grade 3 or 4 diarrhea:** Withhold treatment until improved to Grade 1 or 0, then resume at reduced dose level.

Pulmonary Toxicity
Interstitial lung disease (ILD) of any grade: Permanently discontinue.

Other Toxicities
Any other Grade 3 or 4 toxic reactions: Withhold treatment until improved to Grade 2 or less, then resume at reduced dose level.

Dosage in Renal/Hepatic Impairment
Mild to moderate impairment: No dose adjustment. **Severe impairment:** Not specified; use caution.

SIDE EFFECTS

Frequent (87%–26%): Diarrhea, rash, paronychia, stomatitis, decreased appetite, dry skin, xerosis, decreased weight. **Occasional (23%–7%):** Alopecia, pruritus, cough, nasal disorder (inflammation, epistaxis, mucosal disorder, rhinitis), conjunctivitis, nausea, extremity pain, constipation, dyspnea, asthenia, musculoskeletal pain, mouth ulceration, insomnia, dermatitis, chest pain, fatigue, vomiting, dysgeusia. **Rare (2%–1%):** Keratitis, dehydration.

ADVERSE EFFECTS/TOXIC REACTIONS

Myelosuppression (anemia, lymphopenia) is an expected response to treatment. Nail reactions including nail infection, nail toxicity, onychoclasis, onycholysis, onychomadesis, paronychia reported in 64% of pts. CTCAE Grade 3 or 4 skin reactions occurred in 21% of pts. Upper respiratory tract infection reported in 12% of pts.

Palmar-plantar erythrodysesthesia syndrome 15% of pts. Severe, sometimes fatal, ILD/pneumonitis reported in 1% of pts.

NURSING CONSIDERATIONS

BASELINE ASSESSMENT
Obtain ANC, CBC, LFT; pregnancy test in females of reproductive potential. Question current breastfeeding status. Confirm compliance of effective contraception. Question history of hepatic impairment, pulmonary disease. Assess skin for open wounds, lesions. Assess hydration status. Receive full medication history and screen for interactions. Offer emotional support.

INTERVENTION/EVALUATION
Monitor CBC, LFT as clinically indicated. Consider ABG, radiologic test if ILD/pneumonitis (excessive cough, dyspnea, hypoxia) is suspected. Monitor daily pattern of bowel activity, stool consistency. Antidiarrheal medication may be needed to manage diarrhea. Assess skin for dermal toxicities, rash; nail toxicities. Monitor for symptoms of hyperglycemia (dehydration, confusion, excessive thirst, Kussmaul respirations, polyuria). Monitor I&Os, hydration status.

PATIENT/FAMILY TEACHING
• Treatment may cause severe diarrhea, which may require antidiarrheal medication. Report worsening of diarrhea or dehydration. • Drink plenty of fluids. • Use effective contraception to avoid pregnancy. Do not breastfeed. • Antacids may interfere with absorption. Take dacomitinib at least 6 hrs before or at least 10 hrs after antacid. • Avoid prolonged sun exposure/tanning beds. Use high SPF sunscreen and lip balm to protect against sunburn. • Report symptoms of liver problems (abdominal pain, bruising, clay-colored stool, amber- or dark-colored urine, yellowing of the skin or eyes); inflammation of the lung (excessive cough, difficulty breathing, chest pain); toxic skin reactions (itching, peeling, rash, redness, swelling), high blood sugar levels (e.g., blurry vision, confusion, frequent urination, increased thirst, fruity breath).

D

dalfampridine

dal-**fam**-pri-deen
(Ampyra, Fampyra ✦)
**Do not confuse Ampyra with
anakinra, or dalfampridine with
desipramine.**

◆CLASSIFICATION

PHARMACOTHERAPEUTIC: Potassium channel blocker. **CLINICAL:** Multiple sclerosis agent.

USES

Indicated to improve ambulation in adults with multiple sclerosis (MS).

PRECAUTIONS

Contraindications: Hypersensitivity to dalfampridine. History of seizures, moderate to severe renal impairment (CrCl equal to or less than 50 mL/min). **Cautions:** Mild renal impairment (CrCl equal to 51–80 mL/min).

ACTION

Improves conduction in demyelinated axons by delaying repolarization and prolonging duration of action potentials. **Therapeutic Effect:** Strengthens skeletal muscle fiber twitch activity; improves peripheral motor neurologic function.

PHARMACOKINETICS

Widely distributed. Minimally metabolized in liver. Protein binding: 97%–99%. Excreted in urine (96%), feces (0.5%). **Half-life:** 5.2–6.5 hrs.

⌛ LIFESPAN CONSIDERATIONS

Pregnancy/Lactation: Unknown if drug crosses placenta or is distributed in breast milk. **Children:** Safety and efficacy not established. **Elderly:** Age-related renal impairment may require dosage adjustment.

INTERACTIONS

DRUG: OCT2 inhibitors (e.g., **cimetidine, clonidine, metformin**) may increase concentration/effect; increase risk of seizures. **HERBAL:** None significant. **FOOD:** None known. **LAB VALUES:** None significant.

AVAILABILITY (Rx)

📎 Tablet, Film-Coated, Extended-Release: 10 mg.

ADMINISTRATION/HANDLING

PO
• Give without regard to food. • Do not break, crush, dissolve, or divide tablets.

INDICATIONS/ROUTES/DOSAGE

Multiple Sclerosis
PO: ADULTS 18 YRS AND OLDER, ELDERLY: 10 mg twice daily. **Maximum:** 20 mg/day.

Dosage in Renal Impairment
CrCl 50 mL/min or less: Contraindicated.

Dosage in Hepatic Impairment
No dose adjustment.

SIDE EFFECTS

Frequent (9%–5%): Insomnia, dizziness, headache, nausea, asthenia, back pain. **Rare (4%–2%):** Paresthesia, nasopharyngitis, constipation, dyspepsia, pharyngolaryngeal pain.

ADVERSE EFFECTS/TOXIC REACTIONS

Seizures may occur at recommended doses and in pts without history of seizures. Severe hypersensitivity reactions, including anaphylaxis, may occur. Urinary tract infection reported in 12% of pts.

NURSING CONSIDERATIONS

BASELINE ASSESSMENT

Obtain BUN, serum creatinine, creatinine clearance. Question history of seizure disorder, renal impairment. Assess motor function, gait, ability to ambulate.

INTERVENTION/EVALUATION

Monitor creatinine clearance. Monitor for urinary, respiratory infection. Assess for therapeutic response (improvement in walking as demonstrated by increase in walking speed). Monitor for hypersensitivity reactions, seizure-like activity (confusion, muscle twitching/jerking, nystagmus, loss of bladder/bowel control).

PATIENT/FAMILY TEACHING

• Avoid tasks that require alertness, motor skills until response to drug is established. • Seizures can occur at prescribed doses. Report confusion, rapid eye movement, twitching/jerking of muscles, loss of bladder/bowel control; staring episodes. • Severe allergic reactions, including anaphylaxis, may occur. Report difficulty breathing, hives, rash, rapid heart rate. • Inform physician if ambulation does not improve or worsens.

---

dalteparin HIGH ALERT

dal-te-par-in
(Fragmin)
■ **BLACK BOX ALERT** ■ Epidural or spinal anesthesia greatly increases potential for spinal or epidural hematoma, subsequent long-term or permanent paralysis.
Do not confuse dalteparin with heparin.

◆CLASSIFICATION

PHARMACOTHERAPEUTIC: Low molecular weight heparin. **CLINICAL:** Anticoagulant.

USES

Non-ST elevation acute coronary syndromes: Prophylaxis of ischemic complications of unstable angina and non–Q-wave myocardial infarction (MI). **Venous thromboembolism prophylaxis:** Prophylaxis of deep vein thrombosis (DVT) in abdominal surgery, hip replacement surgery, or medical pts with severely restricted mobility during acute illness. **Venous thromboembolism treatment in pts with active cancer:** Extended treatment of symptomatic venous thromboembolism (VTE) to reduce recurrence in adults with cancer (begin with the initial VTE treatment and continue for 6 mos). **Venous thromboembolism treatment in pediatric pts:** Treatment of symptomatic VTE to reduce recurrence in pts 1 mos and older. **OFF-LABEL:** Mechanical heart valve (bridging anticoagulation), superficial vein thrombosis, VTE prophylaxis (pts with active cancer, total knee arthroplasty), VTE treatment (DVT/PE).

PRECAUTIONS

Contraindications: Hypersensitivity to dalteparin, heparin, pork products; active major bleeding; concurrent heparin therapy; unstable angina; history of heparin-induced thrombocytopenia (HIT), or HIT with thrombosis; non–Q-wave MI; prolonged venous thromboembolism undergoing epidural/neuraxial anesthesia. **Cautions:** Conditions with increased risk for hemorrhage, bacterial endocarditis, renal/hepatic impairment, uncontrolled hypertension, history of recent GI ulceration/hemorrhage, peptic ulcer disease, pericarditis, preexisting thrombocytopenia, recent childbirth, concurrent use of aspirin.

ACTION

Antithrombin in presence of low molecular weight heparin inhibits factor Xa, thrombin. **Therapeutic Effect:** Produces anticoagulation.

PHARMACOKINETICS

Route	Onset	Peak	Duration
SQ	N/A	4 hrs	N/A

Protein binding: less than 10%. **Half-life:** 3–5 hrs.

⊠ LIFESPAN CONSIDERATIONS

Pregnancy/Lactation: Use with caution, particularly during last trimester, immediate postpartum period (increased risk of maternal hemorrhage). Unknown

---

if distributed in breast milk. **Children:** Safety and efficacy not established. **Elderly:** No age-related precautions noted.

INTERACTIONS

DRUG: NSAIDs (e.g., ibuprofen, ketorolac, naproxen) may increase risk of bleeding. May increase effect of **apixaban, dabigatran, edoxaban, rivaroxaban.** **HERBAL:** Herbals with anticoagulant/antiplatelet properties (e.g., **garlic, ginger, ginkgo biloba**) may increase risk of bleeding. **FOOD:** None known. **LAB VALUES:** May increase serum ALT, AST. May decrease serum triglycerides.

AVAILABILITY (Rx)

Injection, Solution: 2,500 units/0.2 mL, 5,000 units/0.2 mL, 7,500 units/0.3 mL, 10,000 units/mL, 12,500 units/0.5 mL, 15,000 units/0.6 mL, 18,000 units/0.72 mL.

ADMINISTRATION/HANDLING

SQ
• Visually inspect for particulate matter or discoloration. • Subcutaneously insert needle into abdomen, outer thigh, or upper arm region and inject solution. • Do not inject into areas of active skin disease or injury such as sunburns, rashes, inflammation, or infection. Rotate injection sites.

INDICATIONS/ROUTES/DOSAGE

Abdominal Surgery
SQ: **ADULTS, ELDERLY:** 2,500 international units once daily, starting 1–2 hrs prior to surgery, then once daily postoperatively; or 5,000 international units the evening before surgery, then once daily postoperatively; or 2,500 international units 1–2 hrs before surgery, followed by 2,500 international units SQ 12 hrs later, then 5,000 international units once daily postoperatively. Usual duration: 5–10 days.

Total Hip Surgery
SQ: **ADULTS, ELDERLY:** Postoperative start: 2,500 international units 4–8 hrs after surgery, then 5,000 international units once daily. Preoperative start: (day of surgery) 2,500 international units 2 hrs before surgery then 2,500 international units 4–8 hrs after surgery, then 5,000 international units once daily. Preoperative start (evening before surgery): 5,000 international units, then 5,000 international units 4–8 hrs after surgery. Usual duration: 5–10 days.

Unstable Angina, Non–Q-Wave MI
SQ: **ADULTS, ELDERLY:** 120 units/kg q12h. Usual duration: 5–8 days (**maximum:** 10,000 units/dose) given with aspirin. Discontinue dalteparin once clinically stable.

Venous Thromboembolism (Cancer pts)
SQ: **ADULTS, ELDERLY:** Initially (month 1), 200 units/kg (**maximum:** 18,000 units) daily for 30 days. **Maintenance (2–6 mos):** 150 units/kg once daily (**maximum:** 18,000 units). If platelet count 50,000–100,000 cells/mm^3, reduce dose by 2,500 units until platelet count recovers to 100,000 cells/mm^3 or more. If platelet count less than 50,000 cells/mm^3, discontinue until platelet count recovers to more than 50,000 cells/mm^3.

Prevention of DVT, Acutely Ill Pt, Immobile Pt
SQ: **ADULTS, ELDERLY:** 5,000 units once daily. Continue for length of hospital stay or until pt is fully ambulatory and VTE risk has diminished.

Treatment, Symptomatic VTE (Children)
SQ: **CHILDREN 8 TO 16 YRS:** 100 units/kg/dose q12h. **CHILDREN 2 YRS TO YOUNGER THAN 8 YRS:** 125 units/kg/dose q12h. **CHILDREN 4 WKS TO YOUNGER THAN 2 YRS:** 150 units/kg/dose q12h.

Dosage in Renal Impairment
For CrCl less than 30 mL/min, monitor anti-Xa levels to determine appropriate dose.

Dosage in Hepatic Impairment
No dose adjustment.

SIDE EFFECTS

Occasional **(7%–3%):** Hematoma at injection site. **Rare (less than**

1%): Hypersensitivity reaction (chills, fever, pruritus, urticaria, asthma, rhinitis, lacrimation, headache); mild, local skin irritation.

ADVERSE EFFECTS/TOXIC REACTIONS

Overdose may lead to bleeding complications ranging from local ecchymoses to major hemorrhage. Thrombocytopenia occurs rarely.

NURSING CONSIDERATIONS

BASELINE ASSESSMENT
Obtain CBC, aPTT, PT/INR; vital signs.

INTERVENTION/EVALUATION
Periodically monitor CBC, stool for occult blood (no need for daily monitoring in pts with normal presurgical coagulation parameters). Assess for any sign of bleeding (bleeding at surgical site, hematuria, blood in stool, bleeding from gums, petechiae, bruising/bleeding at injection sites).

PATIENT/FAMILY TEACHING
• Usual length of therapy is 5–10 days. • Do not take any OTC medication (esp. aspirin) without consulting physician. • Report bleeding, bruising, dizziness, light-headedness, rash, itching, fever, swelling, breathing difficulty. • Rotate injection sites daily.

dantrolene

dan-troe-leen
(Dantrium, Revonto, Ryanodex)
■ **BLACK BOX ALERT** ■ Potential for hepatotoxicity.
Do not confuse Dantrium with danazol or Daraprim, or Revonto with Revatio.

◆CLASSIFICATION

PHARMACOTHERAPEUTIC: Calcium release blocker. **CLINICAL:** Skeletal muscle relaxant.

USES

PO: Treatment of spasticity associated with upper motor neuron disorder (e.g., spinal cord injuries, CVA, cerebral palsy, multiple sclerosis). **Parenteral:** Management of malignant hyperthermia. **OFF-LABEL:** Neuroleptic malignant syndrome.

PRECAUTIONS

Contraindications: Hypersensitivity to dantrolene. **IV:** None. **PO:** When spasticity used to maintain posture/balance during locomotion or to obtain increased motor function. Active hepatic disease. **Cautions:** Cardiac/pulmonary impairment, history of hepatic disease.

ACTION

Interferes with release of calcium from sarcoplasmic reticulum of skeletal muscle. Prevents/reduces the increase in myoplasmic calcium ion concentration. **Therapeutic Effect:** Dissociates excitation-contraction coupling. Interferes with catabolic process associated with malignant hyperthermia.

PHARMACOKINETICS

Poorly absorbed from GI tract. Protein binding: High. Metabolized in liver. Primarily excreted in urine. **Half-life:** IV: 4–8 hrs; PO: 8.7 hrs.

⧗ LIFESPAN CONSIDERATIONS

Pregnancy/Lactation: Readily crosses placenta. Breastfeeding not recommended. **Children:** No age-related precautions noted in pts 5 yrs and older. **Elderly:** No precautions specified.

INTERACTIONS

DRUG: CNS depressants (e.g., LORazepam, morphine, zolpidem) may increase CNS depression with short-term use. **HERBAL: Herbals with sedative properties (e.g., chamomile, kava kava, valerian)** may increase CNS depression. **FOOD:** None known. **LAB VALUES:** May alter serum ALT, AST.

D

AVAILABILITY (Rx)

Capsules: 25 mg, 50 mg, 100 mg. **Injection, Powder for Reconstitution:** 20-mg vial. **Injection Suspension:** 250 mg powder.

ADMINISTRATION/HANDLING

 IV

Reconstitution • Reconstitute 20-mg vial with 60 mL Sterile Water for Injection (**not** Bacteriostatic Water for Injection). *(Ryanodex):* 250-mg vial with 5 mL Sterile Water for Injection.

Rate of administration • For therapeutic or emergency dose, give IV over 2–3 min. • For IV infusion, administer over 1 hr. • Diligently monitor for extravasation (high pH of IV preparation). May produce severe complications. *(Ryanodex):* Do not dilute; infuse into IV catheter or indwelling catheter. Infuse over 1 min.

Storage • Store at room temperature. • Use within 6 hrs after reconstitution. • Solution is clear, colorless. Discard if cloudy, precipitate forms.

PO
• Give without regard to food.

⬛ IV INCOMPATIBILITIES

D₅W, 0.9% NaCl.

INDICATIONS/ROUTES/DOSAGE

Spasticity
PO: ADULTS, ELDERLY; CHILDREN 5 YRS AND OLDER, ADOLESCENTS: 50 KG OR GREATER: Initially, 25 mg once daily for 7 days; then 25 mg 3 times/day for 7 days; then 50 mg 3 times/day for 7 days; then 100 mg 3 times/day. **Maximum:** 400 mg/day. **CHILDREN 5 YRS AND OLDER, ADOLESCENTS LESS THAN 50 KG:** Initially, 0.5 mg/kg/dose once or twice daily for 7 days; then 0.5 mg/kg/dose 3 times/day for 7 days; then 1 mg/kg/dose 3 times/day for 7 days; then 2 mg/kg/dose 3 times/day.

Maximum: 12 mg/kg/day up to 400 mg/day.

Management of Malignant Hyperthermic Crisis
IV: ADULTS, ELDERLY, CHILDREN: Initially, a minimum of 2.5 mg/kg rapid IV; may repeat up to total cumulative dose of 10 mg/kg. May follow with 1 mg/kg q4–6h or 0.25 mg/kg/hr continuous infusion.

Dosage in Renal/Hepatic Impairment
No dose adjustment. Contraindicated with active hepatic disease.

SIDE EFFECTS

Frequent: Drowsiness, dizziness, weakness, general malaise, diarrhea (mild). **Occasional:** Confusion, diarrhea (severe), headache, insomnia, constipation, urinary frequency. **Rare:** Paradoxical CNS excitement or restlessness, paresthesia, tinnitus, slurred speech, tremor, blurred vision, dry mouth, nocturia, impotence, rash, pruritus.

ADVERSE EFFECTS/TOXIC REACTIONS

Risk of hepatotoxicity, most notably in females, pts 35 yrs and older, pts taking other hepatotoxic medications concurrently. Overt hepatitis noted most frequently between 3rd and 12th mo of therapy. Overdose results in vomiting, muscular hypotonia, muscle twitching, respiratory depression, seizures.

NURSING CONSIDERATIONS

BASELINE ASSESSMENT
Obtain LFT. Record onset, type, location, duration of muscular spasm. Check for immobility, stiffness, swelling.

INTERVENTION/EVALUATION
Assist with ambulation. For pts on long-term therapy, hepatic/renal function tests, CBC should be performed periodically. Assess for therapeutic response: relief of pain, stiffness, spasm.

• Drowsiness usually diminishes with continued therapy. • Avoid tasks that require alertness, motor skills until response to drug is established. • Avoid alcohol/other depressants. • Report continued weakness, fatigue, nausea, diarrhea, skin rash, itching, bloody/tarry stools.

dapagliflozin

dap-a-gli-**floe**-zin
(Farxiga)
Do not confuse dapagliflozin with bexagliflozin, canagliflozin, empagliflozin, or ertugliflozin. Farxiga with Fetzima.

FIXED-COMBINATIONS

Qtern: dapagliflozin/saxagliptin (an antidiabetic): 5 mg/5 mg, 10 mg/5 mg. **Qternmet XR:** dapagliflozin/saxagliptin/metformin (an antidiabetic): 2.5 mg/2.5 mg/1000 mg, 5 mg/2.5 mg/1000 mg, 5 mg/5 mg/1000 mg, 10 mg/5 mg/1000 mg. **Xigduo XR:** dapagliflozin/metformin (an antidiabetic): 2.5 mg/1000 mg, 5 mg/1000 mg, 10 mg/500 mg, 10 mg/1000 mg.

◆CLASSIFICATION

PHARMACOTHERAPEUTIC: Sodium-glucose cotransporter 2 (SGLT2) inhibitor. **CLINICAL:** Antidiabetic.

USES

Diabetes (type 2): Adjunctive treatment to diet and exercise to improve glycemic control in pts with type 2 diabetes mellitus in adults and pts aged 10 yrs and older. **Heart failure (HF) with reduced ejection fraction:** To reduce risk of hospitalization for HF in adults with type 2 diabetes mellitus and either established cardiovascular disease or multiple cardiovascular risk factors. To reduce risk of cardiovascular death, hospitalization for HF, and urgent HF visits in adults with HF. **Chronic kidney disease:** To reduce the risk of sustained eGFR decline, end-stage kidney disease, cardiovascular death, and hospitalization for HF in adults with chronic kidney disease at risk of progression.

PRECAUTIONS

Contraindications: Hypersensitivity to dapagliflozin; pts who are being treated for glycemic control without established cardiovascular disease or multiple cardiovascular risk factors with severe renal impairment (eGFR less than 30 mL/min); ESRD requiring dialysis. **Cautions:** Concomitant use of loop diuretics, other hypoglycemic agents (e.g., insulin, insulin secretagogues), baseline systolic hypotension, renal impairment, hypovolemia/dehydration, recent genital mycotic infection; pts at risk for diabetic ketoacidosis (insulin dose reduction, acute febrile illness, reduced calorie intake, surgery, alcohol abuse, history of pancreatitis). Not recommended in pts with active bladder cancer, diabetic ketoacidosis, type 1 diabetes mellitus.

ACTION

Inhibits SGLT2 in proximal renal tubule, reducing reabsorption of filtered glucose from tubular lumen and lowering renal threshold for glucose. Reduces reabsorption of sodium and increases delivery of sodium to the distal tubule. **Therapeutic Effect:** Increases urinary excretion of glucose; lowers serum glucose levels. Reduces cardiac preload and afterload; downregulates sympathetic activity.

PHARMACOKINETICS

Widely distributed. Metabolized in liver. Protein binding: 91%. Peak plasma concentration: 2 hrs. Eliminated in urine (75%), feces (21%). Unknown if removed by hemodialysis. **Half-life:** 12.9 hrs.

D

⧗ LIFESPAN CONSIDERATIONS

Pregnancy/Lactation: Not recommended during second or third trimester. Unknown if distributed in breast milk. Breastfeeding not recommended. **Children:** Safety and efficacy not established in pts younger than 10 yrs. **Elderly:** May have increased risk for adverse reactions (dehydration, hypotension, syncope).

INTERACTIONS

DRUG: **Insulin, insulin secretagogues (e.g., glyBURIDE)** may increase risk of hypoglycemia. May decrease concentration/effect of **lithium.** **HERBAL:** Maitake may increase hypoglycemic effect. **FOOD:** None known. **LAB VALUES:** May increase serum creatinine; low-density lipoprotein cholesterol (LDL-C); Hct. May decrease serum bicarbonate; eGFR. Expected to result in positive urine glucose test. May interfere with 1,5-anhydrogluitol (1,5-AG) assay.

AVAILABILITY (Rx)

Tablets: 5 mg, 10 mg.

ADMINISTRATION/HANDLING

PO
• Administer in the morning without regard to food.

INDICATIONS/ROUTES/DOSAGE

Type 2 Diabetes Mellitus (Glycemic Control)
PO: ADULTS, ELDERLY, CHILDREN 10 YRS AND OLDER: Initially, 5 mg once daily in AM. May increase to 10 mg once daily after 4–12 wks if needed for additional glycemic control.

Type 2 Diabetes Mellitus (Risk Reduction for HF, Cardiovascular Disease)
PO: ADULTS, ELDERLY: 10 mg once daily.

Heart Failure (Risk Reduction)
PO: ADULTS, ELDERLY: 10 mg once daily.

Chronic Kidney Disease
PO: ADULTS, ELDERLY: 10 mg once daily.

Dose Modification
Concomitant use of insulin, insulin secretagogue: Consider lowering dose of insulin or insulin secretagogue to reduce hypoglycemic events.

Dosage in Renal Impairment
eGFR 45 mL/min or greater: No dose adjustment. **eGFR 25–44 mL/min:** 10 mg daily (except for DM: not recommended). **eGFR less than 25 mL/min:** Initiation not recommended but may continue 10 mg daily to reduce the risk of eGFR decline, ESKD, CV death, and HF.

Dosage in Hepatic Impairment
Mild to moderate impairment: No dose adjustment. **Severe impairment:** No dose adjustment; use caution.

SIDE EFFECTS

Rare (3%–1%): Back pain, increased urination, nausea, constipation, extremity pain, discomfort with urination.

ADVERSE EFFECTS/TOXIC REACTIONS

Symptomatic hypotension (orthostatic hypotension, postural dizziness, syncope) may occur, esp. in pts who are elderly, use concomitant loop diuretics, or have baseline systolic hypotension. Intravascular volume depletion/contraction may cause acute kidney injury requiring dialysis. Fatal cases of ketoacidosis were reported. Hypoglycemic events were reported in pts using concomitant insulin, insulin secretagogues. Infections including influenza, nasopharyngitis, pyelonephritis, urosepsis, UTI, genital mycotic infections (male and female), upper respiratory tract infection may occur. Necrotizing fasciitis of the perineum (Fournier gangrene), a life-threatening necrotizing infection of the genital and perineum region that requires urgent surgical intervention, has been reported. Hypersensitivity reactions including anaphylaxis, angioedema, urticaria have occurred.

NURSING CONSIDERATIONS

BASELINE ASSESSMENT

Obtain BUN, serum creatinine, eGFR, CrCl, blood glucose level, Hgb A1c; B/P. Assess hydration status. Correct volume depletion prior to initiation. Assess pt's understanding of diabetes management, routine home glucose monitoring. Obtain dietary consult for nutritional education. Question history of renal impairment, type 1 diabetes, ketoacidosis. In pts requiring surgery, consider suspending treatment at least 3 days prior to surgery.

INTERVENTION/EVALUATION

Monitor BUN, serum creatinine, eGFR, CrCl, blood glucose level, Hgb A1c; B/P periodically. Monitor for ketoacidosis (e.g., dehydration, confusion, extreme thirst, sweet-smelling breath, Kussmaul respirations, nausea), hypoglycemia (anxiety, confusion, diaphoresis, diplopia, dizziness, headache, hunger, perioral numbness, tachycardia, tremors), hyperglycemia (fatigue, Kussmaul respirations, polyphagia, polyuria, polydipsia, nausea, vomiting). Pts presenting with metabolic acidosis should be screened for ketoacidosis, regardless of serum glucose levels. Concomitant use of beta blockers (e.g., carvedilol, metoprolol) may mask symptoms of hypoglycemia. Monitor for acute kidney injury (dark-colored urine, flank pain, decreased urine output, muscle aches), infections (cough, fatigue, fever), urinary tract infections (dysuria, fever, flank pain, malaise), mycotic infections, Fournier gangrene (perineal necrosis). Screen for glucose-altering conditions (fever, increased activity or stress, surgical procedures). Monitor weight, I&Os. Monitor for hypersensitivity reactions (anaphylaxis, angioedema, urticaria).

PATIENT/FAMILY TEACHING

• Diabetes mellitus requires lifelong control. Diet and exercise are principal parts of treatment; do not skip or delay meals. Test blood sugar regularly. Monitor daily calorie intake. • When taking combination drug therapy or when glucose conditions are altered (excessive alcohol ingestion, insufficient carbohydrate intake, hormone deficiencies, critical illness), have a low blood sugar treatment available (e.g., glucagon, oral dextrose). • Genital itching or discharge may indicate yeast infection. • Report symptoms of perineal necrosis (e.g., discoloration, pain, swelling of the scrotum, penis, or perineum). • Therapy may increase risk for dehydration, low blood pressure, which may cause kidney failure. Report decreased urination, amber-colored urine, flank pain, fatigue, swelling of the hands or feet. Drink enough fluids to maintain adequate hydration. Pts with HF should be cautious of overhydration. • Report symptoms of UTI, kidney infection (back pain, pelvic pain, burning while urinating, cloudy or foul-smelling urine), allergic reactions (difficulty breathing, rash, wheezing; swelling of the face or tongue. • Go slowly from lying to standing. • Do not breastfeed.

DAPTOmycin

dap-toe-mye-sin
(Cubicin RF)
Do not confuse Cubicin with Cleocin, or DAPTOmycin with DACTINomycin.

◆CLASSIFICATION

PHARMACOTHERAPEUTIC: Cyclic lipopeptide antibacterial agent. **CLINICAL:** Antibiotic.

USES

Treatment of adult and pediatric pts (1–17 yrs of age) with complicated skin and skin structure infections (cSSSIs) caused by susceptible isolates of the following gram-positive bacteria: S. aureus (including methicillin-resistant), S. pyogenes, S. agalactiae, S. dysgalactiae, Enterococcus faecalis (vancomycin-susceptible isolates only).

Treatment of adult and pediatric pts (1–17 yrs of age) with *S. aureus* bloodstream infections (bacteremia). **OFF-LABEL:** Diabetic foot infection, bacterial meningitis, osteomyelitis, prosthetic joint infection, septic arthritis.

PRECAUTIONS

Contraindications: Hypersensitivity to daptomycin. **Cautions:** Severe renal impairment (CrCl less than 30 mL/min), concurrent use of other medications associated with myopathy (e.g., statins).

ACTION

Binds to bacterial membranes and causes rapid depolarization. Inhibits intracellular protein, DNA, RNA synthesis. **Therapeutic Effect:** Bactericidal.

PHARMACOKINETICS

Widely distributed. Protein binding: 90%. Primarily excreted unchanged in urine. Moderately removed by hemodialysis. **Half-life:** 7–8 hrs (increased in renal impairment).

⧗ LIFESPAN CONSIDERATIONS

Pregnancy/Lactation: Unknown if distributed in breast milk. **Children:** Pts younger than 12 mos of age may have increased risk of nervous/muscular system effects. **Elderly:** No age-related precautions noted.

INTERACTIONS

DRUG: **HMG-CoA reductase inhibitors (e.g., simvastatin)** may cause myopathy. **HERBAL:** None significant. **FOOD:** None known. **LAB VALUES:** May increase alkaline phosphatase, CPK, serum potassium. May alter LFT results.

AVAILABILITY (Rx)

Injection, Powder for Reconstitution: 500 mg/vial.

ADMINISTRATION/HANDLING

 IV

Reconstitution • Reconstitute 500-mg vial with 10 mL 0.9% NaCl to provide a concentration of 50 mg/mL. May further dilute in 0.9% NaCl. • Do not shake or agitate vial.
Rate of administration • For IV injection, give over 2 min (concentration: 50 mg/mL) (adults only). • For intermittent IV infusion (piggyback), infuse over 30 min. **(Pts 1-6 yrs of age):** Administer over 60 min.
Storage • Refrigerate intact vials. • Appears as pale yellow to light brown lyophilized cake. • Reconstituted solution is stable for 12 hrs at room temperature or up to 48 hrs if refrigerated. • Discard if particulate forms.

▦ IV INCOMPATIBILITIES

Diluents containing dextrose. If same IV line is used to administer different drugs, flush line with 0.9% NaCl.

▦ IV COMPATIBILITIES

0.9% NaCl, lactated Ringer's, heparin.

INDICATIONS/ROUTES/DOSAGE

Complicated Skin/Skin Structure Infections
IV: **ADULTS, ELDERLY:** 4–6 mg/kg q24h. **CHILDREN (12–17 YRS):** 5 mg/kg q24h. **(7–11 YRS):** 7 mg/kg q24h. **(2–6 YRS):** 9 mg/kg q24h. **(12–23 MOS):** 10 mg/kg q24h.

Systemic Infections
IV: **ADULTS, ELDERLY:** 8–10 mg/kg q24h. **CHILDREN (12–17 YRS):** 7 mg/kg q24h. **(7–11 YRS):** 9 mg/kg q24h. **(1–6 YRS):** 12 mg/kg q24h.

Dosage in Renal Impairment
CrCl less than 30 mL/min, hemodialysis (HD), peritoneal dialysis (PD): Dosage is 4 mg/kg q48h for skin and soft tissue infections; 6 mg/kg q48h for staphylococcal bacteremia. **HD:** Give dose after dialysis. **Continuous renal replacement therapy: Continuous venovenous hemodialysis (CVVHD):** 8 mg/kg q48h. **Continuous venovenous hemofiltration (CVVH) or continuous venovenous hemodiafiltration**

(CVVHDF): 8 mg/kg q48h or 4–6 mg/kg q24h.

Dosage in Hepatic Impairment
No dose adjustment.

SIDE EFFECTS

Frequent (6%–5%): Constipation, nausea, peripheral injection site reactions, headache, diarrhea. **Occasional (4%–3%):** Insomnia, rash, vomiting. **Rare (less than 3%):** Pruritus, dizziness, hypotension.

ADVERSE EFFECTS/TOXIC REACTIONS

Myopathy (muscle pain/weakness, particularly in distal extremities) with CPK levels greater than 10 times ULN has occurred. Rhabdomyolysis may cause renal failure. Eosinophilic pneumonia, with symptoms including fever, hypoxia, respiratory insufficiency, pulmonary infiltrates was reported 2–4 wks after initiation. Antibiotic-associated colitis (abdominal cramps, fever, severe diarrhea), other superinfections may result from altered bacterial balance in GI tract. Persisting or relapsing *S. aureus* bacteremia/endocarditis, caused by reduced DAPTOmycin susceptibility, has occurred.

NURSING CONSIDERATIONS

BASELINE ASSESSMENT

Obtain CPK, blood cultures before first dose (therapy may begin before results are known). Question history of renal impairment. Screen for concomitant use of statins.

INTERVENTION/EVALUATION

Assess oral cavity for white patches on mucous membranes, tongue (thrush). Monitor for myopathy (muscle pain, weakness), CPK levels, renal function tests. Monitor daily pattern of bowel activity, stool consistency. Mild GI effects may be tolerable, but increasing severity may indicate onset of antibiotic-associated colitis. Be alert for superinfection: fever, vomiting, diarrhea, anal/genital pruritus, oral mucosal changes (ulceration, pain,

erythema). Monitor for dizziness; institute appropriate measures. Obtain repeat blood cultures in pts with persistent or relapsing *S. aureus* bacteremia/endocarditis or poor response to therapy.

PATIENT/FAMILY TEACHING

• Report rash, headache, nausea, dizziness, constipation, diarrhea, muscle pain, or any other new symptom.

daratumumab

dar-a-**toom**-ue-mab
(Darzalex)
Do not confuse daratumumab with adalimumab, ofatumumab, panitumumab, or necitumumab.

◆CLASSIFICATION

PHARMACOTHERAPEUTIC: Anti-CD38 monoclonal antibody. **CLINICAL:** Antineoplastic.

USES

Multiple myeloma (relapsed/refractory): Monotherapy for the treatment of pts with multiple myeloma who have received at least three prior lines of therapy including a proteasome inhibitor and an immunomodulatory agent or who are double-refractory to a proteasome inhibitor and an immunomodulatory agent. In combination with dexamethasone and bortezomib for treatment of multiple myeloma in pts who have received at least one prior therapy. In combination with pomalidomide and dexamethasone for treatment of multiple myeloma in pts who have received at least two prior therapies including lenalidomide and a proteasome inhibitor. In combination with carfilzomib and dexamethasone in pts with relapsed or refractory multiple myeloma who have received 1–3 prior lines of therapy. **Multiple myeloma (newly diagnosed):** Treatment of newly diagnosed multiple myeloma in combination with bortezomib, melphalan, and predniSONE or in combination with lenalidomide and dexamethasone in pts ineligible for autologous stem cell transplant. In combination with bortezomib, thalidomide, and dexamethasone in newly diagnosed pts who are eligible for autologous stem cell transplant.

PRECAUTIONS

Contraindications: Hypersensitivity to daratumumab. **Cautions:** Obstructive pulmonary disorders (e.g., COPD, emphysema), conditions predisposing to infection (e.g., diabetes, immunocompromised pts, kidney failure, open wounds), baseline cytopenias, herpes zoster infection, elderly.

ACTION

Binds to cell surface glycoprotein CD38 on CD38-expressing tumor cells (highly expressed on myeloma cells). Inhibits tumor cell proliferation and induces apoptosis. **Therapeutic Effect:** Inhibits tumor cell growth. Promotes tumor cell death.

PHARMACOKINETICS

Widely distributed. Metabolism not specified. Steady state reached approx. 5 mos into the q4wk dosing period (by 21st infusion). Elimination not specified. **Half-life:** 18 ± 9 days.

⧗ LIFESPAN CONSIDERATIONS

Pregnancy/Lactation: Avoid pregnancy; may cause fetal harm/malformations. Monoclonal antibodies are known to cross the placenta. Females of reproductive potential should use effective contraception during treatment and up to 3 mos after discontinuation. Unknown if distributed in breast milk. However, human immunoglobulin G is present in breast milk. **Children:** Safety and efficacy not established. **Elderly:** May have higher rates of infections, side effects.

INTERACTIONS

DRUG: May decrease therapeutic effect of **BCG intravesical, vaccines (live).** **HERBAL:** **Echinacea** may decrease

therapeutic effect. **FOOD:** Nonsignificant. **LAB VALUES:** Drug may be detected on both serum protein electrophoresis and immunofixation assays used to monitor multiple myeloma endogenous M protein. May affect the determination of complete response and disease progression of some pts with immunoglobulin G kappa myeloma protein. May cause positive Coombs' test. Expected to decrease Hgb, Hct, lymphocytes, neutrophils, platelets, RBCs.

AVAILABILITY (Rx)

Injection Solution: 100 mg/5 mL, 400 mg/20 mL.

ADMINISTRATION/HANDLING

 IV

Preparation for administration • Calculate the dose required based on weight in kg. • Solution should appear colorless to pale yellow. Do not use if opaque particles, discoloration, or foreign particles are observed. • Remove a volume from the 0.9% NaCl infusion bag that is equal to the required volume of the dose solution. • Dilute in 1000 mL (first infusion) or 500 mL (subsequent infusions) 0.9% NaCl bag. • Mix by gentle inversion. Do not shake or agitate. • Infusion bags must be made of polyvinylchloride, polypropylene, polyethylene, or polyolefin blend. • Diluted solution may develop very small translucent to white proteinaceous particles; do not use if diluted solution is discolored or if visibly opaque or foreign particles are observed. • Discard used portions of vials.

Infusion guidelines • Prior to administration, premedicate with an IV corticosteroid, acetaminophen, and an IV or oral antihistamine approx. 60 min before each infusion (see manufacturer guidelines). • Infuse using an in-line, sterile, nonpyrogenic, low protein-binding polyethersulfone filter (0.22 or 0.2 μm). • Infuse via dedicated line using infusion pump. • Do not administer as IV push or bolus. • Infusion should be completed within 15 hrs. • If infusion cannot be completed for any reason, do not save unused portions for reuse. • Postinfusion, administer an oral corticosteroid on the first and second day after each infusion to reduce risk of delayed infusion reactions (see manufacturer guidelines). • In pts with a history of obstructive pulmonary disease, consider short-acting and long-acting bronchodilators and an inhaled corticosteroid postinfusion (may discontinue if no infusion reaction occurs after the first four infusions).

Rate of administration • **First infusion (1000 mL volume):** Infuse at 50 mL/hr for the first 60 min. Increase in increments of 50 mL/hr q1hr if no infusion reactions occur. **Maximum:** 200 mL/hr. • **Second infusion (500 mL volume):** Infuse at 50 mL/hr for the first 60 min. Increase in increments of 50 mL/hr q1hr if there were no Grade 1 or greater infusion reactions during the first 3 hrs of first infusion. **Maximum:** 200 mL/hr. • **Subsequent infusions (500 mL volume):** Infuse at 100 mL/hr if there were no Grade 1 or greater infusion reactions during a final infusion rate of greater than or equal to 100 mL/hr in the first two infusions. Increase in increments of 50 mL/hr q1hr if tolerated. **Maximum:** 200 mL/hr.

Storage • Refrigerate unused vials. • Do not shake. • May refrigerate diluted solution up to 24 hrs. • If diluted solution is refrigerated, allow solution to warm to room temperature before use. • Protect from light.

❋ IV INCOMPATIBILITIES
Do not mix with other medications.

INDICATIONS/ROUTES/DOSAGE
Note: The initial dose (16 mg/kg on wk 1) may be divided over 2 consecutive days (8 mg/kg/day on days 1 and 2 of wk 1 of therapy) to facilitate administration.

Multiple Myeloma (Relapsed/Refractory)
IV: ADULTS, ELDERLY: (Monotherapy or combination with lenalidomide/ dexamethasone or pomalidomide/ dexamethasone): Wks 1–8: 16 mg/ kg once wkly. **Wks 9–24:** 16 mg/kg once q2wks. **Wk 25 and beyond:** 16 mg/kg once q4wks until disease progression. **(Combination with bortezomib/dexamethasone):** Wks 1–9: 16 mg/kg once wkly. **Wks 10–24:** 16 mg/kg q3wks for 5 doses. **Wk 25 and beyond:** 16 mg/kg q4wks until disease progression. **(Combination with carfilzomib and dexamethasone):** Wk 1: 8 mg/kg on days 1 and 2. **Wks 2–8:** 16 mg/kg wkly. **Wks 9–24:** 16 mg/kg q2wks. **Wk 25 and beyond:** 16 mg/kg q4wks until disease progression.

Multiple Myeloma (Newly Diagnosed)
IV: ADULTS, ELDERLY: (In combination with bortezomib, melphalan and predniSONE): Wks 1–6: 16 mg/kg once wkly. **Wks 7–54:** 16 mg/kg q3wks for 16 doses. **Wk 55 and beyond:** 16 mg/kg q4wks until disease progression. **(In combination with lenalidomide and low-dose dexamethasone):** Wks 1–8: 16 mg/kg once wkly for 8 doses. **Wks 9–24:** 16 mg/kg once q2wks for 8 doses. **Wks 25 and beyond:** 16 mg/kg once q4wks until disease progression. **(In combination with bortezomib, thalidomide, and dexamethasone): Induction:** Wks 1–8: 16 mg/kg once wkly for 8 doses. **Wks 9–24:** 16 mg/kg once q2wks for 8 doses. Stop for high-dose chemotherapy and ASCT. **Consolidation:** Wks 1–8 q2wks.

Dose Modification
Infusion Reactions
Promptly interrupt infusion if any reaction occurs. **Grade 1 or 2:** Once symptoms resolve, resume infusion at a decreased rate that is 50% (or less) of previous rate. If no further reactions are observed, may increase infusion rate

D

as appropriate. **Grade 3:** If symptoms resolve to Grade 2 or less, consider resuming infusion at a decreased rate that is 50% (or less) of previous rate. If no further reactions are observed, may increase rate as appropriate. If a Grade 3 reaction recurs, decrease rate as outlined earlier. If Grade 3 reaction occurs for a third time, permanently discontinue. **Grade 4:** Permanently discontinue.

Dosage in Renal Impairment
No dose adjustment.

Dosage in Hepatic Impairment
Mild impairment: No dose adjustment. **Moderate to severe impairment:** Not specified; use caution.

SIDE EFFECTS

Frequent (37%–14%): Fatigue, back pain, nausea, pyrexia, cough, nasal congestion, arthralgia, diarrhea, dyspnea, decreased appetite, extremity pain, constipation, vomiting. **Occasional (12%–10%):** Headache, musculoskeletal chest pain, chills, hypertension.

ADVERSE EFFECTS/TOXIC REACTIONS

Anemia, leukopenia, neutropenia, thrombocytopenia are expected responses to therapy. Infusion reactions occurred in approx. 50% of pts (mostly during first infusion). Infusion reactions can also occur with subsequent infusions (mainly during the infusion or within 4 hrs of completion). Severe infusion reactions may include cough, dyspnea, bronchospasm, hypertension, hypoxia, laryngeal edema, pulmonary edema, wheezing. Less common reactions may include chills, headache, hypotension, rash, nausea, pruritus, urticaria, vomiting. Infections including pneumonia, upper respiratory tract infection, nasopharyngitis reported in 20%–11% of pts. Herpes zoster reported in 3% of pts. Thrombocytopenia may increase risk of bleeding.

NURSING CONSIDERATIONS

BASELINE ASSESSMENT

Obtain CBC, blood type and screen; vital signs. Obtain pregnancy test in female pts of reproductive potential. Question history of COPD, emphysema, herpes infection; prior hypersensitivity reaction to any drug in treatment regimen; prior infusion reaction. Assess nutritional status. Screen for active infection. Offer emotional support.

INTERVENTION/EVALUATION

Monitor CBC, vital signs periodically. Administer in an environment equipped to monitor for and manage infusion reactions. If infusion reaction of any grade/severity occurs, immediately interrupt infusion and manage symptoms. Accurately record characteristics of infusion reactions (severity, type, time of onset). Reactions may affect future infusion rates. To prevent herpes zoster reactivation in pts with prior history, consider antiviral prophylaxis within 1 wk of starting treatment and continue for 3 mos following discontinuation. Monitor for infection. Monitor daily pattern of bowel activity, stool consistency.

PATIENT/FAMILY TEACHING

• Treatment may depress your immune system and reduce your ability to fight infection. Report symptoms of infection such as body aches, chills, cough, fatigue, fever. Avoid those with active infection. • Use effective contraception to avoid pregnancy. Do not breastfeed. • Severe infusion reactions can occur at any time. Immediately report symptoms of infusion reactions such as chills, cough, difficulty breathing, headache, hives, itching, nausea, rash, stuffy or runny nose, throat tightness, vomiting, wheezing.

daratumumab/ hyaluronidase fihj

dar-a-**toom**-ue-mab **hye**-al-ure-**on**-i-dase

(Darzalex Faspro)

Do not confuse daratumumab with daclizumab, daratumumab, darolutamide, denosumab, dinutuximab, dupilumab, durvalumab, elotuzumab, rituximab/hyaluronidase, trastuzumab/hyaluronidase, or Darzalex Faspro with Darzalex.

◆CLASSIFICATION

PHARMACOTHERAPEUTIC: Anti-CD38 Monoclonal antibody. **CLINICAL:** Antineoplastic.

USES

Multiple myeloma (newly diagnosed): In combination with bortezomib, melphalan, and prednisone in newly diagnosed pts who are ineligible for autologous stem cell transplant; in combination with lenalidomide and dexamethasone in newly diagnosed pts who are ineligible for autologous stem cell transplant; in combination with bortezomib, thalidomide, and dexamethasone in pts who are eligible for autologous stem cell transplant; in combination with bortezomib, lenalidomide, and dexamethasone for induction and consolidation in pts who are eligible for autologous stem cell transplant; **Multiple myeloma (relapsed/refractory):** In combination with lenalidomide and dexamethasone in pts who have received at least one prior therapy. In combination with pomalidomide and dexamethasone in pts who have received at least one prior line of therapy, including lenalidomide and a proteasome inhibitor. In combination with carfilzomib and dexamethasone in pts with relapsed or refractory multiple myeloma who have received 1–3 prior lines of therapy. in combination with bortezomib and dexamethasone in pts who have received at least one prior therapy; as monotherapy in pts who have received at least three prior lines of therapy including a proteasome inhibitor (PI) and an immunomodulatory agent or who are double refractory to a PI and an immunomodulatory agent. **Light chain**

(AL) amyloidosis: Treatment of newly diagnosed light-chain amyloidosis in adults (in combination with bortezomib, cyclophosphamide, and dexamethasone).

PRECAUTIONS

Contraindications: Hypersensitivity to daratumumab, hyaluronidase. Combination treatment with lenalidomide in pregnant women. **Cautions:** Baseline cytopenias, active infection, obstructive pulmonary disorders (e.g., COPD, emphysema), herpes zoster infection, elderly; conditions predisposing to infection (e.g., diabetes, immunocompromised pts, renal failure, open wounds); history of hepatitis B infection.

ACTION

Daratumumab binds to cell surface glycoprotein CD38 on CD38-expressing tumor cells (highly expressed on myeloma cells). Inhibits tumor cell proliferation and induces apoptosis. Hyaluronidase increases permeability of subcutaneous tissue. **Therapeutic Effect:** Inhibits tumor cell growth and survival.

PHARMACOKINETICS

Widely distributed. Peak plasma concentration: 3 days. Eliminated by parallel and nonlinear saturable target mediated clearance. **Half-life:** 20 days.

⬓ LIFESPAN CONSIDERATIONS

Pregnancy/Lactation: Avoid pregnancy; may cause fetal harm. Females of reproductive potential must use effective contraception during treatment and for at least 3 mos after discontinuation. Unknown if distributed in breast milk; however, human immunoglobulin G (IgG) is present in breast milk. Breastfeeding not recommend. **Children:** Safety and efficacy not established. **Elderly:** May have higher risk of infections, side effects.

INTERACTIONS

DRUG: May decrease effect of **BCG intravesical, vaccines (live).** May increase adverse/toxic effect of **natalizumab, Pimecrolimus, tacrolimus**

---

may increase adverse/toxic effects. **HERBAL:** **Echinacea** may decrease therapeutic effect. **FOOD:** None known. **LAB VALUES:** May mask detection of antibodies to minor antigens. Drug may be detected on both serum protein electrophoresis and immunofixation assays used to monitor multiple myeloma endogenous M-protein. May affect the determination of complete response and disease progression of some pts with IgG kappa myeloma protein. May cause positive Coombs test. May increase serum glucose. May decrease serum calcium; Hgb, leukocytes, lymphocytes, neutrophils, platelets.

AVAILABILITY (Rx)

Injection Solution: Daratumumab 1,800 mg/hyaluronidase 30,000 units (120 mg/2,000 units/mL).

ADMINISTRATION/HANDLING

SQ

Premedication • Pretreat with acetaminophen 650–1000 mg PO, diphenhydramine 25–50 mg PO or IV, and a long- or intermediate-acting corticosteroid 1–3 hrs prior to each dose. • See manufacturer guidelines regarding premedication and postmedication corticosteroid therapy.

Preparation • Remove vial from refrigerator and allow solution to warm to room temperature. • Visually inspect for particulate matter or discoloration. Solution should appear colorless to yellow, clear to opalescent. Do not use if solution is cloudy, discolored, or visible particles are observed. • Withdraw 15 mL from vial into syringe. • To avoid clogging, immediately attach a new hypodermic needle or subcutaneous infusion set to syringe.

Administration • Insert needle subcutaneously into abdomen (only), approx. 3 inches (7.5 cm) to the right or left of navel and inject solution. • Do not inject into areas of active skin disease or injury such as sunburns, skin rashes, inflammation, skin infections, or active psoriasis. • Rotate injection sites. • Do not administer IV or intramuscularly. • If a dose is missed, administer as soon as possible and adjust dosing schedule to maintain dosing intervals.

Rate of administration • Inject over 3–5 minutes. • Decrease injection rate or interrupt administration if pain is experienced. If pain is not relieved by slowing or interrupting injection, may choose second injection site on opposite side of abdomen.

Storage • Refrigerate vials in original carton until time of use. • Protect from light. • Do not shake. • Do not freeze or expose to heating sources. • After vial is allowed to warm to room temperature, use within 24 hrs. • May store syringe containing solution at room temperature for up to 4 hrs.

INDICATIONS/ROUTES/DOSAGE

Multiple Myeloma

SQ: **ADULTS:** 1,800 mg/30,000 units/dose according to schedule. Continue until disease progression or unacceptable toxicity.

Dosing Schedule

In combination with lenalidomide, pomalidomide, or carfilzomib and dexamethasone (4-wk cycle) and for monotherapy: Give dose once weekly on wks 1–8, then once q2wks on wks 9–24, then once monthly on wk 25 and thereafter.

In combination with bortezomib, melphalan, prednisone: Give dose once weekly on wks 1–6, then once q3wks on wks 7–54, then once monthly on wk 55 and thereafter.

In combination with bortezomib and dexamethasone: Give dose once weekly on wks 1–9, then once q3wks on wks 10–24, then once monthly on wk 25 and thereafter.

In combination with borezomib, thalidomide, and dexamethasone: Induction: Wks 1–8: Once wkly for 8 doses. **Wks 9–16:** Give doses once q2wks for 8 doses. Stop for high dose chemotherapy and ASCT. **Consolidation: Wks 1–8:** q2wks.

In combination with bortezomib, cyclophosphamide, and dexamethasone: Give dose once wkly on wks 1–8, then once q2wks on wks 9–24, then once monthly on wk 25 and thereafter.

Light-Chain Amyloidosis (Newly Diagnosed)
SQ: ADULTS: In combination with bortezomib, cyclophosphamide, and dexamethasone: Wks 1–8: Give dose once wkly for a total of 8 doses. **Wks 9–24:** Give dose once q2wks (beginning wk 9) for a total of 8 doses. **Wks 25 and beyond:** Give dose once q4wks (beginning week 25). Continue until disease progression or unacceptable toxicity or a maximum of 2 yrs.

Dose Modifications
Myelosuppression
Consider withholding treatment until neutropenia, thrombocytopenia improves.

Hypersensitivity Reactions
Permanently discontinue if anaphylaxis or Grade 4 administration-related reactions occur.

Dosage in Renal Impairment
No dose adjustment.

Dosage in Hepatic Impairment
Mild impairment: No dose adjustment. **Moderate to severe impairment:** Not specified; use caution.

SIDE EFFECTS
Note: Frequency and occurrence of side effects may vary based on treatment as monotherapy or in combination with other therapies. **Occasional (15%–6%):** Diarrhea, fatigue, pyrexia, back pain, injection site reaction, peripheral edema, arthralgia, musculoskeletal chest pain, constipation, vomiting, abdominal pain, decreased appetite, dehydration, insomnia, hypertension, hypotension, dizziness, neuropathy, paresthesia, pruritus, rash, cough, nausea, chills, dyspnea.

ADVERSE EFFECTS/TOXIC REACTIONS
Note: Frequency and occurrence of adverse reactions may vary based on treatment as monotherapy or in combination with other therapies. Myelosuppression (anemia, leukopenia, neutropenia, thrombocytopenia) has occurred. Grade 3 and 4 neutropenia was reported, esp. in pts with lower body weights. Severe systemic reactions including bronchospasm, dyspnea, hypertension, hypoxia, tachycardia wheezing reported in 10% of pts. Other systemic reactions including nasal congestion, cough, throat irritation, allergic rhinitis may occur. Anaphylactic reactions including chest pain, chills, hypotension, nausea, pruritus, pyrexia, vomiting were reported. Infections including upper respiratory tract infection (24% of pts), pneumonia (8% of pts); herpes zoster, UTI, influenza, sepsis (10% of pts) were reported. Atrial fibrillation reported in less than 10% of pts. May cause hepatitis B virus reactivation. Thrombocytopenia may increase risk of bleeding.

NURSING CONSIDERATIONS

BASELINE ASSESSMENT
Obtain CBC, blood type and screen; pregnancy test in females of reproductive potential. Confirm compliance of effective contraception. Inform blood bank of treatment and possible treatment-related interference with serologic testing. In pts with COPD, inhaled corticosteroids and bronchodilators should be considered during the first 4 treatment doses. If pt does not experience a major systemic administration-related reaction after the first 4 doses, consider discontinuation of the additional inhaled corticosteroids and bronchodilators. To prevent herpes zoster reactivation in pts with a history of infection, initiate antiviral prophylaxis within 1 wk of initiation and continue for 3 mos after last dose. Question history of hepatitis B virus infection, COPD, emphysema, herpes zoster infection. Screen for active infection. Administer premedication and postmedication therapy per manufacturer guidelines. Offer emotional support.

D

INTERVENTION/EVALUATION

Monitor CBC periodically for myelosuppression. Diligently observe for hypersensitivity reactions throughout injection and treatment course; early detection is vital. If anaphylactic reaction occurs, initiate appropriate medical care (antipyretics, corticosteroids, oxygen therapy, IV hydration). Monitor for infections (cough, fever, fatigue), herpes zoster or hepatitis B virus reactivation; symptoms of hyperglycemia (blurred vision, confusion, excessive thirst, Kussmaul respirations, polyuria). If serious infection, sepsis occurs, initiate appropriate antimicrobial therapy. Monitor daily pattern of bowel activity, stool consistency. Encourage nutritional intake.

PATIENT/FAMILY TEACHING

• Treatment may depress your immune system and reduce your ability to fight infection. Report symptoms of infection such as body aches, burning with urination, chills, cough, fatigue, fever. Avoid those with active infection. Dormant chronic viral infections such as herpes zoster, hepatitis B infection can become reactivated. • Pretreatment and posttreatment with acetaminophen, antihistamines, or steroidal anti-inflammatories may help reduce allergic reactions. • Life-threatening anaphylaxis may occur. Immediately report serious allergic reactions of any kind, regardless of the time the dose was administered. • Report symptoms of bone marrow depression such as bruising, fatigue, fever, shortness of breath, weight loss; bleeding easily, bloody urine or stool. • Females of childbearing potential must use effective contraception during treatment and for at least 3 mos after last dose. Do not breastfeed. • Diarrhea is a common side effect. Drink plenty of fluids.

darbepoetin alfa   TOP 100

dar-be-poe-**e**-tin **al**-fa
(Aranesp)

■ BLACK BOX ALERT ■

Increased risk of serious cardiovascular events, thromboembolic events, mortality, time-to-tumor progression when administered to a target hemoglobin greater than 11 g/dL. Shortened overall survival and/or increased risk of tumor progression has been reported with breast, cervical, head/neck, NSCL cancers. **Do not confuse Aranesp with Aricept, or darbepoetin with dalteparin or epoetin.**

◆CLASSIFICATION

PHARMACOTHERAPEUTIC: Erythropoiesis stimulating agent (ESA). **CLINICAL:** Hematopoietic agent.

USES

Treatment of anemia associated with chronic renal failure (including pts on dialysis and pts not on dialysis), treatment of anemia caused by concurrent myelosuppressive chemotherapy in pts planned to receive chemotherapy for minimum of 2 additional months. **OFF-LABEL:** Treatment of symptomatic anemia in myelodysplastic syndrome (MDS). Anemia of prematurity.

PRECAUTIONS

Contraindications: Hypersensitivity to darbepoetin. Pure red cell aplasia that begins after treatment with darbepoetin alfa or other erythropoietin protein medication. Uncontrolled hypertension. **Cautions:** History of seizures, hypertension. Not recommended in pts with mild to moderate anemia and HF or CAD.

ACTION

Stimulates division and differentiation of committed erythroid progenitor cells; induces release of reticulocytes from bone marrow into bloodstream. **Therapeutic Effect:** Induces erythropoiesis.

PHARMACOKINETICS

Widely distributed. **Half-life:** 48.5 hrs.

⧗ LIFESPAN CONSIDERATIONS

Pregnancy/Lactation: Unknown if drug crosses placenta or is distributed in breast milk. **Children:** Safety and efficacy not established. **Elderly:** Age-related renal impairment may require dosage adjustment.

INTERACTIONS

DRUG: None significant. **HERBAL:** None significant. **FOOD:** None known. **LAB VALUES:** May decrease serum ferritin, serum transferrin saturation.

AVAILABILITY (Rx)

Injection Solution: 25 mcg/mL, 40 mcg/mL, 60 mcg/mL, 100 mcg/mL, 200 mcg/mL. **Prefilled Syringe:** 10 mcg/0.4 mL, 25 mcg/0.42 mL, 40 mcg/0.4 mL, 60 mcg/0.3 mL, 100 mcg/0.5 mL, 150 mcg/0.3 mL, 200 mcg/0.4 mL, 300 mcg/0.6 mL, 500 mcg/mL.

ADMINISTRATION/HANDLING

 IV

Preparation • Avoid excessive agitation of vial; do not shake (will cause foaming). Do not dilute.
Rate of administration • May be given as IV bolus.
Storage • Refrigerate. • Do not shake. Vigorous shaking may denature medication, rendering it inactive.

SQ
• Use 1 dose per vial; do not reenter vial. Discard unused portion.

🔲 IV INCOMPATIBILITIES

Do not mix with other medications.

INDICATIONS/ROUTES/DOSAGE

Anemia in Chronic Renal Failure
◄ALERT► Individualize dosing and use lowest dose to reduce need for RBC transfusions. IV route is recommended for pts on hemodialysis. **On dialysis:** Initiate when Hgb less than 10 g/dL; reduce or stop dose when Hgb approaches or exceeds 11 g/dL. **Not on dialysis:** Initiate

when Hgb less than 10 g/dL and Hgb decline would likely result in RBC transfusion; reduce dose or stop if Hgb exceeds 10 g/dL.
IV, SQ: ADULTS, ELDERLY: On dialysis: Initially, 0.45 mcg/kg once wkly or 0.75 mcg/kg once q2wks. **Not on dialysis:** 0.45 mcg/kg q4wks. **INFANTS, CHILDREN: On dialysis:** Initially, 0.45 mcg/kg wkly. **Not on dialysis:** Initially, 0.45 mcg/kg wkly **OR** 0.75 mcg/kg q2wks. **Decrease dose by 25%:** If Hgb approaches 12 g/dL or increases greater than 1 g/dL in any 2-wk period. **Increase dose by 25%:** If Hgb does not increase by 1 g/dL after 4 wks of therapy and Hgb is below target range (with adequate iron stores). Do not increase dose more frequently than every 4 wks. **Note:** If pt does not attain Hgb range of 10–12 g/dL after appropriate dosing over 12 wks, do not increase dose and use minimum effective dose to maintain Hgb level that will avoid red blood cell transfusions. Discontinue treatment if responsiveness does not improve.

Anemia Associated With Chemotherapy
◄ALERT► Initiate only if Hgb less than 10 g/dL and anticipated duration of myelosuppression is 2 months or longer. Titrate dose to maintain Hgb level and avoid RBC transfusions. Discontinue upon completion of chemotherapy.
SQ: ADULTS, ELDERLY: 2.25 mcg/kg once wkly or 500 mcg every q3wks. **Increase dose:** If Hgb does not increase by 1 g/dL after 6 wks and remains below 10 g/dL, increase dose to 4.5 mcg/kg once wkly. No dose adjustment if using q3wk dosing.
Decrease dose: Decrease dose by 40% if Hgb increases greater than 1 g/dL in any 2-wk period or Hgb reaches level that will avoid red blood cell transfusions. **Note:** Withhold dose when Hgb exceeds a level needed to avoid RBC transfusions; resume at dose 40% lower when Hgb approaches a level where transfusions may be required.

D

Dosage in Renal/Hepatic Impairment
No dose adjustment.

SIDE EFFECTS

Frequent: Myalgia, hypertension/hypotension, headache, diarrhea. **Occasional:** Fatigue, edema, vomiting, reaction at injection site, asthenia, dizziness.

ADVERSE EFFECTS/TOXIC REACTIONS

Cardiovascular events, including CVA, MI, venous thromboembolism, vascular access device thrombosis, mortality, may occur when given to target hemoglobin greater than 11 g/dL or during rapid rise in hemoglobin. Hypersensitivity reactions, including anaphylaxis, may occur. Cases of anemia and pure red cell aplasia may occur in pts with chronic renal disease when given subcutaneously.

NURSING CONSIDERATIONS

BASELINE ASSESSMENT

Obtain CBC (esp. note Hgb, Hct). Assess B/P before drug administration. B/P often rises during early therapy in pts with history of hypertension. Assess serum iron (transferrin saturation should be greater than 20%), serum ferritin (greater than 100 ng/mL) before and during therapy. Consider supplemental iron therapy.

INTERVENTION/EVALUATION

Monitor CBC, reticulocyte count, serum BUN, creatinine, ferritin, potassium, phosphate. Monitor B/P aggressively for increase (25% of pts taking medication require antihypertension therapy, dietary restrictions).

PATIENT/FAMILY TEACHING

• Frequent blood tests needed to determine correct dose. • Report swollen extremities, breathing difficulty, extreme fatigue, or severe headache. • Avoid tasks requiring alertness, motor skills until response to drug is established.

darifenacin

dare-i-**fen**-a-sin
(Enablex ✿)

◆CLASSIFICATION

PHARMACOTHERAPEUTIC: Muscarinic receptor antagonist. Anticholinergic agent. **CLINICAL:** Urinary antispasmodic.

USES

Management of symptoms of bladder overactivity (urge incontinence, urinary urgency/frequency).

PRECAUTIONS

Contraindications: Hypersensitivity to darifenacin. Pts with or at risk of uncontrolled narrow-angle glaucoma, gastric retention, urine retention. **Cautions:** Bladder outflow obstruction, hepatic impairment, nonobstructive prostatic hyperplasia, decreased GI motility (e.g., severe constipation, ulcerative colitis), GI obstructive disorders, controlled narrow-angle glaucoma, myasthenia gravis, concurrent use of strong CYP3A4 inhibitors. Hot weather and/or exercise.

ACTION

Acts as a direct antagonist at muscarinic receptor sites in cholinergically innervated organs; limits bladder contractions. **Therapeutic Effect:** Reduces symptoms of bladder irritability/overactivity (urge incontinence, urinary urgency/frequency), improves bladder capacity.

PHARMACOKINETICS

Widely distributed. Protein binding: 98%. Metabolized in liver. Excreted in urine (60%), feces (40%). **Half-life:** 13–19 hrs.

⧗ LIFESPAN CONSIDERATIONS

Pregnancy/Lactation: Unknown if drug crosses placenta or is distributed in breast milk. **Children:** Safety and efficacy not established. **Elderly:** No age-related precautions noted.

INTERACTIONS

DRUG: **Strong CYP3A4 inhibitors (e.g., clarithromycin, ketoconazole, ritonavir)** may increase concentration/effect. **Strong CYP3A4 inducers (e.g., carBAMazepine, phenytoin, rifAMPin)** may decrease concentration/effect. **Anticholinergics (e.g., aclidinium, ipratropium, tiotropium, umeclidinium)** may increase anticholinergic effect. May increase concentration/effect of **thioridazine. HERBAL:** None significant. **FOOD:** None known. **LAB VALUES:** None known.

AVAILABILITY (Rx)

 Tablets (Extended-Release): 7.5 mg, 15 mg.

ADMINISTRATION/HANDLING

PO
• Give with water without regard to food. • Administer extended-release tablets whole; do not break, crush, dissolve, or divide tablet.

INDICATIONS/ROUTES/DOSAGE

Overactive Bladder
PO: ADULTS, ELDERLY: Initially, 7.5 mg once daily. If response is not adequate after at least 2 wks, may increase to 15 mg once daily. Do not exceed 7.5 mg once daily in moderate hepatic impairment or concurrent use with strong or potent CYP3A4 inhibitors (e.g., clarithromycin, fluconazole, protease inhibitors).

Dosage in Renal Impairment
No dose adjustment.

Dosage Hepatic Impairment
Moderate impairment: Maximum: 7.5 mg. **Severe impairment:** Not recommended.

SIDE EFFECTS

Frequent (35%–21%): Dry mouth, constipation. **Occasional (8%–4%):** Dyspepsia, headache, nausea, abdominal pain. **Rare (3%–2%):** Asthenia, diarrhea, dizziness, ocular dryness.

ADVERSE EFFECTS/TOXIC REACTIONS

UTI occurs occasionally.

NURSING CONSIDERATIONS

BASELINE ASSESSMENT
Monitor voiding pattern, assess signs/symptoms of overactive bladder prior to therapy as baseline.

INTERVENTION/EVALUATION
Monitor I&O. Palpate bladder and use bladder scanner to assess for urine retention. Monitor daily pattern of bowel activity, stool consistency for evidence of constipation. Dry mouth may be relieved with sips of water. Assess for relief of symptoms of overactive bladder (urge incontinence, urinary frequency/urgency).

PATIENT/FAMILY TEACHING
• Swallow tablet whole; do not chew, crush, dissolve, or divide. • Increase fluid intake to reduce risk of constipation. • Avoid tasks that require alertness, motor skills until response to drug is established.

darolutamide

dar-oh-**loo**-ta-mide
(Nubeqa)
Do not confuse darolutamide with abiraterone, apalutamide, bicalutamide, dutasteride, enzalutamide, flutamide, or nilutamide.

◆**CLASSIFICATION**

PHARMACOTHERAPEUTIC: Androgen receptor inhibitor. **CLINICAL:** Antineoplastic.

D

USES

Treatment of nonmetastatic castration-resistant prostate cancer (nmCRPC). Treatment of metastatic hormone-sensitive prostate cancer (mHSPC) in combination with docetaxel.

PRECAUTIONS

Contraindications: Hypersensitivity to darolutamide. **Cautions:** Hepatic/renal impairment, conditions predisposing to infection (e.g., diabetes, renal failure, immunocompromised pts, open wounds); history of cardiovascular disease (HF, ischemic heart disease). Avoid concomitant use of a combined G-gp and strong or moderate CYP3A4 inducer.

ACTION

Binds directly to ligands of androgen receptor, inhibiting androgen-receptor translocation and androgen receptor-mediated transcription. **Therapeutic Effect:** Decreases proliferation of prostate tumor cells, increases apoptosis (cellular death), resulting decreased tumor volume.

PHARMACOKINETICS

Widely distributed. Metabolized in liver to active metabolite. Protein binding: 92%. Peak plasma concentration: 4 hrs. Steady state reached in 2–5 days. Excreted in feces (32%), urine (63%). **Half-life:** 20 hrs.

⧖ LIFESPAN CONSIDERATIONS

Pregnancy/Lactation: Not indicated in female population. May cause fetal harm if administered in pregnant females. **Males:** Males with female partners of reproductive potential must use effective contraception during treatment and up to 1 wk after discontinuation. May impair fertility. **Children:** Safety and efficacy not established. **Elderly:** No age-related precautions noted.

INTERACTIONS

DRUG: May increase concentration/effect of **alpelisib, cladribine, ozanimod, pazopanib, topotecan.**

Combined P-gp and strong CYP3A4 inducers (e.g., carBAMazepine, phenytoin, riFAMpin) **or moderate CYP3A4 inducers** (e.g., dexamethasone, modafinil, nafcillin). may decrease concentration/effect. **HERBAL:** None significant. **FOOD:** None known. **LAB VALUES:** May increase serum AST, bilirubin. May decrease neutrophils.

AVAILABILITY (Rx)

 Tablets: 300 mg.

ADMINISTRATION/HANDLING

PO
• Give with food. • Swallow tablets whole; do not break, cut, crush, or divide.

INDICATIONS/ROUTES/DOSAGE

Note: Pts should receive a gonadotropin-releasing hormone (GnRH) analog concurrently or have had a bilateral orchiectomy.

nmCRPC
PO: ADULTS, ELDERLY: 600 mg twice daily.

mHSPC
Note: Administer the first cycle of docetaxel within 6 wks of starting darolutamide.
PO: ADULTS, ELDERLY: 600 mg twice daily.

Dose Modification
Based on Common Terminology Criteria for Adverse Effects (CTCAE).
Any Grade 3 toxicity or intolerable side effect: Withhold treatment or reduce to 300 mg twice daily until symptoms improve. Doses less than 300 mg twice daily not recommended.

Dosage in Renal Impairment
Mild to moderate impairment: No dose adjustment. **Severe impairment (eGFR 15–29 mL/min) not undergoing HD:** 300 mg twice daily.

Dosage in Hepatic Impairment
Mild impairment: No dose adjustment. **Moderate impairment:** 300 mg twice

daily. **Severe impairment:** Not specified; use caution.

SIDE EFFECTS

Occasional (16%–6%): Fatigue, asthenia, extremity pain. **Rare (3%–less than 1%):** Rash, hypertension, nausea, diarrhea.

ADVERSE EFFECTS/TOXIC REACTIONS

Cardiovascular events including ischemic heart disease (4% of pts), cardiac failure (2% of pts), cardiac arrest were reported. Other adverse effects may include hematuria, urinary retention, pneumonia.

NURSING CONSIDERATIONS

BASELINE ASSESSMENT

Pts should also receive a concomitant gonadotropin-releasing hormone analog or had a bilateral orchiectomy. Question history of hepatic/renal impairment, cardiac disease. Screen for active infection. Receive full medication history and screen for interactions. Offer emotional support.

INTERVENTION/EVALUATION

Monitor CBC periodically for neutropenia. Monitor for symptoms of HF (dyspnea, exercise intolerance, palpitations, peripheral edema), infection (cough, fever, fatigue).

PATIENT/FAMILY TEACHING

• Treatment may depress your immune system response and reduce your ability to fight infection. Report symptoms of infection such as body aches, chills, cough, fatigue, fever. Avoid those with active infection. • Report symptoms of liver problems (e.g., bruising, confusion; dark, amber-, orange-colored urine; right upper abdominal pain, yellowing of the skin or eyes); heart failure (e.g., chest pain, difficulty breathing, palpitations, swelling of extremities). • Males with female partners of childbearing potential must wear condoms during sexual activity. • There is a high risk of interactions with other medications. Do not take newly prescribed medi-

cations unless approved by prescriber who originally started therapy. • Avoid herbal supplements (esp. St. John's wort).

---

darunavir

dar-**ue**-na-veer
(Prezista)

FIXED-COMBINATION(S)

Prezcobix: Darunavir/cobicistat (antiretroviral booster): 800 mg/150 mg. **Symtuza:** Darunavir/cobicistat (antiretroviral booster)/emtricitabine (reverse transcriptase inhibitor)/tenofovir alafenamide (reverse transcriptase inhibitor): 800 mg/150 mg/200 mg/10 mg.

◆CLASSIFICATION

PHARMACOTHERAPEUTIC: Protease inhibitor (anti-HIV). **CLINICAL:** Antiretroviral.

USES

Treatment of HIV infection in combination with ritonavir and other antiretroviral agents in adults and children 3 yrs and older. **OFF-LABEL:** HIV-1 nonoccupational post-exposure prophylaxis (nPEP).

PRECAUTIONS

Contraindications: Hypersensitivity to darunavir. Concurrent therapy with alfuzosin, colchicine (in pts with renal and/or hepatic impairment), dihydroergotamine, dronedarone, elbasvir/grazoprevir, ergonovine, ergotamine, lovastatin, lurasidone, methylergonovine, oral midazolam, pimozide, ranolazine, rifAMPin, sildenafil (for treatment of PAH), simvastatin, St. John's wort, triazolam. **Cautions:** Diabetes, hemophilia, known sulfonamide allergy, hepatic impairment.

ACTION

Binds to site of HIV-I protease activity, inhibiting cleavage of viral precursors into functional proteins required

D

for infectious HIV. **Therapeutic Effect:** Prevents formation of mature viral cells.

PHARMACOKINETICS

Widely distributed. Metabolized in liver. Protein binding: 95%. Excreted in feces (80%), urine (14%). Not significantly removed by hemodialysis. **Half-life:** 15 hrs.

⧖ LIFESPAN CONSIDERATIONS

Pregnancy/Lactation: Unknown if drug crosses placenta or is distributed in breast milk. Breastfeeding not recommended. **Children:** Safety and efficacy not established in pts younger than 3 yrs. **Elderly:** No age-related precautions noted.

INTERACTIONS

DRUG: May increase concentration/effects of **amiodarone, axitinib, bosutinib, budesonide, colchicine, dronedarone, eletriptan, ergot derivatives** (e.g., **ergotamine**), **fluticasone** (nasal), **lovastatin, midazolam, nimodipine, ranolazine, regorafenib, simvastatin, thioridazine. Strong CYP3A4 inducers** (e.g., **carBAMazepine, phenytoin, rifAMPin**) may decrease concentration/effect. **Strong CYP3A4 inhibitors** (e.g., **carBAMazepine, ketoconazole, ritonavir**) may increase concentration/effect. May decrease effects of **methadone, oral contraceptives. HERBAL:** Garlic, St. John's wort may lead to loss of virologic response, potential resistance to darunavir. **FOOD:** Food increases plasma concentration. **LAB VALUES:** May increase aPTT, PT, serum alkaline phosphatase, bilirubin, amylase, lipase, cholesterol, triglycerides, uric acid. May decrease lymphocytes/neutrophil count, platelets, WBC count; serum bicarbonate, albumin, calcium. May alter serum glucose, sodium.

AVAILABILITY (Rx)

Suspension, Oral: *(Prezista):* 100 mg/mL
🖫 **Tablets:** *(Prezista):* 75 mg, 150 mg, 600 mg, 800 mg.

ADMINISTRATION/HANDLING

PO
• Give with food (increases plasma concentration). • Coadministration with ritonavir required. • Shake suspension prior to each dose. Use provided oral dosing syringe.

INDICATIONS/ROUTES/DOSAGE

Note: Genotypic testing recommended in therapy-experienced pts.

HIV Infection, Treatment Experienced
PO: ADULTS, ELDERLY: (With 1 or more darunavir resistance–associated substitution): 600 mg administered twice daily with 100 mg ritonavir twice daily. **(With no darunavir resistance–associated substitutions):** 800 mg with 100 mg ritonavir or 150 mg cobicistat once daily.

HIV Infection, Treatment Naive
PO: ADULTS, ELDERLY: 800 mg administered with 100 mg ritonavir or 150 mg cobicistat once daily.

Usual Dosage During Pregnancy
PO: ADULTS: 600 mg administered twice daily with 100 mg ritonavir twice daily.

Treatment Naive or Experienced Without Darunavir Resistance–Associated Substitution
PO: (tablet or suspension): CHILDREN WEIGHING 40 KG OR MORE: 800 mg (ritonavir 100 mg) once daily. **WEIGHING 30–39 KG:** 675 mg (ritonavir 100 mg) once daily. **WEIGHING 15–29 KG:** 600 mg (ritonavir 100 mg) once daily.
PO: (suspension only): WEIGHING 14 KG TO LESS THAN 15 KG: 490 mg (ritonavir 96 mg) once daily. **13 KG TO LESS THAN 14 KG:** 455 mg (ritonavir 80 mg) once daily. **12 KG TO LESS THAN 13 KG:** 420 mg (ritonavir 80 mg) once daily. **11 KG TO LESS THAN 12 KG:** 385 mg (ritonavir 64 mg) once daily. **10 KG TO LESS THAN 11 KG:** 350 mg (ritonavir 64 mg) once daily.

Treatment Naive or Experienced With at least 1 Darunavir Resistance–Associated Substitution

PO: (tablet or suspension): CHILDREN WEIGHING 40 KG OR MORE: 600 mg (100 mg ritonavir) twice daily. **WEIGHING 30–39 KG:** 450 mg (60 mg ritonavir) twice daily. **WEIGHING 15–29 KG:** 375 mg (48 mg ritonavir) twice daily.

PO: (suspension only): WEIGHING 14 KG TO LESS THAN 15 KG: 280 mg (48 mg ritonavir) twice daily. **13 KG TO LESS THAN 14 KG:** 260 mg (40 mg ritonavir) twice daily. **12 KG TO LESS THAN 13 KG:** 240 mg (40 mg ritonavir) twice daily. **11 KG TO LESS THAN 12 KG:** 220 mg (32 mg ritonavir) twice daily. **10 KG TO LESS THAN 11 KG:** 200 mg (32 mg ritonavir) twice daily.

Dosage in Renal Impairment
No dose adjustment.

Dosage in Hepatic Impairment
Mild to moderate impairment: No dose adjustment. **Severe impairment:** Not recommended.

SIDE EFFECTS

Frequent (19%–13%): Diarrhea, nausea, headache, nasopharyngitis. **Occasional (3%–2%):** Constipation, abdominal pain, vomiting. **Rare (less than 2%):** Allergic dermatitis, dyspepsia, flatulence, abdominal distention, anorexia, arthralgia, myalgia, paresthesia, memory impairment.

ADVERSE EFFECTS/TOXIC REACTIONS

Hyperglycemia, exacerbation of diabetes, diabetic ketoacidosis, new-onset diabetes have been reported in protease inhibitors. Drug-induced hepatotoxicity was reported, esp. in pts with advanced HIV disease, cirrhosis, hepatitis B or C virus infection, or pts taking multiple medications. May increase risk of bleeding in pts with history of hemophilia A or B. Immune reconstitution syndrome (inflammatory response to dormant opportunistic infections such as *Mycobacterium avium,* cytomegalovirus, PCP, tuberculosis, or acceleration of autoimmune disorders such as Graves' disease, polymyositis, Guillain-Barré) may occur. Skin reactions (including Stevens-Johnson syndrome, toxic epidermal necrolysis) occur rarely. Hypersensitivity reactions including anaphylaxis, angioedema, bronchospasm may occur.

NURSING CONSIDERATIONS

BASELINE ASSESSMENT

Obtain CD4+ count, viral load, HIV RNA level. Confirm HIV genotype. Question history of diabetes, hemophilia, hepatic impairment, prior hypersensitivity reactions. Receive full medication history (including herbal products); screen for contraindications/interactions. Offer emotional support.

INTERVENTION/EVALUATION

Monitor CD4+ count, viral load, HIV RNA level for treatment effectiveness. Monitor BMP, LFT, renal function, serum blood glucose periodically. An increase in serum creatinine greater than 0.4 mg/dL from baseline may indicate renal impairment. Closely monitor for GI discomfort. Monitor daily pattern of bowel activity, stool consistency. Monitor for hepatotoxicity (bruising, hematuria, jaundice, right upper abdominal pain, nausea, vomiting, weight loss), hypersensitivity reactions. Assess skin for rash, other skin reactions. Assess for immune reconstitution syndrome, opportunistic infections (onset of fever, oral mucosa changes, cough, other respiratory symptoms).

PATIENT/FAMILY TEACHING

• Treatment does not cure HIV infection, nor does it reduce risk of transmission. Practice safe sex with barrier methods or abstinence. • There is a high risk of drug interactions with other medications. Do not take newly prescribed medications unless approved by prescriber who

D

originally started treatment. Do not take herbal products, esp. St. John's wort. • If amiodarone therapy cannot be withheld or stopped, immediately report symptoms of slow heart rate such as chest pain, confusion, dizziness, fainting, light-headedness, memory problems, palpitations, weakness. • Report any skin reactions. • Report any signs of decreased urine output, abdominal pain, yellowing of skin or eyes, darkened urine, clay-colored stools, weight loss. • As immune system strengthens, it may respond to dormant infections hidden within the body. Report any new fever, chills, body aches, cough, night sweats, shortness of breath. Antiretrovirals may cause excess body fat in the upper back, neck, breast, and trunk and may cause decreased body fat in legs, arms, and face. • Drug resistance can form if therapy is interrupted for even a short time; do not run out of supply. • Report symptoms of high blood sugar levels (confusion, excessive thirst/hunger, headache, frequent urination).

---

dasatinib   `HIGH ALERT`

da-**sa**-ti-nib
(Sprycel)
Do not confuse dasatinib with erlotinib, imatinib, or lapatinib.

◆**CLASSIFICATION**

PHARMACOTHERAPEUTIC: BCR-ABL tyrosine kinase inhibitor. **CLINICAL:** Antineoplastic.

USES

Adults: Treatment of newly diagnosed Philadelphia chromosome–positive (Ph+) chronic myeloid leukemia (CML) in chronic phase; chronic, accelerated, or myeloid or lymphoid blast phase Ph+ CML with resistance or intolerance to prior therapy, including imatinib; Philadelphia chromosome-positive acute lymphoblastic leukemia (Ph+ ALL) with resistance or intolerance to prior therapy. **Pts 1 yr and older:** Treatment of Ph+ CML in chronic phase; newly diagnosed Ph+ ALL in combination with chemotherapy. **OFF-LABEL:** Gastrointestinal stromal tumors (GIST).

PRECAUTIONS

Contraindications: Hypersensitivity to dasatinib. **Cautions:** Hepatic impairment, myelosuppression (particularly thrombocytopenia), pts prone to fluid retention, pts at risk for QT interval prolongation or torsades de pointes (congenital long QT syndrome, medications that prolong QT interval, hypokalemia, hypomagnesemia); cardiovascular/pulmonary disease. Concomitant use of anticoagulants, CYP3A4 inducers/inhibitors may increase risk of pulmonary arterial hypertension.

ACTION

Reduces activity of proteins responsible for uncontrolled growth of leukemia cells by binding to most imatinib-resistant BCR-ABL mutations of pts with CML or ALL. **Therapeutic Effect:** Inhibits proliferation, tumor growth of CML and ALL cancer cell lines.

PHARMACOKINETICS

Widely distributed. Protein binding: 96%. Metabolized in liver. Eliminated primarily in feces. **Half-life:** 3–5 hrs.

LIFESPAN CONSIDERATIONS

Pregnancy/Lactation: Has potential for severe teratogenic effects, fertility impairment. Breastfeeding not recommended. **Children:** Safety and efficacy not established in pts younger than 1 yr. **Elderly:** No age-related precautions noted.

INTERACTIONS

DRUG: CYP3A4 **inhibitors (e.g., clarithromycin, ketoconazole, ritonavir)** may increase concentration/effect. **CYP3A4 inducers**

(e.g., carBAMazepine, phenytoin, rifAMPin) may decrease concentration/ effect. May decrease therapeutic effect of **BCG (intravesical), vaccines (live)**. **H₂ antagonists (e.g., famotidine), proton pump inhibitors (e.g., omeprazole, pantoprazole)** may decrease concentration/effect; avoid concomitant use. May increase adverse effects of **vaccines (live)**. **HERBAL: Echinacea** may decrease therapeutic effect. **St. John's wort** may decrease concentration/ effect. **FOOD: Grapefruit products** may increase concentration/toxicity (increased risk of torsades, myelotoxicity). **LAB VALUES:** May decrease WBC, platelets, Hgb, Hct, RBC; serum calcium, phosphates. May increase serum ALT, AST, bilirubin, creatinine.

AVAILABILITY (Rx)

Tablets (Film-Coated): 20 mg, 50 mg, 70 mg, 80 mg, 100 mg, 140 mg.

ADMINISTRATION/HANDLING

PO
• Give without regard to food. • Give with food or large glass of water if GI upset occurs. • Do not break, crush, dissolve, or divide film-coated tablets. • Do not give antacids either 2 hrs prior to or within 2 hrs after dasatinib administration.

INDICATIONS/ROUTES/DOSAGE

Concomitant use of CYP3A4 inhibitors: Consider decreasing dose from 100 mg to 20 mg or 140 mg to 40 mg. **Concomitant use of CYP3A4 inducers:** Consider increasing dose with monitoring.

Chronic-Phase CML
PO: ADULTS, ELDERLY: Initially, 100 mg once daily.

Accelerated-Phase CML, Myeloid- or Lymphoid Blast-Phase CML, Ph+ ALL
PO: ADULTS, ELDERLY: Initially, 140 mg once daily.

Ph+ CML in Chronic Phase
PO: CHILDREN 1 YR AND OLDER WEIGHING 45 KG OR GREATER: Initially, 100 mg once daily; **30–44 KG:** 70 mg once daily; **20–29 KG:** 60 mg once daily; **10–19 KG:** 40 mg once daily.

Newly Diagnosed Ph+ ALL (in combination with chemotherapy)
PO: CHILDREN 1 YR AND OLDER WEIGHING 45 KG OR GREATER: Initially, 100 mg once daily. **30–44 KG:** 70 mg once daily. **20–29 KG:** 60 mg once daily. **10–19 KG:** 40 mg once daily.

Dosage in Renal/Hepatic Impairment
No dose adjustment.

SIDE EFFECTS

Frequent (50%–32%): Fluid retention, diarrhea, headache, fatigue, musculoskeletal pain, fever, rash, nausea, dyspnea. **Occasional (28%–12%):** Cough, abdominal pain, vomiting, anorexia, asthenia, arthralgia, stomatitis, dizziness, constipation, peripheral neuropathy, myalgia. **Rare (less than 12%):** Abdominal distention, chills, weight increase, pruritus.

ADVERSE EFFECTS/TOXIC REACTIONS

Pleural effusion occurred in 8% of pts, febrile neutropenia in 7%, GI bleeding, pneumonia in 6%, thrombocytopenia in 5%, dyspnea in 4%; anemia, cardiac failure in 3%.

NURSING CONSIDERATIONS

BASELINE ASSESSMENT
Obtain CBC weekly for first mo, biweekly for second mo, and periodically thereafter. Monitor LFT before treatment begins and monthly thereafter. Obtain baseline weight. Offer emotional support.

INTERVENTION/EVALUATION
Monitor CBC weekly for first mo, biweekly for second mo, then periodically thereafter. Monitor LFT monthly. Weigh daily, monitor for unexpected rapid

weight gain. Offer antiemetics to control nausea, vomiting. Monitor daily pattern of bowel activity, stool consistency. Assess oral mucous membranes for evidence of stomatitis. Monitor CBC for neutropenia, thrombocytopenia; monitor hepatic function tests for hepatotoxicity.

PATIENT/FAMILY TEACHING

• Avoid crowds, those with known infection. • Avoid contact with anyone who recently received live virus vaccine; do not receive vaccinations. • Antacids may be taken up to 2 hrs before or 2 hrs after taking dasatinib. • Avoid grapefruit products. • Do not chew, crush, dissolve, or divide tablets.

DAUNOrubicin   **HIGH ALERT**

daw-noe-**roo**-bi-sin
(Cerubidine)

■ **BLACK BOX ALERT** ■ May cause cumulative, dose-related myocardial toxicity. Severe myelosuppression may lead to infection or hemorrhage. Must be administered by personnel trained in administration/handling of chemotherapeutic agents. Caution in pts with renal impairment or hepatic dysfunction. Extravasation may cause severe local tissue necrosis.

Do not confuse DAUNOrubicin with DACTINomycin, DOXOrubicin, epiRUBicin, IDArubicin, or valrubicin.

FIXED COMBINATION(s)

Vyxeos: daunorubicin/cytarabine (a nucleoside metabolic inhibitor): 44 mg/100 mg.

◆CLASSIFICATION

PHARMACOTHERAPEUTIC: Anthracycline topoisomerase II inhibitor. **CLINICAL:** Antineoplastic.

USES

Remission induction in acute nonlymphocytic leukemia (myelogenous, monocytic, erythroid) of adults and for remission induction in acute lymphocytic leukemia of children and adults.

PRECAUTIONS

Contraindications: Hypersensitivity to DAUNOrubicin. **Cautions:** Preexisting heart disease or bone marrow suppression, hypertension, concurrent chemotherapeutic agents, elderly, infants, radiation therapy.

ACTION

Inhibits DNA and RNA synthesis by intercalation between DNA base pairs and by steric obstruction. Cell cycle–phase nonspecific. **Therapeutic Effect:** Inhibits tumor cell growth and survival.

PHARMACOKINETICS

Widely distributed. Protein binding: High. Does not cross blood-brain barrier. Metabolized in liver. Excreted in urine (40%); biliary excretion (40%). **Half-life:** 18.5 hrs; metabolite: 26.7 hrs.

⊠ LIFESPAN CONSIDERATIONS

Pregnancy/Lactation: Avoid pregnancy; may cause fetal harm. Breastfeeding not recommended. **Children:** Cardiotoxicity may be more frequent and occur at lower cumulative doses. **Elderly:** Cardiotoxicity may be more frequent; reduced bone marrow reserves require caution. Age-related renal impairment may require dosage adjustment.

INTERACTIONS

DRUG: Bevacizumab, cyclophosphamide may increase risk of cardiotoxicity. **Bone marrow depressants (e.g., cladribine)** may enhance myelosuppression. May decrease therapeutic effect of **BCG (intravesical). Live virus vaccines** may potentiate virus replication, increase vaccine side effects, decrease pt's antibody response to vaccine. **HERBAL: Echinacea** may decrease therapeutic effect. **FOOD:** None known. **LAB VALUES:** May increase serum alkaline phosphatase, bilirubin, uric acid, AST.

AVAILABILITY (Rx)
Injection Solution: 5 mg/mL.

ADMINISTRATION/HANDLING
 IV (Cerubidine)

Give by IV push or IV infusion.
Reconstitution • May further dilute with 100 mL D_5W or 0.9% NaCl.
Rate of administration • For IV push, withdraw desired dose into syringe containing 10–15 mL 0.9% NaCl. Inject over 1–5 min into tubing of rapidly infusing IV solution of D_5W or 0.9% NaCl. • For IV infusion, further dilute with 100 mL D_5W or 0.9% NaCl. Infuse over 15–30 min. • Extravasation produces immediate pain, severe local tissue damage. Aspirate as much infiltrated drug as possible, then infiltrate area with hydrocortisone sodium succinate injection (50–100 mg hydrocortisone) and/or isotonic sodium thiosulfate injection or ascorbic acid injection (1 mL of 5% injection). Apply cold compresses.
Storage • Refrigerate intact vials. • Protect from light. • Solutions prepared for infusion stable for 24 hrs at room temperature.

⚙ IV COMPATIBILITIES
Granisetron, ondansetron.

INDICATIONS/ROUTES/DOSAGE
◄ALERT► Refer to individual protocols. Cumulative dose should not exceed 550 mg/m² in adults (increased risk of cardiotoxicity) or 400 mg/m² in those receiving chest irradiation.

Acute Lymphocytic Leukemia (Remission Induction)
IV: **ADULTS, ELDERLY:** 45 mg/m² on days 1, 2, and 3 (in combination with vin-CRIStine, predniSONE, asparaginase). **CHILDREN 2 YRS AND OLDER AND BODY SURFACE AREA 0.5 m² OR GREATER:** 25 mg/m² on day 1 of every wk for up to 4–6 cycles (in combination with vinCRIStine, predniSONE). **CHILDREN YOUNGER THAN 2 YRS, OR BODY SURFACE AREA LESS THAN 0.5 m²:** 1 mg/kg/dose on day 1 of every wk for up to 4 to 6 cycles (in combination with vinCRIStine, predniSONE).

Acute Non-Lymphocytic Leukemia (Remission Induction)
IV: **ADULTS YOUNGER THAN 60 YRS:** 45 mg/m² on days 1, 2, and 3 of induction course, then on days 1 and 2 of subsequent courses (in combination with cytarabine). **ADULTS 60 YRS AND OLDER:** 30 mg/m² on days 1, 2, and 3 of induction course, then on days 1 and 2 of subsequent courses (in combination with cytarabine).

Dosage in Renal Impairment
Serum creatinine greater than 3 mg/dL: 50% of normal dose.

Dosage in Hepatic Impairment
Bilirubin 1.2–3 mg/dL: 75% of normal dose. **Bilirubin 3.1–5 mg/dL:** 50% of normal dose. **Bilirubin greater than 5 mg/dL:** DAUNOrubicin is not recommended for use in this pt population.

SIDE EFFECTS
Frequent: Complete alopecia (scalp, axillary, pubic), nausea, vomiting (beginning a few hrs after administration and lasting 24–48 hrs). **Occasional:** Diarrhea, abdominal pain, esophagitis, stomatitis, transverse pigmentation of fingernails, toenails. **Rare:** Transient fever, chills.

ADVERSE EFFECTS/TOXIC REACTIONS
Myelosuppression (severe leukopenia, anemia, thrombocytopenia) is expected. Decreases in platelet count, WBC count occur in 10–14 days, then return to normal level by third week. Cardiotoxicity including absolute decrease in LVEF, HF, death may occur, esp. in children and pts with preexisting cardiac disease. ECG findings and/or cardiomyopathy is manifested as HF (risk increases when cumulative dose exceeds 550 mg/m² in adults, 300 mg/m² in children 2 yrs and older, or total dosage greater than 10 mg/kg in children younger than 2 yrs).

Pericarditis-myocarditis may occur. Secondary leukemias were reported in pts exposed to topoisomerase II inhibitors when used concomitantly with other antineoplastics or radiation therapy. Extravasation can cause severe local tissue necrosis.

NURSING CONSIDERATIONS

BASELINE ASSESSMENT

Obtain CBC, LFT, BUN, serum creatinine, CrCl, GFR in pts with renal impairment. Obtain ECG before initiation, esp. in pts with cardiac disease. Antiemetics may be effective in preventing, treating nausea. Ensure patency of IV access. Obtain accurate height and weight for dose calculation. Offer emotional support.

INTERVENTION/EVALUATION

Obtain CBC frequently; BMP, LFT, serum uric acid periodically. Monitor daily pattern of bowel activity, stool consistency. Monitor for hematologic toxicity (fever, sore throat, signs of local infection, unusual bruising/bleeding from any site); symptoms of anemia (excessive fatigue, weakness). Diligently monitor for extravasation, tissue necrosis.

PATIENT/FAMILY TEACHING

• Urine may turn reddish color for 1–2 days after beginning therapy. • Hair loss is reversible, but new hair growth may have different color, texture. New hair growth resumes about 5 wks after last therapy dose • Maintain strict oral hygiene. • Do not have immunizations without physician's approval (drug lowers resistance). • Avoid contact with those who have recently received live virus vaccine. • Promptly report fever, sore throat, signs of local infection, unusual bruising/bleeding from any site, yellowing of whites of eyes/skin, difficulty breathing. • Report persistent nausea, vomiting. • Treatment may impair the heart's ability to pump blood effectively; report difficulty breathing, chest pain, palpitations, swelling of the legs or feet.

denosumab

den-**oh**-sue-mab
(Prolia, Xgeva)
Do not confuse denosumab with daclizumab, or Prolia with Avandia or Zebeta.

◆CLASSIFICATION

PHARMACOTHERAPEUTIC: Monoclonal antibody (with affinity for RANKL).
CLINICAL: Bone-modifying agent.

USES

Prolia: Treatment of osteoporosis in postmenopausal women at high risk for fracture. Treatment of glucocorticoid-induced osteoporosis in pts at high risk of fracture who are receiving an equivalent dose of 7.5 mg or more of predniSONE for duration of at least 6 mos. Treatment to increase bone mass in men with osteoporosis at high risk for fractures; treatment of bone loss in men receiving androgen deprivation therapy for nonmetastatic prostate cancer and in women at high risk for fractures receiving adjuvant aromatase inhibitor therapy for breast cancer. **Xgeva:** Prevention of skeletal-related events (e.g., fracture, spinal cord compression) in pts with bone metastases from solid tumor or multiple myeloma. Treatment of giant cell tumor of bone in adults and skeletally mature adolescents that is unresectable or where surgery is likely to result in severe morbidity. Treatment of hypercalcemia of malignancy refractory to bisphosphonate therapy. **OFF-LABEL:** Treatment of bone destruction caused by rheumatoid arthritis.

PRECAUTIONS

Contraindications: Hypersensitivity to denosumab. **Prolia:** Preexisting hypocalcemia, pregnancy. **Xgeva:** Preexisting hypocalcemia. **Cautions:** History of hypoparathyroidism, thyroid/parathyroid surgery, malabsorption syndromes, excision of small intestine, immunocompromised pts. Pts with severe renal impairment or receiving dialysis (greater risk for developing hypocalcemia). Pts with impaired immune system or immunosuppressive therapy.

ACTION

Binds to RANKL; blocks interaction between RANKL and RANK, preventing osteoclast formation. **Therapeutic Effect:** Decreases bone resorption; increases bone mass in osteoporosis; decreases skeletal-related events and tumor-induced bone destruction in solid tumors, multiple myeloma. Inhibits tumor growth.

PHARMACOKINETICS

Serum level detected 1 hr after administration. **Half-life:** 32 days.

⌛ LIFESPAN CONSIDERATIONS

Pregnancy/Lactation: Avoid pregnancy; may cause fetal harm. Unknown if distributed in breast milk. Breastfeeding not recommended. **Children:** Safety and efficacy not established in adolescents who are not skeletally mature. **Elderly:** No age-related precautions noted.

INTERACTIONS

DRUG: May enhance adverse/toxic effect of **immunosuppressants**. **HERBAL:** None significant. **FOOD:** None known. **LAB VALUES:** May decrease serum calcium. May increase serum cholesterol.

AVAILABILITY (Rx)

Injection, Solution: *(Prolia):* 60 mg/mL. *(Xgeva):* 120 mg/1.7 mL.

ADMINISTRATION/HANDLING

SQ
• Administer in upper arm, upper thigh, or abdomen.
Storage • Refrigerate. Use within 14 days once at room temperature. • Solution appears as clear, colorless to pale yellow.

INDICATIONS/ROUTES/DOSAGE

Note: Administer calcium and vitamin D to prevent/treat hypocalcemia.

Prolia
Bone Loss, Osteoporosis
SQ: ADULTS, ELDERLY: 60 mg every 6 mos.

Xgeva
Prevention of Skeletal-Related Events From Solid Tumors, Multiple Myeloma
SQ: ADULTS, ELDERLY: 120 mg q4wks. Administer calcium and vitamin D as needed to treat or prevent hypocalcemia.

Giant Cell Tumor of Bone
SQ: ADULTS, ELDERLY, MATURE ADOLESCENTS: 120 mg q4wks with additional doses on days 8 and 15 of first mos of therapy. Administer calcium and vitamin D as needed to treat or prevent hypocalcemia.

Hypercalcemia of Malignancy
SQ: ADULTS, ELDERLY, ADOLESCENTS: 120 mg q4wks with additional doses on days 8 and 15 of first mos of therapy.

Dosage in Renal/Hepatic Impairment
No dose adjustment.

SIDE EFFECTS

Frequent (35%–12%): Back pain, extremity pain. **Occasional (8%–5%):** Musculoskeletal pain, vertigo, peripheral edema, sciatica. **Rare (4%–2%):** Bone pain, upper abdominal pain, rash, insomnia, flatulence, pruritus, myalgia, asthenia, GI reflux.

ADVERSE EFFECTS/TOXIC REACTIONS

Life-threatening hypocalcemia may occur in pts with advanced chronic kidney disease. Increases risk of infection, specifically cystitis, UTI, cellulitis, upper respiratory tract infection, pneumonia, pharyngitis, herpes zoster (shingles). Osteonecrosis of the jaw (OJN) was reported. Suppression of bone turnover, pancreatitis have been reported.

❧ Canadian trade name　　　🔰 Non-Crushable Drug　　　🅷🅸 High Alert drug

NURSING CONSIDERATIONS

BASELINE ASSESSMENT

Hypocalcemia must be corrected prior to treatment. Calcium 1,000 mg/day and vitamin D at least 400 international units/day should be given. Dental exam should be provided prior to treatment. Recommend baseline bone density scan.

INTERVENTION/EVALUATION

Monitor serum magnesium, calcium, ionized calcium, phosphate. In pts predisposed with hypocalcemia and disturbances of mineral metabolism, clinical monitoring of calcium, mineral levels is highly recommended. Adequately supplement all pts with calcium and vitamin D. Monitor for delayed fracture healing.

PATIENT/FAMILY TEACHING

• Report rash, new-onset eczema. • Seek prompt medical attention if signs, symptoms of severe infection (rash, itching, reddened skin, cellulitis) occur. • Report muscle stiffness, numbness, cramps, spasms (signs of hypocalcemia); swelling or drainage from jaw, mouth, or teeth.

desmopressin

des-moe-**press**-in
(DDAVP, Nocduma, Stimate)

◆CLASSIFICATION

PHARMACOTHERAPEUTIC: Synthetic vasopressin analog (hormone, posterior pituitary). **CLINICAL:** Antihemophilic. Hemostatic.

USES

Injection: Antidiuretic replacement therapy for management of central (cranial) diabetes insipidus, temporary polyuria/polydipsia following head trauma or surgery in pituitary region. Use in pts with mild hemophilia A or von Willebrand disease to maintain hemostasis. **Intranasal: Stimate:** Use in pts with mild hemophilia A or von Willebrand disease to maintain hemostasis. **DDAVP:** Management of diabetes insipidus in adults and children 4 yrs of age and older. **Oral:** Antidiuretic replacement therapy in the management of central diabetes insipidus. Management of temporary polyuria and polydipsia following head trauma or surgery in the pituitary region. Treatment of nocturia due to nocturnal polyuria in adults who awaken at least 2 times per night to void. Management of primary nocturnal enuresis, either alone or as an adjunct to behavioral conditioning or other nonpharmacologic intervention. **OFF-LABEL:** Deceased organ donor management, intracranial hemorrhage associated with antiplatelet agents, prevention of overly rapid sodium correction in chronic severe hyponatremia, uremic bleeding.

PRECAUTIONS

Contraindications: Hypersensitivity to desmopressin. Hyponatremia, history of hyponatremia, moderate to severe renal impairment. **Cautions:** Predisposition to thrombus formation; conditions with fluid, electrolyte imbalance; coronary artery disease; hypertensive cardiovascular disease, elderly pts, cystic fibrosis, HF, renal impairment, polydipsia. Avoid use in hemophilia A with factor VIII levels less than 5%; hemophilia B; severe type I, type IIB, platelet-type von Willebrand's disease.

ACTION

Increases cAMP in renal tubular cells, which increases water permeability, decreasing urine volume. Increases levels of von Willebrand factor, factor VIII, tissue plasminogen activator (tPA). **Therapeutic Effect:** Shortens activated partial thromboplastin time (aPTT), bleeding time. Decreases urinary output.

PHARMACOKINETICS

Route	Onset	Peak	Duration
PO	1 hr	2–7 hrs	8–12 hrs
IV	15–30 min	1.5–3 hrs	8–12 hrs
Intranasal	15 min–1 hr	1–5 hrs	8–12 hrs

Poorly absorbed after PO, nasal administration. Metabolism: Unknown. **Half-life: PO:** 1.5–2.5 hrs. **Intranasal:** 3.3–3.5 hrs. **IV:** 0.4–4 hrs.

⌛ LIFESPAN CONSIDERATIONS

Pregnancy/Lactation: Unknown if distributed in breast milk. **Children:** Caution in neonates, pts younger than 3 mos (increased risk of fluid balance problems). Careful fluid restrictions recommended in infants. **Elderly:** Increased risk of hyponatremia, water intoxication.

INTERACTIONS

DRUG: CarBAMazepine, lamoTRIgine, NSAIDs (e.g., ibuprofen, ketorolac, naproxen), SSRIs (e.g., citalopram, sertraline), tricyclic antidepressants (e.g., amitriptyline, doxepin, nortriptyline) may increase effect. **Demeclocycline, lithium** may decrease effect. **Corticosteroids** (e.g., **dexamethasone, predniSONE), loop diuretics** (e.g., **furosemide)** may increase hyponatremic effect. **HERBAL:** None significant. **FOOD:** None known. **LAB VALUES:** May decrease serum sodium.

AVAILABILITY (Rx)

Injection Solution: *(DDAVP):* 4 mcg/mL. **Nasal Solution:** 100 mcg/mL (10 mcg/spray). **Nasal Spray:** 1.5 mg/mL (150 mcg/spray). **Tablets:** *(DDAVP):* 0.1 mg, 0.2 mg. **Tablets, Sublingual:** 27.7 mcg, 55.3 mcg.

ADMINISTRATION/HANDLING

 IV

Reconstitution • For IV infusion, dilute in 10–50 mL 0.9% NaCl (10 mL for children 10 kg or less; 50 mL for adults, children greater than 10 kg).
Rate of administration • Infuse over 15–30 min.
Storage • Refrigerate.

PO
• May give without regard to food.

SQ
• Withdraw dose from vial. Further dilution not required.

Intranasal
• Refrigerate DDAVP Rhinal Tube solution, Stimate nasal spray. • Rhinal Tube solution, Stimate nasal spray are stable for 3 wks at room temperature. • DDAVP nasal spray is stable at room temperature. • Calibrated catheter (rhinyle) is used to draw up measured quantity of desmopressin; with one end inserted in nose, pt blows on other end to deposit solution deep in nasal cavity. • For infants, young children, obtunded pts, air-filled syringe may be attached to catheter to deposit solution.

INDICATIONS/ROUTES/DOSAGE

Nocturia
Sublingual: ADULTS, ELDERLY: (Females): 27.7 mcg once daily 1 hr before bedtime. **(Males):** 55.3 mcg once daily 1 hr before bedtime.

Primary Nocturnal Enuresis
PO: CHILDREN 6 YRS AND OLDER: 0.2 mg once before bedtime. May titrate as needed up to a maximum of 0.6 mg/day.

Central Cranial Diabetes Insipidus
◄ **ALERT** ► Fluid restriction should be observed.
PO: ADULTS, ELDERLY: Initially, 0.05–0.2 mg once daily at bedtime. Adjust bedtime dosage in 0.05-mg increments. Assess need for daytime dose based on daytime polyuria. **Maintenance:** 0.1–0.8 mg/day in 2–3 equally divided doses. Maximum: 1.2 mg/day. **CHILDREN 4 YRS AND OLDER, ADOLESCENTS:** Initially, 0.05 mg twice daily. Titrate to desired response. **Daily range:** 0.1–0.8 mg/day in 2–3 divided doses.
IV, SQ: ADULTS, ELDERLY: 0.25–1 mcg q12–24h. **CHILDREN 12 YRS AND OLDER:** 2–4 mcg/day in 2 divided doses or one-tenth of maintenance intranasal dose.
Intranasal: *(Use 100 mcg/mL concentration):* **ADULTS, ELDERLY, CHILDREN OLDER THAN 12 YRS:** 5–40 mcg (0.1–0.4

mL) in 1–3 doses/day. **Usual dose:** 10 mcg 2 times/day. **CHILDREN 3 MOS–12 YRS**: Initially, 10 mcg once daily into one nostril. May titrate up to 30 mcg once daily (or 30 mcg divided into 2 daily doses, usually with 20 mcg given in the morning and 10 mcg given at nighttime).

Hemophilia A, Von Willebrand's Disease (Type I)
Intranasal: *(Use 1.5 mg/mL concentration providing 150 mcg/spray):* **ADULTS, ELDERLY, CHILDREN WEIGHING MORE THAN 50 KG**: 300 mcg; use 1 spray in each nostril. **ADULTS, ELDERLY, CHILDREN WEIGHING 50 KG OR LESS**: 150 mcg as a single spray. Repeat use based on clinical conditions/laboratory work.

Dosage in Renal Impairment
CrCl less than 50 mL/min: Not recommended.

Dosage in Hepatic Impairment
No dose adjustment.

SIDE EFFECTS

Occasional: IV: Pain, redness, swelling at injection site; headache, abdominal cramps, vulvular pain, flushed skin, mild B/P elevation, nausea with high dosages. **Nasal:** Rhinorrhea, nasal congestion, slight B/P elevation.

ADVERSE EFFECTS/TOXIC REACTIONS

Water intoxication, hyponatremia (headache, drowsiness, confusion, decreased urination, rapid weight gain, seizures, coma) may occur in overhydration. Children, elderly pts, infants are esp. at risk.

NURSING CONSIDERATIONS

BASELINE ASSESSMENT
Obtain serum electrolytes, vital signs, urine specific gravity. Check lab values for factor VIII coagulant concentration for hemophilia A, von Willebrand's disease; coagulation profiles.

INTERVENTION/EVALUATION
Check B/P, pulse with IV infusion. Monitor weight, fluid intake; urine volume, urine specific gravity, urine sodium; serum sodium osmolality for diabetes insipidus. Assess factor VIII antigen levels, aPTT, factor VIII activity level for hemophilia.

PATIENT/FAMILY TEACHING
• Avoid overhydration. • Follow guidelines for proper intranasal administration. • Report headache, shortness of breath, heartburn, nausea, abdominal cramps.

deucravacitinib

due-**krav**-a-**sye**-ti-nib
(Sotyktu)
Do not confuse deucravacitinib with upadacitinib or Sotyktu with Sotylize.

◆CLASSIFICATION

PHARMACOTHERAPEUTIC: Tyrosine kinase 2 (TYK2) inhibitor. **CLINICAL:** Antipsoriatic agent.

USES

Treatment of adults with moderate to severe plaque psoriasis who are candidates for systemic therapy or phototherapy.

PRECAUTIONS

Contraindications: Hypersensitivity to deucravacitinib. **Cautions:** Hepatic impairment (not recommended in pts with severe hepatic impairment), conditions predisposing to infection (e.g., diabetes, immunocompromised pts, renal failure, open wounds); chronic opportunistic infections (e.g., herpes virus infection, fungal infections); prior exposure to tuberculosis or use in pts who reside or travel to areas where TB is endemic; history of malignancy. Hepatitis B or C virus infection, rheumatoid arthritis. Concomitant use of live vaccines is not recommended.

ACTION

Binds to and inhibits regulatory domain of TYK2, preventing downstream signaling and activation of Janus kinase (JAK) family, including JAK-STAT pathway. **Therapeutic Effect:** Alters biologic immune response; reduces inflammation of psoriatic lesions.

PHARMACOKINETICS

Widely distributed. Metabolized in liver. Protein binding: 82–90%. Peak plasma concentration: 2–3 hrs. Excreted in feces (26%), urine (13%). Not substantially removed by hemodialysis (5%). **Half-life:** 10 hrs.

⌛ LIFESPAN CONSIDERATIONS

Pregnancy/Lactation: Unknown if distributed in breast milk. **Children:** Safety and efficacy not established. **Elderly:** May have increased risk for adverse effects, serious infections.

INTERACTIONS

DRUG: May decrease therapeutic effect of **vaccines (live), BCG (intravesical).** **HERBAL:** None significant. **FOOD:** None known. **LAB VALUES:** May increase serum ALT, AST, creatine phosphokinase (CPK), triglycerides. May decrease eGFR.

AVAILABILITY (Rx)

🔖 **Tablets:** 6 mg.

ADMINISTRATION/HANDLING

PO
• Give without regard to food. • Administer tablet whole; do not cut or crush. • Tablet cannot be chewed.

INDICATIONS/ROUTES/DOSAGE

◀ **ALERT** ▶ Do not initiate in pts with severe or active infection.

Plaque Psoriasis
PO: ADULTS, ELDERLY: 6 mg once daily.

Dosage in Renal Impairment
No dose adjustment.

Dosage in Hepatic Impairment
Mild to moderate impairment: No dose adjustment. **Severe impairment:** Not recommended.

SIDE EFFECTS

Occasional (16–14%): Mouth ulceration, stomatitis, folliculitis, acne.

ADVERSE EFFECTS/TOXIC REACTIONS

Upper respiratory tract infections (bacterial, viral, unspecified) including nasopharyngitis, pharyngitis, rhinitis, sinusitis, tonsillitis reported in 19% of pts. Rhabdomyolysis, elevated CPK levels were reported. Hypersensitivity reactions including angioedema may occur. May cause viral reactivation of herpes simplex, herpes zoster. May increase risk of serious infections, tuberculosis; new malignancies including lymphomas. Hepatic enzyme elevation greater than 3 times upper limit of normal was reported.

NURSING CONSIDERATIONS

BASELINE ASSESSMENT

Consider completion of all age-appropriate immunizations prior to initiation. Evaluate for active tuberculosis and test for latent infection prior to initiation and periodically during therapy. An induration of 5 mm or greater with tuberculin skin testing should be considered a positive test result when assessing if treatment for latent tuberculosis is necessary. Screen for active infection or chronic opportunistic infections. Question history of hepatic/renal impairment, hepatitis B or C virus infection, herpes viral infection, prior malignancies. Conduct dermatological exam; record characteristics of psoriatic lesions.

INTERVENTION/EVALUATION

Monitor LFT in pts with baseline hepatic impairment. Monitor for hypersensitivity reaction, angioedema, rhabdomyolysis (muscle weakness, myalgia, myopathy decreased urinary output). Obtain CPK level if rhabdomyolysis is suspected. Monitor for symptoms of tuberculosis, including those who tested negative for latent tuberculosis prior to initiation. Monitor for infections (cough, fatigue, fever). If serious infection occurs, interrupt or discontinue treatment and initiate appropriate antimicrobial therapy. Assess skin for improvement of psoriatic lesions.

PATIENT/FAMILY TEACHING

• Treatment may depress your immune system and reduce your ability to fight infection. Report symptoms of infection such as body aches, burning with urination, chills, cough, fatigue, fever. Avoid those with active infection. • Do not receive live vaccines. • Expect frequent tuberculosis screening. • Report travel plans to possible endemic areas. • Rhabdomyolysis, a breakdown of muscle tissue that can result in kidney failure, may occur. Report flank pain, muscle aches, darkened urine, decreased urinary output. • Report liver problems (abdominal pain, bruising, clay-colored stool, amber or dark-colored urine, yellowing of the skin or eyes). • Treatment may cause reactivation of chronic viral infections; new cancers including lymphomas. • Allergic reactions such as swelling of the face, lips, or tongue require immediate medical attention.

dexamethasone

dex-a-**meth**-a-sone
(Dexamethasone Intensol, Maxidex)
Do not confuse dexamethasone with dextroamphetamine, or Maxidex with Maxzide.

FIXED-COMBINATION(S)

Ciprodex Otic: dexamethasone/ciprofloxacin (antibiotic): 0.1%/0.3%.
Dexacidin, Maxitrol: dexamethasone/neomycin/polymyxin (anti-infectives): 0.1%/3.5 mg/10,000 units per g or mL.

◆CLASSIFICATION

PHARMACOTHERAPEUTIC: Glucocorticoid. **CLINICAL:** Anti-inflammatory. Antiemetic.

USES

Used primarily as an anti-inflammatory or immunosuppressant agent in a variety of diseases (e.g., allergic states, edematous states, neoplastic diseases, rheumatic disorders allergic, hematologic, dermatologic, neoplastic, rheumatic, autoimmune, nervous system, renal and respiratory origin). **OFF-LABEL:** Antiemetic, treatment of croup, dexamethasone suppression test (indicator consistent with suicide and/or depression), accelerate fetal lung maturation. Treatment of acute mountain sickness, high-altitude cerebral edema. Asthma (acute exacerbation), COVID-19, migraine (recurrence prevention).

PRECAUTIONS

Contraindications: Hypersensitivity to dexamethasone. Systemic fungal infections. **Cautions:** Thyroid disease, renal/hepatic impairment, cardiovascular disease, diabetes, glaucoma, cataracts, myasthenia gravis, pts at risk for seizures, osteoporosis, post-MI, elderly.

ACTION

Decreases inflammation by suppression of neutrophil migration, decreases production of inflammatory mediators. Reverses increased capillary permeability. Suppresses normal immune response. **Therapeutic Effect:** Decreases inflammation.

PHARMACOKINETICS

Widely distributed. Protein binding: High. Metabolized in liver. Primarily excreted in urine. Minimally removed by hemodialysis. **Half-life:** 3–4.5 hrs.

⌛ LIFESPAN CONSIDERATIONS

Pregnancy/Lactation: Crosses placenta. Distributed in breast milk. **Children:** Prolonged treatment with high-dose therapy may decrease short-term growth rate, cortisol secretion. **Elderly:** Higher risk for developing hypertension, osteoporosis.

INTERACTIONS

DRUG: Amphotericin may increase hypokalemia. **CYP3A4 inducers (e.g., carBAMazepine, phenytoin, rifAMPin)** may decrease concentration/effect. **CYP3A4 inhibitors (e.g., clarithromycin, ketoconazole, ritonavir), macrolide antibiotics** may increase concentration/effect. May decrease therapeutic effects of **vaccines (live). HERBAL: Echinacea** may increase immunosuppressant effect. **FOOD:** Interferes with **calcium** absorption. **LAB VALUES:** May increase serum glucose, lipids, sodium levels. May decrease serum calcium, potassium, thyroxine, WBC.

AVAILABILITY (Rx)

Elixir: 0.5 mg/5 mL. **Injection, Solution:** 4 mg/mL, 10 mg/mL. **Ophthalmic Solution:** 0.1%. **Ophthalmic Suspension:** 0.1%. **Solution, Oral:** 0.5 mg/5 mL. **Solution, Oral Concentrate:** *(Dexamethasone Intensol):* 1 mg/mL. **Tablets:** 0.5 mg, 0.75 mg, 1 mg, 1.5 mg, 2 mg, 4 mg, 6 mg.

ADMINISTRATION/HANDLING

 IV

◀**ALERT**▶ Dexamethasone sodium phosphate may be given by IV push or IV infusion. Rapid injection may cause genital burning sensation in females.
• For IV push, give over 1–4 min if dose is less than 10 mg. • For IV infusion, mix with 50–100 mL 0.9% NaCl or D₅W and infuse over 15–30 min. • For neonates, solution must be preservative free. • IV solution must be used within 24 hrs.

IM
• Give deep IM, preferably in gluteus maximus.

PO
• Give with milk, food (to decrease GI effect).

Ophthalmic Solution, Suspension
• Place gloved finger on lower eyelid and pull out until a pocket is formed between eye and lower lid. • Place prescribed number of drops or 1/4 to 1/2 inch ointment into pocket. • Instruct pt to close eye gently for 1–2 min (so that medication will not be squeezed out of the sac). • Instruct pt to apply digital pressure to lacrimal sac at inner canthus for 1–2 min to minimize systemic absorption.

⚕ IV COMPATIBILITIES

Dexmedetomidine, heparin, potassium chloride, propofol.

INDICATIONS/ROUTES/DOSAGE

Usual Dosage Range
PO, IM, IV: ADULTS, ELDERLY: 4–20 mg/day as a single dose or in 2–4 divided doses. **High dose:** 0.4–0.8 mg/kg/day (usually not exceeding 40 mg/day).

Usual Ophthalmic Dosage, Ocular Inflammatory Conditions
ADULTS, ELDERLY, CHILDREN: *(Solution):* Initially, 1–2 drops q1h while awake and q2h at night for 1 day, then reduce to 3–4 times/day. *(Suspension):* 1–2 drops up to 4–6 times/day.

Dosage in Renal/Hepatic Impairment
No dose adjustment.

SIDE EFFECTS

Frequent: **Inhalation:** Cough, dry mouth, hoarseness, throat irritation. **Intranasal:** Burning, mucosal dryness. **Ophthalmic:** Blurred vision. **Systemic:** Insomnia, facial edema (cushingoid appearance ["moon face"]), moderate abdominal distention, indigestion, increased appetite, nervousness, facial flushing, diaphoresis. **Occasional:** **Inhalation:** Localized fungal infection (thrush). **Intranasal:** Crusting inside nose, epistaxis, sore throat, ulceration of nasal mucosa. **Ophthalmic:**

D

Decreased vision; lacrimation; eye pain; burning, stinging, redness of eyes; nausea; vomiting. **Systemic:** Dizziness, decreased/blurred vision. **Rare: Inhalation:** Increased bronchospasm, esophageal candidiasis. **Intranasal:** Nasal/pharyngeal candidiasis, eye pain. **Systemic:** Generalized allergic reaction (rash, urticaria); pain, redness, swelling at injection site; psychological changes; false sense of well-being; hallucinations; depression.

ADVERSE EFFECTS/TOXIC REACTIONS

Long-term therapy: Muscle wasting (esp. arms, legs), osteoporosis, spontaneous fractures, amenorrhea, cataracts, glaucoma, peptic ulcer disease, HF. **Ophthalmic:** Glaucoma, ocular hypertension, cataracts. **Abrupt withdrawal following long-term therapy:** Severe joint pain, severe headache, anorexia, nausea, fever, rebound inflammation, fatigue, weakness, lethargy, dizziness, orthostatic hypotension.

NURSING CONSIDERATIONS

BASELINE ASSESSMENT

Question for hypersensitivity to any corticosteroids. Obtain baselines for height, weight, B/P, serum glucose, electrolytes. Question medical history as listed in Precautions.

INTERVENTION/EVALUATION

Monitor I&O, daily weight, serum glucose. Assess for edema. Evaluate food tolerance. Report hyperacidity promptly. Check vital signs at least twice daily. Be alert to infection (sore throat, fever, vague symptoms). Monitor serum electrolytes, esp. for hypercalcemia, hypokalemia, paresthesia (esp. lower extremities, nausea/vomiting, irritability). Assess emotional status, ability to sleep. Abrupt withdrawal may cause adrenal insufficiency; taper dose gradually.

PATIENT/FAMILY TEACHING

• Do not change dose/schedule or stop taking drug. • **Must** taper off gradually under medical supervision. • Report fever, sore throat, muscle aches, sudden weight gain, edema, exposure to measles/chickenpox. • Severe stress (serious infection, surgery, trauma) may require increased dosage. • Avoid alcohol, limit caffeine.

---

dexmedetomidine

dex-med-e-**toe**-mye-deen
(Igalmi, Precedex)
Do not confuse Precedex with Percocet or Peridex.

◆CLASSIFICATION

PHARMACOTHERAPEUTIC: Alpha$_2$ agonist. **CLINICAL:** Sedative.

USES

Sedation of initially intubated, mechanically ventilated adults in intensive care setting. Use in nonintubated pts requiring sedation before and/or during surgical and other procedures. **Igalmi:** Acute treatment of adults with agitation associated with schizophrenia or bipolar I or II disorder.

PRECAUTIONS

Contraindications: Hypersensitivity to dexmedetomidine. **Cautions:** Cardiac conduction delay disorders (e.g., AV block), bradycardia, hepatic impairment, hypovolemia, diabetes, hypotension, chronic hypertension, severe ventricular dysfunction, elderly, use of vasodilators or drugs decreasing heart rate.

ACTION

Selective alpha$_2$-adrenergic agonist. Inhibits norepinephrine release. **Therapeutic Effect:** Produces anesthetic, sedative effects.

PHARMACOKINETICS

Protein binding: 94%. Metabolized in liver. Excreted in urine (85%), feces (4%). **Half-life:** 2 hrs.

⏳ LIFESPAN CONSIDERATIONS

Pregnancy/Lactation: Unknown if distributed in breast milk. **Children:** Safety and efficacy not established. **Elderly:** May have increased risk of hypotension.

INTERACTIONS

DRUG: **Sedatives** (e.g., **midazolam**, **LORazepam**), **opioids** (e.g., **fentaNYL**, **morphine**, **HYDROmorphone**), **hypnotics** (e.g., **zolpidem**, **temazepam**) may increase CNS depression. **Antihypertensives** (e.g., **amLODIPine**, **cloNIDine**, **lisinopril**, **valsartan**) may increase risk of hypotension. **Beta blockers** (e.g., **carvedilol**, **metoprolol**), **calcium channel blockers** (e.g., **dilTIAZem**, **verapamil**) may increase risk of bradycardia, hypotension. **QT interval–prolonging medications** (e.g., **amiodarone**, **azithromycin**, **ciprofloxacin**, **haloperidol**, **methadone**, **sotolol**) may increase risk of QT interval prolongation. **Tricyclic antidepressants** (e.g., **amitriptyline**, **doxepin**) may decrease antihypertensive effect. **HERBAL:** **Herbs with hypertensive properties** (e.g., **licorice**, **yohimbe**) **or hypotensive properties** (e.g., **garlic**, **ginger**, **ginkgo biloba**) may alter effects. **FOOD:** None known. **LAB VALUES:** May increase serum alkaline phosphatase, ALT, AST, glucose, potassium. May decrease serum calcium, magnesium; Hgb, Hct, RBC.

AVAILABILITY (Rx)

Injection Solution: 80 mcg/20 mL, 200 mcg/2 mL vials, 4 mcg/mL solutions (50 mL, 100 mL). **Sublingual Film:** *(Igalmi):* 120 mcg, 180 mcg.

ADMINISTRATION/HANDLING

💧 IV

Reconstitution • Visually inspect for particulate matter or discoloration. Solution should appear clear, colorless. • Dilute 2 mL of dexmedetomidine with 48 mL 0.9% NaCl for a final concentration of 4 mcg/mL.

Rate of administration • Individualized, titrated to desired effect. Use controlled infusion pump.

Storage • Store at room temperature.

SL

• May cut film in half for proper dose.
• Place film under tongue or behind lower lip and allow to dissolve. Film cannot be chewed or swallowed. • No eating or drinking for at least 15 min after sublingual or 1 hr after buccal administration.

⚙ IV COMPATIBILITIES

Amiodarone (Cordarone), bumetanide (Bumex), calcium gluconate, magnesium sulfate, norepinephrine, potassium chloride.

INDICATIONS/ROUTES/DOSAGE

ICU Sedation

Note: Loading dose is generally not recommended due to concerns for hemodynamic compromise (e.g., hypertension, hypotension, bradycardia).

IV: ADULTS: Loading dose of 1 mcg/kg over 10 min followed by maintenance infusion of 0.2–1.5 mcg/kg/hr. Titrate by 0.2 mcg/kg/hr q30min to sedation goal or clinical effect. **ELDERLY:** May require decreased dosage.

Agitation (Associated With Schizophrenia, Bipolar Disorder I or II)

SL/Buccal: ADULTS: **(Mild to moderate agitation):** Initially, 120 mcg; optional second and third doses (at least 2 hr apart): 60 mcg. **Maximum total daily dose:** 240 mcg. **(Severe agitation):** Initially, 180 mcg; optional second and third doses (at least 2 hr apart): 90 mcg. **Maximum total daily dose:** 360 mcg. Elderly: Initially, 120 mg. May repeat up to 2 additional doses of 60 mcg given at least 2 hrs apart. **Maximum:** 240 mcg/day.

Dosage in Renal Impairment

No dose adjustment.

Dosage in Hepatic Impairment

SL: Mild to moderate impairment: Initially, 90 mcg for mild to moderate agitation or 120 mcg for severe agitation. May repeat up to 2 additional doses of

---

 Canadian trade name   Non-Crushable Drug   **High** **Alert** High Alert drug

D

60 mcg at least 2 hrs apart (**maximum: 210 mcg** for mild to moderate agitation or 240 mcg for severe agitation). **Severe impairment:** Initially, 60 mcg for mild to moderate agitation or 90 mcg for severe agitation. May repeat up to 2 additional doses of 60 mcg at least 2 hrs apart (**maximum:** 180 mcg for mild to moderate agitation or 210 mcg for severe agitation).

SIDE EFFECTS

Frequent (25%–12%): Hypotension, hypertension. **Occasional (9%–3%):** Nausea, constipation, bradycardia, pyrexia, dry mouth, vomiting, hypovolemia. **Rare (2%–less than 1%):** Agitation, hyperpyrexia, thirst, oliguria, wheezing.

ADVERSE EFFECTS/TOXIC REACTIONS

Significant bradycardia, sinus arrest, cardiac arrest, AV block, SVT, ventricular tachycardia may occur and may be fatal. Transient hypertension was reported during loading doses. Atrial fibrillation, hypoxia, pleural effusion may occur with too-rapid IV infusion. Bradycardia, hypotension may be more pronounced in pts with diabetes, hypovolemia, hypertension, or who are elderly. Acute respiratory distress syndrome (ARDS), respiratory failure, acidosis may occur with prolonged infusion time greater than 24 hrs. When used for ICU sedation, withdrawal symptoms (nausea, vomiting, agitation) may occur after discontinuation. If continuous infusion is used for greater than 24 hrs, tolerance and reduced drug effectiveness may occur.

NURSING CONSIDERATIONS

BASELINE ASSESSMENT

Obtain B/P, heart rate. Recommend continuous cardiac monitoring during use. Assess mental status prior to initiation. Obtain full medication history; screen for medications known to cause hypotension, bradycardia, sedation. Question history of heart block, bradycardia, severe ventricular dysfunction; hepatic impairment.

INTERVENTION/EVALUATION

Assess cardiac monitor for arrhythmia, bradycardia, hypotension. Anticholinergic agents (e.g., glycopyrrolate, atropine) may be effective in treating drug-induced bradycardia. Monitor level of sedation; respiratory rate, rhythm. Monitor ventilator settings. Discontinue once pt is extubated.

PATIENT/FAMILY TEACHING

• B/P, heart will be continuously monitored during infusion. • If infusion is used for more than 6 hrs, agitation, nervousness, headaches may occur for up to 48 hrs. • Report other symptoms that may occur within 48 hrs (abdominal pain, confusion, constipation, dizziness, sweating, weakness, salt cravings, weight loss).

dextroamphetamine and amphetamine

dex-troe-am-**fet**-ah-meen/am-**fet**-ah-meen
(Adderall, Adderall-XR, Mydayis)

■ **BLACK BOX ALERT** ■ High potential for abuse. Due to high risk of abuse, monitor for signs of drug abuse and misuse (e.g., drug-seeking behavior, dependency) at initiation and during treatment. **Do not confuse Adderall with Inderal.**

◆ CLASSIFICATION

PHARMACOTHERAPEUTIC: Amphetamine (Schedule II). **CLINICAL:** CNS stimulant.

USES

Treatment of narcolepsy (immediate-release only); treatment of ADHD.

PRECAUTIONS

Contraindications: Hypersensitivity to dextroamphetamine, amphetamine, or sympathomimetics. Advanced arteriosclerosis, agitated mental states, glaucoma, history of alcohol or drug abuse, hypersensitivity to sympathomimetic amines, hyperthyroidism, moderate to severe hypertension, symptomatic cardiovascular disease, use of MAOIs within 14 days. **Cautions:** Elderly, debilitated pts, history of seizures, mild hypertension; history of drug abuse and misuse, drug-seeking behavior, dependency. Preexisting psychotic or bipolar disorder.

ACTION

Promotes release of primarily dopamine and norepinephrine from storage site in presynaptic nerve terminals. **Therapeutic Effect:** Increases motor activity, mental alertness; decreases drowsiness, fatigue; suppresses appetite.

PHARMACOKINETICS

Widely distributed including CNS. Metabolized in liver. Excreted in urine. Removed by hemodialysis. **Half-life:** 10–13 hrs.

⧗ LIFESPAN CONSIDERATIONS

Pregnancy/Lactation: Distributed in breast milk. **Children:** Safety and efficacy not established in pts younger than 3 yrs. **Elderly:** Age-related cardiovascular, cerebrovascular, hepatic/renal impairment may increase risk of side effects.

INTERACTIONS

DRUG: MAOIs (e.g., phenelzine, selegiline) may prolong, intensify effects. **HERBAL:** None significant. **FOOD:** None known. **LAB VALUES:** May increase plasma corticosteroid.

AVAILABILITY (Rx)

Tablets: *(Adderall)*: 5 mg, 7.5 mg, 10 mg, 12.5 mg, 15 mg, 20 mg, 30 mg.

⧗ **Capsules: *(Extended-Release [Adderall-XR])*:** 5 mg, 10 mg, 15 mg, 20 mg, 25 mg, 30 mg. ***Mydayis:*** 12.5 mg, 25 mg, 37.5 mg, 50 mg.

ADMINISTRATION/HANDLING

PO

• Give immediate-release tablets at least 6 hrs before bedtime to prevent insomnia. • Extended-release capsules should be swallowed whole; do not break, crush, or cut. • Avoid afternoon doses to prevent insomnia. • May open capsules and sprinkle on applesauce. Instruct pt not to chew sprinkled beads; take immediately.

INDICATIONS/ROUTES/DOSAGE

Narcolepsy

PO: ADULTS, CHILDREN OLDER THAN 12 YRS: Initially, 10 mg/day. Increase by 10 mg/day at wkly intervals until therapeutic response is achieved. **Usual range:** 20–60 mg/day given in 1–3 divided doses. **CHILDREN 6–12 YRS:** Initially, 5 mg/day. Increase by 5 mg/day at wkly intervals until therapeutic response is achieved. **Usual range:** 5–60 mg/day given in 1–3 divided doses.

ADHD

ADULTS, ELDERLY: *(Adderall):* Initially, 5 mg 1–2 times/day. May increase by 5- to 10-mg increments in at least wkly intervals. **Maximum:** 40 mg/day in 2–3 divided doses (usual intervals of 4–6 hrs). ***(Adderall-XR):*** Initially, 10–20 mg once daily in the morning. May increase in increments of 10–20 mg by at least wkly intervals. up to 60 mg/day. ***(Mydayis):*** Initially, 12.5 mg once daily in morning. May increase by 12.5 mg no sooner than once wkly. **Maximum:** 50 mg/day. **CHILDREN 13–17 YRS: *(Adderall):*** Initially, 5 mg 1–2 times/day. May increase by 5 mg at wkly intervals. **Maximum:** 40 mg/day in 1–3 divided doses (usual intervals of 4–6 hrs). ***(Adderall-XR):*** Initially, 10 mg once daily in the morning. May increase to 20 mg/day after 1 wk if symptoms are not controlled. May increase up to 60 mg/day. ***(Mydayis):*** Initially, 12.5 mg once daily in morning. May increase by 12.5 mg no sooner than once wkly. **Maximum:** 25 mg/day. **CHILDREN 6–12 YRS: *(Adderall):*** Initially, 5 mg 1–2 times/day. May increase in 5-mg increments at wkly intervals until optimal response is obtained. **Maximum:** 40 mg/day given in 1–3 divided doses (use intervals of 4–6 hrs between additional doses). *(Adderall-XR):* Initially, 5–10 mg once daily in the morning. May increase daily dose in 5- to 10-mg increments at wkly intervals. **Maximum:** 30 mg/day. **CHILDREN 3–5 YRS:** *(Adderall):* Initially, 2.5 mg/day given every morning. May increase daily dose in 2.5-mg increments at wkly intervals until optimal response is obtained. **Maximum:** 40 mg/day given in 1–3 divided doses (use intervals of 4–6 hrs between additional doses). Not recommended in children younger than 3 yrs.

Dosage in Renal/Hepatic Impairment
No dose adjustment.

SIDE EFFECTS
Frequent: Increased motor activity, talkativeness, nervousness, mild euphoria, insomnia. **Occasional:** Headache, chills, dry mouth, GI distress, worsening depression in pts who are clinically depressed, tachycardia, palpitations, chest pain, dizziness, decreased appetite.

ADVERSE EFFECTS/TOXIC REACTIONS
Overdose may produce skin pallor/flushing, arrhythmias, psychosis. Abrupt withdrawal after prolonged use of high doses may produce lethargy (may last for wks). Prolonged administration to children with ADHD may temporarily suppress normal weight/height pattern.

NURSING CONSIDERATIONS

BASELINE ASSESSMENT
Assess attention span, impulse control, interaction with others. Assess risk of drug abuse, misuse, drug-seeking behavior. Obtain baseline B/P. Assess sleep pattern.

INTERVENTION/EVALUATION
Monitor for CNS overstimulation, increase in B/P, growth rate, change in pulse rate, respirations, weight loss. Monitor for misuse, abuse, drug-seeking behavior. **Narcolepsy:** Observe/docu-

ment frequency of narcoleptic episodes. **ADHD:** Observe for improved attention span.

PATIENT/FAMILY TEACHING
• Normal dosage levels may produce tolerance to drug's anorexic mood-elevating effects within a few wks. • Dry mouth may be relieved with sugarless gum, sips of water. • Take early in day. • Do not break, chew, or crush extended-release capsules. • May mask extreme fatigue. • Report pronounced anxiety, dizziness, decreased appetite, dry mouth, new or worsening behavior, chest pain, palpitations. • Avoid alcohol, caffeine.

diazePAM
dye-**az**-e-pam
(Diastat, DiazePAM Intensol, Valium, Valtoco)

■ **BLACK BOX ALERT** ■ Concomitant use of benzodiazepines and opioids may result in profound sedation, respiratory depression, and death. Reserve for pts for whom alternative treatment options are inadequate. Due to high risk of abuse, monitor for symptoms of drug abuse and misuse (drug-seeking behavior, dependency). Continued use may lead to clinically significant physical dependence.
Do not confuse diazePAM with diazoxide, dilTIAZem, Ditropan, or LORazepam, or Valium with Valcyte.

◆CLASSIFICATION
PHARMACOTHERAPEUTIC: Benzodiazepine (Schedule IV). **CLINICAL:** Antianxiety, skeletal muscle relaxant, anticonvulsant.

USES
Alcohol withdrawal syndrome: Symptomatic relief of acute agitation, tremor, impending delirium, delirium tremens,

hallucinations. **Anxiety:** Short-term relief of severe anxiety symptoms. Management of anxiety disorders. **Muscle Spasms:** Adjunct for relief of skeletal muscle spasms. **Seizures:** Adjunct for convulsive disorders, status epilepticus. **OFF-LABEL:** Neuroleptic malignant syndrome, serotonin syndrome, opioid withdrawal, vertigo (acute episodes).

PRECAUTIONS

Contraindications: Hypersensitivity to diazepam. Acute narrow-angle glaucoma, untreated open-angle glaucoma, severe respiratory depression, severe hepatic insufficiency, sleep apnea syndrome, myasthenia gravis. Children younger than 6 mos (oral). **Cautions:** Pts receiving other CNS depressants or psychoactive agents, depression, history of drug and alcohol abuse, renal/hepatic impairment, respiratory disease, impaired gag reflex, concurrent use of strong CYP3A4 inhibitors or inducers.

ACTION

Depresses all levels of CNS by enhancing action of gamma-aminobutyric acid (GABA), a major inhibitory neurotransmitter in the brain. **Therapeutic Effect:** Produces anxiolytic effect, elevates seizure threshold, produces skeletal muscle relaxation.

PHARMACOKINETICS

Widely distributed. Protein binding: 98%. Excreted in urine. Minimally removed by hemodialysis. **Half-life:** 20–70 hrs (increased in hepatic dysfunction, elderly).

⧗ LIFESPAN CONSIDERATIONS

Pregnancy/Lactation: Crosses placenta. Distributed in breast milk. May increase risk of fetal abnormalities if administered during first trimester of pregnancy. Chronic ingestion during pregnancy may produce withdrawal symptoms, CNS depression in neonates. **Children/Elderly:** Use small initial doses with gradual increases to avoid ataxia, excessive sedation. Elderly at

increased risk of impaired cognition, delirium, falls, fractures.

INTERACTIONS

DRUG: Alcohol, CNS depressants (e.g., gabapentin, morphine, zolpidem) may increase CNS depression. **CYP3A4 inducers (e.g., carBAMazepine, rifAMPin)** may decrease concentration. **CYP3A4 inhibitors (e.g., itraconazole, ketoconazole)** may increase concentration/effect. May increase concentration/effects of **OLANZapine. HERBAL:** Herbals with sedative properties (e.g., chamomile, kava kava, valerian) may increase CNS depression. **FOOD:** None significant. **LAB VALUES:** None significant. **Therapeutic serum level:** 0.5–2 mcg/mL; **toxic serum level:** greater than 3 mcg/mL.

AVAILABILITY (Rx)

Injection, Solution: 5 mg/mL. **Nasal:** 5 mg/0.1 mL, 7.5 mg/0.1 mL, 10 mg/0.1 mL. **Oral Concentrate:** *(DiazePAM Intensol):* 5 mg/mL. **Oral Solution:** 5 mg/5 mL. **Rectal Gel:** *(Diastat):* 2.5 mg, 10 mg, 20 mg. **Tablet:** *(Valium):* 2 mg, 5 mg, 10 mg.

ADMINISTRATION/HANDLING

 IV

Rate of administration • Give by IV push into tubing of flowing IV solution as close as possible to vein insertion point. • Administer directly into large vein (reduces risk of thrombosis/phlebitis). Do not use small veins (e.g., wrist/dorsum of hand). • Administer IV at rate not exceeding 5 mg/min for adults. For children, give 1–2 mg/min (too-rapid IV may result in hypotension, respiratory depression). • Monitor respirations q5–15 min for 2 hrs.

Storage • Store at room temperature.

Intranasal
• Do not test or prime before use.
• Administer one spray into one nostril.

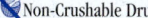

IM

• Injection may be painful. Inject deeply into large muscle mass.

PO

• Give without regard to food. • Dilute oral concentrate with water, juice, carbonated beverages; may be mixed in semisolid food (applesauce, pudding).

Gel

• Insert rectal tip and gently push plunger over 3 sec. Remove tip after 3 additional sec. • Buttocks should be held together for 3 sec after removal.

▨ IV INCOMPATIBILITIES

Acetaminophen, dexmedetomidine, heparin, potassium chloride, propofol.

▨ IV COMPATIBILITIES

DOBUTamine, hydromorphone, morphine.

INDICATIONS/ROUTES/DOSAGE

Anxiety (Acute/Severe)

IM, IV, PO: ADULTS: 2–10 mg q3–6hrs PRN up to 40 mg/day based on response and tolerability.

Anxiety Disorders

PO: Initially, 2–5 mg once or twice daily. May gradually increase based on response and tolerability up to 40 mg/day in 2–4 divided doses.

Muscle Spasm, Spasticity/Rigidity

PO: ADULTS: Initially, 2 mg twice daily or 5 mg at bedtime. May gradually increase up to 40–60 mg/day in 3–4 divided doses based on response and tolerability. **ADOLESCENTS, CHILDREN, INFANTS 6 MOS AND OLDER:** Initially, 1–2.5 mg 3–4 times daily. May gradually increase as needed and tolerated.

Alcohol Withdraw

IV, PO: ADULTS: 5–20 mg PRN until appropriate sedation achieved. Dose and frequency determined by severity of withdrawal symptoms.

Status Epilepticus

IV: ADULTS: 5–10 mg as a single dose given at a maximum infusion rate of 5 mg/min. May repeat in 3–5 min if seizures do not subside. **CHILDREN 5 YRS AND OLDER:** 1 mg slow IV q2–5min up to maximum of 10 mg. May repeat in 2–4 hrs if needed. **30 DAYS TO LESS THAN 5 YRS:** 0.2–0.5 mg slow IV q2–5min up to maximum of 5 mg. May repeat in 2–4 hrs if needed.

Acute Active Seizures

IV: ADULTS: 5–10 mg as a single dose. May repeat at 3- to 5-min intervals up to a total dose of 30 mg. **Intranasal:** 0.2 mg/kg as a single dose. May repeat once based on response and tolerability after 4 or more hrs. **Maximum dose:** 2 doses/episode. Do not use for more than 1 episode q5days or more than 5 episodes/mo.

Control of Increased Seizure Activity (Breakthrough Seizures) in Pts With Refractory Epilepsy Who Are on Stable Regimens of Anticonvulsants

Note: Do not use gel for more than 5 episodes/mo or more than 1 episode q5days. **PO: ADULTS, ELDERLY:** 2–10 mg 2–4 times/day.

Rectal gel: ADULTS, CHILDREN 12 YRS AND OLDER: 0.2–0.5 mg/kg; may be repeated in 4–12 hrs. **CHILDREN 6–11 YRS:** 0.3 mg/kg; may be repeated in 4–12 hrs. **Maximum:** 20 mg. **CHILDREN 2–5 YRS:** 0.5 mg/kg; may be repeated in 4–12 hrs. **Maximum:** 20 mg.

Dosage in Renal Impairment

Use caution.

Dosage in Hepatic Impairment

Use caution. Oral tablets contraindicated in severe hepatic impairment.

SIDE EFFECTS

Frequent: Pain with IM injection, drowsiness, fatigue, ataxia. **Occasional:** Slurred speech, orthostatic hypotension, headache, hypoactivity, constipation, nausea, blurred vision. **Rare:** Paradoxical CNS reactions   (hyperactivity/nervousness in children, excitement/restlessness in elderly/debilitated pts) generally noted during first 2 wks of therapy, particularly in presence of uncontrolled pain.

ADVERSE EFFECTS/TOXIC REACTIONS

IV route may produce pain, swelling, thrombophlebitis, carpal tunnel syndrome. Abrupt or too-rapid withdrawal may result in pronounced restlessness, irritability, insomnia, hand tremor, abdominal/muscle cramps, diaphoresis, vomiting, seizures. Abrupt withdrawal in pts with epilepsy may produce increase in frequency/severity of seizures. Overdose results in drowsiness, confusion, diminished reflexes, CNS depression, coma. **Antidote:** Flumazenil (see Appendix for dosage).

NURSING CONSIDERATIONS

BASELINE ASSESSMENT

Assess B/P, pulse, respirations immediately before administration. Assess risk of drug abuse, misuse, drug-seeking behavior. **Anxiety:** Assess autonomic response (cold, clammy hands; diaphoresis), motor response (agitation, trembling, tension). **Musculoskeletal spasm:** Record onset, type, location, duration of pain. Check for immobility, stiffness, swelling. **Seizures:** Review history of seizure disorder (length, intensity, frequency, duration, LOC). Observe frequently for recurrence of seizure activity. Assess for potential of abuse/misuse (e.g., drug-seeking behavior, mental health conditions, history of substance abuse).

INTERVENTION/EVALUATION

Monitor heart rate, respiratory rate, B/P, mental status. Assess children, elderly for paradoxical reaction, particularly during early therapy. Evaluate for therapeutic response (decrease in intensity/frequency of seizures; calm facial expression, decreased restlessness; decreased intensity of skeletal muscle pain). Screen for misuse, abuse, drug-seeking behavior. **Therapeutic**

serum level: 0.5–2 mcg/mL; **toxic serum level:** greater than 3 mcg/mL.

PATIENT/FAMILY TEACHING

• Avoid alcohol. • Limit caffeine. • May cause drowsiness; avoid tasks that require alertness, motor skills until response to drug is established. • May be habit forming. • Avoid abrupt discontinuation after prolonged use.

diclofenac

dye-**kloe**-fen-ak
(Cambia, Flector, Lofena, Voltaren Gel, Zipsor, Zorvolex)

■ **BLACK BOX ALERT** ■ Increased risk of serious cardiovascular thrombotic events, including myocardial infarction, CVA. Increased risk of severe GI reactions, including ulceration, bleeding, perforation of stomach, intestines. Contraindicated for treatment of perioperative pain in setting of CABG surgery.

Do not confuse diclofenac with Diflucan or Duphalac, or Voltaren with traMADol, Ultram, or Verelan.

FIXED-COMBINATION(S)

Arthrotec: diclofenac/miSOPROStol (an antisecretory gastric protectant): 50 mg/200 mcg, 75 mg/200 mcg.

◆CLASSIFICATION

PHARMACOTHERAPEUTIC: NSAID (nonselective). **CLINICAL:** Analgesic, anti-inflammatory.

USES

Ankylosing spondylitis: Acute or long-term use for relief of signs and symptoms of ankylosing spondylitis. **Dysmenorrhea:** Treatment of primary dysmenorrhea. **Migraine (acute attacks):** Treatment of migraine attacks with or without aura in adults. **Osteoarthritis/**

rheumatoid arthritis: Relief of signs and symptoms of osteoarthritis, rheumatoid arthritis. **Acute pain:** Treatment of mild to moderate acute pain in pts 12 yrs of age and older and adults (Zipsor) and adults (Zorvolex). **Gel (Voltaren):** Relief of pain of osteoarthritis of joints amenable to topical treatment, (e.g., knees, hands). **OFF-LABEL:** Treatment of gout (acute flares). Treatment of juvenile idiopathic arthritis.

PRECAUTIONS

Contraindications: Hypersensitivity to diclofenac. Pts experiencing asthma, urticaria after taking aspirin, other NSAIDs. Pts with moderate to severe renal impairment in perioperative period who are at risk for volume depletion (injection only); perioperative pain in setting of CABG surgery. **Cautions:** HF, hypertension, renal/hepatic impairment, hepatic porphyria, history of GI disease (e.g., bleeding, ulcers), concomitant use of aspirin or anticoagulants, elderly, debilitated pts.

ACTION

Reversibly inhibits cyclo-oxygenase-1 and -2 (COX-1 and COX-2) enzymes, resulting in decreased formation of prostaglandin precursors. **Therapeutic Effect:** Produces analgesic, antipyretic, anti-inflammatory effects.

PHARMACOKINETICS

Route	Onset	Peak	Duration
PO	30 min	2–3 hrs	Up to 8 hrs

Widely distributed. Protein binding: Greater than 99%. Metabolized in liver. Primarily excreted in urine. Minimally removed by hemodialysis. **Half-life:** 1.2–2 hrs.

⏳ LIFESPAN CONSIDERATIONS

Pregnancy/Lactation: Crosses placenta. Unknown if distributed in breast milk. Avoid use during third trimester (may adversely affect fetal cardiovascular system: premature closure of ductus arteriosus). **Children:** Safety and efficacy not established in pts younger than 12 yrs. **Elderly:** GI bleeding, ulceration more likely to cause serious adverse effects. Age-related renal impairment may increase risk of hepatic/renal toxicity; reduced dosage recommended.

INTERACTIONS

DRUG: Aspirin, NSAIDs (e.g., ibuprofen, naproxen) may increase risk of GI side effects/bleeding. May increase **cycloSPORINE** concentration/toxicity. **HERBAL: Herbals with anticoagulant/antiplatelet activity (e.g., garlic, ginger, ginkgo biloba)** may increase adverse effects. **FOOD:** None known. **LAB VALUES:** May increase urine protein, serum BUN, alkaline phosphatase, creatinine, LDH, potassium, ALT, AST. May decrease serum uric acid.

AVAILABILITY (Rx)

Transdermal Patch: *(Flector):* 1.3%. **Transdermal Gel:** *(Voltaren):* 1%. **Capsules:** *(Zipsor):* 25 mg. *(Zorvolex):* 18 mg, 35 mg. **Oral Solution:** *(Cambia):* 50-mg packets. **Tablets:** *(Immediate-Release):* 50 mg.

🔖 **Tablets:** *(Delayed-Release):* 25 mg, 50 mg, 75 mg. 🔖 **Tablets:** *(Extended-Release):* 100 mg.

ADMINISTRATION/HANDLING

PO
• Do not break, crush, dissolve, or divide enteric-coated tablets. • May give with food, milk, antacids if GI distress occurs. • *(Cambia):* Mix one packet in 1–2 oz water, stir well, and instruct pt to drink immediately.

Transdermal Patch
• Apply to intact skin; avoid contact with eyes. • Do not wear when bathing/showering. • Wash hands after handling.

INDICATIONS/ROUTES/DOSAGE

Osteoarthritis
PO: ADULTS, ELDERLY: 100–150 mg/day in 2–4 divided doses for immediate-release and delayed-release or once daily

for extended-release. *(Zorvolex):* 35 mg 3 times/day.

Rheumatoid Arthritis (RA)
PO: ADULTS, ELDERLY: 100 mg/day in 2–4 divided doses for immediate-release and delayed-release once or twice daily for extended-release. **Maximum:** 200 mg/day.

Ankylosing Spondylitis
PO: ADULTS, ELDERLY: 100–150 mg/day in divided doses (may choose immediate-release [given in 2–4 divided doses], delayed-release [given in 2–4 divided doses], once or extended-release [given once daily]). **Maximum:** 150 mg/day

Acute Pain
PO: ADULTS, ELDERLY: 100–150 mg/day in divided doses (may choose immediate-release [given in 2–4 divided doses] or delayed-release [given in 2–4 divided doses] or extended-release [given once daily]). May give 100 mg as an initial loading dose followed by a maintenance dose. **Maximum:** (after day 1): 150 mg/day. *(Zorvolex):* 35 mg 3 times/day. **Maximum:** 105 mg/day. *(Zipsor):* **CHILDREN 12 YRS AND OLDER:** 25 mg 4 times/day.

Dysmenorrhea
Note: Begin at onset of menses or 1–2 days prior to onset of menses for severe symptoms. Usual duration: 1–5 days. **PO: ADULTS:** 150 mg/day in divided doses (may choose immediate-release [given in 2-4 divided doses] or delayed-release [given in 2–4 divided doses]). May give 75–100 mg as an initial loading dose followed by a maintenance dose. **Maximum:** (after day 1): 150 mg/day.

Migraine (Oral Solution or Immediate-Release Tablet)
PO: ADULTS, ELDERLY: 50–100 mg once.

Dosage in Renal Impairment
Not recommended in severe impairment.

Dosage in Hepatic Impairment
May require dose adjustment. Use caution.

SIDE EFFECTS
Frequent (9%–4%): PO: Headache, abdominal cramps, constipation, diarrhea, nausea, dyspepsia. **Ophthalmic:** Burning, stinging on instillation, ocular discomfort. **Occasional (3%–1%): PO:** Flatulence, dizziness, epigastric pain. **Ophthalmic:** Ocular itching, tearing. **Rare (less than 1%): PO:** Rash, peripheral edema, fluid retention, visual disturbances, vomiting, drowsiness.

ADVERSE EFFECTS/TOXIC REACTIONS
Overdose may result in acute renal failure. In pts treated chronically, peptic ulcer, GI bleeding, gastritis, severe hepatic reaction (jaundice), nephrotoxicity (hematuria, dysuria, proteinuria), severe hypersensitivity reaction (bronchospasm, angioedema) occur rarely.

NURSING CONSIDERATIONS

BASELINE ASSESSMENT
Obtain B/P. **Anti-inflammatory:** Assess onset, type, location, duration of pain, inflammation. Inspect appearance of affected joints for immobility, deformities, skin condition.

INTERVENTION/EVALUATION
Monitor CBC, renal function, LFT, urine output, occult blood test, B/P. Monitor for headache, dyspepsia. Monitor daily pattern of bowel activity, stool consistency. Assess for therapeutic response: relief of pain, stiffness, swelling; increased joint mobility; reduced joint tenderness; improved grip strength.

PATIENT/FAMILY TEACHING
• Swallow tablets whole; do not chew, crush, dissolve, or divide. • Avoid aspirin, alcohol during therapy (increases risk of GI bleeding). • If GI upset occurs, take with food, milk. • Report skin rash, itching, weight gain, changes in vision, black stools, bleeding, jaun-

dice, upper quadrant pain, persistent headache. • **Ophthalmic:** Do not use hydrogel soft contact lenses. • **Topical:** Avoid exposure to sunlight, sunlamps. • Report rash.

dilTIAZem

dil-**tye**-a-zem
(Apo-Diltiaz , <u>Cardizem</u>, Cardizem CD, Cardizem LA, Cartia XT, Dilt-XR, Matzim LA, Taztia XT, Tiadylt ER, Tiazac)
Do not confuse Cardizem with Cardene or Cardene SR, Cartia XT with Procardia XL, dilTIAZem with Calan, diazePAM, or Dilantin, or Tiazac with Ziac.

FIXED-COMBINATION(S)

Teczem: dilTIAZem/enalapril (ACE inhibitor): 180 mg/5 mg.

◆CLASSIFICATION

PHARMACOTHERAPEUTIC: Calcium channel blocker. Non-dihydropyridine. **CLINICAL:** Antianginal, antihypertensive, class IV antiarrhythmic.

USES

PO: Treatment of angina due to coronary artery spasm (Prinzmetal's variant angina), chronic stable angina (effort-associated angina). Treatment of hypertension. **Parenteral:** Control of ventricular rate in atrial fibrillation/flutter. Conversion of paroxysmal supraventricular tachycardia (PSVT) to normal sinus rhythm. **OFF-LABEL:** Nonsustained ventricular tachycardia/ventricular premature beats, pulmonary arterial hypertension.

PRECAUTIONS

Contraindications: PO: Hypersensitivity to dilTIAZem, acute MI, pulmonary congestion, second- or third-degree AV block (except in presence of pacemaker), severe hypotension (less than 90 mm Hg, systolic), sick sinus syndrome (except in presence of pacemaker). **IV:** Hypersensitivity to dilTIAZem. Sick sinus syndrome or second- or third-degree block (except with functioning pacemaker), cardiogenic shock, administration of IV beta blocker within several hours, atrial fibrillation/flutter associated with accessory bypass tract, severe hypotension, ventricular tachycardia. **Cautions:** Renal/hepatic impairment, HF, concurrent use with beta blocker, hypertrophic obstructive cardiomyopathy.

ACTION

Inhibits calcium movement across cardiac, vascular smooth-muscle cell membranes (causes dilation of coronary arteries, peripheral arteries, arterioles) during depolarization. **Therapeutic Effect:** Relaxes coronary vascular smooth muscle, and coronary vasodilation increases myocardial oxygen delivery in pts with vasospastic angina.

PHARMACOKINETICS

Route	Onset	Peak	Duration
PO	0.5–1 hr	N/A	N/A
PO (extended-release)	2–3 hrs	N/A	N/A
IV	3 min	N/A	N/A

Widely distributed. Protein binding: 70%–80%. Primarily excreted in urine. Not removed by hemodialysis. **Half-life:** 3–8 hrs.

⧖ LIFESPAN CONSIDERATIONS

Pregnancy/Lactation: Distributed in breast milk. **Children:** No age-related precautions noted. **Elderly:** Age-related renal impairment may require dosage adjustment.

INTERACTIONS

DRUG: Beta blockers (e.g., atenolol, carvedilol, metoprolol) may increase effects; risk of bradycardia.

Strong CYP3A4 inhibitors (e.g., clarithromycin, ketoconazole, ritonavir) may increase concentration/effect. Strong CYP3A4 inducers (e.g., carBAMazepine, phenytoin, rifAMPin) may decrease concentration/effect. May increase concentration/effects of **bosutinib, budesonide, statins (e.g., atorvastatin, simvastatin). HERBAL:** Ephedra, St. John's wort, yohimbe may decrease concentration/effect. **Herbals with hypotensive properties (e.g., garlic, ginger, ginkgo biloba)** may increase effect. **FOOD: Grapefruit products** may increase concentration/effect. **LAB VALUES:** ECG: May increase PR interval.

AVAILABILITY (Rx)

Injection, Solution: 25 mg/5 mL, 50 mg/10 mL, 125 mg/25 mL. **Tablets, Immediate-Release:** 30 mg, 60 mg, 90 mg, 120 mg. **Capsules, Extended-Release, 24 Hour:** 120 mg, 180 mg, 240 mg, 300 mg, 360 mg, 420 mg. **Capsules, Extended-Release, 12 Hour:** 60 mg, 90 mg, 120 mg. **Tablets, Extended-Release, 24 Hour:** 120 mg, 180 mg, 240 mg, 300 mg, 360 mg, 420 mg.

ADMINISTRATION/HANDLING

IV

Reconstitution • Add 125 mg to 100 mL D$_5$W, 0.9% NaCl to provide concentration of 1 mg/mL.
Rate of administration • Infuse per dilution/rate chart provided by manufacturer.
Storage • Refrigerate vials. • After dilution, stable for 24 hrs.

PO

• Give immediate-release tablets before meals and at bedtime. • Tablets may be crushed. • Do not break, crush, dissolve, or divide sustained-release capsules or extended-release capsules or tablets. • Taztia XT capsules may be opened and mixed with applesauce; follow with glass of water. • Cardizem CD, Cardizem LA, Cartia XT, Matzim LA may be given

without regard to food. • Dilt-XR to be given on empty stomach.

IV INCOMPATIBILITIES

Insulin.

IV COMPATIBILITIES

Dexmedetomidine, norepinephrine, potassium chloride, potassium phosphate.

INDICATIONS/ROUTES/DOSAGE

Angina

PO: *(Immediate-Release):* **ADULTS, ELDERLY:** Initially, 30 mg 4 times/day. May increase as needed at 1- to 2-day intervals. **Range:** 240–360 mg/day in 3–4 divided doses.
PO: *(24h once daily):* **ADULTS, ELDERLY:** Initially, 120–180 mg once daily. May increase at 7- to 14-day intervals. **Range:** 240–360 mg.

Hypertension

PO: *(Extended-Release Capsule [once-daily dosing]):* Initially, 120–240 mg/day. May increase at 7- to 14-day intervals. Usual dose: 120–360 mg/day.
PO: *(Extended-Release Capsule [twice-daily dosing]):* **ADULTS, ELDERLY:** Initially, 60–120 mg twice daily. May increase at 7- to 14-day intervals. **Maintenance:** 240–360 mg/day in 2 divided doses.

Temporary Control of Rapid Ventricular Rate in Atrial Fibrillation/Flutter; Rapid Conversion of Paroxysmal Supraventricular Tachycardia to Normal Sinus Rhythm

IV bolus: ADULTS, ELDERLY: Initially, 0.25 mg/kg (average dose: 20 mg) actual body weight over 2 min. May repeat in 15 min at dose of 0.35 mg/kg (**average dose:** 25 mg) actual body weight. Subsequent doses individualized.
IV infusion: ADULTS, ELDERLY: After initial bolus injection, may begin infusion at 5–10 mg/hr; may increase by 5 mg/hr up to a maximum of 15 mg/hr. Continuous infusion longer than 24 hrs or infusion rate greater than 15 mg/hr are not recommended. Attempt conversion to PO therapy as soon as possible.

Dosage in Renal/Hepatic Impairment
Use with caution.

SIDE EFFECTS

Frequent (10%–5%): Peripheral edema, dizziness, light-headedness, headache, bradycardia, asthenia. **Occasional (5%–2%):** Nausea, constipation, flushing, ECG changes. **Rare (less than 2%):** Rash, micturition disorder (polyuria, nocturia, dysuria, frequency of urination), abdominal discomfort, drowsiness.

ADVERSE EFFECTS/TOXIC REACTIONS

Abrupt withdrawal may increase frequency, duration of angina, HF; second- or third-degree AV block occurs rarely. Overdose produces nausea, drowsiness, confusion, slurred speech, profound bradycardia. **Antidote:** Glucagon, insulin drip with continuous calcium infusion (see Appendix for dosage).

NURSING CONSIDERATIONS

BASELINE ASSESSMENT

Record onset, type (sharp, dull, squeezing), radiation, location, intensity, duration of anginal pain, precipitating factors (exertion, emotional stress). Assess baseline renal/hepatic function tests. Assess B/P, apical pulse immediately before drug is administered. Obtain baseline ECG in pts with history of arrhythmia.

INTERVENTION/EVALUATION

Assist with ambulation if dizziness occurs. Assess for peripheral edema. Monitor pulse rate for bradycardia. Assess B/P, renal function, LFT, ECG with IV therapy. Question for asthenia, headache.

PATIENT/FAMILY TEACHING

• Do not abruptly discontinue medication. • Compliance with therapy regimen is essential to control anginal pain. • To avoid postural dizziness, go from lying to standing slowly. • Avoid tasks that require alertness, motor skills until response to drug is established. • Report palpitations, shortness of breath, pronounced dizziness, nausea, constipation. • Avoid alcohol (may increase risk of hypotension or vasodilation).

---

dimethyl fumarate

dye-**meth**-il-**fue**-ma-rate
(Tecfidera)
Do not confuse dimethyl fumarate with dimethyl sulfoxide or monomethyl fumarate.

◆CLASSIFICATION

PHARMACOTHERAPEUTIC: Fumaric acid agent. **CLINICAL:** Multiple sclerosis agent. Immunomodulator.

USES

Treatment of relapsing-remitting multiple sclerosis including clinically isolated syndrome, relapsing-remitting disease, and active secondary progressive disease.

PRECAUTIONS

Contraindications: Hypersensitivity to dimethyl fumarate. **Cautions:** Hepatic impairment (may increase hepatic transaminases), lymphopenia (may decrease lymphocyte count).

ACTION

Exact mechanism of action unknown. May include anti-inflammatory action and cytoprotective properties. **Therapeutic Effect:** Modifies disease progression.

PHARMACOKINETICS

Undergoes rapid hydrolysis into active metabolite, monomethyl fumarate. Peak concentration: 2–212 hrs. Protein binding: 27%–45%. Extensively metabolized by esterases. Primarily eliminated as exhaled carbon dioxide (60%). **Half-life:** 1 hr.

⌛ LIFESPAN CONSIDERATIONS

Pregnancy/Lactation: Unknown if distributed in breast milk. **Children:** Safety and efficacy not established. **Elderly:** No age-related precautions noted.

INTERACTIONS

DRUG: May decrease therapeutic effects; increase adverse effects of **vaccines (live)**. **HERBAL:** None known. **FOOD:** None significant. **LAB VALUES:** May decrease lymphocytes. May increase serum ALT, AST; eosinophils; urine albumin.

AVAILABILITY (Rx)

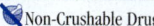 **Capsules, Delayed-Release:** 120 mg, 240 mg.

ADMINISTRATION/HANDLING

PO
• Give capsule whole; do not break, crush, dissolve, or divide. • May give without regard to food. May give with food to decrease flushing reaction and GI effects. • Protect from light.

INDICATIONS/ROUTES/DOSAGE

Relapsing-Remitting Multiple Sclerosis
PO: ADULTS/ELDERLY: Initially, 120 mg twice daily for 7 days. Then, increase to 240 mg twice daily.

Dosage in Renal/Hepatic Impairment
No dose adjustment.

SIDE EFFECTS

Frequent (40%): Flushing. **Occasional (18%–5%):** Abdominal pain, diarrhea, nausea, vomiting, dyspepsia, pruritus, rash, erythema.

ADVERSE EFFECTS/TOXIC REACTIONS

Lymphopenia may increase risk for infection. Severe flushing may lead to non-compliance of therapy.

NURSING CONSIDERATIONS

BASELINE ASSESSMENT

Obtain CBC, CMP, urine pregnancy if applicable. Assess hydration status (urine output, skin turgor). Question history of hepatic impairment, lymphopenia. Assess baseline symptoms of MS (e.g., bladder/bowel dysfunction, cognitive impairment, depression, dysphagia, fatigue, gait disorder, numbness/

tingling, pain, seizures, spasticity, tremors, weakness). Screen for active infection.

INTERVENTION/EVALUATION

Monitor CBC, LFT. Encourage PO intake. Offer antiemetics for nausea, vomiting. Question any episodes of noncompliance due to flushing, GI symptoms. Monitor for infectious process (fever, malaise, chills, body aches, cough). Conduct neurologic assessment. Assess for symptomatic improvement of MS.

PATIENT/FAMILY TEACHING

• Abdominal pain, diarrhea, nausea, and flushing are common. Side effects may decrease over time. • Take with meals to decrease flushing reaction. • Swallow capsule whole; do not chew, crush, dissolve, or divide. • Two dosage strengths will be provided for starting dose and maintenance dose. • Report any yellowing of skin or eyes, upper abdominal pain, bruising, dark-colored urine, fever, body aches, cough, dehydration.

diphenhydrAMINE

dye-fen-**hye**-dra-meen
(Banophen, Benadryl, Diphen)
Do not confuse Benadryl with benazepril, Bentyl, or Benylin, or diphenhydrAMINE with desipramine, dicyclomine, or dimenhyDRINATE.

FIXED-COMBINATION(S)

Advil PM: diphenhydramine/ibuprofen (NSAID): 38 mg/200 mg. With calamine, an astringent, and camphor, a counterirritant **(Caladryl).**

◆CLASSIFICATION

PHARMACOTHERAPEUTIC: Histamine-1 antagonist, first generation. **CLINICAL:** Antihistamine, anticholinergic, antipruritic, antitussive, antiemetic, antidyskinetic.

 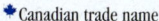

USES

Treatment of allergic reactions, including nasal allergies and allergic dermatoses; prevention/treatment of nausea, vomiting, or vertigo due to motion sickness; antitussive; short-term management of insomnia; adjunct to EPINEPHrine in treatment of anaphylaxis. Topical form used for relief of pruritus from insect bites, skin irritations. **OFF-LABEL:** Allergic angioedema, infusion-related reactions, nausea/vomiting (pregnancy related), acute vertigo.

PRECAUTIONS

Contraindications: Hypersensitivity to diphenhydrAMINE. Neonates or premature infants, breastfeeding. **Cautions:** Narrow-angle glaucoma, stenotic peptic ulcer, prostatic hypertrophy, pyloroduodenal/bladder neck obstruction, asthma, COPD, increased IOP, cardiovascular disease, hyperthyroidism, elderly.

ACTION

Competes with histamine for H-1 receptor site on effector cells in GI tract, blood vessels, respiratory tract. **Therapeutic Effect:** Produces anticholinergic, antipruritic, antitussive, antiemetic, antidyskinetic, sedative effects.

PHARMACOKINETICS

Route	Onset	Peak	Duration
PO	15–30 min	1–4 hrs	4–6 hrs
IV, IM	Less than 15 min	1–4 hrs	4–6 hrs

Widely distributed. Protein binding: 98%–99%. Metabolized in liver. Primarily excreted in urine. **Half-life:** 1–4 hrs. Adults: 7–12 hrs, elderly: 9–18 hrs, children: 4–7 hrs.

⏳ LIFESPAN CONSIDERATIONS

Pregnancy/Lactation: Crosses placenta. Detected in breast milk (may produce irritability in breastfed infants). Increased risk of seizures in neonates, premature infants if used during third trimester of pregnancy. May prohibit lactation. **Children:** Not recommended in newborns, premature infants (increased risk of paradoxical reaction, seizures). **Elderly:** Potentially inappropriate due to potent anticholinergic effects. Increased risk for dizziness, sedation, confusion, hypotension, hyperexcitability.

INTERACTIONS

DRUG: **Alcohol, CNS depressants (e.g., LORazepam, morphine, zolpidem)** may increase CNS depressant effects. **Anticholinergics (e.g., aclidinium, ipratropium, tiotropium, umeclidinium)** may increase anticholinergic effects. **HERBAL:** **Gotu kola, kava kava, valerian** may increase CNS depression. **FOOD:** None known. **LAB VALUES:** May suppress wheal/flare reactions to antigen skin testing unless drug is discontinued 4 days before testing.

AVAILABILITY (OTC)

Capsules: 25 mg, 50 mg. **Cream:** 1%, 2%. **Elixir:** 12.5 mg/5 mL. **Injection Solution:** 50 mg/mL. **Liquid:** 12.5 mg/5 mL. **Tablets:** 25 mg, 50 mg. **Tablets, Chewable:** 12.5 mg.

ADMINISTRATION/HANDLING

 IV

• May be given undiluted. • Give IV injection over at least 1 min. **Maximum rate:** 25 mg/min.

IM

• Give deep IM into large muscle mass.

PO

• Give without regard to food.

▦ IV COMPATIBILITIES

Acetaminophen, dexmedetomidine, granisetron, heparin, ondansetron, potassium chloride, propofol.

INDICATIONS/ROUTES/DOSAGE

Allergic Reaction

PO: **ADULTS, ELDERLY:** 25 mg q4–6h PRN or 50 mg q6–8h PRN. **IM, IV:**

10–50 mg/dose q6hrs PRN. **PO: ADO-
LESCENTS, CHILDREN, INFANTS:** 0.5–1
mg/kg/day q6–8h. **Usual dose: ADOLES-
CENTS:** 25–50 mg. **CHILDREN, INFANTS:**
12.5–25 mg.

Motion Sickness
Note: When used for prophylaxis, give
30 min before motion.
PO: *(Prophylaxis):* **ADULTS, ELDERLY:**
25 mg q4–6h PRN or 50 mg q6–8h
PRN. **ADOLESCENTS:** 12.5–25 mg/dose.
CHILDREN: 0.5–1 mg/kg/day in 3–4
divided doses. **Usual dose:** 12.5–25
mg/dose.
IV/IM: *(Treatment):* **ADULTS, ELDERLY:**
10–50 mg/dose q6h as needed. **INFANTS,
CHILDREN, ADOLESCENTS:** 1.25 mg/kg/
dose q6h. **PO: ADULTS, ELDERLY:** 25
mg q4–6h or 50 mg q6–8h as needed.
INFANTS, CHILDREN, ADOLESCENTS: 5 mg/
kg/day q6–8h as needed. **Usual dose:**
12.5–25 mg. **Maximum:** 50 mg/dose.

Nighttime Sleep Aid
**PO: ADULTS, ELDERLY, CHILDREN 12 YRS
AND OLDER:** 25–50 mg at bedtime.
CHILDREN 2–11 YRS: 0.5–1 mg/kg/dose.
Maximum single dose: 50 mg.

Pruritus
**Topical: ADULTS, ELDERLY, CHILDREN 12
YRS AND OLDER:** Apply 1% or 2% cream
or spray 3–4 times/day. **CHILDREN 2–11
YRS:** Apply 1% cream or spray 3–4
times/day.

Parkinsonism, Dystonic Reaction
PO: ADULTS, ELDERLY: 25–50 mg q4–12h.
Maximum: 300 mg/day. **IM/IV:** 25–50
mg/dose once.

Dosage in Renal/Hepatic Impairment
No dose adjustment.

SIDE EFFECTS
Frequent: Drowsiness, dizziness, muscle
weakness, hypotension, urinary retention, thickening of bronchial secretions,
dry mouth, nose, throat, lips; in elderly:
Sedation, dizziness, hypotension. **Occasional:** Epigastric distress, flushing,
visual/hearing disturbances, paresthesia,
diaphoresis, chills.

ADVERSE EFFECTS/TOXIC REACTIONS
Hypersensitivity reactions (eczema,
pruritus, rash, cardiac disturbances,
photosensitivity) may occur. Overdose
symptoms may vary from CNS depression (sedation, apnea, hypotension,
cardiovascular collapse, death) to severe
paradoxical reactions (hallucinations,
tremors, seizures). Children, infants,
neonates may experience paradoxical reactions (restlessness, insomnia,
euphoria, nervousness, tremors). Overdosage in children may result in hallucinations, seizures, death.

NURSING CONSIDERATIONS

BASELINE ASSESSMENT
If pt is having acute allergic reaction,
obtain history of recently ingested
foods, drugs, environmental exposure, emotional stress. Monitor B/P
rate; depth, rhythm, type of respiration; quality, rate of pulse. Assess lung
sounds for rhonchi, wheezing, rales.

INTERVENTION/EVALUATION
Monitor B/P, esp. in elderly (increased
risk of hypotension). Monitor children
closely for paradoxical reaction. Monitor
for sedation.

PATIENT/FAMILY TEACHING
• Tolerance to antihistaminic effect generally does not occur; tolerance to sedative effect may occur. • Avoid tasks that
require alertness, motor skills until response to drug is established. • Dry
mouth, drowsiness, dizziness may be an
expected response to drug. • Avoid alcohol.

D

diroximel fumarate

dye-**rox**-i-mel **fyoo**-ma-rate
(Vumerity)
**Do not confuse diroximel fuma-
rate with dimethyl fumarate or
monomethyl fumarate.**

◆CLASSIFICATION

PHARMACOTHERAPEUTIC: Fumaric
acid derivative. **CLINICAL:** Multiple
sclerosis agent.

USES

Treatment of relapsing forms of multiple sclerosis (MS) in adults, to include
clinically isolated syndrome, relapsing-
remitting disease, and active secondary
progressive disease.

PRECAUTIONS

Contraindications: Hypersensitivity
reactions to diroximel fumarate or
dimethyl fumarate. Concomitant use with
dimethyl fumarate. **Cautions:** Baseline
lymphopenia, hepatic/renal impairment; conditions predisposing to
infection (e.g., diabetes, renal failure, immunocompromised pts, open
wounds); history of chronic opportunistic infections (esp. fungal/viral infections, tuberculosis).

ACTION

Exact mechanism of action unknown.
May include anti-inflammatory action and
cytoprotective properties via activation
of the nuclear factor (erythroid-derived
2)–like-2 pathway. **Therapeutic
Effect:** Modifies disease progression
of MS.

PHARMACOKINETICS

Undergoes rapid hydrolysis by esterases into active metabolite, monomethyl
fumarate. Protein binding: 27%–45%.
Peak plasma concentration: 2.5–3 hrs.
Primarily eliminated as exhaled carbon
dioxide. **Half-life:** 1 hr.

⧗ LIFESPAN CONSIDERATIONS

Pregnancy/Lactation: Generally not initiated in pts considering a planned pregnancy or during pregnancy. Unknown
if distributed in breast milk. **Children:** Safety and efficacy not established. **Elderly:** Not specified.

INTERACTIONS

DRUG: Alcohol may decrease concen-
tration/effect. **Dimethyl or monomethyl fumarate** may increase
adverse effects. **HERBAL:** None significant. **FOOD: High-fat, high-calorie
meals** may reduce absorption/concen-
tration. **LAB VALUES:** May increase
serum ALT, AST, bilirubin; urine
albumin. May decrease lymphocytes,
eosinophils.

AVAILABILITY (Rx)

🖉 **Capsules, Delayed-Release:** 231 mg.

ADMINISTRATION/HANDLING

PO

• May take with or without food. Avoid
high-fat, high-calorie meals. Meals
should not be more than 700 calories
and contain no more than 30 g of fat.
• Administer capsule whole; do not
crush, open, or sprinkle on food. • Avoid
alcohol at same time of administration.

INDICATIONS/ROUTES/DOSAGE

Multiple Sclerosis (Relapsing)
PO: ADULTS: 231 mg twice daily for
7 days, then increase to a maintenance
dose of 462 mg twice daily.

Dose Modifications
**Unable to tolerate maintenance dose
(GI effects, flushing):** May reduce dose
to 231 mg twice daily for up to 4 wks, then
re-escalate dose to 462 mg twice daily. Consider permanent discontinuation if unable
to tolerate return to maintenance dose.

Hepatotoxicity
Acute hepatic injury: Permanently discontinue if significant hepatic injury occurs.

D

Infections
Bacterial/fungal/viral infections: Consider withholding treatment until infection is resolved.

Lymphopenia
Lymphocyte count less than 500 cells/mm³ for greater than 6 mos: Consider withholding treatment until improved.

Dosage in Renal Impairment
Mild impairment: No dose adjustment. **Moderate to severe impairment:** Not recommended.

Dosage in Hepatic Impairment
Mild to severe impairment: Not specified; use caution.

SIDE EFFECTS

Frequent (40%): Flushing. **Occasional (18%–5%):** Abdominal pain, diarrhea, nausea, vomiting, pruritus, rash, erythema, dyspepsia.

ADVERSE EFFECTS/TOXIC REACTIONS

Hypersensitivity reactions including anaphylaxis, angioedema, dyspnea, urticaria were reported. Progressive multifocal leukoencephalopathy (PML), an opportunistic viral infection of the brain caused by the JC virus, may result in progressive permanent disability and death. Serious herpes zoster infections including disseminated herpes zoster, herpes zoster ophthalmicus, herpes zoster meningoencephalitis, herpes zoster meningomyelitis was reported. Other serious bacterial, fungal, viral infections may occur. Acute hepatic injury with serum aminotransferase greater than 5 times ULN and total bilirubin greater than 2 times ULN was reported. Severe flushing may lead to noncompliance of therapy.

NURSING CONSIDERATIONS

BASELINE ASSESSMENT
Obtain CBC (including lymphocyte count), LFT; pregnancy test in females of reproductive potential. Assess baseline symptoms of MS (e.g., bladder/bowel dysfunction, cognitive impairment, depression, dysphagia, fatigue, gait disorder, numbness/tingling, pain, seizures, spasticity, tremors, weakness). Screen for active infection. Question history of hypersensitivity reactions, hepatic/renal impairment, herpes zoster infection, chronic infection.

INTERVENTION/EVALUATION
Obtain CBC (including lymphocyte count) 6 mos after initiation, then q6–12mos thereafter. Monitor LFT as clinically indicated. Pts with altered mental status, seizures, visual disturbances, generalized or unilateral weakness should be evaluated for herpes zoster meningoencephalitis, herpes zoster meningomyelitis, PML. If herpes zoster infection or other serious infection occurs, initiate treatment as appropriate. To reduce occurrence/severity of flushing, may administer non–enteric-coated aspirin (up to 325 mg) PO 30 min prior to dose. Question for noncompliance due to flushing, GI symptoms. Conduct neurologic assessment. Assess for symptomatic improvement of MS.

PATIENT/FAMILY TEACHING
• Treatment may depress your immune system and reduce your ability to fight infection. Report symptoms of infection such as body aches, burning with urination, chills, cough, fatigue, fever. Avoid those with active infection. Report travel plans to possible endemic areas. • PML, an opportunistic viral infection of the brain, may cause progressive, permanent disabilities or death. Report symptoms of PML or herpes zoster infection of the brain such as confusion, memory loss, paralysis, trouble speaking, vision loss, seizures, weakness. • GI symptoms (e.g., abdominal pain, diarrhea, nausea, vomiting, upset stomach), flushing are common side effects. • Take with meals to decrease flushing reaction. If taken with food, avoid high-fat, high-calorie meal or snack. Do not ingest alcohol with dose. • Report liver problems (abdominal pain, bruising, clay-colored stool, amber- or

D

dark-colored urine, yellowing of the skin or eyes). • Allergic reactions such as difficulty breathing, hives, rash, swelling of the face or tongue, wheezing can happen at any time. If allergic reaction occurs, seek immediate medical attention.

DOBUTamine HIGH ALERT

doe-**bue**-ta-meen
Do not confuse DOBUTamine with DOPamine.

◆ CLASSIFICATION

PHARMACOTHERAPEUTIC: Adrenergic agonist. **CLINICAL:** Cardiac stimulant.

USES

Short-term management of acute cardiac decompensation. **OFF-LABEL:** Inotropic support, stress echocardiography (diagnostic agent).

PRECAUTIONS

Contraindications: Hypersensitivity to dobutamine. Hypertrophic cardiomyopathy with outflow obstruction. **Cautions:** Atrial fibrillation, hypovolemia, post-MI, concurrent use of MAOIs, elderly.

ACTION

Direct-action inotropic agent acting primarily on myocardial $beta_1$-adrenergic receptors. **Therapeutic Effect:** Enhances myocardial contractility, increases heart rate.

PHARMACOKINETICS

Route	Onset	Peak	Duration
IV	1–2 min	10 min	Length of infusion

Metabolized in liver. Primarily excreted in urine. Not removed by hemodialysis. **Half-life:** 2 min.

⧖ LIFESPAN CONSIDERATIONS

Pregnancy/Lactation: Unknown if drug crosses placenta or is distributed in breast milk. **Children/Elderly:** No age-related precautions noted.

INTERACTIONS

DRUG: Sympathomimetics (e.g., norepinephrine, phenylephrine), linezolid may increase effects. **HERBAL:** None significant. **FOOD:** None known. **LAB VALUES:** May decrease serum potassium.

AVAILABILITY (Rx)

Infusion (Ready-to-Use): 1 mg/mL (250 mL), 2 mg/mL (250 mL), 4 mg/mL (250 mL). **Injection Solution:** 12.5-mg/mL vial.

ADMINISTRATION/HANDLING

◀ALERT▶ Correct hypovolemia with volume expanders before DOBUTamine infusion. Pts with atrial fibrillation should be digitalized before infusion. Administer by IV infusion only.

 IV

Reconstitution • Dilute vial in 0.9% NaCl or D_5W to maximum concentration of 5,000 mcg/mL (5 mg/mL).
Rate of administration • Use infusion pump to control flow rate. • Titrate dosage to individual response. • Infiltration causes local inflammatory changes. • Extravasation may cause dermal necrosis.
Storage • Store at room temperature. • Pink discoloration of solution (due to oxidation) does not indicate significant loss of potency if used within recommended time period. • Further diluted solution for infusion is stable for 48 hrs at room temperature, 7 days if refrigerated.

✿ IV COMPATIBILITIES

Calcium chloride, calcium gluconate, dexmedetomidine, diltiazem, dopamine, insulin, nitroglycerin, norepinephrine, potassium chloride, propofol, vasopressin.

INDICATIONS/ROUTES/DOSAGE

◀ALERT▶ Dosage determined by severity of decompensation.

Cardiac Decompensation (Hemodynamic Support)
IV infusion: ADULTS, ELDERLY: Initially, 2–5 mcg/kg/min. **Maintenance:** 2–10

mcg/kg/min titrated to desired response. **Maximum:** 20 mcg/kg/min. **NEONATES, INFANTS, CHILDREN, ADOLESCENTS:** Initially, 0.5–1 mcg/kg/min. Titrate gradually every few minutes until desired response. **Usual range:** 2–20 mcg/kg/minute.

Dosage in Renal/Hepatic Impairment
No dose adjustment.

SIDE EFFECTS

Frequent (greater than 5%): Increased heart rate, B/P. **Occasional (5%–3%):** Pain at injection site. **Rare (3%–1%):** Nausea, headache, anginal pain, shortness of breath, fever.

ADVERSE EFFECTS/TOXIC REACTIONS

Overdose may produce severe tachycardia, severe hypertension.

NURSING CONSIDERATIONS

BASELINE ASSESSMENT

Pt must be on continuous cardiac monitoring. Determine weight (for dosage calculation). Obtain initial B/P, heart rate, respirations. Correct hypovolemia before drug therapy.

INTERVENTION/EVALUATION

Continuously monitor for cardiac rate, arrhythmias. Maintain accurate I&O; measure urinary output frequently. Assess serum potassium, plasma DOBUTamine (therapeutic range: 40–190 ng/mL). Monitor B/P continuously (hypertension risk greater in pts with preexisting hypertension). Check cardiac output, pulmonary wedge pressure/central venous pressure (CVP) frequently. Immediately notify physician of decreased urinary output, cardiac arrhythmias, significant increase in B/P, heart rate, or less commonly, hypotension.

DOCEtaxel [HIGH ALERT]

doe-se-**tax**-el

■ **BLACK BOX ALERT** ■ Avoid use with serum bilirubin more than

upper limit of normal (ULN) or serum ALT, AST more than 1.5 times ULN in conjunction with serum alkaline phosphatase more than 2.5 times ULN. Severe hypersensitivity reaction (rash, hypotension, bronchospasm, anaphylaxis) may occur. Fluid retention syndrome (pleural effusions, ascites, edema, dyspnea at rest) has been reported. Pts with abnormal hepatic function, receiving higher doses, and pts with non–small-cell lung carcinoma (NSCLC) and history of prior platinum treatment receiving DOCEtaxel dose of 100 mg/m^2 at higher risk for mortality. Avoid use with ANC less than 1,500 cells/mm^3. **Do not confuse DOCEtaxel with PACLitaxel.**

◆ CLASSIFICATION

PHARMACOTHERAPEUTIC: Antimicrotubular, taxoid. **CLINICAL:** Antineoplastic.

USES

Breast cancer: Treatment of locally advanced or metastatic breast carcinoma as a single agent after failure of prior chemotherapy. Adjuvant treatment (in combination with doxorubicin and cyclophosphamide) of operable node-positive breast cancer. **Non–small-cell lung cancer (NSCLC):** Treatment of locally advanced or metastatic NSCLC after failure of prior platinum-based chemotherapy. Treatment of previously untreated locally advanced or metastatic NSCLC (in combination with cisplatin). **Prostate cancer:** Treatment of metastatic castration-resistant prostate cancer (in combination with prednisone). **Head and neck cancer:** Treatment (induction) of locally advanced squamous cell head and neck cancer (in combination with cisplatin and fluorouracil). **Gastric adenocarcinoma:** Treatment of advanced gastric adenocarcinoma (in combination with cisplatin and fluorouracil) in pts who have not received prior chemotherapy for advanced disease. **OFF-LABEL:** Anal carcinoma, bladder cancer (advanced/metastatic), esophageal cancer (advanced/metastatic), Ewing sarcoma (recurrent/

---

refractory), osteosarcoma, ovarian cancer, prostate cancer (hormone-sensitive), thyroid carcinoma (anaplastic).

PRECAUTIONS

Contraindications: Hypersensitivity to DOCEtaxel. History of severe hypersensitivity to drugs formulated with polysorbate 80, neutrophil count less than 1,500 cells/mm³. **Cautions:** Hepatic impairment, baseline cytopenias; concomitant CYP3A4 inhibitors/inducers, fluid retention, pulmonary disease, HF, active infection.

ACTION

Promotes assembly of microtubules and inhibits depolymerization of tubulin, which stabilizes microtubules. **Therapeutic Effect:** Inhibits DNA, RNA, protein synthesis. Inhibits tumor cell growth and survival.

PHARMACOKINETICS

Widely distributed. Protein binding: 94%. Extensively metabolized in liver. Excreted in feces (75%), urine (6%). **Half-life:** 11.1 hrs.

⏳ LIFESPAN CONSIDERATIONS

Pregnancy/Lactation: May cause fetal harm. Unknown if distributed in breast milk. Breastfeeding not recommended. **Children:** Safety and efficacy not established in pts younger than 16 yrs. **Elderly:** No age-related precautions noted.

INTERACTIONS

DRUG: **Strong CYP3A4 inhibitors (e.g., clarithromycin, ketoconazole, ritonavir)** may increase concentration/effect. **Strong CYP3A4 inducers (e.g., carBAMazepine, phenytoin, rifAMPin)** may decrease concentration/effect. May decrease therapeutic effects; increase adverse effects of **vaccines (live).** **HERBAL:** Echinacea may decrease therapeutic effect. **St. John's wort** may decrease concentration/effect. **FOOD:** None known. **LAB VALUES:** May increase serum alkaline phosphatase, bilirubin, ALT, AST. Reduces neutrophil, platelet count, Hgb, Hct.

AVAILABILITY (Rx)

Injection Solution: 10 mg/mL.

ADMINISTRATION/HANDLING

 IV

Note: Preparation instructions may vary by manufacturer.

Reconstitution (solution) • Withdraw dose and add to 250–500 mL 0.9% NaCl or D₅W in glass or polyolefin container to provide a final concentration of 0.3–0.74 mg/mL.

Rate of administration • Administer as a 1-hr infusion. • Monitor closely for hypersensitivity reaction (flushing, localized skin reaction, bronchospasm [may occur within a few min after beginning infusion]).

Storage • Store vials between 36°F–77°F. • Protect from bright light. • If refrigerated, stand vial at room temperature for 5 min before administering (do not store in PVC bags). • Diluted solution should be used within 4 hrs (including infusion time).

💠 IV COMPATIBILITIES

Calcium gluconate, granisetron, magnesium sulfate, ondansetron, palonosetron.

INDICATIONS/ROUTES/DOSAGE

◀ **ALERT** ▶ Premedicate with oral corticosteroids (e.g., dexamethasone 16 mg/day for 5 days beginning day 1 before DOCEtaxel therapy); reduces severity of fluid retention, hypersensitivity reaction Usual dosing: Refer to individual protocols.

Breast Carcinoma
IV: **ADULTS:** Locally advanced or metastatic: 60–100 mg/m² given over 1 hr q3wks as a single agent. Operable, node positive: 75 mg/m² q3wks for 6 courses (in combination with DOXOrubicin and cyclophosphamide).

Non–Small-Cell Lung Carcinoma
IV: ADULTS: 75 mg/m^2 q3wks (as monotherapy or in combination with CISplatin).

Prostate Cancer
IV: ADULTS, ELDERLY: 75 mg/m^2 q3wks with concurrent administration of predniSONE.

Head/Neck Cancer
IV: ADULTS, ELDERLY: 75 mg/m^2 q3wks (in combination with CISplatin and fluorouracil) for 3–4 cycles, followed by radiation therapy.

Gastric Adenocarcinoma
IV: ADULTS, ELDERLY: 75 mg/m^2 q3wks (in combination with CISplatin and fluorouracil).

Dose Modification for Gastric or Head/Neck Cancer

ALT, AST 2.5 to 5 times ULN and alkaline phosphatase less than or equal to 2.5 times ULN	80% of dose
ALT, AST 1.5 to 5 times ULN and alkaline phosphatase 2.5 to 5 times ULN	80% of dose
ALT, AST greater than 5 times ULN and/or alkaline phosphatase greater than 5 times ULN	Discontinue DOCEtaxel

Note: Toxicity includes febrile neutropenia, neutrophils less than 500 cells/mm^3 for longer than 1 wk, severe cutaneous reactions. Also, for NSCLC, platelet nadir less than 25,000 cells/mm^3, any CTCAE Grade 3 or 4 nonhematologic toxicity.

Breast Cancer
Reduce dose to 75 mg/m^2; if toxicity persists, reduce to 55 mg/m^2.

Breast Cancer Adjuvant
Administer when neutrophils are less than 1,500 cells/mm^3. If toxicity persists, or Grade 3 or 4 stomatitis, reduce dose to 60 mg/m^2.

Non–Small-Cell Lung Cancer
Monotherapy

Hold dose until toxicity resolves, then reduce dose to 55 mg/m^2. Discontinue if Grade 3 or 4 neuropathy occurs.
Combination Therapy
Reduce dose to 65 mg/m^2; may further reduce to 50 mg/m^2 if needed.

Prostate Cancer
Reduce dose to 60 mg/m^2; discontinue if toxicity persists.

Gastric or Head and Neck Cancer
Reduce dose to 60 mg/m^2; if neutropenic toxicity persists, further reduce to 45 mg/m^2. For Grade 3 or 4 thrombocytopenia, reduce dose from 75 mg/m^2 to 60 mg/m^2; discontinue if toxicity persists.

Dosage in Renal Impairment
No dose adjustment.

Dosage in Hepatic Impairment
Total bilirubin more than ULN, or ALT, AST more than 1.5 times ULN with alkaline phosphatase more than 2.5 times ULN: Use not recommended.

SIDE EFFECTS

Frequent (80%–19%): Alopecia, asthenia, hypersensitivity reaction (e.g., dermatitis), which is decreased in pts pretreated with oral corticosteroids; fluid retention, stomatitis, nausea, diarrhea, fever, nail changes, vomiting, myalgia. **Occasional:** Hypotension, edema, anorexia, headache, weight gain, infection (urinary tract, injection site, indwelling catheter tip), dizziness. **Rare:** Dry skin, sensory disorders (vision, speech, taste), arthralgia, weight loss, conjunctivitis, hematuria, proteinuria.

ADVERSE EFFECTS/TOXIC REACTIONS

In pts with normal hepatic function, neutropenia (ANC count less than 1,500 cells/mm^3), leukopenia (WBC count less than 4,000 cells/mm^3) occur in 96% of pts; anemia (hemoglobin level less than 11 g/dL) occurs in 90% of pts; thrombocytopenia (platelet count less than 100,000 cells/mm^3)

D

occurs in 8% of pts; infection occurs in 28% of pts. Neurosensory, neuromotor disturbances (distal paresthesia, weakness) occur in 54% and 13% of pts, respectively.

NURSING CONSIDERATIONS

BASELINE ASSESSMENT

Obtain ANC, CBC, serum chemistries. Antiemetics may be effective in preventing, treating nausea/vomiting. Pt should be pretreated with corticosteroids to reduce fluid retention, hypersensitivity reaction. Offer emotional support.

INTERVENTION/EVALUATION

Frequently monitor blood counts, particularly ANC count (less than 1,500 cells/mm^3 requires discontinuation of therapy). Monitor LFT, serum uric acid levels. Observe for cutaneous reactions (rash with eruptions, mainly on hands, feet). Assess for extravascular fluid accumulation: Rales in lungs, dependent edema, dyspnea at rest, pronounced abdominal distention (due to ascites).

PATIENT/FAMILY TEACHING

* Hair loss is reversible, but new hair growth may have different color or texture. * New hair growth resumes 2–3 mos after last therapy dose. * Maintain strict oral hygiene. * Do not have immunizations without physician's approval (drug lowers resistance). * Avoid those who have recently taken any live virus vaccine. * Report persistent nausea, diarrhea, respiratory difficulty, chest pain, fever, chills, unusual bleeding, bruising.

---

dofetilide

doe-**fet**-i-lide
(Tikosyn)

■ **BLACK BOX ALERT** ■ Pt must be placed in a setting with continuous cardiac monitoring for minimum of 3 days and monitored by staff familiar with treatment of life-threatening arrhythmias.

◆CLASSIFICATION

PHARMACOTHERAPEUTIC: Potassium channel blocker. **CLINICAL:** Antiarrhythmic: Class III.

USES

Maintenance of normal sinus rhythm (NSR) in pts with chronic atrial fibrillation/atrial flutter of longer than 1-wk duration who have been converted to NSR. Conversion of atrial fibrillation/flutter to NSR. **OFF-LABEL:** Supraventricular tachycardia.

PRECAUTIONS

Contraindications: Hypersensitivity to dofetilide. Congenital or acquired prolonged QT syndrome (do not use if baseline QT interval or QTc is greater than 440 msec), severe renal impairment, concurrent use of drugs that may prolong QT interval, hypokalemia, hypomagnesemia, concurrent use with bictegravir, verapamil, dolutegravir, itraconazole, ketoconazole, prochlorperazine, megestrol, cimetidine, hydroCHLOROthiazide, trimethoprim. Severe renal impairment (CrCl less than 20 mL/min). **Cautions:** Severe hepatic impairment, renal impairment, pts previously taking amiodarone, elderly. Concurrent use of other agents that prolong QT interval. Pts with sick sinus syndrome or second- or third-degree heart block unless functional pacemaker in place.

ACTION

Prolongs repolarization without affecting conduction velocity by blocking one or more time-dependent potassium currents. No effect on sodium channels, alpha-adrenergic, beta-adrenergic receptors. **Therapeutic Effect:** Terminates reentrant tachyarrhythmias, preventing reinduction.

PHARMACOKINETICS

Widely distributed. Minimally metabolized in liver. Protein binding: 60%–70%. Peak plasma concentration: 2–3 hrs. Steady state reached in 2–3 days. Excreted primarily in urine (80%). **Half-life:** 10 hrs.

⏳ LIFESPAN CONSIDERATIONS

Pregnancy/Lactation: Unknown if drug is distributed in breast milk. **Children:** No age-related precautions noted. **Elderly:** Age-related renal impairment may require dosage adjustment.

INTERACTIONS

DRUG: **Lamotrigine, ketoconazole, trimethoprim, verapamil** may increase concentration/effect. **QT interval–prolonging medications (e.g., azithromycin, ceritinib, fingolimod, haloperidol, moxifloxacin)** may increase risk of QT interval prolongation. **HERBAL: Ephedra** may worsen arrhythmias. **FOOD:** None known. **LAB VALUES:** None significant.

AVAILABILITY (Rx)

Capsules: 125 mcg, 250 mcg, 500 mcg.

ADMINISTRATION/HANDLING

PO
• Give without regard to food. • Do not break, crush, or open capsules.

INDICATIONS/ROUTES/DOSAGE

◀**ALERT**▶ ECG interval measurements (esp. Qtc intervals), creatinine clearance, must be determined prior to first dose. Correct hypokalemia, hypomagnesemia prior to starting.

Atrial Fibrillation/Flutter
PO: ADULTS, ELDERLY: Initially, 500 mcg twice daily. Modify dose in response to QTc interval.

Dosage in Renal Impairment

Creatinine Clearance	Dosage
Greater than 60 mL/min	500 mcg twice daily
40–60 mL/min	250 mcg twice daily
20–39 mL/min	125 mcg twice daily
Less than 20 mL/min	Contraindicated

Dosage in Hepatic Impairment
No dose adjustment.

SIDE EFFECTS

Rare (less than 2%): Headache, chest pain, dizziness, dyspnea, nausea, insomnia, back/abdominal pain, diarrhea, rash.

ADVERSE EFFECTS/TOXIC REACTIONS

Serious ventricular arrhythmias, including torsades de pointes, may occur; usually within the first 3 days of therapy.

NURSING CONSIDERATIONS

BASELINE ASSESSMENT

Obtain serum electrolyte levels (esp. potassium, magnesium). Prior to initiating treatment, QTc intervals must be determined. Do not use if heart rate less than 50 beats/min. Provide continuous ECG monitoring, calculation of creatinine clearance, equipment for resuscitation available for minimum of 3 days. Anticipate proarrhythmic events.

INTERVENTION/EVALUATION

Assess for conversion of cardiac arrhythmias and absence of new arrhythmias. Constantly monitor ECG. Provide emotional support. Monitor renal function for electrolyte imbalance (prolonged or excessive diarrhea, sweating, vomiting, thirst).

PATIENT/FAMILY TEACHING

• Instruct pt on need for compliance and requirement for periodic monitoring of ECG and renal function. • Do not break, crush, or open capsule.

dolutegravir

doe-loo-teg-ra-veer
(Tivicay, Tivicay PD)

FIXED COMBINATION(S)

Dovato: dolutegravir/lamivudine (antiretrovirals): 50 mg/300 mg. **Juluca:** dolutegravir/rilopivirine (antiretrovirals): 50 mg/25 mg.

 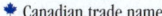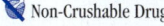

Triumaq: dolutegravir/abacavir/
lamivudine (antiretrovirals): 50 mg/
600 mg/300 mg.

◆CLASSIFICATION

PHARMACOTHERAPEUTIC: Integrase
stand transfer inhibitor (INSTI).
CLINICAL: Antiretroviral.

USES

In combination with other antiretroviral
agents for the treatment of HIV-1 infection in adults (treatment naive or experienced) and pediatric pts (treatment
naive or experienced but integrase strand
transfer inhibitor [INSTI] naive) at least
4 wks of age and weighing at least 3 kg.

PRECAUTIONS

Contraindications: Hypersensitivity
to dolutegravir. Co-administration of
dofetilide. **Cautions:** Diabetes, hepatic/
renal impairment, history of hepatitis
or tuberculosis, prior hypersensitivity
reaction to INSTIs.

ACTION

Inhibits HIV integrase by blocking strand
transfer of retroviral DNA integration
(essential for HIV replication cycle). **Therapeutic Effect:** Interferes with HIV replication, slowing progression of HIV infection.

PHARMACOKINETICS

Widely distributed. Metabolized in liver.
Peak plasma concentration: 2–3 hrs.
Excreted in feces (53%), urine (31%).
Half-life: 14 hrs.

⧖ LIFESPAN CONSIDERATIONS

Pregnancy/Lactation: May increase
risk of neural tube defects when used
at conception and in early pregnancy.
Breastfeeding not recommend due to risk
of postnatal HIV transmission. Unknown
if distributed in human breast milk. **Children:** Safety and efficacy not established
in pts less than 4 wks or weighing under
3 kg or who are INSTI-experienced with

documented or clinically suspected resistance to other INSTIs. **Elderly:** May have
increased risk of adverse effects or worsening hepatic, renal, cardiac function.

INTERACTIONS

**DRUG: Medications containing alumi-
num, calcium, magnesium or iron;
strong CYP3A4 inducers (e.g., car-
BAMazepine, phenytoin, rifAMPin),
nonnucleoside reverse transcriptase
inhibitors (e.g., efavirenz, etravipine,
nevirapine); protease inhibitors (e.g.,
fosamprenavir/ritonavir, tipranavir/
ritonavir, sucralfate)** may decrease con-
centration/effects. May increase concentra-
tion/effect of metFORMIN. **HERBAL:** St
John's wort may decrease therapeutic
effect. **FOOD:** None known. **LAB VALUES:**
May increase serum ALT, AST, bilirubin,
cholesterol, creatinine, creatine kinase
(CK), glucose, lipase, triglycerides. May
decrease creatinine clearance, neutrophils.

AVAILABILITY (Rx)

Tablets: 10 mg, 25 mg, 50 mg. **Tablets,
Soluble (for oral suspension):** 5 mg.

ADMINISTRATION/HANDLING

PO
• Give without regard to food. Administer at
least 2 hrs before or at least 6 hrs after giving
medications containing aluminum, calcium,
iron, magnesium (supplements, antacids,
laxatives). **Soluble tablets:** May be dispersed in water as an oral suspension or
given whole. Do not administer more than
1 tablet at a time to reduce risk of choking.
Do not break, cut, or crush tablets.

INDICATIONS/ROUTES/DOSAGE

HIV Infection
PO: ADULTS/ELDERLY: 50 mg once daily.
Increase to 50 mg twice daily if also receiving efavirenz, fosamprenavir/ritonavir,
tipranavir/ ritonavir, rifAMPin or INSTI-
experienced with certain INSTI-associated
resistance substitutions or clinically suspected INSTI resistance. **INFANTS, CHIL-
DREN, ADOLESCENTS: Tablets: 14–19 KG:**

40 mg once daily. **20 KG OR GREATER:** 50 mg once daily. **Soluble tablets (preferred in pts less than 20 KG): 20 KG OR GREATER:** 30 mg once daily. **14–19 KG:** 25 mg once daily. **10–13 KG** 20 mg once daily. **6–9 KG:** 15 mg once daily. **3–5 KG:** 5 mg once daily.

Dosage in Renal Impairment
CrCl 30 mL/min or less: Use caution.

Dosage in Hepatic Impairment
Mild to severe impairment: No dose adjustment.

SIDE EFFECTS

Rare (3%–1%): Insomnia, headache, nausea.

ADVERSE EFFECTS/ TOXIC REACTIONS

Hypersensitivity reaction including rash, fever, angioedema, difficulty breathing, skin blistering/peeling, arthralgia, lethargy was reported. Pts co-infected with hepatitis B or C have increased risk for viral reactivation, worsening of hepatic function, and may experience hepatic decompensation and/or failure if therapy is discontinued. May cause redistribution/accumulation of body fat (lipodystrophy). May induce immune recovery syndrome (inflammatory response to dormant opportunistic infections such as *Mycobacterium* avium, cytomegalovirus, PCP, tuberculosis, or acceleration of autoimmune disorders such as Graves' disease, polymyositis, Guillain-Barré).

NURSING CONSIDERATIONS

BASELINE ASSESSMENT

Obtain CBC, CMP, CD4+ count, viral load, HIV-1 RNA level; pregnancy test in females of reproductive potential. Screen all pts for hepatitis B or C co-infection. Receive full medication history including herbal products. Offer emotional support.

INTERVENTION/EVALUATION

Monitor CD4+ count, viral load, HIV-1 RNA level for treatment effectiveness. Monitor LFT; assess for hepatic injury (bruising, hematuria, jaundice, right upper abdominal pain, nausea, vomiting, weight loss). If discontinuation of drug regimen occurs, monitor hepatic function for viral reactivation. Initiate anti-HBV therapy if warranted. Monitor renal function as clinically indicated. An increase of serum creatinine greater than 0.4 mg/dL from baseline may indicate renal impairment. Cough, dyspnea, fever, excess band cells on CBC may indicate acute infection (WBC may be unreliable in pts with uncontrolled HIV infection). Assess skin for skin reactions, rash. Monitor for immune recovery syndrome.

PATIENT/FAMILY TEACHING

• Treatment does not cure HIV infection nor reduce risk of transmission. Practice safe sex with barrier methods or abstinence. • Drug resistance can form if treatment is interrupted; do not run out of supply. • As immune system strengthens, it may respond to dormant infections hidden within the body. Report fever, chills, body aches, cough, night sweats, shortness of breath. • Fatal cases of liver inflammation or failure have occurred; report abdominal pain, clay-colored stools, yellowing of skin or eyes, weight loss. • Report symptoms of kidney inflammation or disease (decreased urine output, flank pain, darkened urine); skin reactions (rash, pustules, skin eruptions). • Breastfeeding not recommended. • Antiretrovirals may cause excess body fat in upper back, neck, breast, trunk, while also causing decreased body fat in legs, arms, face. • Do not take newly prescribed medications unless approved by prescriber who originally started treatment. • Do not take herbal products, esp. St. John's wort.

donanemab-azbt

doe-**nan**-e-mab
(Kisunla)
■ **BLACK BOX ALERT** ■ Monoclonal antibodies used for aggregated

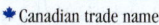 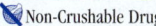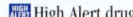

forms of beta amyloid may cause amyloid-related imaging abnormalities (ARIA), characterized as ARIA with edema (ARIA-E) or ARIA with hemosiderin deposition (ARIA-H). Pts with apolipoprotein E (ApoE) ε4 homozygotes (about 15% of Alzheimer's pts) have a higher incidence of ARIA compared to heterozygotes and noncarriers when treated with amyloid beta–directed antibodies. Life-threatening intracranial hemorrhages were reported. ARIA-E may cause focal neurologic deficits that mimic symptoms of stroke.
Do not confuse donanemab with denosumab or lecanemab.

◆CLASSIFICATION

PHARMACOTHERAPEUTIC: Humanized immunoglobulin gamma 1 (IgG1) monoclonal antibody. **CLINICAL:** Anti-Alzheimer's disease agent.

USES

Treatment of Alzheimer's disease in pts with mild cognitive impairment or mild dementia stage of disease.

PRECAUTIONS

Contraindications: Hypersensitivity to donanemab-azbt. **Cautions:** History of or at increased risk for intracranial hemorrhage. Pts who are ApoE ε4 homozygotes. Concomitant use of antithrombotic medications (anticoagulants, antiplatelets, thrombolytics).

ACTION

Targets aggregated forms of amyloid beta protein (accumulates in brain of pt's with Alzheimer's disease). **Therapeutic Effect:** Slows cognitive/functional decline in mild Alzheimer's dementia.

PHARMACOKINETICS

Widely distributed. Degraded by proteolytic enzymes. Steady state reached after a single dose. **Half-life:** 12.1 days.

⧗ LIFESPAN CONSIDERATIONS

Pregnancy/Lactation: Unknown if distributed in breast milk. **Children:** Safety

and efficacy not established. **Elderly:** No age-related precautions noted.

INTERACTIONS

DRUG: Antithrombotics (**anticoagulants** [e.g., **warfarin**], **antiplatelets** [e.g., **aspirin**], **thrombolytics** [e.g., **alteplase**]) may increase risk of intracranial hemorrhage. **HERBAL:** None significant. **FOOD:** None known. **LAB VALUES:** None significant.

AVAILABILITY (Rx)

Injection Solution: 350 mg/20 mL (17.5 mg/mL).

ADMINISTRATION/HANDLING

 IV

Infusion guidelines • Do not administer as IV push or bolus. • Upon completion of infusion, flush infusion line to ensure the entire dose is administered. • If a prior infusion reaction has occurred, consider administration of an antihistamine, acetaminophen, NSAIDs, or corticosteroids for subsequent infusions.

Dilution • Allow vial to warm to room temperature. • Visually inspect for particulate matter or discoloration. Solution should appear clear to opalescent, colorless to slightly yellow or brown. Do not use if solution is cloudy, discolored, or if visible particles are observed. • Dilute the 700 mg dose (40 mL) in 30–135 mL 0.9% NaCl infusion bag. Final infusion volume is equal to 70–175 mL with a final concentration of 700 mg/70 mL (10 mg/mL) to 700 mg/175 mL (4 mg/mL). • Dilute the 1,400 mg dose (80 mL) in 60–270 mL 0.9% NaCl infusion bag. Final infusion volume is equal to 140–350 mL with a final concentration of 1,400 mg/140 mL (10 mg/mL) to 1,400 mg/350 mL (4 mg/mL). • Mix by gentle inversion. Do not shake or agitate.

Rate of administration • Infuse over 30 min.

Storage • Refrigerate unused vials in original carton to protect from light. Do not freeze. • Vials may be stored at room temperature for up to 3 days. • May refrigerate diluted solution for up to 72 hrs or store at room temperature for up to 12 hrs. • If refrigerated, allow diluted solution to warm to room temperature before administration. • Storage times include duration of infusion.

INDICATIONS/ROUTES/DOSAGE

Alzheimer's Disease
IV: **ADULTS, ELDERLY:** 700 mg once q4wks for 3 doses, then 1,400 mg once q4wks thereafter. If amyloid plaques reduce to minimal levels on amyloid PET imaging, may consider stopping treatment.

Dose Modifications
Pts with ARIA-E

Severity of Clinical Symptoms	ARIA-E Severity on MRI		
	Mild	Moderate	Severe
Asymptomatic	Continue treatment	Withhold treatment*	Withhold treatment*
Mild	Continue treatment based on clinical judgement	Withhold treatment*	
Moderate to Severe	Withhold treatment*		

*Withhold treatment until MRI shows radiographic resolution and symptoms resolve. Consider a follow-up MRI 2–4 mos after initial identification. Resume treatment based on clinical judgement.

Pts with ARIA-H

Severity of Clinical Symptoms	ARIA-H Severity on MRI		
	Mild	Moderate	Severe
Asymptomatic	Continue treatment	Withhold treatment*	Withhold treatment†
Symptomatic	Withhold treatment*	Withhold treatment*	

*Withhold treatment until MRI shows radiographic resolution and symptoms resolve. Consider a follow-up MRI 2–4 mos after initial identification. Resume treatment based on clinical judgement.
†Withhold treatment until MRI shows radiographic resolution and symptoms resolve. Consider permanently discontinuation or resuming treatment based on clinical judgement.

Development of Intracranial Hemorrhage (ICH)
ICH greater than 1 cm in diameter during treatment: Withhold treatment until MRI shows radiographic resolution and symptoms resolve. May resume based on clinical judgement.

Dosage in Hepatic/Renal Impairment
No dose adjustment.

SIDE EFFECTS
Occasional: Headache.

ADVERSE EFFECTS/TOXIC REACTIONS
May cause ARIA, ARIA-E, or ARIA-H, including microhemorrhage and superficial siderosis. ARIA can spontaneously occur in pts with Alzheimer's disease and can range from asymptomatic to life-threatening. Pts with ApoE ε4 homozygotes have a higher incidence of ARIA compared to heterozygotes and noncarriers when treated with amyloid beta–directed antibodies. Symptoms of ARIA include confusion, dizziness, focal deficits, headache, nausea, visual changes, gait difficulty. Intracerebral hemorrhage greater than 1 cm in diameter was reported. Hypersensitivity reactions including anaphylaxis, angioedema, bronchospasm may occur. Infusion-related reactions, including body aches, chest pain, chills, dyspnea, erythema, headache, hypertension, hypotension, joint pain, nausea and vomiting, may occur. Intestinal obstruction/perforation occur rarely.

D

NURSING CONSIDERATIONS

BASELINE ASSESSMENT
Test for ApoE ε4 status. Confirm presence of amyloid beta pathology prior to initiation. Obtain MRI of the brain at baseline and periodically during treatment. Question history of hypersensitivity reactions, infusion reactions prior to each infusion. Assess cognitive function (e.g., memory attention, reasoning), activities of daily living.

INTERVENTION/EVALUATION
Obtain MRI of the brain prior to the second, third, fourth, and seventh infusions. Monitor for symptoms of ARIA (aphasia, confusion, dizziness, headache, nausea, weakness, or seizure, vision changes), intracranial hemorrhage (altered mental status, aphasia, blindness, hemiparesis, unequal pupils, seizures) for at least 24 wks after initiation. Consider MRI of the brain if ARIA is suspected. Monitor for hypersensitivity reactions, infusion reactions during each infusion for at least 30 min after completion. Immediately discontinue infusion if reaction occurs. Consider treatment with an antihistamine, acetaminophen, NSAIDs, or corticosteroids (including pretreatment for future doses). Monitor behavior, mood/cognitive function, activities of daily living.

PATIENT/FAMILY TEACHING
• MRIs of the brain will be obtained to assess for ARIA. ARIA may present as swelling in areas of the brain, which usually resolves over time. Some areas may contain small spots of bleeding that that may range from asymptomatic to life-threatening. • Report confusion, difficulty speaking, one-sided weakness, vision changes, seizures, which may indicate life-threatening bleeding of the brain. • Severe allergic reactions, including anaphylaxis, may occur. Difficulty breathing, dizziness, hives, rapid heart rate, rash, swelling of the face or tongue require immediately medical attention. • Treatment is not a cure for Alzheimer's disease, but it may slow the progression of symptoms.

donepezil

doe-**nep**-e-zil
(Aricept RDT ✽, Aricept)
Do not confuse Aricept with Aciphex, Ascriptin, or Azilect.

FIXED-COMBINATION(S)
Namzaric: donepezil/memantine (NMDA receptor antagonist): 10 mg/14 mg, 10 mg/28 mg.

◆CLASSIFICATION
PHARMACOTHERAPEUTIC: Central acetylcholinesterase inhibitor. **CLINICAL:** Cholinergic.

USES
Treatment of mild, moderate, or severe dementia of Alzheimer's disease. **OFF-LABEL:** Treatment of Parkinson's disease dementia, dementia with Lewy bodies, vascular dementia.

PRECAUTIONS
Contraindications: History of hypersensitivity to donepezil, other piperidine derivatives. **Cautions:** Asthma, COPD, bradycardia, bladder outflow obstruction, history of ulcer disease, those taking concurrent NSAIDs, supraventricular cardiac conduction disturbances (e.g., sick sinus syndrome, Wolff-Parkinson-White syndrome), seizure disorder.

ACTION
Reversibly inhibits enzyme acetylcholinesterase, increasing concentration of acetylcholine at cholinergic synapses, enhancing cholinergic function in CNS. **Therapeutic Effect:** Slows progression of Alzheimer's disease.

PHARMACOKINETICS
Widely distributed. Protein binding: 96%. Extensively metabolized. Eliminated in urine, feces. **Half-life:** 70 hrs.

⧗ LIFESPAN CONSIDERATIONS

Pregnancy/Lactation: Unknown if drug is distributed in breast milk. **Children:** Safety and efficacy not established. **Elderly:** No age-related precautions noted.

INTERACTIONS

DRUG: Anticholinergic agents (e.g., **glycopyrrolate, scopolamine**) may decrease therapeutic effect. May increase concentration/effects of **antipsychotic agents** (e.g., **aripiprazole, risperidone**), beta blockers (e.g., **atenolol, carvedilol, metoprolol**). QT interval prolonging medications (e.g., **amiodarone, azithromycin, ciprofloxacin, haloperidol, methadone, sotalol**) may increase risk of QT interval prolongation. **HERBAL:** None significant. **FOOD:** None known. **LAB VALUES:** None significant.

AVAILABILITY (Rx)

Tablets: 5 mg, 10 mg, 23 mg. **Tablets (Orally Disintegrating):** 5 mg, 10 mg. **Transdermal System:** Patch provides 5 mg/day, 10 mg/day.

ADMINISTRATION/HANDLING

PO
• May be given at bedtime without regard to food. • **Tablet (23 mg):** Swallow tablets whole; do not break, crush, dissolve, or divide. • **Orally disintegrating tablet:** Allow tablet to dissolve completely on tongue. Follow dose with water.

TRANSDERMAL
• Allow to reach room temperature before opening. • Apply to back (avoiding the spine). Do not apply to red, irritated, or cut skin. **Storage** • Refrigerate unused patches. Do not freeze.

INDICATIONS/ROUTES/DOSAGE

Alzheimer's Disease
PO: ADULTS, ELDERLY: For mild to moderate, initially 5 mg/day at bedtime. May increase at 4- to 6-wk intervals to 10 mg/day at bedtime. **Range:** 5–10 mg/day. For moderate to severe Alzheimer's, a dose of 23 mg once daily can be administered once pt has been taking 10 mg once daily for at least 3 mos. **Range:** 10–23 mg/day. **Transdermal: (apply patch wkly):** Initially, 5 mg/day. After 4-6 wks, may increase to 10 mg/day.

Dosage in Renal/Hepatic Impairment
No dose adjustment.

SIDE EFFECTS

Frequent (11%–8%): Nausea, diarrhea, headache, insomnia, nonspecific pain, dizziness. **Occasional (6%–3%):** Mild muscle cramps, fatigue, vomiting, anorexia, ecchymosis. **Rare (3%–2%):** Depression, abnormal dreams, weight loss, arthritis, drowsiness, syncope, frequent urination.

ADVERSE EFFECTS/TOXIC REACTIONS

Overdose may result in cholinergic crisis (severe nausea, increased salivation, diaphoresis, bradycardia, hypotension, flushed skin, abdominal pain, respiratory depression, seizures, cardiorespiratory collapse). Increasing muscle weakness may occur, resulting in death if muscles of respiration become involved. **Antidote:** Atropine sulfate 1–2 mg IV with subsequent doses based on therapeutic response.

NURSING CONSIDERATIONS

BASELINE ASSESSMENT
Assess cognitive function (e.g., memory, attention, reasoning). Obtain baseline vital signs. Assess history for peptic ulcer, urinary obstruction, asthma, COPD, seizure disorder, cardiac conduction disturbances.

INTERVENTION/EVALUATION
Monitor behavior, mood/cognitive function, activities of daily living. Monitor for cholinergic reaction (GI discomfort/cramping, feeling of facial warmth, excessive salivation/diaphoresis), lacrimation, pallor, urinary urgency, dizziness. Monitor for nausea, diarrhea, headache, insomnia.

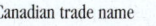 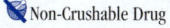

D

• Report nausea, vomiting, diarrhea, diaphoresis, increased salivary secretions, severe abdominal pain, dizziness. • May take without regard to food (best taken at bedtime). • Not a cure for Alzheimer's disease but may slow progression of symptoms.

DOPamine

HIGH ALERT

dope-a-meen

■ BLACK BOX ALERT ■ If extravasation occurs, infiltrate area with phentolamine (5–10 mL 0.9% NaCl) as soon as possible, no later than 12 hrs after extravasation.

Do not confuse DOPamine with DOBUTamine or Dopram.

◆CLASSIFICATION

PHARMACOTHERAPEUTIC: Sympathomimetic (adrenergic agonist). **CLINICAL:** Cardiac stimulant, vasopressor.

USES

Adjunct in treatment of severe hypotension or shock (e.g., septic shock, cardiogenic shock, decompensated heart failure, post-cardiac arrest), persisting after adequate fluid volume replacement. **OFF-LABEL:** Symptomatic bradycardia or heart block unresponsive to atropine or cardiac pacing.

PRECAUTIONS

Contraindications: Hypersensitivity to dopamine, sulfites. Pheochromocytoma, ventricular fibrillation. Uncorrected tachyarrhythmias. **Cautions:** Ischemic heart disease, occlusive vascular disease, hypovolemia, recent use of MAOIs (within 2–3 wks), ventricular arrhythmias, post-MI.

ACTION

Stimulates adrenergic and dopaminergic receptors. Effects are dose dependent. Lower dosage stimulates dopaminergic receptors, causing renal vasodilation. Higher doses stimulate both dopaminergic and beta$_1$-adrenergic receptors, causing cardiac stimulation and renal vasodilation. Higher doses stimulate alpha-adrenergic receptors, causing vasoconstriction, increased B/P. **Therapeutic Effect: Low dosage (1–5 mcg/kg/min):** Increases renal blood flow, urinary flow, sodium excretion. **Low to moderate dosage (5–10 mcg/kg/min):** Increases myocardial contractility, stroke volume, cardiac output. **High dosage (greater than 10 mcg/kg/min):** Increases peripheral resistance, vasoconstriction, B/P.

PHARMACOKINETICS

Route	Onset	Peak	Duration
IV	1–2 min	N/A	Less than 10 min

Widely distributed. Does not cross blood-brain barrier. Metabolized in liver, kidneys, plasma. Primarily excreted in urine. Not removed by hemodialysis. **Half-life:** 2 min.

⧖ LIFESPAN CONSIDERATIONS

Pregnancy/Lactation: Unknown if drug crosses placenta or is distributed in breast milk. **Children:** Recommended close hemodynamic monitoring (gangrene due to extravasation reported). **Elderly:** No age-related precautions noted.

INTERACTIONS

DRUG: Ergot derivatives (e.g., ergotamine), MAOIs (e.g., phenelzine, selegiline), tricyclic antidepressants (e.g., amitriptyline) may increase hypertensive effects. **HERBAL:** None significant. **FOOD:** None known. **LAB VALUES:** None significant.

AVAILABILITY (Rx)

Injection Solution: 40 mg/mL. **Injection (Premix With Dextrose):** 0.8 mg/mL (250

---

mL, 500 mL), 1.6 mg/mL (250 mL, 500 mL), 3.2 mg/mL (250 mL).

ADMINISTRATION/HANDLING

◄ALERT► Fluid volume depletion must be corrected before administering DOPamine (may be used concurrently with fluid replacement).

 IV

Reconstitution • Available prediluted in 250 or 500 mL D_5W or dilute in 250–500 mL 0.9% NaCl or D_5W, to maximum concentration of 3,200 mcg/mL (3.2 mg/mL).
Rate of administration • Administer into large vein (antecubital fossa, central line preferred) to prevent extravasation. • Use infusion pump to control flow rate. • Titrate drug to desired hemodynamic, renal response (optimum urinary flow determines dosage).
Storage • Do not use solutions darker than slightly yellow or discolored to yellow, brown, pink to purple (indicates decomposition of drug). • Stable for 24 hrs after dilution.

⊞ IV INCOMPATIBILITIES

Ibuprofen, insulin.

⊞ IV COMPATIBILITIES

Amiodarone, argatroban, dexmedetomidine, diltiazem, heparin, norepinephrine, potassium chloride, propofol, vasopressin.

INDICATIONS/ROUTES/DOSAGE

◄ALERT► Effects of DOPamine are dose dependent. Titrate to desired response. Doses greater than 20 mcg/kg/min may not have beneficial effect on BP and may increase risk of tachyarrhythmias.

Hemodynamic Support
IV infusion: ADULTS, ELDERLY, CHILDREN: NEONATES: Initially, 2–5 mcg/kg/min. Increase gradually in 5–10 mcg/kg/min increments until optimal response is achieved. **Range:** 2–20 mcg/kg/min.

SIDE EFFECTS

Frequent: Headache, arrhythmias, tachycardia, anginal pain, palpitations, vasoconstriction, hypotension, nausea, vomiting, dyspnea. **Occasional:** Piloerection (goose bumps), bradycardia, widening of QRS complex.

ADVERSE EFFECTS/TOXIC REACTIONS

High doses may produce ventricular arrhythmias, tachycardia. Pts with occlusive vascular disease are at high risk for further compromise of circulation to extremities, which may result in gangrene. Tissue necrosis with sloughing may occur with extravasation of IV solution.

NURSING CONSIDERATIONS

BASELINE ASSESSMENT

Continuous cardiac monitoring is required. Determine weight (for dosage calculation). Obtain initial B/P, heart rate, respirations. Assess patency of IV access.

INTERVENTION/EVALUATION

Continuously monitor for cardiac arrhythmias. Measure urinary output frequently. If extravasation occurs, immediately infiltrate affected tissue with 10–15 mL 0.9% NaCl solution containing 5–10 mg phentolamine mesylate. Monitor B/P, heart rate, respirations q15min during administration (more often if indicated). Assess cardiac output, pulmonary wedge pressure, or central venous pressure (CVP) frequently. Assess peripheral circulation (palpate pulses, note color/temperature of extremities). Immediately notify physician of decreased urinary output, cardiac arrhythmias, significant changes in B/P, heart rate, or failure to respond to increase or decrease in infusion rate, decreased peripheral circulation (cold, pale, mottled extremities). Taper dosage before discontinuing (abrupt cessation of therapy may result in marked hypotension). Be alert to excessive vasoconstriction (decreased urine output, increased heart rate, arrhythmias, disproportionate increase in diastolic B/P, decrease in pulse pressure); slow or temporarily stop infusion, notify physician.

doxazosin

dox-a-**zoe**-sin
(Apo-Doxazosin ✦, Cardura,
Cardura XL)
**Do not confuse Cardura with
Cardene, Cordarone, Coumadin,
K-Dur, or Ridaura, or doxazo-
sin with doxapram, doxepin, or
DOXOrubicin.**

◆**CLASSIFICATION**

PHARMACOTHERAPEUTIC: Alpha-
adrenergic blocker. **CLINICAL:** Antihypertensive.

USES

Cardura: Treatment of mild to moderate hypertension. Used alone or in combination with other antihypertensives.
Treatment of urinary outflow obstruction and/or obstruction and irritation
associated with benign prostatic hyperplasia **(BPH)**. **Cardura XL:** Treatment
of urinary outflow obstruction and/or
obstruction and irritation associated
with benign prostatic hyperplasia. **OFF-
LABEL:** Facilitate distal ureteral stone
expulsion.

PRECAUTIONS

Contraindications: Hypersensitivity to
doxazosin or other quinazolines (prazosin, terazosin). **Cautions:** Constipation, ileus, GI obstruction, hepatic
impairment.

ACTION

Hypertension: Selectively blocks
alpha$_1$-adrenergic receptors, decreasing peripheral vascular resistance. **BPH:**
Inhibits postsynaptic alpha-adrenergic
receptors in prostatic stromal and
bladder neck tissues. **Therapeutic
Effect: Hypertension:** Causes peripheral vasodilation, lowering B/P. **BPH:**
Relaxes smooth muscle of bladder, prostate, reducing BPH symptoms.

PHARMACOKINETICS

Route	Onset	Peak	Duration
PO (antihy- pertensive)	1–2 hrs	2–6 hrs	24 hrs

Well absorbed from GI tract. Protein
binding: 98%–99%. Metabolized in
liver. Primarily eliminated in feces.
Not removed by hemodialysis. **Half-
life:** 19–22 hrs.

⧖ LIFESPAN CONSIDERATIONS

Pregnancy/Lactation: Unknown if
drug crosses placenta or is distributed
in breast milk. **Children:** Safety and
efficacy not established. **Elderly:** May
be more sensitive to hypotensive
effects.

INTERACTIONS

DRUG: **Strong CYP3A4 inducers (e.g.,
carBAMazepine, phenytoin, rifAMPin)**
may decrease concentration/effect. **Strong
CYP3A4 inhibitors (e.g., clarithromycin, ketoconazole, ritonavir)** may
increase concentration/effect. **HERBAL:
Herbs with hypertensive properties
(e.g., licorice, yohimbe) or hypotensive
properties (e.g., garlic, ginger, ginkgo
biloba)** may alter effects. **FOOD:** None
known. **LAB VALUES:** None significant.

AVAILABILITY (Rx)

Tablets: 1 mg, 2 mg, 4 mg, 8 mg.

Tablets, Extended-Release: 4 mg, 8 mg.

ADMINISTRATION/HANDLING

PO
• Give without regard to food. • Do not
break, crush, dissolve, or divide extended-
release tablet. • Immediate-release tablets
given morning or evening; extended-release
tablets given with morning meal.

INDICATIONS/ROUTES/DOSAGE

Hypertension
PO: *(Immediate-Release):* **ADULTS,
ELDERLY:** Initially, 1 mg once daily. May
increase to 2 mg once daily. Thereafter,

may increase upward over several wks to a maximum of 16 mg/day.

Benign Prostatic Hyperplasia
PO: *(Immediate-Release):* **ADULTS, ELDERLY:** Initially, 1 mg/day. May titrate at intervals of 1–2 wks by doubling daily dose to 2 mg, 4 mg, and 8 mg. **Maximum:** 8 mg/day. *(Extended-Release):* Initially, 4 mg/day. May increase to 8 mg in 3–4 wks. **Maximum:** 8 mg/day. **Note:** When switching to extended-release, omit evening dose prior to starting morning dose.

Dosage in Renal Impairment
No dose adjustment.

Dosage in Hepatic Impairment
Mild to moderate Impairment: Use caution. **Severe impairment:** Avoid use.

SIDE EFFECTS

Frequent (20%–10%): Dizziness, asthenia, headache, edema. **Occasional (9%–3%):** Nausea, pharyngitis, rhinitis, pain in extremities, drowsiness. **Rare (2%–1%):** Palpitations, diarrhea, constipation, dyspnea, myalgia, altered vision, anxiety.

ADVERSE EFFECTS/TOXIC REACTIONS

First-dose syncope (hypotension with sudden loss of consciousness) may occur 30–90 min after initial dose of 2 mg or greater, too-rapid increase in dosage, addition of another antihypertensive agent to therapy. First-dose syncope may be preceded by tachycardia (pulse rate 120–160 beats/min).

NURSING CONSIDERATIONS

BASELINE ASSESSMENT
Give first dose at bedtime. If initial dose is given during daytime, pt must remain recumbent for 3–4 hrs. Assess B/P, pulse immediately before each dose and q15–30min until B/P is stabilized (be alert to fluctuations).

INTERVENTION/EVALUATION
Monitor B/P, I&O. Monitor pulse diligently (first-dose syncope may be preceded by tachycardia). Assess for edema, headache. Assist with ambulation if dizziness, light-headedness occurs.

PATIENT/FAMILY TEACHING
• Full therapeutic effect may not occur for 3–4 wks. • May cause syncope (fainting); go from lying to standing slowly. • Avoid tasks that require alertness, motor skills until response to drug is established.

doxepin

dox-e-pin
(Prudoxin, Silenor, Sinequan , Zonalon)

■ **BLACK BOX ALERT** ■ Increased risk of suicidal ideation and behavior in children, adolescents, young adults 18–24 yrs with major depressive disorder, other psychiatric disorders.
Do not confuse doxepin with digoxin, doxapram, doxazosin, Doxidan, or doxycycline, or SINEquan with SEROquel, or Singulair.

◆CLASSIFICATION
PHARMACOTHERAPEUTIC: Tricyclic. **CLINICAL:** Antidepressant, antianxiety, antineuralgic, antipruritic.

USES
Treatment of depression including psychotic and bipolar depression. **Silenor (only):** Treatment of insomnia in pts with difficulty staying asleep. **Topical:** Treatment of pruritus associated with atopic dermatitis.

PRECAUTIONS
Contraindications: Hypersensitivity to doxepin. Glaucoma, hypersensitivity to other tricyclic antidepressants, urinary retention, use of MAOIs within 14 days.

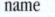 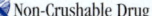

Cautions: Cardiac/hepatic/renal disease, pts at risk for suicidal ideation, respiratory compromise, sleep apnea, history of bowel obstruction, increased IOP, glaucoma, history of seizures, history of urinary retention/obstruction, hyperthyroidism, prostatic hypertrophy, hiatal hernia, elderly.

ACTION

Increases synaptic concentrations of norepinephrine, serotonin by inhibiting reuptake. **Therapeutic Effect:** Produces antidepressant, anxiolytic effects.

PHARMACOKINETICS

PO: Widely distributed. Protein binding: 80%–85%. Metabolized in liver. Primarily excreted in urine. Not removed by hemodialysis. **Half-life:** 6–8 hrs. **Topical:** Absorbed through skin. Distributed to body tissues. Metabolized to active metabolite. Excreted in urine.

⌛ LIFESPAN CONSIDERATIONS

Pregnancy/Lactation: Crosses placenta. Distributed in breast milk. **Children:** Safety and efficacy not established in pts younger than 12 yrs. **Elderly:** Increased risk of toxicity (lower dosages recommended). Avoid doses greater than 6 mg/day due to anticholinergic effects, sedation, and orthostatic hypotension.

INTERACTIONS

DRUG: Alcohol, **CNS depressants (e.g., LORazepam, morphine, zolpidem)** may increase CNS, respiratory depression. **MAOIs (e.g., phenelzine, selegiline)** may increase risk of seizures, hyperpyrexia, hypertensive crisis (discontinue at least 2 wks prior to starting doxepin). **Anticholinergic agents (e.g., aclidinium, ipratropium, umeclidinium)** may increase anticholinergic effect. May increase QT interval-prolonging effect of **dronedarone. Strong CYP2D6 inhibitors (e.g., buPROPion, PARoxetine)** may increase concentration/effect.

HERBAL: Herbals with sedative properties (e.g., chamomile, kava kava, valerian) may increase CNS depression. **St. John's wort** may decrease concentration/effect. **FOOD:** None known. **LAB VALUES:** May alter serum glucose, ECG readings. **Therapeutic serum level:** 110–250 ng/mL; **toxic serum level:** Greater than 300 ng/mL.

AVAILABILITY (Rx)

Capsules: 10 mg, 25 mg, 50 mg, 75 mg, 100 mg, 150 mg. **Cream:** *(Prudoxin, Zonalon):* 5%. **Oral Concentrate:** 10 mg/mL. **Tablets:** *(Silenor):* 3 mg, 6 mg.

ADMINISTRATION/HANDLING

PO
• Give with food, milk if GI distress occurs. • Dilute concentrate in 4-oz glass of water, milk, or grapefruit, orange, tomato, prune, pineapple juice. Incompatible with carbonated drinks. • Give larger portion of daily dose at bedtime. **Insomnia:** Administer within 30 min prior to bedtime.

Topical
• Apply thin film of cream on affected areas of skin. • Do not use for more than 8 days. • Do not use occlusive dressing.

INDICATIONS/ROUTES/DOSAGE

Depression
Note: Gradually taper dose upon discontinuation of antidepressant therapy. **PO: ADULTS:** Initially, 25–50 mg/day at bedtime. May increase gradually in 25–50 mg increments at intervals of 3 days or longer to usual dose of 100 mg–300 mg/day (single dose should not exceed 150 mg). **ELDERLY:** Initially, 10–25 mg at bedtime. May increase by 10–25 mg/day every 3–7 days.

Insomnia (Silenor Only)
PO: ADULTS: 3–6 mg (give within 30 min of bedtime). **ELDERLY:** 3 mg (give within 30 min of bedtime). May increase to 6 mg once daily.

Pruritus Associated With Atopic Dermatitis

Topical: ADULTS, ELDERLY: Apply thin film 4 times/day at 3- to 4-hr intervals. Not recommended for more than 8 days.

Dosage in Renal Impairment

No dose adjustment.

Dosage in Hepatic Impairment

Use lower initial dose; adjust gradually. *(Silenor):* Initially, 3 mg once daily.

SIDE EFFECTS

Frequent: PO: Orthostatic hypotension, drowsiness, dry mouth, headache, increased appetite, weight gain, nausea, unusual fatigue, unpleasant taste. **Topical:** Edema, increased pruritus, eczema, burning, tingling, stinging at application site, altered taste, dizziness, drowsiness, dry skin, dry mouth, fatigue, headache, thirst. **Occasional: PO:** Blurred vision, confusion, constipation, hallucinations, difficult urination, eye pain, irregular heartbeat, fine muscle tremors, nervousness, impaired sexual function, diarrhea, diaphoresis, heartburn, insomnia. **Silenor:** Nausea, upper respiratory infection. **Topical:** Anxiety, skin irritation/cracking, nausea. **Rare: PO:** Allergic reaction, alopecia, tinnitus, breast enlargement. **Topical:** Fever, photosensitivity.

ADVERSE EFFECTS/TOXIC REACTIONS

Abrupt or too-rapid withdrawal may result in headache, malaise, nausea, vomiting, vivid dreams. Overdose may produce confusion, severe drowsiness, agitation, tachycardia, arrhythmias, shortness of breath, vomiting.

NURSING CONSIDERATIONS

BASELINE ASSESSMENT

Assess B/P, pulse, ECG (those with history of cardiovascular disease). Obtain CBC, serum electrolyte tests before long-term therapy. Assess pt's appearance, behavior, level of interest, mood, suicidal ideation, sleep pattern.

INTERVENTION/EVALUATION

Monitor B/P, pulse, weight. Perform CBC, serum electrolyte tests periodically to assess renal/hepatic function. Monitor mental status, suicidal ideation. Supervise suicidal-risk pt closely during early therapy (as depression lessens, energy level improves, increasing suicide potential). Assess appearance, behavior, speech pattern, level of interest, mood. **Therapeutic serum level:** 110–250 ng/mL; **toxic serum level:** Greater than 300 ng/mL.

PATIENT/FAMILY TEACHING

• Do not discontinue abruptly. • Change positions slowly to avoid dizziness. • Avoid tasks that require alertness, motor skills until response to drug is established. • Do not cover affected area with occlusive dressing after applying cream. • Avoid alcohol, limit caffeine. • May increase appetite. • Avoid exposure to sunlight/artificial light source. • Therapeutic effect may be noted within 2–5 days, maximum effect within 2–3 wks. • Report worsening depression, suicidal ideation, unusual changes in behavior (esp. at initiation of therapy or with changes in dosage).

DOXOrubicin

dox-o-**rue**-bi-sin
(Adriamycin, Caelyx ✦, Doxil)

■ **BLACK BOX ALERT** ■ May cause concurrent or cumulative myocardial toxicity. Acute allergic or anaphylaxis-like infusion reaction may be life-threatening. Severe myelosuppression may occur. Must be administered by personnel trained in administration/handling of chemotherapeutic agents. Secondary acute myelogenous leukemia and myelodysplastic syndrome have been reported. Potent vesicant.

Do not confuse DOXOrubicin with dactinomycin, DAUNOrubicin, doxazosin, epiRUBicin, IDArubicin, or valrubicin, or

D

Adriamycin with Aredia or Idamycin.

◆CLASSIFICATION

PHARMACOTHERAPEUTIC: Anthracycline, topoisomerase II inhibitor. **CLINICAL:** Antineoplastic.

USES

Adriamycin: Treatment of acute lymphoblastic lymphoma, acute myeloid leukemia, bladder cancer, bone sarcoma, Hodgkin's lymphoma, non-Hodgkin's lymphoma, neuroblastoma, ovarian cancer, soft tissue sarcoma, Wilms tumor. **Doxil:** Treatment of AIDS-related Kaposi's sarcoma, advanced ovarian cancer. Used with bortezomib to treat multiple myeloma in pts who have not previously received bortezomib and have received at least one previous treatment. **OFF-LABEL: Adriamycin:** Hepatocellular cancer, renal carcinoma, neuroendocrine tumors, pancreatic cancer, Waldenstrom macroglobulinemia, multiple myeloma, endometrial carcinoma, uterine sarcoma. **Doxil:** Metastatic breast cancer, Hodgkin's lymphoma, cutaneous T-cell lymphomas, advanced soft tissue sarcomas, recurrent or metastatic cervical cancer, advanced or metastatic uterine sarcoma.

PRECAUTIONS

Contraindications: Hypersensitivity to DOXOrubicin. **Adriamycin:** Severe hepatic impairment, severe myocardial insufficiency, recent MI (within 4–6 wks), severe arrhythmias. Previous or concomitant treatment with high accumulative doses of DOXOrubicin, DAUNOrubicin, IDArubicin, or other anthracyclines or anthracenediones; severe, persistent drug-induced myelosuppression or baseline ANC count less than 1,500 cells/mm³. **Doxil:** Breastfeeding (Canada). **Cautions:** Hepatic impairment. Cardiomyopathy, preexisting myelosuppression, severe HF. Pts who received radiation therapy.

ACTION

Inhibits DNA, RNA synthesis by binding with DNA strands. Liposomal encapsulation increases uptake by tumors, prolongs drug action, may decrease toxicity. **Therapeutic Effect:** Prevents cell division.

PHARMACOKINETICS

Widely distributed. Metabolized in liver. Protein binding: 74%–76%. Excreted in feces (40%), urine (5%–12%). **Half-life:** 20–48 hrs.

⧗ LIFESPAN CONSIDERATIONS

Pregnancy/Lactation: If possible, avoid use during pregnancy, esp. first trimester. Breastfeeding not recommended. **Children/Elderly:** Cardiotoxicity may be more frequent in pts younger than 2 yrs or older than 70 yrs.

INTERACTIONS

DRUG: Bevacizumab may increase risk of cardiotoxicity. **Bone marrow depressants (e.g., cladribine)** may increase myelosuppression. **Strong CYP3A4 inducers (e.g., carBAMazepine, phenytoin, rifAMPin)** may decrease concentration/effect. **Strong CYP3A4 inhibitors (e.g., clarithromycin, ketoconazole, ritonavir)** may increase concentration/effect. May decrease therapeutic effects; increase adverse effects of **vaccines (live).** **HERBAL:** Echinacea may decrease therapeutic effect. **FOOD:** None known. **LAB VALUES:** May cause ECG changes, increase serum uric acid. May decrease neutrophils, RBCs.

AVAILABILITY (Rx)

Injection, Powder for Reconstitution: 10 mg, **Injection Solution:** *(Adriamycin):* 2 mg/mL (5-mL, 10-mL, vial). **Lipid Complex:** *(Doxil):* 2 mg/mL (10 mL, 25 mL).

ADMINISTRATION/HANDLING

◀**ALERT**▶ Wear gloves. If powder or solution comes into contact with skin, wash thoroughly. Avoid small veins; swollen/edematous extremities; areas overlying joints, tendons. • *(Doxil):* Do not use with in-line filter or mix with any diluent except D₅W. May be carcinogenic, mutagenic, teratogenic. Handle with extreme care during preparation/administration.

 IV

Reconstitution • Dilute with 50–1,000 mL D₅W or 0.9% NaCl and give as continuous infusion. • *(Doxil):* Dilute each dose in 250 mL D₅W (doses greater than 90 mg in 500 mL D₅W).
Rate of administration • *(Adriamycin):* For IV push, administer into tubing of freely running IV infusion of D₅W or 0.9% NaCl, preferably via butterfly needle over 3–5 min (avoids local erythematous streaking along vein and facial flushing). • Must test for flashback q30sec to be certain needle remains in vein during injection. IV piggyback over 15–60 min or continuous infusion. • Extravasation produces immediate pain, severe local tissue damage. Terminate administration immediately; withdraw as much medication as possible, obtain extravasation kit, follow protocol. • *(Doxil):* Give as infusion over 60 min. Do not use in-line filter.
Storage • *(Adriamycin solution):* Refrigerate vials. Solutions diluted in D₅W or 0.9% NaCl stable for 48 hrs at room temperature. • *(Doxil):* Refrigerate unopened vials. After solution is diluted, use within 24 hrs.

🟦 IV INCOMPATIBILITIES

DOXOrubicin: Heparin. Doxil: Do not mix with any other medications.

🟦 IV COMPATIBILITIES

Granisetron, leucovorin, ondansetron.

INDICATIONS/ROUTES/DOSAGE

◀**ALERT**▶ Refer to individual protocols.

Usual Dosage
IV: *(Adriamycin):* ADULTS: **(Single-agent therapy):** 60–75 mg/m² as a single dose

every 21 days, 20 mg/m² once wkly. **(Combination therapy):** 40–75 mg/m² q21–28 days. Because of risk of cardiotoxicity, do not exceed cumulative dose of 550 mg/m² (400–450 mg/m² for those previously treated with related compounds or irradiation of cardiac region). CHILDREN: **(Single-agent therapy):** 60–75 mg/m² q3wks. **(Combination therapy):** 40–75 mg/m² q21–28 days.

Kaposi's Sarcoma
IV: *(Doxil):* ADULTS: 20 mg/m² q3wks infused over 30 min. Continue until disease progression or unacceptable toxicity.

Ovarian Cancer
IV: *(Doxil):* ADULTS: 50 mg/m² q4wks. Continue until disease progression or unacceptable toxicity.

Multiple Myeloma
IV: *(Doxil):* ADULTS: 30 mg/m²/dose on day 4 q3wks (in combination with bortezomib) for 8 cycles. Continue until disease progression or unacceptable toxicity.

Dosage in Renal Impairment
No dose adjustment.

Dose Modifications
Adriamycin
Neutropenic fever/Infection: Reduce dose to 75%. **ANC less than 1,000 cells/mm³:** Delay treatment until ANC 1,000 cells/mm³ or more. **Platelets less than 100,000/mm³:** Delay treatment until platelets 100,000 cells/mm³ or more.
Doxil
Adjustments for hand-foot syndrome, stomatitis, hematologic toxicities: Refer to manufacturer's guidelines.

Dosage in Hepatic Impairment

ADRIAMYCIN

Hepatic Function	Dosage
ALT, AST 2–3 times ULN	75% of normal dose

Hepatic Function	Dosage
ALT, AST greater than 3 times ULN or bilirubin 1.2–3 mg/dL	50% of normal dose
Bilirubin 3.1–5 mg/dL	25% of normal dose
Bilirubin greater than 5 mg/dL	Not recommended

ULN = upper limit of normal.

DOXIL

Hepatic Function	Dosage
Bilirubin 1.2–3 mg/dL	50% of normal dose
Bilirubin greater than 3 mg/dL	25% of normal dose

SIDE EFFECTS

Frequent: Alopecia, nausea, vomiting, stomatitis, esophagitis (esp. if drug is given on several successive days), reddish urine. **Doxil:** Nausea. **Occasional:** Anorexia, diarrhea; hyperpigmentation of nailbeds, phalangeal, dermal creases. **Rare:** Fever, chills, conjunctivitis, lacrimation.

ADVERSE EFFECTS/TOXIC REACTIONS

Myelosuppression (anemia, leukopenia, thrombocytopenia) generally occurs within 10–15 days, returns to normal levels by third wk. Cardiotoxicity (either acute, manifested as transient ECG abnormalities, or chronic, manifested as HF) may occur.

NURSING CONSIDERATIONS

BASELINE ASSESSMENT

Obtain ANC, CBC before and at frequent intervals during therapy. Obtain ECG before therapy, LFT before each dose. Antiemetics may be effective in preventing, treating nausea. Offer emotional support.

INTERVENTION/EVALUATION

Monitor for stomatitis (burning or erythema of oral mucosa at inner margin of lips, difficulty swallowing). Observe IV injection site for infiltration, vein irritation. May lead to ulceration of mucous membranes within 2–3 days. Monitor hematologic status, renal/hepatic function studies, serum uric acid levels. Monitor daily pattern of bowel activity, stool consistency. Monitor for hematologic toxicity (fever, sore throat, signs of local infection, unusual bruising/bleeding from any site), symptoms of anemia (excessive fatigue, weakness).

PATIENT/FAMILY TEACHING

• Treatment may depress your immune system and reduce your ability to fight infection. Report symptoms of infection such as body aches, burning with urination, chills, cough, fatigue, fever. Avoid those with active infection. • Report symptoms of bone marrow depression (e.g., bruising, fatigue, fever, shortness of breath, weight loss; bleeding easily, bloody urine or stool). • Maintain strict oral hygiene. • Do not have immunizations without physician's approval (drug lowers resistance). • Avoid contact with those who have recently received live virus vaccine. • Report persistent nausea/vomiting. • Avoid alcohol (may cause GI irritation, a common side effect with liposomal DOXOrubicin).

---

doxycycline

dox-i-**sye**-kleen
(Apo-Doxy ✦, Avidoxy, Doryx, Doxy-100, Oracea, Vibramycin)
Do not confuse doxycycline with dicyclomine, doxepin, omadacycline, minocycline, tetracycline, or Oracea with Orencia, or Vibramycin with Vancomycin or Vibativ.

◆CLASSIFICATION

PHARMACOTHERAPEUTIC: Tetracycline. **CLINICAL:** Antibiotic.

USES

Treatment of infections including acne, acute intestinal amebiasis, *Clostridium*, malaria (prophylaxis), *Mycoplasma pneumoniae*, respiratory tract

---

infections, rickettsial infections, sexually transmitted infections caused by susceptible microorganisms including *H. influenzae, Klebsiella* spp., *S. pneumoniae, M. pneumoniae, Chlamydia trachomatis, N. gonorrhoeae, E. coli, E. aerogenes, Shigella* species, *Acinetobacter* species. **Oracea:** Treatment of inflammatory lesions in adults with rosacea. **OFF-LABEL:** Bite wound infection, COPD (acute exacerbation), Lyme disease, otitis media, surgical prophylaxis.

PRECAUTIONS

Contraindications: Hypersensitivity to doxycycline, other tetracyclines. **Cautions:** History or predisposition to oral candidiasis (Oracea); recent *Clostridium difficile* infection or antibiotic-associated colitis; history of pancreatitis. Avoid use during pregnancy, during tooth development in children. Avoid prolonged exposure to sunlight.

ACTION

Inhibits bacterial protein synthesis by binding to ribosomes. May cause alterations in the cytoplasmic membrane. **Therapeutic Effect:** Bacteriostatic.

PHARMACOKINETICS

Widely distributed. Partially inactivated in GI tract by chelate formation. Protein binding: greater than 90%. Peak plasma concentration: 1.5–4 hrs (immediate-release); 2.8–3 hrs (delayed-release). Excreted in feces (30%), urine (23%–40%). **Half-life:** 15–24 hrs.

⧖ LIFESPAN CONSIDERATIONS

Pregnancy/Lactation: Crosses placenta; distributed in breast milk. **Children:** May cause permanent discoloration of teeth, enamel hypoplasia. **Elderly:** No age-related precautions noted.

INTERACTIONS

DRUG: **Antacids containing aluminum, calcium, magnesium; laxatives containing magnesium, oral iron preparations** decrease absorption. **Barbiturates, carBAMazepine** may decrease concentration/effect. **Bile acid sequestrants** may decrease absorption. **HERBAL:** None significant. **FOOD:** None known. **LAB VALUES:** May increase serum alkaline phosphatase, amylase, bilirubin, ALT, AST. May alter CBC.

AVAILABILITY (Rx)

Capsules: 40 mg, 50 mg, 75 mg, 100 mg, 150 mg. **Injection, Powder for Reconstitution:** 100 mg. **Oral Suspension:** 25 mg/5 mL. **Tablets:** 20 mg, 50 mg, 75 mg, 100 mg, 150 mg.

🦥 **Tablets, Delayed-Release:** 50 mg, 75 mg, 100 mg, 150 mg, 200 mg.

ADMINISTRATION/HANDLING

◀**ALERT**▶ Do not administer IM or SQ. Space doses evenly around clock.

🩸 **IV**

Reconstitution • Reconstitute each 100-mg vial with 10 mL Sterile Water for Injection for concentration of 10 mg/mL. • Further dilute each 100 mg with at least 100 mL D₅W, 0.9% NaCl, lactated Ringer's.
Rate of administration • Infuse over 1–4 hrs.
Storage • Stability based on solution (see manufacturer guidelines). • Protect from direct sunlight. Discard if precipitate forms.

PO
• Oral suspension is stable for 2 wks at room temperature. • Give with full glass of fluid. • Instruct pt to sit up for 30 min after taking to reduce risk of esophageal irritation and ulceration. • In general, give with meals to decrease GI upset. • Avoid concurrent use of antacids, milk; separate by 2 hrs.

⬛ IV INCOMPATIBILITIES

Heparin.

⬛ IV COMPATIBILITIES

Amiodarone, dexmedetomidine, diltiazdem, magnesium sulfate, propofol.

INDICATIONS/ROUTES/DOSAGE

Usual Dosage
PO: ADULTS, ELDERLY: 100–200 mg/day in 1–2 divided doses. **IV:** 100 mg q12h.
IV/PO: CHILDREN OLDER THAN 8 YRS: 2.2 mg/kg/dose. (**Maximum:** 100 mg/dose, 200 mg/day).

Dosage in Renal/Hepatic Impairment
No dose adjustment.

SIDE EFFECTS

Frequent: Decreased appetite, nausea, vomiting, diarrhea, dysphagia, photosensitivity (may be severe). **Occasional:** Rash, urticaria.

ADVERSE EFFECTS/TOXIC REACTIONS

Superinfection (esp. fungal), benign intracranial hypertension (headache, visual changes) may occur. Hepatotoxicity, fatty degeneration of liver, pancreatitis occur rarely.

NURSING CONSIDERATIONS

BASELINE ASSESSMENT
Question for history of allergies, esp. to tetracyclines, sulfites.

INTERVENTION/EVALUATION
Monitor daily pattern of bowel activity, stool consistency. Assess skin for rash. Be alert for superinfection: fever, vomiting, diarrhea, anal/genital pruritus, oral mucosal changes (ulceration, pain, erythema).

PATIENT/FAMILY TEACHING
• Avoid unnecessary exposure to sunlight. • Do not take with antacids, iron products. • Complete full course of therapy. • After application of dental gel, avoid brushing teeth, flossing the treated areas for 7 days. • Report severe diarrhea. • May cause nausea, vomiting. If GI upset occurs, may take with small amount food; however, Oracea should be taken on an empty stomach.

dulaglutide

doo-la-**gloo**-tide
(Trulicity)

■ **BLACK BOX ALERT** ■ Contraindicated in pts with a personal/family history of medullary thyroid carcinoma (MTC) or in pts with multiple endocrine neoplasia syndrome type 2 (MEN2). Unknown if dulaglutide causes thyroid cell tumors in humans.
Do not confuse dulaglutide with albiglutide or liraglutide.

◆**CLASSIFICATION**

PHARMACOTHERAPEUTIC: GLP-1 receptor agonist. **CLINICAL:** Antidiabetic.

USES

Adjunct to diet and exercise to improve glycemic control in adults and pts 10 yrs of age and older with type 2 diabetes mellitus. Reduce risk of major adverse cardiovascular events in adults with type 2 diabetes mellitus who have established cardiovascular disease or multiple cardiovascular risk factors.

PRECAUTIONS

Contraindications: Hypersensitivity to dulaglutide, other GLP-1 receptor agonists. Personal/family history of medullary thyroid carcinoma or multiple endocrine neoplasia syndrome type 2. **Cautions:** Pts with increased serum calcitonin, thyroid nodules, hx pancreatitis, renal/hepatic impairment. Not recommended in pts with severe GI disease, diabetic ketoacidosis, or type 1 diabetes.

ACTION

Activates GLP-1 receptors in pancreatic beta cells. **Therapeutic Effect:** Augments glucose-dependent insulin release, slows gastric emptying. Improves glycemic control.

PHARMACOKINETICS

Widely distributed. Degraded into amino acids by general protein catabolism. Peak plasma concentration: 24–72 hrs. Steady state reached in 2–4 wks. Elimination not specified. **Half-life:** 5 days.

⧗ LIFESPAN CONSIDERATIONS

Pregnancy/Lactation: Unknown if distributed in breast milk. Must either discontinue drug or discontinue breast-feeding. **Children:** Safety and efficacy not established in pts younger than 10 yrs. **Elderly:** No age-related precautions noted.

INTERACTIONS

DRUG: Insulin, insulin secreta-gogues (e.g., glyBURIDE) may increase risk of hypoglycemia. **Lira-glutide, semaglutide** may enhance adverse/toxic effects. **HERBAL:** None significant. **FOOD:** None known. **LAB VALUES:** Expected to decrease serum glucose, Hgb A1c. May increase amylase, lipase.

AVAILABILITY (Rx)

Prefilled Injector Pen: 0.75 mg/0.5 mL, 1.5 mg/0.5 mL, 3 mg/0.5 mL, 4.5 mg/0.5 mL.

ADMINISTRATION/HANDLING

SQ

Guidelines • Administer any time of day, without regard to food, on same day each week. • May change administration day if last dose was given more than 3 days prior. If dose missed, administer within 3 days of missed dose. If more than 3 days have passed after missed dose, wait until next regularly scheduled dose to administer.
Administration • Subcutaneously insert needle into abdomen, thigh, or upper arm region and inject solution. • Do not reuse needle. • Rotate injection sites each week.
Storage • Refrigerate unused pens/syringes; do not freeze. • May store at

room temperature for up to 14 days. • Protect from light.

INDICATIONS/ROUTES/DOSAGE

Type 2 Diabetes Mellitus, Reduce Risk of Major Adverse CV Events

SQ: ADULTS/ELDERLY: Initially, 0.75 mg once wkly. May increase to 1.5 mg once wkly after 4-8 wks. May further increase to 3 mg once wkly after at least 4 wks on 1.5 mg wkly dose. **Maximum:** 4.5 mg once wkly after at least 4 wks on 3 mg once wkly.

Type 2 Diabetes Mellitus

CHILDREN 10 YRS AND OLDER: Initially, 0.75 mg once wkly. May increase dose to maximum of 1.5 mg once wkly after at least 4 wks.

Dose Modification

Concomitant use with insulin secre-tagogue (e.g., sulfonylurea) or insu-lin: Consider reduced dose of insulin secretagogue or insulin based on glyce-mic goal.

Dosage in Renal Impairment

No dose adjustment.

Dosage in Hepatic Impairment

Use caution.

SIDE EFFECTS

Occasional (12%–6%): Nausea, diarrhea, vomiting, abdominal pain. **Rare (4% or less):** Decreased appetite, dyspepsia, fatigue, asthenia.

ADVERSE EFFECTS/TOXIC REACTIONS

May increase risk of acute renal failure or worsening of chronic renal impair-ment (esp. with dehydration), severe gastroparesis, pancreatitis, thyroid C-cell tumors. May increase risk of hypoglyce-mia when used with other hypoglycemic agents or insulin. Dyspnea, pruritus, rash may indicate hypersensitivity reaction. May prolong PR interval by 2–3 msec or may rarely cause first-degree AV block, tachycardia.

D

NURSING CONSIDERATIONS

BASELINE ASSESSMENT

Obtain fasting glucose level, Hgb A1c, BMP. Question history of medullary thyroid carcinoma, multiple endocrine neoplasia syndrome type 2, pancreatitis, renal impairment; first-degree AV block, PR interval prolongation. Receive full medication history and screen for use of other hypoglycemic agents or insulin. Assess pt's understanding of diabetes management, routine home glucose monitoring, medication self-administration. Assess hydration status.

INTERVENTION/EVALUATION

Monitor capillary blood glucose levels, Hgb A1c; renal function test in pts with renal impairment reporting severe GI reactions, including diarrhea, gastroparesis, vomiting. Screen for thyroid tumors (dysphagia, dyspnea, persistent hoarseness, neck mass). If tumor suspected, consider endocrinologist consultation. Clinical significance of serum calcitonin level or thyroid ultrasound with GLP-1–associated thyroid tumors is debated/unknown. Assess for hypoglycemia, hyperglycemia, hypersensitivity/allergic reaction. Screen for glucose-altering conditions: fever, stress, surgical procedures, trauma. Obtain dietary consult for nutritional education. Encourage PO intake.

PATIENT/FAMILY TEACHING

• Diabetes requires lifelong control. Diet and exercise are principal parts of treatment; do not skip or delay meals. Test blood sugar regularly. Monitor daily calorie intake. • When taking additional medications to lower blood sugar or when glucose demands are altered (fever, infection, stress, trauma), have low blood sugar treatment available (glucagon, oral dextrose). • Report suspected pregnancy or plans for breastfeeding. • Therapy may increase risk of thyroid cancer; report lumps or swelling of the neck; hoarseness, shortness of breath, trouble swallowing. • Persistent, severe abdominal pain that radiates to the back (with or without vomiting) may indicate acute pancreatitis. • Rash, itching, hives may indicate allergic reaction.

DULoxetine   TOP 100

du-**lox**-e-teen
(Cymbalta, Drizalma Sprinkle)

■ **BLACK BOX ALERT** ■ Increased risk of suicidal thinking and behavior in children, adolescents, young adults 18–24 yrs with major depressive disorder, other psychiatric disorders.
Do not confuse DULoxetine with FLUoxetine or PARoxetine.

◆CLASSIFICATION

PHARMACOTHERAPEUTIC: Serotonin norepinephrine reuptake inhibitor (SNRI). **CLINICAL:** Antidepressant.

USES

Major depressive disorder (MDD): Treatment of major depressive disorder (unipolar) (MDD) in adults. **Neuropathic pain associated with diabetes:** Management of pain associated with diabetic neuropathy in adults. **Musculoskeletal pain:** Management of chronic musculoskeletal pain including osteoarthritis of knee and low back pain in adults. **Generalized anxiety disorder:** Treatment of generalized anxiety disorder (GAD) in adults and children 7 yrs and older. **Fibromyalgia:** Treatment of fibromyalgia in adults and children 13 yrs of age and older. **OFF-LABEL:** Treatment of stress urinary incontinence in women. Chemotherapy-induced peripheral neuropathy.

PRECAUTIONS

Contraindications: Hypersensitivity to DULoxetine. Uncontrolled narrow-angle

---

glaucoma. Use of MAOI intended to treat psychiatric disorder (concurrent or within 14 days of discontinuing MAOI). Initiation of MAOI intended to treat psychiatric disorder within 5 days of discontinuing DULoxetine. Initiation of DULoxetine in pt receiving linezolid or IV methylene blue. **Cautions:** Renal impairment, history of alcoholism, chronic hepatic disease, history of mania, pts with suicidal ideation or behavior. Concurrent use with inhibitors of CYP1A2 or thioridazine, CNS depressants. Hypertension, controlled narrow-angle glaucoma, impaired GI motility. Concomitant use of NSAIDs (may increase risk of bleeding), history of seizures. Use of medications that lower seizure threshold; elderly; pts at high risk for suicide.

ACTION

Appears to inhibit serotonin and norepinephrine reuptake at CNS neuronal presynaptic membranes; is a less potent inhibitor of DOPamine reuptake. **Therapeutic Effect:** Produces antidepressant effect.

PHARMACOKINETICS

Widely distributed. Protein binding: greater than 90%. Metabolized in liver. Excreted in urine (70%), feces (20%). **Half-life:** 8–17 hrs.

⚕ LIFESPAN CONSIDERATIONS

Pregnancy/Lactation: May produce neonatal adverse reactions (constant crying, feeding difficulty, hyperreflexia, irritability). Unknown if distributed in breast milk. Breastfeeding not recommended. **Children:** Safety and efficacy not established. **Elderly:** Caution required when increasing dosage.

INTERACTIONS

DRUG: Alcohol increases risk of hepatic injury. **CYP1A2** and **CYP2D6 inhibitors (e.g., FLUoxetine, fluvoxaMINE, PARoxetine)** may increase plasma concentration. **MAOIs** may cause serotonin syndrome (autonomic hyperactivity,

coma, diaphoresis, excitement, hyperthermia, rigidity). **Aspirin, NSAIDs (e.g., ibuprofen, ketorolac, naproxen)** may increase risk of bleeding. May increase concentration, potential toxicity of **tricyclic antidepressants. HERBAL:** Glucosamine, herbs with anticoagulant/antiplatelet properties (e.g., garlic, ginger, ginkgo biloba)** may increase effect. **St. John's wort, Syrian rue** may enhance the serotonergic effect resulting in serotonin syndrome. **FOOD:** None known. **LAB VALUES:** May increase serum bilirubin, ALT, AST, alkaline phosphatase.

AVAILABILITY (Rx)

🖊 **Capsules (Delayed-Release, Enteric-Coated Pellets):** 20 mg, 30 mg, 40 mg, 60 mg. *(Drizalma Sprinkle):* 20 mg, 30 mg, 40 mg, 60 mg delayed-release capsules.

ADMINISTRATION/HANDLING

◄**ALERT**► Allow at least 14 days to elapse between use of MAOIs and DULoxetine.

PO
• Give without regard to food. Give with food, milk if GI distress occurs. • Do not break, crush, cut delayed-release capsules. • Contents of capsule may be sprinkled on applesauce or mixed in apple juice and swallowed (without chewing) immediately.

INDICATIONS/ROUTES/DOSAGE

Fibromyalgia
PO: ADULTS, ELDERLY, ADOLESCENTS 13 YRS OF AGE OR OLDER: Initially, 30 mg/day for 1 wk. Increase to 60 mg/day as tolerated.

Major Depressive Disorder
PO: ADULTS, ELDERLY: Initially, 40–60 mg/day in 1 or 2 divided doses. For doses greater than 60 mg/day, titrate in increments of 30 mg/day over 1 wk. **Maximum:** 120 mg/day.

Diabetic Neuropathy Pain
PO: ADULTS, ELDERLY: 60 mg once daily. **Maximum:** 60 mg/day. Consider lower dose with renal impairment or if tolerability is a concern.

D

Generalized Anxiety Disorder

PO: ADULTS, ELDERLY: Initially, 30–60 mg once daily. May increase up to 120 mg/day in 30-mg increments wkly. **CHILDREN 7–17 YRS:** Initially, 30 mg once daily. After 2 wks, may increase to 60 mg once daily. May further increase in increments of 30 mg/day at wkly intervals. **Maximum:** 120 mg/day.

Chronic Musculoskeletal Pain

PO: ADULTS, ELDERLY: 30 mg once daily for 1 wk, then increase to 60 mg once daily. **Maximum:** 60 mg/day.

Dosage in Renal Impairment

Mild to moderate impairment: No dose adjustment. **Severe impairment (GFR less than 30 mL/min):** Not recommended.

Dosage in Hepatic Impairment

Avoid use in pts with chronic hepatic disease or cirrhosis.

SIDE EFFECTS

Frequent (20%–11%): Nausea, dry mouth, constipation, insomnia. **Occasional (9%–5%):** Dizziness, fatigue, diarrhea, drowsiness, anorexia, diaphoresis, vomiting. **Rare (4%–2%):** Blurred vision, erectile dysfunction, delayed or failed ejaculation, anorgasmia, anxiety, decreased libido, hot flashes.

ADVERSE EFFECTS/TOXIC REACTIONS

May slightly increase heart rate. Colitis, dysphagia, gastritis, irritable bowel syndrome occur rarely.

NURSING CONSIDERATIONS

BASELINE ASSESSMENT

Assess appearance, behavior, speech pattern, level of interest, mood, sleep pattern, suicidal tendencies. Question pain level, intensity, location of pain.

INTERVENTION/EVALUATION

For pts on long-term therapy, serum chemistry profile to assess hepatic/renal function should be performed periodically. Supervise suicidal-risk pt closely during early therapy (as depression lessens, energy level improves, increasing suicide potential). Monitor B/P, mental status, anxiety, social functioning, serum glucose levels.

PATIENT/FAMILY TEACHING

• Therapeutic effect may be noted within 1–4 wks. • Do not abruptly discontinue medication. • Avoid tasks that require alertness, motor skills until response to drug is established. • Inform physician of intention of pregnancy or if pregnancy occurs. • Report anxiety, agitation, panic attacks, worsening of depression. • Avoid heavy alcohol intake (associated with severe hepatic injury).

dupilumab

doo-**pil**-ue-mab
(Dupixent)
Do not confuse dupilumab with belimumab, daclizumab, denosumab or durvalumab.

◆CLASSIFICATION

PHARMACOTHERAPEUTIC: Interleukin-4 alpha antagonist. Monoclonal antibody. **CLINICAL:** Antiasthmatic.

USES

Atopic dermatitis: Treatment of moderate to severe atopic dermatitis with moderate to severe hand and foot involvement in adults and pediatric pts 6 mos and older whose disease is not adequately controlled with topical prescription therapies or when those therapies are not advisable. May be used with or without corticosteroids. **Asthma:** Add-on maintenance treatment of moderate to severe asthma in adults and pts 6 yrs and older with an eosinophilic phenotype or corticosteroid-dependent asthma. **Chronic rhinosinusitis with nasal polyposis:** Add-on maintenance treatment in adults with inadequately controlled chronic rhinosinusitis with nasal polyposis. **Eosinophilic esophagitis:** Treatment of adults and children 1 yr of age and older, weighing at least 15 kg, with eosinophilic esophagitis. **Prurigo nodularis (PN):** Treatment of adults with PN. **Chronic obstructive pulmonary disease (COPD):** Add-on maintenance treatment of adults with inadequately controlled COPD and an eosinophilic phenotype.

PRECAUTIONS

Contraindications: Hypersensitivity to dupilumab. **Cautions:** History of herpes simplex infection, parasitic (helminth) infection. Avoid use of live vaccines.

ACTION

Binds to the IL-4Ra subunit inhibiting interleukin-4 (IL-4) and interleukin-13 (IL-13), signaling cytokine-induced responses, including release of pro-inflammatory cytokines. Mechanism of action in asthma not established. **Therapeutic Effect:** Reduces skin inflammation.

PHARMACOKINETICS

Widely distributed. Degraded into small peptides and amino acids via catabolic pathway. Peak plasma concentration: 7 days. Steady state reached by wk 16. Excretion/clearance: Time to nondetectable concentration: 10 wks. **Half-life:** Not specified.

⌛ LIFESPAN CONSIDERATIONS

Pregnancy/Lactation: Unknown if distributed in breast milk. However, human immunoglobulin G (IgG) is present in breast milk and is known to cross the placenta. **Children:** Safety and efficacy not established in pts younger than 6 mos. **Elderly:** No age-related precautions noted.

INTERACTIONS

DRUG: May decrease therapeutic effects; increase adverse effects of **vaccines (live). HERBAL:** None significant. **FOOD:** None known. **LAB VALUES:** May increase eosinophils.

AVAILABILITY (Rx)

Injection, Solution: 100 mg/0.67 mL 200 mg/1.14 mL, 300 mg/2 mL in prefilled syringe. **Solution, Pen Injector:** 200 mg/1.14 mL. 300 mg/2 mL (2 mL).

ADMINISTRATION/HANDLING
SQ

Preparation • Remove prefilled syringe from refrigerator and allow to warm to room temperature (approx. 45 min) with needle cap intact. • Visually inspect for particulate matter or discoloration. Solution should appear clear to slightly opalescent, colorless to pale yellow in color. Do not use if solution is cloudy, discolored, or if visible particles are observed.

Administration • Insert needle subcutaneously into upper arms, outer thigh, or abdomen, and inject solution. • Do not inject into areas of active skin disease or injury such as sunburns, skin rashes, inflammation, skin infections, or active psoriasis. • Rotate injection sites.

Storage • Refrigerate in original carton until time of use. • May be stored at room temperature for up to 14 days. • Protect from light. • Do not freeze or expose to external heat sources. • Do not shake.

INDICATIONS/ROUTES/DOSAGE
Atopic Dermatitis

SQ: ADULTS, ELDERLY: Initially, 600 mg (two 300-mg injections at different sites), then 300 mg every other week. If a dose is missed, administer within 7 days of missed dose, then resume normal schedule. If missed dose is not within 7 days, wait until next scheduled dose. **CHILDREN 6 YRS AND OLDER, ADOLESCENTS 17 YRS OR YOUNGER, WEIGHING 60 KG OR MORE:** Initially, 600 mg once (administered as two 300-mg injections), followed by a maintenance dose of 300 mg q2wks. **WEIGHING 30–59 KG:** Initially, 400 mg once (administered as two 200-mg injections), followed by a maintenance dose of 200 mg q2wks. **WEIGHING 15–29 KG:** Initially, 600 mg once (given as two 300-mg injections). **Maintenance:** 300 mg q4wks. **CHILDREN 6 MOS TO 5 YRS WEIGHING 15–29 KG:** 300 mg q4wks. **WEIGHING 5–14 KG:** 200 mg q4wks.

Asthma (Moderate to Severe)
SQ: ADULTS, ELDERLY, CHILDREN 12 YRS AND OLDER: Initially, 400 mg (give as two 200-mg injections) or 600 mg (give as two 300-mg injections). **Maintenance:** 200 mg (following initial 400-mg dose) or 300 mg (following initial 600-mg dose) every other wk. **CHILDREN 6-11 YRS: (Note):** An initial loading dose is not necessary. If patient has atopic dermatitis comorbidity, the dosing for atopic dermatitis (including the initial loading dose) should be used to determine dupilumab therapy. **30 KG OR GREATER:** 200 mg q2wks. **15–29 KG:** 100 mg q2wks or 300 mg q4wks.

Asthma (Steroid-Dependent or With Atopic Dermatitis)
SQ: ADULTS, ELDERLY, CHILDREN 12 YRS AND OLDER: Initially, 600 mg, then 300 mg every other wk.

Rhinosinusitis (Chronic) With Nasal Polyposis
SQ: ADULTS, ELDERLY: 300 mg every other wk. If a dose is missed, administer within 7 days of missed dose, then resume usual schedule. If a dose is missed by more than 7 days, skip dose and give at next regularly scheduled time.

Eosinophilic Esophagitis
SQ: ADULTS, ELDERLY, CHILDREN 1 YR AND OLDER WEIGHING AT LEAST 40 KG: 300 mg wkly. **30 TO LESS THAN 40 KG:** 300 mg every other wk. **15 TO LESS THAN 30 KG:** 200 mg every other wk.

Prurigo Nodularis
SQ: ADULTS, ELDERLY: Initially, 600 mg, then 300 mg every other wk.

COPD
SQ: ADULTS, ELDERLY: 300 mg every other week.

Dosage in Renal/Hepatic Impairment
No dose adjustment (not studied).

SIDE EFFECTS
Occasional (10%): Injection site reactions, eye inflammation/irritation. **Rare (1%):** Eye pruritus, dry eye.

ADVERSE EFFECTS/TOXIC REACTIONS
Hypersensitivity reactions including serum sickness (arthralgia, itching, glomerulonephritis, hypotension, lymphadenopathy, malaise, proteinuria, pyrexia, rash, shock, splenomegaly), urticaria reported in less than 1% of pts, which correlated with high antibody titers. Blepharitis, conjunctivitis (allergic, bacterial, giant papillary, viral), keratitis (ulcerative, allergic, atopic keratoconjunctivitis), herpes simplex infection (genital, otitis externa, herpes virus infection) may occur. Unknown if treatment will influence the immunologic response to helminth (parasite) infection.

NURSING CONSIDERATIONS

BASELINE ASSESSMENT
Question history of herpes zoster infection, parasitic infection, hypersensitivity reaction. Question recent administration of live virus vaccine. Pts with preexisting helminth (parasite) infection should be treated prior to first dose. Inhaled or systemic corticosteroids should not be suddenly discontinued upon initiation. Conduct dermatologic exam; record characteristics of psoriatic lesions. Consider administration of age-appropriate immunizations (if applicable) before initiation. Assess pt's willingness to self-inject medication.

INTERVENTION/EVALUATION
Interrupt or discontinue treatment if hypersensitivity reaction, opportunistic infection (esp. parasite infection, herpes zoster infection), worsening of asthma-related symptoms (esp. in pts tapering off corticosteroids) occurs. Concomitant use of topical calcineurin inhibitors is allowed, but only for areas that remain problematic (face, neck, genitals, skin folds). Assess for improvement of skin lesions.

• A healthcare provider will show you how to properly prepare and inject your medication. You must demonstrate correct preparation and injection techniques before using medication at home. • Inject medication into your outer thigh or abdomen; caregivers may also inject medication in the outer arm. • Immediately report allergic reactions such as difficulty breathing, itching, hives, rash, swelling of the face or tongue. • Report infections of any kind. • Do not stop corticosteroid therapy unless directed by prescriber. • Do not receive live vaccines. • Do not interrupt or stop asthma medications or treatments.

durvalumab

dur-**val**-ue-mab
(Imfinzi)
Do not confuse durvalumab with daclizumab, dupilumab, or nivolumab.

◆ CLASSIFICATION

PHARMACOTHERAPEUTIC: Anti-programmed death ligand-1 (PD-L1). Monoclonal antibody. **CLINICAL:** Antineoplastic.

USES

Non–small-cell lung cancer (NSCLC): Treatment of unresectable stage III NSCLC that has not progressed following concurrent platinum-based chemotherapy and radiation therapy. Treatment of adults with metastatic NSCLC with no sensitizing epidermal growth factor receptor (EGFR) mutations or anaplastic lymphoma kinase (ALK) genomic tumor aberrations (in combination with tremelimumab-acti and platinum-based chemotherapy). In combination with platinum-containing chemotherapy as neoadjuvant treatment, followed as a single agent as adjuvant treatment after surgery, for the treatment of adults with resectable (tumors greater than or equal to 4 cm and/or node positive) NSCLC and no known EGFR mutations or ALK rearrangements. **Extensive-stage small-cell lung cancer (ES-SCLC):** First-line treatment of adults with ES-SCLC in combination with etoposide and either CARBOplatin or CISplatin. **Limited-stage small cell lung cancer (LS-SCLC):** Single agent, for the treatment of adults with LS-SCLC, whose disease has not progressed following concurrent platinum-based chemotherapy and radiation therapy. **Biliary tract cancer (BTC):** Treatment of adults with locally advanced or metastatic BTC in combination with gemcitabine and CISplatin. **Unresectable hepatocellular carcinoma (uHCC):** Treatment of adults with uHCC in combination wth tremelimumab-acti. **Endometrial cancer:** In combination with carboplatin and paclitaxel followed by durvalumab as a single agent, for the treatment of adults with primary advanced or recurrent edometrial cancer that is mismatch repair deficient (dMMR).

PRECAUTIONS

Contraindications: Hypersensitivity to durvalumab. **Cautions:** Active infection, conditions predisposing to infection (e.g., diabetes, immunocompromised pts, renal failure, open wounds); corticosteroid intolerance, baseline hematologic cytopenias, elderly pts, hepatic impairment, interstitial lung disease, renal insufficiency; history of autoimmune disorders (Crohn's disease, demyelinating polyneuropathy, Guillain-Barré syndrome, Hashimoto's thyroiditis, hyperthyroidism, myasthenia gravis, rheumatoid arthritis, Type 1 diabetes, vasculitis); diabetes, pancreatitis.

ACTION

Blocks programmed cell death ligand 1 (PD-L1) binding to PD-1 and CD80 (B7.1). PD-L1 blockade increases T-cell activation allowing T-cells to kill tumor cells. Restores antitumor T-cell function. **Therapeutic Effect:** Inhibits tumor cell growth and metastasis.

D

PHARMACOKINETICS

Widely distributed. Metabolism not specified. Steady state reached in 16 wks. Excretion not specified. **Half-life:** 17 days.

⌛ LIFESPAN CONSIDERATIONS

Pregnancy/Lactation: Avoid pregnancy; may cause fetal harm. Females of reproductive potential should use effective contraception during treatment and for at least 3 mos after discontinuation. Unknown if distributed in breast milk; however, human immunoglobulin G (IgG) is present in breast milk and is known to cross the placenta. Breastfeeding not recommended during treatment and for at least 3 mos after discontinuation. **Children:** Safety and efficacy not established. **Elderly:** May have increased risk of toxic reactions; use caution.

INTERACTIONS

DRUG: Corticosteroids (Systemic) may decrease therapeutic effect. **HERBAL:** None significant. **FOOD:** None known. **LAB VALUES:** May increase serum albumin, alkaline phosphatase, ALT, AST, bilirubin, calcium, creatinine, glucose, magnesium. May decrease serum sodium; Hgb, Hct, lymphocytes, neutrophils, RBCs. May increase or decrease serum potassium.

AVAILABILITY (Rx)

Injection: 120 mg/2.4 mL (50 mg/mL), 500 mg/10 mL (50 mg/mL).

ADMINISTRATION/HANDLING

 IV

Preparation • Visually inspect vial for particulate matter or discoloration. Solution should appear clear to opalescent, colorless to slightly yellow in color. • Do not use if solution is cloudy, discolored, or if visible particles are observed. • Do not shake. • Withdraw proper volume from vial and dilute in 0.9% NaCl or D_5W to a final concentration of 1–15 mg/mL. • Gently invert to mix; do not shake. • Diluted solution should appear clear, colorless, and free of particles.

Rate of administration • Infuse over 60 min via dedicated IV line using a sterile, low protein-binding 0.2- or 0.22-micron in-line filter. • When given in combination with tremelimumab-acti, administer tremelimumab-acti over 60 min followed by a 60 min observation period. Then, administer durvalumab as a separate IV infusion over 60 min on the same day. Use separate infusion bags and filters for each infusion.

Storage • Refrigerate unused vials in original carton. • Protect from light. May refrigerate diluted solution for no more than 28 days or store at room temperature for no more than 8 hrs. If refrigerated, allow diluted solution to warm to room temperature before use. • Do not freeze or shake.

⚕ IV INCOMPATIBILITIES

Do not infuse with other medications.

INDICATIONS/ROUTES/DOSAGE

BTC

IV: ADULTS, ELDERLY: 30 KG OR GREATER: 1,500 mg (in combination with gemcitabine and CISplatin) q3wks up to 8 cycles, then 1,500 mg q4wks as a single agent. **LESS THAN 30 KG:** 20 mg/kg (in combination with gemcitabine and CISplatin q3wks [21 days]) up to 8 cycles, then 20 mg/kg q4wks as a single agent. Continue until disease progression or unacceptable toxicity.

NSCLC Stage III

IV: ADULTS, ELDERLY: 30 KG OR GREATER: 10 mg/kg q2wks or 1,500 mg q4wks. **LESS THAN 30 KG:** 10 mg/kg q2wks. Continue until disease progression or unacceptable toxicity or a maximum of 12 mos.

LS-SCLC

IV: ADULTS, ELDERLY: (following concurrent platinum-based chemotherapy and radiation therapy): **PTS GREATER THAN 30 KG OR GREATER:** 1,500 mg q4wks. **PTS LESS THAN 30 KG:** 20 mg/kg q4wks.

ES-SCLC

IV: ADULTS, ELDERLY: 30 KG OR GREATER: 1,500 mg q3wks (in combination with etoposide and either CARBOplatin or CISplatin) for 4 cycles, then q4wks as single therapy. **LESS THAN 30 KG:** 20 mg/kg q3wks (in combination with etoposide and either CARBO platin or CISplatin) for 4 cycles, then 10 mg/kg q2wks as a single agent. Continue until disease progression or unacceptable toxicity.

uHCC

IV: ADULTS, ELDERLY: ADULTS, ELDERLY: 30 KG OR GREATER: 1,500 mg following a single dose of tremelimumab-acti 300 mg at day 1 of cycle 1, then 1,500 mg as a single agent q4wks. **LESS THAN 30 KG:** 20 mg/kg following a single dose of tremelimumab-acti 4 mg/kg at day 1 of cycle 1, then 20 mg/kg as a single agent q4wks. After cycle 1 of combination therapy, administer as a single agent q4wks until disease progression or unacceptable toxicity.

NSCLC Metastatic

IV: ADULTS, ELDERLY: 30 KG OR GREATER: 1,500 mg q3wks (in combination w/ tremelimumab-actl and platinum-based chemotherapy) for 4 cycles, then 1,500 mg q4wks as a single agent with peme-trexed maintenance therapy q4wks, and a fifth dose of tremelimumab-actl in combination with durvalumab dose 6 at wk 16. **LESS THAN 30 KG:** 20 mg/kg q3wks (in combination with tremelimumab-actl 1 mg/kg and platinum-based chemo-therapy), and then 20 mg/kg q4wks as a single agent with pemetrexed therapy q4wks, and a fifth dose of tremelimumab-actl 1 mg/kg, in combination with dur-valumab dose 6 at week 16.

Neoadjuvant and Adjuvant Treatment of Resectable NSCLC

IV: ADULTS, ELDERLY: PTS WEIGHING GREATER THAN 30 KG: (Neoadjuvant): 1,500 mg, in combination with chemotherapy, q3wks for up to 4 cycles prior to surgery. **(Adjuvant):** 1,500 mg, as a single agent, q4wks for up to 12 cycles after surgery. **PTS WEIGHING LESS THAN 30 KG: (Neoadjuvant):** 20 mg/kg q3wks, in combination with chemotherapy, for up to 4 cycles prior to surgery. **(Adjuvant):** 20 mg/kg q4wks, as a single agent, for up to 12 cycles after surgery.

Endometrial Cancer

IV: ADULTS, ELDERLY, 30 KG OR GREATER: 1,120 mg in combination with carboplatin and paclitaxel q3wks for 6 cycles, followed by durvalumab 1,500 mg q4 wks as a single agent. **LESS THAN 30 KG:** 15 mg/kg in com-bination with carboplatin and paclitaxel q3wks for 6 cycles, followed by durvalumab 20 mg/kg q4wks as a single agent.

Dose Modification

Note: Withhold and/or discontinue dur-valumab to manage adverse reactions. Based on severity of adverse reactions, withhold durvalumab and administer systemic corti-costeroids. Initiate corticosteroid taper when adverse reactions improve to below Grade 1, and continue taper over at least 1 mo. If treatment is not permanently discontinued due to adverse reactions, resume therapy when adverse reactions return to Grade 1 or lower and the corticosteroid dose has been reduced to less than 10 mg predniSONE (or equivalent) per day. No dose reductions of durvalumab are recommended.

Colitis (GI toxicity)

Grade 2 diarrhea or colitis: Withhold dose. Start predniSONE 1–2 mg/kg/day (or equivalent) followed by taper. **Grade 3 or 4 diarrhea or colitis:** Permanently discontinue. Start predniSONE 1–2 mg/kg/day (or equivalent), followed by taper.

Dermatitis

Grade 2 rash or dermatitis (for greater than 1 wk); Grade 3 rash or dermati-tis: Withhold dose. Consider starting pred-niSONE 1–2 mg/kg/day (or equivalent), followed by taper. **Grade 4 rash or der-matitis:** Permanently discontinue. Con-sider starting predniSONE 1–2 mg/kg/day (or equivalent), followed by taper.

Endocrinopathies

Grade 2–4 adrenal insufficiency (hypophysitis, hypopituitarism): With-hold dose until clinically stable. Start pred-niSONE 1–2 mg/kg/day (or equivalent), followed by taper. Consider hormone replacement therapy as clinically indicated. **Grade 2–4 hyperthyroidism:** Withhold

D

dose until clinically stable and manage symptoms. **Grade 2–4 hypothyroidism:** Consider hormone replacement therapy. **Grade 2–4 type 1 diabetes:** Withhold dose until clinically stable. Start insulin therapy as clinically indicated.

Hepatotoxicity

Grade 2 hepatitis (serum ALT or AST greater than 3 and up to 5 times upper limit of normal [ULN] or serum bilirubin greater than 1.5 and up to 3 times ULN); Grade 3 hepatitis (serum ALT or AST less than or equal to 8 times ULN or serum bilirubin less than or equal to 5 times ULN): Withhold dose. Start predniSONE 1–2 mg/kg/day (or equivalent), followed by taper. **Grade 3 hepatitis (serum ALT or AST greater than 8 times ULN or serum bilirubin greater than 5 times ULN; transaminase elevation (concurrent serum ALT or AST greater than 3 times ULN and serum bilirubin greater than 2 times ULN) with no known cause:** Permanently discontinue. Start predniSONE 1–2 mg/kg/day (or equivalent), followed by taper.

Infection

Grade 3 or 4 infection: Withhold dose and manage symptoms. Start anti-infectives for suspected or confirmed infections.

Infusion-Related Reactions

Grade 1 or 2: Interrupt or decrease rate of infusion. Consider premedication for subsequent infusions. **Grade 3 or 4:** Permanently discontinue.

Nephritis (Renal toxicity during treatment)

Grade 2 nephritis (serum creatinine greater than 1.5 and up to 3 times ULN): Withhold dose. Start predniSONE 1–2 mg/kg/day (or equivalent), followed by taper. **Grade 3 nephritis (serum creatinine greater than 3 and up to 6 times ULN); Grade 4 nephritis (serum creatinine greater than 6 times ULN):** Permanently discontinue. Start predniSONE 1–2 mg/kg/day (or equivalent), followed by taper.

Other Toxic Reactions

Any other Grade 3 reactions: Withhold dose and manage symptoms. **Any other Grade 4 reactions:** Permanently discontinue. Start predniSONE 1–4 mg/kg/day (or equivalent), followed by taper.

Pneumonitis

Grade 2 pneumonitis: Withhold dose. Start predniSONE 1–2 mg/kg/day (or equivalent), followed by taper. **Grade 3 or Grade 4 pneumonitis:** Permanently discontinue. Start predniSONE 1–4 mg/kg/day (or equivalent) followed by taper.

Dosage in Renal/Hepatic Impairment

Not specified; use caution.

SIDE EFFECTS

Frequent (39%–19%): Fatigue, asthenia, malaise, back/musculoskeletal/neck pain, myalgia, constipation, decreased appetite. **Occasional (16%–11%):** Nausea, peripheral edema, scrotal edema, lymphedema, abdominal/flank pain, diarrhea, pyrexia, dyspnea, cough, dermatitis, dermatitis acneiform, dermatitis psoriasiform, psoriasis, maculopapular rash, pustular rash, eczema, erythema, erythema multiforme, erythematous rash, acne, lichen planus.

ADVERSE EFFECTS/TOXIC REACTIONS

Myelosuppression (anemia, neutropenia, lymphopenia) is an expected response to therapy. May cause severe, sometimes fatal immune-mediated reactions such as adrenal insufficiency, colitis, hepatitis, hypothyroidism, hyperthyroidism, hypophysitis, nephritis, pneumonitis, type 1 diabetes, rash; aseptic meningitis, hemolytic anemia, keratitis, myocarditis, myositis, thrombocytopenic purpura, uveitis. Urinary tract infections including candiduria, cystitis, urosepsis occurred in 15% of pts.

NURSING CONSIDERATIONS

BASELINE ASSESSMENT

Obtain CBC, BMP, LFT, thyroid function test; pregnancy test in females of repro-

---

ductive potential; vital signs. Question medical history as listed in Precautions; prior infusion reactions. Question intolerance to corticosteroids. Screen for active infection. Assess nutritional/hydration status. Conduct neurologic/dermatologic exam. Offer emotional support.

INTERVENTION/EVALUATION

Monitor CBC, BMP, LFT, serum ionized calcium, magnesium; thyroid function test periodically. Monitor for infusion reactions including angioedema, back or neck pain, dyspnea, flushing, pruritus, pyrexia, rash, syncope. Consider increasing corticosteroid dose if toxic effects worsen or do not improve. Assess skin for rash, lesions. Diligently monitor for immune-mediated adverse effects as listed in Adverse Effects/Toxic Reactions. If immune-mediated reactions occur, consider referral to specialist. Obtain CXR if interstitial lung disease, pneumonitis suspected. Interrupt or discontinue treatment if serious infection, opportunistic infection, sepsis occurs, and initiate appropriate antimicrobial therapy. If corticosteroid therapy is started, monitor capillary blood glucose and screen for corticosteroid side effects or intolerance. Report neurologic changes including nuchal rigidity with fever, positive Kernig's sign, positive Brudzinski's sign, altered mental status, seizures (related to aseptic meningitis). Strictly monitor I&O. Encourage fluid intake.

PATIENT/FAMILY TEACHING

• Treatment may depress your immune system and reduce your ability to fight infection. Report symptoms of infection such as body aches, chills, cough, fatigue, fever. Avoid those with active infection. • Use effective contraception to avoid pregnancy. Do not breastfeed. • Treatment may cause serious or life-threatening inflammatory reactions. Report symptoms of treatment-related inflammatory events in the following body systems: brain (confusion, headache, fever, rigid neck, seizures), colon (severe abdominal pain or diarrhea), eye (blurry vision, double vision, unequal pupil size, sensitivity to light, drooping eyelid), lung (chest pain, cough, shortness of breath), liver (bruising easily, amber-colored urine, clay-colored/tarry stools, yellowing of skin or eyes), nerves (severe nerve pain or loss of motor function), pituitary (persistent or unusual headache, dizziness, extreme weakness, fainting, vision changes), thyroid (trouble sleeping, high blood pressure, fast heart rate [overactive thyroid] or fatigue, goiter, weight gain [underactive thyroid]). Immediately report infusion reactions such as neck or back pain, dizziness, fever, flushing, itching, shortness of breath, swelling of the face. • Treatment may cause severe diarrhea. Drink plenty of fluids.

efbemalenograstim alfa-vuxw

ef-**bem**-a-**len**-oh-**gra**-stim **al**-fa
(Ryzneuta)
Do not confuse efbemalenogras-tim with filgrastim or pegfil-grastim.

◆CLASSIFICATION

PHARMACOTHERAPEUTIC: Hemat-opoietic agent. **CLINICAL:** Human granulocyte stimulating factor (G-CSF).

USES

To decrease the incidence of infection, as manifested by febrile neutropenia, in adults with nonmyeloid malignancies receiving myelosuppressive anticancer drugs associated with a clinically significant incidence of febrile neutropenia.

PRECAUTIONS

Contraindications: Hypersensitivity to efbemalenograstim alfa; other human granulocyte colony-stimulating factors (e.g., filgrastim, pegfilgrastim). **Cautions:** Sickle cell disease, baseline thrombocytopenia; concomitant use of drugs that cause thrombocytopenia. Not indicated for mobilization of blood progenitor cells for hematopoietic stem cell transplantation; in pts with malignancies with myeloid characteristics (due to G-CSF's potential to act as growth factor). Contains natural rubber latex (do not administer to pts with latex allergy).

ACTION

Colony stimulating factor acts on hematopoietic cells, binding to cell surface receptors. **Therapeutic Effect:** Stimulates proliferation, differentiation, commitment, and end cell functional activation.

PHARMACOKINETICS

Widely distributed. Metabolized into small peptides via catabolic pathway. Peak plasma concentration: 9–48 hrs. **Half-life:** 35.6 hrs.

⧖ LIFESPAN CONSIDERATIONS

Pregnancy/Lactation: Unknown if distributed in breast milk. **Children:** Safety and efficacy not established. **Elderly:** No age-related precautions noted.

INTERACTIONS

DRUG: None significant. **HERBAL:** None significant. **FOOD:** None known. **LAB VALUES:** May decrease Hgb, RBCs, platelets.

AVAILABILITY (Rx)

Injection, Prefilled Syringe: 20 mg/mL.

ADMINISTRATION/HANDLING

SQ
Preparation • Remove carton from refrigerator and allow solution to warm to room temperature (approx. 30 min) without removing prefilled syringe (protects solution from light). Do not shake or agitate. • Visually inspect for particulate matter or discoloration. Solution should appear clear and colorless. Do not use if solution is cloudy, discolored, or visible particles are observed.
Administration • Insert needle subcutaneously into outer thigh, abdomen, or back of upper arm and inject solution. • Do not inject within 2 inches (5 cm) of navel or into areas of active skin disease or injury such as sunburns, skin rashes, inflammation, skin infections, or psoriatic lesions. • Rotate injection sites. • Do not administer IV or intramuscularly. • If a dose is delayed, administer as soon as possible.
Storage • Refrigerate in original carton to protect from light. Do not freeze. • Discard prefilled syringes that have remained at room temperature for more than 48 hrs.

INDICATIONS/ROUTES/DOSAGE

Chemotherapy-Induced Neutropenia
SQ: ADULTS, ELDERLY: 20 mg once per chemotherapy cycle at least 24 hrs after cytotoxic chemotherapy. Do not give within 14 days before or less than 24 hrs after cytotoxic chemotherapy.

Dosage in Renal/Hepatic Impairment
No dose adjustment.

SIDE EFFECTS

Frequent (51%): Nausea. **Occasional (15%–12%):** Anemia, thrombocytopenia.

ADVERSE EFFECTS/TOXIC REACTIONS

Acute respiratory distress syndrome, aortitis, capillary leak syndrome, glomerulonephritis, leukocytosis, thrombocytopenia, sickle cell crisis, splenic rupture may occur. Myelodysplastic syndrome and acute myeloid leukemia were reported in pts being treated for breast or lung cancer with chemotherapy and radiation therapy, or with radiation therapy alone. May cause tumor growth stimulatory effects on malignant cells. Hypersensitivity reactions including dyspnea, facial edema, hypotension, tachycardia, wheezing were reported. Life-threatening capillary leak syndrome (hypoalbuminemia, hypotension, fluid overload, leukocytosis, hemoconcentration) may occur.

NURSING CONSIDERATIONS

BASELINE ASSESSMENT
Obtain CBC. Question for prior hypersensitivity reactions other human granulocyte colony-stimulating factors (e.g., filgrastim, pegfilgrastim); history of sickle cell disease. Verify schedule of cytotoxic chemotherapy. Dose should not be given within 14 days before or less than 24 hrs after cytotoxic chemotherapy.

INTERVENTION/EVALUATION
Monitor CBC as clinically indicated. Monitor for acute respiratory distress syndrome (dyspnea, fever, lung infiltrates), aortitis (abdomen/back/chest pain, fatigue, fever; elevated C-reactive protein, WBC), glomerulonephritis (edema, fatigue, hematuria, hypertension, muscle cramps, nausea/vomiting; decreased urinary output, foamy urine), hypersensitivity reactions, splenic rupture (dizziness, hypotension, left shoulder pain, upper abdominal pain). Pts with sickle cell disease should be routinely assessed for sickle cell crisis (dyspnea, hypoxia, generalized pain [extreme], jaundice, weakness, vision changes). If weight has increased by 2.5 kg or 5% (or greater) from baseline and pt is hypotensive, check for cough, dyspnea, hypoalbuminemia, peripheral edema (may indicate capillary leak syndrome).

PATIENT/FAMILY TEACHING
• Report chills, fever, severe bone pain, difficulty breathing. • Life-threatening rupture of the spleen can occur. Report dizziness, left shoulder pain, low blood pressure, upper abdominal pain. • Report symptoms of capillary leak syndrome (dizziness, fatigue, sudden weight gain, shortness of breath, swelling of face or extremities); inflammation of the aorta (e.g., abdomen/back/chest pain, fatigue, fever), kidney problems (decreased urine output, dark-colored urine), allergic reactions (difficulty breathing, fast heartbeat, low pressure, wheezing). • Treatment may cause life-threatening sickle cell crisis in pts with history of sickle cell disease.

elacestrant

el-a-**kes**-trant
(Orserdu)
Do not confuse elacestrant with eliglustat or fulvestrant.

◆CLASSIFICATION

PHARMACOTHERAPEUTIC: Estrogen receptor antagonist. **CLINICAL:** Antineoplastic.

E

USES

Treatment of postmenopausal females or adult males with estrogen receptor (ER)–positive, human epidermal growth factor receptor 2 (HER2)–negative, estrogen receptor 1 gene (ESR1)–mutated advanced or metastatic breast cancer with disease progression following at least one line of endocrine therapy.

PRECAUTIONS

Contraindications: Hypersensitivity to elacestrant. **Cautions:** Mild to moderate hepatic impairment, dyslipidemia. Not recommended in pts with severe hepatic impairment. Avoid concomitant use of strong or moderate CYP3A4 inhibitors or inducers.

ACTION

Binds to estrogen receptor (ER)-alpha. In ER-positive, human epidermal growth factor receptor 2 (HER2)–negative breast cancer cells, inhibits 17-beta estradiol–mediated cell proliferation via proteasomal pathway. **Therapeutic Effect:** Inhibits tumor cell growth.

PHARMACOKINETICS

Widely distributed. Metabolized in liver. Protein binding: (greater than 99%). Peak plasma concentration: 1–4 hrs. Steady state reached in 6 days. Excreted in feces (82%), urine (7.5%). **Half-life:** 30–50 hrs.

⧖ LIFESPAN CONSIDERATIONS

Pregnancy/Lactation: Not indicated in female pts prior to menopause; however, fetal harm may occur when given during pregnancy. Males with female partners of reproductive potential must use effective contraception during treatment and for at least 7 days after discontinuation. Unknown if distributed in breast milk. Breastfeeding not recommended during treatment and for at least 7 days after discontinuation. May impair fertility. **Children:** Safety and efficacy not established. **Elderly:** No age-related precautions noted.

INTERACTIONS

DRUG: Strong CYP3A4 inhibitors (e.g., clarithromycin, ketoconazole, ritonavir), moderate CYP3A4 inhibitors (e.g., dilTIAZem, fluconazole, verapamil) may increase concentration/effect. Strong CYP3A4 inducers (e.g., carBAMazepine, phenytoin, riFAMPin), moderate CYP3A4 inducers (e.g., dexamethasone, modafinil, nafcillin) may decrease concentration/effect. May increase concentration effect of BCRP substrates (e.g., methotrexate, pravastatin, topotecan), P-gp substrates (e.g., digoxin, dilTIAZem, tacrolimus). **HERBAL:** St. John's wort may decrease concentration/effect. **FOOD:** Grapefruit products may increase concentration/effect. **LAB VALUES:** May increase serum ALT, AST, cholesterol, creatinine, triglycerides. May decrease Hgb; serum sodium.

AVAILABILITY (Rx)

 Tablets: 86 mg, 345 mg.

ADMINISTRATION/HANDLING

PO
• Give with food (may reduce nausea/vomiting) at the same each day. • Administer tablet whole; do not break, crush, or divide. Tablet cannot be chewed. Do not give if tablet is broken, cracked, or not intact. • If vomiting occurs after administration, give next dose at the regularly scheduled time the following day (do not give additional dose). • If a dose is missed by more than 6 hrs, skip the dose and resume at the next regularly scheduled time the following day.

INDICATIONS/ROUTES/DOSAGE

Breast Cancer (ESR1-Mutated, Advanced, or Metastatic)
PO: ADULTS, ELDERLY: 345 mg once daily until disease progression or unacceptable toxicity.

Dose Reduction Schedule for Adverse Events
First dose reduction: 258 mg (three 86 mg tablets) once daily. **Second dose reduction:** 172 mg (two 86 mg tablets) once daily. **Unable to tolerate 172 mg dose:** Permanently discontinue.

Dose Modification
Based on Common Terminology Criteria for Adverse Events (CTCAE).

Grade 1 Adverse Reactions
Continue treatment at same dose.

Grade 2 Adverse Reactions
Consider withholding treatment until improved to Grade 1 or 0 (or baseline), then resume at same dose.

Grade 3 Adverse Reactions
Withhold treatment until improved to Grade 1 or 0 (or baseline), then resume at reduced dose. If Grade 3 adverse reactions recur, withhold treatment until improved to Grade 1 or 0 (or baseline), then resume at next reduced dose level.

Grade 4 Adverse Reactions
Withhold treatment until improved to Grade 1 or 0 (or baseline), then resume at reduced dose. If adverse reaction is intolerable or Grade 4 adverse reactions recur, permanently discontinue.

Dosage in Renal Impairment
Not specified; use caution.

Dosage in Hepatic Impairment
Mild impairment: No dose adjustment. **Moderate impairment:** Reduce starting dose to 258 mg once daily. **Severe impairment:** Not recommended.

SIDE EFFECTS

Frequent (41–19%): Musculoskeletal pain, nausea, fatigue, vomiting. **Occasional (15% to less than 10%):** Decreased appetite, diarrhea, constipation, headache, abdominal pain, hot flush, dyspepsia, rash, insomnia, dyspnea, dizziness, stomatitis, gastroesophageal reflux disease.

ADVERSE EFFECTS/TOXIC REACTIONS

Dyslipidemia reported in 27–30% of pts.

NURSING CONSIDERATIONS

BASELINE ASSESSMENT
Obtain CBC, LFT, lipid profile. Educate compliance of effective contraception in males with female partners of reproductive potential. Verify presence of ESR1 mutation in plasma specimen. Question history hepatic impairment, dyslipidemia. Receive full medication history and screen for interactions. Offer emotional support.

INTERVENTION/EVALUATION
Monitor LFT in pts with hepatic impairment; lipid profile periodically. Assess for adverse reactions of any grade following CTCAE criteria. Offer antiemetic for nausea/vomiting. Assess skin for rash. Monitor daily pattern of bowel activity, stool consistency.

PATIENT/FAMILY TEACHING
• Take with food to reduce vomiting.
• There is a high risk of interactions with other medications. Do not take

---

newly prescribed medications unless approved by prescriber who originally started treatment. Do not take herbal products or ingest grapefruit products. • Males with female partners who can become pregnant must use effective contraception to avoid pregnancy. • Treatment may increase cholesterol and triglyceride levels. • Report side effects that worsen despite medical management.

elbasvir/grazoprevir

el-bas-vir/graz-**oh**-pre-vir
(Zepatier)

■ BLACK BOX ALERT ■ Hepatitis B virus reactivation may cause fulminant hepatitis, hepatic failure, and death.

Do not confuse elbasvir with daclatasvir, ombitasvir or grazoprevir with boceprevir or simeprevir.

◆CLASSIFICATION

PHARMACOTHERAPEUTIC: NS5A inhibitor/NS3/4A protease inhibitor.
CLINICAL: Antihepaciviral.

USES

Treatment of chronic hepatitis C virus (HCV) genotype 1 or 4 infection in adults and pts 12 yrs of age and older or weighing at least 30 kg.

PRECAUTIONS

Contraindications: Hypersensitivity to elbasvir or grazoprevir, decompensated hepatic cirrhosis, moderate or severe hepatic impairment; concomitant use of organic anion transporting polypeptides 1B1/3 (OATP1B1/3) inhibitors, strong CYP3A4 inducers. Concomitant use of atazanavir, carBAMazepine, cycloSPORINE, darunavir, efavirenz, lopinavir, phenytoin, rifAMPin, saquinavir, St. John's

wort, tipranavir. Any contraindications or hypersensitivity to ribavirin (if used with treatment regimen). **Cautions:** HIV infection, mild hepatic impairment. Safety and efficacy not established in pts with hepatitis B virus coinfection, liver transplant recipients.

ACTION

Elbasvir inhibits hepatitis C virus (HCV) NS5A protein, which is essential for viral RNA replication and virion assembly. Grazoprevir inhibits HCV NS3/4A protease needed for processing HCV-encoded polyproteins, which is essential for viral replication. **Therapeutic Effect:** Inhibits viral replication of hepatitis C virus.

PHARMACOKINETICS

Widely distributed. Metabolized in liver. Protein binding: elbasvir (99.9%), grazoprevir (98.8%). Peak plasma concentration: 3 hrs. Steady state reached in approx. 6 days. Excreted in feces (greater than 90%), urine (less than 1%). **Half-life:** elbasvir: 24 hrs; grazoprevir: 31 hrs.

⧖ LIFESPAN CONSIDERATIONS

Pregnancy/Lactation: Use caution in pregnancy. Unknown if distributed in breast milk. When used with ribavirin, breastfeeding and pregnancy are contraindicated during treatment and up to 6 mos after discontinuation. **Children:** Safety and efficacy not established in pts younger than 12 yrs. **Elderly:** May have increased risk of hepatotoxicity.

INTERACTIONS

DRUG: **Atazanavir, darunavir, cycloSPORINE** may significantly increase risk of hepatotoxicity; use contraindicated. **Strong CYP3A4 inducers (e.g., carbamazepine, phenytoin, rifampin),**

moderate CYP3A4 inducers (e.g., dexamethasone, modafinil, nafcillin) may decrease concentration/effect. Strong CYP3A4 inhibitors (e.g., clarithromycin, ketoconazole, ritonavir) may increase concentration/effect. May increase concentration/effects of atorvastatin, fluvastatin, lovastatin, niMODipine, rosuvastatin, simvastatin, tacrolimus. HERBAL: St. John's wort may decrease concentration/effect; use contraindicated. FOOD: None known. LAB VALUES: May decrease Hgb. May increase serum ALT, bilirubin.

AVAILABILITY (Rx)

Fixed-Dose Combination Tablets: elbasvir 50 mg/grazoprevir 100 mg.

ADMINISTRATION/HANDLING

PO
• Give without regard to food.

INDICATIONS/ROUTES/ DOSAGE

Note: NS5A resistance testing recommended in HCV genotype 1a infected pts prior to initiating treatment with Zepatier.

Chronic Hepatitis C Virus Infection
PO: ADULTS, ELDERLY, CHILDREN 12 YRS OR OLDER OR 30 KG OR GREATER: 1 tablet once daily.

Treatment Regimen and Duration
PO: ADULTS, ELDERLY: Genotype 1a: Treatment-naive or peginterferon alfa (PegIFN)/ribavirin (RBV)–experienced without baseline NS5A polymorphisms: 1 tablet once daily for 12 wks. Genotype 1a: Treatment-naive or PegIFN/RBV–experienced with baseline NS5A polymorphisms: 1 tablet once daily with ribavirin for 16 wks. Genotype 1b: Treatment-naive or PegIFV/RBV–experienced: 1 tablet once daily for 12 wks. Genotype 1a or 1b: PegIFV/RBV/protease inhibitor–experienced: 1 tablet once daily with ribavirin for 12 wks. Genotype 4: Treatment-naive: 1 tablet once daily for 12 wks. Genotype 4: PegIFN/RBV–experienced: 1 tablet once daily with ribavirin for 16 wks.

Treatment-Induced Hepatotoxicity
Consider discontinuation in pts with persistent serum ALT elevation greater than 10 times upper limit of normal (ULN). Permanently discontinue if serum ALT elevation is accompanied with elevated alkaline phosphatase, conjugated bilirubin, prolonged INR, or signs of acute hepatic inflammation.

Dosage in Renal Impairment
No dose adjustment.

Dosage in Hepatic Impairment
Mild impairment: No dose adjustment. Moderate to severe impairment: Contraindicated.

SIDE EFFECTS

Occasional (11%–3%): Fatigue, headache, diarrhea, nausea, insomnia, dyspnea, rash, pruritus, irritability. Rare (2%): Abdominal pain, arthralgia.

ADVERSE EFFECTS/TOXIC REACTIONS

Serum ALT elevation up to 5 times ULN reported in 1% of pts. Serum bilirubin elevation greater than 2.5 times ULN occurred in 6% of pts. Serum ALT elevation occurred more frequently in the elderly, female pts, and pts of Asian ancestry.

NURSING CONSIDERATIONS

BASELINE ASSESSMENT

Obtain CBC, LFT, HCV-RNA level; pregnancy test in female pts of reproductive potential. Confirm hepatitis C genotype. In pts with HCV genotype 1a, recommend testing for the presence of NS5A resistance-associated polymorphisms prior to initiation. Receive full medication history including herbal products; screen for contraindications. Question history of chronic anemia, hepatitis B virus infection, HIV infection, liver transplantation.

INTERVENTION/EVALUATION

Obtain LFT at wk 8, then as clinically indicated. For pts receiving 16 wks of therapy, obtain additional LFT at wk 12. Monitor CBC periodically; HCV-RNA levels at wks 4, 8, 12, 16 and as clinically indicated. Monitor for hepatotoxicity. Assess for anemia-related dizziness, exertional dyspnea, fatigue, weakness, syncope. Encourage nutritional intake. Assess for decreased appetite, weight loss. Obtain monthly pregnancy tests in females of reproductive potential if treated with ribavirin.

PATIENT/FAMILY TEACHING

• Treatment may be used in combination with ribavirin (inform pt of side effects/toxic reactions). If therapy includes ribavirin, female pts of reproductive potential should avoid pregnancy during treatment and up to 6 mos after last dose. • Do not take newly prescribed medication unless approved by the doctor who originally started treatment. • Do not take herbal products, esp. St. John's wort. • Avoid alcohol, grapefruit products. • Report signs of treatment-induced liver injury such as abdominal pain, clay-colored stool, dark amber urine, decreased appetite, fatigue, weakness, yellowing of the skin or eyes. • Maintain proper nutritional intake.

eletriptan

el-e-**trip**-tan
(Relpax)

♦**CLASSIFICATION**

PHARMACOTHERAPEUTIC: Serotonin receptor agonist. **CLINICAL:** Antimigraine.

USES

Treatment of acute migraine headache with or without aura.

PRECAUTIONS

Contraindications: Hypersensitivity to eletriptan. Arrhythmias associated with conduction disorders, cerebrovascular syndrome including strokes and transient ischemic attacks (TIAs), coronary artery disease, hemiplegic or basilar migraine, ischemic heart disease, peripheral vascular disease including ischemic bowel disease, severe hepatic impairment, uncontrolled hypertension; use within 24 hrs of treatment with another 5-HT$_1$ agonist, an ergotamine-containing or ergot-type medication such as dihydroergotamine (DHE) or methysergide. Recent use (within 72 hrs) of strong CYP3A4 inhibitors (e.g., clarithromycin, ketoconazole, itraconazole, ritonavir). **Cautions:** Mild to moderate renal/hepatic impairment, controlled hypertension, history of CVA.

ACTION

Selective agonist for serotonin in cranial arteries; causes vasoconstriction and reduces inflammation. **Therapeutic Effect:** Relieves migraine headache.

PHARMACOKINETICS

Widely distributed. Metabolized by liver. Excreted in urine. **Half-life:** 4.4 hrs (increased in hepatic impairment, elderly [older than 65 yrs]).

⏳ LIFESPAN CONSIDERATIONS

Pregnancy/Lactation: May decrease possibility of ovulation. Distributed in breast milk. **Children:** Safety and efficacy not established. **Elderly:** Increased risk of hypertension in those older than 65 yrs.

INTERACTIONS

DRUG: Ergot derivatives (e.g., ergotamine) may increase vasoconstrictive effect. **Strong CYP3A4 inhibitors (e.g., clarithromycin, ketoconazole, ritonavir)** may increase concentration/effect. **MAOIs (e.g., phenelzine, selegiline)** may cause serotonin syndrome. **HERBAL:** None significant. **FOOD:** None known. **LAB VALUES:** None significant.

AVAILABILITY (Rx)

 Tablets: 20 mg, 40 mg.

ADMINISTRATION/HANDLING

PO

• Give without regard to food. • Administer as soon as symptoms appear.

INDICATIONS/ROUTES/DOSAGE

Acute Migraine Headache
PO: ADULTS, ELDERLY: Initially, 20–40 mg as a single dose. **Maximum:** 40 mg/dose. If headache improves but then returns, dose may be repeated after 2 hrs. **Maximum:** 80 mg/day.

Dosage in Renal/Hepatic Impairment
No dose adjustment. Not recommended in severe hepatic impairment.

SIDE EFFECTS

Occasional (6%–5%): Dizziness, drowsiness, asthenia, nausea. **Rare (3%–2%):** Paresthesia, headache, dry mouth, warm or hot sensation, dyspepsia, dysphagia.

ADVERSE EFFECTS/TOXIC REACTIONS

Cardiac reactions (ischemia, coronary artery vasospasm, MI), noncardiac vasospasm-related reactions (hemorrhage, CVA) occur rarely, particularly in pts with hypertension, obesity, diabetes, strong family history of coronary artery disease; smokers; males older than 40 yrs; postmenopausal women. May cause GI ischemia, bowel infarction, non–cardiac-related vasospasms including peripheral vascular ischemia, Raynaud's syndrome. Overuse may increase frequency, occurrence of headaches.

NURSING CONSIDERATIONS

BASELINE ASSESSMENT

Question characteristics of migraine headaches (onset, location, duration, possible precipitating symptoms). Obtain baseline B/P for evidence of uncontrolled hypertension (contraindication).

INTERVENTION/EVALUATION

Evaluate for relief of migraine headaches (photophobia, phonophobia, nausea, vomiting, pain, dizziness, fogginess). Monitor for cardiac arrhythmia, coronary events, hypertension, hypersensitivity reaction.

PATIENT/FAMILY TEACHING

• Take a single dose as soon as symptoms of an actual migraine attack appear. • Medication is intended to relieve migraine headaches, not to prevent or reduce number of attacks. • Avoid tasks that require alertness, motor skills until response to drug is established. • Immediately report palpitations, pain/tightness in chest/throat, sudden or severe abdominal pain, pain/weakness of extremities.

elexacaftor/ tezacaftor/ivacaftor

e-lex-a-**kaf**-tor/tez-a-**kaf**-tor/eye-va-**kaf**-tor
(Trikafta)
Do not confuse elexacaftor/ tezacaftor/ivacaftor (Trikafta)

E

with lumacaftor/ivacaftor (Orkambi).

◆**CLASSIFICATION**

PHARMACOTHERAPEUTIC: Cystic fibrosis transmembrane conductance regulator (CFTR) modulator. **CLINICAL:** Cystic fibrosis agent.

USES

Treatment of cystic fibrosis (CF) in pts aged 2 yrs and older who have at least one F508del mutation in the CFTR gene.

PRECAUTIONS

Contraindications: Hypersensitivity to elexacaftor, tezacaftor, ivacaftor. **Cautions:** Moderate hepatic impairment, concomitant use of CYP3A4 inhibitors. Avoid use of concomitant strong CYP3A inducers. Not recommended in severe hepatic impairment.

ACTION

Mutations in the CFTR gene (encodes the CFTR protein) are the cause of cystic fibrosis. The Phe508del mutation (most common CFTR mutation) causes abnormal CFTR trafficking, reducing the quantity of CFTR protein at the cell surface and disrupting channel gating. Elexacaftor and tezacaftor improve cellular processing/trafficking of Phe508del-CFTR, increasing CFTR at the cell surface. Ivacaftor increases chloride channel transport by augmenting channel gating. **Therapeutic Effect:** Improves lung/organ function, decreases respiratory exacerbations.

PHARMACOKINETICS

Widely distributed. Metabolized in liver. Protein binding: elexacaftor: Greater than 99%, tezacaftor: 99%, ivacaftor: 99%. Peak plasma concentration: elexacaftor: 4–12 hrs, tezacaftor: 2–4 hrs, ivacaftor: 3–6 hrs. Steady state reached within 14 days (elexacaftor), 8 days (tezacaftor), 3–5 days (ivacaftor). Excretion: elexacaftor: Feces (87%), urine (less than 1%); tezacaftor: Feces (72%), urine

(14%); ivacaftor: Feces (89%), urine (7%). **Half-life:** elexacaftor: 29.8 ± 10.6 hrs, tezacaftor: 17.4 ± 3.66 hrs, ivacaftor: 15 ± 3.92 hrs.

⧖ LIFESPAN CONSIDERATIONS

Pregnancy/Lactation: Unknown if distributed in breast milk. Hormonal contraceptives may increase incidence of rash events. **Children:** Safety and efficacy not established in pts younger than 2 yrs. **Elderly:** Safety and efficacy not established.

INTERACTIONS

DRUG: **Strong CYP3A4 inhibitors (e.g., clarithromycin, ketoconazole, ritonavir), moderate CYP3A4 inhibitors (e.g., erythromycin, fluconazole)** may increase concentration/effect. **Strong CYP3A4 inducers (e.g., carBAMazepine, phenytoin, rifAMPin)** may decrease concentration/effect. **HERBAL: St. John's wort** may decrease concentration/effect. **FOOD: Grapefruit products** may increase concentration/effect. **LAB VALUES:** May increase serum ALT, AST, bilirubin, CPK. May decrease serum glucose.

AVAILABILITY (Rx)

Fixed-Dose Combination (Copackaged With Ivacaftor): Tablets: elexacaftor 100 mg/tezacaftor 50 mg/ivacaftor 75 mg copackaged with ivacaftor 150 mg; elexacaftor 50 mg/tezacaftor 25 mg/ivacaftor 37.5 mg copackaged with ivacaftor 75 mg. **Oral granules:** elexacaftor 100 mg/tezacaftor 50 mg/ivacaftor 75 mg copackaged with ivacaftor 75 mg; elexacaftor 80 mg/tezacaftor 40 mg ivacaftor 60 mg copackaged with ivacaftor 59.5 mg.

ADMINISTRATION/HANDLING

PO
• Give with fat-containing food (e.g., eggs, butter, peanut butter, whole-milk dairy products [e.g., whole milk, cheese, yogurt]). • Administer tablets whole;

---

do not break, crush, or divide. • If a morning dose is missed by more than 6 hrs, give as soon as possible, but do not give evening dose. If an evening dose is missed by more than 6 hrs, skip the evening dose and administer the morning dose at usual scheduled time. Do not give morning and evening doses at same time. **Oral granules:** Mix entire contents of oral granules with 1 tsp soft food or liquid that is at or below room temperature. Once mixed, use within 1 hr.

INDICATIONS/ROUTES/DOSAGE

Cystic Fibrosis
PO: ADULTS, CHILDREN 6 YRS AND OLDER: 30 kg or greater: 2 fixed-dose combination tablets (elexacaftor 100 mg, tezacaftor 50 mg, ivacaftor 75 mg per tablet) in the morning and 1 tablet of ivacaftor (150 mg) in the evening (approx. 12 hrs apart). **6–11 YRS, LESS THAN 30 KG:** Two tablets of elexacaftor 50 mg/tezacaftor 25 mg/ivacaftor 37.5 mg (total dose of elexacaftor 100 mg/ tezacaftor 50 mg/ivacaftor 75 mg) in the morning and ivacaftor 75 mg in the evening. **2–5 YRS, 14 KG OR GREATER:** One packet (containing elexacaftor 100 mg/ tezacaftor 50 mg/ivacaftor 75 mg) in the morning and one packet ivacaftor 75 mg in the evening. **LESS THAN 14 KG:** One packet (containing elexacaftor 80 mg/ tezacaftor 40 mg/ivacaftor 60 mg) in the morning and one packet ivacaftor 59.5 mg in the evening.

Dose Modification
Concomitant Use of Moderate CYP3A4 Inhibitors
Note: Do not give evening dose of ivacaftor.
Dosing schedule for day 1: 2 fixed-dose combination tablets (elexacaftor 100 mg, tezacaftor 50 mg, ivacaftor 75 mg per tablet) in the morning. **Day 2:** 1 tablet of ivacaftor (150 mg) in the morning. **Day 3:** 2 fixed-dose combination tablets (elexacaftor 100 mg, tezacaftor 50 mg, ivacaftor 75 mg per tablet) in the morning. **Day 4:** 1 tablet of ivacaftor

(150 mg) in the morning. Repeat the 4-day cycle thereafter.

Concomitant Use of Strong CYP3A4 Inhibitors
Note: Do not give evening dose of ivacaftor.
Dosing schedule for day 1: 2 fixed-dose combination tablets (elexacaftor 100 mg, tezacaftor 50 mg, ivacaftor 75 mg per tablet) in the morning. **Day 2 and 3:** No dose. **Day 4:** 2 fixed-dose combination tablets (elexacaftor 100 mg, tezacaftor 50 mg, ivacaftor 75 mg per tablet) in the morning. Repeat the 4-day cycle thereafter.

Hepatotoxicity
Serum ALT/AST greater than 5 times ULN, serum ALT/AST greater than 3 times ULN with bilirubin greater than 2 times ULN: Withhold treatment until resolved. Consider the risk versus benefit of resuming treatment.

Rash
Rash in females taking hormonal contraception: Consider withholding treatment and hormonal contraceptive until rash is resolved, then consider resuming treatment without hormonal contraceptive. If rash does not recur, may consider resuming hormonal contraceptive.

Dosage in Renal Impairment
Mild to moderate impairment: No dose adjustment. **Severe impairment, ESRD:** Not specified; use caution.

Dosage in Hepatic Impairment
Mild impairment: No dose adjustment. **Moderate impairment:** 2 fixed-dose combination tablets (elexacaftor 100 mg, tezacaftor 50 mg, ivacaftor 75 mg per tablet) in the morning only (do not give evening ivacaftor dose). **Severe impairment:** Not recommended.

SIDE EFFECTS

Occasional (17%–7%): Headache, abdominal pain, diarrhea, rash, nasal congestion, rhinorrhea, rhinitis. **Rare (5%–2%):** Flatulence, abdominal distention, dizziness, dysmenorrhea, acne, eczema, pruritus.

ADVERSE EFFECTS/TOXIC REACTIONS

Elevated transaminases may occur. Worsening of hepatic function was reported in pts with baseline hepatic impairment. Cataracts were reported in pediatric pts taking ivacaftor. Infections including upper respiratory tract infection (16% of pts), influenza (7% of pts), sinusitis (5% of pts), conjunctivitis, pharyngitis, tonsillitis, UTI were reported. Rash events were reported more frequently in females, which may be related to concomitant use of hormonal contraceptives.

NURSING CONSIDERATIONS

BASELINE ASSESSMENT

Obtain LFT. If pt's genotype is unknown, a CF mutation test should be obtained to confirm presence of at least one F508del mutation. Assess baseline symptoms of cystic fibrosis (abdominal discomfort/gas, persistent cough, inability to mobilize secretions, poor weight gain, lung infections, dyspnea). Question history of hepatic impairment. Receive full medication history and screen for drug interactions.

INTERVENTION/EVALUATION

Monitor LFT q3mos for 12 mos, then annually thereafter (or more frequently in pts with baseline hepatic impairment). Assess respiratory function, organ function for treatment effectiveness. Assess sputum production; ability to mobilize secretions. If concomitant use of strong or moderate CYP3A4 inhibitors is unavoidable, monitor for toxicities. Monitor for rash in females taking hormonal contraception.

PATIENT/FAMILY TEACHING

• Always take medication with fatty foods. • There is a high risk of interactions with other medications. Do not take newly prescribed medications unless approved by prescriber who originally started therapy. • Avoid vitamins, grapefruit products, herbal supplements (esp. St. John's wort). • Report symptoms of liver problems (e.g., bruising, confusion; dark, amber, orange-colored urine; right upper abdominal pain, yellowing of the skin or eyes). • Report vision changes, cataracts; signs of respiratory infection (e.g., cough, fever, shortness of breath). • Rashes are more common in female pts taking hormonal contraception.

elotuzumab

el-oh-**tooz**-ue-mab
(Empliciti)
Do not confuse elotuzumab with alemtuzumab, eculizumab, evolocumab, pertuzumab, gemtuzumab, trastuzumab.

◆CLASSIFICATION

PHARMACOTHERAPEUTIC: Anti-SLAMF7. Monoclonal antibody. **CLINICAL:** Antineoplastic.

USES

Multiple myeloma: Treatment of multiple myeloma (in combination with lenalidomide and dexAMETHasone) in pts who have received one to three prior therapies or (in combination with pomalidomide and dexAMETHasone) in pts who have received at least two prior therapies including lenalidomide and a proteasome inhibitor.

PRECAUTIONS

Contraindications: Hypersensitivity to elotuzumab. **Cautions:** Diabetes, baseline cytopenias, hypertension; history of chronic opportunistic infections (esp. viral infections, fungal infections), conditions predisposing to infection (e.g., diabetes, kidney failure, open wounds). Concomitant use of medications known to cause bradycardia (e.g., antiarrhythmics, beta blockers, calcium channel blockers). Concomitant use of live vaccines not recommended during treatment and up to 3 mos after discontinuation. Avoid use during severe active infection.

ACTION

Binds to and specifically targets signaling lymphocytic activation molecule family member 7 (SLAMF7), a protein that is expressed on most myeloma and natural killer cells. Directly activates natural killer cells and facilitates cellular death. **Therapeutic Effect:** Inhibits tumor cell growth and metastasis.

PHARMACOKINETICS

Widely distributed. Metabolism not specified. Elimination not specified. **Half-life:** Not specified; 97% of steady-state concentration is expected to be eliminated within 82 days.

LIFESPAN CONSIDERATIONS

Pregnancy/Lactation: Avoid pregnancy; may cause fetal harm/malformations/fetal demise when used with lenalidomide. Unknown if distributed in breast milk. However, immunoglobulin G (IgG) is present in breast milk. Breastfeeding contraindicated when used with concomitant lenalidomide. **Men:** Lenalidomide is present in semen. Recommend use of barrier methods during sexual activity. **Children:** Safety and efficacy not established. **Elderly:** No age-related precautions noted.

INTERACTIONS

DRUG: May increase immunosuppressant/toxic effects of **immunosuppressants (e.g., fingolimod, leflunomide, nivolumab)**. **Roflumilast** may increase immunosuppressant effect. May enhance adverse/toxic effect of **live vaccines;** may decrease therapeutic effect of **vaccines (live), BCG (intravesical)**. **HERBAL:** Echinacea may decrease effect. **FOOD:** None known. **LAB VALUES:** May be detected on both serum protein electrophoresis and immu-

nofixation assays used to monitor multiple myeloma endogenous M-protein. May affect the determination of complete response and disease progression of some pts with IgG kappa myeloma protein. Expected to decrease lymphocytes, leukocytes, platelets. May decrease serum albumin, bicarbonate, calcium. May increase serum alkaline phosphatase, ALT, AST, glucose, potassium.

AVAILABILITY (Rx)

Injection, Powder for Reconstitution: 300 mg, 400 mg.

ADMINISTRATION/HANDLING

 IV

Reconstitution • Calculate the dose and number of vials required based on weight in kg. • Reconstitute the 300-mg vial with 13 mL of Sterile Water for Injection or the 400-mg vial with 17 mL of Sterile Water for Injection using an 18-g or lower (e.g., 17, 16, or 15) needle. • Gently roll vial upright to mix. To dissolve any powder left on top of vial or stopper, gently invert vial several times. • Do not shake or agitate. • The powder should dissolve in less than 10 min. • After dissolution, allow vials to stand for 5–10 min. • Visually inspect solution for particulate matter or discoloration. Solution should appear clear, colorless to slightly yellow. Discard if solution is cloudy or discolored or if foreign particles are observed. Each vial contains an overfill volume to allow for a specific withdrawal of 12 mL (300-mg vial) or 16 mL (400-mg vial). • Final concentration of withdrawn volume (without overfill) will equal 25 mg/mL. • Dilute in 230 mL of 0.9% NaCl or 5% Dextrose injection in polyvinyl chloride or polyolefin infusion bag. • Mix by gentle inversion; do not shake or agitate. • The volume may be adjusted in order to not exceed 5 mL/kg of pt weight at any given dose.

Infusion guidelines • Prior to administration, premedicate with dexAMETHasone, acetaminophen, antihistamine (H_1 antagonist, plus H_2 antagonist) approx. 45–90 min before each infusion (see

E

manufacturer guidelines). • Use an in-line, sterile, nonpyrogenic, low protein-binding filter (0.2–1.2 mm). • Infuse via dedicated line using an infusion pump.

Rate of administration • **First infusion (cycle 1, dose 1) 10 mg/mL:** Infuse at 0.5 mL/min for the first 30 min. If no infusion reactions occur, may increase to 1 mL/min for next 30 min. If tolerated, may increase to 2 mL/min. • **Second infusion (cycle 1, dose 2):** Initiate at 3 mL/min for first 30 min if no infusion reactions occurred during first infusion. If tolerated, may increase to 4 mL/min until infusion completed. • **Subsequent infusions (cycle 1, doses 3 and 4, all subsequent infusions):** Initiate at 5 mL/min until completion if no infusion reactions occurred during prior infusion. **20 mg/mL: (Dose 1):** Initiate at 3 mL/min for the first 30 min. If no infusion reactions occur, may increase to 4 mL/min. **(Dose 2 and all subsequent doses):** 5 mL/min.

Storage • Refrigerate intact vials until time of use. • Do not freeze or shake. • Refrigerate diluted solution up to 24 hrs. • May store at room temperature up to 8 hrs (of the total 24 hrs). • Diluted solution must be administered within 24 hrs of reconstitution. • Protect from light.

▨ IV INCOMPATIBILITIES

Do not mix with other medications.

INDICATIONS/ROUTES/DOSAGE

Multiple Myeloma

Note: Premedicate with dexAMETHasone, H_1 or H_2 blocker, and acetaminophen 45–90 mins before infusion.

IV: ADULTS, ELDERLY: *(In combination with lenalidomide and dexAMETHasone):* **Cycles 1 and 2:** 10 mg/kg once wkly on days 1, 8, 15, 22 of 28-day cycle. **Cycles 3 and beyond:** 10 mg/kg once q2wks on days 1 and 15 of 28-day cycle. Continue until disease progression or unacceptable toxicity. *(In combination with pomalidomide and dexA-*

METHasone): **Cycles 1 and 2:** 10 mg/kg once wkly on days 1, 8, 15, 22 of 28-day cycle. **Cycles 3 and beyond:** 20 mg/kg once q4wks on day 1 of 28-day cycle. Continue until disease progression or unacceptable toxicity.

Dose Modification
Infusion Reactions
Grade 2 or higher reaction: Interrupt infusion until symptoms improve. Once resolved to Grade 1 or 0, resume infusion at 0.5 mL/min. If tolerated, increase in increments of 0.5 mL/min q30mins back to previous rate. May further increase rate as indicated if no reaction recurs. If infusion reaction recurs, stop infusion and do not restart for that day.

Dosage in Renal/Hepatic Impairment
Not specified; use caution.

SIDE EFFECTS

Frequent (61%–20%): Fatigue, diarrhea, pyrexia, constipation, cough, peripheral neuropathy, decreased appetite. **Occasional (16%–10%):** Extremity pain, headache, vomiting, decreased weight, oropharyngeal pain, hypoesthesia, mood change, night sweats.

ADVERSE EFFECTS/TOXIC REACTIONS

Infusion reactions reported in 10% of pts. Most infusion reactions were Grade 3 and lower. Lymphopenia, leukopenia, thrombocytopenia are expected responses to therapy. Infections were reported in 81% of pts. Grade 3 or 4 infections occurred in 28% of pts. Nasopharyngitis (25% of pts), upper respiratory tract infection (23% of pts), opportunistic infection (22% of pts), herpes zoster (14% of pts), fungal infection (10% of pts), influenza; second primary malignancies, skin malignancies, solid tumors, malignant neoplasms; tachycardia, bradycardia, systolic or diastolic hypertension, hypotension; pulmonary embolism may occur. Hepatotoxicity with elevation of serum alkaline phosphatase greater than

2 times upper limit of normal (ULN), serum ALT/AST greater than 3 times ULN, total bilirubin greater than 2 times ULN reported in 3% of pts. Other adverse effects may include cataracts (12% of pts), hyperglycemia (89% of pts), hypersensitivity reaction (greater than 5% of pts). Thrombocytopenia may increase risk of bleeding.

NURSING CONSIDERATIONS

BASELINE ASSESSMENT

Obtain CBC, BMP, LFT; serum ionized calcium; capillary blood glucose, vital signs; pregnancy test in female pts of reproductive potential. Obtain baseline ECG in pts concurrently using medications known to cause bradycardia. Question history of chronic opportunistic infections, diabetes, hepatic impairment, pulmonary embolism; prior infusion or hypersensitivity reactions. Screen for medications known to cause bradycardia, hyperglycemia. Screen for active infection. Offer emotional support.

INTERVENTION/EVALUATION

Obtain CBC, BMP, LFT, ionized calcium periodically. Administer in an environment equipped to monitor for and manage infusion reactions. If infusion reaction of any grade/severity occurs, immediately interrupt infusion and manage symptoms. Accurately record characteristics of infusion reactions (severity, type, time of onset). Infusion reactions may affect future infusion rates. Monitor HR, BP q30mins during infusion and for at least 2 hrs after completion in pts with prior hemodynamic reactions. Cough, dyspnea, hypoxia, tachycardia may indicate pulmonary embolism. Monitor for bradycardia, cataracts, hyperglycemia, hyperkalemia, hypersensitivity reaction, hepatotoxicity, neuropathy, tachycardia. Assess for new primary malignancies (solid tumors, skin cancers); skin for new lesions, moles. Monitor daily pattern bowel activity, stool consistency.

PATIENT/FAMILY TEACHING

• Treatment may depress your immune system and reduce your ability to fight infection. Report symptoms of infection such as body aches, chills, cough, fatigue, fever. Avoid those with active infection. • Therapy may decrease your heart rate, esp. in those taking medications that lower heart rate; report dizziness, chest pain, palpitations, or fainting. • Avoid pregnancy. Do not breastfeed. • Male pts should use condoms during sexual activity. • Treatment includes a steroid that may raise blood sugar levels; report dehydration, blurry vision, confusion, frequent urination, increased thirst, fruity breath. • Report allergic reactions of any kind. • Abdominal pain, easy bruising, clay-colored stools, dark-amber urine, fatigue, loss of appetite, yellowing of skin or eyes may indicate liver problem.

empagliflozin

em-pa-gli-**floe**-zin
(Jardiance)
Do not confuse empagliflozin with bexagliflozin, canagliflozin, dapagliflozin, or ertugliflozin.

FIXED-COMBINATION(S)

Glyxambi: empagliflozin/linagliptin (an antidiabetic): 10 mg/5 mg, 25 mg/5 mg. **Synjardy:** Empagliflozin/metFORMIN (an antidiabetic): 5 mg/500 mg, 5 mg/1000 mg, 12.5 mg/500 mg, 12.5 mg/1000 mg. **Trijardy XR:** empagliflozin/linagliptin (an antidiabetic)/metFORMIN (an antidiabetic): 10 mg/5 mg/1,000 mg; 25 mg/5 mg/1,000 mg; 5mg/ 2.5 mg/1,000 mg; 12.5 mg/2.5 mg/1,000 mg.

◆CLASSIFICATION

PHARMACOTHERAPEUTIC: Sodium-glucose co-transporter 2 (SGLT2) inhibitor. **CLINICAL:** Antidiabetic.

E

USES

Diabetes mellitus: Adjunctive treatment to diet and exercise to improve glycemic controls in adults and pts 10 yrs and older with type 2 diabetes mellitus. **Risk reduction:** Reduce risk of cardiovascular death in pts with type 2 diabetes and cardiovascular disease. Reduce risk of cardiovascular death and hospitalization for adults with HF. **Chronic kidney disease:** Reduce risk of sustained decline in eGFR, end-stage kidney disease, cardiovascular death, and hospitalization in adults with chronic kidney disease at risk of progression.

PRECAUTIONS

Contraindications: History of hypersensitivity to empagliflozin, other SGLT2 inhibitors, severe renal impairment (eGFR less than 30 mI/min), end-stage renal disease, dialysis. **Cautions:** Concomitant use of loop diuretics, other hypoglycemic agents (e.g., insulin, insulin secretagogues), baseline systolic hypotension, renal impairment, hypovolemia/dehydration, recent genital mycotic infection; pts at risk for diabetic ketoacidosis (insulin dose reduction, acute febrile illness, reduced calorie intake, surgery, alcohol abuse, history of pancreatitis). Not recommended in pts with active bladder cancer, diabetic ketoacidosis, type 1 diabetes mellitus.

ACTION

Inhibits SGLT2 in proximal renal tubule, reducing reabsorption of filtered glucose from tubular lumen and lowering renal threshold for glucose. Reduces reabsorption of sodium and increases delivery of sodium to the distal tubule. **Therapeutic Effect:** Increases urinary excretion of glucose; lowers serum glucose levels. Reduces cardiac preload and afterload; downregulates sympathetic activity.

PHARMACOKINETICS

Widely distributed. Metabolized in liver. Peak plasma concentration: 1.5 hrs. Protein binding: 86%. Excreted in urine (54%) and feces (41%). **Half-life:** 12.4 hrs.

⧗ LIFESPAN CONSIDERATIONS

Pregnancy/Lactation: Avoid use during second or third trimester. Unknown if distributed in breast milk. Breastfeeding not recommended during treatment. **Children:** Safety and efficacy not established. **Elderly:** May have increased risk for adverse reactions (e.g., hypotension, syncope, dehydration).

INTERACTIONS

DRUG: Insulin, **insulin secretagogues (e.g., glyBURIDE)** may increase risk of hypoglycemia. May increase concentration/effects of **loop diuretics (e.g., furosemide)**. **HERBAL: Herbals with hypoglycemic properties (e.g., fenugreek, flaxseed, ginseng, gotu kola)** may increase hypoglycemic effect. **FOOD:** None known. **LAB VALUES:** May increase serum creatinine; low-density lipoprotein cholesterol (LDL-C); Hct. May decrease serum bicarbonate; eGFR. Expected to result in positive urine glucose test. May interfere with 1,5-anhydroglucitol (1,5-AG) assay.

AVAILABILITY (Rx)

Tablets: 10 mg, 25 mg.

ADMINISTRATION/HANDLING

PO
• Give without regard to food in the morning.

INDICATIONS/ROUTES/DOSAGE

Reduce Risk of Cardiovascular Death, Heart Failure, Chronic Kidney Disease
PO: ADULTS, ELDERLY: 10 mg once daily in the morning.

Type 2 Diabetes Mellitus
PO: ADULTS, ELDERLY, CHILDREN 10 YRS AND OLDER: Initially, 10 mg once daily in the morning. May increase to 25 mg once daily after 4–12 wks.

Dosage in Renal Impairment
GFR 30 mL/min or greater: No dose adjustment. **GFR less than 30 mL/min:** Not recommended.

Dosage in Hepatic Impairment

No dose adjustment.

SIDE EFFECTS

Rare (4%–1.1%): Increased urination, dyslipidemia, arthralgia, nausea.

ADVERSE EFFECTS/TOXIC REACTIONS

Symptomatic hypotension (orthostatic hypotension, postural dizziness, syncope) may occur, esp. in pts who are elderly, use concomitant loop diuretics, or have baseline systolic hypotension. Intravascular volume depletion/contraction may cause acute kidney injury requiring dialysis. Fatal cases of ketoacidosis were reported. Hypoglycemic events were reported in pts using concomitant insulin, insulin secretagogues. Infections including influenza, nasopharyngitis, pyelonephritis, urosepsis, UTI, genital mycotic infections (male and female), upper respiratory tract infection may occur. Necrotizing fasciitis of the perineum (Fournier gangrene), a life-threatening necrotizing infection of the genital and perineum region that requires urgent surgical intervention, has been reported. Hypersensitivity reactions including anaphylaxis, angioedema, urticaria have occurred.

NURSING CONSIDERATIONS

BASELINE ASSESSMENT

Obtain BUN, serum creatinine, eGFR, CrCl, blood glucose level, Hgb A1c; B/P. Assess hydration status. Correct volume depletion prior to initiation. Assess pt's understanding of diabetes management, routine home glucose monitoring. Obtain dietary consult for nutritional education. Question history of renal impairment, type 1 diabetes, ketoacidosis. In pts requiring surgery, consider suspending treatment at least 3 days before surgery. Receive full medication history and screen for interactions.

INTERVENTION/EVALUATION

Monitor BUN, serum creatinine, eGFR, CrCl, blood glucose level, Hgb A1c; B/P periodically. Monitor for ketoacidosis (e.g.,

dehydration, confusion, extreme thirst, sweet-smelling breath, Kussmaul respirations, nausea), hypoglycemia (anxiety, confusion, diaphoresis, diplopia, dizziness, headache, hunger, perioral numbness, tachycardia, tremors), hyperglycemia (fatigue, Kussmaul respirations, polyphagia, polyuria, polydipsia, nausea, vomiting). Pts presenting with metabolic acidosis should be screened for ketoacidosis, regardless of serum glucose levels. Concomitant use of beta blockers (e.g., carvedilol, metoprolol) may mask symptoms of hypoglycemia. Monitor for acute kidney injury (dark-colored urine, flank pain, decreased urine output, muscle aches), infections (cough, fatigue, fever), urinary tract infections (dysuria, fever, flank pain, malaise), mycotic infections, Fournier gangrene (perineal necrosis). Screen for glucose-altering conditions (fever, increased activity or stress, surgical procedures). Monitor weight, I&Os. Monitor for hypersensitivity reactions (anaphylaxis, angioedema, urticaria).

PATIENT/FAMILY TEACHING

• Diabetes mellitus requires lifelong control. Diet and exercise are principal parts of treatment; do not skip or delay meals. Test blood sugar regularly. Monitor daily calorie intake. • When taking combination drug therapy or when glucose conditions are altered (excessive alcohol ingestion, insufficient carbohydrate intake, hormone deficiencies, critical illness), have a low blood sugar treatment available (e.g., glucagon, oral dextrose). • Genital itching or discharge may indicate yeast infection. • Report symptoms of perineal necrosis (e.g., discoloration, pain, swelling of the scrotum, penis, or perineum). • Therapy may increase risk for dehydration, low blood pressure, which may cause kidney failure. Report decreased urination, amber-colored urine, flank pain, fatigue, swelling of the hands or feet. Drink enough fluids to maintain adequate hydration. Pts with HF should be cautious of overhydration. • Report symptoms of UTI, kidney infection (back pain, pelvic pain, burning while urinating, cloudy or foul-smelling urine), allergic reactions (difficulty breathing, rash, wheezing; swelling of the face or tongue. • Go slowly from lying to standing. • Do not breastfeed.

E

emtricitabine

em-tri-**sye**-ta-bine (Emtriva)

■ **BLACK BOX ALERT** ■ Serious, sometimes fatal, lactic acidosis and severe hepatomegaly with steatosis (fatty liver) have been reported. Severe exacerbations of hepatitis B virus (HBV) reported in pts co-infected with HIV-1 and HBV following discontinuation. If discontinuation of therapy occurs, monitor hepatic function for at least several mos. Initiate anti-HBV therapy if warranted.

FIXED-COMBINATION(S)

Atripla: emtricitabine/efavirenz (an antiretroviral)/tenofovir disoproxil fumarate (TDF) (an antiretroviral): 200 mg/600 mg/300 mg. **Complera:** emtricitabine/rilpivirine (an antiretroviral)/tenofovir disoproxil fumarate (TDF) (an antiretroviral): 200 mg/25 mg/300 mg. **Descovy:** emtricitabine/tenofovir alafenamide (TAF) (a nucleotide reverse transcriptase inhibitor): 200 mg/25 mg. **Genvoya:** emtricitabine/elvitegravir (an integrase inhibitor)/cobicistat (a pharmacokinetic enhancer)/tenofovir alafenamide (TAF) (a nucleotide reverse transcriptase inhibitor): 200 mg/150 mg/150 mg/10 mg. **Odefsey:** emtricitabine/rilpivirine (nonnucleoside reverse transcrip-tase inhibitor [NNRTI])/tenofovir alafenamide (TAF) (a nucleotide reverse transcriptase inhibitor): 200 mg/25 mg/25 mg. **Stribild:** emtricitabine/elvitegravir (an integrase inhibitor)/cobicistat (a pharmacokinetic enhancer)/tenofovir disoproxil fumarate (TDF) (a nucleotide reverse transcriptase inhibitor): 200 mg/150 mg/150 mg/300 mg. **Truvada:** emtricitabine/

tenofovir disoproxil fumarate (TDF) (an antiretroviral): 200 mg/300 mg.

◆Classification

PHARMACOTHERAPEUTIC: Nucleoside reverse transcriptase inhibitor. **CLINICAL:** Antiretroviral agent.

USES

Used in combination with at least two other antiretroviral agents for treatment of HIV-1 infection. **OFF-LABEL:** Occupational/nonoccupational HIV post-exposure prophylaxis.

PRECAUTIONS

Contraindications: Hypersensitivity to emtricitabine. **Cautions:** Renal impairment; history of hepatitis, hepatic impairment.

ACTION

Emtricitabine is phosphorylated intracellularly to emtricitabine 5′-triphosphate, which interferes with HIV viral RNA-dependent DNA polymerase. **Therapeutic Effect:** Impairs HIV replication, slowing progression of HIV infection.

PHARMACOKINETICS

Widely distributed. Metabolized via phosphorylated by cellular enzymes. Protein binding: less than 4%. Excreted in urine (86%), feces (14%). **Half-life:** 10 hrs.

⧗ LIFESPAN CONSIDERATIONS

Pregnancy/Lactation: Breastfeeding not recommended due to risk of postnatal transmission of HIV infection. **Children:** No age-related precautions noted. **Elderly:** Age-related renal impairment may require dosage adjustment.

INTERACTIONS

DRUG: None significant. **HERBAL:** None significant. **FOOD:** None known. **LAB VALUES:** May increase serum amylase,

ALT, AST, lipase, triglycerides. May alter serum glucose.

AVAILABILITY (Rx)

Capsules: 200 mg. **Oral Solution:** 10 mg/mL.

ADMINISTRATION/HANDLING

PO

• Give without regard to food.

INDICATIONS/ROUTES/DOSAGE

HIV

PO: ADULTS, ELDERLY, ADOLESCENTS 18 YRS AND OLDER: (Capsules): 200 mg once daily. **(Solution):** 240 mg once daily. **ADOLESCENTS 17 YRS OR YOUNGER, CHILDREN, INFANTS 3 MOS AND OLDER: (Solution):** 6 mg/kg/dose once daily. **Maximum:** 240 mg/day. **(Capsules): PTS WEIGHING 33 KG OR MORE AND ABLE TO SWALLOW CAPSULE WHOLE:** 200 mg once daily. **1 TO LESS THAN 3 MOS: (Solution):** 3 mg/kg once daily.

Dosage in Renal Impairment

Creatinine Clearance	Capsule	Oral Solution
30–49 mL/ min	200 mg q48h	120 mg q24h
15–29 mL/ min	200 mg q72h	80 mg q24h
Less than 15 mL/ min; hemodialysis pts	200 mg q96h	60 mg q24h (administer after dialysis)

Administer after dialysis on dialysis days.

Dosage in Hepatic Impairment

No dose adjustment.

SIDE EFFECTS

Frequent (23%–13%): Headache, rhinitis, rash, diarrhea, nausea. **Occasional (14%–4%):** Cough, vomiting, abdominal pain, insomnia, depression, paresthesia, dizziness, peripheral neuropathy, dyspepsia, myalgia. **Rare (3%–2%):** Arthralgia, abnormal dreams.

ADVERSE EFFECTS/TOXIC REACTIONS

Fatal cases of lactic acidosis, severe hepatomegaly with steatosis have occurred. A majority of cases occurred in women. If therapy is discontinued, pts co-infected with hepatitis B virus have an increased risk for viral replication, worsening of hepatic function, and may experience hepatic decompensation and/or failure. May induce immune reconstitution syndrome (inflammatory response to dormant opportunistic infections such as *Mycobacterium avium*, cytomegalovirus, PCP, tuberculosis, or acceleration of autoimmune disorders such as Graves' disease, polymyositis, Guillain-Barré). Acute renal failure or worsening renal impairment may occur. May cause redistribution or accumulation of body fat (lipodystrophy).

NURSING CONSIDERATIONS

BASELINE ASSESSMENT

CD4+ count, viral load, HIV-1 RNA level; pregnancy test in females of reproductive potential. Test all pts for HBV infection. Offer emotional support. Question history of hepatic disease.

INTERVENTION/EVALUATION

Monitor CD4+ count, viral load, HIV-1 RNA level for treatment effectiveness. An increase of serum creatinine greater than 0.4 mg/dL from baseline may indicate renal impairment. Cough, dyspnea, fever, excess band cells on CBC may indicate acute infection (WBC may be unreliable in pts with uncontrolled HIV infection). Obtain serum lactate level if lactic acidosis suspected. Monitor daily pattern of bowel activity, stool consistency. Question for evidence of nausea, pruritus. Assess skin for rash, urticaria. Monitor for immune reconstitution syndrome, hepatitis B virus reactivation.

PATIENT/FAMILY TEACHING

• Treatment does not cure HIV infection nor reduce risk of transmission. Practice safe sex with barrier methods or abstinence. • Drug resistance can form if treatment is interrupted; do not run out of supply. • As immune system strengthens, it may respond to dormant infections hidden within the body. Report any new fever, chills, body aches, cough, night sweats, shortness of breath. • Do not breastfeed. • Antiretrovirals may cause excess body fat in upper back, neck, breast, trunk; and may cause decreased body fat in legs, arms, face. Report new-onset or worsening of depression. • Report persistent or severe abdominal pain, nausea, vomiting, numbness.

enalapril

en-**al**-a-pril
(Epaned, Vasotec)

■ **BLACK BOX ALERT** ■ May cause fetal injury. Discontinue as soon as possible once pregnancy is detected.

Do not confuse enalapril with Anafranil, Elavil, Eldepryl, lisinopril, or ramipril.

FIXED-COMBINATION(S)

Lexxel: enalapril/felodipine (calcium channel blocker): 5 mg/2.5 mg, 5 mg/5 mg. **Teczem:** enalapril/dilTIAZem (calcium channel blocker): 5 mg/180 mg. **Vaseretic:** enalapril/hydroCHLOROthiazide (diuretic): 5 mg/12.5 mg, 10 mg/25 mg.

◆CLASSIFICATION

PHARMACOTHERAPEUTIC: Angiotensin-converting enzyme (ACE) inhibitor. **CLINICAL:** Antihypertensive.

USES

Treatment of hypertension alone or in combination with other antihypertensives in adults and children older than 1 mo. Treatment of symptomatic congestive HF with reduced ejection fraction (improves symptoms, increases survival, decreases frequency of hospitalization). In pts with stable asymptomatic left ventricular dysfunction (decreases the risk of development of overt HF and incidence of hospitalization for HF). **OFF-LABEL:**

Proteinuria in steroid-resistant nephrotic syndrome, proteinuric chronic kidney disease, acute coronary syndrome.

PRECAUTIONS

Contraindications: Hypersensitivity to enalapril. History of angioedema from previous treatment with ACE inhibitors. Idiopathic/hereditary angioedema. Concomitant use of aliskiren in pts with diabetes. Coadministration with or within 36 hrs of switching to or from a neprilysin inhibitor (e.g., sacubitril). **Cautions:** Renal impairment, hypertrophic cardiomyopathy with outflow tract obstruction; severe aortic stenosis; before, during, or immediately after major surgery. Concomitant use of potassium supplement; unstented unilateral or bilateral renal artery stenosis.

ACTION

Suppresses renin-angiotensin-aldosterone system (prevents conversion of angiotensin I to angiotensin II, a potent vasoconstrictor; may inhibit angiotensin II at local vascular, renal sites). Decreases plasma angiotensin II, increases plasma renin activity, decreases aldosterone secretion. **Therapeutic Effect:** In hypertension, reduces peripheral arterial resistance. In HF, increases cardiac output; decreases peripheral vascular resistance, B/P, pulmonary capillary wedge pressure, heart size.

PHARMACOKINETICS

Route	Onset	Peak	Duration
PO	1 hr	4–6 hrs	24 hrs
IV	15 min	1–4 hrs	6 hrs

Widely distributed. Undergoes hepatic biotransformation to enalaprilat. Protein binding: 50%–60%. Primarily excreted in urine. Removed by hemodialysis. **Half-life:** 11 hrs (increased in renal impairment).

⌛ LIFESPAN CONSIDERATIONS

Pregnancy/Lactation: Crosses placenta. Distributed in breast milk. May cause fetal/neonatal mortality, morbidity. **Children:** Safety and efficacy not established in pts younger than 1 mo. **Elderly:** May be more susceptible to hypotensive effects.

INTERACTIONS

DRUG: Aliskiren may increase hyperkalemic effect. May increase potential for hypersensitivity reactions to **allopurinol.** Angiotensin receptor blockers (e.g., **losartan, valsartan**) may increase adverse effects. May increase adverse effects of **lithium, sacubitril.** **HERBAL:** Herbals with hypertensive properties (e.g., **licorice, yohimbe**) or hypotensive properties (e.g., **garlic, ginger, ginkgo biloba**) may alter effects. **FOOD:** None known. **LAB VALUES:** May increase serum BUN, alkaline phosphatase, bilirubin, creatinine, potassium, ALT, AST. May decrease serum sodium. May cause positive ANA titer.

AVAILABILITY (Rx)

Injection Solution: 1.25 mg/mL. **Oral Solution:** *(Epaned):* 1 mg/mL. **Tablets:** 2.5 mg, 5 mg, 10 mg, 20 mg.

ADMINISTRATION/HANDLING

 IV

Reconstitution • May give undiluted or dilute with D₅W or 0.9% NaCl.
Rate of administration • For IV push, give undiluted over 5 min. • For IV piggyback, infuse over 10–15 min.
Storage • Store parenteral form at room temperature. • Use only clear, colorless solution. • Diluted IV solution is stable for 24 hrs at room temperature.

PO
• Give without regard to food. • **Oral Solution:** May store refrigerated or at room temperature. If stored at room temperature, discard after 60 days.

IV COMPATIBILITIES

Calcium gluconate, dexmedetomidine, heparin, magnesium sulfate, potassium chloride, potassium phosphate.

INDICATIONS/ROUTES/DOSAGE

Hypertension
PO: ADULTS, ELDERLY: Initially, 5 mg/day. Evaluate after 2–4 wks. Titrate as needed up to 40 mg/day in 1 or 2 divided doses. **CHILDREN 1 MO–16 YRS:** Initially, 0.08 mg/kg **(maximum dose:** 5 mg) once daily. Adjust dose based on pt response.

Adjunctive Therapy for HF
PO: ADULTS, ELDERLY: Initially, 2.5 mg twice daily. Titrate slowly at 1–2 wk intervals. **Target:** 10–20 mg twice daily.

Dosage in Renal Impairment
CrCl greater than 30 mL/min: No dosage adjustment. **CrCl 30 mL/min or less: (HTN):** Initially, 2.5 mg/day. Titrate until B/P controlled. **(HF):** Initially, 2.5 mg twice daily. May increase by 2.5 mg/dose at greater than 4-day intervals. **Maximum:** 40 mg/day. **Hemodialysis:** Initially, 2.5 mg on dialysis days; adjust dose on nondialysis days depending on B/P.

Dosage in Hepatic Impairment
No dose adjustment.

SIDE EFFECTS

Frequent (7%–5%): Headache, dizziness. **Occasional (3%–2%):** Orthostatic hypotension, fatigue, diarrhea, cough, syncope. **Rare (less than 2%):** Angina, abdominal pain, vomiting, nausea, rash, asthenia.

ADVERSE EFFECTS/TOXIC REACTIONS

Excessive hypotension ("first-dose syncope") may occur in pts with HF, severe salt or volume depletion. Angioedema (facial, lip swelling), hyperkalemia occur rarely. Agranulocytosis, neutropenia may be noted in pts with renal impairment, collagen vascular diseases (scleroderma, systemic lupus erythematosus). Nephrotic syndrome may be noted in those with history of renal disease.

E

NURSING CONSIDERATIONS

BASELINE ASSESSMENT

Obtain BUN, serum creatinine, CrCL. Receive full medication history, esp. potassium-sparing diuretics. Obtain B/P immediately before each dose (be alert to fluctuations). In pts with renal impairment, autoimmune disease, or taking drugs that affect leukocytes/immune response, CBC should be performed before beginning therapy, q2wks for 3 mos, then periodically thereafter.

INTERVENTION/EVALUATION

Assist with ambulation if dizziness occurs. Monitor B/P. Monitor daily pattern of bowel activity, stool consistency.

PATIENT/FAMILY TEACHING

• To reduce hypotensive effect, go from lying to standing slowly. • Several wks may be needed for full therapeutic effect of B/P reduction. • Skipping doses or voluntarily discontinuing drug may produce severe rebound hypertension. • Limit alcohol intake. • Report vomiting, diarrhea, diaphoresis, persistent cough, difficulty in breathing; swelling of face, lips, tongue.

encorafenib

en-koe-**raf**-e-nib
(Braftovi)
Do not confuse encorafenib with binimetinib, cobimetinib, dabrafenib, dasatinib, erlotinib, trametinib, or vemurafenib, or Braftovi with Mektovi.

◆CLASSIFICATION

PHARMACOTHERAPEUTIC: BRAF kinase inhibitor. **CLINICAL:** Antineoplastic.

USES

Melanoma: Treatment of pts with unresectable or metastatic melanoma with a BRAF V600E or V600K mutation (in combination with binimetinib). **Colorectal cancer (CRC):** Treatment of metastatic CRC in adults with a BRAF V600E mutation (in combination with cetuximab) after prior therapy. **Non–small-cell lung cancer (NSCLC):** Treatment of adults with metastatic NSCLC with a BRAF V600E mutation (in combination with binimetinib).

PRECAUTIONS

Contraindications: Hypersensitivity to encorafenib. **Cautions:** Baseline cytopenias; active infection; conditions predisposing to infection (e.g., diabetes, renal failure, immunocompromised pts, open wounds), diabetes, hepatic/renal impairment; pts at risk for QTc interval prolongation (congenital long QT syndrome, HF, mediations that prolong QTc interval, hypokalemia, hypomagnesemia); concomitant use of strong or moderate CYP3A4 inhibitors or strong or moderate CYP3A4 inducers.

ACTION

An ATP-competitive inhibitor of protein kinase BRAF, which suppresses the MAPK pathway. **Therapeutic Effect:** Inhibits tumor cell growth.

PHARMACOKINETICS

Widely distributed. Metabolized in liver. Protein binding: 86%. Peak plasma concentration: 2 hrs. Steady state reached in 15 days. Excreted in urine (47%), feces (47%). **Half-life:** 3.5 hrs.

⧗ LIFESPAN CONSIDERATIONS

Pregnancy/Lactation: Avoid pregnancy; may cause fetal harm. Female pts of reproductive potential must use effective nonhormonal contraception (e.g., barrier methods) during treatment and for at least 2 wks after discontinuation. Unknown if distributed in breast milk. Breastfeeding not recommended during treatment and for at least 2 wks after discontinuation. **Males:** May impair fertility. **Children:** Safety and efficacy not established. **Elderly:** No age-related precautions noted.

INTERACTIONS

DRUG: Strong CYP3A4 inhibitors (e.g., **clarithromycin, ketoconazole**), moderate CYP3A4 inhibitors (e.g., **cip-**

rofloxacin, dilTIAZem, fluconazole, verapamil) may increase concentration/effect. **Strong CYP3A4 inducers (e.g., carBAMazepine, phenytoin, rifAMPin)** may decrease concentration/effect. May decrease concentration/effect of **oral contraceptives. QT interval–prolonging medications (e.g., amiodarone, azithromycin, haloperidol, sotalol)** may increase risk of QTc interval prolongation. **HERBAL:** None significant. **FOOD: Grapefruit products** may increase concentration/effect; avoid use. **LAB VALUES:** May increase serum alkaline phosphatase, ALT, AST, creatinine, GGT, glucose, magnesium. May decrease serum sodium; Hct, Hgb, leukocytes, lymphocytes, neutrophils, RBCs.

AVAILABILITY (Rx)

 Capsules: 75 mg.

ADMINISTRATION/HANDLING

PO
• Give without regard to food. • If a dose is missed or vomiting occurs after administration, give next dose at regularly scheduled time • Do not give a missed dose within 12 hrs of next dose. • Administer whole; do not break, cut, or open capsule. Capsule cannot be chewed.

INDICATIONS/ROUTES/DOSAGE

Metastatic Melanoma, Non-Small Cell Lung Cancer
PO: ADULTS, ELDERLY: 450 mg once daily (in combination with binimetinib). Continue until disease progression or unacceptable toxicity. If binimetinib withheld, reduce encorafenib dose to 300 mg until binimetinib is restarted.

Dose Reduction for Adverse Reactions (Metastatic)
First dose reduction: 300 mg once daily. **Second dose reduction:** 225 mg once daily. **Unable to tolerate 225-mg dose:** Permanently discontinue.

Colorectal Cancer, Metastatic (With BRAF V600E Mutation)
PO: ADULTS, ELDERLY: 300 mg once daily (in combination with cetuximab). Con-

tinue until disease progression or unacceptable toxicity.

Dose Reduction for Adverse Reactions (CRC)
First dose reduction: 225 mg once daily. **Second dose reduction:** 150 mg once daily. **Unable to tolerate 150-mg dose:** Permanently discontinue.

Dose Modification
Based on Common Terminology Criteria for Adverse Events (CTCAE). See prescribing information for binimetinib for recommended dose modification.

Dermatologic Reactions
Grade 2 skin reaction: If not improved within 2 wks, withhold treatment until improved to Grade 1 or 0, then resume at same dose. **Grade 3 skin reaction:** Withhold treatment until improved to Grade 1 or 0, then resume at same dose for first occurrence or at reduced dose for subsequent occurrence. **Grade 4 skin reaction:** Permanently discontinue.

Hepatotoxicity
Grade 2 serum ALT, AST elevation: Maintain dose. If not improved within 4 wks, withhold treatment until improved to Grade 1 or 0 (or to pretreatment baseline), then resume at same dose. **Grade 3 or 4 serum ALT, AST elevation:** See Other Adverse Reactions.

New Primary Malignancies
Noncutaneous RAS mutation–positive malignancies: Permanently discontinue.

QTc Interval Prolongation
QTcF interval greater than 500 msec and less than or equal to 60 msec from baseline: Withhold treatment until QTcF is less than or equal to 500 msec, then resume at reduced dose. **QTcF interval greater than 500 msec and greater than 60 msec from baseline:** Permanently discontinue.

Uveitis
Grade 1 or 2 uveitis that does not respond to ocular therapy; Grade

E

3 uveitis: Withhold treatment for up to 6 wks. If symptoms improve, resume at same or reduced dose. If not improved, permanently discontinue.

Other Adverse Reactions (Including Hemorrhage)

Any recurrent Grade 2 reaction; first occurrence of any Grade 3 reaction: Withhold treatment for up to 4 wks. If improved to Grade 1 or 0 (or to pretreatment baseline), resume at reduced dose. If not improved, permanently discontinue. **First occurrence of any Grade 4 reaction:** Permanently discontinue or withhold treatment for up to 4 wks. If improved to Grade 1 or 0 (or to pretreatment baseline), resume at reduced dose. If not improved, permanently discontinue. **Recurrent Grade 3 reaction:** Consider permanent discontinuation. **Recurrent Grade 4 reaction:** Permanently discontinue.

Concomitant Use With CYP3A4 Inhibitors

If strong CYP3A4 inhibitor cannot be discontinued, reduce dose to one-third of the dose prior to use of strong CYP3A4 inhibitor. If moderate CYP3A4 inhibitor cannot be discontinued, reduce dose to one-half of the dose prior to use of moderate CYP3A4 inhibitor. If CYP3A4 inhibitor is discontinued for 3–5 half-lives, may resume dose prior to starting CYP3A4 inhibitor.

Dosage in Renal Impairment

Mild impairment: No dose adjustment. **Moderate to severe impairment:** Not specified; use caution.

Dosage in Hepatic Impairment

Mild to moderate impairment: No dose adjustment. **Severe impairment:** Not specified; use caution.

SIDE EFFECTS

Frequent (43%–14%): Fatigue, nausea, vomiting, abdominal pain, arthralgia, hyperkeratosis, myopathy, rash, headache, constipation, pyrexia, dry skin, dizziness, alopecia. **Occasional (13%–**3%):** Pruritus, peripheral neuropathy, extremity pain, dysgeusia, acneiform dermatitis.

ADVERSE EFFECTS/TOXIC REACTIONS

Myelosuppression (anemia, leukopenia, lymphopenia, neutropenia) is an expected response to therapy. In pts receiving combination therapy, new primary cutaneous malignancies including cutaneous squamous cell carcinoma (including keratoacanthoma) (3% of pts), basal cell carcinoma (2% of pts) have occurred. In pts receiving single-agent therapy, new primary cutaneous malignancies including cutaneous squamous cell carcinoma (including keratoacanthoma) (8% of pts), basal cell carcinoma (1% of pts), new primary melanoma (5% of pts) have occurred. May increase potential for new primary noncutaneous malignancies associated with activation of RAS through mutation. May increase cellular proliferation of BRAF wild-type cells and activate MAP-kinase signaling. Serious hemorrhagic events including GI bleeding, rectal bleeding (4% of pts), hematochezia (3% of pts), hemorrhoidal hemorrhage (1% of pts) were reported. Fatal intracranial hemorrhage reported in 2% of pts in the setting of new or progressive brain metastasis. Uveitis, including iritis and iridocyclitis, occurred in 4% of pts. QTc interval prolongation reported in 1% of pts. Grade 3 or 4 dermatologic toxicities reported in 21% of pts when used as a single agent. Other reactions occurring in less than 10% of pts include facial paresis, pancreatitis, panniculitis, drug hypersensitivity.

NURSING CONSIDERATIONS

BASELINE ASSESSMENT

Obtain CBC, BMP, LFT; pregnancy test in female pts of reproductive potential. Confirm compliance of effective non-hormonal contraception. Correct hypokalemia, hypomagnesemia prior to and during treatment. Confirm presence of BRAF V600E or V600K mutation in tumor specimen. Perform full dermatologic exam; assess skin for moles, lesions, papillomas. Consider baseline ECG in pts at risk for QTc interval prolongation. Receive full medication history and screen for interactions (esp. QTc interval–prolonging medications). Question history of diabetes, hepatic/renal impairment, HF. Screen for active infection. Offer emotional support.

INTERVENTION/EVALUATION

Monitor CBC for anemia, leukopenia, lymphopenia, neutropenia; LFT for hepatotoxicity (bruising, hematuria, jaundice, right upper abdominal pain, nausea, vomiting, weight loss); serum potassium, magnesium in pts with QTc interval prolongation. Assess skin for new lesions, toxicities q2mos during treatment and up to 6 mos after discontinuation. Assess for eye pain/redness, visual changes at each office visit and at regular intervals. Monitor for toxicities if discontinuation of CYP3A4 inhibitor or CYP3A inducer is unavoidable. Monitor for signs of hyperglycemia (thirst, polyuria, confusion, dehydration). If QT interval–prolonging medications cannot be withheld, diligently monitor ECG for QT interval prolongation, cardiac arrhythmias. Monitor for GI bleeding, bloody stool; symptoms of intracranial bleeding (aphasia, blindness, confusion, facial droop, hemiplegia, seizures). Diligently screen for infections.

PATIENT/FAMILY TEACHING

• Treatment may depress your immune system and reduce your ability to fight infection. Report symptoms of infection such as body aches, chills, cough, fatigue, fever. Avoid those with active infection. • Expect frequent eye exams, skin exams. • Report any vision changes, eye redness. • Treatment may cause new skin cancers. Report new warts, moles. • Report symptoms of liver problems (bruising, confusion; dark, amber- or orange-colored urine; right upper abdominal pain, yellowing of the skin or eyes); hemorrhagic stroke (confusion, difficulty speaking, one-sided weakness or paralysis, loss of vision), GI bleeding such (bloody stools, rectal bleeding). • Use effective contraception to avoid pregnancy. Do not breastfeed. • Avoid grapefruit products, herbal supplements (esp. St. John's wort). • Report palpitations, chest pain, shortness of breath, dizziness, fainting; may indicate arrhythmia. •

enfortumab vedotin-ejfv

en-**fort**-ue-mab ve-**doe**-tin
(Padcev)
Do not confuse enfortumab with brentuximab vedotin, or elotuzumab.

◆CLASSIFICATION

PHARMACOTHERAPEUTIC: Anti-Nectin-4, antibody-drug conjugate (ADC), monoclonal antibody. **CLINICAL:** Antineoplastic.

USES

As a single agent for treatment of adults with locally advanced or metastatic bladder cancer (urothelial) who have previously received a programmed death receptor-1 (PD-1) or programmed death-ligand 1 (PD-L1) inhibitor and a platinum-containing chemotherapy or are ineligible for cisplatin-containing chemotherapy and have previously received one or more prior lines of therapy. In combination with pembrolizumab for the treatment of adults with locally advanced or metastatic urothelial cancer who are not eligible for cisplatin-containing chemotherapy.

E

PRECAUTIONS

Contraindications: Hypersensitivity to enfortumab vedotin-ejfv. **Cautions:** Baseline cytopenias, diabetes, pts at risk for hyperglycemia (e.g., diabetes, chronic use of corticosteroids); conditions predisposing to infection (e.g., diabetes, renal failure, immunocompromised pts, open wounds); dermatologic disease; history of herpes zoster infection; concomitant use of CYP3A4 inhibitors. Not recommended in pts with moderate to severe hepatic impairment.

ACTION

Binds to and internalizes Nectin-4 antibody conjugated to a microtubule-disrupting agent, monomethyl auristatin E (MMAE). MMAE binds to and disrupts cellular microtubule network, causing cell cycle arrest and apoptosis (cellular death). **Therapeutic Effect:** Inhibits tumor cell growth.

PHARMACOKINETICS

Widely distributed. Metabolized via catabolism to small peptides, amino acids, unconjugated MMAE, unconjugated MMAE-related catabolites. Protein binding: 68%–82%. Peak plasma concentration: ADC: At end of infusion; MMAE: 2 days. Excreted in feces (17%), urine (6%). **Half-life:** ADC: 3.4 days; MMAE: 2.4 days.

⧗ LIFESPAN CONSIDERATIONS

Pregnancy/Lactation: Avoid pregnancy; may cause fetal harm. Females of reproductive potential must use effective contraception during treatment and for at least 2 mos after discontinuation. Unknown if distributed in breast milk. Breastfeeding not recommended during treatment and for at least 3 wks after discontinuation. May impair fertility. **Males:** Males with females of reproductive potential must use effective contraception during treatment and for at least 4 mos after discontinuation. **Children:** Safety and efficacy not established. **Elderly:** No age-related precautions noted.

INTERACTIONS

DRUG: **Strong CYP3A4 inhibitors (e.g., clarithromycin, ketoconazole, ritonavir)** may increase concentration/effect. **Strong CYP3A4 inducers (e.g., carBAMazepine, phenytoin, rifAMPin)** may decrease concentration/effect. **HERBAL:** None significant. **FOOD:** None known. **LAB VALUES:** May increase serum creatinine, glucose, lipase, uric acid. May decrease serum phosphate, potassium, sodium; Hgb, leukocytes, lymphocytes, neutrophils, platelets.

AVAILABILITY (Rx)

Injection, Powder for Reconstitution: 20 mg, 30 mg.

ADMINISTRATION/HANDLING
🖤 **IV**

Reconstitution • Must be prepared by personnel trained in aseptic manipulations and admixing of cytotoxic drugs. • Calculate the number of vials needed for reconstitution based on weight in kg. • Directing stream toward glass wall of vial, reconstitute 20-mg vial with 2.3 mL or 30-mg vial with 3.3 mL of Sterile Water for Injection to a final concentration of 10 mg/mL. • To prevent foaming, swirl vial gently until powder is completely dissolved. • Allow contents to settle until all bubbles are gone (at least 1 min). Do not shake or agitate. • Visually inspect for particulate matter or discoloration. Solution should appear clear to slightly opalescent, colorless to slightly yellow in color. Do not use if solution is cloudy or discolored or if visible particles are observed. • Dilute in infusion bag of 5% Dextrose, 0.9%

NaCl, or lactated Ringer's to a final concentration of 0.3–4 mg/mL. • Do not shake or agitate diluted solution. • Discard unused portions of vial.

Rate of administration • Give over 30 min via dedicated IV line. • Do not infuse as IV push or bolus.

Storage • Refrigerate unused vials in original carton. • May refrigerate reconstituted vials for up to 4 hrs. • May refrigerate diluted solution for up to 8 hrs. • Protect from light. • Do not shake, agitate, or freeze.

⊞ IV INCOMPATABILITIES

Do not mix with other medications or other infusion solutions that contain medications.

INDICATIONS/ROUTES/DOSAGE

Bladder Cancer (Urothelial)
IV: ADULTS, ELDERLY: (Single Agent): 1.25 mg/kg (up to a maximum of 125 mg) on days 1, 8, and 15 of a 28-day cycle. Continue until disease progression or unacceptable toxicity. **In combination with pembrolizumab:** 1.25 mg/kg (up to a maximum dose of 125 mg) on days 1 and 8 of a 21-day cycle. Continue until disease progression or unacceptable toxicity.

Dose Reduction Schedule for Adverse Events
First dose reduction: 1 mg/kg up to 100 mg. **Second dose reduction:** 0.75 mg/kg up to 75 mg. **Third dose reduction:** 0.5 mg/kg up to 50 mg.

Dose Modification
Based on Common Terminology Criteria for Adverse Events (CTCAE).

Hyperglycemia
Serum blood glucose greater than 250 mg/dL: Withhold treatment until serum blood glucose level is less than or equal to 250 mg/dL, then resume at same dose.

Peripheral Neuropathy
Grade 2 peripheral neuropathy: Withhold treatment until improved to Grade 1 or 0, then resume at same dose. If neuropathy recurs, withhold treatment until improved to Grade 1 or 0, then resume at reduced dose level. **Grade 3 or 4 peripheral neuropathy:** Permanently discontinue.

Thrombocytopenia
Grade 2 or 3 thrombocytopenia: Withhold treatment until improved to Grade 1 or 0, then resume at same dose or reduced dose level. **Grade 4 thrombocytopenia:** Permanently discontinue.

Skin Toxicity
Grade 3 rash, pruritus, cutaneous reactions: Withhold treatment until improved to Grade 1 or 0, then resume at same dose or reduced dose level. **Grade 4 or recurrent Grade 3 rash, pruritus, cutaneous reactions:** Permanently discontinue.

Other Nonhematologic Toxicity
Grade 3 nonhematologic toxicity: Withhold treatment until improved to Grade 1 or 0, then resume at same dose or reduced dose level. **Grade 4 nonhematologic toxicity:** Permanently discontinue.

Dosage in Renal Impairment
Mild to severe impairment: No dose adjustment.

Dosage in Hepatic Impairment
Mild impairment: No dose adjustment. **Moderate to severe impairment:** Not recommended.

SIDE EFFECTS

Frequent (56%–26%): Fatigue, asthenia, decreased appetite, nausea, dysgeusia, diarrhea, dry eye, eye irritation, increased lacrimation, ocular discomfort, rash, erythema, skin exfoliation, urticaria, alopecia, dry skin, pruritus. **Occasional (18%):** Vomiting.

♣ Canadian trade name   🦬 Non-Crushable Drug   ⬛ High Alert drug

E

ADVERSE EFFECTS/TOXIC REACTIONS

Myelosuppression (anemia, leukopenia, lymphopenia, neutropenia) is an expected response to therapy. Fatal cases of hyperglycemia, diabetic ketoacidosis (DKA) were reported in pts regardless of history of diabetes. Grade 3 or 4 hyperglycemia was reported in 8% of pts, and more prevalent in pts with higher body mass index and in pts with elevated hemoglobin A1c. Peripheral neuropathy including hypoesthesia, gait disturbance, muscular weakness, paresthesia, peripheral motor/sensorimotor neuropathy reported in 49% of pts. Ocular disorders including keratitis, blurred vision, limbal stem cell deficiency, and other events associated with dry eyes have occurred. Grade 3 or 4 skin reactions including symmetrical drug-related intertriginous and flexural exanthema, bullous dermatitis, exfoliative dermatitis, palmar-plantar erythrodysesthesia (redness, swelling, numbness, skin sloughing of the hands and feet) reported in 10% of pts. Skin and soft tissue infusion site extravasation with secondary cellulitis, bullae, exfoliation reported in 1% of pts. Other serious reactions including UTI (6% of pts), cellulitis (5% of pts), febrile neutropenia (4% of pts), sepsis (3% of pts), acute kidney injury (3% of pts); acute respiratory failure, aspiration pneumonia, cardiac disorder (less than 1% of pts) may occur. GI events including colitis, enterocolitis were reported. Herpes zoster infection reported in 3% of pts.

NURSING CONSIDERATIONS

BASELINE ASSESSMENT

Obtain weight in kilograms. Obtain CBC, LFT, blood glucose level, pregnancy test in females of reproductive potential. Verify compliance of effective contraception in females and males with female partners of reproductive potential. Obtain visual acuity. Screen for active infection. Question history of dermatological disease, hepatic impairment, optic disorders. Receive full medication history and screen for interactions. Offer emotional support.

INTERVENTION/EVALUATION

Monitor CBC, LFT, blood glucose levels periodically. Monitor for hyperglycemia (blurred vision, confusion, excessive thirst, Kussmaul respirations, polyuria); new onset or worsening peripheral neuropathy. Assess skin for dermatologic toxicities, palmar-plantar erythrodysesthesia. Consider topical corticosteroid if dermatologic effects occur. Consider artificial tears for dry eye prophylaxis. If symptoms do not resolve, consider treatment with topical steroids and referral to ophthalmologist. Monitor for drug toxicities if discontinuation or dose reduction of concomitant CYP3A4 inhibitor is unavoidable. If extravasation occurs, stop infusion and monitor for adverse reactions. Monitor daily pattern of bowel activity, stool consistency. Monitor for infections (cough, fatigue, fever). If serious infection, sepsis occurs, initiate appropriate antimicrobial therapy.

PATIENT/FAMILY TEACHING

• Treatment may depress your immune system and reduce your ability to fight infection. Report symptoms of infection such as body aches, burning with urination, chills, cough, fatigue, fever. Avoid those with active infection. • Report symptoms of bone marrow depression (e.g., bruising, fatigue, fever, shortness of breath, weight loss; bleeding easily, bloody urine or stool). • Report change of vision, blurry vision, dry eye symptoms not relieved by artificial tears. • Report symptoms of toxic skin reactions (e.g., itching, peeling, rash, redness, swelling); high blood sugar levels (e.g., blurred vision, excessive thirst/hunger, headache, frequent urination); or nervous system changes (e.g., altered memory, confusion, delirium, difficulty speaking, gait disturbance, numbness, tremors). • Females of childbearing potential must use effective contraception during treatment and for at least 2 mos after last dose. Do not breastfeed. Males with female partners of childbearing potential must use effective contraception during treatment and for at least 4 mos after last dose. • There is a high risk of interactions with other medications. Do not

---

take any newly prescribed medications unless approved by prescriber who originally started treatment. Avoid grapefruit products, herbal supplements (esp. St. John's wort). • Diarrhea is a common side effect. Drink plenty of fluids.

---

enoxaparin   TOP 100   HIGH ALERT

en-**ox**-a-par-in
(Lovenox)

■ **BLACK BOX ALERT** ■ Epidural or spinal anesthesia greatly increases potential for spinal or epidural hematoma, subsequent long-term or permanent paralysis.

Do not confuse Lovenox with Lasix, Levaquin, Lotronex, or Protonix, or enoxaparin with dalteparin or heparin.

◆CLASSIFICATION

PHARMACOTHERAPEUTIC: Low molecular weight heparin. **CLINICAL:** Anticoagulant.

USES

Prophylaxis of deep vein thrombosis (DVT): DVT prophylaxis following hip or knee replacement surgery, abdominal surgery, or pts with severely restricted mobility during acute illness. **Unstable angina and non–Q-wave myocardial infarction:** Prophylaxis of ischemic complications of unstable angina and non–Q-wave MI when administered with aspirin. **Treatment of acute ST-segment elevation myocardial infarction (STEMI):** When administered with aspirin, to reduce rate of recurrent MI or death in pts receiving thrombolysis and being managed medically or w/percutaneous coronary intervention (PCI). **Acute DVT:** Treatment of DVT with or without pulmonary embolism (PE) (inpatient); without PE (outpatient) (in conjunction with warfarin). **OFF-LABEL:** DVT prophylaxis following moderate-risk general surgery, gynecologic surgery; management of venous thromboembolism (VTE) during pregnancy. Bariatric surgery, mechanical heart valve to bridge anticoagulation, percutaneous coronary intervention (PCI) adjunctive therapy, frostbite (adjunctive), hemodialysis anticoagulation of circuit, superficial vein thrombosis.

PRECAUTIONS

Contraindications: Hypersensitivity to enoxaparin. Active major bleeding, concurrent heparin therapy, hypersensitivity to heparin, pork products. History of heparin-induced thrombocytopenia (HIT) in past 100 days or in the presence of circulating antibodies. **Cautions:** Conditions with increased risk of hemorrhage, platelet defects, renal impairment (renal failure), elderly, uncontrolled arterial hypertension, history of recent GI ulceration or hemorrhage. When neuraxial anesthesia (epidural or spinal anesthesia) or spinal puncture is used, pts anticoagulated or scheduled to be anticoagulated with enoxaparin for prevention of thromboembolic complications are at risk for developing an epidural or spinal hematoma that can result in long-term or permanent paralysis. Bacterial endocarditis, hemorrhagic stroke, history of heparin-induced thrombocytopenia (HIT), severe hepatic disease.

ACTION

Enhances the inhibition rate of clotting proteases by antithrombin III. Impairs normal hemostasis and inhibition of factor Xa. **Therapeutic Effect:** Produces anticoagulation. Does not significantly influence PT, aPTT.

PHARMACOKINETICS

Route	Onset	Peak	Duration
SQ	N/A	3–5 hrs	12 hrs

Widely distributed. Excreted primarily in urine. Not removed by hemodialysis. **Half-life:** 4.5–7 hrs.

⊠ LIFESPAN CONSIDERATIONS

Pregnancy/Lactation: Use with caution, particularly during third trimester, immediate postpartum period (increased risk of maternal hemorrhage). Unknown if distributed in breast milk. Pregnant women with mechanical heart valves (and their fetuses) may have increased risk of bleeding. **Children:** Safety and efficacy not established in pts younger than 1 mo. **Elderly:** May be more susceptible to bleeding.

INTERACTIONS

DRUG: Anticoagulants (e.g., **apixaban, dabigatran, edoxaban, rivaroxaban), antiplatelets (e.g., aspirin, clopidogrel, ticagrelor), NSAIDs (ibuprofen, ketorolac, naproxen), thrombolytics (e.g., alteplase), warfarin** may increase anticoagulant effect; risk of bleeding. **HERBAL:** Herbals with **anticoagulant/antiplatelet activity (e.g., garlic, ginger, ginkgo biloba)** may increase adverse effects. **FOOD:** None known. **LAB VALUES:** Increases serum alkaline phosphatase, ALT, AST. May decrease Hgb, Hct, platelets, RBCs.

AVAILABILITY (Rx)

Injection Solution: 30 mg/0.3 mL, 40 mg/0.4 mL, 60 mg/0.6 mL, 80 mg/0.8 mL, 100 mg/mL, 120 mg/0.8 mL, 150 mg/mL in prefilled syringes.

ADMINISTRATION/HANDLING

◄**ALERT**► Do not mix with other injections, infusions. Do not give IM.

SQ
Preparation • Visually inspect for particulate matter or discoloration. Solution should appear clear, colorless to pale yellow in color. Do not use if solution is cloudy, discolored, or if visible particles are observed.
Administration • Flick syringe so that the air bubble rises toward the plunger. • Insert needle subcutaneously into abdomen or outer thigh and inject

solution (including air bubble). • Do not inject into areas of active skin disease or injury such as sunburns, skin rashes, inflammation, skin infections, or active psoriasis. • Rotate injection sites. **Storage** • Store at room temperature.

INDICATIONS/ROUTES/DOSAGE

Prevention of Deep Vein Thrombosis (DVT) After Hip and Knee Surgery
SQ: ADULTS, ELDERLY: Knee surgery: 30 mg twice daily or 40 mg once daily, generally for 10–14 days or up to 35 days, with initial dose given 12 hrs or more pre-operatively or 12 hrs or more post-operatively once hemostasis achieved. **Hip surgery: (Once daily):** An initial dose of 40 mg, given 12 hrs or more pre-operatively or 12 hrs or more post-operatively once hemostasis achieved. Following hip surgery, recommend continuing 40 mg once daily for at least 10–14 days or up to 35 days post-op. **(Twice daily):** 30 mg q12h with initial dose, 12 hrs or more pre-operatively or 12 hrs or more post-operatively once hemostasis achieved and q12h for at least 10–14 days or up to 35 days.

Prevention of DVT After Non-Orthopedic Surgery
SQ: ADULTS, ELDERLY: 40 mg once daily, with initial dose given at least 2 hrs before abdominal surgery or approximately 12 hrs before other non-orthopedic surgery. Continue until fully ambulatory and risk of VTE has diminished (usually 10–14 days).

Prevention of DVT After Bariatric Surgery
Note: Optimal duration unknown (usually until hospital discharge or up to 6 wks based on VTE risk). **BMI 50 kg/m² or less:** 40 mg q12h. **BMI greater than 50 kg/m²:** 60 mg q12h.

Prevention of Long-Term DVT in Nonsurgical Acute Illness
SQ: ADULTS, ELDERLY: 40 mg once daily; continue until risk of DVT has diminished (usually for length of hospital stay or when pt is fully ambulatory and VTE risk has diminished).

Prevention of Ischemic Complications of Unstable Angina, Non–Q-Wave MI (With Oral Aspirin Therapy)
SQ: **ADULTS, ELDERLY:** 1 mg/kg q12h (with oral aspirin).

STEMI
SQ: **ADULTS YOUNGER THAN 75 YRS:** 30 mg IV once plus 1 mg/kg q12h (**maximum:** 100 mg first 2 doses only). **ADULTS 75 YRS OR OLDER:** 0.75 mg/kg (**maximum:** 75 mg first 2 doses only) q12h.

Acute DVT
SQ: **ADULTS, ELDERLY: (inpatient):** 1 mg/kg q12h or 1.5 mg/kg once daily. (**outpatient):** 1 mg/kg q12h.

Usual Pediatric Dosage
SQ: **CHILDREN 2 MOS AND OLDER:** 0.5 mg/kg q12h (prophylaxis); 1 mg/kg q12h (treatment). **NEONATES, INFANTS YOUNGER THAN 2 MOS:** 0.75/mg/kg/dose q12h (prophylaxis); 1.5 mg/kg/dose q12h (treatment).

Dosage in Renal Impairment
Elimination is decreased when CrCl is less than 30 mL/min. Monitor and adjust dosage as necessary.

Use	Dosage
Abdominal surgery, pts with acute illness	30 mg once/day
Hip, knee surgery	30 mg once/day
DVT, angina, MI	1 mg/kg once/day
STEMI: (younger than 75 yrs)	30 mg IV once plus 1 mg/kg q24h
STEMI (75 yrs or older)	1 mg/kg q24h
NSTEMI	1 mg/kg q24h

Dosage in Hepatic Impairment
Use caution.

SIDE EFFECTS

Occasional (4%–1%): Injection site hematoma, nausea, peripheral edema.

ADVERSE EFFECTS/TOXIC REACTIONS

May lead to bleeding complications ranging from local ecchymoses to major hemorrhage. May cause heparin-induced thrombocytopenia (HIT). **Antidote:** IV injection of protamine sulfate (1% solution) equal to dose of enoxaparin injected. 1 mg protamine sulfate neutralizes 1 mg enoxaparin. One additional dose of 0.5 mg protamine sulfate per 1 mg enoxaparin may be given if aPTT tested 2–4 hrs after first injection remains prolonged.

NURSING CONSIDERATIONS

BASELINE ASSESSMENT

Obtain CBC. Note platelet count. Question medical history as listed in Precautions. Ensure that pt has not received spinal anesthesia, spinal procedures. Assess for active bleeding. Assess pt's willingness to self-inject medication. Assess potential risk of bleeding.

INTERVENTION/EVALUATION

Periodically monitor CBC, stool for occult blood (no need for daily monitoring in pts with normal presurgical coagulation parameters). A decrease in the platelet count of more than 50% from baseline may indicate heparin-induced thrombocytopenia. Ensure active hemostasis of puncture site following PCI. Assess for any sign of bleeding (bleeding at surgical site, hematuria, blood in stool, bleeding from gums, petechiae, bruising, bleeding from injection sites).

PATIENT/FAMILY TEACHING

• Usual length of therapy is 7–10 days.
• A healthcare provider will show you how to properly prepare and inject your medication. You must demonstrate correct preparation and injection techniques before using medication at home. • Do not discontinue current blood thinning regimen or take any newly prescribed medications unless approved by the prescriber who originally started treatment. • Suddenly stopping therapy may increase the risk of blood clots or stroke. • Report bleeding of any kind (bloody urine, stool; nosebleeds; in-

creased menstrual bleeding). If bleeding occurs, it may take longer to stop bleeding. • Immediately report signs of stroke (confusion, headache, numbness, one-sided weakness, trouble speaking, loss of vision). • Minor blunt force trauma to the head, chest, or abdomen can be life-threatening. • Do not take aspirin, herbal supplements, OTC nonsteroidal anti-inflammatories (may increase risk of bleeding). • Consult physician before any surgery/dental work. • Use electric razor, soft toothbrush to prevent bleeding.

entrectinib

en-**trek**-ti-nib
(Rozlytrek)
Do not confuse entrectinib with alectinib, enasidenib, encorafenib, erdafitinib, erlotinib, fedratinib, or larotrectinib.

◆**Classification**

PHARMACOTHERAPEUTIC: Tropomyosin receptor kinase (TRK) inhibitor. **CLINICAL:** Antineoplastic.

USES

Non–small-cell lung cancer (NSCLC): Treatment of adults with metastatic non–small-cell lung cancer (NSCLC) whose tumors are ROS1 positive. **Solid tumors:** Treatment of adult and pediatric pts (1 mo and older) with solid tumors that have a neurotrophic receptor tyrosine kinase (NTRK) gene fusion without a known acquired resistance mutation; are metastatic or where surgical resection is likely to result in severe morbidity; or have no satisfactory alternative treatment or that have progressed following treatment.

PRECAUTIONS

Contraindications: Hypersensitivity to entrectinib. **Cautions:** Baseline cytopenias, hepatic impairment, cardiac disease (cardiomyopathy, HF), conditions predisposing to infection (e.g., diabetes, immunocom-

promised pts), renal failure, open wounds), pts at risk for bone fractures (e.g., fall risk, osteoporosis, chronic use of corticosteroids), pts at risk for QTc interval prolongation, cardiac arrhythmias (congenital long QT syndrome, HF, concomitant use of QT interval–prolonging medications, hypokalemia, hypomagnesemia); pts at high risk for suicide ideation and behavior (e.g., history of depression, mood disorder, psychiatric disorder). History of hyperuricemia, gout. Avoid concomitant use of moderate or strong CYP3A4 inhibitors/inducers.

ACTION

Inhibits activation of tropomyosin receptor kinase (TRK) proteins encoded by NTRK gene fusions. Inhibits proto-oncogenic tyrosine-protein kinase ROS1 and anaplastic lymphoma kinase (ALK). **Therapeutic Effect:** Inhibits tumor cell proliferation.

PHARMACOKINETICS

Widely distributed. Metabolized in liver. Protein binding: 99%. Peak plasma concentration: 4–6 hrs. Excreted in feces (83%), urine (3%). **Half-life:** 20–40 hrs.

⧖ LIFESPAN CONSIDERATIONS

Pregnancy/Lactation: Avoid pregnancy; may cause fetal harm. Females of reproductive potential should use effective contraception during treatment and for at least 5 wks after discontinuation. Unknown if distributed in breast milk. Breastfeeding not recommended during treatment and up to 7 days after discontinuation. **Males:** Males with female partners of reproductive potential should use effective contraception during treatment and for at least 3 mos after discontinuation. **Children:** Safety and efficacy not established in pts younger than 1 mo. **Elderly:** Safety and efficacy not established.

INTERACTIONS

DRUG: Strong CYP3A4 inhibitors (e.g., clarithromycin, ketoconazole, ritonavir), moderate CYP3A4 inhibitors (e.g., dilTIAZem, verapamil) may increase concentration/effect. Strong CYP3A4 inducers (e.g., carBAMazepine, phenytoin, rifAMPin), moderate CYP3A4 inducers (e.g., dexamethasone, modafinil, nafcillin) may decrease concentration/effect. QT interval-prolonging medications (e.g., amiodarone, azithromycin, ciprofloxacin, haloperidol, methadone, sotalol) may increase risk of QT interval prolongation, torsades de pointes. **HERBAL:** None significant. **FOOD:** Grapefruit products may increase concentration/effect. **LAB VALUES:** May increase serum alkaline phosphatase, ALT, AST, amylase, creatinine, lipase, potassium, sodium, uric acid. May decrease serum albumin, calcium, phosphate; Hgb, RBC, lymphocytes, neutrophils.

AVAILABILITY (Rx)

Pellets: 50 mg per packet.

Capsules: 100 mg, 200 mg.

ADMINISTRATION/HANDLING

PO

• Give without regard to food. Administer capsules whole for pts who can swallow whole capsules and whose doses are multiples of 100 mg. • Capsules prepared as an oral suspension are indicated for pts having difficulty or unable to swallow capsules, require enteral administration, or for dose increments of 10 mg. • **Pellets:** Indicated for pts having difficulty or unable to swallow capsules but can swallow soft food and whose doses are multiples of 50 mg. • Capsules cannot be chewed. • If a dose is missed, give as soon as possible unless next dose is due within 12 hrs. • If vomiting occurs immediately after administration, repeat the dose.

INDICATIONS/ROUTES/DOSAGE

NSCLC (ROS1-Positive)

PO: ADULTS: 600 mg once daily. Continue until disease progression or unacceptable toxicity.

Solid Tumors (NTRK Gene Fusion Positive)

PO: ADULTS: CHILDREN WITH BODY SURFACE AREA (BSA) GREATER THAN 1.5 m²: 600 mg once daily. **CHILDREN OLDER THAN 6 MOS:** BSA 1.11–1.50 m²: 400 mg; BSA 0.81–1.10 m²: 300 mg; BSA 0.51–0.80 m²: 200 mg; BSA 0.50 m² or less: 300 mg/m². **CHILDREN GREATER THAN 1 MO TO 6 MOS:** 250 mg/m² once daily. Continue until disease progression or unacceptable toxicity.

Dose Reduction Schedule

Dose Reduction for Adverse Reactions	Adults/ Children 12 yrs and Older With BSA Greater Than 1.5 m²	Children 12 yrs and Older With BSA 1.11–1.5 m²	Children 12 yrs and Older With BSA 0.91–1.1 m²
First reduction	400 mg once daily	400 mg once daily	300 mg once daily
Second reduction	200 mg once daily	200 mg once daily	200 mg once daily

Permanently discontinue if unable to tolerate two dose reductions.

Dose Modification

Based on Common Terminology Criteria for Adverse Events (CTCAE).

Cardiotoxicity

Grade 2 or 3 HF: Withhold treatment until improved to Grade 1 or 0, then resume at reduced dose level. **Grade 4 HF:** Permanently discontinue. **QTc interval greater than 500 msec:** Withhold treatment until QTc interval recovers to baseline. Resume at the same dose if risk factors for QT interval prolongation are identified and corrected. Resume at a reduced dose if risk factors for QT interval prolongation risk factors are not identified. **Torsades de pointes, polymorphic ventricular tachycardia, symptoms of serious arrhythmia:** Permanently discontinue.

Central Nervous System (CNS) Toxicity

Intolerable Grade 2 CNS effects: Withhold treatment until improved to Grade 1 or baseline, then resume at same dose or reduced dose level. **Grade 3 CNS effects:** Withhold treatment until improved to Grade 1 or baseline, then resume at reduced dose level. **Grade 4 CNS effects:** Permanently discontinue.

Hematologic Toxicity
Grade 3 or 4 anemia or neutropenia: Withhold treatment until improves to Grade 2 or less, then resume at the same or reduced dose.

Hepatotoxicity
Grade 3 hepatotoxicity: Withhold treatment until improved to Grade 1 or baseline. Resume at same dose if resolved within 4 wks. Permanently discontinue if not resolved within 4 wks. **Recurrence of Grade 3 hepatotoxicity:** Resume at reduced dose if resolved within 4 wks. **Grade 4 hepatotoxicity:** Withhold treatment until improved to Grade 1 or baseline. Resume at reduced dose if resolved within 4 wks. Permanently discontinue if not resolved within 4 wks or if Grade 4 hepatotoxicity recurs. **Serum ALT/AST greater than 3 times ULN with bilirubin greater than 1.5 times ULN (without cholestasis or hemolysis):** Permanently discontinue.

Hyperuricemia
Grade 4 or symptomatic hyperuricemia: Start urate-lowering medication. Withhold treatment until improved, then resume at same or reduced dose.

Ocular Toxicity
Grade 2 (or greater) vision disorders: Withhold treatment until improved or stabilized, then resume at the same or reduced dose.

Other Toxicities
Any other Grade 3 or 4 toxicity: Withhold treatment until toxicity improves to Grade 1 or baseline, then resume at the same or reduced dose if resolved within 4 wks. Permanently discontinue if not resolved within 4 wks or if Grade 4 toxicity recurs.

Concomitant Use of CYP3A4 Inhibitor
If strong CYP3A4 inhibitor cannot be avoided, reduce entrectinib dose to 100 mg. If moderate CYP3A4 inhibitor cannot be avoided, reduce entrectinib dose to 200 mg. If strong or moderate CYP3A4 inhibitor is discontinued for 3–5 half-lives, resume entrectinib dose prior to use of CYP3A4 inhibitor.

Dosage in Renal Impairment
Mild to moderate impairment: No dose adjustment. **Severe impairment:** Not specified; use caution.

Dosage in Hepatic Impairment
Mild impairment: No dose adjustment. **Moderate to severe impairment:** Not specified; use caution.

SIDE EFFECTS

Frequent (48%–21%): Fatigue, asthenia, constipation, dysgeusia, edema (facial, generalized, localized, peripheral), dizziness, vertigo, postural dizziness, diarrhea, nausea, dysesthesia, paresthesia, hyperesthesia, hypoesthesia, dysesthesia, oral hypoesthesia, dyspnea, myalgia, musculoskeletal pain, increased weight, cough, vomiting, pyrexia, arthralgia. **Occasional (18%–10%):** Headache, hypotension, abdominal pain, sleep disorder, hypersomnia, insomnia, somnolence, decreased appetite, muscular weakness, back pain, rash, extremity pain, dysphagia, dehydration. **Rare (4%):** Hypoxia, syncope.

ADVERSE EFFECTS/TOXIC REACTIONS

Myelosuppression (anemia, lymphopenia, neutropenia) is an expected response to therapy. HF reported in 3% of pts. Median onset of HF was approx. 2 mos. Myocarditis in the absence of HF reported in less than 1% of pts. CNS effects including altered mental status, aphasia, amnesia, ataxia, balance disorder, cognitive impairment, confusion, delirium, disturbance in attention, hallucinations, memory impairment, peripheral neuropathy reported in 27% of pts. Mood disorders including affect lability, affective disorder, agitation, anxiety, depression, euphoria, irritability, mood swings, psychomotor dysfunction, suicide reported in 10% of pts. Bone fractures (hip, femoral, bilateral femoral neck, tibial shaft) reported in 5% of adults and 23% of pediatric pts. Hepatotoxicity (serum ALT/AST elevation) reported in 36%–42% of pts; Grade 3 or 4 transaminase elevation reported in 3% of pts. Hyperuricemia reported in 9% of pts. QTc interval prolongation of greater than 60 msec (3% of pts) and greater than 500 msec (less than 1% of pts) has occurred. Ocular toxicities including adhesions, blindness, blurry vision, cataract, corneal erosion, diplopia, visual impairment, photophobia, photopsia, retinal hemorrhage, vitreous detachment, vitreous floaters may occur. Infections including respiratory tract infection, lung infection, pneumonia (10% of pts), UTI (13% of pts), sepsis were reported. Other reactions may include pulmonary embolism, falls, GI perforation.

NURSING CONSIDERATIONS

BASELINE ASSESSMENT

Obtain CBC, LFT, uric acid level; pregnancy test in females of reproductive potential. Verify use of effective contraception in females of reproductive potential. Confirm presence of NTRK gene fusion or ROS1 rearrangements in tumor specimen. Assess risk of QT interval prolongation, fractures, falls. Question history of cardiac disease, HF, gout, hyperuricemia; depression, mood disorder, suicidal ideation and behavior. Obtain ECG; echocardiogram for baseline LVEF. Screen for active infection. Receive full medication history and screen for interactions. Offer emotional support.

INTERVENTION/EVALUATION

Monitor CBC, uric acid level periodically. Monitor LFT for hepatotoxicity (bruising, hematuria, jaundice, right upper abdominal pain, nausea, vomiting, weight loss) q2wks for 1 mo, then monthly thereafter. Monitor for symptoms of HF (dyspnea, edema, fatigue, palpitations). Assess LVEF by echocardiogram if cardiotoxicity, HF is suspected. Monitor ECG periodically. Diligently assess for suicidal ideation and behavior; new-onset or worsening of anxiety, depression, mood disorder. Consult mental health professional if mood disorder is suspected. Monitor for symptoms of tumor lysis syndrome (acute renal failure, electrolyte imbalance, hyperuricemia, cardiac arrhythmias, seizures); bone fractures (pain, deformity, changes in mobility), hyperuricemia (joint pain/inflammation/redness), PE (chest pain, dyspnea, tachycardia); infections (cough, fatigue, fever). If serious infection or sepsis occurs, initiate appropriate antimicrobial therapy. Assess for visual changes at each office visit. If change of vision occurs, consider referral to ophthalmologist. Assess for CNS effects. Monitor for toxicities if discontinuation of CYP3A4 inhibitor is unavoidable. If QT interval–prolonging medications cannot be withheld, diligently monitor ECG for QT interval prolongation, cardiac arrhythmias. Monitor daily pattern of bowel activity, stool consistency, I&Os.

PATIENT/FAMILY TEACHING.

• Treatment may depress your immune system and reduce your ability to fight infection. Report symptoms of infection such as body aches, burning with urination, chills, cough, fatigue, fever. Avoid those with active infection. • Report symptoms of bone marrow depression such as bruising, fatigue, fever, shortness of breath, weight loss; bleeding easily, bloody urine or stool. • Therapy may cause vision changes or decrease the heart's ability to pump blood effectively. • Report symptoms of liver problems (bruising, confusion; dark, amber-, orange-colored urine; right upper abdominal pain, yellowing of the skin or eyes); HF (shortness of breath, palpitations; swelling of legs, ankle, feet); bone fractures (e.g., pain, deformity, changes in mobility), gout (joint pain/swelling/redness/warmth), nervous system changes (altered memory, confusion, delirium, difficulty speaking, gait disturbance, numbness, tremors), lung embolism (difficulty breathing, chest pain, rapid heart rate). • Seek immediate medical attention if thoughts of suicide, new onset or worsening of anxiety, depression, or changes in mood occur. • Avoid tasks that require alertness, motor skills until response to drug is established. • Use effective contraception. Do not breastfeed. • There is a high risk of interactions with other medications. Do not take any newly prescribed medications unless approved by prescriber who originally started treatment. Avoid grapefruit products, herbal supplements. • Diarrhea is a common side effect. Drink plenty of fluids.

enzalutamide

en-za-**loo**-ta-mide
(Xtandi)
Do not confuse enzalutamide with bicalutamide, flutamide, or nilutamide.

◆CLASSIFICATION

PHARMACOTHERAPEUTIC: Antiandrogen renal inhibitor. **CLINICAL:** Antineoplastic.

USES

In combination with talazoparib for treatment of adults with HRR gene-mutated metastatic castration-resistant prostate cancer (mCRPC). Treatment of metastatic castration-sensitive prostate cancer (mCSPC). Treatment of non-metastatic castration-sensitive prostate cancer (nmC-SPC) with biochemical recurrence (BCR) at high risk for metastasis.

PRECAUTIONS

Contraindications: Hypersensitivity to enzalutamide. Women who are pregnant or may become pregnant (not indicated in female population). **Cautions:** History of seizure disorder, underlying brain injury with loss of consciousness, transient ischemic attack within past 12 mos, CVA, brain metastases, brain arteriovenous abnormality, ischemic heart disease; pts at risk for fractures (e.g., osteoporosis, osteopenia), falls; conditions predisposing to infection (e.g., diabetes, renal failure, immunocompromised pts, open wounds), use of concurrent medications that may lower seizure threshold.

ACTION

Inhibits androgen binding to androgen receptors in target tissue, and inhibits interaction with DNA. **Therapeutic Effect:** Decreases proliferation, induces cell death of prostate cancer cells.

PHARMACOKINETICS

Widely distributed. Maximum plasma concentration achieved in 0.5–3 hrs. Metabolized in liver. Protein binding: (97%–98%). Primarily excreted in urine. **Half-life:** 5.8 days (**Range:** 2.8–10.2 days).

⧗ LIFESPAN CONSIDERATIONS

Pregnancy/Lactation: Not used in female population. **Children:** Safety and efficacy not established. **Elderly:** No age-related precautions noted.

INTERACTIONS

DRUG: Strong CYP2C8, CYP3A4 inhibitors (e.g., gemfibrozil, itraconazole) may increase concentration/effect. **Strong CYP3A4 inducers (e.g., carBAMazepine, phenytoin, rifAMPin)** may decrease concentration/effect. May decrease concentration/effect of **cycloSPORINE, sirolimus. HERBAL:** None significant. **FOOD:** None known. **LAB VALUES:** May increase serum ALT, AST, bilirubin. May decrease Hgb, Hct, platelets, WBC count.

AVAILABILITY (Rx)

Capsules: 40 mg. **Tablet:** 40 mg, 80 mg.

ADMINISTRATION/HANDLING

PO
• May give with or without food. Take at same time each day. Capsule or tablet should be swallowed whole. • Do not break, crush, dissolve, or open capsules. Do not cut, crush, or allow the tablets to be chewed.

INDICATIONS/ROUTES/DOSAGE

Note: MCRP and mCSPC pts should also receive a gonadotropin-releasing hormone (GnRH) analog concurrently or have had bilateral orchiectomy. Pts with nmCSPC with high-risk BCR may be treated with or without a GnRH analog.

mCRPC, mCSPC, nmCSPC

PO: ADULTS, ELDERLY: 160 mg once daily, continue until disease progression or unacceptable toxicity.

Dose Modification

If CTCAE Grade 3 or greater toxicity or an intolerable side effect occurs, withhold treatment for 1 week or until symptoms improve to Grade 2 or less, then resume at same dose or a reduced dose (120 mg or 80 mg). **Concurrent use of strong CYP2C8 inhibitors:** Avoid use (if possible). If concurrent use is necessary, reduce the enzalutamide dose to 80 mg once daily. **Concurrent use of strong CYP3A4 inducers:** Increase dose to 240 mg once daily.

Dosage in Renal/Hepatic Impairment

No dose adjustment.

SIDE EFFECTS

Common (51%): Asthenia. **Frequent (26%–15%):** Back pain, diarrhea, arthralgia, hot flashes, peripheral edema, musculoskeletal pain. **Occasional (12%–6%):** Headache, dizziness, insomnia, hematuria, paresthesia, anxiety, hypertension. **Rare (4%–2%):** Mental impairment disorders (includes amnesia, memory impairment, cognitive disorder, attention deficit), hematuria (includes pollakiuria, pruritus, dry skin).

ADVERSE EFFECTS/TOXIC REACTIONS

Upper respiratory tract infection occurs in 11% of pts; lower respiratory tract and lung infection (includes pneumonia, bronchitis) occur in slightly less (9% of pts). Spinal cord compression and cauda equina syndrome occur in 7% of pts. Life-threatening ischemic heart disease reported in 3% of pts. May increase risk of cardiovascular disease. Fall and fractures were reported.

Reversible posterior leukoencephalopathy syndrome (RPLS) may present as aphasia, altered mental status, paralysis, vision loss, weakness. Hypersensitivity reactions including angioedema, anaphylaxis may occur. May increase risk of seizures.

NURSING CONSIDERATIONS

BASELINE ASSESSMENT

Obtain LFT. Assess risk for falls/fractures. Screen for active infection. Question history of seizures, ischemic heart disease, cerebrovascular disease. Optimize cardiovascular risk factors (diabetes, hypertension, dyslipidemia) to reduce risk of treatment-induced ischemic heart disease. Obtain full medication history and screen for interactions. Offer emotional support.

INTERVENTION/EVALUATION

Monitor LFT periodically. Monitor B/P for hypertension. Obtain echocardiogram if ischemic heart disease (dyspnea, edema, exercise intolerance, palpitations) is suspected. Monitor for hypersensitivity reactions, seizure activity. Monitor for infections (cough, fatigue, fever). RPLS should be considered in pts with altered mental status, confusion, headache, seizures, visual disturbances. Altered gait, paralysis, numbness/weakness/pain of extremities may indicate spinal cord compression or cauda equina syndrome. Question incidence of falls.

PATIENT/FAMILY TEACHING

• Treatment may depress your immune system and reduce your ability to fight infection. Report symptoms of infection such as body aches, burning with urination, chills, cough, fatigue, fever. Avoid those with active infection. • There is a high risk of interactions with other medications. Do not take any newly prescribed medications unless approved by prescriber who originally started treatment. Avoid herbal supplements (esp. St. John's wort). • Treatment may increase risk of falls/fractures, seizures. • Life-threatening heart disease may occur. Report difficulty breathing, palpitations, swelling of ankles or feet. • Nervous system changes including confusion, seizures, headache, blurry vision, trouble speaking may indicate life-threatening brain dysfunction/swelling. • Sexually active men must wear condom during treatment and for 1 wk after treatment due to potential risks to fetus. • Women who are pregnant or are planning pregnancy may not touch medication without gloves.

epcoritamab-bysp

ep-koe-**rit**-a-mab
(Epkinly)

■ **BLACK BOX ALERT** ■ Life-threatening cytokine release syndrome (CRS) can occur. Treatment must be initiated in a step-up dosing schedule to reduce incidence/severity of CRS. If CRS occurs, withhold treatment until resolved or permanently discontinue based on severity. Immune effector cell-associated neurotoxicity syndrome (ICANS) may occur (can be life threatening). If ICANS occurs, withhold treatment until resolved or permanently discontinue based on severity.

Do not confuse epcoritamab with encorafenib or elranata-mab.

◆CLASSIFICATION

PHARMACOTHERAPEUTIC: Bispecific CD20-directed CD3 T-cell engager. **CLINICAL:** Antineoplastic.

USES

Diffuse large B-cell lymphoma (DLBCL). Treatment of adults with relapsed or refractory DLBCL, not otherwise specified, including DLBCL arising from indolent lymphoma, and high-grade B-cell lymphoma after two or more lines of systemic therapy. **Follicular lymphoma (FL):** Treatment of adults with relapsed or refractory FL after 2 or more lines of systemic therapy.

PRECAUTIONS

Contraindications: Hypersensitivity to epcoritamab-bysp. **Cautions:** Baseline cytopenias, dehydration, conditions predisposing to infection (e.g., diabetes, renal failure, immunocompromised pts, open wounds). Avoid administration of live vaccines.

ACTION

Binds to CD3 receptor expressed on surface of T cells and CD20 expressed on surface of lymphoma cells. **Therapeutic Effect:** Activates T cells causing release of proinflammatory cytokines and induces lysis of B cells.

PHARMACOKINETICS

Widely distributed. Metabolized into small peptides by catabolic pathways. Excretion not specified. **Half-life:** 22 days at the end of Cycle 3.

⧗ LIFESPAN CONSIDERATIONS

Pregnancy/Lactation: Avoid pregnancy; may cause fetal harm. Females of reproductive potential must use effective contraception during treatment and for at least 4 mos after discontinuation. Unknown if distributed in breast milk. Breastfeeding not recommended during treatment and for at least 4 mos after discontinuation. May impair fertility. **Children:** Safety and efficacy not established. **Elderly:** No age-related precautions noted.

INTERACTIONS

DRUG: May decrease therapeutic effects of **BCG (intravesical), vaccines (live). HERBAL:** None significant. **FOOD:** None known. **LAB VALUES:** May increase serum ALT, AST, creatinine. May decrease Hgb, lymphocytes, platelets, neutrophils, WBC; serum sodium, magnesium, phosphate. May increase or decrease serum potassium.

AVAILABILITY (Rx)

Injection Solution: 4 mg/0.8 mL, 48 mg/0.8 mL.

ADMINISTRATION/HANDLING
SQ

Administration guidelines • Must be administered at a facility with medical support by a healthcare professional trained in management of CRS and ICANS. • Hospitalization is recommended for 24 hrs after administration of the 48 mg dose on Cycle 1, Day 15. • Pts must be adequately hydrated.

Premedication • Premedicate all pts with diphenhydrAMINE 50 mg PO or IV (or equivalent) and acetaminophen 650–1,000 mg PO approximately 30–120 min prior to each wkly dose, in addition to prednisoLONE 100 mg PO or IV or dexAMETHasone 15 mg PO or IV (or equivalent) approximately 30–120 min prior to each wkly dose and for 3 consecutive days after each wkly dose during Cycle 1. • In pts who experienced Grade 2 or 3 CRS with previous dose during Cycle 2 and beyond, premedicate with prednisoLONE 100 mg PO or IV or dexAMETHasone 15 mg PO or IV (or equivalent) approximately 30–120 min prior to next dose and for 3 consecutive days after the next dose. Continue until a dose is given without subsequent Grade 2 or greater CRS.

Preparation • Preparation guidelines are highly specific. Some doses require dilution. • Vials removed from refrigerator should be allowed to warm to room temperature for no more than 1 hr. After warming, gently swirl vial; do not shake, vortex, or invert. • Visually inspect for particulate matter or discoloration. Solution should appear clear to slightly opalescent, colorless to slightly yellow. Do not use if solution is discolored. • **0.16 mg dose preparation:** Transfer solution from the 4 mg/0.8 mL vial into a separate empty vial labeled "Dilution A," then dilute with 4.2 mL 0.9% NaCl. Gently swirl for 30–45 sec. Transfer 2 mL of diluted solution from Dilution A vial into a new vial labeled "Dilution B," then further dilute Dilution B with 8 mL 0.9% NaCl to a final concentration of 0.16 mg/mL. Gently swirl for 30–45 sec. Withdraw 1 mL of diluted solution from Dilution B vial into syringe for the 0.16 mg dose. Discard remaining unused diluted solutions. • **0.8 mg dose preparation:** Transfer solution from the 4 mg/0.8 mL vial into a separate empty vial labeled "Dilution A," then dilute with 4.2 mL 0.9% NaCl to a final concentration of 0.8 mg/mL. Gently swirl for 30–45 sec. Withdraw 1 mL of diluted solution from Dilution A vial into syringe for the 0.8 mg dose. Discard remaining unused diluted solutions. • **48 mg dose preparation:** Withdraw solution from the 48 mg/0.8 mL vial into a syringe for 48 mg dose.

Administration • Insert needle subcutaneously into outer thigh or lower part of the abdomen (preferred site) and inject solution. • Do not inject into areas of active skin disease or injury such as sunburns, skin rashes, inflammation, skin infections, or active psoriasis. • Rotate injection sites. • Do not administer IV or intramuscularly.

Storage • Refrigerate unused vials in original carton until time of use. Protect from light. • Do not shake. • May refrigerate diluted solution for up to 24 hrs or store at room temperature for up to 12 hrs. Protect from direct sunlight.

INDICATIONS/ROUTES/DOSAGE

Note: Dosing schedule based on a 28-day cycle and continued until disease progression or unacceptable toxicity. If treatment is withheld for CRS or ICANS, restart alternate therapy schedule per manufacturer guidelines.

DLBCL (Relapsed or Refractory)
SQ: **ADULTS, ELDERLY:** *(Step-up Schedule):* **Cycle 1:** 0.16 mg on day 1, then 0.8 mg on day 8, then 48 mg on days 15 and 22. **Cycles 2 and 3:** 48 mg on days 1, 8, 15, and 22. **Cycles 4–9:** 48 mg on days 1 and 15. **(Maintenance): Cycle 10 and Beyond:** 48 mg on day 1.

Follicular Lymphoma (Relapsed or Refractory)
SQ: ADULTS, ELDERLY: *(Step-up Schedule):* **Cycle 1:** 0.16 mg on day 1, then 0.8 mg on day 8, then 3 mg on day 15, then 48 mg on day 22. **Cycles 2 and 3:** 48 mg on days 1, 8, 15, and 22. **Cycles 4–9:** 48 mg

on days 1 and 15. (**Maintenance**): **Cycle 10 and Beyond:** 48 mg on day 1.

Dose Modification and Symptom Management

Based on Common Terminology Criteria for Adverse Events (CTCAE).

CRS

Grade 1: Withhold treatment and mange symptoms. Verify CRS symptoms are resolved prior to next dose. **Grade 2:** Withhold treatment and mange symptoms. Prior to next dose, verify CRS symptoms are resolved, then premedicate per guidelines and monitor more frequently (or consider hospitalization). **Grade 3:** Withhold treatment and mange symptoms. Admission to intensive care unit may be required. Prior to next dose, verify CRS symptoms are resolved, then premedicate per guidelines and hospitalize for next dose. **Grade 4:** Permanently discontinue treatment and mange symptoms. Admission to intensive care unit may be required.

ICANS

Note: Neurology consultation should be considered for evaluation and management of any grade ICANS. Evaluate for other causes of neurologic symptoms. Seizure prophylaxis may be required. If indicated, give dexAMETHasone 10 mg IV q6h until symptoms improve to Grade 1 or 0, then taper.
Grade 1: Withhold treatment until resolved. **Grade 2:** Withhold treatment until resolved. Start dexAMETHasone therapy. **Grade 3:** *(First occurrence):* Withhold treatment until resolved. Start dexAMETHasone therapy. Admission to intensive care may be required. *(Recurrent Grade 3):* Permanently discontinue treatment. Start dexAMETHasone therapy. Admission to intensive care may be required. **Grade 4:** Permanently discontinue treatment. Start dexAMETHasone therapy or treat with methylPREDNISolone 1,000 mg IV daily for 2 or more days. Admission to intensive care may be required.

Infection

Grade 2–4 infection: Withhold treatment until resolved. Consider permanent discontinuation for Grade 4 infection.

Neutropenia

ANC less than 500 cells/mm³: Withhold treatment until ANC is 500 cells/mm³ or greater.

Thrombocytopenia

Platelet count less than 50,000 cells/mm³: Withhold treatment until platelets count is 50,000 cells/mm³ or greater.

Other Adverse Reactions

Any other Grade 3 adverse reactions: Withhold treatment until improved to Grade 1 or baseline.

Dosage in Renal Impairment
Mild to moderate impairment: No dose adjustment. **Severe impairment:** Not specified; use caution.

Dosage in Hepatic Impairment
Mild impairment: No dose adjustment. **Moderate to severe impairment:** Not specified; use caution.

SIDE EFFECTS

Frequent (29–23%): Fatigue, asthenia, lethargy, musculoskeletal pain, injection site reactions (erythema, inflammation, pain, pruritus, rash, swelling), pyrexia, abdominal pain. **Occasional (20–12%):** Diarrhea, nausea, rash, dermatitis, skin exfoliation, edema (facial, generalized, peripheral), headache, vomiting, decreased appetite.

ADVERSE EFFECTS/TOXIC REACTIONS

Myelosuppression (anemia, leukopenia, lymphopenia, neutropenia, thrombocytopenia) is an expected response to therapy, but more severe reactions including bone marrow depression, febrile neutropenia may occur. Life-threatening CRS reported in 51% of pts. Symptoms of CRS may include fatigue, headache, hypotension, hypoxia, nausea, pyrexia, tachycardia; serious events may include acute respiratory distress syndrome, atrial fibrillation, capillary leak syndrome, disseminated intravascular coagulation (DIC), hepatocellular injury, hemophagocytic lymphohistiocytosis/macrophage activation syndrome (HLM/MAS), multiorgan dysfunction, pulmonary edema. Life-threatening neurological tox-icities including ICANS, cerebral edema, leukoencephalopathy, seizures may occur. Life-threatening infections, including pneumonia, upper respiratory tract infection, urinary tract infection may occur. Cardiac arrhythmias, including bradycardia, supraventricular extrasystoles, supraventricular tachycardia, tachycardia, were reported. May cause herpes zoster reactivation.

NURSING CONSIDERATIONS

BASELINE ASSESSMENT
Obtain CBC, BMP, LFT, pregnancy test in females of reproductive potential. Confirm compliance with effective contraception. Administer in an environment equipped to manage symptoms of CRS, neurological toxicities. Pts should be hospitalized for at least 24 hrs following the first 48 mg dose. Premedicate all pts per administration guidelines. Recommend prophylaxis therapy for *Pneumocystis jirovecii* pneumonia, herpes virus prior to initiation. Ensure pt is adequately hydrated prior to each dose. Conduct baseline neurological assessment. Screen for active infection. Offer emotional support.

INTERVENTION/EVALUATION
Monitor CBC for myelosuppression (bleeding, bruising, dyspnea, fever, petechiae, weakness) as clinically indicated. Diligently monitor for symptoms of CRS, neurological toxicities throughout treatment, esp. during the step-up phase and the first 48 mg dose. Severe symptoms may require intensive care. Conduct routine neurological assessments. Aphasia, confusion, lethargy, tremor, seizures may indicate neurological toxicity, ICANS. Be alert for infections, esp. respiratory tract infections including *P. jirovecii* pneumonia, bacterial/fungal/pneumococcal/viral pneumonia (cough, dyspnea, hypoxia, pleuritic chest pain). Monitor daily pattern of bowel activity, stool consistency.

PATIENT/FAMILY TEACHING
• Treatment may depress your immune system response and reduce your ability to fight infection. Report symptoms of infection such as body aches, chills, cough, fatigue, fever. Avoid those with active infection. • Report symptoms of bone marrow depression such as bruising, fatigue, fever, shortness of breath, weight loss; bleeding easily, bloody urine or stool. • Treatment may cause life-threatening effects that must be immediately treated by medical personnel. Report symptoms of CRS (chills, facial swelling, fever, low blood pressure, nausea, vomiting, or weakness), ICANS (confusion, difficulty speaking or slurred speech, loss of consciousness, loss of balance, or seizures). Severe symptoms may require hospitalization. • Avoid tasks that require alertness, motor skills such as driving or operating machinery until response to drug is established.

EPINEPHrine

ep-i-**nef**-rin
(Adrenalin, EpiPen, EpiPen Jr., Neffy)
Do not confuse EPINEPHrine with ePHEDrine.

FIXED-COMBINATION(S)
LidoSite: EPINEPHrine/lidocaine (anesthetic): 0.1%/10%.

◆CLASSIFICATION
PHARMACOTHERAPEUTIC: Sympathomimetic (alpha-, beta-adrenergic agonist). **CLINICAL:** Antiglaucoma, bronchodilator, cardiac stimulant, antiallergic, antihemorrhagic, priapism reversal agent.

USES
Allergic reactions: Treatment of type 1 allergic reactions, including anaphylactic reactions. **Hypotension/shock:** Treatment of hypotension associated with septic shock in adults to increase mean arterial BP. **OFF-LABEL:** Asthma (acute severe), bradycardia or AV block (symptomatic), post cardiac arrest shock, inotropic support, sudden cardiac arrest (due to asystole, pulseless electrical activity, ventricular fibrillation, or pulseless ventricular tachycardia).

E

PRECAUTIONS

Contraindications: Hypersensitivity to EPINEPHrine. **Note:** There are no absolute contraindications with injectable EPINEPHrine in a life-threatening situation. **IV:** Narrow-angle glaucoma, thyrotoxicosis, diabetes, hypertension, other cardiovascular disorders. **Inhalation:** Concurrent use or within 2 wks of MAOIs. **Cautions:** Elderly, diabetes mellitus, hypertension, Parkinson's disease, thyroid disease, cerebrovascular or cardiovascular disease, concurrent use of tricyclic antidepressants. History of prostate enlargement, urinary retention.

ACTION

Stimulates alpha-adrenergic receptors (vasoconstriction, pressor effects), beta$_1$-adrenergic receptors (cardiac stimulation), beta$_2$-adrenergic receptors (bronchial dilation, vasodilation). **Therapeutic Effect:** Relaxes smooth muscle of bronchial tree, produces cardiac stimulation, dilates skeletal muscle vasculature.

PHARMACOKINETICS

Route	Onset	Peak	Duration
IM	5–10 min	20 min	1–4 hrs
SQ	5–10 min	20 min	1–4 hrs
Inhalation	3–5 min	20 min	1–3 hrs

Well absorbed after parenteral administration; minimally absorbed after inhalation. Metabolized in liver, other tissues, sympathetic nerve endings. Excreted in urine. Ophthalmic form may be systemically absorbed as a result of drainage into nasal pharyngeal passages. Mydriasis occurs within several min and persists several hrs; vasoconstriction occurs within 5 min and lasts less than 1 hr.

⧖ LIFESPAN CONSIDERATIONS

Pregnancy/Lactation: Crosses placenta. Distributed in breast milk. **Children/Elderly:** No age-related precautions noted.

INTERACTIONS

DRUG: Ergot derivatives (e.g., ergonovine, ergotamine, methylergonovine), MAOIs (e.g., phenelzine, selegiline), tricyclic antidepressants (e.g., amitriptyline) may increase concentration/effect. Beta blockers (e.g., atenolol, carvedilol, metoprolol) may decrease concentration/effect. **HERBAL:** Ephedra, yohimbe may increase CNS stimulation. **FOOD:** None known. **LAB VALUES:** May decrease serum potassium.

AVAILABILITY (Rx)

Injection, Solution (Prefilled Syringes): (EpiPen): 0.3 mg/0.3 mL. **(EpiPen Jr.):** 0.15 mg/0.3 mL. **Injection, Solution:** 0.1 mg/mL (1:10,000), 1 mg/mL (1:1,000). **Nasal Spray:** 2 mg nasal spray device.

Solution for Oral Inhalation: (Adrenalin): 2.25% (0.5 mL).

ADMINISTRATION/HANDLING

 IV

Reconstitution • For injection, dilute each 1 mg of 1:1,000 solution with 10 mL 0.9% NaCl to provide 1:10,000 solution and inject each 1 mg or fraction thereof over 1 min or more (except in cardiac arrest). • For infusion, further dilute with 250–500 mL D$_5$W. Maximum concentration 64 mcg/mL.
Rate of administration • For IV infusion, give at 1–10 mcg/min (titrate to desired response).
Storage • Store parenteral forms at room temperature. • Do not use if solution appears discolored or contains a precipitate.

SQ
• Shake ampule thoroughly. • Use tuberculin syringe for injection into lateral deltoid region. • Massage injection site (minimizes vasoconstriction effect). Use only 1:1,000 solution.

IM
• Administer in anterolateral aspect of middle third of thigh. Do not inject into the buttocks, digits, hands or feet.

❂ IV INCOMPATIBILITIES

Clevidipine.

❂ IV COMPATIBILITIES

Calcium chloride, calcium gluconate, dexmedetomidine, heparin, norepinephrine, potassium chloride, vasopressin.

INDICATIONS/ROUTES/DOSAGE

Hypersensitivity Reactions (Including Anaphylaxis)

IM: ADULTS, ELDERLY: 0.3–0.5 mg (use 0.5 mg in pts greater than 50 kg) using the 1 mg/mL solution. May repeat q5–15min for adequate response. **ADOLESCENTS, CHILDREN, INFANTS:** 0.01 mg/kg (0.01 mL/kg/dose of the 1 mg/mL solution) not to exceed: **(PREPUBERTAL CHILD):** 0.3 mg/dose; **(ADOLESCENT):** 0.5 mg/dose administered q5–15min.

Self-treatment using auto-injector IM (preferred), SQ: 0.3–0.5 mg may repeat q5–15min **Self-treatment using nasal spray:** One 2 mg spray. May repeat 5 min later if symptoms do not improve.

Hypotension (Shock)

IV infusion: ADULTS, ELDERLY: Initially, 0.01–0.5 mcg/kg/min. Titrate to desired response. **ADOLESCENTS, CHILDREN, INFANTS:** Initially, 0.1–1 mcg/kg/min. Titrate to desired response.

Dosage in Renal/Hepatic Impairment

No dose adjustment.

SIDE EFFECTS

Frequent: Systemic: Tachycardia, palpitations, anxiety. **Nasal:** Throat irritation, headache, nasal discomfort, jittery sensation, tremor, rhinorrhea. **Ophthalmic:** Headache, eye irritation, watering of eyes. **Occasional: Systemic:** Dizziness, lightheadedness, facial flushing, headache, diaphoresis, increased B/P, nausea, trembling, insomnia, vomiting, fatigue. **Ophthalmic:** Blurred/decreased vision, eye pain. **Rare: Systemic:** Chest discomfort/pain, arrhythmias, bronchospasm, dry mouth/throat.

ADVERSE EFFECTS/TOXIC REACTIONS

Excessive doses may cause acute hypertension, arrhythmias. Prolonged/excessive use may result in metabolic acidosis due to increased serum lactic acid. Metabolic acidosis may cause disorientation, fatigue, hyperventilation, headache, nausea, vomiting, diarrhea.

NURSING CONSIDERATIONS

INTERVENTION/EVALUATION

Monitor changes of B/P, HR. Assess lung sounds for rhonchi, wheezing, rales. Monitor ABGs. In cardiac arrest, adhere to ACLS protocols.

PATIENT/FAMILY TEACHING

• Avoid excessive use of caffeine. • Report any new symptoms (tachycardia, shortness of breath, dizziness) immediately: May be systemic effects.

eplerenone

ep-**ler**-e-none
(Inspra)
Do not confuse Inspra with Spiriva.

◆CLASSIFICATION

PHARMACOTHERAPEUTIC: Aldosterone receptor antagonist. **CLINICAL:** Antihypertensive.

USES

Hypertension: Treatment of hypertension alone or in combination with other antihypertensive agents. **Post myocardial infarction:** Improve survival of pts with symptomatic heart failure (HF) with reduced ejection fraction (HFrEF) after an acute myocardial infarction (AMI). **OFF-LABEL:** HF with preserved or reduced ejection fraction, primary aldosteronism.

PRECAUTIONS

Contraindications: Hypersensitivity to eplerenone. Concurrent use with strong

CYP3A4 inhibitors (e.g., ketoconazole, itraconazole), CrCl less than 30 mL/min, serum potassium level greater than 5.5 mEq/L at initiation. Use in pts with Addison's disease. **Hypertension (additional):** Type 2 diabetes with microalbuminuria; CrCl less than 50 mL/min; serum creatinine greater than 2 mg/dL in men, greater than 1.8 mg/dL in women; concomitant use of potassium supplements or potassium-sparing diuretics. **Cautions:** Hyperkalemia, HF, post-MI, diabetes, mild renal impairment.

ACTION

Binds to mineralocorticoid receptors in kidney, heart, blood vessels, brain, blocking binding of aldosterone. **Therapeutic Effect:** Reduces B/P. Prevents myocardial and vascular fibrosis.

PHARMACOKINETICS

Widely distributed. Protein binding: 50%. Metabolized in liver. Excreted in urine (67%), feces (32%). Not removed by hemodialysis. **Half-life:** 4–6 hrs.

⧗ LIFESPAN CONSIDERATIONS

Pregnancy/Lactation: Unknown if drug crosses placenta or is distributed in breast milk. **Children:** Safety and efficacy not established. **Elderly:** No age-related precautions noted.

INTERACTIONS

DRUG: **ACE inhibitors (e.g., enalapril, lisinopril), angiotensin II antagonists (e.g., losartan, valsartan), potassium-sparing diuretics (e.g., spironolactone), potassium supplements** increase risk of hyperkalemia. May increase the hyperkalemic effect of **cycloSPORINE. Strong CYP3A4 inhibitors (e.g., clarithromycin, ketoconazole, ritonavir)** may increase concentration/effect. **Strong CYP3A4 inducers (e.g., carBAMazepine, phenytoin, rifAMPin)** may decrease concentration/effect. **NSAIDs (e.g., diclofenac, meloxicam, naproxen)** may decrease antihyper-

tensive effect. **HERBAL: Herbals with hypertensive properties (e.g., licorice, yohimbe) or hypotensive properties (e.g., garlic, ginger, ginkgo biloba)** may alter effects. **FOOD: Grapefruit products** may increase potential for hyperkalemia, arrhythmias. **LAB VALUES:** May increase serum potassium, ALT, AST, cholesterol, triglycerides, serum creatinine, uric acid. May decrease serum sodium.

AVAILABILITY (Rx)

 Tablets: 25 mg, 50 mg.

ADMINISTRATION/HANDLING

• May give without regard to food.

INDICATIONS/ROUTES/DOSAGE

Hypertension
PO: **ADULTS, ELDERLY:** Initially, 50 mg once daily. Evaluate response after 2–4 wks. If 50 mg once daily produces an inadequate B/P response, may increase dosage to a maximum dose of 50 mg twice daily.

HF Following MI
PO: **ADULTS, ELDERLY:** Initially, 25 mg once daily. May double the dose after 4 wks if serum potassium and kidney function are stable. **(Maximum):** 50 mg once daily.

Dosage Adjustment for Serum Potassium Concentrations in HF
Less than 5 mEq/L: Increase dose from 25 mg daily to 50 mg daily or increase dose from 25 mg every other day to 25 mg daily. **5–5.4 mEq/L:** No adjustment needed. **5.5–5.9 mEq/L:** Decrease dose from 50 mg daily to 25 mg daily or from 25 mg daily to 25 mg every other day. Decrease dose from 25 mg every other day to withhold medication. **6 mEq/L or greater:** Withhold medication until potassium is less than 5.5 mEq/L, then restart at 25 mg every other day.

Dosage in Renal Impairment
Contraindicated in pts with hypertension with CrCl less than 50 mL/min or serum creatinine greater than 2 mg/dL in males

or greater than 1.8 mg/dL in females. All other indications, CrCl less than 30 mL/min, use is contraindicated.

Dosage in Hepatic Impairment
No dose adjustment.

SIDE EFFECTS
Rare (3%–1%): Dizziness, diarrhea, cough, fatigue, flu-like symptoms, abdominal pain.

ADVERSE EFFECTS/TOXIC REACTIONS
Hyperkalemia may occur, particularly in pts with type 2 diabetes mellitus and microalbuminuria.

NURSING CONSIDERATIONS

BASELINE ASSESSMENT
Obtain serum potassium level. Obtain B/P, apical pulse immediately before each dose, in addition to regular monitoring (be alert to fluctuations). If excessive reduction in B/P occurs, place pt in supine position, feet slightly elevated.

INTERVENTION/EVALUATION
Monitor serum potassium. Assist with ambulation if dizziness occurs. Assess B/P for hypertension/hypotension. Assess for evidence of flu-like symptoms.

PATIENT/FAMILY TEACHING
• Avoid tasks that require alertness, motor skills until response to drug is established (possible dizziness effect). • Hypertension requires lifelong control. • Avoid exercising during hot weather (risk of dehydration, hypotension). • Do not use salt substitutes containing potassium.

epoetin alfa
TOP 100

e-**poe**-e-tin **al**-fa
(Epogen, Eprex ✤, Procrit, Retacrit)

■ **BLACK BOX ALERT** ■ Increased risk of serious cardiovascular events, thromboembolic events, mortality, time-to-tumor progression in pts with head and neck cancer, metastatic breast cancer, non–small-cell lung cancer when administered to a target hemoglobin of more than 11 g/dL. Increases rate of deep vein thrombosis in perioperative pts not receiving anticoagulant therapy.
Do not confuse epoetin with darbepoetin, or Epogen with Neupogen.

◆ CLASSIFICATION
PHARMACOTHERAPEUTIC: Erythropoiesis-stimulating agent (ESA). **CLINICAL:** Erythropoietin.

USES
Anemia due to chronic kidney disease (CKD): Treatment of anemia due to CKD, including pts on dialysis and not on dialysis, to decrease the need for red blood cell (RBC) transfusion. **Anemia due to zidovudine in pts with HIV infection:** Administered at less than or equal to 4,200 mg/wk in pts with HIV infection with endogenous serum erythropoietin levels of less than or equal to 500 units/mL. **Anemia due to chemotherapy in pts with cancer:** Pts with nonmyeloid malignancies where anemia is due to the effect of myelosuppressive chemotherapy, and there is a minimum of 2 additional mos of chemotherapy. **Reduction of allogeneic RBC transfusions in pts undergoing elective, noncardiac, nonvascular surgery:** Pts with perioperative hemoglobin greater than 10 to less than or equal to 13 g/dL at high risk for blood loss from surgery. **OFF-LABEL:** Anemia in myelodysplastic syndromes.

PRECAUTIONS
Contraindications: Hypersensitivity to epoetin. Pure red cell aplasia that begins after treatment, uncontrolled hypertension. Use of multiple dose vial containing benzyl alcohol in neonates, infants, pregnant females, and lactating females. **Cautions:** History of seizures or controlled hypertension. **Cancer pts:** Tumor growth, shortened survival

may occur when Hgb levels of 11 g/dL or greater are achieved with epoetin alfa. **Chronic renal failure pts:** Increased risk for serious cardiovascular reactions (e.g., stroke, MI) when Hgb levels greater than 11 g/dL are achieved with epoetin alfa.

ACTION

Stimulates division, differentiation of erythroid progenitor cells in bone marrow. **Therapeutic Effect:** Induces erythropoiesis, releases reticulocytes from bone marrow into blood, where they mature into erythrocytes.

PHARMACOKINETICS

Well absorbed after SQ administration. Following administration, an increase in reticulocyte count occurs within 10 days, and increases in Hgb, Hct, and RBC count are seen within 2–6 wks. **Half-life:** 4–13 hrs.

⏳ LIFESPAN CONSIDERATIONS

Pregnancy/Lactation: Unknown if drug crosses placenta or is distributed in breast milk. **Children:** Use of multiple dose vial containing benzyl alcohol in neonates, infants i s contraindicated. **Elderly:** No age-related precautions noted.

INTERACTIONS

DRUG: None significant. **HERBAL:** None significant. **FOOD:** None known. **LAB VALUES:** May increase serum BUN, phosphorus, potassium, creatinine, uric acid, sodium. May decrease bleeding time, iron concentration, serum ferritin.

AVAILABILITY (Rx)

Injection Solution: *(Epogen, Procrit):* 2,000 units/mL, 3,000 units/mL, 4,000 units/mL, 10,000 units/mL, 20,000 units/mL, 40,000 units/mL.

ADMINISTRATION/HANDLING

◄**ALERT**► Avoid excessive agitation of vial; do not shake (foaming).

 IV

Reconstitution • No reconstitution necessary.
Rate of administration • May be given as an IV bolus.
Storage • Refrigerate. • Vigorous shaking may denature medication, rendering it inactive.

SQ

• Mix in syringe with bacteriostatic 0.9% NaCl with benzyl alcohol 0.9% (bacteriostatic saline) at a 1:1 ratio (benzyl alcohol acts as local anesthetic; may reduce injection site discomfort). • Use 1 dose per vial; do not reenter vial. Discard unused portion.

▦ IV INCOMPATIBILITIES

Do not mix injection form with other medications.

INDICATIONS/ROUTES/DOSAGE

Anemia Associated With Chemotherapy

◄**ALERT**► Begin therapy only if Hgb less than 10 g/dL and anticipated duration of myelosuppressive chemotherapy is greater than 2 mos. Use minimum effective dose to maintain Hgb level that will avoid red blood cell transfusions. Discontinue upon completion of chemotherapy.
SQ: ADULTS, ELDERLY: Initially, 150 units/kg 3 times/wk or 40,000 units once wkly. **IV: CHILDREN 5 YRS AND OLDER:** 600 units/kg once wkly. Titrate dose to maintain Hgb level sufficient enough to avoid RBC transfusions.
Increase dose: ADULTS, ELDERLY: If Hgb does not increase by greater than 1 g/dL and remains below 10 g/dL after initial 4 wks, may increase to 300 units/kg 3 times/wk or 60,000 units once wkly. **CHILDREN:** If Hgb does not increase by greater than 1 g/dL and remains less than 10 g/dL after initial 4 wks of once-wkly dosing, may increase dose to 900 units/kg/wk. **Maximum:** 60,000 units once wkly.

Decrease dose: Decrease dose by 25% if Hgb increases greater than 1 g/dL in any 2-wk period or Hgb level reaches level that will avoid red blood cell transfusions.

Reduction of Allogenic Blood Transfusions in Elective Surgery
SQ: ADULTS, ELDERLY: 300 units/kg/day for 15 days total, 10 days before surgery, on the day of surgery, and 4 days after surgery or 600 units/kg once weekly for 4 doses given 21, 14, 7 days before surgery and on the day of surgery.

Anemia in Chronic Renal Failure
◄ **ALERT** ► Individualize dose, using lowest dose to reduce need for RBC transfusions. **On dialysis:** Initiate when Hgb less than 10 g/dL; reduce dose or discontinue if Hgb approaches or exceeds 11 g/dL (IV route recommended for pts on hemodialysis). **Not on dialysis:** Initiate when Hgb less than 10 g/dL; reduce dose or stop if Hgb exceeds 10 g/dL.
IV, SQ: ADULTS, ELDERLY, ADOLESCENTS OLDER THAN 16 YRS: 50–100 units/kg 3 times/wk. **CHILDREN 16 YRS AND YOUNGER:** 50 units/kg 3 times/wk. **Maintenance: Decrease dose by 25%:** If Hgb increases greater than 1 g/dL in any 2-wk period. **Increase dose by 25%:** If Hgb does not increase by greater than 1 g/dL after 4 wks of therapy. Do not increase dose more frequently than every 4 wks. **Note:** If pt does not attain adequate response after appropriate dosing over 12 wks, do not continue to increase dose, and use minimum effective dose to maintain Hgb level that will avoid red blood cell transfusions.

HIV Infection in Pts Treated With Zidovudine (AZT)
IV, SQ: ADULTS: Initially, 100 units/kg 3 times/wk for 8 wks; may increase by 50–100 units/kg 3 times/wk. Evaluate response q4–8wks thereafter. Adjust dosage by 50–100 units/kg 3 times/wk. If dosages larger than 300 units/kg 3 times/wk are not eliciting response,

it is unlikely pt will respond. **Maintenance:** Titrate to maintain desired Hgb level. Hgb levels should not exceed 12 g/dL. If Hgb greater than 12 g/dL, resume treatment with 25% dose reduction when Hgb drops below 11 g/dL. Discontinue if Hgb increase not attained with 300 units/kg for 8 wks.

Dosage in Renal/Hepatic Impairment
No dose adjustment.

SIDE EFFECTS

Pts Receiving Chemotherapy
Frequent (20%–17%): Fever, diarrhea, nausea, vomiting, edema. **Occasional (13%–11%):** Asthenia, shortness of breath, paresthesia. **Rare (5%–3%):** Dizziness, trunk pain.

Pts With Chronic Renal Failure
Frequent (24%–11%): Hypertension, headache, nausea, arthralgia. **Occasional (9%–7%):** Fatigue, edema, diarrhea, vomiting, chest pain, skin reactions at administration site, asthenia, dizziness.

Pts With HIV Infection Treated With AZT
Frequent (38%–15%): Fever, fatigue, headache, cough, diarrhea, rash, nausea. **Occasional (14%–9%):** Shortness of breath, asthenia, skin reaction at injection site, dizziness.

ADVERSE EFFECTS/TOXIC REACTIONS

Hypertensive encephalopathy, thrombosis, cerebrovascular accident, MI, seizures, pure red cell aplasia may occur. Hyperkalemia occurs occasionally in pts with chronic renal failure, usually in those who do not comply with medication regimen, dietary guidelines, frequency of dialysis regimen. May increase risk of tumor progression or recurrence in pts with cancer. Severe cutaneous reactions including Erythema multiform, Stevens-Johnson syndrome, toxic epidermal necrolysis were reported.

E

NURSING CONSIDERATIONS

BASELINE ASSESSMENT

Assess B/P before initiation (80% of pts with chronic renal failure have history of hypertension). B/P often rises during early therapy in pts with history of hypertension. Consider that all pts eventually need supplemental iron therapy. Assess serum iron (should be greater than 20%), serum ferritin (should be greater than 100 ng/mL) before and during therapy. Establish baseline CBC (esp. note Hct).

INTERVENTION/EVALUATION

Assess CBC routinely (esp. Hgb, Hct). Monitor aggressively for increased B/P (25% of pts require antihypertensive therapy, dietary restrictions). Monitor temperature, esp. in cancer pts on chemotherapy and zidovudine-treated HIV pts. Monitor serum BUN, uric acid, creatinine, phosphorus, potassium, esp. in chronic renal failure pts.

PATIENT/FAMILY TEACHING

• Frequent laboratory assessments needed to determine correct dosage. • Immediately report any severe headache. • Avoid potentially hazardous activity during first 90 days of therapy (increased risk of seizures in pts with chronic renal failure during first 90 days). • Specific dietary regimen must be maintained.

---

erdafitinib

er-da-**fi**-ti-nib
(Balversa)
Do not confuse erdafitinib with enasidenib, encorafenib, erlotinib or gefitinib, or Balversa with Balziva.

◆CLASSIFICATION

PHARMACOTHERAPEUTIC: Fibroblast growth factor receptor (FGFR) inhibitor. Tyrosine kinase inhibitor.
CLINICAL: Antineoplastic.

USES

Treatment of adult pts with locally advanced or metastatic bladder cancer (urothelial) that has susceptible FGFR3 or FGFR2 genetic mutation alterations and progressed during or following at least one line of prior platinum-containing chemotherapy including within 12 mos of neoadjuvant or adjuvant platinum-containing chemotherapy.

PRECAUTIONS

Contraindications: Hypersensitivity to erdafitinib. **Cautions:** Baseline hemoglobinemia, neutropenia, leukopenia, thrombocytopenia; conditions predisposing to infection (e.g., diabetes, renal failure, immunocompromised pts, open wounds), hepatic/renal impairment, optic disorders, pts at risk for hyperphosphatemia (hypoparathyroidism, concomitant use of phosphorus-containing medications, chronic kidney disease), CYP2C9 poor metabolizers (pts with CYP2C9*3/*3 genotype); concomitant use of CYP3A4 inhibitors or inducers, CYP2C9 inducers or inhibitors, CYP34A substrates, OAT2 substrates, or P-gp substrates.

ACTION

Binds to and inhibits fibroblast growth factor receptor (FGFR) enzyme activity. Decreases FGFR-related signaling and cell viability. **Therapeutic Effect:** Inhibits tumor cell growth and metastasis. Induces cellular death of tumor cells.

PHARMACOKINETICS

Widely distributed. Metabolized in liver. Protein binding: 99.8%. Peak plasma concentration: 2.5 hrs. Steady state reached in 2 wks. Excreted in feces (69%), urine (19%). **Half-life:** 59 hrs.

⧗ LIFESPAN CONSIDERATIONS

Pregnancy/Lactation: Avoid pregnancy; may cause fetal harm. Females and males with female partners of reproductive potential should use effective contraception during treatment and up to 1 mo after discontinuation. Unknown if distributed in breast milk. Breastfeeding not recommended during treatment and for at least 1 mo after discontinua-

---

tion. May impair fertility in female pts. **Children:** Safety and efficacy not established. **Elderly:** No age-related precautions noted.

INTERACTIONS

DRUG: **Strong CYP3A4 inhibitors (e.g., clarithromycin, ketoconazole), moderate CYP3A4 inhibitors (e.g., ciprofloxacin, dilTIAZem, fluconazole, verapamil)** may increase concentration/effect. **Strong CYP3A4 inducers (e.g., carBAMazepine, phenytoin, rifAMPin)** may decrease concentration/effect. **Phosphate-altering drugs (e.g., ergocalciferol, K-phos, PhosLo, Renagel)** may alter phosphate level; may affect dose modifications. **HERBAL:** None significant. **St. John's wort** may decrease concentration/effect. **FOOD:** **Phosphorus-containing foods (e.g., dairy products, deli meats, nuts, peanut butter)** may increase serum phosphate; may affect dose modifications. Restrict phosphate intake to 600–800 mg daily. **LAB VALUES:** May increase serum alkaline phosphatase, ALT, AST, calcium, creatinine, glucose, potassium. May decrease serum albumin, sodium; Hgb, leukocytes, neutrophils, platelets. May increase or decrease serum phosphate.

AVAILABILITY (Rx)

 Tablets: 3 mg, 4 mg, 5 mg.

ADMINISTRATION/HANDLING

PO
• Give without regard to food. Administer tablets whole; do not break, cut, crush, or divide. Tablets should not be chewed. • If a dose is missed, give as soon as possible. If vomiting occurs after administration, give next dose at regularly scheduled time.

INDICATIONS/ROUTES/DOSAGE

Note: Assess serum phosphate levels 14–21 days after therapy initiation. Restrict phosphate intake to 600–800 mg daily

Bladder Cancer (Urothelial)
PO: ADULTS, ELDERLY: Initially, 8 mg once daily. After 14–21 days, increase dose to 9 mg once daily if serum phosphate is less than 5.5 mg/dL and there are no ocular toxicities or Grade 2 (or higher) adverse reactions. Continue until disease progression or unacceptable toxicity.

Dose Reduction Schedule for Adverse Reactions

Dose	First Dose Reduction	Second Dose Reduction	Third Dose Reduction	Fourth Dose Reduction	Fifth Dose Reduction
9 mg	8 mg	6 mg	5 mg	4 mg	Discontinue
8 mg	6 mg	5 mg	4 mg	Discontinue	N/A

Dose Modification
Based on Common Terminology Criteria for Adverse Events (CTCAE).

Hyperphosphatemia
Serum phosphate 5.6–6.9 mg/dL (1.8–2.3 mmol/L): Maintain dose. **7–9 mg/dL (2.3–2.9 mmol/L):** Withhold treatment until serum phosphate is less than 5.5 mg/dL (or baseline), then resume at same dose. May reduce dose if hyperphosphatemia lasts greater than 1 wk. **Greater than 9 mg/dL and less than 10 mg/dL (greater than 2.9 mmol/L):** Withhold treatment until serum phosphate is less than 5.5 mg/dL (or baseline), then resume at next lower dose level. **Greater than 10 mg/dL (greater than 3.2 mmol/L); significant change of baseline renal function; Grade 3 hypercalcemia:** Withhold treatment until serum phosphate is less than 5.5 mg/dL (or baseline), then resume at 2 lower dose levels.

Serious Retinopathy/Retinal Pigment Epithelial Detachment
Asymptomatic; clinical of diagnostic observation: Withhold treatment until resolved. Resume at next lower dose level if resolved within 4 wks. Consider re-esca-

lation of dose if symptoms do not recur for 1 mo. If stable but not resolved for 2 consecutive eye exams, resume at next lower dose level. **Visual acuity 20/40 (or better) or greater than or equal to 3 lines of decreased vision from baseline:** Withhold treatment until resolved. Resume at next lower dose level if resolved within 4 wks. **Visual acuity worse than 20/40 or greater than 3 lines of decreased vision from baseline:** Withhold treatment until resolved. Resume at 2 lower dose levels if resolved within 4 wks. Consider permanent discontinuation if recurrent. **Visual acuity 20/200 or worse in affected eye:** Permanently discontinue.

Other Adverse Reactions

Any Grade 3 reaction: Withhold treatment until improved to Grade 1 or 0, then resume at next lower dose level. **Any Grade 4 reaction:** Permanently discontinue.

Dosage in Renal Impairment

Mild to moderate impairment: No dose adjustment. **Severe impairment:** Not specified; use caution.

Dosage in Hepatic Impairment

Mild impairment: No dose adjustment. **Moderate to severe impairment:** Not specified; use caution.

SIDE EFFECTS

Frequent (56%–20%): Stomatitis, fatigue, asthenia, lethargy, malaise, diarrhea, dry mouth, onycholysis, onychoclasis, nail disorder, nail dystrophy, nail ridging, decreased appetite, dysgeusia, constipation, dry eye, alopecia, abdominal pain, nausea, musculoskeletal pain, back/chest/neck pain. **Occasional (17%–10%):** Blurry vision, decreased weight, cachexia, pyrexia, vomiting, nail discoloration, oropharyngeal pain, arthralgia, increased lacrimation, dyspnea.

ADVERSE EFFECTS/TOXIC REACTIONS

Hemoglobinemia, leukopenia, neutropenia, thrombocytopenia are expected responses to therapy. Ocular toxicities including serious retinopathy/retinal pigment epithelial detachment reported in 25% of pts. Ocular disorders including keratitis, foreign body sensation, corneal erosion reported in 28% of pts. Grade 3 serious retinopathy/retinal pigment epithelial detachment reported in 3% of pts. Hyperphosphatemia reported in 76% of pts with 32% of pts requiring oral phosphate binders. Palmar-plantar erythrodysesthesia syndrome reported in 26% of pts. Hematuria reported in 11% of pts. Infections including paronychia (17% of pts), urinary tract infection (17% of pts), conjunctivitis (11% of pts) may occur.

NURSING CONSIDERATIONS

BASELINE ASSESSMENT

Obtain CBC, BMP, LFT, pregnancy test in female pts of reproductive potential. Confirm presence of susceptible FGFR genetic alterations in tumor specimens. Verify compliance of effective contraception in female pts and male pts with female partners of reproductive potential. Obtain visual acuity. Screen for active infection. Question history of hepatic/renal impairment, optic disorders. Receive full medication history and screen for interactions. Offer emotional support.

INTERVENTION/EVALUATION

Monitor CBC, BMP, LFT, serum ionized calcium periodically. Obtain serum phosphate level 14–21 days after initiation. Restrict phosphorus intake to 600–800 mg daily. If serum phosphate is greater than 7 mg/dL, consider administration of an oral phosphate binder until serum phosphate is less than 5.5 mg/dL. Obtain weekly serum phosphate levels in pts who develop hyperphosphatemia. Monitor for symptoms of hyperphosphatemia, which may mimic symptoms of hypocalcemia (facial twitching, muscle cramps, numbness of hand, feet, lips; seizures). Assess skin for dermal toxicities. Monthly ophthalmologic exams (including visual acuity, slit lamp examination, fundoscopy, optical coherence tomography) should be performed by a specialist for the first 4 mos, then q3mos thereafter, or emergently if new symptoms occur. Obtain urinalysis if UTI is suspected (dysuria, fever, foul-smelling or cloudy urine, urinary frequency). Diligently monitor for infections.

PATIENT/FAMILY TEACHING

• Treatment may depress your immune system and reduce your ability to fight infection. Report symptoms of infection such as body aches, burning with urination, chills, cough, fatigue, fever. Avoid those with active infection. • Report symptoms of bone marrow depression such as bruising, fatigue, fever, shortness of breath, weight loss; bleeding easily, bloody urine or stool. • Expect frequent eye exams, skin exams. Immediately report vision changes of any kind. • Use effective contraception to avoid pregnancy. Do not breast-feed. • Limit intake of phosphorus-containing food unless blood tests verify acceptable phosphate levels. • Report liver problems such as bruising, confusion, dark or amber-colored urine, right upper abdominal pain, or yellowing of the skin or eyes; symptoms of UTI (burning with urination, fever, urinary frequency, foul-smelling or cloudy urine). • There is a high risk of interactions with other medications. Do not take any newly prescribed medications unless approved by prescriber who originally started treatment. • Avoid grapefruit products, herbal supplements (esp. St. John's wort).

---

eriBULin

er-i-**bue**-lin
(Halaven)
Do not confuse eriBULin with epiRUBicin or erlotinib.

◆CLASSIFICATION

PHARMACOTHERAPEUTIC: Microtubule inhibitor. **CLINICAL:** Antineoplastic.

USES

Breast cancer: Treatment of metastatic breast cancer in pts who previously received at least 2 chemotherapeutic regimens for treatment (therapy should have included an anthracycline and a taxane in either the adjuvant or metastatic setting). **Liposarcoma:** Treatment of metastatic or unresectable liposarcoma in pts who received a prior anthracycline-containing regimen. **OFF-LABEL:** Uterine leiomyosarcoma (refractory).

PRECAUTIONS

Contraindications: Hypersensitivity to eriBULin. **Cautions:** Pts at risk for QT interval prolongation (e.g., congenital long QT syndrome, QT interval–prolonging medications, hypokalemia, hypomagnesemia); hepatic/renal impairment, moderate to severe neuropathy, HF; conditions predisposing to infection (e.g., diabetes, renal failure, immunocompromised pts, open wounds).

ACTION

Inhibits growth phase of microtubule by inhibiting formation of mitotic spindles. Causes mitotic blockage and arrests the cell cycle. **Therapeutic Effect:** Blocks cells in mitotic phase of cell division, leading to tumor cell death.

PHARMACOKINETICS

Widely distributed. Metabolism is negligible. Protein binding: 49%–65%. Excreted in feces (82%), urine (9%). **Half-life:** 40 hrs.

⌛ LIFESPAN CONSIDERATIONS

Pregnancy/Lactation: Avoid pregnancy; may cause fetal harm. Females of reproductive potential must use effective contraception during treatment and for at least 2 wks after discontinuation. Unknown if distributed in breast milk. **Males:** Males with female partners of reproductive potential must use effective contraception during treatment and for at least 3.5 mos after discontinuation. May impair fertility. **Children:** Safety and efficacy not established. **Elderly:** No age-related precautions noted.

INTERACTIONS

DRUG: May decrease levels/effects of **BCG (intravesical). May increase QT**

E

interval–prolonging effect of amiodarone, azithromycin, ciprofloxacin, haloperidol. **HERBAL:** None significant. **FOOD:** None known. **LAB VALUES:** May decrease WBC, Hgb, Hct, platelet count, potassium. May increase ALT.

AVAILABILITY (Rx)

Injection, Solution: 1 mg/2 mL (0.5 mg/mL).

ADMINISTRATION/HANDLING

 IV

Reconstitution • May administer undiluted or dilute in 100 mL 0.9% NaCl. **Rate of administration** • Administer over 2–5 min. **Storage** • Store at room temperature. • Once diluted, syringe or diluted solution may be stored for up to 4 hrs at room temperature or up to 24 hrs if refrigerated.

⚙ IV INCOMPATIBILITIES

Do not dilute with D₅W or administer through IV line containing solutions with dextrose or in same IV line with other medications.

INDICATIONS/ROUTES/DOSAGE

Metastatic Breast Cancer, Liposarcoma
IV: ADULTS, ELDERLY: 1.4 mg/m² on days 1 and 8 of 21-day cycle.

Recommended Dose Delays

Do not administer day 1 or day 8 of treatment for any of the following: ANC less than 1,000 cells/mm³, platelets less than 75,000 cells/mm³, Grade 3 or 4 nonhematologic toxicities. Day 8 dose may be delayed for maximum of 1 wk. If toxicities do not resolve or improve to Grade 2 severity by day 15, omit dose. If toxicities resolve or improve to Grade 2 severity by day 15, continue treatment at reduced dose and initiate next cycle no sooner than 2 wks later. Do not re-escalate dose after it has been reduced.

Dosage in Renal Impairment

Mild impairment: No dose adjustment. **Moderate to severe impairment:** CrCl 15–49 mL/min: 1.1 mg/m²/dose.

Dosage in Hepatic Impairment

Mild impairment: 1.1 mg/m²/dose. **Moderate impairment:** 0.7 mg/m²/dose. **Severe impairment:** Use not recommended.

SIDE EFFECTS

Common (54%–35%): Fatigue, asthenia, alopecia, peripheral sensory neuropathy, nausea. **Frequent (25%–18%):** Constipation, arthralgia/myalgia, decreased weight, anorexia, pyrexia, headache, diarrhea, vomiting. **Occasional (16%–9%):** Back pain, dyspnea, cough, bone pain, extremity pain, urinary tract infection, oral mucosal inflammation.

ADVERSE EFFECTS/TOXIC REACTIONS

Neutropenia occurs in 82% of pts, with 57% developing Grade 3 neutropenia. Severe neutropenia (ANC less than 500 cells/mm³) lasting more than 1 wk occurred in 12%. Anemia occurs in 58% of pts. Peripheral neuropathy occurs in 8% of pts. Prolonged QTc interval may be noted on or after day 8 of treatment.

NURSING CONSIDERATIONS

BASELINE ASSESSMENT

Obtain CBC (prior to each dose); pregnancy test in females of reproductive potential. Screen for active infection, QT interval–prolonging medications. Offer emotional support.

INTERVENTION/EVALUATION

Monitor for infections (cough, fatigue, fever). Monitor for symptoms of neuropathy (burning sensation, hyperesthesia, hypoesthesia, paresthesia, discomfort, neuropathic pain). Assess hands, feet for erythema. Monitor CBC for evidence of neutropenia, thrombocytopenia. Assess mouth for stomatitis (erythema, ulceration, mucosal burning).

PATIENT/FAMILY TEACHING

• Treatment may depress your immune system response and reduce your ability to fight infection. Report symptoms of infection such as body aches, chills, cough, fatigue, fever. Avoid those with active infection. • Report symptoms of bone marrow depression such as bruising, fatigue, fever, shortness of breath, weight loss; bleeding easily, bloody urine or stool. • Report liver problems (abdominal pain, bruising, clay-colored stool, amber- or dark-colored urine, yellowing of the skin or eyes), kidney problems (decreased urine output, flank pain, darkened urine). • Use effective contraception to avoid pregnancy. Do not breastfeed.

erlotinib HIGH ALERT

er-**loe**-ti-nib
(Tarceva)
Do not confuse erlotinib with dasatinib, eriBULin, gefitinib, imatinib, or lapatinib.

◆CLASSIFICATION

PHARMACOTHERAPEUTIC: Epidermal growth factor receptor (EGFR) inhibitor; tyrosine kinase inhibitor. **CLINICAL:** Antineoplastic.

USES

Non–small-cell lung cancer (NSCLC): Treatment of locally advanced or metastatic NSCLC after failure of at least one prior chemotherapy regimen (as monotherapy). **Pancreatic cancer:** First-line treatment of locally advanced, unresectable, or metastatic pancreatic cancer (in combination with gemcitabine). **OFF-LABEL:** Renal cell carcinoma (papillary advanced).

PRECAUTIONS

Contraindications: Hypersensitivity to erlotinib. **Cautions:** Severe hepatic/renal impairment, cardiovascular disease. Concurrent use of strong CYP3A4 inhibitors and inducers or CYP1A2 inhibitors, pts at risk for GI perforation (e.g., peptic ulcer disease, diverticular disease), conditions predisposing to infection (e.g., diabetes, renal failure, immunocompromised pts, open wounds).

ACTION

Reversibly inhibits overall epidermal growth factor receptor (EGFR)–tyrosine kinase activity. Inhibits intracellular phosphorylation. **Therapeutic Effect:** Produces tumor cell death.

PHARMACOKINETICS

Widely distributed. Metabolized in liver. Protein binding: 93%. Excreted in feces (83%), urine (8%). **Half-life:** 24–36 hrs.

⚠ LIFESPAN CONSIDERATIONS

Pregnancy/Lactation: Unknown if drug crosses placenta or is distributed in breast milk. **Children:** Safety and efficacy not established. **Elderly:** No age-related precautions noted.

INTERACTIONS

DRUG: Strong CYP3A4 inhibitors (e.g., clarithromycin, ketoconazole, ritonavir) may increase concentration/effects. **Strong CYP3A4 inducers (e.g., carBAMazepine, phenytoin, rifAMPin)** may decrease concentration/effect. **Antacids, proton pump inhibitors (e.g., omeprazole, pantoprazole), H₂ antagonists (e.g., famotitdine)** may decrease absorption/effect. **Warfarin** may increase risk of bleeding. **Statins (e.g., atorvastatin, simvastatin)** may increase risk of myopathy, rhabdomyolysis. **HERBAL: St. John's wort** may decrease concentration/effect. **FOOD: Grapefruit products** may increase potential for myelotoxicity. **LAB VALUES:** May increase serum bilirubin, ALT, AST.

AVAILABILITY (Rx)

Tablets: 25 mg, 100 mg, 150 mg.

ADMINISTRATION/HANDLING

PO
• Give at least 1 hr before or 2 hrs after ingestion of food. • Avoid grapefruit products. • May dissolve in 3–4 oz water and give orally or via feeding tube. • Give 10 hrs after or 2 hrs before H₂ antagonists (e.g., famotidine)

Avoid proton inhibitors (e.g., pantoprazole), if possible.

INDICATIONS/ROUTES/DOSAGE

NSCLC
PO: ADULTS, ELDERLY: 150 mg/day until
disease progression or unacceptable toxicity occurs.

Pancreatic Cancer
PO: ADULTS, ELDERLY: 100 mg/day, in
combination with gemcitabine, until disease
progression or unacceptable toxicity occurs.

Dose Modification
Permanently discontinue treatment in pts
with interstitial lung disease (ILD); severe
hepatotoxicity that does not significantly
improve or resolve within 3 wks; GI perforation; severe bullous, blistering, or exfoliative skin conditions; corneal perforation
or severe ulceration. Withhold treatment
and consider discontinuation in pts with
preexisting hepatic impairment or biliary
obstruction for doubling or tripling of
transaminase values over baseline; severe
renal toxicity, acute or worsening ocular
disorders. Withhold treatment in pts with
severe rash or persistent diarrhea not
responsive to medical management; Grade
3 or 4 keratitis or Grade 2 keratitis lasting
longer than 2 wks; or pt being investigated
for ILD. Once improved to Grade 1 or 0,
then resume at reduced 50-mg dose increments.

Dosage in Renal Impairment
Interrupt treatment for Grade 3 or 4
renal toxicity during treatment.

Dosage in Hepatic Impairment
Use extreme caution. Reduce starting
dose to 75 mg and individualize dose
escalation if tolerated.

SIDE EFFECTS
Frequent (85%–21%): Rash, diarrhea,
decreased appetite, fatigue, cough, dyspnea, pyrexia, nausea, dry skin. **Occasional (19%–11%):** Back pain, chest pain,
mucosal inflammation, stomatitis, pruritus,
cough, headache, paronychia, arthralgia,
musculoskeletal pain.

ADVERSE EFFECTS/TOXIC REACTIONS
Severe, life-threatening pneumonitis, ILD,
respiratory failure reported in 9% of pts.
Life-threatening hepatorenal syndrome
reported in less than 1% of pts. Fatal cases
of GI perforation; blistering, and exfoliative
skin reactions, including Stevens-Johnson
syndrome/toxic epidermal necrolysis;
ocular disorders including dry eye, keratoconjunctivitis, keratitis, leading to corneal
perforation or ulceration, were reported.
CVA reported in 3% of pts. Microangiopathic
hemolytic anemia with thrombocytopenia
was reported. Fatal hemorrhagic events
were reported in pts taking concomitant
warfarin. Myopathy, rhabdomyolysis was
reported in pts taking concomitant statin
therapy. Depression reported in 19% of pts.

NURSING CONSIDERATIONS

BASELINE ASSESSMENT
Obtain CBC, BMP, LFT; pregnancy test in
females of reproductive potential. Confirm
compliance of effective contraception. Question history of CVA, optic disorders, pulmonary disease, hepatic/renal impairment, GI
perforation. Screen for active infection. Receive full medication history and screen for
interactions. Offer emotional support.

INTERVENTION/EVALUATION
Monitor CBC, LFT, renal function periodically. An increase of serum creatinine
greater than 0.4 mg/dL from baseline may
indicate renal impairment. Consider ABG,
radiologic test if ILD/pneumonitis (excessive cough, dyspnea, fever, hypoxia) is
suspected. Consider treatment with corticosteroids if ILD/pneumonitis is confirmed.
Monitor for infections (cough, fatigue,
fever). If serious infection occurs, initiate
appropriate antimicrobial therapy. Monitor
daily pattern of bowel activity, stool consistency. Abdominal pain, fever, melena may
indicate GI perforation. Monitor for toxic
skin reactions, rash. Assess for symptoms of

CVA (aphasia, blindness, confusion, facial droop, hemiplegia, seizures). Monitor for ocular toxicities. Monitor for depression.

PATIENT/FAMILY TEACHING

• Treatment may depress your immune system response and reduce your ability to fight infection. Report symptoms of infection such as body aches, chills, cough, fatigue, fever. Avoid those with active infection. • Report symptoms of lung inflammation (excessive coughing, difficulty breathing, chest pain); liver problems (abdominal pain, bruising, clay-colored stool, amber or dark colored urine, yellowing of the skin or eyes), eye problems (dry eye, eye pain/swelling/redness), kidney problems (decreased urine output, flank pain, darkened urine); toxic skin reactions (rash, skin eruptions), stroke (confusion, difficulty speaking, one-sided weakness or paralysis, loss of vision), intestinal tear (abdominal pain, bloody stool, fever). • Use effective contraception to avoid pregnancy. Do not breastfeed. • There is a high risk of interactions with other medications. Do not take newly prescribed medications unless approved by prescriber who originally started treatment. • Report changes in mood, depression.

erythromycin

er-**ith**-roe-**mye**-sin
(Akne-Mycin, EES, Erybid ✦, Eryc, EryDerm, EryPed, Ery-Tab, Erythrocin)
Do not confuse Eryc with Emcyt, or erythromycin with azithromycin or clarithromycin.

FIXED-COMBINATION(S)

Eryzole, Pediazole: erythromycin/sulfiSOXAZOLE (sulfonamide): 200 mg/600 mg per 5 mL.

◆CLASSIFICATION

PHARMACOTHERAPEUTIC: Macrolide. **CLINICAL:** Antibiotic, anti-acne.

USES

Treatment of susceptible infections due to *S. pyogenes, S. pneumoniae, S. aureus, M. pneumoniae, Legionella, Chlamydia,* other susceptible bacterial infections including infections of upper and lower respiratory tract, non-gonococcal urethritis, diphtheria, pertussis, gastroenteritis, syphillis. Surgical prophylaxis. Skin and soft tissue infections, intestinal amebiasis, pelvic inflammatory disease, urogenital infections, Legionnaire's disease. **Topical:** Treatment of acne vulgaris. **Ophthalmic:** Prevention of gonococcal ophthalmia neonatorum, superficial ocular infections. **OFF-LABEL: Systemic:** Treatment of acne vulgaris, COPD (prevention of exacerbation), gastroparesis. **Topical:** Treatment of minor bacterial skin infections. **Ophthalmic:** Treatment of blepharitis, conjunctivitis, keratitis, chlamydial trachoma.

PRECAUTIONS

Contraindications: Hypersensitivity to erythromycin. Concomitant administration with ergot derivatives, lovastatin, pimozide, simvastatin. **Cautions:** Elderly, myasthenia gravis, strong CYP3A4 inhibitor, hepatic impairment, pts with prolonged QT intervals, uncorrected hypokalemia or hypomagnesemia, concurrent use of class IA or III antiarrhythmics.

ACTION

Penetrates bacterial cell membranes, reversibly binds to bacterial ribosomes, inhibiting RNA-dependent protein synthesis. **Therapeutic Effect:** Bacteriostatic.

PHARMACOKINETICS

Variably absorbed from GI tract (depending on dosage form used). Protein binding: 70%–90%. Widely distributed. Metabolized in liver. Primarily eliminated in feces by bile. Not removed by hemodialysis. **Half-**

E

E

life: 1.4–2 hrs (increased in renal impairment).

⧗ LIFESPAN CONSIDERATIONS

Pregnancy/Lactation: Crosses placenta. Distributed in breast milk. Erythromycin estolate may increase hepatic enzymes in pregnant women. **Children/Elderly:** No age-related precautions noted. High dosage in pts with decreased hepatic/renal function increases risk of hearing loss.

INTERACTIONS

DRUG: May increase concentration/effect of **bosutinib, budesonide, busPIRone, cycloSPORINE, statins (e.g., atorvastatin, simvastatin). Amiodarone, dronedarone, fluconazole** may increase QT interval–prolonging effect. **Strong CYP3A4 inducers (e.g., carBAMazepine, phenytoin, rifAMPin)** may decrease concentration/effect. **HERBAL:** None significant. **FOOD:** None known. **LAB VALUES:** May increase serum alkaline phosphatase, bilirubin, ALT, AST.

AVAILABILITY (Rx)

Gel, Topical: 2%. **Injection, Powder for Reconstitution:** 500 mg. **Ointment, Ophthalmic:** 0.5%. **Ointment, Topical:** *(Akne-Mycin):* 2%. **Oral Suspension:** *(EES, EryPed):* 200 mg/5 mL, 400 mg/5 mL. **Tablet as Base:** 250 mg, 500 mg. **Tablet as Ethylsuccinate:** *(EES):* 400 mg.

 Capsules, Delayed-Release: 250 mg. **Tablets, Delayed-Release** *(Ery-Tab):* 250 mg, 333 mg, 500 mg.

ADMINISTRATION/HANDLING

🖉 IV

Reconstitution • Reconstitute each 500 mg with 10 mL Sterile Water for Injection without preservative to provide a concentration of 50 mg/mL. • Further dilute with 100–250 mL D₅W or 0.9% NaCl to maximum concentration of 5 mg/mL.

Rate of administration • For intermittent IV infusion (piggyback), infuse over 20–60 min.

Storage • Store parenteral form at room temperature. • Initial reconstituted solution in vial is stable for 2 wks refrigerated or 24 hrs at room temperature. • Diluted IV solution stable for 8 hrs at room temperature or 24 hrs if refrigerated. • Discard if precipitate forms.

PO

• May give with food to decrease GI upset. • Oral suspension is stable for 35 days at room temperature. • Do not crush delayed-release capsules, enteric-coated tablets.

Ophthalmic

• Place gloved finger on lower eyelid and pull out until a pocket is formed between eye and lower lid. • Place 1/4–1/2 inch of ointment into pocket. • Instruct pt to close eye gently for 1–2 min (so that medication will not be squeezed out of the sac) and to roll eyeball to increase contact area of drug to eye.

▒ IV COMPATIBILITIES

Amiodarone, dexmedetomidine, diltiazem, heparin, magnesium sulfate, morphine, multivitamins, potassium chloride.

INDICATIONS/ROUTES/DOSAGE

Usual Dosage Range

PO: ADULTS, ELDERLY: *(Base):* 250–500 mg q6–12h. **Maximum:** 4 g/day. **CHILDREN:** 40–50 mg/kg/day in divided doses q6–8h. **Maximum:** 4 g/day. *(Ethylsuccinate):* **ADULTS, ELDERLY:** 400–800 mg q6–12h. **Maximum:** 4 g/day. **CHILDREN:** 40–50 mg/kg/day in divided doses q6–8h. **Maximum:** 4 g/day. **NEONATES:** 10 mg/kg/dose q8–12h.

IV: ADULTS, ELDERLY: 15–20 mg/kg/day divided q6h. **Maximum:** 4 g/day. **ADOLESCENTS, CHILDREN, INFANTS:** 15–20 mg/kg/day divided q6h. **Maximum:** 4 g/day. **NEONATES:** 10 mg/kg/dose q8–12h.

Dosage in Renal/Hepatic Impairment
No dose adjustment.

SIDE EFFECTS

Frequent: IV: Abdominal cramping/discomfort, phlebitis/thrombophlebitis. **Topical:** Dry skin (50%). **Occasional:** Nausea, vomiting, diarrhea, rash, urticaria. **Rare: Ophthalmic:** Sensitivity reaction with increased irritation, burning, itching, inflammation. **Topical:** Urticaria.

ADVERSE EFFECTS/TOXIC REACTIONS

Antibiotic-associated colitis, other superinfections (abdominal cramps, severe watery diarrhea, fever), reversible cholestatic hepatitis may occur. High dosage in pts with renal impairment may lead to reversible hearing loss. Anaphylaxis occurs rarely. Ventricular arrhythmias, prolonged QT interval occur rarely with IV form.

NURSING CONSIDERATIONS

BASELINE ASSESSMENT

Question for history of allergies (particularly erythromycins), hepatitis. Receive full medication history and screen for interactions.

INTERVENTION/EVALUATION

Monitor daily pattern of bowel activity, stool consistency. Assess skin for rash. Assess for hepatotoxicity (malaise, fever, abdominal pain, GI disturbances). Be alert for superinfection: fever, vomiting, diarrhea, anal/genital pruritus, oral mucosal changes (ulceration, pain, erythema). Check for phlebitis (heat, pain, red streaking over vein). Monitor for high-dose hearing loss.

PATIENT/FAMILY TEACHING

• Continue therapy for full length of treatment. • Doses should be evenly spaced. • Take medication with 8 oz water 1 hr before or 2 hrs following food or beverage. • **Ophthalmic:** Report burning, itching, inflammation. • **Topical:** Report excessive skin dryness, itching, burning. • Improvement of acne may not occur for 1–2 mos; maximum

benefit may take 3 mos; therapy may last mos or yrs. • Use caution if using other topical acne preparations containing peeling or abrasive agents, medicated or abrasive soaps, cosmetics containing alcohol (e.g., astringents, aftershave lotion).

escitalopram

es-sye-**tal**-o-pram
(Cipralex ✦, Lexapro)
■ **BLACK BOX ALERT** ■ Increased risk of suicidal ideation and behavior in children, adolescents, young adults 18–24 yrs with major depressive disorder, other psychiatric disorders.

◆ CLASSIFICATION

PHARMACOTHERAPEUTIC: Selective serotonin reuptake inhibitor. **CLINICAL:** Antidepressant.

USES

Treatment of major depressive disorder in adults and children 12–17 yrs of age. Treatment of generalized anxiety disorder (GAD). **OFF-LABEL:** Social anxiety disorder, obsessive compulsive disorder, panic disorder, posttraumatic stress disorder, binge eating disorder, bulimia nervosa, pervasive developmental disorders (e.g., autism), vasomotor symptoms associated with menopause.

PRECAUTIONS

Contraindications: Hypersensitivity to escitalopram. Use of MAOI intended to treat psychiatric disorders (concurrent or within 14 days of discontinuing either escitalopram or MAOI). Initiation in pts receiving linezolid or IV methylene blue. Concurrent use with pimozide. **Cautions:** Hepatic/renal impairment, history of seizure disorder, concurrent use of CNS depressants, pts at high risk of suicide, concomitant aspirin, NSAIDs, warfarin (may potentiate bleeding risk), elderly, metabolic disease; recent history of MI, cardiovascular disease.

ACTION

Blocks uptake of neurotransmitter serotonin at neuronal presynaptic membranes, increasing its availability at postsynaptic receptor sites. **Therapeutic Effect:** Antidepressant effect.

PHARMACOKINETICS

Widely distributed. Protein binding: 56%. Primarily metabolized in liver. Primarily excreted in feces, with a lesser amount eliminated in urine. **Half-life:** 35 hrs.

⌛ LIFESPAN CONSIDERATIONS

Pregnancy/Lactation: Distributed in breast milk. **Children:** May cause increased anticholinergic effects or hyperexcitability. **Elderly:** More sensitive to anticholinergic effects (e.g., dry mouth), more likely to experience dizziness, sedation, confusion, hypotension, hyperexcitability.

INTERACTIONS

DRUG: Alcohol, **CNS depressants (e.g., LORazepam, morphine, zolpidem)** may increase CNS depression. **Aspirin, NSAIDs (e.g., ibuprofen, ketorolac, naproxen), warfarin** may increase risk of bleeding. **MAOIs (e.g., phenelzine, selegiline)** may cause serotonin syndrome (autonomic hyperactivity, diaphoresis, excitement, hyperthermia, rigidity, neuroleptic malignant syndrome, coma). **SUMAtriptan** may cause weakness, hyperreflexia, poor coordination. **Strong CYP3A4 inducers (e.g., carBAMazepine, phenytoin, rifAMPin)** may decrease concentration/effect. **HERBAL:** St. John's wort, Syrian rue may enhance serotonergic effect of serotonergic agents. **Herbals with anticoagulant/antiplatelet properties (e.g., garlic, ginger, ginkgo biloba)** may increase risk of bleeding. **FOOD:** None known. **LAB VALUES:** May decrease serum sodium.

AVAILABILITY (Rx)

Oral Solution: 5 mg/5 mL.

🞱 **Tablets:** 5 mg, 10 mg, 20 mg.

ADMINISTRATION/HANDLING

PO
• Administer once daily (morning or evening) without regard to food.

INDICATIONS/ROUTES/DOSAGE

Depression
PO: **ADULTS:** Initially, 10 mg once daily in the morning or evening. May increase to 20 mg after a minimum of 1 wk. **ELDERLY:** 5–10 mg/day. **ADOLESCENTS 12–17 YRS:** Initially, 10 mg once daily. May increase to 20 mg/day after at least 3 wks. **Maximum:** 20 mg once daily.

Generalized Anxiety Disorder
PO: **ADULTS:** Initially, 10 mg once daily in morning or evening. May increase to a maximum of 20 mg after minimum of 1 wk. **ELDERLY:** 10 mg/day.

Dosage in Renal Impairment
Mild to moderate impairment: No dose adjustment. **Severe impairment:** Use caution in pts with CrCl less than 20 mL/min.

Dosage in Hepatic Impairment
10 mg/day.

SIDE EFFECTS

Frequent (21%–11%): Nausea, dry mouth, drowsiness, insomnia, diaphoresis. **Occasional (8%–4%):** Tremor, diarrhea, abnormal ejaculation, dyspepsia, fatigue, anxiety, vomiting, anorexia. **Rare (3%–2%):** Sinusitis, sexual dysfunction, menstrual disorder, abdominal pain, agitation, decreased libido.

ADVERSE EFFECTS/TOXIC REACTIONS

May increase risk of suicidal thoughts and behavior in adolescents and young adults. Life-threatening serotonin syndrome may include mental status changes (agitation, hallucinations, delirium, coma), autonomic instability (tachycardia, labile blood pressure, dizziness, sweating, flushing, hyperthermia), neuromuscular symptoms (tremor, rigidity, myoclonus hyperactive reflexes, incoordination). May cause hyponatremia as a result of syndrome of inappropriate antidiuretic hormone (SIADH). May increase risk of bleeding; narrow angle glaucoma; seizures.

NURSING CONSIDERATIONS

BASELINE ASSESSMENT
For pts on long-term therapy, LFT, renal function tests, blood counts should be performed periodically. Observe, record behavior. Assess psychological status, thought content, sleep pattern, appearance, interest in environment.

INTERVENTION/EVALUATION
Supervise suicidal-risk pt closely during early therapy (as depression lessens, energy level improves, suicide potential increases). Assess appearance, behavior, speech pattern, level of interest, mood. Monitor for suicidal ideation (esp. at beginning of therapy or when doses are increased or decreased), social interaction, mania, panic attacks.

PATIENT/FAMILY TEACHING
• Do not stop taking medication or increase dosage. • Avoid alcohol. • Avoid tasks that require alertness, motor skills until response to drug is established. • Report worsening depression, suicidal ideation, unusual changes in behavior.

---

esmolol **HIGH ALERT**

es-moe-lol
(Brevibloc)
Do not confuse Brevibloc with Bumex or Buprenex, or esmolol with Osmitrol.

◆CLASSIFICATION

PHARMACOTHERAPEUTIC: Beta$_1$-adrenergic blocker. **CLINICAL:** Antiarrhythmic, antihypertensive.

USES
Rapid, short-term control of ventricular rate in supraventricular tachycardia (SVT),

atrial fibrillation or flutter; treatment of tachycardia and/or hypertension (esp. intraop or postop). Treatment of noncompensatory sinus tachycardia. **OFF-LABEL:** Thyroid storm, hypertensive emergencies, ventricular tachycardia.

PRECAUTIONS

Contraindications: Hypersensitivity to esmolol. Cardiogenic shock, uncompensated cardiac failure, second- or third-degree heart block (except in pts with pacemaker), severe sinus bradycardia, sick sinus syndrome, IV administration of calcium blockers in close proximity to esmolol, pulmonary hypertension. **Cautions:** Compensated HF; concurrent use of digoxin, verapamil, dilTIAZem. Diabetes, myasthenia gravis, renal impairment, history of anaphylaxis to allergens. Hypovolemia, hypertension, bronchospastic disease, peripheral vascular disease, Raynaud's disease.

ACTION
Selectively blocks beta$_1$-adrenergic receptors. **Therapeutic Effect:** Slows sinus heart rate, decreases cardiac output, reducing B/P.

PHARMACOKINETICS
Rapidly metabolized primarily by esterase in cytosol of red blood cells. Protein binding: 55%. Less than 1%–2% excreted in urine. **Half-life:** 9 min.

LIFESPAN CONSIDERATIONS
Pregnancy/Lactation: Crosses placenta; distributed in breast milk. **Children:** Safety and efficacy not established. **Elderly:** No age-related precautions noted.

INTERACTIONS
DRUG: **Alpha-2 agonists** (e.g., **norepinephrine**), **calcium channel blockers** (e.g., **dilTIAZem, verapamil**), **dronedarone, rivastigmine** may increase the concentration/effect. May increase bradycardic effect of **fingolimod.** May increase vasoconstricting effect of **ergot derivatives** (e.g., **ergotamine**). **HERBAL:**

Herbals with hypotensive properties (e.g., garlic, ginger, ginkgo biloba) may increase effect. Herbals with hypertensive properties (e.g., yohimbe) may decrease effect. **FOOD:** None known. **LAB VALUES:** None significant.

AVAILABILITY (Rx)

Injection Solution: 10 mg/mL (10 mL, 250 mL), 20 mg/mL (100 mL).

ADMINISTRATION/HANDLING

◀**ALERT**▶ Give by IV infusion. Avoid butterfly needles, very small veins (can cause thrombophlebitis).

 IV

Rate of administration • Administer by controlled infusion device; titrate to tolerance and response. • Infuse IV loading dose over 1–2 min.
Storage • Use only clear and colorless to light yellow solution. • Discard solution if discolored or precipitate forms.

🔲 IV INCOMPATIBILITIES

Ibuprofen.

🔲 IV COMPATIBILITIES

Acetaminophen, amiodarone, dexmedetomidine, diltiazem, heparin, insulin, magnesium sulfate, norepinephrine, potassium chloride, potassium phosphate.

INDICATIONS/ROUTES/DOSAGE

Rate Control in Supraventricular Arrhythmias
IV: ADULTS, ELDERLY: Initially, loading dose of 500 mcg/kg/min for 1 min, followed by 50 mcg/kg/min for 4 min. If optimum response is not attained, may increase to 100 mcg/kg/min for 4 min. If necessary, may futher increase to 150 mcg/kg/min for 4 min, then to 200 mcg/kg/min.

Intraop/Postop Tachycardia Hypertension (Immediate Control)
IV: ADULTS, ELDERLY: Initially, 1,000 mcg/kg over 30 sec, then 150 mcg/kg/min infusion up to 300 mcg/kg/min to maintain desired heart rate and/or blood pressure.

Dosage in Renal/Hepatic Impairment
No dose adjustment.

SIDE EFFECTS

Generally well tolerated, with transient, mild side effects. **Frequent:** Hypotension (systolic B/P less than 90 mm Hg) manifested as dizziness, nausea, diaphoresis, headache, cold extremities, fatigue. **Occasional:** Anxiety, drowsiness, flushed skin, vomiting, confusion, inflammation at injection site, fever.

ADVERSE EFFECTS/TOXIC REACTIONS

Overdose may produce profound hypotension, bradycardia, dizziness, syncope, drowsiness, breathing difficulty, bluish fingernails or palms of hands, seizures. May potentiate insulin-induced hypoglycemia in diabetic pts.

NURSING CONSIDERATIONS

BASELINE ASSESSMENT

Assess B/P, apical pulse immediately before drug is administered (if pulse is 60 or less/min or systolic B/P is 90 mm Hg or less, withhold medication, contact physician).

INTERVENTION/EVALUATION

Monitor B/P for hypotension, ECG, heart rate, respiratory rate, development of diaphoresis, dizziness (usually first sign of impending hypotension). Assess pulse for quality, irregular rate, bradycardia, extremities for coldness. Assist with ambulation if dizziness occurs. Assess for nausea, diaphoresis, headache, fatigue.

---

esomeprazole

es-o-**mep**-ra-zole
(NexIUM, NexIUM 24 HR, NexIUM IV)
Do not confuse esomeprazole with ARIPiprazole or omeprazole, or NexIUM with NexAVAR.

FIXED-COMBINATION(S)

Vimovo: esomeprazole/naproxen (NSAID): 20 mg/375 mg, 20 mg/500 mg.

◆CLASSIFICATION

PHARMACOTHERAPEUTIC: Proton pump inhibitor. **CLINICAL:** Gastric acid inhibitor.

USES

PO: Gastroesophageal reflux disease (GERD): Short-term treatment (4–8 wks) of erosive esophagitis; maintenance treatment of healing of erosive esophagitis; symptomatic gastroesophageal reflux disease (GERD). **Pathological hypersecretory conditions:** Treatment of pathologic hypersecretory conditions, including Zollinger-Ellison syndrome. **H. pylori eradication:** Used in triple therapy with amoxicillin and clarithromycin for treatment of H. pylori infection in pts with duodenal ulcer. **NSAID-associated gastric ulcer:** Reduces risk of NSAID-induced gastric ulcer. **OTC:** Treatment of frequent heartburn (2 or more days/wk). **IV:** Treatment of GERD with erosive esophagitis. Reduce risk of ulcer re-bleeding postprocedures. **OFF-LABEL:** Eosinophilic esophagitis, NSAID-induced gastric ulcers, peptic ulcer disease (treatment of complicated ulcers).

PRECAUTIONS

Contraindications: Hypersensitivity to esomeprazole, other proton pump inhibitors. Concomitant use with rilpivirine. **Cautions:** May increase risk of hip, wrist, spine fractures; hepatic impairment; elderly; Asian populations. Concurrent use of CYP3A4 inducers (e.g., rifAMPin).

ACTION

Inhibits H^+/K^+-ATPase on surface of gastric parietal cells. **Therapeutic Effect:** Reduces gastric acid secretion.

PHARMACOKINETICS

Widely distributed. Protein binding: 97%. Extensively metabolized in liver.

Primarily excreted in urine. **Half-life:** 1–1.5 hrs.

⧖ LIFESPAN CONSIDERATIONS

Pregnancy/Lactation: Unknown if drug crosses placenta or is distributed in breast milk. **Children:** Safety and efficacy not established. **Elderly:** No age-related precautions noted.

INTERACTIONS

DRUG: May decrease concentration/effect of **acalabrutinib, cefuroxime, erlotinib, neratinib, pazopanib. Strong CYP2C19 inducers (e.g., FLUoxetine)** may decrease concentration/effect. **CYP3A4 inducers (e.g., carBAMazepine, phenytoin, rifAMPin)** may decrease concentration/effect. **HERBAL:** St. John's wort may decrease concentration/effect. **FOOD:** None known. **LAB VALUES:** None significant.

AVAILABILITY (Rx)

Injection, Powder for Reconstitution: 40 mg. **Oral Suspension, Delayed-Release Packets:** 2.5 mg, 5 mg, 10 mg, 20 mg, 40 mg.

 Capsules (Delayed-Release: [NexIUM]): 20 mg, 40 mg. **[NexIUM 24 HR]:** 20 mg. **Tablets: (Delayed-Release):** 20 mg.

ADMINISTRATION/HANDLING

🖳 IV

Reconstitution • For IV push, add 5 mL of 0.9% NaCl to esomeprazole vial.
Infusion • For IV infusion, dissolve contents of one vial in 50 mL 0.9% NaCl, or D_5W.
Rate of administration • For IV push, administer over not less than 3 min. For intermittent infusion (piggyback) infuse over 10–30 min. • Flush line with 0.9% NaCl, or D_5W, both before and after administration.
Storage • Use only clear and colorless to very slightly yellow solution. • Discard solution if particulate forms. • IV infusion stable for 12 hrs

---

in 0.9% NaCl or lactated Ringer's; 6 hrs in D₅W.

PO (Capsules)
• Give 1 hr or more before eating (best before breakfast). • Do not crush, cut capsule; administer whole. • For pts with difficulty swallowing capsules, open capsule and mix pellets with 1 tbsp applesauce. Swallow immediately without chewing.

PO (Oral Suspension)
• Empty contents into 5 mL water for 2.5 mg, 5 mg; 15 mL for 10 mg, 20 mg, 40 mg and stir. • Let stand 2–3 min to thicken. • Stir and drink within 30 min.

PO (Tablets)
• Administer whole (do not crush or allow chewing). • Give with full glass of water before breakfast.

▨ IV INCOMPATIBILITIES
Do not mix esomeprazole with any other medications through the same IV line or tubing.

INDICATIONS/ROUTES/DOSAGE

Erosive Esophagitis (Treatment)
PO: ADULTS, ELDERLY, CHILDREN 12 YRS AND OLDER: 20–40 mg once daily for 4–8 wks. May continue for additional 4–8 wks. **CHILDREN 1–11 YRS, WEIGHING 20 KG OR MORE:** 10–20 mg/day for up to 8 wks. **WEIGHING LESS THAN 20 KG:** 10 mg/day for up to 8 wks. **CHILDREN 1–11 MOS, WEIGHING MORE THAN 7.5 KG–12 KG:** 10 mg/day for up to 6 wks. **6–7.5 KG:** 5 mg/day for up to 6 wks. **3–5 KG:** 2.5 mg/day for up to 6 wks.

Maintenance Therapy for Erosive Esophagitis (Healing)
PO: ADULTS, ELDERLY: 20 mg/day.

Treatment of NSAID-Induced Gastric Ulcers
PO: ADULTS, ELDERLY: 20 mg/day for 8 wks.

Prevention of NSAID-Induced Gastric Ulcer
PO: ADULTS, ELDERLY: 20–40 mg once daily for up to 6 mos.

Gastroesophageal Reflux Disease (GERD)
IV: ADULTS, ELDERLY: 20 or 40 mg once daily for up to 10 days. **CHILDREN 1–17 YRS, WEIGHING 55 KG OR MORE:** 20 mg once daily; **1–17 YRS, WEIGHING LESS THAN 55 KG:** 10 mg once daily; **1 MO TO LESS THAN 1 YR:** 0.5 mg/kg once daily. **PO: ADULTS, ELDERLY, CHILDREN, 12–17 YRS:** 20 mg once daily for up to 8 wks. **CHILDREN 1–11 YRS:** 10 mg/day for up to 8 wks.

Zollinger-Ellison Syndrome
PO: ADULTS, ELDERLY: 40 mg 2 times/day.

Duodenal Ulcer Caused by *Helicobacter pylori*
PO: ADULTS, ELDERLY: 40 mg once daily (as part of multidrug regimen).

Heartburn (OTC)
PO: ADULTS, ELDERLY: 20 mg/day for 14 days. May repeat after 4 mos if needed.

Dosage in Renal Impairment
No dose adjustment.

Dosage in Hepatic Impairment
Mild to moderate impairment: No dose adjustment. **Severe impairment:** Doses should not exceed 20 mg/day.

SIDE EFFECTS

Frequent (7%): Headache. **Occasional (3%–2%):** Diarrhea, abdominal pain, nausea. **Rare (less than 2%):** Dizziness, asthenia, vomiting, constipation, rash, cough.

ADVERSE EFFECTS/TOXIC REACTIONS

Pancreatitis, hepatotoxicity, interstitial nephritis occur rarely.

NURSING CONSIDERATIONS

BASELINE ASSESSMENT
Assess epigastric/abdominal pain. Question history of hepatic impairment, pathologic bone fractures.

INTERVENTION/EVALUATION
Evaluate for therapeutic response (relief of GI symptoms). Question if GI

discomfort, nausea, diarrhea occur. Monitor for occult blood, observe for hemorrhage in pts with peptic ulcer.

PATIENT/FAMILY TEACHING

• Report headache. • Take at least 1 hr before eating. • If swallowing capsules is difficult, open capsule and mix pellets with 1 tbsp applesauce. Swallow immediately without chewing.

estradiol

es-tra-**dye**-ole
(Alora, Climara, Delestrogen, Depo-Estradiol, Divigel, Dotti, Elestrin, Estrogel, Evamist, Femring, Menostar, Minivelle, Vivelle-Dot)

■ BLACK BOX ALERT ■ Increased risk of dementia when given to women 65 yrs and older. Use of estrogen without progestin increases risk of endometrial cancer in postmenopausal women with intact uterus. Increased risk of invasive breast cancer in postmenopausal women using conjugated estrogens with medroxyPROGESTERone. Do not use to prevent cardiovascular disease or dementia.
Do not confuse Alora with Aldara, or Estraderm with Testoderm.

FIXED-COMBINATION(S)

Activella: estradiol/norethindrone (hormone): 1 mg/0.5 mg. **Climara PRO:** estradiol/levonorgestrel (progestin): 0.045 mg/24 hr, 0.015 mg/24 hr. **Combi-patch:** estradiol/norethindrone (hormone): 0.05 mg/0.14 mg, 0.05 mg/0.25 mg. **Femhrt:** estradiol/norethindrone (hormone): 5 mcg/1 mg. **Lunelle:** estradiol/medroxyprogesterone (progestin): 5 mg/25 mg per 0.5 mL.

◆CLASSIFICATION

PHARMACOTHERAPEUTIC: Estrogen derivative. **CLINICAL:** Estrogen, antineoplastic.

USES

Treatment of moderate to severe vasomotor symptoms associated with menopause, vulvar and vaginal atrophy associated with menopause, secondary amenorrhea, hypoestrogenism (due to castration, hypogonadism, primary ovarian failure), metastatic breast cancer (palliation) in men and postmenopausal women, advanced prostate cancer (palliation), prevention of osteoporosis in postmenopausal women.

PRECAUTIONS

Contraindications: Hypersensitivity to estradiol, angioedema, hepatic dysfunction or disease, undiagnosed abnormal vaginal bleeding, active or history of arterial thrombosis, estrogen-dependent cancer (known, suspected, or history of), known or suspected breast cancer (except for pts being treated for metastatic disease), pregnancy, thrombophlebitis or thromboembolic disorders (current or history of), known protein C, protein S, antithrombin deficiency or other known thrombophilic disorder. **Cautions:** Renal insufficiency, diabetes mellitus, endometriosis, severe hypocalcemia, hyperlipidemias, asthma, epilepsy, migraines, SLE, hypertension, hypocalcemia, hypothyroidism, history of jaundice due to past estrogen use or pregnancy, cardiovascular disease, obesity, porphyria, severe hypocalcemia.

ACTION

Modulates pituitary secretion of gonadotropins; follicle-stimulating hormone (FSH), luteinizing hormone (LH). **Therapeutic Effect:** Promotes normal growth/development of female sex organs. Reduces elevated levels of FSH, LH.

PHARMACOKINETICS

Well absorbed from GI tract. Widely distributed. Protein binding: 50%–80%. Metabolized in liver. Primarily excreted in urine. **Half life:** Unknown.

E

⧗ LIFESPAN CONSIDERATIONS

Pregnancy/Lactation: Contraindicated during pregnancy. Breastfeeding not recommended. **Children:** Caution in pts for whom bone growth is not complete (may accelerate epiphyseal closure). **Elderly:** May increase risk of new-onset dementia.

INTERACTIONS

DRUG: **CYP3A4 inducers** (e.g., carBAMazepine, rifAMPin) may decrease concentration/effects. **CYP3A4 inhibitors** (e.g., clarithromycin, ketoconazole, ritonavir) may increase concentration/effect. May decrease therapeutic effect of **anastrozole**, **exemestane**. **HERBAL:** Herbals with estrogenic properties (e.g., dong quai, ginkgo biloba, ginseng, red clover) may increase adverse effects. **FOOD:** None known. **LAB VALUES:** May increase serum glucose, calcium, HDL, triglycerides. May decrease serum cholesterol, LDL. May affect metapyrone testing, thyroid function tests.

AVAILABILITY (Rx)

Cream, Topical: 0.4%, 0.6%. **Emulsion, Topical:** *(Estrasorb):* 4.35 mg estradiol/1.74 g pouch (contents of 2 pouches deliver estradiol 0.05 mg/day). **Gel, Topical:** *(Divigel):* 0.1% (0.25-g packet delivers estradiol 0.25 mg, 0.5-g packet delivers estradiol 0.5 mg, 1-g packet delivers 1 mg). *(Elestrin):* 0.06% delivers 0.52 mg estradiol/actuation. *(Estrogel):* 0.06% delivers 0.75 mg/actuation. **Injection (Cypionate):** *Depo-Estradiol:* 5 mg/mL. **(Valerate):** *Delestrogen:* 10 mg/mL, 20 mg/mL, 40 mg/mL. **Tablets:** 0.5 mg, 1 mg, 2 mg. **Topical Spray:** *(Evamist):* 1.53 mg/spray. **Transdermal System:** *(Alora):* twice wkly: 0.025 mg/24 hrs, 0.05 mg/24 hrs, 0.075 mg/24 hrs, 0.1 mg/24 hrs. *(Climara):* once wkly: 0.025 mg/24 hrs, 0.0375 mg/24 hrs, 0.05 mg/24 hrs, 0.06 mg/24 hrs, 0.075 mg/24 hrs, 0.1 mg/24 hrs. *(Menostar):* once wkly: 0.014 mg/24 hrs. *(Minivelle, Vivelle-Dot):* Twice wkly: 0.025 mg/24 hrs, 0.0375 mg/24 hrs, 0.05 mg/24 hrs, 0.075 mg/24 hrs, 0.1 mg/24 hrs. **Vaginal Cream:** *(Estrace):* 0.1 mg/g. **Vaginal Ring:** *(Estring):* 2 mg (releases 7.5 mcg/day over 90 days). *(Femring):* 0.05 mg/day (total estradiol 12.4 mg release 0.05 mg/day over 3 mos); 0.1 mg/day (total estradiol 24.8 mg release 0.1 mg/day over 3 mos). **Vaginal Tablet:** *(Vagifem):* 10 mcg.

ADMINISTRATION/HANDLING

IM
• Rotate vial to disperse drug in solution. • Inject deep IM in large muscle mass.

PO
• Administer at same time each day.
• Administer with food.

Transdermal
• Remove old patch; select new site (buttocks are alternative application site). • Peel off protective strip to expose adhesive surface. • Apply to clean, dry, intact skin on trunk of body (area with as little hair as possible). • Press in place for at least 10 sec (do not apply to breasts or waistline).

Vaginal
• Apply at bedtime for best absorption. • Insert end of filled applicator into vagina, directed slightly toward sacrum; push plunger down completely. • Avoid skin contact with cream (prevents skin absorption).

INDICATIONS/ROUTES/DOSAGE

Prostate Cancer
IM: *(Delestrogen):* **ADULTS, ELDERLY:** 30 mg or more q1–2wks.
PO: **ADULTS, ELDERLY:** 1–2 mg 3 times/day.

Breast Cancer (Metastatic)
PO: **ADULTS, ELDERLY:** 10 mg 3 times/day.

Osteoporosis Prophylaxis in Postmenopausal Females

PO: ADULTS, ELDERLY: 0.5 mg/day cyclically (3 wks on, 1 wk off).

Transdermal: *(Climara):* **ADULTS, ELDERLY:** Initially, 0.025 mg/24 hrs wkly; adjust dose as needed.

Transdermal: *(Alora, Minivelle, Vivelle-Dot):* **ADULTS, ELDERLY:** Initially, 0.025 mg/24 hrs patch twice wkly; adjust dose as needed.

Transdermal: *(Menostar):* **ADULTS, ELDERLY:** 0.014 mg/24 hrs patch wkly (also administer a progestin for 14 days q6–12 mos).

Secondary Amenorrhea, Hypoestrogenism

PO: ADULTS, ELDERLY: 1–2 mg/day; adjust dose as needed.

IM: *(Depo-Estradiol):* **ADULTS, ELDERLY:** 1.5–2 mg monthly.

IM: *(Delestrogen):* **ADULTS, ELDERLY:** 10–20 mg q4wks.

Transdermal: *(Alora):* Initially, 0.1 mg/day twice wkly. *(Climara):* 0.1 mg/day once wkly. *(Vivelle-Dot):* 0.1 mg/day twice wkly.

Vasomotor Symptoms Associated With Menopause

PO: ADULTS, ELDERLY: Initially, 0.5–1 mg once daily. **Range:** 0.5–2 mg once daily.

IM: *(Depo-Estradiol):* **ADULTS, ELDERLY:** 1–5 mg q3–4wks.

IM: *(Delestrogen):* **ADULTS, ELDERLY:** 10–20 mg q4wks.

Topical gel: *(Estrogel):* **ADULTS, ELDERLY:** 1.25 g/day. *(Divigel):* Initially, 0.25 g/day (range: 0.25–1.25 g/day). *(Elestrin):* 0.87 g/day.

Transdermal spray: *(Evamist):* Initially, 1 spray daily. May increase to 2–3 sprays daily.

Transdermal: *(Climara):* **ADULTS, ELDERLY:** 0.025 mg/24 hrs wkly. Adjust dose as needed. **Range:** 0.025–0.1 mg.

Transdermal: ADULTS, ELDERLY: *(Alora, Vivelle-Dot):* 0.025–0.05 mg/24 hrs twice wkly. **Range:** 0.025–0.1 mg.

Vaginal ring: *(Femring):* **ADULTS, ELDERLY:** Initially, 0.05 mg/day intravaginally q3mos. **Range:** 0.05–0.1 intravaginally q3mos.

Vulvar and Vaginal Atrophy Associated With Menopause

IM: *(Delestrogen):* **ADULTS, ELDERLY:** 10–20 mg q4wks.

Vaginal ring: *(Femring):* Initially 0.05 mg/day intravaginally q3mos. **Range:** 0.05–0.1 mg q3mos.

PO: *(Estrace):* 0.5–1 mg/day.

Topical gel: *(Estrogel):* 1.25 g/day at same time each day.

Transdermal: *(Alora):* 0.05 mg twice wkly. *(Climara):* 0.025 mg once weekly. *(Vivelle-Dot):* 0.0375 mg twice weekly.

Vaginal ring: *(Estring):* **ADULTS, ELDERLY:** 2 mg. Ring to remain in place for 90 days.

Vaginal cream: *(Estrace):* Insert 2–4 g/day intravaginally for 2 wks, then reduce dose to half of initial dose for 2 wks, then maintenance dose of 1 g 1–3 times/wk.

Vaginal tablet: *(Vagifem):* **ADULTS, ELDERLY:** Initially, 1 tablet/day for 2 wks. **Maintenance:** 1 tablet twice wkly.

Dosage in Renal Impairment

No dose adjustment.

Dosage in Hepatic Impairment

Contraindicated.

SIDE EFFECTS

Frequent: Anorexia, nausea, swelling of breasts, peripheral edema marked by swollen ankles and feet. **Transdermal:** Skin irritation, redness. **Occasional:** Vomiting (esp. with high doses), headache (may be severe), intolerance to contact lenses, hypertension, glucose intolerance, brown spots on exposed skin. **Vaginal:** Local irritation, vaginal discharge, changes in vaginal bleeding (spotting, breakthrough, prolonged bleeding). **Rare:** Chorea (involuntary movements), hirsutism (abnormal hairiness), loss of scalp hair, depression.

E

ADVERSE EFFECTS/TOXIC REACTIONS

Prolonged administration increases risk of gallbladder disease, thromboembolic disease, breast/cervical/vaginal/endometrial/hepatic carcinoma. Cholestatic jaundice occurs rarely.

NURSING CONSIDERATIONS

BASELINE ASSESSMENT

Assess frequency/severity of vasomotor symptoms. Question medical history as listed in Precautions. Question for possibility of pregnancy (contraindicated).

INTERVENTION/EVALUATION

Monitor B/P, weight, serum calcium, glucose, LFT. Monitor for loss of vision, sudden onset of proptosis, diplopia, migraine, thromboembolic disorders.

PATIENT/FAMILY TEACHING

• Limit alcohol, caffeine. • Avoid grapefruit products. • Immediately report sudden headache, vomiting, disturbance of vision/speech, numbness/weakness of extremities, chest pain, calf pain, shortness of breath, severe abdominal pain, mental depression, unusual bleeding. • Avoid smoking. • Report abnormal vaginal bleeding. • Never place patch on breast or waistline.

---

etanercept

e-**tan**-er-sept
(Enbrel, Enbrel SureClick, Enbrel Mini)

■**BLACK BOX ALERT** ■ Serious, potentially fatal infections, including bacterial sepsis, tuberculosis, have occurred. Lymphomas, other malignancies may occur (reported in children/adolescents).
Do not confuse Enbrel with Levbid.

◆**CLASSIFICATION**

PHARMACOTHERAPEUTIC: Protein, TNF inhibitor. **CLINICAL:** Antiarthritic.

USES

Rheumatoid arthritis (RA): Treatment of moderate to severely active RA. **Polyarticular juvenile idiopathic arthritis (JIA):** Treatment of moderately to severely active polyarticular JIA in pts 2 yrs or older. **Ankylosing spondylitis (AS):** Reduce signs/symptoms in pts with active AS. **Psoriatic arthritis:** Reduce signs/symptoms, inhibiting the progression of structural damage of active arthritis and improve physical function in pts with psoriatic arthritis. **Juvenile psoriatic arthritis (JPsA):** Treatment of active JPsA in pediatric pts 2 yrs of age and older. **Plaque psoriasis:** Treatment of chronic, moderate to severe plaque psoriasis in pts 4 yrs or older. **OFF-LABEL:** Treatment of acute graft-versus-host disease. Nonradiographic axial spondyloarthritis, Stevens-Johnson syndrome.

PRECAUTIONS

Contraindications: Hypersensitivity to etanercept. Serious active infection or sepsis. **Cautions:** History of recurrent infections, conditions predisposing to infection (e.g., diabetes, renal failure, immunocompromised pts, open wounds). History of HF, decreased left ventricular function, significant hematologic abnormalities; moderate to severe alcoholic hepatitis, elderly, preexisting or recent-onset CNS demyelinating disorder.

ACTION

Binds to tumor necrosis factor (TNF), blocking its interaction with cell surface receptors. Elevated levels of TNF, involved in inflammatory processes and the resulting joint pathology of rheumatoid arthritis, JIA, AS, and plaque psoriasis. **Therapeutic Effect:** Relieves symptoms of arthritis, psoriasis, spondylitis.

PHARMACOKINETICS

Widely distributed. Metabolism not specified. Peak plasma concentration: 69 hrs. **Half-life:** 72–132 hrs.

⧗ LIFESPAN CONSIDERATIONS

Pregnancy/Lactation: Unknown if distributed in breast milk. **Children:** No age-related precautions noted in pts 2 yrs and older. **Elderly:** No age-related precautions noted.

INTERACTIONS

DRUG: Anakinra, anti-TNF agents, baricitinib, pimecrolimus, tacrolimus (topical), tocilizumab may alter concentration/effects; increase adverse/toxic effects of **vaccines (live). HERBAL: Echinacea** may decrease effects. **FOOD:** None known. **LAB VALUES:** May increase serum alkaline phosphatase, ALT, AST, bilirubin.

AVAILABILITY (Rx)

Injection Solution (Cartridge): 50 mg/mL.
Injection, Solution (Prefilled Syringe): 25 mg/0.5 mL, 50 mg/mL.

ADMINISTRATION/HANDLING

◄ **ALERT** ► Do not add other medications to solution. Do not use filter during reconstitution or administration.

SQ

• Refrigerate prefilled syringes. • Inject into thigh, abdomen, upper arm. Rotate injection sites. • Give new injection at least 1 inch from an old site and never into area where skin is tender, bruised, red, hard. • Once reconstituted, may be stored in vial for up to 14 days refrigerated.

INDICATIONS/ROUTES/DOSAGE

Rheumatoid Arthritis (RA), Psoriatic Arthritis, Ankylosing Spondylitis
SQ: ADULTS, ELDERLY: 25 mg twice wkly given 72–96 hrs apart or 50 mg once wkly. **Maximum:** 50 mg/wk.

Juvenile Psoriatic Arthritis (JPsA)
SQ: CHILDREN 2–17 YRS: (63 kg or greater): 50 mg once wkly. **(Less than 63 kg):** 0.8 mg/kg once wkly. **Maximum:** 50 mg/dose.

Juvenile Rheumatoid Arthritis (JIA)
SQ: CHILDREN 2–17 YRS: (63 kg or greater): 50 mg once wkly. **(Less than 63 kg):** 0.8 mg/kg once wkly. **Maximum:** 50 mg/dose.

Plaque Psoriasis
SQ: ADULTS, ELDERLY: 50 mg twice wkly (give 3–4 days apart) for 3 mos. (25 mg or 50 mg once wkly have also been used.) **Maintenance:** 50 mg once wkly. **CHILDREN 4–17 YRS: (63 KG OR GREATER):** 50 mg once wkly. **(LESS THAN 63 KG):** 0.8 mg/kg once wkly. **Maximum:** 50 mg/wk.

Dosage in Renal/Hepatic Impairment
No dose adjustment.

SIDE EFFECTS

Frequent (37%): Injection site erythema, pruritus, pain, swelling; abdominal pain, vomiting (more common in children than adults). **Occasional (16%–4%):** Headache, rhinitis, dizziness, pharyngitis, cough, asthenia, abdominal pain, dyspepsia. **Rare (less than 3%):** Sinusitis, allergic reaction.

ADVERSE EFFECTS/TOXIC REACTIONS

Infection (pyelonephritis, cellulitis, osteomyelitis, wound infection, leg ulcer, septic arthritis, diarrhea, bronchitis, pneumonia) occurs in 29%–38% of pts. Rare adverse effects include heart failure, hypertension, hypotension, pancreatitis, GI hemorrhage.

NURSING CONSIDERATIONS

BASELINE ASSESSMENT

Assess onset, type, location, duration of pain, inflammation. If significant exposure to varicella virus has occurred during treatment, therapy should be temporarily discontinued and treatment with varicella-zoster immune globulin should be considered. Screen for active infection. Question history as listed in Precautions. Question travel history. Screen for active infection.

INTERVENTION/EVALUATION

Assess for improvement of joint swelling, pain, tenderness. Monitor erythrocyte sedimentation rate (ESR), C-reactive protein level, CBC with differential, platelet count. Observe for signs of infection.

PATIENT/FAMILY TEACHING

• A healthcare provider will show you how to properly prepare and inject medication. You must demonstrate correct preparation and injection techniques before using medication at home. • Treatment may depress your immune system response and reduce your ability to fight infection. Report symptoms of infection such as body aches, chills, cough, fatigue, fever. Avoid those with active infection. • Report travel plans to endemic areas. • Injection site reaction generally occurs in first mo of treatment and decreases in frequency during continued therapy. • Do not receive live vaccines during treatment. • Report persistent fever, bruising, bleeding, pallor.

---

etoposide, VP-16   [HIGH ALERT]

e-**toe**-poe-side
(Etopophos, Toposar, VePesid ✦)

■ **BLACK BOX ALERT** ■ Severe myelosuppression with resulting infection, bleeding may occur. Must be administered by personnel trained in administration/handling of chemotherapeutic agents.

Do not confuse etoposide with etidronate, or VePesid with Pepcid or Versed.

◆CLASSIFICATION

PHARMACOTHERAPEUTIC: Topoisomerase II inhibitor. **CLINICAL:** Antineoplastic.

USES

Testicular tumors (refractory): Combination therapy in pts who have surgical, chemotherapeutic, radiotherapeutic therapy. **Small-cell lung carcinoma:** First-line treatment in combination with other chemotherapeutic agents. **OFF-LABEL:** Acute lymphoblastic leukemia, acute myeloid leukemia, adrenocortical carcinoma, AIDS-related Kaposi sarcoma, breast cancer (metastatic), Hodgkin's lymphoma, multiple myeloma neuroendocrine tumors (metastatic), non-Hodgkin's lymphomas, non–small-cell lung cancer, ovarian cancer (refractory), prostate cancer (castration resistant), metastatic, sarcomas.

PRECAUTIONS

Contraindications: Hypersensitivity to etoposide. **Cautions:** Hepatic/renal impairment, myelosuppression, elderly, pts with low serum albumin.

ACTION

Induces single- and double-stranded breaks in DNA. Cell cycle–dependent and phase-specific; most effective in S and G_2 phases of cell division. **Therapeutic Effect:** Inhibits, alters DNA synthesis.

PHARMACOKINETICS

Variably absorbed from GI tract. Rapidly distributed, low concentrations in CSF. Protein binding: 97%. Metabolized in liver. Primarily excreted in urine. Not removed by hemodialysis. **Half-life:** 3–12 hrs.

⧖ LIFESPAN CONSIDERATIONS

Pregnancy/Lactation: If possible, avoid use during pregnancy, esp. first trimester. May cause fetal harm. Breastfeeding not recommended. **Children:** Safety and efficacy not established. **Elderly:** Age-related renal impairment may require dosage adjustment.

INTERACTIONS

DRUG: Bone marrow depressants (e.g., **cladribine**) may increase myelosuppression. May increase concentration/adverse effects of **vaccines (live)**. **Vaccines (live)** may decrease concentration effect. Strong CYP3A4 inducers (e.g., **carBAMazepine, phenytoin, rifAMPin**) may decrease concentration/effect. May

---

decrease therapeutic effect of **BCG (intravesical)**, **vaccines (live)**. **HERBAL:** None significant. **FOOD: Grapefruit juice** may decrease concentration/effect. **LAB VALUES:** Expected decrease of leukocytes, platelets, RBC, Hgb, Hct.

AVAILABILITY (Rx)

Capsules: 50 mg. **Injection Solution:** *(Toposar):* 20 mg/mL (5 mL, 25 mL, 50 mL). **(Etopophos):** 100 mg.

ADMINISTRATION/HANDLING

◄ALERT► Administer by slow IV infusion. Wear gloves when preparing solution. If powder or solution comes in contact with skin, wash immediately and thoroughly with soap, water. May be carcinogenic, mutagenic, teratogenic. Handle with extreme care during preparation, administration.

 IV

Reconstitution • *(Toposar):* Dilute to a concentration of 0.2–0.4 mg/mL in D₅W or 0.9% NaCl. *(Etopophos):* Dilute to concentration of 10-20 mg/mL in D5W or 0.9% NaCl.
Rate of administration • *(Toposar):* Infuse slowly, at least 30–60 min (rapid IV may produce marked hypotension). • Monitor for anaphylactic reaction during infusion (chills, fever, dyspnea, diaphoresis, lacrimation, sneezing, throat, back, chest pain). *(Etopophos):* Administer over 5 min to 3.5 hrs.
Storage • *(Toposar):* Store injection at room temperature before dilution. • Concentrate for injection is clear, yellow. • Diluted solution is stable at room temperature for 96 hrs at 0.2 mg/mL, 24 hrs at 0.4 mg/mL. • Discard if crystallization occurs. *(Etopophos):* Refrigerate vials. Following reconstitution, may further dilute to concentration as low as 0.1 mg/mL. Solutions further diluted can be refrigerated or stored at room temperature for 24 hrs.

PO
• May give without regard to food.
Storage • Refrigerate gelatin capsules.

▦ IV COMPATIBILITIES

Granisetron, ondansetron.

INDICATIONS/ROUTES/DOSAGE

◄ALERT► Dosage individualized based on clinical response, tolerance to adverse effects. Treatment repeated at 3- to 4-wk intervals. Refer to individual protocols.

Refractory Testicular Tumors
IV: ADULTS: 50–100 mg/m² per day on days 1–5 of each 21-day (or 28-day cycle), or 100 mg/m² on days 1, 3, and 5 of each 21-day (or 28-day) cycle.

Small-Cell Lung Carcinoma
IV: ADULTS: 35 mg/m²/day for 4 days or 50 mg/m²/day for 5 days.

Dosage in Renal Impairment

Creatinine Clearance	Dosage
15–50 mL/min	75% of normal dose
Less than 15 mL/min	Consider further dose reduction

Dosage in Hepatic Impairment
No dose adjustment.

SIDE EFFECTS

Frequent (66%–43%): Mild to moderate nausea/vomiting, alopecia. **Occasional (13%–6%):** Diarrhea, anorexia, stomatitis. **Rare (2% or less):** Hypotension, peripheral neuropathy.

ADVERSE EFFECTS/TOXIC REACTIONS

Myelosuppression manifested as hematologic toxicity, principally anemia, leukopenia (occurring 7–14 days after drug administration), thrombocytopenia (occurring 9–16 days after administration), and, to lesser extent, pancytopenia. Bone marrow recovery occurs by day 20. Hepatotoxicity occurs occasionally. Amenorrhea, angioedema, cortical blindness (transient), cyanosis, dysphagia, erythema, esophagitis, extravasation (induration/necrosis), hyperpigmentation, hypersensitivity reaction, pneumonitis, heart disease (ischemic), laryngospasm, maculopapular rash, malaise, metabolic acidosis, mucositis, MI, optic neuritis, ovarian failure, pruritic erythematous rash, pruritus, pulmonary fibrosis, radiation-recall phenomenon (dermatitis), reversible posterior leukoencephalopathy syndrome (RPLS), seizure, Stevens-Johnson syndrome, tongue edema, toxic epidermal necrolysis, toxic megacolon reported in less than 1% of pts.

NURSING CONSIDERATIONS

BASELINE ASSESSMENT
Obtain CBC before and at frequent intervals during therapy. Antiemetics readily control nausea, vomiting. Screen for active infection. Offer emotional support.

INTERVENTION/EVALUATION
Monitor CBC, B/P, hepatic/renal function tests. Monitor daily pattern of bowel activity, stool consistency. Monitor for hematologic toxicity (fever, sore throat, signs of local infection, unusual bruising/bleeding from any site), symptoms of anemia (excessive fatigue, weakness). Assess for paresthesia (peripheral neuropathy). Monitor for infection (cough, fatigue, fever).

PATIENT/FAMILY TEACHING
• Treatment may depress your immune system response and reduce your ability to fight infection. Report symptoms of infection such as body aches, chills, cough, fatigue, fever. Avoid those with active infection. • Avoid pregnancy. • Promptly report fever, sore throat, signs of local infection, unusual bruising or bleeding from any site, burning or pain with urination, numbness in extremities, yellowing of skin or eyes.

etrasimod

e-**tras**-i-mod
(Velsipity)
Do not confuse etrasimod with fingolimod, ozanimod, ponesimod, or siponimod.

◆CLASSIFICATION

PHARMACOTHERAPEUTIC: Sphingosine 1-phosphate receptor modulator.
CLINICAL: Immunomodulatory GI agent.

USES
Treatment of moderately to severely active ulcerative colitis in adults.

PRECAUTIONS
Contraindications: Hypersensitivity to etrasimod. Recent (within 6 mos) MI, unstable angina, TIA, decompensated HF requiring hospitalization, NYHA class III/IV HF; sick sinus syndrome, Mobitz type II second- or third-degree AV block, sinoatrial block (unless pt has a functioning pacemaker). **Cautions:** Conditions predisposing to infection (e.g., diabetes, immunocompromise, renal failure, open wounds), baseline sinus bradycardia, hepatic impairment, hypertension, altered pulmonary function, pts at risk for developing AV block (e.g., congenital heart disease, ischemic heart disease, HF), pts at risk for macular edema (e.g., diabetes, history of uveitis). Concomitant use of antiarrhythmics, beta blockers, calcium channel blockers, immunosuppressants, immune modulators, antineoplastics, QT interval-prolonging medications. Not recommended in pts with severe active infection; CYP2C9 poor metabolizers using moderate to strong CYP2C8 or CYP3A4 inhibitors; history of cardiac arrest, cerebrovascular disease, HF, ischemic heart disease, uncontrolled hypertension, recurrent cardiogenic syncope, severe sleep apnea (untreated) unless approved by a cardiologist.

ACTION

Binds with high affinity to S1P receptors 1, 4, and 5, blocking capacity of lymphocytes to move out from lymphoid organs, reducing the number of lymphocytes in peripheral blood. **Therapeutic Effect:** Reduces lymphocyte migration into the intestine, reducing inflammation.

PHARMACOKINETICS

Widely distributed. Metabolized in liver. Protein binding: 97.9%. Peak plasma concentration: 4 hrs. Steady-state reached in 7 days. Excreted in feces (82%), urine (5%). **Half-life:** 30 hrs.

⧗ LIFESPAN CONSIDERATIONS

Pregnancy/Lactation: Avoid pregnancy; may cause fetal harm. Females of reproductive potential should use effective contraception during treatment and for 1 wk after discontinuation. Unknown if distributed in human breast milk. **Children:** Safety and efficacy not established. **Elderly:** No age-related precautions noted.

INTERACTIONS

DRUG: Strong CYP3A4 inhibitors (e.g., clarithromycin, ketoconazole, ritonavir), moderate CYP3A4 inhibitors (e.g., dilTIAZem, verapamil), CYP2C9 inhibitors (e.g., amiodarone, fluconazole) may increase concentration/effect. **Beta blockers (e.g., atenolol, carvedilol, metoprolol), calcium channel blockers (e.g., dilTIAZem, verapamil)** may increase risk of AV block, bradycardia. **Class III antiarrhythmics (e.g., amiodarone, sotalol)** may increase risk of torsades de pointes in pts with baseline sinus bradycardia. **QT interval-prolonging medications (e.g., amiodarone, azithromycin, ciprofloxacin, haloperidol, sotalol)** may increase risk of QT interval prolongation, torsades de pointes. May decrease levels/effects of **vaccines (live).** May increase levels/adverse effects of **alemtuzumab, leflunomide, natalizumab, tacrolimus.** **HERBAL:** None significant. **FOOD:** None

known. **LAB VALUES:** May increase serum alkaline phosphatase, ALT, AST, bilirubin, GGT, cholesterol. Expected to reduce peripheral lymphocyte count from baseline value.

AVAILABILITY (Rx)

Tablets: 2 mg.

ADMINISTRATION/HANDLING

PO
• Give without regard to food. • Administer tablet whole; do not break, crush, or allow chewing. • If a dose is missed, skip it and give next dose at the regular scheduled time. Do not double the next dose.

INDICATIONS/ROUTES/DOSAGE

Ulcerative Colitis (Active, Moderate to Severe)
PO: ADULTS: 2 mg once daily.

Dosage in Renal/Hepatic Impairment
No dose adjustment.

SIDE EFFECTS

Occasional (9%–6%): Headache, migraine. **Rare (5%–2%):** Dizziness, arthralgia, hypertension, nausea, bradycardia.

ADVERSE EFFECTS/TOXIC REACTIONS

Life-threatening infections may occur. Fatal cases of cryptococcal meningitis, disseminated cryptococcal infections were reported. Herpes zoster infections reported in less than 1% of pts. Reactivation of herpes viral infection may cause herpes simplex encephalitis and varicella zoster meningitis. Progressive multifocal leukoencephalopathy (PML), an opportunistic viral infection of the brain caused by the JC virus, may result in progressive, permanent disability and death. Urinary tract infection (UTI) reported in 3% of pts. Posterior reversible encephalopathy syndrome, a dysfunction of the brain that may evolve into an ischemic CVA or cerebral hemorrhage, may occur. Macular edema may occur. Pts with diabetes or history of uveitis are at an increased

E

risk for developing macular edema. AV conduction delays, bradycardia was reported. Reduction of pulmonary function (absolute forced expiratory volume over 1 second) may occur in as early as 3 mos after initiation. Cutaneous malignancies including basal cell carcinoma, melanoma, squamous cell carcinoma were reported. Hepatotoxicity reported in 5% of pts. Use of concomitant immunosuppressants after stopping etrasimod may have additive immune system effects.

NURSING CONSIDERATIONS

BASELINE ASSESSMENT

Obtain CBC, LFT, ECG, vital signs. Consultation with a cardiologist is advised in pts with QT interval prolongation, cardiac arrhythmias requiring treatment with class Ia or class III antiarrhythmic; ischemic heart disease, HF, uncontrolled hypertension, history of cardiac arrest, CVA or TIA (greater than 6 mos); history of Mobitz type II second- or third-degree AV block, sick sinus syndrome, sinoatrial heart block. Pts with preexisting cardiac conditions should be closely monitored, esp. during initiation. Pts without a documented history of vaccination against varicella zoster or a confirmed history of varicella infection (chickenpox) should be tested for antibodies prior to initiation. A full vaccination course for varicella in antibody-negative pts is recommended. Obtain baseline ophthalmologic evaluation of the fundus (including the macula). Receive full medication history and screen for interaction. Question history as listed in PRECAUTIONS. Screen for active infection. Assess skin for lesions prior to or shortly after initiation. Assess symptoms of ulcerative colitis (abdominal pain, diarrhea, fatigue, fever, rectal bleeding, urgency to defecate, weight loss).

INTERVENTION/EVALUATION

Monitor LFT for hepatotoxicity (bruising, jaundice, right upper abdominal pain, nausea, vomiting, weight loss). Initiation of therapy will cause a transient reduction in heart rate, AV conduction. In pts with preexisting cardiac conditions, monitor for symptomatic bradycardia, hypotension. Obtain ECG if chest pain, dizziness, dyspnea, palpitations, syncope occurs. Obtain ophthalmic examination with any change of vision. Pts with altered mental status, seizures, visual disturbances, unilateral weakness should be evaluated for cryptococcal meningitis, varicella zoster meningitis, posterior reversible encephalopathy syndrome, PML. Persistent immunosuppressive effects may occur after discontinuation. Closely monitor for adverse effects if other immunosuppressants are initiated after discontinuation. Monitor for infections (cough, fatigue, fever), UTI (dysuria, fever, flank pain, malaise). herpetic infections, respiratory tract infections, sepsis. Monitor B/P for hypertension. Assess skin for malignancies, new lesions. Assess for improvement of ulcerative colitis symptoms.

PATIENT/FAMILY TEACHING

• Treatment may depress your immune system and reduce your ability to fight infection. Report symptoms of infection such as body aches, burning with urination, chills, cough, fatigue, fever. Avoid those with active infection. • Any change of vision will require an immediate eye examination. • PML, an opportunistic viral infection of the brain, may cause progressive, permanent disabilities or death. Report symptoms of PML such as confusion, memory loss, paralysis, trouble speaking, vision loss, seizures, weakness. • Treatment may worsen high blood pressure. • Report liver problems (abdominal pain, bruising, clay-colored stool, amber or dark colored urine, yellowing of the skin or eyes), lung problems (reduced lung function, shortness of breath), heart arrhythmias (chest pain, dizziness, fainting, palpitations, slow or irregular heart rate). • Posterior reversible encephalopathy syndrome, a dysfunction of the brain that may cause a stroke or bleeding in the brain, may

---

E

occur. • Use effective contraception to avoid pregnancy. Do not breastfeed. • Due to high risk of interactions, do not take newly prescribed medications unless approved by the prescriber who originally started treatment. • Do not receive live vaccines within 4 wks of initiation. • Treatment may cause skin cancers. Avoid prolonged sun exposure/tanning beds. Use high SPF sunscreen, lip balm, clothing to protect against sunburn/skin irritation. • Worsening symptoms of ulcerative colitis may occur after stopping treatment.

everolimus

e-veer-oh-li-mus
(Afinitor, Afinitor Disperz, Zortress)

■ **BLACK BOX ALERT** ■ Immunosuppressant (may result in infection, malignancy including lymphoma or skin cancer); increased risk of nephrotoxicity in renal transplants (avoid standard doses of cycloSPORINE); increased risk of renal arterial or venous thrombosis in renal transplants.

Do not confuse Afinitor with Lipitor, or everolimus with sirolimus, tacrolimus, or temsirolimus.

◆CLASSIFICATION

PHARMACOTHERAPEUTIC: mTOR kinase inhibitor. **CLINICAL:** Antineoplastic, immunosuppressant.

USES

Afinitor: Renal cell carcinoma: Treatment of advanced renal cell carcinoma after failure of treatment with SUNItinib or SORAfenib. **Tuberous sclerosis complex (TSC) with subependymal giant cell astrocytoma (SEGA):** Treatment of SEGA associated with tuberous sclerosis. **Neuroendocrine tumors (NET):** Treatment of progressive neuroendocrine tumors of pancreatic origin and progressive, well-differentiated, nonfunctional neuroendocrine tumors of GI or lung origin. **Breast cancer:** Treatment of advanced hormone receptor–positive, HER2-negative breast cancer in postmenopausal women. **Tuberous sclerosis complex (TSC):** Treatment of TSC not requiring immediate surgery. **Afinitor Disperz: TSC with SEGA:** Treatment of SEGA associated with TSC requiring intervention but that cannot be curatively resected. **Seizures:** Treatment of TSC-associated partial-onset seizures. **Zortress: Transplant prophylaxis:** Prophylaxis of organ rejection after kidney/liver transplant at low to moderate immunologic risk. **OFF-LABEL:** Carcinoid tumors (advanced), heart/lung transplants, Hodgkin lymphoma (relapsed/refractory), Waldenstrom macroglobnulinema (relapsed/refractory).

PRECAUTIONS

Contraindications: Hypersensitivity to everolimus, sirolimus, other rapamycin derivatives. **Cautions:** Conditions predisposing to infection (e.g., diabetes, renal failure, immunocompromised pts, open wounds). Hereditary galactose intolerance; renal/hepatic impairment; hyperlipidemia; concurrent use of CYP3A4 inducers and inhibitors. Medications known to cause angioedema.

ACTION

Binds to the FK binding protein to form a complex that inhibits activation of mTOR. Inhibits vascular endothelial growth factor (VEGF). **Therapeutic Effect:** Reduces cell proliferation, produces cell death. Has antiproliferative and antiangiogenic properties.

PHARMACOKINETICS

Peak concentration occurs in 1–2 hrs following administration, with steady-state levels achieved in 2 wks. Undergoes extensive hepatic metabolism. Protein binding: 74%. Eliminated in feces (80%), urine (5%). **Half-life:** 30 hrs.

⧗ LIFESPAN CONSIDERATIONS

Pregnancy/Lactation: Avoid pregnancy during treatment and for up to 8 wks

---

E

after discontinuation. Breastfeeding not recommended during treatment and for up to 2 wks after discontinuation. May cause fetal harm. Unknown if distributed in breast milk. **Children:** Safety and efficacy not established. **Elderly:** No age-related precautions noted.

INTERACTIONS

DRUG: CYP3A4 inhibitors (e.g., **clarithromycin, ketoconazole, ritonavir), P-gp inhibitors (e.g., amiodarone, azithromycin, carvedilol, cycloSPORINE, dilTIAZem, verapamil)** may increase concentration/effect. **CYP3A4 inducers (e.g., carBAMazepine, phenytoin, rifAMPin)** may decrease concentration/effect. May decrease therapeutic effect of **BCG (intravesical), vaccines (live).** **HERBAL:** Echinacea may decrease therapeutic effect. **St. John's wort** may decrease concentration/effect. **FOOD: High-fat meals** may reduce plasma concentration. **Grapefruit products** may increase concentration/effect (potential for myelotoxicity, nephrotoxicity). **LAB VALUES:** May increase serum BUN, creatinine, glucose, triglycerides, lipids. May decrease neutrophils, Hgb, platelets.

AVAILABILITY (Rx)

Tablets: *(Zortress):* 0.25 mg, 0.5 mg, 0.75 mg, 1 mg. Tablets: *(Afinitor):* 2.5 mg, 5 mg, 7.5 mg, 10 mg. Tablets for Oral Suspension: *(Afinitor Disperz):* 2 mg, 3 mg, 5 mg.

ADMINISTRATION/HANDLING

• Give without regard to food. • Swallow tablets whole; do not crush/cut Afinitor or Zortress. • If pt unable to swallow Afinitor tablets, may disperse in water with gentle stirring; give immediately. • Administer Afinitor Disperz as suspension only. Disperse in water until dissolved. • Avoid direct contact of dispersed tablet or oral solution with skin or mucous membranes.

INDICATIONS/ROUTES/DOSAGE

◄**ALERT**► If pt requires coadministration of a strong CYP3A4 inducer (e.g.,

carBAMazepine, dexAMETHasone, PHENobarbital, phenytoin, rifabutin, rifAMPin), consider doubling the dose. If strong inducer is discontinued, reduce everolimus to dose used prior to initiation. If moderate CYP3A4 inhibitors are required, reduce dose by 50%.

Renal Carcinoma, Neuroendocrine Tumors, Breast Cancer (in Combination With exemestane), TSC
PO: ADULTS, ELDERLY: *(Afinitor):* 10 mg once daily. **Coadministration with CYP3A4 inhibitors or P-gp inhibitors:** 2.5 mg once daily. May increase to 5 mg/day. **Coadministration with CYP3A4 inducers:** Increase by 5-mg increments up to 20 mg/day.

Renal Transplant Rejection Prophylaxis
PO: ADULTS, ELDERLY: *(Zortress):* Initially, 0.75 mg 2 times/day. Adjust dose at 4- to 5-day intervals based on serum concentration, tolerability, and response. Give in combination with basiliximab and concurrently cycloSPORINE (reduced dose required) and corticosteroids.

Liver Transplant Rejection Prophylaxis (Begin at Least 30 Days Post-transplant)
PO: ADULTS, ELDERLY: *(Zortress):* Initially, 1 mg 2 times/day (in combination with tacrolimus [reduced dose required] and a corticosteroid). Adjust dose at 4- to 5-day intervals based on serum concentration, tolerability, and response.

SEGA
PO: ADULTS, ELDERLY: *(Afinitor Disperz):* Initially, 4.5 mg/m^2 once daily, titrated to attain trough concentration of 5–15 ng/mL. **If trough greater than 15 ng/mL:** Reduce dose by 2.5 mg/day (tablets) or 2 mg/day (tablets for oral suspension). **If trough less than 15 ng/mL:** Increase dose by 2.5 mg/day (tablets) or 2 mg/day (tablets for oral suspension).

TSC-Associated Partial-Onset Seizures
PO: ADULTS, ELDERLY, CHILDREN 2 YRS AND OLDER: *(Afinitor Disperz):* Ini-

tially, 5 mg/m² once daily, titrated to attain trough concentration of 5–15 ng/mL. Maximum dose increment at any titration must not exceed 5 mg.

Dosage in Renal Impairment
No dose adjustment.

Dosage in Hepatic Impairment

	Mild	Moderate	Severe
Breast Cancer PNET, RCC, renal angiomyolipoma	7.5 mg/day or 5 mg/day	5 mg/day or 2.5 mg/day	2.5 mg/day
Liver/Renal transplant	Reduce dose by 33%	Reduce dose by 50%	Reduce dose by 50%
SEGA	No change	No change	Initial dose 2.5 mg/m²/day

SIDE EFFECTS

Common (44%–26%): Stomatitis, asthenia. Diarrhea, cough, rash, nausea. **Frequent (25%–20%):** Peripheral edema, anorexia, dyspnea, vomiting, pyrexia. **Occasional (19%–10%):** Mucosal inflammation, headache, epistaxis, pruritus, dry skin, epigastric distress, extremity pain. **Rare (less than 10%):** Abdominal pain, insomnia, dry mouth, dizziness, paresthesia, eyelid edema, hypertension, nail disorder, chills.

ADVERSE EFFECTS/TOXIC REACTIONS

Noninfectious pneumonitis characterized as hypoxia, pleural effusion, cough, or dyspnea was reported in 14% of pts; Grade 3 noninfectious pneumonitis reported in 4%. Localized and systemic infections, including pneumonia, other bacterial infections, and invasive fungal infections, have occurred due to everolimus immunosuppressive properties. Renal failure occurs in 3% of pts.

NURSING CONSIDERATIONS

BASELINE ASSESSMENT
Assess medical history, esp. renal function, use of other immunosuppressants. Obtain CBC, BMP, LFT before treatment begins and routinely thereafter. Screen for active infection. Offer emotional support.

INTERVENTION/EVALUATION
Offer antiemetics to control nausea, vomiting. Monitor daily pattern of bowel activity, stool consistency. Assess skin for evidence of rash, edema. Monitor CBC, particularly Hgb, platelet, neutrophil count; BUN, creatinine, LFT. Monitor for shortness of breath, fatigue, hypertension. Monitor for infection (cough, fatigue, fever).

PATIENT/FAMILY TEACHING
• Treatment may depress your immune system and reduce your ability to fight infection. Report symptoms of infection such as body aches, burning with urination, chills, cough, fatigue, fever. Avoid those with active infection. • Report symptoms of bone marrow depression (e.g., bruising, fatigue, fever, shortness of breath, weight loss; bleeding easily, bloody urine or stool). • Avoid direct contact of crushed tablets with skin or mucous membrane (wash thoroughly if contact occurs). • Avoid grapefruit products.

---

exemestane

ex-e-**mes**-tane
(Aromasin)
Do not confuse Aromasin with Arimidex, or exemestane with estramustine.

◆CLASSIFICATION

PHARMACOTHERAPEUTIC: Aromatase inhibitor. **CLINICAL:** Antineoplastic.

 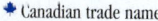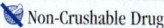

E

USES

Treatment of advanced breast cancer in postmenopausal women whose disease has progressed following tamoxifen therapy. Adjuvant treatment of postmenopausal women with estrogen receptor–positive early breast cancer after 2–3 yrs of tamoxifen therapy for completion of 5 consecutive yrs of adjuvant hormonal therapy.

PRECAUTIONS

Contraindications: Hypersensitivity to exemestane. **Cautions:** Not indicated for use in premenopausal women. Concomitant use of estrogen-containing agents, strong CYP3A4 inducers.

ACTION

Irreversibly inactivates aromatase, the principal enzyme that converts androgens to estrogens in both premenopausal and postmenopausal women, lowering circulating estrogen level. **Therapeutic Effect:** Inhibits growth of breast cancers stimulated by estrogens.

PHARMACOKINETICS

Widely distributed. Protein binding: 90%. Metabolized in liver. Excreted in urine and feces. **Half-life:** 24 hrs.

⌛ LIFESPAN CONSIDERATIONS

Pregnancy/Lactation: Indicated for postmenopausal women. **Children:** Not indicated for use in this pt population. **Elderly:** No age-related precautions noted.

INTERACTIONS

DRUG: **CYP3A4 inducers (e.g., PHENobarbital, rifAMPin)** may decrease concentration/effect. **Estrogen derivatives** may decrease therapeutic effect. **HERBAL:** **St. John's wort** may decrease concentration. **FOOD:** None known. **LAB VALUES:** May increase serum alkaline phosphatase, ALT, AST.

AVAILABILITY (Rx)

Tablets: 25 mg.

ADMINISTRATION/HANDLING

PO
• Give after meals.

INDICATIONS/ROUTES/DOSAGE

Breast Cancer (Adjuvant Treatment)
PO: POSTMENOPAUSAL WOMEN: 25 mg once daily after a meal (following 2–3 yrs tamoxifen therapy) for total duration of 5 yrs of endocrine therapy (in absence of recurrence or contralateral breast cancer).

Breast Cancer (Advanced)
PO: POSTMENOPAUSAL WOMEN: 25 mg once daily after a meal. 50 mg/day when used concurrently with potent CYP3A4 inducers (e.g., rifAMPin, phenytoin). Continue until tumor progression.

Dosage in Renal/Hepatic Impairment
No dose adjustment.

SIDE EFFECTS

Frequent (22%–10%): Fatigue, nausea, depression, hot flashes, pain, insomnia, anxiety, dyspnea. **Occasional (8%–5%):** Headache, dizziness, vomiting, peripheral edema, abdominal pain, anorexia, flu-like symptoms, diaphoresis, constipation, hypertension. **Rare (4%):** Diarrhea.

ADVERSE EFFECTS/TOXIC REACTIONS

MI has been reported.

NURSING CONSIDERATIONS

BASELINE ASSESSMENT

Question history of cardiac disease. Receive full medication history and screen for interactions. Offer emotional support.

INTERVENTION/EVALUATION

Monitor for onset of depression. Assess sleep pattern. Monitor for and assist with ambulation if dizziness occurs. Assess for headache. Offer antiemetic for nausea/vomiting.

PATIENT/FAMILY TEACHING

• Report if nausea, hot flashes become unmanageable. • Avoid tasks that re-

---

quire alertness, motor skills until response to drug is established. • Best taken after meals and at same time each day.

ezetimibe [TOP 100]

e-**zet**-i-mib
(Ezetrol ✦, Zetia)
Do not confuse Zetia with Zebeta or Zestril.

FIXED-COMBINATION(S)

Roszet: ezetimibe/rosuvastatin (statin): 10 mg/5 mg, 10 mg/10 mg, 10 mg/20 mg, 10 mg/40 mg. **Vytorin:** ezetimibe/simvastatin (statin): 10 mg/10 mg, 10 mg/20 mg, 10 mg/40 mg, 10 mg/80 mg.

◆CLASSIFICATION

PHARMACOTHERAPEUTIC: Antihyperlipidemic. **CLINICAL:** Anticholesterol agent.

USES

Primary hyperlipidemia: In combination with a statin, or alone when additional low density lipoprotein cholesterol (LDL-C) lowering therapy is not possible. As an adjunct to diet to reduce elevated LDL-C in adults with primary hyperlipidemia. **Heterozygous familial hypercholesterolemia (HeFH):** In combination with a statin as an adjunct to diet to reduce elevated LDL-C in pts 10 yrs and older with HeFH. **Mixed hyperlipidemia:** In combination with fenofibrate as an adjunct to diet to reduce elevated LDL-C in adults with mixed hyperlipidemia. **Homozygous familial hypercholesterolemia (HoFH):** In combination with a statin, and other LDL-C lowering therapies, to reduce elevated LDL-C levels in adults and in pts 10 yrs and older with HoFH. **Homozygous familial sitosterolemia:** As an adjunct to diet for the reduction of elevated sitos-

terol and campesterol levels in adults and pts 9 yrs and older.

PRECAUTIONS

Contraindications: Hypersensitivity to ezetimibe. Concurrent use of an HMG-CoA reductase inhibitor (atorvastatin, fluvastatin, lovastatin, pravastatin, simvastatin) in pts with active hepatic disease or unexplained persistent elevations in serum transaminase; pregnancy and breastfeeding (when used with a statin). **Cautions:** Severe renal or mild hepatic impairment. Not recommended in those with moderate or severe hepatic impairment.

ACTION

Inhibits cholesterol absorption in brush border of small intestine, leading to decrease in delivery of intestinal cholesterol to liver. Reduces hepatic cholesterol stores and increases clearance of cholesterol from the blood. **Therapeutic Effect:** Reduces total serum cholesterol, LDL, triglycerides; increases HDL.

PHARMACOKINETICS

Widely distributed. Protein binding: Greater than 90%. Metabolized in small intestine and liver. Excreted in feces (78%), urine (11%). **Half-life:** 22 hrs.

⌛ LIFESPAN CONSIDERATIONS

Pregnancy/Lactation: Unknown if drug crosses placenta or is distributed in breast milk. **Children:** Safety and efficacy not established in younger than 9 yrs. **Elderly:** Age-related mild hepatic impairment may require dosage adjustment.

INTERACTIONS

DRUG: **Bile acid sequestrants (e.g., cholestyramine)** may decrease absorption/effect. May increase concentration/effect of **cycloSPORINE**. **Fenofibrate and derivatives, gemfibrozil** may increase adverse effects. **HERBAL:** None

 ✦ Canadian trade name   🐋 Non-Crushable Drug   [HIGH ALERT] High Alert drug

significant. **FOOD:** None known. **LAB VALUES:** May increase serum alkaline phosphatase, bilirubin, ALT, AST.

AVAILABILITY (Rx)

Tablets: 10 mg.

ADMINISTRATION/HANDLING

• Give without regard to food. • May give at same time as statins. Give at least 2 hrs before or 4 hrs after bile acid sequestrants.

INDICATIONS/ROUTES/DOSAGE

Primary Hyperlipidemia, HeFH, Mixed Hyperlipidemia, HoFH, Homozygous Familial Sitosterolemia

PO: ADULTS, ELDERLY, CHILDREN 10 YRS AND OLDER: Initially, 10 mg once daily, given with or without food. If pt is also receiving a bile acid sequestrant, give ezetimibe at least 2 hrs before or at least 4 hrs after bile acid sequestrant.

Dosage in Renal Impairment
No dose adjustment.

Dosage in Hepatic Impairment
Mild impairment: No dose adjustment.
Moderate to severe impairment: Not recommended.

SIDE EFFECTS

Occasional (4%–3%): Back pain, diarrhea, arthralgia, sinusitis, abdominal pain. **Rare (2%):** Cough, pharyngitis, fatigue, depression.

ADVERSE EFFECTS/TOXIC REACTIONS

Hepatitis, hypersensitivity reaction, myopathy, rhabdomyolysis occur rarely.

NURSING CONSIDERATIONS

BASELINE ASSESSMENT

Obtain diet history, esp. fat consumption. Obtain serum cholesterol, triglycerides, hepatic function tests, blood counts during initial therapy and periodically during treatment. Treatment should be discontinued if hepatic enzyme levels persist more than 3 times normal limit. Receive full medication history and screen for interactions. Question history of hepatic/renal impairment.

INTERVENTION/EVALUATION

Monitor daily pattern of bowel activity, stool consistency. Question pt for signs/symptoms of back pain, abdominal disturbances. Monitor serum cholesterol, triglycerides for therapeutic response.

PATIENT/FAMILY TEACHING

• Periodic laboratory tests are essential part of therapy. • Do not stop medication without consulting physician. • Report muscular or bone pain. • May take at same time as statins. Take at least 2 hrs before or 4 hrs after cholestyramine, colestipol, colesevelam.

famciclovir

fam-**sye**-klo-veer
(Apo-Famciclovir 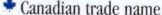, Famvir 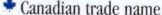)
Do not confuse famciclovir with acyclovir, ganciclovir, or valGAN-ciclovir; or Famvir with Femara.

◆CLASSIFICATION

PHARMACOTHERAPEUTIC: Synthetic nucleoside. **CLINICAL:** Antiviral.

USES

Treatment of acute herpes zoster (shingles) in immunocompetent pts, treatment and suppression of recurrent genital herpes in immunocompetent pts, treatment of recurrent orolabial/genital (mucocutaneous herpes simplex) in adults with HIV. Treatment of herpes labialis (cold sores) in immunocompetent pts. **OFF-LABEL:** Herpes simplex prevention in solid organ transplants, chickenpox (HIV pts). Initial treatment of genital herpes in immunocompetent pts; initial and suppressive treatment of genital herpes in immunocompromised pts.

PRECAUTIONS

Contraindications: Hypersensitivity to famciclovir, penciclovir. **Cautions:** Renal impairment. Avoid use in galactose intolerance, severe lactose deficiency, or glucose-galactose malabsorption syndromes.

ACTION

Inhibits HSV-2 polymerase, inhibiting herpes viral DNA synthesis and replication. **Therapeutic Effect:** Suppresses replication of herpes simplex virus, varicella-zoster virus. Shortens healing time of herpes zoster lesions. Reduces symptom severity of genital herpes.

PHARMACOKINETICS

Widely distributed. Protein binding: 20%–25%. Rapidly metabolized to penciclovir by enzymes in GI tract, liver, plasma. Excreted unchanged in urine. Removed by hemodialysis. **Half-life:** 2–3 hrs (increased in severe renal failure).

⧗ LIFESPAN CONSIDERATIONS

Pregnancy/Lactation: Unknown if excreted in breast milk. **Children:** Safety and efficacy not established. **Elderly:** Age-related renal impairment may require dosage adjustment.

INTERACTIONS

DRUG: May decrease therapeutic effect of **live vaccines, varicella vaccines**. **HERBAL:** None significant. **FOOD:** None known. **LAB VALUES:** May increase serum ALT, AST, amylase, bilirubin, lipase. May decrease neutrophils, platelets.

AVAILABILITY (Rx)

Tablets: 125 mg, 250 mg, 500 mg.

ADMINISTRATION/HANDLING
PO
• Give without regard to food. • Give with food to decrease GI distress.

INDICATIONS/ROUTES/DOSAGE

Herpes Zoster (Shingles)
PO: ADULTS: Immunocompetent: 500 mg q8h for 7 days. Begin as soon as possible after diagnosis and within 72 hrs of rash onset.

Genital Herpes Simplex (Initial)
PO: ADULTS: 250 mg 3 times/day for 7–10 days. **HIV PTS:** 500 mg twice daily for 7–10 days.

Genital Herpes Simplex (Recurrence)
PO: ADULTS: Immunocompetent: 1,000 mg twice daily for 1 day.

Genital Herpes Simplex (Suppression)
PO: ADULTS: Immunocompetent: 250 mg twice daily (reassess annually).

Herpes Labialis (Cold Sores)
PO: ADULTS, ELDERLY: Immunocompetent: (Recurrent): 1,500 mg as single dose.

Recurrent Orolabial/Genital Herpes (HIV)
PO: ADULTS, ELDERLY: 500 mg 2 times/day for 7 days.

F

 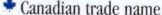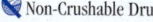

Creatinine Clearance	Herpes Zoster	Recurrent Genital Herpes (single-day regimen)	Recurrent Genital Herpes (suppression)	Recurrent Herpes Labialis Treatment (single-day regimen)	Recurrent Orolabial or Genital Herpes in HIV Pts
40–59 mL/min	500 mg q12h	500 mg q12h	—	750 mg	—
20–39 mL/min	500 mg q24h	500 mg	125 mg q12h	500 mg	500 mg q24h
Less than 20 mL/min	250 mg q24h	250 mg	125 mg q24h	250 mg	250 mg q24h
Hemodialysis	250 mg after each hemodialysis session	250 mg after each hemodialysis session	125 mg after each hemodialysis session	250 mg after each hemodialysis session	250 mg after each hemodialysis session

Dosage in Renal Impairment

Dosage and frequency are modified based on creatinine clearance and disease process.

Dosage in Hemodialysis Pts

Herpes zoster: 250 mg after each dialysis treatment. **Genital herpes:** 125 mg after each dialysis treatment.

Dosage in Hepatic Impairment

No dose adjustment.

SIDE EFFECTS

Frequent (23%–12%): Headache, nausea. **Occasional (10%–2%):** Dizziness, drowsiness, paresthesia (esp. feet), diarrhea, vomiting, constipation, decreased appetite, fatigue, fever, pharyngitis, sinusitis, pruritus. **Rare (less than 2%):** Insomnia, abdominal pain, dyspepsia, flatulence, back pain, arthralgia.

ADVERSE EFFECTS/TOXIC REACTIONS

Urticaria, severe skin rash, hallucinations, confusion (delirium, disorientation occur predominantly in elderly) has been reported.

NURSING CONSIDERATIONS

BASELINE ASSESSMENT

Question history of galactose intolerance, severe lactose deficiency, glucose-galactose malabsorption, renal impairment. Assess herpetic lesions.

INTERVENTION/EVALUATION

Monitor herpetic lesions. Be alert to neurologic effects: headache, dizziness. Provide analgesics, comfort measures.

PATIENT/FAMILY TEACHING

• Do not touch lesions with fingers to avoid spreading infection to new site. • **Genital herpes:** Continue therapy for full length of treatment. • Avoid contact with lesions during duration of outbreak to prevent cross-contamination. • Use condoms during sexual activity. • Report if lesions recur or do not improve. • Avoid tasks that require alertness, motor skills until response to drug is established.

famotidine

fa-**moe**-ta-deen
(Acid Reducer, Apo-Famotidine ✦, Pepcid)
Do not confuse famotidine with cimetidine, fluoxetine, or furosemide.

FIXED-COMBINATION(S)

Duexis: famotidine/ibuprofen (an NSAID): 26.6 mg/800 mg. **Pepcid Complete:** famotidine/calcium chloride/magnesium hydroxide (antacids): 10 mg/800 mg/165 mg.

◆CLASSIFICATION

PHARMACOTHERAPEUTIC: H_2 receptor antagonist. **CLINICAL:** Antiulcer, gastric acid secretion inhibitor.

USES

Duodenal ulcer: (Active therapy): Short-term treatment (4-8 wks) of active duodenal ulcer. **(Maintenance Therapy):** Treatment of duodenal ulcer at reduced dosage after healing of an active ulcer. **Gastric ulcer:** Short-term treatment (6–8 wks) of active benign gastric ulcer. **Gastroesophageal reflux disease (GERD):** Short-term treatment of pts with symptoms of GERD and esophagitis due to GERD (including erosive or ulcerative disease). **Hypersecretory conditions:** Treatment of pathological hypersecretory conditions (e.g., Zollinger-Ellison syndrome). **OTC:** Relief of heartburn, acid indigestion, sour stomach. **OFF-LABEL:** Stress ulcer prophylaxis in critically ill pts, chronic spontaneous urticaria, mastocytosis (adjunct).

PRECAUTIONS

Contraindications: Hypersensitivity to famotidine, other H$_2$ antagonists. **OTC:** Avoid use in pts with dysphagia, odynophagia, hematemesis, melena, hematochezia, renal impairment. **Cautions:** Renal/hepatic impairment, elderly, thrombocytopenia.

ACTION

Inhibits histamine action of H$_2$ receptors of parietal cells. **Therapeutic Effect:** Inhibits gastric acid secretion (fasting, nocturnal, or stimulated by food, caffeine, insulin).

PHARMACOKINETICS

Route	Onset	Peak	Duration
PO	1 hr	1–4 hrs	10–12 hrs
IV	0.5 hr	0.5–3 hrs	10–12 hrs

Rapidly, incompletely absorbed from GI tract. Protein binding: 15%–20%. Partially metabolized in liver. Primarily excreted in urine. Not removed by hemodialysis. **Half-life:** 2.5–3.5 hrs (increased in renal impairment).

⏳ LIFESPAN CONSIDERATIONS

Pregnancy/Lactation: Unknown if drug crosses placenta or is distributed in breast milk. **Children:** No age-related precautions noted. **Elderly:** Confusion more likely to occur, esp. in pts with renal/hepatic impairment.

INTERACTIONS

DRUG: May decrease absorption of **atazanavir, cefuroxime, itraconazole, ketoconazole.** May decrease concentration/effect of **bosutinib, dasatinib, erlotinib, gefitinib, neratinib, pazopanib.** May increase concentration/effect of **risedronate.** **HERBAL:** None significant. **FOOD:** None known. **LAB VALUES:** Interferes with skin tests using allergen extracts. May increase serum alkaline phosphatase, ALT, AST. May decrease platelet count.

AVAILABILITY (Rx)

Infusion, Premix: 20 mg in 50 mL 0.9% NaCl. **Injection, Solution:** 10 mg/mL (2-mL vial). **Powder for Oral Suspension:** 40 mg/5 mL. **Tablets:** 10 mg, 20 mg, 40 mg.

ADMINISTRATION/HANDLING

 IV

Reconstitution • For IV push, dilute 20 mg with 5–10 mL 0.9% NaCl. • For intermittent IV infusion (piggyback), dilute with 50–100 mL D$_5$W, or 0.9% NaCl. **Rate of administration** • Give IV push over at least 2 min. • Infuse piggyback over 15–30 min. **Storage** • Refrigerate unused vials. • IV solution appears clear, colorless. • After dilution, IV solution is stable for 48 hrs if refrigerated.

PO

• Store tablets, suspension at room temperature. • Following reconstitution, oral suspension is stable for 30 days at room temperature. • Give without regard to meals. • Shake suspension well before use.

⊞ IV COMPATIBILITIES

Calcium gluconate, dexmedetomidine, insulin, magnesium sulfate, potassium phosphate.

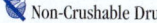

INDICATIONS/ROUTES/DOSAGE

Duodenal Ulcer

PO: ADULTS, ELDERLY: ADOLESCENTS, CHILDREN WEIGHING MORE THAN 40 KG: (Tablets): 40 mg once/day at bedtime or 20 mg twice daily. **CHILDREN 1–16 YRS:** (Suspension): 0.5 mg/kg at bedtime or divided twice daily. **Maximum:** 40 mg/day.

Prevention of Duodenal Ulcer Recurrence

PO: ADULTS, ELDERLY: 20 mg once daily at bedtime.

Gastric Ulcer

PO: ADULTS, ELDERLY: 40 mg/day at bedtime for up to 8 wks.

Gastroesophageal Reflux Disease (GERD)

Note: A proton pump inhibitor is recommended for more severe or more frequent initial symptoms (with or without evidence of erosive esophagitis).
PO: ADULTS, ELDERLY (Mild/intermittent symptoms without evidence of erosive esophagitis): Initially, 20 mg twice daily. **CHILDREN 1–16 YRS:** 1 mg/kg/day in 2 divided doses up to 40 mg in 2 divided doses. **CHILDREN 3–11 MOS:** 0.5 mg/kg/dose twice daily. **0–3 MOS:** 0.5 mg/kg/dose once daily. **ADULTS, ELDERLY: (Esophagitis including erosions and ulcerations):** 20–40 mg 2 times/day for up to 12 wks.

Pathological Hypersecretory Conditions

PO ADULTS, ELDERLY: Initially, 20 mg q6h up to 160 mg q6h.

Acid Indigestion, Heartburn (OTC Use)

PO: ADULTS, ELDERLY, CHILDREN 12 YRS AND OLDER: 10–20 mg q12h. May take 15–60 min before eating. **Maximum:** 40 mg/day.

Usual Parenteral Dosage

IV: ADULTS, ELDERLY, CHILDREN OLDER THAN 12 YRS: 20 mg q12h. **CHILDREN 1–12 YRS:** 0.25–0.5 mg/kg q12h. **Maximum:** 40 mg/day (20 mg/dose).

Dosage in Renal Impairment

Creatinine

Clearance	Dosage
Less than 50 mL/min	50% normal dose or increase dosing interval to 48 hrs

Dosage in Hepatic Impairment

No dose adjustment.

SIDE EFFECTS

Occasional (5%): Headache. **Rare (2% or less):** Confusion, constipation, diarrhea, dizziness.

ADVERSE EFFECTS/TOXIC REACTIONS

Agranulocytosis, pancytopenia, thrombocytopenia occur rarely.

NURSING CONSIDERATIONS

BASELINE ASSESSMENT

Assess epigastric/abdominal pain. Verify platelet count in critically ill pts.

INTERVENTION/EVALUATION

Monitor daily pattern of bowel activity, stool consistency. Monitor for headache. Assess for confusion in elderly. Consider interrupting treatment in pts who develop thrombocytopenia.

PATIENT/FAMILY TEACHING

• Report headache. • Avoid excessive amounts of coffee, aspirin. • Report persistent symptoms of heartburn, acid indigestion, sour stomach.

fam-trastuzumab deruxtecan-nxki

fam tras-**tu**-zoo-mab de-**rux**-the-can (Enhertu)

■ **BLACK BOX ALERT** ■ Serious and fatal cases of interstitial lung disease (ILD), pneumonitis were reported. Monitor for symptoms of ILD, pneumonitis including cough, dyspnea, fever, worsening of respiratory symptoms. Permanently discontinue in pts with Grade 2 (or higher) ILD, pneumonitis occurs. Treatment may cause fetal harm. Recommend effective contraception.
Do not confuse fam-trastuzumab deruxtecan-nxki with ado-trastuzumab emtansine, bren-

tuximab vedotin, pertuzumab, trastuzumab (or biosimilars), or trastuzumab/hyaluronidase.

◆CLASSIFICATION

PHARMACOTHERAPEUTIC: Human epidermal growth factor receptor 2 (HER2)–directed; Antibody drug conjugate; topoisomerase inhibitor. Humanized IgG1 monoclonal antibody. **CLINICAL:** Antineoplastic.

USES

Breast cancer: Treatment of adults with unresectable or metastatic HER2-positive breast cancer who have received a prior anti-HER2-based regimen either in the metastatic setting or in the neoadjuvant or adjuvant setting and have developed disease recurrence during or within 6 mos of completing therapy. Treatment of adults with unresectable or metastatic HER2-low breast cancer who have received prior chemotherapy in the metastatic setting or developed disease recurrence during or within 6 mos of completing adjuvant chemotherapy. **Gastric cancer:** Treatment of locally advanced or metastatic HER2-positive gastric or gastroesophageal junction adenocarcinoma in adults who have received a prior trastuzumab-based regimen. **Non–small-cell lung cancer (NSCLC):** Treatment of adults with unresectable or metastatic NSCLC whose tumors have activating HER2 (ERBB2) mutations who have received prior systemic therapy. **Solid tumors:** Adults with unresectable or metastatic HER2-positive (IHC 3+) solid tumors having received prior systemic treatment and no satisfactory alternative treatment options.

PRECAUTIONS

Contraindications: Hypersensitivity to fam-trastuzumab deruxtecan-nxki, trastuzumab. **Cautions:** Baseline cytopenias, hepatic impairment, pulmonary disease, cardiovascular disease, HF; conditions predisposing to infection (e.g., diabetes, renal failure, immunocompromised pts, open wounds). Do not substitute with trastuzumab or ado-trastuzumab.

ACTION

Composed of a cleavable tetrapeptide-based linker (trastuzumab) and cytotoxic topoisomerase I inhibitor, DXd (an exatecan derivative). Binds to HER2 receptor and undergoes internalization and intracellular linker cleavage by lysosomal enzymes, resulting in DNA damage and apoptosis (cellular death). **Therapeutic Effect:** Inhibits tumor cell growth.

PHARMACOKINETICS

Widely distributed. Degrades into small peptides and amino acids via catabolic pathway. DXd is metabolized in liver. Protein binding: 97%. Excretion not specified. **Half-life:** 5.7 days, (DXd): 5.8 days.

⏳ LIFESPAN CONSIDERATIONS

Pregnancy/Lactation: Avoid pregnancy; may cause fetal harm. Females of reproductive potential should use effective contraception during treatment and for at least 7 mos after discontinuation. Unknown if distributed in breast milk. Breastfeeding not recommended during treatment and for at least 7 mos after discontinuation. **Males:** Males with female partners of reproductive potential should use effective contraception during treatment and for at least 4 mos after discontinuation. May impair fertility. **Children:** Safety and efficacy not established. **Elderly:** No age-related precautions noted.

INTERACTIONS

DRUG: May decrease effect of **BCG (intravesical).** May increase cardiotoxic effects of **anthracyclines (e.g., DOXO-rubicin). Cladribine** may increase myelosuppressive effect. **HERBAL:** None significant. **FOOD:** None known. **LAB VALUES:** May increase serum ALT, AST. May decrease serum potassium; Hgb, Hct, leukocytes, lymphocytes, neutrophils, platelets, RBCs, WBCs.

AVAILABILITY (Rx)

Injection, Powder for Reconstitution: 100 mg.

ADMINISTRATION/HANDLING

 IV

Reconstitution • Must be prepared by personnel trained in aseptic manipulations and admixing of cytotoxic drugs. • Calculate the number of vials needed for reconstitution based on weight in kg. • Direct stream toward glass wall of vial. • Reconstitute 100 mg vial with 5 mL of Sterile Water for Injection to a final concentration of 20 mg/mL. • Swirl vial gently until powder is completely dissolved. Do not shake or agitate. • Visually inspect for particulate matter or discoloration. Solution should appear clear and colorless to light yellow in color. Do not use if solution is cloudy, discolored, or if visible particles are observed. • Dilute in 100 mL infusion bag of D₅W. Infusion bag must be made of polyvinyl chloride (PVC) or polyolefin. • Mix by gentle inversion. • Do not shake or agitate diluted solution.

Infusion guidelines • If diluted solution was refrigerated, allow solution to warm to room temperature before infusion. • Infuse via dedicated IV line using an infusion set made of polyolefin or polybutadiene, and a 0.2 or 0.22 micron in-line filter made of polyethersulfone or polysulfone. • Do not administer as IV push or bolus. • If a dose is missed, do not wait until next cycle; administer as soon as possible. Adjust schedule to maintain q3wk cycle.

Rate of administration • Give initial infusion over 90 min. Give subsequent infusions over 30 min if prior infusions were tolerated. May slow or interrupt infusion if infusion reactions occur.

Storage • Refrigerate unused vials in original carton. • May refrigerate reconstituted vials for up to 24 hrs. • May refrigerate diluted solution for up to 24 hrs or store at room temperature for up to 4 hrs. • Protect from light. • Do not shake, agitate, or freeze.

⊞ IV INCOMPATABILITIES

Do not mix with solutions containing NaCl or other medications.

INDICATIONS/ROUTES/DOSAGE

Breast Cancer (HER2-Positive, HER2-Low)
IV: ADULTS: 5.4 mg/kg q3wks (21-day cycle) until disease progression or unacceptable toxicity.

Gastric Cancer (HER2-Positive)
IV: ADULTS: 6.4 mg/kg q3wks. Continue until disease progression or unacceptable toxicity.

NSCLC (HER2 Mutation)
IV: ADULTS: 5.4 mg/kg q3wks. Continue until disease progression or unacceptable toxicity.

Solid Tumors
IV: ADULTS: 5.4 mg/kg q3wks. Continue until disease progression or unacceptable toxicity.

Dose Reduction for Adverse Events
Note: Do not re-escalate if a dose reduction is made.
First dose reduction: 4.4 mg/kg.
Second dose reduction: 3.2 mg/kg.
Unable to tolerate 3.2 mg/kg: Permanently discontinue.

Dose Modification
Based on Common Terminology Criteria for Adverse Events (CTCAE).

Interstitial Lung Disease (ILD)
Grade 1 ILD/pneumonitis (asymptomatic): Withhold treatment until resolved. If resolved within 28 days, resume at same dose. If resolved in greater than 28 days, resume at reduced dose level.
Grade 2 ILD/pneumonitis (symptomatic):
Permanently discontinue.

Neutropenia
Grade 3 neutropenia (500–999 cells/mm³): Withhold treatment until improved to Grade 2 or less, then resume at same dose. **Grade 4 neutropenia (less than 500 cells/mm³):** Withhold treatment until improved to Grade 2 or less, then resume at reduced dose level. **Febrile neutropenia (less than 1,000 cells/mm³ and temperature greater than 38.3°C or**

sustained temperature 38°C for more than 1 hr): Withhold treatment until resolved, then resume at reduced dose level.

Left Ventricular Dysfunction
Left ventricular ejection fraction (LVEF) greater than 45% and an absolute decrease from baseline of 10%–20%: Maintain the same dose. **LVEF 40%–45% and an absolute decrease from baseline of less than 10%:** Maintain same dose and assess LVEF within 3 wks. **LVEF 4%–45% and an absolute decrease from baseline of 10%–20%:** Withhold treatment and assess LVEF within 3 wks. If LVEF improves to within 10% from baseline, resume at same dose. If LVEF does not improve to within 10% from baseline, permanently discontinue. **LVEF less than 40% or an absolute decrease from baseline of greater than 20%:** Withhold treatment and assess LVEF within 3 wks. If LVEF of less than 40% or an absolute decrease from baseline of greater than 20% is confirmed, permanently discontinue. **Symptomatic HF:** Permanently discontinue.

Dosage in Renal Impairment
Mild to moderate impairment: No dose adjustment. **Severe impairment:** Not specified; use caution.

Dosage in Hepatic Impairment
Mild to moderate impairment: No dose adjustment. **Severe impairment:** Not specified; use caution.

SIDE EFFECTS

Frequent (79%–29%): Nausea, fatigue, asthenia, vomiting, alopecia, constipation, decreased appetite, diarrhea. **Occasional (20%–10%):** Cough, abdominal pain, headache, stomatitis, aphthous ulcer, mouth ulceration, oral mucosa erosion/blistering, dyspnea, dyspepsia, dry eye, rash, dizziness.

ADVERSE EFFECTS/TOXIC REACTIONS

Myelosuppression (anemia, leukopenia, lymphopenia, neutropenia, thrombocytopenia) is an expected response to therapy, but more severe reactions including severe neutropenia, febrile neutropenia may be life-threatening. Grade 3 or 4 neutropenia reported in 16% of pts. Severe, life-threatening pneumonitis, ILD, respiratory failure reported in 9% of pts. Left ventricular dysfunction (reduced ejection fraction) may occur. Epistaxis reported in 13% of pts. Upper respiratory tract infections reported in 15% of pts.

NURSING CONSIDERATIONS

BASELINE ASSESSMENT
Obtain CBC; pregnancy test in females of reproductive potential. Confirm compliance of effective contraception. Confirm HER2-mutation status. Obtain weight in kilograms. Assess LVEF by echocardiogram. Question history of hepatic impairment, pulmonary disease, cardiovascular disease, HF. Screen for active infection. Assess hydration/nutritional status. Offer emotional support.

INTERVENTION/EVALUATION
Monitor CBC for myelosuppression prior to each dose. Consider ABG, radiologic test if ILD/pneumonitis (excessive cough, dyspnea, fever, hypoxia) is suspected. Consider treatment with corticosteroids if ILD/pneumonitis is confirmed. Assess LVEF by echocardiogram at regular intervals. If treatment is withheld due to change in LVEF, monitor LVEF within 3 wks. Monitor for infections (cough, fatigue, fever). If serious infection occurs, initiate appropriate antimicrobial therapy. Monitor daily pattern of bowel activity, stool consistency. Offer antiemetic if nausea/vomiting occurs.

PATIENT/FAMILY TEACHING
• Treatment may depress your immune system response and reduce your ability to fight infection. Report symptoms of infection such as body aches, chills, cough, fatigue, fever. Avoid those with active infection. • Report symptoms of bone marrow depression (e.g., bruising, fatigue, fever, shortness of breath, weight loss; bleeding easily, bloody urine or stool). • Report symptoms of lung inflammation (excessive coughing, difficulty

F

breathing, chest pain); heart failure (e.g., chest pain, difficulty breathing, palpitations, swelling of extremities). • Treatment may reduce the heart's ability to pump effectively; expect routine echocardiograms. • Use effective contraception to avoid pregnancy. Do not breastfeed. • Nausea/vomiting is a common side effect. • Maintain proper hydration and nutrition.

---

febuxostat

fe-**bux**-oh-stat
(Uloric)
Do not confuse febuxostat with panobinostat or Femstat.

◆CLASSIFICATION

PHARMACOTHERAPEUTIC: Xanthine oxidase inhibitor. **CLINICAL:** Anti-gout agent.

USES

Management of hyperuricemia in adults with gout having an inadequate response to maximum dose of allopurinol, intolerant to allopurinol, or when allopurinol is not advisable. **OFF-LABEL:** Prevention of tumor lysis syndrome.

PRECAUTIONS

Contraindications: Hypersensitivity to febuxostat. Concomitant use with azaTHIOprine, mercaptopurine. **Cautions:** Severe renal/hepatic impairment, history of cardiac disease or stroke. Hypersensitivity to allopurinol. Pts at risk for urate formation.

ACTION

Decreases uric acid production by selectively inhibiting the enzyme xanthine oxidase. **Therapeutic Effect:** Reduces uric acid concentrations in serum and urine.

PHARMACOKINETICS

Widely distributed. Protein binding: 99%. Metabolized in liver. Excreted in urine (49%), feces (45%). Removed by hemodialysis. **Half-life:** 5–8 hrs.

⧗ LIFESPAN CONSIDERATIONS

Pregnancy/Lactation: Unknown if drug crosses placenta or is distributed in breast milk. **Children:** Safety and efficacy not established. **Elderly:** No age-related precautions noted.

INTERACTIONS

DRUG: May increase concentration, toxicity of **azaTHIOprine, didanosine, mercaptopurine. HERBAL:** None significant. **FOOD:** None known. **LAB VALUES:** May increase serum alkaline phosphatase, ALT, AST, LDH, amylase, sodium, potassium, cholesterol, triglycerides, BUN, creatinine. May decrease platelets, Hgb, Hct, neutrophils. May prolong prothrombin time.

AVAILABILITY (Rx)

Tablets: 40 mg, 80 mg.

ADMINISTRATION/HANDLING

PO
• Give without regard to food or antacids.

INDICATIONS/ROUTES/DOSAGE

◀**ALERT**▶ Recommended concomitant NSAID or colchicine with initiation of therapy and continue for up to 6 mos to prevent exacerbations of gout.

Hyperuricemia
PO: ADULTS, ELDERLY: Initially, 40 mg once daily. If pt does not achieve serum uric acid level less than 6 mg/dL after 2 wks with 40 mg, may give 80 mg once daily. **Maximum:** 120 mg/day.

Dosage in Renal/Hepatic Impairment
Mild to moderate impairment: No dose adjustment. **Severe impairment:** Use caution.

SIDE EFFECTS

Rare (1%): Nausea, arthralgia, rash, dizziness.

ADVERSE EFFECTS/TOXIC REACTIONS

Hepatic function abnormalities occur in 6% of pts. May increase risk of thromboembolic events including CVA, MI.

NURSING CONSIDERATIONS

BASELINE ASSESSMENT

Assess renal function, LFT; concomitant use with azaTHIOprine, mercaptopurine, theophylline (contraindicated).

INTERVENTION/EVALUATION

Discontinue medication immediately if rash appears. Encourage high fluid intake (3,000 mL/day). Monitor I&O (output should be at least 2,000 mL/day). Monitor CBC, serum uric acid, renal function, LFT. Assess urine for cloudiness, unusual color, odor. Assess for therapeutic response (reduced joint tenderness, swelling, redness, limitation of motion). Monitor for symptoms of CVA, MI.

PATIENT/FAMILY TEACHING

• Encourage drinking 8–10 (8-oz) glasses of fluid daily while taking medication. • Report rash, chest pain, shortness of breath, symptoms suggestive of stroke. • Gout attacks may occur for several months after starting treatment (medication is not a pain reliever). • Continue taking even if gout attack occurs.

fenofibrate (and derivatives)

TOP 100

fen-o-**fye**-brate
(Antara, Fenoglide, Fibricor, Lipofen, Lipidil EZ ✦, Tricor, Trilipix)
Do not confuse Tricor with Fibricor or Tracleer.

◆CLASSIFICATION

PHARMACOTHERAPEUTIC: Fibric acid derivative. **CLINICAL:** Antihyperlipidemic.

USES

Primary hypercholesterolemia/ mixed dyslipidemia: Adjunct to diet for reduction of low-density lipoprotein cholesterol (LDL-C), total cholesterol, triglycerides (types IV and V hyperlipidemia), apo-lipoprotein B, and to increase high-density lipoprotein cholesterol (HDL-C) in pts with primary hypercholesterolemia, mixed dyslipidemia. **Severe hypertriglyceridemia:** Adjunctive therapy to diet for treatment of severe hypertriglyceridemia (Fredrickson types IV and V). **OFF-LABEL:** Primary biliary cholangitis.

PRECAUTIONS

Contraindications: Hypersensitivity to fenofibrate. Active hepatic disease, preexisting gallbladder disease, severe renal/hepatic dysfunction (including primary biliary cirrhosis, unexplained persistent hepatic function abnormality), breastfeeding, end-stage renal disease (ESRD). **Cautions:** Anticoagulant therapy (e.g., warfarin), history of hepatic disease, venous thromboembolism, mild to moderate renal impairment, substantial alcohol consumption, statin or colchicine therapy (increased risk of myopathy, rhabdomyolysis), elderly.

ACTION

Downregulates apoprotein C-III and upregulates synthesis of apoprotein A-I, fatty acid transport protein, and lipoprotein lipase, increasing VLDL catabolism. **Therapeutic Effect:** Decreases triglycerides, VLDL levels, modestly increases HDL.

PHARMACOKINETICS

Widely distributed. Absorption increased when given with food. Protein binding: 99%. Metabolized in liver. Excreted in urine (60%), feces (25%). Not removed by hemodialysis. **Half-life:** 10–35 hrs.

⧖ LIFESPAN CONSIDERATIONS

Pregnancy/Lactation: Safety in pregnancy not established. Breastfeeding not recommended. **Children:** Safety and efficacy not established. **Elderly:** No age-related precautions noted.

✦ Canadian trade name   🦺 Non-Crushable Drug   🟥 High Alert drug

F

INTERACTIONS

DRUG: May increase effects of **anticoagulants** (**e.g., warfarin**); increase risk of bleeding. **Bile acid sequestrants** may reduce absorption. **CycloSPORINE** may increase concentration/effect, risk of nephrotoxicity. **Colchicine, HMG-CoA reductase inhibitors** (**e.g., atorvastatin, simvastatin**) may increase risk of severe myopathy, rhabdomyolysis, acute renal failure. **HERBAL:** None significant. **FOOD:** **All foods** increase absorption. **LAB VALUES:** May increase serum creatine kinase (CK), ALT, AST. May decrease Hgb, Hct, WBC; serum uric acid.

AVAILABILITY (Rx)

Capsules: 43 mg, 50 mg, 67 mg, 90 mg, 130 mg, 134 mg, 150 mg, 200 mg. **Capsules, Delayed-Release:** 45 mg, 135 mg. **Tablets:** 35 mg, 40 mg, 48 mg, 54 mg, 105 mg, 120 mg, 145 mg, 160 mg.

ADMINISTRATION/HANDLING

PO

• Give Fenoglide, Lipofen, Lofibra with meals. • Antara, Fibricor, Tricor, Triglide, and Trilipix may be given without regard to food. Antara, Fenoglide, Lipofen: Swallow whole; do not open (capsules), crush, dissolve, or cut.

INDICATIONS/ROUTES/DOSAGE

Hypertriglyceridemia

PO: *(Antara):* ADULTS, ELDERLY: 30–90 mg/day. *(Generic):* ADULTS, ELDERLY: 43–130 mg/day. *(Fenoglide):* ADULTS, ELDERLY: 40–120 mg/day with meals. *(Fibricor):* ADULTS, ELDERLY: 35–105 mg/day. *(Lipofen):* ADULTS, ELDERLY: 50–150 mg/day with meals. *(Lofibra):* ADULTS, ELDERLY: (micronized) 67–200 mg/day with meals; (tablets): 54–160 mg/day. *(Tricor):* ADULTS, ELDERLY: 48–145 mg/day. *(generic):* ADULTS, ELDERLY: 160 mg/day. *(Trilipix):* ADULTS, ELDERLY: 45–135 mg/day.

Hypercholesterolemia, Mixed Hyperlipidemia

PO: *(Antara):* ADULTS, ELDERLY: 90 mg/day. *(Fenofibrate):* ADULTS, ELDERLY: 130 mg/day. *(Fenoglide):* ADULTS, ELDERLY: 120 mg/day with meals. *(Fibricor):* ADULTS, ELDERLY: 105 mg/day. *(Lipofen):* ADULTS, ELDERLY: 150 mg/day with meals. *(Lofibra):* ADULTS, ELDERLY: (micronized) 200 mg/day with meals; (tablets): 160 mg/day. *(Tricor):* ADULTS, ELDERLY: 145 mg/day. *(generic):* ADULTS, ELDERLY: 160 mg/day. *(Trilipix):* ADULTS, ELDERLY: 135 mg/day.

Dose Modification
Discontinuation of Treatment

Discontinue treatment in pts with cholelithiasis, increased CPK level, suspected or diagnosed myopathy/myositis. Permanently discontinue if HDL-C is severely depressed.

Dosage in Renal Impairment

Monitor renal function before adjusting dose. Decrease dose or increase dosing interval for pts with renal failure.

Initial doses:	Antara: 30 mg/day	Lofibra: 67 mg/day
	Fenoglide: 40 mg/day	Tricor: 48 mg/day
	Lipofen: 50 mg/day	Triglide: 50 mg/day

Dosage in Hepatic Impairment
Contraindicated.

SIDE EFFECTS

Frequent (8%–4%): Pain, rash, headache, asthenia, fatigue, flu-like symptoms, dyspepsia, nausea/vomiting, rhinitis. **Occasional (3%–2%):** Diarrhea, abdominal pain, constipation, flatulence, arthralgia, decreased libido, dizziness, pruritus. **Rare (less than 2%):** Increased appetite, insomnia, polyuria, cough, blurred vision, eye floaters, earache.

ADVERSE EFFECTS/TOXIC REACTIONS

May increase cholesterol excretion into bile, leading to cholelithiasis. Hypersensitivity reactions, including angioedema and anaphylaxis, were reported. Severe cutaneous reactions, including Stevens-Johnson syndrome, toxic epidermal necrolysis, drug reaction and eosinophilia and systemic symptoms (DRESS) may occur. Serious muscle toxicities, including myopathy and rhabomyolysis; venous thromboembolic events (e.g., deep vein thrombosis [DVT], pulmonary embolism [PE], thrombophlebitis) have occurred in pts taking fibric acid derivatives. Pancreatitis, hepatitis, thrombocytopenia, agranulocytosis occur rarely.

NURSING CONSIDERATIONS

BASELINE ASSESSMENT
Obtain diet history, esp. fat consumption. Obtain serum cholesterol, triglycerides, LFT during initial therapy and periodically during treatment. Treatment should be discontinued if hepatic enzyme levels persist greater than 3 times normal limit. Question medical history as listed in Precautions.

INTERVENTION/EVALUATION
For pts on concurrent therapy with HMG-CoA reductase inhibitors, monitor for complaints of myopathy (muscle pain, weakness). Monitor serum creatine kinase (CK). Monitor serum cholesterol, triglyceride for therapeutic response.

PATIENT/FAMILY TEACHING
• Report severe diarrhea, constipation, nausea. • Report skin rash/irritation, insomnia, muscle pain, tremors, dizziness.

fentaNYL   TOP 100   HIGH ALERT

fen-ta-nil
(Actiq, Fentora, Subsys)

■ **BLACK BOX ALERT** ■ Physical and psychological dependence may occur with prolonged use. Must be alert to abuse, misuse, or diversion. May cause life-threatening hypoventilation, respiratory depression, or death. Use with strong or moderate CYP3A4 inhibitors may result in potentially fatal respiratory depression. **Buccal:** Tablet and lozenge contain enough medication to potentially be fatal to children. **Transdermal patch:** Serious or life-threatening hypoventilation has occurred. Limit use to children 2 yrs of age and older. Exposure to direct heat source increases drug release, resulting in overdose/death. **Do not confuse fentaNYL with alfentanil or SUFentanil.**

◆ CLASSIFICATION

PHARMACOTHERAPEUTIC: Opioid, narcotic agonist (Schedule II). **CLINICAL:** Analgesic.

USES

Injection: (FentaNYL): Pain relief, preop medication; adjunct to general or regional anesthesia. **Transdermal patch:** Management of pain in opioid-tolerant pts that is severe enough to require daily, around-the-clock, long-term opioid treatment. **Transdermal device (e.g., Ionsys):** Short-term management of acute postoperative pain. **Transmucosal lozenge, buccal tablet, intranasal (Lazanda), sublingual liquid: Cancer pain, breakthrough:** Management of breakthrough cancer pain in opioid-tolerant patients. **OFF-LABEL:** Pain/sedation (critically ill pts), procedural sedation/analgesia outside operating room, rapid sequence intubation (pretreatment).

PRECAUTIONS

Contraindications: Hypersensitivity to fentaNYL. **Transdermal device (additional):** Significant respiratory depression, acute/severe bronchial asthma, paralytic ileus, GI obstruction. **Transdermal patch (additional):** Significant respiratory depression, acute/severe bronchial asthma, paralytic ileus, short-term therapy for acute or postoperative pain, pts who are not opioid tolerant. **Transmucosal buccal, buccal films, lozenges, sublingual tablets/spray, nasal spray (additional):** Management of acute or postoperative pain, pts who are not opioid tolerant. GI obstruction, significant respiratory depression (Actiq, Fentora only), acute or severe bronchial asthma. **Cautions:** Bradycardia; renal, hepatic, respiratory disease; head injuries;

F

altered LOC; biliary tract disease; acute pancreatitis; cor pulmonale; significant COPD; increased ICP; use of MAOIs within 14 days; elderly; morbid obesity; history of drug abuse and misuse, drug-seeking behavior, dependency.

ACTION

Binds to opioid receptors in CNS, reducing stimuli from sensory nerve endings; inhibits ascending pain pathways. **Therapeutic Effect:** Alters pain reception, increases pain threshold.

PHARMACOKINETICS

Route	Onset	Peak	Duration
IV	1–2 min	3–5 min	0.5–1 hr
IM	7–15 min	20–30 min	1–2 hrs
Transder-mal	6–8 hrs	24 hrs	72 hrs
Transmu-cosal	5–15 min	20–30 min	1–2 hrs

Well absorbed after IM or topical administration. Transmucosal form absorbed through buccal mucosa and GI tract. Protein binding: 80%–85%. Metabolized in liver. Primarily excreted by biliary system. **Half-life:** 2–4 hrs IV; 17 hrs transdermal; 6.6 hrs transmucosal.

⌛ LIFESPAN CONSIDERATIONS

Pregnancy/Lactation: Readily crosses placenta. Unknown if distributed in breast milk. May prolong labor if administered in latent phase of first stage of labor or before cervical dilation of 4–5 cm has occurred. Respiratory depression may occur in neonate if mother received opiates during labor. **Children:** Neonates more susceptible to respiratory depressant effects. Patch: Safety and efficacy not established in pts younger than 12 yrs. **Elderly:** May be more susceptible to respiratory depressant effects. Age-related renal impairment may require dosage adjustment.

INTERACTIONS

DRUG: Strong CYP3A4 inhibitors (e.g., clarithromycin, ketoconazole, ritonavir) may increase concentration/effect; risk for respiratory depression. **Strong CYP3A4 inducers (e.g., carBA-Mazepine, phenytoin, rifAMPin)** may decrease concentration/effect. **Alcohol, CNS depressants (e.g., LORazepam, haloperidol, zolpidem)** may increase CNS depression. May increase serotonergic effect of **MAOIs (e.g., phenelzine, selegiline)**. **HERBAL: Herbals with sedative properties (e.g., chamomile, kava kava, valerian)** may increase CNS depression. **St. John's wort** may enhance serotonergic effect. **FOOD:** None known. **LAB VALUES:** May increase serum amylase, lipase.

AVAILABILITY (Rx)

Buccal Tablet: 100 mcg, 200 mcg, 400 mcg, 600 mcg, 800 mcg. **Injection Solution:** 50 mcg/mL. **Sublingual Spray: (Subsys):** 800 mcg, 1,200 mcg, 1,600 mcg. **Transdermal Patch:** 12 mcg/hr, 25 mcg/hr, 37.5 mcg/hr, 50 mcg/hr, 62.5 mcg/hr, 75 mcg/hr, 87.5 mcg/hr, 100 mcg/hr. **Transmucosal Lozenges:** 200 mcg, 400 mcg, 600 mcg, 800 mcg, 1,200 mcg, 1,600 mcg.

ADMINISTRATION/HANDLING

 IV

Rate of administration • Give by slow IV injection (over 1–2 min). • Too-rapid injection increases risk of severe adverse reactions (skeletal/thoracic muscle rigidity resulting in apnea, laryngospasm, bronchospasm, peripheral circulatory collapse, anaphylactoid effects, cardiac arrest). **Storage** • Store parenteral form at room temperature. • Opiate antagonist (naloxone) should be readily available.

Transdermal
• Apply to hairless area of intact skin of upper torso. • Use flat, nonirritated site. • Firmly press evenly and hold for 30 sec, ensuring that adhesion is in full contact with skin and that edges are completely sealed. • Use only water to cleanse site before application (soaps, oils may irritate

skin). • Rotate sites of application. • Carefully fold used patches so that system adheres to itself; discard in toilet. • If patch becomes loose, cover with a transparent adhesive dressing; if patch comes off, apply new patch, rotating sites (this starts a new dosing interval). Normal exposure to water may loosen the adhesive.

Buccal Tablets
• Place tablet above a rear molar between upper cheek and gum. • Dissolve over 30 min. • Swallow remaining pieces with water. • Do not split tablet.

Sublingual Spray
• Open blister pack with scissors immediately prior to use. • Spray contents underneath tongue.

Sublingual Tablets
• Place under tongue. • Dissolves rapidly. • Do not suck, chew, or swallow tablet.

Transmucosal
• Suck lozenge vigorously. • Allow to dissolve over 15 min. • Do not chew.

IV COMPATIBILITIES
Acetaminophen, amiodarone, dexmedetomidine, norepinephrine, potassium chloride, propofol.

Usual Buccal Dose (Fentora)
ADULTS, ELDERLY: Initially, 100 mcg. Titrate dose up to 800 mcg single dose, providing adequate analgesia with tolerable side effects.

Usual Sublingual Spray Dose (Subsys)
ADULTS, ELDERLY: Initially, 100 mcg. May repeat with same dose in 30 min if pain not relieved. Must wait at least 4 hours before treating another episode of pain. May titrate to 200 mcg to 400 mcg to 600 mcg to 800 mcg to 1,200 mcg to 1,600 mcg.

Usual Transdermal Dose
ADULTS, ELDERLY, CHILDREN 12 YRS AND OLDER: Initially, 12–25 mcg/hr. May increase after 3 days. Do not titrate more frequently than q3days following initial application or q6days thereafter.

Usual Transmucosal Dose (Actiq)
ADULTS, CHILDREN: 200–1,200 mcg for breakthrough pain. Limit to 4 applications/day. Must wait at least 4 hrs before treating another episode. Titrate to provide adequate analgesia while minimizing adverse effects.

Dosage in Renal/Hepatic Impairment
Injection: No dose adjustment.
Transdermal patch: MILD TO MODERATE IMPAIRMENT: Reduce dose by 50%.
SEVERE IMPAIRMENT: Not recommended.

SIDE EFFECTS
Frequent: IV: Postop drowsiness, nausea, vomiting. **Transdermal (10%–3%):** Headache, pruritus, nausea, vomiting, diaphoresis, dyspnea, confusion, dizziness, drowsiness, diarrhea, constipation, decreased appetite. **Occasional: IV:** Postop confusion, blurred vision, chills, orthostatic hypotension, constipation, difficulty urinating. **Transdermal (3%–1%):** Chest pain, arrhythmias, erythema, pruritus, syncope, agitation, skin irritations.

ADVERSE EFFECTS/TOXIC REACTIONS
Overdose or too-rapid IV administration may produce severe respiratory depression, skeletal/thoracic muscle rigidity (may lead to apnea, laryngospasm, bronchospasm, cold/clammy skin, cyanosis, coma). Tolerance to analgesic effect may occur with repeated use. **Antidote:** Naloxone (see Appendix H for dosage). Abrupt stoppage of prolonged high-dose, continuous infusions may induce opiate withdrawal. Concomitant use with benzodiazepines may result in profound sedation, respiratory depression, coma, and death.

NURSING CONSIDERATIONS
BASELINE ASSESSMENT
Resuscitative equipment, opiate antagonist (naloxone 0.5 mcg/kg) should be available for initial use. Es-

tablish baseline B/P, respirations. Assess type, location, intensity, duration of pain. Determine daily morphine equivalency in cancer pts who are being transitioned to chronic therapy. Assess risk of drug abuse, misuse, drug-seeking behavior.

INTERVENTION/EVALUATION

Assist with ambulation. Encourage postop pt to turn, cough, deep breathe q2h. Monitor respiratory rate, B/P, heart rate, oxygen saturation. Assess for relief of pain. In pts with prolonged high-dose, continuous infusions (critical care, ventilated pts), consider weaning drip gradually or transition to a fentaNYL patch to decrease symptoms of opiate withdrawal. Screen for misuse, abuse, drug-seeking behavior.

PATIENT/FAMILY TEACHING

* Avoid alcohol; do not take other medications without consulting physician. * Avoid tasks that require alertness, motor skills until response to drug is established. * Teach pt proper transdermal, buccal, lozenge administration. * **Transdermal:** Avoid saunas (increases drug release time). * Use as directed to avoid overdosage; potential for physical dependence with prolonged use. * Report constipation, absence of pain relief. * Taper slowly after long-term use.

ferric carboxymaltose

fer-ik kar-box-ee-**mawl**-tose
(Injectafer)

ferric gluconate

fer-ick **gloo**-koe-nate
(Ferrlecit)

ferrous fumarate

fer-us **fue**-ma-rate
(Ferrocite, Palafer ✤)

ferrous gluconate

fer-us **gloo**-koe-nate
(Apo-Ferrous Gluconate ✤, Ferate)

ferrous sulfate

fer-us **sul**-fate
(Fer-In-Sol, Fer-Iron, Slow-Fe)

ferumoxytol

fer-ue **mox**-i-tol
(Feraheme)

Iron Dextran

(Infed)

Iron sucrose

(Venofer)

◆**CLASSIFICATION**

PHARMACOTHERAPEUTIC: Enzymatic mineral. **CLINICAL:** Iron preparation.

USES

Ferric carboxymaltose: Treatment of iron deficiency in adults and pts 1 yr of age and older who have either intolerance or an unsatisfactory response to oral iron; adults with non-dialysis-dependent chronic kidney disease; iron deficiency in adults with HF class II/III to improve exercise capacity. **Ferumoxytol:** Treatment of iron deficiency in adults. **Ferrous fumarate, gluconate, sulfate:** Prevention, treatment of iron-deficiency anemia. **Ferric gluconate:** Treatment of iron-deficiency anemia in combination with erythropoietin in HD pts. **Iron dextran:** Treatment of iron deficiency in adults and pediatric pts 4 mos of age or older. **Iron sucrose:** Treatment of iron-deficiency anemia in chronic kidney disease.

PRECAUTIONS

Contraindications: Hypersensitivity to iron salts. Hemochromatosis, hemolytic anemias. **Cautions:** Peptic ulcer, regional enteritis, ulcerative colitis, pts receiving frequent blood transfusions.

ACTION

Essential component in formation of Hgb, myoglobin, enzymes. Promotes effective erythropoiesis and transport, utilization of oxygen. **Therapeutic Effect:** Prevents iron deficiency.

PHARMACOKINETICS

Absorbed in duodenum and upper jejunum. Ten percent absorbed in pts with normal iron stores; increased to 20%–30% in pts with inadequate iron stores. Primarily bound to serum transferrin. Excreted in urine, sweat, sloughing of intestinal mucosa, menses. **Half-life:** 6 hrs.

⏳ LIFESPAN CONSIDERATIONS

Pregnancy/Lactation: Crosses placenta; distributed in breast milk. **Children/Elderly:** No age-related precautions noted.

INTERACTIONS

DRUG: Antacids may decrease absorption of ferrous compounds. May decrease absorption of **bisphosphonates (e.g., risedronate), cefdinir, quinolones, tetracyclines. HERBAL:** None significant. **FOOD: Cereal, coffee, dietary fiber, eggs, milk, tea** decrease absorption. **LAB VALUES:** May increase serum bilirubin, iron. May decrease serum calcium.

AVAILABILITY

Ferric Carboxymaltose
Injection, Solution: 750 mg/15 mL.

Ferric Gluconate
Injection, Solution: 12.5 mg/mL.

Ferrous Fumarate
Tablets: 90 mg (29.5 mg elemental iron), 324 mg (106 mg elemental iron).

Ferrous Gluconate
Tablets: 240 mg (27 mg elemental iron) (Fergon), 325 mg (36 mg elemental iron).

Ferrous Sulfate
Oral Solution: 75 mg/mL (15 mg/mL elemental iron). **Tablets:** 325 mg (65 mg elemental iron). **Syrup:** 300 mg/5 mL (60 mg elemental iron per 5 mL). **Solution, Injection:** *(Infed):* 50 mg/mL. *(Venofer):* 20 mg/mL. *(Feraheme):* 510 mg/17 mL.

🐚 **Tablets:** *(Timed-Release):* 160 mg (50 mg elemental iron). **Ferumoxytol:** 510 mg/17 mL.

ADMINISTRATION/HANDLING

PO
• Store all forms (tablets, capsules, suspension, drops) at room temperature. • Ideally, give between meals with water or juice but may give with meals if GI discomfort occurs. • Transient staining of mucous membranes, teeth occurs with liquid iron preparation. To avoid staining, place liquid on back of tongue with dropper or straw. • Do not give with milk or milk products. • Do not break, crush, dissolve, or divide timed-release tablets.

INDICATIONS/ROUTES/DOSAGE

Iron-Deficiency Anemia
Dosage is expressed in terms of milligrams of elemental iron. Assess degree of anemia, pt weight, presence of any bleeding. Expect to use periodic hematologic determinations as guide to therapy.
IV: *(Ferric Carboxymaltose):* **ADULTS, ELDERLY: (50 KG OR GREATER):** 750 mg on day 1; repeat dose after at least 7 days. **(LESS THAN 50 KG):** 15 mg/kg on day 1; repeat dose after at least 7 days. *(Ferric Gluconate):* **ADULTS, ELDERLY:** 125 mg/dose. Usual dose: 1,000 mg given over 8 sessions. *(Ferumoxytol):* **ADULTS, ELDERLY:** 510 mg (as IV infusion). May repeat dose 3–8 days after initial dose.
PO: *(Ferrous Fumarate):* **ADULTS, ELDERLY:** 65–200 mg/day in 2–3 divided doses. **CHILDREN:** 3–6 mg/kg/day in 2–3 divided doses. *(Ferrous Gluconate):* **ADULTS, ELDERLY:** 65–200 mg/day in 2–3 divided doses. **CHILDREN:** 3–6 mg/kg/day

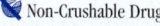

in 2–3 divided doses. *(Ferrous Sulfate):* **ADULTS, ELDERLY:** 65–200 mg/day in 2–3 divided doses. **CHILDREN:** 3–6 mg/kg/day in 2–3 divided doses.

IV: *(Iron Dextran):* **ADULTS, ELDERLY, CHILDREN WEIGHING MORE THAN 15 KG:** Dose in mL (50 mg elemental iron/mL) = 0.0442 (desired Hgb less observed Hgb) × lean body weight (in kg) + (0.26 × lean body weight). Give 2 mL or less once daily until total dose reached. **IV: ADULTS, ELDERLY, CHILDREN WEIGHING MORE THAN 15 KG:** Dose in mL (50 mg elemental iron/mL) = 0.0442 (desired Hgb less observed Hgb) × lean body weight (in kg) + (0.26 × lean body weight). Give 2 mL or less once daily until total dose reached. **CHILDREN WEIGHING 5–15 KG:** Dose in mL (50 mg elemental iron/mL) = 0.0442 (desired Hgb less observed Hgb) × body weight (in kg) + (0.26 × body weight). Give 2 mL or less once daily until total dose reached.

IV: *(Iron Sucrose):* **ADULTS, ELDERLY (HEMODIALYSIS-DEPENDENT PTS):** 5 mL iron sucrose (100 mg elemental iron) delivered during dialysis; administer 1–3 times/wk to total dose of 1,000 mg in 10 doses. Give no more than 3 times/wk. **CHILDREN 2 YRS AND OLDER:** 0.5 mg/kg/dose (**maximum:** 100 mg) q2wks for 6 doses. **(PERITONEAL DIALYSIS–DEPENDENT PTS): ADULTS, ELDERLY:** Two infusions of 300 mg over 90 min 14 days apart, followed by a single 400-mg dose over 2.5 hrs 14 days later. **CHILDREN 2 YRS AND OLDER:** 0.5 mg/kg/dose (**maximum:** 100 mg) q4wks for 3 doses. **(NON–DIALYSIS-DEPENDENT PTS): ADULTS, ELDERLY:** 200 mg over 2–5 min on 5 different occasions within 14 days. **CHILDREN 2 YRS AND OLDER:** 0.5 mg/kg/dose (**maximum:** 100 mg) q4wks for 3 doses.

Prevention of Iron Deficiency

PO: *(Ferrous Fumarate):* **ADULTS, ELDERLY:** 30–60 mg/day. **CHILDREN: (5–12 YRS):** 30–60 mg/day. **(2–4 YRS):** 30 mg/day. **(6 MOS–1 YR):** 10–12.5 mg/day. *(Ferrous Gluconate):* **ADULTS, ELDERLY:** 30–60 mg/day. **CHILDREN: (5–12 YRS):** 30–60 mg/day.

(2–4 YRS): 30 mg/day. **(6 MOS–1 YR):** 10–12.5 mg/day. *(Ferrous Sulfate):* **ADULTS, ELDERLY:** 30–60 mg/day. **CHILDREN: (5–12 YRS):** 30–60 mg/day. **(2–4 YRS):** 30 mg/day. **(6 MOS–1 YR):** 10–12.5 mg/day.

SIDE EFFECTS

Occasional: Mild, transient nausea. **Rare:** Heartburn, anorexia, constipation, diarrhea.

ADVERSE EFFECTS/TOXIC REACTIONS

Large doses may aggravate existing GI tract disease (peptic ulcer, regional enteritis, ulcerative colitis). Severe iron poisoning occurs most often in children, manifested as vomiting, severe abdominal pain, diarrhea, dehydration, followed by hyperventilation, pallor, cyanosis, cardiovascular collapse.

NURSING CONSIDERATIONS

BASELINE ASSESSMENT

Assess nutritional status, dietary history. Question history of hemochromatosis, hemolytic anemia, ulcerative colitis. Question use of antacids, calcium supplements.

INTERVENTION/EVALUATION

Monitor serum iron, total iron-binding capacity, reticulocyte count, Hgb, ferritin. Monitor daily pattern of bowel activity, stool consistency. Assess for clinical improvement, record relief of iron-deficiency symptoms (fatigue, irritability, pallor, paresthesia of extremities, headache).

PATIENT/FAMILY TEACHING

• Expect stool color to darken. • Oral liquid may stain teeth. • To prevent mucous membrane and teeth staining with liquid preparation, use dropper or straw and allow solution to drop on back of tongue. • If GI discomfort occurs, take after meals or with food. • Do not take within 2 hrs of other medication or eggs, milk, tea, coffee, cereal. • Do not take antacids or OTC calcium supplements.

fesoterodine

fes-oh-**ter**-oh-deen
(Toviaz)
Do not confuse fesoterodine with fexofenadine or tolterodine.

◆CLASSIFICATION

PHARMACOTHERAPEUTIC: Muscarinic receptor antagonist. **CLINICAL:** Anticholingergic.

USES

Overactive bladder: Treatment of adults with overactive bladder with symptoms including urinary incontinence, urgency, frequency. **Neurogenic detrusor overactivity (NDO):** Treatment of NDO in pts 6 yrs of age and older and weighing more than 25 kg.

PRECAUTIONS

Contraindications: Hypersensitivity to fesoterodine. Gastric retention, uncontrolled narrow-angle glaucoma, urinary retention. **Cautions:** Severe renal impairment, severe hepatic impairment, clinically significant bladder outflow obstruction (risk of urinary retention), GI obstructive disorders (e.g., pyloric stenosis [risk of gastric retention]), treated narrow-angle glaucoma, myasthenia gravis, concurrent therapy with strong CYP3A4 inhibitors, elderly, use in hot weather.

ACTION

Exhibits antimuscarinic activity by interceding via cholinergic muscarinic receptors, thereby mediating urinary bladder contraction. **Therapeutic Effect:** Decreases urinary frequency, urgency.

PHARMACOKINETICS

Widely distributed. Protein binding: 50%. Rapidly and extensively hydrolyzed to its active metabolite. Primarily excreted in urine. **Half-life:** 7 hours.

⧗ LIFESPAN CONSIDERATIONS

Pregnancy/Lactation: Unknown if distributed in breast milk. **Children:** Safety and efficacy not established in pts younger than 6 yrs. **Elderly:** Increased incidence of antimuscarinic adverse events, including dry mouth, constipation, dyspepsia; increase in residual urine, dizziness, urinary tract infections higher in pts 75 yrs of age and older.

INTERACTIONS

DRUG: **CYP3A4 inhibitors** (e.g., **clarithromycin, ketoconazole, ritonavir**) may increase concentration/effect. **Aclidinium, ipratropium, tiotropium, umeclidinium** may increase anticholinergic effect. **Strong CYP3A4 inducers** (e.g., **carBAMazepine, phenytoin, rifAMPin**) may decrease concentration/effect. **HERBAL:** **St. John's wort** may decrease concentration/effect. **FOOD:** None known. **LAB VALUES:** May increase serum ALT, GGT.

AVAILABILITY (Rx)

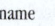 **Tablets, Extended-Release:** 4 mg, 8 mg.

ADMINISTRATION/HANDLING

PO
• May be administered with or without food. • Swallow whole; do not break, crush, dissolve, or divide tablet.

INDICATIONS/ROUTES/DOSAGE

Overactive Bladder
PO: ADULTS, ELDERLY: Initially, 4 mg once daily. May increase to 8 mg once daily. **Maximum dose** for pts with concurrent use of strong CYP3A4 inhibitors (e.g., erythromycin, ketoconazole) is 4 mg once daily.

NDO
PO: CHILDREN WEIGHING 26–35 KG: 4 mg once daily. May increase to 8 mg once daily after 7 days. **GREATER THAN 35 KG:** 4 mg once daily, then increase dose to 8 mg once daily after 7 days.

 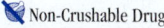

F

F

Dosage in Renal Impairment
PO: ADULTS, ELDERLY: Maximum: 4 mg with CrCl less than 30 mL/min.

Dosage in Hepatic Impairment
Mild to moderate impairment: No dose adjustment. **Severe impairment:** Not recommended.

SIDE EFFECTS
Frequent (34%–18%): Dry mouth. **Occasional (6%–3%):** Constipation, urinary tract infection, dry eyes. **Rare (2% or less):** Nausea, dysuria, back pain, rash, insomnia, peripheral edema.

ADVERSE EFFECTS/TOXIC REACTIONS
Severe anticholinergic effects including abdominal cramps, facial warmth, excessive salivation/lacrimation, diaphoresis, pallor, urinary urgency, blurred vision.

NURSING CONSIDERATIONS

BASELINE ASSESSMENT
Assess urinary pattern (e.g., urinary frequency, urgency). Question history as listed in Precautions. Receive full medication history and screen for interactions.

INTERVENTION/EVALUATION
Assist with ambulation if dizziness occurs. Question for visual changes. Monitor incontinence, postvoid residuals. Monitor daily pattern of bowel activity, stool consistency.

PATIENT/FAMILY TEACHING
• May cause constipation and urinary retention. • Blurred vision may occur; use caution until drug effects are established. • Heat prostration (due to decreased sweating) can occur if used in a hot environment. • Do not ingest grapefruit products.

fexofenadine

fex-oh-**fen**-a-deen
(Allegra Allergy, Allegra Allergy Children's)

Do not confuse Allegra with Viagra, or fexofenadine with fesoterodine.

FIXED-COMBINATION(S)
Allegra-D 12 Hour: fexofenadine/pseudoephedrine (sympathomimetic): 60 mg/120 mg. **Allegra-D 24 Hour:** fexofenadine/pseudoephedrine (sympathomimetic): 180 mg/240 mg.

◆CLASSIFICATION
PHARMACOTHERAPEUTIC: Histamine H_1 antagonist (second generation). **CLINICAL:** Antihistamine.

USES
Relief of symptoms associated with hayfever or other upper respiratory allergies (e.g., runny nose, sneezing, itching of nose/throat). **OFF-LABEL:** Urticaria (new onset, chronic spontaneous).

PRECAUTIONS
Contraindications: Hypersensitivity to fexofenadine. **Cautions:** Renal impairment, hypertension (if drug combined with pseudoephedrine). Orally disintegrating tablet not recommended in children younger than 6 yrs.

ACTION
Competes with histamine-1 receptor site on effector cells in GI tract, blood vessels, and respiratory tract. **Therapeutic Effect:** Relieves hayfever/upper respiratory symptoms.

PHARMACOKINETICS

	Onset	Peak	Duration
PO	60 min	—	12 hrs or greater

Widely distributed. Protein binding: 60%–70%. Does not cross blood-brain barrier. Minimally metabolized. Excreted in feces (80%), urine (11%). Not removed by hemodialysis. **Half-life:** 14.4 hrs (increased in renal impairment).

⧗ LIFESPAN CONSIDERATIONS

Pregnancy/Lactation: Unknown if drug crosses placenta or is distributed in breast milk. **Children:** Safety and efficacy not established in pts younger than 2 yrs. **Elderly:** No age-related precautions noted.

INTERACTIONS

DRUG: **Aluminum-** and **magnesium-containing antacids** may decrease absorption. **Aclidinium, ipratropium, tiotropium, umeclidinium** may increase anticholinergic effect. **CNS depressants (e.g., alcohol, morphine, oxyCODONE, zolpidem)** may increase CNS depression. **HERBAL:** Herbals with **sedative properties (e.g., chamomile, kava kava, valerian)** may increase CNS depression. **FOOD:** **Grapefruit products** may decrease concentration/effect. **LAB VALUES:** May suppress wheal, flare reactions to antigen skin testing unless drug is discontinued at least 4 days before testing.

AVAILABILITY (Rx)

Oral Suspension: 30 mg/5 mL. **Tablets:** 60 mg, 180 mg. **Tablets (Orally Disintegrating):** 30 mg.

ADMINISTRATION/HANDLING

PO
• **Suspension (regular tablet):** Give without regard to food. • Avoid giving with fruit juices (apple, grapefruit, orange). Administer with water only. • Shake suspension well before use.

PO (Orally-Disintegrating Tablet)
• Take on empty stomach. • Remove from blister pack; immediately place on tongue. • May take with or without liquid. • Do not split or cut.

PO (Once-Daily Formulation)
• Give whole with water (avoid fruit juices).

INDICATIONS/ROUTES/DOSAGE

Hayfever, Upper Respiratory Symptoms
PO: **ADULTS, ELDERLY:** 60 mg twice daily or 180 mg once daily. **CHILDREN 12 YRS AND OLDER:** 60 mg twice daily. **CHILDREN 2–11 YRS:** 30 mg twice daily.

Dosage in Renal Impairment
PO: **ADULTS, ELDERLY, CHILDREN 12 YRS AND OLDER:** 60 mg once daily. **CHILDREN 2–11 YRS:** 30 mg once daily. **CHILDREN 6 MOS–LESS THAN 2 YRS:** 15 mg once daily.

Dosage in Hepatic Impairment
No dose adjustment.

SIDE EFFECTS

Rare (less than 2%): Drowsiness, headache, fatigue, nausea, vomiting, abdominal distress, dysmenorrhea.

ADVERSE EFFECTS/TOXIC REACTIONS

Hypersensitivity reaction occurs rarely.

NURSING CONSIDERATIONS

BASELINE ASSESSMENT
Assess severity of congestion, rhinitis, urticaria, watery eyes. Monitor rate, depth, rhythm, type of respiration; quality, rate of pulse. Assess lung sounds for rhonchi, wheezing, rales.

INTERVENTION/EVALUATION
Assess for therapeutic response; relief from allergy: itching, red, watery eyes, rhinorrhea, sneezing.

PATIENT/FAMILY TEACHING
• Avoid tasks that require alertness, motor skills until response to drug is established. • Avoid alcohol during antihistamine therapy. • Coffee, tea may help reduce drowsiness. • Do not take with any fruit juices.

fidaxomicin

fye-**dax**-oh-**mye**-sin
(Dificid)
Do not confuse fidaxomicin with azithromycin, clindamycin, erythromycin, gentamicin, plazomicin, or tobramycin.

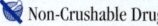 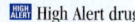

◆CLASSIFICATION

PHARMACOTHERAPEUTIC: Macrolide.
CLINICAL: Antibiotic.

USES

Treatment of *Clostridioides difficile*–associated diarrhea in adults and children 6 mos and older.

PRECAUTIONS

Contraindications: Hypersensitivity to fidaxomicin. **Cautions:** History of anemia, neutropenia, macrolide allergy.

ACTION

Binds to ribosomal sites of susceptible organisms, inhibiting RNA-dependent protein synthesis by RNA polymerase. **Therapeutic Effect:** Bactericidal against *C. difficile*.

PHARMACOKINETICS

Minimal systemic absorption after PO administration. Mainly confined to GI tract. Excreted primarily in feces (92%). **Half-life:** 9 hrs.

⧗ LIFESPAN CONSIDERATIONS

Pregnancy/Lactation: Unknown if distributed in breast milk. **Children:** Safety and efficacy not established in pts younger than 6 mos. **Elderly:** No age-related precautions noted.

INTERACTIONS

DRUG: None significant. **HERBAL:** None known. **FOOD:** None significant. **LAB VALUES:** May increase serum alkaline phosphatase, ALT, AST, bilirubin. May decrease serum bicarbonate; platelets.

AVAILABILITY (Rx)

Tablets: 200 mg. **Oral suspension:** 40 mg/mL.

ADMINISTRATION/HANDLING

• Give without regard to food. • **Suspension:** May refrigerate oral suspension for up to 12 days. • Remove from refrigerator 15 min prior to each dose. Shake well. Use oral dosing syringe.

INDICATIONS/ROUTES/DOSAGE

Clostridioides difficile–**Associated Diarrhea**
PO: ADULTS: 200 mg twice daily for 10 days. **ADOLESCENTS, CHILDREN, INFANTS 6 MOS AND OLDER: (WEIGHING 12.5 KG OR MORE):** 200 mg twice daily for 10 days. **(9 KG TO LESS THAN 12.5 KG):** *Oral suspension:* 160 mg twice daily for 10 days. **(7 KG TO LESS THAN 9 KG):** 120 mg twice daily for 10 days. **(4 KG TO LESS THAN 7 KG):** 80 mg twice daily for 10 days.

Dosage in Renal/Hepatic Impairment
No dose adjustment.

SIDE EFFECTS

Occasional (13%–6%): Pyrexia, nausea, vomiting, abdominal pain. **Rare (less than 2%):** Abdominal distension, abdominal tenderness, dyspepsia, dysphagia, flatulence, hyperglycemia.

ADVERSE EFFECTS/TOXIC REACTIONS

Hypersensitivity reactions including angioedema, dyspnea, pruritus, rash were reported. May increase risk of development of drug-resistant bacteria or superinfection when used in the absence of proven or strongly suspected *C. difficile* infection. GI hemorrhage reported in 4% of pts. Other reactions include drug eruption, metabolic acidosis.

NURSING CONSIDERATIONS

BASELINE ASSESSMENT

Verify positive *C. difficile* toxin test before initiating treatment. Initiate contact precautions. Assess bowel sounds, stool characteristics (color, frequency, consistency). Assess hydration status.

INTERVENTION/EVALUATION

Monitor for volume loss, dehydration, hypotension, abdominal pain, pyrexia. Encourage nutrition/fluid intake. Monitor daily pattern of bowel activity, stool consistency. Routinely assess bowel sounds. Screen for intestinal obstruction (increased nausea, abdominal pain, hyperactive bowel sounds) and consider radiologic test if suspected. Monitor for hypersensitivity reactions, GI bleeding (melena, rectal bleeding).

PATIENT/FAMILY TEACHING

• It is essential to complete drug therapy despite improvement of symptoms. Early discontinuation may result in antibacterial resistance and increased risk of recurrent infection. • Report GI bleeding; symptoms of bowel obstruction (e.g., abdominal pain, fever, nausea, vomiting). Report allergic reactions such as itching, rash; swelling of the face or tongue. • *C. difficile* infection is extremely contagious to others. Wash hands frequently with soap and water, esp. after bowel movements. *C. difficile* spores can live on objects for months. Use bleach products to cleanse bathroom, doorknobs, other high-touch surfaces. If possible, use a separate bathroom away from others. • Drink plenty of fluids.

---

filgrastim

fil-**gras**-tim
(Granix, Neupogen, Nivestym, Releuko, Zarxio)
Do not confuse Neupogen with Epogen, Neulasta, Neumega, or Nutramigen.

◆CLASSIFICATION

PHARMACOTHERAPEUTIC: Hematopoietic agent. **CLINICAL:** Granulocyte colony-stimulating factor (G-CSF).

USES

Granix: Decreases duration of severe neutropenia in adults and children 1 mo and older with nonmyeloid malignancies receiving chemotherapy associated with severe neutropenia, fever. **Neupogen, Zarxio:** Reduces neutropenia duration, sequelae in pts with nonmyeloid malignancies having myeloablative therapy followed by bone marrow transplant (BMT). Mobilization of hematopoietic progenitor cells into

peripheral blood for collection by apheresis. Reduces incidence and duration of severe neutropenia (e.g., fever, infections, oropharyngeal ulcers) in symptomatic pts with congenital neutropenia, cyclic neutropenia, or idiopathic neutropenia. Decreases incidence of infection in pts with malignancies receiving chemotherapy associated with increased incidence of severe neutropenia with fever. Reduces time to neutrophil recovery/duration of fever after induction/consolidation chemotherapy in AML pts. **Neupogen:** Increases survival in pts acutely exposed to myelosuppressive doses of radiation. **OFF-LABEL:** Treatment of alcoholic hepatitis, neutropenia in advanced HIV infection, anemia in myelodysplastic syndrome, hepatitis C virus infection treatment-associated neutropenia. Hematopoietic cell mobilization in healthy donors for peripheral blood stem cell allogenic transplantation.

PRECAUTIONS

Contraindications: Hypersensitivity to filgrastim. **Neupogen, Zarxio (additional):** History of serious allergic reaction to human granulocyte colony-stimulating factors. **Cautions:** Malignancy with myeloid characteristics (due to G-CSF's potential to act as growth factor), gout, psoriasis, neutrophil count greater than 50,000 cells/mm^3, sickle cell disease, concomitant use of other drugs that may result in thrombocytopenia. Do not use 24 hrs before or after cytotoxic chemotherapy.

ACTION

Stimulates production, maturation, activation of neutrophils. **Therapeutic Effect:** Increases migration and cytotoxicity of neutrophils.

PHARMACOKINETICS

Widely distributed. Onset of action: 24 hrs (plateaus in 3–5 days). WBC returns to normal in 4–7 days. Not removed by hemodialysis. **Half-life:** 3.5 hrs.

⧗ LIFESPAN CONSIDERATIONS

Pregnancy/Lactation: Unknown if drug crosses placenta or is distributed in

---

 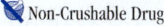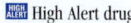

breast milk. **Children/Elderly:** No age-related precautions noted.

INTERACTIONS

DRUG: May increase concentration/effects of **bleomycin, cyclophosphamide, topotecan. HERBAL:** None significant. **FOOD:** None known. **LAB VALUES:** May increase LDH, leukocyte alkaline phosphatase (LAP) scores, serum alkaline phosphatase, uric acid.

AVAILABILITY (Rx)

Injection Solution: *(Granix, Neupogen):* 300 mcg/mL, 480 mcg/1.6 mL **Injection, Prefilled Syringe:** *(Granix, Neupogen, Zarxio):* 300 mcg/0.5 mL, 480 mcg/0.8 mL.

ADMINISTRATION/HANDLING

◄**ALERT**► May be given by SQ injection, short IV infusion (15–30 min), or continuous IV infusion. Do not dilute with normal saline.

 IV

Reconstitution • Allow vial to warm to room temperature (approx. 30 min). • Visually inspect for particulate matter or discoloration. • Dilute in D₅W from concentration of 300 mcg/mL to 5 mcg/mL (do not dilute to a final concentration less than 5 mcg/mL). Diluted solutions of 5–15 mcg/mL should have addition of albumin to a final concentration of 2 mg/mL. • Do not dilute with saline.
Rate of administration • For intermittent infusion (piggyback), infuse over 15–30 min. • For continuous infusion, give single dose over 4–24 hrs. • In all situations, flush IV line with D₅W before and after administration.
Storage • Refrigerate vials and syringes. • Stable for up to 24 hrs at room temperature (provided vial contents are clear and contain no particulate matter).

SQ

• Insert needle subcutaneously into upper arm, outer thigh, abdomen (except the 2-inch area around navel), or upper outer area of buttocks and inject solu-

tion. • Do not inject into areas of active skin disease or injury such as sunburns, skin rashes, inflammation, skin infections, or active psoriasis. • Rotate injection sites. • Do not administer IV or intramuscularly.
Storage • Refrigerate unused solutions. • Allow refrigerated solutions to warm to room temperature before administation. Store in refrigerator, but remove before use and allow to warm to room temperature.

⚙ IV COMPATIBILITIES

Calcium gluconate, potassium chloride.

INDICATIONS/ROUTES/DOSAGE

◄**ALERT**► Begin therapy at least 24 hrs after last dose of chemotherapy and at least 24 hrs after bone marrow infusion. Dosing based on actual body weight.

Chemotherapy-Induced Neutropenia
IV or SQ infusion, SQ injection: *(Neupogen and biosimilars):* **ADULTS, ELDERLY, CHILDREN:** Initially, 5 mcg/kg/day. May increase by 5 mcg/kg for each chemotherapy cycle based on duration/severity of neutropenia; continue for up to 14 days or until absolute neutrophil count (ANC) reaches 10,000 cells/mm³.
Granix
SQ: ADULTS, ELDERLY: 5 mcg/kg/day. Continue until nadir has passed and neutrophil count recovered to normal range.

Bone Marrow Transplant
IV or SQ infusion: *(Neupogen and biosimilars):* **ADULTS, ELDERLY, CHILDREN:** 10 mcg/kg/day. Administer the first dose at least 24 hrs after cytotoxic chemotherapy and at least 24 hrs after bone marrow infusion. Adjust dosage daily during period of neutrophil recovery based on neutrophil response.

Mobilization of Progenitor Cells
IV or SQ infusion: *(Neupogen and biosimilars):* **ADULTS:** 10 mcg/kg/day in donors beginning at least 4 days before first leukapheresis and continuing until last leukapheresis (usually for 6–7 days).

Discontinue for WBC greater than 100,000 cells/mm³.

Chronic Neutropenia, Congenital Neutropenia
SQ: *(Neupogen and biosimilars):* **ADULTS, CHILDREN:** Initially, 6 mcg/kg/dose twice daily. Adjust dose based on ANC/clinical response.

Idiopathic or Cyclic Chronic Neutropenia
SQ: *(Neupogen and biosimilars):* **ADULTS, CHILDREN:** Initially, 5 mcg/kg/dose once daily. Adjust dose based on ANC/clinical response.

Radiation Injury Syndrome
SQ: *(Neupogen only):* **ADULTS, ELDERLY:** 10 mcg/kg once daily. Continue until ANC remains greater than 1,000 cells/mm³ for 3 consecutive CBCs or ANC exceeds 10,000 cells/mm³ after radiation-induced nadir.

Dosage in Renal/Hepatic Impairment
No dose adjustment.

SIDE EFFECTS
Frequent (57%–11%): Nausea/vomiting, mild to severe bone pain (more frequent with high-dose IV form, less frequent with low-dose SQ form), alopecia, diarrhea, fever, fatigue. **Occasional (9%–5%):** Anorexia, dyspnea, headache, cough, rash. **Rare (less than 5%):** Psoriasis, hematuria, proteinuria, osteoporosis.

ADVERSE EFFECTS/TOXIC REACTIONS
Long-term administration occasionally produces chronic neutropenia, splenomegaly. Acute respiratory distress syndrome, alveolar hemorrhage and hemoptysis (pts undergoing peripheral blood progenitor cell collection mobilization), capillary leak syndrome, cutaneous vasculitis, glomerulonephritis, leukocytosis, MI, thrombocytopenia, sickle cell crisis, splenic rupture may occur.

NURSING CONSIDERATIONS

BASELINE ASSESSMENT
Obtain CBC prior to initiation and twice wkly thereafter.

INTERVENTION/EVALUATION
In septic pts, be alert for adult respiratory distress syndrome. Closely monitor those with preexisting cardiac conditions. Monitor B/P (transient decrease in B/P may occur), temperature, CBC with differential, platelet count, serum uric acid, hepatic function tests.

PATIENT/FAMILY TEACHING
• Report fever, chills, severe bone pain, chest pain, palpitations, difficulty breathing; left upper abdominal pain/tightness; flank pain.

finasteride

fin-**as**-ter-ide
(Propecia, <u>Proscar</u>)
Do not confuse finasteride with furosemide, or Proscar with ProSom, Provera, or PROzac.

FIXED-COMBINATION(S)
Entadfi: finasteride/tadalafil (PDE5 inhibitor): 5 mg/5 mg.

♦CLASSIFICATION
PHARMACOTHERAPEUTIC: 5-alpha-reductase inhibitor. **CLINICAL:** Benign prostatic hyperplasia agent.

USES
Proscar: Treatment (monotherapy) of symptomatic benign prostatic hyperplasia (BPH) to improve symptoms, reduce risk of acute urinary retention, or reduce the need for surgery, including transurethral resection of the prostate (TURP) and prostatectomy. Used in combination with an alpha-blocker (e.g., doxazosin) to reduce risk of symptomatic progression of BPH. **Propecia:** Treatment of male pattern hair loss. **OFF-LABEL:** Treatment of female hirsutism.

PRECAUTIONS
Contraindications: Hypersensitivity to finasteride, pregnancy or women

---

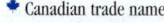 Canadian trade name   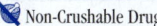 Non-Crushable Drug   **High Alert** High Alert drug

F

of child-bearing potential. **Cautions:** Hepatic impairment, urinary outflow obstruction, urinary retention. Women who are attempting to conceive should avoid exposure to crushed or broken tablets.

ACTION

Inhibits 5-alpha reductase, an intracellular enzyme that converts testosterone into dihydrotestosterone (DHT) in prostate gland, resulting in decreased serum DHT. **Therapeutic Effect:** Reduces size of prostate gland.

PHARMACOKINETICS

Route	Onset	Peak	Duration
PO (reduction of DHT)	8 hrs	—	24 hrs

Widely distributed. Protein binding: 90%. Metabolized in liver. Excreted in feces (57%), urine (39%). **Half-life:** 6–8 hrs. Onset of clinical effect: 3–6 mos of continued therapy.

⧗ LIFESPAN CONSIDERATIONS

Pregnancy/Lactation: Physical handling of tablet by those who are or may become pregnant may produce abnormalities of external genitalia of male fetus. **Children:** Not indicated for use in children. **Elderly:** No age-related precautions noted.

INTERACTIONS

DRUG: None significant. **HERBAL:** None significant. **FOOD:** None known. **LAB VALUES:** Decreases serum prostate-specific antigen (PSA) level, even in presence of prostate cancer. Decreases dihydrotestosterone (DHT). Increases follicle-stimulating hormone (FSH), luteinizing hormone (LH), testosterone.

AVAILABILITY (Rx)

🖊 **Tablets:** 1 mg (Propecia), 5 mg (Proscar).

ADMINISTRATION/HANDLING

PO
• Do not break, crush, dissolve, or divide film-coated tablets. • Give without regard to food.

INDICATIONS/ROUTES/DOSAGE

Benign Prostatic Hyperplasia (BPH)
PO: ADULTS,   ELDERLY: (Proscar): 5 mg once daily. Use as single agent or in combination with an alpha-1 adrenergic antagonist (e.g., doxazosin) (6–12 mos of treatment usually needed to assess benefit).

Hair Loss
PO: ADULTS: (Propecia): 1 mg/day (daily use for at least 12 mos or more is necessary before benefit is observed).

Dosage in Renal Impairment
No dose adjustment.

Dosage in Hepatic Impairment
Use caution.

SIDE EFFECTS

Rare (4%–2%): Gynecomastia, sexual dysfunction (impotence, decreased libido, decreased volume of ejaculate).

ADVERSE EFFECTS/TOXIC REACTIONS

Hypersensitivity reaction, circumoral swelling, testicular pain occur rarely.

NURSING CONSIDERATIONS

BASELINE ASSESSMENT
Digital rectal exam, serum prostate-specific antigen (PSA) determination should be performed in pts with benign prostatic hyperplasia (BPH) before initiating therapy and periodically thereafter. Assess usual urinary characteristics (frequency, ability to empty bladder, urinary flow). Assess degree of urinary retention with bladder scan.

INTERVENTION/EVALUATION
Diligently monitor urinary output, esp. in pts with large residual urinary volume,

severely diminished urinary flow, or obstructive uropathy. Obtain periodic bladder scan to assess treatment effectiveness (or to assess for acute urinary retention).

PATIENT/FAMILY TEACHING

• Treatment may cause impotence, decreased volume of ejaculate. • May not notice improved urinary flow even if prostate gland shrinks. • Must take medication longer than 6 mos, and it is unknown if medication decreases need for surgery. • Because of potential risk to fetus, women who are or may become pregnant should not handle tablets or be exposed to pt's semen. • Immediately report inability to urinate or severe bladder pain.

finerenone

fin-**er**-e-none
(Kerendia)
Do not confuse finerenone with drospirenone, eplerenone, or propafenone or Kerendia with Avandia.

◆**CLASSIFICATION**

PHARMACOTHERAPEUTIC: Nonsteroidal mineralocorticoid receptor (MR) antagonist. **CLINICAL:** Anti-inflammatory agent.

USES

To reduce the risk of sustained estimated glomerular filtration rate (eGFR) decline, end-stage kidney disease, cardiovascular death, nonfatal myocardial infarction (MI), and hospitalization for HF in adults with chronic kidney disease (CKD) associated with type 2 diabetes.

PRECAUTIONS

Contraindications: Hypersensitivity to finerenone. Concomitant use of strong CYP3A4 inhibitors (e.g., clarithromycin, ketoconazole, ritonavir). Adrenal insufficiency. **Cautions:** Mild to moderate hepatic impairment. Avoid use in pts with

severe hepatic impairment. Avoid concomitant use of mild to moderate CYP3A4 inhibitors or strong or moderate CYP3A4 inducers.

ACTION

Selectively blocks MR-mediated sodium reabsorption and MR overactivation in both epithelial (kidney) and nonepithelial (heart, blood vessels) tissues. **Therapeutic Effect:** Reduces inflammation and fibrosis in epithelial and nonepithelial tissues.

PHARMACOKINETICS

Widely distributed. Metabolized in liver. Protein binding: 92%. Peak plasma concentration: 0.5–1.25 hrs. Excreted in feces (20%), urine (80%). Unlikely to be removed by hemodialysis. **Half-life:** 2–3 hrs.

LIFESPAN CONSIDERATIONS

Pregnancy/Lactation: Unknown if distributed in breast milk. Breastfeeding not recommended during treatment and for at least 1 day after discontinuation. **Children:** Safety and efficacy not established. **Elderly:** No age-related precautions noted.

INTERACTIONS

DRUG: Strong CYP3A4 inhibitors (e.g., clarithromycin, ketoconazole, ritonavir) may increase concentration/effect; use contraindicated. Moderate CYP3A4 inhibitors (e.g., dilTIAZem, fluconazole, verapamil) may increase concentration/effect; risk of hyperkalemia. Strong CYP3A4 inducers (e.g., carBAMazepine, phenytoin, rifAMPin), moderate CYP3A4 inducers (e.g., bosentan, nafcillin) may decrease concentration/effect. **HERBAL:** St. John's wort may decrease concentration/effect. Herbals containing potassium (e.g., alfalfa, milkweed, nettle, turmeric) may increase risk of hyperkalemia. **FOOD:** Grapefruit products may increase concentration/

F

effect. **Potassium-containing foods (e.g., fresh or dry fruits; vegetables; beef, certain fish)** may increase risk of hyperkalemia. **LAB VALUES:** May increase serum potassium. May decrease serum sodium.

AVAILABILITY (Rx)

Tablets: 10 mg, 20 mg.

ADMINISTRATION/HANDLING

PO

• Give without regard to food. • If unable to swallow, tablet may be crushed and mixed with water or soft food (e.g., applesauce) and given immediately. • If a dose is missed, give as soon as possible that day. Do not double the next dose.

INDICATIONS/ROUTES/DOSAGE

Risk Reduction for HF and CKD Associated With Diabetes Mellitus

PO: ADULTS, ELDERLY: 10 mg or 20 mg once daily based on eGFR and serum potassium level. **eGFR 60 mL/min/1.73m² or greater:** 20 mg once daily. **eGFR 25-59 mL/min/1.73m²:** 10 mg once daily. **(Daily target dose):** 20 mg once daily.

Dose Modification

Serum Potassium Level	Current Finerenone Dose	
	10 mg once daily	**20 mg once daily**
4.8 mEq/L or less	Increase to 20 mg once daily. If eGFR has decreased by more than 30%, continue 10 mg dose.	Continue 20 mg dose
4.9–5.5 mEq/L	Continue 10 mg dose	Continue 20 mg dose
Greater than 5.5 mEq/L	Withhold dose and consider restarting when serum potassium level is 5 mEq/L or less	Withhold dose until serum potassium level is 5 mEq/L or less

Dosage in Renal Impairment

Not recommended in pts with eGFR less than 25 mL/min/1.73m².

Dosage in Hepatic Impairment

Mild to moderate impairment: No dose adjustment. **Severe impairment:** Not recommended.

SIDE EFFECTS

Moderate (18%): Hyperkalemia. **Rare (5%–1%):** Hypotension, hyponatremia.

ADVERSE EFFECTS/TOXIC REACTIONS

May cause hyperkalemia. Overdose may further increase risk of hyperkalemia.

NURSING CONSIDERATIONS

BASELINE ASSESSMENT

Obtain serum potassium, eGFR; pregnancy test in females of reproductive potential. Do not initiate treatment if serum potassium is >5.0 mEq/L. Question history of hepatic impairment. Obtain full medication history and screen for interactions.

INTERVENTION/EVALUATION

Obtain serum potassium level 4 wks after initiation and with any dose adjustment. Consider more frequent monitoring if serum potassium level is 4.8–5 mEq/L upon initiation or in pts with history of moderate hepatic impairment. Monitor for symptoms of hyperkalemia (cardiac arrhythmia, chest pain, palpitations, muscle weakness, nausea, tingling, vomiting).

PATIENT/FAMILY TEACHING

• Treatment may cause high potassium levels; report (chest pain, palpitations, muscle weakness, nausea, tingling, vomiting). Limit intake of potassium-rich foods. • There is a high risk of interactions with other medications. Do not take newly prescribed medications unless approved by prescriber who originally started treatment. Avoid herbal supplements, grapefruit products. • Do not breastfeed.

fingolimod   TOP 100

fin-**goe**-li-mod
(Gilenya, Tascenso ODT)

◆ CLASSIFICATION

PHARMACOTHERAPEUTIC: Sphingosine 1-phosphate (S1P) receptor modulator. **CLINICAL:** Multiple sclerosis agent.

USES

Treatment of relapsing forms of multiple sclerosis (MS), including clinically isolated syndrome, relapsing-remitting disease, and active secondary progressive disease, in pts 10 yrs of age and older.

PRECAUTIONS

Contraindications: Hypersensitivity to fingolimod. Sick sinus syndrome, second-degree or higher conduction block (unless pt has functioning pacemaker). Baseline QT interval 500 msec or greater. Concurrent use of class Ia or III antiarrhythmic. Recent (within 6 mos) MI, unstable angina, stroke, TIA, decompensated requiring hospitalization or NYHA class III/IV HF. **Cautions:** Concomitant use of antiarrhythmics, beta blockers, calcium channel blockers, immunosuppressants, immune modulators, antineoplastics, QT interval–prolonging medications (e.g., amiodarone, ciprofloxacin); bradycardia, severe hepatic impairment, ischemic heart disease, diabetes, hypokalemia, hypomagnesemia; history of syncope, uveitis; pts at risk for developing bradycardia or heart block.

ACTION

Blocks capacity of lymphocytes to move out from lymph nodes, reducing number of lymphocytes available to the CNS. **Therapeutic Effect:** May involve reduction of lymphocyte migration into central nervous system, which reduces central inflammation.

PHARMACOKINETICS

Metabolized by the enzyme sphingosine kinase to active metabolite. Highly distributed in red blood cells (85%). Minimally metabolized in liver. Protein binding: 99.7%. Primarily excreted in urine. **Half-life:** 6–9 days.

⌛ LIFESPAN CONSIDERATIONS

Pregnancy/Lactation: May cause fetal harm. Unknown if distributed in breast milk. **Children:** Safety and efficacy not established in pts younger than 10 yrs. **Elderly:** Age-related severe hepatic impairment may increase risk of adverse reactions.

INTERACTIONS

DRUG: Beta blockers (e.g., **carvedilol**, **metoprolol**), calcium channel blockers (e.g., **dilTIAZem**, **verapamil**), **ceritinib**, **esmolol** may increase risk of bradycardia. May increase effects of QT interval–prolonging medications (e.g., **amiodarone**, **azithromycin**, **ciprofloxacin**, **haloperidol**). May increase toxic effects of **leflunomide**, **natalizumab**. May decrease effect of **sipuleucel-T**. May increase immunosuppressive effect of **tofacitinib**, **other immunosuppressants**. May decrease therapeutic effect of **vaccines**, increase toxic effects of **live vaccines**. **HERBAL:** Echinacea may decrease therapeutic effect. **FOOD:** None known. **LAB VALUES:** Expect decrease in neutrophil count. May increase serum alkaline phosphatase, ALT, AST, bilirubin, triglycerides. May reduce diagnostic effect of *Coccidioides immitis* skin test.

AVAILABILITY (Rx)

Capsules: 0.25 mg, 0.5 mg. **Tablet ODT:** 0.25 mg, 0.5 mg.

ADMINISTRATION/HANDLING

PO
• May give without regard to food. • **ODT tablet:** Peel back foil covering one blister and gently remove orally disintegrating tablet (ODT). Do not push ODT through the foil • Remove

---

ODT and place on the tongue, allowing it to dissolve before swallowing. May be taken with our without water.

INDICATIONS/ROUTES/DOSAGE

Multiple Sclerosis
PO: ADULTS 18 YRS AND OLDER, ELDERLY: 0.5 mg once daily. **CHILDREN 10 YRS AND OLDER, ADOLESCENTS WEIGHING MORE THAN 40 KG:** 0.5 mg once daily. **WEIGHING 40 KG OR LESS:** 0.25 mg once daily.

Dosage in Renal/Hepatic Impairment
Mild to moderate impairment: No dose adjustment. **Severe impairment:** Use caution.

SIDE EFFECTS

Frequent (25%–10%): Headache, diarrhea, back pain, cough. **Occasional (8%–5%):** Dyspnea, clinical depression, dizziness, hypertension, migraine, paresthesia, decreased weight. **Rare (4%–2%):** Blurred vision, alopecia, eye pain, asthenia, eczema, pruritus.

ADVERSE EFFECTS/TOXIC REACTIONS

Infections (influenza, herpes viral infection, bronchitis, sinusitis, gastroenteritis, ear infection) reported in 13%–4% of pts. Pts with diabetes or history of uveitis are at increased risk for developing macular edema. Cases of skin cancer, lymphoma, basal cell carcinoma have been reported. Progressive multifocal leukoencephalopathy (PML) (weakness, paralysis, vision loss, aphasia, cognition impairment) may occur. Neurotoxicity, posterior reversible encephalopathy may evolve into cerebral hemorrhage, CVA. May increase risk of hypertension.

NURSING CONSIDERATIONS

BASELINE ASSESSMENT

Obtain CBC, serum chemistries prior to initial treatment. At initial treatment (within first 4–6 hrs after dose), medication reduces heart rate, AV conduction, followed by progressive increase after first day of treatment. Obtain baseline vitals, with particular attention to pulse rate. Perform ophthalmologic evaluation prior to treatment and 3–4 mos after initiation of treatment. Question medical history as listed in Precautions. Obtain full medication history and screen for interactions.

INTERVENTION/EVALUATION

Monitor for bradycardia for 6 hrs after first dose, then as appropriate. Periodically monitor CBC, serum chemistries, particularly lymphocyte count (expected to decrease approximately 80% from baseline with continued treatment). Monitor for signs of systemic or local infection. Diligently monitor for hypersensitivity reaction, neurological changes, symptoms of posterior reversible encephalopathy (altered mental status, seizures, visual disturbances), PML, QT interval prolongation. Assess for new skin lesions, malignancies. Conduct ophthalmologic exams q3–4 mos after initiation, during treatment, and with any changes in vision.

PATIENT/FAMILY TEACHING

• Obtain regular eye examinations during and for 2 mos following treatment. • Use effective contraception to avoid pregnancy. Do not breastfeed. • Immediately report neurological changes such as confusion, severe headache, seizure activity, vision changes, trouble speaking, one-sided weakness, paralysis. • Treatment may increase risk of certain cancers; report new skin lesions, fever, chills, night sweats, generalized weakness, weight loss, or pain or swelling of the lymph nodes. • Report allergic reactions such as itching, rash, swelling of the face or tongue. • Report symptoms of infection, visual changes, yellowing of skin, eyes, dark urine. • Due to high risk for drug interactions, do not take newly prescribed medication unless approved by prescriber who originally started treatment.

fluconazole

flu-**kon**-a-zole
(Diflucan)
**Do not confuse Diflucan
with diclofenac, Diprivan, or
disulfiram, or fluconazole with
itraconazole, ketoconazole,
omeprazole, or pantoprazole.**

♦**CLASSIFICATION**

PHARMACOTHERAPEUTIC: Synthetic
azole. **CLINICAL:** Antifungal agent.

USES

Antifungal prophylaxis in pts undergoing bone marrow transplant; candidiasis
(esophageal, oropharyngeal, peritoneal,
urinary tract, vaginal); systemic *Candida* infections (e.g., candidemia, disseminated candidiasis, pneumonia);
treatment of cryptococcal meningitis.
OFF-LABEL: Blastomyocosis, coccidioidomycosis (prophylaxis/treatment), cryptococcosis (pulmonary), onychomycosis,
tinea infections.

PRECAUTIONS

Contraindications: Hypersensitivity to fluconazole. Concomitant administration of
QT-prolonging medications (e.g., erythromycin, pimozide). **Cautions:** Hepatic/renal
impairment, hypokalemia, hypersensitivity
to other triazoles (e.g., itraconazole, ter-
conazole), imidazoles (e.g., butoconazole,
ketoconazole). Medications or conditions
known to cause arrhythmias.

ACTION

Interferes with fungal cytochrome P-450
activity, an enzyme necessary for ergosterol formation (principal sterol in
fungal cell membrane). **Therapeutic
Effect:** Directly damages fungal membrane, altering its function. Fungistatic.

PHARMACOKINETICS

Widely distributed, including to CSF. Protein binding: 11%. Partially metabolized
in liver. Excreted unchanged primarily
in urine. Partially removed by hemodialysis. **Half-life:** 20–30 hrs (increased
in renal impairment).

⌛ LIFESPAN CONSIDERATIONS

Pregnancy/Lactation: Secreted in human
breast milk. Use caution in breastfeeding
females. **Children:** No age-related precautions noted. **Elderly:** Age-related renal
impairment may require dosage adjustment.

INTERACTIONS

DRUG: May increase concentration/
effect of **budesonide, calcium channel
blockers (e.g., amLODIPine, NIFE-
dipine, verapamil), cycloSPORINE,
ivabradine, methadone, rifabutin,
sirolimus, tacrolimus, tofacitinib.**
May decrease effect of *Saccharomyces
boulardii.* May increase concentration/
effect, risk of myopathy of **HMG-CoA
reductase inhibitors (e.g., atorvastatin, simvastatin). HERBAL:** None
significant. **FOOD:** None known. **LAB
VALUES:** May increase serum alkaline
phosphatase, bilirubin, ALT, AST.

AVAILABILITY (Rx)

Injection, Solution, Pre-Mix: 400 mg
(200 mL). **Powder for Oral Suspension:** 10 mg/mL, 40 mg/mL. **Tablets:** 50 mg, 100 mg, 150 mg, 200 mg.

ADMINISTRATION/HANDLING
 IV

Rate of administration • Do not exceed maximum flow rate of 200 mg/hr.
Storage • Store at room temperature. • Do not remove from outer
wrap until ready to use. • Squeeze
inner bag to check for leaks. • Do
not use parenteral form if solution is
cloudy, precipitate forms, seal is not
intact, or it is discolored. • Do not
add supplementary medication.

PO
• Give without regard to food.

▓ IV INCOMPATIBILITIES

Calcium gluconate.

▓ IV COMPATIBILITIES

Amiodarone, dexmedetomidine.

INDICATIONS/ROUTES/DOSAGE

◄ALERT► PO and IV therapy equally effective; IV therapy recommended for pts intolerant of drug or unable to take orally. Oral suspension stable for 14 days at room temperature or refrigerated.

Usual Dosage

Note: Duration and dose dependent on location/severity of infection.
PO/IV: ADULTS, ELDERLY: (Loading dose): 200–800 mg. **(Maintenance dose):** 100–400 mg/day. **ADOLESCENTS, CHILDREN, INFANTS: Loading dose:** 6–12 mg/kg. **Maintenance dose:** 3–12 mg/kg once daily. **Maximum:** 600 mg/day. **NEONATES: (Prophylaxis):** 3–6 mg/kg/dose twice weekly. **(Treatment):** Initially, 25 mg/kg on day 1, then 12 mg/kg once daily.

Dosage in Renal Impairment

After a loading dose of 400 mg, daily dosage is based on creatinine clearance.

Creatinine Clearance	Dosage
Greater than 50 mL/min	100%
50 mL/min or less	50%
Dialysis	50%
CCRT	400–800 mg as loading dose
CVVH	then 200–800 mg/day
CVVHDF	400–800 mg as loading dose, then 400–800 mg/day

Dosage in Hepatic Impairment

Use caution.

SIDE EFFECTS

Occasional (4%–1%): Hypersensitivity reaction (chills, fever, pruritus, rash), dizziness, drowsiness, headache, constipation, diarrhea, nausea, vomiting, abdominal pain.

ADVERSE EFFECTS/TOXIC REACTIONS

Exfoliative skin disorders, serious hepatic injury, blood dyscrasias (eosinophilia, thrombocytopenia, anemia, leukopenia) have been reported rarely. May increase risk of QT prolongation, torsades de pointes. Skin disorders including Stevens-Johnson syndrome, toxic epidermal necrolysis may occur.

NURSING CONSIDERATIONS

BASELINE ASSESSMENT

Obtain CBC, LFT; serum potassium in critically ill pts. Receive full medication history and screen for interactions. Assess areas of infection. Assess infected area.

INTERVENTION/EVALUATION

Monitor hepatic function in critically ill pts. Assess for hypersensitivity reaction (chills, fever). Report rash, itching promptly. Monitor daily pattern of bowel activity, stool consistency. Assess for dizziness; provide assistance as needed.

PATIENT/FAMILY TEACHING

• Report dark urine, pale stool, jaundiced skin or sclera of eyes, rash, pruritus. • Pts with oropharyngeal infections should maintain fastidious oral hygiene. • Consult physician before taking any other medication.

---

fluorouracil, 5-FU `HIGH ALERT`

flure-oh-**ue**-ra-sil
(Carac, Efudex, Fluoroplex, Tolak)
■ **BLACK BOX ALERT** ■ Must be administered by personnel trained in administration/handling of chemotherapeutic agents.
Do not confuse Efudex with Efidac.

◆CLASSIFICATION

PHARMACOTHERAPEUTIC: Antimetabolite. **CLINICAL:** Antineoplastic.

USES

Parenteral: Treatment of breast, colon/rectal, gastric, pancreatic cancers. **Topical:** Treatment of multiple actinic or solar keratoses, superficial basal cell carcinomas. **OFF-LABEL: Parenteral:** Anal carcinoma; biliary tract, bladder (muscle invasive), cervical, esophageal, head and neck (squamous cell) cancers; neuroendocrine tumors; small bowel adenocarcinoma; glaucoma surgery (adjunctive therapy).

PRECAUTIONS

Contraindications: Hypersensitivity to fluorouracil. Myelosuppression, poor nutritional status, potentially serious infections. **Cautions:** History of high-dose pelvic irradiation, hepatic/renal impairment, palmar-plantar erythrodysesthesia syndrome (hand and foot syndrome), previous use of alkylating agents. Pts with widespread metastatic marrow involvement.

ACTION

Blocks formation of thymidylic acid. Cell cycle–specific for S phase of cell division. **Therapeutic Effect:** Inhibits DNA, RNA synthesis. **Topical:** Destroys rapidly proliferating cells.

PHARMACOKINETICS

Widely distributed. Crosses blood-brain barrier. Metabolized in liver. Primarily excreted by lungs as carbon dioxide. Removed by hemodialysis. **Half-life:** 16 min.

⌛ LIFESPAN CONSIDERATIONS

Pregnancy/Lactation: If possible, avoid use during pregnancy, esp. first trimester. May cause fetal harm. Unknown if distributed in breast milk. Breastfeeding not recommended. **Children:** No age-related precautions noted. **Elderly:** Age-related renal impairment may require dosage adjustment.

INTERACTIONS

DRUG: Bone marrow depressants (e.g., cladribine) may increase risk of myelosuppression. May decrease the therapeutic effect of **BCG (intravesical), vaccines (live).** May increase adverse/toxic effects of **vaccines (live). HERBAL: Echinacea** may decrease therapeutic effect. **FOOD:** None known. **LAB VALUES:** May decrease serum albumin. **Topical:** May cause eosinophilia, leukocytosis, thrombocytopenia, toxic granulation.

AVAILABILITY (Rx)

Cream: 0.5%, 1%, 4%, 5%, **Injection Solution:** 50 mg/mL. **Solution, Topical:** 2%, 5%.

ADMINISTRATION/HANDLING

◄ALERT► Give by IV injection or IV infusion. Do not add to other IV infusions. Avoid small veins, swollen/edematous extremities, areas overlying joints, tendons. May be carcinogenic, mutagenic, teratogenic. Handle with extreme care during preparation/administration.

 IV

Reconstitution • IV push does not need to be diluted or reconstituted. • Inject through Y-tube or 3-way stopcock of free-flowing solution. • For IV infusion, further dilute with 50–1,000 mL D₅W or 0.9% NaCl. **Rate of administration** • Give IV push slowly over 1–2 min. • IV infusion is administered over 30 min–24 hrs (refer to individual protocols). • Extravasation produces immediate pain, severe local tissue damage.

Storage • Store at room temperature. • Solution appears colorless to faint yellow. Slight discoloration does not adversely affect potency or safety. • If precipitate forms, redissolve by heating, shaking vigorously; allow to cool to body temperature. • Diluted solutions stable for 72 hrs at room temperature.

🚫 IV INCOMPATIBILITIES

Ondansetron.

🚫 IV COMPATIBILITIES

Granisetron, palonosetron, potassium chloride,

F

INDICATIONS/ROUTES/DOSAGE

Note: Refer to individual protocols.

Usual Range

IV bolus: ADULTS, ELDERLY: 200–1,000 mg/m²/day for 1–21 days or 500–600 mg/m²/dose q3–4wks.

IV infusion: ADULTS, ELDERLY: 15 mg/kg/day or 500 mg/m²/day over 4 hrs for 5 days or 800–1,200 mg/m² over 24–120 hrs.

Breast Cancer

IV: ADULTS, ELDERLY: 500–600 mg/m² on days 1 and 8 q28days (in combination with cyclophosphamide and epirubicin or methotrexate).

Colorectal Cancer

IV: ADULTS, ELDERLY: 400 mg/m² bolus on day 1, then 2,400–3,000 mg/m² over 46 hrs (as a continuous infusion) q2wks (in combination with leucovorin ± either oxaliplatin or irinotecan).

Gastric Cancer

IV: ADULTS, ELDERLY: Continuous infusion (as part of a platinum containing regimen). The dose, duration, and frequency of each cycle varies based on the regimen.

Pancreatic Cancer

IV: ADULTS, ELDERLY: 2,400 mg/m² as a continuous infusion over 46 hrs q14 days for 24 wks (in combination with leucovorin, irinotecan, and oxaliplatin).

Multiple Actinic or Solar Keratoses

Topical: *(0.5%):* **ADULTS, ELDERLY:** Apply once daily for up to 4 wks. *(5%):* **ADULTS, ELDERLY:** Apply twice daily for 2–4 wks. *(1%):* Apply twice daily for 2–6 wks. *(4%):* Apply once daily for 4 wks.

Basal Cell Carcinoma

Topical: *(5%):* **ADULTS, ELDERLY:** Apply twice daily for 3–6 wks up to 10–12 wks.

Dosage in Renal Impairment

No dose adjustment.

Dosage in Hepatic Impairment

Use extreme caution.

SIDE EFFECTS

Parenteral: Frequent (greater than 10%): Alopecia, dermatitis, anorexia, diarrhea, esophagitis, dyspepsia, stomatitis. **Occasional (10%–1%):** Cardiotoxicity (angina, ECG changes), skin dryness, epithelial fissuring, nausea, vomiting, excessive lacrimation, blurred vision. **Rare (less than 1%):** Headache, photosensitivity, somnolence, allergic reaction, dyspnea, hypotension, MI, pulmonary edema. **Topical: Occasional:** Erythema, skin ulceration, pruritus, hyperpigmentation, dermatitis, insomnia, stomatitis, irritability, photosensitivity, excessive lacrimation, blurred vision.

ADVERSE EFFECTS/TOXIC REACTIONS

Earliest sign of toxicity (4–8 days after beginning therapy) is stomatitis (dry mouth, burning sensation, mucosal erythema, ulceration at inner margin of lips). Most common dermatologic toxicity is pruritic rash (generally on extremities, less frequently on trunk). Leukopenia (WBC less than 3,500 cells/mm³) generally occurs within 9–14 days after drug administration but may occur as late as 25th day. Thrombocytopenia (platelets less than 100,000 cells/mm³) occasionally occurs within 7–17 days after administration. Pancytopenia, agranulocytosis occur rarely.

NURSING CONSIDERATIONS

BASELINE ASSESSMENT

Obtain CBC, renal function, LFT and monitor during therapy. Question history of hypersensitivity reaction, hepatic/renal impairment. Offer emotional support.

INTERVENTION/EVALUATION

Monitor for rapidly falling WBC, platelet count; intractable diarrhea, GI bleeding (bright red or tarry stool). Assess oral mucosa for stomatitis. Drug should be discontinued if intractable diarrhea, stomatitis, GI bleeding occurs. Assess skin for rash.

PATIENT/FAMILY TEACHING

• Maintain strict oral hygiene. • Report signs/symptoms of infection (cough, fatigue, fever), unusual bruising/bleeding, visual changes, nausea, vomiting, diarrhea, chest pain, palpitations. • Avoid sunlight, artificial light sources; wear protective clothing, sunglasses, sunscreen. • **Topical:** Apply only to affected area. • Do not use occlusive coverings. • Be careful near eyes, nose, mouth. • Wash hands thoroughly after application. • Treated areas may be unsightly for several weeks after therapy.

FLUoxetine

floo-**ox**-e-teen
(PROzac)
■ **BLACK BOX ALERT** ■ Increased risk of suicidal thinking and behavior in children, adolescents, young adults 18–24 yrs of age with major depressive disorder, other psychiatric disorders.
Do not confuse FLUoxetine with DULoxetine, famotidine, fluvastatin, fluvoxaMINE, furosemide, or PARoxetine, or PROzac with Paxil, PriLOSEC, Prograf, Proscar, or ProSom.

FIXED-COMBINATION(S)

Symbyax: FLUoxetine/OLANZapine (an antipsychotic): 25 mg/6 mg, 25 mg/12 mg, 50 mg/6 mg, 50 mg/12 mg.

✦CLASSIFICATION

PHARMACOTHERAPEUTIC: Selective serotonin reuptake inhibitor (SSRI). **CLINICAL:** Antidepressant.

USES

Treatment of major depressive disorder (MDD) in adults and children 8 yrs and older, obsessive-compulsive disorder (OCD) in adults and children 7 yrs and older, binge-eating and vomiting in moderate to severe bulimia nervosa in adults, premenstrual dysphoric disorder (PMDD) in adults, panic disorder with or without agoraphobia in adults. Treatment of resistant or bipolar 1 depression (with OLAN-Zapine) in adults and children 10 yrs and older. **OFF-LABEL:** Treatment of fibromyalgia, posttraumatic stress disorder (PTSD), social anxiety disorder, binge eating disorder, premenstrual dysphoric disorder, generalized anxiety disorder (GAD).

PRECAUTIONS

Contraindications: Hypersensitivity to FLUoxetine. Use of MAOIs within 5 wks of discontinuing FLUoxetine or within 14 days of discontinuing MAOIs. Initiation in pts receiving linezolid or methylene blue. Use with pimozide or thioridazine. **Note:** Do not initiate thioridazine until 5 wks after discontinuing FLUoxetine. **Cautions:** Seizure disorder, cardiac dysfunction (e.g., history of MI), diabetes, pts at risk for QT interval prolongation, cardiac arrhythmias (congenital long QT syndrome, HF, QT interval–prolonging medications, hypokalemia, hypomagnesemia), renal/hepatic impairment, pts at high risk for suicide, in pts where weight loss is undesirable, elderly. Pts at risk of acute narrow-angle glaucoma or with increased intraocular pressure.

ACTION

Selectively inhibits serotonin uptake in CNS, enhancing serotonergic function. **Therapeutic Effect:** Relieves depression; reduces obsessive-compulsive, bulimic behavior.

PHARMACOKINETICS

Widely distributed. Crosses blood-brain barrier. Protein binding: 94%. Metabolized in liver. Primarily excreted in urine. Not removed by hemodialysis. **Half-life:** 2–3 days; metabolite, 7–9 days.

⧖ LIFESPAN CONSIDERATIONS

Pregnancy/Lactation: Unknown whether drug crosses placenta or is distributed in breast milk. **Children:** May be more sensitive to behavioral side effects (e.g., insomnia, restlessness). **Elderly:** No age-related precautions noted.

INTERACTIONS

DRUG: NSAIDs (e.g., **ibuprofen, ketorolac, naproxen**), **antiplatelets** (e.g., **clopidogrel**), **anticoagulants** (e.g., **warfarin**) may increase risk of bleeding. **Alcohol, other CNS depressants** (e.g., **LORazepam, morphine, zolpidem**) may increase CNS depression. **MAOIs** (e.g., **phenelzine, selegiline**) may produce serotonin syndrome and neuroleptic malignant syndrome. **Strong CYP2D6 inhibitors** (e.g., **bupropion**) may increase concentration/effect. May decrease concentration/effect of **tamoxifen.** QT interval–prolonging medications (e.g., **amiodarone, azithromycin, ciprofloxacin, haloperidol, methadone, sotalol**) may increase risk of QT interval prolongation. May increase adverse effects of **tricyclic antidepressants** (e.g., **amitriptyline**). **HERBAL:** Herbals with sedative properties (e.g., **chamomile, kava kava, valerian**) may increase CNS depression. **St. John's wort, Syrian rue** may decrease concentration/effect, enhance serotonergic effect. **FOOD:** None known. **LAB VALUES:** May decrease serum sodium. May increase serum ALT, AST.

AVAILABILITY (Rx)

Capsules: 10 mg, 20 mg, 40 mg. **Oral Solution:** 20 mg/5 mL. **Tablets:** 10 mg, 20 mg, 60 mg.

Capsules (Delayed-Release): 90 mg.

ADMINISTRATION/HANDLING

PO

• Give without regard to food, but give with food, milk if GI distress occurs. • **Bipolar disorder:** Give once daily in evening. • **Depression, OCD:** Give once daily in morning or twice daily (morning and noon). • **Bulimia:** Give once daily in morning.

INDICATIONS/ROUTES/DOSAGE

◄ALERT► Use lower or less frequent doses in pts with renal/hepatic impairment, pts with concurrent disease or multiple medications, the elderly. Decrease gradually to minimize withdrawal symptoms and to allow for detection of re-emerging symptoms.

Depression

PO: **ADULTS, ELDERLY:** Initially, 20 mg each morning. May increase after several wks by 20 mg/day. **Maximum:** 80 mg/day as single or 2 divided doses. **CHILDREN 8–18 YRS:** Initially, 10–20 mg/day. Lower-weight children may be started at 10 mg/day and increased to 20 mg/day after several wks if needed. **Maximum: 12–18 YRS:** 60 mg/day. **8–11 YRS:** 40 mg/day.

Panic Disorder

PO: **ADULTS, ELDERLY:** Initially, 5–10 mg/day. After 3–7 days, may increase dose in 5–10 mg increments at intervals of at least 1 wk to usual dose of 20–40 mg/day. **Maximum:** 60 mg/day.

Bulimia Nervosa

PO: **ADULTS:** Initially, 20 mg/day. May increase by 20 mg increments at intervals of at least 1 wk. **Maximum:** 60 mg/day.

Obsessive-Compulsive Disorder (OCD)

PO: **ADULTS, ELDERLY:** Initially, 10–20 mg once daily. May increase by 20 mg increments at intervals of at least 1 wk. **Range:** 40–80 mg/day. **Maximum:** 80 mg/day. **CHILDREN 7–18 YRS:** Initially, 10 mg/day. May increase to 20 mg/day after 2 wks. **Range:** 20–60 mg/day. **Maximum:** 60 mg/day.

Depression Associated With Bipolar Disorder

PO: **ADULTS, ELDERLY, CHILDREN 10–17 YRS:** *(With Olanzapine):* Initially, 20 mg/day in evening. May increase gradually in 10–20 mg increments. **Range:** 20–50 mg/day.

Premenstrual Dysphoric Disorder (PMDD) (Sarafem)

PO: **ADULTS:** **(Continuous daily dosing):** Initially, 10 mg once daily. Increase to 20 mg/day over first month. In a subsequent menstrual cycle, a further increase to 30 mg/

day may be necessary. **(Intermittent dosing):** Initially, 10 mg once daily during luteal phase of menstrual cycle only. Over first month, may increase to 20 mg once daily during luteal phase. In a subsequent menstrual cycle, a further increase to 30 mg/day during luteal phase may be necessary.

Dosage in Renal/Hepatic Impairment
Use caution.

SIDE EFFECTS

Frequent (greater than 10%): Headache, asthenia, insomnia, anxiety, drowsiness, nausea, diarrhea, decreased appetite. **Occasional (9%–2%):** Dizziness, tremor, fatigue, vomiting, constipation, dry mouth, abdominal pain, nasal congestion, diaphoresis, rash. **Rare (less than 2%):** Flushed skin, light-headedness, impaired concentration.

ADVERSE EFFECTS/TOXIC REACTIONS

May increase risk of suicide. Agitation, coma, diarrhea, delirium, hallucinations, hyperreflexia, hyperthermia, tachycardia, seizures may indicate life-threatening serotonin syndrome.

NURSING CONSIDERATIONS

BASELINE ASSESSMENT
Assess appearance, behavior, mood, suicidal tendencies. For pts on long-term therapy, baseline renal function, LFT, blood counts should be performed at baseline and periodically thereafter.

INTERVENTION/EVALUATION
Supervise suicidal-risk pt closely during early therapy (as depression lessens, energy level improves, increasing suicide potential). Monitor mental status, anxiety, social functioning, appetite, nutritional intake. Monitor daily pattern of bowel activity, stool consistency. Assess skin for rash. Monitor serum LFT, glucose, sodium; weight.

PATIENT/FAMILY TEACHING
• Maximum therapeutic response may require 4 or more wks of therapy. • Do not abruptly discontinue medication. • Avoid tasks that require alertness, motor skills until response to drug is established. • Avoid alcohol. • To avoid insomnia, take last dose of drug before 4 PM. • Seek immediate medical attention if thoughts of suicide, new-onset or worsening of anxiety, depression, or changes in mood occur.

fluticasone   TOP 100

floo-**tik**-a-sone
(Arnuity Ellipta, Cutivate ✦, Flonase, ✦ Flonase Allergy Relief, Flovent Diskus, Xhance, Flonase Sensimist)
Do not confuse Cutivate with Ultravate, or Flonase with Flovent, Beconase.

FIXED-COMBINATION(S)

Advair, Advair Diskus, Advair HFA: fluticasone/salmeterol (bronchodilator): 100 mcg/50 mcg, 250 mcg/50 mcg, 500 mcg/50 mcg. **Breo Ellipta:** fluticasone/vilanterol (bronchodilator): 100 mcg/25 mcg. **Dymista:** fluticasone/azelastine (an antihistamine): 50 mcg/137 mcg per spray. **Trelegy Ellipta:** fluticasone/umeclidinium (anticholinergic)/vilanterol (bronchodilator): 100 mcg/62.5 mcg/25 mcg.

◆CLASSIFICATION

PHARMACOTHERAPEUTIC: Corticosteroid. **CLINICAL:** Anti-inflammatory, antipruritic.

USES

Nasal: Management of nasal symptoms of perennial nonallergic rhinitis in adults and children 4 yrs and older. Management of seasonal and perennial allergic rhinitis in adults, children 2 yrs and older. **(Xhance):** Treatment of chronic rhinosinusitis with or without nasal polyps in pts 18 yrs and older. **(OTC):** Relief of hayfever/other upper respiratory allergies. **Topical:** Relief of inflammation/pruritus associated with steroid-responsive disorders (e.g., contact dermatitis, eczema), atopic dermatitis in adults and children 3 mos of age and older. **Inhalation:** Maintenance treatment of bronchial asthma as prophylactic therapy in adults and children 12 yrs and older (ArmonAir), children 5 yrs and older (Arnuity Ellipta), children 4 yrs and older (Flovent). **OFF-LABEL:** Inhalation: COPD maintenance, eosinophilic esophagitis. **Nasal:** Rhinosinusitis without polyps.

PRECAUTIONS

Contraindications: Hypersensitivity to fluticasone. (Arnuity Ellipta, Flovent Diskus): Severe hypersensitivity to milk proteins or lactose. **Inhalation:** Primary treatment of status asthmaticus, acute exacerbation of asthma, other acute asthmatic conditions. **Cautions:** Untreated systemic ocular herpes simplex; untreated fungal, bacterial infection; active or quiescent tuberculosis. Thyroid disease, cardiovascular disease, diabetes, glaucoma, hepatic/renal impairment, cataracts, myasthenia gravis, seizures, GI disease, risk for osteoporosis, untreated localized infection of nasal mucosa. Following acute MI; concurrent use with strong CYP3A4 inhibitors.

ACTION

Direct local effect as potent vasoconstrictor, anti-inflammatory. **Therapeutic Effect:** Prevents, controls inflammation.

PHARMACOKINETICS

Inhalation/intranasal: Protein binding: 91%. Metabolized in liver. Excreted in urine. **Half-life:** 3–7.8 hrs. **Topical:** Amount absorbed depends on affected area and skin condition (absorption increased with fever, hydration, inflamed or denuded skin).

⧗ LIFESPAN CONSIDERATIONS

Pregnancy/Lactation: Unknown if drug crosses placenta or is distributed in breast milk. **Children:** Safety and efficacy not established. Children may experience growth suppression with prolonged or high doses. **Elderly:** No age-related precautions noted.

INTERACTIONS

DRUG: **Strong CYP3A4 inhibitors (e.g., clarithromycin, ketoconazole, ritonavir)** may increase concentration/effect. **HERBAL:** None significant. **FOOD:** None known. **LAB VALUES:** None significant.

AVAILABILITY (Rx)

Aerosol for Oral Inhalation: *(Flovent HFA):* 44 mcg/inhalation, 110 mcg/inhalation, 220 mcg/inhalation. **Cream:** 0.05%. **Ointment:** 0.005%. **Powder for Oral Inhalation:** *(Flovent Diskus):* 50 mcg/blister, 100 mcg/blister, 250 mcg/blister. *(Arnuity Ellipta):* 50 mcg/actuation, 100 mcg/actuation, 200 mcg/actuation. **Suspension Intranasal Spray:** *(Flonase Allergy Relief):* 50 mcg/inhalation. *(Flonase Sensimist):* 27.5 mcg/spray. *(Xhance):* 93 mcg/actuation.

ADMINISTRATION/HANDLING

Inhalation
• *(Flovent HFA):* Shake container well. Prime before first use. Instruct pt to exhale completely. Place mouthpiece fully into mouth, inhale, and hold breath as long as possible before exhaling. • Allow 30–60 seconds between inhalations. • Rinsing mouth after each use decreases dry mouth, hoarseness. • *(Flovent Diskus):* Do not shake or prime before use. Place mouthpiece fully into mouth, inhale quickly and deeply, remove device, and hold breath up to 10 seconds. • *(Arnuity Ellipta):* Do not shake or prime before use; put mouthpiece between lips, breathe deeply and slowly through the mouth,

remove inhaler, and hold breath for 3–4 seconds.

Intranasal
• Instruct pt to clear nasal passages as much as possible before use (topical nasal decongestants may be needed 5–15 min before use). • Tilt head slightly forward. • Insert spray tip into 1 nostril, pointing toward inflamed nasal turbinates, away from nasal septum. • Pump medication into 1 nostril while pt holds other nostril closed, concurrently inspires through nose.

INDICATIONS/ROUTES/DOSAGE
Nonallergic Rhinitis
Intranasal: (Flonase): ADULTS, ELDERLY: Initially, 200 mcg (2 sprays in each nostril once daily or 1 spray in each nostril q12h). **Maintenance:** 1 spray in each nostril once daily. May increase to 100 mcg (2 sprays) in each nostril. **Maximum:** 200 mcg/day. CHILDREN 4 YRS AND OLDER: Initially, 100 mcg (1 spray in each nostril once daily). **Maximum:** 200 mcg/day (2 sprays each nostril). **(Flonase Sensimist):** ADULTS, ELDERLY, CHILDREN 12 YRS AND OLDER: 110 mcg (2 sprays in each nostril) once daily. **Maintenance:** 55 mcg (1 spray in each nostril) once daily. CHILDREN 2–11 YRS: 55 mcg (1 spray in each nostril) once daily.

Allergic Rhinitis
(Flonase Sensimist): ADULTS, ELDERLY, CHILDREN 12 YRS AND OLDER: 110 mcg (2 sprays in each nostril) once daily. **Maintenance:** 55 mcg (1 spray in each nostril) once daily. CHILDREN 2–11 YRS: 55 mcg (1 spray in each nostril) once daily.

Usual Topical Dosage
Note: Ointment for adults only.
Topical: ADULTS, ELDERLY, CHILDREN 3 MOS AND OLDER: Apply sparingly to affected area once or twice daily.

Chronic Rhinosinusitis (With or Without Nasal Polyps)
(Xhance): ADULTS, ELDERLY: 186 mcg (1 spray per nostril) or 372 mcg (2 sprays per nostril) twice daily.

Maintenance Treatment of Asthma
Inhalation powder: (Arnuity Ellipta): ADULTS, ELDERLY, CHILDREN 12 YRS AND OLDER: 100–200 mcg once daily. **Maximum:** 200 mcg/day. CHILDREN 5–11 YRS: 50 mcg once daily. **(Flovent Diskus):** ADULTS, ELDERLY, CHILDREN 12 YRS AND OLDER: Initially, 100 mcg twice daily. **Maximum:** 1,000 mcg twice daily. **(Flovent HFA):** ADULTS, ELDERLY, CHILDREN 12 YRS AND OLDER: 88 mcg twice daily. **Maximum:** 880 mcg twice daily. USUAL PEDIATRIC DOSE (4–11 YRS): **(Flovent Diskus):** Initially, 50 mcg twice daily. May increase to 100 mcg twice daily. **(Flovent HFA):** 88 mcg twice daily.

Dosage in Renal/Hepatic Impairment
No dose adjustment. **(Arnuity Ellipta):** Use caution in hepatic impairment.

SIDE EFFECTS
Frequent: Inhalation: Throat irritation, hoarseness, dry mouth, cough, temporary wheezing, oropharyngeal candidiasis (particularly if mouth is not rinsed with water after each administration). **Intranasal:** Mild nasopharyngeal irritation, nasal burning, stinging, dryness, rebound congestion, rhinorrhea, altered sense of taste. **Occasional: Inhalation:** Oral candidiasis. **Intranasal:** Nasal/pharyngeal candidiasis, headache. **Topical:** Stinging, burning of skin.

ADVERSE EFFECTS/TOXIC REACTIONS
When pts are switched from systemic corticosteroids to orally inhaled fluticasone, life-threatening exacerbation of asthma or adrenal insufficiency may occur due to systemic corticosteroid withdraw. May cause paradoxical bronchospasm, wheezing. Hypersensitivity reactions

including anaphylaxis, angioedema, bronchospasm, rash, urticaria may occur. Cataracts, glaucoma, increased intraocular pressure reported rarely. Long-term use may result in loss of bone mineral density (BMD). May cause local *Candida* infections of the mouth and throat. Respiratory tract infections, pneumonia reported in pts with COPD receiving inhaled corticosteroids.

NURSING CONSIDERATIONS

BASELINE ASSESSMENT

Obtain history of skin disorder, asthma, rhinitis. Question hypersensitivity, esp. milk products or lactose. Question medical history as listed in Precautions.

INTERVENTION/EVALUATION

Monitor rate, depth, rhythm, type of respiration; quality/rate of pulse. Assess lung sounds for rhonchi, wheezing, rales. Assess oral mucous membranes for evidence of candidiasis. Monitor growth in pediatric pts. **Topical:** Assess involved area for therapeutic response to irritation.

PATIENT/FAMILY TEACHING

• Pts receiving bronchodilators by inhalation concomitantly with steroid inhalation therapy should use bronchodilator several min before corticosteroid aerosol (enhances penetration of steroid into bronchial tree). • Do not change dose/schedule or stop taking drug; must taper off gradually under medical supervision. • Maintain strict oral hygiene. • Rinse mouth and gargle with water immediately after inhalation (prevents mouth/throat dryness, oral fungal infection). • Use of an inhaler spacer can help with delivery of medication and reduce the incidence of thrush. • Increase fluid intake (decreases lung secretion viscosity). • **Intranasal:** Clear nasal passages before use. • Report if no improvement in symptoms or if sneezing/nasal irritation occurs. • Improvement noted in several days to weeks. • **Topical:** Rub thin film gently into affected area. • Use only for prescribed area and no longer than ordered. • Avoid contact with eyes.

fondaparinux

fon-**dap**-a-rin-ux
(Arixtra)

■ **BLACK BOX ALERT** ■ Epidural or spinal anesthesia greatly increases potential for spinal or epidural hematoma, subsequent long-term or permanent paralysis.

◆CLASSIFICATION

PHARMACOTHERAPEUTIC: Factor Xa inhibitor. **CLINICAL:** Antithrombotic.

USES

Prophylaxis of deep vein thrombosis (DVT): Prevention of DVT, which may lead to pulmonary embolism (PE) in pts undergoing total hip replacement, hip fracture surgery, knee replacement surgery, abdominal surgery. **Treatment of acute DVT:** Treatment of acute DVT when administered in conjunction with warfarin. **Treatment of acute PE:** Treatment of acute PE when administered in conjunction with warfarin sodium (when initial therapy is administered in the hospital). **OFF-LABEL:** Treatment of heparin-induced thrombocytopenia (HIT), acute symptomatic superficial vein thrombosis of the legs, acute coronary syndrome. Venous thromboembolism (VTE) prophylaxis in medical pts with acute illness with risk of VTE.

PRECAUTIONS

Contraindications: Hypersensitivity to fondaparinux, active major bleeding, bacterial endocarditis, prophylaxis treatment in pts with body weight less than 50 kg, severe renal impairment (CrCl less than 30 mL/min), thrombocytopenia associated with antiplatelet antibody formation in presence of fondaparinux. **Cautions:** Conditions with increased risk of bleeding, bacterial endocarditis, active ulcerative GI disease, hemorrhagic stroke; shortly after brain, spinal, or ophthalmologic surgery; concurrent platelet inhibitors, severe uncontrolled hypertension, history of CVA, history of heparin-induced thrombocytopenia, renal/hepatic impairment, elderly, indwelling epidural catheter use.

ACTION

Factor Xa inhibitor that selectively binds to antithrombin and increases its affinity for factor Xa, inhibiting factor Xa, stopping blood coagulation cascade. **Therapeutic Effect:** Indirectly prevents formation of thrombin and subsequently fibrin clot.

PHARMACOKINETICS

Widely distributed. Undergoes minimal, if any, metabolism. Highly bound to antithrombin III. Distributed mainly in blood and to a minor extent in extravascular fluid. Excreted unchanged in urine. Removed by hemodialysis. **Half-life:** 17–21 hrs (increased in renal impairment).

LIFESPAN CONSIDERATIONS

Pregnancy/Lactation: Use with caution, particularly during third trimester, immediate postpartum period (increased risk of maternal hemorrhage). Unknown if excreted in breast milk. **Children:** Safety and efficacy not established. **Elderly:** Age-related renal impairment may increase risk of bleeding.

INTERACTIONS

DRUG: Anticoagulants (e.g., **heparin, warfarin**), **aspirin, NSAIDs** (e.g., **ibuprofen, ketorolac, naproxen**) may increase risk of bleeding. May increase effect of **apixaban, dabigatran, edoxaban, rivaroxaban.** **HERBAL:** Herbals with anticoagulant/antiplatelet properties (e.g., **garlic, ginger, ginkgo biloba**) may increase effect. **FOOD:** None known. **LAB VALUES:** May cause reversible increases in

serum creatinine, ALT, AST. May decrease Hgb, Hct, platelet count.

AVAILABILITY (Rx)

Injection, Solution: 2.5 mg/0.5 mL, 5 mg/0.4 mL, 7.5 mg/0.6 mL, 10 mg/0.8 mL.

ADMINISTRATION/HANDLING

SQ
• Parenteral form appears clear, colorless. Discard if discoloration or particulate matter is noted. • Store at room temperature. • Do not expel air bubble from prefilled syringe before injection. • Insert needle subcutaneously into upper arm, outer thigh, or abdomen and inject solution. • Do not inject into areas of active skin disease or injury such as sunburns, rashes, inflammation, skin infections, or active psoriasis. • Rotate injection sites.

INDICATIONS/ROUTES/DOSAGE

◄**ALERT**► For SQ administration only.
Prevention of Venous Thromboembolism
SQ: ADULTS WEIGHING 50 KG OR MORE: 2.5 mg once daily for 5–9 days after surgery (up to 10 days following abdominal surgery; optimal duration in orthopedic surgery is unknown, but usually given for a minimum of 10–14 days and extended for up to 35 days. Initial dose should be given no earlier than 6–8 hrs after surgery. Initiate dose once hemostasis established. **WEIGHING LESS THAN 50 KG:** Contraindicated.

Treatment of DVT, PE
Note: Start warfarin on first treatment day and continue fondaparinux until INR reaches 2 to 3 for at least 24 hr. Usual duration of fondaparinux: 5–9 days (up to 26 days).
SQ: ADULTS, ELDERLY WEIGHING MORE THAN 100 KG: 10 mg once daily. **ADULTS, ELDERLY WEIGHING 50–100 KG:** 7.5 mg once daily. **ADULTS, ELDERLY WEIGHING LESS THAN 50 KG:** 5 mg once daily.

Dosage in Renal Impairment
CrCl greater than 50 mL/min: No dose adjustment. **CrCl 30–50 mL/min:** Use caution (50% dose reduction or use of

low-dose heparin). **CrCl less than 30 mL/min:** Contraindicated.

Dosage in Hepatic Impairment
Mild to moderate impairment: No dose adjustment. **Severe impairment:** Use caution.

SIDE EFFECTS

Frequent (19%–11%): Anemia, fever, nausea. **Occasional (10%–4%):** Edema, constipation, rash, vomiting, insomnia, increased wound drainage, hypokalemia. **Rare (less than 4%):** Dizziness, hypotension, confusion, urinary retention, injection site hematoma, diarrhea, dyspepsia, headache.

ADVERSE EFFECTS/TOXIC REACTIONS

Accidental overdose may lead to bleeding complications ranging from local ecchymoses to major hemorrhage. Thrombocytopenia occurs rarely.

NURSING CONSIDERATIONS

BASELINE ASSESSMENT

Obtain CBC, renal function test. Evaluate potential risk for bleeding. Question history of recent surgery, trauma, intracranial hemorrhage, GI bleeding. Question medical history as listed in Precautions. Ensure that pt has not received spinal anesthesia, spinal procedures.

INTERVENTION/EVALUATION

Periodically monitor CBC, esp. platelet count, stool for occult blood (no need for daily monitoring in pts with normal presurgical coagulation parameters). Assess for any signs of bleeding: bleeding at surgical site, hematuria, blood in stool, bleeding from gums, petechiae, ecchymosis, bleeding from injection sites. Monitor B/P, pulse; hypotension, tachycardia may indicate bleeding, hypovolemia.

PATIENT/FAMILY TEACHING

• Usual length of therapy is 5–9 days. • Do not take any OTC medication (esp. aspirin, NSAIDs). • Report swelling of hands/feet, unusual back pain, unusual bleeding/bruising, weakness. Treatment may increase risk of bleeding into the brain; report confusion, one-sided weakness, trouble speaking, seizures. Treatment may increase risk of GI bleeding; report bloody stool, vomiting up blood; dark, tarry stools.

fosphenytoin

fos-**fen**-i-toyn
(Cerebyx)
■ **BLACK BOX ALERT** ■ The rate of fosphenytoin intravenous (IV) administration should not exceed 150 mg phenytoin sodium equivalent (PE)/min due to risk of severe hypotension and cardiac arrhythmias. Cardiac monitoring is recommended.
Do not confuse Cerebyx with CeleBREX or CeleXA, or fosphenytoin with fospropofol.

◆CLASSIFICATION

PHARMACOTHERAPEUTIC: Hydantoin. **CLINICAL:** Anticonvulsant.

USES

Control of generalized tonic-clonic status epilepticus. Prevention, treatment of seizures occurring during neurosurgery. Short-term substitution for oral phenytoin. **OFF-LABEL:** Traumatic brain injury (seizure prevention), trigeminal neuralgia (rescue therapy).

PRECAUTIONS

Contraindications: Hypersensitivity to fosphenytoin, phenytoin, other hydantoins. Adams-Stokes syndrome; second- or third-degree AV block; sinus bradycardia; SA block; concurrent use of delavirdine. History of hepatotoxicity attributed to fosphenytoin or phenytoin. **Cautions:** Porphyria, diabetes, hypothyroidism, hypotension, severe myocardial insufficiency, renal/hepatic disease, hypoalbuminemia.

ACTION

Stabilizes neuronal membranes, limits spread of seizure activity by increasing efflux or decreasing influx of sodium ions across cell membranes in the motor cortex during nerve impulse generation. **Therapeutic Effect:** Decreases seizure activity.

PHARMACOKINETICS

Widely distributed. Protein binding: 95%–99%. Rapidly and completely hydrolyzed to phenytoin after IM or IV administration. Time of complete conversion to phenytoin: 4 hrs after IM injection; 2 hrs after IV infusion. **Half-life:** 8–15 min (for conversion to phenytoin). (Phenytoin: 12–29 hrs.)

⧗ LIFESPAN CONSIDERATIONS

Pregnancy/Lactation: May increase frequency of seizures during pregnancy. Increased risk of congenital malformations. Unknown if excreted in breast milk. **Children:** Safety and efficacy not established. **Elderly:** Lower dosage recommended.

INTERACTIONS

DRUG: Alcohol, other CNS depressants (e.g., **LORazepam, morphine, zolpidem**) may increase CNS depression. May decrease concentration/effect of **apixaban, axitinib, dabigatran, dronedarone, itraconazole, ivabradine, nimodipine, rivaroxaban. HERBAL:** Herbals with sedative properties (e.g., **chamomile, kava kava, valerian**) may increase CNS depression. **FOOD:** None known. **LAB VALUES:** May increase serum glucose, GGT, alkaline phosphatase.

AVAILABILITY (Rx)

Injection Solution: 100 mg PE/2 mL, 500 mg PE/10 mL.

ADMINISTRATION/HANDLING
🖐 IV

Reconstitution • Dilute in D_5W or 0.9% NaCl to a concentration ranging from 1.5–25 mg PE/mL.

Rate of administration • Administer at rate less than 150 mg PE/min (decreases risk of hypotension, arrhythmias). **Children:** 2 mg PE/kg/min. **Maximum:** 150 mg PE/min.
Storage • Refrigerate unused vials. • Do not store at room temperature for longer than 48 hrs.

▦ IV INCOMPATIBILITIES
Midazolam.

▦ IV COMPATIBILITIES
Lorazepam, phenobarbital.

INDICATIONS/ROUTES/DOSAGE
◀ALERT▶ 150 mg fosphenytoin yields 100 mg phenytoin. Dosage, concentration solution, infusion rate of fosphenytoin are expressed in terms of phenytoin equivalents (PE).

Status Epilepticus
IV: ADULTS: **Loading dose:** 15–20 mg PE/kg infused at rate of 100–150 mg PE/min. May give an additional 5–10 mg PE/kg 10 min after loading dose. **Maximum total loading dose:** 30 mg PE/kg. **Maintenance dose:** Initially, 4–7 mg PE/kg/day (**usual daily dose:** 300–400 mg PE) given in 2–4 divided doses. ADOLESCENTS, CHILDREN: **Loading dose:** 15–20 mg PE/kg. **Maximum dose:** 1,500 mg PE. **Maintenance dose:** 2–4 mg PE/kg given 12 hrs after loading dose, then q12h (4–8 mg PE/kg/day in divided doses).

Short-Term Substitution for Oral Phenytoin
IV, IM: ADULTS: May substitute for oral phenytoin at same total daily dose.

Dosage in Renal/Hepatic Impairment
No dose adjustment.

SIDE EFFECTS
Frequent: Dizziness, paresthesia, tinnitus, pruritus, headache, drowsiness. **Occasional:** Morbilliform rash.

ADVERSE EFFECTS/TOXIC REACTIONS
Toxic fosphenytoin serum concentration may produce ataxia (muscular

incoordination), nystagmus (rhythmic oscillation of eyes), diplopia, lethargy, slurred speech, nausea, vomiting, hypotension. As drug level increases, extreme lethargy may progress to coma.

NURSING CONSIDERATIONS

BASELINE ASSESSMENT
Review history of seizure disorder (intensity, frequency, duration, LOC). Initiate seizure precautions. Obtain vital signs, medication history (esp. use of phenytoin, other anticonvulsants). Observe clinically.

INTERVENTION/EVALUATION
Monitor ECG, cardiac function, respiratory function, B/P during and immediately following infusion (10–20 min). Discontinue if skin rash appears. Interrupt or decrease rate if hypotension, arrhythmias occur. Monitor free and total Dilantin levels (2 hrs after IV infusion or 4 hrs after IM injection).

PATIENT/FAMILY TEACHING
• If noncompliance is cause of acute seizures, discuss and address reasons for noncompliance. • Avoid tasks that require alertness, motor skills until response to drug is established.

frovatriptan

froe-va-**trip**-tan
(Frova)

◆**CLASSIFICATION**

PHARMACOTHERAPEUTIC: Serotonin 5-HT$_1$ receptor agonist. **CLINICAL:** Antimigraine.

USES
Acute treatment of migraine headache with or without aura in adults.

PRECAUTIONS
Contraindications: Hypersensitivity to frovatriptan. Management of basilar or hemiplegic migraine, cerebrovascular or peripheral vascular disease, coronary artery disease, ischemic heart disease (angina pectoris, history of MI, silent ischemia, Prinzmetal's angina), severe hepatic impairment (Child-Pugh Grade C), uncontrolled hypertension, use within 24 hrs of ergotamine-containing preparations or another serotonin receptor agonist. **Cautions:** Mild to moderate hepatic impairment, history of seizures or structural brain lesions.

ACTION
Selective agonist for serotonin in cranial arteries causing vasoconstriction and reduction of inflammation. **Therapeutic Effect:** Relieves migraine headache.

PHARMACOKINETICS
Widely distributed. Protein binding: 15%. Metabolized in liver. Eliminated in feces (62%), urine (32%). **Half-life:** 26 hrs (increased in hepatic impairment).

⧗ LIFESPAN CONSIDERATIONS
Pregnancy/Lactation: Unknown if excreted in breast milk. **Children:** Safety and efficacy not established. **Elderly:** Not recommended in this population.

INTERACTIONS
DRUG: May increase concentration effects of **ergot derivatives (e.g., ergonovine, ergotamine, methylergonovine), MAOIs (e.g., phenelzine, selegine), triptans (e.g., sumatriptan).** **HERBAL:** None significant. **FOOD:** None known. **LAB VALUES:** None significant.

AVAILABILITY (Rx)
Tablets: 2.5 mg.

ADMINISTRATION/HANDLING
PO
• Give with fluids as soon as symptoms appear.

INDICATIONS/ROUTES/DOSAGE
Acute Migraine Headache
PO: ADULTS, ELDERLY: Initially, 2.5 mg. If headache improves but then returns,

dose may be repeated after at least 2 hrs. **Maximum:** 5 mg/day.

Dosage in Renal Impairment
No dose adjustment.

Dosage in Hepatic Impairment
Mild to moderate impairment: No dose adjustment. **Severe impairment:** Use caution.

SIDE EFFECTS

Occasional (8%–4%): Dizziness, paresthesia, fatigue, flushing. **Rare (3%–2%):** Hot/cold sensation, dry mouth, dyspepsia.

ADVERSE EFFECTS/TOXIC REACTIONS

Cardiac reactions (ischemia, coronary artery vasospasm, MI), noncardiac vasospasm-related reactions (cerebral hemorrhage, CVA) occur rarely, particularly in pts with hypertension, obesity, smokers, diabetes, strong family history of coronary artery disease; males older than 40 yrs; postmenopausal women.

NURSING CONSIDERATIONS

BASELINE ASSESSMENT

Question history of peripheral vascular disease, renal/hepatic impairment, possibility of pregnancy, cardiac disease. Question regarding onset, location, duration of migraine, possible precipitating factors.

INTERVENTION/EVALUATION

Assess for relief of migraine headache, potential for photophobia, phonophobia (sound sensitivity), nausea, vomiting.

PATIENT/FAMILY TEACHING

• Take a single dose as soon as symptoms of an actual migraine attack appear. • Medication is intended to relieve migraine headaches, not to prevent or reduce number of attacks. • Avoid tasks that require alertness, motor skills until response to drug is established. • Immediately report palpitations, pain, tightness in chest or throat, sudden or severe abdominal pain, pain or weakness of extremities.

fruquintinib

frue-**kwin**-ti-nib
(Fruzaqla)

◆CLASSIFICATION

PHARMACOTHERAPEUTIC: Vascular endothelial growth factor receptor (VEGFR) inhibitor, kinase inhibitor. **CLINICAL:** Antineoplastic.

USES

Treatment of adults with metastatic colorectal cancer (mCRC) who have been previously treated with fluoropyrimidine-, oxaliplatin-, and irinotecan-based chemotherapy, an anti-VEGF therapy, and, if RAS wild-type and medically appropriate, an anti-EGFR therapy.

PRECAUTIONS

Contraindications: Hypersensitivity to fruquintinib. **Cautions:** Baseline cytopenias, hepatic/renal impairment, hypertension; conditions predisposing to infection (e.g., diabetes, renal failure, immunocompromised pts, open wounds); pts at risk for bleeding (e.g., history of intracranial/GI/GU bleeding, coagulation disorders, recent trauma; concomitant use of anticoagulants, antiplatelet medication, chronic NSAIDs); history of arterial thrombosis (e.g., CVA, MI, pulmonary embolism), GI perforation. Hypersensitivity reaction to yellow No. 5 or 6 (food coloring). Avoid concomitant use of strong or moderate CYP3A4 inducers.

ACTION

Inhibits phosphorylation of VEGFR-1, VEGFR-2, and VEGFR-3, preventing angiogenesis and tumor cell proliferation. **Therapeutic Effect:** Inhibits tumor growth.

F

PHARMACOKINETICS

Widely distributed. Metabolized in liver. Protein binding: 95%. Peak plasma concentration: 2 hrs. Steady-state reached in 14 days. Excreted in urine (60%), feces (30%). **Half-life:** 42 hrs.

⧗ LIFESPAN CONSIDERATIONS

Pregnancy/Lactation: Avoid pregnancy; may cause fetal harm. Females and males with female partners of reproductive potential should use effective contraception during treatment and for at least 2 wks after discontinuation. Unknown if distributed in breast milk. Breastfeeding not recommended during treatment and for at least 2 wks after discontinuation. **Children:** Safety and efficacy not established. **Elderly:** No age-related precautions noted.

INTERACTIONS

DRUG: Anticoagulants (e.g., **heparin, warfarin**), antiplatelets (e.g., **aspirin, clopidogrel**), chronic use of NSAIDS (e.g., **diclofenac, meloxicam, naproxen**) may increase risk of bleeding. **Strong CYP3A4 inducers** (e.g., **carBAMazepine, phenytoin, riFAMpin**), moderate CYP3A4 inducers (e.g., **dexamethasone, modafinil, nafcillin**) may decrease concentration/effect. **HERBAL:** Herbals with anticoagulant/antiplatelet properties (e.g., **dong quai, feverfew garlic, ginger, ginko biloba, white willow**) may increase risk of bleeding. **St. John's wort** may decrease concentration/effect. **FOOD:** None known. **LAB VALUES:** May increase serum alkaline phosphatase, ALT, AST, bilirubin, creatinine, glucose, uric acid. May decrease Hgb, lymphocytes, platelets; serum calcium, magnesium, potassium, sodium. May increase activated partial thromboplastin time (aPTT).

AVAILABILITY (Rx)

Capsules: 1 mg, 5 mg.

ADMINISTRATION/HANDLING

PO

• Give without regard to food. • Administer capsule whole; do not break, cut, or open. Capsule cannot be chewed. • If a dose is missed by more than 12 hrs, skip the dose and resume at the next regularly scheduled time. • If vomiting occurs after administration, do not readminister dose; give next dose at the regularly scheduled time (do not give an additional dose).

INDICATIONS/ROUTES/DOSAGE

Colorectal Cancer (Metastatic)

PO: **ADULTS:** 5 mg once daily for the first 21 days of each 28-day cycle. Continue until disease progression or unacceptable toxicity.

Dose Reduction Schedule for Adverse Events

First dose reduction: 4 mg once daily. **Second dose reduction:** 3 mg once daily. **Unable to tolerate 3 mg dose:** Permanently discontinue.

Dose Modification

Based on Common Terminology Criteria for Adverse Events (CTCAE).

Hepatotoxicity

Serum ALT/AST greater than 3 times upper limit of normal (ULN) with total bilirubin less than or equal to 2 times ULN: Withhold treatment until improved to grade 1 or baseline, then resume at reduced dose. **Permanent discontinuation:** Permanently discontinue treatment in pts with serum ALT/AST greater than 3 times ULN with total bilirubin greater than 2 times ULN (with cholestasis or hemolysis); serum ALT/AST greater than 20 times ULN; bilirubin greater than 10 times ULN.

Hemorrhagic Events

Grade 2 hemorrhage: Withhold treatment until improved to grade 1 or bleeding has fully resolved, then resume at reduced dose. **Grade 3 or 4 hemorrhage:** Permanently discontinue.

Hypertension

Grade 3 hypertension (despite optimal **hypertensive therapy):** Withhold treatment until improved to grade 1 or 0, then resume at reduced dose. **Grade 4 hypertension:** Permanently discontinue.

Palmar-Plantar Erythrodysesthesia Syndrome (PPES)

Grade 2 PPES: Withhold treatment until improved to grade 1 or 0, then resume at same dose. **Grade 3 PPES:** Withhold treatment until improved to grade 1 or 0, then resume at reduced dose.

Proteinuria

Urine protein level greater than 2 g/24 hrs: Withhold treatment until urine protein level is less than 1 g/24 hrs or fully resolved, then resume at reduced dose. **Nephrotic syndrome; urine protein that does not improve to less than 1 g/24 hrs:** Permanently discontinue.

Other Adverse Reactions

Any other grade 3 adverse reaction: Withhold treatment until improved to grade 1, then resume at reduced dose. **Any other grade 4 adverse reaction:** Discontinue treatment. If adverse reaction is not life-threatening and fully resolves or improves to grade 1, may consider resuming treatment at reduced dose based on clinical judgement.

Dosage in Renal Impairment

Mild to moderate impairment: No dose adjustment. **Severe impairment:** Not specified; use caution.

Dosage in Hepatic Impairment

Mild impairment: No dose adjustment. **Moderate impairment:** Not specified; use caution. **Severe impairment:** Treatment not recommended.

SIDE EFFECTS

Frequent (61%–21%): Hypertension, dysphonia, stomatitis, abdominal pain, diarrhea, fatigue, musculoskeletal pain, decreased appetite. **Occasional (15%–10%):** Back pain, arthralgia, throat pain.

ADVERSE EFFECTS/TOXIC REACTIONS

Myelosuppression (anemia, lymphopenia, thrombocytopenia) is an expected response to therapy. Severe hypertension, hypertensive crisis may occur. Hypertension reported in 49% of pts with median onset occurring 14 days after initiation. Hypertensive crisis reported in less than 1% of pts. May increase risk of arterial thromboembolic events. Severe, sometimes fatal, hemorrhagic events may occur. GI bleeding reported in 6% of pts. May cause impaired wound healing or wound dehiscence requiring medical intervention. Proteinuria may indicate acute renal injury or nephrotic syndrome. GI perforation reported in 1% of pts. Infections including respiratory tract infection, pneumonia, bacterial infection, sepsis were reported. Reversible posterior leukoencephalopathy syndrome (RPLS), a dysfunction of the brain that may evolve into an ischemic CVA or cerebral hemorrhage, may occur. Palmar-plantar erythrodysesthesia syndrome (PPES), a chemotherapy-induced skin condition that presents with skin redness, swelling, numbness, sloughing of the hands and feet may occur. Elevated hepatic enzymes (transaminitis) reported in up to 48% of pts. Coloring of capsules (yellow No. 5 or 6) may cause hypersensitivity reactions. Other adverse reactions may include fistula formation, hypothyroidism, intestinal obstruction, rash.

NURSING CONSIDERATIONS

BASELINE ASSESSMENT

Obtain CBC, BMP, LFT, thyroid panel, vital signs; pregnancy test in females of reproductive potential. Question for recent surgeries, dental procedures. Question history of thromboembolism (CVA, MI, pulmonary embolism), hypertension, hemorrhagic events, hypersensitivity to yellow No. 5 or 6. Verify baseline hypertension is adequately controlled prior to initiation. Screen for active infection. Receive full medication history and screen for interactions. Assess skin for open wounds, lesions, surgical incisions. Consider withholding treatment prior to elective surgery or after major surgery until wound is fully healed. Offer emotional support.

INTERVENTION/EVALUATION

Monitor CBC for myelosuppression (bleeding, bruising, dyspnea, fever, petechiae, weakness); LFT for hepatotoxicity (bruising, jaundice, right upper abdominal pain, nausea, vomiting, weight loss); thyroid panel, vital signs as clinically indicated. Persistent diastolic hypertension may indicate hypertensive crisis. If urine dipstick is greater than or equal to 2+, obtain 24 hr urine protein test. Monitor for decreased urine output, renal dysfunction, nephrotic syndrome. Due to risk for arterial occlusions, monitor for MI (chest pain, diaphoresis, left arm/jaw pain, increased serum troponin, ST segment elevation), CVA (altered mental status, aphasia, facial droop, hemiparesis, seizures, loss of vision), pulmonary embolism (chest pain, dyspnea, hypoxia, tachycardia). Monitor for hemorrhagic events including intracranial hemorrhage (altered mental status, aphasia, facial droop, hemiparesis, unequal pupils, seizures, loss of vision), GI/GU bleeding (hematemesis, melena, rectal bleeding), epistaxis; bleeding of any kind. RPLS should be considered in pts with altered mental status, confusion, headache, seizures, visual disturbances. Assess skin for impaired wound healing, rash; symptoms of PPES. Report abdominal pain, fever, hemoptysis, melena, (may indicate GI perforation/fistula formation). Monitor daily pattern of bowel activity,

stool consistency. Monitor for infections (cough, fatigue, fever), UTI (dysuria, fever, flank pain, malaise).

PATIENT/FAMILY TEACHING

• Treatment may depress your immune system response and reduce your ability to fight infection. Report symptoms of infection such as body aches, chills, cough, fatigue, fever. Avoid those with active infection. • Life-threatening arterial blood clots may occur; report symptoms of heart attack (chest pain, difficulty breathing, jaw pain, nausea, pain that radiates to the left arm, sweating), stroke (blindness, confusion, facial paralysis, one-sided weakness, loss of consciousness, trouble speaking, seizures), lung embolism (difficulty breathing, chest pain, rapid heart rate). • Life-threatening bleeding may occur; report bloody stool, urine; rectal bleeding, nosebleeds, vomiting up blood. • Treatment may cause or worsen high blood pressure. Blurry vision, confusion, chest pain, headache, seizures may indicate life-threatening high blood pressure crisis. • Report liver problems (abdominal pain, bruising, clay-colored stool, amber or dark colored urine, yellowing of the skin or eyes); thyroid dysfunction (fatigue, goiter, weight gain), kidney problems (decreased urine output, flank pain, darkened urine), toxic skin reactions (sloughing, rash, redness, swelling; poor healing of wounds). • Nervous system changes including altered mental status, seizures, headache, blurry vision, high blood pressure, trouble speaking, one-sided weakness may indicate life threatening brain dysfunction/swelling that can lead to stroke. • Use effective contraception to avoid pregnancy. Do not breastfeed. • Do not take newly prescribed medications unless approved by prescriber who originally started treatment. • Notify physician before any planned surgeries/dental procedures.

furosemide

HIGH ALERT

fur-**oh**-se-myde
(Apo-Furosemide , Furoscix, Lasix)

■ **BLACK BOX ALERT** ■ Large doses can lead to profound diuresis with water and electrolyte depletion. **Do not confuse furosemide with famotidine, finasteride, fluconazole, FLUoxetine, loperamide, or torsemide, or Lasix with Lidex, Lovenox, Luvox, or Luxiq.**

◆CLASSIFICATION

PHARMACOTHERAPEUTIC: Loop diuretic. **CLINICAL:** Diuretic. Antihypertensive.

USES

Treatment of edema associated with heart failure (HF), cirrhosis of liver (e.g., ascites), renal disease (e.g., nephrotic syndrome), acute pulmonary edema (PE). **Furoscix:** At home treatment of congestion due to fluid overload in NYHA Class II/III chronic HF.

PRECAUTIONS

Contraindications: Hypersensitivity to furosemide. Anuria. **Cautions:** Hepatic cirrhosis, hepatic coma, severe electrolyte depletion, systemic lupus erythematosus, prostatic hyperplasia/urinary stricture.

ACTION

Inhibits reabsorption of sodium, chloride in ascending loop of Henle and proximal/distal renal tubules. **Therapeutic Effect:** Increases excretion of water, sodium, chloride, magnesium, calcium.

PHARMACOKINETICS

Route	Onset	Peak	Duration
PO	30–60 min	1–2 hrs	6–8 hrs
IV	5 min	20–60 min	2 hrs
IM	30 min	N/A	N/A

Moderately absorbed from GI tract. Protein binding: greater than 98%. Partially metabolized in liver. Primarily excreted in urine (nonrenal clearance increases in severe renal impairment). Not removed by hemodialysis. **Half-life:** 30–90 min (increased in renal/hepatic impairment, neonates).

⧗ LIFESPAN CONSIDERATIONS

Pregnancy/Lactation: Crosses placenta. Distributed in breast milk. **Children:** Half-life increased in neonates; may require increased dosage interval. **Elderly:** May be more sensitive to hypotensive, electrolyte effects, developing circulatory collapse, thromboembolic effect. Age-related renal impairment may require dosage adjustment.

INTERACTIONS

DRUG: Bile acid sequestrants (e.g., cholestyramine), sucralfate may decrease absorption/effect. May increase hyponatremic effect of **desmopressin.** May increase QT interval–prolonging effect of **dofetilide.** May increase concentration/effects of **aminoglycosides (e.g., gentamicin, tobramycin), iodinated contrast agents, lithium. Hypokalemia-causing medications (e.g., HCTZ, laxatives)** may increase risk of hypokalemia. **HERBAL: Herbals with hypertensive properties (e.g., licorice, yohimbe)** or **hypotensive properties (e.g., garlic, ginger, ginkgo biloba)** may alter effects. **FOOD:** None known. **LAB VALUES:** May increase serum glucose, BUN, uric acid. May decrease serum calcium, chloride, magnesium, potassium, sodium.

AVAILABILITY (Rx)

Injection Solution: 10 mg/mL (2 mL, 4 mL, 10 mL). *(Furoscix):* 80 mg/10 mL in single dose prefilled cartridge for use only with co-packaged, single-use on-body infusor. **Oral Solution:** 10 mg/mL, 40 mg/5 mL. **Tablets:** 20 mg, 40 mg, 80 mg.

F

ADMINISTRATION/HANDLING

IV

Rate of administration • May give undiluted but is compatible with D$_5$W or 0.9% NaCl. • May be diluted for infusion to 1–2 mg/mL (**Maximum:** 10 mg/mL). • Administer each 40 mg or fraction by IV push over 1–2 min. Do not exceed administration rate of 4 mg/min for short-term intermittent infusion.

Storage • Solution appears clear, colorless. • Discard yellow solutions. • Stable for 24 hrs at room temperature when mixed with 0.9% NaCl or D$_5$W.

IM
• Temporary pain at injection site may be noted.

PO
• Administer without regard to food.

⬛ IV INCOMPATIBILITIES

Diltiazem, vasopressin.

⬛ IV COMPATIBILITIES

Bumetanide, dexmedetomidine, heparin, ibuprofen, norepinephrine, potassium chloride.

INDICATIONS/ROUTES/DOSAGE

Edema
PO: ADULTS, ELDERLY: Initially, 20–40 mg once, then titrate as needed. **Maximum effective single dose:** 80–200 mg. **Maximum recommended total daily dose:** 600 mg. **INFANTS, CHILDREN, ADOLESCENTS:** Initially, 2 mg/kg/dose. May increase by 1–2 mg/kg/dose at 6–8 hr intervals. **Maximum:** 6 mg/kg/day (not to exceed maximum adult dose of 600 mg/day). **NEONATES:** 1 mg/kg/dose 1–2 times/day. **Range:** 0.5–2 mg/kg/dose.

IV: ADULTS, ELDERLY: 20–40 mg once, then titrate as needed. **Maximum effective dose:** 80–200 mg. **Maximum recommended total daily dose:** 600 mg. **INFANTS, CHILDREN, ADOLESCENTS:** Initially, 0.5–2 mg/kg/dose. May increase by 1 mg/kg/dose no sooner than 2 hrs after previous dose. **Maximum:** 6 mg/kg/dose. (Not to exceed maximum adult dose of 200 mg/dose.) **NEONATES:** 1 mg/kg/dose 1–2 times/day. **Range:** 0.5–2 mg/kg/dose.

IV infusion: ADULTS, ELDERLY: (bolus dose): 1–2.5 times total daily maintenance dose and begin initial infusion rate of 5 mg/hr; repeat loading dose before increasing infusion rate. **Maximum:** 40 mg/hr. **CHILDREN:** Bolus loading dose of 0.1–2 mg/kg, then initial infusion rate of 0.05–0.4 mg/kg/hr; titrate to desired effect. **NEONATES: Bolus dose:** 1–2 mg/kg then initial infusion rate of 0.1–0.2 mg/kg/hr. May increase by 0.1 mg/kg/hr q12–24h. **Maximum:** 0.4 mg/kg/hr.

SQ infusion: ADULTS, ELDERLY: On-body infusor delivers 30 mg over 1st hr, then 12.5 mg/hr for subsequent 4 hrs.

Dosage in Renal Impairment
Avoid use in oliguric states.

Dosage in Hepatic Impairment
No dose adjustment. Decreased effect, increased sensitivity to hypokalemia/volume depletion in cirrhosis.

SIDE EFFECTS

Expected: Increased urinary frequency/volume. **Frequent:** Nausea, dyspepsia, abdominal cramps, diarrhea or constipation, electrolyte disturbances. **Occasional:** Dizziness, light-headedness, headache, blurred vision, paresthesia, photosensitivity, rash, fatigue, bladder spasm, restlessness, diaphoresis. **Rare:** Flank pain.

ADVERSE EFFECTS/TOXIC REACTIONS

Vigorous diuresis may lead to profound water loss/electrolyte depletion, resulting in hypokalemia, hyponatremia, dehydration. Sudden volume depletion may result in increased risk of thrombosis, circulatory collapse, sudden death. Acute hypotensive episodes may occur, sometimes several days after beginning therapy. Ototoxicity (deafness, vertigo, tinnitus) may occur, esp. in pts with severe renal impairment. Can exacerbate diabetes mellitus, systemic lupus erythematosus, gout, pancreatitis. Blood dyscrasias have been reported.

NURSING CONSIDERATIONS

BASELINE ASSESSMENT
Check vital signs, esp. B/P, pulse, for hypotension before administration. Assess renal function, serum electrolytes, esp. serum sodium, potassium. Assess skin turgor, mucous membranes for hydration status; observe for edema. Obtain baseline weight. Initiate I&O monitoring. Auscultate lung sounds. In pts with hepatic cirrhosis and ascites, consider giving initial doses in a hospital setting.

INTERVENTION/EVALUATION
Monitor B/P, vital signs, serum electrolytes, I&O, weight. Monitor urine output. Watch for symptoms of electrolyte imbalance: Hypokalemia may result in changes in muscle strength, tremor, muscle cramps, altered mental status, cardiac arrhythmias; hyponatremia may result in confusion, thirst, cold/clammy skin. Consider potassium supplementation if hypokalemia occurs.

PATIENT/FAMILY TEACHING
• Expect increased frequency, volume of urination. • Report palpitations, signs of electrolyte imbalances (noted previously), hearing abnormalities (sense of fullness in ears, tinnitus). • Eat foods high in potassium such as whole grains (cereals), legumes, meat, bananas, apricots, orange juice, potatoes (white, sweet), raisins. • Avoid sunlight, sunlamps.

F

gabapentin

ga-ba-**pen**-tin
(Gralise, Horizant, <u>Neurontin</u>)
**Do not confuse Neurontin with
Motrin, Neoral, nitrofurantoin,
Noroxin, or Zarontin.**

G

◆CLASSIFICATION

PHARMACOTHERAPEUTIC: Gamma-
aminobutyric acid analogue. **CLINI-
CAL:** Anticonvulsant, antineuralgic.

USES

Neurontin: Adjunct in treatment of focal
(partial) seizures (with or without secondary
generalized seizures) in children 3 yrs and
older and adults. Management of postherpetic
neuralgia (PHN). **Horizant:** Treatment of
moderate to severe primary restless legs syndrome (RLS), PHN. **Gralise:** Management of
PHN. **OFF-LABEL:** Treatment of alcohol use
disorder, alcohol withdrawal, fibromyalgia,
generalized anxiety disorder (GAD), seasonal
anxiety disorder (SAD), vasomotor symptoms
associated with menopause. Cough (chronic),
hiccups, pruritus (chronic)

PRECAUTIONS

Contraindications: Hypersensitivity to gabapentin. **Cautions:** Severe renal impairment, elderly, history of suicidal behavior; substance abuse. Risk of respiratory
depression in pts with respiratory risk
factors (e.g., COPD, elderly).

ACTION

Binds to gabapentin binding sites in brain
and may modulate release of excitatory
neurotransmitters, which participate in
epileptogenesis and nociception. **Therapeutic Effect:** Reduces seizure activity,
neuropathic pain.

PHARMACOKINETICS

Widely distributed. Protein binding: less
than 5%. Crosses blood-brain barrier. Primarily excreted unchanged in urine. Removed by hemodialysis. **Half-life:** 5–7 hrs
(increased in renal impairment, elderly).

⧖ LIFESPAN CONSIDERATIONS

Pregnancy/Lactation: Crosses placenta,
excreted in breast milk. **Children:** Safety
and efficacy not established in pts 3 yrs and
younger. **Elderly:** Age-related renal impairment may require dosage adjustment.
May increase risk of respiratory depression.

INTERACTIONS

**DRUG: Alcohol, other CNS depres-
sants (e.g., LORazepam, oxyCO-
DONE, zolpidem)** may increase CNS
depression. **HERBAL: Herbals with
sedative properties (e.g., chamomile, kava kava, valerian)** may increase CNS depression. **FOOD:** None
known. **LAB VALUES:** May alter serum
glucose; WBC. May increase serum alkaline phosphatase, ALT, AST, bilirubin.

AVAILABILITY (Rx)

Capsules: 100 mg, 300 mg, 400 mg. **Oral
Solution:** 250 mg/5 mL. **Tablets:** 600 mg,
800 mg. **Tablets: *(Gralise):*** 300 mg, 600 mg.

🖏 **Tablets: *(Extended-Release [Horizant]):***
300 mg, 600 mg.

ADMINISTRATION/HANDLING

PO

Immediate-release/solution • Give
without regard to food • Give first dose
on first day at bedtime (avoids somnolence, dizziness) • Capsules may be
opened and sprinkled on food. **Extended-
Release** • Administer with evening meal.
Administer tablet whole. Do not cut, crush,
divide, allow chewing of tablet.

INDICATIONS/ROUTES/DOSAGE

Note: When given 3 times/day, maximum time between doses should not exceed 12 hrs. If treatment is discontinued
or anticonvulsant therapy is added, do so
gradually over at least 1 wk (reduces risk
of loss of seizure control).

Adjunctive Therapy for Seizure Control
**PO: ADULTS, ELDERLY, CHILDREN 12 YRS AND
OLDER: *(Immediate-Release):*** Initially, 300 mg
3 times/day. May titrate up to 600 mg 3 times/
day. **CHILDREN 3–11 YRS:** Initially, 10–15 mg/

kg/day in 3 divided doses. May titrate up to 25–35 mg/kg/day (for children 5–11 yrs) and 40 mg/kg/day (for children 3–4 yrs).

Adjunctive Therapy for Neuropathic Pain
PO: ADULTS, ELDERLY: *(Immediate-Release):* Initially, 100–300 mg 1–3 times/day. May increase up to 1,200 mg 3 times/day. *(Extended-Release):* Initially, 300 mg at bedtime. May increase up to target dose of 900–3,600 mg once daily.

Postherpetic Neuralgia
PO: ADULTS, ELDERLY: *(Immediate-Release):* 300 mg once on day 1, 300 mg twice daily on day 2, and 300 mg 3 times/day on day 3 as needed. **Range:** up to 1,800 mg/day. *(Extended-Release) (Gralise):* 300 mg once on day 1; 600 mg once on day 3, then daily thereafter. May further decrease as needed up to 1,800 mg once daily. *(Horizant):* 600 mg once daily in AM for 3 days, then increase to 600 mg twice daily.

RLS
PO: ADULTS, ELDERLY: *(Horizant):* 300–600 mg once daily at about 5 PM.

Dosage in Renal Impairment
Dosage and frequency are modified based on creatinine clearance.

Creatinine Clearance	Neurontin Dosage (Immediate-Release)	Gralise Dosage (Extended-Release)	Horizant Dosage	
			RLS	**PHN**
30–59 mL/min	200–700 mg q12h	600–1,800 mg once/day	300–600 mg/day	Same
16–29 mL/min	200–700 mg once daily	Not recommended	300 mg/day	Same
Less than 16 mL/min	100–300 mg once daily	Not recommended	300 mg q48h	Same
Hemodialysis	125–350 mg following HD	Not recommended	Not recommended	300–600 mg following HD

Dosage in Hepatic Impairment
No dose adjustment.

SIDE EFFECTS
Frequent (19%–10%): Fatigue, drowsiness, dizziness, ataxia. **Occasional (8%–3%):** Nystagmus, tremor, diplopia, rhinitis, weight gain, peripheral edema. **Rare (less than 2%):** Anxiety, dysarthria, memory loss, dyspepsia, pharyngitis, myalgia.

ADVERSE EFFECTS/TOXIC REACTIONS
Abrupt withdrawal may increase seizure frequency, increase risk of suicidal behavior/thoughts. Overdosage may result in slurred speech, drowsiness, lethargy, diarrhea. Drug reaction with eosinophilia and systemic symptoms (multiorgan hypersensitivity) was reported. Hypersensitivity reaction, including anaphylaxis and angioedema, can occur at any time.

NURSING CONSIDERATIONS

BASELINE ASSESSMENT
Review history of seizure disorder (type, onset, intensity, frequency, duration, LOC). Assess location, intensity of neuralgia/neuropathic pain. Question history of renal impairment.

INTERVENTION/EVALUATION
Provide safety measures as needed. Monitor seizure frequency/duration, renal function, weight, behavior in children. Monitor for signs/symptoms of depression, suicidal ideation and behavior; hypersensitivity reaction.

PATIENT/FAMILY TEACHING
• Do not abruptly stop taking drug (may increase seizure frequency). • Avoid

G

tasks that require alertness, motor skills until response to drug is established. • Avoid alcohol. • Report suicidal ideation, depression, unusual behavioral changes (esp. with changes in dosage), worsening of seizure activity or loss of seizure control. • Seek medical attention for allergic reactions including difficulty breathing, coughing, wheezing, throat tightness, swelling of face or tongue.

galantamine

gal-**an**-ta-meen
(Razadyne ER)
Do not confuse Razadyne with Rozerem.

◆CLASSIFICATION

PHARMACOTHERAPEUTIC: Acetylcholinesterase inhibitor (central). **CLINICAL:** Antidementia.

USES

Treatment of mild to moderate dementia of Alzheimer's type. **OFF-LABEL:** Alzheimer's disease (severe), dementia with Lewy bodies and Parkinson disease. Vascular dementia.

PRECAUTIONS

Contraindications: Hypersensitivity to galantamine. **Cautions:** Moderate renal/hepatic impairment (not recommended in severe impairment), history of ulcer disease, asthma, COPD, bladder outflow obstruction, supraventricular cardiac conduction conditions (except with pacemaker), seizure disorder, concurrent medications that slow cardiac conduction through SA or AV node. Elderly with low body weight and/or serious comorbidities.

ACTION

Elevates acetylcholine concentrations in cerebral cortex by slowing degeneration of acetylcholine released by still intact cholinergic neurons. May increase serotonin/glutamate levels. **Therapeutic Effect:** Slows progression of Alzheimer's disease.

PHARMACOKINETICS

Widely distributed. Protein binding: 18%. Distributed to blood cells; binds to plasma proteins, mainly albumin. Metabolized in liver. Excreted in urine. **Half-life:** 7 hrs.

⌛ LIFESPAN CONSIDERATIONS

Pregnancy/Lactation: Unknown if crosses placenta or is distributed in breast milk. **Children:** Not indicated in children. **Elderly:** No age-related precautions noted, but use is not recommended in pts with severe hepatic/renal impairment (CrCl less than 9 mL/min).

INTERACTIONS

DRUG: Anticholinergic agents (e.g., hyoscyamine, glycopyrrolate) may decrease levels/effects. **Strong CYP3A4 inhibitors (e.g., clarithromycin, ketoconazole, ritonavir)** may increase concentration/effect. May increase bradycardiac effect of **beta blockers (e.g., carvedilol, metoprolol). HERBAL:** None significant. **FOOD:** None known. **LAB VALUES:** None significant.

AVAILABILITY (Rx)

Oral Solution: 4 mg/mL. **Tablets:** 4 mg, 8 mg, 12 mg.

Capsules: *(Extended-Release)*: 8 mg, 16 mg, 24 mg.

ADMINISTRATION/HANDLING

PO
• **Immediate-release:** Give tablet or solution with morning and evening meals. • Mix oral solution with nonalcoholic beverage, take immediately. • **Extended Release:** Capsule etc Give with breakfast. Swallow whole. Do not break, crush, cut, or divide.

INDICATIONS/ROUTES/DOSAGE

Note: If therapy interrupted for 3 or more days, restart at lowest dose; then increase gradually.

Alzheimer's Disease

PO: *(Immediate-Release Tablets, Oral Solution):* **ADULTS, ELDERLY:** Initially, 4 mg twice daily (8 mg/day). After a minimum of 4 wks (if well tolerated), may increase to 8 mg twice daily (16 mg/day). After another 4 wks, may increase to 12 mg twice daily (24 mg/day). **Range:** 16–24 mg/day in 2 divided doses.

PO: *(Extended-Release):* **ADULTS, ELDERLY:** Initially, 8 mg once daily for 4 wks; then increase to 16 mg once daily for 4 wks or longer. If tolerated, may increase to 24 mg once daily. Range: 16–24 mg once daily.

Dosage in Renal/Hepatic Impairment

Moderate impairment: Maximum dosage is 16 mg/day. **Severe impairment:** Not recommended.

SIDE EFFECTS

Frequent (17%–7%): Nausea, vomiting, diarrhea, anorexia, weight loss. **Occasional (5%–4%):** Abdominal pain, insomnia, depression, headache, dizziness, fatigue, rhinitis. **Rare (less than 3%):** Tremors, constipation, confusion, cough, anxiety, urinary incontinence.

ADVERSE EFFECTS/TOXIC REACTIONS

Overdose may cause cholinergic crisis (increased salivation, lacrimation, urination, defecation, bradycardia, hypotension, muscle weakness). Treatment aimed at generally supportive measures, use of anticholinergics (e.g., atropine). Toxic skin reactions including Stevens-Johnson syndrome, acute generalized exanthematous pustulosis, erythema multiforme were reported. Vagotonic effects may cause bradycardia, heart block.

NURSING CONSIDERATIONS

BASELINE ASSESSMENT

Assess cognitive, behavioral, functional deficits of pt. Obtain baseline serum renal function, LFT. Question history as listed in Precautions, esp. cardiac conduction disorders.

INTERVENTION/EVALUATION

Monitor cognitive, behavioral, functional status of pt. Evaluate ECG, periodic rhythm strips in pts with underlying arrhythmias. Assess for evidence of GI disturbances (nausea, vomiting, diarrhea, anorexia, weight loss). Monitor for toxic skin reactions; cardiac effects (bradycardia).

PATIENT/FAMILY TEACHING

• Take with meals (reduces risk of nausea). • Avoid tasks that require alertness, motor skills until response to drug is established. • Report persistent GI disturbances, excessive salivation, diaphoresis, excessive tearing, excessive fatigue, insomnia, depression, dizziness, increased muscle weakness, palpitations.

gefitinib

ge-fi-ti-nib
(Iressa)
Do not confuse gefitinib with erlotinib, dasatinib, imatinib, or lapatinib.

◆CLASSIFICATION

PHARMACOTHERAPEUTIC: Epidermal growth factor receptor (EGFR) inhibitor. Tyrosine kinase inhibitor. **CLINICAL:** Antineoplastic.

G

USES

First-line treatment of metastatic non–small-cell lung cancer (NSCLC) whose tumors have epidermal growth factor receptor (EGFR) exon 19 deletions or exon 21 substitution mutations.

PRECAUTIONS

Contraindications: Hypersensitivity to gefitinib. **Cautions:** Hepatic impairment, pts at risk for interstitial lung disease (e.g., COPD, sarcoidosis, connective disease); pts at risk for GI perforation (e.g., Crohn's disease, diverticulitis, GI tract or abdominal malignancies, GI ulcers). Ocular disease, concurrent administration of CYP3A4 inducers and inhibitors.

ACTION

Reversibly inhibits epidermal growth factor receptor–tyrosine kinase (EGFR-TK), a key driver in tumor cell growth. EGFR is expressed on cell surfaces of cancer cells. **Therapeutic Effect:** Inhibits tumor cell proliferation and growth.

PHARMACOKINETICS

Widely distributed. Peak plasma levels in 3–7 hrs. Protein binding: 90%. Metabolized in liver. Excreted primarily in feces (86%). **Half-life:** 48 hrs.

⌛ LIFESPAN CONSIDERATIONS

Pregnancy/Lactation: Avoid pregnancy. Use effective contraception during treatment and for at least 2 wks after discontinuation. Unknown if crosses placenta or distributed in breast milk. **Children:** Safety and efficacy not established. **Elderly:** No age-related precautions noted.

INTERACTIONS

DRUG: **CYP3A4 inhibitors (e.g., clarithromycin, ketoconazole, ritonavir)** may increase concentration. **CYP3A4 inducers (e.g., carBAMazepine, phenytoin, rifAMPin)** may decrease concentration. **H$_2$ antagonists (e.g., famotidine), proton pump inhibitors (e.g., pantoprazole)** may decrease concentration. May increase bleeding risk with **warfarin. Antacids** may decrease concentration/effect. **HERBAL:** None significant. **FOOD: Grapefruit products** may increase concentration/adverse effects. **LAB VALUES:** May increase serum AST, ALT, bilirubin, urine protein.

AVAILABILITY (Rx)

Tablets: 250 mg.

ADMINISTRATION/HANDLING

• May give without regard to food. • Avoid grapefruit products. • Do not crush or cut. • Administer whole or dispersed in water. Gently swirl glass for up to 20 min and immediately ingest once dispersed. • If a dose is missed, administer as soon as possible. Do not give a missed dose within 12 hrs of next dose.

INDICATIONS/ROUTES/DOSAGE

NSCLC
PO: ADULTS, ELDERLY: 250 mg once daily. Continue until disease progression or unacceptable toxicity.

Dose Modification
Hepatotoxicity
Withhold treatment for worsening of hepatic function. Consider discontinuation in pts who develop severe hepatic impairment.

Severe or Persistent Diarrhea
Withhold treatment in pts with severe or persistent (up to 14 days) diarrhea.

Ocular Toxicities
Withhold treatment or discontinue treatment in pts with severe or worsening ocular toxicities.

Permanent Discontinuation
Permanently discontinue in pts with confirmed interstitial lung disease, GI perforation.

Concomitant Use of CYP3A4 Inducers
Consider increasing dose to 500 mg once daily if use of CYP3A4 is unavoidable. If CYP3A4 inducer is discontinued, reduce dose to 250 mg 7 days after discontinuation.

Dosage in Renal Impairment
No dose adjustment.

Dosage in Hepatic Impairment

Mild impairment: No dose adjustment. **Moderate to severe impairment:** Use with caution.

SIDE EFFECTS

Frequent (47%–15%): Skin reactions (e.g., acne, pruritus, rash, xeroderma), diarrhea, decreased appetite, vomiting. **Occasional (7%–5%):** Stomatitis, nail disorders (e.g., infection).

ADVERSE EFFECTS/TOXIC REACTIONS

Interstitial lung disease (ILD)/pneumonitis reported in 1% of pts. Grade 3 or 4 hepatotoxicity reported in 5% of pts. GI perforation reported in less than 1% of pts. Grade 3 or 4 diarrhea reported in 3% of pts. Ocular disorders including aberrant eyelash growth, blepharitis, corneal erosion, dry eye, conjunctivitis may occur. Severe cutaneous reactions, including toxic epidermal necrolysis, Stevens-Johnson syndrome, erythema multiforme, were reported. Hemorrhagic events, including epistaxis, hematuria, reported in 4% of pts. Hypersensitivity reactions, including angioedema, may occur.

NURSING CONSIDERATIONS

BASELINE ASSESSMENT

Obtain LFT; pregnancy test in females of reproductive potential. Verify EGRF mutation serostatus. Question history of hepatic impairment, pulmonary disease. Assess risk of GI perforation. Receive full medication history and screen for interactions. Assess usual bowel movement patterns, stool characteristics. Offer emotional support.

INTERVENTION/EVALUATION

Periodically monitor LFT for hepatotoxicity (bruising, jaundice, right upper abdominal pain, nausea, vomiting, weight loss). Consider ABG, radiologic test if ILD/pneumonitis (excessive cough, dyspnea, fever, hypoxia) is suspected. Consider treatment with corticosteroids if ILD/pneumonitis is confirmed. Monitor for symptoms of GI perforation (abdominal pain, fever, melena, hematemesis).

Consider referral to ophthalmologic if ocular toxicities occur. Assess skin for cutaneous reactions, skin toxicities. Monitor daily pattern of bowel activity, stool consistency; I&O, hydration status.

PATIENT/FAMILY TEACHING

• Report liver problems (abdominal pain, bruising, clay-colored stool, amber or dark-colored urine, yellowing of the skin or eyes); symptoms of lung inflammation (excessive cough, difficulty breathing, chest pain); toxic skin reactions (itching, peeling, rash, redness, swelling). • Treatment may cause severe diarrhea, which may require antidiarrheal medication. Report worsening of diarrhea or dehydration. • Drink plenty of fluids. • Allergic reactions, including swelling of face, lips, tongue, may occur. If allergic reaction occurs, seek immediate medical attention. • Treatment may cause severe rashes, peeling, or blistering of the skin. • Severe, persistent diarrhea may cause dehydration. Drink plenty of fluids. • Use effective contraception to avoid pregnancy. Do not breastfeed. • Do not take newly prescribed medications unless approved by prescriber who originally started treatment. Do not ingest grapefruit products.

gemcitabine

jem-**sye**-ta-been
(Infugem)
Do not confuse gemcitabine with gemtuzumab.

◆CLASSIFICATION

PHARMACOTHERAPEUTIC: Antimetabolite. **CLINICAL:** Antineoplastic.

USES

Breast cancer: First-line treatment of metastatic breast cancer in combination with PACLitaxel after failure of adjuvant chemotherapy. **Pancreatic cancer:** Treatment of locally ad-

G

vanced (stage II, III) or metastatic (stage IV) adenocarcinoma of pancreas. **Non–small-cell lung cancer (NSCLC): First-line treatment:** In combination with CISplatin for inoperable, locally advanced stage IIIA or IIIB or metastatic stage IV NSCLC. **Ovarian cancer:** Treatment of advanced ovarian cancer (in combination with CARBOplatin) that has relapsed at least 6 mos after completion of platinum-based therapy. **OFF-LABEL:** Treatment of biliary tract carcinoma, bladder carcinoma, germ cell tumors (e.g., testicular), Hodgkin's lymphoma, non-Hodgkin's lymphoma, cervical cancer, malignant pleural mesothelioma, sarcomas. Head and neck cancer, pancreatic cancer (adjuvant), renal carcinoma (metastatic), small-cell lung cancer, uterine sarcoma.

PRECAUTIONS

Contraindications: Hypersensitivity to gemcitabine. **Cautions:** Renal/hepatic impairment, baseline cytopenias, elderly, concurrent radiation therapy, impaired pulmonary function.

ACTION

Inhibits ribonucleotide reductase, the enzyme necessary for catalyzing DNA synthesis. Cell-cycle specific for the S-phase. **Therapeutic Effect:** Produces death of cells undergoing DNA synthesis.

PHARMACOKINETICS

Not extensively distributed after IV infusion (increased with length of infusion). Protein binding: less than 10%. Metabolized intracellularly by nucleoside kinases. Excreted primarily in urine. **Half-life:** Influenced by duration of infusion. Infusion 1 hr or less: 42–94 min; infusion 3–4 hrs: 4–10.5 hrs.

⧗ LIFESPAN CONSIDERATIONS

Pregnancy/Lactation: Avoid pregnancy; may cause fetal harm. Females of reproductive potential must use effective contraception during treatment and for at least 6 mos after discontinuation. Breastfeeding not recommended during treatment and for at least 1 wk after discontinuation. **Males:** Males with female partners of reproductive potential must use effective contraception during treatment and for at least 3 mos after last dose. May impair fertility. **Children:** Safety and efficacy not established. **Elderly:** Increased risk of hematologic toxicity.

INTERACTIONS

DRUG: **Bone marrow depressants (e.g., cladribine)** may increase risk of myelosuppression. May increase adverse/toxic effect of **vaccines (live).** May diminish the therapeutic effect of **BCG (intravesical), vaccines (live).** **HERBAL:** **Echinacea** may decrease therapeutic effect. **FOOD:** None known. **LAB VALUES:** May increase serum BUN, alkaline phosphatase, bilirubin, creatinine, ALT, AST. May decrease Hgb, Hct, leukocyte count, platelet count.

AVAILABILITY (Rx)

Injection, Powder for Reconstitution: 200-mg, 1-g, 2-g vials. **Injection, Solution:** 38 mg/mL, 100 mg/mL. **Injection, Premixed Infusion Bags Containing 10 mg/mL of Gemcitabine in 0.9% NaCl:** 1,200 mg in 120 mL, 1,300 mg in 130 mL, 1,400 mg in 140 mL, 1,500 mg in 150 mL, 1,600 mg in 160 mL, 1,700 mg in 170 mL, 1,800 mg in 180 mL, 1,900 mg in 190 mL, 2,000 mg in 200 mL, 2,200 mg in 220 mL.

ADMINISTRATION/HANDLING

 IV

Reconstitution • Use gloves when handling/preparing. • Reconstitute with 0.9% NaCl injection without preservative to provide concentration of 38 mg/mL. • Shake to dissolve. Further diluted with 50–500 mL 0.9% NaCl to a concentration as low as 0.1 mg/mL.
Rate of administration • Infuse over 30 min. • Infusion time greater than 60 min increases toxicity.
Storage • Store at room temperature (refrigeration may cause crystallization). • Reconstituted vials or diluted

---

solutions are stable for 24 hrs at room temperature. Do not refrigerate.

▓ IV INCOMPATIBILITIES

Furosemide.

▓ IV COMPATIBILITIES

Calcium gluconate, granisetron, ondansetron, palonesetron, potassium chloride.

INDICATIONS/ROUTES/DOSAGE

◄**ALERT**► Dosage is individualized based on clinical response, tolerance to adverse effects. When used in combination therapy, consult specific protocols for optimum dosage, sequence of drug administration. See manufacturer guidelines regarding dose modifications.

Breast Cancer (Metastatic)
IV: ADULTS, ELDERLY: (in combination with PACLitaxel): 1,250 mg/m^2 over 30 min on days 1 and 8 of each 21-day cycle. Continue until disease progression or unacceptable toxicity.

Non–Small-Cell Lung Cancer (NSCLC) (Inoperable, Locally Advanced, or Metastatic)
IV: ADULTS, ELDERLY, CHILDREN: (in combination with CISplatin): 1,000 mg/m^2 on days 1, 8, and 15, repeated every 28 days; or 1,250 mg/m^2 on days 1 and 8. Repeat every 21 days.

Ovarian Cancer (Advanced)
IV: ADULTS, ELDERLY: (in combination with CARBOplatin): 1,000 mg/m^2 on days 1 and 8 of each 21-day cycle.

Pancreatic Cancer (Locally Advanced or Metastatic)
IV: ADULTS: 1,000 mg/m^2 once wkly for up to 7 wks (or until toxicity necessitates decreasing dosage or withholding the dose), followed by 1 wk of rest. Subsequent cycles should consist of once-wkly dose for 3 consecutive wks out of every 4 wks (days 1, 8, 15 q28days).

Dosage in Renal/Hepatic Impairment
No dose adjustment.

Dosage Reduction
Pancreatic Cancer, Non–Small-Cell Lung Cancer
Dosage adjustments should be based on granulocyte count and platelet count, as follows:

Absolute Granulocyte Counts (cells/mm^3)	Platelet Count (cells/mm^3)	% of Full Dose
1,000	100,000	100
500–999	50,000–99,000	75
Less than 500 or	Less than 50,000	Hold

Breast Cancer

Absolute Granulocyte Counts (cells/mm^3)	Platelet Count (cells/mm^3)	% of Full Dose
Equal to or greater than 1,200 and	Greater than 75,000	100
1,000–1,199 or	50,000–75,000	75
700–999 and	Equal to or greater than 50,000	50
Less than 700 or	Less than 50,000	Hold

Ovarian Cancer

Absolute Granulocyte Counts (cells/mm^3)	Platelet Count (cells/mm^3)	% of Full Dose
1,500 or greater and	100,000 or greater	100
1,000–1,499 and/or	75,000–99,999	50
Less than 1,000 and/or	Less than 75,000	Hold

SIDE EFFECTS

Frequent (69%–20%): Nausea, vomiting, generalized pain, fever, mild to moderate pruritic rash, mild to moderate dyspnea, constipation, peripheral edema. **Occasional (19%–10%):** Diarrhea, petechiae, alopecia, stomatitis, infection, drowsiness, paresthesia. **Rare:** Diaphoresis, rhinitis, insomnia, malaise.

G

ADVERSE EFFECTS/TOXIC REACTIONS

Myelosuppression (anemia, neutropenia, thrombocytopenia) is an expected response to therapy. Severe, life-threatening toxicity may occur when given during or within 7 days of radiation therapy. Prolongation of infusion time beyond 60 min or doses given more frequently than every wk may increase risk of asthenia, hypotension, severe flu-like symptoms. Pulmonary toxicity including pneumonitis, pulmonary fibrosis, pulmonary edema, acute respiratory distress syndrome (ARDS) was reported. Life-threatening hemolytic uremic syndrome may lead to renal failure, dialysis, and death. Drug-induced hepatic injury, including hepatic failure and death, has occurred. Posterior reversible encephalopathy syndrome, a dysfunction of the brain caused by swelling, may evolve into an ischemic CVA or cerebral hemorrhage. May cause capillary leak syndrome.

NURSING CONSIDERATIONS

BASELINE ASSESSMENT

Obtain CBC, BMP, LFT; pregnancy test in females of reproductive potential. Confirm compliance of effective contraception. Screen for active infection. Drug should be suspended or dosage modified if myelosuppression is detected. Question history of pulmonary disease, hepatic/renal impairment. Offer emotional support.

INTERVENTION/EVALUATION

Monitor CBC with differential prior to each dose; LFT, renal function periodically. An increase of serum creatinine greater than 0.4 mg/dL from baseline may indicate renal impairment. Monitor pulmonary status, pulse oximeter readings. Consider ABG, radiologic test if ILD/pneumonitis (excessive cough, dyspnea, fever, hypoxia) is suspected. Consider treatment with corticosteroids if ILD/pneumonitis is confirmed. Monitor for infections (cough, fatigue, fever). If serious infection occurs, initiate appropriate antimicrobial therapy. Monitor daily pattern of bowel activity,

stool consistency. Assess skin for rash. RPLS should be considered in pts with altered mental status, confusion, headache, seizures, visual disturbances.

PATIENT/FAMILY TEACHING

• Treatment may depress your immune system response and reduce your ability to fight infection. Report symptoms of infection such as body aches, chills, cough, fatigue, fever. Avoid those with active infection. • Report symptoms of lung inflammation (excessive coughing, difficulty breathing, chest pain); liver problems (abdominal pain, bruising, clay-colored stool, amber- or dark-colored urine, yellowing of the skin or eyes), kidney problems (decreased urine output, flank pain, darkened urine). • Therapy may cause kidney failure, requiring treatment with dialysis. • Nervous system changes including confusion, headache, seizures may indicate life-threatening brain dysfunction/swelling. • Use effective contraception to avoid pregnancy. Do not breastfeed.

gentamicin

jen-ta-**mye**-sin

■ **BLACK BOX ALERT** ■ Aminoglycoside antibiotics may cause neurotoxicity, nephrotoxicity. Risk of ototoxicity directly proportional to dosage, duration of treatment; ototoxicity usually is irreversible, precipitated by tinnitus, vertigo. May cause fetal harm if given during pregnancy.

Do not confuse gentamicin with azithromycin, clindamycin, fidaxomicin, plazomicin, tobramycin, or vancomycin.

◆CLASSIFICATION

PHARMACOTHERAPEUTIC: Aminoglycoside. **CLINICAL:** Antibiotic.

USES

Parenteral: Treatment of serious infections including sepsis, meningitis, UTIs, respiratory tract infections, peritonitis, bone infections, skin and soft tissue infections caused by susceptible microorganisms including *P. aeruginosa*, *Proteus* species (indole-positive and indole-negative), *E. coli, Klebsiella-Enterobacter-Serratia* species, *Citrobacter* species, and *Staphylococcus* species (coagulase-positive and coagulase-negative). **Ophthalmic:** Ophthalmic infections caused by susceptible bacteria. **OFF-LABEL:** Surgical (preoperative) prophylaxis, brucellosis, osteomyelitis (prevention), pelvic infections, peritonitis, tularemia.

PRECAUTIONS

Contraindications: Hypersensitivity to gentamicin, other aminoglycosides (cross-sensitivity) or their components. **Cautions:** Elderly, neonates due to renal insufficiency or immaturity, neuromuscular disorders (potential for respiratory depression), vestibular or cochlear impairment, renal impairment, hypocalcemia, myasthenia gravis. Pediatric pts on extracorporeal membrane oxygenation.

ACTION

Interferes with bacterial protein synthesis. Binds to 30S ribosomal subunit, causing a defective cell membrane. **Therapeutic Effect:** Bactericidal.

PHARMACOKINETICS

Rapid, complete absorption after IM administration. Protein binding: Less than 30%. Widely distributed (does not cross blood-brain barrier, low concentrations in CSF). Excreted unchanged in urine. Removed by hemodialysis. **Half-life:** 2–4 hrs (increased in renal impairment, neonates; decreased in cystic fibrosis, burn, or febrile pts).

⏳ LIFESPAN CONSIDERATIONS

Pregnancy/Lactation: Readily crosses placenta; unknown if distributed in breast milk. **Children:** Caution in neonates: Immature renal function increases half-life and toxicity. **Elderly:** Age-related renal impairment may require dosage adjustment.

INTERACTIONS

DRUG: Nephrotoxic (e.g., furosemide, IV contrast dye), ototoxic medications (e.g., CISplatin, cycloSPORINE, foscarnet, furosemide, mannitol) may increase risk of nephrotoxicity, ototoxicity. **HERBAL:** None significant. **FOOD:** None known. **LAB VALUES:** May increase serum BUN, creatinine, bilirubin, LDH, ALT, AST. May decrease serum calcium, magnesium, potassium, sodium. **Therapeutic serum level:** Peak: 4–10 mcg/mL; trough: 0.5–2 mcg/mL. **Toxic serum level:** Peak: Greater than 10 mcg/mL; trough: Greater than 2 mcg/mL.

AVAILABILITY (Rx)

Injection, Infusion: 60 mg/50 mL, 80 mg/50 mL, 80 mg/100 mL, 100 mg/50 mL, 100 mg/100 mL, 120 mg/100 mL. **Injection, Solution:** 10 mg/mL, 40 mg/mL. **Ointment, Ophthalmic:** 0.3%. **Solution, Ophthalmic:** 0.3%.

ADMINISTRATION/HANDLING

 IV

Reconstitution • Dilute with 50–100 mL D$_5$W or 0.9% NaCl. Amount of diluent for infants, children depends on individual needs.
Rate of administration • Infuse over 30–60 min for adults, older children; over 60–120 min for infants, young children.
Storage • Store vials at room temperature. • Solution appears clear or slightly yellow. • Intermittent IV infusion (piggyback) is stable for 48 hrs at room temperature or refrigerated. • Discard if precipitate forms.

IM

• To minimize discomfort, give deep IM slowly. • Less painful if injected into gluteus maximus than lateral aspect of thigh.

Ophthalmic

• Place gloved finger on lower eyelid and pull out until a pocket is formed between eye and lower lid. • Place prescribed number of drops or ointment into pocket.

G

Instruct pt to close eye gently for 1–2 min (so that medication will not be squeezed out of the sac). • **Solution:** Instruct pt to apply digital pressure to lacrimal sac at inner canthus for 1 min to minimize systemic absorption. • **Ointment:** Instruct pt to roll eyeball to increase contact area of drug to eye. • Remove excess solution or ointment around eye with tissue.

 ## IV INCOMPATIBILITIES

Furosemide.

 ## IV COMPATIBILITIES

Amiodarone, dexmedetomidine, diltiazem, insulin, magnesium sulfate, potassium chloride, propofol.

INDICATIONS/ROUTES/DOSAGE

◄**ALERT**► Space parenteral doses evenly around the clock. Peak, trough levels are determined periodically to maintain desired serum concentrations and minimize risk of toxicity. Target peak concentrations based on indication and site of infection (e.g., 4–6 mcg/mL for UTI; 7–10 mcg/mL for serious infection). Trough concentrations should be less than 2 mcg/mL.

Usual Parenteral Dosage

IM, IV: ADULTS, ELDERLY: (Conventional): 3–5 mg/kg/day in divided doses q8h. **(Once daily):** 5–7 mg/kg/dose q24h. **ADOLESCENTS, CHILDREN, INFANTS:** 2–2.5 mg/kg/dose q8h.
Note: Higher doses and different dosing intervals may be required to achieve target concentrations if MIC is 1 mg/L or less.

Gestational Age	Postnatal Age	Dose
<30 wks	≤14 days	5 mg/kg q48h
	≥15 days	5 mg/kg q36h
30–34 wks	≤10 days	5 mg/kg q36h
	11–60 days	5 mg/kg q24h
≥35 wks	≤7 days	4 mg/kg q24h
	8–60 days	5 mg/kg q24h

Hemodialysis (HD)

Note: Administer after HD on dialysis days.
Loading dose: 2–3 mg/kg, then 1 mg/kg q48–72h for mild UTI or synergy (consider redose for pre- or post-HD concentrations less than 1 mg/L); 1–1.5 mg/kg q48–72h for moderate to severe UTI (consider redose for pre-HD concentration less than 1.5–2 mg/L or post-HD concentrations less than 1 mg/L); 1.5–2 mg/kg q48–72h for systemic gram-negative rod infection (consider redose for pre-HD concentration less than 3–5 mg/L or post-HD concentrations less than 2 mg/L).

Continuous Renal Replacement Therapy (CRRT)

Loading dose: 2–3 mg/kg, then 1 mg/kg q24–36h for mild UTI or synergy (redose when concentration less than 1 mg/L); 1–1.5 mg/kg q24–36h for moderate to severe UTI (redose when concentration less than 1.5–2 mg/L); 1.5–2.5 mg/kg q24–48h for systemic gram-negative infection (redose when concentration less than 3–5 mg/L).

Usual Ophthalmic Dosage

Ophthalmic ointment: ADULTS, ELDERLY: Apply 1/2-inch strip to conjunctival sac 2–3 times/day.
Ophthalmic solution: ADULTS, ELDERLY, CHILDREN: 1–2 drops q2–4h up to 2 drops/hr.

Dosage in Renal Impairment

Adults

Creatinine Clearance	Conventional Dosage	Once-Daily Dosage
Greater than 60 mL/mil	q8h	q24h
41–60 mL/min	q12h	q36h
20–40 mL/min	q24h	q48h
Less than 20 mL/min	Loading dose, then monitor levels to determine dosage interval	Monitor levels

Children

Creatinine Clearance	Conventional Dosage
Greater than 50 mL/min	q8h
30–50 mL/min	q12–18h
10–29 mL/min	q18–24h
Less than 10 mL/min	q48–72h

Dosage in Hepatic Impairment
Monitor plasma concentrations.

SIDE EFFECTS

Occasional: IM: Pain, induration at injection site. **IV:** Phlebitis, thrombophlebitis, hypersensitivity reactions (fever, pruritus, rash, urticaria). **Ophthalmic:** Burning, tearing, itching, blurred vision. **Rare:** Alopecia, hypertension, fatigue.

ADVERSE EFFECTS/TOXIC REACTIONS

Nephrotoxicity may be reversible if drug is stopped at first sign of symptoms. Irreversible ototoxicity (tinnitus, dizziness, diminished hearing), neurotoxicity (headache, dizziness, lethargy, tremor, visual disturbances) occur occasionally. Risk increases with higher dosages, prolonged therapy, or if solution is applied directly to mucosa. Superinfections, particularly with fungi, may result from bacterial imbalance via any route of administration. Ophthalmic application may cause paresthesia of conjunctiva, mydriasis.

NURSING CONSIDERATIONS

BASELINE ASSESSMENT

Dehydration must be treated before beginning parenteral therapy. Establish baseline hearing acuity. Question for history of allergies, esp. aminoglycosides, sulfites (parabens for topical/ophthalmic routes). Screen for risk of acute kidney injury, esp. pts at risk for renal failure (baseline renal insufficiency, elderly, HF, hypertension, septic shock).

INTERVENTION/EVALUATION

Monitor I&O (maintain hydration), urinalysis, BUN, creatinine. Be alert to ototoxic, neurotoxic symptoms (see Adverse Effects/ Toxic Reactions). Check IM injection site for induration. Evaluate IV site for phlebitis (heat, pain, red streaking over vein). Assess for rash (**Ophthalmic:** redness, burning, itching, tearing). Be alert for superinfection (genital/anal pruritus, changes in oral mucosa, diarrhea). When treating pts with neuromuscular disorders, assess respiratory response carefully. **Therapeutic serum level:** Peak: 4–10 mcg/mL; peak levels are 2–3 times greater with once-daily dosing; trough: 0.5–2 mcg/mL. **Toxic serum level:** Peak: Greater than 10 mcg/mL; trough: Greater than 2 mcg/mL.

PATIENT/FAMILY TEACHING

• Discomfort may occur with IM injection. • Blurred vision, tearing may occur briefly after each ophthalmic dose. • Report any hearing, visual, balance, urinary problems, even after therapy is completed. • **Ophthalmic:** Report if tearing, redness, irritation continues.

gepirone

je-**pye**-rone
(Exxua)

■ **BLACK BOX ALERT** ■ May increase risk of suicidal thoughts and behavior. Monitor closely for emergence or worsening of symptoms.
Do not confuse gepirone with buspirone or bupropion, or Exxua with Euflexxa.

◆CLASSIFICATION

PHARMACOTHERAPEUTIC: 5-HT1A receptor agonist. **CLINICAL:** Antidepressant.

USES

Treatment of major depressive disorder (MDD) in adults.

PRECAUTIONS

Contraindications: Hypersensitivity to gepirone. Baseline QTc interval greater than 450 msec; severe hepatic impairment; concomitant use of strong CYP3A4 inhibitors, monoamine oxidase inhibitors

(MAOI) or within 14 days of discontinuing MAOI; history of congenital long QT syndrome. **Cautions:** Hepatic/renal impairment; pts at risk for QT interval prolongation or torsades de pointes (e.g., cardiac disease, congenital long QT syndrome, HF, QT interval-prolonging medications, hypokalemia, hypomagnesemia). Concomitant use of strong CYP3A4 inducers, QT interval-prolonging medications, other serotonergic medications. Not recommended in pts with history of bipolar disorder, mania, hypomania.

ACTION

Selective agonist activity at 5-HT1A receptors, modulating serotonergic activity in the central nervous system. **Therapeutic Effect:** Produces antidepressant effect.

PHARMACOKINETICS

Widely distributed. Metabolized in liver. Protein binding: 72%. Peak plasma concentration: 6 hrs. Steady-state reached in 2–4 days. Excreted in urine (81%), feces (13%). **Half-life:** 5 hrs.

⌛ LIFESPAN CONSIDERATIONS

Pregnancy/Lactation: May cause fetal harm. Neonates exposed to serotonergic antidepressants during the third trimester have an increased risk of drug withdrawal syndrome after birth. Unknown if distributed in breast milk. **Children:** Safety and efficacy not established. **Elderly:** Maximum daily dose is reduced due to increased concentration/effect; decreased clearance of drug.

INTERACTIONS

DRUG: MAOIs (e.g., **phenelzine, selegiline**), potent inhibitors of monoamine oxidase (e.g., **linezolid, methylene blue**), SSRIs (e.g., **escitalopram, sertraline**), SNRIs (e.g., **duloxetine, venlafaxine**), tricyclic antidepressants (e.g., **amitriptyline, desipramine, doxepin**) may increase risk of serotonin syndrome. QT interval prolonging medications (e.g., **amiodarone, azithromycin, certinib,**

haloperidol, moxifloxacin, sotalol) may increase risk of QTc interval prolongation, torsades de pointes. **Strong CYP3A4 inhibitors (e.g., clarithromycin, ketoconazole, ritonavir)** may increase concentration/effect; use contraindicated. **Moderate CYP3A4 inhibitors (e.g., dilTIAZem, verapamil)** may increase concentration/effect. **Strong CYP3A4 inducers (e.g., carBAMazepine, phenytoin, riFAMpin)** may decrease concentration/effect. **HERBAL:** St. John's wort may decrease concentration/effect. **FOOD:** None known. **LAB VALUES:** None significant.

AVAILABILITY (Rx)

💊 Tablets, Extended-Release: 18.2 mg, 36.3 mg, 54.5 mg, 72.6 mg.

ADMINISTRATION/HANDLING

PO
• Give with food at the same time each day. • Administer tablet whole; do not break, cut, or dissolve. Tablet cannot be chewed. • Do not give an extra dose if the previous dose was missed.

INDICATIONS/ROUTES/DOSAGE

Major Depressive Disorder
PO: ADULTS: Initially, 18.2 mg once daily. Based on response and tolerability, may increase to 36.3 mg once daily on day 4, then 54.5 mg once daily after day 7, then 72.6 mg once daily after an additional week. **Maximum:** 72.6 mg once daily. **ELDERLY:** Initially, 18.2 mg once daily. Based on response and tolerability, may increase to 36.3 mg once daily after day 7. **Maximum:** 36.3 mg once daily.

Concomitant Use of Moderate CYP3A4 Inhibitor
Note: Concomitant use of a strong CYP3A4 inhibitor is contraindicated. If concomitant use of a moderate CYP3A4 inhibitor is unavoidable, reduce gepirone dose by 50%.

Dosage in Renal Impairment
Creatinine clearance (CrCl) 50 mL/min or greater: No dose adjustment.

CrCl less than 50 mL/min: Initially, 18.2 mg once daily. Based on response and tolerability, may increase to 36.3 mg once daily after day 7. **Maximum:** 36.3 mg once daily.

Dosage in Hepatic Impairment

Mild impairment: No dose adjustment. **Moderate impairment:** Initially, 18.2 mg once daily. Based on response and tolerability, may increase to 36.3 mg once daily after day 7. **Maximum:** 36.3 mg once daily. **Severe impairment:** Contraindicated.

SIDE EFFECTS

Frequent (20%): Headache. **Occasional (14%–7%):** Fatigue, sedation, somnolence, nausea, dizziness, diarrhea. **Rare (5%–1%):** Insomnia, dry mouth, vomiting, abdominal pain, dyspepsia, increased appetite, constipation, nasal congestion, paresthesia, increased weight.

ADVERSE EFFECTS/TOXIC REACTIONS

May increase risk of suicidal ideation and behavior. QTc interval prolongation may increase risk of torsades de pointes. Life-threatening serotonin syndrome may occur when given with concomitant SSRIs, SNRIs, tricyclic antidepressants, or within 14 days of an MAOI. Symptoms of serotonin syndrome include mental status change (agitation, hallucinations, delirium, coma), autonomic instability (tachycardia, labile blood pressure, dizziness, sweating, flushing, hyperthermia), neuromuscular symptoms (tremor, rigidity, myoclonus [localized muscle twitching], hyperactive reflexes, incoordination). May cause hypomania, mania, mixed episodes in pts with history of bipolar disorder. Infections, including upper respiratory tract infection, nasopharyngitis, may occur. Hypersensitivity reactions including pruritus, rash, urticaria were reported. Other reactions may include breast tenderness, confusion, dyspnea, peripheral edema, increased energy, feeling abnormal, hypoesthesia, abnormal thinking.

NURSING CONSIDERATIONS

BASELINE ASSESSMENT

Obtain BMP, serum magnesium; ECG; vital signs. Do not initiate in pts with QTc interval greater than 450 msec at baseline. Question history hepatic/renal impairment, congenital long QT syndrome; bipolar disorder, mania, hypomania; suicidal ideation and behavior. Receive full medication history and screen for interactions (esp. use of MAOIs, serotonergic medications). Assess appearance, behavior, speech pattern, level of interest, mood, sleep pattern. Offer emotional support.

INTERVENTION/EVALUATION

Closely monitor for suicidal ideation and behavior; worsening of depression, mood disorder. Consult mental health professional if worsening of mood disorder is suspected. Monitor for symptoms of QT interval prolongation (chest pain, dizziness, dyspnea, palpitations, syncope). Monitor ECG more frequently in pts taking concomitant QT interval–prolonging medications. Monitor for serotonin syndrome, esp. in pts taking concomitant serotonergic medications. Assess for improvement of depression (improved self-care, social interaction, level of interest, mood; establishment of personal goals).

PATIENT/FAMILY TEACHING

• Seek immediate medical attention if thoughts of suicide, new-onset or worsening of anxiety, depression, or changes in mood occurs. • Report symptoms of serotonin overproduction, including confusion, excessive talking, hallucinations, headache, hyperactivity, insomnia, racing thoughts, seizure activity, tremors; sexual dysfunction, fever. • There is a high risk of interactions with other medications. Do not take newly prescribed medications unless approved by prescriber who originally started treatment. • Treatment may affect the electrical conduction of the heart, which may lead to life-threatening heart arrhythmias; report chest pain, dizziness, fainting, palpitations, shortness of breath. • Avoid tasks that require alertness, motor skills until response to drug is established.

gilteritinib

gil-te-ri-ti-nib
(Xospata)

■ **BLACK BOX ALERT** ■ Life-threatening and/or fatal differentiation syndrome with symptoms including fever, dyspnea, hypoxia, pulmonary infiltrates, pleural or pericardial effusion, rapid weight gain or peripheral edema, hypotension, renal dysfunction may occur. Initiate corticosteroid therapy and hemodynamic monitoring in pts suspected of differentiation syndrome until symptoms resolve.
Do not confuse gilteritinib with gefitinib, Gilotrif, or glasdegib.

◆CLASSIFICATION

PHARMACOTHERAPEUTIC: FMS-like tyrosine kinase 3 (FLT3) inhibitor. Tyrosine kinase inhibitor. **CLINICAL:** Antineoplastic.

USES

Treatment of adults who have relapsed or refractory acute myeloid leukemia (AML) with an FMS-like tyrosine kinase 3 (FLT3) mutation.

PRECAUTIONS

Contraindications: Hypersensitivity to gilteritinib. **Cautions:** Baseline neutropenia, hypotension; active infection, cardiac disease, hepatic/renal impairment, electrolyte imbalance, conditions predisposing to infection (e.g., diabetes, renal failure, immunocompromised pts, open wounds); pts at risk for QTc interval prolongation (congenital long QT syndrome, HF, QT interval–prolonging medications, hypokalemia, hypomagnesemia); concomitant use of P-gp inhibitors, strong CYP3A4 in-

hibitors, strong CYP3A4 inducers; history of GI perforation, pancreatitis.

ACTION

Inhibits multiple tyrosine kinases including FLT3 receptor signaling and proliferation in cells expressing FLT3 mutation. **Therapeutic Effect:** Induces apoptosis in mutant-expressing leukemic cells.

PHARMACOKINETICS

Widely distributed. Metabolized in liver. Protein binding: 94%. Peak plasma concentration: 4–6 hrs. Steady state reached in 15 days. Excreted in feces (65%), urine (16%). **Half-life:** 113 hrs.

⧗ LIFESPAN CONSIDERATIONS

Pregnancy/Lactation: Avoid pregnancy; may cause fetal harm. Females of reproductive potential must use effective contraception during treatment and for at least 6 mos after discontinuation. Unknown if distributed in breast milk. Breastfeeding not recommended during treatment and for at least 2 mos after discontinuation. **Males:** Males with female partners of reproductive potential must use effective contraception during treatment and for at least 4 mos after discontinuation. **Children:** Safety and efficacy not established. **Elderly:** No age-related precautions noted.

INTERACTIONS

DRUG: Strong **CYP3A4 inhibitors (e.g., clarithromycin, ketoconazole)** may increase concentration/effect. **CYP3A4 inducers** used concomitantly with **P-gp inducers, strong CYP3A4 inducers (e.g., carBAMazepine, phenytoin, rifAMPin)** may decrease concentration/effect. **QT interval–prolonging medications (e.g., amiodarone, azithromycin, citalopram, escitalopram, haloperidol, sotalol)** may increase risk of QTc interval prolongation. May decrease therapeutic effect of **selective serotonin receptor inhibitors (SSRIs) (e.g., escitalopram, FLUoxetine, sertraline). HERBAL:** None significant. **FOOD:** High-fat meals may delay absorption. **LAB VALUES:** May increase serum alkaline phosphatase, ALT, AST, creatine kinase, triglycerides. May decrease serum calcium, phosphate, sodium; neutrophils.

AVAILABILITY (Rx)

 Tablets: 40 mg.

ADMINISTRATION/HANDLING

PO
* Give without regard to meals. • Administer whole; do not break, cut, crush, or divide tablets. • Tablets cannot be chewed. • If vomiting occurs after administration, give next dose at regularly scheduled time. • If a dose is missed, administer as soon as possible. • Do not give a missed dose within 12 hrs of next dose.

INDICATIONS/ROUTES/DOSAGE

Acute Myeloid Leukemia
PO: ADULTS: 120 mg once daily for at least 6 mos (in absence of disease progression or unacceptable toxicity). Continue until disease progression or unacceptable toxicity.

Dose Modification
Based on Common Terminology Criteria for Adverse Events (CTCAE).

Differentiation Syndrome
Withhold treatment if symptoms are severe and persist for more than 48 hrs after initiation of corticosteroids. Resume treatment when symptoms improve to Grade 2 or less.

QT Interval Prolongation
QTc interval greater than 500 msec: Withhold treatment until QTc interval returns to within 30 msec of baseline or 480 msec or less, then resume at reduced dose of 80 mg.
QTc interval increased by greater than 30 msec on ECG on day 8 of cycle 1: Confirm with ECG on day 9. If confirmed, consider reducing dose to 80 mg.

Other Adverse Reactions
Any Grade 3 or higher toxicity: Withhold treatment until improved to Grade 1, then resume at reduced dose of 80 mg.

Pancreatitis
Withhold treatment until pancreatitis is resolved, then resume at reduced dose of 80 mg.

Reversible Posterior Leukoencephalopathy Syndrome
Permanently discontinue.

Dosage in Renal/Hepatic Impairment
Mild to moderate impairment: No dose adjustment. **Severe impairment:** Not specified; use caution.

SIDE EFFECTS

Frequent (50%–21%): Myalgia, arthralgia, pain (back, bone, chest, extremity, musculoskeletal, neck), asthenia, fatigue, malaise, fever, mucositis, edema (face, generalized, localized, peripheral), rash, diarrhea, dyspnea, nausea, cough, constipation, eye disorder, headache, dizziness, hypotension, vomiting. **Occasional (18%–11%):** Abdominal pain, neuropathy, insomnia, dysgeusia.

ADVERSE EFFECTS/TOXIC REACTIONS

Life-threatening and/or fatal differentiation syndrome, a condition with rapid proliferation and differentiation of myeloid cells, reported in 3% of pts. Reversible posterior leukoencephalopathy syndrome reported in 1% of pts. QT interval prolongation with QTc interval greater than 500 msec and QTc interval greater than 60 msec from baseline have occurred. Pancreatitis reported in 4% of pts. Other significant adverse effects may include renal impairment (21% of pts), cardiac failure (4% of pts), pericardial effusion (4% of pts), pericarditis (2% of pts), large intestine perforation (1% of pts).

NURSING CONSIDERATIONS

BASELINE ASSESSMENT

Obtain CBC, BMP, LFT, ECG; pregnancy test in female pts of reproductive potential. Replete electrolytes if applicable. Confirm presence of FLT3-positive mutation. Screen for active infection. Confirm compliance of effective contraception. Question history of cardiac/hepatic/renal disease, GI perforation, pancreatitis. Assess risk for QT interval prolongation. Receive full medication history and screen for interactions. Offer emotional support.

INTERVENTION/EVALUATION

Monitor CBC, BMP, LFT, CPK at least wkly for 4 wks, then every other week for 4 wks, then monthly until discontinuation. If QT interval–prolonging medications cannot be withheld, diligently monitor ECG; serum potassium, magnesium for QT interval prolongation, cardiac arrhythmias. An increase of serum creatinine greater than 0.4 mg/dL from baseline may indicate renal impairment. Obtain ECG on days 8 and 15 of cycle 1 and prior to the start of next two subsequent cycles. Monitor B/P for hypotension, esp. in pts taking antihypertensives. Monitor for symptoms of differentiation syndrome (dyspnea, fever hypotension, hypoxia, pulmonary infiltrates, pleural or pericardial effusion, rapid weight gain or peripheral edema, renal dysfunction, or concomitant febrile neutropenic dermatosis). If differentiation syndrome is suspected, initiate corticosteroids and hemodynamic monitoring until symptoms resolve for at least 3 days. Reversible posterior leukoencephalopathy syndrome should be considered in pts with altered mental status, headache, seizures, visual disturbances. Report abdominal pain, fever, melena (may indicate GI perforation). Monitor daily pattern of bowel activity, stool consistency. Assess skin for toxic skin reactions, rash. Monitor for pancreatitis (severe, steady abdominal pain often radiating to the back [with or without vomiting]). Ensure adequate hydration, nutrition.

PATIENT/FAMILY TEACHING

• Treatment may depress your immune system response and reduce your ability to fight infection. Report symptoms of infection such as body aches, chills, cough, fatigue, fever. Avoid those with active infection. • Report symptoms of bone marrow depression such as bruising, fatigue, fever, shortness of breath, weight loss; bleeding easily, bloody urine or stool. • Treatment may cause life-threatening differentiation syndrome as early as 2 days after starting therapy. Report difficulty breathing, fever, low blood pressure, rapid weight gain, swelling of the hands or feet, decreased urine output. • Nervous system changes including confusion, headache, seizures may indicate life-threatening brain dysfunction/swelling. • Use effective contraception to avoid pregnancy. Do not breastfeed. • Report liver problems (abdominal pain, bruising, clay-colored stool, amber- or dark-colored urine, yellowing of the skin or eyes); heart problems (chest tightness, dizziness, fainting, palpitations, shortness of breath skin), kidney problems (decreased urine output, flank pain, darkened urine); toxic skin reactions (rash, skin eruptions). • Persistent, severe abdominal pain that radiates to the back (with or without vomiting) may indicate acute inflammation of the pancreas. • There is a high risk of interactions with other medications. Do not take newly prescribed medications unless approved by prescriber who originally started treatment. • Do not take herbal products or ingest grapefruit products. • Report dizziness, chest pain, fainting, palpitations, shortness of breath); may indicate heart arrhythmia.

glasdegib

glas-**deg**-ib
(Daurismo)

■ **BLACK BOX ALERT** ■ May cause severe birth defects, embryo-fetal death in pregnant females. Obtain pregnancy test in females of reproductive potential prior to

---

initiation. Females of reproductive potential must use effective contraception during treatment and for at least 30 days after discontinuation. Due to potential exposure through semen, males with female partners of reproductive potential or a pregnant partner must use effective contraception (e.g., condoms) during treatment and for at least 30 days after discontinuation despite prior vasectomy.

Do not confuse glasdegib with gefitinib, gilteritinib, sonidegib, or vismodegib.

◆CLASSIFICATION

PHARMACOTHERAPEUTIC: Hedgehog pathway inhibitor. **CLINICAL:** Antineoplastic.

USES

Treatment of newly diagnosed acute myeloid leukemia in adults who are 75 yrs or older or who have comorbidities that preclude use of intensive induction chemotherapy (in combination with low-dose cytarabine).

PRECAUTIONS

◀**ALERT**▶ Do not donate blood products or sperm during treatment and for at least 30 days after discontinuation. **Contraindications:** Hypersensitivity to glasdegib. **Cautions:** Baseline cytopenias; active infection, cardiac disease, hepatic/renal impairment, electrolyte imbalance; conditions predisposing to infection (e.g., diabetes, renal failure, immunocompromised pts, open wounds); pts at risk for QTc interval prolongation, cardiac arrhythmias (congenital long QT syndrome, HF, QT interval–prolonging medications, hypokalemia, hypomagnesemia); concomitant use of anticoagulants, strong CYP3A4 inhibitors, strong CYP3A4 inducers.

ACTION

Blocks translocation of Smoothened (SMO) into cilia, preventing SMO-mediated activation of downstream Hedge-hog targets. **Therapeutic Effect:** Inhibits tumor cell growth and reduces the number of blast cells in marrow.

PHARMACOKINETICS

Widely distributed. Metabolized in liver. Protein binding: 91%. Peak plasma concentration: 1.3–1.8 hrs. Steady state reached in 8 days. Excreted in urine (49%), feces (42%). **Half-life:** 17.4 hrs.

⧖ LIFESPAN CONSIDERATIONS

Pregnancy/Lactation: Avoid pregnancy; may cause fetal harm. Females of reproductive potential must use effective contraception during treatment and for at least 30 days after discontinuation. Unknown if distributed in breast milk. Breastfeeding not recommended during treatment and for at least 30 days after discontinuation. **Males:** May impair fertility. Males with female partners of reproductive potential or a pregnant partner must use effective contraception during treatment and for at least 30 days after discontinuation despite prior vasectomy. **Children:** Safety and efficacy not established. **Elderly:** No age-related precautions noted.

INTERACTIONS

DRUG: Strong CYP3A4 inhibitors (e.g., clarithromycin, ketoconazole) may increase concentration/effect. **Strong CYP3A4 inducers (e.g., carBAMazepine, phenytoin, rifAMPin)** may decrease concentration/effect. **QT interval–prolonging medications (e.g., amiodarone, azithromycin, haloperidol, sotalol)** may increase risk of QT interval prolongation. **HERBAL:** None significant. **FOOD:** None known. **LAB VALUES:** May increase serum alkaline phosphatase, ALT, AST, bilirubin, CPK, creatinine, potassium. May decrease Hgb, neutrophils, platelets; serum calcium, magnesium, phosphate.

AVAILABILITY (Rx)

Tablets: 25 mg, 100 mg.

G

ADMINISTRATION/HANDLING

PO

• Give without regard to meals. • Administer whole; do not break, cut, crush, or divide tablets. • Tablets cannot be chewed. • If vomiting occurs after administration, give next dose at regularly scheduled time. • If a dose is missed, administer as soon as possible. • Do not give a missed dose within 12 hrs of next dose.

INDICATIONS/ROUTES/DOSAGE

Acute Myeloid Leukemia

PO: ADULTS, ELDERLY: 100 mg once daily on days 1–28 (in combination with cytarabine 20 mg SQ twice daily on days 1–10 of each 28-day cycle) for a minimum of 6 cycles. Continue until disease progression or unacceptable toxicity.

Dose Modification

Based on Common Terminology Criteria for Adverse Events (CTCAE).

Neutropenia

Neutrophils less than 500 cells/mm³ for more than 42 days in absence of disease: Permanently discontinue glasdegib and cytarabine.

Nonhematologic Toxicity

Any Grade 3 nonhematologic toxicity: Withhold treatment (including cytarabine) until improved to Grade 1 or 0, then resume at same dose or reduce to 50 mg (resume cytarabine at same dose or reduce to 15 mg or 10 mg). If toxicity recurs, permanently discontinue glasdegib and cytarabine. If recurrent toxicity is only related to glasdegib, then cytarabine may be continued. **Any Grade 4 nonhematologic toxicity:** Permanently discontinue glasdegib and cytarabine.

QT Interval Prolongation (on at least two separate ECGs)

QTc interval 481–500 msec: Assess and replete electrolyte levels. Assess and adjust concomitant use of medications known to cause QTc interval prolongation. When QTc interval prolongation improves to 480 msec or less, monitor ECG at least wkly for 2 wks. **QTc interval greater 500 msec:** Withhold treatment. Assess and replete electrolyte levels. Assess and adjust concomitant use of medications known to cause QTc interval prolongation. When QTc interval returns to within 30 msec of baseline or 480 msec or less, resume at reduced dose of 50 mg. **QTc interval prolongation with life-threatening arrhythmia:** Permanently discontinue.

Thrombocytopenia

Platelets less than 10,000 cells/mm³ for more than 42 days in absence of disease: Permanently discontinue glasdegib and cytarabine.

Dosage in Renal Impairment

Mild to moderate impairment: No dose adjustment. **Severe impairment:** Not specified; use caution.

Dosage in Hepatic Impairment

Mild impairment: No dose adjustment. **Moderate to severe impairment:** Not specified; use caution.

SIDE EFFECTS

Frequent (36%–18%): Fatigue, asthenia, edema, pain (back, bone, chest, musculoskeletal, neck), myalgia, arthralgia, nausea, dyspnea, mucositis, decreased appetite, dysgeusia, rash, constipation, pyrexia, diarrhea, cough, vomiting, dizziness. **Occasional (15%–12%):** Muscle spasm, headache, toothache, alopecia.

ADVERSE EFFECTS/TOXIC REACTIONS

Myelosuppression (anemia, neutropenia, thrombocytopenia) is an expected response to therapy. Cardiac arrhythmias including atrial fibrillation, ventricular fibrillation, ventricular tachycardia may occur. QT interval prolongation with QTc interval greater than 500 msec (5% of pts) and QTc interval greater than 60 msec from baseline (4% of pts) have occurred. Bleeding events including disseminated intravascular coagulation, epistaxis, hemoptysis, hemorrhage (cerebral, eye, conjunctival, GI, retinal, tracheal), thrombotic thrombocytopenic purpura, subdural hematoma reported in 30% of pts. Febrile neutropenia reported in 31% of pts. Renal insufficiency including acute kidney injury, oliguria, renal failure reported in 19% of pts. Infections including pneumonia (19% of pts), sepsis (7% of pts) may occurred.

NURSING CONSIDERATIONS

BASELINE ASSESSMENT

Obtain CBC, BMP, LFT, ECG; pregnancy test in female pts of reproductive potential. Replete electrolytes if applicable. Screen for active infection. Confirm compliance of effective contraception. Receive full medication history and screen for interactions. Assess risk for QT interval prolongation. Question history of cardiac/pulmonary/renal disease, cardiac arrhythmias. Offer emotional support.

INTERVENTION/EVALUATION

Monitor CBC, BMP, LFT at least wkly for 1 mo, then monitor electrolytes, BUN, serum creatinine, GFR, CrCl monthly thereafter. An increase of serum creatinine greater than 0.4 mg/dL from baseline may indicate renal impairment. Obtain ECG approx. 1 wk after initiation, then monthly for 2 mos (or more frequently if indicated). If QT interval–prolonging medications cannot be withheld, diligently monitor ECG; serum potassium, magnesium for QT interval prolongation, cardiac arrhythmias. Obtain CK level if muscle aches or spasms occur. Serum CK level elevations usually occur before muscle symptoms are reported. Diligently monitor for infections, febrile neutropenia. Monitor for bleeding events of any kind; symptoms of intracranial bleeding (aphasia, blindness, confusion, facial droop, hemiplegia, seizures). Assess skin for toxic skin reactions, rash.

PATIENT/FAMILY TEACHING

• Treatment may depress your immune system response and reduce your ability to fight infection. Report symptoms of infection such as body aches, chills, cough, fatigue, fever. Avoid those with active infection. • Report symptoms of bone marrow depression such as bruising, fatigue, fever, shortness of breath, weight loss; bleeding easily, bloody urine or stool. • Do not donate blood or blood products during treatment and for at least 30 days after last dose. • Treatment may cause muscle damage, which may lead to kidney failure. Report musculoskeletal symptoms such as muscle pain/spasms/tenderness/weakness. • Report liver problems (abdominal pain, bruising, clay-colored stool, amber- or dark-colored urine, yellowing of the skin or eyes), hemorrhagic stroke (confusion, difficulty speaking, one-sided weakness or paralysis, loss of vision), kidney problems (decreased urine output, flank pain, darkened urine), skin reactions (rash, skin eruptions), bleeding of any kind. • Report dizziness, chest pain, fainting, palpitations, shortness of breath); may indicate heart arrhythmia. • Use effective contraception to avoid pregnancy. Do not breastfeed. • There is a high risk of interactions with other medications. Do not take newly prescribed medications unless approved by prescriber who originally started treatment. • Avoid grapefruit products, herbal supplements (esp. St. John's wort).

---

glatiramer TOP 100

gla-**tir**-a-mer
(Copaxone, Glatopa, Glatect)
Do not confuse Copaxone with Compazine.

◆CLASSIFICATION

PHARMACOTHERAPEUTIC: Immunosuppressive. **CLINICAL:** Neurologic agent for multiple sclerosis.

G

USES

Treatment of relapsing forms of multiple sclerosis (MS), including clinically isolated syndrome, relapsing-remitting disease, and active secondary progressive disease, in adults.

PRECAUTIONS

Contraindications: Hypersensitivity to glatiramer, mannitol. **Cautions:** Pts exhibiting immediate postinjection reaction (flushing, chest pain, palpitations, anxiety, dyspnea, urticaria); conditions predisposing to infection (e.g., diabetes, renal failure, immunocompromised pts, open wounds); history of chronic opportunistic infections (esp. fungal/viral infections, tuberculosis).

ACTION

Induces/activates T-lymphocyte suppressor cells specific to myelin antigens. May also interfere with the antigen-presenting function of immune cells. **Therapeutic Effect:** Slows progression of multiple sclerosis.

PHARMACOKINETICS

Substantial fraction of glatiramer is hydrolyzed locally. Some fraction of injected material enters lymphatic circulation, reaching regional lymph nodes; some may enter systemic circulation intact.

⌛ LIFESPAN CONSIDERATIONS

Pregnancy/Lactation: Unknown if distributed in breast milk. **Children/ Elderly:** Safety and efficacy not established.

INTERACTIONS

DRUG: None significant. **HERBAL:** None significant. **FOOD:** None known. **LAB VALUES:** None significant.

AVAILABILITY (Rx)

Injection Solution: *(Copaxone, Glatopa):* 20 mg/mL in prefilled syringes, 40 mg/ mL in prefilled syringes.

ADMINISTRATION/HANDLING

SQ

Preparation • If refrigerated, allow solution to warm to room temperature (approx. 20 min) with needle cap intact. • Visually inspect for particulate matter or discoloration. Solution should appear clear, colorless to slightly yellow in color. Do not use if solution is cloudy, discolored, or visible particles are observed.
Administration • Insert needle subcutaneously into upper arm, outer thigh, hip, or abdomen and inject solution. • Do not inject into areas of active skin disease or injury such as sunburns, skin rashes, inflammation, skin infections, or active psoriasis. • Rotate injection sites. • Do not administer IV or intramuscularly.
Storage • Refrigerate prefilled syringes in original carton until time of use. • Protect from intense light. • Do not freeze or expose to heating sources. • May store at room temperature for 30 days.

INDICATIONS/ROUTES/DOSAGE

Multiple Sclerosis
Note: Dose forms 20 mg/mL and 40 mg/ mL are not interchangeable.
SQ: ADULTS, ELDERLY: 20 mg once daily or 40 mg 3 times/wk at least 48 hrs apart.

Dosage in Renal/Hepatic Impairment
No dose adjustment.

SIDE EFFECTS

Expected (73%–40%): Pain, erythema, inflammation, pruritus at injection site, asthenia. **Frequent (27%–18%):** Arthralgia, vasodilation, anxiety, hypertonia, nausea, transient chest pain, dyspnea, flu-like symptoms, rash, pruritus. **Occasional (17%–10%):** Palpitations, back pain, diaphoresis, rhinitis, diarrhea, urinary urgency. **Rare (less than 9%):** Anorexia, fever, neck pain, peripheral edema, ear pain, facial edema, vertigo, vomiting.

ADVERSE EFFECTS/TOXIC REACTIONS

Immediate postinjection reactions including anxiety, chest pain, dyspnea, flushing, palpitations, tachycardia, throat constriction may occur. Transient chest pain (not associated with immediate postinjection reactions) have occurred. Localized lipoatrophy, skin necrosis reported in 2% of pts. Severe hepatic injury, hepatic failure may occur.

NURSING CONSIDERATIONS

BASELINE ASSESSMENT

Assess baseline symptoms of MS (e.g., bladder/bowel dysfunction, cognitive impairment, depression, dysphagia, fatigue, gait disorder, numbness/tingling, pain, seizures, spasticity, tremors, weakness). Screen for active infection.

INTERVENTION/EVALUATION

Monitor LFT as clinically indicated. Monitor for immediate postreaction symptoms; injection site reactions, necrosis. Conduct neurologic assessment. Assess for symptomatic improvement of MS.

PATIENT/FAMILY TEACHING

• A healthcare provider will show you how to properly prepare and inject your medication. You must demonstrate correct preparation and injection techniques before using medication at home.
• Treatment may depress your immune system and reduce your ability to fight infection. Report symptoms of infection such as body aches, burning with urination, chills, cough, fatigue, fever. Avoid those with active infection. • Report travel plans to possible endemic areas. • Report liver problems (abdominal pain, bruising, clay-colored stool, amber- or dark-colored urine, yellowing of the skin or eyes). • Immediate injections reactions such as anxiety, chest pain, difficulty breathing, fast heart rate, flushing, palpitations, throat constriction may occur.

glecaprevir/ pibrentasvir

glec-**a**-pre-vir/pi-**brent**-as-vir (Mavyret)

■ **BLACK BOX ALERT** ■ Test all pts for hepatitis B virus (HBV) infection before initiation. HBV reactivation was reported in HCV/HBV co-infected pts who were undergoing or had completed treatment with HCV direct-acting antivirals and were not receiving HBV antiviral therapy. HBV reactivation may cause fulminant hepatitis, hepatic failure, and death.

Do not confuse glecaprevir with boceprevir, grazoprevir, fosamprenavir, paritaprevir, simeprevir, telaprevir, or voxilaprevir, or pibrentasvir with daclatasvir, ledipasvir, ombitasvir, or velpatasvir.

FIXED-COMBINATION(S)

Mavyret: glecaprevir/pibrentasvir: 100 mg/40 mg.

◆CLASSIFICATION

PHARMACOTHERAPEUTIC: NS3/4A protease inhibitor, NS5A protein inhibitor. **CLINICAL:** Antihepaciviral.

USES

Treatment of adults and children 3 yrs and older with chronic hepatitis C virus (HCV) genotype 1, 2, 3, 4, 5, or 6 infection without cirrhosis or with compensated cirrhosis (Child-Pugh A). Treatment of adults and pediatric pts 3 yrs and older with HCV genotype 1 infection who have previously been treated with an HCV regimen containing an NS5A inhibitor or an NS5A protease inhibitor, but not both.

PRECAUTIONS

Contraindications: Hypersensitivity to glecaprevir, pibrentasvir. Concomitant

G

G

use with atazanavir, rifAMPin. Severe hepatic impairment. **Cautions:** HIV infection, hepatic disease unrelated to HCV infection, HBV infection. Concomitant use of P-gp substrates or inhibitors, BCRP substrates, CYP3A4 inducers. Not recommended in pts with moderate hepatic impairment.

ACTION

Glecaprevir inhibits NS3/4A protease, necessary for proteolytic cleavage of HCV-encoded polyprotein. Pibrentasvir inhibits the HCV NS5A protein, essential for viral replication. **Therapeutic Effect:** Inhibits viral replication of HCV.

PHARMACOKINETICS

Widely distributed. Glecaprevir metabolized in liver. Pibrentasvir metabolism not specified. Protein binding: (glecaprevir): 98%; (pibrentasvir): greater than 99%. Peak plasma concentration: 5 hrs. Glecaprevir excreted in feces (92%), urine (1%). Pibrentasvir primarily excreted in feces (97%). **Half-life:** (glecaprevir): 6 hrs; (pibrentasvir): 13 hrs.

⏳ LIFESPAN CONSIDERATIONS

Pregnancy/Lactation: Unknown if distributed in breast milk. **Children:** Safety and efficacy not established in pts younger than 3 yrs. **Elderly:** No age-related precautions noted.

INTERACTIONS

DRUG: Atazanavir, cycloSPORINE, darunavir may increase concentration of glecaprevir/pibrentasvir. Glecaprevir/pibrentasvir may increase concentration of **afatinib, atorvastatin, digoxin, lovastatin, simvastatin, topotecan, venetoclax, voxilaprevir.** CYP3A4 inducers (e.g., carBAMazepine, phenytoin, rifAMPin) may decrease concentration/effect. **Ethinyl estradiol–containing hormonal contraceptives** may increase risk of hepatotoxicity. **HERBAL:** St. John's wort may decrease concentration/effect. **FOOD:** None known. **LAB VALUES:** May increase serum bilirubin.

AVAILABILITY (Rx)

Fixed-Dose Combination Tablets: glecaprevir/pibrentasvir: 100 mg/40 mg. **Oral Pellets:** glecaprevir/pibrentasvir 50 mg/20 mg.

ADMINISTRATION/HANDLING

PO
• Give with food. • If dose is missed, administer as soon as possible if no more than 18 hrs have passed since the last dose. If more than 18 hrs have passed, skip the missed dose and administer the next dose at regularly scheduled time. • **Oral pellets:** Give pellets together, with food, once daily. Open packets and mix with a small amount of food (e.g., peanut butter, cream cheese) and give within 15 min. Do not dissolve in food or allow chewing.

INDICATIONS/ROUTES/DOSAGE

Hepatitis C Virus Infection
PO: ADULTS, ELDERLY, CHILDREN 12 YRS AND OLDER, 3 YRS AND OLDER (WEIGHING 45 KG OR MORE): 3 tablets once daily (total dose: glecaprevir 300 mg and pibrentasvir 120 mg). **30–44 KG:** 250 mg/100 mg (five 50 mg/20 mg packets of oral pellets) once daily; **20–29 KG:** 200 mg/80 mg (four 50 mg/20 mg packets of oral pellets) once daily; **Less than 20 KG:** 150 mg/60 mg (three 50 mg/20 mg packets of oral pellets) once daily.

Treatment Regimen and Duration
Treatment-Naive HCV Genotype 1, 2, 3, 4, 5, or 6
Without cirrhosis: glecaprevir/pibrentasvir for 8 wks. **With compensated cirrhosis:** glecaprevir/pibrentasvir for 8 wks.

Treatment-Experienced Genotype 1
Prior treatment with NS5A inhibitor (without NS3/4A protease inhibitor) without cirrhosis or with compensated cirrhosis: glecaprevir/pibrentasvir for 16 wks. Prior treatment with NS3/4A protease inhibitor (without NS5A inhibitor) without cirrhosis or with compensated cirrhosis: glecaprevir/pibrentasvir for 12 wks. Prior treat-

ment with peginterferon, ribavirin, sofosbuvir without cirrhosis: glecaprevir/pibrentasvir for 8 wks. **Prior treatment with peginterferon, ribavirin, sofosbuvir with compensated cirrhosis:** glecaprevir/pibrentasvir for 12 wks.

Treatment-Experienced Genotype 2, 4, 5, or 6
Prior treatment with peginterferon, ribavirin, sofosbuvir without cirrhosis: glecaprevir/pibrentasvir for 8 wks. **Prior treatment with peginterferon, ribavirin, sofosbuvir with compensated cirrhosis:** glecaprevir/pibrentasvir for 12 wks.

Treatment-Experienced Genotype 3
Prior treatment with peginterferon, ribavirin, sofosbuvir without cirrhosis or with compensated cirrhosis: glecaprevir/pibrentasvir for 16 wks.

Liver/Kidney Transplant Recipients
Recommend glecaprevir/pibrentasvir for 12 wks. A treatment duration of 16 wks is recommended in pts with HCV genotype 1 who are treatment-experienced (prior treatment with NS5A inhibitor [without NS3/4A protease inhibitor]) or in pts with HCV genotype 3 who are treatment-experienced (prior treatment with peginterferon, ribavirin, sofosbuvir).

Dosage in Renal Impairment
No dose adjustment.

Dosage in Hepatic Impairment
Mild impairment: No dose adjustment. **Moderate impairment:** Not recommended. **Severe impairment:** Contraindicated.

SIDE EFFECTS

Frequent (16%–11%): Headache, fatigue. **Occasional (9%–7%):** Nausea, diarrhea, pruritus.

ADVERSE EFFECTS/TOXIC REACTIONS

HBV reactivation was reported in pts co-infected with HBV/HVC. HBV reactivation may result in fulminant hepatitis, hepatic failure, death.

NURSING CONSIDERATIONS

BASELINE ASSESSMENT

Obtain LFT, HCV-RNA level. Confirm hepatitis C virus genotype. Test all pts for hepatitis B virus infection. Initiate anti-HBV therapy if warranted. Question history of hepatic disease unrelated to HCV infection, HIV infection; liver/kidney transplantation; concomitant use of other antiretroviral therapy. Receive full medication history and screen for interactions (esp. atazanavir, rifAMPin).

INTERVENTION/EVALUATION

Periodically monitor HCV-RNA level for treatment effectiveness (or upon completion of treatment). Closely monitor for exacerbation of hepatitis or HBV reactivation. Monitor for rhabdomyolysis (muscle weakness, myalgia, myopathy, decreased urinary output) in pts taking HMG-CoA reductase inhibitors.

PATIENT/FAMILY TEACHING

• Take with food. • There is a high risk of drug interactions with other medications. Do not take newly prescribed medications unless approved by prescriber who originally started treatment. Do not take herbal products. • Pts taking statins (lipid medication) may have an increased risk of rhabdomyolysis, a breakdown of muscle tissue that can cause kidney failure. Report flank pain, muscle pain, darkened urine, decreased urinary output. • Ethinyl estradiol–containing hormonal contraceptives may increase risk of liver injury and are not recommended.

golimumab

goe-**lim**-ue-mab
(Simponi, Simponi Aria)

■ **BLACK BOX ALERT** ■ Tuberculosis (TB), invasive fungal infections, other opportunistic infections reported. Discontinue treatment if active infection or sepsis occurs. Test for TB prior to and during treatment, regardless of initial result; if positive, start treatment for TB prior to initiating therapy. Lymphoma, other malignancies reported in pts treated with tumor necrosis factor blockers.

Do not confuse Simponi (SQ) with Simponi Aria (IV)

◆**CLASSIFICATION**

PHARMACOTHERAPEUTIC: Monoclonal antibody. Tumor necrosis factor (TNF) blocking agent. **CLINICAL:** Antipsoriatic agent, antirheumatic, disease-modifying agent.

USES

Simponi: Treatment of adults with active ankylosing spondylitis. Treatment of adults with active psoriatic arthritis (alone or in combination with methotrexate). Treatment of adults with moderate to severe active rheumatoid arthritis (in combination with methotrexate). Treatment of moderate to severe active ulcerative colitis in adults with corticosteroid dependence or are refractory/intolerant to other therapies. **Simponi Aria:** Treatment of adults with active ankylosing spondylitis. Treatment of active psoriatic arthritis in pts 2 yrs of age and older. Treatment of active polyarticular juvenile idiopathic arthritis in pts 2 yrs of age and older. Treatment of adults with moderate to severe active rheumatoid arthritis (in combination with methotrexate). Axial spondyloarthritis (active, nonradiographic).

PRECAUTIONS

Contraindications: Hypersensitivity to golimumab. **Cautions:** Elderly, concomitant immunosuppressants, comorbid conditions predisposing to infections (e.g., diabetes). Residence or travel from areas of endemic mycosis; tuberculosis, underlying hematologic disorders, preexisting or recent-onset demyelinating disorders (e.g., multiple sclerosis, polyneuropathy), pts with HF or decreased left ventricular function. Avoid concomitant use with live vaccines, abatacept, or anakinra (increased incidence of serious infections). Do not start during an active infection.

ACTION

Binds specifically to tumor necrosis factor (TNF) alpha, blocking its interaction with cell surface TNF receptors. **Therapeutic Effect:** Alters biologic activity of TNF alpha, reduces inflammation, may alter pathophysiology of rheumatoid arthritis.

PHARMACOKINETICS

Steady state reached by wk 12. Elimination pathway not specified. **Half-life:** 12–14 days.

⧖ LIFESPAN CONSIDERATIONS

Pregnancy/Lactation: Unknown if distributed in breast milk. Must either discontinue drug or discontinue breastfeeding. **Children:** Safety and efficacy not established. **Elderly:** May have increased risk of serious infections, malignancy.

INTERACTIONS

DRUG: Anakinra, anti-TNF agents, pimecrolimus, tacrolimus (topical), tocilizumab may increase adverse effects. May decrease concentration/therapeutic effect of **BCG (intravesical). Vaccines (live)** may alter concentration/effect. May increase levels, adverse effects of **natalizumab. HERBAL: Echinacea** may decrease therapeutic effect. **FOOD:** None known. **LAB VALUES:** May increase ALT, AST. May decrease Hgb, leukocytes, neutrophils, platelets.

AVAILABILITY (Rx)

Injection Solution: *(Simponi):* 50 mg/0.5 mL, 100 mg/mL in single-dose prefilled autoinjector or prefilled syringe. **Injection Solution:** *(Simponi Aria):* 50 mg/4 mL per single-use vial (12.5 mg/mL).

ADMINISTRATION/HANDLING

Simponi SQ

• Remove prefilled syringe or autoinjector from refrigerator. Allow to sit at room temperature for 30 min; do not warm in any other way. • Avoid areas where skin is scarred, tender, bruised, red, scaly, hard. Recommended injection site is front of middle thighs, although lower abdomen 2 inches below navel or outer, upper arms are acceptable. • Inject within 5 min after cap has been removed.

Autoinjector
• Push open end of autoinjector firmly against skin at 90-degree angle. • Do not pull autoinjector away from skin until a first "click" sound is heard and then a second "click" sound (injection is finished and needle is pulled back). This usually takes 3 to 6 sec but may take up to 15 sec for the second "click" to be heard. If autoinjector is pulled away from skin before injection is completed, full dose may not be administered.

Prefilled Syringe
• Gently pinch skin and hold firmly. Use a quick, dart-like motion to insert needle into pinched skin at a 45-degree angle.
Storage • Refrigerate; do not freeze. • Solution appears slightly opalescent, colorless to light yellow. Discard if cloudy or contains particulate.

Simponi Aria
 ◄ALERT► Use in-line 0.22-micron filter.

IV

Reconstitution • Calculate dosage and number of vials needed based on pt weight. • Visually inspect for particulate matter. • Dilute in 100 mL 0.9% NaCl. • Prior to mixing, withdraw and discard volume of 0.9% NaCl equal to the volume of patient-dosed solution. • Slowly inject solution into bag and gently mix. • Do not shake.
Rate of administration • Infuse over 30 min using an in-line low protein-binding 0.22-micron filter.
Storage • Refrigerate vials, prefilled syringes • Vial solution should be colorless to light yellow and opalescent. • It is normal for solution to develop fine translucent particles since drug is a protein. • Do not use if opaque particles, discoloration, or other foreign particles are present. • May store diluted solution at room temperature up to 4 hrs.

⊞ IV INCOMPATIBILITIES
Do not infuse concomitantly with other drugs.

INDICATIONS/ROUTES/DOSAGE

Active Psoriatic Arthritis
SQ: *(Simponi):* ADULTS, ELDERLY: 50 mg once monthly (alone or in combination with methotrexate or other nonbiologic DMARD).
IV infusion: *(Simponi Aria):* ADULTS, ELDERLY: 2 mg/kg at wk 0, 4 then q8wks thereafter. CHILDREN 2 YRS OF AGE OR OLDER, ADOLESCENTS: 80 mg/m²/dose at wks 0, 4, then q8wks thereafter.

Moderate to Severe Active Rheumatoid Arthritis (With Methotrexate)
SQ: *(Simponi):* ADULTS, ELDERLY: 50 mg once monthly (in combination with methotrexate).
IV infusion: *(Simponi Aria):* ADULTS, ELDERLY: 2 mg/kg at wk 0 and wk 4. Then decrease frequency to q8wks (in combination with methotrexate).

Active Ankylosing Spondylitis
SQ: *(Simponi):* ADULTS, ELDERLY: 50 mg once monthly (may be given with or without methotrexate or other nonbiologic DMARD).
IV infusion: *(Simponi Aria):* ADULTS, ELDERLY: 2 mg/kg at wk 0, 4 then q8wks thereafter.

Ulcerative Colitis
SQ: *(Simponi):* ADULTS, ELDERLY: Initially, 200 mg, then 100 mg 2 wks later, and then 100 mg q4wks thereafter.

Polyarticular Juvenile Idiopathic Arthritis
IV: *(Simponi Aria):* CHILDREN 2 YRS OF AGE OR OLDER, ADOLESCENTS: 80 mg/m²/dose at wks 0, 4, then q8wks thereafter.

Dosage in Renal/Hepatic Impairment
No dose adjustment.

SIDE EFFECTS
Frequent (13%): Laryngitis, nasopharyngitis, pharyngitis, rhinitis, upper re-

G

 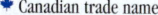

spiratory tract infection. **Occasional (3%–2%):** Bronchitis, hypertension, rash, pyrexia. **Rare (less than 1%):** Dizziness, paresthesia, constipation.

ADVERSE EFFECTS/TOXIC REACTIONS

Neutropenia, lymphopenia may increase risk of infection. New-onset psoriasis, exacerbation of preexisting psoriasis have been reported. Serious infections including sepsis, pneumonia, cellulitis, TB, invasive fungal infections reported. May increase risk of lymphoma, melanoma, new malignancies. New onset or exacerbation of CNS demyelinating disorders, including multiple sclerosis, or worsening of HF have occurred. Viral reactivation of herpes zoster, HIV, hepatitis B virus infection may occur. Pts who receive TNF blockers have risk of autoantibody formation (immunogenicity). Hypersensitivity reactions including anaphylaxis reported. May induce lupus-like symptoms (butterfly rash, new joint pain, peripheral edema, UV sensitivity).

NURSING CONSIDERATIONS

BASELINE ASSESSMENT

Obtain CBC, LFT; pregnancy test in females of reproductive potential. Do not initiate therapy if active infection suspected. Evaluate for active TB and test for latent infection prior to and during treatment. Induration of 5 mm or greater with tuberculin skin test should be considered a positive result when assessing for latent TB. Antifungal therapy should be considered for those who reside or travel to regions where mycoses are endemic. Question history of anemia, HF, CNS disorders, hepatic impairment, HIV, malignancies. Assess skin for moles, lesions. Receive full medication history including herbal products.

INTERVENTION/EVALUATION

Monitor CBC, LFT every 4–8 wks, then periodically. Screen pts for TB (night sweats, hemoptysis, weight loss, fever) regardless of baseline tuberculin skin test result. Monitor hepatitis B virus carriers during treatment and several mos after treatment. If any viral reactivation occurs, interrupt treatment and consider antiviral therapy. Discontinue treatment if acute infection, opportunistic infection, or sepsis occurs, and initiate appropriate antimicrobial therapy. Routinely assess skin for new lesions. Peripheral edema, difficulty breathing, coarse crackles on lung auscultation, elevated BNP may indicate worsening HF. Monitor for hypersensitivity reactions.

PATIENT/FAMILY TEACHING

• Treatment may depress your immune system and reduce your ability to fight infection. Report symptoms of infection such as body aches, chills, cough, fatigue, fever. Avoid those with active infection. • Do not receive live vaccines. • Report history of HIV, fungal infections, HF, hepatitis B, multiple sclerosis, TB, or close relatives who have active TB. Report travel plans to possible endemic areas. Blood levels, TB screening will be routinely monitored. • Hives, swelling of face, difficulty breathing may indicate allergic reaction. • Do not breastfeed. • Abdominal pain, yellowing of skin or eyes, dark-amber urine, clay-colored stools, fatigue, loss of appetite may indicate liver problems. • Decreased platelet count may increase risk of bleeding. • Swelling of hands or feet, difficulty breathing may indicate HF.

---

goserelin HIGH ALERT

goe-se-**rel**-in
(Zoladex, Zoladex LA)

◆CLASSIFICATION

PHARMACOTHERAPEUTIC: Gonadotropin-releasing hormone analogue.
CLINICAL: Antineoplastic.

USES

Breast cancer: Palliative treatment of advanced breast cancer in pre- and perimenopausal women. **Endometrial thinning:** Endometrial thinning before ablation for dysfunctional uterine bleeding. **Endometriosis:** Management of endometriosis, including pain relief and reduction of lesions. **Prostate cancer:** Palliative treatment of advanced carcinoma of the prostate. Management of locally confined prostate cancer (in combination with an antiandrogen). **OFF-LABEL:** Breast cancer (advanced with endocrine-based combination therapy), breast cancer (early-stage premenopausal ovarian preservation during chemotherapy), breast cancer (premenopausal ovarian suppression during adjuvant endocrine therapy).

PRECAUTIONS

Contraindications: Hypersensitivity to goserelin, GnRH, GnRH agonist analogues. Pregnancy (except when used for palliative treatment of advanced breast cancer). **Cautions:** Women of childbearing potential until pregnancy has been excluded. Pts at risk for decreased bone density; diabetes.

ACTION

Initially, stimulates release of luteinizing hormone (LH) and follicle-stimulating hormone (FSH) from anterior pituitary. Chronic administration causes a sustained suppression of pituitary gonadotropins. **Therapeutic Effect:** In females, reduces ovarian, uterine, mammary gland size; regresses hormone-responsive tumors. In males, decreases testosterone level, reduces growth of abnormal prostate tissue.

PHARMACOKINETICS

Protein binding: 27%. Metabolized in liver. Excreted in urine. **Half-life:** 4.2 hrs (male); 2.3 hrs (female).

🕱 LIFESPAN CONSIDERATIONS

Pregnancy/Lactation: Crosses placenta; unknown if distributed in breast milk. **Children:** Safety and efficacy not established. **Elderly:** No age-related precautions noted.

INTERACTIONS

DRUG: Medications prolonging the QT interval (e.g., amiodarone, azithromycin, ceritinib, haloperidol, moxifloxacin) may increase risk of QT interval prolongation, cardiac arrhythmias. **HERBAL:** None significant. **FOOD:** None known. **LAB VALUES:** May increase serum prostatic acid phosphatase, testosterone, calcium; Hgb A1c.

AVAILABILITY (Rx)

Injection, Implant: *(Zoladex):* 3.6 mg, 10.8 mg.

ADMINISTRATION/HANDLING

SQ Implant
• Administer implant by inserting needle at 30- to 45-degree angle into anterior abdominal wall below the navel line. Do not attempt to eliminate air bubbles or aspirate prior to injection. Do not penetrate into muscle or peritoneum.

INDICATIONS/ROUTES/DOSAGE

Prostatic Carcinoma (Advanced)
SQ: ADULTS OLDER THAN 18 YRS, ELDERLY: 3.6 mg every 28 days or 10.8 mg q12wks subcutaneously into upper abdominal wall.

Prostate Carcinoma (Locally Confined)
SQ: ADULTS, ELDERLY: (in combination with an antiestrogen and radiotherapy, begin 8 wks prior to radiotherapy): 3.6 mg once. 28 days after initial dose, give 3.6 mg q28days for 4 doses or 10.8 mg one time.

Breast Carcinoma (Advanced)
SQ: ADULTS: 3.6 mg every 28 days. Subcutaneously into upper abdominal wall.

Endometrial Thinning
SQ: ADULTS: 3.6 mg q28 days for 1 or 2 doses prior to endometrial ablation. Perform surgery at 4 wks (if giving 1 dose) or within 2–4 wks (following administration of second dose).

Endometriosis
SQ: ADULTS: 3.6 mg every 28 days for 6 mos.

G

No dose adjustment.

SIDE EFFECTS

Frequent (60%–13%): Headache, hot flashes, depression, diaphoresis, sexual dysfunction, impotence, lower urinary tract symptoms. **Occasional (10%–5%):** Pain, lethargy, dizziness, insomnia, anorexia, nausea, rash, upper respiratory tract infection, hirsutism, abdominal pain. **Rare:** Pruritus.

ADVERSE EFFECTS/TOXIC REACTIONS

Arrhythmias, HF, hypertension occur rarely. Ureteral obstruction, spinal cord compression have been observed (immediate orchiectomy may be necessary). Hypersensitivity reactions, including anaphylaxis, may occur. Hyperglycemia, new-onset diabetes occurred in men taking GnRH antagonists. Increased risk of MI, sudden cardiac death was reported. Injection site injuries including hematoma, hemorrhage, hemorrhagic shock may require blood transfusion or surgical intervention. May cause decreased mineral bone density, osteoporosis, bone fracture. Pituitary apoplexy, pituitary adenoma were reported. May cause QT interval prolongation.

NURSING CONSIDERATIONS

BASELINE ASSESSMENT

Question history of diabetes, cardiovascular disease, recent MI, prior hypersensitivity reaction. Receive full medication history; screen for QT interval–prolonging medications, anticoagulant medications. Screen for conditions predisposing to QT interval prolongation. In males, question history of urethral obstruction, urinary retention, spinal cord compression, spinal stenosis. Obtain urine pregnancy. If applicable, obtain bone density test.

INTERVENTION/EVALUATION

Monitor pt closely for worsening signs/symptoms of prostatic cancer, esp. during first mo of therapy.

PATIENT/FAMILY TEACHING

• Use nonhormonal methods of contraception during therapy. • Report suspected pregnancy or if regular menstruation does not cease. • Breakthrough menstrual bleeding may occur if dose is missed. • Immediately report sudden weakness, paralysis, numbness, tingling; difficulty urinating, bladder distention. • Do not take newly prescribed medications unless approved by prescriber who originally started treatment. • Severe bleeding may occur at the injection site, esp. in pts who take blood-thinning medication. • Pts with heart disease are at an increased risk of heart attack or sudden death.

---

granisetron

gra-**nis**-e-tron
(Sancuso, Sustol)
Do not confuse granisetron with alosetron, cilansetron, dolasetron, ondansetron, or palonosetron.

◆CLASSIFICATION

PHARMACOTHERAPEUTIC: Selective serotonin receptor antagonist (5-HT$_3$). **CLINICAL:** Antiemetic.

USES

Prevention of nausea/vomiting associated with emetogenic cancer therapy and cancer radiation therapy. **OFF-LABEL:** Prevention, treatment of postop nausea, vomiting.

PRECAUTIONS

Contraindications: Hypersensitivity to granisetron. Hypersensitivity to other 5-HT$_3$ receptor antagonists. **Cautions:** Congenital QT prolongation, concomitant administration of medications that prolong QT interval, electrolyte abnormalities, cumulative high-dose anthracycline therapy. Following abdominal surgery or in chemotherapy-induced nausea, vomiting (may mask progressive ileus or gastric distention), hepatic disease.

ACTION

Selectively blocks serotonin stimulation at receptor sites centrally in chemoreceptor trigger zone, peripherally on vagal nerve terminals. **Therapeutic Effect:** Prevents nausea/vomiting.

PHARMACOKINETICS

Route	Onset	Peak	Duration
IV	1–3 min	N/A	24 hrs

Widely distributed. Protein binding: 65%. Metabolized in liver. Excreted in urine (48%), feces (38%). **Half-life:** 10–12 hrs (increased in elderly).

⏳ LIFESPAN CONSIDERATIONS

Pregnancy/Lactation: Unknown if distributed in breast milk. **Children:** Safety and efficacy not established in pts younger than 2 yrs. **Elderly:** No age-related precautions noted.

INTERACTIONS

DRUG: QT interval–prolonging medications (e.g., **amiodarone**, **azithromycin**, **ciprofloxacin**, **haloperidol**, **methadone**, **sotalol**) may increase risk of QT interval prolongation, cardiac arrhythmias. **SSRIs** (e.g., **escitalopram**, **PARoxetine**, **sertraline**), **SNRIs** (e.g., **DULoxetine**, **venlafaxine**) may increase risk of serotonin syndrome. **HERBAL:** None significant. **FOOD:** None known. **LAB VALUES:** May increase serum ALT, AST.

AVAILABILITY (Rx)

Injection: *(Extended-Release [Sustol]):* 10 mg/0.4 mL single-dose syringe. **Injection Solution:** 1 mg/mL. **Tablets:** 1 mg. **Transdermal Patch:** *(Sancuso):* 52-cm² patch containing 34.3 mg granisetron delivering 3.1 mg/24 hrs.

ADMINISTRATION/HANDLING

 IV

Reconstitution • May be given undiluted or dilute with 20–50 mL 0.9% NaCl or D₅W. Do not mix with other medications.

Rate of administration • May give undiluted as IV push over 30 sec. • For IV piggyback, infuse over 5–10 min depending on volume of diluent used. **Storage** • Appears as a clear, colorless solution. • Store at room temperature. • After dilution, stable for 24 hrs at room temperature. • Inspect for particulates, discoloration.

PO

• Give 30 min up to 1 hr prior to initiating chemotherapy/radiation.

SQ

• Administer in skin of back of upper arm, abdomen (at least 1 inch away from umbilicus). Avoid areas of compromised skin. Administer over 20–30 sec.

Transdermal

• Apply to clean, dry intact skin on upper outer arm. • Remove immediately from pouch before application. • Do not cut patch.

▦ IV COMPATIBILITIES

Acetaminophen, calcium gluconate, dexmedetomidine, furosemide, magnesium sulfate, potassium chloride.

INDICATIONS/ROUTES/DOSAGE

Prevention of Chemotherapy-Induced Nausea/Vomiting
PO: ADULTS, ELDERLY: 2 mg up to 1 hr before chemotherapy or 1 mg up to 1 hr before chemotherapy, with a second dose 12 hrs later.
IV: ADULTS, ELDERLY, CHILDREN 2 YRS AND OLDER: 10 mcg/kg/dose (**Maximum:** 1 mg/dose) within 30 min of chemotherapy. **Maximum:** 1 mg.
SQ: ADULTS, ELDERLY: In combination with dexAMETHasone: 10 mg at least 30 min before chemotherapy. Do not repeat more frequently than 7 days.
Transdermal: ADULTS, ELDERLY: Apply 24–48 hrs prior to chemotherapy. Remove minimum 24 hrs after completion of chemotherapy. May be worn up to 7 days, depending on chemotherapy duration.

G

Prevention of Radiation-Induced Nausea/Vomiting

PO: ADULTS, ELDERLY: (High-emetogenic-risk radiation therapy): 2 mg once daily, given 1 hr before each fraction of radiation (in combination with dexAMETHasone). **Moderate-emetogenic-risk radiation therapy (upper abdomen, craniospinal irradiation):** 2 mg once daily given 1–2 hrs prior to each fraction of radiation. May administer with or without dexamethasone before the first 5 fractions.

Dosage in Renal/Hepatic Impairment

No dose adjustment. *(Sustol):* **Moderate impairment:** No more frequently than 14 days. **Severe impairment:** Not recommended.

SIDE EFFECTS

Frequent (21%–14%): Headache, constipation, asthenia. **Occasional (8%–6%):** Diarrhea, abdominal pain. **Rare (less than 2%):** Altered taste, fever.

ADVERSE EFFECTS/TOXIC REACTIONS

Hypersensitivity reaction, hypertension, hypotension, arrhythmias (sinus bradycardia, atrial fibrillation, AV block, ventricular ectopy), ECG abnormalities occur rarely. Increased risk of serotonin syndrome reported in pts taking concomitant serotonergic drugs (e.g., SSRIs, SNRIs). May prolong QTc interval.

NURSING CONSIDERATIONS

BASELINE ASSESSMENT

Assess hydration status. Ensure that granisetron is given within 30 min of starting chemotherapy. Receive full medication history and screen for interactions. Screen for QT interval–prolonging conditions.

INTERVENTION/EVALUATION

Monitor for therapeutic effect. Assess for headache. Monitor for dehydration due to recurrent vomiting. Monitor daily pattern of bowel activity, stool consistency.

PATIENT/FAMILY TEACHING

• Granisetron is effective shortly following administration; prevents nausea/vomiting. • Transitory taste disorder may occur.

guselkumab

gue-sel-**koo**-mab
(Tremfya)
Do not confuse guselkumab with golimumab, infliximab, secukinumab.

◆CLASSIFICATION

PHARMACOTHERAPEUTIC: Interleukin-23 inhibitor. Monoclonal antibody. **CLINICAL:** Antipsoriasis agent.

USES

Plaque psoriasis: Treatment of moderate to severe plaque psoriasis in adult pts who are candidates for systemic therapy or phototherapy. **Psoriatic arthritis:** Treatment of active psoriatic arthritis in adults. **Ulcerative colitis:** Treatment of adults with moderately to severely active ulcerative colitis.

PRECAUTIONS

Contraindications: Hypersensitivity to guselkumab. **Cautions:** Hepatic impairment, active infection until resolved, history of chronic or recurrent infections, conditions predisposing to infection (e.g., diabetes, immunocompromised pts, open wounds), prior tuberculosis exposure (do not give to pts with active TB infection). Concomitant use of live vaccines not recommended.

ACTION

Selectively binds to interleukin-23 receptor reducing levels of IL-17A, IL-17F, IL-22. IL-23 is a cytokine that is involved in inflammatory and immune responses. **Therapeutic Effect:** Inhibits release of proinflammatory cytokines and chemokines.

PHARMACOKINETICS

Widely distributed. Degraded into small peptides and amino acids via catabolic pathways. Peak plasma concentration: 5.5 days. Elimination not specified. **Half-life:** 15–18 days.

⧗ LIFESPAN CONSIDERATIONS

Pregnancy/Lactation: Unknown if distributed in breast milk. However, human immunoglobulin G (IgG) is present in breast milk and is known to cross placenta. **Children:** Safety and efficacy not established. **Elderly:** No age-related precautions noted.

INTERACTIONS

DRUG: May enhance adverse/toxic effects, diminish therapeutic effects of **natalizumab, pimecrolimus, vaccines (live)**. May decrease therapeutic effect of **BCG (intravesical)**. **HERBAL:** Echinacea may decrease therapeutic effect. **FOOD:** None known. **LAB VALUES:** May increase serum ALT, AST.

AVAILABILITY (Rx)

Injection, Solution: SQ Injection: 100 mg/mL single-dose One-Press patient-controlled injector; 200 mg/2 mL single-dose prefilled pen; 100 mg/mL, 200 mg/2 mL single-dose prefilled syringes. **IV Injection:** 200 mg/20 mL (10 mg/mL) solution in a single-dose vial. 100 mg/mL prefilled syringe, single-dose one-press patient-controlled injector.

ADMINISTRATION/HANDLING

 IV

Preparation • Withdraw 20 mL of the 0.9% NaCl from 250 mL infusion bag. • Add 200 mg to the infusion bag for a final concentration of 0.8 mg/mL.
Rate of Administration • Infuse over at least 1 hr.
Stability • Diluted solution may be kept at room temperature for up to 10 hrs.

SQ
Preparation • Remove prefilled syringe from refrigerator and allow to warm to room temperature (approx. 30 min) with needle cap intact. • Visually inspect for particulate matter or discoloration. Solution should appear clear, colorless to slightly yellow in color; may contain small translucent particles. Do not use if solution is cloudy, discolored, or if large particles are observed. • Discard unused portions.
Administration • Insert needle subcutaneously into back of upper arms, front of thighs, or into lower abdomen (except for 2 inches around navel), and inject solution. • Do not inject into areas of the skin where it is tender, bruised, red, hard, thick, scaly, or affected by psoriasis. • Rotate injection sites.
Storage • Refrigerate prefilled syringes in original carton until time of use. • Do not freeze. • Do not shake. • Protect from light.

INDICATIONS/ROUTES/DOSAGE

Plaque Psoriasis
SQ: ADULTS, ELDERLY: 100 mg at wk 0, wk 4, and then q8wks thereafter.

Psoriatic Arthritis
SQ: ADULTS, ELDERLY: 100 mg at wks 0 and 4, then q8wks thereafter. May administer alone or in combination with conventional disease-modifying antirheumatic drugs (e.g., methotrexate).

Ulcerative Colitis
IV: ADULTS, ELDERLY: (Induction): 200 mg over at least 1 hr at wks 0, 4, and 8. **(Maintenance): SQ:** 100 mg at wk 16, then q8wks thereafter, or 200 mg at wk 12, then q4wks thereafter. Use the lowest effective recommended dosage to maintain therapeutic response.

Dosage in Renal/Hepatic Impairment
Not specified; use caution.

SIDE EFFECTS

Occasional (5%–2%): Headache, tension headache, arthralgia, diarrhea.

ADVERSE EFFECTS/TOXIC REACTIONS

May increase risk of tuberculosis infection. Other infections including upper

 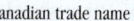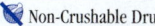

respiratory tract infection, nasopharyngitis, pharyngitis, viral upper respiratory tract infection (14% of pts), gastroenteritis, viral gastroenteritis (1% of pts), tinea infections (1% of pts), herpes simplex virus (1% of pts) may occur. Mild to moderate elevated serum ALT, AST reported in 3% of pts.

NURSING CONSIDERATIONS

BASELINE ASSESSMENT

Obtain LFT in pts with hepatic impairment. Question history of hepatic impairment, herpes zoster infection, parasitic infection. Screen for active infection. Pts should be evaluated for active tuberculosis and tested for latent infection prior to initiating treatment and periodically during therapy. Induration of 5 mm or greater with tuberculin skin testing should be considered a positive test result when assessing if treatment for latent tuberculosis is necessary. Conduct dermatologic exam; record characteristics of psoriatic lesions. Assess pt's willingness to self-inject medication.

INTERVENTION/EVALUATION

Monitor LFT periodically. Monitor for symptoms of tuberculosis, including those who tested negative for latent tuberculosis infection prior to initiating therapy. Interrupt or discontinue treatment if serious infection, opportunistic infection, or sepsis occurs, and initiate appropriate antimicrobial therapy. Assess skin for improvement of lesions.

PATIENT/FAMILY TEACHING

• A healthcare provider will show you how to properly prepare and inject your medication. You must demonstrate correct preparation and injection techniques before using medication at home. • Treatment may depress your immune system response and reduce your ability to fight infection. Report symptoms of infection such as body aches, chills, cough, fatigue, fever. Avoid those with active infection. • Do not receive live vaccines. • Expect frequent tuberculosis screening. Report travel plans to possible endemic areas. • Report liver problems such as abdominal pain, bruising, clay-colored stool, yellowing of the skin or eyes.

haloperidol

hal-o-**per**-i-dol
(Haldol Decanoate, Apo-Peridol ✦)

■ **BLACK BOX ALERT** ■ Increased risk of mortality in elderly pts with dementia-related psychosis with use of injections.

Do not confuse Haldol with Stadol.

◆**CLASSIFICATION**

PHARMACOTHERAPEUTIC: First-generation (typical) antipsychotic. **CLINICAL:** Antipsychotic, antiemetic, antidyskinetic.

USES

Schizophrenia: Treatment of manifestations of psychotic disorders such as schizophrenia. **Tourette's syndrome:** Control of tics and vocal utterances in adults and children. **Behavioral disorders (nonpsychotic):** Treatment of severe behavioral problems in children with combative, explosive hyperexcitability that cannot be accounted for by immediate provocation. **Hyperactivity:** Short-term treatment of hyperactivity in children showing excessive motor activity with some of following symptoms: impulsivity, difficulty sustaining attention, aggression, mood lability, poor frustration tolerance. **OFF-LABEL:** Treatment of acute agitation/aggression, palliative care (nausea/vomiting), bipolar disorder (mania/hyopmania), critical care delirium, chemotherapy-induced breakthrough nausea/vomiting.

PRECAUTIONS

Contraindications: Hypersensitivity to haloperidol, CNS depression, coma, Parkinson's disease. **Cautions:** Renal/hepatic impairment, cardiovascular disease, history of seizures, prolonged QT syndrome, medications that prolong QT interval, hypothyroidism, thyrotoxicosis, electrolyte imbalance (e.g., hypokalemia, hypomagnesemia), EEG abnormalities, narrow–angle glaucoma, elderly, pts at risk for pneumonia, decreased GI motility, urinary retention, BPH, visual disturbances, myelosuppression. Pts at risk for orthostatic hypotension (e.g., cerebrovascular disease).

ACTION

Nonselectively blocks postsynaptic DOP-amine receptors in brain. **Therapeutic Effect:** Produces tranquilizing effect. Strong extrapyramidal, antiemetic effects; weak anticholinergic, sedative effects.

PHARMACOKINETICS

Widely distributed. Protein binding: 92%. Metabolized in liver. Excreted in urine. Not removed by hemodialysis. **Half-life:** 20 hrs.

⌛ LIFESPAN CONSIDERATIONS

Pregnancy/Lactation: Crosses placenta. Distributed in breast milk. **Children:** More susceptible to dystonias; not recommended in pts younger than 3 yrs. **Elderly:** More susceptible to orthostatic hypotension, anticholinergic effects, sedation; increased risk for extrapyramidal effects. Decreased dosage recommended.

INTERACTIONS

DRUG: **Alcohol, other CNS depressants (e.g., diphenhydrAMINE, gabapentin, LORazepam, morphine)** may increase CNS depression. CYP3A4 inducers (e.g., **carBAMazepine, phenytoin, rifAMPin**) may decrease concentration. QT interval–prolonging medications (e.g., amiodarone, azithromycin, ciprofloxacin, haloperidol, methadone, sotalol) may increase risk of QT prolongation. **Aclidinium, ipratropium, tiotropium, umeclidinium** may increase anticholinergic effect. **Metoclopramide may increase adverse effects.** **HERBAL:** **Herbals with sedative properties (e.g., chamomile, kava, kava, valerian)** may increase CNS depression. **FOOD:** None known. **LAB VALUES:** None significant. **Therapeutic serum level:** 0.2–1 mcg/mL; **toxic serum level:** Greater than 1 mcg/mL.

H

AVAILABILITY (Rx)

Injection, Oil: *(Decanoate):* 50 mg/mL, 100 mg/mL. **Injection, Solution:** *(Lactate):* 5 mg/mL. **Oral Concentrate:** 2 mg/mL. **Tablets:** 0.5 mg, 1 mg, 2 mg, 5 mg, 10 mg, 20 mg.

ADMINISTRATION/HANDLING

 IV

◄ALERT► Only haloperidol lactate is given IV.
Note: For IV administration, ECG monitoring for QT prolongation/arrhythmias is recommended.
Reconstitution • May give undiluted. • May add to 50–100 mL of D_5W.
Rate of administration • Give IV push at rate of 5 mg/min. • Infuse IV piggyback over 30 min. • For IV infusion, up to 25 mg/hr has been used (titrated to pt response).
Storage • Discard if precipitate forms, discoloration occurs. • Store at room temperature; do not freeze. • Protect from light.

IM
Parenteral administration • Pt should remain recumbent for 30–60 min to minimize hypotensive effect. • Prepare Decanoate IM injection using 21-gauge needle. • Do not exceed maximum volume of 3 mL per IM injection site. • Inject slow, deep IM into upper outer quadrant of gluteus maximus.

PO
• Give without regard to food. • Scored tablets may be crushed. • Dilute oral concentrate with water or juice. • Avoid skin contact with oral concentrate; may cause contact dermatitis.

🟦 IV COMPATIBILITIES

Acetaminophen, dexmedetomidine, norepinephrine.

INDICATIONS/ROUTES/DOSAGE

Schizophrenia
IV: *(Lactate):* **ADULTS, ELDERLY:** Initially, 2–10 mg/day in 1–3 divided doses. Adjust dose based on response and tolerability. **Maximum:** 20 mg/day. *(Decanoate):* **ADULTS, ELDERLY:** Initially, 10–20 times stabilized oral dose. **Maximum initial dose:** 100 mg (doses greater the 100 mg should be given as 2 separate injections 3–7 days apart). **Maintenance:** 10–15 times daily oral dose. **Maximum:** 450 mg q4wks.
PO: ADULTS, ELDERLY: Initially, 2–10 mg/day in 1–3 divided doses. Adjust dose based on response and tolerability. **Maximum:** 30 mg/day.

Tourette's Disorder
PO: ADULTS: Initially, 1–2 mg/day in 1–3 divided doses. May increase dose in increments of 0.5–2 mg q2–3 days up to 12 mg/day. **Usual dose:** 15 mg/day. **Maximum:** 100 mg/day. **CHILDREN 3–12 YRS, ADOLESCENTS:** Initially, 0.25–0.5 mg/day in 2–3 divided doses. May increase daily dose by 0.25–0.5 mg every 5–7 days to usual maintenance dose of 1–4 mg/day in 2–3 divided doses. **Maximum:** 15 mg/day.

Behavioral Disorders
PO: CHILDREN 3–12 YRS: Initially, 0.5 mg/day in 2–3 divided doses. May increase total daily dose by 0.5 mg/day q5–7 days up to 0.05–0.075 mg/kg/day in 2–3 divided doses. **Maximum:** 6 mg/day.

Dosage in Renal/Hepatic Impairment
No dose adjustment.

SIDE EFFECTS

Frequent: Blurred vision, constipation, orthostatic hypotension, dry mouth, swelling or soreness of female breasts, peripheral edema. **Occasional:** Allergic reaction, difficulty urinating, decreased thirst, dizziness, diminished sexual function, drowsiness, nausea, vomiting, photosensitivity, lethargy.

ADVERSE EFFECTS/TOXIC REACTIONS

Extrapyramidal symptoms (EPS) appear to be dose related and typically occur in first few days of therapy. Marked drowsiness/lethargy, excessive salivation, fixed stare may be mild to severe in intensity. Less frequently noted are severe akathisia (motor restlessness), acute dystonias: torticollis (neck muscle spasm), opisthotonos (rigidity of back muscles), oculogyric crisis (rolling back of eyes). Tardive dyskinesia (tongue protrusion, puffing of cheeks, chewing/puckering of the mouth) may occur during long-term therapy or after drug discontinuance and may be irreversible. Elderly female pts have greater risk of developing this reaction. May increase risk of QT interval prolongation, cardiac arrhythmias.

NURSING CONSIDERATIONS

BASELINE ASSESSMENT

Assess behavior, appearance, emotional status, response to environment, speech pattern, thought content. Assess mental status. Screen for comorbidities as listed in Precautions (esp. seizure disorder, long QT syndrome).

INTERVENTION/EVALUATION

Monitor B/P, heart rate/rhythm. Monitor ECG, QT interval. Supervise suicidal-risk pts closely during early therapy (as depression lessens, energy level improves, increasing suicide potential). Monitor for rigidity, tremor, mask-like facial expression, fine tongue movement. Assess for therapeutic response (interest in surroundings, improvement in self-care, increased ability to concentrate, relaxed facial expression). **Therapeutic serum level:** 0.2–1 mcg/mL; **toxic serum level:** Greater than 1 mcg/mL.

PATIENT/FAMILY TEACHING

• Full therapeutic effect may take up to 6 wks. • Do not abruptly withdraw from long-term drug therapy. • Sugarless gum, sips of water may relieve dry mouth. • Drowsiness generally subsides during continued therapy. • Avoid tasks that require alertness, motor skills until response to drug is established. • Avoid alcohol. • Report muscle stiffness, lip puckering, tongue protrusion, restlessness. • Avoid overheating, dehydration, exposure to sunlight (increased risk of heatstroke).

heparin

hep-a-rin
(Hepalean Leo ✦)
Do not confuse heparin with Hespan.

◆CLASSIFICATION

PHARMACOTHERAPEUTIC: Blood modifier. **CLINICAL:** Anticoagulant.

USES

Prophylaxis and treatment of thromboembolic disorders (e.g., venous thromboembolism, pulmonary embolism) and thromboembolic complications associated with atrial fibrillation; anticoagulant for extracorporeal and dialysis procedures; maintain patency of IV devices. Prevents clotting in arterial and cardiac surgery. **OFF-LABEL:** Ischemic heart disease (acute coronary syndromes): STEMI, non-STEMI, PCI), mechanical heart valve (anticoagulant bridging, postsurgical management), peripheral arterial occlusion. Frostbite (adjunctive), mechanical heart valve (bridging anticoagulation, postsurgical management).

PRECAUTIONS

Contraindications: Hypersensitivity to heparin. Severe thrombocytopenia, uncontrolled active bleeding (unless secondary to disseminated intravascular coagulation [DIC]), history of heparin-induced thrombocytopenia (HIT), heparin-induced thrombocytopenia with thrombosis (HITT), or pts who test positive for HIT antibody. **Cautions:** Allergy to pork. Pts at risk for bleeding (e.g., congenital/acquired bleeding disorders, active GI ulcerative disease, hemophilia, concomitant platelet inhibitors, severe hypertension, menses, recent lumbar puncture or spinal anesthesia; recent major surgery, trauma). Use of preservative-free heparin recommended in neonates, infants, pregnant or nursing mothers.

ACTION

Potentiates action of antithrombin III. Interferes with blood coagulation by blocking conversion of prothrombin to thrombin and fibrinogen to fibrin. **Therapeutic Effect:** Prevents further extension of existing thrombi or new clot formation. No effect on existing clots.

PHARMACOKINETICS

Well absorbed following SQ administration. Protein binding: Very high. Metabolized in liver. Removed from circulation via uptake by reticuloendothelial system. Primarily excreted in urine. Not removed by hemodialysis. **Half-life:** 1–6 hrs.

⌛ LIFESPAN CONSIDERATIONS

Pregnancy/Lactation: Use with caution, particularly during last trimester, immediate postpartum period (increased risk of maternal hemorrhage). Does not cross placenta. Not distributed in breast milk. **Children:** No age-related precautions noted. Benzyl alcohol preservative may cause gasping syndrome in infants. **Elderly:** More susceptible to hemorrhage. Age-related renal impairment may increase risk of bleeding.

INTERACTIONS

DRUG: Anticoagulants (e.g., apixaban, dabigatran, rivaroxaban, warfarin) may increase anticoagulant effect; risk of bleeding. **platelet aggregation inhibitors (e.g., aspirin), thrombolytics (e.g., tissue plasminogen activator [TPA])** may increase risk of bleeding. **HERBAL: Herbals with anticoagulant/antiplatelet properties (e.g., garlic, ginger, ginkgo biloba)** may increase risk of bleeding. **FOOD:** None known. **LAB VALUES:** May increase free fatty acids, serum ALT, AST; aPTT. May decrease serum cholesterol.

AVAILABILITY (Rx)

Injection Solution: 1,000 units/mL (1 mL, 10 mL, 30 mL), 5,000 units/mL (1 mL, 10 mL), 5,000 units/0.5 mL, 10,000 units/mL (1 mL, 4 mL, 5 mL), 20,000 units/mL (1 mL). **Premix Solution for Infusion:** 1,000 units (500 mL), 12,500 units/250 mL (0.45% NaCl), 25,000 units/250 mL (D5W, 0.45% NaCl).

ADMINISTRATION/HANDLING

◄**ALERT**► Do not give by IM injection (pain, hematoma, ulceration, erythema).

 IV

◄**ALERT**► Used in full-dose therapy. Intermittent IV dosage produces higher incidence of bleeding abnormalities. Continuous IV route preferred.
Reconstitution • Premix solution requires no reconstitution.
Rate of administration • Infuse and titrate per protocol using infusion pump.
Storage • Store at room temperature.

SQ
◄**ALERT**► Used in low-dose therapy. • After withdrawal of heparin from vial, change needle before injection (prevents leakage along needle track). • Inject above iliac crest or in abdominal fat layer. Do not inject within 2 inches of umbilicus or any scar tissue. • Withdraw needle rapidly, apply prolonged pressure at injection site. Do not massage or apply heat/cold to injection site. • Rotate injection sites.

▓ IV COMPATIBILITIES

Acetaminophen, calcium gluconate, clevidipine, dexmedetomidine, furosemide, hydralazine, hydrocortisone, ibuprofen, magnesium sulfate, potassium chloride, propofol.

INDICATIONS/ROUTES/DOSAGE

Note: Variations occur among hospitals with reagents (lot numbers) and corresponding control of aPTT values. Refer to institution-specific nomograms based on current reagent.

Line Flushing
IV: ADULTS, ELDERLY, CHILDREN: 100 units as needed. **INFANTS WEIGHING LESS THAN 10 KG:** 10 units as needed.

Atrial Fibrillation
IV infusion: ADULTS, ELDERLY: 60–80 units/kg bolus (**Maximum:** 5,000 units), then 12–18 units/kg/hr (**Maximum:** 1,000 units/hr). Adjust infusion rate to maintain anticoagulation target based on institutional protocol.

Acute Coronary Syndrome
IV infusion: ADULTS, ELDERLY: 60 units/kg bolus (**Maximum:** 4,000 units), then 12 units/kg/hr (**Maximum:** 1,000 units/hr as continuous infusion). Adjust infusion rate to maintain anticoagulation target based on institutional protocol.

Treatment of DVT/PE
IV infusion: ADULTS, ELDERLY: 80 units/kg bolus (**Maximum:** 5,000 units), then 18 units/kg/hr. Adjust infusion rate to maintain anticoagulation target based on institutional protocol.

Usual Infant/Neonatal Dose
IV infusion: 75 units/kg bolus over 10 min, then initial maintenance dose of 28 units/kg/hr. Adjust dose according to aPTT per protocol.

Usual Adolescent/Children Dose
IV infusion: 75 units/kg bolus over 10 min, then initial maintenance dose of 20 units/kg/hr. Adjust infusion rate to maintain anticoagulation target based on institutional protocol.

Thromboembolic Prophylaxis
SQ: ADULTS, ELDERLY, PTS WEIGHING MORE THAN 120 KG: 7,500 units SQ q8–12h. PTS WEIGHING 50–120 KG: 5,000 units SQ q8–12h. PTS WEIGHING LESS THAN 50 KG: 2,500 units SQ q8–12h.

Dosage in Renal/Hepatic Impairment
No dose adjustment.

SIDE EFFECTS

Occasional: Pruritus, burning (particularly on soles of feet) caused by vasospastic reaction. **Rare:** Pain, cyanosis of extremity 6–10 days after initial therapy lasting 4–6 hrs, hypersensitivity reaction (chills, fever, pruritus, urticaria, asthma, rhinitis, lacrimation, headache).

ADVERSE EFFECTS/TOXIC REACTIONS

Bleeding complications ranging from local ecchymoses to major hemorrhage (cutaneous/GI/genitourinary/intracranial/nasal/oral/pharyngeal/urethral/vaginal bleeding) occur more frequently in high-dose therapy, intermittent IV infusion, women 60 yrs and older. HIT can cause life-threatening thromboembolism such as CVA, MI, DVT, pulmonary embolism, renal artery thrombosis, mesenteric thrombosis. **Antidote:** Protamine sulfate 1–1.5 mg IV for every 100 units heparin SQ within 30 min of overdose, 0.5–0.75 mg for every 100 units heparin SQ if within 30–60 min of overdose, 0.25–0.375 mg for every 100 units heparin SQ if 2 hrs have elapsed since overdose, 25–50 mg if heparin was given by IV infusion.

NURSING CONSIDERATIONS

BASELINE ASSESSMENT
Obtain CBC, PT/INR, aPTT. Cross-check dose with coworker. Assess for bleeding risk. Question history of recent trauma, head injuries, GI/GU bleeding. Ensure that pt has not received spinal anesthesia, spinal procedures.

INTERVENTION/EVALUATION
Monitor CBC, PT/INR daily. Obtain aPTT (or anti-Xa assay) 6 hrs after initiation or any change in dosage (or per clinical standards) until maintenance dose is established, then check aPTT (or anti-Xa assay) q24hrs (or per clinical standards). In long-term therapy, monitor 1–2 times/mo. Diligently assess for bleeding. If platelet count decreases more than 50% from baseline, obtain stat HIT antibody test. If HIT antibody positive, discontinue heparin and consider treatment with direct thrombin inhibitor (e.g., argatroban); avoid all heparin products and place heparin allergy on chart. Monitor urine and stool for occult blood. Assess for decrease in B/P, increase in pulse rate, complaint of abdominal/back pain, severe headache (may be evidence of hem-

H

orrhage). Question for increase in amount of discharge during menses. Assess peripheral pulses; skin for ecchymosis, petechiae. Check for excessive bleeding from minor cuts, scratches. Assess gums for erythema, gingival bleeding. Assess urine output for hematuria. Avoid IM injections due to potential for hematomas. When converting to warfarin (Coumadin) therapy, monitor PT/INR results (will be 10%–20% higher while heparin is given concurrently).

PATIENT/FAMILY TEACHING

• Use electric razor, soft toothbrush to prevent bleeding. • Report red or dark urine, black or red stool, coffee-ground vomitus, blood-tinged mucus from cough, signs of stroke, nosebleeds, or increase in menstruation. • Do not use any OTC medication without physician approval (may interfere with platelet aggregation). • Wear or carry identification that notes anticoagulant therapy. • Inform dentist, other physicians of heparin therapy. • Limit alcohol.

hydrALAZINE

hye-**dral**-a-zeen
(Apresoline ✤)
Do not confuse hydrALAZINE with hydrOXYzine.

FIXED-COMBINATION(S)

BiDil: hydrALAZINE/isosorbide (a nitrate): 37.5 mg/20 mg.

◆CLASSIFICATION

PHARMACOTHERAPEUTIC: Vasodilator. **CLINICAL:** Antihypertensive.

USES

Management of moderate to severe hypertension. **OFF-LABEL:** Hypertensive emergency in pregnancy/postpartum (including acute onset severe hypertension in preeclampsia/eclampsia). Treatment of HF with reduced ejection fraction.

PRECAUTIONS

Contraindications: Hypersensitivity to hydrALAZINE. Coronary artery disease, mitral valvular rheumatic heart disease. **Cautions:** Advanced renal impairment, cerebrovascular accident, suspected coronary artery disease. Pts with mitral valvular disease, positive ANA titer, pulmonary hypertension.

ACTION

Direct vasodilating effects on arterioles. **Therapeutic Effect:** Decreases B/P, systemic vascular resistance.

PHARMACOKINETICS

Route	Onset	Peak	Duration
PO	20–30 min	N/A	Up to 8 hrs
IV	5–20 min	N/A	1–4 hrs

Widely distributed. Protein binding: 85%–90%. Metabolized in liver. Primarily excreted in urine. Not removed by hemodialysis. **Half-life:** 3–7 hrs (increased in renal impairment).

⧖ LIFESPAN CONSIDERATIONS

Pregnancy/Lactation: Drug crosses placenta. Unknown if distributed in breast milk. Thrombocytopenia, leukopenia, petechial bleeding, hematomas have occurred in newborns (resolved within 1–3 wks). **Children:** No age-related precautions noted. **Elderly:** More sensitive to hypotensive effects. Age-related renal impairment may require dosage adjustment.

INTERACTIONS

DRUG: Diuretics (e.g., **furosemide, HCTZ**), other antihypertensives (e.g., **amLODIPine, cloNIDine, lisinopril, valsartan**) may increase hypotensive effect. **HERBAL:** Herbals with hypertensive properties (e.g., **licorice, yohimbe**) or hypotensive properties (e.g., **garlic, ginger, ginkgo biloba**) may alter effects. **FOOD:** Any **foods** may increase absorption. **LAB VALUES:** May produce positive direct Coombs' test.

AVAILABILITY (Rx)

Injection Solution: 20 mg/mL. Tablets: 10 mg, 25 mg, 50 mg, 100 mg.

ADMINISTRATION/HANDLING

 IV

Rate of administration • May give undiluted. • Administer slowly: Maximum rate 5 mg/min (0.2 mg/kg/min for children).
Storage • Store at room temperature.

PO
• May give without regard to food (best given consistently with meals).

⚙ IV INCOMPATIBILITIES

Furosemide.

⚙ IV COMPATIBILITIES

Heparin, potassium chloride.

INDICATIONS/ROUTES/DOSAGE

Hypertension (Chronic)
PO: ADULTS, ELDERLY: Initially, 10 mg 4 times/day for first 2–4 days. May increase to 25 mg 4 times/day balance of first wk. May increase by 10–25 mg/dose gradually q2–5 days to 50 mg 4 times/day. Usual range: 100–200 mg/day in 2–3 divided doses. Maximum: 300 mg/day. CHILDREN, ADOLESCENTS: Initially, 0.75 mg/kg/day in 2–4 divided doses. May increase over 3–4 wks. Maximum: 7.5 mg/kg/day in 2–4 divided doses or 200 mg/day in divided doses, whichever is less.

Hypertensive Emergency
IV, IM: ADULTS, ELDERLY: Initially, 10–20 mg/dose q4–6h. May increase to 40 mg/dose. CHILDREN, ADOLESCENTS: Initially, 0.1–0.2 mg/kg/dose q4–6h. Usual range: 0.2–0.6 mg/kg/dose q4–6h. as needed. Maximum dose: 20 mg.

Dosage in Renal Impairment
Dosage interval is based on creatinine clearance.

Creatinine Clearance	Dosage
10–50 mL/min	q8h
Less than 10 mL/min	q12–24h

Dosage in Hepatic Impairment
No dose adjustment.

SIDE EFFECTS

Occasional: Headache, anorexia, nausea, vomiting, diarrhea, palpitations, tachycardia, angina pectoris. Rare: Constipation, ileus, edema, peripheral neuritis (paresthesia), dizziness, muscle cramps, anxiety, hypersensitivity reactions (rash, urticaria, pruritus, fever, chills, arthralgia), nasal congestion, flushing, conjunctivitis.

ADVERSE EFFECTS/TOXIC REACTIONS

High dosage may produce lupus erythematosus–like reaction (fever, facial rash, muscle/joint aches, glomerulonephritis, splenomegaly). Severe orthostatic hypotension, skin flushing, severe headache, myocardial ischemia, cardiac arrhythmias may develop. Profound shock may occur with severe overdosage.

NURSING CONSIDERATIONS

BASELINE ASSESSMENT
Obtain B/P, heart rate immediately before each dose, in addition to regular monitoring (be alert to fluctuations).

INTERVENTION/EVALUATION
Monitor B/P, heart rate. Monitor for headache, palpitations, tachycardia. Assess for peripheral edema of hands, feet.

PATIENT/FAMILY TEACHING
• To reduce hypotensive effect, go from lying to standing slowly. • Report muscle/joint aches, fever (lupus-like reaction), flu-like symptoms. • Limit alcohol use.

hydroCHLOROthiazide

hye-dro-**klor**-oh-**thy**-ah-zide
(Urozide ✦)

FIXED-COMBINATION(S)

Atacand HCT: hydroCHLOROthiazide/candesartan (an angiotensin II receptor antagonist): 12.5 mg/16 mg, 12.5 mg/32 mg. **Avalide:** hydroCHLOROthiazide/irbesartan (an angiotensin II receptor antagonist): 12.5 mg/150 mg, 12.5 mg/300 mg, 25 mg/300 mg. **Benicar HCT:** hydroCHLOROthiazide/olmesartan (an angiotensin II receptor antagonist): 12.5 mg/20 mg, 12.5 mg/40 mg, 25 mg/40 mg. **Generic:** hydroCHLOROthiazide/captopril (an ACE inhibitor): 15 mg/25 mg, 15 mg/50 mg, 25 mg/25 mg, 25 mg/50 mg. **Diovan HCT:** hydroCHLOROthiazide/valsartan (an angiotensin II receptor antagonist): 12.5 mg/80 mg, 12.5 mg/160 mg. **Maxide:** hydroCHLOROthiazide/triamterene (a potassium-sparing diuretic): 25 mg/37.5 mg, 25 mg/50 mg, 50 mg/75 mg. **Hyzaar:** hydroCHLOROthiazide/losartan (an angiotensin II receptor antagonist): 12.5 mg/50 mg, 12.5 mg/100 mg, 25 mg/100 mg. **Lotensin HCT:** hydroCHLOROthiazide/benazepril (an ACE inhibitor): 6.25 mg/5 mg, 12.5 mg/10 mg, 12.5 mg/20 mg, 25 mg/20 mg. **Micardis HCT:** hydroCHLOROthiazide/telmisartan (an angiotensin II receptor antagonist): 12.5 mg/40 mg, 12.5 mg/80 mg. **Zestoretic:** hydroCHLOROthiazide/lisinopril (an ACE inhibitor): 12.5 mg/10 mg, 12.5 mg/20 mg, 25 mg/20 mg. **Tekturna HCT:** hydroCHLOROthiazide/aliskiren (a renin inhibitor): 12.5 mg/150 mg, 25 mg/300 mg. **Tribenzor:** hydroCHLOROthiazide/olmesartan/amLODIPine: 12.5 mg/20 mg/5 mg, 12.5 mg/40 mg/5 mg, 25 mg/40 mg/5 mg, 12.5 mg/40 mg/10 mg, 25 mg/40 mg/10 mg. **Generic:** hydroCHLOROthiazide/moexipril (an ACE inhibitor): 12.5 mg/7.5 mg, 25 mg/15 mg. **Vaseretic:** hydroCHLOROthiazide/enalapril (an ACE inhibitor): 12.5 mg/5 mg, 25 mg/10 mg. **Ziac:** hydroCHLOROthiazide/bisoprolol (a beta blocker): 6.25 mg/5 mg, 6.25 mg/10 mg.

◆CLASSIFICATION

PHARMACOTHERAPEUTIC: Sulfonamide derivative. Thiazide diuretic. **CLINICAL:** Antihypertensive.

USES

Hypertension (chronic): Treatment of mild to moderate hypertension. **Edema:** Treatment of edema due to HF, renal impairment (e.g., nephrotic syndrome, acute glomerulosclerosis, chronic renal failure), hepatic cirrhosis, sterioid/estrogen therapy. **OFF-LABEL:** Treatment of calcium nephrolithiasis, diabetes insipidus.

PRECAUTIONS

Contraindications: Hypersensitivity to hydroCHLOROthiazide. Anuria, history of hypersensitivity to sulfonamides or thiazide diuretics. **Cautions:** Severe renal/hepatic impairment, prediabetes or diabetes, elderly or debilitated, history of gout, moderate to high serum cholesterol, hypercalcemia, hypokalemia.

ACTION

Inhibits sodium reabsorption in distal renal tubules, causing excretion of sodium, potassium, hydrogen ions, water. **Therapeutic Effect:** Promotes diuresis; reduces B/P.

PHARMACOKINETICS

Route	Onset	Peak	Duration
PO (diuretic)	2 hrs	4–6 hrs	6–12 hrs

Variably absorbed from GI tract. Primarily excreted unchanged in urine. Not removed by hemodialysis. **Half-life:** 5.6–14.8 hrs.

⧖ LIFESPAN CONSIDERATIONS

Pregnancy/Lactation: Crosses placenta. Small amount distributed in breast milk. Breastfeeding not recommended. **Children:** No age-related precautions noted, except jaundiced infants may be at risk for hyperbilirubinemia. **Elderly:** May be more sensitive to hypotensive, electrolyte effects. Age-related renal impairment may require dosage adjustment.

INTERACTIONS

DRUG: Bile acid sequestrants (e.g., cholestyramine) may decrease concentration/effect. **Antihypertensives (e.g., amLODIPine, cloNIDine, lisinopril, valsartan)** may increase hypotensive effect. May increase risk of **lithium** toxicity. **HERBAL:** Herbals with **hypertensive properties (e.g., licorice, yohimbe) or hypotensive properties (e.g., garlic, ginger, ginkgo biloba)** may alter effects. **Licorice** may increase hypokalemic effect. **FOOD:** None known. **LAB VALUES:** May increase serum glucose, cholesterol, LDL, bilirubin, calcium, creatinine, uric acid, triglycerides. May decrease urinary calcium, serum magnesium, potassium, sodium.

AVAILABILITY (Rx)

Capsules: 12.5 mg. **Tablets:** 12.5 mg, 25 mg, 50 mg.

ADMINISTRATION/HANDLING

PO
• May take with or without food. If GI upset occurs, give with food or milk, preferably with breakfast (may prevent nocturia). • Give last dose no later than 6 PM unless instructed otherwise.

INDICATIONS/ROUTES/DOSAGE

Edema
PO: ADULTS: Initially, 25–50 mg/day in 1–2 divided doses. Adjust dose based on response and tolerability. **Maximum:** 200 mg/day in 1–2 divided doses.

Hypertension
PO: ADULTS: Initially, 12.5–25 mg once daily. Evaluate after 2–4 wks. May increase dose up to 50 mg once daily.

Usual Elderly Dose
PO: ADULTS: Initially, 12.5 mg once daily. Titrate in increments of 12.5 mg as necessary. **Maximum:** 50 mg/day in 1–2 divided doses.

Usual Pediatric Dosage (Edema/HTN)
PO: CHILDREN 2–12 YRS: 1–2 mg/kg/day. **Maximum:** 100 mg/day. **CHILDREN 6 MOS–2 YRS:** 1–2 mg/kg/day in 1–2 divided doses. **Maximum:** 37.5 mg/day. **CHILDREN YOUNGER THAN 6 MOS:** 1–3 mg/kg/day in 1–2 divided doses. **Maximum:** Up to 3.3 mg/kg/day PO in 2 divided doses has been recommended by some pediatric experts.

Dosage in Renal Impairment
Creatinine clearance less than 30 mL/min: Generally not effective. Avoid use with creatinine clearance less than 10 mL/min.

Dosage in Hepatic Impairment
Use caution.

SIDE EFFECTS

Expected: Increased urinary frequency (diminishes with continued use), urine volume. **Frequent:** Potassium depletion. **Occasional:** Orthostatic hypotension, headache, GI disturbances, photosensitivity.

ADVERSE EFFECTS/TOXIC REACTIONS

Vigorous diuresis may cause significant water loss/electrolyte depletion, resulting in hypokalemia, hyponatremia, dehydration. Acute hypotension may occur. Hyperglycemia may occur during prolonged therapy. Pancreatitis, blood dyscrasias, pulmonary edema, allergic pneumonitis, dermatologic reactions occur rarely. Overdose can lead to lethargy, coma without changes in electrolytes or hydration.

H

NURSING CONSIDERATIONS

BASELINE ASSESSMENT

Obtain vital signs, serum electrolytes. Evaluate skin turgor, mucous membranes for hydration status. Evaluate for peripheral edema. Assess muscle strength, mental status. Note skin temperature, moisture. Obtain baseline weight. Monitor I&O.

INTERVENTION/EVALUATION

Monitor B/P, vital signs, serum electrolytes, I&O, daily weight. Note extent of diuresis. Watch for changes from initial assessment (hypokalemia may result in weakness, tremor, muscle cramps, nausea, vomiting, altered mental status, tachycardia; hyponatremia may result in confusion, thirst, cold/clammy skin). Be esp. alert for potassium depletion in pts taking digoxin (cardiac arrhythmias). Potassium supplementation should be considered if hypokalemia occurs.

PATIENT/FAMILY TEACHING

• Expect increased frequency (diminishes with continued use), volume of urination. • To reduce hypotensive effect, go from lying to standing slowly. • Eat foods high in potassium, such as whole grains (cereals), legumes, meat, bananas, apricots, orange juice, potatoes (white, sweet), raisins. • Protect skin from sun, ultraviolet light (photosensitivity may occur).

HYDROcodone

hye-droe-**koe**-done

■ **BLACK BOX ALERT** ■ Risk of opioid addiction, abuse, and misuse. Serious, life-threatening, or fatal respiratory depression may occur. Accidental ingestion by children can result in fatal overdose. Prolonged use during pregnancy may result in opioid withdrawal syndrome. Concomitant use of CYP3A4 inhibitors may increase concentration/effect. Discontinuation of CYP3A4 inducers may increase concentration/effect. Concomitant use of CNS depressants (e.g., benzodiazepines) may result in profound sedation, respiratory depression, coma, or death.
Do not confuse Hycodan with Vicodin.

FIXED-COMBINATION(S)

HYDROcodone 5 mg/acetaminophen 300 mg; HYDROcodone 5 mg/acetaminophen 325 mg; HYDROcodone 7.5 mg/acetaminophen 300 mg; HYDROcodone 7.5 mg/acetaminophen 325 mg; HYDROcodone 10 mg/acetaminophen 300 mg HYDROcodone 10 mg/acetaminophen 325 mg.

◆CLASSIFICATION

PHARMACOTHERAPEUTIC: Opioid agonist (Schedule III). **CLINICAL:** Narcotic analgesic.

USES

Relief of moderate to moderately severe pain.

PRECAUTIONS

Contraindications: Hypersensitivity to HYDROcodone. Significant respiratory depression, acute or severe bronchial asthma or hypercarbia, GI obstruction including paralytic ileus (known or suspected). **Cautions:** Adrenal insufficiency, biliary tract disease, pancreatitis, CNS depression/coma, acute alcoholism, hypothyroidism; severe renal, hepatic, or pulmonary impairment; urinary stricture, prostatic hypertrophy, seizures, elderly, debilitated, other CNS depressants, history of drug abuse and misuse, drug-seeking behavior, dependency.

ACTION

Binds with opioid receptors in CNS. **Therapeutic Effect:** Reduces intensity of incoming pain stimuli from sensory nerve endings, altering pain perception, emotional response to pain; suppresses cough reflex.

PHARMACOKINETICS

Route	Onset	Peak	Duration
PO (analgesic)	10–20 min	30–60 min	4–6 hrs
PO (antitussive)	N/A	N/A	4–6 hrs

Widely distributed. Metabolized in liver. Primarily excreted in urine. **Half-life:** 3.8 hrs (increased in elderly).

⌛ LIFESPAN CONSIDERATIONS

Pregnancy/Lactation: Readily crosses placenta. Distributed in breast milk. May prolong labor if administered in latent phase of first stage of labor or before cervical dilation of 4–5 cm has occurred. Respiratory depression may occur in neonate if mother received opiates during labor. Regular use of opiates during pregnancy may produce withdrawal symptoms (irritability, excessive crying, tremors, hyperactive reflexes, fever, vomiting, diarrhea, yawning, sneezing, seizures) in the neonate. **Children:** Pts younger than 2 yrs may be more susceptible to respiratory depression. **Elderly:** May be more susceptible to respiratory depression, may cause paradoxical excitement. Age-related renal impairment, prostatic hypertrophy or obstruction may increase risk of urinary retention; dosage adjustment recommended.

INTERACTIONS

DRUG: CNS depressants (e.g., alcohol, morphine, oxyCODONE, zolpidem) may increase CNS depression. **MAOIs (e.g., phenelzine, selegiline)** may increase adverse effects. **CYP3A4 inhibitors (e.g., clarithromycin, ketoconazole, ritonavir)** may increase or prolong opioid effects. **HERBAL: Herbals with sedative properties (e.g., chamomile, kava, kava, valerian)** may increase CNS depression. **St. John's wort** may decrease concentration/effect. **FOOD:** None known. **LAB VALUES:** May increase serum amylase, lipase.

AVAILABILITY (Rx)

Solution, Oral: HYDROcodone 7.5 mg/acetaminophen 325 mg/15 mL; HYDROcodone 10 mg/acetaminophen 325 mg/15 mL. **Tablet:** Hydrocodone 5 mg/acetaminophen 325 mg, hydrocodone 7.5 mg/acetaminophen 325 mg, hydrocodone 10 mg/acetaminophen 325 mg.

ADMINISTRATION/HANDLING

PO
• Give without regard to food.

INDICATIONS/ROUTES/DOSAGE

Analgesia (Combination Products)
PO: ADULTS, CHILDREN WEIGHING 50 KG OR MORE: Initially, 5–10 mg q3–4h as needed. **ADULTS, CHILDREN WEIGHING LESS THAN 50 KG:** Initially, 0.1–0.2 mg/kg q4–6h as needed. **ELDERLY:** 2.5–5 mg q4–6h.

Dosage in Renal Impairment
No dose adjustment.

Dosage in Hepatic Impairment
Use caution.

SIDE EFFECTS

Frequent: Lethargy, hypotension, diaphoresis, facial flushing, dizziness, drowsiness. **Occasional:** Urine retention, blurred vision, constipation, dry mouth, headache, nausea, vomiting, difficult/painful urination, euphoria, dysphoria.

ADVERSE EFFECTS/TOXIC REACTIONS

Overdose results in respiratory depression, skeletal muscle flaccidity, cold/clammy skin, cyanosis, extreme drowsiness progressing to seizures, stupor, coma. Tolerance to analgesic effect, physical dependence may occur with repeated use. Prolonged duration of action, cumulative effect may occur in those with hepatic/renal impairment. Concomitant use with benzodiazepines may result in profound sedation,

H

respiratory depression, coma, and death. **Antidote:** Naloxone (see Appendix H).

NURSING CONSIDERATIONS

BASELINE ASSESSMENT

Obtain vital signs. If respirations are 12/min or less (20/min or less in children), withhold medication, contact physician. Assess for potential of abuse/misuse (e.g., drug-seeking behavior, mental health conditions, history of substance abuse). **Analgesic:** Assess onset, type, location, duration of pain. Effect of medication is reduced if full pain recurs before next dose. **Antitussive:** Assess type, severity, frequency of cough.

INTERVENTION/EVALUATION

Palpate bladder for urinary retention. Monitor daily pattern of bowel activity, stool consistency. Initiate deep breathing and coughing exercises, particularly in pts with pulmonary impairment. Assess for clinical improvement; record onset of relief of pain, cough. Screen for misuse, abuse, drug-seeking behavior.

PATIENT/FAMILY TEACHING

• Go from lying to standing slowly to avoid orthostatic hypotension. • Avoid tasks that require alertness, motor skills until response to drug is established. • Avoid alcohol. • Tolerance or dependence may occur with prolonged use at high dosages. • Report nausea, vomiting, constipation, shortness of breath, difficulty breathing. • Taper slowly after long-term use.

hydrocortisone

hye-droe-**kor**-ti-sone
(Anusol HC, Cortaid, Cortef, SOLU-Cortef, Cortenema, Preparation H, Proctocort)
Do not confuse hydrocortisone with hydroCHLOROthiazide, HYDROcodone, or hydroxychlo-

roquine, **Cortef with Coreg, or SOLU-Cortef with SOLU-medrol.**

FIXED-COMBINATION(S)

Cortisporin: hydrocortisone/neomycin/polymyxin (an anti-infective): 5 mg/10,000 units/5 mg, 10 mg/10,000 units/5 mg. **Lipsovir:** hydrocortisone/acyclovir (an antiviral): 1%/5%.

◆CLASSIFICATION

PHARMACOTHERAPEUTIC: Corticosteroid. **CLINICAL:** Glucocorticoid.

USES

Systemic: Allergic states: e.g., perennial/seasonal allergic rhinitis, transfusion reactions. **Dermatologic diseases:** e.g., atopic/contact dermatitis, severe psoriasis. **Endocrine disorders:** e.g., adrenocortical insufficiency, hypercalcemia associated with cancer. **Hematologic diseases:** e.g., acquired (autoimmune) hemolytic anemia, immune thrombocytopenia. **Respiratory diseases:** e.g., bronchial asthma, aspiration pneumonia. **Rheumatic disorders:** e.g., rheumatoid arthritis, systemic lupus erythematosus. **Topical:** Inflammatory dermatoses, adjunctive treatment of ulcerative colitis, atopic dermatitis, inflamed hemorrhoids. **OFF-LABEL:** Systemic: Asthma (acute exacerbation), COVID-19 infection, septic shock, thyroid storm.

PRECAUTIONS

Contraindications: Hypersensitivity to hydrocortisone. Systemic fungal infections. Use in premature infants. Administration of live or attenuated virus vaccines. IM administration in idiopathic thrombocytopenia purpura. Intrathecal administration. **Cautions:** Thyroid dysfunction, cirrhosis, hypertension, osteoporosis, thromboembolic tendencies or thrombophlebitis, HF, seizure disorders, diabetes, respiratory tuberculosis, untreated systemic infections, renal/hepatic impairment, acute MI, myasthenia gravis, glaucoma, cataracts, increased intraocular pressure, elderly, immunocompromised pts (e.g., diabetes, renal failure, open wounds).

ACTION

Inhibits accumulation of inflammatory cells at inflammation sites, phagocytosis, lysosomal enzyme release, synthesis and/or release of mediators of inflammation. Reverses increased capillary permeability. **Therapeutic Effect:** Prevents/suppresses cell-mediated immune reactions. Decreases/prevents tissue response to inflammatory process.

PHARMACOKINETICS

Route	Onset	Peak	Duration
IV	N/A	4–6 hrs	8–12 hrs

Widely distributed. Metabolized in liver. **Half-life:** Plasma, 1.5–2 hrs; biologic, 8–12 hrs.

⧗ LIFESPAN CONSIDERATIONS

Pregnancy/Lactation: Crosses placenta; distributed in breast milk. May produce cleft palate if used chronically during first trimester. Breastfeeding not recommended. **Children:** Prolonged treatment or high dosages may decrease short-term growth rate, cortisol secretion. **Elderly:** May be more susceptible to developing hypertension or osteoporosis.

INTERACTIONS

DRUG: CYP3A4 inducers (e.g., car-BAMazepine, phenytoin, rifAMPin) may decrease effects. **Live virus vaccines** may decrease pt's antibody response to vaccine, increase vaccine side effects, potentiate virus replication. May decrease therapeutic effect of **aldesleukin, BCG (intravesical).** May increase hyponatremic effect of **desmopressin. HERBAL:** Echinacea may decrease therapeutic effect. **FOOD:** None known. **LAB VALUES:** May increase serum glucose, lipids, sodium. May decrease serum calcium, potassium, thyroxine; WBC count.

AVAILABILITY (Rx)

Cream, Rectal: *(Anusol HC, Preparation H Hydrocortisone):* 1%, 2.5%. **Cream, Topical:** 0.5%, 1%, 2.5%. **Injection, Powder for Reconstitution:** *(Solu-Cortef):* 100 mg, 250 mg, 500 mg, 1 g. **Ointment, Topical:** 0.5%, 1%, 2.5%. **Suppository** *(Anusol HC):* 25 mg. **Suspension, Rectal:** *(Cortenema):* 100 mg/60 mL. **Tablets:** *(Cortef):* 5 mg, 10 mg, 20 mg.

ADMINISTRATION/HANDLING

 IV

Hydrocortisone Sodium Succinate
Reconstitution • Initially, reconstitute vial per manufacturer's instructions. • May further dilute with D_5W or 0.9% NaCl. For IV push, dilute to 50 mg/mL; for intermittent infusion, dilute to 1 mg/mL. **Note:** 100–3,000 mg may be added to 50 mL D_5W or 0.9% NaCl.
Rate of administration • Administer IV push over 3–5 min (over 10 min for doses 500 mg or greater). Give intermittent infusion over 20–30 min.
Storage • Store at room temperature. • Once reconstituted, stable for 3 days at room temperature. Once further diluted with 0.9% NaCl or D_5W, stability is concentration dependent: 1 mg/mL (24 hrs), 2–60 mg/mL (4 hrs).

PO
• Give with food or milk if GI distress occurs.

Rectal
• Shake homogeneous suspension well. • Instruct pt to lie on left side with left leg extended, right leg flexed. • Gently insert applicator tip into rectum, pointed slightly toward navel (umbilicus). Slowly instill medication.

Topical
• Gently cleanse area before application. • Use occlusive dressings only as ordered. • Apply sparingly; rub into area thoroughly.

H

❖ IV COMPATIBILITIES

Acetaminophen, calcium gluconate, dexmedetomidine, ibuprofen, magnesium sulfate, propofol.

INDICATIONS/ROUTES/DOSAGE

Note: Dosage is variable and must be individualized based on disease treated and response.

Usual Dosage

IV, IM: **ADULTS, ELDERLY, ADOLESCENTS:** 100–500 mg/dose. May repeat at intervals of 2, 4, or 6 hrs as indicated by pt's response/clinical condition. **CHILDREN:** 1–5 mg/kg/day in divided doses based on response and disease being treated.

PO: **ADULTS, ELDERLY, ADOLESCENTS:** 20–240 mg/day in divided doses. based on response and disease being treated. **CHILDREN:** 2.5–10 mg/kg/day in divided doses based on response and disease being treated.

Adjunctive Treatment of Ulcerative Colitis

Rectal: *(Enema):* **ADULTS, ELDERLY:** 100 mg 1 or 2 times/day. Continue for 3–4 wks. Once improved, may taper gradually to a nightly regimen.

(Rectal Foam): **ADULTS, ELDERLY:** 1 applicator 1–2 times/day. Continue for 3–4 wks. Once improved, may taper gradually to a nightly regimen.

Usual Topical Dose

ADULTS, ELDERLY: Apply sparingly 2–4 times/day.

Dosage in Renal/Hepatic Impairment

No dose adjustment.

SIDE EFFECTS

Frequent: Insomnia, heartburn, anxiety, abdominal distention, diaphoresis, acne, mood swings, increased appetite, facial flushing, delayed wound healing, increased susceptibility to infection, diarrhea, or constipation. **Occasional:** Headache, edema, change in skin color, frequent urination. **Topical:** Pruritus, redness, irritation.

Rare: Tachycardia, allergic reaction (rash, hives), psychological changes, hallucinations, depression. **Topical:** Allergic contact dermatitis, purpura. **Systemic:** Absorption more likely with use of occlusive dressings or extensive application in young children.

ADVERSE EFFECTS/TOXIC REACTIONS

Long-term therapy: Hypocalcemia, hypokalemia, muscle wasting (esp. arms, legs), osteoporosis, spontaneous fractures, amenorrhea, cataracts, glaucoma, peptic ulcer, HF. **Abrupt withdrawal after long-term therapy:** Nausea, fever, headache, sudden severe joint pain, rebound inflammation, fatigue, weakness, lethargy, dizziness, orthostatic hypotension.

NURSING CONSIDERATIONS

BASELINE ASSESSMENT

Obtain weight, B/P, serum glucose, cholesterol, electrolytes. Screen for infections including fungal infections, TB, viral skin lesions. Question medical history as listed in Precautions.

INTERVENTION/EVALUATION

Assess for edema. Be alert to infection (reduced immune response): sore throat, fever, vague symptoms. Monitor daily pattern of bowel activity, stool consistency. Monitor electrolytes, B/P, weight, serum glucose. Monitor for hypocalcemia (muscle twitching, cramps), hypokalemia (weakness, paresthesia [esp. lower extremities], nausea/vomiting, irritability, ECG changes). Assess emotional status, ability to sleep.

PATIENT/FAMILY TEACHING

• Report fever, sore throat, muscle aches, sudden weight gain, swelling, visual disturbances, behavioral changes. • Do not take aspirin or any other medication without consulting physician. • Limit caffeine; avoid alcohol. • Inform dentist, other physicians of cortisone therapy now or within past 12 mos. • **Topical:** Apply after shower or bath for best absorption. • Do not cover or use occlusive dressings unless ordered by physician; do

H

not use tight diapers, plastic pants, coverings. • Avoid contact with eyes.

HYDROmorphone 🔲HIGH ALERT

hye-droe-**mor**-fone
(Dilaudid, Hydromorph Contin ✦)

■ **BLACK BOX ALERT** ■ High abuse potential, life-threatening respiratory depression risk. Other opioids, alcohol, CNS depressants increase risk of potentially fatal respiratory depression. Highly concentrated form (Dilaudid HP, 10 mg/mL) not to be interchanged with less concentrated form (Dilaudid); overdose, death may result. *Extended-Release Tablets:* For use in opioid-tolerant pts. Do not crush, break, chew, or dissolve. Swallow whole.

Do not confuse Dilaudid with Demerol or Dilantin, or HYDROmorphone with HYDROcodone or morphine.

◆CLASSIFICATION

PHARMACOTHERAPEUTIC: Opioid agonist (Schedule II). **CLINICAL:** Narcotic analgesic.

USES

Immediate-release: (Tablet, oral solution, injection, suppository): Management of moderate to severe pain. **Extended-release:** Management of pain in opioid-tolerant pts to require daily, around-the-clock, long-term opioid treatment. **OFF-LABEL:** Pain/sedation (critically ill puts in ICU).

PRECAUTIONS

Contraindications: Hypersensitivity to HYDROmorphone. Acute or severe bronchial asthma, severe respiratory depression. GI obstruction including paralytic ileus (known or suspected). **Additional Product-Specific Contraindications: Dilaudid HP injection:** Opioid-intolerant pts. **Extended-Release Tablets:** Opioid-intolerant pts, preexisting GI surgery/diseases causing GI

narrowing. **Cautions:** Severe hepatic, renal, respiratory disease; hypothyroidism, adrenal cortical insufficiency, seizures, acute alcoholism, head injury, intracranial lesions, increased intracranial pressure, prostatic hypertrophy, Addison's disease, urethral stricture, pancreatitis, biliary tract disease, cardiovascular disease, morbid obesity, delirium tremens, toxic psychosis, pts with CNS depression or coma, pts with depleted blood volume, obstructive bowel disorder; history of drug abuse and misuse, drug-seeking behavior, dependency.

ACTION

Binds to opioid receptors in CNS, reducing intensity of pain stimuli from sensory nerve endings. **Therapeutic Effect:** Alters perception, emotional response to pain; suppresses cough reflex.

PHARMACOKINETICS

Route	Onset	Peak	Duration
PO	30 min	90–120 min	4 hrs
IV	10–15 min	15–30 min	2–3 hrs
IM	15 min	30–60 min	4–5 hrs
SQ	15 min	30–90 min	4 hrs
Rectal	15–30 min	N/A	N/A

Well absorbed from GI tract after IM administration. Widely distributed. Metabolized in liver. Excreted in urine. **Half-life:** 2.6–4 hrs.

⧗ LIFESPAN CONSIDERATIONS

Pregnancy/Lactation: Readily crosses placenta. Unknown if distributed in breast milk. May prolong labor if administered in latent phase of first stage of labor or before cervical dilation of 4–5 cm has occurred. Respiratory depression may occur in neonate if mother receives opiates during labor. Regular use of opiates during pregnancy may produce withdrawal symptoms in the neonate (irritability, excessive crying, tremors, hyperactive reflexes, fever, vomiting, diarrhea, yawning, sneezing, seizures). **Children:** Pts younger than 2 yrs may be more susceptible to respiratory depression. **Elderly:** May be more susceptible to respiratory depression, may cause

H

paradoxical excitement. Age-related renal impairment, prostatic hypertrophy or obstruction may increase risk of urinary retention; dosage adjustment recommended.

INTERACTIONS

DRUG: **CNS depressants (e.g., alcohol, morphine, LORazepam, zolpidem)** may increase CNS depression. **MAOIs (e.g., phenelzine, selegiline)** may increase adverse effects. **HERBAL: Herbals with sedative properties (e.g., chamomile, kava, kava, valerian)** may increase CNS depression. **FOOD:** None known. **LAB VALUES:** May increase serum amylase, lipase.

AVAILABILITY (Rx)

Injection, Solution: 1 mg/mL, 2 mg/mL, 4 mg/mL, 10 mg/mL. **Liquid, Oral:** 1 mg/mL. **Suppository:** 3 mg. **Tablets:** 2 mg, 4 mg, 8 mg.

 Tablets: *(Extended-Release):* 8 mg, 12 mg, 16 mg, 32 mg.

ADMINISTRATION/HANDLING

IV

◄**ALERT**► High-concentration injection (10 mg/mL) should be used only in pts tolerant to opiate agonists, currently receiving high doses of another opiate agonist for severe, chronic pain due to cancer.
Reconstitution • May give undiluted. • May further dilute with 5 mL Sterile Water for Injection or 0.9% NaCl.
Rate of administration • Administer IV push very slowly (over 2–3 min). • Rapid IV increases risk of severe adverse reactions (chest wall rigidity, apnea, peripheral circulatory collapse, anaphylactoid effects, cardiac arrest).
Storage • Store at room temperature; protect from light. • Slight yellow discoloration of parenteral form does not indicate loss of potency.

IM, SQ
• Subcutaneously or intramuscularly insert needle and inject solution. Pulling back the plunger before IM injection may ensure that drug is not delivered directly into bloodstream (however, this topic is currently debated). • Administer slowly; rotate injection sites. • Pts with circulatory impairment experience higher risk of overdosage due to delayed absorption of repeated administration.

PO
• Give without regard to food. • Extended-release tablets must be swallowed whole; do not break, crush, dissolve, or divide. **Oral solution** • Calibrated oral syringe/dosing cup should be used.

Rectal
• Refrigerate suppositories. • Moisten suppository with cold water before inserting well up into rectum.

▦ IV INCOMPATIBILITIES
Clevidipine.

▦ IV COMPATIBILITIES
Acetaminophen, dexmedetomidine, dobutamine, magnesium sulfate, norepinephrine.

INDICATIONS/ROUTES/DOSAGE

Analgesia (Acute, Moderate to Severe)
PO: ADULTS: *(Immediate-Release):* Initially 1–2 mg q4–6h as needed (Usual range): 1–4 mg q4–6h as needed. **ELDERLY:** Initially, 1–2 mg q3–4h as needed. Use with caution; initiating at the low end of the dosage range is recommended. **CHILDREN, ADOLESCENTS WEIGHING MORE THAN 50 KG:** 1–2 mg q3–4h as needed. **CHILDREN OLDER THAN 6 MOS WEIGHING LESS THAN 50 KG:** 0.03–0.08 mg/kg/dose q3–4h as needed.
IV (For use in opiate-naive pts): **ADULTS:** 0.2–0.5 mg q2–4h as needed. **(Usual range):** 0.2–1 mg q2–4h as needed. **ELDERLY:** 0.2 mg q2–3h PRN or 0.25–0.5 mg q3–4 PRN. **CHILDREN, ADOLESCENTS WEIGHING MORE THAN 50 KG:** 0.2–

0.6 mg/dose q2–4h as needed. **CHILDREN WEIGHING 50 KG OR LESS:** 0.015 mg/kg/dose q3–6h as needed.
Rectal: ADULTS, ELDERLY: 3 mg q6–8h. *(Extended-Release):* Unless pain is associated with cancer, palliative care, or sickle cell disease, do NOT use with chronic pain until treated for at least 1 wk with immediate-release dosage form.

Dosage in Renal/Hepatic Impairment
Decrease initial dose; use with caution.

SIDE EFFECTS

Frequent: Drowsiness, dizziness, hypotension (including orthostatic hypotension), decreased appetite. **Occasional:** Confusion, diaphoresis, facial flushing, urinary retention, constipation, dry mouth, nausea, vomiting, headache, pain at injection site. **Rare:** Allergic reaction, depression.

ADVERSE EFFECTS/TOXIC REACTIONS

Overdose results in respiratory depression, skeletal muscle flaccidity, cold/clammy skin, cyanosis, extreme drowsiness progressing to seizures, stupor, coma. Tolerance to analgesic effect, physical dependence may occur with repeated use. Prolonged duration of action, cumulative effect may occur in those with hepatic/renal impairment. Concomitant use with benzodiazepines may result in profound sedation, respiratory depression, coma, and death. **Antidote:** Naloxone (see Appendix H).

NURSING CONSIDERATIONS

BASELINE ASSESSMENT

Obtain vital signs. If respirations are 12/min or less (20/min or less in children), withhold medication, contact physician. Assess risk of drug abuse, misuse, drug-seeking behavior. **Analgesic:** Assess onset, type, location, duration of pain. Effect of medication is reduced if full pain recurs before next dose. **Antitussive:** Assess type, severity, frequency of cough. Screen for misuse, abuse, drug-seeking behavior.

INTERVENTION/EVALUATION

Monitor vital signs; assess for pain relief, cough. To prevent pain cycles, instruct pt to request pain medication as soon as discomfort begins. Monitor daily pattern of bowel activity, stool consistency (esp. in long-term use). Initiate deep breathing and coughing exercises, particularly in pts with pulmonary impairment. Assess for clinical improvement; record onset of relief of pain, cough. Screen for misuse, abuse, drug-seeking behavior.

PATIENT/FAMILY TEACHING

• Avoid alcohol. • Avoid tasks that require alertness/motor skills until response to drug is established. • Tolerance or dependence may occur with prolonged use at high dosages. • Change positions slowly to avoid orthostatic hypotension. • Do not chew, crush, dissolve, or divide extended-release tablets.

H

ibandronate

eye-**ban**-droe-nate
(Boniva)

◆CLASSIFICATION

PHARMACOTHERAPEUTIC: Bisphosphonate. **CLINICAL:** Calcium regulator.

USES

Treatment/prevention of osteoporosis in
postmenopausal women. **OFF-LABEL:** Hypercalcemia of malignancy; reduces bone
pain and skeletal complications from metastatic bone disease due to breast cancer.
Prostate cancer, metastatic, bone pain.

PRECAUTIONS

Contraindications: Hypersensitivity   to
ibandronate,   other   bisphosphonates;
oral tablets in pts unable to stand or sit
upright for at least 60 min; pts with abnormalities of the esophagus that would
delay emptying (e.g., stricture, achala-
sia), hypocalcemia. **Cautions:** GI diseases (duodenitis, dysphagia, esophagitis, gastritis, ulcers [drug may exacerbate
these conditions]), renal impairment
with CrCl less than 30 mL/min.

ACTION

Inhibits bone resorption via activity on
osteoclasts or osteoclast precursors.
Therapeutic Effect: Reduces rate of
bone resorption, resulting in indirect increased bone mineral density.

PHARMACOKINETICS

Absorbed in upper GI tract. Extent of
absorption impaired by food, beverages
(other than plain water). Protein binding:
85%–99%. Rapidly binds to bone. Unabsorbed portion excreted in urine. **Half-
life: PO:** 37–157 hrs; **IV:** 5–25 hrs.

⧗ LIFESPAN CONSIDERATIONS

Pregnancy/Lactation: May cause fetal
harm/malformations. Unknown if distributed in breast milk. Breastfeeding not

recommended. **Children:** Safety and efficacy not established. **Elderly:** No age-
related precautions noted.

INTERACTIONS

**DRUG: Antacids, calcium, magne-
sium, proron pump inhibitors
(PPIs) (e.g., omeprazole, pantoprazole)** may decrease concentra-
tion/effect. **HERBAL:** None significant.
**FOOD: Beverages (other than plain
water), dietary supplements, dairy
products, food** interfere with absorption. **LAB VALUES:** May decrease serum
alkaline phosphatase. May increase serum cholesterol.

AVAILABILITY (Rx)

Injection Solution: 3 mg/3 mL syringe.

Tablets: 150 mg.

ADMINISTRATION/HANDLING

PO
• Give 60 min before first food or beverage of the day, on an empty stomach with
6–8 oz plain water (not mineral water)
while pt is standing or sitting in upright
position. • Pt cannot lie down for 60
min following   administration. • Instruct pt to swallow whole; do not break,
crush, dissolve, or divide tablet (potential for oropharyngeal ulceration).

IV
• Give over 15–30 sec.

INDICATIONS/ROUTES/DOSAGE

Note: May consider discontinuing after
3–5 yrs in pts at low risk for fracture.
Consider supplemental calcium and vitamin D if dietary intake is inadequate.

Osteoporosis
**PO (Prevention/Treatment): ADULTS,
ELDERLY:** 150 mg once monthly.
IV (Treatment): ADULTS, ELDERLY: 3 mg
q3mos.

Dosage in Renal Impairment
Not recommended for pts with CrCl less
than 30 mL/min.

ibrutinib

Dosage in Hepatic Impairment
No dose adjustment.

SIDE EFFECTS

Frequent (13%–6%): Back pain, dyspepsia, peripheral discomfort, diarrhea, headache, myalgia. **IV:** Abdominal pain, dyspepsia, constipation, nausea, diarrhea. **Occasional (4%–3%):** Dizziness, arthralgia, asthenia. **Rare (2% or less):** Vomiting, hypersensitivity reaction.

ADVERSE EFFECTS/TOXIC REACTIONS

Upper respiratory infection occurs occasionally. Overdose results in hypocalcemia, hypophosphatemia, significant GI disturbances.

NURSING CONSIDERATIONS

BASELINE ASSESSMENT

Obtain serum calcium, vitamin D level. Hypocalcemia, vitamin D deficiency must be corrected before beginning therapy. Obtain results of bone density study.

INTERVENTION/EVALUATION

Monitor serum calcium, phosphate. Monitor renal function tests.

PATIENT/FAMILY TEACHING

• Expected benefits occur only when medication is taken with full glass (6–8 oz) of plain water, first thing in the morning and at least 60 min before first food, beverage, medication of the day. Any other beverage (mineral water, orange juice, coffee) significantly reduces absorption of medication. • Do not chew, crush, dissolve, or divide tablets; swallow whole. • Do not lie down for at least 60 min after taking medication (potentiates delivery to stomach, reduces risk of esophageal irritation). • Report swallowing difficulties, pain when swallowing, chest pain, new/worsening heartburn. • Consider weight-bearing exercises; modify behavioral factors (e.g., cigarette smoking, alcohol consumption). • Calcium and vitamin D supplements should be taken if dietary intake inadequate.

ibrutinib

eye-**broo**-ti-nib
(Imbruvica)
Do not confuse ibrutinib with axitinib, dasatinib, erlotinib, gefitinib, imatinib, nilotinib, PONATinib, SORAfenib, SUNItinib, or vandetanib.

◆ CLASSIFICATION

PHARMACOTHERAPEUTIC: Bruton tyrosine kinase inhibitor. **CLINICAL:** Antineoplastic.

USES

Chronic lymphocytic leukemia/ small lymphocytic lymphoma (CLL/ SLL): Treatment of adults with CLL/SLL or CLL/SLL with 17p deletion (as monotherapy or in combination with riTUXimab or obinutuzumab or in combination with bendamustine and riTUXimab): **Waldenstrom's macroglobulinemia (WM)** Treatment of WM as monotherapy or in combination with riTUXimab. **Chronic graft-versus-host disease (cGVHD):** Treatment of adults and children 1 yr and older with cGVHD after failure of at least one line of systemic therapy.

PRECAUTIONS

Contraindications: Hypersensitivity to ibrutinib. **Cautions:** Hepatic/renal impairment, hypertension, elderly, pregnancy, history of GI disease (e.g., bleeding, ulcers); pts at high risk for tumor lysis syndrome (high tumor burden).

ACTION

Inhibits enzymatic activity of Bruton's tyrosine kinase (BTK), a signaling molecule that promotes malignant B-cell proliferation and survival. **Therapeutic Effect:** Decreases malignant B-cell proliferation and survival.

PHARMACOKINETICS

Widely distributed. Metabolized in liver. Peak plasma concentration: 1–2 hrs.

Protein binding: 97%. Excreted in feces (80%), urine (10%). **Half-life:** 4–6 hrs.

⧗ LIFESPAN CONSIDERATIONS

Pregnancy/Lactation: Avoid pregnancy; may cause fetal harm. Females of reproductive potential must use effective contraception during treatment and for at least 1 mo after discontinuation. Unknown if distributed in breast milk. **Males:** Males with female partners of reproductive potential must use effective conception during treatment and for at least 1 mo after discontinuation. **Children:** Safety and efficacy not established. **Elderly:** Increased risk of cardiac events (atrial fibrillation, hypertension), infections (pneumonia, cellulitis), GI events (diarrhea, dehydration, bleeding).

INTERACTIONS

DRUG: Strong CYP3A4 inhibitors (e.g., **ketoconazole, clarithromycin**) may increase plasma concentration/effect; avoid use. **Strong CYP3A4 inducers** (e.g., **car-BAMazepine, rifAMPin, phenytoin**) may decrease plasma concentration/effect; avoid use. **Anticoagulants** (e.g., **warfarin**), **antiplatelets** (e.g., **aspirin, clopidogrel**), **NSAIDs** may increase risk of bleeding. May decrease the therapeutic effect of **BCG** (intravesical), **vaccines** (live). May increase adverse/toxic effects of **natalizumab, vaccines** (live). **HERBAL:** St. John's wort may decrease concentration/effect. **FOOD:** Grapefruit products, Seville oranges may increase concentration/effect. **Bitter orange** may increase concentration/effect. **LAB VALUES:** May decrease Hgb, Hct, neutrophils, platelets.

AVAILABILITY (Rx)

Oral Suspension: 70 mg/mL.

🔖 **Capsules:** 70 mg, 140 mg. **Tablets:** 140 mg, 280 mg, 420 mg.

ADMINISTRATION/HANDLING

PO

• Give with water. • Swallow capsules/tablets whole. Do not break, cut, or open capsules. Do not break, cut, crush, or divide tablets. Capsules/tablets cannot be chewed. **Oral suspension** • Only give oral dosing syringes provided. • Discard 60 days after opening. • Shake well before use.

INDICATIONS/ROUTES/DOSAGE

WM

PO: ADULTS, ELDERLY: 420 mg once daily (as monotherapy or in combination with riTUXimab). Continue until disease progression or unacceptable toxicity.

CLL/SLL

PO: ADULTS, ELDERLY: 420 mg once daily (as monotherapy or in combination with riTUXimab). Continue until disease progression or unacceptable toxicity.

GVHD

PO: ADULTS, ELDERLY, CHILDREN 12 YRS OF AGE AND OLDER: 420 mg once daily. **CHILDREN 1 TO LESS THAN 12 YRS OF AGE:** 240 mg/m^2 once daily (up to 420 mg). Continue until cGVHD progression, recurrence of underlying malignancy or unacceptable toxicity.

Dose Modification

Based on Common Terminology Criteria for Adverse Events (CTCAE).

Any Grade 3 or Greater Nonhematologic Event, Grade 3 or Greater Neutropenia With Infection or Fever, or Any Grade 4 Hematologic Toxicities

Interrupt treatment until resolution to Grade 1 or baseline, then restart at initial dose. If toxicity recurs, interrupt treatment until resolution to Grade 1 or baseline, then reduce dose to 420 mg daily (one capsule less). If toxicity recurs, interrupt treatment until resolution to Grade 1 or baseline, then reduce dose to 280 mg once daily (one capsule less). If toxicity still occurs at 280 mg dose, discontinue treatment.

Concomitant Use of Moderate CYP3A4 Inhibitors (e.g., fluconazole, dilTIAZem, verapamil)

Start at reduced dose of 140 mg daily. If toxicity occurs, either discontinue treatment or find alternate agent with less CYP3A4 inhibition.

Concomitant Short-Term Use of Strong CYP3A4 Inhibitors (7 days or less) (e.g., antifungals, antibiotics)
Interrupt treatment until strong CYP3A4 medications no longer needed.

Concomitant Chronic Use of Strong CYP3A4 Inhibitors or Inducers
Treatment not recommended.

Dosage in Renal Impairment
No dose adjustment.

Dosage in Hepatic Impairment
Mild impairment: Decrease dose to 140 mg. **Moderate to severe impairment:** Avoid use.

SIDE EFFECTS

Frequent (51%–23%): Diarrhea, fatigue, musculoskeletal pain, peripheral edema, nausea, bruising, dyspnea, constipation, rash, abdominal pain, vomiting. **Occasional (21%–11%):** Decreased appetite, cough, pyrexia, stomatitis, asthenia, dizziness, muscle spasms, dehydration, headache, dyspepsia, petechiae, arthralgia.

ADVERSE EFFECTS/TOXIC REACTIONS

Anemia, lymphopenia, neutropenia, thrombocytopenia are expected responses to therapy. Severe myelosuppression (Grade 3–4 CTCAE) reported in 41% of pts: Neutropenia (29%), thrombocytopenia (17%), anemia (9%). Infections including upper respiratory tract infection, UTI, pneumonia, skin infection, sinusitis were reported. Hemorrhagic events including epistaxis, GI bleeding, hematuria, intracranial hemorrhage, subdural hematoma reported in 5% of pts. Serious and fatal cases of renal toxicity reported: Increased serum creatinine 1.5 times upper limit of normal (ULN) (67% of pts), increased serum creatinine 1.53 times ULN (9% of pts). Second primary malignancies including skin cancer (4%), other carcinomas (1%) occurred. Fatal cardiac arrhythmias (ventricular tachycardia, atrial fibrillation, atrial flutter) may occur. Tumor lysis syndrome may present as acute renal failure, hypocalcemia, hyperuricemia, hyperphosphatemia.

NURSING CONSIDERATIONS

BASELINE ASSESSMENT

Obtain vital signs, CBC, serum chemistries, LFT, PT/INR if on anticoagulants. Question history of arrhythmias, HF, GI bleed, hepatic/renal impairment, peripheral edema, pulmonary disease. Obtain negative pregnancy test before initiating treatment. Assess hydration status. Receive full medication history including herbal products. Assess skin for open/unhealed wounds, lesions, moles. Assess risk of tumor lysis syndrome. Conduct baseline neurologic exam. Offer emotional support.

INTERVENTION/EVALUATION

Monitor CBC monthly; LFT, serum chemistries, renal function routinely. Monitor stool frequency, consistency, characteristics. Immediately report hemorrhagic events: epistaxis, hematuria, hemoptysis, melena. Monitor serum uric acid level if tumor lysis syndrome (acute renal failure, electrolyte imbalance, cardiac arrhythmias, seizures) is suspected. Obtain ECG for arrhythmias, dyspnea, palpitations. Screen for possible intracranial hemorrhage: altered mental status, aphasia, hemiparesis, unequal pupils, homonymous hemianopsia (blindness of one half of vision on same side of both eyes). Monitor for renal toxicity (anuria, hypertension, generalized edema, flank pain). Assess skin for new lesions.

PATIENT/FAMILY TEACHING

• Treatment may depress your immune system response and reduce your ability to fight infection. Report symptoms of infection such as body aches, chills, cough, fatigue, fever. Avoid those with active infection. • Report symptoms of bone marrow depression such as bruising, fatigue, fever, shortness of breath, weight loss; bleeding easily, bloody urine or stool. • Report palpitations, chest pain, shortness of breath, dizziness, fainting; may indicate arrhythmia. • Therapy may cause life-threatening tumor lysis syndrome (a condition caused by the rapid breakdown of cancer cells), which can cause kidney failure. Report decreased urination, amber-colored urine; confusion, difficulty breathing, fatigue, fever, muscle or joint pain, palpitations, seizures, vomiting. • Report any black/tarry stools, bruising, nausea, RUQ abdominal pain, yellowing of skin or eyes, palpitations, nose bleeds, blood in urine or stool, decreased urine output. • Avoid alcohol. • Do not take herbal products. • Do not ingest grape-fruit products. • Severe diarrhea may lead to dehydration. • Contact physician before any planned surgical/dental procedures. • Immediately report neurological changes: confusion, one-sided paralysis, difficulty speaking, partial blindness. • Do not receive live vaccines. • Do not break, crush, or open capsule. • Use effective contraception to avoid pregnancy.

ibuprofen

eye-bue-**pro**-fen
(Advil, Caldolor, Motrin, NeoProfen)

■**BLACK BOX ALERT** ■Increased risk of serious cardiovascular thrombotic events, including myocardial infarction, CVA. Contraindicated in setting of CABG surgery. Increased risk of severe GI reactions, including ulceration, bleeding, perforation.
Do not confuse Motrin with Neurontin or Advil with Aleve.

FIXED-COMBINATION(S)

Children's Advil Cold: ibuprofen/pseudoephedrine (a nasal decongestant): 100 mg/15 mg per 5 mL. **Combunox:** ibuprofen/oxyCODONE (a narcotic analgesic): 400 mg/5 mg. **Duexis:** ibuprofen/famotidine (an H₂ antagonist): 800 mg/26.6 mg. **Reprexain CIII:** ibuprofen/HYDROcodone (a narcotic analgesic): 200 mg/5 mg. **Vicoprofen:** ibuprofen/HYDROcodone (a narcotic analgesic): 200 mg/7.5 mg. **Combogesic IV: Injection:** Ibuprofen/acetaminophen 300 mg/1,000 mg in 100 mL vials.

◆CLASSIFICATION

PHARMACOTHERAPEUTIC: NSAID. **CLINICAL:** Antirheumatic, analgesic, antipyretic, antidysmenorrheal, vascular headache suppressant.

USES

Oral: Treatment of fever, inflammatory disease, and rheumatoid disorders, osteoarthritis, mild to moderate pain, primary dysmenorrhea. **OTC:** Reduce fever; manage pain due to headache, physical or athletic overexertion (e.g., sprains/strains), dental pain, minor muscle/bone/joint pain, backache, acute migraine, sore throat. **Caldolor:** Indicated in adults and children aged 3 mos and older for management of mild to moderate pain and moderate to severe pain as an adjunct to opioid analgesics, reduction of fever. **Neo-Profen:** To close a clinically significant patent ductus arteriosus (PDA) in premature infants weighing between 500 and 1,500 g who are no more than 32 wks gestational age when usual medical management is ineffective. **OFF-LABEL:** Treatment of cystic fibrosis, pericarditis. Juvenile idiopathic arthritis. Gout (acute flares). Abnormal uterine bleeding.

PRECAUTIONS

Contraindications: History of hypersensitivity to ibuprofen, aspirin, other NSAIDs. Treatment of perioperative pain in coronary artery bypass graft (CABG) surgery. Aspirin triad (bronchial asthma, aspirin intolerance, rhinitis). **NeoProfen:** Preterm neonates with proven or suspected untreated infection, elevated total bilirubin, congenital heart disease in whom patency of the patent ductus arteriosus is necessary for satisfactory pulmonary or systemic blood flow (e.g., pulmonary atresia), bleeding, thrombocytopenia, coagulation defects, proven or suspected necrotizing enterocolitis, significant renal impairment. **Cautions:** Pts with fluid retention, HF, dehydration, coagulation disorders, concurrent use with aspirin, anticoagulants, steroids; history of GI disease (e.g., bleeding, ulcers), smoking, use of alcohol, elderly, debilitated pts, hepatic/renal impairment, asthma.

ACTION

Reversibly inhibits COX-1 and COX-2 enzymes, resulting in decreased formation of prostaglandin precursors. **Therapeutic Effect:** Produces analgesic, anti-inflammatory effects; decreases fever.

PHARMACOKINETICS

Route	Onset	Peak	Duration
PO (analgesic)	0.5 hr	N/A	4–6 hrs
PO (antirheumatic)	2 days	1–2 wks	N/A

Widely distributed. Protein binding: 90%–99%. Metabolized in liver. Primarily excreted in urine. Not removed by hemodialysis. **Half-life:** 2–4 hrs.

LIFESPAN CONSIDERATIONS

Pregnancy/Lactation: Unknown if drug crosses placenta or is distributed in breast milk. Avoid use during third trimester (may adversely affect fetal cardiovascular system: premature closure of ductus arteriosus). **Children:** Safety and efficacy not established in pts younger than 3 mos. **Elderly:** GI bleeding, ulceration more likely to cause serious adverse effects. Age-related renal impairment may increase risk of hepatic/renal toxicity; reduced dosage recommended.

INTERACTIONS

DRUG: May decrease concentration/effects of **angiotensin II receptor blockers (ARBs)** (e.g., **losartan, valsartan), angiotensin-converting enzyme (ACE) inhibitors** (e.g., **enalapril, lisinopril), loop diuretics** (e.g., **furosemide). Aspirin, other salicylates** may increase risk of GI side effects, bleeding. May increase effect of **apixaban, dabigatran, rivaroxaban, warfarin. Bile acid sequestrants** (e.g., **cholestyramine)** may decrease absorption/effect. May increase nephrotoxic effect of **cycloSPORINE.** May

increase concentration, risk of toxicity of **lithium, methotrexate. HERBAL: Glucosamine, herbs with anticoagulant/ antiplatelet properties (e.g., garlic, ginger, ginseng, ginkgo biloba)** may increase concentration/effect. **FOOD:** None known. **LAB VALUES:** May prolong bleeding time. May alter serum glucose level. May increase serum BUN, creatinine, potassium, ALT, AST. May decrease serum calcium, glucose; Hgb, Hct, platelets.

AVAILABILITY (Rx)

Capsules: 200 mg. **Injection, Solution: *(Neo-Profen)*:** 10 mg/mL (2 mL). *(Caldolor)*: 100 mg/mL, 800 mg/200 mL. **Suspension, Oral:** 100 mg/5 mL. **Suspension, Oral Drops:** 40 mg/mL. **Tablets:** 200 mg, 400 mg, 600 mg, 800 mg. **Tablets, Chewable:** 100 mg.

ADMINISTRATION/HANDLING

IV (Caldolor)

Reconstitution • Dilute with D_5W or 0.9% NaCl to final concentration of 4 mg/ mL or less.
Rate of administration • Infuse over at least 30 min.
Storage • Store at room temperature. • Stable for 24 hrs after dilution.

IV (NeoProfen)

Reconstitution • Dilute to appropriate volume with D_5W or 0.9% NaCl. • Discard any remaining medication after first withdrawal from vial.
Rate of administration • Administer via IV port nearest the insertion site. • Infuse continuously over 15 min.
Storage • Store at room temperature. • Stable for 30 min after dilution.

PO
• Give with food or milk.

INDICATIONS/ROUTES/DOSAGE

Fever

PO: ADULTS, ELDERLY: 200–400 mg q4–6h prn. May titrate up to 600–800 mg q6h. **Maximum:** 3,200 mg/day.
CHILDREN 12 YRS AND OLDER, ADOLESCENTS: 200–400 mg q4–6h prn. **Maximum**

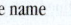 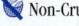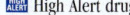

daily dose: 2,400 mg/day IV, 1,200 mg/day OTC oral. **CHILDREN 6 MOS AND OLDER:**

Weight		Dosage	
kg	lbs	Age	(mg)
5.4–8.1	12–17	6–11 mos	50
8.2–10.8	18–23	12–23 mos	75
10.9–16.3	24–35	2–3 yrs	100
16.4–21.7	36–47	4–5 yrs	150
21.8–27.2	48–59	6–8 yrs	200
27.3–32.6	60–71	9–10 yrs	250
32.7–43.2	72–95	11 yrs	300

IV: ADULTS, ELDERLY: 200–400 mg q4–6h prn. May titrate up to 600–800 mg q6h. **Maximum:** 3,200 mg/day. **CHILDREN 12–17 YRS:** 400 mg q4–6h prn. **Maximum:** 2,400 mg/day. **CHILDREN 6 MOS–11 YRS:** 10 mg/kg q4–6h prn. **Maximum:** 400 mg/dose. **Maximum:** 40 mg/kg/day up to 2,400 mg/day. **CHILDREN 3–5 MOS:** Single dose of 10 mg/kg up to a maximum of 100 mg. Infusion time must be at least 10 min.

Osteoarthritis, Rheumatoid Disorders
PO: ADULTS, ELDERLY: 400–800 mg q6–8h. **Maximum:** 3,200 mg/day.

Pain
PO: ADULTS, ELDERLY: 200–400 mg q4–6h prn or 600–800 mg q6–8h PRN. **Maximum:** 3,200 mg/day. **CHILDREN 12 YRS AND OLDER, ADOLESCENTS:** 200–400 mg q4–6h prn. **Maximum daily dose:** 2,400 mg/day. **CHILDREN 6 MOS–11 YRS:** See chart under Fever dosing.
IV: ADULTS, ELDERLY: 200–400 mg q4–6h PRN or 600–800 mg q6–8h PRN. **Maximum:** 3.2 g/day. **CHILDREN, ADOLESCENTS: (12–17 YRS):** 400 mg q4–6h prn. **Maximum:** 2,400 mg/day. **(6 MOS–12 YRS):** 10 mg/kg (**Maximum dose:** 400 mg) q4–6h prn. **Maximum:** 40 mg/kg/day or 2,400 mg, whichever is less. **CHILDREN 3–5 MOS:** Single dose of 10 mg/kg up to a maximum of 100 mg. Infusion time must be at least 10 min.
OTC PO: ADULTS, ELDERLY: 200 mg q4–6h as needed. May increase to 400 mg q4–6 as needed. **Maximum:** 1,200 mg/day.

Primary Dysmenorrhea
PO: ADULTS: Initially, 400 mg q4h PRN or 600–800 mg q6–8h PRN. **Maximum:** 3.2 g/day. For severe symptoms, begin at onset of menses or 1–2 days prior to onset of menses. Usual duration: 1–5 days.

Patent Ductus Arteriosus (PDA)
IV, Oral Suspension: INFANTS: Initially, 10 mg/kg followed by 2 doses of 5 mg/kg at 24 hrs and 48 hrs. All doses based on birth weight.

Dosage in Renal Impairment
Hold if anuria or oliguria is evident. Avoid use in severe impairment.

Dosage in Hepatic Impairment
Avoid use in severe impairment.

SIDE EFFECTS

Occasional (9%–3%): Nausea, vomiting, dyspepsia, dizziness, rash. **Rare (less than 3%):** Diarrhea or constipation, flatulence, abdominal cramps or pain, pruritus, increased B/P.

ADVERSE EFFECTS/TOXIC REACTIONS

Overdose may result in metabolic acidosis. Rare reactions with long-term use include peptic ulcer, GI bleeding, gastritis, severe hepatic reaction (cholestasis, jaundice), nephrotoxicity (dysuria, hematuria, proteinuria, nephrotic syndrome), severe hypersensitivity reaction (particularly in pts with systemic lupus erythematosus or other collagen diseases). **NeoProfen:** Hypoglycemia, hypocalcemia, respiratory failure, UTI, edema, atelectasis may occur. **Caldolor:** Abdominal pain, anemia, cough, dizziness, dyspnea, edema, hypertension, nausea, vomiting have been reported.

NURSING CONSIDERATIONS

BASELINE ASSESSMENT

Assess onset, type, location, duration of pain, inflammation. Inspect appearance of affected joints for immobility, deformities, skin condition. Assess temperature. Question medical history as listed in Precautions.

INTERVENTION/EVALUATION

Monitor for evidence of nausea, dyspepsia. Assess skin for rash. Observe for bleeding, bruising, occult blood loss. Evaluate for therapeutic response: Relief of pain, stiffness, swelling; increased joint mobility; reduced joint tenderness; improved grip strength. Monitor for fever.

PATIENT/FAMILY TEACHING

Avoid aspirin, alcohol during therapy (increases risk of GI bleeding). • If GI upset occurs, take with food, milk, antacids. • May cause dizziness. • Report ringing in ears, persistent stomach pain, respiratory difficulty, unusual bruising/bleeding, swelling of extremities, chest pain/palpitations.

---

ifosfamide   █ HIGH ALERT █

eye-**fos**-fa-mide
(Ifex)

■ BLACK BOX ALERT ■ Hemorrhagic cystitis may occur. Severe myelosuppressant. May cause CNS toxicity, including confusion, coma. Must be administered by personnel trained in administration/handling of chemotherapeutic agents. May cause severe nephrotoxicity, resulting in renal failure.
Do not confuse ifosfamide with cyclophosphamide.

◆CLASSIFICATION

PHARMACOTHERAPEUTIC: Alkylating agent. **CLINICAL:** Antineoplastic.

USES

Treatment of germ cell testicular carcinoma (used in combination with other chemotherapy agents and with concurrent mesna for prophylaxis of hemorrhagic cystitis). **OFF-LABEL:** Neuroblastoma, rhabdomyocarcoma, soft tissue sarcomas, Hodgkin's, non-Hodgkin's lymphoma; osteosarcoma; Ewing's sarcoma.

PRECAUTIONS

Contraindications: Hypersensitivity to ifosfamide. Urinary outflow obstruction. **Cautions:** Renal/hepatic impairment, compromised bone marrow reserve, active urinary tract infection, preexisting cardiac disease, prior radiation therapy, conditions predisposing to infection (e.g., diabetes, renal failure, immunocompromised pts, open wounds). Avoid use in pts with WBC less than 2,000 cells/mm^3 and platelets less than 50,000 cells/mm^3.

ACTION

Inhibits DNA, protein synthesis by cross-linking with DNA strands, preventing cell growth. **Therapeutic Effect:** Produces cellular death (apoptosis).

PHARMACOKINETICS

Metabolized in liver. Protein binding: negligible. Crosses blood-brain barrier (to a limited extent). Primarily excreted in urine. Removed by hemodialysis. **Half-life:** 11–15 hrs (high dose); 4–7 hrs (low dose).

⌛ LIFESPAN CONSIDERATIONS

Pregnancy/Lactation: If possible, avoid use during pregnancy, esp. first trimester. Males must use effective contraception and not conceive a child during treatment and for at least 6 months after discontinuation. May cause fetal harm. Distributed in breast milk. Breastfeeding not recommended. **Children:** Not intended for this pt population. **Elderly:** Age-related renal impairment may require dosage adjustment.

INTERACTIONS

DRUG: Bone marrow depressants (e.g., cladribine) may increase myelosuppression. May decrease therapeutic effect of **BCG (intravesical)**. **Live virus vaccines** may potentiate virus replication, increase vaccine side effects, decrease pt's antibody response to vaccine. **HERBAL: Echinacea** may decrease therapeutic effect. **FOOD:** None known. **LAB VALUES:** May increase serum BUN, bilirubin, creatinine, uric acid, ALT, AST.

AVAILABILITY (Rx)

Injection, Powder for Reconstitution: *(Ifex):* 1 g, 3 g. **Injection, Solution:** 50 mg/mL (20 mL, 60 mL quantity of diluent).

ADMINISTRATION/HANDLING

◄**ALERT**► Hemorrhagic cystitis occurs if mesna is not given concurrently. Mesna should always be given with ifosfamide.

 IV

Reconstitution • Reconstitute vial with Sterile Water for Injection or Bacteriostatic Water for Injection to provide concentration of 50 mg/mL. Shake to dissolve. • Further dilute with 50–1,000 mL D_5W or 0.9% NaCl to provide concentration of 0.6–20 mg/mL.
Rate of administration • Infuse over minimum of 30 min. • Give with at least 2,000 mL PO or IV fluid (prevents bladder toxicity). • Give with protectant against hemorrhagic cystitis (i.e., mesna).
Storage • Store vials of powder at room temperature. • Refrigerate vials of solution. • After reconstitution with Bacteriostatic Water for Injection, vials and diluted solutions stable for 24 hrs if refrigerated.

⚙ IV COMPATIBILITIES

Granisetron, ondansetron, palonosetron.

INDICATIONS/ROUTES/DOSAGE

◄**ALERT**► Dosage individualized based on clinical response, tolerance to adverse effects. When used in combination therapy, consult specific protocols for optimum dosage, sequence of drug administration.

Germ Cell Testicular Carcinoma
IV: ADULTS: 1.2–2 g/m^2/day for 5 consecutive days. Repeat q3wks or after recovery from hematologic toxicity. Administer with mesna and hydration (to prevent bladder toxicity).

Dosage in Renal/Hepatic Impairment
Use caution.

SIDE EFFECTS

Frequent (83%–58%): Alopecia, nausea, vomiting. **Occasional (15%–5%):** Confusion, drowsiness, hallucinations, infection. **Rare (less than 5%):** Dizziness, seizures, disorientation, fever, malaise, stomatitis (mucosal irritation, glossitis, gingivitis).

ADVERSE EFFECTS/TOXIC REACTIONS

Hemorrhagic cystitis with hematuria, dysuria occurs frequently if protective agent (mesna) is not used. Myelosuppression (leukopenia, thrombocytopenia) occurs frequently. Pulmonary toxicity, hepatotoxicity, nephrotoxicity, cardiotoxicity, CNS toxicity (confusion, hallucinations, drowsiness, coma) may require discontinuation of therapy. Secondary malignancies including lymphoma, thyroid cancer, sarcoma were reported. Veno-occlusive hepatic disease may occur. May impair healing of wounds.

NURSING CONSIDERATIONS

BASELINE ASSESSMENT

Obtain urinalysis before each dose. If hematuria occurs (greater than 10 RBCs per field), therapy should be withheld until resolution occurs. Obtain WBC, platelet count, Hgb before each dose. Question history of hepatic/renal impairment, cardiac disease. Screen for active infection. Offer emotional support.

INTERVENTION/EVALUATION

Monitor CBC, urinalysis, renal function, LFT. Assess for fever, sore throat, signs of local infection, unusual bruising/bleeding from any site, symptoms of anemia (excessive fatigue, weakness). Monitor for toxicities.

PATIENT/FAMILY TEACHING

• Treatment may depress your immune system response and reduce your ability to fight infection. Report symptoms of infection such as body aches, chills, cough, fatigue, fever. Avoid those with active infection. • Drink plenty of fluids (protects against cystitis). • Do not have immunizations without physician's approval (drug lowers resistance). • Avoid contact with those who have recently received live virus vaccine. • Avoid crowds, those with infections. • Report unusual bleeding/bruising, fever, chills, sore throat, joint pain, sores in mouth or on lips, yellowing skin or eyes.

iloperidone

eye-loe-**per**-i-doan
(Fanapt, Fanapt Titration Pack)

■ **BLACK BOX ALERT** ■ Elderly pts with dementia-related psychosis are at increased risk for mortality due to cerebrovascular events. **Do not confuse iloperidone with amiodarone or dronedarone.**

◆ CLASSIFICATION

PHARMACOTHERAPEUTIC: Second-generation (atypical) antipsychotic. **CLINICAL:** Antipsychotic.

USES

Acute treatment of schizophrenia in adults. Acute treatment of manic or mixed episodes associated with bipolar I disorder in adults.

PRECAUTIONS

Contraindications: Hypersensitivity to iloperidone. **Cautions:** Cardiovascular disease (HF, history of MI, ischemia, cardiac conduction abnormalities), cerebrovascular disease (increases risk of CVA in pts with dementia, seizure disorders). Pts at risk for orthostatic hypotension. Pts with bradycardia, hypokalemia, hypomagnesemia may be at greater risk for torsades de pointes. History of seizures, conditions lowering sci-

zure threshold, high risk of suicide, risk of aspiration pneumonia, congenital QT syndrome, concurrent use of medications that prolong QT interval, decreased GI motility, urinary retention, BPH, xerostomia, visual problems, hepatic impairment, narrow-angle glaucoma, diabetes, elderly.

ACTION

Mixed combination of DOPamine type 2 (D_2) and serotonin type 2 (5-HT$_2$) antagonisms (thought to improve negative symptoms of psychosis). **Therapeutic Effect:** Diminishes symptoms of schizophrenia and reduces incidence of extrapyramidal side effects.

PHARMACOKINETICS

Widely distributed. Metabolized in liver. Protein binding: 92–97%. Excreted in urine (45%–58%), feces (20%). **Half-life:** 18–33 hrs.

⧗ LIFESPAN CONSIDERATIONS

Pregnancy/Lactation: Unknown if drug crosses placenta or is excreted in breast milk. Breastfeeding not recommended. **Children:** Safety and efficacy not established. **Elderly:** More susceptible to postural hypotension. Increased risk of cerebrovascular events, mortality, including stroke in elderly pts with psychosis.

INTERACTIONS

DRUG: **Alcohol, CNS depressants** (e.g., **diphenhydrAMINE,** **LORazepam, morphine**) may increase CNS depression. **Strong CYP3A4 inhibitors** (e.g., **clarithromycin, ketoconazole, ritonavir), strong CYP2D6 inhibitors** (e.g., **FLUoxetine, PARoxetine**) may increase concentration/effect. **QT interval–prolonging medications** (e.g., **amiodarone, azithromycin, ciprofloxacin, haloperidol, methadone, sotalol**) may increase risk of QT interval prolongation, torsades de pointes. **HERBAL:** Herbals with **sedative properties** (e.g., **chamomile, kava kava, valerian**) may increase CNS depression. **FOOD:** None known. **LAB VALUES:** May increase serum prolactin levels.

AVAILABILITY (Rx)

Tablets: 1 mg, 2 mg, 4 mg, 6 mg, 8 mg, 10 mg, 12 mg.

ADMINISTRATION/HANDLING

PO
• Give without regard to food.

INDICATIONS/ROUTES/DOSAGE

Note: Titrate to the proper dose range with dosage adjustments not to exceed 2 mg twice daily (4 mg/day). Reduce dose by 50% when receiving strong CYP2D6 or CYP3A4 inhibitors or poor metabolizers of CYP2D6 (see Interactions).

Schizophrenia
PO: ADULTS: To avoid orthostatic hypotension, begin with 1 mg twice daily, then adjust dosage to 2 mg twice daily, 4 mg twice daily, 6 mg twice daily, 8 mg twice daily, 10 mg twice daily, and 12 mg twice daily on days 2, 3, 4, 5, 6, and 7, respectively, to reach target daily dose of 12–24 mg/day in 2 divided doses.

Bipolar I Disorder (Manic or Mixed)
Note: Reduce dose by 50% when given concomitantly with strong CYP2D6 or CYP3A4 inhibitors or in pts who are poor metabolizers of CYP2D6 (see Interactions).
PO: ADULTS, ELDERLY: (day 1): 1 mg twice daily. **(day 2):** 3 mg twice daily. **(day 3):** 6 mg twice daily. **(day 4):** 9 mg twice daily. **(day 5):** 12 mg twice daily. **Recommended dose:** 12 mg twice daily.

Dosage in Renal Impairment
No dose adjustment.

Dosage in Hepatic Impairment
Mild impairment: No dose adjustment. **Moderate impairment:** Use caution. **Severe impairment:** Not recommended.

SIDE EFFECTS

Frequent (20%–12%): Dizziness, drowsiness, tachycardia. **Occasional (10%–4%):** Nausea, dry mouth, nasal congestion, weight increase, diarrhea, fatigue, orthostatic hypotension. **Rare (3%–1%):** Arthralgia, musculoskeletal stiffness, abdominal discomfort, nasopharyngitis, tremor, hypotension, rash, ejaculatory failure, dyspnea, blurred vision, lethargy.

ADVERSE EFFECTS/TOXIC REACTIONS

Extrapyramidal disorders, including tardive dyskinesia (protrusion of tongue, puffing of cheeks, chewing/puckering of the mouth), occur in 4% of pts. Upper respiratory infection occurs in 3% of pts. QT interval prolongation may produce torsades de pointes, a form of ventricular tachycardia. Neuroleptic malignant syndrome (e.g., hyperpyrexia, muscle rigidity, altered mental status, irregular pulse or B/P) has been noted.

NURSING CONSIDERATIONS

BASELINE ASSESSMENT
Assess pt's behavior, appearance, emotional status, response to environment, speech pattern, thought content. ECG should be obtained to assess for QT prolongation before instituting medication. Question medical history as listed in Precautions.

INTERVENTION/EVALUATION
Monitor for orthostatic hypotension; assist with ambulation. Monitor for fine tongue movement (may be first sign of tardive dyskinesia, possibly irreversible). Monitor serum potassium, magnesium in pts at risk for electrolyte disturbances. Assess for therapeutic response (greater interest in surroundings, improved self-care, increased ability to concentrate, relaxed facial expression).

PATIENT/FAMILY TEACHING
• Avoid tasks that require alertness, motor skills until response to drug is established. • Be alert to symptoms of orthostatic hypotension; slowly go from lying to standing. • Report if feeling faint, if experiencing heart palpitations, or if fever or muscle rigidity occurs. • Report extrapyramidal symptoms (e.g., involuntary muscle movements, tics) immediately.

---

imatinib

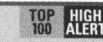 TOP 100 HIGH ALERT

im-**at**-in-ib
(Gleevec)
Do not confuse imatinib with dasatinib, erlotinib, lapatinib, nilotinib, SORAfenib, or SUNItinib.

◆CLASSIFICATION

PHARMACOTHERAPEUTIC: BCR-ABL tyrosine kinase inhibitor. **CLINICAL:** Antineoplastic.

USES

Philadelphia positive chronic myeloid leukemia (Ph+ CML): Newly diagnosed pts with Ph+ CML in chronic phase. **Ph+ CML in blast crisis (BC), accelerated phase (AP) or chronic phase (CP):** Pts with Ph+ CML in blast crisis, accelerated phase, or in chronic phase after failure of interferon-alpha therapy. **Ph+ acute lymphoblastic leukemia (ALL):** Adults with relapsed or refractory Ph+ ALL. Children with newly diagnosed Ph+ ALL in combination with chemotherapy. **Myelodysplastic/myeloproliferative diseases (MDS/MPD):** Adults with MDS/MPD associated with platelet-derived growth factor receptor (PDGFR) gene rearrangements. **Aggressive systemic mastocytosis (ASM):** Adults with ASM without the D816V c-Kit mutation or with c-Kit mutational status unknown. **Hypereosinophilic syndrome (HES) and/or chronic eosinophilic leukemia (CEL):** Adults with HES and/or CEL who have the FIP1L1-PDGFRα fusion kinase (mutational analysis or fluorescence in situ hybridization [FISH] demonstration of CHIC2 allele deletion) and for pts with HES and/or CEL who are FIP1L1-PDGFRα fusion kinase negative or unknown. **Dermatofibrosarcoma protuberans (DFSP):** Adults with unresectable, recurrent and/or metastatic DFSP. **Kit+ gastrointestinal stromal tumors (GIST):** Pts with Kit (CD117) positive unresectable and/or metastatic malignant GIST. **Adjuvant treatment Of GIST:** Adjuvant treatment of adults following complete gross resection of Kit (CD117) positive GIST. **OFF-LABEL:** Treatment of desmoid tumors (soft tissue sarcoma). Post–stem cell transplant (allogeneic), follow-up treatment in recurrent CML. Treatment of advanced or metastatic melanoma.

PRECAUTIONS

Contraindications: Hypersensitivity to imatinib. **Cautions:** Hepatic/renal impairment, thyroidectomy pts, hypothyroidism, gastric surgery pts. history of effusions or edema (pleural effusion, pericardial effusion, generalized edema); conditions predisposing to infection (e.g., diabetes, renal failure, immunocompromised pts, open wounds), pts at risk for GI perforation (e.g., Crohn's disease, diverticulitis, GI tract or abdominal malignancies, GI ulcers), pts at high risk for tumor lysis syndrome (high tumor burden)

ACTION

Inhibits Bcr-Abl tyrosine kinase, an enzyme created by Philadelphia chromosome abnormality found in pts with chronic myeloid leukemia. **Therapeutic Effect:** Blocks tumor cell proliferation and induces cellular death (apoptosis).

PHARMACOKINETICS

Widely distributed. Protein binding: 95%. Metabolized in liver. Eliminated in feces (68%), urine (13%). **Half-life:** 18 hrs; metabolite, 40 hrs.

⧗ LIFESPAN CONSIDERATIONS

Pregnancy/Lactation: May cause fetal harm. Breastfeeding not recommended. **Children:** Safety and efficacy not established. **Elderly:** Increased frequency of fluid retention.

 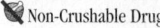

INTERACTIONS

DRUG: Strong CYP3A4 inducers (e.g., **carBAMazepine, phenytoin, rifAMPin**) may decrease concentration/ effect. **Strong CYP3A4 inhibitors (e.g., clarithromycin, ketoconazole, ritonavir)** may increase concentration/ effect. **Bone marrow depressants (e.g., cladribine)** may increase myelosuppression. **Live virus vaccines** may potentiate virus replication, increase vaccine side effects, decrease pt's antibody response to vaccine. May increase concentration/effect of **warfarin. HERBAL: Echinacea** may decrease therapeutic effect. **FOOD: Grapefruit products** may increase concentration. **LAB VALUES:** May increase serum bilirubin, ALT, AST, creatinine. May decrease platelet count, RBC, WBC count; serum potassium, albumin, calcium.

AVAILABILITY (Rx)

Tablets: 100 mg, 400 mg.

ADMINISTRATION/HANDLING

PO
• Give with a meal and large glass of water. • Tablets may be dispersed in water or apple juice (stir until dissolved; give immediately). Do not crush or chew tablets. • Doses of 600 mg or less should be given once daily; doses of 800 mg should be given as 400 mg twice daily.

INDICATIONS/ROUTES/DOSAGE

Ph+ Chronic Myeloid Leukemia (CML) (Chronic Phase), Newly Diagnosed
PO: ADULTS, ELDERLY: 400 mg once daily; may increase to 600 mg/day. **Maximum:** 600 mg. **CHILDREN:** 340 mg/m²/day. **Maximum:** 600 mg.

Ph+ CML (Accelerated Phase), Blast Crisis
PO: ADULTS, ELDERLY: 600 mg once daily. May increase to 800 mg/day in 2 divided doses (400 mg twice daily).

Ph+ Acute Lymphoblastic Leukemia (ALL)
PO: ADULTS, ELDERLY: 600 mg once daily. **CHILDREN:** 340 mg/m²/day (in combination with chemotherapy). **Maximum:** 600 mg.

Gastrointestinal Stromal Tumors (GIST) (Following Complete Resection)
PO: ADULTS, ELDERLY: 400 mg once daily for 3 yrs.

GIST (Unresectable)
PO: ADULTS, ELDERLY: 400 mg once daily. May increase up to 400 mg twice daily.

Aggressive Systemic Mastocytosis (ASM) With Eosinophilia
PO: ADULTS, ELDERLY: Initially, 100 mg/ day. May increase up to 400 mg/day.

ASM Without Mutation of the D816V C-Kit or Unknown Mutation Status of C-Kit
PO: ADULTS, ELDERLY: 400 mg once daily.

Dermatofibrosarcoma Protuberans (DFSP)
PO: ADULTS, ELDERLY: 400 mg twice daily.

Hypereosinophilic Syndrome (HES)/ Chronic Eosinophilic Leukemia (Negative or Unknown Mutational State)
PO: ADULTS, ELDERLY: 400 mg once daily.

HES/CEL With Positive FIP1L1-PDGFR Fusion Kinase
PO: ADULTS, ELDERLY: Initially, 100 mg/ day. May increase up to 400 mg/day.

Myelodysplastic/Myeloproliferative Disease (MDS/MPD)
PO: ADULTS, ELDERLY: 400 mg once daily.

Usual Dosage for Children (2 yrs and older)
Ph+ CML (Chronic Phase, Recurrent, or Resistant)
PO: 340 mg/m²/day. **Maximum:** 600 mg/day.
Ph+ CML (Chronic Phase, Newly Diagnosed, Ph+ ALL)
PO: 340 mg/m²/day. **Maximum:** 600 mg/day.

Dosage With Strong CYP3A4 Inducers
Increase dose by 50% with careful monitoring.

Dosage in Renal Impairment

Creatinine Clearance	Maximum Dose
40–59 mL/min	600 mg
20–39 mL/min	400 mg
Less than 20 mL/min	100 mg

Dosage in Hepatic Impairment

Mild to moderate impairment: No adjustment. **Severe impairment:** Reduce dosage by 25%.

SIDE EFFECTS

Frequent (68%–24%): Nausea, diarrhea, vomiting, headache, fluid retention, rash, musculoskeletal pain, muscle cramps, arthralgia. **Occasional (23%–10%):** Abdominal pain, cough, myalgia, fatigue, fever, anorexia, dyspepsia, constipation, night sweats, pruritus, dizziness, blurred vision, somnolence. **Rare (less than 10%):** Nasopharyngitis, petechiae, asthenia, epistaxis.

ADVERSE EFFECTS/TOXIC REACTIONS

Severe fluid retention (pleural effusion, pericardial effusion, pulmonary edema, ascites), hepatotoxicity occur rarely. Neutropenia, thrombocytopenia are expected responses to the therapy. Respiratory toxicity is manifested as dyspnea, pneumonia. Heart damage (left ventricular dysfunction, HF) may occur. Grade 3 hemorrhage reported in 2% of pts. May increase risk of GI perforation. Dermal toxicities, including erythema multiforme, Stevens-Johnson syndrome, may occur. May retard growth in children and adolescents. Tumor lysis syndrome may present as acute renal failure, hypocalcemia, hyperuricemia, hyperphosphatemia, which may be fatal. May cause renal toxicity.

NURSING CONSIDERATIONS

BASELINE ASSESSMENT

Obtain CBC, BMP, LFT; pregnancy test in females of reproductive potential. Question history of hepatic impairment/renal impairment, hypothyroidism, HF, edema. Due to increased risk of tumor lysis syndrome, assess hydration status prior to each treatment. Assess risk of GI perforation. Receive full medication history and screen for interactions. Screen for active infection. Receive full medication history and screen for interactions. Offer emotional support.

INTERVENTION/EVALUATION

Monitor CBC for myelosuppression wkly for 4 wks, then biweekly for 4 wks, then periodically thereafter. Obtain LFT if hepatotoxicity (bruising, jaundice, right upper abdominal pain, nausea, vomiting, weight loss) is suspected. Obtain serum calcium, phosphate, uric acid if tumor lysis syndrome is suspected (presents as acute renal failure, electrolyte imbalance, cardiac arrhythmias, seizures). Diligently monitor for infections (cough, fatigue, fever). If serious infection occurs, initiate appropriate antimicrobial therapy. If dyspnea occurs, obtain radiologic exam to assess for effusions/pleurisy. Monitor for edema (third spacing, dyspnea, weight gain), symptoms of GI perforation (abdominal pain, fever, melena, hematemesis). Assess skin for cutaneous reactions, skin toxicities. Monitor daily pattern of bowel activity, stool consistency; I&Os, hydration status; be alert for unexpected weight gain.

PATIENT/FAMILY TEACHING

• Treatment may depress your immune system response and reduce your ability to fight infection. Report symptoms of infection such as body aches, chills, cough, fatigue, fever. Avoid those with active infection. • Report symptoms of bone marrow depression such as bruising, fatigue, fever, shortness of breath, weight loss; bleeding easily, bloody urine or stool. • Report liver problems (abdominal pain, bruising, clay-colored stool, amber or dark-colored urine, yellowing of the skin or eyes), toxic skin reactions (blistering, peeling, rash, skin eruptions); symptoms of edema (shortness of breath, swelling of extremities, weight gain), lung effusion (chest pain, dry cough, shortness of breath). • Use effective contraception to avoid pregnancy. Do not breastfeed. • Therapy may cause tumor lysis syndrome (a condition caused by the rapid breakdown of cancer cells), which can cause kidney failure and can be fatal. Report decreased urination, amber-colored urine; confusion, difficulty breathing, fatigue, fever, muscle or joint pain, palpitations, seizures, vomiting. • Report severe or persistent abdominal pain, bloody stool, fever, vomiting; may indicate rupture in GI tract. • Avoid tasks that require alertness, motor skills until response to drug is established.

immune globulin IV (IGIV)

im-**mune glob**-u-lin
(Asceniv, Bivigam, Flebogamma DIF, Gammagard Liquid, Gammagard S/D, Gammaplex, Gamunex-C, Hizentra, Octagam 5%, Privigen, Xembify)

■ **BLACK BOX ALERT** ■ Acute renal impairment characterized by increased serum creatinine, oliguria, acute renal failure, osmotic nephrosis, particularly pts with any degree of renal insufficiency, diabetes mellitus, volume depletion, sepsis, and those older than age 65 yrs. Thrombosis may occur (administer at the minimum dose and minimum infusion rate; ensure adequate hydration).

◆**CLASSIFICATION**

PHARMACOTHERAPEUTIC: Immune globulin, blood product. **CLINICAL:** Immunizing agent.

USES
Treatment of pts with primary humoral immunodeficiency syndromes, acute/chronic immune idiopathic thrombocytopenic purpura (ITP), prevention of coronary artery aneurysms associated with Kawasaki disease, prevention of bacterial infections in pts with hypogammaglobulinemia and/or recurrent bacterial infections associated with B-cell chronic lymphocytic leukemia (CLL) or primary humoral immunodeficiency disorders. Treatment of chronic inflammatory demyelinating polyneuropathies. Treatment of dermatomyositis multifocal motor neuropathy. **OFF-LABEL:** Encephalomyelitis (acute), Guillain-Barre syndrome, hematopoetic stem cell transplantation (HSCT), chronic graft versus host disease (GVHD), systemic lupus erythematosus (SLE), pure red cell aplasia related to human parvovirus B19 infection, myasthenia gravis (acute exacerbation).

PRECAUTIONS
Contraindications: Hypersensitivity to immune globulin. Selective IgA deficiency, hyperprolinemia (Hizentra, Privigen), severe thrombocytopenia, coagulation disorders where IM injections contraindicated. Hypersensitivity to corn (Octagam); infants/neonates for whom sucrose or fructose tolerance has not been established (Gammaplex). **Cautions:** Cardiovascular disease, history of thrombosis, renal impairment.

ACTION
Replacement therapy for primary/secondary immunodeficiencies and IgG antibodies against bacteria, viral antigens; interferes with receptors on cells of reticuloendothelial system for autoimmune cytopenias/idiopathic thrombocytopenia purpura (ITP); increases antibody titer and antigen-antibody reaction potential. **Therapeutic Effect:** Provides passive immunity replacement for immunodeficiencies, increases antibody titer.

PHARMACOKINETICS

Evenly distributed between intravascular and extravascular space. **Half-life:** 21–23 days.

⏳ LIFESPAN CONSIDERATIONS

Pregnancy/Lactation: Unknown if drug crosses placenta or is distributed in breast milk. **Children/Elderly:** No age-related precautions noted.

INTERACTIONS

DRUG: May decrease concentration/therapeutic effects of **vaccines (live).** **HERBAL:** None significant. **FOOD:** None known. **LAB VALUES:** None significant.

AVAILABILITY (Rx)

Injection, Powder for Reconstitution: *(Gammagard S/D):* 5 g, 10 g. **Injection, Solution:** *(Asceniv, Bivigam 10%, Flebogamma DIF 5%, 10%, Gammagard Liquid 10%, Gammaplex 5%, Gamunex-C 10%, Octagam 5%, Privigen 10%).*

ADMINISTRATION/HANDLING
📲 IV

◀**ALERT**▶ Monitor vital signs, B/P diligently during and immediately after IV administration (precipitous fall in B/P may indicate anaphylactic reaction). Stop infusion immediately. EPINEPHrine should be readily available.
Reconstitution • Reconstitute only with diluent provided by manufacturer. • Discard partially used or turbid preparations.
Rate of administration • Give by infusion only. • After reconstitution, administer via separate tubing. • Rate of infusion varies with product used.
Storage • Refer to individual IV preparations for storage requirements, stability after reconstitution.

🔲 IV INCOMPATIBILITIES

Do not mix with any other medications.

INDICATIONS/ROUTES/DOSAGE
Primary Immunodeficiency Syndrome

IV: ADULTS, ELDERLY, CHILDREN: 400–600 mg/kg as single dose q3–4wks. Dosage range: 200–800 mg

Idiopathic Thrombocytopenic Purpura (ITP)

IV: ADULTS, ELDERLY, CHILDREN: 1 g/kg once daily for 1–2 days (may withhold second dose if adequate platelet response is achieved in 24 hrs) **OR** 400 mg/kg once daily for 5 days.

Kawasaki Disease

Note: Must be used with aspirin.
IV: CHILDREN: American Heart Association guidelines: 2,000 mg/kg as a single dose given over 10–12 hrs within 10 days of disease onset.

Hypogammaglobulinemia

IV: ADULTS, ELDERLY, CHILDREN: (Secondary to malignancy): 200–400 mg/kg/dose q3–4wks.

Primary Humoral Immunodeficiency Disorders

400–600 mg/kg as single dose q3–4wks.

Chronic Inflammatory Demyelinating Polyneuropathy

IV: ADULTS, ELDERLY, CHILDREN: Loading Dose: 2 g/kg divided over 2–5 days (consecutive). **Maintenance:** 1 g/kg/day q3wks or 500 mg/kg for 2 consecutive days q3wks.

Dermatomyositis

IV: ADULTS, ELDERLY: 1 g/kg/day on 2 consecutive days q4wks or 2 g/kg as single dose q4wks.

Multifocal Motor Neuropathy

IV: ADULTS, ELDERLY: Initially, 2 g/kg in divided doses over 2–5 consecutive days. Maintenance: 1–2 g/kg q2–6qwks.

Dosage in Renal Impairment

Caution when giving IV.

Dosage in Hepatic Impairment

No dose adjustment.

SIDE EFFECTS

Frequent: Tachycardia, backache, headache, arthralgia, myalgia. **Occasional:** Fatigue, wheezing, injection site rash/pain, leg cramps, urticaria, bluish color of lips/nailbeds, light-headedness.

ADVERSE EFFECTS/TOXIC REACTIONS

Anaphylactic reactions occur rarely, but incidence increases with repeated injections. EPINEPHrine should be readily available. Overdose may produce chest tightness, chills, diaphoresis, dizziness, facial flushing, nausea, vomiting, fever, hypotension. Hypersensitivity reaction (anxiety, arthralgia, dizziness, flushing, myalgia, palpitations, pruritus) occurs rarely.

NURSING CONSIDERATIONS

BASELINE ASSESSMENT

Question history of cardiac disease, thrombosis. Have EPINEPHrine readily available. Pt should be well hydrated prior to administration.

INTERVENTION/EVALUATION

Control rate of IV infusion carefully; too-rapid infusion increases risk of precipitous fall in B/P, signs of anaphylaxis (facial flushing, chest tightness, chills, fever, nausea, vomiting, diaphoresis). Assess pt closely during infusion, esp. first hr; monitor vital signs continuously. Stop infusion if aforementioned signs noted. For treatment of idiopathic thrombocytopenic purpura (ITP), monitor platelet count.

PATIENT/FAMILY TEACHING

• Report sudden weight gain, fluid retention, edema, decreased urine output, shortness of breath.

inFLIXimab   TOP 100

in-**flix**-i-mab
(Avsola, Inflectra, <u>Remicade</u>, Renflexis)
 BLACK BOX ALERT ■ Risk of severe/fatal opportunistic infec-tions (tuberculosis, sepsis, fungal), reactivation of latent infections. Rare cases of very aggressive, usually fatal hepatosplenic T-cell lymphoma reported in adolescents, young adults with Crohn's disease. **Do not confuse inFLIXimab with riTUXimab, or Remicade with Reminyl.**

◆CLASSIFICATION

PHARMACOTHERAPEUTIC: Tumor necrosis factor (TNF) blocking agent. Monoclonal antibody. **CLINICAL:** Antirheumatic, disease-modifying, GI, immunosuppressant agent.

USES

Rheumatoid arthritis: In combination with methotrexate, reduces signs/symptoms, inhibits progression of structural damage, improves physical function in moderate to severe active rheumatoid arthritis (RA). **Psoriatric arthritis:** Treatment of psoriatic arthritis. **Crohn's disease:** Reduces signs/symptoms, induces and maintains remission in moderate to severe active Crohn's disease in adults and children 6 yrs and older. Reduces number of draining enterocutaneous/rectovaginal fistulas, maintains fistula closure in fistulizing Crohn's disease in adults. **Ankylosing spondylitis:** Reduces sign/symptoms of active ankylosing spondylitis. **Plaque psoriasis:** Treatment of chronic severe plaque psoriasis as alternative to other systemic therapy. **Ulcerative colitis:** Reduces sign/symptoms, induces and maintains clinical remission and mucosal healing, eliminates corticosteroid use in moderate to severe active ulcerative colitis in adults and children 6 yrs and older. **OFF-LABEL:** Colitis, pustular psoriasis, sarcoidosis (refractory).

PRECAUTIONS

Contraindications: Hypersensitivity to inFLIXimab. Moderate to severe HF (doses greater than 5 mg/kg should be avoided). Sensitivity to murine proteins, sepsis, serious active infection. **Cautions:** Hematologic abnormalities, history of COPD, preexisting or recent-onset CNS demyelinating disorders, seizures, mild HF, history of chronic opportunistic infections (esp. bacterial, invasive fungal, mycobacterial, protozoal, viral, tuberculosis); conditions predisposing to infection (e.g., diabetes, immunocompromised pts, renal failure, open wounds); elderly; chronic hepatitis B virus infection.

ACTION

Binds to tumor necrosis factor (TNF), inhibiting functional activity of TNF (induction of proinflammatory cytokines, enhanced leukocytic migration, activation of neutrophils/eosinophils). **Therapeutic Effect:** Prevents disease and allows diseased joints to heal.

PHARMACOKINETICS

Widely distributed. Metabolism not specified. **Half-life:** 8–9.5 days.

⌛ LIFESPAN CONSIDERATIONS

Pregnancy/Lactation: Unknown if distributed in breast milk. **Children:** Safety and efficacy not established. **Elderly:** Use cautiously due to higher rate of infection.

INTERACTIONS

DRUG: May increase concentration/effects of **anakinra, anti-TNF agents, baricitinib, pimecrolimus, tacrolimus (topical), tocilizumab**. May decrease therapeutic effect of **BCG (intravesical). Belimumab, tocilizumab** may increase concentration/effect. Concentration/effect may be altered by **vaccines (live). HERBAL:** Echinacea may decrease effects. **FOOD:** None known. **LAB VALUES:** May increase serum alkaline phosphatase, ALT, AST, bilirubin.

AVAILABILITY (Rx)

Injection, Powder for Reconstitution: 100 mg.

ADMINISTRATION/HANDLING

 IV

Reconstitution • Reconstitute each vial with 10 mL Sterile Water for Injection, using 21-gauge or smaller needle. Direct stream of Sterile Water for Injection to glass wall of vial. • Swirl vial gently to dissolve contents (do not shake). • Allow solution to stand for 5 min and inject into 250-mL bag 0.9% NaCl; gently mix. Concentration should range between 0.4 and 4 mg/mL. • Begin infusion within 3 hrs after reconstitution.
Rate of administration • Administer IV infusion over at least 2 hrs using a low protein-binding filter.
Storage • Refrigerate vials. • Solution should appear colorless to light yellow and opalescent; do not use if discolored or if particulate forms.

🔃 IV INCOMPATIBILITIES

Do not infuse in same IV line with other agents.

INDICATIONS/ROUTES/DOSAGE

◀ALERT▶ Premedicate with antihistamines, acetaminophen, steroids to prevent/manage infusion reactions.
Rheumatoid Arthritis (RA)
IV: **ADULTS, ELDERLY: In combination with methotrexate:** 3 mg/kg followed by additional doses at 2 and 6 wks after first infusion, then q8wks thereafter. **Range:** 3–10 mg/kg repeated at 4- to 8-wk intervals.

Crohn's Disease
IV: **ADULTS, ELDERLY, CHILDREN 6 YRS AND OLDER:** 5 mg/kg followed by additional doses at 2 and 6 wks after first infusion, then q8wks thereafter. For adults who respond then lose response, consideration may be given to treatment with 10 mg/kg.

Ankylosing Spondylitis
IV: **ADULTS, ELDERLY:** 5 mg/kg followed by additional doses at 2 and 6 wks after first infusion, then q6wks thereafter.

Psoriatic Arthritis

IV: **ADULTS, ELDERLY:** 5 mg/kg followed by additional doses at 2 and 6 wks after first infusion, then q8wks thereafter. May be used with or without methotrexate.

Plaque Psoriasis

IV: **ADULTS, ELDERLY:** 5 mg/kg followed by additional doses at 2 and 6 wks after first infusion, then q8wks thereafter. May require 10 mg/kg and/or dosing as q4wks in maintenance phase.

Ulcerative Colitis

IV: **ADULTS, ELDERLY, CHILDREN 6 YRS AND OLDER:** 5 mg/kg followed by additional doses at 2 and 6 wks after first infusion, then q8wks thereafter.

Dosage in Renal/Hepatic Impairment

No dose adjustment.

SIDE EFFECTS

Frequent (22%–10%): Headache, nausea, fatigue, fever. **Occasional (9%–5%):** Fever/chills during infusion, pharyngitis, vomiting, pain, dizziness, bronchitis, rash, rhinitis, cough, pruritus, sinusitis, myalgia, back pain. **Rare (4%–1%):** Hypotension or hypertension, paresthesia, anxiety, depression, insomnia, diarrhea, UTI.

ADVERSE EFFECTS/TOXIC REACTIONS

Leukopenia, neutropenia, thrombocytopenia, pancytopenia were reported. Serious, sometimes fatal, infections (bacterial, mycobacterial, viral, invasive fungal, other opportunistic infections) may occur. Serious infections may include aspergillosis, blastomycosis, coccidioidomycosis, cryptococcosis, cytomegalovirus, esophageal candidiasis, herpes zoster, histoplasmosis, listeriosis, pneumocystosis, pneumocystosis, salmonellosis, pneumonia, tuberculosis, sepsis. Lymphomas (Hodgkin's disease, non-Hodgkin's lymphoma), other malignancies (basal cell carcinoma, breast/colorectal/hepatic/renal cancer, leukemia, leiomyosarcoma, melanoma, solid organ cancers) were reported. Hypersensitivity reactions including anaphylaxis, urticaria, dyspnea, hypotension may occur. May cause reactivation of hepatitis B virus infection. Other serious reactions may including cardiovascular events (cardiac arrhythmias, hypotension, hypertension, MI, HF (or worsening of HF); neurological events (seizures, systemic vasculitis), exacerbation of nervous system demyelinating disorders (Guillain-Barré syndrome, multiple sclerosis, optic neuritis).

NURSING CONSIDERATIONS

BASELINE ASSESSMENT

Assess hydration status (skin turgor urinary status). Question history of CNS disorders, COPD, HF. Screen for active infection. Pts should be evaluated for active tuberculosis and tested for latent infection prior to initiating treatment and periodically during therapy. Induration of 5 mm or greater with tuberculin skin test should be considered a positive test result when assessing if treatment for latent tuberculosis is necessary. Verify that pt has not received live vaccines prior to initiation.

INTERVENTION/EVALUATION

Monitor urinalysis, erythrocyte sedimentation rate (ESR), B/P. Monitor for signs of infection. Monitor daily pattern of bowel activity, stool consistency. **Crohn's disease:** Monitor C-reactive protein, frequency of stools. Assess for abdominal pain. **Rheumatoid arthritis (RA):** Monitor C-reactive protein. Assess for decreased pain, swollen joints, stiffness.

PATIENT/FAMILY TEACHING

• Treatment may depress your immune system and reduce your ability to fight infection. • Report symptoms of infection such as body aches, chills, cough, fatigue, fever. Avoid those with active infection. • Do not receive live vaccines. • Expect frequent tuberculosis screening. • Report travel plans to possible endemic areas.

inotuzumab ozogamicin

in-oh-**tooz**-ue-mab **oh**-zoe-ga-**mye**-sin
(Besponsa)

■ **BLACK BOX ALERT** ■ Hepatotoxicity, including fatal hepatic veno-occlusive disease may occur, esp. in pts who underwent hematopoietic stem cell transplant (HSCT) or underwent HSCT conditioning regimens containing two alkylating agents and had a total bilirubin level greater than ULN. Other risk factors for hepatic veno-occlusive disease may include advanced age, prior hepatic disease, later salvage lines, greater number of treatment cycles. Permanently discontinue in pts who develop hepatic veno-occlusive disease. LFT elevations may require treatment interruption, dose reduction, or permanent discontinuation. Increased occurrence of post-HSCT nonrelapse mortality was reported.

Do not confuse inotuzumab with ado-trastuzumab, alemtuzumab, atezolizumab, benralizumab, dinutuximab, elotuzumab, gemtuzumab, ipilimumab, obinutuzumab, pertuzumab, trastuzumab.

◆CLASSIFICATION

PHARMACOTHERAPEUTIC: Anti-CD22. Antibody drug conjugate (ADC). Monoclonal antibody. **CLINICAL:** Antineoplastic.

USES

Treatment of relapsed or refractory CD22-positive B-cell precursor acute lymphoblastic leukemia (ALL) in adults and children 1 year and older.

PRECAUTIONS

Contraindications: Hypersensitivity to inotuzumab. **Cautions:** Conditions predisposing to infection (e.g., diabetes, immunocompromised pts, renal failure, open wounds), elderly. Pts at risk for hepatic veno-occlusive disease (e.g., advanced age, prior HSCT, prior hepatic disease (e.g., cirrhosis, hepatitis), later salvage lines, greater number of treatment cycles). Pts at risk for QT interval prolongation or torsades de pointes (congenital long QT syndrome, medications that prolong QT interval, hypokalemia, hypomagnesemia). Pts at risk for hemorrhage (e.g., history of intracranial/GI bleeding, coagulation disorders, recent trauma; concomitant use of anticoagulants, antiplatelets, NSAIDS). Pts at risk for tumor lysis syndrome (high tumor burden).

ACTION

Binds to and internalizes ADC-CD22 complex in CD22-expressing tumor cells, promoting cellular release of N-acetyl-gamma-calicheamicin dimethyl hydrazide (a cytotoxic agent). Activation of N-acetyl-gamma-calicheamicin dimethyl hydrazide induces breakage of double-strand DNA, resulting in cell cycle arrest and apoptosis. **Therapeutic Effect:** Inhibits tumor cell growth and metastasis in ALL.

PHARMACOKINETICS

Widely distributed. N-acetyl-gamma-calicheamicin dimethyl hydrazide metabolized by nonenzymatic reduction. Protein binding: 97%. Steady state reached by treatment cycle 4. Excretion not specified. **Half-life:** 12.3 days.

⌛ LIFESPAN CONSIDERATIONS

Pregnancy/Lactation: Avoid pregnancy; may cause fetal harm. Unknown if distributed in breast milk. Females of reproductive potential must use effective contraception during treatment and for at least 8 mos after discontinuation. Males with female partners of reproductive potential must use effective contraception during treatment and for at least 5 mos after discontinuation. Breastfeeding not recommended during treatment and for at least 2 mos after discontinuation. May impair fertility in females. **Children:** Safety and efficacy not established in pts younger than 1 yr. **Elderly:** No age-related precautions noted.

INTERACTIONS

DRUG: QT interval–prolonging medications (e.g., **amiodarone, azithromycin, ciprofloxacin, haloperidol, sotalol**) may increase risk of QT interval prolongation, torsades de pointes. May increase adverse effects of **natalizumab, vaccines (live).** May decrease therapeutic effect of **BCG (intravesical), vaccines (live). HERBAL:** Echinacea may decrease concentration/effect. **FOOD:** None known. **LAB VALUES:** May decrease Hgb, leukocytes, lymphocytes, neutrophils, platelets. May increase serum alkaline phosphatase, ALT, amylase AST, bilirubin, GGT, lipase, uric acid. May decrease diagnostic effect of *Coccidioides immitis* skin test.

AVAILABILITY (Rx)

Injection, Powder for Reconstitution: 0.9 mg.

ADMINISTRATION/HANDLING

 IV

Premedication • Premedicate with a corticosteroid, antipyretic, and antihistamine before each dose.
Reconstitution • Must be prepared by personnel trained in aseptic manipulations and admixing of cytotoxic drugs. • Calculate the number of vials required for dose. • Reconstitute each vial with 4 mL Sterile Water for Injection for a final concentration of 0.25 mg/mL that delivers 3.6 mL (0.9 mg). • Gently swirl vial until completely dissolved. • Do not shake or agitate. • Visually inspect for particulate matter or discoloration. Solution should appear clear to opalescent, colorless to slightly yellow in color. Do not use if solution is cloudy or discolored, or if visible particles are observed. • Calculate required volume of reconstituted solution according to body surface

area. • Dilute in 50 mL 0.9% NaCl polyvinyl chloride (PVC) infusion bag made of (DEHP or non-DEHP), polyolefin, or ethylene vinyl acetate. • Mix by gently inversion. Do not shake or agitate. • Discard unused portions.
Rate of administration • Infuse over 60 min via dedicated IV line. • In-line filters are not required. However, if an in-line filter is used, filters made of polyethersulfone (PES), polyvinylidene fluoride (PVDF), or hydrophilic polysulfone (HPS) are recommended. Do not use filters made of nylon or mixed cellulose ester (MCE). • Do not administer as IV push or bolus.
Storage • Refrigerate unused vials in original carton. • Protect vial, reconstituted solution, diluted solution from light. • Do not freeze. • Reconstitution solution must be diluted within 4 hrs. • Diluted solution may be stored at room temperature for up to 4 hrs or refrigerated for up to 3 hrs. • If refrigerated, allow diluted solution to warm to room temperature (approx. 1 hr). • Infusion must be completed within 8 hrs of reconstitution.

INDICATIONS/ROUTES/DOSAGE

ALL (Relapsed or Refractory)

IV: ADULTS, ELDERLY, CHILDREN 1 YR AND OLDER: Induction cycle 1: 0.8 mg/m² on day 1, then 0.5 mg/m² on day 8 and day 15 of 21-day cycle (total cycle dose: 1.8 mg/m² per cycle, given in 3 divided doses). May extend duration of induction cycle to 28 days if pt achieves complete remission (CR), complete remission with incomplete hematologic recovery (CRi), or to allow time for recovery of toxicity. **Subsequent cycles in pts with CR or CRi:** 0.5 mg/m² on days 1, 8, and 15 of 28-day cycle (total cycle dose: 1.5 mg/m² per cycle, given in 3 divided doses). **Subsequent cycles in pts who have not achieved CR or CRi:** 0.8 mg/m² on day 1, then 0.5 mg/m² on day 8 and day 15 of 28-day cycle (total cycle dose: 1.8 mg/m² per cycle, given in 3 divided doses). Recommend discontinuation in pts who do not achieve CR or CRi within 3 cycles. **Proceeding to HCST:** Treatment duration of 2 cycles. May consider a third cycle in pts who do not achieve CR or Cri and minimal residual disease after 2 cycles. **Not proceeding to HCST:** May consider up to a maximum of 6 cycles.

Dose Modification

Note: Doses within a treatment cycle (e.g., day 8, day 15) do not require interruption if related to neutropenia or thrombocytopenia. Treatment interruptions within a cycle are recommended for nonhematological toxicities. Do not re-escalate reduced doses that are related to toxicity.

Duration of Dose Interruption (Nonhematological toxicities)
Less than 7 days within a cycle: Interrupt the next dose (ensure a minimum of 6 days between doses). **7 days or more:** Skip the next dose within the cycle. **14 days or more:** Once toxicity is adequately resolved, decrease total dose of subsequent cycle by 25%. May further reduce to 2 doses per cycle for subsequent cycles if further dose modification is required. If unable to tolerate a total dose reduction of 25%, followed by a reduction to 2 doses per cycle, permanently discontinue. **More than 28 days:** Consider permanent discontinuation.

Hematologic Toxicities
ANC greater than or equal to 1,000 cells/mm³ (prior to treatment): If ANC decreases, interrupt next cycle until ANC is greater than or equal to 1,000 cells/mm³. Discontinue treatment if ANC is less than 1,000 cells/mm³ for more than 28 days (and related to treatment). **Platelet count greater than or equal to 50,000 cells/mm³ (prior to treatment):** If platelet count decreases, interrupt next cycle until platelet count is greater than or equal to 50,000 cells/mm³. Discontinue treatment if platelet count is less than 50,000 cells/mm³ for more than 28 days (and related to treatment). **ANC less than 1,000**

cells/mm³ and/or platelet count less than 50,000 cells/mm³ (prior to treatment): If ANC or platelet count decreases, interrupt next cycle until one of following occurs: ANC and platelet count recover to at least baseline of the prior cycle; ANC is greater than or equal to 1,000 cells/mm³ and platelet count is greater than or equal to 50,000 cells/mm³; disease is improved or stable, and the decrease of ANC and platelet count is not related to treatment.

Hepatotoxicity
Serum ALT/AST greater than 2.5 times ULN and serum bilirubin greater than 1.5 times ULN: Interrupt treatment until serum ALT/AST is less than or equal to 2.5 times ULN and serum bilirubin is less than 1.5 times ULN prior to each dose (unless related to Gilbert's syndrome or hemodialysis). Permanently discontinue if serum ALT/AST does not recover to less than or equal to 2.5 times ULN or serum bilirubin does not recover to less than 1.5 times ULN. **Hepatic veno-occlusive disease, severe liver injury:** Permanently discontinue.

Other Nonhematologic Toxicities
Any CTCAE Grade 2 nonhematologic toxicities: Withhold treatment until recovery to Grade 1 or pretreatment grade levels before each dose.

Dosage in Renal Impairment
Mild impairment: No dose adjustment to initial dose. **Severe to moderate impairment:** Not specified; use caution.

Dosage in Hepatic Impairment
Mild to moderate impairment: No dose adjustment to initial dose. **Severe impairment, ESRD, HD:** Use caution.

SIDE EFFECTS

Frequent (35%–17%): Fatigue, asthenia, headache, migraine, sinus headache, pyrexia, nausea, abdominal pain, esophageal pain, abdominal tenderness, hepatic pain. **Occasional (16%–11%):** Constipation, vomiting, stomatitis, aphthous ulcer, mucosal inflammation, mouth ulceration, oral pain, oropharyngeal pain, chills.

ADVERSE EFFECTS/TOXIC REACTIONS

Anemia, leukopenia, lymphopenia, neutropenia, thrombocytopenia are expected responses to therapy, but more severe reactions, including bone marrow failure, febrile neutropenia, may be life-threatening. Hemorrhagic events including contusion, ecchymosis, epistaxis, gingival bleeding, hematemesis, hematochezia, hematotympanum, hematuria, metrorrhagia, subdural hematoma, postprocedural hematoma, hemorrhagic shock, hemorrhage (conjunctival, gastric, GI, hemorrhoidal, intra-abdominal, intracranial, lip, mesenteric, mouth, muscle, rectal, SQ, vaginal) have occurred. Hepatotoxicity, including fatal hepatic veno-occlusive disease, may occur, esp. in pts who underwent HSCT or underwent HSCT conditioning regimens containing two alkylating agents and had a total bilirubin level greater than ULN. An increased occurrence of post-HSCT non-relapse mortality was reported. Serious, sometimes fatal, infections including neutropenic sepsis, pneumonia, sepsis, pseudomonal sepsis occurred in 5% of pts. Tumor lysis syndrome may present as acute renal failure, hypocalcemia, hyperuricemia, hyperphosphatemia. May cause QT interval prolongation, esp. in pts with history of long QTc prolongation or in pts taking medications known to prolong QT interval.

NURSING CONSIDERATIONS

BASELINE ASSESSMENT

Obtain ANC, CBC, LFT, ECG before each dose. Calculate body surface area. Obtain pregnancy test in females of reproductive potential. Screen for active infection. Assess risk for bleeding, hemorrhage, hepatic veno-occlusive disease, infection, QT prolongation. Due to risk of tumor lysis syndrome, assess adequate hydration before initiation. Receive full medication history and screen for interactions. Offer emotional support.

INTERVENTION/EVALUATION

Monitor ANC, CBC for myelosuppression. Monitor ECG for QT interval prolongation. LFTs should be obtained before each dose and correlated with symptoms of hepatic veno-occlusive disease (ascites, serum bilirubin elevation, hepatomegaly, rapid weight gain). Diligently monitor pts who underwent HSCT or are planning HSCT. Monitor for infusion-related reactions (e.g., chills, dyspnea, fever, rash) during infusion and for at least 1 hr after infusion is completed. If infusion-related reaction occurs during administration, interrupt infusion and provide medical support. Severe reactions may require administration of antihistamines, corticosteroids. Permanently discontinue treatment if severe or life-threatening reactions occur. Be alert for serious infection, opportunistic infection, sepsis (fever, decreased urinary output, hypotension, tachycardia, tachypnea). If infection occurs, provide anti-infective therapy as appropriate. Monitor for hemorrhagic events including intracranial hemorrhage (altered mental status, aphasia, blindness, hemiparesis, unequal pupils, seizures), GI bleeding (hematemesis, melena, rectal bleeding), epistaxis. Tumor lysis syndrome may present as acute renal failure, hypocalcemia, hyperuricemia, hyperphosphatemia. Monitor daily pattern of bowel activity, stool consistency.

PATIENT/FAMILY TEACHING

• Treatment may depress your immune system response and reduce your ability to fight infection. Report symptoms of infection such as body aches, chills, cough, fatigue, fever. Avoid those with active infection. • Report symptoms of bone marrow depression such as bruising, fatigue, fever, shortness of breath, weight loss; bleeding easily, bloody urine or stool. • Therapy may cause life-threatening tumor lysis syndrome (a condition caused by the rapid breakdown of cancer cells), which can cause kidney failure. Report decreased urination, amber-colored urine; confusion, difficulty breathing, fatigue, fever, muscle or joint pain, palpitations, seizures, vomiting. • Avoid pregnancy using effective contraception. Treatment may cause fetal harm. Do not breastfeed during treatment and for at least 2 mos after last dose. • Life-threatening bleeding may occur; report bloody stool, bloody urine; rectal bleeding, nosebleeds, vomiting up blood; symptoms of hemorrhagic stroke (confusion, blindness, difficulty speaking, paralysis, seizures). • Do not take any newly prescribed medications unless approved by doctor who originally started treatment. • Report symptoms of long QT syndrome such as chest pain, dizziness, fainting, palpitations, shortness of breath. • Report liver problems such as abdominal pain, bruising, clay-colored stool, amber or dark-colored urine, yellowing of the skin or eyes. • Pts who have had HSCT or are planning HSCT have an increased risk of mortality.

---

insulin

in·su·lin
Do not confuse NovoLOG with HumaLOG or NovoLIN.

■ **BLACK BOX ALERT** ■ (Afrezza): Acute bronchospasms reported in pts with asthma and COPD.

FIXED-COMBINATION(S)

HumaLOG Mix 75/25: lispro suspension 75% and lispro solution 25%. **HumuLIN Mix 50/50:** NPH 50% and regular 50%. **HumuLIN 70/30, NovoLIN 70/30:** NPH 70% and rapid-

acting regular 30%. **NovoLOG Mix 70/30:** aspart suspension 70% and aspart solution 30%. **Ryzodeg 70/30:** degludec suspension 70% and aspart solution 30%. **Soliqua 100/33:** glargine 100 units/mL and lixisenatide (a glucagon-like peptide 1 [GLP-1] receptor agonist) 33 mcg/mL. **Xultophy 100/3.6:** degludec 100 units/mL and liraglutide (a GLP-1 receptor agonist) 3.6 mg/mL.

✦CLASSIFICATION

PHARMACOTHERAPEUTIC: Exogenous insulin. **CLINICAL:** Antidiabetic.

USES

Treatment of type 1 diabetes (insulin-dependent) and type 2 diabetes (non–insulin-dependent) to improve glycemic control. **OFF-LABEL: Insulin aspart, insulin lispro, insulin regular:** Gestational diabetes, mild to moderate diabetic ketoacidosis, mild to moderate hyperosmolar hyperglycemic state. **Insulin NPH:** Gestational diabetes.

PRECAUTIONS

Contraindications: Hypersensitivity to insulin, use during episodes of hypoglycemia. **Afrezza only:** Chronic lung disease. **Cautions:** Pts at risk for hypokalemia; renal/hepatic impairment, elderly. **Afrezza only:** Must be used with a long-acting insulin in type 1 diabetes. Not recommended for use in diabetic ketoacidosis or in smokers. Pts with active lung cancer, history of lung cancer, or at risk for lung cancer.

ACTION

Acts via specific receptor to regulate metabolism of carbohydrates, protein, and fats. Acts on liver, skeletal muscle, and adipose tissue. **Liver:** Stimulates hepatic glycogen synthesis, synthesis of fatty acids. **Muscle:** Increases protein, glycogen synthesis. **Adipose tissue:** Stimulates lipoproteins to provide free fatty acids, triglyceride synthesis. **Therapeutic Effect:** Controls serum glucose levels.

PHARMACOKINETICS

Rapid-Acting

	Onset (min)	Peak (hrs)	Duration (hrs)
Aspart (NovoLOG)	10–20	1–3	3–5
Glulisine (Apidra)	5–15	0.75–1.25	2–4
Insulin Human (Afrezza)	15–30	1	2
Lispro (HumaLOG, Lyumjev)	15–30	0.5–2.5	3–6.5

Short-Acting

	Onset (min)	Peak (hrs)	Duration (hrs)
Regular (HumuLIN R)	30–60	1–5	6–10
Regular (NovoLIN R)	30–60	1–5	6–10

Intermediate-Acting

	Onset (hrs)	Peak (hrs)	Duration (hrs)
NPH (HumuLIN N)	1–2	6–14	16–24+
NPH (NovoLIN N)	1–2	6–14	16–24+

Long-Acting

	Onset (hrs)	Peak (hrs)	Duration (hrs)
Degludec (Tresiba)	0.5–1.5	12	42
Detemir (Levemir)	3–4	3–9	6–23
Glargine (Lantus, Rezvoglar, Semglee)	3–4	No peak	24
Glargine (Toujeo)	Over 6	No peak	Over 24

⧖ LIFESPAN CONSIDERATIONS

Pregnancy/Lactation: Insulin is the drug of choice for diabetes in pregnancy; close medical supervision is needed. Following delivery, insulin needs may drop for 24–72 hrs, then rise to pre-pregnancy levels. Not distributed in breast milk; lactation may decrease insulin requirements. **Children:** No age-related precautions noted. **Elderly:** Decreased vision, fine motor tremors may lead to inaccurate self-dosing.

INTERACTIONS

DRUG: **Beta blockers (e.g., carvedilol, metoprolol)** may alter effects; may mask signs, prolong periods of hypoglycemia. **Glucagon-like peptide 1 (GLP-1) agents (e.g., liraglutide), dipeptidyl peptidase (DPP)-4 agents (e.g., linagliptin), thiazolidinediones (e.g., pioglitazone), pramlintide** may increase hypoglycemic effect. **HERBAL:** **Herbals with hypoglycemic properties (e.g., fenugreek)** may increase hypoglycemic effect. **FOOD:** None known. **LAB VALUES:** May decrease serum magnesium, phosphate, potassium.

AVAILABILITY (Rx)

Rapid-Acting
Inhalation Powder: *(Afrezza):* 4 units, 8 units, 12 units as single-use inhalation cartridges. ***Aspart (NovoLOG):*** 100 units/mL vial, 3-mL cartridge, 3-mL Flex-Pen. **Glulisine (Apidra):** 100 units/mL vial, 3-mL cartridge. **Lispro (Admelog, Lyumjev, HumaLOG):** 100 units/mL vial, 3-mL cartridge, 3-mL pen.

Short-Acting
Regular: *(HumuLIN R):* 100 units/mL vial, U-500 Kwik Pen. **Regular:** *(NovoLIN R):* 100 units/mL vial, 3-mL cartridge, 3-mL Innolet prefilled syringe.

Intermediate-Acting
NPH: *(HumuLIN N):* 100 units/mL vial, 3-mL pen. **NPH:** *(NovoLIN N):* 100 units/mL vial, 3-mL cartridge, 3-mL Innolet prefilled syringe.

Long-Acting
Detemir: *(Levemir):* 100 units/mL vial, 3-mL Flex-Pen. **Glargine:** *(Lantus, Semglee):* 100 units/mL vial, 3-mL cartridge. **Glargine:**

(Toujeo SoloStar): 300 units/mL. *(Basaglar KwikPen):* 100 units/mL.

Intermediate- and Short-Acting Mixtures: HumuLIN 50/50, HumuLIN 70/30, HumaLOG Mix 75/25, HumaLOG Mix 50/50, NovoLIN 70/30, NovoLOG Mix 70/30.

Solution, IV *(Myxredlin):* 100 units/100 mL in NaCl 0.9% (100 mL).

ADMINISTRATION/HANDLING

 IV

Regular and Insulin Glulisine
• *(Apidra):* Use only if solution is clear.
• May give undiluted.

Rapid-Acting
• *(Afrezza):* Administer using a single inhalation/cartridge. Give at beginning of a meal. • *(Aspart [NovoLOG]):* May give SQ, IV infusion. • Can mix with NPH (draw aspart into syringe first; inject immediately after mixing). • After first use, stable at room temperature for 28 days. • Administer 5–10 min before meals. • *(Glulisine [Apidra]):* May mix with NPH (draw glulisine into syringe first; inject immediately after mixing). • After first use, stable at room temperature for 28 days. • Administer 15 min before or within 20 min after starting a meal. • *(Lispro [HumaLOG]):* For SQ use only. • May mix with NPH. Stable for 28 days at room temperature; syringe is stable for 14 days if refrigerated. • After first use, stable at room temperature for 28 days. • Administer 15 min before or immediately after meals.

Short-Acting
Regular • *(HumuLIN R, NovoLIN R):* May give SQ, IM, IV. • May mix with NPH for immediate use or for storage for future use. Stable for 1 mo at room temperature, 3 mos if refrigerated. • Can mix with Sterile Water for Injection or 0.9% NaCl. • After first use, stable at room temperature for 28 days. • Administer 30 min before meals.

Intermediate-Acting
NPH • *(HumuLIN N, NovoLIN N):* For SQ use only. • May mix with aspart (NovoLOG) or lispro (HumaLOG). Draw aspart or lispro first and use immediately. • May mix with regular (HumuLIN R, NovoLIN R) insulin. Draw regular insulin first, use immediately or may store for future use (up to 28 days). • After first use, stable at room temperature for 28 days. • Administer 15 min before meals when mixed with aspart or lispro; 30 min before meals when mixed with regular insulin.

Long-Acting
• *(Degludec [Tresiba]):* For SQ use only. • Do not mix with other insulins. • After first use, stable at room temperature for 56 days. • May take once daily any time of day. • *(Detemir [Levemir]):* For SQ use only. • Do not mix with other insulins. • After first use, stable at room temperature for 42 days. • Evening dose given at dinner or at bedtime. Twice-daily regimens can be given 12 hrs after morning dose. • *(Glargine [Lantus, Toujeo]):* For SQ use only. • Do not mix with other insulins. • After first use, stable at room temperature for 28 days. • Administer once daily at same time. Meal timing is not applicable.

SQ
• Check serum glucose concentration before administration; dosage highly individualized. • SQ injections may be given in thigh, abdomen, upper arm, buttocks, upper back if there is adequate adipose tissue. • Rotation of injection sites is essential; maintain careful record. • Prefilled syringes should be stored in vertical or oblique position to avoid plugging; plunger should be pulled back slightly and syringe rocked to remix solution before injection.

▓ IV INCOMPATIBILITIES
Norepinephrine.

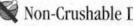

❖ IV COMPATIBILITIES

Dobutamine, heparin, ibuprofen, magnesium sulfate, propofol.

INDICATIONS/ROUTES/DOSAGE

Note: Insulin requirements vary dramatically among pts, requiring dosage adjustment.

Type 1 Diabetes

Multiple daily injections, guided by glucose monitoring or continuous SQ insulin infusions, is standard of care. **Usual initial dose:** 0.4–0.5 unit/kg/day in divided doses (consider initial doses of 0.2–0.4 units/kg/day to avoid hypoglycemia). **Usual maintenance:** 0.4–1 units/kg/day in divided doses.

Type 2 Diabetes

Initially, 10 units/day or 0.1–0.2 units/kg/day as a single dose (usually at bedtime). **Maximum initial dose:** 15–20 units/day. Pts with Hgb A1c greater then 8%, fasting plasma glucose greater than 250 mg/dL, or insulin resistance, 0.2–0.3 units/kg/day (15–20 units/day is recommended).

Dosage in Renal Impairment

Creatinine Clearance	Dose
10–50 mL/min	75% normal dose
Less than 10 mL/min	25%–50% normal dose

Dosage in Hepatic Impairment

Insulin requirement may be reduced.

SIDE EFFECTS

Occasional: Localized redness, swelling, itching (due to improper insulin injection technique), allergy to insulin cleansing solution. **Infrequent:** Somogyi effect (rebound hyperglycemia) with chronically excessive insulin dosages. Systemic allergic reaction (rash, angioedema, anaphylaxis), lipodystrophy (depression at injection site due to breakdown of adipose tissue), lipohypertrophy (accumulation of SQ tissue at injection site due to inadequate site rotation). **Rare:** Insulin resistance.

ADVERSE EFFECTS/TOXIC REACTIONS

Severe hypoglycemia (due to hyperinsulinism) may occur with insulin overdose, decrease/delay of food intake, excessive exercise, pts with brittle diabetes. Diabetic ketoacidosis may result from stress, illness, omission of insulin dose, longterm poor insulin control.

NURSING CONSIDERATIONS

BASELINE ASSESSMENT

Obtain serum glucose level, Hgb A1c. Discuss lifestyle to determine extent of learning, emotional needs. If given IV, obtain serum chemistries (esp. serum potassium).

INTERVENTION/EVALUATION

Assess for hypoglycemia (refer to pharmacokinetics table for peak times and duration): cool, wet skin, tremors, dizziness, headache, anxiety, tachycardia, numbness in mouth, hunger, diplopia. Assess sleeping pt for restlessness, diaphoresis. Check for hyperglycemia: polyuria (excessive urine output), polyphagia (excessive food intake), polydipsia (excessive thirst), nausea/vomiting, dim vision, fatigue, deep and rapid breathing (Kussmaul respirations). Be alert to conditions altering glucose requirements: fever, trauma, increased activity/stress, surgical procedure.

PATIENT/FAMILY TEACHING

• Diet and exercise are essential parts of treatment; do not skip/delay meals. • Carry candy, sugar packets, other sugar supplements for immediate response to hypoglycemia. • Wear or carry medical alert identification. • Check with physician when insulin demands are altered (e.g., fever, infection, trauma, stress, heavy physical activity). • Do not take other medication without consulting physician. • Weight control, exercise, hygiene (including foot care) are integral parts of therapy. • Protect skin, limit sun exposure. • Inform dentist, physician, surgeon of medication before any treatment is given.

ipilimumab

ip-i-**lim**-ue-mab
(Yervoy)

◆CLASSIFICATION

PHARMACOTHERAPEUTIC: Human cytotoxic T-lymphocyte antigen 4 (CTLA-4)–blocking antibody. Monoclonal antibody. **CLINICAL:** Antineoplastic.

USES

Melanoma: Treatment of unresectable or metastatic melanoma in adults and pediatric pts 12 yrs and older as a single agent or in combination with nivolumab. Adjuvant treatment of pts with cutaneous melanoma with pathologic involvement of regional lymph nodes of more than 1 mm who have undergone complete resection, including total lymphadenectomy. **Renal cell carcinoma (RCC):** Treatment of adults with intermediate- or poor-risk advanced renal cell carcinoma, as first-line treatment in combination with nivolumab. **Colorectal cancer:** Treatment of adults and pediatric pts 12 yrs and older with microsatellite instability-high (MSI-H) or mismatch repair deficient (dMMR) metastatic colorectal cancer that has progressed following treatment with fluoropyrimidine, oxaliplatin, and irinotecan in combination with nivolumab. **Hepatocellular carcinoma:** Treatment of pts with hepatocellular carcinoma who have been previously treated with SORAfenib, in combination with nivolumab. **Non–small-cell lung cancer (NSCLC):** Treatment of adults with metastatic NSCLC expressing PD-L1 with no EGFR or ALK genomic tumor aberra-

tions as first-line treatment in combination with nivolumab. Treatment of adults with metastatic or recurrent NSCLC with no EGFR or ALK genomic tumor aberrations as first-line treatment in combination with nivolumab and 2 cycles of platinum-doublet chemotherapy. **Malignant pleural mesothelioma:** Treatment of adults with unresectable malignant pleural mesothelioma as first-line treatment in combination with nivolumab. **Esophageal cancer:** Treatment of adult patients with unresectable advanced or metastatic esophageal squamous cell carcinoma as first-line treatment in combination with nivolumab. **OFF-LABEL:** Melanoma (with brain metastases).

PRECAUTIONS

Contraindications: Hypersensitivity to ipilimumab. **Cautions:** Hepatic impairment, chronic peripheral neuropathy, thyroid/adrenal/pituitary dysfunction, autoimmune disorders (ulcerative colitis, Crohn's disease, lupus, sarcoidosis).

ACTION

Augments T-cell activation and proliferation. Binds to cytotoxic T-lymphocyte–associated antigen 4 (CTLA-4) and blocks interaction of CTLA-4 with its ligands, allowing for enhanced T-cell activation and proliferation. **Therapeutic Effect:** May indirectly mediate T-cell immune responses against tumors.

PHARMACOKINETICS

Metabolized in liver. Steady state reached by third dose. **Half-life:** 14.7 days.

⌛ LIFESPAN CONSIDERATIONS

Pregnancy/Lactation: May cause fetal harm. Use effective contraception during treatment and for at least 3 mos after discontinuation. Unknown if distributed in breast milk. **Children:** Safety and efficacy not established in pts younger than 12 yrs. **Elderly:** No age-related precautions noted.

INTERACTIONS

DRUG: None significant. **HERBAL:** None significant. **FOOD:** None known. **LAB**

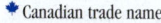 ◆ Canadian trade name   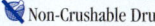 Non-Crushable Drug   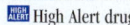 High Alert drug

VALUES: May increase serum ALT, AST, bilirubin; eosinophils.

AVAILABILITY (Rx)

Injection, Solution: 5 mg/mL (10 mL, 40 mL vials).

ADMINISTRATION/HANDLING
🖱 IV

◄**ALERT**► Use sterile, nonpyrogenic, low protein-binding in-line filter. Use dedicated line only.

Reconstitution • Calculate number of vials needed for injection. • Inspect for particulate matter or discoloration. • Allow vials to stand at room temperature for approximately 5 min. • Withdraw proper volume and transfer to infusion bag. Dilute in NaCl or D₅W with final concentration ranging from 1–2 mg/mL. • Mix by gentle inversion. Do not shake or agitate.
Rate of administration • Infuse over 30–90 min (based on indication). Flush with 0.9% NaCl or D₅W at end of infusion.
Storage • Solution should be translucent to white or pale yellow with amorphous particles. • Discard vial if cloudy or discolored. • Refrigerate vials until time of use. • May store diluted solution either under refrigeration or at room temperature for no more than 24 hrs.

INDICATIONS/ROUTES/DOSAGE

Melanoma
IV: ADULTS, ELDERLY, CHILDREN 12 YRS AND OLDER: (Single agent): 3 mg/kg q3wks. Maximum: 4 doses. **(In combination with nivolumab):** 3 mg/kg q3wks for maximum of 4 doses or until unacceptable toxicity, whichever occurs first. After completing 4 doses of combination therapy, administer nivolumab as a single agent until disease progression or unacceptable toxicity. **Adjuvant treatment: (Single agent):** 10 mg/kg q3wks up to a maximum of 4 doses, then 10 mg/kg q12wks for up to 3 yrs.

Renal Cell Carcinoma (RCC)
IV: ADULTS, ELDERLY: 1 mg/kg q3wks, in combination with nivolumab, for a maximum of 4 doses, then give nivolumab as a single agent until disease progression or unacceptable toxicity.

Colorectal Cancer
IV: ADULTS, ELDERLY: 1 mg/kg q3wks, in combination with nivolumab, for a maximum of 4 doses, then give nivolumab as a single agent until disease progression or unacceptable toxicity.

Hepatocellular Carcinoma
IV: ADULTS, ELDERLY: 3 mg/kg q3wks, in combination with nivolumab, for a maximum of 4 doses, then give nivolumab as a single agent until disease progression or unacceptable toxicity.

Non–Small-Cell Lung Cancer (NSCLC)
IV: ADULTS, ELDERLY: (Metastatic expressing PD-L1): 1 mg/kg q6wks with nivolumab until disease progression or unacceptable toxicity, or up to 2 yrs in pts without disease progression. **(Metastatic or recurrent):** 1 mg/kg q6wks (with nivolumab 360 mg q3wks and histology-based platinum-doublet chemotherapy q3wks for 2 cycles), in combination with nivolumab, until disease progression or unacceptable toxicity, or up to 2 yrs in pts without disease progression.

Malignant Pleural Mesothelioma
IV: ADULTS, ELDERLY: 1 mg/kg q6wks (with nivolumab q3wks) until disease progression or unacceptable toxicity, or up to 2 yrs in pts without disease progression.

Esophageal Cancer
IV: ADULTS, ELDERLY: 1 mg/kg q6wks (with nivolumab q2wks or q3wks) until disease progression or unacceptable toxicity, or up to 2 yrs.

Dosage Modification
Hold scheduled dose for moderate immune-mediated adverse reactions. Pts with complete or partial resolution of adverse reactions and who are receiving less than 7.5 mg/day of predniSONE may resume

scheduled doses. Permanently discontinue for persistent moderate adverse reactions or inability to reduce corticosteroid dose to 7.5 mg/day, failure to complete full treatment course in 16 wks, any severe or life-threatening adverse reactions.

Hepatotoxicity

ALT/AST greater than 2.5 times upper limit of normal (ULN) or bilirubin greater than 1.5–3 times ULN: Withhold treatment. **ALT/AST greater than 5 times ULN or bilirubin greater than 3 times ULN:** Permanently discontinue.

Dosage in Renal/Hepatic Impairment

No dose adjustment.

SIDE EFFECTS

Frequent (42%): Fatigue. **Occasional (32%–29%):** Diarrhea, pruritus, rash, colitis.

ADVERSE EFFECTS/TOXIC REACTIONS

Severe and fatal immune-mediated adverse reactions have occurred. Enterocolitis (7% of pts) may present with fever, ileus, abdominal pain, GI bleeding, intestinal perforation, severe dehydrating diarrhea. Endocrinopathies (4% of pts), including hypopituitarism, adrenal insufficiency, hypogonadism, hypothyroidism, may present with fatigue, headache, mental status change, unusual bowel habits, hypotension and may require emergent hormone replacement therapy. Dermatitis including toxic epidermal necrolysis (2% of pts) may present with full-thickness ulceration or necrotic, bullous, hemorrhagic manifestations. Hepatotoxicity (1% of pts), defined as LFT greater than 2.5–5 times ULN, may present with right upper abdominal pain, jaundice, black/tarry stools, bruising, dark-colored urine, nausea, vomiting. Neuropathy (1% of pts), including Guillain-Barré syndrome or myasthenia gravis, may present with weakness, sensory alterations, paresthesia, paralysis. Other serious adverse reactions such as pneumonitis, meningitis, nephritis, eosinophilia, pericarditis, myocarditis, angiopathy, temporal arteritis, vasculitis, polymyalgia rheumatica, conjunctivitis, blepharitis, episcleritis, scleritis, leukocy toclastic vasculitis, erythema multiforme, psoriasis, pancreatitis, arthritis, autoimmune thyroiditis reported. Anti-ipilimumab antibodies reported in 1.1% of pts. All severe immune-mediated adverse reactions require immediate high-dose corticosteroid therapy.

NURSING CONSIDERATIONS

BASELINE ASSESSMENT

Obtain CBC, BMP, LFT; pregnancy test in females of reproductive potential. Screen for history of hepatic impairment, chronic neuropathy, thyroid/adrenal/pituitary dysfunction, autoimmune disorders. Screen for active infection. Receive full medication history including herbal products. Offer emotional support.

INTERVENTION/EVALUATION

Monitor vital signs, LFT, thyroid panel before each dose. Continue focused assessment and screen for life-threatening immune-mediated adverse reactions. If adverse reactions occur, immediately notify physician and initiate proper treatment. Report suspected pregnancy. Obtain CBC, blood cultures for fever, suspected infection. ECG for palpitations, chest pain, difficulty breathing, dizziness. If predniSONE therapy initiated, monitor capillary blood glucose and screen for side effects.

PATIENT/FAMILY TEACHING

• Serious and fatal adverse reactions indicate inflammation to certain systems: intestines (diarrhea, dark/tarry stools, abdominal pain), liver (yellowing of the skin, dark-colored urine, right upper quadrant pain, bruising), skin (rash, mouth sores, blisters, ulcers), nerves (weakness, numbness, tingling, difficulty breathing, paralysis), hormonal glands (headaches, weight gain, palpitations, changes in mood or behavior, dizziness), eyes (blurry vision, double vision, eye pain/redness). • PredniSONE therapy may be started if adverse reactions occur. • May cause fetal harm, stillbirth, premature delivery. • Report any chest pain, palpitations, fever, swollen glands, stomach pain, vomiting, or any sign of adverse reactions.

ipratropium

TOP 100

ip-ra-**troe**-pee-um
(Atrovent HFA, Apo-Ipravent 🍁)
**Do not confuse Atrovent with
Alupent or Serevent, or ipratro-
pium with tiotropium.**

FIXED-COMBINATION(S)

Combivent, DuoNeb: ipratropium/
albuterol (a bronchodilator): *Aerosol:*
18 mcg/90 mcg per actuation. *Solution:* 0.5 mg/2.5 mg per 3 mL.

◆CLASSIFICATION

PHARMACOTHERAPEUTIC: Anticholinergic. **CLINICAL:** Bronchodilator.

USES

Inhalation, nebulization: Maintenance
treatment of bronchospasm associated with
COPD, including bronchitis, emphysema.
Not indicated for immediate bronchospasm
relief. **Nasal spray:** Symptomatic relief
of rhinorrhea associated with allergic
and nonallergic perennial rhinitis (in
adults and children 6 yrs and older) and
associated with seasonal allergic rhinitis
(in adults and children 5 yrs and older).
Symptomatic relief of rhinorrhea associated
with common cold (in adults and children
5 yrs and older). **OFF-LABEL:** Acute asthma
(exacerbation).

PRECAUTIONS

Contraindications: History of
hypersensitivity to ipratropium, atropine.
Cautions: Narrow-angle glaucoma,
prostatic hypertrophy, bladder neck
obstruction, myasthenia gravis.

ACTION

Blocks action of acetylcholine at
parasympathetic sites in bronchial
smooth muscle. Application to nasal
mucosa inhibits serous/seromucous
gland secretions. **Therapeutic
Effect:** Causes bronchodilation,
inhibits nasal secretions.

PHARMACOKINETICS

Route	Onset	Peak	Duration
Inhalation	1–3 min	1.5–2 hrs	Up to 4 hrs
Nasal	5 min	1–4 hrs	4–8 hrs

Minimal systemic absorption after
inhalation. Metabolized in liver (systemic
absorption). Primarily excreted in feces.
Half-life: 1.5–4 hrs (nasal).

⌛ LIFESPAN CONSIDERATIONS

Pregnancy/Lactation: Unknown if
distributed in breast milk. **Children/El-
derly:** No age-related precautions noted.

INTERACTIONS

DRUG: Anticholinergics (e.g.,
**aclidinium, ipratropium, tiotropium,
umeclidinium**), **medications
with anticholinergic properties**
may increase toxicity. **HERBAL:** None
significant. **FOOD:** None known. **LAB
VALUES:** None significant.

AVAILABILITY (Rx)

Aerosol for Oral Inhalation: *(Atrovent
HFA):* 17 mcg/actuation. **Solution, Intra-
nasal Spray:** 0.03%; 0.06%. **Solution for
Nebulization:** 0.02% (500 mcg).

ADMINISTRATION/HANDLING

Inhalation
• Does not require shaking. Prime before first use or if not used for more than
3 days. • Instruct pt to exhale completely, place mouthpiece between lips,
inhale deeply through mouth while fully
depressing top of canister. Hold breath as
long as possible before exhaling
slowly. • Allow at least 1 minute between inhalations. • Rinse mouth with
water immediately after inhalation (prevents mouth/throat dryness).

Nebulization
• May be administered with or without
dilution in 0.9% NaCl. • Stable for 1 hr
when mixed with albuterol. • Give over
5–15 min.

Nasal
• Store at room temperature. • Initial pump priming requires 7 actua-

tions of pump. • If used regularly as recommended, no further priming is required. If not used for more than 4 hrs, pump will require 2 actuations, or if not used for more than 7 days, the pump will require 7 actuations to reprime.

INDICATIONS/ROUTES/DOSAGE
COPD
Inhalation: ADULTS, ELDERLY: (Acute exacerbation): 2 inhalations q4–6h as needed. (Intermittent symptom relief): 2 inhalations q4–6h as needed. (Maintenance): 2 inhalations q6h. (Hospital-based care): 2–4 inhalations q1hr for up to 3 doses, then q2–4h as needed. **Nebulization: ADULTS, ELDERLY,** (Acute exacerbation): 500 mcg q6–8h as needed. (Intermittent symptom relief): 500 mcg q4–8h as needed. (Maintenance): 500 mcg q6–8h. (Hospital-based care): 500 mcg q1h for up to 3 doses, then q2–4h as needed.

Rhinorrhea (Perennial Allergic/ Nonallergic Rhinitis)
Intranasal: *(0.03%):* **ADULTS, ELDERLY, CHILDREN 6 YRS AND OLDER:** 2 sprays (21 mcg/spray) per nostril 2–3 times/day. **Maximum:** 168–252 mcg/day.

Rhinorrhea (Common Cold)
Intranasal: *(0.06%):* **ADULTS, ELDERLY, CHILDREN 12 YRS AND OLDER:** 2 sprays (42 mcg/spray) per nostril 3–4 times/day for up to 4 days. **Maximum:** 504–672 mcg/day. **CHILDREN 5–11 YRS:** 2 sprays per nostril 3 times/day for up to 4 days. **Maximum:** 504 mcg/day.

Rhinorrhea (Seasonal Allergy)
Intranasal: *(0.06%):* **ADULTS, ELDERLY, CHILDREN 5 YRS AND OLDER:** 2 sprays (42 mcg/spray) per nostril 4 times/day for up to 3 wks. Total dose: 672 mcg/day.

Dosage in Renal/Hepatic Impairment
No dose adjustment.

SIDE EFFECTS
Frequent: Inhalation (6%–3%): Cough, dry mouth, headache, nausea. **Nasal:** Dry nose/mouth, headache, nasal irritation. **Occasional: Inhalation (2%):** Dizziness, transient increased bronchospasm. **Rare (less than 1%): Inhalation:** Hypotension, insomnia, metallic/unpleasant taste, palpitations, urinary retention. **Nasal:** Diarrhea, constipation, dry throat, abdominal pain, nasal congestion.

ADVERSE EFFECTS/TOXIC REACTIONS
Worsening of angle-closure glaucoma, acute eye pain, hypotension occur rarely.

NURSING CONSIDERATIONS
BASELINE ASSESSMENT
Auscultate lung sounds. Question history of glaucoma, urinary retention, myasthenia gravis.

INTERVENTION/EVALUATION
Monitor rate, depth, rhythm, type of respiration; quality, rate of pulse. Assess lung sounds for rhonchi, wheezing, rales. Monitor ABGs. Observe for retractions (clavicular, sternal, intercostal), hand tremor. Evaluate for clinical improvement (quieter, slower respirations, relaxed facial expression, cessation of retractions). Monitor for improvement of rhinorrhea.

PATIENT/ FAMILY TEACHING
• Increase fluid intake (decreases lung secretion viscosity). • Do not take more than 2 inhalations at any one time (excessive use may produce paradoxical bronchoconstriction, decreased bronchodilating effect). • Rinsing mouth with water immediately after inhalation may prevent mouth and throat dryness. • Avoid excessive use of caffeine derivatives (chocolate, coffee, tea, cola, cocoa).

irbesartan

ir-be-**sar**-tan
(Avapro)

■ BLACK BOX ALERT ■ May cause fetal injury, mortality if used during second or third trimester of pregnancy. Discontinue as soon as possible once pregnancy is detected.
Do not confuse Avapro with Anaprox.

FIXED-COMBINATION(S)

Avalide: irbesartan/hydroCHLOROthiazide (a diuretic): 150 mg/12.5 mg, 300 mg/12.5 mg, 300 mg/25 mg.

◆CLASSIFICATION

PHARMACOTHERAPEUTIC: Angiotensin II receptor antagonist. **CLINICAL:** Antihypertensive.

USES

Hypertension: Treatment of hypertension alone or in combination with other antihypertensives. **Diabetic nephropathy:** Treatment of diabetic nephropathy in pts with an elevated serum creatinine and proteinuria (greater than 300 mg/day) in pts with type 2 diabetes and hypertension. **OFF-LABEL:** Acute coronary syndrome (STEMI, non-STEMI), proteinuric chronic kidney disease (non-diabetic).

PRECAUTIONS

Contraindications: Hypersensitivity to irbesartan. Concomitant use with aliskiren in pts with diabetes. **Cautions:** Renal impairment, unstented unilateral or bilateral renal artery stenosis, dehydration, HF, idiopathic or hereditary angioedema or angioedema associated with ACE inhibitor therapy.

ACTION

Blocks vasoconstriction, aldosterone-secreting effects of angiotensin II, inhibiting binding of angiotensin II to AT_1 receptors. **Therapeutic Effect:** Produces vasodilation, decreases peripheral resistance, decreases B/P.

PHARMACOKINETICS

Route	Onset	Peak	Duration
PO	—	1–2 hrs	Greater than 24 hrs

Widely distributed. Protein binding: 90%. Metabolized in liver. Excreted in feces (80%), urine (20%). Not removed by hemodialysis. **Half-life:** 11–15 hrs.

⧗ LIFESPAN CONSIDERATIONS

Pregnancy/Lactation: Unknown if distributed in breast milk. May cause fetal or neonatal morbidity or mortality. **Children:** Safety and efficacy not established. **Elderly:** No age-related precautions noted.

INTERACTIONS

DRUG: May increase adverse of **ACE inhibitors** (e.g., **benazepril, lisinopril**). **NSAIDs** (e.g., **ibuprofen, ketorolac, naproxen**) may decrease antihypertensive effect. **HERBAL:** Herbals with hypertensive properties (e.g., **licorice, yohimbe**) or hypotensive properties (e.g., **garlic, ginger, ginkgo biloba**) may alter effects. **FOOD:** None known. **LAB VALUES:** May slightly increase serum BUN, creatinine. May decrease Hgb.

AVAILABILITY (Rx)

Tablets: 75 mg, 150 mg, 300 mg.

ADMINISTRATION/HANDLING

PO
• Give without regard to food.

INDICATIONS/ROUTES/DOSAGE

Hypertension
PO: ADULTS, ELDERLY, CHILDREN 13 YRS AND OLDER: Initially, 75–150 mg/day. May increase to 300 mg/day. **CHILDREN 6–12 YRS:** Initially, 75 mg/day. May increase to 150 mg/day.

Diabetic Nephropathy
PO: ADULTS, ELDERLY: Initially, 75 mg once daily. Titrate based on B/P response and tolerability. **Maximum:** 300 mg once daily.

Dosage in Renal/Hepatic Impairment
No dose adjustment.

SIDE EFFECTS

Occasional (9%–3%): Upper respiratory tract infection, fatigue, diarrhea, cough. **Rare (2%–1%):** Heartburn, dizziness, headache, nausea, rash.

ADVERSE EFFECTS/TOXIC REACTIONS

Overdose may manifest as hypotension, syncope, tachycardia. Bradycardia occurs less often.

NURSING CONSIDERATIONS

BASELINE ASSESSMENT

Obtain B/P, pulse immediately before each dose in addition to regular monitoring (be alert to fluctuations). Question possibility of pregnancy. Assess medication history (esp. diuretic therapy).

INTERVENTION/EVALUATION

Maintain hydration (offer fluids frequently). Assess for evidence of upper respiratory infection. Assist with ambulation if dizziness occurs. Monitor B/P, pulse. Assess for hypotension.

PATIENT/ FAMILY TEACHING

• May cause fetal or neonatal morbidity or mortality. • Report any sign of infection (sore throat, fever). • Avoid exercising during hot weather (risk of dehydration, hypotension).

irinotecan

eye-ri-noe-tee-kan
(Camptosar, Onivyde)

■ **BLACK BOX ALERT** ■ **(Camptosar, Onivyde):** Can induce both early and late forms of severe diarrhea. Early diarrhea (during or shortly after administration) accompanied by salivation, rhinitis, lacrimation, diaphoresis, flushing. Late diarrhea (occurring more than 24 hrs after administration) can be prolonged and life-threatening. **(Camptosar):** May produce severe, profound myelosuppression. Administer under supervision of experienced cancer chemotherapy physician. **(Onivyde):** Severe, life-threatening, or fatal neutropenic fever/sepsis occurred. Withhold for ANC below 1,500 cells/mm³ or neutropenic fever. Monitor blood cell counts.

◆CLASSIFICATION

PHARMACOTHERAPEUTIC: Topoisomerase-I inhibitor. **CLINICAL:** Antineoplastic.

USES

Camptosar: First-line therapy in combination with 5-fluorouracil and leucovorin in pts with metastatic carcinoma of the colon or rectum. Pts with metastatic carcinoma of the colon or rectum whose disease has recurred or progressed following initial fluorouracil-based therapy. **Onivyde:** First-line treatment of adults with metastatic pancreatic adenocarcinoma in combination with oxaliplatin, fluorouracil, and leucovorin. Treatment of metastatic adenocarcinoma of the pancreas (in combination with 5-fluorouracil and leucovorin) after disease progression following gemcitabine-based therapy. **OFF-LABEL: Camptosar:** Cervical cancer, CNS tumor (recurrent glioblastoma), esophageal cancer (metastatic/locally advanced), Ewing sarcoma, gastric cancer, NSCLC (advanced), ovarian cancer, pancreatic cancer (advanced/metastatic), rhabdomyosarcoma, small-cell lung cancer.

PRECAUTIONS

Contraindications: Hypersensitivity to irinotecan. **Cautions:** Pt previously receiving pelvic, abdominal irradiation (increased risk of myelosuppression), pts older than 65 yrs, hepatic dysfunction, hyperbilirubinemia, renal impairment, preexisting pulmonary disease, conditions predisposing to infection (e.g., diabetes, renal failure, immunocompromised pts, open wounds).

ACTION

Binds reversibly with topoisomerase I, an enzyme that relieves torsional strain in DNA by inducing reversible single-strand breaks Prevents religation of these single-stranded breaks, resulting in damage to double-strand DNA, cell death. **Therapeutic Effect:** Produces cytotoxic effect on cancer cells.

PHARMACOKINETICS

Widely distributed. Metabolized in liver. Protein binding: 95% (metabolite). Excreted in urine and eliminated by biliary route. **Half-life:** 6–12 hrs; metabolite, 10–20 hrs.

⧗ LIFESPAN CONSIDERATIONS

Pregnancy/Lactation: Avoid pregnancy; may cause fetal harm. Females of reproductive potential must use effective contraception during treatment and for at least 6 mos after discontinuation. Breastfeeding not recommended during treatment and for at least 7 days after discontinuation. May impair fertility. **Males:** Males with female partners of reproductive potential must use effective contraception during treatment and for at least 3 mos after discontinuation. May impair fertility. **Children:** Safety and efficacy not established. **Elderly:** Risk of diarrhea significantly increased.

INTERACTIONS

DRUG: Strong CYP3A4 inducers (e.g., carBAMazepine, phenytoin, rifAMPin), vaccines (live) may decrease concentration/effect. **Strong CYP3A4 inhibitors (e.g., clarithromycin, ketoconazole, ritonavir)** may increase concentration/effect. May increase concentration/effects of **vaccines (live).** May decrease the therapeutic effect of **BCG (intravesical). UGT1A1 inhibitors (e.g., erlotinib, nilotinib)** may increase concentration/effect. **HERBAL: Echinacea** may decrease therapeutic effect. **St. John's wort** may decrease concentration/effect. **FOOD:** None known. **LAB VALUES:** May increase serum alkaline phosphatase, AST. May decrease Hgb, leukocytes, platelets.

AVAILABILITY (Rx)

Injection Solution: *(Conventional):* 20 mg/mL (2 mL, 5 mL, 15 mL, 25 mL). **_(Liposomal):_** 43 mg/10 mL.

ADMINISTRATION/HANDLING

 IV

Camptosar

Reconstitution • Dilute in D_5W (preferred) or 0.9% NaCl to concentration of 0.12–2.8 mg/mL. **Rate of administration** • Administer all doses as IV infusion over 30–90 min. • Assess for extravasation (flush site with Sterile Water for Injection, apply ice if extravasation occurs). **Storage** • Store vials at room temperature, protect from light. • Solution diluted with D_5W is stable for 24 hrs at room temperature or 48 hrs if refrigerated. • Solution diluted with 0.9% NaCl is stable for 24 hrs at room temperature. • Do not refrigerate solution if diluted with 0.9% NaCl.

Onivyde

Reconstitution • Withdraw dose from vial and dilute with 500 mL D_5W or 0.9% NaCl. Mix gently. **Rate of administration** • Infuse over 90 min. **Storage** • Refrigerate vials; do not freeze. • Protect from light. • Stable for 4 hrs at room temperature or 24 hrs refrigerated.

INDICATIONS/ROUTES/DOSAGE

Carcinoma of the Colon, Rectum (Camptosar)

IV: *(Single-Agent Therapy):* **ADULTS, ELDERLY: (WEEKLY REGIMEN):** Initially, 125 mg/m^2 once wkly for 4 wks, followed by a rest period of 2 wks. Additional courses may be repeated q6wks. Dosage may be adjusted in 25–50 mg/m^2 increments/decrements to as high as 150 mg/m^2 or as low as 50 mg/m^2. **(3-WEEK REGIMEN):** 350 mg/m^2 q3wks. Dosage may be adjusted to as low as 200 mg/m^2 in decrements of 25–50 mg/m^2. **_(In Combination With Leucovorin and 5-Fluorouracil):_** (Leucovorin given immediately following irinotecan, then 5-fluorouracil immediately following leucovorin.) **REGIMEN 1:** 125 mg/m^2 on days 1, 8, 15, 22. Dose may be adjusted to 100 mg/m^2, then 75 mg/m^2, then decrements of approximately 20%. **REGIMEN 2**: 180 mg/m² on days 1, 15, 29. Dose may be adjusted to 150 mg/m², then 120 mg/m², then decrements of approximately 20%.

Pancreatic Cancer (Onivyde)

IV infusion: **ADULTS, ELDERLY**: **(In combination with fluorouracil and leucovoran)**: 70 mg/m² once q2wks. Reduce initial starting dose to 50 mg/m² in pts homozygous for the UGT1A1*28 allele. May increase dose to 70 mg/m² as tolerated. **(In combination with oxaliplatin, fluorouracil, and leucovorin)**: 50 mg/m² once q2wks. Starting dose in pts homozygous for the UGT1A1*28 allele is 50 mg/m².

Dosage in Renal Impairment

No dose adjustment.

Dosage in Hepatic Impairment

Serum Bilirubin	Dose
Greater than ULN to 2 mg/dL:	Reduce dose one level
Greater than 2 mg/dL:	Not recommended

SIDE EFFECTS

Frequent (64%–22%): Nausea, alopecia, vomiting, diarrhea, constipation, fatigue, fever, asthenia, skeletal pain, abdominal pain, dyspnea. **Occasional (19%–16%)**: Anorexia, headache, stomatitis, rash.

ADVERSE EFFECTS/TOXIC REACTIONS

Myelosuppression is an expected response to therapy, but more severe reactions including febrile neutropenia may be life threatening. Pts who are homozygous for the UGT1A1*28 allele are at increased risk for neutropenia. Hypersensitivity reactions including anaphylaxis may occur. Fatal pulmonary toxicities, interstitial pulmonary disease were reported. Diarrhea may cause severe dehydration, renal failure, which can be fatal. Cholinergic reactions including rhinitis, increased salivation, miosis, lacrimation, diaphoresis, flushing, and intestinal hyperperistalsis may occur.

NURSING CONSIDERATIONS

BASELINE ASSESSMENT

Obtain CBC (prior to each dose), LFT; pregnancy test in females of reproductive potential. Due to risk of severe dehydration related to diarrhea, ensure adequate hydration prior to each dose. Question history pulmonary disease, hepatic/renal impairment. Screen for active infection. Receive full medication history and screen for interactions. Premedicate with antiemetics on day of treatment, starting at least 30 min before administration. Offer emotional support.

INTERVENTION/EVALUATION

Monitor CBC as indicated. Monitor pulmonary status, pulse oximeter readings. Consider ABG, radiologic test if ILD/pneumonitis (excessive cough, dyspnea, fever, hypoxia) is suspected. Consider treatment with corticosteroids if ILD/pneumonitis is confirmed. Monitor for infections (cough, fatigue, fever). If serious infection occurs, initiate appropriate antimicrobial therapy. Monitor daily pattern of bowel activity, stool consistency. Severe diarrhea may be life-threatening. Monitor for hypersensitivity reactions, anaphylaxis. Assess skin for rash.

PATIENT/ FAMILY TEACHING

• Treatment may depress your immune system response and reduce your ability to fight infection. Report symptoms of infection such as body aches, chills, cough, fatigue, fever. Avoid those with active infection. • Report symptoms of lung inflammation (excessive coughing, difficulty breathing, chest pain); liver problems (abdominal pain, bruising, clay-colored stool, amber- or dark-colored urine, yellowing of the skin or eyes). • Diarrhea may cause severe dehydration, which can be life-threatening. Report diarrhea of any severity. • Allergic reactions, including anaphylaxis, can occur. • Use effective contraception to avoid pregnancy. Do not breastfeed. • There is a high risk of interactions with other medications. Do not take newly prescribed medications unless ap-

I

proved by prescriber who originally started treatment. • Report diarrhea, vomiting, fever, light-headedness, dizziness. • Do not have immunizations without physician's approval (drug lowers resistance). • Avoid contact with those who have recently received live virus vaccine. • Avoid crowds, those with infections.

isatuximab-irfc

eye-sa-**tux**-i-mab
(Sarclisa)
Do not confuse isatuximab with daratumumab, dinutuximab, elotuzumab, ipilimumab, ixabepilone, ixazomib or riTUXimab.

◆CLASSIFICATION

PHARMACOTHERAPEUTIC: Anti-CD38 immunoglobulin G1–derived monoclonal antibody. **CLINICAL:** Antineoplastic.

USES

Treatment of multiple myeloma (in combination with pomalidomide and dexamethasone) in adults who have received at least two prior therapies including lenalidomide and a proteasome inhibitor. Treatment of relapsed or refractory multiple myeloma (in combination with carfilzomib and dexAMETHasone) in adults who have received 1–3 prior lines of therapy. Treatment of adults with newly diagnosed multiple myeloma (in combination with bortezomib, lenalidomide and dexamethasone), who are not eligible for autologous stem cell transplant (ASCT).

PRECAUTIONS

Contraindications: Hypersensitivity to isatuximab. **Cautions:** Baseline cytopenias, conditions predisposing to infection (e.g., diabetes, renal failure, immunocompromised pts, open wounds).

ACTION

Binds to and inhibits cell surface glycoprotein CD38 on CD38-expressing tumor cells (highly expressed on myeloma cells). Promotes antibody-dependent cellular phagocytosis and cell-mediated cytotoxicity. Suppresses CD38-positive T-regulatory cells and activates natural killer cells in the absence of CD38-positive target tumor cells. **Therapeutic Effect:** Inhibits tumor cell growth.

PHARMACOKINETICS

Widely distributed. Metabolized into small peptides via catabolic pathway. Steady state reached in 8 wks. **Half-life:** Not specified.

⧗ LIFESPAN CONSIDERATIONS

Pregnancy/Lactation: Avoid pregnancy; may cause fetal harm. Females of reproductive potential must use effective contraception during treatment and for at least 5 mos after discontinuation. Unknown if distributed in breast milk. However, human immunoglobulin G (IgG) is present in breast milk and is known to cross the placenta. Breastfeeding not recommended. **Children:** Safety and efficacy not established. **Elderly:** No age-related precautions noted.

INTERACTIONS

DRUG: May decrease effect of **BCG intravesical, vaccines (live).** May increase adverse/toxic effect of **leflunomide, natalizumab. Cladribine, upadacitinib** may enhance the immunosuppressive effect. **Pimecrolimus, tacrolimus (topical)** may increase adverse/toxic effects **HERBAL:** Echinacea may decrease therapeutic effect. **FOOD:** None known. **LAB VALUES:** May mask detection of antibodies to minor antigens. Drug may be detected on both serum protein electrophoresis and immunofixation assays used to monitor multiple myeloma endogenous M-protein. May affect the determination of complete response and disease progression of some pts with IgG kappa myeloma protein. May cause positive Coombs test. May decrease Hgb, Hct, lymphocytes, neutrophils, platelets, RBCs.

AVAILABILITY (Rx)

Injection Solution: 100 mg/5 mL (20 mg/mL), 500 mg/25 mg/mL (20 mg/mL).

ADMINISTRATION/HANDLING
IV

Premedication • Give dexAMETHasone 40 mg PO or IV (20 mg PO or IV in pts 75 yrs or older), acetaminophen 650–1000 mg PO (or equivalent), an H_2 antagonist, and diphenhydrAMINE 25–50 mg PO or IV (or equivalent) 15–60 min prior to infusion. DiphenhydrAMINE IV is preferred for the first 4 treatments.

Infusion guidelines • Infusion bag must be made of polyolefins, polyethylene, polypropylene, polyvinyl chloride (PVC) with di-(2-ethylhexyl) phthalate (DEHP), or ethyl vinyl acetate (EVA). • Infuse via dedicated IV line with a 0.22 micron in-line filter. • Do not administer as IV push or bolus. • Do not administer with other infusions. • If a dose is missed, give as soon as possible and adjust schedule to maintain treatment interval.

Preparation • Must be prepared by personnel trained in aseptic manipulations and admixing of cytotoxic drugs. • Calculate the number of vials needed for dose based on weight in kg. • Visually inspect for particulate matter or discoloration. Solution should appear clear to slightly opalescent, colorless to slightly yellow in color. Do not use if solution is cloudy, discolored, or if visible particles are observed. • Remove a volume from a 250 mL NaCl or D_5W infusion bag that is equal to the required volume of vial for dose. • Dilute in 250 mL NaCl or D_5W infusion bag. • Gently invert to mix. Do not shake or agitate.

Rate of administration • **First infusion:** Infuse at 25 mL/hr for 60 min. May increase rate in increments of 25 mL/hr q30min up to a maximum rate of 150 mL/hr if no infusion reactions occur. • **Second infusion:** Infuse at 50 mL/hr for the first 30 min. May increase rate in increments of 100 mL/hr q30min up to a maximum rate of 200 mL/hr if no infusion reactions occur. • **Subsequent infusions:** Infuse at 200 mL/hr if previous infusion rates were tolerated. **Maximum rate:** 200 mL/hr.

Infusion reactions • If Grade 1 or 2 infusion-related reactions occur, interrupt infusion and treat symptoms. If symptoms improve, resume infusion at half of the initial infusion rate. If symptoms do not recur after 30 min, may increase to initial rate, and then follow usual titration protocol. • Permanently discontinue in pts with a Grade 3 or 4 infusion-related reaction or if symptoms do not improve or recur after interrupting infusion.

Storage • Refrigerate unused vials in original carton. • Protect from light. • May refrigerate diluted solution for up to 48 hrs or store at room temperature for up to 8 hrs. • Do not shake, agitate, or freeze.

⚙ IV INCOMPATABILITIES

Do not mix with solutions containing other medications.

INDICATIONS/ROUTES/DOSAGE
Multiple Myeloma (Previously Treated)

IV: **ADULTS:** **Cycle 1:** 10 mg/kg actual body weight on days 1, 8, 15, and 22 of a 28-day cycle (in combination with pomalidomide and dexAMETHasone, or in combination with carfilzomib and dexAMETHasone). **Cycle 2 and thereafter:** 10 mg/kg actual body weight on days 1 and 15 of 28-day cycle (in combination with pomalidomide and dexAMETHasone, or in combination with carfilzomib and dexAMETHasone). Continue until disease progression or unacceptable toxicity. If hematological toxicity occurs, may consider withholding treatment until blood counts improve.

Multiple Myeloma (Newly Diagnosed)

IV: **ADULTS:** (in combination with bortezomib, lenalidomide, and dexamethasone) **Cycle 1:** (42-day cycle) Days 1, 8, 15, 22, and 29. **Cycles 2–4:** (42-

day cycles) Days 1, 15, and 29 (q2wks). **Cycles 5–17:** (28-day cycles) Days 1 and 15 (q2 wks). **Cycles 18 and beyond:** (28-day cycles) Day 1 (q4wks).

Dose Modification
Neutropenia
Grade 4 neutropenia: Withhold treatment until neutrophil count improves to 1,000 cells/mm^3, then resume at same dose.

Dosage in Renal Impairment
No dose adjustment.

Dosage in Hepatic Impairment
Mild impairment: No dose adjustment. **Moderate to severe impairment:** Not specified; use caution.

SIDE EFFECTS
Frequent (26%): Diarrhea. **Occasional (17%–12%):** Dyspnea, nausea, vomiting.

ADVERSE EFFECTS/TOXIC REACTIONS
Myelosuppression (anemia, lymphopenia, neutropenia, thrombocytopenia) is an expected response to therapy, but more severe reactions including severe neutropenia, febrile neutropenia may be life threatening. Grade 3 or 4 neutropenia reported in 85% of pts. Infusion-related reactions including chills, cough, dyspnea, nausea reported in 39% of pts. Grade 3 or 4 infusion reactions including dyspnea, hypertension, bronchospasm reported in 1% of pts. Infections including pneumonia (bronchopulmonary aspergillosis, *Haemophilus* pneumonia, influenza, *Pneumocystis jiroveci* pneumonia; bacterial/candidal/streptococcal/viral pneumonia), respiratory tract infections (bronchiolitis, bronchitis, viral bronchitis, nasopharyngitis, laryngitis, pharyngitis, parainfluenza virus infection, rhinitis, tracheitis, bacterial infection), UTI were reported. Secondary malignancies including skin squamous cell carcinoma, breast angiosarcoma, myelodysplastic syndrome were reported.

NURSING CONSIDERATIONS

BASELINE ASSESSMENT
Obtain CBC, blood type and screen; pregnancy test in females of reproductive potential. Confirm compliance of effective contraception. Inform blood bank of treatment and possible treatment-related interference with serologic testing. Administer in an environment equipped to monitor for and manage infusion-related reactions. Obtain weight in kilograms. Screen for active infection. Question for prior infusion-related reactions before each infusion. Offer emotional support.

INTERVENTION/EVALUATION
Monitor CBC periodically for myelosuppression. Monitor vital sign during infusion. If infusion-related reaction occurs, interrupt infusion and manage symptoms. Infusion reactions were usually reported during the first infusion. Most infusion reactions resolve on the same day of administration. Monitor for infections (cough, fatigue, fever), new malignancies. If serious infection occurs, initiate appropriate antimicrobial therapy. Monitor daily pattern of bowel activity, stool consistency. Offer antiemetic if nausea/vomiting occurs.

PATIENT/FAMILY TEACHING
• Treatment may depress your immune system and reduce your ability to fight infection. Report symptoms of infection such as body aches, burning with urination, chills, cough, fatigue, fever. Avoid those with active infection. • Report symptoms of bone marrow depression (e.g., bruising, fatigue, fever, shortness of breath, weight loss; bleeding easily, bloody urine or stool). • Immediately report symptoms of infusion-related reactions such as chills, cough, difficulty breathing, nausea, throat tightness. • Pretreatment with acetaminophen, antihistamines, steroidal anti-inflammatories

may help reduce infusion reactions. • Due to pretreatment with a corticosteroid, pts with diabetes may experience a transient rise in blood sugar levels. • Use effective contraception to avoid pregnancy. Do not breastfeed. • Treatment may cause new cancers.

isavuconazonium

eye-sa-vue-**kon**-a-**zoe**-nee-um (Cresemba)

◆**CLASSIFICATION**

PHARMACOTHERAPEUTIC: Azole antifungal derivative. **CLINICAL:** Antifungal.

USES

Treatment of invasive aspergillosis and invasive mucormycosis. **Injection:** adults and pts 1 yr of age and older. **Capsules:** adults and pts 6 yrs of age and older weighing 16 kg or greater. **OFF-LABEL:** Candidiasis: Esophageal (fluconazole refractory), invasive fungal infections (prophylaxis).

PRECAUTIONS

Contraindications: Hypersensitivity to isavuconazonium or isavuconazole, concomitant use of strong CYP3A4 inhibitors (e.g., ketoconazole, high-dose ritonavir), strong CYP3A4 inducers (e.g., carBAMazepine, rifAMPin, St. John's wort), history of short QT syndrome. **Cautions:** Renal/hepatic impairment, hypersensitivity to other azoles. Pts at risk for acute pancreatitis; concomitant use of nephrotoxic medications; pts at risk for hypokalemia, hypomagnesemia. Concomitant use of medications that prolong QT interval.

ACTION

Isavuconazonium is the prodrug of isavuconazole. Interferes with fungal cyto-chrome activity, decreasing ergosterol synthesis, inhibiting fungal cell membrane formation. **Therapeutic Effect:** Damages fungal cell wall membrane.

PHARMACOKINETICS

Widely distributed. Metabolized in liver. Protein binding: greater than 99%. Peak plasma concentration: 2–3 hrs. Excreted in feces (46%), urine (46%). **Half-life:** 130 hrs.

⧗ LIFESPAN CONSIDERATIONS

Pregnancy/Lactation: May cause fetal harm. Avoid pregnancy. Breastfeeding not recommended. **Children:** Safety and efficacy not established. **Elderly:** No age-related precautions noted.

INTERACTIONS

DRUG: Strong **CYP3A4 inhibitors (e.g., clarithromycin, ketoconazole, ritonavir)** may increase concentration/effect. Strong **CYP3A4 inducers (e.g., carBAMazepine, rifAMPin)** may decrease concentration/effect. May increase concentration/effects of **cycloSPORINE, digoxin, eplerenone, everolimus, midazolam, mycophenolate sirolimus, tacrolimus.** May decrease therapeutic effect of *Saccharomyces boulardii.* **HERBAL:** St. John's wort may decrease concentration/effect. **FOOD:** None known. **LAB VALUES:** May increase serum alkaline phosphatase, ALT, AST, bilirubin. May decrease serum potassium, magnesium.

AVAILABILITY (Rx)

Injection Powder: 372 mg/vial (equivalent to 200 mg isavuconazole). **Capsules:** 74.5 mg (equivalent to 40 mg of isavuconazole), 186 mg (equivalent to 100 mg isavuconazole).

ADMINISTRATION/HANDLING

❄ IV

Reconstitution • Reconstitute vial with 5 mL Sterile Water for Injection. • Gently shake until completely dissolved. • Visually inspect for particulate matter or discoloration. Solution may contain visible translucent to white particles. • Inject reconstituted solution into 250 mL 0.9% NaCl or 5% Dextrose injection. • Gently invert bag to mix. Do not shake or agitate. Do not use pneumatic transport system. • Diluted solution may also contain visible translucent to white particles (which will be removed by in-line filter).

Administration • Do not give as IV push or bolus. Flush IV line with 0.9% NaCl or 5% Dextrose injection prior to and after infusion.

Rate of administration • Infuse over 60 min (minimum) using 0.2- to 1.2-micron in-line filter.

Storage • Refrigerate unused vials. • Diluted solution may be stored at room temperature up to 6 hrs or refrigerated up to 24 hrs. • Do not freeze.

PO
• Give without regard to food. • Do not cut, crush, divide, or open capsules.

INDICATIONS/ROUTES/DOSAGE

Note: 372 mg is equivalent to 200 mg isavuconazole. Duration of therapy: minimum of 6–12 wks.

Invasive Aspergillosis, Invasive Mucormycosis
IV: ADULTS, ELDERLY, CHILDREN 3–17 YRS OF AGE WEIGHING 37 KG OR GREATER: Loading dose: 372 mg q8h for 6 doses (48 hrs). **Maintenance:** 372 mg once daily. Start maintenance dose 12–24 hrs after last loading dose. **3–17 YRS OF AGE WEIGHING LESS THAN 37 KG: Loading Dose:** 10 mg/kg q8h for 6 doses (48 hrs). **Maintenance:** 10 mg/kg once daily. **1 TO LESS THAN 3 YRS OF AGE WEIGHING LESS THAN 18 KG: Loading dose:** 15 mg/kg q8h for 6 doses (48 hrs). **Maintenance:** 15 mg/kg IV once daily.
PO: ADULTS, ELDERLY, CHILDREN 6–17 YRS OF AGE WEIGHING 32 KG OR GREAT: Loading dose: 372 mg q8h for 6 doses (48 hrs). **25–31 KG:** 298 mg q8h for 6 doses (48 hrs). **18–24 KG:**

223.5 mg q8h for 6 doses (48 hrs). **16–17 KG:** 149 mg q8h for 6 doses (48 hrs). **Maintenance:** 372 mg once daily. **25–31 KG:** 298 mg once daily. **18–24 KG:** 223.5 mg once daily. **16–17 KG:** 149 mg once daily. Start maintenance dose 12–24 hrs after last loading dose.

Dosage in Renal Impairment
No dose adjustment.

Dosage in Hepatic Impairment
Mild to moderate impairment: No dose adjustment. **Severe impairment:** Not specified; use caution.

SIDE EFFECTS

Frequent (28%–17%): Nausea, vomiting, diarrhea, abdominal pain, headache, dyspnea. **Occasional (15%–6%):** Peripheral edema, constipation, fatigue, insomnia, back pain, delirium, agitation, confusion, disorientation, chest pain, rash, pruritus, hypotension, anxiety, dyspepsia, injection site reaction, decreased appetite.

ADVERSE EFFECTS/TOXIC REACTIONS

Severe hepatic injury including cholestasis, hepatitis, hepatic failure reported in pts with underlying medical conditions (e.g., hematologic malignancies). Infusion-related reactions including chills, dizziness, dyspnea, hypoesthesia, hypotension, paresthesia may occur. Acute respiratory failure, renal failure, Stevens-Johnson syndrome, serious hypersensitivity reaction (including anaphylaxis) were reported.

NURSING CONSIDERATIONS

BASELINE ASSESSMENT
Obtain LFT, pregnancy test in females of reproductive potential Specimens for fungal culture, histopathology should be obtained prior to initiating therapy. Receive full medication history and screen for interactions/contraindications.

Question history of hypersensitivity reaction, hepatic impairment.

INTERVENTION/EVALUATION

Monitor LFT periodically. Monitor for infusion-related reactions, hypersensitivity reactions, anaphylaxis. Monitor I&O. Report worsening of hepatic/renal function.

PATIENT/FAMILY TEACHING

• Swallow capsule whole; do not chew, crush, cut, or open capsules. • Use effective contraception to avoid pregnancy. • Do not take herbal products such as St. John's wort. • Report liver problems such as upper abdominal pain, bleeding, dark or amber-colored urine, nausea, vomiting, or yellowing of the skin or eyes. • Report decreased urinary output, extremity swelling, dark-colored urine; skin changes such as rash, skin bubbling, or sloughing.

isosorbide dinitrate

eye-soe-**sor**-bide
(ISDN 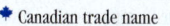, Isordil)

isosorbide mononitrate

(Apo-ISMN 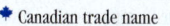, Imdur 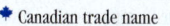)
Do not confuse Imdur with Imuran, Inderal, or K-Dur, Isordil with Inderal, Isuprel, or Plendil.

FIXED-COMBINATION(S)

BiDil: isosorbide dinitrate/hydrALA-ZINE (a vasodilator): 20 mg/37.5 mg.

◆CLASSIFICATION

PHARMACOTHERAPEUTIC: Nitrate.
CLINICAL: Antianginal.

USES

Dinitrate: Prevention of angina pectoris due to coronary artery disease. **Mononitrate:** Treatment (immediate-release only) and prevention of angina pectoris due to coronary artery disease. **OFF-LABEL: Dinitrate:** HF with reduced ejection fraction.

PRECAUTIONS

Contraindications: Hypersensitivity to nitrates, concurrent use of sildenafil, tadalafil, vardenafil, or riociguat. **Cautions:** Inferior wall MI, head trauma, increased intracranial pressure (ICP), orthostatic hypotension, blood volume depletion from diuretic therapy, systolic B/P less than 90 mm Hg, hypertrophic cardiomyopathy, alcohol consumption.

ACTION

Forms free radical nitric oxide which activates intracellular cyclic guanosine monophosphate, leading to smooth muscle relaxation. **Therapeutic Effect:** Relaxes vascular smooth muscle of arterial, venous vasculature. Decreases preload, afterload, cardiac oxygen demand.

PHARMACOKINETICS

Route	Onset	Peak	Duration
Dinitrate			
Sublingual	3 min	N/A	1–2 hrs
PO	45–60 min	N/A	up to 8 hrs
Mononitrate			
PO (extended-release)	30–60 min	N/A	12–24 hrs

Dinitrate poorly absorbed and metabolized in liver to its active metabolite isosorbide mononitrate. Mononitrate well absorbed after PO administration. Primarily excreted in urine. **Half-life:** Dinitrate, 1–4 hrs; mononitrate, 4 hrs.

⧗ LIFESPAN CONSIDERATIONS

Pregnancy/Lactation: Unknown if drug crosses placenta or is distributed in breast milk. **Children:** Safety and efficacy not established. **Elderly:** May be more sensitive to hypotensive effects. Age-related renal impairment may require dosage adjustment.

 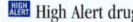

INTERACTIONS

DRUG: Alcohol, riociguat, sildenafil, tadalafil, vardenafil may potentiate hypotensive effects (concurrent use of these agents is contraindicated). **Strong CYP3A4 inhibitors (e.g., clarithromycin, ketoconazole/ritonavir)** may increase concentration/effect. **HERBAL:** None significant. **FOOD:** None known. **LAB VALUES:** May increase urine catecholamine, urine vanillylmandelic acid levels.

AVAILABILITY (Rx)

Dinitrate
Tablets: 5 mg, 10 mg, 20 mg, 30 mg, 40 mg.

Mononitrate
Tablets: 10 mg, 20 mg.

Tablets, Extended-Release: 30 mg, 60 mg, 120 mg.

ADMINISTRATION/HANDLING

PO *(Dinitrate):* • Do not administer around the clock (to prevent tolerance to nitrate effect). • Allow nitrate-free interval of at least 14 hrs.
PO *(Mononitrate):* • Do not administer around the clock. IR tablet should be scheduled twice daily with doses 7 hrs apart. • Administer ER tablet once daily in the morning (do not crush or allow chewing).

INDICATIONS/ROUTES/DOSAGE

Angina
Note: Dinitrate used only for prevention.
PO: *(Isosorbide Dinitrate) (Immediate-Release):* ADULTS, ELDERLY: Initially, 5–20 mg 2–3 times/day. **Maintenance:** 10–40 mg 2–3 times/day.
PO: *(Isosorbide Mononitrate) (Immediate-Release):* ADULTS, ELDERLY: 10–20 mg twice daily given 7 hrs apart to decrease tolerance development. In pts with small stature, may start at 5 mg twice daily and titrate to at least 10 mg twice daily in first 2–3 days of therapy. *(Sustained-Release):* Initially, 30–60 mg/day in morning as a single dose. May increase dose at several-day intervals to 120 mg once daily. **Maximum daily single dose:** 240 mg.

Dosage in Renal/Hepatic Impairment
No dose adjustment.

SIDE EFFECTS

Frequent: Headache (may be severe) occurs mostly in early therapy, diminishes rapidly in intensity, usually disappears during continued treatment. **Sublingual:** Burning, tingling at oral point of dissolution. **Occasional:** Transient flushing of face/neck, dizziness, weakness, orthostatic hypotension, nausea, vomiting, restlessness. GI upset, blurred vision, dry mouth.

ADVERSE EFFECTS/TOXIC REACTIONS

Discontinue if blurred vision occurs. Severe orthostatic hypotension manifested by syncope, pulselessness, cold/clammy skin, diaphoresis has been reported. Tolerance may occur with repeated, prolonged therapy, but may not occur with extended-release form. Minor tolerance with intermittent use of sublingual tablets. High dosage tends to produce severe headache.

NURSING CONSIDERATIONS

BASELINE ASSESSMENT
Record onset, type (sharp, dull, squeezing), radiation, location, intensity, duration of anginal pain; precipitating factors (exertion, emotional stress). If headache occurs during management therapy, administer medication with meals.

INTERVENTION/EVALUATION
Assist with ambulation if light-headedness, dizziness occurs. Assess for facial/neck flushing. Monitor number of anginal episodes, orthostatic B/P.

PATIENT/FAMILY TEACHING
• Do not chew, crush, dissolve, or divide sublingual, extended-release, sustained-release forms. • Take sublingual tablets while sitting down. • Go from lying to standing slowly (prevents dizziness effect). • Take oral form on empty stomach (however, if headache occurs during

management therapy, take medication with meals). • Dissolve sublingual tablet under tongue; do not swallow. • Avoid alcohol (intensifies hypotensive effect). • If alcohol is ingested soon after taking nitrates, possible acute hypotensive episode (marked drop in B/P, vertigo, pallor) may occur. • Report signs/symptoms of hypotension, angina.

itraconazole

it-ra-**kon**-a-zole
(Sporanox, Tolsura)

■ **BLACK BOX ALERT** ■ Serious cardiovascular events, including HF, ventricular tachycardia, torsades de pointes, death, have occurred due to concurrent use with colchicine (pts with renal/hepatic impairment), dofetilide, dronedarone, eplerenone, ergot alkaloids, felodipine, fesoterodine, irinotecan, ivabradine, levomethadyl, lovastatin, lurasidone, methadone, midazolam (oral), pimozide, quiNIDine, ranolazine, simvastatin, solifenacin, ticagrelor, or triazolam. Negative inotropic effects observed following IV administration. Contraindicated for treatment of onychomycosis in pts with HF, ventricular dysfunction.

Do not confuse itraconazole with fluconazole, ketoconazole, miconazole, posaconazole, voriconazole, or Sporanox with Suprax or Topamax.

◆CLASSIFICATION

PHARMACOTHERAPEUTIC: Azole-derivative antifungal. **CLINICAL:** Antifungal.

USES

Oral capsules: Treatment of blastomycosis (pulmonary and extrapulmonary), histoplasmosis (including chronic cavitary pulmonary disease and disseminated, nonmeningeal histoplasmosis), aspergillosis, pulmonary and extrapulmonary, in pts who are intolerant of or who are refractory to amphotericin B therapy. Treatment of onychomycosis of the toenail (with or without fingernail involvement) due to dermatophytes (*tinea unguium*), and onychomycosis of the fingernail due to dermatophytes (*tinea unguium*). **Oral solution:** Treatment of oral and esophageal candidiasis. **OFF-LABEL:** Coccidioidomycosis, paracoccidioidomycosis, invasive fungal infections (prophylaxis), sporotrichosis, tinea infections.

PRECAUTIONS

Contraindications: Hypersensitivity to itraconazole, other azoles. Treatment of onychomycosis in pts with evidence of ventricular dysfunction (e.g., HF or history of HF); concurrent use of dofetilide, dronedarone, eplerenone, ergot derivatives, felodipine, irinotecan, lovastatin, lurasidone, methadone, midazolam (oral), pimozide, ranolazine, simvastatin, ticagrelor, triazolam, quiNIDine; concurrent use with colchicine, fesoterodine, solifenacin in pts with renal/hepatic impairment; treatment of onychomycosis in women who are pregnant or are intending to become pregnant. **Cautions:** Preexisting hepatic impairment (not recommended in pts with active hepatic disease, elevated LFTs), renal impairment, pts with risk factors for HF (e.g., COPD, myocardial ischemia).

ACTION

Inhibits synthesis of ergosterol (vital component of fungal cell formation). **Therapeutic Effect:** Damages fungal cell membrane, altering its function. Fungistatic.

PHARMACOKINETICS

Widely distributed. Absorption is increased when taken with food. Protein binding: 99%. Widely distributed, primarily in fatty tissue, liver, kidneys. Metabolized in liver. Primarily excreted in urine. Not removed by hemodialysis. **Half-life:** 16–26 hrs.

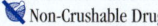

◆ Canadian trade name   Non-Crushable Drug   HIGH ALERT High Alert drug

⌛ LIFESPAN CONSIDERATIONS

Pregnancy/Lactation: Distributed in breast milk. **Children:** Safety and efficacy not established. **Elderly:** Age-related renal impairment may require dosage adjustment.

INTERACTIONS

DRUG: May increase concentration/toxicity of **aliskiren, calcium channel–blocking agents** (e.g., **felodipine, NIFEdipine**), **cycloSPORINE, docetaxel, dofetilide, eplerenone, ergot alkaloids, HMG-CoA reductase inhibitors** (e.g., **lovastatin, simvastatin**), **midazolam, sirolimus, tacrolimus, warfarin. Strong CYP3A4 inhibitors** (e.g., **clarithromycin, ketoconazole, ritonavir**) may increase concentration/effect. **Strong CYP3A4 inducers** (e.g., **carBAMazepine, phenytoin, rifAMPin**) may decrease concentration/effect. **Antacids, H₂ antagonists** (e.g. **famotidine**), **proton pump inhibitors** (e.g., **pantoprazole**) may decrease absorption. **HERBAL:** None significant. **FOOD:** Grapefruit products may alter absorption. **LAB VALUES:** May increase serum alkaline phosphatase, bilirubin, ALT, AST, LDH. May decrease serum potassium.

AVAILABILITY (Rx)

Capsules: *(Sporanox):* 100 mg. *(Tolsura):* 65 mg. **Oral Solution:** *(Sporanox):* 10 mg/mL.

ADMINISTRATION/HANDLING

PO
• Give capsules with food (increases absorption). Administer capsules whole; do not crush, break, or allow chewing. • Give solution on empty stomach. Swish vigorously in mouth, then swallow.

INDICATIONS/ROUTES/DOSAGE

Note: Capsules/tablets are not bioequivalent with oral solution.

Blastomycosis, Histoplasmosis

PO: ADULTS, ELDERLY: *(Sporanox Capsule):* 200 mg 3 times/day for 3 days, then 200 mg twice daily. *(Tolsura):* 130 mg once daily; if no improvement or evidence of progressive fungal infection, increase dose in 65 mg increments to a maximum of 260 mg/day given in 2 divided doses. May give a loading dose of 130 mg 3 times/day for the first 3 days of treatment. Treatment should be continued for 6–12 mos (blastomycosis), 6–12 wks (histoplasmosis).

Aspergillosis

PO: ADULTS, ELDERLY: *(Sporanox Capsule):* 200 mg 2 times/day for minimum of 16 wks. May give loading dose of 200 mg 3 times/day for 3 days. *(Tolsura):* 130 mg 1–2 times/day. May give a loading dose of 130 mg 3 times/day for the first 3 days of treatment. Treatment should be continued for minimum of 6–12 wks.

Esophageal Candidiasis

PO: ADULTS, ELDERLY: *(Oral Solution):* FDA-approved dosage is 100–200 mg PO once daily for a minimum of 3 weeks and for 2 weeks after resolution of symptoms.

Oropharyngeal Candidiasis

PO: ADULTS, ELDERLY: *(Oral Solution):* 200 mg (10 mL) swish and swallow once daily for 7–14 days up to 28 days for refractory disease.

Onychomycosis (Fingernail)

PO: ADULTS, ELDERLY: *(Sporanox Capsule):* *(Continuous dosing):* 200 mg once daily for 6 wks. *(Pulse dosing):* 200 mg twice daily for 7 days, off for 21 days, repeat 200 mg twice daily for 7 days.

Onychomycosis (Toenail)

PO: ADULTS, ELDERLY: *(Sporanox Capsule):* *(Continuous dosing):* 200 mg once daily for 12 wks. *(Pulse dosing):* 200 mg twice daily for 7 days. Repeat q4wks for a total of 3 mos.

Dosage in Renal/Hepatic Impairment

Use caution.

SIDE EFFECTS

Frequent (11%–9%): Nausea, rash. **Occasional (5%–3%):** Vomiting, headache, diarrhea, hypertension, peripheral edema, fatigue, fever. **Rare (2% or less):** Abdominal pain, dizziness, anorexia, pruritus.

ADVERSE EFFECTS/TOXIC REACTIONS

Hepatotoxicity (anorexia, abdominal pain, unusual fatigue/weakness, jaundiced skin/sclera, dark urine) occurs rarely.

NURSING CONSIDERATIONS

BASELINE ASSESSMENT

Obtain LFT. Assess allergies. Receive full medication history (numerous contraindications/cautions).

INTERVENTION/EVALUATION

Monitor for hepatotoxicity (abdominal pain, jaundice, nausea, vomiting). Monitor LFT in pts with preexisting hepatic impairment.

PATIENT/ FAMILY TEACHING

• Take capsules with food, liquids if GI distress occurs. • Therapy will continue for at least 3 mos, until lab tests, clinical presentation indicate infection is controlled. • Report liver problems (abdominal pain, bruising, clay-colored stool, amber- or dark-colored urine, yellowing of the skin or eyes). • Avoid grapefruit products.

---

ivabradine

eye-**vab**-ra-deen
(Corlanor)

◆CLASSIFICATION

PHARMACOTHERAPEUTIC: Hyperpolarization-activated cyclic nucleotide-gated (HCN) channel blocker. **CLINICAL:** Reduces risk of worsening HF.

USES

To reduce the risk of hospitalization for worsening HF in adults with stable, symptomatic chronic HF with reduced left ventricular ejection fraction of 35% or less, who are in sinus rhythm with resting heart rate 70 beats/min or more and either are on maximally tolerated doses of beta-blockers or have a contraindication to use of a beta-blocker. Treatment of stable symptomatic HF due to dilated cardiomyopathy in pts 6 mos and older who are in sinus rhythm with an elevated heart rate. **OFF-LABEL:** Stable angina.

PRECAUTIONS

Contraindications: Hypersensitivity to ivabradine. Acute decompensated HF, B/P less than 90/50 mm Hg, sick sinus syndrome; sinoatrial block or third-degree AV block (unless a functional pacemaker is present), resting heart rate less than 60 bpm prior to initiation, severe hepatic impairment, pacemaker dependence (heart rate maintained exclusively by a pacemaker), concomitant use of strong CYP3A4 inhibitors. **Cautions:** History of atrial fibrillation, hypertension. Avoid concomitant use of dilTIAZem or verapamil. Avoid use in pts with second-degree heart block (unless a functioning pacemaker is present). Pts at risk for bradycardia. Not recommended with pacemakers set to rate of 60 bpm or greater.

ACTION

Reduces spontaneous pacemaker activity of the cardiac sinus node by blocking HCN channels that are responsible for cardiac current, which regulates heart rate. Does not affect ventricular repolarization or myocardial contractility. Also inhibits retinal current involved in reducing bright light in retina. **Therapeutic Effect:** Reduces heart rate.

PHARMACOKINETICS

Widely distributed. Metabolized in liver and intestines. Protein binding: 70%. Peak plasma

---

concentration: 1 hr. Eliminated in feces, urine (% not specified). **Half-life:** 6 hrs.

⧗ LIFESPAN CONSIDERATIONS

Pregnancy/Lactation: May cause fetal harm. Females of reproductive potential should use effective contraception. Unknown if distributed in breast milk. If treatment is decided to be absolutely necessary, pregnant pts should be closely monitored for destabilizing HF, esp. during the first trimester. Pregnant women with chronic HF in the third trimester should be closely monitored for preterm birth. **Children:** Safety and efficacy not established in pts younger than 6 mos. **Elderly:** No age-related precautions noted.

INTERACTIONS

DRUG: **Bradycardia-causing agents (e.g., dilTIAZem, verapamil)** may increase concentration/effect; may further increase risk of bradycardia. **Strong CYP3A4 inhibitors (e.g., clarithromycin, ketoconazole, ritonavir)** may increase concentration/effect. **Strong CYP3A4 inducers (e.g., carBAMazepine, phenytoin, rifAMPin)** may decrease concentration/effect. **HERBAL:** None significant. **FOOD:** **Grapefruit products** may increase concentration/effect. **LAB VALUES:** None significant.

AVAILABILITY (Rx)

Oral Solution: 5 mg/5 mL (1 mg/mL). **Tablets:** 5 mg, 7.5 mg.

ADMINISTRATION/HANDLING

PO
• Give with food. **Oral solution**
• Empty entire contents of ampule into medication cup. Use calibrated oral syringe to measure dose.

INDICATIONS/ROUTES/DOSAGE

HF

PO: **ADULTS, ELDERLY:** Initially, 5 mg twice daily for 14 days, then adjust dose to resting heart rate of 50–60 bpm. Fur-

ther adjustments based on resting heart rate and tolerability. **Maximum:** 7.5 mg twice daily. (See Dose Modification). **Pts with history of conduction defects, pts in whom bradycardia could lead to hemodynamic compromise:** Initiate therapy at 2.5 mg twice daily. **CHILDREN 40 KG AND GREATER:** Initially, 2.5 mg twice daily. Assess pt at 2-wk intervals and adjust dose by 2.5 mg to target a heart rate (HR) reduction of at least 20%. **Maximum:** 7.5 mg twice daily. **CHILDREN LESS THAN 40 KG:** *(Oral Solution):* Initially, 0.05 mg/kg twice daily. Assess pt at 2-wk intervals and adjust dose by 0.05 mg/kg to target a heart rate (HR) reduction of at least 20%. **Maximum: (CHILDREN 6 MOS TO LESS THAN 1 YR OLD):** 0.2 mg/kg twice daily. **(CHILDREN 1 YR OLD AND OLDER):** 0.3 mg/kg twice daily (up to a total of 7.5 mg twice daily).

Dose Modification

Adjust dose to maintain a resting heart between 50–60 bpm as follows:

Heart Rate	Dose Adjustment
Greater than 60 bpm	Increase by 2.5 mg (given twice daily) up to maximum dose of 7.5 mg daily.
50–60 bpm	Maintain dose.
Less than 50 bpm or symptomatic bradycardia	Decrease by 2.5 mg (given twice daily); if current dose is 2.5 mg twice daily, permanently discontinue.

Dosage in Renal Impairment

CrCl 15 mL/min or greater: No dose adjustment. **CrCl less than 15 mL/min:** Use caution.

Dosage in Hepatic Impairment

Mild to moderate impairment: No dose adjustment. **Severe impairment:** Contraindicated.

SIDE EFFECTS

Occasional   (10%–3%): Bradycardia, hypertension, phosphenes (visual disturbances, luminous phenomena), visual brightness.

ADVERSE EFFECTS/TOXIC REACTIONS

May increase risk of atrial fibrillation (8.3% of pts). Bradycardia, sinus arrest, or heart block may occur. Bradycardia occurred in 10% of pts. Risk factors for bradycardia may include sinus node dysfunction, conduction defects (e.g., first- or second-degree AV block, bundle branch block), ventricular dyssynchrony, or use of negative chronotropic drugs. Phosphenes, a transient enhanced brightness in the visual field (which may include halos, stroboscopic or kaleidoscopic effect, colored bright lights, or multiple images) may occur. Phosphenes are usually triggered by sudden variations in light intensity and generally occur within the first 2 mos of treatment. Other adverse reactions such as angioedema, diplopia, erythema, hypotension, pruritus, rash, syncope, urticaria, vertigo, visual impairment occur rarely. Overdose may lead to severe and prolonged bradycardia requiring temporary cardiac pacing or infusion of IV beta-stimulating agents.

NURSING CONSIDERATIONS

BASELINE ASSESSMENT

Obtain heart rate, B/P. Confirm negative pregnancy test before initiating therapy. Receive full medication history and screen for interactions. Screen for contraindications as listed in Precautions. Question history of atrial fibrillation, bradycardia, hypertension.

INTERVENTION/EVALUATION

Monitor heart rate, B/P. Diligently monitor for atrial fibrillation, bradycardia, syncope. If symptomatic bradycardia occurs, temporary cardiac pacing or infusion of beta-stimulating agents may be warranted. Monitor for hypersensitivity reaction. Monitor for visual changes. Initiate fall precautions.

PATIENT/FAMILY TEACHING

• Take medication with meals. • Avoid grapefruit products, herbal supplements such as St. John's wort. • Use effective contraception to avoid pregnancy. • Report symptoms of low heart rate such as confusion, dizziness, fatigue, fainting, low blood pressure, pallor. • Report symptoms of atrial fibrillation such as chest pressure, palpitations, shortness of breath. • Treatment may cause luminous phenomena (phosphenes), a transient visual brightness that may include halos, light sensitivity, or colored bright lights. • Avoid tasks that require alertness, motor skills until response to drug is established. • Report allergic reactions such as hives, itching, rash, tongue swelling.

ivosidenib

eye-voe-**sid**-e-nib
(Tibsovo)

■ **BLACK BOX ALERT** ■
Life-threatening and/or fatal differentiation syndrome with symptoms including fever, dyspnea, hypoxia, pulmonary infiltrates, pleural or pericardial effusion, rapid weight gain or peripheral edema, hypotension, renal dysfunction may occur. Initiate corticosteroid therapy and hemodynamic monitoring in pts suspected of differentiation syndrome until symptoms resolve. **Do not confuse ivosidenib with enasidenib, ibrutinib, idelalisib, imatinib, or ixazomib.**

◆**CLASSIFICATION**

PHARMACOTHERAPEUTIC: Isocitrate dehydrogenase-1 (IDH1) inhibitor. **CLINICAL:** Antineoplastic.

USES

Acute myeloid leukemia (AML): Treatment as monotherapy or in

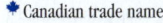 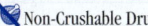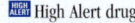

combination with azacitidine of AML with a susceptible IDH1 mutation in adults with newly diagnosed AML who are 75 yrs or older or who have comorbidities that preclude use of intensive induction chemotherapy. Treatment of adults with relapsed or refractory AML with a susceptible isocitrate dehydrogenase-1 (IDH1) mutation. **Myelodysplastic syndromes (MDS):** Treatment of adults with relapsed or refractory MDS with a susceptible IDH1 mutation. **Cholangiocarcinoma:** Treatment of adults with locally advanced or metastatic IDH1-mutated cholangiocarcinoma who have been previously treated.

PRECAUTIONS

Contraindications: Hypersensitivity to ivosidenib. **Cautions:** Baseline leukopenia, hypotension; active infection, cardiac disease, hepatic/renal impairment, electrolyte imbalance; conditions predisposing to infection (e.g., diabetes, renal failure, immunocompromised pts, open wounds); pts at risk for QTc interval prolongation, cardiac arrhythmias (congenital long QT syndrome, HF, QT interval–prolonging medications, hypokalemia, hypomagnesemia); concomitant use strong or moderate CYP3A4 inhibitors, strong CYP3A4 inducers; dehydration; pts at high risk for tumor lysis syndrome (high tumor burden).

ACTION

Inhibits IDH1 enzymes on mutant IDH1 variants, decreasing 2-hydroxyglutarate (2-HG) levels and restoring myeloid differentiation. **Therapeutic Effect:** Reduces blast counts; increases percentage of myeloid cells. Inhibits tumor growth and proliferation.

PHARMACOKINETICS

Widely distributed. Metabolized in liver. Protein binding: 92%–96%. Peak plasma concentration: 3 hrs. Steady state reached in 14 days. Excreted in feces (77%), urine (17%). **Half-life:** 93 hrs.

⧗ LIFESPAN CONSIDERATIONS

Pregnancy/Lactation: Avoid pregnancy; may cause fetal harm. Unknown if distributed in breast milk. Breastfeeding not recommended during treatment and for at least 30 days after discontinuation. **Children:** Safety and efficacy not established. **Elderly:** No age-related precautions noted.

INTERACTIONS

DRUG: **Strong CYP3A4 inhibitors (e.g., clarithromycin, ketoconazole), moderate CYP3A4 inhibitors (e.g., erythromycin, dilTIAZem, fluconazole)** may increase concentration/effect. **Strong CYP3A4 inducers (e.g., carBAMazepine, phenytoin, rifAMPin)** may decrease concentration/effect. **QT interval–prolonging medications (e.g., amiodarone, azithromycin, citalopram, clarithromycin, escitalopram, haloperidol)** may increase risk of QTc interval prolongation. May increase QT prolongation effect of **dronedarone. May decrease effect of oral contraceptives. HERBAL:** None significant. **FOOD:** High-fat meals may increase concentration/effect. **LAB VALUES:** May increase serum alkaline phosphatase, ALT, AST, bilirubin, creatinine, uric acid. May decrease Hgb, WBCs; serum magnesium, phosphate, potassium, sodium.

AVAILABILITY (Rx)

Tablets: 250 mg.

ADMINISTRATION/HANDLING

PO
• Give without regard to food. • Do not give with a high-fat meal. • Administer whole; do not break, cut, crush, or divide tablets. • Tablets cannot be chewed. • If vomiting occurs after administration, give next dose at regularly scheduled time. • If a dose is missed, administer as soon as possible • Do not give a missed dose within 12 hrs of next dose.

INDICATIONS/ROUTES/DOSAGE

Acute Myeloid Leukemia (Newly Diagnosed)

PO: ADULTS, ELDERLY: (as monotherapy or in combination with azacitidine) 500 mg once daily for at least 6 mos in pts without disease progression or unacceptable toxicity. Continue until disease progression or unacceptable toxicity.

Acute Myeloid Leukemia, Myelodysplastic Syndromes (Relapsed or Refractory)

PO: ADULTS, ELDERLY: (monotherapy) 500 mg once daily. Continue until disease progression or unacceptable toxicity. For pts without disease progression or unacceptable toxicity, continue for a minimum of 6 mos.

Cholangiocarcinoma

PO: ADULTS, ELDERLY: (as monotherapy) 500 mg once daily. Continue until disease progression or unacceptable toxicity.

Dose Modification

Based on Common Terminology Criteria for Adverse Events (CTCAE).

Differentiation Syndrome

Withhold treatment if symptoms are severe and persist for more than 48 hrs after initiation of corticosteroids. Resume treatment when symptoms improve to Grade 2 or less.

Guillain-Barré Syndrome

Permanently discontinue.

Noninfectious Leukocytosis

WBC count greater than 25,000 cells/mm³ or absolute increase in total WBC count greater than 15,000 cells/mm³ from baseline: If indicated, treat with hydroxyurea and leukapheresis. Taper hydroxyurea after leukocytosis improves or resolves. If leukocytosis does not improve with hydroxyurea, withhold treatment until resolved, then resume at same dose.

QT Interval Prolongation

QTc interval 481–500 msec: Withhold treatment. Assess and replete electrolyte levels. Assess and adjust concomitant use of medications known to cause QTc interval prolongation. When QTc interval prolongation improves to 480 msec or less, resume at same dose and monitor ECG at least wkly for 2 wks. **QTc interval greater than 500 msec:** Withhold treatment. Assess and replete electrolyte levels. Assess and adjust concomitant use of medications known to cause QTc interval prolongation. When QTc interval returns to within 30 msec of baseline or 480 msec or less, resume at reduced dose of 250 mg. **QTc interval prolongation with life-threatening arrhythmia:** Permanently discontinue.

Other Adverse Reactions

Any Grade 3 or higher toxicity: Withhold treatment until improved to Grade 2, then resume at reduced dose of 250 mg. May increase to 500 mg if toxicities further improve to Grade 1 or 0. **Recurrent Grade 3 or higher toxicity:** Permanently discontinue.

Concomitant Use of CYP3A4 Inhibitor

If concomitant CYP3A4 inhibitor cannot be discontinued, reduce ivosidenib dose to 250 mg. If CYP3A4 inhibitor is discontinued for 3–5 half-lives, increase ivosidenib dose to 500 mg.

Dosage in Renal/Hepatic Impairment

Mild to moderate impairment: No dose adjustment. **Severe impairment:** Not specified; use caution.

SIDE EFFECTS

Frequent (39%–18%): Fatigue, asthenia, arthralgia, diarrhea, dyspnea, edema, nausea, abdominal pain, mucositis, rash, pyrexia, cough, constipation, vomiting, decreased appetite, myalgia. **Occasional (16%–12%):** Chest pain, headache, neuropathy, hypotension.

ADVERSE EFFECTS/TOXIC REACTIONS

Anemia, leukopenia are expected responses to therapy. Life-threatening and/

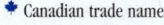 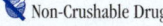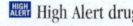

or fatal differentiation syndrome, a condition with rapid proliferation and differentiation of myeloid cells, reported in 19%–25% of pts. QT interval prolongation with QTc interval greater than 500 msec (9% of pts) and QTc interval greater than 60 msec from baseline (14% of pts) have occurred. Guillain-Barré syndrome occurred in less than 1% of pts. Noninfectious leukocytosis reported in 12% of pts. Tumor lysis syndrome may present as acute renal failure, hypocalcemia, hyperuricemia, hyperphosphatemia.

NURSING CONSIDERATIONS

BASELINE ASSESSMENT

Obtain CBC, BMP, LFT; ECG; pregnancy test in female pts of reproductive potential. Replete electrolytes if applicable. Confirm presence of IDH1 mutations in the blood or bone marrow. Assess adequate hydration prior to initiation due to increased risk of tumor lysis syndrome, diarrhea, vomiting. Screen for active infection. Receive full medication history and screen for interactions. Concomitant use of other medications may need to be adjusted. Assess risk for QT interval prolongation, tumor lysis syndrome. Question history of cardiac/hepatic/renal disease, cardiac arrhythmias. Offer emotional support.

INTERVENTION/EVALUATION

Monitor CBC, BMP, LFT at least wkly for 4 wks, then every other wk for 4 wks, then monthly until discontinuation. Monitor CK levels wkly for at least 4 wks. An increase of serum creatinine greater than 0.4 mg/dL from baseline may indicate renal impairment. Monitor serum uric acid level if tumor lysis syndrome (acute renal failure, electrolyte imbalance, cardiac arrhythmias, seizures) is suspected. Monitor ECG at least wkly for 3 wks, then monthly until discontinuation. If QT interval–prolonging medications cannot be withheld, diligently monitor ECG; serum potassium, magnesium for QT interval prolongation, cardiac arrhythmias. Monitor B/P for hypotension, esp. in pts taking antihypertensives. Monitor for symptoms of differentiation syndrome (dyspnea, fever hypotension, hypoxia, pulmonary infiltrates, pleural or pericardial effusion, rapid weight gain or peripheral edema, renal dysfunction, or concomitant febrile neutropenic dermatosis). If differentiation syndrome is suspected, initiate corticosteroids and hemodynamic monitoring until symptoms resolve for at least 3 days. Monitor for symptoms of Guillain-Barré syndrome (dysphagia, dysarthria, dyspnea, motor weakness, paresthesia, sensory alterations). Diligently monitor for infection. Assess skin for skin reactions, rash. Monitor daily pattern of bowel activity, stool consistency. Ensure adequate hydration, nutrition.

PATIENT/FAMILY TEACHING

• Treatment may depress your immune system response and reduce your ability to fight infection. Report symptoms of infection such as body aches, chills, cough, fatigue, fever. Avoid those with active infection. • Report symptoms of bone marrow depression such as bruising, fatigue, fever, shortness of breath, weight loss; bleeding easily, bloody urine or stool. • Report palpitations, chest pain, shortness of breath, dizziness, fainting; may indicate arrhythmia. • Therapy may cause life-threatening tumor lysis syndrome (a condition caused by the rapid breakdown of cancer cells), which can cause kidney failure. Report decreased urination, amber-colored urine; confusion, difficulty breathing, fatigue, fever, muscle or joint pain, palpitations, seizures, vomiting. • Treatment may cause life-threatening differentiation syndrome as early as 2 days after starting therapy. Report difficulty breathing, fever, low blood pressure, rapid weight gain, swelling of the hands or feet, decreased urine output. • Report liver problems (abdominal pain, bruising, clay-colored stool, amber- or dark-colored urine, yellowing of the skin or eyes), kidney problems (decreased urine output, flank pain, darkened urine), skin reactions (rash, skin eruptions). • There is a high risk of interactions with other medications. Do not take newly prescribed

---

medications unless approved by prescriber who originally started treatment. • Avoid grapefruit products, herbal supplements (esp. St. John's wort). • Report suspected pregnancy. Do not breastfeed. • Drink plenty of fluids. • Avoid high-fat meals during administration.

ixabepilone

ix-ab-**ep**-i-lone
(Ixempra)

■ **BLACK BOX ALERT** ■ Combination therapy with capecitabine is contraindicated in pts with serum ALT or AST greater than 2.5 times upper limit of normal (ULN) or bilirubin greater than 1 times ULN due to increased risk of toxicity, neutropenia-related mortality.

◆**CLASSIFICATION**

PHARMACOTHERAPEUTIC: Epothilone microtubule inhibitor, antimitotic agent. **CLINICAL:** Antineoplastic.

USES

Combination therapy with capecitabine for treatment of metastatic or locally advanced breast cancer in pts after failure of anthracycline, taxane therapy, or is taxane-resistant and further anthracycline therapy is contraindicated. As monotherapy, treatment of metastatic or locally advanced breast cancer in pts after failure of anthracycline, taxane, and capecitabine therapy. **OFF-LABEL:** Recurrence therapy for platinum-resistant epithelial ovarian/fallopian tube/primary peritoneal cancer who have been previously treated with taxanes.

PRECAUTIONS

Contraindications: Hypersensitivity to ixabepilone. Severe hypersensitivity reaction (Grade 3 or 4) to Cremophor, baseline neutrophil count less than 1,500 cells/mm³ or platelet count less than 100,000

cells/mm³. **Combination capecitabine therapy:** Serum ALT or AST greater than 2.5 times the upper limit of normal, bilirubin greater than 1 times the upper limit of normal. **Cautions:** Diabetes, existing moderate to severe neuropathy, history of cardiovascular disease. **Monotherapy:** Serum ALT or AST greater than 5 times upper limit of normal bilirubin greater than 3 times upper limit of normal.

ACTION

Binds directly on microtubules during active stage of G2 and M phases of cell cycle, preventing formation of microtubules, an essential part of the process of separation of chromosomes. **Therapeutic Effect:** Blocks cells in mitotic phase of cell division, leading to cell death.

PHARMACOKINETICS

Metabolized in liver. Protein binding: 77%. Excreted in feces (65%), urine (21%). **Half-life:** 52 hrs.

⧗ LIFESPAN CONSIDERATIONS

Pregnancy/Lactation: May cause fetal harm. Unknown if distributed in breast milk. **Children:** Safety and efficacy not established. **Elderly:** Higher incidence of severe adverse reactions in those older than 65 yrs.

INTERACTIONS

DRUG: Strong CYP3A4 inhibitors (e.g., **clarithromycin, ketoconazole, ritonavir**) may increase concentration/effect. Strong CYP3A4 inducers (e.g., **carBAMazepine, phenytoin, rifAMPin**) may decrease concentration/effect. **HERBAL:** None significant. **FOOD:** Grapefruit products may increase concentration/effect. **LAB VALUES:** May increase serum ALT, AST, bilirubin. May decrease WBCs, Hgb, platelets.

AVAILABILITY (Rx)

Injection, Solution: Kit: 15-mg kit supplied with diluent for Ixempra, 8 mL; 45 mg supplied with diluent for Ixempra, 23.5 mL.

ADMINISTRATION/HANDLING

 IV

Reconstitution • Withdraw diluent and slowly inject into vial. • Gently swirl and invert until powder is completely dissolved. • Further dilute with 250 mL lactated Ringer's. • Solution may be stored in vial for a maximum of 1 hr at room temperature. • Final concentration for infusion is between 0.2 mg/mL and 0.6 mg/mL. • Mix infusion bag by manual rotation.

Rate of administration • Administer through an in-line filter of 0.2 to 1.2 microns. • Infuse over 3 hrs. Administration must be completed within 6 hrs of reconstitution.

Storage • Refrigerate kit. • Prior to reconstitution, kit should be removed from refrigerator and allowed to stand at room temperature for approximately 30 min. • When vials are initially removed from refrigerator, a white precipitate may be observed in the diluent vial. • This precipitate will dissolve to form a clear solution once diluent warms to room temperature. • Once diluted with lactated Ringer's, solution is stable at room temperature and room light for a maximum of 6 hrs.

INDICATIONS/ROUTES/DOSAGE

◀**ALERT**▶ An H_1 antagonist (diphenhydrAMINE 50 mg PO or equivalent) and an H_2 antagonist (famotidine 20–40 mg PO or equivalent) must be given prior to beginning treatment with ixabepilone. Pts who experienced a previous hypersensitivity reaction to ixabepilone require pretreatment with corticosteroids (e.g., dexAMETHasone 20 mg IV 30 min before infusion, or PO 1 hr before infusion) in addition to pretreatment with H_1 and H_2 antagonists.

Breast Cancer (Monotherapy or in Combination With Capecitabine)
IV: ADULTS, ELDERLY: 40 mg/m² infused over 3 hrs q3 wks. Calculate doses for pts with body surface area (BSA) greater than 2.2 m² based on 2.2 m². Continue until disease progression or unacceptable toxicity.

Monotherapy Dosage Adjustments for Hepatic Impairment

Mild Hepatic Impairment (ALT and AST less than 2.5 times upper limit of normal [ULN] and bilirubin less than 1 time ULN)
IV: ADULTS, ELDERLY: 40 mg/m² infused over 3 hrs q3 wks.

Mild Hepatic Impairment (ALT and AST greater than 2.5 times ULN and less than 10 times ULN and bilirubin greater than 1 time ULN and less than 1.5 times ULN)
IV: ADULTS, ELDERLY: 32 mg/m² infused over 3 hrs q3 wks.

Moderate Hepatic Impairment (ALT and AST less than 10 times ULN and bilirubin greater than 1.5 times ULN and less than 3 times ULN)
IV infusion: ADULTS, ELDERLY: 20–30 mg/m² infused over 3 hrs q3 wks (initiate at 20 mg/m²; may increase up to a maximum of 30 mg/m² in subsequent cycles if tolerated).

Dosage With Strong CYP3A4 Inhibitors/Inducers
Inhibitors: Consider dose reduction to 20 mg/m². **Inducers:** Consider dose increase to 60 mg/m².

Dosage in Renal Impairment
No dose adjustment.

Dose Modification
Dosage adjustment based on grade of neuropathy, hematologic conditions.

Hematologic
Neutrophils less than 500 cells/mm³ for 7 days or longer: Reduce dose by 20%. **Neutropenic fever:** Reduce dose by 20%. **Platelets less than 25,000 cells/mm³ (less than 50,000 cells/mm³ with bleeding):** Reduce dose by 20%.

Neuropathy
Grade 2 for 7 days or longer or Grade 3 for less than 7 days: Reduce dose by 20%. **Grade 3 for 7 days or lon-**

ger: Discontinue treatment. **Grade 3 (other than neuropathy):** Reduce dose by 20%. **Grade 4:** Discontinue treatment.

SIDE EFFECTS

Common (62%): Peripheral sensory neuropathy. **Frequent (56%–46%):** Fatigue, asthenia, myalgia, arthralgia, alopecia, nausea. **Occasional (29%–11%):** Vomiting, stomatitis, mucositis, diarrhea, musculoskeletal pain, anorexia, constipation, abdominal pain, headache. **Rare (9%–5%):** Skin rash, nail disorder, edema, hand-foot syndrome (blistering/rash/peeling of skin on palms of hands, soles of feet), pyrexia, dizziness, pruritus, gastroesophageal reflux disease (GERD), hot flashes, taste disorder, insomnia.

ADVERSE EFFECTS/TOXIC REACTIONS

Neuropathy occurs early during treatment; 75% of new-onset or worsening neuropathy occurred during first 3 cycles. Diabetics may be at increased risk for severe neuropathy manifested as Grade 4 neutropenia. Neutropenia, leukopenia occur commonly; anemia, thrombocytopenia occur rarely. Hypersensitivity reactions including bronchospasm, flushing, rash, dyspnea may occur. Severe hypersensitivity reactions may require emergent intervention (e.g., epinephrine, corticosteroids).

NURSING CONSIDERATIONS

BASELINE ASSESSMENT

Obtain CBC, BMP, LFT; pregnancy in females of reproductive potential. Question history of hepatic impairment, cardiac disease. Offer emotional support.

INTERVENTION/EVALUATION

Monitor for symptoms of neuropathy (burning sensation, hyperesthesia, hypoesthesia, paresthesia, discomfort, neuropathic pain). Assess skin for erythema. Monitor CBC for evidence of neutropenia, thrombocytopenia; LFT for hepatotoxicity. Assess mouth for stomatitis, mucositis. If hypersensitivity reactions occur, provide immediate supportive measures.

PATIENT/FAMILY TEACHING

• Treatment may depress your immune system response and reduce your ability to fight infection. Report symptoms of infection such as body aches, chills, cough, fatigue, fever. Avoid those with active infection. • Report allergic reactions such as bronchospasm, difficulty breathing, flushing.

ixazomib

ix-**az**-oh-mib
(Ninlaro)
Do not confuse ixazomib with bortezomib, carfilzomib, idelalisib, or ixekizumab.

◆CLASSIFICATION

PHARMACOTHERAPEUTIC: Proteasome inhibitor. **CLINICAL:** Antineoplastic.

USES

Treatment of multiple myeloma (in combination with lenalidomide and dexamethasone) in pts who have received at least 1 prior therapy.

PRECAUTIONS

Contraindications: Severe hypersensitivity to ixazomib. **Cautions:** Baseline neutropenia, thrombocytopenia; hepatic/renal impairment, chronic peripheral edema, predisposing factors to infection (e.g., diabetes, renal failure, open wounds). Concomitant use of strong CYP3A4 inducers not recommended.

ACTION

Reversibly inhibits activity of beta 5 subunit of the 20S proteasome, leading to cell cycle arrest and tumor cell death (apoptosis). **Therapeutic Effect:** Inhibits tumor cells growth and metastasis.

◆ Canadian trade name   🔹 Non-Crushable Drug   🔲 High Alert drug

PHARMACOKINETICS

Widely distributed. Metabolized in liver. Protein binding: 99%. Peak plasma concentration: 1 hr. Excreted in urine (62%), feces (22%). Not removed by hemodialysis. **Half-life:** 9.5 days.

⧗ LIFESPAN CONSIDERATIONS

Pregnancy/Lactation: Avoid pregnancy; may cause fetal harm/malformations. Female and male pts of reproductive potential should use effective contraception during treatment and up to 3 mos after discontinuation. Unknown if distributed in breast milk. Breastfeeding not recommended. **Children:** Safety and efficacy not established. **Elderly:** No age-related precautions noted.

INTERACTIONS

DRUG: Strong CYP3A4 inducers (e.g., carBAMazepine, phenytoin, rifAMPin) may decrease concentration/effect; avoid use. **HERBAL: St. John's wort** may decrease concentration/effect. **FOOD: High-fat meals** may decrease absorption/concentration. **LAB VALUES:** Expected to decrease neutrophils, platelets.

AVAILABILITY (Rx)

Capsules: 2.3 mg, 3 mg, 4 mg.

ADMINISTRATION/HANDLING

PO
• Capsule contents are hazardous; use cytotoxic precautions during handling and disposal. • Administer capsule whole; do not break, cut, crush, or open. • Give at least 1 hr before or 2 hrs after food. • Give on the same day each wk and at the same time that day. If a dose is missed, do not administer within 72 hrs of next scheduled dose. • If vomiting occurs after dosing, do not readminister; give dose at next scheduled time.

INDICATIONS/ROUTES/DOSAGE

Multiple Myeloma
Note: ANC should be 1,000 cells/mm^3 or greater, platelets 75,000 cells/mm^3 or greater, nonhematologic toxicities at baseline or Grade 1 or less prior to initiating a new cycle of therapy.
PO: ADULTS, ELDERLY: 4 mg once wkly on days 1, 8, and 15 of 28-day cycle, in combination with lenalidomide 25 mg daily (on days 1–21 of 28-day cycle) and dexamethasone 40 mg (on days 1, 8, 15, and 22 of 28-day cycle). Continue until disease progression or unacceptable toxicity.

Dose Reduction Schedule
Initial dose: 4 mg. **First dose reduction:** 3 mg. **Second dose reduction:** 2.3 mg. **Unable to tolerate 2.3-mg dose:** Permanently discontinue.

Dose Modification
Based on Common Terminology Criteria for Adverse Events (CTCAE).

Thrombocytopenia
Platelet count less than 30,000 cells/mm^3: Withhold ixazomib and lenalidomide until platelet count is 30,000 cells/mm^3 or greater, then resume ixazomib at the same dose and resume lenalidomide at reduced dose level (see manufacturer guidelines). **Recurrence of platelet count less than 30,000 cells/mm^3:** Withhold ixazomib and lenalidomide until platelet count is 30,000 cells/mm^3 or greater, then resume ixazomib at reduced dose level and resume lenalidomide at the same dose. **Additional occurrences:** Alternate dose modification of ixazomib and lenalidomide.

Neutropenia
Absolute neutrophil count (ANC) less than 500 cells/mm^3: Withhold ixazomib and lenalidomide until ANC is 500 cells/mm^3 or greater, then resume ixazomib at the same dose and resume lenalidomide at reduced dose level (see manufacturer guidelines). **Recurrence of ANC less than 500 cells/mm^3:** Withhold ixazomib and lenalidomide until ANC is 500 cells/mm^3 or greater, then resume ixazomib

at reduced dose level and resume lenalidomide at the same dose. **Additional occurrences:** Alternate dose modification of ixazomib and lenalidomide.

Rash
Grade 2 or 3: Withhold lenalidomide until resolved to Grade 1 or 0, then resume lenalidomide at next lower dose level (see manufacturer guidelines) and resume ixazomib at the same dose. **Recurrence of Grade 2 or 3:** Withhold ixazomib and lenalidomide until recovery to Grade 1 or 0, then resume ixazomib at reduced dose level and resume lenalidomide at the same dose. **Grade 4:** Permanently discontinue. **Additional occurrences:** Alternate dose modification of ixazomib and lenalidomide.

Peripheral Neuropathy
Grade 1 (with pain) or Grade 2: Withhold ixazomib until resolved to baseline or improved to Grade 1 or 0 without pain (at prescriber's discretion), then resume ixazomib at the same dose. **Grade 2 (with pain) or Grade 3:** Withhold ixazomib until resolved to baseline or improved to Grade 1 or 0 without pain (at prescriber's discretion), then resume ixazomib at reduced dose level. **Grade 4:** Permanently discontinue.

Any Other Nonhematologic Toxicity
Grade 3 or 4: Withhold ixazomib until resolved to baseline or improved to Grade 1 or 0 (at physician's discretion), then resume ixazomib at reduced dose level.

Dosage in Renal Impairment
Mild to moderate impairment: Not specified; use caution. **Severe impairment (CrCl less than 30 mL/min), end-stage renal disease:** Reduce starting dose to 3 mg.

Dosage in Hepatic Impairment
Mild impairment: No dose adjustment. **Moderate to severe impairment:** Reduce starting dose to 3 mg.

SIDE EFFECTS

Frequent (42%–26%): Diarrhea, constipation, nausea. **Occasional (22%–5%):** Vomiting, back pain, blurry vision, dry eye.

ADVERSE EFFECTS/TOXIC REACTIONS

Neutropenia, thrombocytopenia are expected responses to therapy. Thrombocytopenia reported in 78% of pts; neutropenia in 67% of pts. Severe diarrhea may lead to discontinuation of treatment. Peripheral neuropathy reported in 28% of pts (sensory neuropathies were the most common type). Peripheral edema occurred in 28% of pts. Dermatologic toxicities including maculopapular and macular rash may occur. Infectious processes including upper respiratory tract infection (19% of pts), conjunctivitis (6% of pts) may occur. Other toxic reactions including neutrophilic dermatosis, posterior reversible encephalopathy, Stevens-Johnson syndrome, thrombotic thrombocytopenic purpura, transverse myelitis, treatment-induced hepatotoxicity, tumor lysis syndrome, occur rarely.

NURSING CONSIDERATIONS

BASELINE ASSESSMENT

Obtain ANC, CBC (esp. platelet count), renal function test (in pts with renal impairment), LFT; pregnancy test in female pts of reproductive potential. Screen for active infection. Question history of peripheral neuropathy, peripheral edema, hepatic/renal impairment, current hemodialysis status. Receive full medication history and screen for interactions. Assess hydration status. Obtain baseline visual acuity. Obtain dietary consult for nutritional support. Offer emotional support.

INTERVENTION/EVALUATION

Monitor ANC, platelet count at least monthly, more frequently during first 3 cycles; LFT in pts with hepatic impairment. Consider concomitant

---

granulocyte colony-stimulating factor (e.g., filgrastim, pegfilgrastim) in pts with neutropenia. Monitor for dehydration, electrolyte imbalance if diarrhea occurs. Offer antiemetics for nausea, antidiarrheals for diarrhea. Monitor for infection (esp. in pts with neutropenia); dermal toxicity, skin rashes, petechiae; peripheral neuropathy (with or without pain); peripheral edema. Monitor daily pattern bowel activity, stool consistency. Monitor for side effects of dexamethasone (e.g., hyperglycemia, weight loss, decreased appetite), lenalidomide (see prescribing information). Reversible posterior leukoencephalopathy syndrome should be considered in pts with altered mental status, confusion, headache, seizures, visual disturbances. Obtain visual acuity if vision becomes blurry.

PATIENT/FAMILY TEACHING

• Treatment may depress your immune system and reduce your ability to fight infection. Report symptoms of infection such as body aches, chills, cough, fatigue, fever. Avoid those with active infection. • Use effective contraception to avoid pregnancy. Do not breastfeed. • Do not take ixazomib and dexamethasone at the same time. Take dexamethasone with food to minimize GI upset. • Do not expose the capsule contents to the skin or eyes. If eyes are exposed to the capsule powder, thoroughly flush eyes with water. If skin is exposed to the capsule powder, thoroughly wash skin with soap and water. • Treatment may cause nerve pain; extreme sensitivity to touch; muscle weakness; or prickling, tingling, numbness in your hands and feet. • Report neurologic changes such as blurry vision, confusion, headache, seizures; may indicate life-threatening brain swelling. • Treatment may increase risk of bleeding. • Do not take herbal supplements, esp. St. John's wort.

ixekizumab

ix-ee-**kiz**-ue-mab
(Taltz)
Do not confuse ixekizumab with daclizumab, eculizumab, gevokizumab, secukinumab, or ustekinumab.

◆CLASSIFICATION

PHARMACOTHERAPEUTIC: Human interleukin-17A antagonist. Monoclonal antibody. **CLINICAL:** Antipsoriasis agent.

USES

Plaque psoriasis: Treatment of moderate to severe plaque psoriasis in adults and children 6 yrs and older who are candidates for systemic therapy or phototherapy. **Psoriatic arthritis:** Treatment of active psoriatic arthritis in adults. **Ankylosing spondylitis:** Treatment of active ankylosing spondylitis in adults. **Axial spondyloarthritis:** Treatment of active nonradiographic axial spondyloarthritis with objective signs of inflammation in adults.

PRECAUTIONS

Contraindications: Hypersensitivity to ixekizumab. **Cautions:** Baseline neutropenia, thrombocytopenia; inflammatory bowel disease (Crohn's disease, ulcerative colitis), HIV infection, concomitant immunosuppressant therapy, conditions predisposing to infection (e.g., diabetes, renal failure, open wounds), pts who have been exposed to tuberculosis. Concomitant use of live vaccines not recommended.

ACTION

Selectively binds to and inhibits interaction of interleukin-17A receptor, a naturally occurring cytokine that is involved in inflammatory and immune response. **Therapeutic Effect:** Alters biologic immune response; inhibits release of pro-inflammatory cytokines and chemokines.

PHARMACOKINETICS

Widely distributed. Degraded into small peptides and amino acids via catabolic pathway. Peak plasma concentration: 4 days. Steady state reached in 8–10 wks. Elimination not specified. **Half-life:** 13 days.

⏳ LIFESPAN CONSIDERATIONS

Pregnancy/Lactation: Unknown if distributed in breast milk. However, human immunoglobulin G is present in breast milk and is known to cross placenta. **Children:** Safety and efficacy not established in pts younger than 6 yrs. **Elderly:** No age-related precautions noted.

INTERACTIONS

DRUG: None significant. **HERBAL:** None significant. **FOOD:** None known. **LAB VALUES:** May decrease neutrophils, platelets. May decrease diagnostic effect of *Coccidioides immitis* skin test.

AVAILABILITY (Rx)

Auto-injector Pen: 80 mg/mL. **Prefilled Syringe:** 20 mg/0.25 mL, 40 mg/0.5 mL, 80 mg/mL.

ADMINISTRATION/HANDLING

SQ

• Follow instructions for preparation according to manufacturer guidelines. • Remove auto-injector or prefilled syringe from refrigerator and allow to warm to room temperature (approx. 30 min) with needle cap intact. • Visually inspect for particulate matter or discoloration. Solution should appear clear, colorless to slightly yellow in color. Do not use if solution is cloudy, discolored, or if visible particles are observed.

Administration • Insert needle subcutaneously into upper arm, outer thigh, or abdomen, and inject solution. • Do not inject into areas of active skin disease or injury such as sunburns, skin rashes, inflammation, skin infections, or active psoriasis. • Rotate injection sites. **Storage** • Refrigerate until time of use. • Do not freeze. • Do not shake. • Protect from light.

INDICATIONS/ROUTES/DOSAGE

Ankylosing Spondylitis

SQ: ADULTS, ELDERLY: 160 mg (two 80-mg injections) once, then 80 mg q4wks.

Plaque Psoriasis

SQ: ADULTS, ELDERLY: Initially, 160 mg (two injections of 80 mg) once, then 80 mg at wks 2, 4, 6, 8, 10, 12, then 80 mg once q4wks. **ADOLESCENTS, CHILDREN 6 YRS AND OLDER: (WEIGHING 50 KG OR MORE):** 160 mg (two 80-mg injections) once, then 80 mg q4wks. **(25–50 KG):** 80 mg once, then 40 mg q4wks. **(LESS THAN 25 KG):** 40 mg once, then 20 mg q4wks.

Psoriatic Arthritis

Note: For pts with coexisting plaque psoriasis, use dosage for plaque psoriasis. **SQ: ADULTS, ELDERLY:** 160 mg (two 80-mg injections) once, then 80 mg q4wks. May give alone or in combination with conventional disease-modifying antirheumatic drugs (e.g., methotrexate).

Nonradiographic Axial Spondyloarthritis

SQ: ADULTS, ELDERLY: 80 mg q4wks.

Dosage in Renal/Hepatic Impairment

Not specified; use caution.

SIDE EFFECTS

Occasional (17%): Injection site reactions (pain, erythema). **Rare (2%):** Nausea.

ADVERSE EFFECTS/TOXIC REACTIONS

May increase risk of infection including tuberculosis. Infections including upper respiratory tract infection (14% of pts), nasopharyngitis (14% of pts), tinea infections (2% of pts) have occurred. Cytopenias including neutropenia (11% of pts), thrombocytopenia (3% of pts)

---

were reported. May cause exacerbation of Crohn's disease and ulcerative colitis. Hypersensitivity reactions, including angioedema, occur rarely.

NURSING CONSIDERATIONS

BASELINE ASSESSMENT

Obtain CBC in pts with known history of neutropenia, thrombocytopenia. Screen for active infection. Pts should be evaluated for active tuberculosis and tested for latent infection prior to initiating treatment and periodically during therapy. Induration of 5 mm or greater with tuberculin skin testing should be considered a positive test result when assessing if treatment for latent tuberculosis is necessary. Consider administration of age-appropriate immunizations (if applicable) before initiation. Question history of Crohn's disease, ulcerative colitis, hypersensitivity reaction. Conduct dermatologic exam; record characteristics of psoriatic lesions.

INTERVENTION/EVALUATION

Monitor for symptoms of tuberculosis, including pts who tested negative for latent tuberculosis infection prior to initiating therapy. Interrupt or discontinue treatment if serious infection, opportunistic infection, or sepsis occurs, and initiate appropriate antimicrobial therapy. Assess skin for improvement of lesions. Monitor for hypersensitivity reaction, symptoms of inflammatory bowel disease.

PATIENT/FAMILY TEACHING

• A healthcare provider will show you how to properly prepare and inject your medication. You must demonstrate correct preparation and injection techniques before using medication at home. • Treatment may depress your immune system response and reduce your ability to fight infection. Report symptoms of infection such as body aches, chills, cough, fatigue, fever. Avoid people with active infection. • Do not receive live vaccines. • Expect frequent tuberculosis screening. • Report travel plans to possible endemic areas. • Immediately report difficulty breathing, itching, hives, rash, swelling of the face or tongue; may indicate allergic reaction. • Treatment may cause worsening of Crohn's disease or cause inflammatory bowel disease. Report abdominal pain, diarrhea, weight loss.

ketorolac

kee-**toe**-role-ak
(Acular, Acular LS, Acuvail, Apo-
Ketorolac ✦, Sprix, Toradol ✦)

■ **BLACK BOX ALERT** ■ Increased
risk of serious cardiovascular
thrombotic events, including myocardial infarction, CVA. Increased
risk of severe GI reactions, including ulceration, bleeding, perforation. Indicated for the short-term
(up to 5 days in adults) management
of moderately severe, acute pain
that requires analgesia at the opioid
level. Oral ketorolac is indicated
as continuation treatment after IV/
IM ketorolac. The total combined
duration of use should not exceed 5
days. Not indicated for use in pediatric pts, nor indicated for minor or
chronic painful conditions.
**Do not confuse Acular with
Acthar or Ocular, ketorolac
with Ketalar, or Toradol with
Foradil, Inderal, TEGretol, or
traMADol.**

◆**CLASSIFICATION**

PHARMACOTHERAPEUTIC: NSAID.
CLINICAL: Analgesic, intraocular anti-
inflammatory.

USES

PO, injection, nasal: Short-term (5 days
or less) relief of mild to moderate pain.
Ophthalmic: Relief of ocular itching
due to seasonal allergic conjunctivitis.
Postoperative ocular pain/inflammation
following cataract surgery. Reduction
of ocular pain and burning/stinging
following corneal refractive surgery. **OFF-
LABEL:** Migraine, severe, acute treatment
(injection, nasal).

PRECAUTIONS

Contraindications: Hypersensitivity to ketorolac, aspirin, or other NSAIDs. Intracranial bleeding, hemorrhagic diathesis,
incomplete hemostasis, high risk of bleeding; concomitant use of aspirin, NSAIDs,
probenecid, or pentoxifylline; labor and

delivery, advanced renal impairment or
risk of renal failure, active or history of
peptic ulcer disease, chronic inflammation
of GI tract, recent or history of GI bleeding/
ulceration. Perioperative pain in setting of
CABG surgery. Prophylaxis before major
surgery. **Cautions:** Hepatic impairment,
history of GI tract disease, asthma, coagulation disorders, receiving anticoagulants,
fluid retention, HF, renal impairment, inflammatory bowel disease, smoking, use of
alcohol, elderly, debilitated.

ACTION

Inhibits COX-1 and COX-2 enzymes, resulting in decreased prostaglandin synthesis;
reduces prostaglandin levels in aqueous humor. **Therapeutic Effect:** Produces analgesic, antipyretic, anti-inflammatory effect;
reduces intraocular inflammation.

PHARMACOKINETICS

Widely distributed. Protein binding: 99%.
Metabolized in liver. Primarily excreted
in urine. Not removed by hemodialysis.
Half-life: 5–9 hrs (increased in renal
impairment, in elderly).

⧖ LIFESPAN CONSIDERATIONS

Pregnancy/Lactation: Unknown if distributed in breast milk. Avoid use during
third trimester (may adversely affect fetal
cardiovascular system: premature closure
of ductus arteriosus). **Children:** Safety
and efficacy not established, but doses of
0.5 mg/kg have been used. **Elderly:** GI
bleeding, ulceration more likely to cause serious adverse effects. Age-related renal impairment may increase risk of hepatic/renal
toxicity; decreased dosage recommended.

INTERACTIONS

DRUG: May decrease effects of **antihypertensives (e.g., amLODIPine, lisinopril), diuretics (e.g., furosemide,
HCTZ).** Aspirin, NSAIDs, other salicylates may increase risk of GI side effects,
bleeding. May increase risk of bleeding
with **heparin, oral anticoagulants
(e.g., warfarin).** May increase concentration, risk of toxicity of **lIthium.** May

K

increase effect of **apixaban, dabigatran, edoxaban, rivaroxaban. Bile acid sequestrants (e.g., cholestyramine)** may decrease absorption/effect. May increase nephrotoxic effect of **cycloSPORINE. HERBAL:** **Glucosamine, herbs with anticoagulant/antiplatelet properties (e.g., garlic, ginger, ginseng, ginkgo biloba)** may increase concentration/effect. **FOOD:** None known. **LAB VALUES:** May prolong bleeding time. May increase serum ALT, AST, BUN, potassium, creatinine.

AVAILABILITY (Rx)

Injection Solution: 15 mg/mL, 30 mg/mL. **Nasal Spray:** *(Sprix):* 1.7-g bottle provides 8 sprays (15.75 mg/spray). **Ophthalmic Solution:** *(Acular LS):* 0.4%, *(Acuvail):* 0.45%, *(Acular):* 0.5%. **Tablets:** 10 mg.

ADMINISTRATION/HANDLING

IV

• Give undiluted as IV push. • Give over at least 15 sec.

IM
• Give deep IM slowly into large muscle mass.

PO
• Give with food, milk, antacids if GI distress occurs.

Nasal
• Blow nose gently to clear nostrils. Tilt head slightly forward and insert the tip of the container into right nostril. Point container away from the center of nose. While pt is holding breath, spray once into right nostril, pressing down evenly on both sides. Immediately after administration, pt should resume breathing through mouth to reduce expelling the product.

Ophthalmic
• Place gloved finger on lower eyelid and pull out until pocket is formed between eye and lower lid. Place prescribed number of drops into pocket. • Instruct

pt to close eye gently for 1–2 min (so that medication will not be squeezed out of the sac) and to apply digital pressure to lacrimal sac at inner canthus for 1 min to minimize system absorption.

⊞ IV COMPATIBILITIES

Acetaminophen.

INDICATIONS/ROUTES/DOSAGE

Note: Total duration is 5 days (parenteral and oral). Do not increase dose/frequency; supplement with low-dose opioids if needed.

Pain Management
Note: Avoid use in the elderly. **Maximum duration:** 5 days combined (parenteral, oral, and nasal). PO only as continuation of IM or IV therapy.
Weighing 50 kg or More and Less Than 65 Yrs of Age
IV: **ADULTS:** 30 mg as single dose or 15–30 mg q6h PRN. **Maximum:** 120 mg/day.
IM: **ADULTS:** 30–60 mg as single dose or 15–30 mg q6h or 10–30 mg q4–6h PRN. **Maximum:** 120 mg/day.
Weighing Less Than 50 kg or 65 Yrs or Older
IV: **ADULTS:** 15 mg as single dose or 15 mg q6h PRN. **Maximum:** 60 mg/day.
IM: **ADULTS:** 30 mg as single dose or 15 mg q6h or 10 mg q4–6h PRN. **Maximum:** 60 mg/day.
PO: **ADULTS:** Initially, 20 mg (10 mg for elderly), then 10 mg q4–6h. **Maximum:** 40 mg/24 hrs.
Nasal spray: ADULTS WEIGHING 50 KG OR MORE AND LESS THAN 65 YRS OF AGE: One spray (15.75 mg) in each nostril (total dose: 31.5 mg) q6–8h. **Maximum dose:** Eight sprays (126 mg/day). ADULTS WEIGHING LESS THAN 50 KG OR 65 YRS OF AGE OR OLDER: One spray (15.75 mg) in only one nostril (total dose: 15.75 mg) q6–8h. **Maximum dose:** Four sprays (63 mg/day).

Allergic Conjunctivitis

Ophthalmic: **ADULTS, ELDERLY, CHILDREN 2 YRS AND OLDER:** 1 drop into affected eye(s) (0.5%) 4 times/day.

Cataract Extraction

Ophthalmic: **ADULTS, ELDERLY:** *(Acular):* 1 drop (0.5%) 4 times/day into affected eye(s). Begin 24 hrs after surgery and continue for 2 wks. *(Acuvail):* 1 drop (0.45%) into affected eye(s) 2 times/day beginning 24 hrs before surgery, on the day of surgery, then continue for 2 wks.

Corneal Refractive Surgery

Ophthalmic: **ADULTS, ELDERLY:** *(Acular LS):* 1 drop (0.4%) 4 times/day as needed for up to 4 days after surgery.

Dosage in Renal Impairment

Contraindicated in advanced renal impairment or risk of renal failure; use caution in renal impairment.

Dosage in Hepatic Impairment

Use caution.

SIDE EFFECTS

Frequent (17%–12%): Headache, nausea, abdominal cramps/pain, dyspepsia. **Occasional (9%–3%):** Diarrhea. **Nasal:** Nasal discomfort, rhinalgia, increased lacrimation, throat irritation, rhinitis. **Ophthalmic:** Transient stinging, burning. **Rare (3%–1%):** Constipation, vomiting, flatulence, stomatitis. **Ophthalmic:** Ocular irritation, allergic reactions

(manifested by pruritus, stinging), superficial ocular infection, keratitis.

ADVERSE EFFECTS/TOXIC REACTIONS

Peptic ulcer, GI bleeding, gastritis, severe hepatic reaction (cholestasis, jaundice) occur rarely. Nephrotoxicity (glomerular nephritis, interstitial nephritis, nephrotic syndrome) may occur in pts with preexisting renal impairment. Acute hypersensitivity reaction (fever, chills, joint pain) occurs rarely.

NURSING CONSIDERATIONS

BASELINE ASSESSMENT

Assess onset, type, location, duration of pain. Obtain baseline renal/hepatic function tests.

INTERVENTION/EVALUATION

Monitor renal function, LFT, urinary output. Monitor daily pattern of bowel activity, stool consistency. Observe for occult blood loss. Assess for therapeutic response: relief of pain, stiffness, swelling; increased joint mobility; reduced joint tenderness; improved grip strength. Monitor for bleeding (may also occur with ophthalmic route due to systemic absorption).

PATIENT/FAMILY TEACHING

• Avoid aspirin, alcohol. • Report abdominal pain, bloody stools, or vomiting blood. • If GI upset occurs, take with food, milk. • Ophthalmic: Transient stinging, burning may occur upon instillation. • Do not administer while wearing soft contact lenses.

K

L

labetalol

la-**bayt**-a-lol
(Apo-Labetalol ✦, Trandate ✦)
Do not confuse labetalol with atenolol, betaxolol, metoprolol or propranolol, or Trandate with traMADol or trental.

FIXED-COMBINATION(S)

Normozide: labetalol/hydroCHLO-ROthiazide (a diuretic): 100 mg/25 mg, 200 mg/25 mg, 300 mg/25 mg.

◆CLASSIFICATION

PHARMACOTHERAPEUTIC: Alpha-, beta-adrenergic blocker. **CLINICAL:** Antihypertensive.

USES

Management of hypertension. IV for severe hypertension. **OFF-LABEL:** Acute aortic syndromes (dissection), acute ischemic stroke, hypertensive emergency in pregnancy/post-partum (including preeclampsia/eclampsia, intracerebral/subarachnoid hemorrhage (acute BP management).

PRECAUTIONS

Contraindications: Hypersensitivity to labetalol. Bronchial asthma, history of obstructive airway disease, cardiogenic shock, uncompensated HF, second- or third-degree heart block (except in pts with functioning pacemaker), severe bradycardia, conditions associated with severe, prolonged hypotension. **Cautions:** Compensated HF, severe anaphylaxis to allergens, myasthenia gravis, psychiatric disease, hepatic impairment, pheochromocytoma, diabetes; concurrent use with digoxin, verapamil, or dilTIAZem; arterial obstruction, elderly. Pts with peripheral vascular disease, Raynaud's disease.

ACTION

Blocks alpha-1, beta-1, beta-2 (large doses) adrenergic receptor sites. **Therapeutic Effect:** Decreases peripheral vascular resistance, B/P.

PHARMACOKINETICS

Route	Onset	Peak	Duration
PO	0.5–2 hrs	2–4 hrs	8–12 hrs
IV	2–5 min	5–15 min	2–4 hrs

Widely distributed. Protein binding: 50%. Metabolized in liver. Primarily excreted in urine. Not removed by hemodialysis. **Half-life:** 6–8 hrs.

⧗ LIFESPAN CONSIDERATIONS

Pregnancy/Lactation: Drug crosses placenta. Small amount distributed in breast milk. **Children:** Safety and efficacy not established. **Elderly:** Age-related peripheral vascular disease may increase susceptibility to decreased peripheral circulation. May have increased risk of orthostatic hypotension.

INTERACTIONS

DRUG: May decrease therapeutic effects of **beta$_2$-adrenergic agonists** (e.g., arformoterol, salmeterol), **theophylline. Dronedarone, rivastigmine** may increase bradycardic effect. May increase bradycardic effect of **fingolimod, ponesimod. HERBAL: Herbals with hypertensive properties** (e.g., licorice, yohimbe) or **hypotensive properties** (e.g., garlic, ginger, ginkgo biloba) may alter effects. **FOOD:** None known. **LAB VALUES:** May increase serum antinuclear antibody titer (ANA), BUN, LDH, alkaline phosphatase, bilirubin, creatinine, potassium, triglycerides, lipoprotein, uric acid, ALT, AST.

AVAILABILITY (Rx)

Injection Solution: 5 mg/mL. **Prefilled Syringe:** 20 mg/4 mL. **Tablets:** 100 mg, 200 mg, 300 mg.

ADMINISTRATION/HANDLING

 IV

◀**ALERT**▶ Prolonged duration of action: Monitor several hrs after administration. Excessive administration may result in prolonged hypotension and/or bradycardia.

Reconstitution • For IV infusion, dilute in D₅W to provide concentration of 1–2 mg/mL.
Rate of administration • For IV push, administer at a rate of 10 mg/min. • For IV infusion, administer at rate of 2 mg/min initially. Rate is adjusted according to B/P. • Monitor B/P immediately before and q5–10min during IV administration (maximum effect occurs within 5 min).
Storage • Store at room temperature. • After dilution, IV solution is stable for 72 hrs. • Solution appears clear, colorless to light yellow. • Discard if discolored or precipitate forms.

PO
• Give without regard to food. • If administering with meals, give in a consistent manner.

❋ IV INCOMPATIBILITIES
Furosemide, ibuprofen.

❋ IV COMPATIBILITIES
Acetaminophen, amiodarone, calcium gluconate, dexmedetomidine, diltiazem, heparain, magnesium sulfate, norepinephrine, potassium chloride, potassium phosphate, propofol.

INDICATIONS/ROUTES/DOSAGE
Hypertension
PO: ADULTS, ELDERLY: Initially, 100 mg twice daily. Adjust in increments of 100 mg twice daily q2–3days. Usual dose: 200–800 mg/day in 2 divided doses. **Maximum:** 2,400 mg/day. **CHILDREN:** Initially, 1–3 mg/kg/day in 2 divided doses up to 10–12 mg/kg/day. **Maximum:** 1,200 mg/day.

Severe Hypertension, Hypertensive Crisis
IV: ADULTS: Initially, 10–20 mg (bolus over 1–2 min). Additional doses of 20–80 mg may be given at 10-min intervals until target BP reached. **Maximum cumulative dose:** 300 mg. **CHILDREN:** 0.2–1 mg/kg/dose. **Maximum:** 40 mg/dose.
IV infusion: ADULTS: Initially, 0.5–2 mg/min up to 10 mg/min. **Maximum cumulative dose:** 300 mg. **CHILDREN:** 0.25–3 mg/kg/hr (initiate at lower end, then titrate slowly).

Dosage in Renal Impairment
No dose adjustment.

Dosage in Hepatic Impairment
Use caution.

SIDE EFFECTS
Frequent (20%–11%): Drowsiness, dizziness, excessive fatigue. **Occasional (10% or less):** Dyspnea, peripheral edema, depression, anxiety, constipation, diarrhea, nasal congestion, weakness, diminished sexual function, transient scalp tingling, insomnia, nausea, vomiting, abdominal discomfort. **Rare:** Altered taste, dry eyes, increased urination, paresthesia.

ADVERSE EFFECTS/TOXIC REACTIONS
May cause, aggravate HF due to decreased myocardial stimulation. Abrupt withdrawal may cause myocardial ischemia, producing chest pain, diaphoresis, palpitations, headache, tremor. May mask signs of acute hypoglycemia (tachycardia, B/P changes) in diabetic pts. Rapid reduction of blood pressure may cause CVA, optic nerve infarction, ischemic changes on ECG. May cause severe orthostatic hypotension.

NURSING CONSIDERATIONS

BASELINE ASSESSMENT
Assess B/P, heart rate immediately before drug administration (if pulse is 60/min or less or systolic B/P is lower than 90 mm Hg, withhold medication, contact physician). Question history of bradycardia, HF, second- or third-degree heart block, myasthenia gravis.

INTERVENTION/EVALUATION
Monitor B/P for hypotension; heart rate. Assist with ambulation if dizziness occurs. Assess for evidence of HF: Dyspnea (particularly on exertion or lying down), night cough, peripheral edema, distended neck veins. Monitor I&O (increase in weight, decrease in urine output may indicate HF).

PATIENT/FAMILY TEACHING
• Do not prematurely stop treatment (may cause or worsen HF) • Slowly go

L

from lying to standing. • Compliance with therapy regimen is essential to control hypertension, arrhythmias. • Avoid tasks that require alertness, motor skills until response to drug is established. • Report shortness of breath, excessive fatigue, weight gain, prolonged dizziness, headache. • Do not use nasal decongestants, OTC cold preparations (stimulants) without physician approval. • Limit alcohol.

lacosamide

la-**koe**-sa-myde
(Motpoly XR, Vimpat)
Do not confuse lacosamide with zonisamide, or Vimpat with Venofer, Vfend, or Vimovo.

◆ CLASSIFICATION

PHARMACOTHERAPEUTIC: Succinimide **(Schedule V). CLINICAL:** Anticonvulsant.

USES

Monotherapy or adjunctive therapy for treatment of focal (partial) onset seizures in adults and children 1 mo and older. Adjunctive therapy in treatment of primary generalized tonic-clonic seizures in adults and children 4 years of age and older. **OFF-LABEL:** Status epilepticus.

PRECAUTIONS

Contraindications: Hypersensitivity to lacosamide. **Cautions:** Renal/hepatic impairment, cardiac conduction problems (e.g., marked first-degree AV block, second-degree or higher AV block, sick sinus syndrome without pacemaker), myocardial ischemia, HF, pts at risk of suicide.

ACTION

Selectively enhances slow inactivation of sodium channels, stabilizing hyperexcitable neuronal membranes and inhibits neuronal firing. **Therapeutic Effect:** Reduces seizure frequency.

PHARMACOKINETICS

Widely distributed. Protein binding: 15%. Peak plasma concentration: (PO): 1–4 hrs; (IV): At end of infusion. Primarily excreted in urine. Steady-state reached in 3 days. Removed by hemodialysis. **Half-life:** 13 hrs.

LIFESPAN CONSIDERATIONS

Pregnancy/Lactation: Use in pregnancy if benefits outweigh risk. Unknown if distributed in breast milk. **Children:** Safety and efficacy not established in pts younger than 1 mo. **Elderly:** No age-related precautions noted.

INTERACTIONS

DRUG: None significant. **HERBAL:** None significant. **FOOD:** None known. **LAB VALUES:** May increase serum ALT; proteinuria.

AVAILABILITY (Rx)

Injection Solution: 10 mg/mL (20 mL).
Oral Solution: 10 mg/mL.
Tablets: 50 mg, 100 mg, 150 mg, 200 mg.

ADMINISTRATION/HANDLING

PO

• Give without regard to food. • Give tablets whole; do not divide. • Oral solution should be administered with a calibrated measuring device. • Discard any unused portion after 6 mos.

IV

• Appears as a clear, colorless solution. • Discard unused portion or if precipitate or discoloration is present. May give without further dilution. • If mixing with diluent, may be stored for 4 hrs at room temperature. Infuse over 30–60 min.

IV COMPATIBILITIES

0.9% NaCl, D$_5$W, lactated Ringer's.

INDICATIONS/ROUTES/DOSAGE

Note: IV dose is same as oral dose. May give undiluted or mixed in compatible diluent and infused over 30–60 min.

Focal (Partial) Onset Seizures

Monotherapy

PO/IV: ADULTS, ELDERLY: Initially, 50–100 mg twice daily. May increase by 50 mg twice daily at wkly intervals. **Maintenance:** 150–200 mg twice daily. **INFANTS, CHILDREN, ADOLESCENTS (1 MO–17 YRS): WEIGHING 50 KG OR MORE:** Initially, 50 mg twice daily. May increase by 50 mg twice daily at wkly intervals. **Maintenance:** 150–200 mg twice daily. **WEIGHING 30–49 KG:** Initially, 1 mg/kg/dose twice daily. May increase by 1 mg/kg/dose twice daily at wkly intervals. **Maintenance:** 2–4 mg/kg/dose twice daily. **WEIGHING 6–29 KG:** Initially, 1 mg/kg/dose twice daily. May increase by 1 mg/kg/dose twice daily at wkly intervals. **Maintenance:** 3–6 mg/kg/dose twice daily. **LESS THAN 6 KG: (IV):** Initially, 0.66 mg/kg/dose 3 times/day. May increase by 0.66 mg/kg/dose at wkly intervals. **Maintenance:** 2.5–5 mg/kg/dose 3 times/day. **PO:** Initially, 1 mg/kg/dose 2 times/day. May increase by 1 mg/kg/dose at wkly intervals. **Maintenance:** 3.75–7.5 mg/kg/dose 3 times/day.

Adjunctive Therapy

PO/IV: ADULTS, ELDERLY: Initially, 50 mg twice daily. May increase by 50 mg twice daily at wkly intervals. **Maintenance:** 100–200 mg twice daily. **Maximum:** 400 mg/day. **INFANTS, CHILDREN, ADOLESCENTS (1 MO–17 YRS): WEIGHING 50 KG OR MORE:** Initially, 50 mg twice daily. **Maintenance:** 100–200 mg twice daily. **WEIGHING 30–49 KG:** Initially, 1 mg/kg/dose twice daily. **Maintenance:** 2–4 mg/kg/dose twice daily. **WEIGHING 6–29 KG:** Initially, 1 mg/kg/dose twice daily. **Maintenance:** 3–6 mg/kg/dose twice daily. **LESS THAN 6 KG:** Same as monotherapy.

Primary Generalized Tonic-Clonic Seizures

PO/IV: ADULTS, ELDERLY, ADOLESCENTS 17 YRS OF AGE OR OLDER: Initially, 50 mg twice daily. May increase at wkly intervals by 50 mg twice daily. Alternatively, may give 200 mg loading dose, followed 12 hrs later by 100 mg twice daily with same titration schedule. **Maintenance:** 100–200 mg twice daily. **CHILDREN 4–16 YRS: (50 KG OR GREATER):** Initially, 50 mg twice daily. May increase at wkly intervals of 50 mg twice daily. **Maintenance:** 100–200 mg twice daily. **(30–49 KG):** Initially, 1 mg/kg/dose twice daily. May increase at wkly intervals by 1 mg/kg/dose twice daily. **Maintenance:** 2–4 mg/kg/dose twice daily. **(11–29 KG):** Initially, 1 mg/kg/dose twice daily; may be increased at wkly intervals by 1 mg/kg/dose twice daily. **Maintenance:** 3–6 mg/kg/dose twice daily.

Switch From IV to PO

When switching from IV to PO form, use same equivalent daily dosage and frequency as IV administration.

Switch From PO to IV

When switching from PO to IV form, initial total daily IV dosage should be equivalent to total daily dosage and frequency of PO form and should be infused IV over 30–60 min.

Dosage in Renal Impairment

Use caution when titrating. **Mild to moderate impairment:** No dose adjustment. **Severe impairment, end-stage renal disease: Maximum:** 300 mg/day.

Dosage in Hepatic Impairment

Use caution when titrating. **Mild to moderate impairment: Maximum:** 300 mg/day. **Severe impairment:** Not recommended.

SIDE EFFECTS

Frequent (31%–13%): Dizziness, headache. **Occasional (11%–5%):** Nausea, double vision, vomiting, fatigue, blurred vision, ataxia, tremor, nystagmus. **Rare**

L

(4%–2%): Vertigo, diarrhea, gait disturbances, memory impairment, depression, pruritus, injection site discomfort.

ADVERSE EFFECTS/TOXIC REACTIONS

May increase risk of suicidal ideation, behavior. PR interval prolongation, AV block, ventricular tachyarrhythmias may occur. Sudden discontinuation may increase risk of seizures. Drug reaction with eosinophilia and systemic symptoms (DRESS), also known as multiorgan hypersensitivity, has been reported. DRESS may present with facial swelling, eosinophilia, fever, lymphadenopathy, rash, which may be associated with other organ systems, such as hepatitis, hematologic abnormalities, myocarditis, nephritis. Psychiatric conditions (aggression, agitation, hallucinations, psychotic disorder) may occur. Leukopenia, anemia, thrombocytopenia occur rarely.

NURSING CONSIDERATIONS

BASELINE ASSESSMENT

Obtain LFT, renal function test. Review history of seizure disorder (intensity, frequency, duration, level of consciousness). Initiate seizure precautions. Question history of cardiac conduction disorders, depression, suicidal ideation and behavior.

INTERVENTION/EVALUATION

Monitor LFT, renal function periodically. Observe for recurrence of seizure activity. Assess for clinical improvement (decrease in intensity/frequency of seizures). Assist with ambulation if dizziness occurs. Assess for suicidal ideation, depression, behavioral changes. Drug should be withdrawn gradually (over a minimum of 1 wk) to minimize potential for increased seizure frequency. Monitor ECG for QT prolongation. Monitor for symptoms of DRESS; cardiac effects.

PATIENT/FAMILY TEACHING

• Strict compliance is essential for seizure control. • Avoid tasks that require alertness, motor skills until response to drug is established. • Do not abruptly discontinue medication (may cause seizures; symptoms of withdrawal syndrome). • Treatment may affect the electrical properties of the heart; report palpitations, loss of consciousness. • Seek immediate medical attention if thoughts of suicide, new-onset or worsening of anxiety, depression, or changes in mood occurs. • Avoid alcohol, nervous system depressants. • Report symptoms of drug-induced hypersensitivity syndrome (e.g., fever, swollen face/lymph nodes; skin rash/peeling/inflammation).

lamiVUDine

la-**miv**-yoo-deen
(Apo-LamiVUDine, ✦ Epivir, Epivir-HBV)

■ **BLACK BOX ALERT** ■ Serious, sometimes fatal lactic acidosis, severe hepatomegaly with steatosis (fatty liver) have occurred. Severe acute exacerbation of hepatitis B virus (HBV) infection was reported in pts coinfected with HBV and HIV-1 after discontinuation. Monitor hepatic function for several mos after discontinuation. Do not use Epivir-HBV for treatment of HIV infection. Epivir contains a higher dose of active ingredient compared to Epivir-HBV. Pts with HIV-1 infection must receive dosage form that is appropriate for treatment.
Do not confuse Epivir with Combivir, or lamiVUDine with lamoTRIgine.

FIXED-COMBINATION(S)

Cimduo: lamiVUDine/tenofovir (antiviral): 300 mg/300 mg. **Combivir:** lamiVUDine/zidovudine (an antiviral): 150 mg/300 mg. **Delstrigo:** lamiVUDine/doravirine/tenofovir (antivirals): 300 mg/100 mg/300 mg. **Dovato:** lamiVUDine/dolutegravir (antiviral): 300 mg/50 mg. **Epzicom:** lamiVUDine/abacavir (an antiviral): 300 mg/600 mg. **Symfi:** lamiVUDine/efavirenz/tenofovir: 300 mg/400 mg/300 mg. **Triumeq:** lamiVUDine/abacavir (antiretroviral)/ dolutegravir (integrase inhibitor): 300 mg/600 mg/50 mg. **Trizivir:** lamiVUDine/zidovudine/abacavir (an antiviral): 150 mg/300 mg/300 mg.

◆CLASSIFICATION

PHARMACOTHERAPEUTIC: Nucleoside reverse transcriptase inhibitor, Antihepadnaviral. **CLINICAL:** Antiviral.

USES

Epivir: Treatment of HIV infection in combination with at least two other antiretroviral agents in adults and children 3 mos and older. **Epivir-HBV:** Treatment of chronic hepatitis B virus infection associated with evidence of hepatitis B viral replication and active hepatic inflammation in adults and children 2 yrs and older. **OFF-LABEL:** HIV-1 nonoccupational postexposure prophylaxis (nPEP).

PRECAUTIONS

Contraindications: Hypersensitivity to lamiVUDine. **Cautions:** Hepatic impairment. Use in children with history of pancreatitis or risk factors for developing pancreatitis autoimmune disease, genetic mutations, pancreas divisum [congenital]). Use in combination with interferon alfa with or without ribavirin in pts coinfected with HIV/HBV.

ACTION

Inhibits HIV reverse transcriptase by viral DNA chain termination. Inhibits RNA-, DNA-dependent DNA polymerase, an enzyme necessary for HIV, hepatitis B virus replication. **Therapeutic Effect:** Slows HIV replication; reduces progression of HIV infection, chronic hepatitis B virus infection.

PHARMACOKINETICS

Widely distributed. Protein binding: less than 36%. Primarily excreted unchanged in urine. Not removed by hemodialysis or peritoneal dialysis. **Half-life:** Children: 2 hrs. **Adults:** 5–7 hrs.

⧖ LIFESPAN CONSIDERATIONS

Pregnancy/Lactation: Drug crosses placenta. Unknown if distributed in breast milk. Breastfeeding not recommended due to risk of postnatal HIV transmission. **Children:** Safety and efficacy not established in pts younger than 3 mos. **Elderly:** Age-related renal impairment may require dosage adjustment.

INTERACTIONS

DRUG: None significant. **HERBAL:** None significant. **FOOD:** None known. **LAB VALUES:** May increase serum amylase, ALT, AST, bilirubin. May decrease absolute neutrophil count, Hgb, platelets. May increase serum lipase in children.

AVAILABILITY (Rx)

Oral Solution: 10 mg/mL. **Tablets:** 100 mg, 150 mg, 300 mg.

ADMINISTRATION/HANDLING
PO
• Give without regard to food.

INDICATIONS/ROUTES/DOSAGE
HIV Infection

PO: ADULTS, ELDERLY: 150 mg twice daily or 300 mg once daily. **CHILDREN 3 YRS AND OLDER: 25 KG OR MORE:** 150 mg twice daily. **20–24 KG:** 75 mg (1/2 tablet) in the morning and 150 mg in the evening. **14–19 KG:** 75 mg (1/2 tablet) twice daily. **INFANTS 3 MOS TO CHILDREN LESS THAN 3 YRS:** *(Oral solution):* 5 mg/kg/dose twice daily. **Maximum:** 150 mg/dose.

Chronic Hepatitis B

PO: ADULTS: 100 mg/day. **CHILDREN 2–17 YRS:** 3 mg/kg/day. **Maximum:** 100 mg/day.

Dosage in Renal Impairment

Dosage and frequency are modified based on creatinine clearance.

Creatinine Clearance	Dosage HIV	Dosage Hepatitis B
30–49 mL/min	150 mg once/daily	100 mg first dose, then 50 mg once/daily
15–29 mL/min	150 mg first dose, then 100 mg once/daily	100 mg first dose, then 25 mg once/daily
5–14 mL/min	150 mg first dose, then 50 mg once/daily	35 mg first dose, then 15 mg once/daily
Less than 5 mL/min	50 mg first dose, then 25 mg once/daily	35 mg first dose, then 10 mg once/daily

Hemodialysis: Dosing post-HD recommended.

Dosage in Hepatic Impairment

No dose adjustment.

SIDE EFFECTS

Frequent (35%–10%): Headache, nausea, malaise, fatigue, nasal disturbances, diarrhea, cough, musculoskeletal pain, neuropathy, insomnia, anorexia, dizziness, fever, chills. **Occasional (9%–5%):** Depression, myalgia, abdominal cramps, dyspepsia, arthralgia.

ADVERSE EFFECTS/TOXIC REACTIONS

Lactic acidosis, severe hepatomegaly with steatosis have occurred. If therapy is discontinued, pts coinfected with HBV have an increased risk for viral replication, worsening of hepatic function, and may experience hepatic decompensation and/or failure. Hepatitis B virus–resistant variants have occurred in pts coinfected with HIV-1/HBV. May increase risk of pancreatitis in children. May induce immune recovery syndrome (inflammatory response to dormant opportunistic infections such as *Mycobacterium avium*, cytomegalovirus, PCP, tuberculosis or acceleration of autoimmune disorders, including Graves' disease, polymyositis, Guillain-Barre). May cause redistribution/accumulation of body fat (lipodystrophy). Lymphadenopathy, splenomegaly reported in children. Paresthesia, peripheral neuropathy reported in 15% of pts.

NURSING CONSIDERATIONS

BASELINE ASSESSMENT

Obtain BUN, serum creatinine, CrCl, eGFR; CD4+ count, viral load, HIV-1 RNA level in pts infected with HIV. Test for HBV infection in pts being treated for HIV-1 infection. Question history of hepatic/renal impairment. Screen for risk factors of developing pancreatitis in children. Offer emotional support.

INTERVENTION/EVALUATION

Monitor CD4+ count, viral load, HIV-1 RNA level for treatment effectiveness in pts treated for HIV-1 infection. Monitor for immune recovery syndrome, esp. after initiating treatment. Cough, dyspnea, fever, excess band cells on CBC may indicate acute infection (WBC may be unreliable in pts with uncontrolled HIV infection). Obtain serum lactate level if lactic acidosis is suspected (confusion, dyspnea, muscle cramps, tachypnea). Obtain serum amylase, lipase level if acute pancreatitis (abdominal pain, fever, nausea, steatorrhea, tachycardia, vomiting) is suspected. Monitor daily pattern of bowel activity, stool consistency.

PATIENT/FAMILY TEACHING

• Treatment does not cure HIV infection nor reduce risk of transmission. Practice safe sex with barrier methods or abstinence. • Drug resistance can form if treatment is interrupted; do not run out of supply. • Fatal cases of liver inflammation or failure have occurred; report abdominal pain, clay-colored stools, yellowing of skin or eyes, weight loss. • Pancreatitis can occur in children; report any new or worsening abdominal pain that radiates to the back or shoulder, with or without nausea/vomiting. • As immune system strengthens, it may respond to dormant infections hidden within the body. Report any new fever, chills, body aches, cough, night sweats, shortness of breath. • Antiretrovirals may cause excess body fat in upper back, neck, breast, trunk, while also causing decreased body fat in legs, arms, face. • Do not breastfeed.

---

lamoTRIgine

la-**moe**-tri-jeen
(<u>LaMICtal</u>, LaMICtal ODT, LaMICtal XR, Subvenite)

■ **BLACK BOX ALERT** ■Severe, potentially life-threatening skin rashes have been reported, including Stevens-Johnson syndrome, toxic epidermal necrolysis. Risk increased with coadministration with valproic acid and rapid-dose titration.

Do not confuse LaMICtal with labetalol, LamISIL, or Lomotil, or lamoTRIgine with labetalol, levETIRAcetam, lamiVUDine, or levothyroxine.

◆ CLASSIFICATION

PHARMACOTHERAPEUTIC: Phenyltriazine. **CLINICAL:** Anticonvulsant.

USES

Focal (partial) onset seizures and generalized onset seizures: (Immediate-release): Adjunctive therapy for pts 2 yrs of age and older for focal (partial) onset seizures, primary generalized tonic-clonic seizures, generalized seizures of Lennox-Gastaut syndrome. Monotherapy for pts 16 yrs of age and older with focal (partial) onset seizures receiving treatment with carbamazepine, phenobarbital, phenytoin, primidone, or valproate as the single AED. **(Extended-release):** Adjunctive therapy for primary generalized tonic-clonic seizures, focal (partial) onset seizures with or without secondary generalization in pts 13 yrs and older. Conversion to monotherapy in pts 13 yrs and older with focal (partial) onset seizures who are receiving treatment with a single antiseizure drug. **Bipolar disorder:** Treatment of pts 18 yrs of age and older as maintenance treatment or to delay the time to occurrence of mood episodes (e.g., depression, mania, hypomania, episodes with mixed features) in pts treated for acute mood episodes with standard therapy. **OFF-LABEL:** Short-lasting unilateral neuralgiform headaches (prophylaxis), trigeminal neuralgia.

PRECAUTIONS

Contraindications: Hypersensitivity to lamoTRIgine. **Cautions:** Renal/hepatic impairment, pts at high risk of suicide, pts taking estrogen-containing oral contraceptives, history of adverse hematologic reaction.

ACTION

Inhibits voltage-sensitive sodium channels, stabilizing neuronal membranes. Inhibits release of glutamide (an excitatory amino acid). **Therapeutic Effect:** Reduces frequency of seizure activity. Delays time to occurrence of acute mood episodes (mania, depression, hypomania).

⧖ LIFESPAN CONSIDERATIONS

Pregnancy/Lactation: Distributed in breast milk. Breastfeeding not recommended. Increased fetal risk of oral cleft formation has been noted with use during pregnancy. **Children:** Safety and efficacy not established in pts younger than 18 yrs with bipolar disorder or in pts younger than 2 yrs with epilepsy. **Elderly:** Age-related renal impairment may require dosage adjustment.

INTERACTIONS

DRUG: Strong CYP3A4 inducers (e.g., carBAMazepine phenytoin riFAMPin) may decrease concentration/

effect. **Valproic acid** may increase concentration/effect. May increase adverse effects of **dofetilide. Estrogen (contraceptive)** may decrease concentration/effect. **CNS depressants (e.g., alcohol, morphine, zolpidem)** may increase CNS depression. **HERBAL:** Herbals with sedative properties (e.g., chamomile, kava kava, valerian) may increase CNS depression. **FOOD:** None known. **LAB VALUES:** None significant.

AVAILABILITY (Rx)

Tablets: 25 mg, 100 mg, 150 mg, 200 mg. **Tablets, Chewable:** 5 mg, 25 mg. **Tablets, Orally Disintegrating:** 25 mg, 50 mg, 100 mg, 200 mg.

Tablets, Extended-Release: 25 mg, 50 mg, 100 mg, 200 mg, 250 mg, 300 mg.

ADMINISTRATION/HANDLING

PO

• Give without regard to food. • Chewable tablets may be dispensed in water or diluted fruit juice, or swallowed whole. • Extended-release tablets must be swallowed whole; do not break, crush, dissolve, or divide. • Place orally disintegrating tablet on tongue, allow to dissolve. Pt must not break, cut, or chew. Can be swallowed without regard to food or water.

INDICATIONS/ROUTES/DOSAGE

Adjunctive Therapy
Lennox-Gastaut, Primary Generalized Tonic-Clonic Seizures, Focal (Partial) Seizures (Not Taking Interacting Medications)
PO: ADULTS, ELDERLY, CHILDREN OLDER THAN 12 YRS: Initially, 25 mg/day for 2 wks, then increase to 50 mg/day for 2 wks. After 4 wks, may increase by 50 mg/day at 1- to 2-wk intervals. **Maintenance:** 225–375 mg/day in 2 divided doses. **CHILDREN 2–12 YRS: Note:** Only whole tablets should be used for dosing. Round dose down to nearest whole tablet. Initially, 0.3 mg/kg/day in 1–2

divided doses for 2 wks, then increase to 0.6 mg/kg/day in 1–2 divided doses for 2 wks. After 4 wks, may increase by 0.6 mg/kg/day at 1- to 2-wk intervals. **Maintenance:** 4.5–7.5 mg/kg/day in 2 divided doses. **Maximum:** 300 mg/day in 2 divided doses.

Adjusted Dosage With Antiepileptic Drugs Containing Valproic Acid
PO: ADULTS, ELDERLY, CHILDREN OLDER THAN 12 YRS: Initially, 12.5–25 mg every other day for 2 wks, then increase to 25 mg/day for 2 wks. After 4 wks, may increase by 25–50 mg/day at 1- to 2-wk intervals. **Maintenance:** 100–400 mg/day in 2 divided doses (100–200 mg/day when taking lamoTRIgine with valproic acid alone). **CHILDREN 2–12 YRS: Note:** Only whole tablets should be used for dosing. Round dose down to nearest whole tablet. Initially, 0.15 mg/kg/day in 1–2 divided doses for 2 wks, then increase to 0.3 mg/kg/day in 1–2 divided doses for 2 wks. After 4 wks, may increase by 0.3 mg/kg/day at 1- to 2-wk intervals. **Maintenance:** 1–5 mg/kg/day in 1–2 divided doses. **Maximum:** 200 mg/day in 1–2 divided doses.

Adjusted Dosage With EIAED Without Valproic Acid
PO: ADULTS, ELDERLY, CHILDREN OLDER THAN 12 YRS: Initially, 50 mg/day for 2 wks, then increase to 100 mg/day in 2 divided doses for 2 wks. After 4 wks, may increase by 100 mg/day at 1- to 2-wk intervals. **Maintenance:** 300–500 mg/day in 2 divided doses. **CHILDREN 2–12 YRS: Note:** Only whole tablets should be used for dosing. Round dose down to nearest whole tablet. Initially, 0.6 mg/kg/day in 2 divided doses for 2 wks, then increase to 1.2 mg/kg/day in 2 divided doses for 2 wks. After 4 wks, may increase by 1.2 mg/kg/day at 1- to 2-wk intervals. **Maintenance:** 5–15 mg/kg/day in 2 divided doses. **Maximum:** 400 mg/day in 2 divided doses.

Usual Maintenance Range for Extended-Release Tablets
Note: Refer to manufacturer for dose escalation regimen. **Pts Taking Valproic**

Acid: 200–250 mg once daily. **Pts Taking Eiaed Without Valproic Acid:** 400–600 mg once daily. **Pts not Taking Eiaed:** 300–400 mg once daily.

Conversion to Monotherapy for Pts Receiving EIAEDs

PO: ADULTS, ELDERLY, CHILDREN: *(Immediate-Release):* After achieving a dose of 500 mg/day, the concomitant AED should be withdrawn in 20% decrements each wk over a 4-wk period. *(Extended-Release):* After achieving a dose of 500 mg/day, the concomitant enzyme-inducing AED should be withdrawn in 20% decrements each week over a 4-wk period. 2 wks after completion of withdrawal of the enzyme-inducing AED, the dosage of Lamictal XR may be decreased no faster than 100 mg/day each wk to achieve the monotherapy maintenance dosage range of 250–300 mg/day.

Conversion to Monotherapy for Pts Receiving Valproic Acid

PO: ADULTS, ELDERLY, CHILDREN: *(Immediate-Release):* (Step 1): Achieve a dose of Lamictal of 200 mg/day (if not already on 200 mg/day). Maintain previous stable dose. (Step 2): Maintain at 200 mg/day. Decrease valproate to 500 mg/day by decrements no greater than 500 mg/day/wk, then maintain the dose of 500 mg/day for 1 wk. (Step 3): Increase Lamictal to 300 mg/day and maintain for 1 wk. Simultaneously decrease valproate to 250 mg/day and maintain for 1 wk. (Step 4): Increase Lamictal by 100 mg/day every week to achieve maintenance dose of 500 mg/day. Discontinue valproate. *(Extended-Release):* (Step 1): Achieve with a (Lamictal XR) dose of 150 mg/day according to escalation guidelines. (Step 2): Maintain at 150 mg/day. Decrease valproate dose by decrements no greater than 500 mg/day/wk to 500 mg/day, then maintain for 1 wk. (Step 3): Increase Lamictal XR to 200 mg/day. Simultaneously decrease valproate to 250 mg/day and maintain for 1 wk. (Step 4): Increase Lamictal XR to 250-300 mg/day, then discontinue valproate.

Bipolar Disorder

PO: ADULTS, ELDERLY: Initially, 25 mg/day for 2 wks, then 50 mg/day for 2 wks, then 100 mg/day for 1 wk, then 200 mg/day beginning with wk 6.

Bipolar Disorder in Pts Receiving EIAEDs (Without Valproic Acid)

PO: ADULTS, ELDERLY: 50 mg/day for 2 wks, then 100 mg/day for 2 wks, then 200 mg/day for 1 wk, then 300 mg/day for 1 wk, then up to usual maintenance dose 400 mg/day in divided doses.

Bipolar Disorder in Pts Receiving Valproic Acid

PO: ADULTS, ELDERLY: 25 mg/day every other day for 2 wks, then 25 mg/day for 2 wks, then 50 mg/day for 1 wk, then 100 mg/day. **Usual maintenance dose with valproic acid:** 100 mg/day.

Usual Dosage for LaMICtal XR

Adjunct therapy: Range: 200–600 mg/day.
Conversion to monotherapy: Range: 250–500 mg/day.

Discontinuation Therapy

◄**ALERT**► A dosage reduction of approximately 50%/wk over at least 2 wks is recommended.

Dosage in Renal Impairment

◄**ALERT**► Decreased dosage may be effective in pts with significant renal impairment.

Dosage in Hepatic Impairment

Mild impairment: No dose adjustment. **Moderate to severe impairment without ascites:** Reduce dose by 25%. **Severe impairment with ascites:** Reduce dose by 50%.

SIDE EFFECTS

Frequent (38%–14%): Dizziness, headache, diplopia, ataxia, nausea, blurred vision, drowsiness, rhinitis. **Occasional (10%–5%):** Rash, pharyngitis, vomiting, cough, flu-like symptoms, diarrhea, dysmenorrhea, fever, insomnia, dyspepsia. **Rare:** Constipation, tremor, anxiety, pruritus, vaginitis, hypersensitivity reaction.

ADVERSE EFFECTS/TOXIC REACTIONS

Abrupt withdrawal may increase seizure frequency. Serious rashes, including Stevens-Johnson syndrome, have been reported. May increase risk of suicidal thoughts and behavior. Hemophagocytic lymphohistiocytosis, a life-threatening syndrome of extreme systemic inflammation characterized by hepatosplenomegaly, lymphadenopathy, fever, rash, organ dysfunction, has occurred. Life-threatening eosinophilia and systemic symptoms (DRESS) may occur. May increase risk of aseptic meningitis. Abrupt withdrawal may increase frequency of seizures.

NURSING CONSIDERATIONS

BASELINE ASSESSMENT

Review history of seizure disorder (type, onset, intensity, frequency, duration, LOC), medication history (esp. other anticonvulsants), other medical conditions (e.g., renal impairment). Initiate seizure precautions. Assess baseline mood, behavior. Question history of suicidal ideation and behavior.

INTERVENTION/EVALUATION

Report occurrence of rash (drug discontinuation may be necessary). Assist with ambulation if dizziness, ataxia occurs. Assess for clinical improvement (decreased intensity/frequency of seizures). Assess for visual abnormalities, headache. Monitor for suicidal ideation, depression, behavioral changes. Monitor for symptoms of DRESS.

PATIENT/ FAMILY TEACHING

• Do not abruptly discontinue medication after long-term therapy. • Avoid alcohol. • Avoid tasks that require alertness, motor skills until response to drug is established. • Carry identification card/bracelet to note anticonvulsant therapy. • Strict compliance is essential for seizure control. • Report any rash, fever, swelling of glands, worsening depression, suicidal ideation, unusual changes in behavior,

worsening of seizure control. • May cause photosensitivity reaction; avoid exposure to sunlight, ultraviolet light.

lansoprazole

lan-**soe**-pra-zole
(<u>Prevacid</u>, Prevacid Solu-Tab)
Do not confuse lansoprazole with ARIPiprazole or dexlansoprazole, or Prevacid with Pravachol, PriLOSEC, or Prinivil.

FIXED-COMBINATION(S)

Prevacid NapraPac: lansoprazole/naproxen (an NSAID): 15 mg/375 mg, 15 mg/500 mg. **Prevpac:** Combination card containing amoxicillin 500 mg (4 capsules), lansoprazole 30 mg (2 capsules), clarithromycin 500 mg (2 tablets).

◆ CLASSIFICATION

PHARMACOTHERAPEUTIC: Proton pump inhibitor. **CLINICAL:** Anti-ulcer agent.

USES

Duodenal ulcer: Short-term treatment (for 4 wks) for healing and symptom relief of active duodenal ulcer. Maintain healing of duodenal ulcers. *H. pylori* **eradication:** Eradication of *H. pylori* to reduce risk of duodenal ulcer recurrence. **Gastric ulcer:** Short-term treatment (for up to 8 wks) for healing and symptom relief of active benign gastric ulcer. Treatment of NSAID-associated gastric ulcer. To reduce risk of NSAID-associated gastric ulcers in pts requiring the use of an NSAID. **Treatment of symptomatic gastroesophageal reflux disease (GERD):** Short-term treatment in adults and pts 12–17 yrs of age (for up to 8 wks) and pts 1–11 yrs of age (for up to 12 wks) for the treatment of heartburn and other symptoms associated with GERD. Healing and symptom relief of all grades of erosive esophagitis (EE). **Pathological**

hypersecretory conditions: Long-term treatment of pathological hypersecretory conditions, including Zollinger-Ellison syndrome. **OTC:** Relief of frequent heartburn (2 or more days/wk). **OFF-LABEL:** Stress ulcer prophylaxis in critically ill. Eosinophilic esophagitis, dyspepsia.

PRECAUTIONS

Contraindications: Hypersensitivity to lansoprazole, other proton pump inhibitors. Concomitant use with rilpivirine. **Cautions:** Hepatic impairment. May increase risk of hip, wrist, spine fractures; GI infections.

ACTION

Inhibits the (H^+, K^+)–ATPase enzyme system, blocking the final step in gastric acid secretion. **Therapeutic Effect:** Suppresses gastric acid secretion.

PHARMACOKINETICS

Rapid, complete absorption (food may decrease absorption) once drug has left stomach. Protein binding: 97%. Distributed primarily to gastric parietal cells. Metabolized in liver. Excreted in bile and urine. Not removed by hemodialysis. **Half-life:** 1.5 hrs (increased in hepatic impairment, elderly).

⧗ LIFESPAN CONSIDERATIONS

Pregnancy/Lactation: Unknown if distributed in breast milk. **Children:** Safety and efficacy not established in pts younger than 1 yr. **Elderly:** No age-related precautions noted, but doses greater than 30 mg not recommended.

INTERACTIONS

DRUG: May decrease concentration/effect of **acalabrutinib, atazanavir, cefuroxime, clopidogrel, erlotinib, neratinib, pazopanib, risedronate.** May increase effect of **warfarin.** Strong CYP2C19 inducers (e.g., **FLUoxetine**), strong CYP3A4 inducers (e.g., **carBAMazepine, phenytoin, rifAMPin**) may decrease concentration/effect. **HERBAL:** St. John's wort may decrease concentration/effect. **FOOD:** **Food** may decrease absorption. **LAB VALUES:** May increase serum LDH, alkaline phosphatase, bilirubin, cholesterol, creatinine, ALT, AST, triglycerides, uric acid; Hgb, Hct. May produce abnormal albumin/globulin ratio, electrolyte balance, platelet, RBC, WBC.

AVAILABILITY (Rx)

Tablets, Orally Disintegrating: 15 mg, 30 mg.

🦫 **Capsules, Delayed-Release:** 15 mg, 30 mg.

ADMINISTRATION/HANDLING
PO

• Administer 30–60 min before a meal. Intact granules should not be chewed or crushed. • Capsules may be opened and sprinkled on applesauce or mixed with apple, orange, or tomato juice and swallowed immediately. • SoluTab should not be swallowed whole, broken, cut or chewed. Place on tongue and allow to dissolve with or without water..

INDICATIONS/ROUTES/DOSAGE

Duodenal Ulcer

PO: ADULTS, ELDERLY: 15 mg/day, for up to 4 wks. **Maintenance:** 15 mg/day.

Erosive Esophagitis

PO: ADULTS, ELDERLY: 30 mg/day, for up to 8 wks. If healing does not occur within 8 wks may give for additional 8 wks. **Maintenance:** 15 mg/day. **CHILDREN 1–11 YRS, WEIGHING MORE THAN 30 KG:** 30 mg/day for up to 12 wks; **WEIGHING 30 KG OR LESS:** 15 mg/day for up to 12 wks.

Gastric Ulcer

PO: ADULTS: 30 mg/day for up to 8 wks.

NSAID Gastric Ulcer

PO: ADULTS, ELDERLY: Healing: 30 mg/day for up to 8 wks. **Prevention:** 15 mg/day for up to 12 wks.

Gastroesophageal Reflux Disease (GERD)

PO: ADULTS: 15 mg/day for up to 8 wks. If symptoms persist after 8 wks, may increase to 30 mg once daily. Once

L

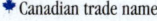 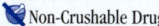

symptoms are controlled, continue treatment for at least 8 wks. **CHILDREN 12–17 YRS:** 30 mg/day up to 8 wks. **CHILDREN 1–11 YRS, WEIGHING MORE THAN 30 KG:** 30 mg/day for up to 8 wks; **WEIGHING 30 KG OR LESS:** 15 mg/day for up to 8 wks.

H. pylori Infection
PO: ADULTS, ELDERLY: (triple drug therapy including amoxicillin, clarithromycin) 30 mg q12h for 10–14 days or (with amoxicillin) 30 mg 3 times/day for 14 days.

Pathologic Hypersecretory Conditions (Including Zollinger-Ellison Syndrome)
PO: ADULTS, ELDERLY: Initially, 60 mg/day. Individualize dosage according to pt needs and for as long as clinically indicated. Administer doses greater than 120 mg/day in divided doses.

Heartburn (OTC)
PO: ADULTS, ELDERLY: 15 mg once daily for 14 days. May repeat q4mos.

Dosage in Renal Impairment
No dose adjustment.

Dosage in Hepatic Impairment
Consider dose reduction in severe impairment.

SIDE EFFECTS
Occasional (3%–2%): Diarrhea, abdominal pain, rash, pruritus, altered appetite. **Rare (1%):** Nausea, headache.

ADVERSE EFFECTS/TOXIC REACTIONS
Bilirubinemia, eosinophilia, hyperlipidemia occur rarely. May increase risk of *C. difficile* infection. Chronic use may increase risk of osteoporosis, fractures.

NURSING CONSIDERATIONS

BASELINE ASSESSMENT
Assess for epigastric/abdominal pain, evidence of GI bleeding.

INTERVENTION/EVALUATION
Assess for therapeutic response (relief of GI symptoms). Question if diarrhea, abdominal pain, nausea occurs. Obtain *C. difficile* PCR test in pts with persistent diarrhea, fever, abdominal pain.

PATIENT/ FAMILY TEACHING
• Do not chew, crush delayed-release capsules. • For pts who have difficulty swallowing capsules, open capsules, sprinkle granules on 1 tbsp of applesauce, swallow immediately.

lapatinib
la-**pa**-tin-ib
(Tykerb)
■ **BLACK BOX ALERT** ■ Hepatotoxicity (serum ALT or AST more than 3 times upper limit of normal [ULN] and total bilirubin more than 2 times ULN), possibly severe, has occurred. **Do not confuse lapatinib with dasatinib, erlotinib, or imatinib.**

◆CLASSIFICATION
PHARMACOTHERAPEUTIC: Epidermal growth factor receptor (EGFR) inhibitor. Tyrosine kinase inhibitor. **CLINICAL:** Antineoplastic.

USES
Combination treatment with capecitabine for the treatment of human epidermal growth receptor type 2 (HER2)–overexpressing advanced or metastatic breast cancer in pts who have received prior therapy including an anthracycline, a taxane, and trastuzumab. Combination treatment with letrozole for treatment of postmenopausal women with *HER2*-overexpressing hormone receptor–positive metastatic breast cancer for whom hormonal therapy is indicated. **OFF-LABEL:** Treatment (in combination with trastuzumab) of *HER2*-overexpressing metastatic breast cancer that progressed on prior trastuzumab-containing therapy. Treatment of *HER2*-overexpressing metastatic breast cancer with brain metastasis.

PRECAUTIONS

Contraindications: Hypersensitivity to lapatinib. **Cautions:** Baseline cytopenias, conditions predisposing to infection (e.g., diabetes, renal failure, immunocompromised pts, open wounds), hepatic impairment, cardiac disease, HF; pts at risk for QT interval prolongation (congenital long QT syndrome, HF, medications that prolong QT interval, hypokalemia, hypomagnesemia); History of treatment with anthracyclines, chest wall irradiation. Avoid concurrent use with strong CYP3A4 inhibitors or inducers.

ACTION

Reversible inhibitory action against kinases targeting intracellular components of epidermal growth factor receptor ErbB1 and a second receptor, human epidermal receptor (HER2 [ErbB2]). **Therapeutic Effect:** Inhibits tumor cell growth and metastasis.

PHARMACOKINETICS

Route	Onset	Peak	Duration
PO	30 min	4 hrs	—

Steady-state level reached within 6–7 days. Incomplete and variable oral absorption. Metabolized in liver. Protein binding: 99%. Minimally excreted in feces and plasma. **Half-life:** 24 hrs.

LIFESPAN CONSIDERATIONS

Pregnancy/Lactation: Avoid pregnancy; may cause fetal harm. Females and males with female partners of reproductive potential must use effective contraception during treatment and for at least 1 wk after discontinuation. Breastfeeding not recommended during treatment and for at least 1 wk after discontinuation. **Children:** Safety and efficacy not established. **Elderly:** No age-related precautions noted.

INTERACTIONS

DRUG: QT interval–prolonging medications (e.g., amiodarone, azithromycin, ceritinib, haloperidol, moxifloxacin) may increase risk of QT interval prolongation, cardiac arrhythmias. **CYP3A4 inhibitors (e.g., clarithromycin, ketoconazole, ritonavir)**, **dexamethasone** may increase concentration/effect. **CYP3A4 inducers (e.g., carBAMazepine, phenytoin, rifAMPin)** may decrease concentration/effect. **HERBAL:** St. John's wort decreases concentration/effect. **FOOD: Grapefruit products** may increase concentration/effect. (potential for torsades, myelotoxicity). **LAB VALUES:** May increase serum ALT, AST, bilirubin. May decrease neutrophils, Hgb, platelets.

AVAILABILITY (Rx)

Tablets: 250 mg.

ADMINISTRATION/HANDLING

PO
• Do not break, crush, dissolve, or divide film-coated tablets. • Give at least 1 hr before or 1 hr after food. Take full dose at same time each day.

INDICATIONS/ROUTES/DOSAGE

Breast Cancer

PO: ADULTS, ELDERLY: With capecitabine: 1,250 mg (5 tablets) once daily. **With letrozole:** 1,500 mg (6 tablets) once daily continuously with letrozole. Continue until disease progresses or unacceptable toxicity.

Dose Modification

Cardiac Toxicity

Discontinue with decreased left ventricular ejection fraction Grade 2 or higher, or in pts with an ejection fraction that drops to lower limit of normal. May be started at a reduced dose (1,000 mg/day) at a minimum of 2 wks when ejection fraction returns to normal and pt is asymptomatic.

Pulmonary Toxicity

Discontinue with symptoms indicative of interstitial lung disease or pneumonitis Grade 3 or higher.

Severe Hepatic Impairment

With capecitabine: 750 mg/day. **With letrozole:** 1,000 mg/day.

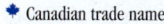 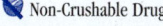 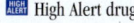

Concomitant Use of CYP3A4 Inhibitors/Inducers

Concomitant use of CYP3A4 inhibitors may require dose reduction of lapatinib (e.g., decrease to 500 mg/day with careful monitoring); CYP3A4 inducers may require dose increase of lapatinib (e.g., increase to 4,500 mg with capecitabine or 5,500 mg with letrozole).

Dosage in Renal Impairment

No dose adjustment.

Dosage in Hepatic Impairment

Mild to moderate impairment: No dose adjustment. **Severe impairment:** See dose modification.

SIDE EFFECTS

Common (65%–44%): Diarrhea, hand-foot syndrome (blistering/rash/peeling of skin on palms of hands, soles of feet), nausea. **Frequent (28%–26%):** Rash, vomiting. **Occasional (15%–10%):** Mucosal inflammation, stomatitis, extremity pain, back pain, dry skin, insomnia.

ADVERSE EFFECTS/TOXIC REACTIONS

May cause cardiac toxicity, decreased LVEF, ILD/pneumonitis. Life-threatening hepatotoxicity may occur days to several mos after initiation. Grade 3 or 4 diarrhea reported in less than 10% and less than 15% of pts, respectively. Concentration-dependent QT interval prolongation may occur. Life-threatening cutaneous reactions including erythema multiforme, Stevens-Johnson syndrome, toxic epidermal necrolysis were reported.

NURSING CONSIDERATIONS

BASELINE ASSESSMENT

Obtain CBC, BMP, LFT, ECG; pregnancy test in females of reproductive potential. Confirm compliance of effective contraception. Assess LVEF by echocardiogram. Confirm *HER2*-positive status. Question history pulmonary disease, hepatic/renal impairment, cardiac disease, HF. Screen for active infection. Assess hydration status. Receive full medication history and screen for interactions. Offer emotional support.

INTERVENTION/EVALUATION

Monitor CBC for myelosuppression; LFT for hepatotoxicity (abdominal pain, nausea, jaundice, weight loss); ECG for QT interval prolongation. Monitor serum electrolytes if severe diarrhea occurs. Diarrhea must be treated promptly. Consider ABG, radiologic test if ILD/pneumonitis (excessive cough, dyspnea, fever, hypoxia) is suspected. Consider treatment with corticosteroids if ILD/pneumonitis is confirmed. Assess LVEF by echocardiogram as clinically indicated. Monitor for infections (cough, fatigue, fever). If serious infection occurs, initiate appropriate antimicrobial therapy. Monitor daily pattern of bowel activity, stool consistency. Monitor for toxicities if discontinuation or dose reduction of strong CYP3A4 inhibitor is avoidable. Assess skin for cutaneous toxicities.

PATIENT/FAMILY TEACHING

• Treatment may depress your immune system response and reduce your ability to fight infection. Report symptoms of infection such as body aches, chills, cough, fatigue, fever. Avoid those with active infection. • Report symptoms of bone marrow depression (e.g., bruising, fatigue, fever, shortness of breath, weight loss; bleeding easily, bloody urine or stool). • Report symptoms of lung inflammation (excessive coughing, difficulty breathing, chest pain); heart failure (e.g., chest pain, difficulty breathing, palpitations, swelling of extremities); liver problems (abdominal pain, bruising, clay-colored stool, amber- or dark-colored urine, yellowing of the skin or eyes). • Treatment may reduce the heart's ability to pump effectively; expect routine echocardiograms. • Use effective contraception to avoid pregnancy. Do not breastfeed. • Diarrhea is a common side effect. • Maintain proper hydration and nutrition. • There is a high risk of interactions with other medications. Do not take newly prescribed medications unless approved by prescriber who originally started treatment.

larotrectinib

lar-oh-**trek**-ti-nib
(Vitrakvi)
**Do not confuse larotrectinib
with alectinib, lapatinib, lenvatinib, or lorlatinib.**

◆CLASSIFICATION

PHARMACOTHERAPEUTIC: Tropomy-
osin receptor kinase (TRK) inhibitor.
Tyrosine kinase inhibitor. **CLINICAL:**
Antineoplastic.

USES

Treatment of adult and pediatric pts with
solid tumors that have a neurotrophic
receptor tyrosine kinase *(NTRK)* gene fusion without a known acquired resistance
mutation; are metastatic or where surgical resection is likely to result in severe
morbidity; and have no satisfactory alternative treatment or that have progressed
following treatment.

PRECAUTIONS

Contraindications: Hypersensitivity to
larotrectinib. **Cautions:** Baseline anemia,
neutropenia; hepatic impairment, active
infection, conditions predisposing to infection (e.g., diabetes, renal failure, immunocompromised pts, open wounds);
concomitant use of strong CYP3A4 provided oral syringe when measuring dose
inhibitors, strong CYP3A4 inducers.

ACTION

Inhibits activation of tropomyosin receptor kinase (TRK) proteins resulting from
NTRK gene fusions, deletion of protein
regulatory domain, or in cells with overexpression of TRK proteins. **Therapeutic
Effect:** Inhibits tumor cell proliferation.

PHARMACOKINETICS

Widely distributed. Metabolized in liver.
Protein binding: 70%. Excreted in feces
(58%), urine (39%). **Half-life:** 2.9 hrs.

⧖ LIFESPAN CONSIDERATIONS

Pregnancy/Lactation: Avoid pregnancy; may cause fetal harm. Females and
males with female partners of reproductive potential must use effective contraception during treatment and for at least
1 wk after discontinuation. Unknown if
distributed in breast milk. Breastfeeding
not recommended during treatment and
for at least 1 wk after discontinuation. May
impair fertility. **Children:** May have increased risk of increased weight, neutropenia. **Elderly:** Not specified; use caution.

INTERACTIONS

**DRUG: Strong CYP3A4 inhibitors
(e.g., clarithromycin, ketoconazole)**
may increase concentration/effect.
**Strong CYP3A4 inducers (e.g., car-
BAMazepine, phenytoin, rifAMPin)**
may decrease concentration/effect.
HERBAL: None significant. **FOOD: Grapefruit products** may increase concentra-
tion/effect. **LAB VALUES:** May increase
serum alkaline phosphatase, ALT, AST.
May decrease serum albumin; Hgb, neutrophils, RBCs.

AVAILABILITY (Rx)

Capsules: 25 mg, 100 mg. **Solution, Oral:**
20 mg/mL.

ADMINISTRATION/HANDLING

PO
• Give without regard to food. • Cap-
sules/oral solution may be used interchangeably. • If vomiting occurs after
administration, give next dose at regularly
scheduled time. • Do not give a missed
dose within 6 hrs of next dose. **Capsules:**
Administer capsules whole with water; do
not break, cut, or open. • Capsules cannot be chewed. **Solution, Oral:** Refrigerate glass bottle. Do not freeze. • Discard
unused contents after 90 days of first
opening bottle. • See manufacturer
guidelines regarding preparation and administration of oral solution. Use provided
oral syringe when measuring dose.

L

◆ Canadian trade name   Non-Crushable Drug   HIGH ALERT High Alert drug

L

INDICATIONS/ROUTES/DOSAGE

Solid Tumors

PO: ADULTS, CHILDREN WITH BODY SUR-FACE AREA OF AT LEAST 1 m²: 100 mg twice daily. Continue until disease progression or unacceptable toxicity. **CHILDREN WITH BODY SURFACE AREA LESS THAN 1 m²:** 100 mg/m² twice daily. Continue until disease progression or unacceptable toxicity.

Dose Reduction Schedule

Dose Reduction for Adverse Reactions	Adults/ Children With Body Surface Area of at Least 1 m²	Children With Body Surface Area Less Than 1 m²
First	75 mg twice daily	75 mg/m² twice daily
Second	50 mg twice daily	50 mg/m² twice daily
Third	100 mg once daily	25 mg/m² twice daily

Dose Modification

Based on Common Terminology Criteria for Adverse Events (CTCAE).

Any Grade 3 or 4 Adverse Reaction

Note (includes hepatotoxicity and neurotoxicity): Withhold treatment until resolved or improved to Grade 1, then resume at reduced dose level. If not resolved within 4 wks, permanently discontinue.

Concomitant Use of Strong CYP3A4 Inhibitor

If strong CYP3A44 inhibitor cannot be discontinued, reduce larotrectinib dose by 50%. If strong CYP3A4 inhibitor is discontinued for 3–5 half-lives, resume larotrectinib dose prior to use of strong CYP3A4 inhibitor.

Concomitant Use of Strong CYP3A4 Inducer

If strong CYP3A4 inducer cannot be discontinued, double the larotrectinib dose. If strong CYP3A4 inducer is discontinued for 3–5 half-lives, resume larotrectinib dose prior to use of strong CYP3A4 inducer.

Dosage in Renal Impairment

No dose adjustment.

Dosage in Hepatic Impairment

Mild impairment: No dose adjustment. **Moderate to severe impairment:** Reduce starting dose by 50%.

SIDE EFFECTS

Frequent (37%–15%): Fatigue, nausea, dizziness, cough, vomiting, constipation, diarrhea, pyrexia, dyspnea, increased weight, peripheral edema. **Occasional (14%–11%):** Arthralgia, myalgia, muscular weakness, headache, abdominal pain, decreased appetite, back pain, extremity pain, nasal congestion, hypertension.

ADVERSE EFFECTS/TOXIC REACTIONS

Myelosuppression (anemia, neutropenia) is an expected response to therapy. Neurotoxic events including delirium, dysarthria, dizziness, gait disturbance, memory impairment, paresthesia, tremor occurred in 53% of pts. Grade 4 encephalopathy reported in less than 1% of pts. Hepatotoxicity with transaminase elevations of any grade reported in 45%. Grade 3 hepatotoxicity reported in 6% of pts. Falls reported in 10% of pts.

NURSING CONSIDERATIONS

BASELINE ASSESSMENT

Obtain CBC, LFT; pregnancy test in females of reproductive potential. Confirm presence of *NTRK* gene fusion in tumor specimen. Screen for active infection. Confirm compliance of effective contraception. Question history of hepatic impairment. Receive full medication history and screen for interactions. Initiate fall precautions. Offer emotional support.

INTERVENTION/EVALUATION

Monitor CBC for anemia, neutropenia periodically; LFT for hepatotoxicity (bruising, hematuria, jaundice, right upper abdominal pain, nausea, vomiting, weight loss) q2wks for 4 wks, then monthly thereafter (or as clinically indicated). Monitor for neurotoxicities. If concomitant use of strong CYP3A4 inhibitor or strong CYP3A4 inducer is unavoidable, monitor for drug toxicities. Closely screen for infections (cough, fatigue, fever).

PATIENT/FAMILY TEACHING

• Treatment may depress your immune system response and reduce your ability to fight infection. Report symptoms of infection such as body aches, chills, cough, fatigue, fever. Avoid those with active infection. • Nervous system changes including altered memory, confusion, delirium, difficulty speaking, gait disturbance, numbness, tremors may occur. Avoid tasks that require alertness, motor skills if neurologic effects are occurring. • Use effective contraception to avoid pregnancy. Do not breastfeed. • Report liver problems (abdominal pain, bruising, clay-colored stool, amber- or dark-colored urine, yellowing of the skin or eyes). • There is a high risk of interactions with other medications. Do not take newly prescribed medications unless approved by prescriber who originally started treatment. • Avoid grapefruit products, herbal supplements (esp. St. John's wort).

---

lecanemab-irmb

lek-**an**-e-mab-irmb
(Leqembi)

■ **BLACK BOX ALERT** ■ Monoclonal antibodies used for aggregated forms of beta amyloid may cause amyloid-related imaging abnormalities (ARIAs), characterized as ARIA with edema (ARIA-E) or ARIA with hemosiderin deposition (ARIA-H). Pts with apolipoprotein E (ApoE) e4 homozygotes have a higher incidence of ARIA compared to heterozygotes and noncarriers when treated with amyloid beta–directed antibodies. Life-threatening intracranial hemorrhages were reported.
Do not confuse lecanemab with donanemab.

◆ CLASSIFICATION

PHARMACOTHERAPEUTIC: Amyloid beta–directed antibody. **CLINICAL:** Immunoglobulin gamma 1 (IgG1) monoclonal antibody; anti–Alzheimer's disease agent.

USES

Treatment of Alzheimer's disease in pts with mild cognitive impairment or mild dementia stage of disease.

PRECAUTIONS

Contraindications: Hypersensitivity to lecanemab. **Cautions:** History of intracranial hemorrhage. Concomitant use of antithrombotic medications.

ACTION

Targets aggregated forms of amyloid beta proteins (accumulates in brain of pts with Alzheimer's disease). **Therapeutic Effect:** Slows cognitive/functional decline in mild Alzheimer's disease dementia.

PHARMACOKINETICS

Widely distributed. Degraded by proteolytic enzymes. Steady state reached in 6 wks. **Half-life:** 5–7 days.

⌛ LIFESPAN CONSIDERATIONS

Pregnancy/Lactation: Unknown if distributed in breast milk. **Children:** Safety and efficacy not established. **Elderly:** No age-related precautions noted.

INTERACTIONS

DRUG: Anticoagulants (e.g., heparin, rivaroxaban, warfarin), thrombolytic agents (e.g., tissue plasminogen activator) may increase risk of

L

---

intracranial hemorrhage. **HERBAL:** None significant. **FOOD:** None known. **LAB VALUES:** May decrease lymphocytes, neutrophils.

AVAILABILITY (Rx)

Injection Solution: 500 mg/5 mL (100 mg/mL), 200 mg/2 mL (100 mg/mL).

ADMINISTRATION/HANDLING

🛢 IV

Infusion Guidelines • Infuse via a dedicated IV line using a sterile, non-protein-binding 0.2 micron in-line filter. • Do not administer as IV push or bolus. • Upon completion of infusion, flush infusion line to ensure the entire dose is administered. • Consider administration of an antihistamine, acetaminophen, NSAIDs, or corticosteroids for future infusions if an infusion reaction has occurred.

Dilution • Calculate the number of vials needed for solution based on weight in kg. • Visually inspect for particulate matter or discoloration. Solution should appear clear to slightly opalescent, colorless to pale yellow. Do not use if solution is cloudy, discolored, or if visible particles are observed. • Dilute in a 250-mL infusion bag containing 0.9% NaCl. • Mix by gentle inversion. Do not shake or agitate. • Discard used portions of vial(s).

Rate of Administration • Infuse over 1 hr. Infusion rate may be slowed or interrupted based on infusion reactions.

Storage • Refrigerate unused vials in original carton. Do not freeze. Protect from light. • Diluted solution may be refrigerated or stored at room temperature for up to 4 hrs. Do not freeze. • Allow diluted solution bag to warm to room temperature before administration.

INDICATIONS/ROUTES/DOSAGE

Alzheimer's Disease

IV: ADULTS, ELDERLY: 10 mg/kg once q2wks.

Dose Modifications

Pts With ARIA-E

Severity of Clinical Symptoms	ARIA-E Severity on MRI		
	Mild	Moderate	Severe
Asymptomatic	Continue treatment	Withhold treatment	Withhold
Mild	Continue treatment based on clinical judgment	Withhold treatment	Withhold treatment
Moderate to Severe	Withhold treatment		

Pts With ARIA-H

Severity of Clinical Symptoms	ARIA-H Severity on MRI		
	Mild	Moderate	Severe
Asymptomatic	Continue treatment	Withhold treatment	Withhold treatment
Symptomatic	Withhold treatment	Withhold treatment	

Dosage in Hepatic/Renal Impairment

No dose adjustment.

SIDE EFFECTS

Occasional (14%–6%): Headache, cough, diarrhea, rash.

ADVERSE EFFECTS/TOXIC REACTIONS

May cause ARIA, ARIA-E, or ARIA-H, including microhemorrhage and superficial siderosis. ARIA can spontaneously occur in pts with Alzheimer's disease and can range from asymptomatic to life-threatening. Pts with apolipoprotein E e4 homozygotes have a higher incidence of ARIA compared to heterozygotes and noncarriers when treated with amyloid beta–directed antibodies. Symptoms of ARIA include confusion, dizziness, focal deficits, headache, nausea, visual changes, and gait difficulty. Intracerebral hemorrhage greater than 1 cm in diameter reported in less than 1% of pts. Hypersensitivity reactions including anaphylaxis, angioedema, broncho-spasm were reported. Infusion-related reactions including body aches, chills, hypertension, hypotension, joint pain, oxygen desaturation, nausea, vomiting may occur.

rapid heart rate, rash, swelling of the face or tongue requires immediately medical attention. • Treatment is not a cure for Alzheimer's disease, but may slow the progression of symptoms.

NURSING CONSIDERATIONS

BASELINE ASSESSMENT
Obtain weight in kg. Test for ApoE e4 homozygotes and confirm presence of amyloid beta pathology prior to initiation. Obtain MRI of brain at baseline and prior to 5th, 7th, and 14th infusion to monitor for ARIA. Question history of hypersensi-tivity reactions, infusion reactions prior to each infusion. Assess cognitive func-tion (e.g., memory attention, reasoning), activities of daily living.

INTERVENTION/EVALUATION
Monitor for symptoms of ARIA (aphasia, confusion, dizziness, headache, nausea, weakness, or seizure, vision changes), intracranial hemorrhage (altered mental status, aphasia, blindness, hemiparesis, unequal pupils, seizures). Monitor for hypersensitivity reactions, infusion re-actions during each infusion. Decrease the infusion rate or discontinue infusion if reactions occur. Consider treatment with an antihistamine, acetaminophen, NSAIDs, or corticosteroids (including pretreatment for future doses). Monitor behavior, mood/cognitive function, activi-ties of daily living.

PATIENT/FAMILY TEACHING
• MRIs of the brain will be obtained to assess for ARIA. ARIA may present as swelling in areas of the brain, which usually resolves over time. Some areas may contain small spots of bleeding that may be asymptomatic or life-threatening. • Life-threatening bleeding in the brain may occur; report confusion, difficulty speaking, one-sided weakness, vision changes, seizures. • Severe allergic re-actions, including anaphylaxis, may oc-cur. Difficulty breathing, dizziness, hives,

ledipasvir/sofosbuvir

le-**dip**-as-vir/soe-**fos**-bue-vir
(Harvoni)

■ **BLACK BOX ALERT** ■ Test all pts for hepatitis B virus (HBV) infection prior to initiation. HBV reactivation was reported in HCV/HBV coinfected pts who were undergoing or had completed treat-ment with HCV direct-acting anti-virals and were not receiving HBV antiviral therapy. HBV reactivation may cause fulminant hepatitis, hepatic failure, and death.
Do not confuse ledipasvir with daclatasvir, elbasvir, or ombitas-vir, or sofosbuvir with dasabuvir.

◆CLASSIFICATION

PHARMACOTHERAPEUTIC: Combi-nation nucleotide analog NS5A in-hibitor and nucleotide analog NS5B polymerase inhibitor. **CLINICAL:** An-tihepaciviral.

USES
Treatment of chronic hepatitis C virus (HCV) in adults and children 3 yrs of age and older with genotype 1, 4, 5, or 6 infec-tion without cirrhosis or with compensated cirrhosis; genotype 1 infection in adults and children 3 yrs of age and older with decompensated cirrhosis, in combination with ribavirin; genotype 1 or 4 infection in adults and children 3 yrs of age and older who are liver transplant recipients without cirrhosis or with compensated cirrhosis, in combination with ribavirin.

PRECAUTIONS
Note: If used with ribavirin, the Contra-indications and Cautions for the use of ribavirin also apply.

L

Contraindications: Hypersensitivity to ledipasvir, sofosbuvir. **Cautions:** Advanced hepatic disease, HIV infection, hepatitis B virus infection. Concomitant use of amiodarone (with or without beta blockers) in pts with underlying cardiac disease. Concomitant use of P-glycoprotein (P-gp) inducers not recommended.

ACTION

Ledipasvir inhibits HCV NS5A protein, essential for viral replication. Sofosbuvir is converted to its active form and inhibits NS5B RNA-dependent RNA polymerase, also essential for viral replication. **Therapeutic Effect:** Inhibits viral replication of HCV.

PHARMACOKINETICS

Widely absorbed. Ledipasvir is metabolized by oxidative processes. Sofosbuvir is metabolized in liver. Protein binding: 99.8% (ledipasvir), 61%–65% (sofosbuvir). Peak plasma concentration: 4–4.5 hrs (ledipasvir), 0.8–1 hr (sofosbuvir). Ledipasvir is excreted in feces (87%) and urine (1%). Sofosbuvir is excreted in urine (80%), feces (14%). **Half-life:** 47 hrs (ledipasvir), 0.4 hr (sofosbuvir).

⌛ LIFESPAN CONSIDERATIONS

Pregnancy/Lactation: Unknown if ledipasvir or sofosbuvir is distributed in breast milk. When administered with ribavirin, therapy is contraindicated in pregnant women and in men whose female partners are pregnant. **Children:** Safety and efficacy not established in pts younger than 3 yrs of age or weigh less than 35 kg. **Elderly:** No age-related precautions noted.

INTERACTIONS

DRUG: May enhance bradycardic effect of **amiodarone**. May increase concentration of **rosuvastatin**. **Aluminum- or magnesium-containing antacids, H₂-receptor antagonists (e.g., famotidine), proton pump inhibitors (e.g., omeprazole), anticonvulsants** (e.g., **carBAMazepine, oxcarbazepine, phenobarbital, primidone**), **antimycobacterials** (e.g., **rifAMPin**) may decrease concentration/effects. **HERBAL:** None significant. **FOOD:** None known. **LAB VALUES:** May increase serum bilirubin.

AVAILABILITY (Rx)

Tablets, Fixed-Dose Combination: 90 mg (ledipasvir)/400 mg (sofosbuvir). **Oral Pellets:** 45 mg (ledipasvir)/200 mg (sofosbuvir); 33.75 mg (ledipasvir)/150 mg (sofosbuvir).

ADMINISTRATION/HANDLING

PO
• Give without regard to food. • **Pellets:** Do not allow chewing. • If administered with food, sprinkle on one or more spoonfuls of nonacidic, soft food at or below room temperature. • Give within 30 min after gently mixing with food.

INDICATIONS/ROUTES/DOSAGE

Hepatitis C Virus Infection

PO: ADULTS, ELDERLY, CHILDREN 3 YRS OF AGE AND OLDER, WEIGHING 35 KG OR MORE: 90 mg/400 mg once daily; **17–34 KG:** 45 mg/200 mg once daily; **LESS THAN 17 KG:** 33.75 mg/150 mg once daily. See manufacturer guidelines for treatment with ribavirin.

Treatment Regimen and Duration for Adults, Elderly, Pts 3 Yrs of Age and Older
Genotype 1
Treatment-naive without cirrhosis or with compensated cirrhosis (Child-Pugh A): Ledipasvir/sofosbuvir for 12 wks. Treatment for 8 wks may be considered. **Treatment-experienced without cirrhosis:** Ledipasvir/sofosbuvir for 12 wks. **Treatment-experienced with compensated cirrhosis (Child-Pugh A):** Ledipasvir/sofosbuvir for 24 wks. **Treatment-naive and treatment-experienced with decompensated cirrhosis (Child-Pugh B or C):** Ledipasvir/sofosbuvir plus ribavirin for 12 wks.

Genotype 1 or 4
Treatment-naive and treatment-experienced liver transplant recipients without cirrhosis or with compensated cirrhosis (Child-Pugh A): Ledipasvir/sofosbuvir plus ribavirin for 12 wks.

Genotype 4, 5, or 6
Treatment-naive and treatment-experienced without cirrhosis or with compensated cirrhosis (Child-Pugh A): Ledipasvir/sofosbuvir for 12 wks.

Dosage in Renal Impairment
Mild to moderate impairment: No dose adjustment. **Severe impairment:** Not specified; use caution.

Dosage in Hepatic Impairment
No dose adjustment.

SIDE EFFECTS

Occasional (16%–4%): Fatigue, headache, nausea, diarrhea. **Rare (3%):** Insomnia. **Ribavirin: Frequent (31%–29%):** Asthenia, headache. **Occasional (18%–5%):** Fatigue, myalgia, irritability, dizziness. **Rare (3%):** Dyspnea.

ADVERSE EFFECTS/TOXIC REACTIONS

HBV reactivation was reported in pts co-infected with HBV/HCV; may result in fulminant hepatitis, hepatic failure, death. Cardiac arrest, symptomatic bradycardia, pacemaker implantation was reported in pts taking concomitant amiodarone. Bradycardia usually occurred within hrs to days, but may occur up to 2 wks after initiation. Pts with underlying cardiac disease, advanced hepatic disease, or pts taking concomitant beta blockers are at an increased risk for bradycardia when used concomitantly with amiodarone. Psychiatric disorders including depression may occur.

NURSING CONSIDERATIONS

BASELINE ASSESSMENT

Obtain LFT, HCV-RNA level; pregnancy test in females of reproductive potential; CBC for pts treated with ribavirin. Confirm HCV genotype. Test all pts for HBV infection prior to initiation. Receive full medication history and screen for contraindications/interactions, esp. concomitant use of amiodarone. Question for history of chronic anemia, HBV infection, HIV infection, liver transplantation.

INTERVENTION/EVALUATION

Periodically monitor LFT, HCV-RNA level for treatment effectiveness. Closely monitor for exacerbation of hepatitis or HBV reactivation. If unable to discontinue amiodarone, consider inpatient cardiac monitoring for at least 48 hrs, followed by outpatient or self-monitoring of heart rate for at least 2 wks after initiation. Cardiac monitoring is also recommended in pts who discontinue amiodarone just prior to initiation. In females of reproductive potential who are taking concomitant ribavirin, reinforce birth control compliance and obtain monthly pregnancy tests. Monitor for new-onset or worsening of depression

PATIENT/FAMILY TEACHING

• Pts who take amiodarone (an antiarrhythmic) during therapy may require inpatient and outpatient cardiac monitoring (and in some cases pacemaker implantation) due to an increased risk of slow heart rate or cardiac arrest. If amiodarone therapy cannot be withheld or stopped, immediately report symptoms of slow heart rate such as chest pain, confusion, dizziness, fainting, light-headedness, memory problems, palpitations, weakness. • Treatment may be used in combination with ribavirin (inform pt of contraindications/adverse effects of ribavirin therapy). If therapy includes treatment with ribavirin, use effective contraception to avoid pregnancy. Do not breastfeed. • There is a high risk of interactions with other medications. Do not take newly prescribed medications unless approved by prescriber who originally started treatment. • Do not take herbal products. • Avoid alcohol. • Report signs of depression.

L

lenalidomide

len-a-**lid**-o-myde
(Revlimid)

■ **BLACK BOX ALERT** ■ Analogue to thalidomide. High potential for significant birth defects. Hematologic toxicity (thrombocytopenia, neutropenia) occurs in 80% of pts. Greatly increases risk for DVT, pulmonary embolism in multiple myeloma pts.
Do not confuse lenalidomide with thalidomide.

◆**CLASSIFICATION**

PHARMACOTHERAPEUTIC: Angiogenesis inhibitor. **CLINICAL:** Antineoplastic.

USES

Myelodysplastic syndrome (MDS): Treatment of low- to intermediate-risk myelodysplastic syndrome (MDS) in pts with deletion 5q cytogenetic abnormality with transfusion-dependent anemia. **Mantle cell lymphoma:** Treatment of pts with mantle cell lymphoma that has relapsed or progressed after 2 prior therapies (one of which included bortezomib). **Multiple myeloma:** Treatment of multiple myeloma (in combination with dexA-METHasone). Maintenance treatment for multiple myeloma (following autologous stem cell transplant). **Follicular lymphoma:** Treatment of previously treated follicular lymphoma (in combination with riTUXimab). **Marginal zone lymphoma:** Treatment of previously treated marginal zone lymphoma (in combination with riTUXimab). **OFF-LABEL:** Chronic lymphocytic leukemia, diffuse large B-cell lymphoma, multiple myeloma (newly diagnosed), myelodysplastic syndrome (without deletion 5q), smoldering myeloma, systemic light chain amyloidosis.

PRECAUTIONS

Contraindications: Hypersensitivity to lenalidomide. Pregnancy. **Cautions:** Renal/hepatic impairment, conditions predisposing to infection (e.g., diabetes, renal failure, immunocompromised pts, open wounds); pts at risk for tumor lysis syndrome (high tumor burden); pts at risk for thrombosis (immobility, indwelling venous catheter/access device, morbid obesity, underlying atherosclerosis, genetic hypercoagulable conditions); history of venous or arterial thrombosis (e.g., CVA, DVT, MI, pulmonary embolism). Avoid use in pts with glucose intolerance, lactase deficiency.

ACTION

Inhibits secretion of pro-inflammatory cytokines, increases secretion of anti-inflammatory cytokines. Enhances cell-mediated immunity by stimulation of T cells. **Therapeutic Effect:** Inhibits myeloma cell growth; induces cell cycle arrest and cell death.

PHARMACOKINETICS

Widely distributed. Protein binding: 30%. Excreted in urine. **Half-life:** 3 hrs (increased in renal impairment).

⧗ LIFESPAN CONSIDERATIONS

Pregnancy/Lactation: Contraindicated in pregnancy; may cause fetal harm/demise. Females of reproductive potential must have two negative pregnancy tests prior to initiation; must either remain abstinent or use two reliable forms of effective contraception, starting 4 wks prior to initiation, during treatment, and for at least 4 wks after discontinuation. Unknown if distributed in breast milk. Breastfeeding not recommended. **Males:** Distributed in semen. Males with female partners of reproductive potential must use latex or synthetic condoms with sexual activity during treatment and up to 4 wks after discontinuation. **Children:** Safety and efficacy not established. **Elderly:** Age-related renal impairment may require caution in dosage selection. Risk of toxic reactions greater in those with renal insufficiency.

INTERACTIONS

DRUG: May increase toxic effects of **abatacept, anakinra, bisphosphonate derivatives, canakinumab, leflunomide, natalizumab, rilonacept, tofacitinib, vedolizumab.** May increase immunosuppressive effects of **certolizumab, ocrelizumab. Denosumab, dipyrone, pimecrolimus** may increase risk of toxicity. **DexAMETHasone, erythropoiesis-stimulating agents, estrogens** may increase risk of thrombosis. **Ocrelizumab** may increase immunosuppressive effect. May increase adverse effects/decrease therapeutic of **vaccines (live). HERBAL:** Echinacea may decrease therapeutic effect. **FOOD:** None known. **LAB VALUES:** May decrease WBC count, Hgb, Hct platelets, troponin I, serum creatinine, sodium, T_3, T_4. May decrease serum bilirubin, glucose, potassium, magnesium.

AVAILABILITY (Rx)

Capsules: 2.5 mg, 5 mg, 10 mg, 15 mg, 20 mg, 25 mg.

ADMINISTRATION/HANDLING

• Administer at the same time each day with water. • May give without regard to food. Administer whole; do not break, open, or allow chewing. • May administer missed dose if within 12 hrs of usual dosing time.

INDICATIONS/ROUTES/DOSAGE

Myelodysplastic Syndrome

PO: **ADULTS, ELDERLY:** 10 mg once daily. Continue until disease progression or unacceptable toxicity.

Dose Modification for Myelodysplastic Syndrome

Thrombocytopenia

Thrombocytopenia within 4 wks with 10 mg/day: BASELINE PLATELETS 100,000 CELLS/mm³ OR GREATER: If platelets less than 50,000 cells/mm³, hold treatment. Resume at 5 mg/day when platelets return to 50,000 cells/mm³ or

greater. **BASELINE PLATELETS LESS THAN 100,000 CELLS/mm³:** If platelets fall to 50% of baseline, hold treatment. Resume at 5 mg/day if baseline is 60,000 cells/mm³ or greater and platelets return to 50,000 cells/mm³ or greater. Resume at 5 mg/day if baseline is less than 60,000 cells/mm³ and platelets return to 30,000 cells/mm³ or greater.

Thrombocytopenia after 4 wks with 10 mg/day: If platelets less than 30,000 cells/mm³ OR less than 50,000 cells/mm³ with platelet transfusion, hold treatment. Resume at 5 mg/day when platelets return to 30,000 cells/mm³ or greater.

Thrombocytopenia developing with 5 mg/day: If platelets less than 30,000 cells/mm³ OR less than 50,000 cells/mm³ with platelet transfusion, hold treatment. Resume at 5 mg every other day when platelets return to 30,000 cells/mm³ or greater.

Neutropenia

Neutropenia within 4 wks with 10 mg/day: BASELINE ABSOLUTE NEUTROPHIL COUNT (ANC) 1,000/MCL OR GREATER: If ANC less than 750 cells/mm³, hold treatment. Resume at 5 mg/day when ANC 1,000 cells/mm³ or greater. **BASELINE ANC LESS THAN 1,000 CELLS/MM³:** If ANC less than 500 cells/mm³, hold treatment. Resume at 5 mg/day when ANC 500 cells/mm³ or greater.

Neutropenia after 4 wks with 10 mg/day: If ANC less than 500 cells/mm³ for 7 days or longer or associated with fever, hold treatment. Resume at 5 mg/day when ANC 500 cells/mm³ or greater.

Neutropenia developing with 5 mg/day: If ANC less than 500 cells/mm³ for 7 days or longer or associated with fever, hold treatment. Resume at 5 mg every other day when ANC 500 cells/mm³ or greater.

Follicular Lymphoma, Marginal Zone Lymphoma

PO: **ADULTS, ELDERLY:** 20 mg once daily for 21 days of 28-day cycle (in combination with riTUXimab) for up to 12 cycles.

⬥ Canadian trade name   Non-Crushable Drug   **HIGH ALERT** High Alert drug

Mantle Cell Lymphoma
PO: ADULTS, ELDERLY: 25 mg once daily on days 1–21 of repeated 28-day cycle. Continue until disease progression or unacceptable toxicity.

Multiple Myeloma
PO: ADULTS, ELDERLY: 25 mg/day on days 1–21 of repeated 28-day cycle (in combination with dexAMETHasone). Continue until disease progression or unacceptable toxicity. If eligible for transplant, HSCT mobilization should occur within 4 cycles of lenalidomide-containing therapy.

Multiple Myeloma Following Auto-HSCT
PO: ADULTS, ELDERLY: 10 mg once daily continuously on days 1–28 of repeated 28-day cycle. If tolerated, may increase to 15 mg once daily after 3 cycles.

Dosage Adjustments for Multiple Myeloma
Thrombocytopenia: If platelets fall to less than 30,000 cells/mm³, hold treatment, monitor CBC. Resume at 15 mg/day when platelets 30,000 cells/mm³ or greater. For each subsequent fall to less than 30,000 cells/mm³, hold treatment and resume at 5 mg/day less than previous dose when platelets return to 30,000 cells/mm³ or greater. Do not dose to less than 5 mg/day.
Neutropenia: If neutrophils fall to less than 1,000 cells/mm³, hold treatment, add G-CSF, follow CBC wkly. Resume at 25 mg/day when neutrophils return to 1,000 cells/mm³ and neutropenia is the only toxicity. Resume at 15 mg/day if other toxicity is present. For each subsequent fall to less than 1,000 cells/mm³, hold treatment and resume at 5 mg/day less than previous dose when neutrophils return to 1,000 cells/mm³ or greater. Do not dose to less than 5 mg/day.

Dosage in Hepatic Impairment
No dose adjustment.

SIDE EFFECTS
Frequent (49%–31%): Diarrhea, pruritus, rash, fatigue. **Occasional (24%–12%):** Constipation, nausea, arthralgia, fever, back pain, peripheral edema, cough, dizziness, headache, muscle cramps, epistaxis, asthenia, dry skin, abdominal pain. **Rare (10%–5%):** Extremity pain, vomiting, generalized edema, anorexia, insomnia, night sweats, myalgia, dry mouth, ecchymosis, rigors, depression, dysgeusia, palpitations.

ADVERSE EFFECTS/TOXIC REACTIONS
Myelosuppression (anemia, leukopenia, lymphopenia, neutropenia, thrombocytopenia) is an expected response to therapy, but more severe reactions, including bone marrow depression, febrile neutropenia, may be life-threatening. May increase risk of venous thromboembolism (DVT, pulmonary embolism) and arterial thromboembolism (CVA, myocardial infarction), esp. in pts being treated for multiple myeloma. Life-threatening tumor lysis syndrome, hepatotoxicity may occur. May increase mortality in pts with multiple myeloma when pembrolizumab is added to a thalidomide analogue and dexamethasone. Severe hypersensitivity reactions, including anaphylaxis, may occur. May cause secondary malignancies, including acute myeloid leukemia, basal or squamous cell carcinoma, myelodysplastic syndrome. Other reactions may include tumor flare reaction, impaired stem cell mobilization, hyperthyroidism, hypothyroidism. Infections, including bronchitis, cellulitis, herpes

Dosage in Renal Impairment	Creatinine Clearance 30–59 mL/min	Creatinine Clearance Less Than 30 mL/min (Non-Dialysis Dependent)	Creatinine Clearance Less Than 30 mL/min (Dialysis Dependent)
Myelodysplastic syndrome	5 mg once daily	2.5 mg once daily	2.5 mg once daily (give after dialysis)
Multiple myeloma	10 mg once daily	15 mg q48h	5 mg once daily (give after dialysis)

zoster, influenza, gastroenteritis, naso-pharyngitis, pneumonia, respiratory tract infection, sepsis, sinusitis, UTI, were reported. Tumor lysis syndrome may present as acute renal failure, hypocal-cemia, hyperuricemia, hyperphosphate-mia. Dermatologic toxicities, including Stevens-Johnson syndrome, toxic epider-mal necrolysis, may occur. Drug reaction with eosinophilia and systemic symptoms (DRESS), also known as multiorgan hy-persensitivity, has been reported. DRESS may present with facial swelling, eosino-philia, fever, lymphadenopathy, and rash, which may be associated with other organ systems, such as hepatitis, hematological abnormalities, myocarditis, nephritis.

NURSING CONSIDERATIONS

BASELINE ASSESSMENT

Obtain ANC, CBC, BMP, LFT, thyroid func-tion. Obtain two negative pregnancy tests in females of reproductive potential. The first pregnancy test should be obtained within 10–14 days and the second test within 24 hrs of initiation. Confirm com-pliance of abstinence or two forms of ef-fective contraception. Due to increased risk of tumor lysis syndrome, assess hydration status routinely. Question his-tory of CVA, DVT, pulmonary embolism, recent MI; prior hypersensitivity reac-tions. Screen for active infection. Offer emotional support.

INTERVENTION/EVALUATION

Monitor CBC for myelosuppression weekly (duration based on indica-tion); LFT for hepatotoxicity (bruising, jaundice, right upper abdominal pain, nausea, vomiting, weight loss) as appro-priate; thyroid function periodically. Ob-tain pregnancy test wkly for 4 wks, then either q4wks (normal menstrual cycle) or q2wks (irregular menstrual cycle). Obtain serum uric acid level if tumor lysis syndrome (acute renal failure, elec-trolyte imbalance, cardiac arrhythmias, seizures) is suspected. Diligently moni-tor for infections (cough, fatigue, fever,

urinary urgency). Assess skin for rash, new lesions, dermatological toxicities; symptoms of drug reaction with eosino-philia and systemic symptoms. Monitor for symptoms of DVT (leg or arm pain/swelling), CVA (aphasia, altered mental status, hemiplegia, vision loss, seizures); MI (arm/jaw pain, chest pain, diaphore-sis, dyspnea), PE (chest pain, dyspnea, tachycardia).

PATIENT/FAMILY TEACHING

• Treatment may depress immune sys-tem response and reduce ability to fight infection. Report symptoms of infection such as body aches, chills, cough, fa-tigue, fever. Avoid those with active infec-tion. • Report symptoms of bone marrow depression such as bruising, fatigue, fe-ver, shortness of breath, weight loss; bleeding easily, bloody urine or stool. • Therapy may cause tumor lysis syndrome (a condition caused by the rapid break-down of cancer cells), which can cause kidney failure and can be fatal. Report decreased urination, amber-colored urine; confusion, difficulty breathing, fa-tigue, fever, muscle or joint pain, palpita-tions, seizures, vomiting. • Report liver problems (abdominal pain, bruising, clay-colored stool, amber or dark-col-ored urine, yellowing of the skin or eyes), toxic skin reactions (inflamma-tion, peeling, rash, sloughing). • Abstain from sexual activity or use reliable forms of effective contraception. Do not breast-feed. • New secondary primary cancers may occur. • Allergic reactions, includ-ing anaphylaxis, may occur. • Treatment may cause blood clots in an artery or vein. Report symptoms of DVT (swelling, pain, hot feeling in the arms or legs; dis-coloration of extremity), heart attack (chest pain, difficulty breathing, jaw pain, nausea, pain that radiates to the arm, sweating), lung embolism (diffi-culty breathing, chest pain, rapid heart rate), stroke (confusion, difficulty speak-ing, one-sided weakness or paralysis, loss of vision).

L

lenvatinib

len-**va**-ti-nib
(Lenvima)
Do not confuse lenvatinib with dasatinib, ibrutinib, imatinib.

◆CLASSIFICATION

PHARMACOTHERAPEUTIC: Vascular endothelial growth factor (VEGF) inhibitor. Tyrosine kinase inhibitor. **CLINICAL:** Antineoplastic.

USES

Differentiated thyroid cancer (DTC): Treatment of locally recurrent or metastatic, progressive, radioactive iodine–refractory differentiated thyroid cancer. **Renal cell carcinoma (RCC):** Treatment of advanced RCC in combination with everolimus after one course of another antineoplastic; in combination with pembrolizumab, for the first-line treatment of adults. **Hepatocellular carcinoma (HCC):** First-line treatment of unresectable HCC. **Endometrial carcinoma (EC):** Treatment of advanced EC (in combination with pembrolizumab) that is mismatch repair proficient (pMMR or not microsatellite instability-high (MSI-H), who have disease progression following prior systemic therapy in any setting and are not candidates for curative surgery or radiation.

PRECAUTIONS

Contraindications: Hypersensitivity to lenvatinib. **Cautions:** Electrolyte imbalance (hypokalemia, hypomagnesemia), hepatic/renal impairment, conditions predisposing to infection (e.g., diabetes, renal failure, immunocompromised pts, open wounds). History of cardiac dysfunction (HF, pulmonary edema, right or left ventricular dysfunction), GI perforation/hemorrhage, hypertension, pts at risk for QT interval prolongation (congenital long QT syndrome, HF, medications that prolong QTc interval, hypokalemia, hypomagnesemia), thromboembolic events (e.g., CVA, DVT), pituitary/thyroid disease.

ACTION

Inhibits tyrosine kinase receptor activity of vascular endothelial growth factor (VEGF) receptors. Inhibits tumor angiogenesis, growth, progression. **Therapeutic Effect:** Decreases tumor cell growth, slows cancer progression.

PHARMACOKINETICS

Widely distributed. Metabolized in liver. Protein binding: 98%–99%. Peak plasma concentration: 1–4 hrs. Excreted in feces (64%), urine (25%). Not removed by dialysis. **Half-life:** 28 hrs.

⏳ LIFESPAN CONSIDERATIONS

Pregnancy/Lactation: Avoid pregnancy; may cause fetal harm. Females of reproductive potential must use effective contraception during treatment for at least 2 wks after discontinuation. Potentially distributed in breast milk. May reduce fertility in both females and males. **Children:** Safety and efficacy not established. **Elderly:** No age-related precautions noted.

INTERACTIONS

DRUG: **Strong CYP3A4 inhibitors (e.g., clarithromycin, ketoconazole, ritonavir)** may increase concentration/effect. May increase QT-prolonging effects of **amiodarone, citalopram, clarithromycin, moxifloxacin, nilotinib, QUEtiapine, ribociclib, thioridazine.** **HERBAL:** None significant. **FOOD:** None known. **LAB VALUES:** May increase serum alkaline phosphatase, ALT/AST, amylase, bilirubin, cholesterol, creatinine, lipase. May decrease serum albumin, glucose, magnesium; platelets. May increase or decrease serum calcium, potassium.

AVAILABILITY (Rx)

Capsules: 4 mg, 10 mg.

---

underlined – top prescribed drug

ADMINISTRATION/HANDLING

PO

• Give without regard to food. • Do not cut, crush, divide, or open capsules. • Should be swallowed whole. May be dissolved with 15 mL water or apple juice by first adding whole capsule to liquid; leave for 10 min, stir for 3 min, then administer. Then add 15 mL to glass, swirl, swallow additional liquid.

INDICATIONS/ROUTES/DOSAGE

Thyroid Cancer

PO: ADULTS, ELDERLY: 24 mg once daily. Continue until disease progression or unacceptable toxicity.

RCC

PO: ADULTS, ELDERLY: 18 mg once daily (in combination with everolimus) 20 mg once daily (in combination with pembrolizumab). Continue until disease progression or unacceptable toxicity.

HCC

PO: ADULTS, ELDERLY: (60 KG OR GREATER): 12 mg once daily. **(LESS THAN 60 KG):** 8 mg once daily. Continue until disease progression or unacceptable toxicity.

Endometrial Carcinoma (Advanced)

PO: ADULTS, ELDERLY: 20 mg once daily (in combination with pembrolizumab). Continue until disease progression or unacceptable toxicity.

Dose Modification

Based on Common Terminology Criteria for Adverse Events (CTCAE).

Adverse Reaction	Modification	Adjusted Dose (Thyroid Cancer)
First occurrence	Interrupt until resolved to Grade 0 or 1 or baseline	20 mg once daily
Second occurrence	Interrupt until resolved to Grade 0 or 1 or baseline	14 mg once daily
Third occurrence	Interrupt until resolved to Grade 0 or 1 or baseline	10 mg once daily

Adjusted dose for RCC is lower. 14 mg for first occurrence, 10 mg for second occurrence, 8 mg for third occurrence.

Arterial Thrombotic Event

Discontinue treatment.

Cardiac Dysfunction

Grade 3 cardiac dysfunction: Withhold treatment until improved to Grade 1 or 0 (or baseline). Either resume at reduced dose or discontinue (depending on the severity and persistence). Discontinue for Grade 4 event.

GI Perforation/Fistula Formation

Discontinue treatment.

Hemorrhagic Events

Grade 3 hemorrhage: Withhold treatment until improved to Grade 1 or 0 (or baseline), then either reduce dose or discontinue (based on severity or persistence). Discontinue for Grade 4 hemorrhage.

Hypertension

Grade 3 hypertension: Withhold treatment until improved with hypertensive therapy, then resume at reduced dose when hypertension is controlled at less than or equal to Grade 2. Discontinue for life-threatening hypertension.

Proteinuria

Urine protein greater than or equal to 2 g/24 hrs: Withhold treatment until improved to less than 2 g/24 hrs. Discontinue if nephrotic syndrome occurs.

QT Prolongation

Grade 3 or 4 QT interval prolongation: Withhold treatment until improved to Grade 1 or 0 (or baseline), then resume at reduced dose.

Renal Failure/Impairment or Hepatotoxicity

Grade 3 or 4 renal dysfunction or hepatotoxicity: Withhold treatment until resolved to Grade 0 or 1 or baseline. Either resume at reduced dose or discontinue (depending on the severity and persistence). Discontinue if hepatic failure occurs.

Reversible Posterior Leukoencephalopathy Syndrome (RPLS)

Withhold treatment until resolved, then resume at reduced dose or discontinue (depending on the severity and persistence of neurologic symptoms).

Other Adverse Reactions

Other persistent or intolerable Grade 2 or 3 reactions; Grade 4 laboratory abnormality: Withhold treatment until improved to Grade 1 or 0 (or baseline), then resume at reduced dose. **Other Grade 4 reactions:** Permanently discontinue.

Dosage in Renal/Hepatic Impairment

Mild to moderate impairment: No dose adjustment. **Severe impairment:** 14 mg once daily.

SIDE EFFECTS

Frequent (73%–29%): Hypertension, diarrhea, fatigue, asthenia, malaise, arthralgia, myalgia, decreased appetite, weight decreased, nausea, stomatitis, glossitis, mouth ulceration, mucosal inflammation, headache, vomiting, dysphonia, abdominal pain, constipation. **Occasional (25%–7%):** Oral pain, glossodynia, cough, peripheral edema, rash, dysgeusia, dry mouth, dizziness, dyspepsia, insomnia, alopecia, hypotension, dehydration, hyperkeratosis.

ADVERSE EFFECTS/TOXIC REACTIONS

Serious adverse effects may include arterial thromboembolic events (5% of pts); cardiac dysfunction (7% of pts); dental and oral infections including gingivitis, parotitis, pericoronitis, periodontitis, sialoadenitis, tooth abscess, tooth infection (10% of pts); GI perforation/fistula formation (2% of pts); hemorrhagic events (35% of pts); hepatotoxicity (4% of pts); hypertension (73% of pts); Grade 3 or greater hypocalcemia (9% of pts); impairment of thyroid-stimulating hormone (57% of pts); palmar-plantar erythrodysesthesia (32% of pts); proteinuria (34% of pts); QT interval prolongation (9% of pts); renal failure (14% of pts); urinary tract infection (11% of pts). Reverse posterior leukoencephalopathy occurs rarely. The median onset of hypertension was 16 days. The most frequently reported hemorrhagic event was epistaxis. The primary risk factor for renal failure was dehydration and hypovolemia related to diarrhea and vomiting.

NURSING CONSIDERATIONS

BASELINE ASSESSMENT

Obtain CBC, BMP, LFT; urinalysis for proteinuria. Confirm negative pregnancy status before initiating treatment. Receive full medication history and screen for interactions. Question history of cardiac/pituitary/thyroid disease, CVA/DVT, hypertension, hepatic/renal impairment, long QT interval syndrome. Assess oral cavity for lesions, poor dentation. Ensure that B/P is controlled prior to initiation. Assess hydration status. Offer emotional support.

INTERVENTION/EVALUATION

Monitor B/P after 1 wk, then q2wks for the first 2 mos, then at least monthly thereafter. Monitor LFT every 2 wks for the first 2 mos, then at least monthly thereafter. Monitor for proteinuria periodically. If urine dipstick proteinuria is greater than or equal to 2+, obtain a 24-hr urine protein test. Monitor blood calcium levels at least monthly and replace as needed depending on severity, presence of ECG changes, persistence of hypocalcemia. Monitor and correct other electrolyte abnormalities as needed. Reversible posterior leukoencephalopathy syndrome should be considered in pts with altered mental status, confusion, headache, seizures, visual disturbances. Immediately report abdominal pain, GI bleeding, hemoptysis (may indicate GI perforation/fistula formation). Obtain cardiac echocardiogram, ECG if cardiac decompensation is suspected.

PATIENT/FAMILY TEACHING

• Report liver problems such as upper abdominal pain, bruising, dark or amber-colored urine, nausea, vomiting, or yellowing of the skin or eyes; heart problems such as chest tightness, dizziness, fainting, palpitations, shortness of breath; kidney problems such as dark-colored urine, decreased urine output, extremity swelling, flank pain; skin changes such as rash, skin bubbling, sloughing. • Neurologic changes including blurry vision, confusion, headache, one-sided weakness, seizures, trouble speaking may indicate high blood pressure crisis, stroke, or life-threatening brain swelling. • Report mouth ulceration, jaw pain. • Swallow capsules whole; do not chew, crush, cut, or open capsules. • Treatment may increase risk of GI bleeding, nosebleeds. • Drink plenty of fluids. • Use effective contraception to avoid pregnancy. Do not breastfeed.

---

letrozole

let-roe-zole
(Femara)
Do not confuse Femara with Famvir, Femhrt, or Provera, or letrozole with anastrozole.

◆CLASSIFICATION

PHARMACOTHERAPEUTIC: Aromatase inhibitor, hormone. **CLINICAL:** Antineoplastic.

USES

First-line treatment of postmenopausal women with hormone receptor–positive or hormone receptor unknown locally advanced or metastatic breast cancer. Second-line treatment of advanced breast cancer in postmenopausal women with disease progression following antiestrogen therapy. Adjuvant treatment of postmenopausal women with hormone receptor–positive early breast cancer. Extended adjuvant treatment of early breast cancer in postmenopausal women having received 5 yrs of tamoxifen therapy. **OFF-LABEL:** Treatment of ovarian (epithelial), endometrial cancer. Infertility/ovulation stimulation, delayed puberty and growth (males), McCune-Albright syndrome, short stature (idiopathic males).

PRECAUTIONS

Contraindications: Hypersensitivity to letrozole, other aromatase inhibitors. Use in women who are or may become pregnant. **Cautions:** Hepatic impairment, hyperlipidemia.

ACTION

Decreases circulating estrogen by inhibiting aromatase, an enzyme that catalyzes the final step in estrogen production (inhibits conversion of androgens to estrogens). **Therapeutic Effect:** Inhibits growth of breast cancers stimulated by estrogens.

PHARMACOKINETICS

Widely distributed. Metabolized in liver. Primarily excreted in urine. Unknown if removed by hemodialysis. **Half-life:** Approx. 2 days.

⌛ LIFESPAN CONSIDERATIONS

Pregnancy/Lactation: Unknown if distributed in breast milk. May cause fetal harm. **Children:** Safety and efficacy not established. **Elderly:** No age-related precautions noted.

L

INTERACTIONS

DRUG: Tamoxifen may reduce concentration. **HERBAL:** None significant. **FOOD:** None known. **LAB VALUES:** May increase serum calcium, cholesterol, GGT, ALT, AST, bilirubin.

AVAILABILITY (Rx)

Tablets: 2.5 mg.

ADMINISTRATION/HANDLING

PO
• Give without regard to food.

INDICATIONS/ROUTES/DOSAGE

Advanced Breast Cancer (First- and Second-Line Treatment)
PO: ADULTS, ELDERLY: 2.5 mg/day. Continue until tumor progression is evident.

Adjuvant Treatment of Early Breast Cancer
PO: ADULTS, ELDERLY: 2.5 mg/day for planned duration of 5 yrs. Discontinue at relapse.

Extended Adjuvant Treatment of Early Breast Cancer
PO: ADULTS, ELDERLY: 2.5 mg/day for planned duration of 5 yrs (after 5 yrs of tamoxifen). Discontinue at relapse.

Dosage in Renal Impairment
No dose adjustment.

Dosage in Severe Hepatic Impairment
PO: ADULTS, ELDERLY: 2.5 mg every other day.

SIDE EFFECTS

Frequent (21%–9%): Musculoskeletal pain (back, arm, leg), nausea, headache. **Occasional (8%–5%):** Constipation, arthralgia, fatigue, vomiting, hot flashes, diarrhea, abdominal pain, cough, rash, anorexia, hypertension, peripheral edema. **Rare (4%–1%):** Asthenia, drowsiness, dyspepsia, weight gain, pruritus.

ADVERSE EFFECTS/TOXIC REACTIONS

Pleural effusion, pulmonary embolism, bone fracture, thromboembolic disorder, MI occur rarely.

BASELINE ASSESSMENT
Obtain CBC, BMP, LFT. Obtain pregnancy test prior to beginning therapy. Offer emotional support.

INTERVENTION/EVALUATION
Monitor CBC, thyroid function, electrolytes, renal function, LFT. Assist with ambulation if asthenia, dizziness occurs. Assess for headache. Offer antiemetic for nausea, vomiting. Monitor for evidence of musculoskeletal pain; offer analgesics for pain relief.

PATIENT/FAMILY TEACHING
• Report if nausea, asthenia, hot flashes become unmanageable. • Discuss importance of negative pregnancy test prior to beginning therapy; discuss nonhormonal methods of birth control. • Explain possible risk to fetus if pt is or becomes pregnant before or during therapy.

leucovorin

loo-**koe**-vor-in
Do not confuse leucovorin with Leukeran.

◆CLASSIFICATION

PHARMACOTHERAPEUTIC: Rescue agent (chemotherapy). **CLINICAL:** Antidote.

USES

Injection: Treatment of megaloblastic anemias when folate deficient. Palliative treatment of advanced colon cancer (with fluorouracil). IV rescue therapy after high-dose methotrexate for osteosarcoma or orally to diminish toxicity and impaired methotrexate elimination. **OFF-LABEL:** Bladder, esophageal, gastric cancers; graft versus host disease, non-Hodgkin's lymphoma. Adjunctive cofactor therapy in methanol toxicity. Prevents pyrimethamine hematologic toxicity in HIV-positive pts.

underlined – top prescribed drug

PRECAUTIONS

Contraindications: Hypersensitivity to leucovorin. Pernicious anemia, other megaloblastic anemias secondary to vitamin B_{12} deficiency. **Cautions:** Renal impairment.

ACTION

Actively competes with methotrexate for same transport processes into cells, displaces methotrexate from intracellular binding sites, and restores active folate stores necessary for DNA/RNA synthesis. **Therapeutic Effect:** Reverses toxic effects of folic acid antagonists. Reverses folic acid deficiency.

PHARMACOKINETICS

Widely distributed. Metabolized in liver, intestinal mucosa. Primarily excreted in urine. **Half-life:** 15 min; metabolite, 30–35 min.

⧗ LIFESPAN CONSIDERATIONS

Pregnancy/Lactation: Unknown if drug crosses placenta or is distributed in breast milk. **Children:** May increase risk of seizures by counteracting anticonvulsant effects of **barbiturates, hydantoins.** **Elderly:** Age-related renal impairment may require dosage adjustment when used for rescue from effects of high-dose methotrexate therapy.

INTERACTIONS

DRUG: May increase concentration/effect of **5-fluorouracil.** May decrease concentration/effects of **fosphenytoin, phenobarbital, phenytoin, primidone, trimethorprim. HERBAL:** None significant. **FOOD:** None known. **LAB VALUES:** May decrease platelets, WBCs (when used in combination with 5-fluorouracil).

AVAILABILITY (Rx)

Injection, Powder for Reconstitution: 50 mg, 100 mg, 200 mg, 350 mg, 500 mg. **Injection, Solution:** 10 mg/mL. **Tablets:** 5 mg, 10 mg, 15 mg, 25 mg.

ADMINISTRATION/HANDLING

 IV

◄ALERT► Strict adherence to timing of 5-fluorouracil following leucovorin therapy must be maintained.

Reconstitution • Reconstitute each 50-mg vial with 5 mL Sterile Water for Injection or Bacteriostatic Water for Injection containing benzyl alcohol to provide concentration of 10 mg/mL. • Due to benzyl alcohol in 1-mg ampule and in Bacteriostatic Water for Injection, reconstitute doses greater than 10 mg/m² with Sterile Water for Injection. • Further dilute with 100–1,000 mL D_5W or 0.9% NaCl.

Rate of administration • Do not exceed 160 mg/min if given by IV infusion (due to calcium content).

Storage • Store powdered vials for parenteral use at room temperature. • Refrigerate solution for injection vials. • Injection appears as clear, yellowish solution. • Use immediately if reconstituted with Sterile Water for Injection; stable for 7 days if reconstituted with Bacteriostatic Water for Injection. Diluted solutions stable for 24 hrs at room temperature or 4 days refrigerated.

▦ IV COMPATIBILITIES

5-Fluorouracil, granisetron.

INDICATIONS/ROUTES/DOSAGE

Rescue in High-Dose Methotrexate Therapy

PO, IV, IM: ADULTS, ELDERLY, CHILDREN: 15 mg (approximately 10 mg/m²) started 24 hrs after starting methotrexate infusion; continue q6h for 10 doses, until methotrexate level is less than 0.05 micromole/L. Additional dose adjusted based on methotrexate levels.

Folic Acid Antagonist Overdose

PO: ADULTS, ELDERLY, CHILDREN: 5–15 mg/day.

Megaloblastic Anemia Secondary to Folate Deficiency

IM/IV: ADULTS, ELDERLY, CHILDREN: 1 mg or less per day.

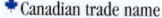 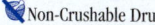

L

Colon Cancer

◀ **ALERT** ▶ For rescue therapy in cancer chemotherapy, refer to specific protocols used for optimal dosage and sequence of leucovorin administration.

IV: ADULTS, ELDERLY: *(In Combination With 5-Fluorouracil):* 200 mg/m² daily for 5 days. Repeat course at 4-wk intervals for 2 courses, then 4- to 5-wk intervals or 20 mg/m² daily for 5 days. Repeat course at 4-wk intervals for 2 courses, then 4- to 5-wk intervals.

Dosage in Renal/Hepatic Impairment
No dose adjustment.

SIDE EFFECTS

Frequent: When combined with chemotherapeutic agents: diarrhea, stomatitis, nausea, vomiting, lethargy, malaise, fatigue, alopecia, anorexia. **Occasional:** Urticaria, dermatitis.

ADVERSE EFFECTS/TOXIC REACTIONS

Excessive dosage may negate chemotherapeutic effects of folic acid antagonists. Anaphylaxis occurs rarely. Diarrhea may cause rapid clinical deterioration.

NURSING CONSIDERATIONS

BASELINE ASSESSMENT
Obtain CBC, LFT, renal function. Give as soon as possible, preferably within 1 hr, for treatment of accidental overdosage of folic acid antagonists.

INTERVENTION/EVALUATION
Monitor for vomiting (may need to change from oral to parenteral therapy). Observe elderly, debilitated closely due to risk for severe toxicities. Assess CBC, BMP, LFT.

PATIENT/FAMILY TEACHING
• Educate purpose of medication in treatment of cancer. • Report allergic reaction, vomiting.

leuprolide

loo-proe-lide
(Camcevi, Eligard, Fensolvi, Lupron ❋, Lupron Depot, Lupron Depot-Ped)

◆ CLASSIFICATION

PHARMACOTHERAPEUTIC: Gonadotropin-releasing hormone (GnRH) analogue. **CLINICAL:** Antineoplastic.

USES

Prostate cancer: Treatment of advanced prostate cancer. **Endometriosis:** Management of endometriosis, including pain relief and reduction of endometriotic lesions. **Central precocious puberty:** Treatment of central precocious puberty in children 2 yrs and older. **Uterine leiomyomata:** Treatment (preoperative) of anemia caused by uterine leiomyomata (fibroids).

PRECAUTIONS

Contraindications: Hypersensitivity to leuprolide, GnRH, GnRH-agonist analogue. Pregnancy or women who may become pregnant, breastfeeding (Lupron Depot 3.75 mg and 11.25 mg), abnormal, undiagnosed vaginal bleeding (Lupron Depot 3.75 mg and 11.25 mg). 22.5 mg, 30 mg, 45 mg Lupron Depot and Eligard (all strengths) not indicated for use in women. **Cautions:** History of psychiatric illness, QTc prolongation or medications that prolong QTc interval, preexisting cardiac disease, chronic alcohol use, steroid therapy, seizures or medications that decrease seizures threshold.

ACTION

Inhibits gonadotropin secretion; produces an initial increase in LH and FSH, causing a transient increase in testosterone (males) and estrone/estradione in premenopausal women. Continuous administration results in decreased levels of testosterone (male) and estrogen (females). **Therapeutic Effect:** Produces pharmacologic castration, decreases growth of abnormal prostate tissue in males; causes endometrial tissue to become inactive, atrophic in females; decreases rate of pubertal development in children with central precocious puberty.

PHARMACOKINETICS

Widely distributed. Protein binding: 43%–49%. **Half-life:** 3–4 hrs.

⧗ LIFESPAN CONSIDERATIONS

Pregnancy/Lactation: Depot: Contraindicated in pregnancy. May cause spontaneous abortion. **Children:** Long-term safety not established. **Elderly:** No age-related precautions noted.

INTERACTIONS

DRUG: None significant. **HERBAL:** None significant. **FOOD:** None known. **LAB VALUES:** May increase serum prostatic acid phosphatase (PAP). Initially increases, then decreases serum testosterone. May increase serum ALT, AST, alkaline phosphatase, glucose, LDH, LDL, cholesterol, triglycerides. May decrease platelets, WBC.

AVAILABILITY (Rx)

Injection Depot Formulation: *(Eligard):* 7.5 mg, 22.5 mg, 30 mg, 45 mg. *(Fensolvi) (6-month):* 45 mg (Ped). *(Lupron Depot-Ped):* (Monthly): 7.5 mg, 11.25 mg, 15 mg, (3 Month): 11.25 mg, 30 mg. *(Lupron Depot):* (Monthly): 3.75 mg, (3-Month): 11.25 mg, 22.5 mg, (4-Month): 30 mg, (6-Month): 45 mg. **Prefilled Syringe:** *(Camcevi):* 42 mg.

ADMINISTRATION/HANDLING

◀**ALERT**▶ May be carcinogenic, mutagenic, teratogenic. Handle with extreme care during preparation/administration.

IM

• *(Lupron Depot, Lupron-Ped Depot):* Store at room temperature. Upon reconstitution, discard if not used within 2 hr. Administer into gluteal area, anterior thigh, or deltoid.

SQ

• *(Camcevi):* Refrigerate. • Do not shake. • Allow to sit at room temperature for 30 min prior to administration (may store at 77°F up to 6 days for excursions). • Select injection site in upper or mid-abdominal area. *(Eligard, Fensolvi):* • Refrigerate. • Allow to reach room temperature. • May be stored outside of refrigerator for up to 8 wks prior to mixing (once mixed, use within 30 min). • Inject into upper or mid abdomen or upper buttock. *(Leuprolide acetate):* • Store at room temperature. • Excursions permitted. • Upon reconstitution, use immediately. • Administer in areas on arm, thigh or abdomen.

INDICATIONS/ROUTES/DOSAGE

Advanced Prostatic Carcinoma

IM: *(Lupron Depot):* **ADULTS, ELDERLY:** 7.5 mg q1mo, 22.5 mg q3mos, 30 mg q4mos, or 45 mg q6mos.
SQ: *(Eligard):* **ADULTS, ELDERLY:** 7.5 mg every mo, 22.5 mg q3mos, 30 mg q4mos, or 45 mg q6mos.
SQ: *(Lupron):* **ADULTS, ELDERLY:** 1 mg/day.
SQ: *(Camcevi):* **ADULTS, ELDERLY:** 42 mg q6mos.

Endometriosis

IM: *(Lupron Depot):* **ADULTS, ELDERLY:** 3.75 mg/mo for up to 6 mos or 11.25 mg q3mos for up to 2 doses (as monotherapy or in combination with norethindrone).

Uterine Leiomyomata

IM: *(Lupron Depot):* **ADULTS, ELDERLY:** 3.75 mg/mo for up to 3 mos or 11.25 mg as a single injection. Give in combination with iron.

Precocious Puberty

IM: *(Lupron Depot-Ped 1-month):* **CHILDREN WEIGHING MORE THAN 37.5 KG:** 15 mg q1mo. **WEIGHING 26 KG TO 37.5 KG:** 11.25 mg q1mo. **WEIGHING 25 KG OR LESS:** 7.5 mg q1mo. Titrate dose

L

upward by 3.75 mg/mo if down regulation not achieved. **LUPRON DEPOT-PED (3 MOS):** 11.25 mg or 30 mg q12wks. **SQ: CHILDREN: Long-acting formulation:** *(Fensolvi):* 45 mg q6mos.

Dosage in Renal/Hepatic Impairment
No dose adjustment.

SIDE EFFECTS

Frequent: Hot flashes (ranging from mild flushing to diaphoresis), migraines, hyperhidrosis. **Females:** Amenorrhea, spotting. **Occasional:** Arrhythmias, palpitations, blurred vision, dizziness, edema, headache, burning, pruritus, swelling at injection site, nausea, insomnia, weight gain. **Females:** Deepening voice, hirsutism, decreased libido, increased breast tenderness, vaginitis, altered mood. **Males:** Constipation, decreased testicle size, gynecomastia, impotence, decreased appetite, angina. **Rare: Males:** Thrombophlebitis.

ADVERSE EFFECTS/TOXIC REACTIONS

Occasionally, signs/symptoms of prostatic carcinoma worsen 1–2 wks after initial dosing (subsides during continued therapy). Increased bone pain and, less frequently, dysuria, hematuria, weakness, paresthesia of lower extremities may be noted. MI, pulmonary embolism occur rarely.

NURSING CONSIDERATIONS

BASELINE ASSESSMENT
Obtain pregnancy test in females of reproductive potential. Obtain serum testosterone, prostatic acid phosphates (PAP) periodically during therapy. Question medical history as listed in Precautions. Offer emotional support.

INTERVENTION/EVALUATION
Monitor for arrhythmias, palpitations. Assess for peripheral edema. Assess sleep pattern. Monitor for visual difficulties.

Assist with ambulation if dizziness occurs. Offer antiemetics if nausea occurs. Serum testosterone, PAP should increase during first wk of therapy. Serum testosterone then should decrease to baseline level or less within 2 wks, PAP within 4 wks.

PATIENT/ FAMILY TEACHING
• Hot flashes tend to decrease during continued therapy. • Temporary exacerbation of signs/symptoms of disease may occur during first few wks of therapy. • Use contraceptive measures. • Report persistent, regular menstruation; pregnancy. • Avoid tasks that require alertness, motor skills until response to drug is established (potential for dizziness).

levalbuterol

lee-val-**bue**-ter-ole
(Xopenex HFA)
Do not confuse Xopenex with Xanax.

◆CLASSIFICATION
PHARMACOTHERAPEUTIC: Beta₂ agonist. **CLINICAL:** Bronchodilator.

USES
Treatment, prevention of bronchospasm due to reversible obstructive airway disease (e.g., asthma, bronchitis, emphysema) in adults, adolescents, and children 4 yrs of age and older.

PRECAUTIONS
Contraindications: History of hypersensitivity to albuterol or levalbuterol. **Cautions:** Cardiovascular disorders (cardiac arrhythmias, HF), seizures, hypertension, hyperthyroidism, diabetes, glaucoma, hypokalemia.

ACTION
Stimulates beta₂-adrenergic receptors in lungs, resulting in relaxation of bronchial smooth muscle. **Therapeutic**

Effect: Relieves bronchospasm, reduces airway resistance.

PHARMACOKINETICS

Route	Onset	Peak	Duration
Inhalation	5–10 min	1.5 hrs	5–6 hrs
Nebulization	10–17 min	1.5 hrs	5–8 hrs

Half-life: 3.3–4 hrs.

⧗ LIFESPAN CONSIDERATIONS

Pregnancy/Lactation: Crosses placenta. Unknown if distributed in breast milk. **Pregnancy category C. Children:** Safety and efficacy not established in pts younger than 4 yrs. **Elderly:** Lower initial dosages recommended.

INTERACTIONS

DRUG: **Beta blockers** (e.g., **carvedilol, metoprolol**) antagonize effects; may produce severe bronchospasm. **MAOIs** (e.g., **phenelzine, tranylcypromine**), **tricyclic antidepressants** (e.g., **amitriptyline, desipramine**) may potentiate cardiovascular effects. **Linezolid** may enhance the hypertensive effect. May increase adverse effects of **loxapine. HERBAL:** None significant. **FOOD:** None known. **LAB VALUES:** May decrease serum potassium.

AVAILABILITY (Rx)

Inhalation Aerosol: 45 mcg/activation. **Solution for Nebulization:** 0.31 mg in 3-mL vials, 0.63 mg in 3-mL vials, 1.25 mg in 3-mL vials, 1.25 mg in 0.5-mL vials.

ADMINISTRATION/HANDLING

Nebulization
• Protect from light, excessive heat. Store at room temperature. • Once foil is opened, use within 2 wks. • Use within 1 wk and protect from light after removal from pouch • Discard if solution is not colorless. • Do not mix with other medications. • Concentrated solution (1.25 mg in 0.5 mL) should be diluted with 2.5 mL 0.9% NaCl prior to use. • Give over 5–15 min.

Inhalation
• Shake well before inhalation. • Prime with 4 test sprays before initial use or if not used for more than 3 days. • Following first inhalation, wait 2 min before inhaling second dose (allows for deeper bronchial penetration). • Rinsing mouth with water immediately after inhalation prevents mouth/throat dryness.

INDICATIONS/ROUTES/DOSAGE

Treatment/Prevention of Bronchospasm (Reversible Obstructive Airway Disease)
Nebulization: ADULTS, ELDERLY, CHILDREN 12 YRS AND OLDER: Initially, 0.63 mg 3 times/day 6–8 hrs apart. May increase to 1.25 mg 3 times/day with close monitoring. **CHILDREN 6–11 YRS:** Initially, 0.31 mg 3 times/day. May increase up to 0.63 mg 3 times/day.
Metered Dose Inhalation: ADULTS, ELDERLY, CHILDREN 4 YRS AND OLDER: 2 inhalations q4–6h or 1 inhalation q4h.

Dosage in Renal/Hepatic Impairment
No dose adjustment.

SIDE EFFECTS

Occasional (11%–4%): Nervousness, tremor, rhinitis, flu-like illness. **Rare (less than 3%):** Tachycardia, dizziness, anxiety, viral infection, dyspepsia, dry mouth, headache, chest pain.

ADVERSE EFFECTS/TOXIC REACTIONS

Excessive sympathomimetic stimulation may cause palpitations, premature heart contraction, tachycardia, chest pain, slight increase in B/P followed by substantial decrease, chills, diaphoresis, blanching of skin. Too-frequent or excessive use may decrease bronchodilating effectiveness, lead to severe, paradoxical bronchoconstriction.

NURSING CONSIDERATIONS

BASELINE ASSESSMENT

Assess lung sounds, oxygen saturation. Note color, amount of sputum.

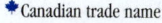 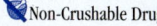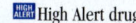

INTERVENTION/EVALUATION

Monitor rate, depth, rhythm, type of respiration; quality/rate of pulse, ECG, serum potassium. Assess lung sounds for wheezing (bronchoconstriction). Observe for paradoxical bronchospasm.

PATIENT/ FAMILY TEACHING

• Increase fluid intake (decreases lung secretion viscosity). • Rinsing mouth with water immediately after inhalation may prevent mouth/throat dryness. • Avoid excessive use of caffeine derivatives (chocolate, coffee, tea, cola, cocoa). • Report if palpitations, tachycardia, chest pain, tremors, dizziness, headache occurs or shortness of breath is not relieved.

levETIRAcetam

lee-ve-tye-**ra**-se-tam
(Elepsia XR, Keppra, Keppra XR, Roweepra, Spritam)
Do not confuse Keppra with Kaletra, Keflex, or Keppra XR, or levETIRAcetam with levoFLOXacin.

◆ CLASSIFICATION

PHARMACOTHERAPEUTIC: Pyrrolidine derivative. **CLINICAL:** Anticonvulsant.

USES

Focal (partial) onset seizures: (Immediate-release tablets, oral solution, IV): Treatment of focal (partial) onset seizures in adults, adolescents, children, and infants 1 mo of age and older. **(Tablets for oral suspension):** Treatment of focal (partial) onset seizures in pts 4 yrs of age and older weighing more than 20 kg. **(ER tablets):** Treatment of focal (partial) onset seizures in adults and pts 12 yrs of age and older. **Juvenile myoclonic seizures: (Immediate-release tablets, oral solution, tablets for oral suspension, IV):** Adjunctive therapy for the treatment of juvenile myoclonic seizures in adults and pts 12 yrs of age and older. **Tonic-clonic seizures: (Immediate-release tablets, oral solution, tablets for oral suspension, IV):** Adjunctive therapy for treatment of primary generalized tonic-clonic seizures in adults and pts 6 yrs of age and older. **OFF LABEL:** Status epilepticus. Seizure prophylaxis for craniotomy, subarachnoid hemorrhage, traumatic brain injury.

PRECAUTIONS

Contraindications: Hypersensitivity to levETIRAcetam. **Cautions:** Renal impairment, pts with depression at high risk for suicide.

ACTION

Exact mechanism unknown. May inhibit voltage-dependent calcium channels, facilitate GABA inhibitory transmission, reduce potassium current, or bind to synaptic proteins that modulate neurotransmitter release. **Therapeutic Effect:** Prevents seizure activity.

PHARMACOKINETICS

Widely distributed. Protein binding: less than 10%. Metabolized primarily by enzymatic hydrolysis. Primarily excreted in urine as unchanged drug. **Half-life:** 6–8 hrs.

⧗ LIFESPAN CONSIDERATIONS

Pregnancy/Lactation: Distributed in breast milk. Breastfeeding not recommended. **Children:** Safety and efficacy not established in pts younger than 1 mo. **Elderly:** Age-related renal impairment may require dosage adjustment.

INTERACTIONS

DRUG: **CNS depressants** (e.g., **alcohol, morphine, zolpidem**) may increase CNS depression. **HERBAL:** Herbals with sedative properties (e.g., **chamomile, kava kava, valerian**) may increase CNS depression. **FOOD:** None known. **LAB VALUES:** May decrease Hgb, Hct, RBC, WBC.

AVAILABILITY (Rx)

Injection, Solution: 100 mg/mL. **Oral Solution:** 100 mg/mL. **Tablets:** 250 mg, 500 mg, 750 mg, 1,000 mg.

 Tablets, Extended-Release: 500 mg, 750 mg, 1,000 mg, 1,500 mg. **Tablets (ODT):** 250 mg, 500 mg, 750 mg, 1,000 mg.

ADMINISTRATION/HANDLING

IV

Rate of infusion • Infuse over 15 min. **Reconstitution** • Dilute with 100 mL 0.9% NaCl or D_5W.
Storage • Store at room temperature. • Stable for 24 hrs following dilution.

PO

• Give without regard to food. • **Oral solution:** Use a calibrated measuring device. • **Tablet (immediate-release, extended-release):** Administer tablet whole; do not cut, break, or crush. • **Tablet (ODT):** Place whole tablet on tongue and follow with sip of liquid. Swallowing allowed only after tablet has disintegrated. • Use oral solution for pts weighing 20 kg or less. • Use tablets or oral solution for pts weighing more than 20 kg.

INDICATIONS/ROUTES/DOSAGE

Focal (Partial) Onset Seizures

IV/PO: ADULTS, ELDERLY, CHILDREN 17 YRS AND OLDER: *(Immediate-Release Tablets, Oral Solution, Tablets for Oral Suspension):* Initially, 500 mg q12h. May increase by 1,000 mg/day q2wks. **Maximum:** 3,000 mg/day in 2 divided doses. *(Extended-Release Tablets):* Initially, 1,000 mg once daily. May increase in increments of 1,000 mg/day q2wks. **Maximum:** 3,000 mg once daily.
IV/PO: CHILDREN 4–16 YRS: *(Oral Solution, Tablets):* 20 mg/kg/day in 2 divided doses. May increase q2wks by 10 mg/kg/dose up to 60 mg/kg/day in 2 divided doses. **Maximum:** 3,000 mg/day. *(Tablets):* **WEIGHING MORE THAN 40 KG:** 500 mg twice daily. May increase q2wks

by 500 mg/dose. **Maximum:** 1,500 mg twice daily. **20–40 KG:** 250 mg twice daily. May increase q2wks by 250 mg/dose. **Maximum:** 750 mg twice daily. **CHILDREN 6 MOS TO YOUNGER THAN 4 YRS:** *(Oral Solution):* 20 mg/kg/day in 2 divided doses. May increase q2wks by 10 mg/kg/dose. **Maximum:** 50 mg/kg/day in 2 divided doses. **CHILDREN 1 MO TO YOUNGER THAN 6 MOS:** *(Oral Solution):* 14 mg/kg/day in 2 divided doses. May increase q2wks by 7 mg/kg/dose. **Maximum:** 42 mg/kg/day in 2 divided doses.

Myoclonic Seizures

PO, IV: ADULTS, CHILDREN 12 YRS AND OLDER: *(Immediate-Release Tablets, Oral Solution, Tablets for Oral Suspension):* Initially, 500 mg q12h. May increase by 1,000 mg/day q2wks. **Maximum:** 3,000 mg/day in 2 divided doses.

Generalized Tonic-Clonic Seizures

PO, IV: ADULTS, ELDERLY, CHILDREN 16 YRS AND OLDER: *(Immediate-Release Tablets, Oral Solution, Tablets for Oral Suspension):* Initially, 500 mg twice daily. May increase by 1,000 mg/day q2wks up to recommended dose of 1,500 mg 2 times/day. **CHILDREN 6–15 YRS:** Initially, 10 mg/kg twice daily. May increase by 20 mg/kg/day q2wks up to recommended dose of 30 mg/kg 2 times/day.

Dosage in Renal Impairment

Dosage is modified based on creatinine clearance. **CrCl less than 50 mL/min:** Not recommended with Keppra XR.

Creatinine Clearance	Dosage (Immediate-Release, IV)	Dosage (Extended-Release)
Greater than 80 mL/min:	500–1,500 mg q12h	1,000–3,000 mg q24h
50–80 mL/min:	500–1,000 mg q12h	1,000–2,000 mg q24h
30–49 mL/min:	250–750 mg q12h	500–1,500 mg q24h
Less than 30 mL/min:	250–500 mg q12h	500–1,000 mg q24h

L

 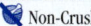

Creatinine Clearance	Dosage (Immediate-Release, IV)	Dosage (Extended-Release)
End-stage renal disease using dialysis:	500–1,000 mg q24h; after dialysis, a 250-to 500-mg supplemental dose is recommended	NA
CRRT	250–750 mg q12h	

Dosage in Hepatic Impairment

No dose adjustment.

SIDE EFFECTS

Frequent (15%–10%): Drowsiness, asthenia, headache, infection. **Occasional (9%–3%):** Dizziness, pharyngitis, pain, depression, anxiety, vertigo, rhinitis, anorexia. **Rare (less than 3%):** Amnesia, emotional lability, cough, sinusitis, anorexia, diplopia.

ADVERSE EFFECTS/TOXIC REACTIONS

Acute psychosis, agitation, delirium, impulsivity have been reported. Sudden discontinuance increases risk of seizure activity. Serious dermatological reactions, including Stevens-Johnson syndrome and toxic epidermal necrolysis, have been reported.

NURSING CONSIDERATIONS

BASELINE ASSESSMENT

Obtain renal function test. Review history of seizure disorder (intensity, frequency, duration, LOC). Initiate seizure precautions. Question prior hypersensitivity reaction.

INTERVENTION/EVALUATION

Observe for recurrence of seizure activity. Assess for clinical improvement (decrease in intensity/frequency of seizures). Monitor renal function tests. Observe for suicidal ideation, depression, behavioral changes. Assist with ambulation if dizziness occurs.

PATIENT/ FAMILY TEACHING

• Drowsiness usually diminishes with continued therapy. • Avoid tasks that require alertness, motor skills until response to drug is established. • Avoid alcohol. • Do not abruptly discontinue medication (may precipitate seizures). • Strict maintenance of drug therapy is essential for seizure control. • Report mood swings, hostile behavior, suicidal ideation, unusual changes in behavior.

levoFLOXacin

lee-voe-**flox**-a-sin

■ **BLACK BOX ALERT** ■ May increase risk of tendonitis, tendon rupture. (Risk increased with concurrent corticosteroids, organ transplant, pts older than 60 yrs.) May exacerbate myasthenia gravis. **Do not confuse levoFLOXacin with levETIRAcetam or levothyroxine.**

◆CLASSIFICATION

PHARMACOTHERAPEUTIC: Fluoroquinolone. **CLINICAL:** Antibiotic.

USES

Treatment of susceptible infections due to *S. pneumoniae, S. aureus, E. faecalis, H. influenzae, M. catarrhalis, Serratia marcescens, K. pneumoniae, E. coli, P. mirabilis, P. aeruginosa, C. pneumoniae, Legionella pneumophila, Mycoplasma pneumoniae,* including acute bacterial exacerbation of chronic bronchitis, acute bacterial sinusitis, community-acquired pneumonia, nosocomial pneumonia, complicated and uncomplicated UTI, acute pyelonephritis, complicated and uncomplicated mild to moderate skin/skin structure infections, prostatitis. Inhalation anthrax (postexposure); plague. **Ophthalmic:** Treatment of superficial infections to conjunctiva (0.5%), cornea (1.5%). **OFF-LABEL:** Bite wound infection, diabetic foot infection, *H. pylori* eradication, neutropenia, osteomyelitis, prostatitis, sexually transmitted infections, PID, *Shigella* infection, surgical prophylaxis.

PRECAUTIONS

Contraindications: Hypersensitivity to levoFLOXacin, other fluoroquinolones. **Cautions:** Known or suspected CNS disorders, seizure disorder, renal impairment, bradycardia, rheumatoid arthritis, elderly, myasthenia gravis, severe cerebral arteriosclerosis, pts at risk for QT interval prolongation (congenital long QT syndrome, HF, medications that prolong QT interval, hypokalemia, hypomagnesemia), diabetes, pts at risk for tendon rupture, tendonitis (e.g., renal failure, concomitant use of corticosteroids, organ transplant recipient, rheumatoid arthritis, elderly, strenuous physical activity or exercise).

ACTION

Inhibits DNA enzyme gyrase in susceptible microorganisms, interfering with bacterial cell replication, repair. **Therapeutic Effect:** Bactericidal.

PHARMACOKINETICS

Widely distributed. Protein binding: 50%. Excreted unchanged in urine. Partially removed by hemodialysis. **Half-life:** 6–8 hrs.

⧗ LIFESPAN CONSIDERATIONS

Pregnancy/Lactation: Distributed in breast milk. Avoid use in pregnancy. **Children:** Safety and efficacy not established. **Elderly:** Age-related renal impairment may require dosage adjustment.

INTERACTIONS

DRUG: May decrease therapeutic effect of **BCG (intravesical)**. **Antacids (calcium, magnesium, iron preparations); sucralfate, zinc** decrease absorption. **NSAIDs (e.g., ibuprofen, ketorolac, naproxen)** may increase risk of CNS stimulation, seizures. **QT interval–prolonging medications (e.g., amiodarone, haloperidol, sotalol)** may increase risk of arrhythmias. May increase anticoagulant effect of **warfarin**. **HERBAL:** None significant. **FOOD:** None known. **LAB VALUES:** May alter serum glucose.

AVAILABILITY (Rx)

Infusion Premix: 250 mg/50 mL, 500 mg/100 mL, 750 mg/150 mL. **Injection, Solution:** 25 mg/mL. **Ophthalmic Solution:** 0.5%, 1.5%. **Oral Solution:** 25 mg/mL. **Tablets:** 250 mg, 500 mg, 750 mg.

ADMINISTRATION/HANDLING

 IV

L

Reconstitution • For infusion using single-dose vial, withdraw desired amount (10 mL for 250 mg, 20 mL for 500 mg). Dilute each 10 mL (250 mg) with minimum 40 mL 0.9% NaCl, D₅W, providing a concentration of 5 mg/mL.
Rate of administration • Administer no less than 60 min for 250 mg or 500 mg; 90 min for 750 mg.
Storage • Available in single-dose 20-mL (500-mg) vials and premixed with D₅W, ready to infuse. • Diluted vials stable for 72 hrs at room temperature, 14 days if refrigerated.

PO

• Do not administer antacids (aluminum, magnesium), sucralfate, iron, or multivitamin preparations with zinc within 2 hrs of administration (significantly reduces absorption). • Give tablets without regard to food. • Give oral solution 1 hr before or 2 hrs after meals.

Ophthalmic

• Place a gloved finger on lower eyelid and pull out until a pocket is formed between eye and lower

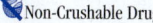

lid. • Place prescribed number of drops into pocket. • Instruct pt to close eye gently (so that medication will not be squeezed out of the sac) and to apply digital pressure to lacrimal sac for 1–2 min to minimize systemic absorption.

⚙ IV INCOMPATIBILITIES

Furosemide, heparin.

⚙ IV COMPATIBILITIES

DexmedeTOMIDine, magnesium sulfate, norepinephrine, potassium chloride.

INDICATIONS/ROUTES/DOSAGE

Usual Dosage Range

PO, IV: ADULTS, ELDERLY: 250–750 mg q24h; 750 mg q24h for severe or complicated infections.

Bacterial Conjunctivitis

Ophthalmic: ADULTS, ELDERLY, CHILDREN 1 YR AND OLDER: 1–2 drops q2h for 2 days while awake (up to 8 times/day), then 1–2 drops q4h while awake up to 4 times/day.

Dosage in Renal Impairment

Normal renal function dosage of 250 mg/day:

Creatinine Clearance	Dosage
20–49 mL/min	No change
10–19 mL/min	250 mg initially, then 250 mg q48h

Normal renal function dosage of 500 mg/day:

Creatinine Clearance	Dosage
50–80 mL/min	No change
20–49 mL/min	500 mg initially, then 250 mg q24h
10–19 mL/min	500 mg initially, then 250 mg q48h

For pts undergoing dialysis, 500 mg initially, then 250 mg q48h.
Normal renal function dosage of 750 mg/day:

Creatinine Clearance	Dosage
50–80 mL/min	No change
20–49 mL/min	Initially, 750 mg, then 750 mg q48h
10–19 mL/min	Initially, 750 mg, then 500 mg q48h
Dialysis	500 mg q48h (administer after dialysis on dialysis days)
Continuous renal replacement therapy	
CVVH	500–750 mg once, then 250 mg q24h
CVVHD	500–750 mg once, then 250–500 mg q24h
CVVHDT	500–750 mg once, then 250–750 mg q24h

Dosage in Hepatic Impairment

No dose adjustment.

SIDE EFFECTS

Occasional (3%–1%): Diarrhea, nausea, abdominal pain, dizziness, drowsiness, headache. **Ophthalmic:** Local burning/discomfort, margin crusting, crystals/scales, foreign body sensation, ocular itching, altered taste. **Rare (less than 1%):** Flatulence; pain, inflammation, swelling in calves, hands, shoulder; chest pain, difficulty breathing, palpitations, edema, tendon pain. **Ophthalmic:** Corneal staining, keratitis, allergic reaction, eyelid swelling, tearing, reduced visual acuity.

ADVERSE EFFECTS/TOXIC REACTIONS

Antibiotic-associated colitis, other superinfections (abdominal cramps, severe watery diarrhea, fever) may occur. Superinfection (genital/anal pruritus, ulceration/changes in oral mucosa, moderate to severe diarrhea) may occur from altered bacterial balance in GI tract. Hypersensitivity reactions, including photosensitivity (rash, pruritus, blisters, edema, sensation of burning skin), have occurred in pts receiving fluoroquinolones. May increase risk of tendonitis, tendon rupture, peripheral neuropathy; CNS effects including agitation, anxiety,

levothyroxine 655

confusion, depression, dizziness, hallucinations, nightmares, paranoia, tremors, vertigo. May exacerbate muscle weakness in pts with myasthenia gravis.

NURSING CONSIDERATIONS

BASELINE ASSESSMENT
Question for hypersensitivity to levoFLOXacin, other fluoroquinolones. Question history as listed in Precautions. Receive full medication history, and screen for interactions, esp. medications that prolong QT interval. Obtain baseline ECG.

INTERVENTION/EVALUATION
Monitor serum glucose, renal function, LFT. Monitor daily pattern of bowel activity, stool consistency. Promptly report hypersensitivity reaction: skin rash, urticaria, pruritus, photosensitivity. Be alert for superinfection: fever, vomiting, diarrhea, anal/genital pruritus, oral mucosal changes (ulceration, pain, erythema). Monitor for muscle weakness, voice dystonia in pts with myasthenia gravis; pain, swelling, bruising, popping of tendons.

PATIENT/FAMILY TEACHING
• It is essential to complete drug therapy despite symptom improvement. Early discontinuation may result in antibacterial resistance or increase risk of recurrent infection. • Report any episodes of diarrhea, esp. the first few mos after final dose. Frequent diarrhea, fever, abdominal pain, blood-streaked stool may indicate infectious diarrhea, which may be contagious to others. • Severe allergic reactions, such as hives, palpitations, rash, shortness of breath, tongue swelling, may occur. • Tendon inflammation/swelling, tendon rupture may occur; report bruising, pain, swelling in tendon areas or snapping, popping of tendons. • Immediately report nervous system problems such as anxiety, confusion, dizziness, nervousness, nightmares, thoughts of suicide, seizures, tremors, trouble sleeping. • Treatment may cause heart problems such as low heart rate, palpitations; permanent nerve damage such as burning, numbness, tingling, weakness. • Do not take aluminum- or magnesium-containing antacids, multivitamins, zinc or iron products at least 2 hrs before or 6 hrs after dose. • Drink plenty of fluids.

levothyroxine [TOP 100]

lee-voe-thy-**rox**-een
(Eltroxin ✦, Euthyrox, Levoxyl, Synthroid, Thyquidity, Tirosint, Unithroid)

■ **BLACK BOX ALERT** ■ Ineffective, potentially toxic for weight reduction. High doses increase risk of serious, life-threatening toxic effects, especially when used with some anorectic drugs.
Do not confuse levothyroxine with lamoTRIgine, Lanoxin, levoFLOXacin or liothyronine, or Levoxyl with Lanoxin, Levaquin, or Luvox, or Synthroid with Symmetrel.

FIXED-COMBINATION(S)
With liothyronine, T_3 **(Thyrolar).**

◆CLASSIFICATION
PHARMACOTHERAPEUTIC: Synthetic isomer of thyroxine. **CLINICAL:** Thyroid hormone (T_4).

USES
PO: Hypothyroidism: Replacement therapy in primary (thyroidal), secondary (pituitary), and tertiary (hypothalamic) congenital or acquired hypothyroidism. **Pituitary thyrotropin (thyroid-stimulating hormone [TSH]) suppression:** Adjunct to surgery and radioiodine therapy for management of thyrotropin-dependent well-differentiated thyroid cancer. **IV:** Treatment of myxedema coma.

PRECAUTIONS
Contraindications: Hypersensitivity to levo thyroxine. Acute MI, untreated subclinical

 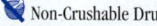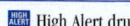

or overt thyrotoxicosis, uncorrected adrenal insufficiency. **Capsule:** Inability to swallow capsules. **Cautions:** Elderly pts, angina pectoris, hypertension, cardiovascular disease, adrenal insufficiency, myxedema, diabetes mellitus and insipidus, swallowing disorders.

ACTION

Converts to T_3, then binds to thyroid receptor proteins exerting metabolic effects through control of DNA transcription and protein synthesis. **Therapeutic Effect:** Involved in normal metabolism, growth and development. Increases basal metabolic rate, enhances gluconeogenesis, stimulates protein synthesis.

PHARMACOKINETICS

Widely distributed. Protein binding: greater than 99%. Deiodinated in peripheral tissues, minimal metabolism in liver. Eliminated by biliary excretion. **Half-life:** 6–7 days.

⧖ LIFESPAN CONSIDERATIONS

Pregnancy/Lactation: Does not cross placenta. Minimal distribution in breast milk. **Children:** No age-related precautions noted. Caution in neonates in interpreting thyroid function tests. **Elderly:** May be more sensitive to thyroid effects; individualized dosage recommended.

INTERACTIONS

DRUG: **Cholestyramine, colestipol, aluminum-** and **magnesium-containing antacids, calcium, iron** may decrease absorption (do not administer within 4 hrs). **Estrogens** may decrease therapeutic effect. May enhance effects of **oral anticoagulants (e.g., warfarin).** **HERBAL:** None significant. **FOOD:** None known. **LAB VALUES:** None known.

AVAILABILITY (Rx)

Capsules: 13 mcg, 25 mcg, 50 mcg, 75 mcg, 88 mcg, 100 mcg, 112 mcg, 125 mcg, 137 mcg, 150 mcg, 175 mcg, 200 mcg. **Injection, Powder for Reconstitution:** 100

mcg, 200 mcg, 500 mcg. **Solution, Oral: (Ermeza):** 150 mcg/5 mL. **(Thyquidity):** 100 mcg/5 mL. **(Tirosint):** 13 mcg/mL, 25 mcg/mL, 37.5 mcg/mL, 44 mcg/mL, 50 mcg/mL, 62.5 mcg/mL, 75 mcg/mL, 88 mcg/mL, 100 mcg/mL, 112 mcg/mL, 125 mcg/mL, 137 mcg/mL, 150 mcg/mL, 175 mcg/mL, 200 mcg/mL. **Tablets:** 25 mcg, 50 mcg, 75 mcg, 88 mcg, 100 mcg, 112 mcg, 125 mcg, 137 mcg, 150 mcg, 175 mcg, 200 mcg, 300 mcg.

ADMINISTRATION/HANDLING

◄**ALERT**► Do not interchange brands (known issues with bioequivalence between manufacturers).

 IV

Reconstitution • Reconstitute 200-mcg or 500-mcg vial with 5 mL 0.9% NaCl to provide concentration of 40 or 100 mcg/mL, respectively; shake until clear. **Rate of administration** • Use immediately; discard unused portions. • Give each 100 mcg or less over 1 min. **Storage** • Store vials at room temperature.

PO

• Administer in the morning on an empty stomach, 30–60 min before food. Give with a full glass of water. • Tablets may be crushed and suspended in 5–10 mL water (use immediately). • Take 4 hrs apart from antacids, iron, calcium supplements. Capsules must be swallowed whole (do not cut, crush, or chew). • **Oral solution:** To administer in water, squeeze the contents into a glass/cup containing water. • To administer directly, either squeeze into mouth or onto a spoon and administer immediately.

▦ IV INCOMPATIBILITIES

Do not use or mix with other IV solutions.

INDICATIONS/ROUTES/DOSAGE

Note: Doses based on clinical response and laboratory parameters. IV dose is 75–80% of oral dose once daily.

Hypothyroidism

Note: Adjust dose q3–6wks based on clinical response and serum TSH and/or free T4 concentrations.

PO: ADULTS 60 YRS OR YOUNGER WITHOUT EVIDENCE OF CORONARY HEART DISEASE: 1.6 mcg/kg/day as single daily dose. **Average dose:** 100–200 mcg/day. **ADULTS OLDER THAN 60 YRS WITHOUT EVIDENCE OF CORONARY HEART DISEASE:** Initially, 25–50 mcg once daily. **ADULTS WITH CARDIAC DISEASE:** Initially, 12.5–50 mcg/day. **CHILDREN OLDER THAN 12 YRS, GROWTH AND PUBERTY INCOMPLETE:** 2–3 mcg/kg/day. **CHILDREN 6–12 YRS:** 4–5 mcg/kg/day. **CHILDREN 1–5 YRS:** 5–6 mcg/kg/day. **CHILDREN 7–12 MOS:** 6–8 mcg/kg/day. **CHILDREN 3–6 MOS:** 8–10 mcg/kg/day. **CHILDREN YOUNGER THAN 3 MOS:** 10–15 mcg/kg/day.

Myxedema Coma

IV: ADULTS, ELDERLY: Initially, 200–400 mcg, then 50–100 mcg once daily until able to tolerate PO administration.

Pituitary Thyroid-Stimulating Hormone (TSH) Suppression

PO: ADULTS, ELDERLY: Initially, 1.6–2 mcg/kg/day immediately after surgery. Adjust dose after 6 wks based on TSH suppression goals.

Dosage in Renal/Hepatic Impairment

No dose adjustment.

SIDE EFFECTS

Occasional: Reversible hair loss at start of therapy in children. **Rare:** Dry skin, GI intolerance, rash, urticaria, pseudotumor cerebri, severe headache in children.

ADVERSE EFFECTS/TOXIC REACTIONS

Excessive dosage produces signs/symptoms of hyperthyroidism (weight loss, palpitations, increased appetite, tremors, anxiety, tachycardia, hypertension, headache, insomnia, menstrual irregularities). Cardiac arrhythmias occur rarely. Long-term therapy may decrease bone mineral density.

NURSING CONSIDERATIONS

BASELINE ASSESSMENT

Obtain TSH, T_3, T_4, weight, vital signs. Signs/symptoms of diabetes, diabetes insipidus, adrenal insufficiency, hypopituitarism. Treat with adrenocortical steroids before thyroid therapy in coexisting hypothyroidism and hypoadrenalism.

INTERVENTION/EVALUATION

Monitor pulse for rate, rhythm (report pulse greater than 100 or marked increase). Observe for tremors, anxiety. Assess appetite, sleep pattern. **Children: (Undertreatment):** May decrease intellectual development, linear growth. **(Overtreatment):** Adversely affects brain maturation, accelerates bone age. Monitor thyroid function tests.

PATIENT/FAMILY TEACHING

• Do not discontinue therapy; replacement for hypothyroidism is lifelong. • Follow-up office visits, thyroid function tests are essential. • Take medication at the same time each day, preferably in the morning. • Monitor pulse for rate, rhythm; report irregular rhythm or pulse rate over 100 beats/min. • Promptly report chest pain, weight loss, anxiety, tremors, insomnia. • Children may have reversible hair loss, increased aggressiveness during first few mos of therapy. • Full therapeutic effect may take 1–3 wks.

linagliptin

lin-a-**glip**-tin
(Tradjenta)
Do not confuse linagliptin with SAXagliptin or SITagliptin.

FIXED-COMBINATION(S)

Glyxambi: linagliptin/empagliflozin (an antidiabetic): 5 mg/10 mg, 5 mg/25 mg. **Jentadueto:** linagliptin/metFORMIN (an antidiabetic): 2.5 mg/500 mg; 2.5 mg/850 mg; 2.5

L

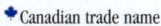 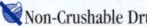

mg/1,000 mg. **Jentadueto XR:** linagliptin/metFORMIN (extended-release): 2.5 mg/1,000 mg; 5 mg/1,000 mg. **Trijardy XR:** empagliflozin (an antidiabetic)/linagliptin (an antidiabetic)/metFORMIN (an antidiabetic): 10 mg/5 mg/1,000 mg; 25 mg/5 mg/1,000 mg; 5mg/2.5 mg/1,000 mg; 12.5 mg/2.5 mg/1,000 mg.

◆ CLASSIFICATION

PHARMACOTHERAPEUTIC: Dipeptidyl peptidase-4 (DDP-4) inhibitor (gliptin). **CLINICAL:** Antidiabetic agent.

USES

Adjunctive treatment to diet and exercise to improve glycemic control in pts with type 2 diabetes alone or in combination with other antidiabetic agents.

PRECAUTIONS

Contraindications: Hypersensitivity to linagliptin, other DD4 inhibitors. **Cautions:** Concurrent use of other hypoglycemics. Not recommended for use in type 1 diabetes, diabetic ketoacidosis, history of pancreatitis, HF.

ACTION

Prolongs active incretin levels by inhibiting DDP-4 enzyme. **Therapeutic Effect:** Incretin hormones increase insulin synthesis/release from pancreatic beta cells and decrease glucagon secretion from pancreatic alpha cells. Lowers serum glucose levels.

PHARMACOKINETICS

Widely distributed. Peak plasma concentration: 1.5 hrs. Extensive tissue distribution. Protein binding: 70%–99%. Minimal metabolism (90% excreted as unchanged metabolite). Excreted primarily in enterohepatic system (80%), urine (5%). **Half-life:** 12 hrs.

⏳ LIFESPAN CONSIDERATIONS

Pregnancy/Lactation: Unknown if distributed in breast milk. **Children:** Safety and efficacy not established. **Elderly:** No age-related precautions noted.

INTERACTIONS

DRUG: **Strong CYP3A4 inducers (e.g., carBAMazepine, phenytoin, rifAMPin)** may decrease concentration/effect. **Antidiabetic agents (e.g., insulin, metFORMIN, SAXagliptin, SITagliptin, sulfonylureas)** may increase risk of hypoglycemia. **HERBAL:** **Ginseng, ginger, other herbs with hypoglycemic activity** may increase risk of hypoglycemia. **FOOD:** None known. **LAB VALUES:** Decreases serum glucose. May increase serum uric acid.

AVAILABILITY (Rx)

Tablets: 5 mg.

ADMINISTRATION/HANDLING

PO
* May give without regard to food.

INDICATIONS/ROUTES/DOSAGE

Note: Dose reduction of insulin and/or insulin secretagogues may be needed.

Type 2 Diabetes Mellitus
PO: **ADULTS, ELDERLY:** 5 mg once daily.

Dosage in Renal/Hepatic Impairment
No dose adjustment.

SIDE EFFECTS

Occasional (5%): Nasopharyngitis. **Rare (less than 2%):** Cough, headache.

ADVERSE EFFECTS/TOXIC REACTIONS

Hypoglycemia reported in 7% of pts. Concomitant use of hypoglycemic medication may increase hypoglycemic risk. Pancreatitis, hypersensitivity reactions (angioedema, rash, urticaria, pruritus, bronchospasm) occur rarely.

NURSING CONSIDERATIONS

BASELINE ASSESSMENT
Obtain blood glucose, hemoglobin A1c level. Assess pt's understanding of diabetes management, routine glucose

monitoring. Receive full medication history including herbal products.

INTERVENTION/EVALUATION

Monitor blood glucose, hemoglobin A1c level. Assess for hypoglycemia (diaphoresis, tremors, dizziness, anxiety, headache, tachycardia, perioral numbness, hunger, diplopia, difficulty concentrating), hyperglycemia (polyuria, polyphagia, polydipsia, nausea, vomiting, fatigue, Kussmaul breathing). Screen for glucose-altering conditions: fever, increased activity or stress, surgical procedures. Dietary consult for nutritional education.

PATIENT/FAMILY TEACHING

• Diabetes requires lifelong control.
• Diet and exercise are principal parts of treatment; do not skip or delay meals.
• Test blood glucose regularly. • When taking combination drug therapy or when glucose demands are altered (excessive alcohol ingestion, insufficient carbohydrate intake, hormone deficiencies, critical illness), have hypoglycemic treatment available (glucagon, oral dextrose). • Monitor daily calorie intake.

---

linezolid

lin-**ez**-oh-lid
(Apo-Linezolid ✣, Zyvox, Zyvoxam ✣)
Do not confuse Zyvox with Zosyn or Zovirax.

◆ CLASSIFICATION

PHARMACOTHERAPEUTIC: Oxazolidinone. **CLINICAL:** Antibiotic.

USES

Pneumonia: Treatment of nosocomial pneumonia caused by *S. aureus* (methicillin-susceptible and -resistant isolates) or *S. pneumoniae;* community-acquired pneumonia caused by *S. pneumoniae* or *S. aureus* (methicillin-susceptible isolates only). **Skin and skin structure**

infections: Caused by *S. aureus* (methicillin-susceptible and -resistant isolates), *S. pyogenes,* or *S. agalactiae.* **VRE:** Treatment of vancomycin-resistant *Enterococcus faecium* infections. **OFF-LABEL:** Anthrax, CNS infection, cystic fibrosis (acute pulmonary exacerbation), endocarditis, intracranial abscess, meningitis (bacterial), osteomyelitis, prosthetic joint infection, septic arthritis, toxic shock syndrome, tuberculosis (drug resistant).

PRECAUTIONS

Contraindications: Hypersensitivity to linezolid. Concurrent use or within 2 wks of MAOIs. **Cautions:** History of seizures, preexisting myelosuppression, medications that may cause bone marrow depression, uncontrolled hypertension, pheochromocytoma, carcinoid syndrome, untreated hyperthyroidism, diabetes, chronic infection; concurrent use of SSRIs, SNRIs, tricyclic antidepressants, triptans, buPROPion.

ACTION

Inhibits bacterial protein synthesis by binding to bacterial ribosomal RNA sites, preventing formation of a functional initiation complex that is essential for bacterial translation. **Therapeutic Effect:** Bacteriostatic against enterococci, staphylococci; bactericidal against streptococci.

PHARMACOKINETICS

Widely distributed. Protein binding: 31%. Metabolized in liver by oxidation. Excreted in urine. **Half-life:** 4–5.4 hrs.

⏳ LIFESPAN CONSIDERATIONS

Pregnancy/Lactation: Unknown if distributed in breast milk. **Children:** No age-related precautions noted. **Elderly:** No age-related precautions noted.

INTERACTIONS

DRUG: **Adrenergic medications (sympathomimetics)** may increase effects. **SSRIs** (e.g., **escitalopram, PARoxetine, sertraline**), **SNRIs** (e.g., **DULoxetine,**

---

venlafaxine) may increase risk of serotonin syndrome. **Alcohol, carBAMazepine, maprotiline, tapentadol** may increase adverse effects. **HERBAL:** Supplements containing **caffeine, tyrosine,** or **tryptophan** may precipitate hypertensive crisis. **FOOD:** Excessive amounts of **tyramine-containing foods, beverages** may cause significant hypertension. **LAB VALUES:** May decrease Hgb, neutrophils, platelets, WBC. May increase serum ALT, AST, alkaline phosphatase, amylase, bilirubin, BUN, creatinine, LDH, lipase.

AVAILABILITY (Rx)

Injection Premix: 2 mg/mL in 100-mL, 300-mL bags. **Powder for Oral Suspension:** 100 mg/5 mL. **Tablets:** 600 mg.

ADMINISTRATION/HANDLING

 IV

Rate of administration • Infuse over 30–120 min. • Should be administered without further dilution.
Storage • Store at room temperature. • Protect from light. • Yellow color does not affect potency.

PO
• Give without regard to food. • Use suspension within 21 days after reconstitution. Gently invert 3–5 times before administration. • Do not shake.

⚙ IV COMPATIBILITIES

Calcium gluconate, dexmedeTOMIDine, heparin, magnesium sulfate, potassium chloride.

INDICATIONS/ROUTES/DOSAGE

Vancomycin-Resistant Infections (VRE)
PO, IV: ADULTS, ELDERLY, CHILDREN OLDER THAN 11 YRS: 600 mg q12h. **CHILDREN 11 YRS AND YOUNGER:** 10 mg/kg q8–12h. **Maximum:** 600 mg/dose.

Pneumonia, Complicated Skin/Skin Structure Infections
PO, IV: ADULTS, ELDERLY, CHILDREN OLDER THAN 11 YRS: 600 mg q12h. **CHILDREN 11**

YRS AND YOUNGER: 10 mg/kg q8h. **Maximum:** 600 mg/dose.

Uncomplicated Skin/Skin Structure Infections
PO: ADULTS, ELDERLY: 600 mg q12h. **CHILDREN OLDER THAN 11 YRS:** 600 mg q12h. **CHILDREN 5–11 YRS:** 10 mg/kg/dose q12h. **Maximum:** 600 mg/dose. **CHILDREN YOUNGER THAN 5 YRS:** 10 mg/kg q8h. **Maximum:** 600 mg/dose.

Usual Neonate Dosage
PO, IV: NEONATES: 10 mg/kg/dose q8–12h.

Dosage in Renal/Hepatic Impairment
No dose adjustment. Administer after HD on dialysis days.

SIDE EFFECTS

Occasional (9%–2%): Diarrhea, nausea, vomiting, insomnia, constipation, rash, dizziness, fever, headache. **Rare (less than 2%):** Altered taste, vaginal candidiasis, fungal infection, tongue discoloration.

ADVERSE EFFECTS/TOXIC REACTIONS

Thrombocytopenia, myelosuppression occur rarely. Antibiotic-associated colitis, other superinfections (abdominal cramps, severe watery diarrhea, fever) may result from altered bacterial balance in GI tract.

NURSING CONSIDERATIONS

BASELINE ASSESSMENT
Obtain appropriate culture specimens for sensitivity testing prior to therapy. Obtain baseline CBC, chemistries. Question medical history as listed in Precautions. Receive full medication history and screen for interactions.

INTERVENTION/EVALUATION
Monitor daily pattern of bowel activity, stool consistency. Mild GI effects may be tolerable, but increasing severity may indicate onset of antibiotic-associated colitis. Be alert for superinfection: fever, vomiting, diarrhea, anal/genital pruritus, oral muco-

sal changes (ulceration, pain, erythema). Monitor CBC, platelets, Hgb, chemistries.

PATIENT/ FAMILY TEACHING
• Continue therapy for full length of treatment. • Doses should be evenly spaced. • May cause GI upset (may take with food, milk). • Excessive amounts of tyramine-containing foods (red wine, aged cheese) may cause severe reaction (severe headache, neck stiffness, diaphoresis, palpitations). • Avoid alcohol. • Report persistent diarrhea, nausea, vomiting.

---

liraglutide

leer-a-**gloo**-tide
(Saxenda, Victoza)
■ **BLACK BOX ALERT** ■ Causes dose-dependent and treatment duration–dependent thyroid C-cell tumors, including medullary thyroid cancer.

FIXED-COMBINATION(S)

Xultophy: liraglutide 3.6 mg/mL and insulin degludec 100 units/mL.

◆CLASSIFICATION

PHARMACOTHERAPEUTIC: Antihyperglycemic (glucagon-like peptide-1 [GLP-1]) receptor agonist. **CLINICAL:** Antidiabetic agent.

USES

Saxenda: Adjunct to diet and increased physical activity for chronic weight management in adults with body mass index (BMI) of 30 kg/m² or greater, or 27 kg/m² or greater, with at least one co-morbid condition (e.g., hypertension, diabetes, dyslipidemia) and pts 12 yrs of age and older with a body weight above 60 kg and an initial BMI corresponding to 30 kg/m2 for adults (obese) by international cutoffs. **Victoza:** Adjunct to diet and exercise to improve glycemic control in adults and children 10 yrs of age and older with type 2 diabetes. Reduce risk of major cardiovascular events (e.g., MI, stroke) in adults with type 2 diabetes and established cardiovascular (CV) disease.

PRECAUTIONS

Contraindications: Hypersensitivity to liraglutide. Personal or family history of medullary thyroid carcinoma (MTC), pts with multiple endocrine neoplasia syndrome type 2 (MEN2). **Saxenda (additional):** Pregnancy. **Cautions:** History of pancreatitis, cholelithiasis, alcohol abuse, renal/hepatic impairment. History of angioedema to other GLP-1 receptor agonists. Do not use in type 1 diabetes or diabetic ketoacidosis. Medications requiring a narrow therapeutic index or requiring rapid GI absorption. Pulmonary aspiration in pts undergoing elective procedures requiring general anesthesia or deep sedation having residual gastric contents despite fasting.

ACTION

Stimulates release of insulin from pancreatic beta cells, mimics enhancement of glucose-dependent insulin secretion, decreases inappropriate glucagon secretion, slows gastric emptying, decreases food intake. **Therapeutic Effect:** Improves glycemic control by increasing postmeal insulin secretion, emptying, increasing satiety.

PHARMACOKINETICS

Metabolized into large proteins without a specific organ as a major route of elimination. Protein binding: greater than 98%. Peak plasma concentration: 8–12 hrs. Excreted in urine (6%), feces (5%). **Half-life:** 13 hrs.

⧗ LIFESPAN CONSIDERATIONS

Pregnancy/Lactation: Unknown if distributed in breast milk. **Children:** Safety and efficacy not established. **Elderly:** No age-related precautions noted.

INTERACTIONS

DRUG: May increase concentration/effects of **glucagon-like peptides** (e.g., **dula-glutide, semaglutide**), hypoglycemia-associated agents (e.g., **glyburide**,

L

 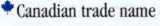 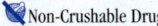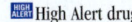

metformin), insulin. **HERBAL:** None significant. **FOOD:** None known. **LAB VALUES:** Decreases glucose serum levels (when used in combination with insulin secretagogues [e.g., sulfonylureas]).

AVAILABILITY (Rx)

SQ, Solution (Prefilled Pen): *(Victoza):* 18 mg/3 mL. *(Saxenda):* 18 mg/3 mL. Delivers doses of 0.6 mg, 1.2 mg, 1.8 mg, 2.4 mg, or 3 mg.

ADMINISTRATION/HANDLING

• Insert needle subcutaneously into upper arms, outer thigh, or abdomen, and inject solution. • Do not inject into areas of active skin disease or injury such as sunburns, skin rashes, inflammation, skin infections, or active psoriasis. • Rotate injection sites.
Storage • Refrigerate prefilled pens. • Discard if freezing occurs. • Discard pen 30 days after initial use.

INDICATIONS/ROUTES/DOSAGE

Diabetes (Victoza) With or Without CV Disease
SQ: ADULTS, ELDERLY, CHILDREN 10 YRS AND OLDER: Initial dose: 0.6 mg once daily for at least 1 wk. (**Note:** This dose is intended to reduce GI symptoms during initial titration; it is not effective for glycemic control.) After 1 wk, increase dose to 1.2 mg. If 1.2-mg dose does not result in acceptable glycemic control, dose can be increased to 1.8 mg.

Weight Management (Saxenda)
SQ: ADULTS, ELDERLY: Initially, 0.6 mg once daily for 1 week. Increase wkly by 0.6 mg/day to a target dose of 3 mg once daily. **Note:** Evaluate change in body weight after 12 wks at maximum tolerated dose or 16 wks after initiation. Discontinue if less than 4% of baseline weight not achieved. **CHILDREN 12 YRS AND OLDER:** Initially, 0.6 mg once daily for 1 wk. Increase by 0.6 mg/day in increments at wkly intervals to 3 mg once daily. If the 3-mg target daily dose is not tolerated, reduce dose to 2.4 mg daily. Discontinue if 2.4-mg dose is not tolerated.

Discontinue therapy if BMI has not reduced at least 1% from baseline after 12 wks on maintenance dose.

Dosage in Renal/Hepatic Impairment
Use caution.

SIDE EFFECTS

Frequent (greater than 13%): Headache, nausea, diarrhea, liraglutide antibody resistance. **Occasional (13%–6%):** Diarrhea, vomiting, dizziness, nervousness, dyspepsia. **Rare (less than 6%):** Weakness, decreased appetite.

ADVERSE EFFECTS/TOXIC REACTIONS

Serious hypoglycemia may occur when used concurrently with insulin analogue (e.g., sulfonylurea); consider lowering dose. May increase risk of thyroid C-cell tumors. Hypersensitivity reactions, including anaphylaxis, angioedema, were reported. Due to delayed gastric emptying effect, may increase risk of aspiration during general anesthesia. Life-threatening pancreatitis may occur. May increase risk of acute gallbladder disease.

NURSING CONSIDERATIONS

BASELINE ASSESSMENT
Obtain blood glucose, hemoglobin A1c level. Discuss pt's lifestyle to determine extent of learning, emotional needs. Ensure follow-up instruction if pt/family does not thoroughly understand diabetes management or glucose testing technique. Dose is gradually increased to improve GI tolerance.

INTERVENTION/EVALUATION
Monitor blood glucose level, food intake. Assess for hypoglycemia (cool wet skin, tremors, dizziness, anxiety, headache, tachycardia, numbness in mouth, hunger, diplopia) or hyperglycemia (polyuria, polyphagia, polydipsia, nausea, vomiting, dim vision, fatigue, deep rapid breathing). Be alert to conditions that alter glucose requirements (fever, increased activity/stress, surgical procedures). Consider lowering dose of insulin analogue to reduce risk of hypoglycemia.

PATIENT/FAMILY TEACHING

• A healthcare provider will show you how to properly prepare and inject your medication. You must demonstrate correct preparation and injection techniques before using medication at home. • Diabetes requires lifelong control. • Prescribed diet, exercise are principal parts of treatment; do not skip/delay meals. • Continue following dietary instructions, regular exercise program, regular testing of blood glucose level. • Serious hypoglycemia may occur when used concurrently with insulin analogue (e.g., sulfonylurea). • Have source of glucose available to treat symptoms of low blood sugar. • Serious allergic reactions, including anaphylaxis and swelling of the face, mouth, and tongue, may occur. • Treatment may cause gallbladder disease or inflammation of the pancreas. Report abdominal pain, fever, nausea, vomiting; yellowing of the skin or eyes.

---

lisinopril
TOP
100

lye-**sin**-o-pril
(Qbrelis, Zestril)

■ **BLACK BOX ALERT** ■ May cause fetal injury, mortality. Discontinue as soon as possible once pregnancy is detected.
Do not confuse lisinopril with fosinopril, Lipitor, or RisperDAL or Zestril with Desyrel, Restoril, Vistaril, Zetia, Zostrix, or Zyprexa.
Do not confuse lisinopril's combination form Zestoretic with PriLOSEC.

FIXED-COMBINATION(S)

Prinzide/Zestoretic: lisinopril/hydroCHLOROthiazide (a diuretic): 10 mg/12.5 mg, 20 mg/12.5 mg, 20 mg/25 mg.

◆ CLASSIFICATION

PHARMACOTHERAPEUTIC: ACE inhibitor. **CLINICAL:** Antihypertensive.

USES

Hypertension: Treatment of hypertension in adults and children 6 yrs and older. **HF with reduced ejection fraction:** Adjunctive therapy to reduce signs/symptoms of systolic HF. **ST elevation MI:** Treatment of acute ST elevation MI within 24 hrs in hemodynamically stable pts to improve survival. **OFF-LABEL:** Non-ST elevation MI, proteinuric chronic kidney disease. Migraine (prevention).

PRECAUTIONS

Contraindications: Hypersensitivity to lisinopril, other ACE inhibitors. History of angioedema from treatment with ACE inhibitors, idiopathic or hereditary angioedema. Concomitant use with aliskiren in pts with diabetes. Coadministration with or within 36 hrs of switching to or from a neprilysin inhibitor (e.g., sacubitril). **Cautions:** Renal impairment, unstented unilateral/bilateral renal artery stenosis, volume depletion, ischemic heart disease, cerebrovascular disease, severe aortic stenosis, hypertrophic cardiomyopathy, HF, systolic B/P less than 100, dialysis, hyponatremia; before, during, or immediately after major surgery. Concomitant use of potassium supplements.

ACTION

Competitive inhibitor of angiotensin-converting enzyme (ACE) (prevents conversion of angiotensin I to angiotensin II, a potent vasoconstrictor; may inhibit angiotensin II at local vascular, renal sites). Decreases plasma angiotensin II, increases plasma renin activity, decreases aldosterone secretion. **Therapeutic Effect:** Reduces blood pressure.

PHARMACOKINETICS

Route	Onset	Peak	Duration
PO	1 hr	6 hrs	24 hrs

Widely distributed. Protein binding: 25%. Primarily excreted unchanged in urine. Removed by hemodialysis. **Half-life:** 12 hrs (increased in renal impairment).

⧖ LIFESPAN CONSIDERATIONS

Pregnancy/Lactation: Crosses placenta. Unknown if distributed in breast milk. **Children:** Safety and efficacy not established. **Elderly:** May be more sensitive to hypotensive effects.

INTERACTIONS

DRUG: **Aliskiren** may increase hyperkalemic effect. May increase potential for allergic reactions to **allopurinol. Angiotensin receptor blockers (e.g., losartan, valsartan)** may increase adverse effects. May increase adverse effects of **lithium, sacubitril. HERBAL:** **Herbals with hypertensive properties (e.g., licorice, yohimbe)** or **hypotensive properties (e.g., garlic, ginger, ginkgo biloba)** may alter effects. **Green tea** may decrease concentration/effect. **FOOD:** None known. **LAB VALUES:** May increase serum BUN, alkaline phosphatase, bilirubin, creatinine, potassium, ALT, AST. May decrease serum sodium. May cause positive ANA titer.

AVAILABILITY (Rx)

Solution, Oral: *(Qbrelis)* 1 mg/mL. **Tablets:** 2.5 mg, 5 mg, 10 mg, 20 mg, 30 mg, 40 mg.

ADMINISTRATION/HANDLING
PO
• Administer as a single daily dose without regard to food.

INDICATIONS/ROUTES/DOSAGE
Hypertension
PO: ADULTS: Initially, 5–10 mg once daily. Evaluate response q2–4wks and titrate dose (e.g., increase the daily dose by doubling), up to 80 mg once daily. **ELDERLY:** Initially, 2.5–5 mg once daily. Evaluate response q2–4wks and titrate dose (e.g., increase the daily dose by doubling), up to 40 mg once daily. **CHILDREN 6 YRS OR OLDER:** Initially, 0.07 mg/kg once daily (up to 5 mg). Titrate at 1- to 2-wk intervals. **Maximum:** 0.6 mg/kg/day or 40 mg/day.

HF
PO: ADULTS, ELDERLY: Initially, 2.5–5 mg/day. May increase by no more than 10 mg/day at intervals of at least 1–2 wks to a target dose of 20–40 mg once daily.

Acute MI (to Improve Survival)
PO: ADULTS, ELDERLY: Hemodynamically stable: 5 mg PO q24hrs for 2 doses, then after 48 hrs, 10 mg PO once daily. **With low systolic blood pressure (100–120 mm Hg):** 2.5 mg PO once daily for 3 days, then 2.5 or 5 mg PO once daily.

Dosage in Renal Impairment
CrCl less than 30 mL/min: Not recommended in children. Titrate to pt's needs after giving the following initial dose:

Hypertension
Creatinine Clearance	Initial Dose
10–30 mL/min	5 mg
Less than 10 mL/min or Dialysis	2.5 mg

HF
CrCl less than 30 mL/min or serum creatinine greater than 3 mg/dL: Initial dose: 2.5 mg.

Acute MI
CrCl 30 mL/min or less: Initial dose: 2.5 mg.

Dosage in Hepatic Impairment
No dose adjustment.

SIDE EFFECTS
Frequent (12%–5%): Headache, dizziness, postural hypotension. **Occasional (4%–2%):** Chest discomfort, fatigue, rash, abdominal pain, nausea, diarrhea, upper respiratory infection. **Rare (1% or less):** Palpitations, tachycardia, peripheral edema, insomnia, paresthesia, confusion, constipation, dry mouth, muscle cramps.

ADVERSE EFFECTS/TOXIC REACTIONS

Excessive hypotension (first-dose syncope) may occur in pts with HF, severe salt/volume depletion. Angioedema (swelling of face and lips), hyperkalemia occur rarely. Agranulocytosis, neutropenia may be noted in pts with collagen vascular disease (scleroderma, systemic lupus erythematosus). Nephrotic syndrome may be noted in pts with history of renal disease.

NURSING CONSIDERATIONS

BASELINE ASSESSMENT

Obtain BMP (esp. serum BUN, creatinine, sodium, potassium; CrCl, GFR). Obtain B/P, apical pulse immediately before each dose in addition to regular monitoring (be alert to fluctuations). In pts with renal impairment, autoimmune disease, taking drugs that affect leukocytes or immune response, CBC and differential count should be performed before beginning therapy and q2wks for 3 mos, then periodically thereafter. Question history of aortic stenosis, cardiac disease, cardiomyopathy, renal impairment or stenosis.

INTERVENTION/EVALUATION

Monitor B/P, renal function tests, serum potassium. Assess for edema. Monitor I&O; weigh daily. Monitor daily pattern of bowel activity, stool consistency. Assist with ambulation if dizziness occurs.

PATIENT/ FAMILY TEACHING

• To reduce hypotensive effect, go from lying to standing slowly. • Limit alcohol intake. • Report vomiting, diarrhea, diaphoresis, swelling of face/lips/tongue, difficulty in breathing, persistent cough. • Limit salt intake. • Maintain adequate hydration. • Report decreased urinary output, dark-colored urine, swelling of the hands and feet. • Immediately report allergic reactions, esp. life-threatening swelling of the face or tongue.

lithium

lith-ee-um
(Carbolith ♣, Lithobid, Lithane ♣, Lithmax ♣)

■ **BLACK BOX ALERT** ■ Lithium toxicity is closely related to serum lithium levels and can occur at therapeutic doses. Routine determination of serum lithium levels is essential during therapy.

Do not confuse Lithobid with Levbid or Lithostat.

◆CLASSIFICATION

PHARMACOTHERAPEUTIC: Mood-stabilizing agent. **CLINICAL:** Antimanic.

USES

Bipolar disorder: (Immediate-release): Treatment of acute mania, acute episodes with mixed features, and maintenance treatment in pts 7 yrs of age and older. **(Extended-release):** Treatment of manic episodes and maintenance treatment in pts 12 yrs of age and older. **OFF-LABEL:** Major depressive disorder (unipolar). Bipolar disorder (acute hypomania, acute major depression).

PRECAUTIONS

Contraindications: Hypersensitivity to lithium. **Immediate-release capsule, solution and tablet:** Severely debilitated pts, severe cardiovascular disease, concurrent use with diuretics, severe dehydration, severe renal disease, severe sodium depletion or dehydration. **Cautions:** Mild to moderate cardiovascular disease, thyroid disease, elderly, mild to moderate renal impairment, medications altering sodium excretion, pregnancy, pts at risk for suicide, hypovolemia, pts receiving neuromuscular blocking agents.

ACTION

Alters cation transport across cell membrane in nerve/muscle cells; influences reuptake of serotonin/norepinephrine. **Therapeutic Effect:** Stabilizes mood, reducing episodes of mania.

PHARMACOKINETICS

Widely distributed. Protein binding: None. Primarily excreted unchanged in urine. Removed by hemodialysis.

L

Half-life: 18–24 hrs (increased in elderly).

⧖ LIFESPAN CONSIDERATIONS

Pregnancy/Lactation: Freely crosses placenta. Distributed in breast milk. **Children:** May increase bone formation or density (alter parathyroid hormone concentrations). **Elderly:** More susceptible to develop lithium-induced goiter or clinical hypothyroidism, CNS toxicity. Increased thirst, urination noted more frequently; lower dosage recommended.

INTERACTIONS

DRUG: Diuretics (e.g., **furosemide, hydroCHLOROthiazide**), NSAIDs (e.g., **ibuprofen, naproxen, ketorolac**), **metroNIDAZOLE,** ACE inhibitors (e.g., **enalapril, lisinopril**), angiotensin II antagonists (e.g., **losartan, valsartan**), SSRIs (e.g., **escitalopram, PARoxetine, sertraline**), calcium channel blockers (e.g., **amLODIPine, dilTIAZem, verapamil**) may increase lithium concentration, risk of toxicity. May increase neurotoxic effect of **tricyclic antidepressants** (e.g., **amitriptyline**). MAOIs (e.g., **phenelzine, selegiline**) may enhance serotonergic effect. **HERBAL: St. John's wort** may alter concentration/effect. **Syrian rue** may increase concentration/effect. **FOOD:** None known. **LAB VALUES:** May increase serum glucose, immunoreactive parathyroid hormone, calcium.

AVAILABILITY (Rx)

Capsules: 150 mg, 300 mg, 600 mg.
Tablets: 300 mg.
Tablets (Extended-Release): 300 mg, 450 mg.

ADMINISTRATION/HANDLING

PO
• Administer with meals, milk to decrease GI upset. • Do not break, crush, dissolve, or divide extended-release tablets.

INDICATIONS/ROUTES/DOSAGE

◄ **ALERT** ► During acute phase, a therapeutic serum lithium concentration of 0.8–1.2 mEq/L is required. For long-term control, desired level is 0.6–1 mEq/L. Monitor serum drug concentration, clinical response to determine proper dosage.

Usual Dosage
PO: ADULTS, ELDERLY, CHILDREN OLDER THAN 12 YRS: Initially, 600–900 mg/day in 2–3 divided doses. May increase by 300–600 mg increments q1–5days based on response and tolerability. **Usual dose:** 900–1,800 mg /day in 1–3 divided doses.

Dosage in Renal Impairment

Creatinine Clearance	Dosage
10–50 mL/min	50%–75% normal dose
Less than 10 mL/min	25%–50% normal dose
End-stage renal disease with HD	Dose after HD

Dosage in Hepatic Impairment
No dose adjustment.

SIDE EFFECTS

◄ **ALERT** ► Side effects are dose related and seldom occur at lithium serum levels less than 1.5 mEq/L. **Occasional:** Fine hand tremor, polydipsia, polyuria, mild nausea. **Rare:** Weight gain, bradycardia, tachycardia, acne, rash, muscle twitching, peripheral cyanosis, pseudotumor cerebri (eye pain, headache, tinnitus, vision disturbances).

ADVERSE EFFECTS/TOXIC REACTIONS

Lithium serum concentration of 1.5–2.0 mEq/L may produce vomiting, diarrhea, drowsiness, confusion, incoordination, coarse hand tremor, muscle twitching, T-wave depression on ECG. Lithium serum concentration of 2.0–2.5 mEq/L may result in ataxia, giddiness, tinnitus, blurred vision, clonic movements, severe hypotension. Acute toxicity may be characterized by seizures, oliguria, circulatory failure, coma, death.

L

NURSING CONSIDERATIONS

BASELINE ASSESSMENT

Question history of cardiac/thyroid disease, renal impairment. Assess hydration status. Assess mental status (e.g., mood, behavior). Serum lithium levels should be tested q3–4days during initial phase of therapy, q1–2mos thereafter, and wkly if there is no improvement of disorder or adverse effects occur.

INTERVENTION/EVALUATION

Clinical assessment of therapeutic effect, tolerance to drug effect is necessary for correct dosing-level management. Assess behavior, appearance, emotional status, response to environment, speech pattern, thought content. Monitor serum lithium concentrations, CBC with differential, urinalysis, creatinine clearance. Monitor renal, hepatic, thyroid, cardiovascular function; serum electrolytes. Assess for increased urinary output, persistent thirst. Report polyuria, prolonged vomiting, diarrhea, fever to physician (may need to temporarily reduce or discontinue dosage). Monitor for signs of lithium toxicity. Assess for therapeutic response (interest in surroundings, improvement in self-care, increased ability to concentrate, relaxed facial expression). Monitor lithium levels q3–4days at initiation of therapy (then q1–2mos). Obtain lithium levels 8–12 hrs postdose. **Therapeutic serum level:** 0.6–1.2 mEq/L; **toxic serum level:** greater than 1.5 mEq/L.

PATIENT/ FAMILY TEACHING

• Limit alcohol, caffeine intake. • Avoid tasks requiring coordination until CNS effects of drug are known. • May cause dry mouth. • Maintain adequate salt, fluid intake (avoid dehydration). • Report vomiting, diarrhea, muscle weakness, tremors, drowsiness, ataxia. • Monitoring of serum level is necessary to determine proper dose.

loratadine

lor-**at**-a-deen
(Claritin, Claritin Reditabs, Loradamed)
Do not confuse loratadine with cloNIDine, or Claritin with clarithromycin.

FIXED-COMBINATION(S)

Alavert Allergy and Sinus, Claritin-D: loratadine/pseudoephedrine (a sympathomimetic): 5 mg/120 mg, 10 mg/240 mg.

◆CLASSIFICATION

PHARMACOTHERAPEUTIC: H_1 antagonist, second generation. **CLINICAL:** Antihistamine.

USES

Allergic rhinitis/conjunctivitis: Relief of nasal and non-nasal symptoms of seasonal allergies. **OTC:** Therapy for symptoms of hay fever, other upper respiratory symptoms. **Urticaria (new onset/chronic spontaneous):** Treatment of itching due to hives.

PRECAUTIONS

Contraindications: Hypersensitivity to loratadine. **Cautions:** Renal/hepatic impairment.

ACTION

Competes with histamine for H_1 receptor sites on effector cells. **Therapeutic Effect:** Prevents allergic responses mediated by histamine (e.g., rhinitis, urticaria, pruritus).

PHARMACOKINETICS

Route	Onset	Peak	Duration
PO	1–3 hrs	8–12 hrs	Longer than 24 hrs

Distributed mainly to liver, lungs, GI tract, bile. Protein binding: 97%; metabolite, 73%–77%. Metabolized in liver. Excreted in urine (40%) and feces (40%). Not removed by hemodialysis. **Half-life:** 8.4 hrs; metabolite, 28 hrs (increased in elderly, hepatic impairment).

⌛ LIFESPAN CONSIDERATIONS

Pregnancy/Lactation: Distributed in breast milk. **Children:** Safety and efficacy not established in pts younger than 2 yrs. **Elderly:** More sensitive to anticholinergic effects (e.g., dry mouth, nose, throat).

INTERACTIONS

DRUG: Aclidinium, ipratropium, tiotropium, umeclidinium may increase anticholinergic effect. **HERBAL: Herbals with sedative properties (e.g., chamomile, kava kava, valerian)** may increase CNS depression. **FOOD:** None known. **LAB VALUES:** May suppress wheal, flare reactions to antigen skin testing unless drug is discontinued 4 days before testing.

AVAILABILITY (Rx)

Capsule:10 mg. **Solution, Oral:** 5 mg/5 mL. **Syrup:** 5 mg/5 mL. **Tablets:** 10 mg. **Tablets, Chewable:** 5 mg. **Tablets, Orally Disintegrating:** 5 mg, 10 mg.

ADMINISTRATION/HANDLING

PO
• May take without regard to food.

Orally Disintegrating Tablets
• Place under tongue. • Disintegration occurs within seconds, after which tablet contents may be swallowed with or without water.

INDICATIONS/ROUTES/DOSAGE

Allergic Rhinitis
PO: ADULTS, ELDERLY, CHILDREN 6 YRS AND OLDER: 10 mg once daily or 5 mg twice daily. **CHILDREN 2–5 YRS:** 5 mg once daily.

Urticaria
PO: ADULTS, ELDERLY: Initially, 10 mg once daily. **Maximum:** 10 mg/day. **CHILDREN 6 YRS OF AGE AND OLDER:** 10 mg once daily. **CHILDREN 2–5 YRS:** 5 mg once daily.

Dosage in Renal Impairment
(CrCl less than 30 mL/min)
PO: ADULTS, ELDERLY, CHILDREN 6 YRS AND OLDER: 10 mg every other day. **CHILDREN 2–5 YRS:** No dose adjustment.

Dosage in Hepatic Impairment
No dose adjustment.

SIDE EFFECTS

Frequent (12%–8%): Headache, fatigue, drowsiness. **Occasional (3%):** Dry mouth, nose, throat. **Rare:** Photosensitivity.

ADVERSE EFFECTS/TOXIC REACTIONS

None significant.

NURSING CONSIDERATIONS

BASELINE ASSESSMENT
Assess lung sounds for wheezing; skin for urticaria, other allergy symptoms.

INTERVENTION/EVALUATION
For upper respiratory allergies, increase fluids to decrease viscosity of secretions, offset thirst, replenish loss of fluids from increased diaphoresis. Monitor symptoms for therapeutic response.

PATIENT/FAMILY TEACHING
• Drink plenty of water (may cause dry mouth). • Avoid alcohol. • Avoid tasks that require alertness, motor skills until response to drug is established (may cause drowsiness). • May cause photosensitivity reactions (avoid direct exposure to sunlight).

LORazepam

lor-**az**-e-pam
(Ativan, LORazepam Intensol, Loreev XR)

■ BLACK BOX ALERT ■ Concomitant use of benzodiazepines and opioids may result in profound sedation, respiratory depression, coma, and death. Reserve concomitant prescribing of these drugs for use in pts for whom alternative treatment options are inadequate. Limit dosages and durations to the minimum required. Follow pts for signs and symptoms of respiratory depression and sedation. Exposes users to risks of abuse, misuse, and addiction, which can lead to overdose/death. Continued use for several days to wks may lead to clinically significant addiction/physical dependence.
Do not confuse Ativan with Ambien or Atarax, or LORazepam with ALPRAZolam, diazePAM, Lovaza, temazepam, or zolpidem.

◆CLASSIFICATION

PHARMACOTHERAPEUTIC: Benzodiazepine (Schedule IV). **CLINICAL:** Antianxiety, sedative-hypnotic, antiemetic, skeletal muscle relaxant, amnesiac, anticonvulsant, antitremor.

USES

PO: Management of anxiety disorders, short-term relief of symptoms of anxiety, anxiety associated with depressive symptoms. **(Loreev XR):** Treatment of anxiety disorders in adults receiving stable, evenly divided, three times daily dosing with LORazepam tablets. **IV:** Status epilepticus, preanesthesia for amnesia, sedation. **OFF-LABEL:** Akathisia (antipsychotic induced), catatonia, chemotherapy-induced nausea/vomiting, mechanically ventilated pts in ICU (sedation), neuroleptic malignant syndrome, acute active seizures (non-epilepticus), serotonin syndrome,

substance withdrawal (alcohol, opioids), vertigo (acute).

PRECAUTIONS

Contraindications: Hypersensitivity to LORazepam, other benzodiazepines. Acute narrow-angle glaucoma, severe respiratory depression (except during mechanical ventilation). **Cautions:** Neonates, renal/hepatic impairment, compromised pulmonary function, depression, concomitant use of CNS depressants; pts at high risk for suicidal ideation and behavior; history of drug abuse and misuse, drug-seeking behavior, dependency.

ACTION

Enhances action of inhibitory neurotransmitter gamma-aminobutyric acid (GABA) in CNS, affecting memory, motor, sensory, cognitive function. **Therapeutic Effect:** Produces anxiolytic, anticonvulsant, sedative, muscle relaxant, antiemetic effects.

PHARMACOKINETICS

Route	Onset	Peak	Duration
PO	30–60 min	N/A	6–8 hrs
IV	5–20 min	N/A	6–8 hrs
IM	20–30 min	N/A	6–8 hrs

Widely distributed. Protein binding: 85%. Metabolized in liver. Primarily excreted in urine. Not removed by hemodialysis. **Half-life:** 10–20 hrs.

⧖ LIFESPAN CONSIDERATIONS

Pregnancy/Lactation: May cross placenta. May be distributed in breast milk. May increase risk of fetal abnormalities if administered during first trimester of pregnancy. Chronic ingestion during pregnancy may produce fetal toxicity, withdrawal symptoms, CNS depression in neonates. **Children:** Safety and efficacy not established in pts younger than 12 yrs. **Elderly:** Use small initial doses with gradual increases to avoid ataxia,

L

 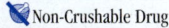

excessive sedation, or paradoxical CNS restlessness, excitement. May be more susceptible to cognitive impairment, delirium, falls, fractures.

INTERACTIONS

DRUG: **Valproic acid** may increase concentration/effects. **Alcohol, other CNS depressants** (e.g., **morphine, PHENobarbital, zolpidem**) may increase CNS depression. **HERBAL:** **Herbals with sedative properties** (e.g., **chamomile, kava kava, valerian**) may increase CNS depression. **FOOD:** None known. **LAB VALUES:** None significant. **Therapeutic serum level:** 50–240 ng/mL; **toxic serum level:** unknown.

AVAILABILITY (Rx)

Injection Solution: 2 mg/mL, 4 mg/mL. **Oral Solution:** *(LORazepam Intensol):* 2 mg/mL. **Tablets:** 0.5 mg, 1 mg, 2 mg.

 Capsules, Extended-Release: 1 mg, 1.5 mg, 2 mg, 3 mg.

ADMINISTRATION/HANDLING

IV

Reconstitution • Dilute with equal volume of Sterile Water for Injection, D_5W, or 0.9% NaCl.
Rate of administration • Give by IV push into tubing of free-flowing IV infusion (0.9% NaCl, D_5W) at a rate not to exceed 2 mg/min.
Storage • Refrigerate parenteral form. • Do not use if discolored or precipitate forms. • Avoid freezing.

IM
• Give deep IM into large muscle mass.

PO
• Give without regard to food (may give with food to decrease GI distress). • Dilute oral solution in water, juice, soda, or semisolid food. Extended-release capsule: Administer whole. Do not crush. Capsules cannot be chewed. May open and mix with applesauce.

IV COMPATIBILITIES

Acetaminophen, amiodarone, dexmedetomidine, heparin, norepinephrine, potassium chloride, propofol.

INDICATIONS/ROUTES/DOSAGE

Anxiety
PO: **ADULTS, ELDERLY:** Initially, 0.5–1 mg 2–3 times/day. May increase q2–3 days in increments of 1 mg up to 6 mg/day in 2–4 divided doses. **ER capsule:** Determine stable daily dose with immediate-release tablets. May convert to extended-release as once-daily dose in morning. **ADOLESCENTS, CHILDREN 12 YRS AND OLDER:** 0.25–2 mg/dose 2–3 times/day. **Maximum dose:** 2 mg.

Status Epilepticus
IV: **ADULTS, ELDERLY:** 0.1 mg/kg/dose. **Maximum:** 4 mg/dose. If seizures continue or recur after 10–15 min, may repeat 4 mg dose.

Dosage in Renal/Hepatic Impairment
PO: No dose adjustment.
IM, IV: **Mild to moderate impairment:** Use caution. Not recommended in severe impairment.

SIDE EFFECTS

Frequent (16%–7%): Drowsiness, dizziness. **Rare (less than 4%):** Weakness, ataxia, headache, hypotension, nausea, vomiting, confusion, injection site reaction.

ADVERSE EFFECTS/TOXIC REACTIONS

Abrupt or too-rapid withdrawal may result in pronounced restlessness, irritability, insomnia, hand tremor, abdominal cramping, muscle cramps, diaphoresis, vomiting, seizures. Overdose results in drowsiness, confusion, diminished reflexes, coma. **Antidote:** Flumazenil (see Appendix H for dosage).

NURSING CONSIDERATIONS

BASELINE ASSESSMENT

Offer emotional support to anxious pt. Pt must remain recumbent following parenteral administration to reduce hypotensive effect. Assess motor responses (agitation, trembling, tension), autonomic responses (cold or clammy hands, diaphoresis). Assess for drug-seeking behavior; risk of drug abuse and misuse.

INTERVENTION/EVALUATION

Monitor B/P, respiratory rate, heart rate. Diligently screen for suicidal ideation and behavior; new onset or worsening of anxiety, depression, mood disorder. Screen for drug abuse and misuse, drug-seeking behavior. Assess for paradoxical reaction, particularly during early therapy. Evaluate for therapeutic response: calm facial expression, decreased restlessness, insomnia, decrease in seizure-related symptoms. **Therapeutic serum level:** 50–240 ng/mL; **toxic serum level:** N/A.

PATIENT/FAMILY TEACHING

• Drowsiness usually subsides during continued therapy. • Avoid tasks that require alertness, motor skills until response to drug is established. • Smoking reduces drug effectiveness. • Do not abruptly discontinue medication after long-term therapy. • Do not use alcohol, CNS depressants. • Contraception recommended for long-term therapy. • Seek immediate medical attention if thoughts of suicide, new onset or worsening of anxiety, depression, or changes in mood occur.

lorlatinib

lor-**la**-ti-nib
(Lorbrena)
Do not confuse lorlatinib with alectinib, brigatinib, ceritinib, crizotinib, erlotinib, lapatinib, neratinib, lenvatinib, loratadine, or LORazepam.

◆CLASSIFICATION

PHARMACOTHERAPEUTIC: Anaplastic lymphoma kinase inhibitor. Tyrosine kinase inhibitor. **CLINICAL:** Antineoplastic.

USES

First-line treatment of metastatic non–small-cell lung cancer (NSCLC) in adults whose tumors are anaplastic lymphoma kinase (ALK)–positive.

PRECAUTIONS

Contraindications: Hypersensitivity to lorlatinib. Concomitant use of strong CYP3A4 inducers. **Cautions:** Baseline cytopenias, hyperlipidemia, cardiac or pulmonary disease, hepatic impairment, concomitant use of strong or moderate CYP3A4 inhibitors, moderate CYP3A4 inducers; pts at risk for atrioventricular (AV) block (idiopathic cardiac conduction disorders), ischemic heart disease, increased vagal tone, concomitant use of antiarrhythmics, beta blockers, calcium channel blockers); history of anxiety, depression, suicidal ideation and behavior, mood disorder.

ACTION

A reversible, potent, third-generation tyrosine kinase inhibitor that is highly selective at targeting ALK and ROS1. Overcomes known ALK resistance mutations. **Therapeutic Effect:** Has anti-tumor activity against multiple mutant forms of the ALK enzyme, including mutations detected in tumors at the time of disease progression on crizotinib and other ALK inhibitors. Anti-tumor activity is dose-dependent correlating with inhibition of ALK phosphorylation.

PHARMACOKINETICS

Widely distributed. Penetrates blood-brain barrier. Metabolized in liver. Protein binding: 66%. Peak plasma concentration: 1.2–2 hrs. Excreted in urine (48%), feces (41%). **Half-life:** 24 hrs.

⧖ LIFESPAN CONSIDERATIONS

Pregnancy/Lactation: Avoid pregnancy; may cause fetal harm. Females of reproductive potential must use effective non-hormonal contraception during treatment and for at least 6 mos after discontinuation. Hormonal contraception may become ineffective with treatment. Unknown if distributed in breast milk. Breastfeeding not recommended during treatment and for at least 7 days after discontinuation. **Males:**

◆ Canadian trade name　　　🐋 Non-Crushable Drug　　　▦ High Alert drug

L

Males with female partners of reproductive potential must use barrier methods during treatment and for at least 3 mos after discontinuation. May impair fertility. **Children:** Safety and efficacy not established. **Elderly:** No age-related precautions noted.

INTERACTIONS

DRUG: Strong CYP3A4 inhibitors (e.g., **clarithromycin, ketoconazole**) may increase concentration/effect. **Strong CYP3A4 inducers (e.g., carBAMazepine, phenytoin, rifAMPin)** may decrease concentration/effect; use contraindicated due to risk of severe hepatotoxicity. **Moderate CYP3A4** at the same time each day **inducers (e.g., bosentan, nafcillin)** may decrease concentration/effect. **HERBAL:** None significant. **FOOD:** None known. **LAB VALUES:** May increase serum alkaline phosphatase, ALT, AST, amylase, cholesterol, glucose, lipase, potassium, triglycerides. May decrease Hgb, lymphocytes, platelets, RBCs; serum albumin, phosphate, magnesium.

AVAILABILITY (Rx)

Tablets: 25 mg, 100 mg.

ADMINISTRATION/HANDLING

PO
• Give without regard to food at the same time each day. • Administer tablets whole; do not break, crush, cut, or divide. Tablets cannot be chewed. Do not give is tablet is broken, cracked, or not intact. • If vomiting occurs after administration, give next dose at regularly scheduled time. • If a dose is missed, administer as soon as possible. • Do not give a missed dose within 4 hrs of next dose.

INDICATIONS/ROUTES/DOSAGE

Non–Small-Cell Lung Cancer (ALK-Positive)
PO: ADULTS, ELDERLY: 100 mg once daily. Continue until disease progression or unacceptable toxicity.

Dose Reduction Schedule
First reduction: 75 mg once daily.
Second reduction: 50 mg once daily.

Unable to tolerate 50-mg dose: Permanently discontinue.

Dose Modification
Based on Common Terminology Criteria for Adverse Events (CTCAE).

Atrioventricular (AV) Block
Second-degree AV block: Withhold treatment until PR interval is less than 200 msec, then resume at reduced dose. **First occurrence of complete AV block:** Withhold treatment until PR interval is less than 200 msec or pacemaker is placed. If pacemaker is placed, resume at same dose. If pacemaker is not placed, resume at reduced dose. **Recurrent complete AV block:** Place pacemaker or permanently discontinue.

Central Nervous System (CNS) Effects
Grade 1 CNS effects: Maintain dose or withhold treatment until improved to baseline, then resume at same dose or reduced dose. **Grade 2 or 3 CNS effects:** Withhold treatment until improved to Grade 1 or 0, then resume at reduced dose. **Grade 4 CNS effects:** Permanently discontinue.

Hyperlipidemia
Grade 4 hypercholesterolemia or hypertriglyceridemia: Withhold treatment until improved to Grade 2 or less, then resume at same dose. **Recurrent severe hypercholesterolemia or hypertriglyceridemia:** Resume at reduced dose.

Interstitial Lung Disease (ILD)
Any grade treatment-related ILD: Permanently discontinue.

Other Adverse Reactions
Other Grade 1 or Grade 2 reaction: Maintain dose or reduce dose.
Other Grade 3 or Grade 4 reaction: Withhold treatment until improved to Grade 2 or less (or baseline), then resume at reduced dose.

Concomitant Use of Strong CYP3A4 Inhibitors
If strong CYP3A4 inhibitor cannot be discontinued, reduce dose to 75 mg. If dose was reduced to 75 mg due to adverse reactions and a CYP3A4 inhibitor is started,

reduce dose to 50 mg. If CYP3A4 inhibitor is discontinued for 3 half-lives, may resume dose prior to starting CYP3A4 inhibitor.

Concomitant Use of Moderate CYP3A4 Inducers

Note: Concomitant use of strong CYP3A4 inducers is contraindicated. If moderate CYP3A4 inducer cannot be discontinued, consider discontinuing CYP3A4 inducer or discontinuing treatment if Grade 2 or higher hepatotoxicity occurs.

Dosage in Renal Impairment

Mild to moderate impairment: No dose adjustment. **Severe impairment:** Not specified; use caution.

Dosage in Hepatic Impairment

Mild impairment: No dose adjustment. **Moderate to severe impairment:** Not specified; use caution.

SIDE EFFECTS

Frequent (57%–18%): Edema (generalized, peripheral), peripheral neuropathy, cognitive effects (amnesia, memory impairment, disorientation), dyspnea, fatigue, asthenia, weight gain, mood effects (aggression, agitation, anxiety, depression, mood swings), arthralgia, diarrhea, headache, cough, nausea. **Occasional (17%–10%):** Myalgia, dizziness, vision disorder, constipation, rash, back pain, extremity pain, vomiting, speech effects (aphasia, dysarthria), pyrexia, sleep effects (abnormal dreams, insomnia, nightmares, sleep talking).

ADVERSE EFFECTS/TOXIC REACTIONS

Myelosuppression (anemia, lymphopenia, thrombocytopenia) is an expected response to therapy. CNS reactions including hallucinations, seizures, suicidal ideation, and changes in cognitive function, mental status, mood, sleep, speech reported in 54% of pts. Grade 3 or 4 elevations in total cholesterol, triglycerides reported in 18% of pts. AV block and PR internal prolongation reported in 1% of pts. Life-threatening ILD/pneumonitis reported in 2% of pts. Other adverse effects, including pneumonia, pulmonary edema, myocardial infarction, embolism, peripheral artery occlusion, respiratory failure, occur rarely.

NURSING CONSIDERATIONS

BASELINE ASSESSMENT

Obtain CBC, LFT, serum cholesterol, triglycerides, ECG; pregnancy test in female pts of reproductive potential. Confirm compliance of effective contraception. Verify ALK-positive NSCLC status. Discontinue strong CYP3A4 inducers for 3 half-lives prior to initiation. Consider initiating or increasing dose of antihyperlipidemic agents. Screen for active infection. Question history of anxiety, depression, mood disorder, suicidal ideation and behavior; cardiac or pulmonary disease, hepatic impairment. Receive full medication history and screen for interactions/contraindications. Conduct baseline neurologic exam. Offer emotional support.

INTERVENTION/EVALUATION

Monitor CBC, LFT periodically. Monitor serum cholesterol, triglycerides monthly for 2 mos, then periodically thereafter. Monitor ECG periodically (or more frequently if symptoms of AV block occur [dizziness, chest pain, syncope]). If moderate CYP3A4 inducer cannot be discontinued, monitor LFT 48 hrs after initiation and for at least 3 times during the first week after initiation. Diligently monitor for suicidal ideation and behavior; new-onset or worsening of anxiety, depression, mood disorder. Consider mental health consultation if psychiatric disorder suspected. Conduct regular neurologic exams to rule out CNS effects. Consider ABG, radiologic test if ILD/pneumonitis (excessive cough, dyspnea, hypoxia) is suspected. If treatment related toxicities occur, consider referral to specialist. Assess skin for rash, dermatitis.

PATIENT/FAMILY TEACHING

• Treatment may depress your immune system response and reduce your ability to fight infection. Report symptoms of infection such as body aches, chills, cough, fatigue, fever. Avoid those with active infection. • Seek immediate medical attention if thoughts of suicide, new-onset or worsening of anxiety, depression, or changes in mood occurs. • Neurologic events including altered speech, hallucinations, seizures may occur. • Report symptoms of heart block (dizziness, chest pain, fainting); liver problems (abdominal pain, bruising, clay-colored stool, amber or dark colored urine, yellowing of the skin or eyes); lung inflammation (excessive cough, difficulty breathing, chest pain); skin reactions (rash). • Use effective contraception to avoid pregnancy. Do not breastfeed. • There is a high risk of interactions with other medications. Do not take newly prescribed medications unless approved by prescriber that originally started therapy. • Avoid grapefruit products, herbal supplements (esp. St. John's wort).

losartan

loe-**sar**-tan
(Cozaar)
■ **BLACK BOX ALERT** ■ May cause fetal injury, mortality. Discontinue as soon as possible once pregnancy is detected.
Do not confuse Cozaar with Colace, Coreg, Hyzaar, or Zocor, or losartan with lorcaserin, valsartan.

FIXED-COMBINATION(S)

Hyzaar: losartan/hydroCHLOROthiazide (a diuretic): 50 mg/12.5 mg, 100 mg/12.5 mg, 100 mg/25 mg.

◆CLASSIFICATION

PHARMACOTHERAPEUTIC: Angiotensin II receptor antagonist. **CLINICAL:** Antihypertensive.

USES

Hypertension: Treatment of hypertension in adults and children 6 yrs and older. Used alone or in combination with other antihypertensives. **Proteinuric**

Chronic kidney disease: Treatment of diabetic nephropathy with an elevated creatinine and proteinuria (in pts with type 2 diabetes and history of hypertension). **OFF-LABEL:** Acute coronary syndrome (STEMI, non-STEMI), HF with reduced ejection fraction, Marfan syndrome with aortic aneurysm; proteinuric chronic kidney disease (non-diabetic), post-transplant erythrocytosis.

PRECAUTIONS

Contraindications: Hypersensitivity to losartan. Concomitant use of aliskiren in pts with diabetes. **Cautions:** Renal/hepatic impairment, unstented renal arterial stenosis, significant aortic/mitral stenosis. Concurrent use of potassium supplements. Pts with history of angioedema.

ACTION

Blocks vasoconstrictor, aldosterone-secreting effects of angiotensin II, inhibiting binding of angiotensin II to AT_1 receptors. **Therapeutic Effect:** Causes vasodilation, decreases peripheral resistance, decreases B/P.

PHARMACOKINETICS

Route	Onset	Peak	Duration
PO	N/A	6 hrs	24 hrs

Widely distributed. Protein binding: 98%. Metabolized in liver. Excreted in feces (60%), urine (35%). Not removed by hemodialysis. **Half-life:** 2 hrs; metabolite, 6–9 hrs.

⧗ LIFESPAN CONSIDERATIONS

Pregnancy/Lactation: Has caused fetal/neonatal morbidity, mortality. Potential for adverse effects on breastfed infant. Breastfeeding not recommended. **Children:** Safety and efficacy not established. **Elderly:** May be more sensitive to hypotensive effects.

INTERACTIONS

DRUG: NSAIDs (e.g., ibuprofen, ketorolac, naproxen) may decrease effects. **Aliskiren** may increase hyperkalemic effect. May increase adverse/toxicity of **ACE inhibitors (e.g., benazepril, lisinopril).** May increase levels/effects of **lithium. HERBAL: Herbals with hypertensive properties (e.g., licorice, yohimbe) or hypotensive properties (e.g., garlic, ginger, ginkgo biloba)** may alter effects. **FOOD:** None known. **LAB VALUES:** May increase serum bilirubin, ALT, AST, Hgb, Hct. May decrease serum glucose.

AVAILABILITY (Rx)

Tablets: 25 mg, 50 mg, 100 mg.

ADMINISTRATION/HANDLING

PO
• May give without regard to food.

INDICATIONS/ROUTES/DOSAGE

Hypertension
PO: ADULTS, ELDERLY: Initially, 25–50 mg once daily. Evaluate response after 2–4 wks. May increase as needed to 100 mg/day in 1–2 divided doses. **CHILDREN 6–16 YRS:** Initially, 0.7 mg/kg (**maximum:** 50 mg) once daily. Adjust dose to BP response. **Maximum:** 1.4 mg/kg or 100 mg/day in 1 or 2 divided doses.

Diabetic Nephropathy
PO: ADULTS, ELDERLY: Initially, 25–50 mg/day. May increase to 100 mg/day based on B/P response and tolerability.

Dosage in Renal Impairment
Not recommended if glomerular filtration rate (GFR) less than 30 mL/min.

Dosage in Hepatic Impairment
PO: ADULTS, ELDERLY: Initially, 25 mg/day. May increase up to 100 mg/day.

SIDE EFFECTS

Frequent (8%): Upper respiratory tract infection. **Occasional (4%–2%):** Dizziness, diarrhea, cough. **Rare (1% or less):** Insomnia, dyspepsia, heartburn, back/leg pain, muscle cramps, myalgia, nasal congestion, sinusitis, depression.

ADVERSE EFFECTS/TOXIC REACTIONS

Overdosage may manifest as hypotension and tachycardia. Bradycardia occurs less often. Institute supportive measures.

NURSING CONSIDERATIONS

BASELINE ASSESSMENT
Obtain B/P, heart rate immediately before each dose, in addition to regular monitoring (be alert to fluctuations). Question for possibility of pregnancy. Assess medication history (esp. diuretics).

INTERVENTION/EVALUATION
Maintain hydration (offer fluids frequently). Assess for evidence of upper respiratory infection, cough. Monitor B/P, heart rate. Assist with ambulation if dizziness occurs. Monitor daily pattern of bowel activity, stool consistency.

PATIENT/FAMILY TEACHING
• Use effective contraception to avoid pregnancy. • Avoid tasks that require alertness, motor skills until response to drug is established (possible dizziness effect). • Report any sign of infection (sore throat, fever), chest pain. • Do not take OTC cold preparations, nasal decongestants. • Do not stop taking medication. • Limit salt intake.

lovastatin

loe-va-stat-in
(Altoprev)
Do not confuse lovastatin with atorvastatin, Leustatin, Lotensin, nystatin, pitavastatin, or pravastatin.

FIXED-COMBINATION(S)

Advicor: lovastatin/niacin: 20 mg/500 mg, 20 mg/750 mg, 20 mg/1,000 mg.

◆CLASSIFICATION

PHARMACOTHERAPEUTIC: HMG-CoA reductase inhibitor. **CLINICAL:** Antihyperlipidemic.

✦ Canadian trade name   🛇 Non-Crushable Drug   🟥 High Alert drug

USES

Primary prevention of coronary heart disease: (Pts without symptomatic cardiovascular disease with average to moderately elevated total cholesterol and LDL-C and below average HDL-C): to reduce the risk of myocardial infarction, unstable angina, coronary revascularization procedures. **Coronary heart disease:** To slow the progression of coronary atherosclerosis. **Hypercholesterolemia:** Adjunct to diet to reduce elevated total cholesterol and LDL-C levels in pts with primary hypercholesterolemia (types IIa and IIb) when the response to diet, restricted in saturated fat and cholesterol, and to other measures alone has been inadequate. **Heterozygous familial hypercholesterolemia (heFH):** Adjunct to diet to reduce total cholesterol, LDL-C, and apolipoprotein B levels in males and postmenarcheal (at least 1 yr) females ages 10–17 yrs with heFH who, despite an adequate trial of diet therapy, have the following findings: LDL-C remains greater than 189 mg/dL or LDL-C remains greater than 160 mg/dL and there is a positive family history of premature cardiovascular disease (CVD) or 2 or more other CVD risk factors present.

PRECAUTIONS

Contraindications: Hypersensitivity to lovastatin. Active hepatic disease, unexplained persistent elevations of serum transaminases. Pregnancy, breastfeeding. Concomitant use of strong CYP3A4 inhibitors. **Cautions:** History of heavy/chronic alcohol use, renal impairment, hepatic disease; concomitant use of amiodarone, cycloSPORINE, fibrates, gemfibrozil, niacin, verapamil (increased risk of myopathy), elderly.

ACTION

Inhibits HMG-CoA reductase, the enzyme that catalyzes the early step in cholesterol synthesis. **Therapeutic Effect:** Decreases LDL, VLDL, triglycerides; increases HDL.

PHARMACOKINETICS

Route	Onset	Peak	Duration
PO (LDL, cholesterol reduction)	3 days	N/A	N/A

Incompletely absorbed from GI tract (increased on empty stomach). Protein binding: 95%. Hydrolyzed in liver. Primarily excreted in feces. Not removed by hemodialysis. **Half-life:** 1.1–1.7 hrs.

⧗ LIFESPAN CONSIDERATIONS

Pregnancy/Lactation: Contraindicated in pregnancy (suppression of cholesterol biosynthesis may cause fetal toxicity) and lactation. Unknown if drug is distributed in breast milk. **Children:** Safety and efficacy not established in pts younger than 10 yrs. **Elderly:** No age-related precautions noted.

INTERACTIONS

DRUG: **Strong CYP3A4 inhibitors (e.g., clarithromycin, ketoconazole, ritonavir)** may increase concentration, risk of myopathy, rhabdomyolysis. **Colchicine, gemfibrozil** may increase risk of myopathy. **HERBAL:** **St. John's wort** may decrease concentration/effect. **FOOD:** **Grapefruit products** may increase concentration/effect. **Red yeast rice** may increase concentration (2.4 mg lovastatin/600 mg rice). **LAB VALUES:** May increase serum ALT, AST, creatine kinase (CK).

AVAILABILITY (Rx)

Tablets: 10 mg, 20 mg, 40 mg.

⬥ **Tablets: (Extended-Release [Altoprev]):** 20 mg, 40 mg, 60 mg.

ADMINISTRATION/HANDLING

PO
• Immediate-release tablet given with evening meal; extended-release at bedtime. • Do not break, crush, dissolve, or divide extended-release tablets.

INDICATIONS/ROUTES/DOSAGE

Hypercholesterolemia, Primary Prevention of CAD

PO: *(Immediate-Release):* **ADULTS, ELDERLY:** Initially, 20 mg/day with the

evening meal. Usual dose: 40–80 mg/day.
Maximum: 80 mg/day.
PO: *(Extended-Release):* **ADULTS, ELDERLY:** Initially, 20–60 mg once daily at bedtime. Adjust at 4-wk intervals. **Maximum:** 60 mg once daily at bedtime.

Heterozygous Familial Hypercholesterolemia
PO: *(Immediate-Release):* **CHILDREN 10–17 YRS:** Initially, 10 mg once daily. May increase in 10-mg increments q3mos until target LDL is achieved. Range: 10–40 mg daily. **Maximum:** 80 mg/day.

Dosage With Concurrent Medication
Amiodarone: Maximum: 40 mg/day.
DilTIAZem, dronedarone, verapamil: Maximum: *(Immediate-Release):* 10 mg/day. *(Extended-Release):* 20 mg/day.
Lomitapide: Consider reduction in dose.

Dosage in Renal Impairment
Use caution.

Dosage in Hepatic Impairment
No dose adjustment.

SIDE EFFECTS

Generally well tolerated. Side effects usually mild and transient. **Frequent (9%–5%):** Headache, flatulence, diarrhea, abdominal pain, abdominal cramping, rash, pruritus. **Occasional (4%–3%):** Nausea, vomiting, constipation, dyspepsia. **Rare (2%–1%):** Dizziness, heartburn, myalgia, blurred vision, eye irritation.

ADVERSE EFFECTS/TOXIC REACTIONS

Potential for cataract development. Occasionally produces myopathy manifested as muscle pain, tenderness, weakness with elevated creatine kinase (CK). Severe myopathy may lead to rhabdomyolysis.

NURSING CONSIDERATIONS

BASELINE ASSESSMENT

Obtain LFT, serum cholesterol, triglycerides; pregnancy test in females of reproductive potential. Receive full medication history and screen for interactions. Obtain diet history.

INTERVENTION/EVALUATION

Monitor LFT. Monitor daily pattern of bowel activity, stool consistency. Monitor for headache, dizziness, blurred vision. Assess for rash, pruritus. Monitor serum cholesterol, triglycerides for therapeutic response. Be alert for malaise, muscle cramping/weakness.

PATIENT/FAMILY TEACHING

• Follow special diet (important part of treatment). • Periodic lab tests are essential part of therapy. • Maintain appropriate birth control measures. • Avoid grapefruit juice, alcohol. • Report severe gastric upset, vision changes, myalgia, weakness, changes in color of urine/stool, yellowing of eyes/skin, unusual bruising.

lurasidone

loo-**ras**-i-done
(Latuda)

■ **BLACK BOX ALERT** ■ Elderly pts with dementia-related psychosis are at increased risk for mortality due to cardiovascular events, infectious diseases. Increased risk of suicidal thinking/behavior in children, adolescents, young adults.

◆CLASSIFICATION

PHARMACOTHERAPEUTIC: DOPamine, serotonin receptor antagonist. **CLINICAL:** Second-generation (atypical) antipsychotic.

USES

Schizophrenia: Treatment of schizophrenia in adults and adolescents (13–17 yrs). **Bipolar major depression:** Treatment of depression associated with bipolar I disorder as monotherapy (children 10 yrs and older, adults) and as adjunctive therapy (adults) with lithium or valproate. **OFF-LABEL:** Major depressive disorder (unipolar) with mixed features (monotherapy).

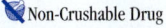

PRECAUTIONS

Contraindications: Hypersensitivity to lurasidone. Concurrent use with strong CYP3A4 inhibitors (e.g., ketoconazole) and inducers (e.g., rifAMPin). **Cautions:** Cardiovascular disease (HF, history of MI, ischemia, conduction abnormalities), cerebrovascular disease (history of CVA in pts with dementia, seizure disorders), diabetes, Parkinson's disease, renal/hepatic impairment, pts at risk for aspiration pneumonia, pts at risk for suicide, disorders where CNS depression is a feature, pts at risk for hypotension, elderly, head trauma, alcoholism, medications that lower seizure threshold.

ACTION

Antagonizes central DOPamine type 2 and serotonin type 2 receptors. **Therapeutic Effect:** Diminishes symptoms of schizophrenia. Reduces incidence of extrapyramidal side effects.

PHARMACOKINETICS

Widely distributed. Steady-state concentration occurs in 7 days. Protein binding: 99%. Metabolized in liver. Excreted in feces (80%), urine (9%). **Half-life:** 18 hrs.

⧗ LIFESPAN CONSIDERATIONS

Pregnancy/Lactation: Unknown if distributed in breast milk. Breastfeeding not recommended. **Children:** Safety and efficacy not established. **Elderly:** More susceptible to postural hypotension. Increased risk of cerebrovascular events (including stroke), mortality, in elderly pts with psychosis.

INTERACTIONS

DRUG: Alcohol, CNS depressants (e.g., LORazepam, morphine, zolpidem) may increase CNS depression. May enhance CNS depressant effect of azelastine (nasal). Strong CYP3A4 inducers (e.g., carBAMazepine, phenytoin, rifAMPin) decrease concentration/effect. Strong CYP3A4 inhibitors (e.g.,

clarithromycin, ketoconazole, ritonavir) may increase concentration/effect. **HERBAL: Herbals with sedative properties (e.g., chamomile, kava kava, valerian)** may increase CNS depression. **St. John's wort** may decrease concentration/effect. **FOOD: Grapefruit products** may increase concentration/effect. **LAB VALUES:** May increase prolactin levels.

AVAILABILITY (Rx)

Tablets: 20 mg, 40 mg, 60 mg, 80 mg, 120 mg.

ADMINISTRATION/HANDLING

PO
• Administer consistently at the same time every day with food. • Do not cut, split, or crush tablets.

INDICATIONS/ROUTES/DOSAGE

Schizophrenia
PO: ADULTS, ELDERLY: Initially, 40 mg once daily in the evening within 30 min of food. May increase in increments of 40 mg/day q3days or longer. Usual dose: 40–80 mg/day. **Maximum:** 160 mg once daily with food. **ADOLESCENTS:** Initially, 40 mg once daily with food. **Maximum:** (less than 18 yrs): 80 mg/day; (18 yrs and older): 160 mg/day.

Bipolar Depression
PO: ADULTS, ELDERLY: (Monotherapy or adjunct to lithium or divalproex): Initially, 20 mg once daily, alone or in combination with lithium or divalproex. May increase in 20 mg increments every 2 or more days. **Maximum:** 120 mg/day. **CHILDREN 10 YRS AND OLDER: (Monotherapy):** Initially, 20 mg once daily. May increase dose after 1 wk. Usual dose: 20–40 mg/day. **Maximum:** 80 mg/day.

Dosage in Renal Impairment
CrCl less than 50 mL/min: Initially, 20 mg/day. **Maximum:** 80 mg/day.

Dosage in Hepatic Impairment
Mild impairment: No dose adjustment. **Moderate impairment:** Initially,

20 mg/day. **Maximum:** 80 mg/day. **Severe impairment:** Initially, 20 mg/day. **Maximum:** 40 mg/day.

SIDE EFFECTS

Frequent (15%–7%): Drowsiness, sedation, insomnia (paradoxical reaction). **Occasional (6%–3%):** Nausea, vomiting, dyspepsia, fatigue, back pain, akathisia, dizziness, agitation, anxiety. **Rare (2%–1%):** Restlessness, salivary hypersecretion, tongue spasm, torticollis, trismus.

ADVERSE EFFECTS/TOXIC REACTIONS

Extrapyramidal disorder (including cogwheel rigidity, drooling, bradykinesia, tardive dyskinesia, tremors) occurs in 5% of pts. Neuroleptic malignant syndrome (fever, muscle rigidity, irregular B/P or pulse, altered mental status, visual changes, dyspnea) occurs rarely.

NURSING CONSIDERATIONS

BASELINE ASSESSMENT

Question history as listed in Precautions. Assess behavior, appearance, emotional status, response to environment, speech pattern, thought content. Renal function, LFT should be obtained before therapy as dose adjustment is required when initiating therapy.

INTERVENTION/EVALUATION

Supervise suicidal risk pt closely during early therapy (as depression lessens, energy level improves, increasing suicide potential). Monitor for potential neuroleptic malignant syndrome. Assess for therapeutic response (greater interest in surroundings, improved self-care, increased ability to concentrate, relaxed facial expression).

PATIENT/FAMILY TEACHING

• Avoid tasks that may require alertness, motor skills until response to drug is established (may cause drowsiness, dizziness). • Avoid alcohol. • Report trembling in fingers, altered gait, unusual muscle/skeletal movements, palpitations, severe dizziness, fainting, visual changes, rash, difficulty breathing. • Report suicidal ideation, unusual changes in behavior.

lurbinectedin

loor-bin-**ek**-te-din
(Zepzelca)
Do not confuse lurbinectedin with trabectedin or Zepzelca with Zejula, Zelboraf, Zoladex, or Zydelig.

◆**Classification**

PHARMACOTHERAPEUTIC: Alkylating agent. **CLINICAL:** Antineoplastic.

USES

Treatment of adults with metastatic small-cell lung cancer (SCLC) with disease progression on or after platinum-based chemotherapy.

PRECAUTIONS

Contraindications: Hypersensitivity to lurbinectedin. **Cautions:** Baseline cytopenias, hepatic/renal impairment, pulmonary disease, conditions predisposing to infection (e.g., diabetes, renal failure, immunocompromised pts, open wounds); concomitant use of strong or moderate CYP3A4 inhibitors or strong or moderate CYP3A4 inducers.

ACTION

Selective inhibitor of oncogenic transcription, which binds preferentially to guanine residues in the minor groove of DNA, forming adducts, and bends the DNA helix towards the major groove. Adduct formation affects the activities of DNA binding proteins, including some transcription factors and DNA repair pathways. **Therapeutic Effect:** Inhibition of oncogenic transcription results in tumor cell apoptosis.

PHARMACOKINETICS

Widely distributed. Metabolized in liver. Protein binding: 99%. Excreted in feces (89%), urine (6%). **Half-life:** 51 hrs.

⌛ LIFESPAN CONSIDERATIONS

Pregnancy/Lactation: Avoid pregnancy; may cause fetal harm. Females of reproductive potential must use effective contraception during treatment and for at least 6 mos after discontinuation. Unknown if distributed in breast milk. Breastfeeding not recommended during treatment and for at least 2 wks after discontinuation. **Males:** Males with female partners of reproductive potential should use effective contraception during therapy and for 4 months after discontinuation. **Children:** Safety and efficacy not established. **Elderly:** May have increased risk of serious adverse effects; myelosuppression.

INTERACTIONS

DRUG: Strong CYP3A4 inhibitors (e.g., clarithromycin, ketoconazole, ritonavir), moderate CYP3A4 inhibitors (e.g., dilTIAZem, fluconazole, verapamil) may increase concentration/effect. **Strong CYP3A4 inducers (e.g., carBAMazepine, phenytoin, rifAMPin), moderate CYP3A4 inducers (e.g., bosentan, nafcillin)** may decrease concentration/effect. May increase the immunosuppressive effect of **baricitinib, tofacitinib, upadacitinib.** May increase the adverse/toxic effect of **natalizumab.** May increase the adverse/toxic effect and diminish the therapeutic effect of **vaccines (live). HERBAL: Herbals with anticoagulant/antiplatelet properties (e.g., garlic, ginger, ginkgo biloba)** may increase risk of bleeding in pts with thrombocytopenia. **Echinacea** may diminish the therapeutic effect. **FOOD: Grapefruit products** may increase concentration/effect. **LAB VALUES:** May increase serum ALT, AST, creatinine, glucose. May decrease serum albumin, magnesium, sodium; absolute neutrophil count, Hgb, leukocytes, lymphocytes, neutrophils, platelets.

AVAILABILITY (RX)

Injection, Powder for Reconstitution: 4 mg.

ADMINISTRATION/HANDLING

 IV

Premedication • Consider premedication with dexamethasone 8 mg IV (or equivalent) and ondansetron 8 mg IV (or equivalent).
Reconstitution • Must be prepared by personnel trained in aseptic manipulations and admixing of cytotoxic drugs. • Calculate the dose needed for reconstitution based on body surface area. • Reconstitute vial with 8 mL of Sterile Water for Injection to a final concentration of 0.5 mg/mL. • Shake vial until powder is completely dissolved. • Visually inspect for particulate matter or discoloration. Solution should appear clear, colorless to slightly yellow. Do not use if solution is cloudy, discolored, or if visible particles are observed. • **Administration via central venous line (CVL):** Dilute in 100 mL 0.9% NaCl or D5W infusion bag. • **Administration via peripheral IV:** Dilute in 250 mL bag of 0.9% NaCl or D5W infusion bag.
Rate of administration • Infuse over 60 min.
Storage • Refrigerate unused vials in original carton. • Diluted solution may be refrigerated or stored at room temperature for up to 24 hrs.

INDICATIONS/ROUTES/DOSAGE

Small-Cell Lung Cancer (Metastatic)
IV: ADULTS, ELDERLY: 3.2 mg/m^2 q3wks if absolute neutrophil count is at least 1,500 cells/mm^3 *and* platelet count is at least 100,000 cells/mm^3. Continue until

disease progression or unacceptable toxicity.

Dose Reduction Schedule
First dose reduction: 2.6 mg/m² q3wks. **Second dose reduction:** 2 mg/m² q3wks.

Dose Modification
Based on Common Terminology Criteria for Adverse Events (CTCAE).

Hepatotoxicity
Grade 2 hepatotoxicity: Withhold treatment until improved to Grade 1 or 0, then resume at same dose. **Grade 3 or 4 hepatotoxicity:** Withhold treatment until improved to Grade 1 or 0, then resume at reduced dose.

Neutropenia
Grade 4 neutropenia or febrile neutropenia: Withhold treatment until improved to Grade 1 or 0, then resume at reduced dose. Consider granulocyte colony-stimulating factor in pts with neutrophil count less than 500 cells/mm³.

Thrombocytopenia
Grade 3 thrombocytopenia with bleeding: Withhold treatment until platelet count improves to greater than or equal to 100,000 cells/mm³. **Grade 4 thrombocytopenia:** Withhold treatment until platelet count improves to greater than or equal to 100,000 cells/mm³, then resume at reduced dose.

Dosage in Renal Impairment
Mild to moderate impairment: No dose adjustment. **Severe impairment:** Not specified; use caution.

Dosage in Hepatic Impairment
Mild impairment: No dose adjustment. **Moderate to severe impairment:** Not specified; use caution.

SIDE EFFECTS

Frequent (77%–31%): Fatigue, nausea, musculoskeletal pain (back, bone, chest, extremity, neck), arthralgia, myalgia, decreased appetite, dyspnea, constipation. **Occasional (22%–less than 10%):** Vomiting, constipation, diarrhea, cough, pyrexia, abdominal pain, peripheral neuropathy, neuralgia, hypoesthesia, hyperesthesia, headache, chest pain, dysgeusia.

ADVERSE EFFECTS/TOXIC REACTIONS

Myelosuppression (neutropenia, thrombocytopenia) is an expected response to therapy, but more severe reactions, including bone marrow depression, febrile neutropenia, may be life-threatening. Grade 3 or 4 neutropenia reported in 41% of pts. Grade 3 or 4 thrombocytopenia reported in 10% of pts. Sepsis reported in 2% of pts. Infections, including respiratory tract infection, pneumonia, reported in 18%–10%. Pneumonitis reported in less than 10% of pts. May cause hepatotoxicity.

NURSING CONSIDERATIONS

BASELINE ASSESSMENT
Obtain CBC, LFT; pregnancy test in females of reproductive potential. Verify use of effective contraception. Screen for active infection. Question history of hepatic impairment, pulmonary disease. Receive full medication history and screen for interactions. Offer emotional support.

INTERVENTION/EVALUATION
Monitor CBC for myelosuppression prior to each dose. Monitor LFT if hepatotoxicity (bruising, hematuria, jaundice, right upper abdominal pain, nausea, vomiting, weight loss) periodically. Consider ABG, radiologic test if pneumonitis (excessive cough, dyspnea, fever, hypoxia) is suspected. Consider treatment with corticosteroids if pneumonitis is confirmed. Diligently monitor for infections (cough, fatigue, fever). If serious infection occurs, initiate appropriate antimicrobial therapy. Offer antiemetics if nausea occurs; antidiarrheal agent if

L

diarrhea occurs. Monitor for toxicities if discontinuation of CYP3A4 inhibitor is unavoidable. Monitor daily pattern of bowel activity, stool consistency. Monitor for bleeding of any kind.

PATIENT/FAMILY TEACHING

• Treatment may depress the immune system response and reduce ability to fight infection. Report symptoms of infection such as body aches, chills, cough, fatigue, fever. Avoid those with active infection. • Report symptoms of bone marrow depression such as bruising, fatigue, fever, shortness of breath, weight loss; bleeding easily, bloody urine or stool. • Report liver problems (abdominal pain, bruising, clay-colored stool, amber or dark-colored urine, yellowing of the skin or eyes), inflammation of the lung (excessive cough, difficulty breathing, chest pain). • Use effective contraception to avoid pregnancy. Do not breastfeed. • Do not take newly prescribed medications unless approved by prescriber who originally started therapy. • Avoid grapefruit products, herbal supplements (esp. St John's wort). • Report bleeding of any kind.

magnesium `HIGH ALERT`

mag-**nee**-zee-um

magnesium chloride

(Slow-Mag)

magnesium citrate

(Citroma, Citro-Mag ✦)

magnesium hydroxide

(Milk of Magnesia)

magnesium oxide

(Mag-Ox 400, Uro-Mag)

magnesium sulfate

(Epsom salt, magnesium sulfate injection)
Do not confuse magnesium sulfate with morphine sulfate.

FIXED-COMBINATION(S)

With aluminum and simethicone, an antiflatulent **(Mylanta).**

◆CLASSIFICATION

CLINICAL: Antacid, anticonvulsant, electrolyte, laxative.

USES

Magnesium chloride: Treatment/prevention of hypomagnesemia. Dietary supplement. **Magnesium citrate:** Evacuation of bowel before surgical, diagnostic procedures. Relieves occasional constipation. **Magnesium hydroxide:** Relief of occasional constipation. Temporary relief of heartburn, upset stomach, acid indigestion. **Magnesium oxide:** Relief of acid indigestion and upset stomach, Dietary supplement. **Magnesium sulfate: IV:** Treatment/prevention of hypomagnesemia; prevention and treatment of seizures in severe preeclampsia or eclampsia; pediatric acute nephritis, treatment of arrhythmias due to hypomagnesemia (ventricular fibrillation, ventricular tachycardia, or torsades de pointes). **OFF-LABEL: Magnesium sulfate:** Asthma (severe exacerbation), fetal neuroprotection (imminent preterm birth), torsades de pointes.

PRECAUTIONS

Contraindications: Antacid: Appendicitis, symptoms of appendicitis, ileostomy, intestinal obstruction, severe renal impairment. **Laxative:** Appendicitis, HF, colostomy, hypersensitivity, ileostomy, intestinal obstruction, undiagnosed rectal bleeding. **Systemic:** Heart block, myocardial damage, IV use for pre-eclampsia/eclampsia during the 2 hrs prior to delivery. **Cautions:** Safety in children younger than 6 yrs not known. **Antacids:** Undiagnosed GI/rectal bleeding, ulcerative colitis, colostomy, diverticulitis, chronic diarrhea. **Laxative:** Diabetes, pts on low-salt diet (some products contain sugar, sodium). **Systemic:** Severe renal impairment. Myasthenia gravis or other neuromuscular diseases.

ACTION

Antacid: Acts in stomach to neutralize gastric acid. **Therapeutic Effect:** Increases pH. **Laxative:** Osmotic effect primarily in small intestine, draws water into intestinal lumen. **Therapeutic Effect:** Promotes peristalsis, bowel evacuation. **Systemic (dietary supplement replacement):** Found primarily in intracellular fluids. **Therapeutic Effect:** Essential for enzyme activity, nerve conduction, muscle contraction. Maintains and restores magnesium levels. **Anticonvulsant:** Blocks neuromuscular transmission, amount of acetylcholine released at motor end plate. **Therapeutic Effect:** Produces seizure control.

PHARMACOKINETICS

Antacid, laxative: Minimal absorption through intestine. Absorbed dose primarily excreted in urine. **Systemic:** Widely distributed. Primarily excreted in urine.

M

⌛ LIFESPAN CONSIDERATIONS

Pregnancy/Lactation: Antacid: Unknown if distributed in breast milk. **Parenteral:** Readily crosses placenta. Distributed in breast milk for 24 hrs after magnesium therapy is discontinued. Continuous IV infusion increases risk of magnesium toxicity in neonate. IV administration should not be used 2 hrs preceding delivery. **Children:** No age-related precautions noted. **Elderly:** Increased risk of developing magnesium deficiency (e.g., poor diet, decreased absorption, medications).

INTERACTIONS

DRUG: May decrease absorption of **quinolones (e.g., ciprofloxacin, levoFLOXacin), tetracycline, bisphosphonates. HERBAL:** None significant. **FOOD:** None known. **LAB VALUES: Antacid:** May increase gastrin production, pH. **Laxative:** May decrease serum potassium. **Systemic:** None significant.

AVAILABILITY (Rx)

Magnesium Chloride
Tablets: *(Slow-Mag):* 71 mg.
Magnesium Citrate
Oral Solution: *(Citroma):* 290 mg/5 mL.
Tablets: 100 mg.
Magnesium Hydroxide
Suspension, Oral: *(Milk of Magnesia):* 400 mg/5 mL, 1,200 mg/15 mL.
Tablets: 400 mg.
Magnesium Oxide
Tablets (Chewable): 400 mg.
Magnesium Sulfate
Solution, Injection: (50% [1g equals 8.12 mEq]) 2 mL, 10 mL, 4 g/100 mL, 2 g/50 mL, 20 g/500 mL, 40 g/1,000 mL.

ADMINISTRATION/HANDLING

 IV

Reconstitution • Must dilute to maximum concentration of 20% for IV infusion. May give IV push, IV piggyback, or continuous infusion.

Rate of administration • For IV push (diluted): Give no faster than 150 mg/min. For IV infusion, maximum rate of infusion is 2 g/hr.
Storage • Store at room temperature.

IM
• For adults, elderly, use 250 mg/mL (25%) or 500 mg/mL (50%) magnesium sulfate concentration. • For infants, children, do not exceed 200 mg/mL (20% diluted solution).

PO (Antacid)
• Shake suspension well before use. • Chewable tablets should be chewed thoroughly before swallowing, followed by full glass of water.

PO (Laxative)
• Drink full glass of liquid (8 oz) with each dose (prevents dehydration). • Flavor may be improved by following with fruit juice, citrus carbonated beverage. • Refrigerate citrate of magnesia (retains potency, palatability).

▦ IV INCOMPATIBILITIES

Amiodarone.

▦ IV COMPATIBILITIES

Dexmedetomidine, heparin, insulin, potassium chloride, propofol.

INDICATIONS/ROUTES/DOSAGE

Magnesium Sulfate
Hypomagnesemia
IV: ADULTS, ELDERLY: (Mild): 1–2 g over 1–2 hrs. **(Moderate):** 2–4 g over 2–12 hrs. **(Severe):** 4–8 g over 4–24 hrs.

Usual Dose for Adolescents, Children, Infants
IV: 2.5–5 mg/kg/dose q6h for 2–3 doses.

Usual Dose for Neonates
IV: 2.5–5 mg/kg/dose q8–12h for 2–3 doses.

Eclampsia/Preeclampsia

IV: ADULTS: 4–6 g loading dose over 20–30 min, then 1–2 g/hr continuous infusion. **Maximum:** 40 g/24 hrs.

Magnesium Chloride
Dietary Supplement

PO: ADULTS, ELDERLY: 2 tablets once daily.

Magnesium Citrate
Laxative

PO: ADULTS, ELDERLY, CHILDREN 12 YRS AND OLDER: 195–300 mL once or in divided doses. **6–12 YRS:** 100–150 mL once or in divided doses. **2–5 YRS:** 60–90 mL once or in divided doses.

Magnesium Hydroxide
Antacid

PO: ADULTS, ELDERLY, CHILDREN 12 YRS AND OLDER: (400 mg/5 mL): 5–15 mL as needed up to 4 times/day.

Laxative

PO: ADULTS, ELDERLY, CHILDREN 12 YRS AND OLDER: (400 mg/5 mL): 30–60 mL at HS or in divided doses. **CHILDREN 6–11 YRS: (400 mg/5 mL):** 15–30 mL at HS. **CHILDREN 2–5 YRS:** 5–15 mL at HS.

Magnesium Oxide
Antacid/Dietary Supplement

PO: ADULTS, ELDERLY: 1–2 tablets daily.

Dosage in Renal Impairment
Use caution.

Dosage in Hepatic Impairment
No dose adjustment.

SIDE EFFECTS

Frequent: Antacid: Chalky taste, diarrhea, laxative effect. **Occasional: Antacid:** Nausea, vomiting, stomach cramps. **Antacid, laxative:** Prolonged use or large doses in renal impairment may cause hypermagnesemia (dizziness, palpitations, altered mental status, fatigue, weakness). **Laxative:** Cramping, diarrhea, increased thirst, flatulence. **Systemic (dietary supplement, electrolyte replacement):** Reduced respiratory rate, decreased reflexes, flushing, hypotension, decreased heart rate.

ADVERSE EFFECTS/TOXIC REACTIONS

Magnesium as antacid, laxative has no known adverse reactions. Systemic use may produce prolonged PR interval, widening of QRS interval. Magnesium toxicity may cause loss of deep tendon reflexes, heart block, respiratory paralysis, cardiac arrest. **Antidote:** 10–20 mL 10% calcium gluconate (5–10 mEq of calcium).

NURSING CONSIDERATIONS

BASELINE ASSESSMENT

Assess sensitivity to magnesium. **Antacid:** Assess GI pain/upset (duration, location, quality, time of occurrence, relief with food, causative/exacerbative factors). **Laxative:** Assess for weight loss, nausea, vomiting, history of recent abdominal surgery. **Systemic:** Assess renal function, serum magnesium.

INTERVENTION/EVALUATION

Antacid: Assess for relief of gastric distress. Monitor renal function (esp. if dosing is long term or frequent). **Laxative:** Monitor daily pattern of bowel activity, stool consistency. Maintain adequate fluid intake. **Systemic:** Monitor renal function, magnesium levels, ECG for cardiac function. Test patellar reflexes before giving repeated, rapid parenteral doses (used as indication of CNS depression; suppressed reflexes may be sign of impending respiratory arrest). Patellar reflex must be present, respiratory

M

rate should be 16/min or over before each parenteral dose. Initiate seizure precautions.

PATIENT/FAMILY TEACHING
• **Antacid:** Take at least 2 hrs apart from other medication. • Do not take longer than 2 wks unless directed by physician. • For peptic ulcer, take 1 and 3 hrs after meals and at bedtime for 4–6 wks. • Chew tablets thoroughly, followed by 8 oz of water; shake suspensions well. • Repeat dosing or large doses may have laxative effect. • **Laxative:** Drink full glass (8 oz) liquid to aid stool softening. • Use only for short term. Do not use if abdominal pain, nausea, vomiting is present. • **Systemic:** Report symptoms of hypermagnesemia (altered mental status, difficulty breathing, dizziness, fatigue, palpitations, weakness).

M

---

mannitol

man-it-ol
(Osmitrol)
Do not confuse Osmitrol with esmolol.

◆CLASSIFICATION

PHARMACOTHERAPEUTIC: Polyol (sugar alcohol). **CLINICAL:** Osmotic diuretic.

USES
Reduces increased ICP due to cerebral edema, brain mass, IOP due to acute glaucoma. **OFF-LABEL:** Kidney transplant (intraoperative volume optimization).

PRECAUTIONS
Contraindications: Hypersensitivity to mannitol. Severe dehydration, active intracranial bleeding (except during craniotomy), severe pulmonary edema, congestion, severe renal disease (anuria), progressive HF. **Cautions:** Concurrent nephrotoxic agents, conditions increasing sensitivity to bronchoconstriction (e.g., recent abdominal, thoracic surgery), sepsis, preexisting renal disease, hypernatremia.

ACTION
Increases osmotic pressure of glomerular filtrate, inhibiting tubular reabsorption of water and electrolytes, resulting in increased urine output. Reduces intracranial pressure by decreasing blood viscosity, thereby increasing cerebral blood flow/oxygen transport. **Therapeutic Effect:** Produces diuresis; reduces intraocular pressure (IOP), intracranial pressure (ICP), cerebral edema.

PHARMACOKINETICS

Route	Onset	Peak	Duration
IV (diuresis)	1–3 hrs	N/A	—
IV (reduced ICP)	15–30 min	N/A	1.5–6 hrs

Remains in extracellular fluid. Primarily excreted unchanged in urine. Removed by hemodialysis. **Half-life:** 4.7 hrs.

⧗ LIFESPAN CONSIDERATIONS
Pregnancy/Lactation: Unknown if drug crosses placenta or is distributed in breast milk. **Children:** Safety and efficacy not established in pts younger than 12 yrs. **Elderly:** Age-related renal impairment may require dosage adjustment.

INTERACTIONS
DRUG: May increase nephrotoxic effect of **aminoglycosides** (e.g., **amikacin, gentamicin, tobramycin**). **HERBAL:** None significant. **FOOD:** None known. **LAB VALUES:** May decrease serum phosphate, potassium. May increase serum sodium, osmolality.

AVAILABILITY (Rx)

Injection Solution: 10%, 15%, 20%, 25%.

ADMINISTRATION/HANDLING

◀**ALERT**▶ Assess IV site for patency before each dose. Pain, thrombosis noted with extravasation. Use in-line filter (less than 5 microns) for concentrations over 20%. Central venous access is recommended for repeated or scheduled doses.

 IV

Rate of administration • Administer test dose for pts with oliguria. • Give IV push over 3–5 min; over 30–60 min for cerebral edema, elevated ICP. Maximum concentration: 25%. • Do not add KCl or NaCl to mannitol 20% or greater. Do not add to whole blood for transfusion.

Storage • Store at room temperature. • If crystals are noted in solution, warm bottle in hot water, shake vigorously at intervals. Cool to body temperature before administration. Do not use if crystals remain after warming procedure.

▨ IV COMPATIBILITIES

Acetaminophen, dexmedetomidine, propofol.

INDICATIONS/ROUTES/DOSAGE

Usual Dosage

Elevated Intracranial Pressure

IV: ADULTS, ELDERLY: (20%): 0.5–2g/kg once. May repeat 0.25–1 g/kg/dose q4–6h based on clinical response. **CHILDREN:** 0.25–1 g/kg/dose; repeat to maintain serum osmolality less than 320 mOsm/kg.

IOP Reduction

IV: ADULTS, ELDERLY: 1.5–2 g/kg over 30–60 min 1–1.5 hrs prior to surgery. **CHILDREN:** 1.5–2 g/kg over 30 min or more 1–1.5 hrs prior to surgery.

Dosage in Renal Impairment

Contraindicated with severe impairment; caution with underlying renal disease.

Dosage in Hepatic Impairment

No dose adjustment.

SIDE EFFECTS

Frequent: Dry mouth, thirst. **Occasional:** Blurred vision, increased urinary frequency/volume, headache, arm pain, backache, nausea, vomiting, urticaria, dizziness, hypotension, hypertension, tachycardia, fever, angina-like chest pain.

ADVERSE EFFECTS/TOXIC REACTIONS

Fluid, electrolyte imbalance may occur due to rapid administration of large doses or inadequate urine output resulting in overexpansion of extracellular fluid. Circulatory overload may produce pulmonary edema, HF. Excessive diuresis may produce hypokalemia. Fluid loss in excess of electrolyte excretion may produce hypernatremia, hyperkalemia.

NURSING CONSIDERATIONS

BASELINE ASSESSMENT

Obtain serum osmolality, sodium. Obtain baseline B/P, pulse. Assess skin turgor, mucous membranes, mental status, muscle strength. Obtain baseline weight. Assess hydration status.

INTERVENTION/EVALUATION

Monitor urinary output to assess for therapeutic response. Monitor serum electrolytes, serum osmolality, ICP, renal function, LFT. Assess vital signs, skin turgor, mucous membranes. Weigh daily. Monitor for signs of hypernatremia (confusion, drowsiness, thirst, dry mouth, cold/clammy skin); signs of hypokalemia (changes in muscle strength, tremors, muscle cramps, altered mental status, cardiac arrhythmias). Signs of hyperkalemia include colic, diarrhea, muscle twitching followed by weakness, paralysis, arrhythmias. Inspect IV tubing, in-line filter for crystallization prior to each IV dose.

M

PATIENT/FAMILY TEACHING
• Expect increased urinary frequency/volume. • May cause dry mouth.

margetuximab-cmkb

mar-je-**tux**-i-mab)-cmkb
(Margenza)

■ **BLACK BOX ALERT** ■ May cause reduction in left ventricular ejection fraction (LVEF). Evaluate cardiac function before initiation and during treatment. Discontinue treatment if clinically significant decrease in LVEF is confirmed. Exposure during pregnancy can cause embryofetal harm.

Do not confuse margetuximab with brentuximab, cetuximab, dinutuximab, isatuximab, mepolizumab, rituximab, siltuximab, or trastuzumab.

♦**Classification**

PHARMACOTHERAPEUTIC: HER2/neu receptor antagonist, monoclonal antibody. **CLINICAL:** Antineoplastic.

USES
Treatment of adults with metastatic HER2-positive breast cancer (in combination with chemotherapy) who have received two or more prior anti-HER2 regimens, at least one of which was for metastatic disease.

PRECAUTIONS
Contraindications: Hypersensitivity to margetuximab-cmkb. **Cautions:** Baseline cytopenias, hepatic/renal impairment, conditions predisposing to infection (e.g., diabetes, renal failure, immunocompromised pts, open wounds); cardiomyopathy (treatment not studied in pts with LVEF less than 50%, history of myocardial infarction, unstable angina within 6 mos, or NYHA class II–IV HF).

Due to increased risk of cardiac dysfunction, avoid anthracyclines for up to 4 mos prior to initiation.

ACTION
Binds to extracellular domain of human epidermal growth factor receptor-2 (HER2) protein, inhibiting proliferation of HER2-overexpressing tumor cells and mediating antibody-dependent cellular toxicity. **Therapeutic Effect:** Inhibits tumor cell proliferation.

PHARMACOKINETICS
Widely distributed. Metabolized into small peptides via catabolic pathway. Steady state reached in 2 mos. Excretion not specified.
Half-life: 19.2 days.

⧗ LIFESPAN CONSIDERATIONS
Pregnancy/Lactation: Avoid pregnancy; may cause fetal harm. Females of reproductive potential should use effective contraception during treatment and for at least 4 mos after discontinuation. Unknown if distributed in breast milk. Breastfeeding not recommended during treatment and for at least 7 mos after discontinuation. **Children:** Safety and efficacy not established. **Elderly:** May have increased risk of adverse reactions, cardiotoxicity.

INTERACTIONS
DRUG: None significant. **HERBAL:** None significant. **FOOD:** None known. **LAB VALUES:** May increase serum alkaline phosphatase, ALT, AST, creatinine, international normalized ratio (INR), lipase. May decrease Hgb, leukocytes, lymphocytes, neutrophils. May prolong aPTT.

AVAILABILITY (Rx)
Injection Solution: 250 mg/10 mL (25 mg/mL).

ADMINISTRATION/HANDLING

 IV

Infusion guidelines • Infusion bag must be made of polyvinylchloride (PVC), polyethylene, polypropylene, polyolefins (only), or copolymer of olefins. • Infuse via dedicated IV line using a sterile, nonpyrogenic, low-protein-binding polyethersulfone (PES), 0.2 micron in-line or add-on filter. • If a dose is missed, give as soon as possible and adjust schedule to maintain treatment interval. • If margetuximab-cmkb and chemotherapy regimen are to be given on the same day, may give margetuximab-cmkb immediately after chemotherapy is complete. • Interrupt infusion if dyspnea or significant hypotension occurs. • Consider premedication with antihistamines, antipyretics, corticosteroids for infusion reaction prophylaxis.

Preparation • Must be prepared by personnel trained in aseptic manipulations and admixing of cytotoxic drugs. • Calculate dose based on weight in kg. Round dose volume to the nearest 0.1 mL. • Visually inspect for particulate matter or discoloration. Solution should appear clear to slightly opalescent, colorless to slightly yellow or brown. Translucent, proteinaceous particles may be present. Do not use if solution is cloudy or discolored. • Gently swirl vial. Do not shake or agitate. • Dilute in 100 mL or 250 mL 0.9% NaCl infusion bag to a final concentration between 0.5 and 7.2 mg/mL. • Gently invert to mix. Do not shake or agitate. • Discard unused portions of vial.

Rate of administration • **Initial infusion:** Infuse over 120 min. • **Subsequent infusions:** Infuse over at least 30 min. • **Infusion reactions:** Decrease infusion rate if mild or moderate infusion reactions occur.

Storage • Refrigerate unused vials in original carton. Protect from light. • Diluted solution may be refrigerated for up to 24 hrs or stored at room temperature up to 4 hrs. • Do not freeze. • If refrigerated, allow diluted solution to warm to room temperature.

⊞ IV INCOMPATABILITIES

Do not dilute in D5W. Do mix or infuse with other medications.

INDICATIONS/ROUTES/DOSAGE

Breast Cancer (HER2-Positive, Metastatic)
IV: ADULTS: 15 mg/kg q3wks. Continue until disease progression or unacceptable toxicity.

Dose Modification

Cardiac Toxicity
Withhold treatment for at least 4 wks for an absolute decrease in LVEF that is greater than or equal to 16% from baseline; LVEF below institutional limits of normal (or 50% if no limits are available) and an absolute decrease in LVEF greater than or equal to 10% from baseline. May resume treatment if LVEF returns to normal limits and the absolute decrease from baseline is less than or equal to 15% within 8 wks. Permanently discontinue if treatment is withheld for more than 3 occasions due to cardiotoxicity or decline of LVEF persists for more than 8 wks.

Infusion-Related Reactions
Interrupt infusion for dyspnea or significant hypotension. Permanently discontinue in pts with severe or life-threatening infusion reactions.

Dosage in Renal Impairment

Mild to moderate impairment: No dose adjustment. **Severe impairment, ESRD:** Not specified; use caution.

Dosage in Hepatic Impairment

Mild impairment: No dose adjustment. **Moderate to severe impairment:** Not specified; use caution.

M

SIDE EFFECTS

Frequent (57%–25%): Fatigue, asthenia, nausea, diarrhea. **Occasional (21%–6%):** Vomiting, constipation, pyrexia, headache, alopecia, abdominal pain, peripheral neuropathy, cough, decreased appetite, arthralgia, myalgia, dyspnea, extremity pain, dizziness, stomatitis, decreased weight, dysgeusia, rash, insomnia. **Rare (5%–2%):** Hypertension, syncope.

ADVERSE EFFECTS/TOXIC REACTIONS

Myelosuppression (anemia, leukopenia, lymphopenia, neutropenia) is an expected response to therapy. Left ventricular dysfunction reported in 2% of pts. Infusion reactions, including arthralgia, cough, chills, diaphoresis, dizziness, dyspnea, fatigue, fever, flushing, headache, hypotension, nausea, pruritus, rash, tachycardia, urticaria, vomiting, reported in 13% of pts. Palmar-plantar erythrodysesthesia syndrome (PPES), a chemotherapy-induced skin condition that presents with skin redness, swelling, numbness, sloughing of the hands and feet, reported in 13% of pts.

NURSING CONSIDERATIONS

BASELINE ASSESSMENT

Obtain CBC, LFT; pregnancy test in females of reproductive potential. Verify use of effective contraception. Obtain weight in kg. Verify presence of HER2 protein overexpression in tumor specimen. Question occurrence of infusion-related reactions prior to each dose. Administer in an environment equipped to monitor for and manage infusion-related reactions; verify emergency resuscitation equipment/medications are readily available.

Assess LVEF by echocardiogram or MUGA scan within 4 wks of initiation. Question history of cardiomyopathy, hepatic/renal impairment; recent administration of anthracyclines. Screen for active infection. Offer emotional support.

INTERVENTION/EVALUATION

Monitor CBC, LFT as clinically indicated. Diligently monitor for infusion reactions. Severe infusion reactions may require emergency resuscitation; early detection is vital. Assess for symptoms of HF (chest pain, dyspnea, palpitations, swelling of extremities). Assess LVEF by echocardiogram or MUGA scan q3mos until discontinuation. If treatment is withheld due to change in LVEF, monitor LVEF at 4-wk intervals. Monitor for infections (cough, fatigue, fever). If serious infection occurs, initiate appropriate antimicrobial therapy. Monitor daily pattern of bowel activity, stool consistency. Assess skin for PPES.

PATIENT/FAMILY TEACHING

• Treatment may depress the immune system response and reduce ability to fight infection. Report symptoms of infection such as body aches, chills, cough, fatigue, fever. Avoid those with active infection. • Life-threatening infusion reactions may occur. Immediately report infusion reactions of any kind. • Treatment may reduce the heart's ability to pump effectively; expect routine echocardiograms. • Report heart problems (difficulty breathing, fainting, palpitations, swelling of extremities), toxic skin reactions (itching, peeling, rash, redness, swelling). • Use effective contraception to avoid pregnancy. Do not breastfeed. • Maintain proper hydration and nutrition. • Avoid tasks that require alertness, motor skills until response to drug is established.

medroxyPROGES-TERone

me-**drox**-ee-proe-**jes**-ter-one
(Depo-Provera, Depo-SubQ Provera 104, Provera)

■ **BLACK BOX ALERT** ■ Prolonged use (over 2 yrs) of contraceptive injection form may result in loss of bone mineral density. Limit long-term use (more than 2 yrs). May increase risk of dementia in postmenopausal women. Increased risk of invasive breast cancer in postmenopausal women in combination with conjugated estrogens.

Do not confuse medroxyPRO-GESTERone with HYDROXYprogesterone, methylPREDNISolone, or methylTESTOSTERone, or Provera with Covera, Femara, Parlodel, or Premarin.

◆CLASSIFICATION

PHARMACOTHERAPEUTIC: Hormone. **CLINICAL:** Progestin, antineoplastic, contraceptive hormone.

USES

Oral: Treatment of secondary amenorrhea and abnormal uterine bleeding due to hormonal imbalance in the absence of organic pathology (e.g., fibroids, uterine cancer). Prevention of endometrial hyperplasia in non-hysterectomized postmenopausal women receiving daily oral conjugated estrogens. **Depo-subQ Provera 104:** Prevention of pregnancy, and management of endometriosis-associated pain. **Depo-Provera:** Adjunctive therapy and/or palliative treatment of inoperable, recurrent, or metastatic endometrial carcinoma. **OFF-LABEL:** Treatment of endometrial hyperplasia.

PRECAUTIONS

Contraindications: Hypersensitivity to medroxyPROGESTERone. Breast cancer (known, suspected, or prior history), history of or active thrombotic disorders (thrombophlebitis, DVT, MI, pulmonary embolism), known or suspected pregnancy, severe hepatic impairment, undiagnosed abnormal vaginal bleeding, cerebrovascular disease. **Cautions:** Conditions aggravated by fluid retention (asthma, seizures, migraine, cardiac/renal dysfunction), diabetes, history of mental depression, preexisting hypercholesterolemia, hypertriglyceridemia.

ACTION

Inhibits secretion of pituitary gonadotropins, transforming proliferative endometrium into secretory endometrium. **Therapeutic Effect:** When used for contraception, inhibits secretion of pituitary gonadotropins, prevents follicular maturation and ovulation, causing endometrial thinning. Reduces incidence of endometrial hyperplasia and risk of adenocarcinoma. When used for endometriosis, progestogens (e.g., medroxyPROGESTERone), leads to atrophy of endometrial tissue. Decreases endometriosis-associated pain.

PHARMACOKINETICS

Widely distributed. Slowly absorbed after IM administration. Protein binding: 90%. Metabolized in liver. Primarily excreted in urine. **Half-life: PO:** 12–17 hrs. **IM:** 40–50 days.

⧖ LIFESPAN CONSIDERATIONS

Pregnancy/Lactation: Avoid use during pregnancy, esp. first 4 mos (congenital heart, limb reduction defects may occur). Distributed in breast milk. **Children:** Safety and efficacy not established. **Elderly:** No age-related precautions noted.

INTERACTIONS

DRUG: Strong CYP3A4 None significant. inducers (e.g., carBAMazepine, phenytoin, rifAMPin) may decrease concentration/effect, resulting in contraceptive failure. May decrease therapeutic effect of **anticoagulants (e.g., warfarin). HERBAL:** None significant. **FOOD:** None known. **LAB VALUES:** May

---

M

◆ Canadian trade name   🔻 Non-Crushable Drug   🔲 High Alert drug

alter serum thyroid, LFT, PT, HDL, total cholesterol, triglycerides; metapyrone test. May increase LDL.

AVAILABILITY (Rx)

Injection Suspension: *(Depo-SubQ Provera 104):* 104 mg/0.65 mL prefilled syringe. *(Depo-Provera):* 150 mg/mL, 400 mg/mL. **Tablets:** *(Provera):* 2.5 mg, 5 mg, 10 mg.

ADMINISTRATION/HANDLING
IM

• Shake vial immediately before administering (ensures complete suspension). • Administer deep IM into gluteal or deltoid muscle. • Shake vigorously prior to administration. • Inject in upper thigh or abdomen (avoid bony areas and umbilicus). • Give over 5–7 sec; do not rub injection area.

PO

• Give with food.

INDICATIONS/ROUTES/DOSAGE

Endometrial Hyperplasia (Prevention)
PO: ADULTS: 5–10 mg/day for 12–14 consecutive days each month starting on day 1 or 16 of cycle.

Secondary Amenorrhea
PO: ADULTS: 5–10 mg/day for 5–10 days, beginning at any time during menstrual cycle.

Abnormal Uterine Bleeding
PO: ADULTS: 5–10 mg/day for 5–10 days, beginning on calculated day 16 or day 21 of menstrual cycle.

Endometrial Carcinoma
IM: ADULTS, ELDERLY: Initially, 400–1,000 mg; repeat at 1-wk intervals.

Pregnancy Prevention
IM: *(Depo-Provera):* **ADULTS:** 150 mg q3mos (q13 wks).
SQ: *(Depo-Subq Provera 104):* **ADULTS:** 104 mg q3mos (q12–14wks).

Endometriosis
SQ: *(Depo-Subq Provera 104):* **ADULTS:** 104 mg q3mos (q12–14 wks).

Dosage in Renal Impairment
No dose adjustment.

Dosage in Hepatic Impairment
Contraindicated with severe impairment.

SIDE EFFECTS

Frequent: Transient menstrual abnormalities (spotting, change in menstrual flow/cervical secretions, amenorrhea) at initiation of therapy. **Occasional:** Edema, weight change, breast tenderness, anxiety, insomnia, fatigue, dizziness. **Rare:** Alopecia, depression, dermatologic changes, headache, fever, nausea.

ADVERSE EFFECTS/TOXIC REACTIONS

Thrombophlebitis, pulmonary/cerebral embolism, retinal thrombosis occur rarely.

NURSING CONSIDERATIONS

BASELINE ASSESSMENT

Obtain usual menstrual history. Question for hypersensitivity to progestins. Obtain baseline weight, B/P, pregnancy test in females of reproductive potential.

INTERVENTION/EVALUATION

Check weight daily; report wkly gain of 5 lb or more. Assess B/P periodically. Assess skin for rash, urticaria. Report development of chest pain, sudden shortness of breath, sudden decrease in vision, migraine headache, pain (esp. with swelling, warmth, redness) in calves, numbness of arm/leg (thrombotic disorders) immediately.

PATIENT/FAMILY TEACHING

• Report sudden loss of vision, severe headache, chest pain, coughing up of blood (hemoptysis), numbness in arm/leg, severe pain/swelling in calf, unusually heavy vaginal bleeding, severe abdominal pain/tenderness. • Depo-Provera Contraceptive injection should be used as long-term birth control method (e.g., longer than 2 yrs) only if other birth control methods are inadequate.

M

megestrol

meh-**jes**-trol
Do not confuse megestrol with mesalamine.

◆CLASSIFICATION

PHARMACOTHERAPEUTIC: Synthetic hormone. **CLINICAL:** Antineoplastic, progestin, appetite stimulant.

USES

Palliative treatment of advanced endometrial or breast carcinoma; treatment of anorexia, cachexia, unexplained significant weight loss in pts with AIDS. **OFF-LABEL:** Cancer related cachexia, endometrial hyperplasia.

PRECAUTIONS

Contraindications: Hypersensitivity to megestrol. **Suspension:** Known or suspected pregnancy. **Cautions:** History of thrombophlebitis, elderly.

ACTION

Antiestrogenic; interferes with normal estrogen cycle by decreasing release of luteinizing hormone (LH) from anterior pituitary gland by inhibiting pituitary function. Antineoplastic effect may act through an antiluteinizing effect mediated via the pituitary. May increase appetite by antagonizing metabolic effects of catabolic cytokines. **Therapeutic Effect:** Reduces tumor size. Increases appetite.

PHARMACOKINETICS

Widely distributed. Metabolized in liver. Excreted in urine. **Half-life:** 13–105 hrs (mean 34 hrs).

⧖ LIFESPAN CONSIDERATIONS

Pregnancy/Lactation: If possible, avoid use during pregnancy, esp. first 4 mos. Breastfeeding not recommended.

Children: Safety and efficacy not established. **Elderly:** Use caution.

INTERACTIONS

DRUG: May increase concentration/effects of **dofetilide, warfarin. HERBAL:** Avoid **black cohosh, dong quai** in estrogen-dependent tumors. Avoid **herbs with progestogenic properties (e.g., bloodroot, chasteberry, yucca);** may increase adverse effects. **FOOD:** None known. **LAB VALUES:** May alter serum thyroid, LFT, PT, HDL, total cholesterol, triglycerides. May increase LDL.

AVAILABILITY (Rx)

Oral Suspension: 40 mg/mL, 625 mg/5 mL. **Tablets:** 20 mg, 40 mg.

ADMINISTRATION/HANDLING

PO
• Store tablets, oral suspension at room temperature. • Shake suspension well before use. • Oral suspension compatible with water, orange juice, apple juice. • Administer without regard to food.

INDICATIONS/ROUTES/DOSAGE

Palliative Treatment of Advanced Breast Cancer
PO: ADULTS, ELDERLY: 40 mg 4 times/day or 160 mg/day for at least 2 mos.

Palliative Treatment of Advanced Endometrial Carcinoma
PO: ADULTS, ELDERLY: 40–320 mg/day in divided doses for at least 2 mos.

Anorexia, Cachexia, Weight Loss
PO: ADULTS, ELDERLY: Initially, 625 mg (125 mg/mL suspension) or 800 mg (40 mg/mL suspension) daily.

Dosage in Renal Impairment
Use caution.

Dosage in Hepatic Impairment
No dose adjustment.

M

SIDE EFFECTS

Frequent: Weight gain secondary to increased appetite. **Occasional:** Nausea, breakthrough menstrual bleeding, backache, headache, breast tenderness, carpal tunnel syndrome. **Rare:** Feeling of coldness.

ADVERSE EFFECTS/TOXIC REACTIONS

Thrombophlebitis, pulmonary embolism occur rarely.

NURSING CONSIDERATIONS

BASELINE ASSESSMENT

Obtain pregnancy test in females of reproductive potential. Offer emotional support.

INTERVENTION/EVALUATION

Monitor for tumor response. Monitor pt weight, caloric intake (appetite stimulant).

PATIENT/FAMILY TEACHING

• Contraception is imperative. • Report lower leg (calf) pain, difficulty breathing, vaginal bleeding. • May cause headache, nausea, vomiting, breast tenderness, backache.

meloxicam

mel-**ox**-i-kam
(Anjeso)

■ **BLACK BOX ALERT** ■ Increased risk of serious cardiovascular thrombotic events, including myocardial infarction, CVA. Increased risk of severe GI reactions, including ulceration, bleeding, GI perforation.

FIXED-COMBINATION(S)

Zynrelef: meloxicam/bupivacaine (an anesthetic): 12 mg/400 mg; 9 mg/300 mg; 6 mg/200 mg; 1.8 mg/60 mg.

◆CLASSIFICATION

PHARMACOTHERAPEUTIC: NSAID. **CLINICAL:** Anti-inflammatory, analgesic.

USES

Oral: Relief of signs/symptoms of osteoarthritis, rheumatoid arthritis (RA). Treatment of juvenile idiopathic arthritis (JIA) in pts 2 yrs of age and older (suspension) and weighing 60 kg or more (tablets). **IV:** Management of moderate to severe pain in adults. **OFF-LABEL:** Treatment of gout (acute flares).

PRECAUTIONS

Contraindications: Hypersensitivity to meloxicam. Pts with aspirin triad (asthma, rhinitis, aspirin intolerance). History of asthma, urticaria with NSAIDs, perioperative pain in setting of CABG surgery. **Injection only:** Moderate to severe renal insufficiency in pts at risk for renal failure due to volume depletion. **Cautions:** Renal/hepatic impairment, asthma, coagulation disorders, hypertension, pts at risk for GI perforation (e.g., Crohn's disease, diverticulitis, GI tract malignancies, peptic ulcers, peritoneal malignancies), history of cardiovascular disease, MI; concurrent use of anticoagulants, fluid retention, HF, dehydration, smoking, alcohol use, elderly, debilitated.

ACTION

Produces analgesic, antipyretic, anti-inflammatory effects by inhibiting prostaglandin synthesis. **Therapeutic Effect:** Reduces inflammatory response, intensity of pain.

PHARMACOKINETICS

Route	Onset	Peak	Duration
PO (Analgesic)	30 min	4–5 hrs	N/A

Widely distributed. Protein binding: 99%. Metabolized in liver. Steady-state reached in 5 days. Excreted equally in urine, feces. Not removed by hemodialysis. **Half-life:** 15–20 hrs.

⧗ LIFESPAN CONSIDERATIONS

Pregnancy/Lactation: Avoid use at 30 wks gestation or more (may cause premature closure of ductus arteriosus). Distributed in breast milk. May impair fertility in both females and males. **Children**: Safety and efficacy not established in children younger than 2 yrs. **Elderly**: Age-related renal impairment may require dosage adjustment. More susceptible to GI toxicity; lower dosage recommended.

INTERACTIONS

DRUG: May increase anticoagulant effect of **apixaban, dabigatran, edoxaban, rivaroxaban. Bile acid sequestrants** (e.g., **cholestyramine**) may decrease absorption. May increase nephrotoxic effect of **cycloSPORINE, tacrolimus, tenofovir.** May decrease effect of **loop diuretics** (e.g., **furosemide**). May decrease antihypertensive effect of **ACE inhibitors** (e.g., **enalapril, lisinopril**), **angiotensin receptor blockers** (e.g., **losartan, valsartan**), **beta blockers** (e.g., **carvedilol, metoprolol**). **HERBAL:** Glucosamine, herbals with anticoagulant/antiplatelet properties (e.g., **garlic, ginger, ginkgo biloba, ginseng**), **alfalfa, anise, bilberry.** may increase concentration/effect. **FOOD:** None known. **LAB VALUES:** May increase serum creatinine, ALT, AST.

AVAILABILITY (Rx)

Injection Solution: *(Anjeso):* 30 mg/mL. **Tablets:** 7.5 mg, 15 mg. **Capsules:** 5 mg, 10 mg. 7.5 mg, 15 mg. *(Suspension, Oral):* 7.5 mg/5 mL.

ADMINISTRATION/HANDLING
IV

• Administer undiluted as an IV bolus over 15 sec.

PO

• Administer without regard to meals (give with food or milk to minimize GI irritation). • **Suspension:** Shake gently prior to use.

INDICATIONS/ROUTES/DOSAGE
Rheumatoid Arthritis (RA)

PO: **ADULTS, ELDERLY:** *(Oral Suspension, Tablet):* Initially, 7.5 mg/day. **Maximum:** 15 mg/day.

Osteoarthritis

PO: *(Capsule):* **ADULTS, ELDERLY:** Initially, 5 mg once daily. May increase to 10 mg once daily. *(Oral Suspension, Tablet):* **ADULTS, ELDERLY:** Initially, 7.5 mg once daily. May increase to 15 mg once daily.

Pain (Moderate to Severe)

IV: **ADULTS, ELDERLY:** 30 mg once daily.

JIA

(Oral Suspension): **CHILDREN 2 YRS AND OLDER, ADOLESCENTS:** 0.125 mg/kg once daily. **Maximum:** 7.5 mg. *(Tablet):* **CHILDREN, ADOLESCENTS WEIGHING 60 KG OR GREATER:** 7.5 mg once daily.

Dosage in Renal Impairment

Not recommended with severe impairment.

Dosage in Hepatic Impairment

No dose adjustment.

SIDE EFFECTS

Frequent (9%–7%): Dyspepsia, headache, diarrhea, nausea. **Occasional (4%–3%):** Dizziness, insomnia, rash, pruritus, flatulence, constipation, vomiting. **Rare (less than 2%):** Drowsiness, urticaria, photosensitivity, tinnitus.

ADVERSE EFFECTS/TOXIC REACTIONS

May increase risk of severe HF; cardiovascular thrombotic events, including MI. Life-threatening GI effects including inflammation, GI bleeding, ulceration, and perforation of esophagus, small intestines, stomach, and large intestines were reported. Hepatotoxicity reported in 1% of pts. May cause new onset or worsening of hypertension. Hypersensitivity reactions including anaphylaxis may occur. Cutaneous toxicities including Stevens-Johnson syndrome, toxic epidermal necrolysis, exfoliative dermatitis may occur. May mask symptoms of inflammation and fever. Severe renal injury may cause hyperkalemia. In pts

M

treated chronically, peptic ulcer, GI bleeding, gastritis, severe hepatic toxicity (jaundice), nephrotoxicity (hematuria, dysuria, proteinuria), severe hypersensitivity reaction (bronchospasm, angioedema) occur rarely.

NURSING CONSIDERATIONS

BASELINE ASSESSMENT

Assess onset, type, location, duration of pain/inflammation. Inspect appearance of affected joints for immobility, deformities, skin condition. Question history of GI bleeding, gastric or duodenal ulcers, hepatic/renal impairment, asthma.

INTERVENTION/EVALUATION

Monitor CBC, renal function, LFT. Assess for therapeutic response: relief of pain, stiffness, swelling; increased joint mobility; reduced joint tenderness; improved grip strength. Monitor B/P for hypertension. Immediately report abdominal pain, fever, hematemesis, melena; may indicate GI perforation. Monitor for hypersensitivity reactions; symptoms of MI (chest pain, dyspnea, syncope, diaphoresis, arm/jaw pain). Assess skin for cutaneous toxicities. Monitor for symptoms of HF (dyspnea, edema, fatigue, palpitations). Obtain LVEF by echocardiogram if HF is suspected.

PATIENT/FAMILY TEACHING

- Take with food, milk to reduce GI upset. • Treatment may worsen high blood pressure. • Immediately report severe or persistent abdominal pain, bloody stool, fever, vomiting blood; may indicate rupture in GI tract. • Report liver problems (abdominal pain, bruising, clay-colored stool, amber- or dark-colored urine, yellowing of the skin or eyes); kidney problems (decreased urine output, flank pain, darkened urine); toxic skin reactions (rash, skin eruptions); symptoms of heart attack (chest pain, difficulty breathing, jaw pain, nausea, pain that radiates to the left arm, sweating), HF (difficulty breathing, fatigue, palpitations, extremity swelling). Allergic reactions, including anaphylaxis, may occur. • Avoid use after 30 wks gestation.

memantine

me-**man**-teen
(Ebixa ✦, <u>Namenda</u>, <u>Namenda XR</u>)

FIXED-COMBINATION(S)

Namzaric: memantine/donepezil (a cholinesterase inhibitor): 7 mg/10 mg; 14 mg/10 mg; 21 mg/10 mg; 28 mg/10 mg.

◆CLASSIFICATION

PHARMACOTHERAPEUTIC: NMDA receptor antagonist. **CLINICAL:** Anti-Alzheimer's agent.

USES

Treatment of moderate to severe dementia of Alzheimer's type. **OFF-LABEL:** Treatment of dementia (e.g., Parkinson's disease with Lewy bodies, comorbid vascular dementia).

PRECAUTIONS

Contraindications: Hypersensitivity to memantine. **Cautions:** Moderate to severe renal impairment, severe hepatic impairment, cardiovascular disease, seizure disorder, GU conditions that raise urine pH level.

ACTION

Decreases effects of glutamate, the principal excitatory neurotransmitter in the brain. Persistent CNS excitation by glutamate is thought to cause symptoms of Alzheimer's disease. **Therapeutic Effect:** May slow clinical deterioration in moderate to severe Alzheimer's disease.

PHARMACOKINETICS

Widely distributed. Protein binding: 45%. Undergoes minimal metabolism. Primarily excreted in urine. **Half-life:** 60–80 hrs.

⧖ LIFESPAN CONSIDERATIONS

Pregnancy/Lactation: Unknown if drug crosses placenta or is distributed in breast milk. **Children:** Not prescribed for this pt population.

M

Elderly: No age-related precautions noted, but use is not recommended in pts with severe renal impairment (CrCl less than 9 mL/min).

INTERACTIONS

DRUG: Urine alkalinizers (e.g., carbonic anhydrase inhibitors, sodium bicarbonate) may decrease renal elimination. **HERBAL:** None significant. **FOOD:** None known. **LAB VALUES:** None significant.

AVAILABILITY (Rx)

Oral Solution: 10 mg/5 mL. **Tablets:** 5 mg, 10 mg.

🪶 **Capsules, Extended-Release:** *(Namenda XR):* 7 mg, 14 mg, 21 mg, 28 mg.

ADMINISTRATION/HANDLING
PO
• Give without regard to food. • Administer oral solution using syringe provided. Do not dilute or mix with other fluids. • Give extended-release capsules whole. Do not crush, divide, or allow chewing. May open capsule and sprinkle on applesauce; give immediately.

INDICATIONS/ROUTES/DOSAGE

Alzheimer's Disease
PO: ADULTS, ELDERLY: *(Immediate-Release):* Initially, 5 mg once daily. May increase dose at intervals of at least 1 wk in 5-mg increments to 10 mg/day (5 mg twice daily), then 15 mg/day (5 mg and 10 mg as separate doses), then 20 mg/day (10 mg twice daily). **Target dose:** 20 mg/day. *(Extended-Release):* Initially, 7 mg once daily. May increase at intervals of at least 7 days in increments of 7 mg. **Maximum:** 28 mg once daily. Switching from immediate-release to extended-release: Begin the day following last dose of immediate-release. 10 mg twice daily: 28 mg once daily. 5 mg twice daily: 14 mg once daily.

Dosage in Renal Impairment

Creatinine Clearance	Dosage Immediate-Release	Dosage Extended-Release
30 mL/min or greater	No adjustments	No adjustments
5–29 mL/min	5 mg twice daily or 10 mg once daily	14 mg once daily

Dosage in Hepatic Impairment
Mild to moderate impairment: No dose adjustment. **Severe impairment:** Use caution.

SIDE EFFECTS

Occasional (7%–4%): Dizziness, headache, confusion, constipation, hypertension, cough. **Rare (3%–2%):** Back pain, nausea, fatigue, anxiety, peripheral edema, arthralgia, insomnia.

ADVERSE EFFECTS/TOXIC REACTIONS

None known.

NURSING CONSIDERATIONS

BASELINE ASSESSMENT

Assess cognitive, behavioral, functional deficits. Assess renal function. Question history of cardiovascular disease, hepatic/renal impairment, seizure disorder.

INTERVENTION/EVALUATION

Monitor BUN, CrCl, serum creatinine. Monitor cognitive, behavioral, functional status of pt. Monitor urine pH (alterations of urine pH toward the alkaline condition may lead to accumulation of the drug with possible increase in side effects).

PATIENT/FAMILY TEACHING

• Do not reduce or stop medication; do not increase dosage without physician direction. • Ensure adequate fluid intake. • If therapy is interrupted for several days, restart at lowest dose, titrate to current dose at minimum of 1-wk intervals. • Local chapter of Alzheimer's Disease Association can provide a guide to services.

M

mepolizumab

me-poe-**liz**-ue-mab
(Nucala)
**Do not confuse mepolizumab
with atezolizumab, certolizumab, eculizumab, omalizumab,
pembrolizumab, or Nucala with
Calan or Nucynta.**

◆CLASSIFICATION

PHARMACOTHERAPEUTIC: Interleu-
kin-5 receptor antagonist. Monoclonal antibody. **CLINICAL:** Antiasthmatic.

USES

Asthma, severe eosinophilic: Add-
on maintenance treatment of pts 6 yrs
of age and older with severe asthma and
with an eosinophil phenotype. **Chronic
rhinosinusitis with nasal polyps
(CRSwNP):** Add-on maintenance treatment of CRSwNP in adults with inadequate response to nasal corticosteroids.
**Eosinophilic granulomatosis with
polyangiitis (EGPA):** Treatment of
adults with EGPA. **Hypereosinophilic
syndrome (HES):** Treatment of adults
and children 12 yrs and older with HES
for 6 mos or longer without an identifi-
able nonhematologic secondary cause.

PRECAUTIONS

Contraindications: Hypersensitivity to
mepolizumab. **Cautions:** History of herpes zoster infection, parasitic infection.
Not indicated for treatment of other
eosinophilic conditions; relief of acute
bronchospasm, status asthmaticus, exercise-induced bronchospasm.

ACTION

Inhibits signaling of interleukin-5 cytokine, reducing production and survival
of eosinophils responsible for asthmatic
inflammation and pathogenesis. **Therapeutic Effect:** Prevents inflammatory
process; relieves signs/symptoms of
asthma.

PHARMACOKINETICS

Widely distributed. Degraded into small
peptides and amino acids via proteolytic
enzymes. Excretion not specified. **Half-
life:** 16–22 days.

LIFESPAN CONSIDERATIONS

Pregnancy/Lactation: Unknown if distributed in breast milk. However, human
immunoglobulin G (IgG) is present in
breast milk and is known to cross placenta.
Children: Safety and efficacy not established in pts younger than 6 yrs. **Elderly:**
Safety and efficacy not established.

INTERACTIONS

DRUG: None known. **HERBAL:** None significant. **FOOD:** None known. **LAB VAL-
UES:** None known.

AVAILABILITY (Rx)

Injection Powder: 100 mg. **Injection
Solution:** 100 mg/mL single-dose autoinjector; 100 mg/mL, 40 mg/0.4 mL single-
dose, prefilled glass syringe.

ADMINISTRATION/HANDLING

SQ
Reconstitution • Using a 2- or 3-mL
syringe and 21G needle, reconstitute vial
with 1.2 mL Sterile Water for Injection to a
final concentration of 100 mg/mL. **•** Direct stream vertically onto center of the lyophilized cake. **•** Gently swirl in a circu-
lar motion for 10 sec at 15-sec intervals
until fully dissolved (approx. 5 min or
more). **•** Do not shake (may cause
foaming/precipitate formation). If mechanical reconstitution device is used,
swirl at 450 rpm for up to 10 min or at
1,000 rpm for up to 5 min. **•** Visually
inspect for particulate matter or discoloration. Solution should appear clear to
opalescent, colorless to pale yellow or pale
brown (essentially free of particles). Air
bubbles are expected and allowed. **•** Do
not use if solution is cloudy or discolored
or if visible particles are observed.
Administration • Prior to administration, withdraw 1 mL of solution (100 mg)

M

from vial. (Remove 0.4 mL for 40-mg dose.) • Do not shake or agitate. • Using a polypropylene syringe fitted with a 21G–27G × 0.5 (13-mm) needle, subcutaneously insert needle into upper arms, outer thigh, or abdomen, and inject solution. • Do not inject into areas of active skin disease or injury such as sunburns, skin rashes, inflammation, skin infections, or active psoriasis. • Rotate injection sites.

Autoinjector/Prefilled Syringes: The 100–mg/mL autoinjector and prefilled syringe are for use in adults and children 12 yrs and older. The 40-mg/0.4-mL prefilled syringe is for use in children aged 6–11 yrs. Remove from the refrigerator and allow to sit at room temp for 30 min prior to injection. For EGPA and HES, separate each injection by at least 2 in.

Storage • Store unused vials below 25°C (77°F). • Do not freeze. • Do not shake. • Protect from light. • May store reconstituted solution below 30°C (86°F) up to 8 hrs.

INDICATIONS/ROUTES/DOSAGE

Asthma (Severe)

SQ: ADULTS, ELDERLY, CHILDREN 12 YRS AND OLDER: 100 mg once q4wks. **CHILDREN 6–11 YRS:** 40 mg once q4wks.

CRSwNP

SQ: ADULTS, ELDERLY: 100 mg once q4wks.

EGPA

SQ: ADULTS, ELDERLY: 300 mg (three 100-mg injections) once q4wks.

HES

SQ: ADULTS, ELDERLY, CHILDREN 12 YRS AND OLDER: 300 mg (three 100-mg injections) once q4wks.

Dosage in Renal/Hepatic Impairment
No dose adjustment.

SIDE EFFECTS

Frequent (19%): Headache. **Occasional (8%–3%):** Injection site reaction (pain, erythema, swelling, itching, burning sensation), back pain, fatigue, eczema, abdominal pain, pruritus, muscle spasms,

ADVERSE EFFECTS/TOXIC REACTIONS

Hypersensitivity reactions including angioedema, bronchospasm, hypotension, urticaria, rash were reported. Hypersensitivity reactions typically occurred hrs to days after administration. Infections including herpes zoster, influenza, UTI may occur. Unknown if treatment will influence the immunological response to helminth (parasite) infection.

NURSING CONSIDERATIONS

BASELINE ASSESSMENT

Obtain pulse rate, oxygen saturation. Auscultate lung fields. Question history of herpes zoster infection, parasitic infection, hypersensitivity reaction. Pts with preexisting helminth (parasite) infection should be treated prior to initiation. Consider varicella vaccination before starting therapy. Inhaled or systemic corticosteroids should not be suddenly discontinued upon initiation. Corticosteroids that are not gradually reduced may cause withdrawal symptoms or unmask conditions that were originally suppressed with corticosteroid therapy.

INTERVENTION/EVALUATION

Monitor rate, depth, rhythm of respirations. Assess lungs for wheezing, rales. Monitor oxygen saturation. Interrupt or discontinue treatment if hypersensitivity reaction, opportunistic infection (esp. parasite infection, herpes zoster infection), worsening of asthma-related symptoms (esp. in pts tapering off corticosteroids) occurs. Obtain pulmonary function test to assess disease improvement. Monitor for increased use of rescue inhalers; may indicate deterioration of asthma.

PATIENT/FAMILY TEACHING

• Not indicated for relief of acute asthmatic episodes. • Have a rescue inhaler readily available. • Increased use of rescue inhaler may indicate worsening of asthma. • Seek medical attention if asthma symptoms worsen or remain uncontrolled after starting treatment. • Immediately report allergic reactions such as

M

difficulty breathing, itching, hives, rash, swelling of the face or tongue. • Report infections of any kind, esp. shingles (herpes zoster). • Do not stop corticosteroid therapy unless directed by prescriber.

meropenem

mer-oh-**pen**-em
Do not confuse meropenem with doripenem, ertapenem, or imipenem.

◆CLASSIFICATION

PHARMACOTHERAPEUTIC: Carbapenem. **CLINICAL:** Antibiotic.

USES

Treatment of complicated skin and skin structure infections (cSSSI) in adults and pts 3 mos and older due to *S. aureus* (methicillin-susceptible isolates only), *S. pyogenes, S. agalactiae,* viridans group streptococci, *E. faecalis* (vancomycin-susceptible isolates only), *P. aeruginosa, E. coli, P. mirabilis, B. fragilis,* and *Peptostreptococcus* species. Treatment of complicated appendicitis and peritonitis in adults and children caused by viridans group streptococci, *E. coli, K. pneumoniae, P. aeruginosa, B. fragilis,* and *Peptostreptococcus* species. Treatment of bacterial meningitis in adults and pts 3 mos and older caused by *H. influenzae, N. meningitidis* and penicillin-susceptible isolates of *S. pneumoniae.* **OFF-LABEL:** Bloodstream, diabetic foot, prosthetic joint, urinary tract infections; cystic fibrosis (acute pulmonary exacerbation), intracranial abscess, neutropenic fever, osteomyelitis, pneumonia, sepsis/septic shock.

PRECAUTIONS

Contraindications: Hypersensitivity to meropenem, anaphylactic reactions to penicillins, cephalosporins, other beta-lactams. **Cautions:** Renal impairment, CNS disorders (particularly with history of seizures, concurrent use with valproic acid).

ACTION

Binds to penicillin-binding proteins. Inhibits bacterial cell wall synthesis. **Therapeutic Effect:** Bactericidal.

PHARMACOKINETICS

Widely distributed into tissues and body fluids, including CSF. Protein binding: 2%. Primarily excreted unchanged in urine. Removed by hemodialysis. **Half-life:** 1 hr.

⧗ LIFESPAN CONSIDERATIONS

Pregnancy/Lactation: Unknown if distributed in breast milk. **Children:** Safety and efficacy not established in pts younger than 3 mos. **Elderly:** Age-related renal impairment may require dosage adjustment.

INTERACTIONS

DRUG: May decrease therapeutic effect of **valproic acid. Probenecid** may increase concentration/effect. **HERBAL:** None significant. **FOOD:** None known. **LAB VALUES:** May increase serum BUN, alkaline phosphatase, LDH, ALT, AST, bilirubin. May decrease Hgb, Hct, WBC.

AVAILABILITY (Rx)

Injection, Powder for Reconstitution: 500 mg, 1 g. **Injection (Solution):** 1 g/50 mL, 500 mg/50 mL.

ADMINISTRATION/HANDLING

 IV

Reconstitution • Reconstitute each 500 mg with 10 mL Sterile Water for Injection, 0.9% NaCl, or D_5W to provide concentration of 50 mg/mL. • Shake to dissolve until clear. • May further dilute with 0.9% NaCl or D_5W to a concentration of 1–20 mg/mL.
Rate of administration • May give by IV push or IV intermittent infusion (piggy-

M

back). • If administering as IV intermittent infusion (piggyback), give over 15–30 min (may also give over 3 hrs); if administered by IV push, give over 3–5 min (at a concentration not greater than 50 mg/mL). **Storage** • Store vials at room temperature. • After reconstitution of vials with 0.9% NaCl, stable for 2 hrs at room temperature or 18 hrs if refrigerated (with D_5W, stable for 1 hr at room temperature, 8 hrs if refrigerated). IV infusion with 0.9% NaCl stable for 4 hrs at room temperature or 24 hrs if refrigerated (with D_5W, 1 hr at room temperature or 4 hrs if refrigerated).

▨ IV COMPATIBILITIES

Calcium gluconate, dexmedetomidine, magnesium sulfate, potassium chloride, potassium phosphate.

INDICATIONS/ROUTES/DOSAGE

Usual Dosage

IV: ADULTS, ELDERLY: 500 mg q6h or 1–2 g q8h. *(Extended-Infusion):* 1–2 g over 3 hrs q8h. **CHILDREN 3 MOS AND OLDER, ADOLESCENTS:** 20 mg/kg/dose q8h. **Maximum dose:** 1,000 mg. **NEONATES:** 20–30 mg/kg/dose q8–12h.

Dosage in Renal Impairment

Dosage and frequency are modified based on creatinine clearance.

Creatinine Clearance	Dosage	Interval
26–49 mL/min	Normal dose	q12h
10–25 mL/min	50% of normal dose	q12h
Less than 10 mL/min	50% of normal dose	q24h
Hemodialysis:	500 mg	q24h
Peritoneal dialysis:	Recommended dose (based on indication)	q24h

Continuous Renal Replacement Therapy (CRRT)

	Dosage	Interval
Continuous venovenous hemofiltration	1 gram then 500 mg OR 1 gram	q8h OR q12h
Continuous venovenous hemodialysis/continuous venovenous hemodiafiltration	1 gram then 500 mg OR 1 gram	q6–8h OR q8–12h

Dosage in Hepatic Impairment

No dose adjustment.

SIDE EFFECTS

Frequent (5%–3%): Diarrhea, nausea, vomiting, headache, inflammation at injection site. **Occasional (2%):** Oral candidiasis, rash, pruritus. **Rare (less than 2%):** Constipation, glossitis.

ADVERSE EFFECTS/TOXIC REACTIONS

Antibiotic-associated colitis, other superinfections (abdominal cramps, severe watery diarrhea, fever) may result from altered bacterial balance in GI tract. Anaphylactic reactions have been reported. Seizures may occur in pts with CNS disorders (e.g., brain lesions, history of seizures), bacterial meningitis, renal impairment. Severe cutaneous toxicities including Stevens-Johnson syndrome, toxic epidermal necrolysis, erythema multiforme, acute generalized exanthematous pustulosis, drug reaction with eosinophilia and systemic response (DRESS). DRESS may present with facial swelling, eosinophilia, fever, lymphadenopathy, rash that may be associated with other organ systems, such as hepatitis, hematologic abnormalities, myocarditis, nephritis.

NURSING CONSIDERATIONS

BASELINE ASSESSMENT

Obtain specimen culture. Question history of seizures; hypersensitivity, allergic reaction to penicillins, cephalosporins.

♣ Canadian trade name   ◆ Non-Crushable Drug   ▦ High Alert drug

M

INTERVENTION/EVALUATION

Monitor daily pattern of bowel activity, stool consistency. Monitor for nausea, vomiting. Evaluate for inflammation at IV injection site. Monitor skin for cutaneous toxicities. Assess skin for rash. Evaluate hydration status. Monitor I&O, renal function, LFT. Check mental status; be alert to tremors, possible seizures. Assess temperature, B/P twice daily, more often if necessary. Monitor serum electrolytes, esp. potassium.

PATIENT/FAMILY TEACHING

• Report persistent diarrhea, abdominal cramps, fever.

---

mesalamine

me-**sal**-a-meen
(Apriso, Asacol HD, Canasa, Delzicol, Lialda, Pentasa, Rowasa, Salofalk ✦, sfRowasa)
Do not confuse Asacol with Os-Cal, Lialda with Aldara, or mesalamine with megestrol, memantine, or methenamine.

◆CLASSIFICATION

PHARMACOTHERAPEUTIC: Salicylic acid derivative. **CLINICAL:** Anti-inflammatory agent.

USES

PO: Treatment, maintenance of remission of mild to moderate active ulcerative colitis. **Rectal:** Treatment of active mild to moderate distal ulcerative colitis, proctosigmoiditis, or proctitis. **OFF-LABEL:** Crohn's disease.

PRECAUTIONS

Contraindications: Hypersensitivity to mesalamine, salicylates. **Cautions:** Active peptic ulcer, pyloric stenosis, pericarditis, myocarditis, renal/hepatic impairment, elderly.

ACTION

Exact mechanism unknown. May modulate local mediators of inflammation, may inhibit tumor necrosis factor. **Therapeutic Effect:** Decreases inflammation in colon.

PHARMACOKINETICS

Moderately absorbed from GI tract. Metabolized in liver. Unabsorbed portion excreted in feces; absorbed portion excreted in urine. Unknown if removed by hemodialysis. **Half-life:** 0.5–1.5 hrs; metabolite, 5–10 hrs.

⌛ LIFESPAN CONSIDERATIONS

Pregnancy/Lactation: Unknown if drug crosses placenta or is distributed in breast milk. **Children:** Safety and efficacy not established. **Elderly:** Age-related renal impairment may require dosage adjustment.

INTERACTIONS

DRUG: Antacids may decrease therapeutic effect. **HERBAL:** None significant. **FOOD:** None known. **LAB VALUES:** May increase serum alkaline phosphatase, ALT, AST, bilirubin.

AVAILABILITY (Rx)

Rectal Suspension: *(Rowasa, sfRowasa):* 4 g/60 mL. **Suppositories:** *(Canasa):* 1 g.
🔖 **Capsules, Controlled-Release:** *(Pentasa):* 250 mg, 500 mg. **Extended-Release:** *(Apriso):* 375 mg. **Capsules, Delayed-Release:** *(Delzicol):* 400 mg. 🔖 **Tablets, Delayed-Release:** *(Asacol HD):* 800 mg. *(Lialda):* 1.2 g.

ADMINISTRATION/HANDLING

◀**ALERT**▶ Store rectal suspension, suppository, oral forms at room temperature.

PO

• Give whole; do not break outer coating of tablet. • Give without regard to food. • *(Apriso):* Do not administer with antacids. • *(Lialda):* Administer once daily with meal.

Rectal

• Shake bottle well. • Instruct pt to lie on left side with lower leg extended, upper leg flexed forward. • Knee-chest position may also be used. • Insert applicator tip into rectum, pointing toward umbilicus. • Squeeze bottle steadily until contents are emptied. • Store suppositories at room temperature. Do not refrigerate.

INDICATIONS/ROUTES/DOSAGE

Ulcerative Colitis
PO: *(Capsule [Pentasa]):* **ADULTS, ELDERLY:** 1 g 4 times daily. *(Capsule [Delzicol]):* **ADULTS, ELDERLY:** 800 mg 3 times daily. **CHILDREN 5 YRS AND OLDER, WEIGHING 54–90 KG:** 1,200 mg in morning and evening. **Maximum:** 2,400 mg/day. **33–53 KG:** 1,200 mg in morning and 800 mg in evening. **Maximum:** 2,000 mg/day. **17–32 KG:** 800 mg in morning and 400 mg in evening. **Maximum:** 1,200 mg/day. *(Tablet [Asacol HD]):* **ADULTS, ELDERLY:** 1.6 g 3 times daily. *(Tablet [Lialda]):* **ADULTS, ELDERLY:** 2.4–4.8 g once daily. **ADOLESCENTS, CHILDREN WEIGHING 51 KG OR GREATER:** 4,800 mg once daily for 8 wks, then decrease to 2,400 mg once daily. **WEIGHING 36–50 KG:** 3,600 mg once daily for 8 wks, then decrease to 2,400 mg once daily. **WEIGHING 24–35 KG:** 2,400 mg once daily for 8 wks, then decrease to 1,200 mg once daily.

Maintenance of Remission in Ulcerative Colitis
PO: *(Capsule [Pentasa]):* **ADULTS, ELDERLY:** 1 g 4 times daily. *(Capsule [Delzicol]):* **ADULTS, ELDERLY:** 1.6–2.4 g in 1–4 divided doses/day. *(Capsule, Extended-Release [Apriso]):* **ADULTS, ELDERLY:** 1.5–3 g once daily in the morning. *(Tablet [Lialda]):* 2.4–3.6 g once daily with food.

Distal Ulcerative Colitis, Proctosigmoiditis, Proctitis
Rectal: *(Retention Enema):* **ADULTS, ELDERLY:** 60 mL (4 g) at bedtime; retained overnight for approximately 8 hrs. *(1 G*

Suppository): **ADULTS, ELDERLY:** Once daily at bedtime (retain for 1–3 hrs).
◄**ALERT**► Suppository should be retained for 1–3 hrs for maximum benefit.

Dosage of Renal/Hepatic Impairment
Use caution.

SIDE EFFECTS

Mesalamine is generally well tolerated, with only mild, transient effects. **Frequent (greater than 6%): PO:** Abdominal cramps/pain, diarrhea, dizziness, headache, nausea, vomiting, rhinitis, unusual fatigue. **Rectal:** Abdominal/stomach cramps, flatulence, headache, nausea. **Occasional (6%–2%): PO:** Hair loss, decreased appetite, back/joint pain, flatulence, acne. **Rectal:** Alopecia. **Rare (less than 2%): Rectal:** Anal irritation.

ADVERSE EFFECTS/TOXIC REACTIONS

Sulfite sensitivity may occur in susceptible pts, manifested as cramping, headache, diarrhea, fever, rash, urticaria, pruritus, wheezing. Discontinue drug immediately. Hepatitis, pancreatitis, pericarditis occur rarely with oral forms.

NURSING CONSIDERATIONS

BASELINE ASSESSMENT
Obtain BUN, serum creatinine, LFT. Assess for abdominal pain, discomfort.

INTERVENTION/EVALUATION
Encourage adequate fluid intake. Assess bowel sounds for peristalsis. Monitor daily pattern of bowel activity, stool consistency; record time of evacuation. Assess skin for rash, urticaria. Discontinue medication if rash, fever, cramping, or diarrhea occurs.

PATIENT/FAMILY TEACHING
• Report rash, fever, abdominal pain, significant diarrhea. • Avoid tasks that require alertness, motor skills until response to drug is established. • May discolor urine yellow-brown. • Suppositories stain fabrics.

M

metFORMIN

met-**for**-min
(Glumetza, Glycon ♥, Riomet)

■ **BLACK BOX ALERT** ■ Lactic acidosis occurs very rarely, but mortality rate is 50%. Risk increases with degree of renal impairment, pt's age, those with diabetes, unstable or acute HF.

Do not confuse metFORMIN with metroNIDAZOLE.

FIXED-COMBINATION(S)

Actoplus Met: metFORMIN/pioglitazone (an antidiabetic): 500 mg/15 mg, 850 mg/15 mg. metFORMIN/glyBURIDE (an antidiabetic): 250 mg/1.25 mg, 500 mg/2.5 mg, 500 mg/5 mg. **Janumet, Janumet XR, Zituvimet, Zituvimet XR:** metFORMIN/SITagliptin (an antidiabetic): 500 mg/50 mg, 1,000 mg/50 mg. **Jentadueto, Jentadueto XR:** metFORMIN/linagliptin (an antidiabetic): 500 mg/2.5 mg; 1,000 mg/2.5 mg; 1,000 mg extended-release/2.5 mg; 1,000 mg extended-release/5 mg. **Kombiglyze XR:** metFORMIN/saXagliptin (an antidiabetic): 500 mg/5 mg, 1,000 mg/5 mg, 1,000 mg/2.5 mg. **Generic:** metFORMIN/glipiZIDE (an antidiabetic): 250 mg/2.5 mg, 500 mg/2.5 mg, 500 mg/5 mg. **Qternmet XR:** metFORMIN/dapagliflozin (an antidiabetic)/saXagliptin (an antidiabetic): 1,000 mg/2.5 mg/2.5 mg; 1,000 mg/5 mg/2.5 mg; 1,000 mg/5 mg/5 mg, **Xigduo XR:** metFORMIN/dapagliglozin (an antidiabetic): 1,000 mg/2.5 mg; 500 mg/5 mg; 1,000 mg/5 mg; 500 mg/10 mg; 1,000 mg/10 mg. **Generic:** metFORMIN/repaglinide (an antidiabetic): 500 mg/1 mg, 500 mg/2 mg.

◆CLASSIFICATION

PHARMACOTHERAPEUTIC: Biguanide antihyperglycemic. **CLINICAL:** Antidiabetic agent.

USES

Management of type 2 diabetes mellitus when hyperglycemia is not managed with diet and exercise alone. **OFF-LABEL:** Weight loss in children with severe obesity and insulin resistance; antipsychotic-induced weight gain; prevention of diabetes mellitus type 2, gestational diabetes mellitus

PRECAUTIONS

◀**ALERT**▶ Lactic acidosis is a rare but potentially severe consequence of metFORMIN therapy. Withhold in pts with conditions that may predispose to lactic acidosis (e.g., hypoxemia, dehydration, hypoperfusion, sepsis). **Contraindications:** Hypersensitivity to metFORMIN. Severe renal disease/dysfunction; acute or chronic metabolic acidosis (with or without coma). **Cautions:** HF, hepatic impairment, excessive acute/chronic alcohol intake, elderly. Recommend temporary discontinuation at time of or before iodinated contrast imaging procedures in pts with CrCl of 30–60 mL/min, or with history of hepatic disease, alcoholism.

ACTION

Decreases hepatic production of glucose. Decreases intestinal absorption of glucose, improves insulin sensitivity. **Therapeutic Effect:** Improves glycemic control, stabilizes/decreases body weight, improves lipid profile.

PHARMACOKINETICS

Slowly, incompletely absorbed. Food delays, decreases extent of absorption. Protein binding: Negligible. Primarily distributed to intestinal mucosa, salivary glands. Primarily excreted unchanged in urine. Removed by hemodialysis. **Half-life:** 9–17 hrs.

⏳ LIFESPAN CONSIDERATIONS

Pregnancy/Lactation: Insulin is drug of choice during pregnancy. Distributed in breast milk in animals. **Children:** Safety and efficacy not established in children younger than 10 yrs. **Elderly:** Age-related renal impairment or peripheral vascular disease may require dosage adjustment or discontinuation.

INTERACTIONS

DRUG: Alcohol may increase adverse effects. **Dolutegravir, ranolazine** may increase concentration/effect. **IV contrast dye** may increase risk of metFORMIN-induced lactic acidosis, acute renal failure (discontinue metFORMIN 24–48 hrs prior to and up to 72 hrs after contrast exposure). **HERBAL: Garlic** may cause hypoglycemia. **FOOD:** None known. **LAB VALUES:** May alter cholesterol, LDL, triglycerides, HDL.

AVAILABILITY (Rx)

Oral Solution: *(Riomet):* 100 mg/mL. **Tablets:** 500 mg, 625 mg, 850 mg, 1,000 mg.

🗲 **Tablets, Extended-Release:** 500 mg, 750 mg, 1,000 mg.

ADMINISTRATION/HANDLING

PO
• Administer with a meal (to decrease GI upset). • **Oral solution:** Use a calibrated oral dosing device to measure dose. • **Extended-release tablets:** Administer tablet whole; do not cut, crush or allow chewing. Give once-daily doses with evening meal.

INDICATIONS/ROUTES/DOSAGE

Diabetes Mellitus
PO: *(Immediate-Release Tablets, Solution):* **ADULTS, ELDERLY:** Initially, 500 mg once or twice daily or 850 mg once daily. Titrate in increments of 500 mg or 850 mg q7days. **Usual maintenance dose:** 1,000 mg twice daily or 850 mg twice daily. **Maximum:** 2,550 mg/day in 2 or 3 divided doses. **CHILDREN 10–16 YRS:** Initially, 500–1,000 mg once daily or 500 mg twice daily. May increase in 500–1,000 mg increments q1–2wks. **Maximum:** 1,000 mg twice daily or 850 mg 3 times/day. *(Extended-Release Tablets):* **ADULTS, ELDERLY:** Initially, 500–1,000 mg once daily. May increase by 500 mg at 1-wk intervals **(Range:** 7 days to 6 wks). **Maximum:** 2,000 mg/day.

Dosage in Renal Impairment
Contraindicated in pts with serum creatinine greater than 1.5 mg/dL (males) or greater than 1.4 mg/dL (females). **Alternative recommendation: CrCl 45–60 mL/min:** Continue use; monitor renal function q3–6 mos. **CrCl 30–44 mL/min:** Use caution. Consider dose reduction; monitor renal function q3mos. **CrCL less than 30 mL/min:** Discontinue use.

Dosage in Hepatic Impairment
Avoid use (risk factor for lactic acidosis).

SIDE EFFECTS

Occasional (greater than 3%): GI disturbances (diarrhea, nausea, vomiting, abdominal bloating, flatulence, anorexia) that are transient and resolve spontaneously during therapy. **Rare (3%–1%):** Unpleasant/metallic taste that resolves spontaneously during therapy.

ADVERSE EFFECTS/TOXIC REACTIONS

Lactic acidosis occurs rarely (0.03 cases/1,000 pts) but is a serious and often fatal (50%) complication. Lactic acidosis is characterized by increase in blood lactate levels (greater than 5 mmol/L), decrease in blood pH, electrolyte disturbances. Symptoms include unexplained hyperventilation, myalgia, malaise, drowsiness. May advance to cardiovascular collapse (shock), acute HF, acute MI, prerenal azotemia.

NURSING CONSIDERATIONS

BASELINE ASSESSMENT
Obtain renal function test, fasting serum glucose, Hgb A1c. Verify pt has not received IV contrast dye within last 48 hrs.

INTERVENTION/EVALUATION
Monitor fasting serum glucose, Hgb A1c, renal function. Monitor folic acid, renal function tests for evidence of early lactic acidosis. If pt is on concurrent oral sulfonylureas, assess for hypoglycemia (anxiety, confusion, diaphoresis, diplopia, dizziness, headache, hunger, perioral numbness, tachycardia, tremors). Be alert to conditions that alter glucose requirements: fever, increased activity, stress, surgical procedure. If lactic acidosis occurs, withhold treatment.

PATIENT/FAMILY TEACHING
• Diabetes mellitus requires lifelong control. Diet and exercise is a principal part of treatment; do not skip or delay meals. • Test blood sugar regularly. • Monitor daily calorie intake. • When taking additional medications to lower blood sugar (e.g., insulin, other oral hypoglycemic) have low blood sugar treatment available (e.g., glucagon, oral dextrose). Be alert to conditions that alter glucose levels (e.g., fever, infection, stress, trauma). • Report symptoms of lactic acidosis (unexplained hyperventilation, muscle aches, extreme fatigue, unusual drowsiness). • Do not take dose for at least 48 hrs after receiving IV contrast dye with radiologic testing.

methadone

meth-a-done
(Metadol ✚, Methadone Intensol, Methadose)

■ **BLACK BOX ALERT** ■ May prolong QT interval, which may cause serious arrhythmias. May cause serious, life-threatening, or fatal respiratory depression. Concomitant use with benzodiazepines, other CNS depressants may increase risk of respiratory depression and death. Monitor for signs of misuse, abuse, addiction. Prolonged maternal use may cause neonatal withdrawal syndrome.

Do not confuse methadone with Mephyton, Metadate CD, Metadate ER, methylphenidate, or morphine.

◆CLASSIFICATION

PHARMACOTHERAPEUTIC: Opioid agonist (Schedule II). **CLINICAL:** Opioid analgesic. Opioid dependency management.

USES
Oral: Moderate to severe pain when a continuous around-the-clock analgesic is needed. Detoxification/maintenance treatment of opioid addiction in conjunction with social/medical services. **Injection:** Management of pain severe enough to require an opioid analgesic when alternate options are inadequate.

PRECAUTIONS
Contraindications: Hypersensitivity to methadone. Severe respiratory depression, acute or severe bronchial asthma (in absence of resuscitative equipment or unmonitored setting), hypercarbia, GI obstruction including paralytic ileus (known or suspected). **Cautions:** Renal/hepatic impairment, elderly/debilitated pts, pts at risk for QTc interval prolongation (congenital long QT syndrome, HF, medications that prolong

M

QTc interval, hypokalemia, hypomagnese-mia), cardiovascular disease, pts at high risk for suicidal ideation and behavior; history of drug abuse and misuse, drug-seeking behavior, dependency; respiratory disease, biliary tract dysfunction, acute pancreatitis, hypothyroidism, Addison's disease, head injury, increased intracranial pressure.

ACTION

Binds with opioid receptors within CNS, causing inhibition of ascending pain pathways. **Therapeutic Effect:** Produces generalized CNS depression. Alters processes affecting analgesia, emotional response to pain; reduces withdrawal symptoms from other opioid drugs.

PHARMACOKINETICS

Route	Onset	Peak	Duration
PO	0.5–1 hr	1.5–2 hrs	6–8 hrs
IM	10–20 min	1–2 hrs	4–5 hrs
IV	N/A	15–30 min	3–4 hrs

Widely distributed. Protein binding: 85%–90%. Metabolized in liver. Primarily excreted in urine. Not removed by hemodialysis. **Half-life:** 7–59 hrs.

⌛ LIFESPAN CONSIDERATIONS

Pregnancy/Lactation: Crosses placenta. Distributed in breast milk. Respiratory depression may occur in neonate if mother received opiates during labor. Regular use of opiates during pregnancy may produce withdrawal symptoms in neonate (irritability, excessive crying, tremors, hyperactive reflexes, fever, vomiting, diarrhea, yawning, sneezing, seizures). **Children:** Paradoxical excitement may occur. Pts younger than 2 yrs more susceptible to respiratory depressant effects. **Elderly:** More susceptible to respiratory depressant effects. Age-related renal impairment may increase risk of urinary retention.

INTERACTIONS

DRUG: Alcohol, CNS depressants (e.g., **LORazepam, morphine, zolpidem**) may increase CNS effects, respiratory depression, hypotension. **Strong CYP3A4 inducers** (e.g., **carBAMazepine, phenytoin, rifAMPin**) may decrease concentration/effects. **Strong CYP3A4 inhibitors** (e.g., **rifAMPin, clarithromycin, ketoconazole, ritonavir**) may increase methadone level. **QT interval–prolonging medications** (e.g., **amiodarone, azithromycin, ciprofloxacin, haloperidol, sotalol**) may increase risk of QTc interval prolongation. **MAOIs** (e.g., **phenelzine, selegiline**) may produce serotonin syndrome. **HERBAL: Herbals with sedative properties** (e.g., **chamomile, kava kava, valerian**) may increase CNS depression. **FOOD: Grapefruit products** may alter concentration/effects. **LAB VALUES:** May increase serum amylase, lipase.

AVAILABILITY (Rx)

Injection Solution: 10 mg/mL. **Oral Concentrate:** 10 mg/mL. **Oral Solution:** 5 mg/5 mL, 10 mg/5 mL. **Tablets, Dispersible:** 40 mg. **Tablets:** 5 mg, 10 mg.

ADMINISTRATION/HANDLING

IM, SQ

◄ALERT► IM preferred over SQ route (SQ produces pain, local irritation, induration).
• Do not use if solution appears cloudy or contains a precipitate. • Administer slowly. • Those with circulatory impairment experience higher risk of overdosage due to delayed absorption of repeated administration.

PO

• Give without regard to food. • Oral dose for detoxification and maintenance may be given in fruit juice or water. • Dispersible tablet should not be chewed or swallowed; add to liquid, allow to dissolve before swallowing.

M

M

INDICATIONS/ROUTES/DOSAGE

Analgesia

PO: ADULTS, ELDERLY: Initially, 2.5–5 mg q8–12h. May increase by 2.5 mg/dose q5–7 days (gradual titration) or 2.5–5 mg q3days (faster titration in monitored setting).
IV, IM, SQ: (only for pts unable to take oral medications) 2.5–10 mg q8–12h.

Dosage in Renal Impairment

CrCl less than 10 mL/min: 50%–75% normal dose. Avoid in severe hepatic disease.

Dosage in Hepatic Impairment

Mild to moderate impairment: No dose adjustment. **Severe Impairment:** Avoid use.

Detoxification

PO: ADULTS, ELDERLY: Initially, dose of 20–30 mg. An additional 5–10 mg may be provided if withdrawal symptoms have not been suppressed or if symptoms reappear after 2–4 hrs. Day 1 dose not to exceed 40 mg. **Maintenance range:** Titrate to a dose that prevents withdrawal symptoms for 24 hrs, reduces craving, reduces euphoria effect of self-administered opioids, while ensuring tolerance to sedative effects of methadone. **Usual range:** 60–120 mg/day. Dose reduction should be in increments of less than 10% of the maintenance dose every 10–14 days. **Short-term:** Initially, titrate to 40 mg/day in 2 divided doses. Continue 40-mg dose for 2–3 days. After 2–3 days of stabilization at 40 mg, gradually decrease dose to level keeping withdrawal symptoms tolerable.

SIDE EFFECTS

Frequent: Sedation, orthostatic hypotension, diaphoresis, facial flushing, constipation, dizziness, nausea, vomiting. **Occasional:** Confusion, urinary retention, palpitations, abdominal cramps, visual changes, dry mouth, headache, decreased appetite, anxiety, insomnia. **Rare:** Allergic reaction (rash, pruritus).

ADVERSE EFFECTS/TOXIC REACTIONS

Overdose results in respiratory depression, skeletal muscle flaccidity, cold/clammy skin, cyanosis, extreme drowsiness progressing to seizures, stupor, coma. Early sign of toxicity presents as increased sedation after being on a stable dose. Cardiac toxicity manifested as QT prolongation, torsades de pointes. Tolerance to analgesic effect, physical dependence may occur with repeated use. **Antidote:** Naloxone (see Appendix J for dosage).

NURSING CONSIDERATIONS

BASELINE ASSESSMENT

Obtain ECG. Assess type, location, intensity of pain. **Detoxification:** Assess pt for opioid withdrawal. Pt should be in recumbent position before drug administration by parenteral route. Obtain vital signs before giving medication. If respirations are 12/min or less (20/min or less in children), withhold medication, contact physician. Assess for potential of abuse/misuse (e.g., drug-seeking behavior, mental health conditions, history of substance abuse).

INTERVENTION/EVALUATION

Monitor vital signs 15–30 min after SQ/IM dose, 5–10 min following IV dose. Oral medication is 50% as potent as parenteral. Assess for adequate voiding. Monitor daily pattern of bowel activity, stool consistency. Assess for clinical improvement, record onset of relief of pain. Provide support to pt in detoxification program; monitor for withdrawal symptoms. Diligently assess for suicidal ideation and behavior; new onset or worsening of anxiety, depression, mood disorder. Screen for drug abuse and misuse, drug-seeking behavior.

PATIENT/FAMILY TEACHING

• Methadone may produce drug dependence, has potential for being abused. • Avoid alcohol. • Do not stop taking abruptly after prolonged

---

use. • May cause dry mouth, drowsiness. • Avoid tasks that require alertness, motor skills until response to drug is established. • Report severe drowsiness, respiratory depression.

---

methotrexate

meth-o-**trex**-ate
(Otrexup, Jylamvo, Rasuvo, Redi-Trex, Trexall, Xatmep)

■ **BLACK BOX ALERT** ■ May cause fetal abnormalities, death. May produce potentially fatal chronic hepatotoxicity, dermatologic reactions, acute renal failure, pneumonitis, myelosuppression, malignant lymphoma, aplastic anemia, GI toxicity secondary malignancies, tumor lysis syndrome, opportunistic infections. Do not use for psoriasis or rheumatoid arthritis treatment in pregnant women. Should only be prescribed by healthcare providers whose knowledge and experience include the use of anti-metabolite therapy. **Do not confuse methotrexate with metOLazone, methylPRED-NISolone, or mitoXANTRONE. or Trexall with Paxil. MTX is an error-prone abbreviation; do not use as an abbreviation.**

◆CLASSIFICATION

PHARMACOTHERAPEUTIC: Antimetabolite. **CLINICAL:** Antineoplastic, antirheumatic disease-modifying, immunosuppressant.

USES

Oncology-related: Acute lymphoblastic leukemia, breast cancer, cutaneous T-cell lymphoma (mycosis fungoides), gestational trophoblastic neoplasia, head and neck cancer (sqaumous cell carcinoma), meningeal leukemia (prophylaxis/treatment), non-Hodgkin's lymphomas, osteosarcoma. **Non-oncology uses:** Polyarticular juvenile idiopathic arthritis, psoriasis, rheumatoid arthritis. **OFF-LABEL: Oncology:** Bladder cancer, graft vs host disease, soft tissue sarcoma. **Non-oncology:** Atopic dermatitis, Crohn's disease, systemic lupus erythematosus (SLE), termination of intrauterine pregnancy.

PRECAUTIONS

Contraindications: Hypersensitivity to methotrexate. Breastfeeding. **For pts with psoriasis, juvenile idiopathic arthritis, or rheumatoid arthritis:** Pregnancy, hepatic disease, alcoholism, immunodeficiency syndrome, preexisting blood dyscrasias. **Cautions:** Peptic ulcer, ulcerative colitis, preexisting myelosuppression, history of chronic hepatic disease, alcohol consumption, obesity, diabetes, hyperlipidemia, use with other hepatotoxic medications, concomitant use of proton pump inhibitors. Use of NSAIDs or aspirin with lower methotrexate doses for rheumatoid arthritis.

ACTION

Irreversibly binds to and inhibits dihydrofolate reductase, inhibiting formation of reduced folates and thymidylate synthetase, which inhibits purine/thymidylic acid synthesis. **Therapeutic Effect:** Interferes with DNA synthesis, repair, and cellular replication.

PHARMACOKINETICS

Widely distributed. Protein binding: 50%–60%. Metabolized in liver. Primarily excreted in urine. Removed by hemodialysis but not by peritoneal dialysis. **Half-life:** 3–10 hrs (large doses, 8–15 hrs).

⏳ LIFESPAN CONSIDERATIONS

Pregnancy/Lactation: Avoid pregnancy during therapy and minimum 3 mos after therapy in males or at least one ovulatory cycle after therapy in females. May cause fetal death, congenital anomalies. Distributed in breast milk. Breastfeeding not recommended. **Children/Elderly:** Renal/hepatic impairment may require dosage adjustment.

M

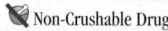

INTERACTIONS

DRUG: Alcohol, hepatotoxic medications (e.g., acetaminophen, acitretin) may increase risk of hepatotoxicity. **Bone marrow depressants (e.g., cladribine)** may increase myelosuppression. May decrease the therapeutic effect of **BCG (intravesical), vaccines (live)**. May increase adverse effects of **natalizumab, BCG (intravesical), vaccines (live). NSAIDs (e.g., ibuprofen, ketorolac, naproxen)** may increase risk of toxicity. **Probenecid, salicylates (e.g., aspirin)** may increase concentration, risk of toxicity. **HERBAL: Echinacea** may decrease therapeutic effect. **FOOD:** None known. **LAB VALUES:** May increase serum uric acid, AST.

AVAILABILITY (Rx)

Injection, Powder for Reconstitution: 1 g. **Injection, Autoinjector:** *(Rasuvo):* 7.5 mg, 10 mg, 12.5 mg, 15 mg, 17.5 mg, 20 mg, 22.5 mg, 25 mg, 27.5 mg, 30 mg. *(Redi-Trex):* 15 mg/0.6 mL, 20 mg/0.8 mL, 25 mg/1 mL. **Injection Solution:** 25 mg/mL. **Injection, Syringe:** *(Otrexup):* 7.5 mg/0.4 mL, 10 mg/0.4 mL, 12.5 mg/0.4 mL, 15 mg/0.4 mL, 17.5 mg/0.4 mL, 20 mg/0.4 mL, 22.5 mg/0.4 mL, 25 mg/0.4 mL. **Solution, Oral:** *(Jylamvo):* 2 mg/mL. *(Xatmep):* 2.5 mg/mL. **Tablets:** 2.5 mg, 5 mg, 7.5 mg, 10 mg, 15 mg.

ADMINISTRATION/HANDLING

◄**ALERT**► May be carcinogenic, mutagenic, teratogenic. Handle with extreme care during preparation/administration. Wear gloves when preparing solution. If powder or solution comes in contact with skin, wash immediately, thoroughly with soap, water. May give IM, IV, intraarterially, intrathecally.

 IV

Reconstitution • Reconstitute powder with D_5W or 0.9% NaCl to provide concentration of 25 mg/mL or less. • For intrathecal use, dilute with preservative-free 0.9% NaCl to provide a concentration not greater than 2–4 mg/mL.

Rate of administration • Give IV push at rate of 10 mg/min. • Give IV infusion at rate of 4–20 mg/hr (refer to specific protocol).

Storage • Store vials at room temperature. Diluted solutions stable for 24 hrs at room temperature.

INDICATIONS/ROUTES/DOSAGE

Oncology Uses

◄**ALERT**► Refer to individual specific protocols for optimum dosage, sequence of administration.

Head/Neck Cancer

PO, IV, IM: ADULTS, ELDERLY: 40 mg/m^2 once wkly. Continue until disease progression or unacceptable toxicity.

Breast Cancer

IV: ADULTS, ELDERLY: 40 mg/m^2 days 1 and 8 q4wks in combination with cyclo-PHOSphamide and fluorouracil.

Mycosis Fungoides

IM, PO: ADULTS, ELDERLY: 25–75 mg PO once wkly (as a single agent) or 10 mg/m^2 PO twice wkly (as part of a combination regimen), **or** 5–50 mg once wkly (for early stage) or 15–37.5 mg twice wkly IM (if poor response to wkly therapy), **or** 25 mg PO once wkly. May increase to 50 mg once wkly.

Rheumatoid Arthritis (RA)

PO: IM, SQ: ADULTS: Initially, 7.5–15 mg once wkly (in combination with folic acid). May increase by 2.5–5 mg/wk q4–12wks up to 25 mg/wk. **ELDERLY:** Initially, 5–7.5 mg/wk.

Juvenile Rheumatoid Arthritis (JRA)

PO, IM, SQ: CHILDREN: Initially, 10–15 mg/m^2 once wkly (in combination with folic acid), then adjust gradually to 20–30 mg/m^2/wk as a single dose. **Usual maximum dose:** 25 mg.

Psoriasis

PO, IM, SQ: ADULTS, ELDERLY: Initially, 10–15 mg once wkly (in combination with folic acid). Adjust dose gradually (q4–8wks) to optimal response. Titrate to lowest effective dose. **Usual range:** 7.5–25 mg/wk.

Dosage in Renal Impairment

Creatinine Clearance	Reduce Dose to
61–80 mL/min	75% of normal
51–60 mL/min	70% of normal
10–50 mL/min	30–50% of normal
Less than 10 mL/min	Avoid use

Dosage in Hepatic Impairment
Use caution.

SIDE EFFECTS

Frequent (10%–3%): Nausea, vomiting, stomatitis, burning/erythema at psoriatic site (in pts with psoriasis). **Occasional (3%–1%):** Diarrhea, rash, dermatitis, pruritus, alopecia, dizziness, anorexia, malaise, headache, drowsiness, blurred vision.

ADVERSE EFFECTS/TOXIC REACTIONS

High potential for various severe toxicities. GI toxicity may produce gingivitis, glossitis, pharyngitis, stomatitis, enteritis, hematemesis. Hepatotoxicity more likely to occur with frequent small doses than with large intermittent doses. Pulmonary toxicity characterized by interstitial pneumonitis. Hematologic toxicity, resulting from marked myelosuppression, may manifest as leukopenia, thrombocytopenia, anemia, hemorrhage. Dermatologic toxicity may produce rash, pruritus, urticaria, pigmentation, photosensitivity, petechiae, ecchymosis, pustules. Severe nephrotoxicity produces azotemia, hematuria, renal failure.

NURSING CONSIDERATIONS

BASELINE ASSESSMENT

Obtain pregnancy test in females of reproductive potential. **Rheumatoid ar-**

thritis: Assess pain, range of motion. Obtain baseline CBC, BMP, LFT, rheumatoid factor. **Psoriasis:** Assess skin lesions. Obtain all functional tests before therapy, repeat throughout therapy. Antiemetics may prevent nausea, vomiting.

INTERVENTION/EVALUATION

Monitor CBC, BMP, LFT, urinalysis, chest X-rays, serum uric acid. Monitor for hematologic toxicity (fever, sore throat, signs of local infection, unusual bruising/bleeding from any site), symptoms of anemia (excessive fatigue, weakness). Assess skin for evidence of dermatologic toxicity. Keep pt well hydrated, urine alkaline. Avoid rectal temperatures, traumas that induce bleeding. Apply 5 full min of pressure to IV sites.

PATIENT/FAMILY TEACHING

• Treatment may depress your immune system response and reduce your ability to fight infection. Report symptoms of infection such as body aches, chills, cough, fatigue, fever. Avoid those with active infection. • Report symptoms of lung inflammation (excessive coughing, difficulty breathing, chest pain); liver problems (abdominal pain, bruising, clay-colored stool, amber- or dark-colored urine, yellowing of the skin or eyes), kidney problems (decreased urine output, flank pain, darkened urine); toxic skin reactions (rash, skin eruptions). • Use effective contraception to avoid pregnancy.

methylergonovine

meth-il-er-**goe**-noe-veen
(Methergine)

◆CLASSIFICATION

PHARMACOTHERAPEUTIC: Ergot alkaloid. **CLINICAL:** Oxytocic agent, uterine stimulant.

USES

Management of uterine atony, hemorrhage and subinvolution of uterus following delivery of placenta. Control uterine hemorrhage following delivery of anterior shoulder in second stage of labor.

PRECAUTIONS

Contraindications: Hypersensitivity to methylergonovine. Hypertension, pregnancy, toxemia. **Cautions:** Renal/hepatic impairment, coronary artery disease, pts at risk for coronary artery disease (diabetes, obesity, smoking, hypercholesterolemia), concurrent use with CYP3A4 inhibitors, occlusive peripheral vascular disease, sepsis, second stage of labor.

ACTION

Increases tone, rate, amplitude of contraction of uterine smooth muscle. **Therapeutic Effect:** Produces sustained contractions, which shortens third stage of labor, reduces blood loss.

PHARMACOKINETICS

Route	Onset	Peak	Duration
PO	5–10 min	N/A	3 hrs
IV	Immediate	N/A	45 min
IM	2–5 min	N/A	3 hrs

Widely distributed. Metabolized in liver. Primarily excreted in urine. **Half-life:** 0.5–2 hrs.

⌛ LIFESPAN CONSIDERATIONS

Pregnancy/Lactation: Contraindicated during pregnancy. Small amounts distributed in breast milk. **Children/Elderly:** Safety and efficacy not established.

INTERACTIONS

DRUG: May increase hypertensive effect of **DOPamine, norepinephrine, phenylephrine, vasopressin. Strong CYP3A4 inhibitors (e.g., clarithromycin, ketoconazole, ritonavir)** may increase concentration/effect. **Beta blockers (e.g., carvedilol, labetalol, metoprolol)** may increase vasoconstrictive effect. May decrease vasodilation effect of **nitroglycerin.** May increase vasoconstricting effect of **serotonin 5-HT$_{1D}$ receptor agonists (e.g., SUMAtriptan). HERBAL:** None significant. **FOOD:** None known. **LAB VALUES:** May decrease serum prolactin.

AVAILABILITY (Rx)

Injection Solution: 0.2 mg/mL. **Tablets:** 0.2 mg.

ADMINISTRATION/HANDLING

Reconstitution • Dilute with 0.9% NaCl to volume of 5 mL.
Rate of administration • Give over at least 1 min, carefully monitoring B/P.
Storage • Refrigerate ampules.

▦ IV COMPATIBILITIES

Heparin, potassium.

INDICATIONS/ROUTES/DOSAGE

Prevention of Hemorrhage
PO: ADULTS: 0.2 mg 3–4 times daily. Continue for up to 7 days.
IV, IM: ADULTS: Initially, 0.2 mg after delivery of anterior shoulder, after delivery of placenta, or during puerperium. May repeat q2–4h for 1–5 doses.
Note: Initial dose may be given parenterally, followed by oral regimen.
IV use in life-threatening emergencies only.

Dosage in Renal/Hepatic Impairment
Use caution.

SIDE EFFECTS

Frequent: Nausea, uterine cramping, vomiting. **Occasional:** Abdominal pain, diarrhea, dizziness, diaphoresis, tinnitus, bradycardia, chest pain. **Rare:** Allergic reaction (rash, pruritus), dyspnea, severe or sudden hypertension.

ADVERSE EFFECTS/TOXIC REACTIONS

Severe hypertensive episodes may result in CVA, serious arrhythmias, seizures. Hypertensive effects are more frequent with pt susceptibility, rapid IV administration, concurrent use of regional anesthesia, vasoconstrictors. Peripheral ischemia may lead to gangrene.

NURSING CONSIDERATIONS

BASELINE ASSESSMENT
Obtain serum calcium level, B/P, pulse. Assess for any evidence of bleeding before administration.

INTERVENTION/EVALUATION
Monitor uterine tone, bleeding, B/P, pulse q15min until stable (about 1–2 hrs). Assess extremities for color, warmth, movement, pain. Report chest pain promptly. Provide support with ambulation if dizziness occurs.

PATIENT/FAMILY TEACHING
• Avoid smoking: Causes increased vasoconstriction. • Report increased cramping, bleeding, foul-smelling lochia. • Report pale, cold hands/feet (possibility of diminished circulation).

methylnaltrexone

meth-il-nal-**trex**-own
(Relistor)
Do not confuse methylnaltrexone with naltrexone.

◆CLASSIFICATION
PHARMACOTHERAPEUTIC: Opioid receptor antagonist. **CLINICAL:** GI agent.

USES
Injection: Treatment of opioid-induced constipation in pts with advanced illness or pain caused by active cancer who require opioid dosage escalation for palliative care. **Injection/tablets:** Treatment of opioid-induced constipation in pts with chronic pain unrelated to cancer including pts with chronic pain related to prior cancer or its treatment not requiring frequent opioid dosage escalation.

PRECAUTIONS
Contraindications: Hypersensitivity to methylnaltrexone. Known or suspected GI obstruction. Pts at increased risk of recurrent GI obstruction. **Cautions:** Renal impairment, history of GI tract lesions (e.g., peptic ulcer disease, GI tract malignancies).

ACTION
Blocks binding of opioids to peripheral opioid receptors within GI tract. Inhibits opioid-induced decreased GI motility and delay in GI transit time. **Therapeutic Effect:** Decreases constipating effect of opioids.

PHARMACOKINETICS
Absorbed rapidly. Undergoes moderate tissue distribution. Protein binding: 11%–15%. Excreted in urine (50%), feces (35%). **Half-life:** 8 hrs.

⧗ LIFESPAN CONSIDERATIONS
Pregnancy/Lactation: Unknown if distributed in breast milk. Breast-feeding not recommended. **Children:** Safety and efficacy not established. **Elderly:** No age-related precautions noted.

INTERACTIONS
DRUG: May increase adverse/toxic effects of **naloxegol, opioid antagonists. HERBAL:** None significant. **FOOD:** None known. **LAB VALUES:** None significant.

AVAILABILITY (Rx)
Injection Solution: 8 mg/0.4 mL, 12 mg/0.6 mL. **Tablets:** 150 mg.

ADMINISTRATION/HANDLING
PO
• Administer with water on an empty stomach at least 30 min before first meal of day.

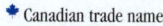 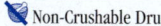

SQ

Preparation • Visually inspect for particulate matter or discoloration. Solution should appear colorless to pale yellow in color. Do not use if solution is cloudy, discolored, or if large particles are observed.

Administration • Insert needle subcutaneously into upper arms, outer thigh, or abdomen, and inject solution. • Do not inject into areas of active skin disease or injury such as sunburns, skin rashes, inflammation, skin infections, or active psoriasis. • Rotate injection sites.

Storage • Once solution is drawn into syringe, may be stored at room temperature. • Administer within 24 hrs.

INDICATIONS/ROUTES/DOSAGE

◀**ALERT**▶ Usual schedule is once every other day, as needed, but no more frequently than once every 24 hrs.

Constipation (Chronic Non-cancer Pain)

PO: ADULTS, ELDERLY: 450 mg once daily in the morning. **SQ: ADULTS, ELDERLY:** 12 mg/day. **Note:** Discontinue all laxatives prior to use (if response is not optimal after 3 days, may resume laxative therapy).

Constipation (Advanced Illness)

Note: Dosage regimen is 1 dose every other day, as needed. Do not administer more frequently than 1 dose per 24-hour period. **SQ: ADULTS, ELDERLY WEIGHING 38 KG TO LESS THAN 62 KG:** 8 mg. **ADULTS, ELDERLY WEIGHING 62–114 KG:** 12 mg. **ADULTS, ELDERLY WHOSE WEIGHT FALLS OUTSIDE THESE RANGES:** Dose at 0.15 mg/kg (round dose up to nearest 0.1 mL of volume).

Dosage in Severe Renal Impairment (CrCl less than 60 mL/min)

SQ: ADULTS, ELDERLY: Administer 50% of recommended dose.

Dosage in Hepatic Impairment

No dose adjustment.

SIDE EFFECTS

Frequent (29%–12%): Abdominal pain, flatulence, nausea. **Occasional (7%–5%):** Diarrhea, dizziness.

ADVERSE EFFECTS/TOXIC REACTIONS

None known.

NURSING CONSIDERATIONS

BASELINE ASSESSMENT

Question characteristics of constipation, frequency of bowel movements. Assess bowel sounds. Question history of GI obstruction, perforation, baseline GI disease; renal impairment. Receive full medication history, including herbal products, and screen for interactions. Assess hydration status.

INTERVENTION/EVALUATION

30% of pts report defecation within 30 min after drug administration. Encourage fluid intake. Assess bowel sounds for peristalsis. Monitor daily pattern of bowel activity, stool consistency. If opioid medication is stopped, drug should be discontinued. Assess for abdominal disturbances.

PATIENT/FAMILY TEACHING

• Laxative effect usually occurs within 30 min but may take up to 24 hrs after medication administration. • Common side effects include transient abdominal pain, nausea, vomiting. • Report persistent or worsening symptoms, or if severe or persistent diarrhea occurs.

methylphenidate

meth-il-**fen**-i-date
(Aptensio XR, Concerta, Cotempla XR-ODT, Daytrana, Jornay PM, Methylin, Quillichew ER, Quillivant XR, Relexxii, Ritalin, Ritalin LA)

■ **BLACK BOX ALERT** ■ Chronic abuse can lead to marked tolerance, psychological dependence. Abrupt withdrawal from prolonged use may lead to severe depression, psychosis.

Do not confuse methylphenidate with methadone, or Ritalin with Rifadin.

◆CLASSIFICATION

PHARMACOTHERAPEUTIC: CNS stimulant (Schedule II). **CLINICAL:** CNS stimulant.

USES

Treatment of attention-deficit hyperactivity disorder (ADHD). Management of narcolepsy (Methylin, Ritalin). **OFF-LABEL:** Severe fatigue (cancer-related or in palliative care setting), major depressive disorder (unipolar) in medically ill, palliative care, terminal illness, or elderly pts.

PRECAUTIONS

Contraindications: Hypersensitivity to methylphenidate. Use during or within 14 days following MAOI therapy; marked anxiety, tension, agitation, motor tics; family history or diagnosis of Tourette's syndrome, glaucoma. **Metadate:** Severe hypertension, HF, arrhythmia, hyperthyroidism, recent MI or angina. **Cautions:** Hypertension, seizures, acute stress reaction, emotional instability, HF, recent MI, hyperthyroidism or thyrotoxicosis, known structural cardiac abnormality, bipolar disorder, cardiomyopathy, arrhythmias, history of drug abuse and misuse, drug-seeking behavior, dependency.

ACTION

Blocks reuptake of norepinephrine, dopamine into presynaptic neurons. Stimulates cerebral cortex and subcortical structures. **Therapeutic Effect:** Decreases motor restlessness, fatigue. Increases motor activity, attention span, mental alertness. Produces mild euphoria.

PHARMACOKINETICS

Onset	Peak	Duration
Immediate-release	2 hrs	3–6 hrs
Sustained-release	4–7 hrs	8 hrs
Extended-release	N/A	12 hrs
Transdermal	2 hrs	N/A

Widely distributed. Protein binding: 15%. Metabolized in liver. Primarily excreted in urine. Unknown if removed by hemodialysis. **Half-life:** 2–4 hrs.

⧗ LIFESPAN CONSIDERATIONS

Pregnancy/Lactation: Unknown if drug crosses placenta or is distributed in breast milk. **Children:** May be more susceptible to developing anorexia, insomnia, stomach pain, decreased weight. Chronic use may inhibit growth. Not approved for children younger than 6 yrs. **Elderly:** No age-related precautions noted.

INTERACTIONS

DRUG: **MAOIs** (e.g., **phenelzine, selegiline**) may increase hypertensive effects. **Other CNS stimulants** (e.g., **caffeine, dextroamphetamine, phentermine**) may have additive effect. **Alcohol** may increase adverse effects. **HERBAL:** **Ephedra** may cause hypertension, arrhythmias. **Yohimbe** may increase CNS stimulation. **FOOD:** None known. **LAB VALUES:** None significant.

AVAILABILITY (Rx)

Oral Solution: *(Methylin):* 5 mg/5 mL, 10 mg/5 mL. **Tablets, Chewable:** 2.5 mg, 5 mg, 10 mg. **Tablets:** *(Ritalin):* 5 mg, 10 mg, 20 mg. **Topical Patch:** *(Daytrana):* 10 mg/9 hrs, 15 mg/9 hrs, 20 mg/9 hrs, 30 mg/9 hrs. **Powder for Suspension, Extended-Release:** *(Quillivant XR):* 25 mg/5 mL.

(Aptensio XR): 10 mg, 15 mg, 20 mg, 30 mg, 40 mg, 50 mg, 60 mg. *(Jornay PM),* 20 mg, 40 mg, 60 mg, 80 mg, 100 mg. *(Ritalin LA):* 10 mg, 20 mg, 30 mg, 40 mg. 🟢 **Tablets, Extended-Release:** *(Concerta):* 18 mg, 27 mg, 36 mg, *(Relexxii):* 63 mg, 72 mg. *(Generic):* 10 mg, 20 mg. **Tablets, Extended-Release ODT:** *(Cotempla XR-ODT):* 8.6 mg, 17.3 mg, 25.9 mg. **Tablets, Chewable, Extended-Release:** *(Quillichew ER):* 20 mg, 30 mg, 40 mg.

ADMINISTRATION/HANDLING

◀**ALERT**▶ Sustained-release, extended-release tablets may be given in place of regular tablets once the daily dose is titrated using regular tablets and the titrated dosage corresponds to sus-

M

tained-release or extended-release tablet strength.

PO

(Aptensio XR) • Give in morning without regard to food. • Do not crush, divide, or allow chewing of capsule contents. Capsule may be opened and sprinkled on a small amount cold applesauce. *(Chewable Tablets)* • Give each dose 30–45 min before a meal. • Administer with 8 or more oz. water or other liquids. *(Concerta)* • Give in the morning; must be taken with water or other fluids. • Do not crush, divide, or allow chewing of tablet. *(Cotempla XR-ODT)* • Give tablet from blister and place on the pt's tongue. • Allow it to disintegrate without chewing or crushing (tablet will disintegrate in saliva and be swallowed). No liquid is needed. *(Jornay PM)* • Give in evening without regard to food. • Do not crush, divide, or allow chewing of capsule contents. Capsule may be opened and a sprinkled on small amount cold applesauce. *(Methylin Oral Solution)* • Give each dose 30–45 min before a meal. *(QuilliCherw ER)* • Give in the morning without regard to food. • Tablets are scored and may be halved. *(Relexxi)* • Give in the morning without regard to food (must be taken with water or other fluids). • Do not crush, divide, or allow chewing of tablet). *(Ritalin LA)* • Give in morning without regard to food. • Do not crush, divide, or allow chewing of capsule contents. Capsule may be opened and sprinkled on a small amount cold applesauce. *(Ritalin)* • Give each dose 30–45 min before a meal. *Quillivant XR)* • Give in the morning without regard to food. • Shake bottle 10 or more sec. prior to administering. Use oral dosing dispenser (provided).

Patch

• To be worn daily for 9 hrs. • Replace daily in morning. • Apply to dry, clean area of hip. • Avoid applying to waistline (clothing may cause patch to rub off). • Alternate application site daily. • Press firmly in place for 30 sec to ensure patch is in good contact with skin. • Do not cut patch.

INDICATIONS/ROUTES/DOSAGE

ADHD

PO: ADULTS: *(Immediate-Release):* Initially, 10–20 mg twice daily, before breakfast and lunch. May increase by 5–10 mg/day at wkly intervals. **Maximum:** 60 mg/day in 2–3 divided doses. **CHILDREN 6 YRS AND OLDER:** Initially, 2.5–5 mg before breakfast and lunch. May increase by 5–10 mg/day at wkly intervals. **Usual dose:** 20–30 mg/day in 2–3 divided doses. **Maximum:** 60 mg/day not to exceed 2 mg/kg/day. *(Aptensio XR):* **ADULTS, CHILDREN 6 YRS AND OLDER:** Initially, 10 mg once daily. May increase at wkly intervals of 10 mg/day. **Maximum:** 60 mg/day. *(Concerta):* **ADULTS 18–65 YRS:** Initially, 18–36 mg once daily. **CHILDREN 6–17 YRS OF AGE:** Initially, 18 mg once daily; may increase by 18 mg/day at wkly intervals. **Maximum:** 54 mg/day in children 6–12 yrs of age, 72 mg or 2 mg/kg/day in children 13–17 yrs of age; 72 mg in adults 18–65 yrs of age. *(Metadate CD):* **ADULTS, CHILDREN 6 YRS AND OLDER:** Initially, 20 mg/day. May increase by 10–20 mg/day at wkly intervals. **Maximum:** 60 mg/day. *(Quillichew ER):* **ADULTS, CHILDREN 6 YRS AND OLDER:** Initially, 20 mg/day. May increase by 10 mg, 15 mg or 20 mg/day at wkly intervals. **Maximum:** 60 mg/day. *(Quillivant XR):* **ADULTS, CHILDREN 6 YRS AND OLDER:** Initially, 20 mg once daily in the morning. May increase in increments of 10–20 mg/day at wkly increments. **Maximum:** 60 mg/day. *(Ritalin LA):* **ADULTS, CHILDREN 6 YRS AND OLDER:** Initially, 10–20 mg/day. May increase by 10 mg/day at wkly intervals. **Maximum:** 60 mg/day. *(Jornay PM):* **ADULTS:** Initially, 20 mg once daily in the evening (between 6:30 PM [1830 hrs] and 9:30 PM [2130 hrs]). May increase by 20 mg/day at wkly intervals. **Maximum:** 100 mg/day. *(Adhansia XR):* **ADULTS:** Initially, 25 mg in the morning. May increase by 10–15 mg at 5-day intervals or more. **Maximum:** 100 mg/day. **CHILDREN 6 YRS OF AGE AND OLDER:** Initially, 25 mg once in morning. May increase by 10–15 mg at 5-day intervals or more. **Maximum:** 85 mg/day. *(Metadate ER):* **CHILDREN**

6 YRS AND OLDER: May replace regular tablets after daily dose is titrated and 8-hr dosage corresponds to sustained-release or extended-release tablet strength. **Maximum:** 60 mg/day. *(Cotempla XR-ODT):* **CHILDREN 6–18 YRS:** Initially, 17.3 mg once daily. May increase in wkly intervals in 8.6 to 17.3 mg increments. **Maximum:** 51.8 mg/day.

Patch: *(Daytrana):* **ADULTS, ADOLESCENTS, CHILDREN 6–17 YRS:** Initially, 10 mg daily (applied and worn for 9 hrs). Remove after 9 hrs (3 hrs before bedtime). Dosage is titrated up to 60 mg/day to desired effect. May increase dose no more frequently than every wk.

Narcolepsy

PO: ADULTS, ELDERLY: *(Immediate-Release):* Initially, 10 mg twice daily, before breakfast and lunch. May increase by 5–10 mg/day at wkly intervals. **Maximum:** 60 mg/day in 2–3 divided doses. **CHILDREN 6 YRS AND OLDER:** *(Immediate-Release):* Initially, 5 mg twice daily (before breakfast and lunch). May increase by 5–10 mg/day at wkly intervals. **Maximum:** 60 mg/day in 2–3 divided doses. *(Extended-Release):* May be given once the immediate-release dose is titrated and the titrated 8-hr dose corresponds to sustained-release or extended-release tablet strength. **Usual dose:** 20 mg 2 times/day. **Maximum:** 60 mg/day.

Dosage in Renal/Hepatic Impairment
No dose adjustment.

SIDE EFFECTS

Frequent: Anxiety, insomnia, anorexia. **Occasional:** Dizziness, drowsiness, headache, nausea, abdominal pain, fever, rash, arthralgia, vomiting. **Rare:** Blurred vision, Tourette's syndrome (uncontrolled vocal outbursts, repetitive body movements, tics), palpitations, priapism.

ADVERSE EFFECTS/TOXIC REACTIONS

Prolonged administration to children with ADHD may delay normal weight gain pattern. Overdose may produce tachycardia, palpitations, arrhythmias, chest pain, psychotic episode, seizures, coma. Hypersensitivity reactions, blood dyscrasias occur rarely.

NURSING CONSIDERATIONS

BASELINE ASSESSMENT
ADHD: Assess attention span, impulsivity, interaction with others, distractibility. **Narcolepsy:** Observe/assess frequency of episodes. Question history of seizures. Assess for potential of abuse/misuse (e.g., drug seeking behavior, mental health conditions, history of substance abuse).

INTERVENTION/EVALUATION
Monitor B/P, pulse, changes in ADHD symptoms. CBC with differential should be performed routinely during therapy. If paradoxical return of attention-deficit occurs, dosage should be reduced or discontinued. Monitor growth. Screen for drug abuse and misuse, drug-seeking behavior.

PATIENT/FAMILY TEACHING
• Avoid tasks that require alertness, motor skills until response to drug is established. • Report any increase in seizures. • Take daily dose early in morning to avoid insomnia. • Report anxiety, palpitations, fever, vomiting, skin rash. • Report new or worsened symptoms (e.g., behavior, hostility, concentration ability). • Avoid caffeine. • Do not stop taking abruptly after prolonged use.

methylPREDNISolone

meth-il-pred-**nis**-oh-lone
(Medrol)

methylPREDNISolone acetate

(DEPO-Medrol)

methylPREDNISolone sodium succinate

M

(SOLU-Medrol)

Do not confuse DEPO-Medrol with SOLU-Medrol, Medrol with Mebaral, or methylPREDNISolone with medroxyPROGESTERone or prednisoLONE.

◆ CLASSIFICATION

PHARMACOTHERAPEUTIC: Adrenal corticosteroid. **CLINICAL:** Anti-inflammatory.

USES

Anti-inflammatory or immunosuppressant in the treatment of hematologic, allergic, neoplastic, dermatologic, endocrine, GI, nervous system, ophthalmic, renal, or rheumatic disorders. **OFF-LABEL:** Graft vs host disease, COVID-19 hospitalized pts, acute respiratory distress syndrome (ARDS), COPD (acute exacerbation), Pneumocystis pneumonia, prostate cancer (metastatic, castration-resistant).

PRECAUTIONS

Contraindications: Hypersensitivity to methylPREDNISolone. Administration of live or attenuated virus vaccines, systemic fungal infection. **IM:** Idiopathic thrombocytopenia purpura. Intrathecal administration. **Cautions:** Respiratory tuberculosis, untreated systemic infections, hypertension, HF, diabetes, GI disease (e.g., peptic ulcer), myasthenia gravis, renal/hepatic impairment, seizures, cataracts, glaucoma, following acute MI, thyroid disorder, thromboembolic tendencies, cardiovascular disease, elderly, psychiatric conditions, osteoporosis.

ACTION

Anti-inflammatory: Suppresses migration of polymorphonuclear leukocytes, reverses increased capillary permeability. Exerts effects on modulating carbohydrate, protein, lipid metabolism. Maintains fluid/electrolyte hemostasis. Influences CV, immunologic, endocrine, musculoskeletal, neurologic physiology. **Therapeutic Effect:** Decreases inflammation.

PHARMACOKINETICS

Route	Onset	Peak	Duration
PO	Rapid	1–2 hrs	30–36 hrs
IM	Rapid	4–8 days	1–4 wks
IV	Rapid	N/A	N/A

Widely distributed. Metabolized in liver. Excreted in urine. Removed by hemodialysis. **Half-life:** 3.5 hrs.

⧖ LIFESPAN CONSIDERATIONS

Pregnancy/Lactation: Crosses placenta. Distributed in breast milk. May cause cleft palate (chronic use in first trimester). Breastfeeding not recommended. **Children:** Prolonged treatment or high dosages may decrease short-term growth rate, cortisol secretion. **Elderly:** No age-related precautions noted.

INTERACTIONS

DRUG: May increase anticoagulant effects of **warfarin. Strong CYP3A4 inducers (e.g., carBAMazepine, phenytoin, rifAMPin)** may decrease concentration/effect. May increase adverse effects; decrease antibody response to **vaccines (live).** May increase concentration/effect of **desmopressin. Strong CYP3A4 inhibitors (e.g., clarithromycin, ketoconazole, ritonavir)** may increase concentration/effect. May decrease therapeutic effect of **BCG (intravesical). HERBAL:** None significant. **FOOD:** None known. **LAB VALUES:** May increase serum glucose, cholesterol, lipids, amylase, sodium. May decrease serum calcium, potassium, thyroxine, hypothalamic-pituitary-adrenal (HPA) axis.

AVAILABILITY (Rx)

Injection, Powder for Reconstitution: (Solu-Medrol): 40 mg, 125 mg, 500 mg, 1 g. **Injection, Suspension: (Depo Medrol):** 20 mg/mL, 40 mg/mL, 80 mg/mL. **Tablets:** 2 mg, 4 mg, 8 mg, 16 mg, 32 mg. **(Dosepak):** 4 mg (21 tablets).

ADMINISTRATION/HANDLING

◄**ALERT**► Do **not** give methylPREDNIsolone acetate IV.

M

IV

Reconstitution • For infusion, add to D$_5$W, 0.9% NaCl.
Rate of administration • Give IV push over 3–15 min. • Give IV piggyback. Dose of 250 mg over 15–30 min; dose of 500–999 mg over at least 30 min; dose of 1 g or greater over 1 hr.
Storage • Store vials at room temperature. Diluted solution is stable for 48 hrs at room temperature or refrigerated.

IM
• MethylPREDNISolone acetate should not be further diluted. • MethylPREDNISolone sodium succinate should be reconstituted with Bacteriostatic Water for Injection. • Give deep IM in gluteus maximus (avoid injection into deltoid muscle).

PO
• Give after meals or with food/milk to decrease GI upset.

▦ IV INCOMPATIBILITIES

Potassium chloride, propofol.

▦ IV COMPATIBILITIES

Acetaminophen, dexmedetomidine, heparin.

INDICATIONS/ROUTES/DOSAGE
Usual Dosage Range
IV: ADULTS, ELDERLY: 40–125 mg/day as a single dose or in divided doses. **CHILDREN:** Initially, 0.11–1.6 mg/kg/day in 3–4 divided doses.
PO: ADULTS, ELDERLY: 16–64 mg/day once daily or in divided doses. **CHILDREN:** Initially, 0.11–1.6 mg/kg/day in 3–4 divided doses.
IM: *(Acetate or Succinate):* ADULTS, ELDERLY: 40–60 mg as a single dose.
Intra-articular: ADULTS, ELDERLY: (Larger joint): 20–80 mg. (Medium joint): 10–40 mg. (Small joint): 4–10 mg.
Intralesional: ADULTS, ELDERLY: Usual range: 20–60 mg.

Dosage in Renal/Hepatic Impairment
No dose adjustment.

SIDE EFFECTS
Frequent: Insomnia, heartburn, anxiety, abdominal distention, diaphoresis, acne, mood swings, increased appetite, facial flushing, GI distress, delayed wound healing, increased susceptibility to infection, diarrhea, constipation. **Occasional:** Headache, edema, tachycardia, change in skin color, frequent urination, depression. **Rare:** Psychosis, increased blood coagulability, hallucinations.

ADVERSE EFFECTS/TOXIC REACTIONS
Long-term therapy: Hypocalcemia, hypokalemia, muscle wasting (esp. in arms, legs), osteoporosis, spontaneous fractures, amenorrhea, cataracts, glaucoma, peptic ulcer, HF. **Abrupt withdrawal after long-term therapy:** Anorexia, nausea, fever, headache, severe arthralgia, rebound inflammation, fatigue, weakness, lethargy, dizziness, orthostatic hypotension.

M

NURSING CONSIDERATIONS

BASELINE ASSESSMENT
Question for hypersensitivity to corticosteroids, components. Obtain height, weight, B/P, serum glucose, electrolytes. Check results of initial tests (tuberculosis [TB] skin test, X-rays, ECG). Question history as listed in Precautions.

INTERVENTION/EVALUATION
Monitor I&O, daily weight; assess for edema. Monitor daily pattern of bowel activity, stool consistency. Check vital signs at least twice daily. Be alert for infection (sore throat, fever, vague symptoms). Monitor serum electrolytes, including B/P, glucose. Monitor for hypocalcemia (muscle twitching, cramps, positive Trousseau's or Chvostek's signs), hypokalemia (weakness, muscle cramps, numbness, tingling [esp. lower extremities], nausea/vomiting, irritability, ECG changes). Assess emotional status, ability to sleep.

PATIENT/FAMILY TEACHING
• Take oral dose with food, milk. • Do not change dose/schedule or stop taking drug; must taper off gradually under medical supervision. • Report fever, sore throat, muscle aches, sudden weight gain or loss, edema, loss of appetite, fatigue. • Severe stress (serious infection, surgery, trauma) may require increased dosage. • Follow-up visits, lab tests are necessary. • Children must be assessed for growth retardation. • Inform dentist, other physicians of methylPREDNISolone therapy now or within past 12 mos.

metOLazone

meh-**toe**-la-zone
(Zaroxolyn ✱)
Do not confuse metOLazone with metaxalone, methotrexate, metoclopramide, or metoprolol, or Zaroxolyn with Zarontin.

◆CLASSIFICATION

PHARMACOTHERAPEUTIC: Thiazide diuretic. **CLINICAL:** Diuretic, antihypertensive.

USES

Treatment of edema due to HF, nephrotic syndrome, or impaired renal function.

PRECAUTIONS

Contraindications: Hypersensitivity to metolazone. Anuria, hepatic coma/precoma. **Cautions:** Hypersensitivity to sulfonamides, thiazide diuretics. Severe renal disease, severe hepatic impairment, gout, prediabetes or diabetes, elevated serum cholesterol, triglycerides.

ACTION

Blocks reabsorption of sodium, potassium, chloride at distal convoluted tubule, increasing excretion of sodium, potassium, water. **Therapeutic Effect:** Reduces B/P, promotes diuresis.

PHARMACOKINETICS

Route	Onset	Peak	Duration
PO (diuretic)	1 hr	—	24 hrs

Incompletely absorbed from GI tract. Protein binding: 95%. Primarily excreted in urine. Not removed by hemodialysis. **Half-life:** 20 hrs.

⧗ LIFESPAN CONSIDERATIONS

Pregnancy/Lactation: Crosses placenta. Small amount distributed in breast milk. Breastfeeding not recommended. **Children:** No age-related precautions noted. **Elderly:** May be more sensitive to hypotensive or electrolyte imbalance. Age-related renal impairment may require dosage adjustment.

INTERACTIONS

DRUG: Bile acid sequestrants (e.g., **cholestyramine**) may decrease absorption. May increase the hypokalemic effect of **topiramate. HERBAL:** Licorice may increase the hypokalemic effect. **Herbals with hypotensive properties (e.g., garlic, ginger, ginkgo biloba) or hypertensive properties (e.g., yohimbe)** may alter effects. **FOOD:** None known. **LAB VALUES:** May increase serum glucose, cholesterol, LDL, bilirubin, calcium, creatinine, uric acid, triglycerides. May decrease urinary calcium, serum magnesium, potassium, sodium.

AVAILABILITY (Rx)

Tablets: 2.5 mg, 5 mg, 10 mg.

ADMINISTRATION/HANDLING

PO
• May give with food, milk if GI upset occurs, preferably with breakfast (may prevent nocturia).

INDICATIONS/ROUTES/DOSAGE

Edema
PO: ADULTS, ELDERLY: Initially, 2.5–5 mg once daily. May increase to a maximum 20 mg/day in 1–2 divided doses.

Dosage in Renal Impairment

Mild to moderate impairment: No dose adjustment. **Severe impairment:** Use caution.

Dosage in Hepatic Impairment

No dose adjustment. Contraindicated with hepatic coma or precoma.

SIDE EFFECTS

Expected: Increased urinary frequency/volume. **Frequent (10%–9%):** Dizziness, light-headedness, headache. **Occasional (6%–4%):** Muscle cramps/spasm, drowsiness, fatigue, lethargy. **Rare (less than 2%):** Asthenia, palpitations, depression, nausea, vomiting, abdominal bloating, constipation, diarrhea, urticaria.

ADVERSE EFFECTS/TOXIC REACTIONS

Vigorous diuresis may lead to profound water loss and electrolyte depletion, resulting in hypokalemia, hyponatremia, dehydration. Acute hypotensive episodes may occur. Hyperglycemia may occur during prolonged therapy. Pancreatitis, paresthesia, blood dyscrasias, pulmonary edema, allergic pneumonitis, dermatologic reactions occur rarely. Overdose can lead to lethargy, coma without changes in electrolytes, hydration.

NURSING CONSIDERATIONS

BASELINE ASSESSMENT

Assess vital signs, esp. B/P for hypotension. Obtain serum electrolytes. Assess skin turgor, mucous membranes for hydration status. Assess for peripheral edema. Obtain baseline weight. Monitor I&O.

INTERVENTION/EVALUATION

Monitor B/P, vital signs, serum electrolytes, I&O, weight. Note extent of diuresis. Monitor for electrolyte disturbances (hypokalemia may result in weakness, tremors, muscle cramps, nausea, vomiting, altered mental status, tachycardia; hyponatremia may result in confusion, thirst, cold/clammy skin).

PATIENT/FAMILY TEACHING

• Expect increased urinary frequency/volume. • Slowly go from lying to standing to reduce hypotensive effect. • Avoid tasks requiring motor skills, mental alertness until response to drug is established. • Eat foods high in potassium, such as whole grains (cereals), legumes, meat, bananas, apricots, orange juice, potatoes (white, sweet), raisins.

---

metoprolol

me-**toe**-pro-lol
(Kaspargo Sprinkle, Lopressor, Toprol XL)

■ **BLACK BOX ALERT** ■ Abrupt withdrawal can produce acute tachycardia, hypertension, ischemia. Drug should be gradually tapered over 1–2 wks.
Do not confuse metoprolol with atenolol, labetalol, nadolol, or stanozolol, or Toprol XL with TEGretol, TEGretol XR, or Topamax.

FIXED-COMBINATION(S)

Dutoprol: metoprolol/hydroCHLOROthiazide (a diuretic): 25 mg/12.5 mg, 50 mg/12.5 mg, 100 mg/12.5 mg. **Lopressor HCT:** metoprolol/hydroCHLOROthiazide (a diuretic): 50 mg/25 mg, 100 mg/25 mg, 100 mg/50 mg.

◆CLASSIFICATION

PHARMACOTHERAPEUTIC: Beta$_1$-adrenergic blocker. **CLINICAL:** Antianginal, antihypertensive, MI adjunct.

USES

Angina: Long-term treatment of angina. **Heart failure (HF) with reduced ejection fraction:** Treatment of stable, symptomatic HF (NYHA class II or III) in pts receiving ACE inhibitors, diuretics. **Hypertension:** Management of hypertension. **Myocardial infarction (MI):** Treatment of hemodynamically

M

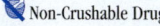

stable MI to reduce cardiovascular mortality. **OFF-LABEL:** Treatment of ventricular arrhythmias, supraventricular tachycardia, migraine prophylaxis, prevent/treat atrial fibrillation/atrial flutter, thyrotoxicosis.

PRECAUTIONS

Contraindications: Hypersensitivity to metoprolol. Second- or third-degree heart block. **Immediate-release: MI:** Severe sinus bradycardia (HR less than 45 beats/min), systolic B/P less than 100 mm Hg, moderate to severe HF, significant first-degree heart block. **Immediate-release: HTN/angina:** Sinus bradycardia, cardiogenic shock, overt HF, sick sinus syndrome (except with pacemaker), severe peripheral arterial disease. **Extended-release:** Severe bradycardia, cardiogenic shock, decompensated HF, sick sinus syndrome (except with functioning pacemaker). **Cautions:** Arterial obstruction, bronchospastic disease, hepatic impairment, peripheral vascular disease, hyperthyroidism, diabetes mellitus, myasthenia gravis, psychiatric disease, history of severe anaphylaxis to allergens. **Extended-release:** Compensated HF.

ACTION

Selectively blocks beta$_1$-adrenergic receptors. **Therapeutic Effect:** Slows heart rate, decreases cardiac output, reduces B/P. Decreases myocardial ischemia severity.

PHARMACOKINETICS

Route	Onset	Peak	Duration
PO	10–15 min	1–2 hrs	N/A
PO (extended-release)	N/A	6–12 hrs	N/A
IV	Immediate	20 min	N/A

Widely distributed. Protein binding: 12%. Metabolized in liver. Primarily excreted in urine. Removed by hemodialysis. **Half-life:** 3–7 hrs.

⧗ LIFESPAN CONSIDERATIONS

Pregnancy/Lactation: Crosses placenta; distributed in breast milk. Avoid use during first trimester. May produce bradycardia, apnea, hypoglycemia, hypothermia during delivery, low-birth-weight infants. **Children:** Safety and efficacy not established. **Elderly:** Age-related peripheral vascular disease may increase susceptibility to decreased peripheral circulation.

INTERACTIONS

DRUG: **Alpha$_2$ agonists (e.g., cloNIDine)** may increase AV-blocking effect. **Strong CYP3A4 inducers (e.g., carBAMazepine, phenytoin, rifAMPin)** may decrease concentration/effect. **Dronedarone, rivastigmine** may increase bradycardic effect. May increase vasoconstriction of **ergot derivatives (e.g., ergotamine). Obinutuzumab** may increase hypotensive effect. **HERBAL: Herbals with hypertensive properties (e.g., licorice, yohimbe) or hypotensive properties (e.g., garlic, ginger, ginkgo biloba)** may alter effects. **FOOD:** None known. **LAB VALUES:** May increase serum antinuclear antibody titer (ANA), serum BUN, lipoprotein, LDH, alkaline phosphatase, bilirubin, creatinine, potassium, uric acid, ALT, AST, triglycerides.

AVAILABILITY (Rx)

Injection Solution: 5 mg/5 mL. **Tablets, Immediate-Release:** 25 mg, 37.5 mg, 50 mg, 75 mg, 100 mg.

Capsules, Extended-Release Sprinkle: 25 mg, 50 mg, 100 mg, 200 mg. **Tablets, Extended-Release:** 25 mg, 50 mg, 100 mg, 200 mg.

ADMINISTRATION/HANDLING

 IV

Rate of administration • May give undiluted. • Administer IV injection over 1 min. • May give by IV piggyback (in 50 mL D$_5$W or 0.9% NaCl) over 30–60 min. • Monitor ECG, B/P during administration.

Storage • Store at room temperature.

PO

• **Immediate-release:** Administer with or immediately following meals. • **Extended-release:** Administer without regard to meals. • Do not crush or allow chewing (may divide tablets in half). • **Sprinkle capsules:** Sprinkle capsules may be given whole or contents may be mixed (1 teaspoonful) on soft food and used within 60 min.

▓ IV COMPATIBILITIES

Acetaminophen, amiodarone, heparin, ibuprofen, norepinephrine.

INDICATIONS/ROUTES/DOSAGE

Hypertension

PO: *(Immediate-Release):* **ADULTS, ELDERLY:** Initially, 50 mg twice daily. Increase at wkly (or longer) intervals. **Usual range:** 100–200 mg/day in 2 divided doses. **Maximum:** 450 mg/day. **CHILDREN:** Initially, 0.5–1 mg/kg/dose twice daily. **Maximum initial dose:** 25 mg twice daily. **Maximum daily dose:** 6 mg/kg/day or 200 mg/day, whichever is less.

PO: *(Extended-Release):* **ADULTS, ELDERLY:** Initially, 25–100 mg/day as single dose. May increase at least at wkly intervals until optimum B/P attained. **Usual range:** 50–200 mg once daily. **Maximum:** 400 mg/day. **CHILDREN 6 YRS OR OLDER:** Initially, 1 mg/kg once daily. **Maximum initial dose:** 50 mg. May increase to 2 mg/kg/day or 200 mg/day, whichever is less.

Angina Pectoris

PO: *(Immediate-Release):* **ADULTS:** Initially, 50 mg twice daily. Increase at wkly (or longer) intervals. **Usual range:** 50–200 mg twice daily. **Maximum:** 400 mg/day. *(Extended-Release):* **ADULTS:** Initially, 100 mg/day as single dose. May increase by at least at wkly intervals until optimum clinical response achieved. **Maximum:** 400 mg/day.

HF

PO: *(Extended-Release):* **ADULTS:** Initially, 12.5–25 mg/day. May titrate gradually by doubling dose q2wks or longer up to target dose of 200 mg/day.

Early Treatment of MI

IV: **ADULTS:** 5 mg q5min for up to 3 doses, followed by 12.5–50 mg q6–12h in acute setting (begin oral 15–30 min after last IV dose). Transition to metoprolol tartrate twice daily or metoprolol succinate once daily. May increase up to a maximum of 200 mg/day.

Dosage in Renal/Hepatic Impairment

No dose adjustment.

SIDE EFFECTS

Frequent: Diminished sexual function, drowsiness, insomnia, unusual fatigue/weakness. **Occasional:** Anxiety, diarrhea, constipation, nausea, vomiting, nasal congestion, abdominal discomfort, dizziness, difficulty breathing, cold hands/feet. **Rare:** Altered taste, dry eyes, nightmares, paresthesia, allergic reaction (rash, pruritus).

ADVERSE EFFECTS/TOXIC REACTIONS

Overdose may produce profound bradycardia, hypotension, bronchospasm. Abrupt withdrawal may result in diaphoresis, palpitations, headache, tremulousness, exacerbation of angina, MI, ventricular arrhythmias. May precipitate HF, MI in pts with heart disease, thyroid storm in those with thyrotoxicosis, peripheral ischemia in those with existing peripheral vascular disease. Hypoglycemia may occur in pts with previously controlled diabetes (may mask signs of hypoglycemia). **Antidote:** Glucagon (see Appendix J for dosage).

NURSING CONSIDERATIONS

BASELINE ASSESSMENT

Assess B/P, heart rate immediately before drug administration (if pulse is 60/min or less or systolic B/P is less than 90 mm Hg, withhold medication, contact physician). **Antianginal:** Record onset, type (sharp, dull, squeezing), radiation, location, intensity, duration of anginal pain, precipitating factors (exertion, emotional stress).

M

 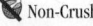

INTERVENTION/EVALUATION

Measure B/P near end of dosing interval (determines whether B/P is controlled throughout day). Monitor B/P for hypotension, respiration for shortness of breath. Assess pulse for quality, rate, rhythm. Assess for evidence of HF: Dyspnea (esp. on exertion, lying down), night cough, peripheral edema, distended neck veins. Monitor I&O (increased weight, decreased urinary output may indicate HF). Therapeutic response to hypertension noted in 1–2 wks.

PATIENT/FAMILY TEACHING

• Do not abruptly discontinue medication. • Compliance with therapy regimen is essential to control hypertension, arrhythmias. • Go from lying to standing slowly. • Report excessive fatigue, dizziness. • Avoid tasks that require alertness, motor skills until response to drug is established. • Do not use nasal decongestants, OTC cold preparations (stimulants) without physician approval. • Monitor B/P, pulse before taking medication. • Restrict salt, alcohol intake.

metroNIDAZOLE

me-troe-**nye**-da-zole
(Flagyl, Likmez, MetroCream, NidaGel ✦, Noritate, Vandazole)
Do not confuse metroNIDAZOLE with meropenem, metFORMIN, methotrexate, or miconazole.

FIXED-COMBINATION(S)

Helidac: metroNIDAZOLE/bismuth/tetracycline (an anti-infective): 250 mg/262 mg/500 mg. **Pylera:** metroNIDAZOLE/bismuth/tetracycline (an anti-infective): 125 mg/140 mg/125 mg.

◆CLASSIFICATION

PHARMACOTHERAPEUTIC: Nitroimidazole derivative. **CLINICAL:** Antibacterial, antiprotozoal, amebicide.

USES

Systemic: (Amebiasis): Treatment of acute intestinal/extraintestinal amebiasis. **(Anaerobic bacterial infections caused by *Bacteroides* species including *B. fragilis*):** Including bone and joint infections (adjunctive), CNS infections, endocarditis, gynecologic infections (also caused by *Clostridium* spp, *Peptococcus* spp, *Peptostreptococcus* spp), intra-abdominal infections (also caused by *Clostridium* spp, *Peptococcus* spp, *Peptostreptococcus* spp), lower respiratory tract infections, sepsis (also caused by *Clostridium* spp), skin and skin structure infections (also caused by *Clostridium* spp, *Peptococcus* spp, *Peptostreptococcus* spp). **Surgical prophylaxis (colorectal). Trichomoniasis:** Treatment of infections caused by *Trichomonas vaginalis* (including asymptomic sexual partners). **Topical:** Treatment of acne rosacea or inflammatory lesions. **Vaginal gel:** Treatment of bacterial vaginosis. OFF-LABEL: Crohn's disease, antibiotic-associated pseudomembranous colitis (AAPC) caused by *C. difficile.* Giardiasis, *H. pylori* eradication. Bite wound infection, sexually transmitted infections.

PRECAUTIONS

Contraindications: Hypersensitivity to metroNIDAZOLE. Pregnancy (first trimester with trichomoniasis), use of disulfiram within 2 wks, use of alcohol during therapy or within 3 days of discontinuing metroNIDAZOLE. **Cautions:** Severe hepatic impairment, end-stage renal disease, seizure disorder, HF, other sodium-retaining states, elderly.

ACTION

Diffuses into organism, interacting with DNA causing a loss of helical DNA structure and strand breakage, inhibiting protein synthesis. **Therapeutic Effect:** Produces bactericidal, antiprotozoal, amebicidal, trichomonacidal effects. Produces

M

anti-inflammatory, immunosuppressive effects when applied topically.

PHARMACOKINETICS

Widely distributed; crosses blood-brain barrier. Minimally absorbed after topical application. Metabolized in liver. Excreted in urine (80%), feces (15%). Removed by hemodialysis. **Half-life:** 8 hrs (increased in cirrhosis, neonates). Active metabolite prolonged in renal failure.

⧖ LIFESPAN CONSIDERATIONS

Pregnancy/Lactation: Readily crosses placenta. Distributed in breast milk. Contraindicated during first trimester in those with trichomoniasis. Topical use during pregnancy, lactation discouraged. **Children:** No age-related precautions noted. **Elderly:** Age-related hepatic impairment may require dosage adjustment.

INTERACTIONS

DRUG: Alcohol may cause disulfiram-type reaction (e.g., abdominal cramps, nausea, vomiting, headache, psychotic reactions). **Disulfiram** may increase risk of toxicity. May increase effects of **oral anticoagulants (e.g., warfarin).** **HERBAL:** None significant. **FOOD:** None known. **LAB VALUES:** May increase serum LDH, ALT, AST.

AVAILABILITY (Rx)

Capsules: 375 mg. **Injection, Infusion:** 500 mg/100 mL. **Suspension, Oral:** 500 mg/5 mL. **Tablets:** 250 mg, 500 mg. **Topical Cream:** *(MetroCream):* 0.75% **(Noritate):** 1%. **Topical Gel:** *(Generic):* 0.75%, 1%. **Vaginal Gel:** *(MetroGel-Vaginal, Vandazole):* 0.75%.

ADMINISTRATION/HANDLING

 IV

Rate of administration • Infuse IV over 30–60 min. Do not give by IV bolus.

Storage • Store at room temperature (ready-to-use infusion bags).

PO

• Give without regard to food. Give with food to decrease GI irritation. **Suspension:** Shake well before use. • Use a calibrated oral dosing device.

▦ IV COMPATIBILITIES

DexmedeTOMIDine, dilTIAZem, magnesium sulfate.

INDICATIONS/ROUTES/DOSAGE

Amebiasis

PO: ADULTS, ELDERLY: 500–750 mg q8h for 5–10 days. **CHILDREN:** 35–50 mg/kg/day in divided doses q8h for 10 days. **Maximum:** 750 mg/dose.

Usual Dosage for Anaerobic Infections

PO, IV: ADULTS, ELDERLY: 500 mg q6–8h. **Maximum:** 4 g/24 hrs. **PO: CHILDREN, INFANTS:** 15–50 mg/kg/day in divided doses q8h. **Maximum:** 2,250 mg/day. **IV: CHILDREN, INFANTS:** 22.5–40 mg/kg/day in 3 divided doses. **Maximum:** 4 g/24 hrs.

Pseudomembranous Colitis

PO: ADULTS, ELDERLY: 500 mg 3 times/day for 10 days. **CHILDREN, ADOLESCENTS:** 7.5 mg/kg/dose 3–4 times/day for 10 days. **Maximum:** 500 mg/dose.

Trichomoniasis:

PO: ADULTS, ELDERLY: 1-Day treatment: 2 g as a single dose or 1 g in 2 divided doses given on the same day. **7-Day treatment:** 250 mg 3 times daily for 7 days.

Bacterial Vaginosis

Intravaginal: ADULTS: 0.75% apply once daily for 5 days. 1.3% apply once as a single dose.
PO: 500 mg twice daily for 7 days.

Rosacea

Topical: ADULTS, ELDERLY: (1%): Apply to affected area once daily. **(0.75%):** Apply to affected area twice daily.

M

 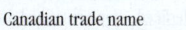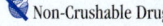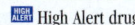

Dosage in Renal Impairment
No dose adjustment.

Dosage in Hepatic Impairment
Mild to moderate impairment: Use caution. No dose adjustment. **Severe impairment:** Reduce dose by 50% for immediate-release; not recommended for extended-release.

SIDE EFFECTS

Frequent: Systemic: Anorexia, nausea, dry mouth, metallic taste. **Vaginal:** Symptomatic cervicitis/vaginitis, abdominal cramps, uterine pain. **Occasional: Systemic:** Diarrhea, constipation, vomiting, dizziness, erythematous rash, urticaria, reddish-brown urine. **Topical:** Transient erythema, mild dryness, burning, irritation, stinging, tearing when applied too close to eyes. **Vaginal:** Vaginal, perineal, vulvar itching; vulvar swelling. **Rare:** Mild, transient leukopenia; thrombophlebitis with IV therapy.

ADVERSE EFFECTS/TOXIC REACTIONS

Oral therapy may result in furry tongue, glossitis, cystitis, dysuria, pancreatitis. Peripheral neuropathy (manifested as numbness, tingling of hands/feet) usually is reversible if treatment is stopped immediately upon appearance of neurologic symptoms. Seizures occur occasionally.

NURSING CONSIDERATIONS

BASELINE ASSESSMENT

Obtain CBC, LFT. Question for history of hypersensitivity to metroNIDAZOLE, other nitroimidazole derivatives (and parabens with topical). Obtain specimens for diagnostic tests, cultures before giving first dose (therapy may begin before results are known).

INTERVENTION/EVALUATION

Monitor daily pattern of bowel activity, stool consistency. Monitor I&O, assess for urinary problems. Be alert to neurologic symptoms (dizziness, paresthesia of extremities). Assess for rash, urticaria. Monitor for onset of superinfection (ulceration/change of oral mucosa, furry tongue, vaginal discharge, genital/anal pruritus).

PATIENT/FAMILY TEACHING

• Urine may be red-brown or dark. • Avoid alcohol, alcohol-containing preparations (cough syrups, elixirs) for at least 48 hrs after last dose. • If taking metroNIDAZOLE for trichomoniasis, refrain from sexual intercourse until full treatment is completed. • For amebiasis, frequent stool specimen checks will be necessary. • **Topical:** Avoid contact with eyes. • May apply cosmetics after application. • MetroNIDAZOLE acts on erythema, papules, pustules but has no effect on rhinophyma (hypertrophy of nose), telangiectasia, ocular problems (conjunctivitis, keratitis, blepharitis). • Other recommendations for rosacea include avoidance of hot/spicy foods, alcohol, extremes of hot/cold temperatures, excessive sunlight.

micafungin

mye-ka-**fun**-jin
Do not confuse micafungin with anidulafungin, caspofungin, or rezafungin. (Mycamine)

◆CLASSIFICATION

PHARMACOTHERAPEUTIC: Echinocandin antifungal. **CLINICAL:** Antifungal.

USES

Candidemia/*Candida* infections: Treatment of candidemia, acute disseminated candidiasis, Candida peritonitis, and abscesses in adults and pts 4 mos of age and older. Treatment of esophageal candidiasis in adults and pts 4 mos of age and older. Prophylaxis of *Candida* infections in adults and pts 4 mos of age and older undergoing hematopoietic stem cell transplantation (HSCT). **OFF-LABEL:** Treatment of infections due to *Aspergillus* spp, endocarditis, oropharyngeal (refactory disease), osteoarticular infection (e.g., osteomyelitis), neutropenic fever (empiric therapy). Solid organ transplant.

PRECAUTIONS

Contraindications: Hypersensitivity to micafungin. **Cautions:** Hepatic/renal impairment, concomitant hepatotoxic medications.

ACTION

Inhibits synthesis of glucan (vital component of fungal cell formation), damaging fungal cell membrane. **Therapeutic Effect:** Decreased glucan content leads to cellular lysis.

PHARMACOKINETICS

Metabolized in liver. Protein binding: Greater than 99%. Primarily excreted in feces. Not removed by hemodialysis. **Half-life:** 11–21 hrs.

⧗ LIFESPAN CONSIDERATIONS

Pregnancy/Lactation: May cause fetal harm. Unknown if distributed in breast milk. **Males:** May reduce sperm count. **Children:** Safety and efficacy not established in pts younger than 4 mos. **Elderly:** No age-related precautions noted.

INTERACTIONS

DRUG: May decrease therapeutic effect of *Saccharomyces boulardii*. May increase concentration/effect of **sirolimus**. **HERBAL:** None significant. **FOOD:** None known. **LAB VALUES:** May increase serum creatinine, alkaline phosphatase, LDH, ALT, AST.

AVAILABILITY (Rx)

Injection, Powder for Reconstitution: 50 mg, 100 mg.

ADMINISTRATION/HANDLING

 IV

Reconstitution • Add 5 mL 0.9% NaCl (preservative free) or D5W to each 50-mg vial (10 mL to 100-mg vial) to yield micafungin 10 mg/mL. • Gently swirl to dissolve; do not shake. • Further dilute in 0.9% NaCl or D$_5$W to final concentration of 0.5–1.5 mg/mL. • Flush existing IV line with 0.9% NaCl before infusion.
Rate of administration • Infuse over 60 min.
Storage • Reconstituted solution is stable for 24 hrs at room temperature. • Discard if precipitate is present.

⊞ IV INCOMPATIBILITIES

Amiodarone, nicardipine.

⊞ IV COMPATIBILITIES

Magnesium sulfate, potassium chloride, potassium/sodium phosphate.

INDICATIONS/ROUTES/DOSAGE

Esophageal Candidiasis
IV: ADULTS, ELDERLY: 150 mg/day for 14–28 days. **CHILDREN 4 MOS OR OLDER WEIGHING MORE THAN 30 KG:** 2.5 mg/kg for 14–21 days. **Maximum:** 150 mg daily. **30 KG OR LESS:** 3 mg/kg for 14–21 days.

Candida Prophylaxis in Stem Cell Pts
IV: ADULTS, ELDERLY: 50 mg/day. **CHILDREN 4 MOS OR OLDER:** 1 mg/kg/day. **Maximum:** 50 mg/day.

Candidemia
IV: ADULTS, ELDERLY: 100 mg/day for for 14 or more days after first negative blood culture; continue until signs/symptoms of candidemia/neutropenia have resolved.

M

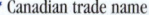

CHILDREN 4 MOS OR OLDER: 2 mg/kg/day. **Maximum:** 100 mg daily.

Dosage in Renal/Hepatic Impairment
No dose adjustment.

SIDE EFFECTS

Occasional (3%–2%): Nausea, headache, diarrhea, vomiting, fever. **Rare (1%):** Dizziness, drowsiness, pruritus, abdominal pain, dyspepsia.

ADVERSE EFFECTS/TOXIC REACTIONS

Hypersensitivity reaction characterized by rash, pruritus, facial edema occurs rarely. Anaphylaxis, hemoglobinuria, hemolytic anemia have been reported.

NURSING CONSIDERATIONS

BASELINE ASSESSMENT
Obtain renal function, LFT.

INTERVENTION/EVALUATION
Monitor BUN, serum creatinine, CrCl, LFT. Monitor for hepatotoxicity.

PATIENT/FAMILY TEACHING
• Report liver problems such as bruising, confusion; dark amber or orange-colored urine; right upper abdominal pain; yellowing of the skin or eyes. • Report decreased urine output; dark, amber urine; swelling of the hands or feet. • Do not take OTC medications that are toxic to the liver (e.g., acetaminophen).

---

midazolam

mye-**da**-zoe-lam
(Nayzilam)

■ **BLACK BOX ALERT** ■ May cause severe respiratory depression, respiratory arrest, apnea. Initial doses in elderly should be conservative. Do not administer by rapid IV injection in neonates (may cause severe hypotension/seizures). Use with opioids may cause profound sedation, respiratory depression, coma, or death. Exposes users to risks of abuse, misuse, and addiction, which can lead to overdose or death. Chronic use may cause clinically significant physical dependence. **Do not confuse midazolam with, ALPRAZolam or LORazepam.**

◆CLASSIFICATION

PHARMACOTHERAPEUTIC: Benzodiazepine (Schedule IV). **CLINICAL:** Sedative, anxiolytic.

USES

Sedation, anxiolytic, amnesia before procedure or induction of anesthesia, conscious sedation before diagnostic/radiographic procedure, continuous IV sedation of intubated or mechanically ventilated pts. Status epilepticus in adults. **Nasal:** Acute treatment of seizure clusters that are distinct from pts' usual seizure pattern in pts 12 yrs of age and older. **OFF-LABEL:** Status epilepticus (refractory), agitation (acute/severe), palliative and end-of-life sedation.

PRECAUTIONS

Contraindications: Hypersensitivity to midazolam. Acute narrow-angle glaucoma, concurrent use of protease inhibitors (e.g., atazanavir, darunavir). **Cautions:** Renal/hepatic/pulmonary impairment, impaired gag reflex, HF, treated open-angle glaucoma, concurrent CNS depressants, obesity, elderly, debilitated.

ACTION

Enhances action of gamma-aminobutyric acid (GABA), one of the major inhibitory neurotransmitters in the brain. **Therapeutic Effect:** Produces anxiolytic, hypnotic, anticonvulsant, muscle relaxant, amnestic effects.

PHARMACOKINETICS

Route	Onset	Peak	Duration
PO	10–20 min	N/A	N/A
IV	1–5 min	5–7 min	20–30 min
IM	5–15 min	30–60 min	2–6 hrs

Widely distributed. Metabolized in liver. Protein binding: 97%. Primarily excreted in urine. Not removed by hemodialysis. **Half-life:** 1–5 hrs.

⌛ LIFESPAN CONSIDERATIONS

Pregnancy/Lactation: Crosses placenta. Unknown if distributed in breast milk. **Children:** Neonates more likely to have respiratory depression. **Elderly:** Age-related renal impairment may require dosage adjustment.

INTERACTIONS

DRUG: **Alcohol, other CNS depressants (e.g., LORazepam, morphine, zolpidem)** may increase CNS effects, respiratory depression, hypotensive effect. **Strong CYP3A4 inhibitors (e.g., clarithromycin, ketoconazole, ritonavir)** may increase concentration/effect. **Strong CYP3A4 inducers (e.g., carBAMazepine, phenytoin, rifAMPin)** may decrease concentration/effect. **HERBAL:** **Herbals with sedative properties (e.g., chamomile, kava kava, valerian)** may increase CNS depression. **FOOD:** **Grapefruit products** increase oral absorption, systemic availability. **LAB VALUES:** None significant.

AVAILABILITY (Rx)

Injection Solution: 1 mg/mL, 5 mg/mL. Nasal Spray: 5 mg/0.1 mL. Syrup: 2 mg/mL.

ADMINISTRATION/HANDLING

 IV

Rate of administration • May give undiluted or as infusion. • Resuscitative equipment, O₂ must be readily available before IV administration. • Administer by slow IV injection over at least 2–5 min at concentration of 1–5 mg/mL. • Reduce IV rate in those older than 60 yrs, debilitated pts with chronic disease states, pulmonary impairment. • Too-rapid IV rate, excessive doses, or single large dose increases risk of respiratory depression/arrest.

Storage • Store vials at room temperature.

IM
• Give deep IM into large muscle mass. **Maximum concentration:** 1 mg/mL.

Nasal
Do not prime before use.

PO
• Do not mix with grapefruit juice. Administer on an empty stomach.

▦ IV INCOMPATIBILITIES

Ibuprofen.

▦ IV COMPATIBILITIES

Calcium gluconate, dexmedetomidine, heparin, insulin, norepinephrine, potassium chloride.

INDICATIONS/ROUTES/DOSAGE

Continuous Sedation During Mechanical Ventilation

IV: ADULTS, ELDERLY: Initially, 0.5–5 mg or 0.01–0.05 mg/kg over at least 2 min. May repeat at 10–15 min intervals until adequate sedation achieved or continuous infusion rate of 0.01–0.1 mg/kg/hr and titrated to desired effect. **CHILDREN:** Initially, 0.05–0.2 mg/kg followed by continuous infusion of 0.05–1.2 mg/kg/hr (0.8–2 mcg/kg/min) titrated to desired effect. **Usual range:** 0.4–6 mcg/kg/min. **Maximum initial dose:** 10 mg/hr.

Seizure Clusters

Nasal: ADULTS, CHILDREN 12 YRS AND OLDER: Initially, one spray (5-mg dose) into one nostril. One additional spray (5-mg dose) into the opposite nostril may be administered after 10 min. **Maximum dose:** 10 mg (2 sprays) per episode. **Maximum frequency:** 1 episode q3days;

M

5 episodes/mos.

Dosage in Renal Impairment
No dose adjustment.

Dosage in Hepatic Impairment
Use caution.

SIDE EFFECTS

Frequent (10%–4%): Decreased respiratory rate, tenderness at IM or IV injection site, pain during injection, oxygen desaturation, hiccups. **Occasional (3%–2%):** Hypotension, paradoxical CNS reaction. **Rare (less than 2%):** Nausea, vomiting, headache, coughing.

ADVERSE EFFECTS/TOXIC REACTIONS

Inadequate or excessive dosage, improper administration may result in cerebral hypoxia, agitation, involuntary movements, hyperactivity, combativeness. Too-rapid IV rate, excessive doses, or single large dose increases risk of respiratory depression/arrest. Respiratory depression/apnea may produce hypoxia, cardiac arrest.

NURSING CONSIDERATIONS

BASELINE ASSESSMENT

Resuscitative equipment, oxygen must be available. Obtain vital signs before administration. Assess level of consciousness. Question history of narrow-angle glaucoma, untreated or uncontrolled open-angle glaucoma.

INTERVENTION/EVALUATION

Monitor respiratory rate, oxygen saturation continuously during administration for underventilation, apnea. Monitor vital signs, level of sedation q3–5min during recovery period. Assess level of consciousness for effectiveness. Monitor for decrease of seizure activity.

midostaurin

mye-doe-**staw**-rim
(Rydapt)
Do not confuse midostaurin with midodrine.

◆CLASSIFICATION

PHARMACOTHERAPEUTIC: FLT inhibitor. Tyrosine kinase inhibitor. **CLINICAL:** Antineoplastic.

USES

Acute myeloid leukemia: Treatment of adult pts with newly diagnosed acute myeloid leukemia (AML) who are FLT3 mutation–positive, as detected by an FDA-approved test (in combination with standard cytarabine and DAUNOrubicin induction and cytarabine consolidation chemotherapy). **Systemic mastocytosis:** Treatment of adult pts with aggressive systemic mastocytosis (ASM), systemic mastocytosis with associated hematologic neoplasm (SM-AHN). **Mast cell leukemia (MCL):** Treatment of patients with MCL.

PRECAUTIONS

Contraindications: Hypersensitivity to midostaurin. **Cautions:** Baseline cytopenias; concomitant use of strong CYP3A4 inhibitors, strong CYP3A4 inducers; pts at risk for hemorrhage (e.g., history of GI bleeding, coagulation disorders, recent trauma; concomitant use of anticoagulants, NSAIDs, antiplatelet medication).

ACTION

Inhibits multiple receptors including FLT3 receptor signaling, and cell proliferation. **Therapeutic Effect:** Induces apoptosis in ITD and ITD mutant expressing leukemic cells.

PHARMACOKINETICS

Widely distributed. Metabolized in liver. Protein binding: 99.8%. Peak plasma concentration: 1–3 hrs. Steady state reached in 28 days. Excreted in feces (95%), urine (5%). **Half-life:** 21 hrs.

⧗ LIFESPAN CONSIDERATIONS

Pregnancy/Lactation: Avoid pregnancy; may cause fetal harm. Females and males with female partners of reproductive potential should use effective contraception during treatment and for at least 4 mos after discontinuation. Unknown if distributed in breast milk. Breastfeeding not recommended. May impair fertility in both females and males. **Children:** Safety and efficacy not established. **Elderly:** No age-related precautions noted.

INTERACTIONS

DRUG: **Moderate CYP3A4 inhibitors (e.g., ciprofloxacin, fluconazole, verapamil), strong CYP3A4 inhibitors (e.g., clarithromycin, ketoconazole, ritonavir)** may increase concentration/effect. **Strong CYP3A4 inducers (e.g., carBAMazepine, phenytoin, rifAMPin)** may decrease concentration/effect. **QT-prolonging agents (e.g., amiodarone, haloperidol, moxifloxacin, sotalol)** may enhance QT-prolonging effect. May decrease therapeutic effect of **BCG (intravesical).** **HERBAL:** St. John's wort may decrease concentration/effect. **FOOD:** **Grapefruit products** may increase concentration/effect. **LAB VALUES:** May increase serum alkaline phosphatase, ALT, AST, bilirubin, creatinine, GGT, glucose, lipase, sodium, uric acid. May decrease Hgb, Hct, lymphocytes, leukocytes, neutrophils, platelets, RBCs; serum albumin, magnesium, phosphate, potassium. May increase or decrease serum calcium or sodium. May prolong aPTT.

AVAILABILITY (Rx)

🐋 **Capsules:** 25 mg.

ADMINISTRATION/HANDLING

PO
• Give with food. • Administer whole; do not cut, crush, open capsules.

INDICATIONS/ROUTES/DOSAGE

Acute Myeloid Leukemia (FLT Positive)
PO: ADULTS, ELDERLY: **Induction:** 50 mg twice daily (at 12-hr intervals) on days 8–21 of each induction in combination with cytarabine and DAUNOrubicin. **Consolidation:** 50 mg twice daily on days 8–21 of each 28-day cycle of consolidation with high-dose cytarabine. **Maintenance:** 50 mg twice daily on days 1–28 of each 28-day cycle for 12 cycles or until relapse (whichever occurs first).

Systemic Mastocytosis, Mast Cell Leukemia
PO: ADULTS, ELDERLY: 100 mg twice daily. Continue until disease progression or unacceptable toxicity.

DOSE MODIFICATION FOR SYSTEMIC MASTOCYTOSIS
Neutropenia
ANC less than 1,000 cells/mm^3 in pts without MCL; ANC less than 500 cells/mm^3 in pts with baseline ANC 500–1,500 cells/mm^3: Withhold treatment until ANC greater than or equal to 1,000 cells/mm^3, then resume at 50 mg twice daily. May increase to 100 mg twice daily if 50 mg dose is tolerated. If neutropenia persists for more than 21 days, permanently discontinue.

Thrombocytopenia
Platelet count less than 50,000 cells/mm^3 in pts without MCL; platelet count less than 25,000 cells/mm^3 in pts with baseline platelet count 25,000–75,000 cells/mm^3: Withhold treatment until platelet count greater than or equal to 50,000 cells/mm^3, then resume at 50 mg twice daily. May increase to 100 mg twice daily if 50-mg dose is tolerated. If thrombocytopenia persists for more than 21 days, permanently discontinue.

M

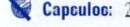

Anemia

Hgb less than 8 g/dL in pts without MCL; life-threatening anemia with baseline Hgb 8–10 g/dL: Withhold treatment until Hgb greater than or equal to 8 g/dL, then resume at 50 mg twice daily. May increase to 100 mg twice daily if 50-mg dose is tolerated. If treatment-induced anemia persists for more than 21 days, permanently discontinue.

Nausea, Vomiting

Grade 3 or 4 nausea, vomiting despite antiemetic therapy: Withhold treatment for 3 days (6 doses), then resume at 50 mg twice daily. May increase to 100 mg twice daily if 50-mg dose is tolerated.

Nonhematologic Toxicities

Any other grade toxicities: Withhold treatment until resolved to Grade 2 or less, then resume at 50 mg twice daily. May increase to 100 mg twice daily if 50-mg dose is tolerated.

Dosage in Rena/Hepatic Impairment
Not specified; use caution.

SIDE EFFECTS

AML: Frequent (83%–24%): Nausea, mucositis, stomatitis, laryngeal pain, vomiting, headache, petechiae, musculoskeletal pain. **Occasional (20%–7%):** Hyperglycemia, hemorrhoids, arthralgia, hyperhidrosis, insomnia, hypertension, dry skin, increased weight. **Rare (4%–3%):** Tremor, eyelid edema. **Systemic mastocytosis: Frequent (82%–23%):** Nausea, vomiting, diarrhea, edema, peripheral edema, fatigue, asthenia, musculoskeletal pain, back pain, extremity pain, abdominal pain, constipation, pyrexia, headache, dyspnea, bronchospasm. **Occasional (19%–6%):** Arthralgia, cough, rash, dizziness, insomnia, hypotension, dyspepsia. **Rare (5%–4%):** Vertigo, chills, mental status change.

ADVERSE EFFECTS/TOXIC REACTIONS

Myelosuppression (anemia, leukopenia, lymphopenia, neutropenia, thrombocytopenia) is an expected response to therapy. Hypersensitivity reactions including anaphylaxis, angioedema, dyspnea, itching, flushing may occur. Infections including bronchitis, bronchopulmonary aspergillosis, colitis, cellulitis, device-related infection, erysipelas, fungal pneumonia, gastroenteritis, hepatic candidiasis, herpes zoster, nasopharyngitis, oral herpes, pneumonia, sepsis, sinusitis, splenic fungal infection, upper respiratory tract infection, UTI have occurred. Renal failure, acute kidney injury may occur. Other adverse effects including angina pectoris, cardiac failure, contusion, duodenal ulcer hemorrhage, epistaxis, gastritis, febrile neutropenia, GI bleeding, hematoma, interstitial lung disease, myocardial infarction, myocardial ischemia, pericardial effusion, pneumonitis, pulmonary congestion, pulmonary edema, thrombosis were reported. May prolong QT interval.

NURSING CONSIDERATIONS

BASELINE ASSESSMENT

Obtain ANC, CBC, BMP, LFT; serum magnesium; vital signs. Ensure electrolytes are corrected prior to initiation. In females of reproductive potential, obtain pregnancy test within 7 days of initiation. Screen for active infection. To reduce risk of nausea/vomiting, administer antiemetic before treatment. Obtain ECG in pts taking QT interval–prolonging medications. Receive full medication history and screen for interactions. Question history as listed in Precautions. Confirm compliance of effective contraception. Offer emotional support.

INTERVENTION/EVALUATION

Monitor ANC, CBC for myelosuppression. Monitor BMP for renal insufficiency, electrolyte imbalance (esp. in pts with diarrhea, vomiting, malnutrition); LFT for transaminitis, hepatotoxicity. Diligently screen for infections, sepsis; provide appropriate antimicrobial therapy if indicated. Obtain ABG, radiologic test if interstitial lung disease or pneumonitis suspected. Monitor for toxicities at least wkly for 4 wks, then every other wk for 8 wks, then monthly thereafter. If treatment-related toxicities occur, consider referral to specialist. Monitor for hemorrhage, melena, hematuria; hypersensitivity reactions; myocardial infarction, pulmonary disease, thrombosis. Monitor I&O.

PATIENT/FAMILY TEACHING

• Treatment may depress your immune system and reduce your ability to fight infection. Report symptoms of infection such as body aches, burning with urination, chills, cough, fatigue, fever. Avoid those with active infection.• Report symptoms of kidney failure (decreased urination, amber-colored urine, flank pain, fatigue, swelling of the hands or feet); liver problems (bruising, confusion; amber, dark, orange-colored urine; right upper abdominal pain, yellowing of the skin or eyes); lung problems (severe cough, difficulty breathing, lung pain, shortness of breath). • Use effective contraception to avoid pregnancy. • Avoid grapefruit products, herbal supplements. • Do not take newly prescribed medications unless approved by the prescriber who originally started treatment. • Heart attacks have occurred; immediately report chest pain, sweating, fainting, palpitations, jaw pain, pain that radiates to the left arm. • Report bleeding of any kind, esp. nosebleeds, blood in stool or urine. • Allergic reactions such as anaphylaxis, difficulty breathing, itching, flushing, rash may occur.

---

milrinone **HIGH ALERT**

mil-ri-none

◆CLASSIFICATION

PHARMACOTHERAPEUTIC: Cardiac inotropic agent. **CLINICAL:** Vasodilator (phosphodiesterase-3 enzyme inhibitor).

USES

Short-term management of acute decompensated HF with reduced ejection fraction. **OFF-LABEL:** Postoperative inotropic support in heart transplant recipients.

PRECAUTIONS

Contraindications: Hypersensitivity to milrinone. **Cautions:** Severe obstructive aortic or pulmonic valvular disease, history of ventricular arrhythmias, atrial fibrillation/flutter, renal impairment. Not recommended in pts with acute MI.

ACTION

Inhibits phosphodiesterase in cardiac and vascular tissue. **Therapeutic Effect:** Relaxes vascular muscle, causing vasodilation. Increases cardiac output, decreases pulmonary capillary wedge pressure, vascular resistance.

PHARMACOKINETICS

Route	Onset	Peak	Duration
IV	5–15 min	N/A	N/A

Protein binding: 70%. Metabolized in liver. Primarily excreted in urine. **Half-life:** 1.7–2.7 hrs.

LIFESPAN CONSIDERATIONS

Pregnancy/Lactation: Unknown if drug crosses placenta or is distributed in breast milk. **Children:** Safety and efficacy not established. **Elderly:** Age-related renal impairment may require dosage adjustment.

INTERACTIONS

DRUG: None significant. **HERBAL:** None significant. **FOOD:** None known. **LAB VALUES:** None significant.

AVAILABILITY (Rx)

Injection Solution: 1 mg/mL, 10-mL vial. **Injection Solution, Premix:** 200 mcg/mL (100 mL, 200 mL).

M

ADMINISTRATION/HANDLING

 IV

Reconstitution • For IV infusion, dilute 20-mg (20-mL) vial with 80 mL 0.9% NaCl or D₅W to provide concentration of 0.2 mg/mL (200 mcg/mL).
Rate of administration • For IV injection (loading dose), administer undiluted slowly over 10 min. • Monitor for arrhythmias, hypotension during IV therapy; reduce or temporarily discontinue infusion until condition stabilizes. Infuse via infusion pump.
Storage • Diluted solutions stable for 72 hrs at room temperature.

IV COMPATIBILITIES

Amiodarone, calcium gluconate, dexmedetomidine, magnesium sulfate, norepinephrine, potassium chloride, vasopressin.

INDICATIONS/ROUTES/DOSAGE

Note: Loading doses are usually not recommended due to risk of hypotension.

HF (With Reduced Ejection Fraction)
IV infusion: ADULTS, ELDERLY: Initially, 0.125–0.25 mcg/kg/min. **Range:** 0.125–0.75 mcg/kg/min. Titrate based on clinical goal.

Dosage in Renal Impairment
CrCl 10–50 mL/min: Initially, 0.0625–0.125 mcg/kg/min. Titrate cautiously esp. in pts with worsening renal function.

Dosage in Hepatic Impairment
No dose adjustment.

SIDE EFFECTS

Occasional (3%–1%): Headache, hypotension. **Rare (less than 1%):** Angina, chest pain.

ADVERSE EFFECTS/TOXIC REACTIONS

Supraventricular/ventricular arrhythmias, nonstained ventricular tachycardia, sustained ventricular tachycardia may occur. Ventricular fibrillation (0.2% of pts) has been documented.

NURSING CONSIDERATIONS

BASELINE ASSESSMENT
Obtain BN peptide. Assess B/P, heart rate before treatment begins and during IV therapy. Assess lung sounds; observe for edema.

INTERVENTION/EVALUATION
Monitor B/P, heart rate, cardiac output, ECG, serum potassium, renal function, signs/symptoms of HF.

mirabegron

mir-a-**beg**-ron
(Myrbetriq)

◆**CLASSIFICATION**

PHARMACOTHERAPEUTIC: Beta₃-adrenergic agonist. **CLINICAL:** Smooth muscle relaxant.

USES

Overactive bladder: Treatment of overactive bladder in adults with symptoms of urinary incontinence, urgency, frequency as monotherapy or in combination with antimuscarinic agent. **Neurogenic detrusor overactivity:** Treatment of neurogenic detrusor overactivity in pts 3 yrs of age and older and weighing 35 kg or greater.

PRECAUTIONS

Contraindications: Hypersensitivity to mirabegron. **Cautions:** Bladder outlet obstruction, pts taking antimuscarinic medications (increases urinary retention), mild to moderate hepatic/renal impairment, pts at risk for QTc interval prolongation (congenital long QT syndrome, HF, medications that prolong QTc interval, hypokalemia, hypomagnesemia). Not recommended in pts with severe uncontrolled hypertension (SBP equal to or greater than 180 mm Hg and/or DBP equal to or greater than 110 mm Hg).

ACTION

Relaxes detrusor smooth muscle of bladder through beta$_3$ stimulation during storage phase of urinary bladder fill–void cycle. **Therapeutic Effect:** Increases bladder capacity, reduces symptoms of urinary urgency, increased voiding frequency, urge incontinence, nocturia.

PHARMACOKINETICS

Widely distributed. Protein binding: 71%. Eliminated in urine (55%), feces (35%). **Half-life:** 50 hrs.

⧗ LIFESPAN CONSIDERATIONS

Pregnancy/Lactation: Unknown if distributed in breast milk. **Children:** Safety and efficacy not established. **Elderly:** No age-related precautions noted.

INTERACTIONS

DRUG: May increase concentration/effects of **aripiprazole, iloperidone, risperidone.** May decrease concentration/effect of **metoprolol, tamoxifen.** **HERBAL:** None significant. **FOOD:** None known. **LAB VALUES:** May increase GGT, LDH; temporarily increase ALT, AST.

AVAILABILITY (Rx)

🐚 **Tablets, Extended-Release:** 25 mg, 50 mg. **Oral Suspension, Extended-Release:** 8 mg/mL after reconstitution.

ADMINISTRATION/HANDLING

PO
Tablets: • Give without regard to food. • Give whole with water. Do not crush, divide, or allow chewing. • **Oral Suspension:** • Give with food. • Use an appropriate dosing device. • Store suspension at room temperature for up to 28 days.

INDICATIONS/ROUTES/DOSAGE

Overactive Bladder
PO: ADULTS, ELDERLY: Initially, 25 mg once daily. May increase to 50 mg once daily after 4–8 wks.

Neurogenic Detrusor Overactivity
PO: CHILDREN 3 YRS OR OLDER WEIGHING 35 KG OR MORE: *(Tablet):* 25 mg once daily. After 4–8 wks, may increase to 50 mg once daily. *(Oral Suspension):* 6 mL (48 mg) once daily. After 4–8 wks, increase to 10 mL (80 mg) once daily. **22–34 KG:** *(Oral Suspension):* Initially, 32 mg once daily. After 4–8 wks, may increase up to 64 mg/day. **11–21 KG:** *(Oral Suspension):* Initially, 24 mg once daily. After 4–8 wks, may increase up to 48 mg/day.

Dosage in Renal Impairment
Mild to moderate impairment: No dosage adjustment. **Severe impairment:** Do not exceed 25 mg once daily.

Dosage in Hepatic Impairment
Mild impairment: No dosage adjustment. **Moderate impairment:** Do not exceed 25 mg once daily. **Severe impairment:** Not recommended.

SIDE EFFECTS

Occasional (9%–4%): Hypertension, headache, nasopharyngitis. **Rare (2%–1%):** Constipation, arthralgia, diarrhea, tachycardia, fatigue.

ADVERSE EFFECTS/TOXIC REACTIONS

Worsening of preexisting hypertension reported infrequently. UTI occurred in 6% of pts, influenza in 3%, and upper respiratory infection in 1.5%.

NURSING CONSIDERATIONS

BASELINE ASSESSMENT
Obtain B/P. Receive full medication history, and screen for possible drug interactions. Monitor I&O (particularly in pts with history of urinary retention).

INTERVENTION/EVALUATION
Obtain bladder scan and palpate bladder to monitor for urinary retention. Measure B/P near end of dosing interval (determines whether B/P is controlled throughout day). Monitor B/P periodically especially in hypertensive pts. For

pts taking digoxin, monitor digoxin serum level for therapeutic effect (very narrow line between therapeutic and toxic level). Assess pulse for quality, irregular rate, bradycardia. Question for evidence of headache.

PATIENT/FAMILY TEACHING
• Report urinary retention. • Do not use nasal decongestants, over-the-counter cold preparations without doctor approval. • Restrict salt, alcohol intake.

---

mirikizumab-mrkz

mir-i-**kiz**-ue-mab
(Omvoh)
Do not confuse mirikizumab with bimekizumab, ixekizumab, risankizumab, tildarkizumab, ustekinumab, or Omvoh with Entyvio.

◆CLASSIFICATION

PHARMACOTHERAPEUTIC: Interleukin-23 antagonist, immunoglobulin G4 (IgG4) monoclonal antibody. **CLINICAL:** Anti ulcerative colitis agent.

USES
Treatment of moderately to severely active ulcerative colitis in adults.

PRECAUTIONS
Contraindications: Hypersensitivity to mirikizumab. **Cautions:** Hepatic impairment, conditions predisposing to infection (e.g., diabetes, immunocompromised pts, renal failure, open wounds), chronic opportunistic infections (e.g., herpesvirus infection, fungal infections); prior exposure to tuberculosis (TB) or use in pts who reside or travel to areas where TB is endemic. Avoid use during active infection or active TB infection. Concomitant use of live vaccines is not recommended. Consider other treatment options in pts with hepatic cirrhosis.

ACTION
Selectively binds to p19 subunit of interleukin-23 (IL-23) (proinflammatory cytokine involved in pathogenesis of ulcerative colitis) preventing downstream release of proinflammatory cytokines. **Therapeutic Effect:** Reduces inflammation, ulceration of the colon and rectum.

PHARMACOKINETICS
Widely distributed. Degraded into small peptides and amino acids via catabolic pathway. Peak plasma concentration: 5 days (subcutaneous route). **Half-life:** 9.3 days.

⧗ LIFESPAN CONSIDERATIONS
Pregnancy/Lactation: Unknown if distributed in breast milk. However, human immunoglobulin G (IgG) is present in breast milk and is known to cross the placenta. **Children:** Safety and efficacy not established. **Elderly:** No age-related precautions noted.

INTERACTIONS
DRUG: **Vaccines (live)** may increase risk of infection following administration (avoid use). **HERBAL:** None significant. **FOOD:** None known. **LAB VALUES:** May increase serum ALT, AST, bilirubin.

AVAILABILITY (Rx)
Injection Solution: 300 mg/15 mL (20 mg/mL). **Injection Solution (Prefilled Syringe, Injector Pen):** 100 mg/mL.

ADMINISTRATION/HANDLING
 IV

Infusion Guidelines • Do not administer as IV push or bolus. • Infuse via dedicated IV access. Do not mix or infuse with other medications or IV solutions other than 0.9% NaCl or D5W. • Upon completion of

---

infusion, flush the infusion line with 0.9% NaCl or D5W at the same rate as infusion to ensure the entire dose is administered. Total time to flush the IV line is in addition to the 30-min infusion time.

Preparation • Visually inspect the vial solution for particulate matter or discoloration. Solution should appear clear to opalescent, colorless to slightly yellow or slightly brown. Do not use if solution is cloudy, discolored, or visible particles are observed. • Dilute in 50-250 mL 0.9% NaCl or D5W infusion bag. • Mix by gentle inversion. Do not shake. • Discard unused portions.

Rate of administration • Infuse over 30 min. **Storage** • Refrigerate unused vials in original carton to protect from light. Do not freeze. • May refrigerate diluted solution for up to 48 hrs or store at room temperature for up to 5 hrs (includes time of vial puncture). Do not shake.

SQ

Preparation • Remove prefilled syringe or injector pen from refrigerator and allow solution to warm to room temperature (approx. 30 min). Do not shake or agitate. • Visually inspect for particulate matter or discoloration. Solution should appear clear to opalescent, colorless to slightly yellow or slightly brown. Do not use if solution is cloudy, discolored, or visible particles are observed.

Administration • Dose requires 2 consecutive injections at different sites. • Insert needle subcutaneously into outer thigh, abdomen, or back of upper arm and inject solution. • Do not inject within 2 inches (5 cm) of navel or into areas of active skin disease or injury such as sunburns, skin rashes, inflammation, skin infections, or psoriatic lesions. • Rotate injection sites. • Do not administer IV or intramuscularly. • If a dose is missed, administer as soon as possible, then give next dose at regularly scheduled time.

Storage • Refrigerate unused prefilled syringe or injector pen in original carton to protect from light. Do not freeze. • May store at room temperature for up to 2 wks. Once stored at room temperature, do not return to refrigerator.

INDICATIONS/ROUTES/DOSAGE

Ulcerative Colitis

IV, SQ: **ADULTS:** **(Induction phase):** 300 mg IV at week 0, 4, and 8. **(Maintenance phase):** 200 mg SQ (given as 2 consecutive injections of 100 mg each) at week 12, then q4wks thereafter.

Dosage in Renal Impairment

Mild to moderate impairment: No dose adjustment. **Severe impairment:** Not specified; use caution.

Dosage in Hepatic Impairment

Not specified; use caution.

SIDE EFFECTS

Occasional (9%–7%): Injections site reactions (erythema, hypersensitivity, pain, urticaria), arthralgia. **Rare (4%):** Rash.

ADVERSE EFFECTS/TOXIC REACTIONS

Hypersensitivity reactions including anaphylaxis, mucocutaneous erythema, pruritus may occur. May increase risk of infections, including herpes viral infection, tuberculosis, upper respiratory tract infections. Hepatotoxicity (serum ALT/AST elevation up to 8–10 times upper limited of normal [ULN] with total serum bilirubin level 2.4 times ULN) was reported.

NURSING CONSIDERATIONS

BASELINE ASSESSMENT

Obtain LFT. Complete age-appropriate immunizations per guidelines prior to initiation. Evaluate for active tuberculosis

M

and test for latent infection prior to initiation and periodically during therapy. An induration of 5 mm or greater with tuberculin skin testing should be considered a positive test result when assessing if treatment for latent tuberculosis is necessary. Screen for active or chronic infections. Question history of hepatic impairment. Assess pt's willingness to self-inject medication. Teach proper injection techniques. Establish baseline symptoms of ulcerative colitis (abdominal pain, diarrhea, fatigue, fever, rectal bleeding, urgency to defecate, weight loss).

INTERVENTION/EVALUATION

Monitor LFT for hepatotoxicity (bruising, jaundice, fatigue, right upper abdominal pain, nausea, vomiting, weight loss) for at least 24 wks as clinically indicated. Monitor for symptoms of tuberculosis (cough, fatigue, fever, hemoptysis, nocturnal sweating, weight loss), including those who tested negative for latent tuberculosis infection prior to initiation. Monitor for infections (body aches, cough, fatigue, fever), herpetic infections, upper respiratory tract infections. Interrupt or discontinue treatment if serious infection, opportunistic infection, or sepsis occurs and initiate appropriate antimicrobial therapy. Assess for improvement of ulcerative colitis symptoms.

PATIENT/FAMILY TEACHING

• Treatment may depress your immune system and reduce your ability to fight infection. Report symptoms of infection such as body aches, burning with urination, chills, cough, fatigue, fever. Avoid those with active infection. • Do not receive live vaccines. • Expect frequent tuberculosis screening. • Report travel plans to possible endemic areas. • A healthcare provider will show you how to properly prepare and inject your medication. You must demonstrate correct preparation and injection techniques before using medication at home. • Immediately report difficulty breathing, itching, hives, rash, swelling of the face or tongue; may indicate an allergic reaction. • Report liver problems (abdominal pain, bruising, clay-colored stool, fatigue, amber or dark colored urine, yellowing of the skin or eyes). • Worsening symptoms of ulcerative colitis may occur after stopping treatment.

mirtazapine

mir-**taz**-a-peen
(Remeron, Remeron Soltab)

■ **BLACK BOX ALERT** ■ Increased risk of suicidal thinking and behavior in pediatric and young adult pts (18–24 yrs) with major depressive disorder, other psychiatric disorders. Closely monitor all antidepressant-treated pts for clinical worsening and emergence of suicidal ideation behaviors.
Do not confuse Remeron with Premarin, Rozerem, or Zemuron.

◆CLASSIFICATION

PHARMACOTHERAPEUTIC: Alpha 2-antagonist. **CLINICAL:** Antidepressant.

USES

Treatment of unipolar major depressive disorder (MDD) in adults. **OFF-LABEL:** Prophylaxis of chronic tension-type headache, panic disorder.

PRECAUTIONS

Contraindications: Hypersensitivity to mirtazapine. Use of MAOIs to treat psychiatric disorders (concurrently or within 14 days of discontinuing either MAOI or mirtazapine), initiation of mirtazapine in pts receiving linezolid or IV methylene blue. **Cautions:** Renal/hepatic impairment, elderly, seizure disorder, suicidal ideation or behavior, alcoholism, concurrent medications that lower seizure threshold, cardiovascular disease, pts at risk for QTc interval prolongation (congenital long QT syndrome, HF, medications that prolong QTc interval, hypokalemia, hypomagnesemia).

ACTION

Acts as antagonist at presynaptic alpha$_2$-adrenergic receptors, increasing norepinephrine, serotonin neurotransmission. Has low anticholinergic activity. **Therapeutic Effect:** Relieves depression.

PHARMACOKINETICS

Widely distributed. Protein binding: 85%. Metabolized in liver. Primarily excreted in urine. Unknown if removed by hemodialysis. **Half-life:** 20–40 hrs (longer in males [37 hrs] than females [26 hrs]).

⧗ LIFESPAN CONSIDERATIONS

Pregnancy/Lactation: Unknown if distributed in breast milk. **Children:** Safety and efficacy not established. **Elderly:** Age-related renal impairment may require dosage adjustment.

INTERACTIONS

DRUG: **Alcohol, CNS depressant medications** (e.g., **LORazepam, morphine, zolpidem**) may increase impairment of cognition, motor skills. **Serotonergic drugs** (e.g., **venlafaxine**) may increase risk of serotonin syndrome. **Strong CYP3A4 inducers** (e.g., **carBAMazepine, phenytoin, rifAMPin**) may decrease concentration/effect. **Strong CYP3A4 inhibitors** (e.g., **clarithromycin, ketoconazole, ritonavir**) may increase concentration/effect. **MAOIs** (e.g., **phenelzine, selegiline**) may increase risk of neuroleptic malignant syndrome, hypertensive crisis, severe seizures. **QT interval–prolonging medications** (e.g., **amiodarone, azithromycin, ciprofloxacin, haloperidol, methadone, sotalol**) may increase risk of QTc interval prolongation. **HERBAL:** **Herbals with sedative properties** (e.g., **chamomile, kava kava, valerian**) may increase CNS depression. **St. John's wort** may decrease concentration/effects, may increase risk of serotonin syndrome. **FOOD:** None known. **LAB VALUES:** May increase serum cholesterol, triglycerides, ALT.

AVAILABILITY (Rx)

Tablets: 7.5 mg, 15 mg, 30 mg, 45 mg. **Tablets, Orally Disintegrating:** 15 mg, 30 mg, 45 mg.

ADMINISTRATION/HANDLING

PO
• Give without regard to food.

Orally Disintegrating Tablets
• Give without regard to food. • Do not split tablet. • Place on tongue; dissolves without water.

INDICATIONS/ROUTES/DOSAGE

Depression
Note: When discontinuing, gradually taper dose to minimize withdrawal symptoms and to allow detection of re-emerging symptoms. **PO: ADULTS:** Initially, 15 mg at bedtime. May increase by 15 mg/day q1–2wks. **Maximum:** 45 mg/day. **ELDERLY:** Initially, 7.5 mg at bedtime. May increase by 7.5–15 mg/day q1–2wks. **Maximum:** 45 mg/day.

Dosage in Renal/Hepatic Impairment
Use caution.

SIDE EFFECTS

Frequent (54%–12%): Drowsiness, dry mouth, increased appetite, constipation, weight gain. **Occasional (89%–4%):** Asthenia, dizziness, flu-like symptoms, abnormal dreams. **Rare:** Abdominal discomfort, vasodilation, paresthesia, acne, dry skin, thirst, arthralgia.

ADVERSE EFFECTS/TOXIC REACTIONS

Higher incidence of seizures than with tricyclic antidepressants (esp. in pts with no

M

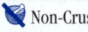

history of seizures). Overdose may produce cardiovascular effects (severe orthostatic hypotension, dizziness, tachycardia, palpitations, arrhythmias). Abrupt discontinuation from prolonged therapy may produce headache, malaise, nausea, vomiting, vivid dreams. Agranulocytosis occurs rarely.

NURSING CONSIDERATIONS

BASELINE ASSESSMENT

Assess mental status, appearance, behavior, speech pattern, level of interest, mood. Obtain baseline weight. Obtain full medication history and screen for interactions. Question history of hepatic/renal impairment, seizure disorder, cardiovascular disease, suicidal behavior and ideation.

INTERVENTION/EVALUATION

For pts on long-term therapy, renal function, LFT, CBC should be performed periodically. Supervise suicidal-risk pt closely during early therapy (as depression lessens, energy level improves, increasing suicide potential). Children, adolescents are at increased risk for suicidal thoughts/behavior and worsening of depression, esp. during first few mos of therapy. Assess appearance, behavior, speech pattern, level of interest, mood. Monitor for hypotension, arrhythmias.

PATIENT/FAMILY TEACHING

• Take as single bedtime dose. • Avoid alcohol, depressant/sedating medications. • Avoid tasks requiring alertness, motor skills until response to drug established. • Report worsening depression, suicidal ideation, unusual changes in behavior. • There is a high risk of interactions with other medications. Do not take newly prescribed medications unless approved by prescriber who originally started treatment. Do not take herbal products. • Treatment may affect the electrical conduction of the heart, which may lead to arrhythmias; report chest pain, dizziness, fainting, palpitations.

mirvetuximab soravtansine-gynx

mir-ve-**tux**-i-mab soe-rav-**tan**-seen (Elahere)

■ **BLACK BOX ALERT** ■ Severe ocular toxicities, including dry eye, eye pain, keratopathy, photophobia, uveitis, visual impairment, may occur. An ophthalmic examination with a slit lamp and visual acuity should be performed at baseline, every other cycle for the first eight cycles, and as clinically indicated. Administer prophylactic artificial tears and ophthalmic topical steroids as recommended. Reduce dose, withhold, or permanently discontinue treatment based on clinical severity of ocular toxicities. **Do not confuse mirvetuximab soravtansine with brentuximab, cetuximab, dinutuximab, or margetuximab or Elahere with Eliquis.**

◆CLASSIFICATION

PHARMACOTHERAPEUTIC: Folate receptor alpha (FRa)–directed antibody/microtubular inhibitor conjugate (ADC). **CLINICAL:** Antineoplastic.

USES

Treatment of adults with folate receptor-alpha–positive, platinum-resistant epithelial ovarian, fallopian tube, or primary peritoneal cancer who have received one to three prior systemic treatment regimens.

PRECAUTIONS

Contraindications: Hypersensitivity to mirvetuximab soravtansine-gynx. **Cautions:** Baseline cytopenias, mild hepatic impairment (avoid use in pts with moderate to severe hepatic impairment), interstitial lung disease (e.g., COPD, sarcoidosis, connective disease disease), conditions predisposing to infection (e.g., diabetes, renal failure, immunocompromised pts, open wounds). History of peripheral neuropathy.

ACTION

An antibody/drug conjugate. Antibody is directed against folate receptor alpha (FR*a*), a protein highly expressed in ovarian cancer, and a conjugate (DM4), a microtubule inhibitor attached to the antibody. Upon binding to FR*a*, mirvetuximab is internalized followed by intracellular release of DM4, disrupting the microtubule network within the cell. **Therapeutic Effect:** Cell cycle arrest and apoptosis (cell death).

PHARMACOKINETICS

Widely distributed. Portions of monoclonal antibody are metabolized via catabolism into small peptides. Portions of DM4 are metabolized in liver. Protein binding: Greater than 99%. Peak plasma concentration: 3 days. Steady state reached in 24 days. Excretion not specified (DM4 detected in urine within 24 hrs of infusion). **Half-life:** 5 days.

⧗ LIFESPAN CONSIDERATIONS

Pregnancy/Lactation: Avoid pregnancy; may cause fetal harm. Females of reproductive potential must use effective contraception during treatment and for at least 7 mos after discontinuation. Unknown if distributed in breast milk. Breastfeeding not recommended during treatment and for at least 1 mo after discontinuation. **Children:** Safety and efficacy not established. **Elderly:** No age-related precautions noted.

INTERACTIONS

DRUG: Strong **CYP3A4 inhibitors (e.g., clarithromycin, ketoconazole, ritonavir)** may increase concentration/effect. **HERBAL:** None significant. **FOOD:** **Grapefruit products** may increase concentration/effect. **LAB VALUES:** May increase serum alkaline phosphatase, ALT, AST. May decrease Hgb, leukocytes, lymphocytes, neutrophils, platelets; serum albumin, magnesium, potassium.

AVAILABILITY (Rx)

Injection Solution: 100/20 mL (5 mg/mL).

ADMINISTRATION/HANDLING

 IV

Infusion guidelines • Must be administered by a healthcare professional trained in the management of infusion reactions. • Do not infuse with other medications or IV solutions except D5W. • Infuse via a dedicated IV line using a sterile 0.2- or 022-micron polyethersulfone (PES) in-line filter. • If no infusion reactions occur with previous dose, may initiate subsequent infusions at the rate previously tolerated.

Premedication • Premedicate with dexAMETHasone 10 mg IV, diphenhydrAMINE 25–50 mg PO or IV, acetaminophen 325–650 mg PO or IV approx. 30 mins prior to each dose and a 5-HT$_3$ serotonin receptor antagonist (or equivalent) prior to each dose and as needed thereafter. • Consider administration of a corticosteroid the day before infusion in pts who experienced an infusion-related reaction. • Administer one drop of topical corticosteroid eye drops in each eye 6 times/day starting the day before each infusion until day 4, then one drop in each eye 4 times/day for days 5–8 of each cycle. Give lubricating eye drops at least 4 times/day (and as needed) during treatment.

Dilution • Must be prepared by personnel trained in aseptic manipulations and admixing of hazardous drugs. • Calculate dose based on adjusted ideal body weight (AIBW). • Allow refrigerated vials to warm to room temperature. • Visually inspect for particulate matter or discoloration. Solution should appear clear to slightly opalescent and colorless. Do not use if solution is cloudy or discolored. • Gently swirl each vial prior to dilution. • Dilute in an infusion bag containing D5W to a final concentration of 1–2 mg/mL. • Gently invert to

M

mix. Do not shake or agitate. • Discard unused portions of vial.

Rate of administration • Infuse at 1 mg/min. • If no reactions occur after 30 mins, may increase infusion rate to 3 mg/min. May further increase infusion rate to 5 mg/min after an additional 30 mins if no infusion reactions occur. **Maximum infusion rate:** 5 mg/min.

Infusion reactions • **Grade 1 reactions:** Continue same infusion rate. • **Grade 2 reactions:** Interrupt infusion and provide supportive measures. When symptoms improve, resume infusion at 50% of the previous rate. May increase infusion rate as appropriate if infusion reactions do not recur. **Grade 3 or 4 reactions:** Discontinue infusion and provide supportive measures.

Storage • Refrigerate unused vials in original carton. Protect from light. Do not freeze. • Diluted solution may be refrigerated for up to 12 hrs or stored at room temperature up to 8 hrs. Do not freeze. • If refrigerated, allow diluted solution to warm to room temperature.

 IV INCOMPATABILITIES

0.9% NaCl.

INDICATIONS/ROUTES/DOSAGE

Epithelial Ovarian, Fallopian Tube, or Primary Peritoneal Cancer (Folate Receptor-Alpha Positive, Platinum-Resistant)

IV: **ADULTS, ELDERLY:** 6 mg/kg adjusted ideal body weight (AIBW) once q3wks of 21-day cycle until disease progression or unacceptable toxicity.

Dose Reduction Schedule

First dose reduction: 5 mg/kg AIBW. **Second dose reduction:** 4 mg/kg AIBW. **Unable to tolerate 4 mg/kg dose AIBW:** Permanently discontinue.

Dose Modification

Based on Common Terminology Criteria for Adverse Events (CTCAE).

Keratitis/Keratopathy

Nonconfluent superficial keratitis: Monitor and continue same dose. **Confluent superficial keratitis; cornea epithelial defect; three-line or more loss in best corrected visual acuity:** Withhold treatment until improved or resolved, then resume same dose or consider dose reduction. **Corneal ulcer; stromal opacity; best corrected distance visual acuity 20/200 or worse:** Withhold treatment until improved or resolved, then resume at reduced dose. **Corneal perforation:** Permanently discontinue.

Peripheral Neuropathy

Grade 2 peripheral neuropathy: Withhold treatment until improved to Grade 1 or less, then resume at reduced dose. **Grade 3 or 4 peripheral neuropathy:** Permanently discontinue.

Pneumonitis

Grade 1 pneumonitis: Monitor and continue same dose. **Grade 2 pneumonitis:** Withhold treatment until improved to Grade 1 or less, then resume at same dose or consider dose reduction. **Grade 3 or 4 pneumonitis:** Permanently discontinue.

Uveitis

Grade 1 (rare cell in anterior chamber): Monitor and continue same dose. **Grade 2 (1–2+ cell or flare in anterior chamber):** Withhold treatment until improved to Grade 1 or less, then resume at same dose. **Grade 3 (3+ cell or flare in anterior chamber):** Withhold treatment until improved to Grade 1 or less, then resume at reduced dose. **Grade 4 (hypopyon):** Permanently discontinue.

Other Adverse Reactions

Any other Grade 3 adverse reactions: Withhold treatment until improved to Grade 1 or less, then resume at reduced dose. **Any other Grade 4 adverse reactions:** Permanently discontinue.

Dosage in Renal Impairment

Mild to moderate impairment: No dose adjustment. **Severe impairment, ESRD:** Not specified; use caution.

Dosage in Hepatic Impairment

Mild impairment: No dose adjustment. **Moderate to severe impairment:** Avoid use.

SIDE EFFECTS

Frequent (50%–27%): Blurred vision, vitreous floaters, reduced visual acuity, diplopia, accommodation disorder, keratitis, presbyopia, corneal deposits, refraction disorder, visual impairment, fatigue, asthenia, nausea, abdominal pain, diarrhea, constipation, dry eye. **Occasional (19%–10%):** Vomiting, decreased appetite, cataract, photophobia, arthralgia, dyspnea, abdominal distension, myalgia.

ADVERSE EFFECTS/TOXIC REACTIONS

Myelosuppression (anemia, leukopenia, lymphopenia, neutropenia, thrombocytopenia) is an expected response to therapy. Ocular toxicities including corneal epithelial microcysts, dry eye, eye pain, keratopathy, photophobia, uveitis, visual impairment reported in 61% of pts. Median onset of ocular toxicities was 1.2 mos. Life-threatening interstitial lung disease, pneumonitis reported in 10% of pts. Peripheral neuropathy including hypoesthesia, hyperesthesia, gait disturbance, muscular weakness, paresthesia, peripheral motor/sensorimotor neuropathy, neuropathic pain, polyneuropathy reported in 36% of pts.

NURSING CONSIDERATIONS

BASELINE ASSESSMENT

Obtain CBC, LFT; pregnancy test in females of reproductive potential. Confirm compliance with effective contraception. Verify presence of folate receptor-alpha expression in tumor specimen. Calculate pt's AIBW using formula per manufacturer guidelines. An ophthalmic examination with a slit lamp and visual acuity should be performed at baseline, every other cycle for the first eight cycles, and as clinically indicated. Administer in an environment equipped to monitor for and manage infusion-related reactions. Question for prior infusion-related reactions before each infusion. Question history of hepatic impairment, interstitial lung disease. Receive full medication history and screen for interactions. Screen for active infection. Offer emotional support.

INTERVENTION/EVALUATION

Monitor CBC, LFT as clinically indicated. Ophthalmic exams with a slit lamp should be performed to assess for eye toxicities. Routinely assess visual acuity. Diligently monitor for infusion reactions during each infusion. If reactions occur, interrupt or decrease the infusion rate and treat symptoms; early detection is vital. Continue administration of ophthalmic topical steroids and lubricating eye drops per manufacturer guidelines. Monitor for peripheral neuropathy (gait disturbance, incoordination, neuropathic pain, numbness, weakness). Consider ABG, radiologic test if pneumonitis (excessive cough, dyspnea, fever, hypoxia) is suspected. Consider treatment with corticosteroids if pneumonitis is confirmed. Monitor for infections (cough, fatigue, fever). Monitor daily pattern of bowel activity, stool consistency.

PATIENT/FAMILY TEACHING

• Treatment may depress your immune system response and reduce your ability to fight infection. Report symptoms of infection such as body aches, chills, cough, fatigue, fever. Avoid those with active infection. • Report symptoms of bone marrow depression (e.g., bruising, fatigue, fever, shortness of breath, weight loss; bleeding easily, bloody urine or stool). • Immediately report symptoms of infusion-related reactions such as chills, cough, difficulty breathing, itching, palpitations. Severe reactions may require emergency care. • Pretreatment with acetaminophen, antihistamines, steroidal anti-inflammatories may help reduce infusion reactions. • Treatment may cause severe eye toxicities, which may lead to severe vision loss, irritation, ulcers of the eye. Expect frequent eye examinations. It is essential to stay compliant with steroid eye drops and lubricating eye drops. Immediately report eye symptoms despite preventive care. Avoid wearing contact lenses. Changes of vision may impair driving or reading. Use caution when driving or operating machinery. • Report liver problems (abdominal pain, bruising, clay-colored stool, amber or dark-colored urine, yellowing of the skin or eyes), inflammation of the lung (excessive cough, difficulty breathing, fever, chest pain), nervous system changes (gait disturbance, lack of coordination; numbness, pain, trouble walking). • Use effective contraception to avoid pregnancy. Do not breastfeed. • There is a high risk of interactions with other medications. Do not take newly prescribed medications unless approved by prescriber who originally started treatment.

---

modafinil

TOP 100

moe-**daf**-i-nil
(Alertec ✦, <u>Provigil</u>)

◆CLASSIFICATION

PHARMACOTHERAPEUTIC: Alpha$_1$-agonist, CNS stimulant (Schedule IV). **CLINICAL:** Wakefulness-promoting agent, antinarcoleptic.

USES

Treatment of excessive daytime sleepiness associated with narcolepsy, shift work sleep disorder, adjunct therapy for obstructive sleep apnea/hypopnea syndrome. **OFF-LABEL:** Fatigue related to cancer (receiving active treatment), multiple sclerosis.

Parkinson's disease (excessive daytime sleepiness), major depressive disorder (augments antidepressants).

PRECAUTIONS

Contraindications: Hypersensitivity to modafinil, armodafinil. **Cautions:** History of clinically significant mitral valve prolapse, left ventricular hypertrophy, renal/hepatic impairment, angina, cardiac disease, myocardial ischemia, recent MI, preexisting psychosis or bipolar disorder, Tourette's syndrome.

ACTION

Exact mechanism unknown. Increases dopamine in brain. Increases alpha activity, decreasing delta, theta, brain wave activity. **Therapeutic Effect:** Reduces number of sleep episodes, total daytime sleep. Increases mental alertness.

PHARMACOKINETICS

Widely distributed. Protein binding: 60%. Widely distributed. Metabolized in liver. Excreted by kidneys. Unknown if removed by hemodialysis. **Half-life:** 15 hrs.

⧗ LIFESPAN CONSIDERATIONS

Pregnancy/Lactation: Unknown if excreted in breast milk. Use caution if given to pregnant women. **Children:** Safety and efficacy not established in pts younger than 16 yrs. **Elderly:** Age-related renal/hepatic impairment may require decreased dosage.

INTERACTIONS

DRUG: May decrease concentration/effect of **cycloSPORINE, oral contraceptives. Alcohol** may decrease therapeutic effect. **Strong CYP3A4 inducers (e.g., carBAMazepine, phenytoin, rifAMPin)** may decrease concentration/effect. **HERBAL:** None significant. **FOOD:** None known. **LAB VALUES:** None significant.

AVAILABILITY (Rx)

Tablets: (Provigil): 100 mg, 200 mg.

ADMINISTRATION/HANDLING

PO
• Give without regard to food.

INDICATIONS/ROUTES/DOSAGE

**Narcolepsy, Obstructive Sleep Apnea/
Hypopnea Syndrome**
PO: ADULTS: 200 mg/day in the morning.
ELDERLY: 100 mg/day in the morning.

Shift Work Sleep Disorder
PO: ADULTS: 200 mg about 1 hr before
start of work shift.

Dosage in Renal Impairment
No dose adjustment.

Dosage in Hepatic Impairment
Mild to moderate impairment: No
dose adjustment. Reduce dose 50% with
severe impairment.

SIDE EFFECTS

Generally well tolerated. **Occasional
(5%):** Headache, nausea, dizziness, insomnia, palpitations, diarrhea.

ADVERSE EFFECTS/TOXIC REACTIONS

Agitation, excitation, increased B/P,
insomnia may occur. Psychiatric disturbances (anxiety, hallucinations, suicidal
ideation), serious allergic reactions
(angioedema, Stevens-Johnson syndrome) have been noted.

NURSING CONSIDERATIONS

BASELINE ASSESSMENT
Obtain baseline evidence of narcolepsy
or other sleep disorders, including pattern, environmental situations, length of
sleep episodes. Question for sudden loss
of muscle tone (cataplexy) precipitated
by strong emotional responses before
sleep episode. Assess frequency/severity
of sleep episodes before drug therapy.

INTERVENTION/EVALUATION
Monitor sleep pattern, evidence of restlessness during sleep, length of insomnia

episodes at night. Assess for dizziness,
anxiety; initiate fall precautions.

PATIENT/FAMILY TEACHING
• Avoid alcohol. • Do not increase dose
without physician approval. • Use alternative contraceptives during therapy and 1
mo after discontinuing modafinil (reduces
effectiveness of oral contraceptives).

mometasone

moe-**met**-a-sone
(Asmanex, Asmanex HFA Apo-
Mometasone ♣, Propel, Sinuva)

FIXED-COMBINATION(S)

Dulera: mometasone/formoterol
(beta-adrenergic agonist): 100 mcg/5
mcg, 200 mcg/5 mcg. **Ryaltris:** mo-
metasone/olopatadine (an antihistamine) 25 mcg/665 mcg per spray.

◆CLASSIFICATION

PHARMACOTHERAPEUTIC: Adrenocorticosteroid. **CLINICAL:** Anti-
inflammatory.

USES

Nasal: upper respiratory allergies:
Relief of hay fever, nasal congestion,
runny nose, sneezing, itchy nose in
adults, children 2 yrs and older. **Seasonal allergic rhinitis (prophylaxis):** Prophylaxis of nasal symptoms
from seasonal allergic rhinitis in adults
and children 12 yrs and older. **Nasal
polyps:** Treatment of nasal polyps in
adults. **Inhalation:** Maintenance treatment of asthma as prophylactic therapy
in adults and children 4 yrs and older.
(Asmanex) and children 5 yrs and
older (Asmanex HFA) **Topical:** Relief of
inflammatory, pruritic manifestations of
steroid-responsive dermatoses in adults
and children 2 yrs and older (cream,
ointment), adults and children 12 yrs
and older (lotion, solution). **OFF-LABEL:**

M

Nasal: Nonallergic rhinitis, rhinosinusitis (adjunctive acute treatment), rhinosinusitis (chronic), rhinosinusitis (acute treatment).

PRECAUTIONS

Contraindications: Hypersensitivity to mometasone. Primary treatment of status asthmaticus or acute bronchospasm. **Cautions:** Thyroid/hepatic/renal impairment, elderly, diabetes, cardiovascular disease, glaucoma, cataracts, myasthenia gravis, pts at risk for osteoporosis, seizures, GI disease (e.g., ulcer, colitis); following MI. Untreated systemic fungal, viral, bacterial infections.

ACTION

Inhibits formation, release, and activity of mediators of inflammation (e.g., histamine, kinins). Reverses the dilation and increased nasal permeability of inflammation. **Therapeutic Effect:** Improves symptoms of asthma, rhinitis.

PHARMACOKINETICS

Undetectable in plasma. Protein binding: 98%–99%. Swallowed portion undergoes extensive metabolism. Excreted in bile (74%), urine (8%). **Half-life:** 5 hrs.

⌛ LIFESPAN CONSIDERATIONS

Pregnancy/Lactation: Unknown if drug crosses placenta or is distributed in breast milk. **Children:** Prolonged treatment/high doses may decrease short-term growth rate, cortisol secretion. **Elderly:** No age-related precautions noted.

INTERACTIONS

DRUG: May increase concentration/effect of **desmopressin.** May decrease concentration/effect of **aldesleukin.** **HERBAL:** None significant. **FOOD:** None known. **LAB VALUES:** None significant.

AVAILABILITY (Rx)

Cream: 0.1%. **Lotion:** 0.1%. **Nasal Spray:** 50 mcg/spray. **Ointment:** 0.1%. **Powder for Oral Inhaler:** *(Asmanex):*

110 mcg (delivers 100 mcg/actuation), 220 mcg (delivers 200 mcg/actuation). *(Asmanex HFA):* 50 mcg/actuation, 100 mcg/actuation, 200 mcg/actuation.

ADMINISTRATION/HANDLING

Inhalation

Dry powder inhaler: Hold twisthaler straight up (base) on bottom, remove cap. • Exhale fully. • Firmly close lips around mouthpiece and inhale a fast, deep breath. • Hold breath for 10 sec. **Metered dose inhaler:** Shake well prior to use. • Exhale fully, close lips around mouthpiece, and breathe in deeply and slowly. Hold breath for 10 sec. After use, rinse mouth with water without swallowing.

Intranasal

• Instruct pt to clear nasal passages as much as possible before use. • Tilt head slightly forward. • Insert spray tip into nostril, pointing toward nasal passages, away from nasal septum. • Spray into one nostril while pt holds other nostril closed, concurrently inspiring through nose to permit medication as high into nasal passages as possible.

Topical

• Apply thin layer of cream, lotion, ointment to cover affected area. Rub in gently. • Do not cover area with occlusive dressing.

INDICATIONS/ROUTES/DOSAGE

Allergic Rhinitis (Seasonal)

Nasal spray: **ADULTS, ELDERLY, CHILDREN 12 YRS AND OLDER:** 2 sprays (100 mcg) in each nostril once daily. Total daily dose: 200 mcg. When used to prevent nasal rhinitis, begin 2–4 wks before start of pollen season. **CHILDREN 2–11 YRS:** 1 spray (50 mcg) in each nostril once daily. **Total daily dose:** 100 mcg.

Asthma

Inhalation: **ADULTS, ELDERLY, CHILDREN 12 YRS AND OLDER:** *(Asmanex HFA):* **(No prior treatment with inhaled corticosteroid):** Initially, 200 mcg twice daily. **Maximum:** 400 mcg twice daily (800 mcg/day). **(Previously received oral corticosteroids):** Initially, 400 mcg twice daily. **Maximum:** 400 mcg twice daily (800 mcg/day). **CHILDREN 5–11 YRS:** 100 mcg twice daily. **Maximum:** 200 mcg/day. *(Asmanex):* **(Previously received bronchodilators alone):** Initially, 220 mcg once daily in evening. **Maximum:** 440 mcg/day. **(Previously received inhaled corticosteroids):** Initially: 220 mcg once daily in evening. **Maximum:** 440 mcg/day. **(Previously received oral corticosteroids):** Initially, 440 mcg twice daily. **Maximum:** 880 mcg/day. **CHILDREN 4–11 YRS: (Regardless of prior therapy):** 110 mcg once daily in evening. Reduce predniSONE no faster than 2.5 mg/day beginning after at least 1 wk of mometasone.

Skin Disease
Topical: ADULTS, ELDERLY, CHILDREN 12 YRS AND OLDER: Apply cream, lotion, or ointment sparingly to affected area once daily.

Upper Respiratory Allergies
Nasal Spray: ADULTS, ELDERLY, CHILDREN 12 YRS AND OLDER: 2 sprays (100 mcg) in each nostril once daily. **CHILDREN 2-11 YRS:** 1 spray (50 mcg) in each nostril once daily.

Nasal Polyp
Nasal Spray: ADULTS, ELDERLY: 2 sprays (100 mcg) in each nostril once or twice daily. Total daily dose: 400 mcg.

Dosage in Renal/Hepatic Impairment
No dose adjustment.

SIDE EFFECTS
Occasional: Inhalation: Headache, allergic rhinitis, upper respiratory infection, muscle pain, fatigue. **Nasal:** Nasal irritation, stinging. **Topical:** Burning. **Rare: Inhalation:** Abdominal pain, dyspepsia, nausea. **Nasal:** Nasal/pharyngeal candidiasis. **Topical:** Pruritus.

ADVERSE EFFECTS/TOXIC REACTIONS
Acute hypersensitivity reaction (urticaria, angioedema, severe bronchospasm) occurs rarely. Transfer from systemic to local steroid therapy may unmask previously suppressed bronchial asthma condition.

NURSING CONSIDERATIONS
BASELINE ASSESSMENT
Question for hypersensitivity to any corticosteroids. Auscultate lung sounds. Teach proper use of nasal spray, oral inhaler.

INTERVENTION/EVALUATION
Monitor for relief of rhinitis, asthma symptoms. Assess lung sounds for wheezing, rales.

PATIENT/FAMILY TEACHING
• Do not change dose schedule or stop taking drug; must taper off gradually under medical supervision. **Nasal:** Report if symptoms do not improve; report if sneezing, nasal irritation occur. • Clear nasal passages prior to use. **Inhalation:** Inhale rapidly, deeply; rinse mouth after inhalation. • Not indicated for acute asthma attacks. **Topical:** Do not cover affected area with bandage, dressing.

montelukast

mon-**tee**-loo-kast
(Singulair)
Do not confuse Singulair with SINEquan.

◆CLASSIFICATION
PHARMACOTHERAPEUTIC: Leukotriene receptor inhibitor. **CLINICAL:** Antiasthmatic.

USES
Asthma: Prophylaxis, chronic treatment of asthma (in adults and children 12 mos and older). **Bronchoconstriction (exercise-induced prevention):** Prevention of exercise-induced bronchoconstriction (in adults and children 6 yrs and older). **Allergic rhinitis:** Relief of symptoms of seasonal allergic rhinitis (hay fever), (in adults and children 2 yrs and older), perennial

allergic rhinitis (in adults and children 6 mos and older). **OFF-LABEL:** Aspirin-exacerbated respiratory disease, hypersensitivity reactions, urticaria (chronic adjunct).

PRECAUTIONS

Contraindications: Hypersensitivity to montelukast. **Cautions:** Systemic corticosteroid treatment reduction during montelukast therapy. Concomitant use of CYP3A4 inducers. Not for use in acute asthma attacks.

ACTION

Binds to cysteinyl leukotriene receptors, inhibiting effects of leukotrienes on bronchial smooth muscle. **Therapeutic Effect:** Decreases bronchoconstriction, vascular permeability, mucosal edema, mucus production.

PHARMACOKINETICS

Route	Onset	Peak	Duration
PO	N/A	N/A	24 hrs
PO (chewable)	N/A	N/A	24 hrs

Widely distributed. Protein binding: 99%. Metabolized in liver. Excreted primarily in feces. **Half-life:** 2.7–5.5 hrs (slightly longer in elderly).

⏳ LIFESPAN CONSIDERATIONS

Pregnancy/Lactation: Unknown if distributed in breast milk. **Children:** Safety and efficacy not established in children younger than 6 mos. **Elderly:** No age-related precautions noted.

INTERACTIONS

DRUG: Gemfibrozil may increase concentration/effect. May increase adverse/toxic effect of **loxapine. HERBAL:** None significant. **FOOD:** None known. **LAB VALUES:** May increase serum ALT, AST, eosinophils.

AVAILABILITY (Rx)

Oral Granules: 4 mg per packet. **Tablets:** 10 mg. **Tablets, Chewable:** 4 mg, 5 mg.

ADMINISTRATION/HANDLING

PO
• May take without regard to food. When treating asthma, administer in evening.
• When treating allergic rhinitis, may individualize administration times. • Granules may be given directly in mouth or mixed with carrots, rice, applesauce, ice cream, baby formula, or breast milk (do not add to any other liquid or food). • Give within 15 min of opening packet.

INDICATIONS/ROUTES/DOSAGE

Bronchial Asthma
PO: ADULTS, ELDERLY, CHILDREN 15 YRS AND OLDER: 10-mg tablet daily, taken in the evening. **CHILDREN 6–14 YRS:** 5-mg chewable tablet daily, taken in the evening. **CHILDREN 1–5 YRS:** 4-mg chewable tablet or oral granules daily, taken in the evening.

Seasonal Allergic Rhinitis
PO: ADULTS, ELDERLY, CHILDREN 15 YRS AND OLDER: 10-mg tablet, taken in the evening. **CHILDREN 6–14 YRS:** 5-mg chewable tablet, taken in the evening. **CHILDREN 2–5 YRS:** 4-mg chewable tablet, or oral granules taken in the evening.

Perennial Allergic Rhinitis
PO: ADULTS, ELDERLY, CHILDREN 15 YRS AND OLDER: 10-mg tablet, taken in the evening. **CHILDREN 6–14 YRS:** 5-mg chewable tablet, taken in the evening. **CHILDREN 6 MOS–5 YRS:** 4-mg chewable tablet or oral granules, taken in the evening.

Exercise-Induced Bronchoconstriction Prevention
PO: ADULTS, ELDERLY, CHILDREN 15 YRS AND OLDER: 10 mg 2 or more hrs before exercise. No additional doses within 24 hrs. **CHILDREN 6–14 YRS:** 5 mg (chew tab) 2 or more hrs prior to exercise. No additional doses within 24 hrs.

Dosage in Renal/Hepatic Impairment
No dose adjustment.

SIDE EFFECTS

ADULTS, CHILDREN 15 YRS AND OLDER: Frequent (18%): Headache. **Occasional (4%):** Influenza. **Rare (3%–2%):** Abdominal pain, cough, dyspepsia, dizziness, fatigue, dental pain. **CHILDREN 6–14 YRS: Rare (less than 2%):** Diarrhea, laryngitis, pharyngitis, nausea, otitis media, sinusitis, viral infection.

ADVERSE EFFECTS/TOXIC REACTIONS

Suicidal ideation and behavior, depression have been noted.

NURSING CONSIDERATIONS

BASELINE ASSESSMENT

Chewable tablet contains phenylalanine (component of aspartame); parents of phenylketonuric pts should be informed. Assess lung sounds for wheezing. Assess for allergy symptoms. Question history of depression, suicidal ideation.

INTERVENTION/EVALUATION

Monitor rate, depth, rhythm, type of respirations; quality/rate of pulse. Assess lung sounds for wheezing. Monitor for change in mood, behavior.

PATIENT/FAMILY TEACHING

• Increase fluid intake (decreases lung secretion viscosity). • Take as prescribed, even during symptom-free periods as well as during exacerbations of asthma. • Drug is not for treatment of acute asthma attacks. • Report increased use or frequency of short-acting bronchodilators, changes in behavior, suicidal ideation.

---

morphine

mor-feen
(Duramorph, Infumorph, M-Eslon ✦, Mitigo, MS Contin, MS-IR ✦)

■ **BLACK BOX ALERT** ■ Risk of severe adverse effects when epidural route of administration is used. Ingestion of alcohol with morphine ER may increase risk of overdose. Risk of opioid addiction, abuse, and misuse. Serious, life-threatening, or fatal respiratory depression may occur. Prolonged use during pregnancy may result in neonatal opioid withdrawal syndrome. Accidental ingestion of even one dose may result in a fatal overdose. Concomitant use with benzodiazepines, other CNS depressants may result in profound sedation, respiratory depression, coma, or death.

Do not confuse morphine with HYDROmorphone, or morphine sulfate with magnesium sulfate, MS Contin with OxyCONTIN. MSO₄ and MS are error-prone abbreviations.

FIXED-COMBINATION(S)

Embeda: morphine/naloxone (an opioid antagonist): 20 mg/0.8 mg, 30 mg/1.2 mg, 50 mg/2 mg, 60 mg/2.4 mg, 80 mg/3.2 mg, 100 mg/4 mg.

◆CLASSIFICATION

PHARMACOTHERAPEUTIC: Opioid agonist (Schedule II). **CLINICAL:** Opioid analgesic.

USES

Injection: Management of severe pain. **Oral: (Extended-release):** Management of pain severe enough to require daily, around-the-clock, long-term opioid treatment. **(Immediate-release): Oral solution:** Management of acute pain (adults; pts 2 yrs of age and older) and chronic pain (adults only). **Tablets:** Management of acute pain (pts 50 kg or more and adults) and chronic pain (adults only). **OFF-LABEL:** Dyspnea (palliative care pts).

PRECAUTIONS

Contraindications: Hypersensitivity to morphine. Acute or severe asthma, GI obstruction, known or suspected paralytic ileus, concurrent use of MAOIs or use of MAOIs within 14 days, severe respiratory depression. **Extreme Caution:** COPD, cor pulmonale, hypoxia, hypercapnia, preexisting respiratory depression, head injury, increased ICP, severe hypotension. **Cautions:** Biliary tract disease, pancreatitis, Addison's disease, cardiovascular disease, morbid obesity, adrenal insufficiency, elderly, hypothyroidism, urethral stricture, prostatic hyperplasia, debilitated pts, pts with CNS depression, toxic psychosis, seizure

M

---

disorders, history of drug abuse and misuse, drug-seeking behavior, dependency.

ACTION

Binds with opioid receptors within CNS, inhibiting ascending pain pathways. **Therapeutic Effect:** Alters pain perception, emotional response to pain.

PHARMACOKINETICS

Route	Onset	Peak	Duration
Oral solution	30 min	1 hr	3–5 hrs
Tablets	30 min	1 hr	3–5 hrs
Tablets (extended-release)	N/A	3–4 hrs	8–12 hrs
IV	Rapid	0.3 hr	3–5 hrs
IM	5–30 min	0.5–1 hr	3–5 hrs
Epidural	15–60 min	1 hr	12–20 hrs
SQ	10–30 min	1.1–5 hrs	3–5 hrs
Rectal	20–60 min	0.5–1 hr	3–7 hrs

Variably absorbed from GI tract. Readily absorbed after IM, SQ administration. Protein binding: 20%–35%. Widely distributed. Metabolized in liver. Primarily excreted in urine. Removed by hemodialysis. **Half-life:** 2–4 hrs (increased in hepatic disease).

⏳ LIFESPAN CONSIDERATIONS

Pregnancy/Lactation: Crosses placenta. Distributed in breast milk. May prolong labor if administered in latent phase of first stage of labor or before cervical dilation of 4–5 cm has occurred. Respiratory depression may occur in neonate if mother received opiates during labor. Regular use of opiates during pregnancy may produce withdrawal symptoms in neonate (irritability, excessive crying, tremors, hyperactive reflexes, fever, vomiting, diarrhea, yawning, sneezing, seizures). **Children:** Paradoxical excitement may occur; those younger than 2 yrs are more susceptible to respiratory depressant effects. **Elderly:** Paradoxical excitement may occur. Age-related renal impairment may increase risk of urinary retention.

INTERACTIONS

DRUG: Alcohol, other CNS depressants (e.g., LORazepam, gabapentin, zolpidem) may increase CNS effects, respiratory depression, hypotension. **MAOIs (e.g., phenelzine, selegiline)** may produce serotonin syndrome. (Reduce dosage to one-fourth of usual morphine dose.) **HERBAL: Herbals with sedative properties (e.g., chamomile, kava kava, valerian)** may increase CNS depression. **FOOD:** None known. **LAB VALUES:** May increase serum amylase, lipase.

AVAILABILITY (Rx)

Injection Solution: 2 mg/mL, 4 mg/mL, 5 mg/mL, 10 mg/mL. **Injection Solution (Epidural, Intrathecal, IV Infusion):** *(Duramorph):* 0.5 mg/mL, 1 mg/mL. **Injection Solution, Epidural or Intrathecal:** *(Infumorph):* 10 mg/mL, 25 mg/mL. **Injection Solution:** *(Mitigo):* 10 mg/mL, 25 mg/mL. **Injection Solution, Patient-Controlled Analgesia (PCA) Pump:** 1 mg/mL. **Solution, Oral:** 10 mg/5 mL, 20 mg/5 mL, 20 mg/mL. **Suppository:** 5 mg, 10 mg, 20 mg, 30 mg. **Tablets:** 15 mg, 30 mg.

Capsules, Extended-Release (24 hr): 10 mg, 20 mg, 30 mg, 45 mg, 50 mg, 60 mg, 75 mg, 80 mg, 90 mg, 100 mg, 120 mg. **Tablets, Extended-Release:** 15 mg, 30 mg, 60 mg, 100 mg, 200 mg.

ADMINISTRATION/HANDLING

 IV

Reconstitution • May give undiluted.• For IV injection, may dilute in Sterile Water for Injection or 0.9% NaCl to final concentration of 0.5–5 mg/mL. • For continuous IV infusion, dilute to concentration of 0.1–5 mg/mL in D₅W and give through controlled infusion device.

M

Rate of administration • Always administer very slowly. Rapid IV increases risk of severe adverse reactions (apnea, chest wall rigidity, peripheral circulatory collapse, cardiac arrest, anaphylactoid effects).

Storage • Store at room temperature.

IM, SQ
• Administer slowly, rotating injection sites. • Pts with circulatory impairment experience higher risk of overdosage due to delayed absorption of repeated administration.

PO
• May give without regard to food. • Mix liquid form with fruit juice to improve taste. • Do not break, crush, dissolve, or allow extended-release capsule, tablets. • *(Capsule, Extended-Release 24 hr):* May be opened and mixed with applesauce immediately prior to administration. Do not crush, dissolve, or allow chewing of beads.

Rectal
• If suppository is too soft, chill for 30 min in refrigerator or run cold water over foil wrapper. • Moisten suppository with cold water before inserting well into rectum.

▩ IV COMPATIBILITIES

Aceptaminophen, amiodarone, ibuprofen, magnesium sulfate, norepinephrine, potassium chloride, propofol.

INDICATIONS/ROUTES/DOSAGE

◀ALERT▶ Dosage should be titrated to desired effect.
Analgesia
PO: *(Immediate-Release):* **ADULTS, ELDERLY:** 10–30 mg q4h as needed. **ADOLESCENTS, CHILDREN, INFANTS 6 MOS AND OLDER WEIGHING 50 KG OR MORE:** 10–20 mg q3–4h as needed. **CHILDREN 6 MOS AND OLDER WEIGHING LESS THAN 50 KG:** 0.15–0.3 mg/kg q3–4h as needed. **CHILDREN YOUNGER THAN 6 MOS:** 0.08–0.1 mg/kg/dose q3–4h.
IV: ADULTS, ELDERLY: 1–4 mg q1–4 hrs as needed. May give up to 10 mg q4h as needed. **ADOLESCENTS, CHILDREN, INFANTS WEIGHING 50 KG OR MORE:** Initially, 2–5 mg q2–4h as needed. **ADOLESCENTS, CHILDREN, INFANTS WEIGHING LESS THAN 50 KG:** 0.05–0.1 mg/kg q2–4h as needed. **NEONATES:** Initially, 0.05–0.1 mg/kg/dose q4–8h as needed.

Patient-Controlled Analgesia (PCA)
IV: ADULTS, ELDERLY: Usual concentration: 1 mg/mL. **Demand dose:** 1 mg **(range:** 0.5–2 mg). **Lockout interval:** 10–20 min. **Maximum cumulative dose:** 30 mg within a 4–hr period.

Dosage in Renal Impairment

Creatinine Clearance	Dose
10–50 mL/min, CRRT	75% of normal dose
Less than 10 mL/min, HD, PD	50% of normal dose

Dosage in Hepatic Impairment
No dose adjustment.

SIDE EFFECTS

◀ALERT▶ Ambulatory pts, pts not in severe pain may experience nausea, vomiting more frequently than pts in supine position or who have severe pain. **Frequent:** Sedation, decreased B/P (including orthostatic hypotension), diaphoresis, facial flushing, constipation, dizziness, drowsiness, nausea, vomiting. **Occasional:** Allergic reaction (rash, pruritus), dyspnea, confusion, palpitations, tremors, urinary retention, abdominal cramps, vision changes, dry mouth, headache, decreased appetite, pain/burning at injection site. **Rare:** Paralytic ileus.

M

ADVERSE EFFECTS/TOXIC REACTIONS

Overdose results in respiratory depression, skeletal muscle flaccidity, cold/clammy skin, cyanosis, extreme drowsiness progressing to seizures, stupor, coma. Tolerance to analgesic effect, physical dependence may occur with repeated use. Prolonged duration of action, cumulative effect may occur in those with hepatic/renal impairment. **Antidote:** Naloxone (see Appendix J for dosage).

NURSING CONSIDERATIONS

BASELINE ASSESSMENT

Assess onset, type, location, duration of pain. Obtain vital signs before giving medication. If respirations are 12/min or less (20/min or less in children), withhold medication, contact physician. Effect of medication is reduced if full pain recurs before next dose. Assess for potential of abuse/misuse (e.g., drug-seeking behavior, mental health conditions, history of substance abuse).

INTERVENTION/EVALUATION

Monitor vital signs 5–10 min after IV administration, 15–30 min after SQ, IM. Be alert for decreased respirations, B/P. Check for adequate voiding. Monitor daily pattern of bowel activity, stool consistency; avoid constipation. Initiate deep breathing, coughing exercises, particularly in those with pulmonary impairment. Assess for clinical improvement; record onset of pain relief. Screen for drug abuse and misuse, drug-seeking behavior.

PATIENT/FAMILY TEACHING

• Change positions slowly to avoid orthostatic hypotension. • Avoid tasks that require alertness, motor skills until response to drug is established. • Avoid alcohol, CNS depressants. • Tolerance, dependence may occur with prolonged use of high doses. • Report ineffective pain control, constipation, urinary retention.

mosunetuzumab-axgb

moe-**sun**-e-**tooz**-ue-mab
(Lunsumio)

■ **BLACK BOX ALERT** ■ Life-threatening cytokine release syndrome (CRS) was reported. Treatment must be initiated in a step-up dosing schedule. If CRS occurs, withhold treatment until resolved or permanently discontinue based on severity. Life-threatening neurotoxicities, including immune effector cell–associated neurotoxicity syndrome (ICANS), may occur.

Do not confuse mosunetuzumab-axgb with alemtuzumab, obinutuzumab, or trastuzumab.

◆CLASSIFICATION

PHARMACOTHERAPEUTIC: Bispecific CD20-directed CD3 T-cell engager. **CLINICAL:** Antineoplastic.

USES

Treatment of adults with relapsed or refractory follicular lymphoma after two or more lines of systemic therapy.

PRECAUTIONS

Contraindications: Hypersensitivity to mosunetuzumab-axgb. **Cautions:** Baseline cytopenias, dehydration, conditions predisposing to infection (e.g., diabetes, renal failure, immunocompromised pts, open wounds), chronic opportunistic infections (e.g., herpes virus infection, Epstein-Barr virus infection); pts at high risk for tumor lysis syndrome (high tumor burden).

ACTION

Binds to CD3 receptor–expressing T cells and CD20-expressing malignant and normal B cells, causing T-cell activation, cytokine production, and cellular destruction. **Therapeutic Effect:** Activates release of proinflammatory cytokines and induces lysis of B cells.

PHARMACOKINETICS

Widely distributed. Metabolism not specified. Steady state reached by approx. cycle 4 (63–84 days). Excretion not specified. **Half-life:** 16.1 days.

☒ LIFESPAN CONSIDERATIONS

Pregnancy/Lactation: Avoid pregnancy; may cause fetal harm (including B-cell lymphocytopenia). Females of reproductive potential must use effective contraception during treatment and for at least 3 mos after discontinuation. Unknown if distributed in breast milk; however, human IgG is present in breast milk and is known to cross the placenta. Breastfeeding not recommended during treatment and for at least 3 mos after discontinuation. **Children:** Safety and efficacy not established. **Elderly:** No age-related precautions noted.

INTERACTIONS

DRUG: May increase concentration/effect of **CYP450 substrates (e.g., atorvastatin, fentanyl, midazolam, phenytoin, warfarin).** **HERBAL:** None significant. **FOOD:** None known. **LAB VALUES:** May increase serum ALT, AST, GGT, glucose, uric acid. May decrease Hgb, lymphocytes, platelets, neutrophils, WBC; serum magnesium, phosphate, potassium.

AVAILABILITY (Rx)

Injection Solution: 1 mg/mL, 30 mg/mL.

ADMINISTRATION/HANDLING

IV

Infusion guidelines • Must be administered by a healthcare professional with medical support trained in management of severe reactions including CRS and neurological toxicities. • Infuse via a dedicated IV line.

• Do not use an in-line filter. A drip chamber filter can be used during infusion. • Infusion bags must be made of polyvinyl chloride (PVC) or polyolefin (PO) such as polyethylene (PE) and polypropylene.

Premedication • Cycle 1 and 2: Premedicate all pts with diphenhydrAMINE 50–100 mg PO or IV (or equivalent), acetaminophen 500–1,000 mg PO approx. 30 mins prior to infusion, and methylPREDNISolone 80 mg IV or dexAMETHasone 20 mg IV completed at least 1 hr before infusion. • **Cycle 3 and beyond:** In pts who experience any grade CRS with previous cycles, continue the same premedication treatment as Cycle 1 and 2.

Preparation • Must be prepared by personnel trained in aseptic manipulations and admixing of cytotoxic drugs. • Visually inspect solution for particulate matter or discoloration. Solution should appear clear and colorless. Do not use if solution is cloudy, discolored, or visible particles are observed. • Withdraw and discard the volume from an infusion bag containing 0.9% NaCl or 0.45% NaCl that is equal to the volume of the required dose. Dilute the 1-mg/mL or 2-mg/2 mL dose in a 50-mL or 100-mL infusion bag; 30 mg/30 mL in a 50-mg, 100-mg, or 250-mL infusion bag; 60 mg/60 mL in a 100-mL or 250-mL infusion bag. • Mix by gentle inversion. Do not shake or agitate.

Rate of administration • Cycle 1: Infuse over a minimum of 4 hrs. • **Cycle 2 and 3 (and beyond):** Infuse over 2 hrs if Cycle 1 infusions were well-tolerated.

Storage • Refrigerate unused vials in original carton. Protect from light. Do not shake. • May refrigerate diluted solution for up to 24 hrs or store at room temperature up to 16 hrs (includes infusion time). • Do not shake, agitate, or freeze. • If refrigerated, allow diluted solution to warm to room temperature. Protect from light.

M

⊞ IV INCOMPATABILITIES

Do not mix with other medications.

INDICATIONS/ROUTES/DOSAGE

Follicular Lymphoma (Relapsed or Refractory)

Note: Administer for 8 cycles unless disease progression or unacceptable toxicity occurs. No further cycles are necessary for pts who are complete responders. An additional 9 cycles (17 cycles total) should be given in pts who are partial responders or have stable disease in response to treatment unless disease progression or unacceptable toxicity occurs. If treatment is withheld, restart alternate therapy schedule per manufacturer guidelines.

IV: ADULTS, ELDERLY: (Step-up dosing schedule): Cycle 1: 1 mg on day 1, then 2 mg on day 8, then 60 mg on day 15 of 21-day cycle. **Cycle 2:** 60 mg on day 1 of 21-day cycle. **Cycles 3 and beyond:** 30 mg on day 1 of 21-day cycle.

Dose Modification and Symptom Management

Based on Common Terminology Criteria for Adverse Events (CTCAE).

CRS

Note: Admission to the intensive care unit may be required for Grade 3 or 4 CRS or recurrent Grade 2 or 3 CRS. **Grade 1 CRS:** Interrupt infusion and manage symptoms. If symptoms resolve, restart infusion at the same infusion rate. Prior to next dose, verify CRS symptoms are resolved for at least 72 hrs, then premedicate per guidelines and monitor more frequently. **Grade 2 CRS:** Interrupt infusion and manage symptoms. If symptoms resolve, restart infusion at a rate decreased by 50%. Prior to next dose, verify CRS symptoms are resolved for at least 72 hrs, then premedicate per guidelines and consider hospitalization. Consider starting infusion of the next dose at a rate decreased by 50%. **Recurrent Grade 2 CRS:** Follow Grade 3 CRS guidelines. **Grade 3 CRS:** Interrupt infusion and provide supportive therapy. Prior to next dose, verify CRS symptoms are resolved for at least 72 hrs, then premedicate per guidelines and hospitalize for the next dose. Start infusion of the next dose at a rate decreased by 50%. **Recurrent Grade 3 CRS:** Permanently discontinue and treat symptoms. **Grade 4 CRS:** Permanently discontinue treatment and mange symptoms.

ICANS

Note: Neurology consultation should be considered for evaluation and management of any grade ICANS. Evaluate for other causes of neurologic symptoms. Seizure prophylaxis may be required. Admission to intensive care may be required for Grade 3 or 4 ICANS. **Grade 2 ICANS:** Provide supportive therapy and withhold treatment until improved to Grade 1 or baseline for at least 72 hrs. **Grade 3 ICANS:** Provide supportive therapy and withhold treatment until improved to Grade 1 or baseline for at least 72 hrs. If Grade 3 ICANS recurs, permanently discontinue treatment. **Grade 4 ICANS:** Provide supportive therapy and permanently discontinue treatment.

Infection

Grades 1–4 infection: Withhold treatment until infection resolves. Consider permanent discontinuation for Grade 4 infection.

Neutropenia

Absolute neutrophil count (ANC) less than 500 cells/mm³: Withhold treatment until ANC is 500 cells/mm³ or greater.

Other Adverse Reactions

Any other Grade 3 or 4 adverse reaction: Withhold treatment until improved to Grade 1 or baseline.

Dosage in Renal Impairment

Mild to moderate impairment: No dose adjustment. **Severe impairment:** Not specified; use caution.

Dosage in Hepatic Impairment

Mild impairment: No dose adjustment. **Moderate to severe impairment:** Not specified; use caution.

SIDE EFFECTS

Frequent (42%–21%): Fatigue, asthenia, lethargy, rash, erythema, dermatitis, headache, pyrexia, musculoskeletal pain, cough, pruritus. **Occasional (17% to less than 10%):** Edema (including in the face), fluid overload, fluid retention, peripheral edema, diarrhea, nausea, dry skin, chills, dizziness, vertigo, abdominal pain, insomnia, arthralgia, dyspnea, skin exfoliation, anxiety, mental status change, gait disturbance, ataxia, tremor.

ADVERSE EFFECTS/TOXIC REACTIONS

Myelosuppression (anemia, leukopenia, lymphopenia, neutropenia, thrombocytopenia) is an expected response to therapy, but more severe reactions including bone marrow depression, febrile neutropenia may occur. CRS reported in 39% of pts, some of which were life-threatening. Symptoms of CRS may include fatigue, headache, hypotension, hypoxia, nausea, pyrexia, tachycardia; serious events may include acute respiratory distress syndrome, atrial fibrillation, capillary leak syndrome, disseminated intravascular coagulation (DIC), hepatocellular injury, hemophagocytic lymphohistiocytosis/macrophage activation syndrome (HLM/MAS), multiorgan dysfunction, pulmonary edema. Life-threatening neurological toxicities including ICANS, cerebral edema, leukoencephalopathy, seizures may occur. Life-threatening infections, including pneumonia, opportunistic infections, sepsis, upper respiratory tract infection, urinary tract infection reported in 17% of pts. Tumor flare, manifested as pain/swelling of lymphoma site lesions, new or worsening pleural effusions, tumor inflammation, reported in 4% of pts. May cause Epstein-Barr virus viremia. Tumor lysis syndrome may present as acute renal failure, hypocalcemia, hyperuricemia, hyperphosphatemia.

NURSING CONSIDERATIONS

BASELINE ASSESSMENT

Obtain CBC, LFT; pregnancy test in females of reproductive potential. Confirm compliance with effective contraception. Administer in an environment equipped to manage symptoms of CRS, neurological toxicities. Premedicate all pts per administration guidelines. Question occurrence of infusion-related reactions prior to each dose. Ensure pt is adequately hydrated prior to each dose. Conduct baseline neurological assessment. Question history of hepatic impairment, chronic opportunistic infections. Receive full medication history and screen for interactions. Screen for active infection. Consider granulocyte colony-stimulating factor prophylaxis in pts with neutropenia. Offer emotional support.

INTERVENTION/EVALUATION

Monitor ANC, CBC for myelosuppression (bleeding, bruising, dyspnea, fever, petechiae, weakness) as clinically indicated. Diligently monitor for symptoms of CRS, neurological toxicities throughout treatment, esp. during the step-up phase. Severe symptoms may require hospitalization or intensive care. Monitor for infusion reactions during each infusion. If infusion reactions occur, interrupt infusion and manage symptoms. Conduct routine neurological assessments. Aphasia, confusion, lethargy, tremor, seizures may indicate neurological toxicity, ICANS. During initial treatment, pts with bulky tumors or disease located in close proximity to airways or vital organs should be monitored for symptoms of compression or obstruction due to mass effect related to tumor flare. If airway obstruction or compression occurs, provide supportive measures. Diligently monitor for infections (cough, fatigue, fever, hypoxia). If serious infection occurs, initiate appropriate antimicrobial therapy. Monitor serum uric acid level if tumor lysis syndrome (acute renal failure, electrolyte imbalance, cardiac arrhythmias, seizures) is suspected. Monitor daily pattern of bowel activity, stool consistency.

PATIENT/FAMILY TEACHING

• Treatment may depress your immune system response and reduce your ability to fight infection. Report symptoms of infection such as body aches, chills, cough, fatigue, fever. Avoid those with active infection. • Report symptoms of bone marrow depression such as bruising, fatigue, fever, shortness of breath, weight loss; bleeding easily, bloody urine or stool. • Treatment may cause life-threatening symptoms that must be immediately treated by medical personnel. Report symptoms of CRS (chills, facial swelling, fever, low blood pressure, nausea, vomiting, or weakness), ICANS (confusion, difficulty speaking or slurred speech, loss of consciousness, loss of balance, or seizures). Severe symptoms may require hospitalization. • Avoid tasks that require alertness, motor skills such as driving or operating machinery until response to drug is established. • Therapy may cause tumor lysis syndrome (a condition caused by the rapid breakdown of cancer cells), which can cause kidney failure and can be fatal. Report decreased urination, amber-colored urine; confusion, difficulty breathing, fatigue, fever, muscle or joint pain, palpitations, seizures, vomiting. • Report liver problems (abdominal pain, bruising, clay-colored stool, amber or dark-colored urine, yellowing of the skin or eyes). • Maintain proper hydration and nutrition. • Use effective contraception to avoid pregnancy. Do not breastfeed.

mycophenolate

mye-koe-**fen**-o-late
(CellCept, Myhibbin, Myfortic)

■ BLACK BOX ALERT ■ Increased risk of congenital malformation, spontaneous abortion. Increased risk for development of lymphoma, skin malignancy. Increased susceptibility to infections. Administer under supervision of physician experienced in immunosuppressive therapy.

◆CLASSIFICATION

PHARMACOTHERAPEUTIC: Immunologic agent. **CLINICAL:** Immunosuppressant.

USES

Should be used concurrently with other immunosuppressants **CellCept:**
Prophylaxis of organ rejection in adults and pediatric recipients 3 mos of age and older receiving allogeneic hepatic/renal/cardiac transplant. **Myfortic:** Prophylaxis of organ rejection in adult pts receiving a kidney transplant and pts at least 5 yrs of age who are at least 6 mos post kidney transplant. **OFF-LABEL:** Bullous pemphigoid, dermatomyositis, eosinophilic granulomatosis, glomerulosclerosis, graft-versus-host disease, hepatitis (autoimmune, refractory), interstitial nephritis (acute), lupus erythematosus, myasthenia gravis (chronic immunosuppressive therapy), uveitis (noninfectious).

PRECAUTIONS

Contraindications: Hypersensitivity to mycophenolate, mycophenolic acid or polysorbate 80 (IV formulation). **Cautions:** Active severe GI disease, renal impairment, neutropenia, women of childbearing potential (use caution when handling).

ACTION

Suppresses immunologically mediated inflammatory response by inhibiting inosine monophosphate dehydrogenase, an enzyme that deprives lymphocytes of nucleotides necessary for DNA, RNA synthesis, thus inhibiting proliferation of T and B lymphocytes. **Therapeutic Effect:** Prevents transplant rejection.

PHARMACOKINETICS

Widely distributed. Protein binding: 97%. Metabolized via hydrolysis to active metabolite mycophenolic acid. Primarily excreted in urine. Not removed by hemodialysis. **Half-life:** 17.9 hrs.

⧗ LIFESPAN CONSIDERATIONS

Pregnancy/Lactation: Avoid use; may cause fetal harm. Females of reproductive potential should use effective contraception during treatment and for at least 6 wks after discontinuation. Breastfeeding not recommended. **Children:** Safety and efficacy not established in children younger than 3 mos. **Elderly:** Age-related renal impairment may require dosage adjustment.

INTERACTIONS

DRUG: May increase concentration/effects of **acyclovir, ganciclovir. Antacids (aluminum- and magnesium-containing), cholestyramine** may decrease absorption. **Vaccines (live)** may alter concentration/effect. **RifAMPin** may decrease concentration/effect. May decrease therapeutic effect of **oral contraceptives.** May increase adverse/toxic effect of **natalizumab.** May decrease therapeutic effect of **BCG (intravesical). Tacrolimus (topical)** may increase adverse/toxic effect. **HERBAL:** Echinacea may decrease therapeutic effect. **FOOD:** None significant. **LAB VALUES:** May increase serum cholesterol, alkaline phosphatase, creatinine, ALT, AST. May alter serum glucose, lipids, calcium, potassium, phosphate, uric acid.

AVAILABILITY (Rx)

CellCept
Capsules: 250 mg. **Injection, Powder for Reconstitution:** 500 mg. **Oral Suspension:** 200 mg/mL. **Tablets:** 500 mg.

 Tablets, Delayed-Release: *(Myfortic):* 180 mg, 360 mg.

ADMINISTRATION/HANDLING

IV

Reconstitution • Reconstitute each 500-mg vial with 14 mL D$_5$W. Gently agitate. • For 1-g dose, further dilute with 140 mL D$_5$W; for 1.5-g dose, further dilute with 210 mL D$_5$W, providing a concentration of 6 mg/mL.
Rate of administration • Infuse over at least 2 hrs. • Begin infusion within 4 hrs of reconstitution.
Storage • Store at room temperature.

PO

• Give on empty stomach (1 hr before or 2 hrs after food). • Do not break, crush, or open capsules or break, crush, dissolve, or divide delayed-release tablets. Avoid inhalation of powder in capsules, direct contact of powder on skin/

mucous membranes. If contact occurs, wash thoroughly with soap, water. Rinse eyes profusely with plain water. • May store reconstituted suspension in refrigerator or at room temperature. • Suspension is stable for 60 days after reconstitution. • Suspension can be administered orally or via an NG tube (minimum size 8 French).

IV INCOMPATIBILITIES

Mycophenolate is compatible only with D$_5$W. Do not infuse concurrently with other drugs or IV solutions.

INDICATIONS/ROUTES/DOSAGE

Note: Give in combination with other immunosuppressants.

Prevention of Renal Transplant Rejection
PO, IV: *(CellCept):* **ADULTS, ELDERLY:** 1 g twice daily. **PO: CHILDREN 3 MONTHS AND OLDER:** *(Suspension):* 600 mg/m²/dose twice daily. **Maximum:** 1 g twice daily. *(Tablets, Capsules):* **BSA greater than or equal to 1.5 m²:** 1,000 mg twice daily. **BSA 1.25 m² to less than 1.5 m²:** 750 mg twice daily .

PO: *(Myfortic):* **ADULTS, ELDERLY:** 720 mg twice daily. **CHILDREN 5–16 YRS (at least 6 mos post–kidney transplant):** 400 mg/m² twice daily. **Maximum:** 720 mg twice daily. **BSA greater than 1.58 m²:** 720 mg twice daily. **BSA 1.19–1.58 m²:** 540 mg twice daily.

Prevention of Heart Transplant Rejection
PO, IV: *(CellCept):* **ADULTS, ELDERLY:** 1.5 g twice daily. **PO: CHILDREN 3 MOS AND OLDER:** *Suspension):* Initially, 600 mg/m² twice daily. If tolerated, may increase to 900 mg/m² twice daily. *Tablets, Capsules:* **BSA greater than or equal to 1.5 m²:** 1,000 mg twice daily. **BSA 1.25 to less than 1.5 m²:** 750 mg twice daily.

Prevention of Hepatic Transplant Rejection
PO, IV: *(CellCept):* **ADULTS, ELDERLY:** 1.5 g orally twice daily or give 1 g IV twice daily. **PO: CHILDREN 3 MOS AND OLDER:** *(Suspension):* Initially, 600 mg/m² twice

M

daily. If tolerated, may increase to 900 mg/m^2 twice daily. **Tablets, Capsules: BSA greater than or equal to 1.5 m^2:** 1,000 mg twice daily. **BSA 1.25 to less than 1.5 m^2:** 750 mg twice daily.

Dosage in Renal/Hepatic Impairment
No dose adjustment.

SIDE EFFECTS

Frequent (37%–20%): UTI, hypertension, peripheral edema, diarrhea, constipation, fever, headache, nausea. **Occasional (18%–10%):** Dyspepsia, dyspnea, cough, hematuria, asthenia, vomiting, edema, tremors, oral candidiasis, acne; abdominal, chest, back pain. **Rare (9%–6%):** Insomnia, respiratory tract infection, rash, dizziness.

ADVERSE EFFECTS/TOXIC REACTIONS

Significant anemia, leukopenia, thrombocytopenia, neutropenia, leukocytosis may occur, particularly in pts undergoing renal transplant rejection. Sepsis, infection occur occasionally. GI tract hemorrhage occurs rarely. May increase risk of new malignancies. Immunosuppression results in increased susceptibility to infection.

NURSING CONSIDERATIONS

BASELINE ASSESSMENT
Obtain pregnancy test in females of reproductive potential. Assess medical history, esp. renal function, existence of active digestive system disease, drug history, esp. other immunosuppressants.

INTERVENTION/EVALUATION
CBC should be performed wkly during first mo of therapy, twice monthly during second and third mos of treatment, then monthly throughout the first yr. If rapid fall in WBC occurs, dosage should be reduced or discontinued. Assess for delayed bone marrow suppression. Monitor for infections (cough, fatigue, fever).

PATIENT/FAMILY TEACHING
• Treatment may depress your immune system and reduce your ability to fight infection. Report symptoms of infection such as body aches, chills, cough, fatigue, fever. Avoid those with active infection. • Report unusual bleeding/bruising, sore throat, mouth sores, abdominal pain, fever. • May cause new cancers. • Use effective contraception to avoid pregnancy. Laboratory follow-up while taking medication is important part of therapy.

nafcillin

naf-**sil**-in

◆CLASSIFICATION

PHARMACOTHERAPEUTIC: Penicillin. **CLINICAL:** Antibiotic.

USES

Treatment of infections caused by susceptible penicillinase-producing staphylococci including bloodstream infections, endocarditis (treatment), meningitis (bacterial), osteomyelitis, pneumonia, prosthetic joint infection, skin/soft tissue infections.

PRECAUTIONS

Contraindications: Hypersensitivity to nafcillin, other penicillins. **Cautions:** History of allergies, particularly cephalosporins; severe renal/hepatic impairment, asthma, HF.

ACTION

Binds to bacterial membranes. **Therapeutic Effect:** Inhibits cell wall synthesis. Bactericidal.

PHARMACOKENETICS

Widely distributed. Poor CSF penetration, but may be enhanced by meningeal inflammation. Metabolized in liver. Protein binding: 90%. Peak plasma concentration: 30–60 min. Excreted in feces, urine. **Half-life:** (Adults): 33–61 min; (infants, children aged 1 mo–14 yrs): 0.75–1.9 hrs; (neonates aged less than 3 wks): 2.2–5.5 hrs; (neonates aged 4–9 wks): 12–2.3 hrs.

⌛ LIFESPAN CONSIDERATIONS

Pregnancy/Lactation: Readily crosses placenta; appears in cord blood, amniotic fluid. Distributed in breast milk. May lead to rash, diarrhea, candidiasis in neonate, infant. **Children:** Immature renal function in neonates may delay renal excretion. **Elderly:** Age-related renal impairment may require dosage adjustment.

INTERACTIONS

DRUG: High doses (2 g q4h) may decrease effects of **warfarin.** May decrease effects of **BCG (intravesical), axitinib, bosutinib, cobimetinib, elbasvir, grazoprevir, neratinib, olaparib, ranolazine, sonidegib. HERBAL:** None significant. **FOOD:** None known. **LAB VALUES:** May cause false-positive Coombs' test.

AVAILABILITY (Rx)

Injection, Powder for Reconstitution: 1 g, 2 g. **Infusion, Premix:** 1 g/50 mL, 2g/100 mL.

ADMINISTRATION/HANDLING

◄**ALERT**► Space doses evenly around the clock.

 IV

Reconstitution • Reconstitute each vial with Sterile Water for Injection or 0.9% NaCl. • For direct IV injection, dilute with 15–30 mL. • For intermittent IV infusion (piggyback), further dilute with 50–100 mL 0.9% NaCl or D₅W (not to exceed concentration of 40 mg/mL).
Rate of administration • Infuse piggyback over 30–60 min. • **Direct injection:** Inject over 5–10 min.
Storage • Refrigerate diluted solution for up to 7 days or store at room temperature for up to 24 hrs. • Discard if precipitate forms.

IM

• Reconstitute each 500 mg with Sterile Water for Injection or 0.9% NaCl to provide concentration of 250 mg/mL. • Inject IM into large muscle mass.

⊞ IV INCOMPATIBILITIES

Insulin.

⊞ IV COMPATIBILITIES

Heparin, magnesium sulfate, propofol.

INDICATIONS/ROUTES/DOSAGE

Can give as 24-hour infusion of 12 g over 24 hrs in 500 mL or 1000 mL normal saline.
Usual Dosage
IV: **ADULTS, ELDERLY:** 1–2 g q4–6h. **INFANTS, CHILDREN, ADOLESCENTS:** 100–200 mg/

kg/day in divided doses q4–6h. **Maximum dose:** 2,000 mg. **Maximum:** 12 g/day. **NEONATES**: 25 mg/kg/dose divided q6–12h. Dose based on body weight and postnatal age.

Dosage in Renal/Hepatic Impairment
No dose adjustment.

SIDE EFFECTS

Frequent: Mild hypersensitivity reaction (fever, rash, pruritus), GI effects (nausea, vomiting, diarrhea). **Occasional:** Hypokalemia with high IV dosages, phlebitis, thrombophlebitis (common in elderly). **Rare:** Extravasation with IV administration.

ADVERSE EFFECTS/TOXIC REACTIONS

Potentially fatal antibiotic-associated colitis, superinfections (abdominal cramps, severe watery diarrhea, fever) may result from altered bacterial balance in GI tract. Hematologic effects (esp. involving platelets, WBCs), severe hypersensitivity reactions, anaphylaxis occur rarely.

NURSING CONSIDERATIONS

BASELINE ASSESSMENT

Question for history of allergies, esp. penicillins, cephalosporins.

INTERVENTION/EVALUATION

Hold medication, promptly report rash (possible hypersensitivity), diarrhea (fever, abdominal pain, mucus/blood in stool may indicate antibiotic-associated colitis). Evaluate IV site frequently for phlebitis (heat, pain, red streaking over vein), infiltration (potential extravasation). Be alert for superinfection: fever, vomiting, diarrhea, anal/genital pruritus, oral mucosal changes (ulceration, pain, erythema).

PATIENT/FAMILY TEACHING

• Continue antibiotic for full length of treatment. • Doses should be evenly spaced. • Discomfort may occur with IM injection. • Report IV discomfort immediately. • Report diarrhea, rash, other new symptoms.

naloxone

nal-**ox**-own
(Kloxxado, Narcan, Rezenopy, ReVive, Zimhi)
Do not confuse naloxone with Lanoxin or naltrexone.

FIXED-COMBINATION(S)

Embeda: naloxone/morphine (an opioid agonist): 0.8 mg/20 mg, 1.2 mg/30 mg, 2 mg/50 mg, 2.4 mg/60 mg, 3.2 mg/80 mg, 4 mg/100 mg. **Suboxone (sublingual film):** naloxone/buprenorphine (an analgesic): 0.5 mg/2 mg, 1 mg/4 mg, 2 mg/8 mg, 3 mg/12 mg. **Zubsolv:** naloxone/buprenorphine: 0.36 mg/1.4 mg, 1.4 mg/5.7 mg.

CLASSIFICATION

PHARMACOTHERAPEUTIC: Opioid antagonist. **CLINICAL:** Antidote.

USES

Narcan: Complete or partial reversal of opioid depression including respiratory depression. Diagnosis of suspected opioid tolerance or acute opioid overdose. **Nasal spray:** Emergency treatment of known or suspected opioid overdose. **Zimhi:** Emergency treatment of known or suspected opioid overdose. **OFF-LABEL:** Opioid-induced pruritus.

PRECAUTIONS

Contraindications: Hypersensitivity to naloxone. **Cautions:** Cardiac/pulmonary disease. Medications with potential for adverse cardiovascular effects (e.g., hypotension, arrhythmias).

ACTION

Competes with and displaces opioids at opioid-occupied receptor sites in CNS. **Therapeutic Effect:** Reverses opioid-induced sleep/sedation, increases respiratory rate, raises B/P to normal range.

PHARMACOKINETICS

Route	Onset	Peak	Duration
IV	1–2 min	N/A	20–60 min
IM	2–5 min	N/A	20–60 min
SQ	2–5 min	N/A	20–60 min

Widely distributed. Metabolized in liver. Primarily excreted in urine. **Half-life:** 60–100 min.

⌛ LIFESPAN CONSIDERATIONS

Pregnancy/Lactation: Unknown if drug crosses placenta or is distributed in breast milk. **Children/Elderly:** No age-related precautions noted.

INTERACTIONS

DRUG: **Methylnaltrexone** may increase adverse/toxic effects. May increase adverse/toxic effects of **naldemedine, naloxegol.** **HERBAL:** None significant. **FOOD:** None known. **LAB VALUES:** None significant.

AVAILABILITY (Rx)

Injection Solution: 0.4 mg/mL. **Injection Solution, Prefilled Syringe:** 2 mg/2 mL. *(Zimhi):* 5 mg/0.5 mL. **Liquid, Nasal:** *(Narcan):* 4 mg/0.1 mL. *(Kloxxado):* 8 mg/0.1 mL. *(Rextovy):* 4 mg/ device. *(Rezenopy):* 10 mg/0.11 mL. *(ReVive):* 3 mg/0.1 mL.

ADMINISTRATION/HANDLING

 IV

Reconstitution • For IV push, may give undiluted (0.4 mg/mL or diluted with 9 mL 0.9% NaCl to concentration of 0.04 mg/mL). • For continuous IV infusion, dilute each 2 mg of naloxone with 500 mL of D$_5$W or 0.9% NaCl, producing solution containing 0.004 mg/mL (4 mcg/mL).
Rate of administration • May give IV push over 30 sec.
Storage • Store parenteral form at room temperature. • Use mixture within 24 hrs; discard unused solution. • Protect from light. • Stable in D$_5$W or 0.9% NaCl at 4 mcg/mL for 24 hrs.

IM/SQ

• Administer into anterolateral aspect of thigh with needle facing downward. May inject through clothing.

INDICATIONS/ROUTES/DOSAGE

Note: If no response seen after a total of 10 mg, consider other causes of respiratory depression.

Opioid Overdose
IV, IM, SQ: ADULTS, ELDERLY: 0.4–2 mg q2–3min as needed. After reversal, additional doses may be required at later intervals (e.g., 20–60 min) depending on type/duration of opioid. **Maximum:** 10 mg total dose. **ADOLESCENTS, CHILDREN, INFANTS:** 0.1 mg/kg if no response, repeat q2–3min. May need to repeat doses q20–60min. *(Nasal Spray):* **ADULTS, ELDERLY, CHILDREN:** *(Kloxxado, Narcan, ReVive, Rextovy):* Single spray (3, 4, 8, or 10 mg) into one nostril. May give q2–3min until emergency medical assistance arrives. *(Rezenopy):* Single spray into one nostril. If no response in 2-3 min, an additional dose may be given into the other nostril. **Maximum:** 2 sprays/day.
IM, SQ: *(Zimhi):* **ADULTS, ELDERLY, CHILDREN:** 5 mg. May repeat q2-3 min until emergency medical assistance is available.

Reversal of Respiratory Depression With Therapeutic Opioid Dosing
IV, IM, SQ: ADULTS, ELDERLY: Initially, 0.1–0.2 mg. Titrate to avoid profound withdrawal, seizures, arrhythmias, or severe pain. **CHILDREN:** 0.005–0.01 mg IV at 2–3 min intervals to the desired degree of reversal.

Dosage in Renal/Hepatic Impairment
No dose adjustment.

SIDE EFFECTS

None known; little or no pharmacologic effect in absence of narcotics.

ADVERSE EFFECTS/TOXIC REACTIONS

Too-rapid reversal of narcotic-induced respiratory depression may result in agitation, nausea, vomiting, tremors, increased B/P, tachycardia, seizures. Excessive dosage in postoperative pts may produce significant reversal of analgesia, agitation, tremors Hypotension or hypertension, ventricular

N

tachycardia/fibrillation, pulmonary edema may occur in pts with cardiovascular disease.

NURSING CONSIDERATIONS

BASELINE ASSESSMENT

Maintain patent airway. Obtain weight of children to calculate drug dosage.

INTERVENTION/EVALUATION

Monitor vital signs, esp. rate, depth, rhythm of respiration, during and frequently following administration. Carefully observe pt after satisfactory response (duration of opiate may exceed duration of naloxone, resulting in recurrence of respiratory depression). Assess for increased pain, seizure activity with reversal of opiate.

naproxen

na-**prox**-en
(Aleve, EC-Naprosyn, Naprelan, Naprosyn)

■ BLACK BOX ALERT ■

Increased risk of serious cardiovascular thrombotic events, including myocardial infarction, CVA. Increased risk of severe GI reactions, including ulceration, bleeding, perforation of stomach, intestines.

Do not confuse Aleve with Alesse, or Anaprox with Anaspaz or Avapro.

FIXED-COMBINATION(S)

Prevacid NapraPac: naproxen/lansoprazole (proton pump inhibitor): 375 mg/15 mg, 500 mg/15 mg. **Treximet:** naproxen/SUMAtriptan (an antimigraine): 60 mg/10 mg; 500 mg/85 mg. **Vimovo:** naproxen/esomeprazole (proton pump inhibitor): 375 mg/20 mg, 500 mg/20 mg.

◆CLASSIFICATION

PHARMACOTHERAPEUTIC: NSAID.
CLINICAL: Analgesic, nonopioid.

USES

Anti-inflammatory: Relief of the signs and symptoms of gout, ankylosing spondylitis, bursitis, polyarticular juvenile idiopathic arthritis (excluding ER tablets), osteoarthritis, rheumatoid arthritis, and tendinopathy. **Dysmenorrhea:** Treatment of primary dysmenorrhea. **Pain/fever:** Relief of mild to moderate pain and/or fever. **OFF-LABEL:** Migraine (acute treatment).

PRECAUTIONS

Contraindications: History of asthma, urticaria; hypersensitivity to naproxen, other NSAIDs. Perioperative pain in setting of CABG surgery. **Cautions:** GI disease (bleeding, ulcers), fluid retention, renal/hepatic impairment, asthma, HF, concurrent use of anticoagulants, smoking, use of alcohol, elderly pts, debilitated pts.

ACTION

Reversibly inhibits COX-1 and COX-2 enzymes, resulting in decreased formation of prostaglandin precursors. **Therapeutic Effect:** Reduces inflammatory response, fever, intensity of pain.

PHARMACOKINETICS

Route	Onset	Peak	Duration
PO (analgesic)	1 hr	2–4 hrs	7 hrs or less
PO (anti-inflammatory)	2 wks	2–4 wks	12 hrs

Widely distributed. Protein binding: 99%. Metabolized in liver. Primarily excreted in urine. Not removed by hemodialysis. **Half-life:** 13 hrs.

⌛ LIFESPAN CONSIDERATIONS

Pregnancy/Lactation: Crosses placenta. Distributed in breast milk. Avoid use during third trimester (may cause premature closure of the ductus arteriosus). **Children:** Safety and efficacy not established in pts younger than 2 yrs. Children older than 2 yrs at increased risk for skin rash. **Elderly:** Age-related renal impairment may increase risk of hepatic/renal toxicity; reduced dosage recommended. More likely to have serious adverse effects with GI bleeding/ulceration.

INTERACTIONS

DRUG: May increase effect of **apixaban, dabigatran, edoxaban, rivaroxaban.** Bile acid sequestrants **(e.g., cholestyramine)** may decrease absorption. May increase nephrotoxic effect of **aliskiren, cycloSPORINE. HERBAL:** Glucosamine, herbals with anticoagulant/antiplatelet properties (e.g., garlic, ginger, ginseng, ginkgo biloba) may increase concentration/effect. **FOOD:** None known. **LAB VALUES:** May prolong bleeding time. May increase serum BUN, creatinine, ALT, AST, alkaline phosphatase. May decrease Hgb, Hct, leukocytes, platelets, uric acid.

AVAILABILITY (Rx)

Capsule: 220 mg. **Oral Suspension:** 125 mg/5 mL. **Tablets:** 220 mg, 250 mg, 275 mg, 375 mg, 500 mg, 550 mg.

🐋 **Tablets, Delayed-Release:** 375 mg, 500 mg. **Extended-Release:** 375 mg, 500 mg, 750 mg.

ADMINISTRATION/HANDLING

PO

• Give controlled-release form whole. Do not cut, crush, or allow chewing. • Best taken with food or milk (decreases GI irritation). • Shake suspension well.

INDICATIONS/ROUTES/DOSAGE

Note: Dosage expressed as naproxen base (200 mg naproxen base equivalent to 220 mg naproxen sodium).

Anti-inflammatory (e.g., Rheumatoid Arthritis [RA], Osteoarthritis, Ankylosing Spondylitis)

PO: ADULTS, ELDERLY: *(Immediate-Release)*: 250–500 mg q12h. **Maximum:** 1.5 g/day. **(Extended-Release):** 750 mg–1 g once daily. **Maximum:** 1.5 g/day.

Acute Gouty Arthritis

Note: Start within 24–48 hrs of flareup. Discontinue 2–3 days after clinical signs resolve. **(Usual duration:** 5–7 days.)
PO: ADULTS, ELDERLY: *(Immediate-Release)*: Initially, 500 mg twice daily **(Extended-Release):** Initially 1–1.5 g once, then 1 g once daily.

Dysmenorrhea

Note: Begin at menses onset or 12 days prior to menses onset for severe symptoms. Usual duration: 1–5 days.
PO: ADULTS: *(Immediate-Release)*: Initially, 500 mg once, then 500 mg q12h or 250 mg q6–8h as needed. **Maximum:** 1,250 mg on day 1, then 1,000 mg once daily. **(Extended-Release):** Initially, 1,000 mg once daily. May temporarily increase to 1,500 mg once daily for acute pain, then reduce to 1,000 mg once daily.

Pain

PO: ADULTS, ELDERLY: *(Immediate-Release)*: Initially, 500 mg once, then 500 mg q12h or 250 mg q6–8 as needed. **Maximum:** 1,250 mg on day 1, then 1,000 mg once daily. **(Extended-Release):** Initially 1,000 mg once daily. May temporarily increase to 1,500 mg once daily for acute pain, then reduce to 1,000 mg once daily.

Juvenile Idiopathic Arthritis (JIA)

PO: *(Oral Suspension Recommended)*: CHILDREN 2 YRS AND OLDER: 10–15 mg/kg/day in 2 divided doses. **Maximum:** 1,000 mg/day.

OTC Uses (Pain, Fever)

PO: ADULTS 65 YRS AND YOUNGER, CHILDREN 12 YRS AND OLDER: Initially, 400 mg once, then 200 mg q8–12h. **Maximum:** 400 mg in any 8- to12-hr period or 600 mg/day. **ELDERLY:** Use with caution (consider a lower dose).

Dosage in Renal Impairment

Not recommended with CrCl less than 30 mL/min.

Dosage in Hepatic Impairment

Use caution.

SIDE EFFECTS

Frequent (9%–4%): Nausea, constipation, abdominal cramps/pain, heartburn, dizziness, headache, drowsiness. **Occasional (3%–1%):** Stomatitis, diarrhea, indigestion. **Rare (less than 1%):** Vomiting, confusion.

ADVERSE EFFECTS/TOXIC REACTIONS

Rare reactions with long-term use include peptic ulcer, GI bleeding, gastritis, severe hepatic reactions (cholestasis, jaundice), nephrotoxicity (dysuria, hematuria, proteinuria, nephrotic syndrome), and severe hypersensitivity reaction (fever, chills, bronchospasm).

NURSING CONSIDERATIONS

BASELINE ASSESSMENT

Assess onset, type, location, duration of pain/inflammation. Inspect appearance of affected joints for immobility, deformities, skin condition. Question history of GI bleeding, gastric or duodenal ulcers, hypertension.

INTERVENTION/EVALUATION

Periodically monitor renal function test during chronic use. Monitor daily pattern of bowel activity, stool consistency. Evaluate for therapeutic response: relief of pain, stiffness, swelling; increased joint mobility, reduced joint tenderness, improved grip strength.

PATIENT/FAMILY TEACHING

• Take with food, milk. • Avoid aspirin, alcohol during therapy (increases risk of GI bleeding). • Report headache, rash, visual disturbances, weight gain, black or tarry stools, bleeding, persistent headache.

naratriptan

nar-a-**trip**-tan
Do not confuse naratriptan with eletriptan or almotriptan.

◆ CLASSIFICATION

PHARMACOTHERAPEUTIC: Serotonin receptor agonist. **CLINICAL:** Antimigraine.

USES

Treatment of acute migraine headache with or without aura in adults. **OFF-LABEL:** Prevention of menstrual migraine.

PRECAUTIONS

Contraindications: Hypersensitivity to naratriptan. Basilar/hemiplegic migraine, cerebrovascular disease, peripheral vascular disease, coronary artery disease, ischemic heart disease (including angina pectoris, history of MI, silent ischemia, Prinzmetal's angina), severe hepatic impairment (Child-Pugh Grade C), severe renal impairment (CrCl less than 15 mL/min), uncontrolled hypertension, use within 24 hrs of ergotamine-containing preparations or another serotonin receptor agonist, 5-HT agonist (e.g., SUMAtriptan), MAOI use within 14 days. **Cautions:** Mild to moderate renal/hepatic impairment, elderly.

ACTION

Selectively binds to serotonin receptors, producing vasoconstrictive effect on cranial blood vessels. **Therapeutic Effect:** Relieves migraine headache.

PHARMACOKINETICS

Widely distributed. Protein binding: 28%–31%. Metabolized in liver. Eliminated primarily in urine. **Half-life:** 6 hrs (increased in hepatic/renal impairment).

⧗ LIFESPAN CONSIDERATIONS

Pregnancy/Lactation: Unknown if drug is distributed in breast milk. **Children:** Safety and efficacy not established. **Elderly:** Not recommended in the elderly.

INTERACTIONS

DRUG: **Ergotamine-containing medications** may produce vasospastic reaction. **SSRIs (e.g., escitalopram, paroxetine, sertraline), SNRIs (e.g., duloxetine, venlafaxine)** may cause serotonin syndrome. May increase serotonergic effect of **MAOIs (e.g., phenelzine, selegiline).** **HERBAL:** None significant. **FOOD:** None known. **LAB VALUES:** None significant.

AVAILABILITY (Rx)

 Tablets: 1 mg, 2.5 mg.

ADMINISTRATION/HANDLING

PO
• Give without regard to food. • Do not break, crush, dissolve, or divide tablets. Administer whole with water.

INDICATIONS/ROUTES/DOSAGE

Acute Migraine Attack
PO: ADULTS: 1–2.5 mg. If headache improves but then returns, dose may be repeated after 4 hrs. **Maximum:** 5 mg/24 hrs. **Maximum dose:** 2.5 mg.

Dosage in Renal/Hepatic Impairment

Hepatic Failure	Creatinine Clearance	Dosage
Mild to moderate	15–39 mL/min	Initial, 1 mg; Max: 2.5 mg/24 hrs
Severe	Less than 15 mL/min	Contraindicated

SIDE EFFECTS

Occasional (5%): Nausea. **Rare (2%):** Paresthesia, dizziness, fatigue, drowsiness, feeling of pressure in throat, neck, jaw.

ADVERSE EFFECTS/TOXIC REACTIONS

Corneal opacities, other ocular defects may occur. Cardiac events (ischemia, coronary artery vasospasm, MI), noncardiac vasospasm-related reactions (hemorrhage, cerebrovascular accident [CVA]) occur rarely, particularly in pts with hypertension, diabetes, strong family history of coronary artery disease, obesity, smokers, males older than 40 yrs, postmenopausal women.

BASELINE ASSESSMENT

Question medical history as listed in Precautions. Question characteristics of migraine headaches (onset, location, duration, possible precipitating symptoms). Obtain medication history and screen for interactions.

INTERVENTION/EVALUATION

Evaluate for relief of migraine headaches (photophobia, phonophobia, nausea, vomiting, pain, dizziness, fogginess).

PATIENT/FAMILY TEACHING

• May cause dizziness, fatigue, drowsiness. • Avoid tasks that require alertness, motor skills until response to drug is established. • Report chest pain, palpitations, tightness in throat, rash, hallucinations, anxiety, panic.

N

neratinib

ne-**ra**-ti-nib
(Nerlynx)
Do not confuse neratinib with afatinib, axitinib, bosutinib, cabozantinib, dasatinib, gefitinib, imatinib, ponatinib, tofacitinib.

◆CLASSIFICATION

PHARMACOTHERAPEUTIC: Epidermal growth factor receptor (EGFR) inhibitor (anti-HER2). Tyrosine kinase inhibitor. **CLINICAL:** Antineoplastic.

USES

As a single agent for extended adjuvant treatment of adult pts with early stage HER2-overexpressed/amplified breast cancer, to follow adjuvant trastuzumab-based therapy. Treatment of advanced or metastatic HER2-positive breast cancer (in combination with capecitabine) in pts who have received 2 or more prior anti–HER2-based regimens in the metastatic setting.

PRECAUTIONS

Contraindications: Hypersensitivity to neratinib. **Cautions:** Dehydration, electrolyte imbalance, hepatic impairment, irritable bowel syndrome with diarrhea. Avoid concomitant use of strong or moderate CYP3A4 inhibitors, CYP3A4 inducers; proton pump inhibitors, H_2 receptor antagonists, antacids.

ACTION

Irreversibly binds to epidermal growth factor receptor (EGFR), human epidermal growth factor receptor 2 (HER2), HER4, reducing autophosphorylation and signaling of EGFR and HER2. **Therapeutic Effect:** Exhibits antitumor activity in EGFR and/or HER2 expressing cancer cell lines.

PHARMACOKINETICS

Widely distributed. Metabolized in liver. Protein binding: 99%. Peak plasma concentration: 2–8 hrs. Excreted in feces (97%), urine (1%). **Half-life:** 7–17 hrs.

⌛ LIFESPAN CONSIDERATIONS

Pregnancy/Lactation: Avoid pregnancy; may cause fetal harm/malformations. Unknown if distributed in breast milk. Breastfeeding not recommended during treatment and for at least 1 month after last dose. Females of reproductive potential should use effective contraception during treatment and for at least 1 mo after discontinuation. **Males:** Males with female partners of reproductive potential should use effective contraception during treatment and up to 3 mos after discontinuation. **Children:** Safety and efficacy not established. **Elderly:** May have increased risk of adverse reactions/toxic effects. Use caution.

INTERACTIONS

DRUG: Aluminum-, magnesium-, calcium-containing antacids, H_2 receptor antagonists (e.g., famotidine), proton pump inhibitors (e.g., omeprazole, pantoprazole) may decrease concentration/effect. Strong CYP3A4 inhibitors (e.g., clarithromycin, ketoconazole, ritonavir), moderate CYP3A4 inhibitors (e.g., dilTIAZem, fluconazole, verapamil) may increase concentration/effect. CYP3A4 inducers (e.g., carBAMazepine, phenytoin, rifAMPin) may decrease concentration/effect. May increase concentration of PAZOPanib, topotecan. **HERBAL:** None significant. **FOOD:** Grapefruit products may increase concentration/effect. **LAB VALUES:** May increase serum ALT, AST, bilirubin.

AVAILABILITY (Rx)

Tablets: 40 mg.

ADMINISTRATION/HANDLING

PO
• Give with food at the same time daily. • Administer whole; do not break, cut, crush, or divide tablets. • If a dose is missed or vomiting occurs after administration, do not give extra dose. Administer next dose at regularly scheduled time. • Take 3 hours after aluminum-, magnesium-, or calcium-containing antacids are given. • Avoid concomitant use of proton pump inhibitors (PPI). Separate administration by at least 2 hrs before or 10 hrs after H_2 receptor antagonist.

INDICATIONS/ROUTES/DOSAGE

Note: Recommend antidiarrheal prophylaxis during first 2 cycles (56 days) of therapy. For pts with early stage and metastatic breast cancer, a dose escalation strategy may be used to improve tolerability and decrease the rate, severity, and duration of neratinib-induced diarrhea. **Dose escalation:** Wk 1 (days 1–7): 120 mg once daily. Wk 2 (days 8–14): 160 mg once daily. Wk 3 (day 15 and thereafter): 240 mg once daily.

Breast Cancer (Extended Adjuvant Therapy)
PO: ADULTS, ELDERLY: 240 mg (6 tablets) once daily until disease recurrence or for up to 1 yr.

Breast Cancer (HER2-Positive; Advanced or Metastatic)

PO: ADULTS, ELDERLY: 240 mg once daily on days 1–21 of a 21-day cycle (in combination with capecitabine on days 1–14). Continue until disease progression or unacceptable toxicity.

Loperamide (Antidiarrheal) Prophylaxis

Wks 1–2 (days 1–14): 4 mg three times/day. **Wks 3–8 (days 15–56):** 4 mg twice daily. **Wks 9–52 (days 57–365):** 4 mg as needed (do not exceed 16 mg/day).

Dose Reduction Schedule (Neratinib)

First dose reduction: 200 mg daily. **Second dose reduction:** 160 mg daily. **Third dose reduction:** 120 mg daily.

Dose Modification

Based on Common Terminology Criteria for Adverse Events (CTCAE).

Diarrhea
Grade 1 diarrhea; Grade 2 diarrhea lasting more than 5 days; Grade 3 diarrhea lasting more than 2 days: Adjust antidiarrheal therapy, diet. Maintain fluid intake (approx. 2 L/day). Once improved to Grade 1 or 0, start loperamide 4 mg with each administration. **Any grade diarrhea with complications (fever, hypotension, renal failure, or Grade 3 or 4 neutropenia):** Withhold treatment and adjust antidiarrheal therapy, diet. Maintain fluid intake (approx. 2 L/day). If diarrhea improves to Grade 1 or 0 within 7 days, resume treatment at same dose level. If diarrhea improves to Grade 1 or 0 for more than 7 days, resume treatment at the next reduced dose level. Once improved to Grade 1 or 0, start loperamide 4 mg with each administration. **Grade 4 diarrhea; recurrent Grade 2 diarrhea (or higher) at 120 mg dose:** Permanently discontinue.

Hepatotoxicity
Grade 3 serum ALT elevation; Grade 3 serum bilirubin elevation: Withhold treatment until improved to Grade 1 or 0 and investigate cause. If serum ALT elevation improves to Grade 1 or 0 within 3 wks,
resume treatment at reduced dose level. **Grade 4 serum ALT elevation; Grade 4 serum bilirubin elevation:** Permanently discontinue and investigate cause.

Other Toxicities
Any other Grade 3 toxicity: Withhold treatment until improved to Grade 1 or 0 (or baseline), then resume at reduced dose level. **Any other Grade 4 toxicity:** Permanently discontinue.

Dosage in Renal Impairment

Not specified; use caution.

Dosage in Hepatic Impairment

Mild to moderate impairment: No dose adjustment. **Severe impairment:** Reduce starting dose to 80 mg.

SIDE EFFECTS

Frequent (95%–26%): Diarrhea, nausea, abdominal pain, vomiting. **Occasional (18%–4%):** Rash (erythematous, follicular, generalized, pruritic, pustular, maculopapular, papular, dermatitis, dermatitis acneiform, toxic skin eruption), stomatitis, mouth ulceration, oral mucosal blistering, mucosal inflammation, oropharyngeal pain, oral pain, glossodynia, glossitis, cheilitis, decreased appetite, muscle spasm, dyspepsia, nail disorder (paronychia, onychoclasis, nail discoloration, nail toxicity, abnormal nail growth, nail dystrophy), dry skin, abdominal distention, decreased weight, dehydration. **Rare (3%):** Dry mouth.

ADVERSE EFFECTS/TOXIC REACTIONS

Diarrhea reported in 95% of pts. Grade 3 diarrhea reported in 40% of pts. Grade 4 diarrhea reported in less than 1% of pts. Median time of onset of diarrhea was days to wks. Severe diarrhea, dehydration, hypotension, renal failure may occur. Hepatotoxicity reported in 5%–10% of pts.

NURSING CONSIDERATIONS

BASELINE ASSESSMENT

Obtain LFT, vital signs. Obtain BMP and screen for electrolyte imbalance. Confirm

HER2-positive status. Obtain pregnancy test prior to initiation. Stress the importance of antidiarrheal therapy. Question history of IBS with chronic diarrhea, hepatic impairment. Assess hydration status. Question usual bowel movement patterns, stool characteristics. Receive full medication history and screen for interactions. Offer emotional support.

INTERVENTION/EVALUATION

Monitor LFT monthly for the first 3 mos, then q3mos thereafter. Monitor for hepatotoxicity (abdominal pain, ascites, confusion, dark-colored urine, jaundice). Obtain BMP (note electrolytes) if severe diarrhea occurs. Ensure compliance of antidiarrheal therapy. Additional antidiarrheal medication may be needed to manage diarrhea despite treatment with loperamide. Monitor daily pattern of bowel activity, stool consistency. If treatment-related toxicities occur, consider referral to specialist. Monitor I&O. Assess skin, nails, oral mucosa for toxic reactions.

PATIENT/FAMILY TEACHING

• Treatment may cause severe diarrhea, which may lead to life-threatening dehydration or hospitalization. Take antidiarrheal medication exactly as prescribed (goal is 1–2 bowel movements/day). Report worsening of diarrhea or dehydration. • Drink plenty of fluids (at least 2 L/day if severe diarrhea occurs). • Report liver problems such as bruising; confusion; amber, dark, orange-colored urine; right upper abdominal pain; yellowing of the skin or eyes. • Use effective contraception to avoid pregnancy. Do not breastfeed. • There is a high risk of interactions with other medications. Do not take newly prescribed medications unless approved by prescriber who originally started therapy. • Do not take herbal supplements. Do not ingest grapefruit products. • Acid-reducing medications may interfere with absorption; avoid use. Do not take aluminum-, magnesium-, calcium-containing antacids 3 hrs before or 3 hrs after dose. • Do not take newly prescribed medications unless approved by the prescriber who originally started treatment.

niCARdipine

nye-**kar**-di-peen
(Cardene IV)
Do not confuse niCARdipine with NIFEdipine or niMODipine.

◆CLASSIFICATION

PHARMACOTHERAPEUTIC: Calcium channel blocker. Dihydropyridine. **CLINICAL:** Antianginal, antihypertensive.

USES

PO: Treatment of chronic stable (effort-associated) angina, hypertension. **Parenteral:** Short-term treatment of hypertension when oral therapy not feasible or desirable. **OFF-LABEL:** Acute aortic syndromes, aortic dissection, acute ischemic stroke, hypertensive emergency in pregnancy/postpartum (including preeclampsia/eclampsia), intracerebral hemorrhage, subarachnoid hemorrhage.

PRECAUTIONS

Contraindications: Hypersensitivity to niCARdipine. Advanced aortic stenosis. **Cautions:** Cardiac/renal/hepatic dysfunction, HF, hypertrophic cardiomyopathy with outflow tract obstruction, aortic stenosis, coronary artery disease, portal hypertension.

ACTION

Inhibits calcium ion movement across cell membranes of cardiac, vascular smooth muscle during depolarization. **Therapeutic Effect:** Relaxes coronary vascular smooth muscle. Causes coronary vasodilation, increasing myocardial oxygen delivery in angina.

PHARMACOKINETICS

Route	Onset	Peak	Duration
PO	0.5–2 hrs	—	8 hrs
IV	10 min	—	8 hrs or less

Widely distributed. Protein binding: 95%. Metabolized in liver. Primarily excreted in urine. Not removed by hemodialysis. **Half-life:** 2–4 hrs.

⏳ LIFESPAN CONSIDERATIONS

Pregnancy/Lactation: Unknown if distributed in breast milk. **Children:** Safety and efficacy not established. **Elderly:** Age-related renal impairment may require dosage adjustment.

INTERACTIONS

DRUG: May increase concentration/ effects of **cycloSPORINE. Strong CYP3A4 inhibitors (e.g., clarithromycin, ketoconazole, ritonavir)** may increase concentration/ effect. **Strong CYP3A4 inducers (e.g., carBAMazepine, phenytoin, rifAMPin)** may decrease concentration/effect. **HERBAL: Herbals with hypertensive properties (e.g., licorice, yohimbe) or hypotensive properties (e.g., garlic, ginger, ginkgo biloba)** may alter effects. **FOOD: Grapefruit products** may increase concentration/effect. **LAB VALUES:** None significant.

AVAILABILITY (Rx)

Capsules: 20 mg, 30 mg. **Infusion, Ready to Use:** 20 mg/200 mL, 40 mg/200 mL. **Injection Solution:** 2.5 mg/mL (10-mL vial).

ADMINISTRATION/HANDLING

 IV

Reconstitution • Dilute in 240 mL D₅W, 0.45% NaCl, or 0.9% NaCl to provide concentration of 0.1 mg/mL. **Rate of administration** • Titrate to desired effect. • Peripheral venous

irritation may be reduced by rotating infusion sites q12h. **Storage** • Store at room temperature. • Diluted IV solution is stable for 24 hrs at room temperature.

PO

• Give without regard to food.

▦ IV COMPATIBILITIES

Calcium gluconate, diltiazem, magnesium sulfate, nitroglycerin, potassium chloride, potassium phosphate.

INDICATIONS/ROUTES/DOSAGE

Chronic Stable Angina, Hypertension
PO: ADULTS, ELDERLY: Initially, 20 mg 3 times/day. Range: 20–40 mg 3 times/day (allow at least 3 days between dosage increases).

Acute Hypertension
IV infusion: ADULTS, ELDERLY: Initially, 5 mg/hr. May increase by 2.5 mg/hr q5–15min. **Maximum:** 15 mg/hr. After B/P goal is achieved, adjust dose to maintain desired BP.

Dosage in Renal Impairment
PO: ADULTS, ELDERLY: Initially, give 20 mg q8h (30 mg twice daily [sustained-release capsules]), then titrate. **IV:** No dose adjustment.

Dosage in Hepatic Impairment
PO: ADULTS, ELDERLY: Initially, give 20 mg twice daily, then titrate. **IV:** No dose adjustment.

SIDE EFFECTS

Frequent (10%–7%): Headache, facial flushing, peripheral edema, light-headedness, dizziness. **Occasional (6%–3%):** Asthenia, palpitations, angina, tachycardia. **Rare (less than 2%):** Nausea, abdominal cramps, dyspepsia, dry mouth, rash.

ADVERSE EFFECTS/TOXIC REACTIONS

Overdose produces confusion, slurred speech, drowsiness, marked hypotension, bradycardia.

N

NURSING CONSIDERATIONS

BASELINE ASSESSMENT
Concurrent therapy with sublingual nitroglycerin may be used for relief of anginal pain. Record onset, type (sharp, dull, squeezing), radiation, location, intensity, duration of anginal pain, precipitating factors (exertion, emotional stress).

INTERVENTION/EVALUATION
Monitor B/P, heart rate during and following IV infusion. Assess for peripheral edema, thrombophlebitis. Assess skin for facial flushing, dermatitis, rash. Question for asthenia, headache. Monitor LFT results. Assess ECG, pulse for tachycardia. Rotate infusion sites to decrease occurrence of thrombophlebitis.

PATIENT/FAMILY TEACHING
• Avoid alcohol, grapefruit products; limit caffeine. • Report if anginal pain not relieved or if palpitations, shortness of breath, swelling, dizziness, constipation, nausea, hypotension occurs. • Avoid tasks requiring motor skills, alertness until response to drug is established.

nicotine

nik-o-teen
(GoodSense Nicotine, Habitrol, Nicoderm CQ, Nicorette Mini, Nicorette Starter Kit, Nicorette, Nicotine Mini; Nicotine Step 1, 2, 3; Nicotrol, Nicotrol NS, Thrive)
Do not confuse NicoDerm with Nitroderm or Nicorette with Nordette.

◆CLASSIFICATION
PHARMACOTHERAPEUTIC: Cholinergic-receptor agonist. **CLINICAL:** Smoking deterrent.

USES
Treatment to aid smoking cessation for relief of nicotine withdrawal symptoms (including nicotine craving).

PRECAUTIONS
Contraindications: Hypersensitivity to nicotine. **Cautions:** Smoking post-MI period, severe or worsening angina, active temporomandibular joint disease (gum), pregnancy, hyperthyroidism, pheochromocytoma, insulin-dependent diabetes, severe renal impairment, eczematous dermatitis, oropharyngeal inflammation, esophagitis, peptic ulcer (delays healing in peptic ulcer disease), coronary artery disease, recent MI, serious cardiac arrhythmias, vasospastic disease, angina, hypertension, hepatic impairment, use of oral inhaler/nasal spray with bronchospastic disease.

ACTION
Binds to nicotinic-cholinergic receptors at the autonomic ganglia, in the adrenal medulla, at neuromuscular junction, and in the brain, producing stimulating effect in the cortex and a rewards effect in the limbic system. **Therapeutic Effect:** Provides source of nicotine during nicotine withdrawal, reduces withdrawal symptoms.

PHARMACOKINETICS
Absorbed slowly after transdermal administration. Protein binding: 5%. Metabolized in liver. Excreted primarily in urine. **Half-life:** 4 hrs.

⧗ LIFESPAN CONSIDERATIONS
Pregnancy/Lactation: Distributed in breast milk. Use of cigarettes, nicotine gum associated with decrease in fetal breathing movements. **Children:** Not recommended in this pt population. **Elderly:** Age-related decrease in cardiac function may require dosage adjustment.

INTERACTIONS

DRUG: None significant. **HERBAL:** None significant. **FOOD:** None known. **LAB VALUES:** None significant.

AVAILABILITY (OTC)

Chewing Gum: 2 mg, 4 mg. **Inhalation (Nicotrol Inhaler):** 10-mg cartridge. **Lozenges:** 2 mg, 4 mg. **Nasal Spray (Nicotrol NS):** 0.5 mg/spray. **Transdermal Patch:** 7 mg/24 hrs, 14 mg/24 hrs, 21 mg/24 hrs.

ADMINISTRATION/HANDLING

Gum
• Chew slowly until slight tingling in mouth is perceived, then place gum between cheek and gum until tingle is gone. • Repeat process until most of tingle is gone (about 30 min). • Do not eat or drink 15 min before using or while gum is in mouth.

Inhaler
• Insert cartridge into inhaler and push hard until it pops into place. • Replace mouthpiece and twist top and bottom (so markings do not line up). • Inhale deeply into back of throat or puff in short breaths (about 20 min).

Lozenge
• Do not chew or swallow. • Allow to dissolve between cheek and gum (about 20–30 min). • Move from one side of mouth to other side until completely dissolved. • Do not eat or drink 15 min before using or while lozenge in mouth.

Transdermal
• Apply to non-hairy, clean, dry skin on upper body or upper outer arm. • Rotate sites. • Apply immediately after removing backing from patch. • Do not cut patch or wear more than 1 patch at a time. • Discard by folding adhesive ends together, replace in pouch, and dispose properly in trash.

Nasal Spray
• Prime pump (6–8 times before first use; 1–2 times if not used for 24 hrs). • Blow nose prior to use. • Breath through mouth and spray once in each nostril. Do not sniff, swallow, inhale through nose during administration. • 2–3 min after administration, blow nose. • Avoid contact with skin, eyes, or mouth.

INDICATIONS/ROUTES/DOSAGE

Smoking Cessation Aid to Relieve Nicotine Withdrawal Symptoms

PO: *(Chewing Gum):* **ADULTS, ELDERLY:** 2 mg. Use 4 mg in pts who smoke first cigarette within 30 min of waking. Chew 1 piece of gum when urge to smoke, up to 24/day. Use following schedule: wks 1–6: q1–2h (at least 9 pieces/day); wks 7–9: q2–4h; wks 10–12: q4–8h.

PO: *(Lozenge):*
◄**ALERT**► For pts who smoke the first cigarette within 30 min of waking, administer the 4-mg lozenge; otherwise, administer the 2-mg lozenge.

ADULTS, ELDERLY: One 4-mg or 2-mg lozenge q1–2h for the first 6 wks (use at least 9 lozenges/day first 6 wks); 1 lozenge q2–4h for wks 7–9; and 1 lozenge q4–8h for wks 10–12. **Maximum:** 1 lozenge at a time, 5 lozenges/6 hrs, 20 lozenges/day.

Transdermal:
◄**ALERT**► Apply 1 new patch q24h. **ADULTS, ELDERLY WHO SMOKE MORE THAN 10 CIGARETTES PER DAY:** Follow the guidelines below. **Step 1:** 21 mg/day for 6 wks. **Step 2:** 14 mg/day for 2 wks. **Step 3:** 7 mg/day for 2 wks. **ADULTS, ELDERLY WHO SMOKE 10 OR LESS CIGARETTES PER DAY:** Follow the guidelines below. **Step 1:** 14 mg/day for 6 wks. **Step 2:** 7 mg/day for 2 wks.

Nasal: ADULTS, ELDERLY: Each dose (2 sprays, 1 spray in each nostril) = 1 mg nicotine. Initially, 1–2 doses/hr. **Maximum:** 5 doses/hr (10 sprays), 40 doses/day (80 sprays). For best results, take at least 8 doses/day (16 sprays). Use beyond 6 mos not recommended.

Inhaler: *(Nicotrol):* **ADULTS, ELDERLY:** Initially, 6–16 cartridges/day (at least 6 for first 3–6 wks). Best results with continuous puffing (20 min). **Maximum:** 16 cartridges/day. Use beyond 6 mos not recommended.

N

Dosage in Renal/Hepatic Impairment
No dose adjustment.

SIDE EFFECTS

Frequent: All forms: Hiccups, nausea. **Gum:** Mouth/throat soreness. **Transdermal:** Erythema, pruritus, burning at application site. **Occasional: All forms:** Eructation, GI upset, dry mouth, insomnia, diaphoresis, irritability. **Gum:** Hoarseness. **Inhaler:** Mouth/throat irritation, cough. **Rare: All forms:** Dizziness, myalgia, arthralgia.

ADVERSE EFFECTS/TOXIC REACTIONS

Overdose produces palpitations, tachyarrhythmias, seizures, depression, confusion, diaphoresis, hypotension, rapid/weak pulse, dyspnea. Lethal dose for adults is 40–60 mg. Death results from respiratory paralysis.

NURSING CONSIDERATIONS

BASELINE ASSESSMENT

Screen, evaluate those with coronary heart disease (history of MI, angina pectoris), serious cardiac arrhythmias, Buerger's disease, Prinzmetal's variant angina.

INTERVENTION/EVALUATION

Monitor smoking habits, B/P, pulse, sleep pattern, skin for erythema, pruritus, burning at application site if transdermal system used.

PATIENT/FAMILY TEACHING

• Follow guidelines for proper application of transdermal system. • Chew gum slowly to avoid jaw ache, maximize benefit. • Report persistent rash, pruritus that occurs with patch. • Do not smoke while wearing patch.

NIFEdipine

nye-**fed**-i-peen
(Adalat XL ✦, Procardia XL)
Do not confuse NIFEdipine with niCARdipine or niMODipine, or Procardia XL with Cartia XT.

PHARMACOTHERAPEUTIC: Calcium channel blocker, dihydropyridine. **CLINICAL:** Antianginal, antihypertensive.

USES

Management of chronic stable or vasospastic angina. Management of hypertension (ER products only). **OFF-LABEL:** Anal fissures, high-altitude pulmonary edema, hypertensive emergency in pregnancy/postpartum (including preeclampsia/eclampsia), pulmonary arterial hypertension, Raynaud phenomenon, tocolysis.

PRECAUTIONS

Contraindications: Hypersensitivity to NIFEdipine. ST elevation myocardial infarction (STEMI). **Cautions:** Renal/hepatic impairment, obstructive coronary disease, HF, severe aortic stenosis, edema, severe left ventricular dysfunction, hypertrophic cardiomyopathy, before major surgery, bradycardia, concurrent use with beta blockers or digoxin, CYP3A4 inhibitors/inducers.

ACTION

Inhibits calcium ion movement across cell membranes of vascular smooth muscle and myocardium during depolarization. **Therapeutic Effect:** Relaxes coronary vascular smooth muscle and coronary vasodilation, increases myocardial oxygen delivery (angina), reduces peripheral vascular resistance, reduces arterial B/P.

PHARMACOKINETICS

Widely distributed. Protein binding: 92%–98%. Metabolized in liver. Primarily excreted in urine. Not removed by hemodialysis. **Half-life:** 2–5 hrs.

⧗ LIFESPAN CONSIDERATIONS

Pregnancy/Lactation: Insignificant amount distributed in breast milk. **Children:** Safety and efficacy not established. **Elderly:** Age-related renal

---

impairment may require dosage adjustment. Use lower initial doses and titrate to response.

INTERACTIONS

DRUG: Strong CYP3A4 inducers (e.g., rifAMPin, PHENobarbital, phenytoin, carBAMazepine) may decrease concentration/effect. **Strong CYP3A4 inhibitors (e.g., clarithromycin, ketoconazole)** may increase concentration/effect. **Beta blockers (e.g., carvedilol, metoprolol)** may have additive effect. May increase **digoxin** concentration, risk of toxicity. **HERBAL: Herbals with hypertensive properties (e.g., licorice, yohimbe)** or hypotensive properties (e.g., garlic, ginger, ginkgo biloba)** may alter effects. **FOOD: Grapefruit products** may increase risk for flushing, headache, tachycardia, hypotension. **LAB VALUES:** May cause positive ANA, direct Coombs' test.

AVAILABILITY (Rx)

Capsules: 10 mg, 20 mg.

🜚 **Tablets, Extended-Release:** 30 mg, 60 mg, 90 mg.

ADMINISTRATION/HANDLING

PO
• May give without regard to food. **Extended-Release:** Administer whole; do not crush, split, or allow chewing.

INDICATIONS/ROUTES/DOSAGE

Angina
PO: *(Extended-Release):* **ADULTS, ELDERLY:** Initially, 30–60 mg/day. May increase at 7- to 14-day intervals. **Usual range:** 30–90 mg/day. **Maximum:** 120 mg/day.

Hypertension
PO: *(Extended-Release):* **ADULTS, ELDERLY:** Initially, 30–60 mg once daily. Evaluate response after 2–4 wks. May titrate up to 90 mg once daily.

Dosage in Renal/Hepatic Impairment
No dose adjustment.

SIDE EFFECTS

Frequent (30%–11%): Peripheral edema, headache, flushed skin, dizziness. **Occasional (12%–6%):** Nausea, shakiness, muscle cramps/pain, drowsiness, palpitations, nasal congestion, cough, dyspnea, wheezing. **Rare (5%–3%):** Hypotension, rash, pruritus, urticaria, constipation, abdominal discomfort, flatulence, sexual dysfunction.

ADVERSE EFFECTS/TOXIC REACTIONS

May precipitate HF, MI in pts with cardiac disease, peripheral ischemia. Overdose produces nausea, drowsiness, confusion, slurred speech. **Antidote:** Glucagon (see Appendix H for dosage).

NURSING CONSIDERATIONS

BASELINE ASSESSMENT
Concurrent therapy with sublingual nitroglycerin may be used for relief of anginal pain. Record onset, type (sharp, dull, squeezing), radiation, location, intensity, duration of anginal pain; precipitating factors (exertion, emotional stress). Check B/P for hypotension immediately before giving medication.

INTERVENTION/EVALUATION
Monitor B/P. Assist with ambulation if light-headedness, dizziness occurs. Assess for peripheral edema. Assess skin for flushing. Monitor LFT. Observe for signs/symptoms of HF.

PATIENT/FAMILY TEACHING
• Go from lying to standing slowly. • Report palpitations, shortness of breath, pronounced dizziness, nausea, exacerbations of angina. • Avoid alcohol; concomitant grapefruit product use.

niMODipine

nye-**mode**-i-peen
(Nimotop 🍁, Nymalize)
Do not confuse niMODipine with amlodipine, niCARdipine or NIFEdipine.

◆CLASSIFICATION

PHARMACOTHERAPEUTIC: Calcium channel blocker, dihydropyridine. **CLINICAL:** Cerebral vasospasm agent.

USES

Improvement of neurologic deficits due to cerebral vasospasm following sub-arachnoid hemorrhage from ruptured intracranial aneurysms.

PRECAUTIONS

Contraindications: Hypersensitivity to niMODipine. Concurrent use with strong CYP3A4 inhibitors (e.g., clarithromycin, voriconazole). **Cautions:** Pts with cirrhosis, baseline hypotension, bradycardia.

⏳ LIFESPAN CONSIDERATIONS

Pregnancy/Lactation: Unknown if crosses placenta or is distributed in breast milk. **Children:** Safety and efficacy not established. **Elderly:** Age-related renal impairment may require dosage adjustment. May experience greater hypotensive response, constipation.

ACTION

Inhibits movement of calcium ions across vascular smooth muscle cell membranes during depolarization. Exerts greatest effect on cerebral arteries. **Therapeutic Effect:** Produces favorable effect on severity of neurologic deficits due to dilation of small cerebral resistance vessels. Prevents cerebral vasospasm.

PHARMACOKINETICS

Widely distributed. Protein binding: 95%. Metabolized in liver. Peak plasma concentration: within 1 hr. Excreted in bile (80%), urine (20%). Not removed by hemodialysis. **Half-life:** 1–2 hrs.

INTERACTIONS

DRUG: CYP3A4 **inhibitors** (e.g., **clarithromycin, ketoconazole, ritonavir**) increase concentration/effect. CYP3A4 **inducers** (e.g., carBAMazepine, phenytoin, rifAMPin) may decrease concentration/effect. **HERBAL:** Herbals with hypertensive properties (e.g., licorice, yohimbe) or hypotensive properties (e.g., garlic, ginger, ginkgo biloba) may alter effects. **St. John's wort** may decrease concentration/effect. **FOOD:** Grapefruit products may increase concentration, risk of toxicity. **LAB VALUES:** None significant.

AVAILABILITY (Rx)

Solution, Oral: *(Nymalize):* 6 mg/mL 30 mg/5 mL, 60 mg/10 mL prefilled syringeS; 30 mg/5 mL unit-dose prefilled syringe; 60 mg/10 mL 8 oz bottle.

Capsules: 30 mg.

ADMINISTRATION/HANDLING

PO

• Administer 1 hr before or 2 hrs after meals. • **Capsule:** If pt unable to swallow, place hole in both ends of capsule with 18-gauge needle to extract contents into syringe. **Oral solution:** (6 mg/mL oral syringe in place of capsule). **Nasogastric or gastric tube administration:** Administer with prefilled oral syringe. • Refill syringe with 10mL of 0.9% saline; flush remaining contents from nasogastric or gastric tube into stomach.

INDICATIONS/ROUTES/DOSAGE

Subarachnoid Hemorrhage
PO: ADULTS, ELDERLY: 60 mg q4h for 21 days. Begin within 96 hrs of subarachnoid hemorrhage.

Dosage in Renal Impairment
No dose adjustment.

Dosage in Hepatic Impairment
PO: ADULTS, ELDERLY: Reduce dose to 30 mg q4h in pts with cirrhosis.

SIDE EFFECTS

Occasional (6%–2%): Hypotension, peripheral edema, diarrhea, headache. **Rare (less than 2%):** Allergic reaction (rash, urticaria), tachycardia, flushing of skin.

ADVERSE EFFECTS/TOXIC REACTIONS

Overdose produces nausea, weakness, dizziness, drowsiness, confusion, slurred speech.

NURSING CONSIDERATIONS

BASELINE ASSESSMENT

Assess level of consciousness, neurologic response, initially and throughout therapy. Assess B/P, heart rate immediately before drug administration. Assess hydration status.

INTERVENTION/EVALUATION

The benefit of giving niMODipine for prevention of cerebral vasospasm must be considered if manageable bradycardia or hypotension occurs. Consider administering 30-mg dose q2h if bradycardia; hypotension is a concern in the acute care setting. Monitor heart rate, B/P for evidence of hypotension, bradycardia. Monitor transcranial Doppler results for evidence of vasospasm. Perform frequent neurological assessments. Vasospasm may cause neurological deficits that mimic symptoms of stroke (aphagia, altered mental status, facial droop, hemiplegia, vision loss) and require immediate intervention.

PATIENT/FAMILY TEACHING

• Report palpitations, shortness of breath, swelling, constipation, nausea, dizziness. Immediately report worsening of stroke-like symptoms (blindness, confusion, one-sided weakness, loss of consciousness, trouble speaking, seizures). Drink plenty of fluids to maintain hydration.

niraparib

nye-**rap**-a-rib
(Zejula)
Do not confuse niraparib with FIXED COMBINATION(S) olaparib, neratinib, or rucaparib.
Akkega: niraparib/abiraterone (a CYP17 inhibitor): 50 mg/500 mg, 100 mg/500 mg.

◆CLASSIFICATION

PHARMACOTHERAPEUTIC: Poly(ADP-ribose) polymerase (PARP) inhibitor.
CLINICAL: Antineoplastic.

USES

Maintenance treatment of adults with advanced epithelial, ovarian, fallopian tube, or primary peritoneal cancer who are in a complete or partial response to first-line platinum-based chemotherapy. Maintenance treatment of adults with deleterious or suspected deleterious germline *BRCA*-mutated recurrent epithelial, ovarian, fallopian tube, or primary peritoneal cancer who are in a complete or partial response to platinum-based chemotherapy. **Note:** Akkega is used for deleterious or suspected deleterious *BRCA*-mutated (BRCAm) metastatic castration-resistant prostate cancer (mCRPC).

PRECAUTIONS

Contraindications: Hypersensitivity to niraparib. **Cautions:** Baseline cytopenias; history of hypertension, cardiac disease; pts at risk for hemorrhage (e.g., history of GI bleeding, coagulation disorders, recent trauma; conditions predisposing to infection (e.g., diabetes, renal failure, immunocompromised pts, open wounds); concomitant use of anticoagulants, antiplatelet medication, NSAIDs).

ACTION

Inhibits poly(ADP-ribose) polymerase (PARP) enzymatic activity, resulting in DNA damage, apoptosis, and cellular death. **Therapeutic Effect:** Induces cytotoxicity in tumor cell lines with and without BRCA deficiencies.

PHARMACOKINETICS

Widely distributed. Metabolized by carboxylesterase to inactive metabolite. Protein binding: 83%. Peak plasma concentration: 3 hrs. Excreted in urine (48%), feces (39%). **Half-Life:** 36 hrs.

⌛ LIFESPAN CONSIDERATIONS

Pregnancy/Lactation: Avoid pregnancy; may cause fetal harm/malformations. Females of reproductive potential should use effective contraception during treatment and for at least 6 mos after discontinuation. Unknown if distributed in breast milk. Breastfeeding not recommended during treatment and up to 1 mo after discontinuation. May impair fertility in males. **Children:** Safety and efficacy not established. **Elderly:** No age-related precautions noted.

INTERACTIONS

DRUG: May increase immunosuppressive effects of **baricitinib, fingolimod, tofacitinib, upadacitinib.** May increase the adverse/toxic effect of **natalizumab. Pimecrolimus, tacrolimus (topical)** may increase adverse/toxic effect. May increase adverse/toxic effect, decrease therapeutic effect of **vaccines (live).** May decrease therapeutic effect of **BCG (intravesical). HERBAL: Echinacea** may decrease therapeutic effect. **FOOD:** None known. **LAB VALUES:** May increase serum alkaline phosphatase, ALT, AST, creatinine, GGT. May decrease ANC, Hgb, Hct, leukocytes, neutrophils, RBCs; serum potassium.

AVAILABILITY (Rx)

Tablets: 100 mg, 200 mg, 300 mg.

ADMINISTRATION/HANDLING

PO

• Give with or without food. • Give at the same time each day. • Administer whole; do not crush, split, or allow chewing. • If a dose is missed or vomiting occurs after administration, do not give extra dose. Administer next dose at regularly scheduled time. • Administration at bedtime may decrease occurrence of nausea.

INDICATIONS/ROUTES/DOSAGE

Ovarian Cancer (Recurrent Germline BRCA-Mutated)

PO: ADULTS, ELDERLY: 300 mg once daily, initiated no later than 8 wks after most recent platinum-containing regimen.

Continue until disease progression or unacceptable toxicity.

Ovarian Cancer (Advanced)

Note: Pts should start treatment no later than 12 wks after most recent platinum-containing regimen.

PO: ADULTS, ELDERLY: 200 mg once daily (if weight less than 77 kg or platelet count is less than 150,000 cells/mm³) or 300 mg once daily (if weight greater than or equal to 77 kg and platelet count greater than or equal to 150,000 cells/mm³). Continue until disease progression or unacceptable toxicity.

Dose Reduction Schedule

First dose reduction: 200 mg daily.
Second dose reduction: 100 mg daily.

Dose Modification

Based on Common Terminology Criteria for Adverse Events (CTCAE).
Note: If acute myeloid leukemia or myelodysplastic syndrome is confirmed, permanently discontinue.

Anemia, Neutropenia
ANC less than 1,000 cells/mm³, Hgb less than 8 g/dL: Withhold treatment for maximum of 28 days until ANC improves to greater than or equal to 1,500 cells/mm³ or Hgb level improves to 9 g/dL or greater, then resume at reduced dose level. If ANC or Hgb level does not improve to an acceptable level within 28 days or if dose is already reduced to 100 mg/day, permanently discontinue.

Hematologic Toxicity Requiring Transfusion
Platelet count less than or equal to 10,000 cells/mm³: Consider transfusion, then resume at reduced dose level.

Nonhematologic Toxicity
Any nonhematologic Grade 3 or 4 toxicity when prophylactic treatment is not possible or toxicity persists despite treatment: Withhold treatment for maximum of 28 days until resolved, then resume at next lower dose level.
Any nonhematologic Grade 3 or 4 toxicity lasting more than 28 days with 100 mg/day regimen: Permanently discontinue.

Thrombocytopenia

Platelet count less than 100,000 cells/mm³: First occurrence: Withhold treatment for maximum of 28 days until improved to greater than or equal to 100,000 cells/mm³, then resume at same dose or reduced dose level. If platelet count is less than 75,000 cells/mm³, resume at reduced dose level. **Second occurrence:** Withhold treatment for maximum of 28 days until improved to greater than or equal to 100,000 cells/mm³, then resume at reduced dose level. If platelet count does not improve to an acceptable level within 28 days or if dose is already reduced to 100 mg/day, permanently discontinue.

Dosage in Renal Impairment

Mild to moderate impairment: No dose adjustment. **Severe impairment, ESRD:** Not specified; use caution.

Dosage in Hepatic Impairment

Mild impairment: No dose adjustment. **Moderate to severe impairment:** Not specified; use caution.

SIDE EFFECTS

Frequent (74%–20%): Nausea, fatigue, asthenia, constipation, vomiting, abdominal pain/distention, insomnia, headache, decreased appetite, rash, mucositis, stomatitis, hypertension, dyspnea. **Occasional (19%–10%):** Myalgia, back pain, dizziness, dyspepsia, cough, arthralgia, anxiety, dysgeusia, dry mouth, palpitations, tachycardia, peripheral edema, decreased weight, depression.

ADVERSE EFFECTS/TOXIC REACTIONS

Myelosuppression (anemia neutropenia, leukopenia, thrombocytopenia) is an expected response to therapy, but more severe reactions including bone marrow failure may result in life-threatening event. Fatal cases of acute myeloid leukemia, myelodysplastic syndrome reported in 1% of pts. Hypertension, hypertensive crisis reported in 9% of pts. Infections including bronchitis, conjunctivitis, nasopharyngitis (23% of pts), UTI (13% of pts) may occur. Epistaxis may occur, esp. in pts with treatment-induced thrombocytopenia.

NURSING CONSIDERATIONS

BASELINE ASSESSMENT

Obtain ANC, CBC, BMP, LFT; vital signs. Obtain pregnancy test in females of reproductive potential. Confirm compliance of effective contraception. Question history of cardiac disease, hypertension. Assess hydration status. Screen for active infection. Offer emotional support.

INTERVENTION/EVALUATION

Monitor ANC, CBC for myelosuppression wkly for first 4 wks, then monthly for 11 mos, then periodically thereafter. In pts with platelet count less than 10,000 cells/mm³, consider withholding anticoagulant, antiplatelet drugs or proceed with transfusion (if applicable). Monitor for acute myeloid leukemia, myelodysplastic syndrome (bleeding or bruising easily, fatigue, frequent infections, pyrexia, hematuria, melena, weakness, weight loss, cytopenias, increased requirements for blood transfusion). Diligently screen for infections (cough, fatigue, fever). Monitor vital signs for arrhythmia, hypertension, tachycardia. Offer antiemetic if nausea, vomiting occurs. Assess skin for rash, toxic reactions. Encourage nutritional intake.

PATIENT/FAMILY TEACHING

• Treatment may depress your immune system and reduce your ability to fight infection. Report symptoms of infection such as body aches, burning with urination, chills, cough, fatigue, fever. Avoid those with active infection. • Treatment may cause severe bone marrow depression or new-onset myeloid leukemia; report bruising, fatigue, fever, frequent infections, shortness of breath, weight loss, bleeding easily, blood in urine or stool. • Use effective contraception to avoid pregnancy. Do not breastfeed. • Dose administration at bedtime may decrease occurrence of nausea.

 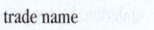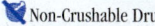

nirmatrelvir/ritonavir

nir-ma-**trel**-vir/rit-**oh**-na-vir
(Paxlovid)

■ **BLACK BOX ALERT** ■

Ritonavir, a strong CYP3A4 inhibitor, may increase concentration/effect of certain concomitant medications, which may result in life-threatening or fatal events. Prescribers must cross-check all home medications for possible drug interactions. Certain home medications may need to be adjusted or interrupted.

Do not confuse nirmatrelvir with molnupiravir or Paxlovid with Paxil or Plavix.

◆CLASSIFICATION

PHARMACOTHERAPEUTIC: Severe acute respiratory syndrome coronavirus 2 (SARS-CoV-2) main protease inhibitor (nirmatrelvir); HIV-1 protease inhibitor, CYP3A4 inhibitor (ritonavir). **CLINICAL:** Antiviral.

USES

Treatment of mild to moderate coronavirus 2019 (COVID-19) infection in adults who are at high risk for progression to severe COVID-19, including hospitalization or death.

PRECAUTIONS

Contraindications: Clinically significant hypersensitivity to nirmatrelvir or ritonavir (e.g., toxic epidermal necrolysis [TEN] or Stevens-Johnson syndrome). Concomitant use of strong CYP3A4 inducers; drugs highly dependent on CYP3A4 metabolism for clearance and for which elevated plasma concentrations are associated with serious and/or life-threatening events (see Interactions). **Cautions:** Hepatic/renal impairment, preexisting liver disease (e.g., hepatitis), hepatic enzyme abnormalities, uncontrolled or undiagnosed HIV-1 infection. Not recommended in pts with severe renal or hepatic impairment. Not approved for pre- or post-exposure prophylaxis for prevention of COVID-19; use for longer than 5 consecutive days; initiating treatment in hospitalized pts due to severe or critical COVID-19 infection.

ACTION

Nirmatrelvir inhibits peptidomimetic activity of SARS-CoV-2 main protease by inhibiting viral polyproteins pp1a and pp1ab, essential for viral replication. Ritonavir inhibits the CYP3A4-mediated metabolism of nirmatrelvir, increasing plasma concentrations of nirmatrelvir (acts as a booster). **Therapeutic Effect:** Inhibits viral replication of COVID-19 infection. Reduces duration of clinical symptoms.

PHARMACOKINETICS

Widely distributed. Nirmatrelvir has minimal metabolic clearance. Ritonavir metabolized in liver. Protein binding: (nirmatrelvir): 69%; (ritonavir) 98%–99%. Peak plasma concentration: 3–4 hrs. Nirmatrelvir excreted in urine (49.6%), feces (35.3%). Ritonavir excreted in feces (86.4%), urine (11.3%). **Half-life:** (nirmatrelvir): 6.05 hrs; (ritonavir) 6.15 hrs.

⧗ LIFESPAN CONSIDERATIONS

Pregnancy/Lactation: No overall difference of birth defects for ritonavir compared to background birth defect rate. Females of reproductive potential using combined hormonal contraceptives must use effective alternative contraception or barriers methods during treatment. Unknown if distributed in breast milk. **Children:** Safety and efficacy not established. **Elderly:** No age-related precautions noted.

INTERACTIONS

DRUG: Concomitant use of the following drugs is contraindicated due to risk of serious or life-threatening event related to increased concentrations/effects: **alpha 1-adrenoreceptor antagonist (e.g., alfuzosin), antianginal (e.g., ranolazine), antiarrhythmic (e.g.,**

N

amiodarone, dronedarone, flecainide, propafenone, quinidine), anti-gout (e.g., colchicine [in pts with renal and/or hepatic impairment]), antipsychotics (e.g., lurasidone, pimozide), benign prostatic hyperplasia agent (e.g., silodosin), cardiovascular agents (e.g., eplerenone, ivabradine), ergot derivatives (e.g., dihydroergotamine, ergotamine, methylergonovine), HMG-CoA reductase inhibitors (e.g., lovastatin, simvastatin), microsomal triglyceride transfer protein inhibitor (e.g., lomitapide), migraine drugs (e.g., eletriptan, ubrogepant), mineralocorticoid receptor antagonist (e.g., finerenone), opioid antagonist (e.g., naloxegol), PDE5 inhibitor (e.g., sildenafil), sedative/hypnotics (e.g., triazolam, oral midazolam), anticancer drugs (e.g., apalutamide), strong CYP3A4 inducers (e.g., carBAMazepine, phenytoin, rifAMPin) may decrease concentration/effect; may cause loss of virologic response and possible resistance; use contraindicated. Anticoagulants (e.g., apixaban, rivaroxaban, warfarin) may increase risk of bleeding. May increase concentration/effect of alpha 1-adrenoreceptor antagonist (e.g., tamsulosin), antiarrhythmics (e.g., lidocaine [systemic], disopyramide), anticancer drugs (e.g., ceritinib, ibrutinib, vinblastine), antifungals (e.g., itraconazole, ketoconazole), anti-HIV drugs (e.g., efavirenz, tenofovir), anti-HIV protease inhibitors (e.g., atazanavir, tipranavir), antipsychotics (e.g., clozapine), bosentan, calcium channel blockers (e.g., amLODIPine, dilTIAZem, verapamil), cardiovascular agents (e.g., ticagrelor), clarithromycin, clonazePAM, corticosteroids (e.g., dexamethasone, methylPREDNISolone), digoxin, ethinyl estradiol, hepatitis C antivirals (e.g., elbasvir/grazoprevir), HMG-CoA reductase inhibitors (e.g., atorvastatin, rosuvastatin), immunosuppressants (e.g., cycloSPORINE, tacrolimus) ivacaftor, Janus kinase (JAK) inhibitors (e.g., tofacitinib, upadacitinib),

muscarinic receptor antagonists (e.g., darifenacin), narcotic analgesics (e.g., fentaNYL, oxyCODONE, methadone), neuropsychiatric agents (e.g., aripiprazole, iloperidone, pimavanserin), PDE5 inhibitors (e.g., sildenafil, tadalafil), pulmonary hypertension agents (e.g., riociguat, tadalafil), rimegepant, sAXagliptin, salmeterol, sedative/hypnotics (e.g., buspirone, diazePAM, zolpidem); avoid use. **HERBAL:** St. John's wort may decrease concentration/effect; may cause loss of virologic response and possible resistance; use contraindicated. **FOOD:** None known. **LAB VALUES:** May increase serum ALT, AST, bilirubin.

AVAILABILITY (Rx)

Co-Packaged Tablets: 300 mg (nirmatrelvir [immediate-release, film-coated]), 100 mg (ritonavir); 150 mg (nirmatrelvir [immediate-release, film-coated]), 100 mg (ritonavir).

ADMINISTRATION/HANDLING

PO
Give without regard to food. • Administer tablets whole; do not break, cut, crush, or divide. Tablets cannot be chewed. • Nirmatrelvir must be co-administered with ritonavir. Failure to correctly co-administer nirmatrelvir with ritonavir may decrease plasma concentrations of nirmatrelvir, causing a decreased therapeutic effect. • If a dose is missed within 8 hrs of regularly scheduled time, give as soon as possible. If a dose is missed by more than 8 hrs, skip the dose and give next dose at regularly scheduled time. Do not double the next dose.

INDICATIONS/ROUTES/DOSAGE

COVID-19 Infection (Mild to Moderate)
Note: Initiate as soon as possible (within 5 days) when COVID-19 infection is diagnosed. If pt is hospitalized due to severe or critical COVID-19 infection after starting treatment, the full 5-day course should be completed at prescriber's discretion. **PO: ADULTS, ELDERLY:** 300 mg of

---

nirmatrelvir (two 150-mg tablets) and 100 mg of ritonavir (one 100-mg tablet) given together twice daily for 5 days.

Dosage in Renal Impairment

Mild impairment (eGFR 60–89 mL/min): No dose adjustment. **Moderate impairment (eGFR 30–59 mL/min):** 150 mg of nirmatrelvir (one 150-mg tablet) and 100 mg of ritonavir (one 100-mg tablet) given together twice daily for 5 days. **Severe impairment (eGFR less than 30mL/min):** Not recommended.

Dosage in Hepatic Impairment

Mild to moderate impairment: No dose adjustment.
Severe impairment: Not recommended.

SIDE EFFECTS

(Frequency not specified): Headache, hypertension, abdominal pain, nausea, vomiting, malaise, altered taste.

ADVERSE EFFECTS/TOXIC REACTIONS

Life-threatening reactions related to drug interactions, including fatal events, have occurred. The most common drug interactions that resulted in serious adverse reactions were calcineurin inhibitors (e.g., tacrolimus, cycloSPORINE) and calcium channel blockers (e.g., dilTIAZem). Severe hypersensitivity reactions, including anaphylaxis, may occur. Dermatologic toxicities including Stevens-Johnson syndrome, toxic epidermal necrolysis may occur. Hepatotoxicity, clinical hepatitis was reported in pts taking ritonavir. Pts with uncontrolled or undiagnosed HIV-1 infection may be at risk for developing resistance to HIV protease inhibitors. Posttreatment viral RNA rebound may occur.

NURSING CONSIDERATIONS

BASELINE ASSESSMENT

Confirm positive test for SARS-CoV-2. Auscultate lung sounds. Assess for symptoms of COVID-19 (anosmia, body aches, congestion, cough, dysgeusia, dyspnea, fever, headache, runny nose). Educate importance of isolation precautions. Receive full medication history (including herbal products) and screen for contraindications/interactions. Concomitant use of other medications may need to be adjusted or withheld. Question history of hepatic/renal impairment, HIV-1 infection.

INTERVENTION/EVALUATION

Monitor for improvement of COVID-19 symptoms. Monitor for skin toxicities, cutaneous reactions; hypersensitivity reactions, anaphylaxis (dyspnea, fever, hypotension, rash, tachycardia). Monitor for hepatotoxicity (bruising, encephalopathy, jaundice, right upper abdominal pain, nausea, vomiting, weight loss) esp. in pts with preexisting liver disease. Ensure the full course of treatment is completed unless an adverse reaction or toxic effect occurs.

PATIENT/FAMILY TEACHING

• Treatment is not a cure, but it may shorten recovery time and reduce symptoms associated with COVID-19 infection. • It is essential to complete the full course of treatment for the best therapeutic response. Do not prematurely stop treatment unless approved by prescriber. • Isolate from others to decrease spread of infection. • Severe allergic reactions such as dizziness, hives, palpitations, rash, shortness of breath may occur. • Report liver problems (abdominal pain, bruising, clay-colored stool, amber or dark-colored urine, yellowing of the skin or eyes), toxic skin reactions (itching, peeling, rash, redness, swelling; blistering of the skin). • Posttreatment viral rebound, a return of symptoms approx. 2–8 days after completion of treatment, may occur. • A bitter, metallic taste is a common side effect that usually subsides after completing treatment. • Drink plenty of fluids. • There is a high risk of interactions with other medications. Do not take newly prescribed medications or restart home medications unless approved by prescriber who originally started treatment. Do not take herbal products (esp. St. John's wort).

nitrofurantoin

nye-troe-fue-**ran**-toyn
(Macrobid, Macrodantin)
**Do not confuse Macrobid with
MicroK or Nitro-Bid, or nitrofuran-
toin with Neurontin or nitroglycerin.**

◆CLASSIFICATION

PHARMACOTHERAPEUTIC: Antibacterial. **CLINICAL:** Antibiotic, UTI
prophylaxis.

USES

Cystitis: (Treatment): Macrobid:
Treatment of acute, uncomplicated cystitis
in adults and children 12 yrs and older
caused by susceptible strains of *E. coli,
S. saprophyticus.* **Macrodantin:** Treatment of acute, uncomplicated cystitis in
adults caused by susceptible strain of *E.
coli,* enterococci, *S. aureus, Klebsiella,
Enterococcus* species. **Cystitis: (Prophylaxis):** Chronic suppression of recurrent UTI.

PRECAUTIONS

Contraindications: Hypersensitivity to
nitrofurantoin. Anuria, oliguria, renal
impairment (CrCl less than 60 mL/min),
infants younger than 1 mo due to risk of
hemolytic anemia. Pregnancy at term, during labor, or delivery, or when onset of labor
is imminent. History of cholestatic jaundice
or hepatic impairment with previous nitrofurantoin therapy. **Cautions:** Renal impairment, diabetes, electrolyte imbalance,
anemia, vitamin B deficiency, debilitated
(greater risk of peripheral neuropathy),
G6PD deficiency (greater risk of hemolytic
anemia), elderly, prolonged therapy (may
cause pulmonary toxicity).

ACTION

Inhibits bacterial enzyme systems,
interfering with protein synthesis,
anaerobic energy metabolism, DNA, RNA,
and cell wall synthesis. **Therapeutic
Effect:** Bactericidal at therapeutic doses.

PHARMACOKINETICS

Microcrystalline form rapidly, completely
absorbed; macrocrystalline form more
slowly absorbed. Food increases absorption. Protein binding: 60%. Primarily
concentrated in urine, kidneys. Metabolized in most body tissues. Primarily
excreted in urine. Removed by hemodialysis. **Half-life:** 20–60 min.

⧗ LIFESPAN CONSIDERATIONS

Pregnancy/Lactation: Readily crosses
placenta. Distributed in breast milk. Contraindicated at term and during lactation
when infant suspected of having G6PD
deficiency. **Children:** No age-related
precautions noted in pts older than 1
mo. **Elderly:** Avoid use. More likely to
develop acute pneumonitis, peripheral
neuropathy. Age-related renal impairment may require dosage adjustment.

INTERACTIONS

**DRUG: Antacids containing mag-
nesium trisilicate** may decrease
absorption. **Probenecid** may alter con-
centration/effect. May decrease effect of
norfloxacin. HERBAL: None significant.
FOOD: None known. **LAB VALUES:** May
increase serum ALT, AST, phosphorus. May
decrease Hgb.

AVAILABILITY (Rx)

**Capsules: *(Macrocrystalline [Macro-
bid]):*** 100 mg. **Capsules: *(Macrocrystalline [Macrodantin]):*** 25 mg, 50 mg,
100 mg. **Oral Suspension: *(Microcrystalline):*** 25 mg/5 mL.

ADMINISTRATION/HANDLING
PO

• Administer with meals (improves
absorption, decreases adverse
effects). • The twice daily formulation
(Macrobid) should not be opened. The
4-times daily formulation (Macrodantin)
may be opened and mixed with food or
juice. May mix suspension with water, milk,
fruit juice; shake well.

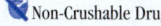

INDICATIONS/ROUTES/DOSAGE

Cystitis

PO: *(Macrodantin):* **ADULTS, ELDERLY:** 50–100 mg q6h; treat males for 7 days or females for 5 days. **Maximum:** 400 mg/day. **CHILDREN, ADOLESCENTS:** 5–7 mg/kg/day in divided doses q6h for 7 days or at least 3 days after obtaining sterile urine. **Maximum:** 400 mg/day (100 mg/dose). **PO:** *(Macrobid):* **ADULTS, ELDERLY, ADOLESCENTS:** 100 mg twice daily; treat males for 7 days or females for 5 days.

Prophylaxis of Recurrent Cystitis

PO: ADULTS, ELDERLY: *(Macrodantin):* 50–100 mg at bedtime. **CHILDREN OLDER THAN 1 MONTH:** 1–2 mg/kg/day in 2 divided doses or single dose at bedtime. **Maximum:** 100 mg/day.

Dosage in Renal Impairment

Contraindicated in pts with CrCl less than 60 mL/min.

Dosage in Hepatic Impairment

No dose adjustment.

SIDE EFFECTS

Frequent: Anorexia, nausea, vomiting, dark urine. **Occasional:** Abdominal pain, diarrhea, rash, pruritus, urticaria, hypertension, headache, dizziness, drowsiness. **Rare:** Photosensitivity, transient alopecia, asthmatic exacerbation in those with history of asthma.

ADVERSE EFFECTS/TOXIC REACTIONS

Superinfection, hepatotoxicity, peripheral neuropathy (may be irreversible), Stevens-Johnson syndrome, permanent pulmonary impairment, anaphylaxis occur rarely.

NURSING CONSIDERATIONS

BASELINE ASSESSMENT

Question for history of asthma. Question medical history as listed in Precautions, and screen for contraindications.

INTERVENTION/EVALUATION

Monitor CBC, BMP, LFT if used long-term; I&O. Monitor daily pattern of bowel activity, stool consistency. Assess skin for rash, urticaria. Be alert for numbness/tingling, esp. of lower extremities (may signal onset of peripheral neuropathy). Observe for signs of hepatotoxicity (fever, rash, arthralgia, hepatomegaly). Monitor respiratory status, esp. in pts with asthma.

PATIENT/ FAMILY TEACHING

• Urine may become dark yellow/brown. • Take with food, milk for best results, to reduce GI upset. • Complete full course of therapy. • Avoid sun, ultraviolet light; use sunscreen, wear protective clothing. • Report cough, fever, chest pain, difficulty breathing, numbness/tingling of fingers, toes. • Rare occurrence of alopecia is transient.

nitroglycerin

nye-troe-**glis**-er-in
(GoNitro, Nitro-Bid, Nitro-Dur, Nitrolingual, NitroMist, Nitrostat, Nitro-Time, Rectiv, Trinipatch ♦)
Do not confuse Nitro-Bid with Macrobid or Nicobid, Nitro-Dur with Nicoderm, nitroglycerin with nitrofurantoin or nitroprusside, or Nitrostat with Nilstat or Nystatin.

◆**CLASSIFICATION**

PHARMACOTHERAPEUTIC: Nitrate. **CLINICAL:** Antianginal, antihypertensive, coronary vasodilator.

USES

Extended-release capsule, topical ointment, transdermal patch: Prevention of angina due to CAD. **Sublingual powder, tablets, spray:** Prevention/treatment of angina due to CAD. **IV solution:** Treatment of angina, acute decompensated HF, perioperative hypertension. Induction of perioperative hypotension. **Rectiv:** Treatment of moderate to severe pain associated with chronic anal fissure. **OFF-LABEL:** Extravasation management (sympathomimetic vasopressors), hypertensive emergency, uterine relaxation.

PRECAUTIONS

Contraindications: Hypersensitivity to nitroglycerin. Allergy to adhesives (transdermal); concurrent use of sildenafil, tadalafil, vardenafil (PDE5 inhibitors). Concurrent use with riociguat. **IV:** Restrictive cardiomyopathy, pericardial tamponade, constrictive pericarditis, increased ICP, uncorrected hypovolemia. **Sublingual, rectal:** Increased intracranial pressure, severe anemia. **Sublingual:** Acute circulatory failure or shock, early MI. **Cautions:** Blood volume depletion, severe hypotension (systolic B/P less than 90 mm Hg), bradycardia (less than 50 beats/min), inferior wall MI and suspected right ventricular involvement.

ACTION

Forms nitric oxide, which increases cGMP, causing dephosphorylation of myosin light chains and smooth muscle relaxation. Produces vasodilation on peripheral veins and arteries (more prominent effect on veins). **Therapeutic Effect:** Decreases myocardial oxygen demand by decreasing preload (LVDP). Improves collateral flow to ischemic areas. **Rectal:** Decreases sphincter tone and intra-anal pressure.

PHARMACOKINETICS

Route	Onset	Peak	Duration
Sublingual	1–3 min	4–8 min	30–60 min
Translingual spray	2 min	4–10 min	30–60 min
Buccal tablet	2–5 min	4–10 min	2 hrs
PO (extended-release)	20–45 min	45–120 min	4–8 hrs

Route	Onset	Peak	Duration
Topical	15–60 min	30–120 min	2–12 hrs
Transdermal patch	40–60 min	60–180 min	18–24 hrs
IV	1–2 min	Immediate	3–5 min

Well absorbed after PO, sublingual, topical administration. Metabolized in liver, by enzymes in bloodstream. Protein binding: 60%. Excreted in urine. Not removed by hemodialysis. **Half-life:** 1–4 min.

⏳ LIFESPAN CONSIDERATIONS

Pregnancy/Lactation: Unknown if drug crosses placenta or is distributed in breast milk. **Children:** Safety and efficacy not established. **Elderly:** More susceptible to hypotensive effects. Age-related renal impairment may require dosage adjustment.

INTERACTIONS

DRUG: Alcohol, other antihypertensives (e.g., amLODIPine, lisinopril, valsartan), vasodilators may increase risk of orthostatic hypotension. Concurrent use of **sildenafil, tadalafil, vardenafil** (PDE5 inhibitors) produces significant hypotension. **Ergot derivatives (e.g., ergotamine)** may decrease effect of vasodilation. May increase hypotensive effect of **riociguat.** **HERBAL:** Herbals with hypertensive properties (e.g., licorice, yohimbe) or hypotensive properties (e.g., garlic, ginger, ginkgo biloba) may alter effects. **FOOD:** None known. **LAB VALUES:** May increase serum methemoglobin, urine catecholamine concentrations.

AVAILABILITY (Rx)

Infusion, Premix: 25 mg/250 mL, 50 mg/250 mL, 100 mg/250 mL. **Injection Solution:** 5 mg/mL. **Ointment: (Nitro-Bid):** 2%. **Ointment, Rectal (Rectiv):** 0.4%. **Translingual Spray:** 0.4 mg/spray. **Transdermal Patch:** 0.1 mg/hr, 0.2 mg/hr, 0.4 mg/hr, 0.6 mg/hr.

🐋 **Capsules, Extended-Release:** 2.5 mg, 6.5 mg, 9 mg. 🐋 **Tablets, Sublingual:** 0.3 mg, 0.4 mg, 0.6 mg.

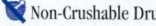 ✦ Canadian trade name 🐋 Non-Crushable Drug 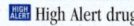 High Alert drug

N

ADMINISTRATION/HANDLING

PO
• Do not break, crush, or open extended-release capsules. • Administer capsule whole with a full glass of water.

Sublingual
• Instruct pt to not swallow, chew, or crush. • Dissolve under tongue. • Administer while seated. • Slight burning sensation under tongue may be lessened by placing tablet in buccal pouch. • Keep sublingual tablets in original container.

Topical
• Spread thin layer on clean, dry, hairless skin of upper arm or body (not below knee or elbow), using applicator or dose-measuring papers. Do not use fingers; do not rub/massage into skin.

Transdermal
• Apply patch on clean, dry, hairless skin of upper arm or body (not below knee or elbow). Remove patch after 12–14 hrs. • May keep patch on when bathing/showering. • Do not cut/trim to adjust dose.

✳ IV COMPATIBILITIES

Clevidipine, dexmedetomidine, heparin, norepinephrine, propofol, vasopressin.

INDICATIONS/ROUTES/DOSAGE
Prevention of Angina
Translingual spray: ADULTS, ELDERLY: 1–2 sprays 5–10 min prior to activities that may provoke angina.
Sublingual: ADULTS, ELDERLY: 0.3 mg or 0.4 mg 5–10 min prior to activities that may provoke angina. **Sublingual Powder:** ADULTS, ELDERLY: 1 packet 5–10 min prior to activities that may provoke angina.
PO: *(Extended-Release):* ADULTS, ELDERLY: 2.5–6.5 mg 3–4 times/day. **Maximum:** 26 mg 4 times/day.

Topical: ADULTS, ELDERLY: Initially, 1/2 inch upon waking and 1/2 inch 6 hrs later. May double dose to 1 inch and double again to 2 inches. **Maximum:** 2 doses/day including nitrate-free interval of 10–12 hrs.
Transdermal patch: ADULTS, ELDERLY: Initially, 0.2–0.4 mg/hr. **Maintenance:** 0.4–0.8 mg/hr. Consider patch on for 12–14 hrs, patch off for 10–12 hrs (prevents tolerance).

Acute Angina
Translingual spray: 1–2 sprays (0.4 mg). Repeat q5min if angina persists. If chest pain does not improve or worsens, call emergency services.
Sublingual tablet: 1 tablet (0.3–0.4 mg) under tongue. If chest pain does not improve or worsens in 3–5 min, call emergency services. After the call, may take additional tablet. A third tablet may be taken 5 min after second dose. **Maximum:** 3 tablets.
Sublingual powder: Initially, 1–2 packets, may repeat q5min.
IV: ADULTS, ELDERLY: Initially, 5–10 mcg/min. Titrate as needed based on response and tolerability in increments of 5–10 mcg/minute q3-5min. **Maximum:** 400 mcg/min.

Anal Fissure
Rectal: ADULTS, ELDERLY: After cleansing, apply around fissure(s) twice daily as directed for 4 wks. If symptoms persist, continue for another 4 wks for a total duration of 8 wks.

Dosage in Renal/Hepatic Impairment
No dose adjustment.

SIDE EFFECTS
Frequent: Headache (possibly severe; occurs mostly in early therapy, diminishes rapidly in intensity, usually disappears during continued treatment), transient flushing of face/neck, dizziness (esp. if pt is standing immobile or is in a warm environment), weakness, orthostatic hypotension. **Sublingual:** Burning, tingling sensation at oral point

of dissolution. **Ointment:** Erythema, pruritus. **Occasional:** GI upset. **Transdermal:** Contact dermatitis.

ADVERSE EFFECTS/TOXIC REACTIONS

Severe orthostatic hypotension may occur, manifested by syncope, pulselessness, cold/clammy skin, diaphoresis. Tolerance may occur with repeated, prolonged therapy; minor tolerance may occur with intermittent use of sublingual tablets. High doses tend to produce severe headache.

NURSING CONSIDERATIONS

BASELINE ASSESSMENT

Record onset, type (sharp, dull, squeezing), radiation, location, intensity, duration of anginal pain; precipitating factors (exertion, emotional stress). Assess B/P, apical pulse before administration and periodically following dose. Pt must have continuous ECG monitoring for IV administration. Rule out right-sided MI, if applicable (may precipitate life-threatening hypotension). Receive full medication history, and screen for interactions, esp. use of PDE5 inhibitors. Question medical history and screen for contraindications.

INTERVENTION/EVALUATION

Monitor B/P, heart rate. Assess for facial, neck flushing. Cardioverter/defibrillator must not be discharged through paddle electrode overlying nitroglycerin (transdermal, ointment) system (may cause burns to pt or damage to paddle via electrical arcing). Consider NS boluses for hypotension.

PATIENT/FAMILY TEACHING

• Go from lying to standing slowly. • Take oral form on empty stomach (however, if headache occurs during therapy, take medication with meals). • Use spray only when lying down. • Dissolve sublingual tablet under tongue; do not swal-low. • Take at first sign of angina. • May take additional dose q5min if needed up to a total of 3 doses. • If not relieved within 5 min, contact physician or immediately go to emergency room. • Do not inhale lingual aerosol but spray onto or under tongue (avoid swallowing after spray is administered). • Expel from mouth any remaining lingual, sublingual, intrabuccal tablet after pain is completely relieved. • Place transmucosal tablets under upper lip or buccal pouch (between cheek and gum); do not chew/swallow tablet. • Avoid alcohol (intensifies hypotensive effect). If alcohol is ingested soon after taking nitroglycerin, possible acute hypotensive episode (marked drop in B/P, vertigo, diaphoresis, pallor) may occur. • Do not use within 48 hrs of sildenafil, tadalafil, vardenafil (PDE5 inhibitors); may cause acute hypotensive episode.

nivolumab

nye-**vol**-ue-mab
(Opdivo)
Do not confuse nivolumab with denosumab, adalimumab, or palivizumab.

◆CLASSIFICATION

PHARMACOTHERAPEUTIC: Anti-PD-1 monoclonal antibody. Immune checkpoint inhibitor. **CLINICAL:** Antineoplastic.

USES

Classical Hodgkin lymphoma (cHL): Treatment of adults with cHL that has relapsed or progressed after autologous hematopoietic stem cell transplantation (HSCT) and brentuximab vedotin, or 3 or more lines of systemic therapy that includes autologous HSCT. **Metastatic**

colorectal cancer (CRC): Treatment of adult and pts 12 yrs and older with microsatellite instability-high (MSI-H) or mismatch repair deficient (dMMR) metastatic CRC that has progressed following treatment with fluoropyrimidine, oxaliplatin, and irinotecan. **Esophageal cancer:** First-line treatment of adults with unresectable advanced or metastatic esophageal squamous cell carcinoma (ESCC) in combination with fluoropyrimidine- and platinum-containing chemotherapy or in combination with ipilimumab. Treatment of adults with unresectable advanced, recurrent, or metastatic ESCC after prior fluoropyrimidine- and platinum-based chemotherapy. Adjuvant treatment of completely resected esophageal or gastroesophageal junction cancer with residual pathologic disease in adults who have received neoadjuvant chemoradiotherapy. **Gastric cancer, gastroesophageal junction cancer, and esophageal adenocarcinoma:** Treatment of adults with advanced or metastatic gastric cancer, gastroesophageal junction cancer, and esophageal adenocarcinoma in combination with fluoropyrimidine- and platinum-containing chemotherapy. **Hepatocellular carcinoma (HCC):** Treatment of adults with HCC who have been previously treated with sorafenib. **Malignant pleural mesothelioma:** First-line treatment of adults with unresectable malignant pleural mesothelioma. **Melanoma:** Treatment of adults and children 12 yrs and older with unresectable or metastatic melanoma, as a single agent or in combination with ipilimumab. Adjuvant treatment of adults and children 12 yrs and older with completely resected Stage IIB, Stace IIC, Stage III, or Stage IV melanoma. **Non–small-cell lung cancer (NSCLC):** First-line treatment of metastatic NSCLC in adults whose tumors express PD-L1. First-line treatment of metastatic or recurrent NSCLC in adults with no EGFR or ALK genomic tumor aberrations. Treatment of metastatic NSCLC with progression on

or after platinum-based chemotherapy. Neoadjuvant treatment of adults with resectable tumors or node-positive NSCLC. Neoadjuvant treatment in adults with resectable (tumors 4 cm or greater or node positive) NSCLC and no known EGFR mutations or ALK rearrangements, in combination with platinum-doublet chemotherapy, followed by single-agent OPDIVO as adjuvant treatment after surgery. **Renal cell carcinoma (RCC):** First-line treatment of adults with intermediate- or poor-risk advanced RCC. First-line treatment of adults with advanced RCC (in combination with cabozantinib). Treatment of adults with advanced RCC (as single agent) who have received prior antiangiogenic therapy. **Squamous cell carcinoma of the head and neck (SCCHN):** Treatment of adults with recurrent or metastatic (SCCHN) with disease progression on or after platinum-based therapy. **Urothelial carcinoma (UC):** Treatment of adults with unresectable or metastatic urothelial carcinoma, as first-line treatment (in combination with cisplatin and gemcitabine). Treatment of adults with locally advanced or metastatic UC who have disease progression during or following platinum-containing chemotherapy or have disease progression within 12 mos of neoadjuvant or adjuvant treatment with platinum-containing chemotherapy. Adjuvant treatment of adults with UC who are at high risk of recurrence after undergoing radical resection.

PRECAUTIONS

Contraindications: Hypersensitivity to nivolumab. **Cautions:** Thyroid/pituitary disease, hepatic/renal impairment, interstitial lung disease, electrolyte imbalance.

ACTION

Binds PD-1 ligands to PD-1 receptor found on T cells, blocking its interaction with the ligands (PD-L1 and PD-L2). Releases PD-1 pathway–mediated inhibition of immune response (including antitumor immune response). **Therapeutic Effect:** Inhibits

T-cell proliferation and cytokine production. Inhibits tumor cell growth and metastasis.

PHARMACOKINETICS

Metabolism not specified. Steady-state concentration reached in 12 wks. Excretion not specified. **Half-life:** 26.7 days.

⏳ LIFESPAN CONSIDERATIONS

Pregnancy/Lactation: Avoid pregnancy; may cause fetal harm. Unknown if distributed in breast milk. Females of reproductive potential should use effective contraception during treatment and up to 5 mos after discontinuation. **Children:** Safety and efficacy not established in pts younger than 12 yrs. **Elderly:** May have increased risk of endocrine/hepatic/pulmonary/optic/renal injury due to age-related diseases.

INTERACTIONS

DRUG: None significant. **HERBAL:** None significant. **FOOD:** None known. **LAB VALUES: Single therapy:** May increase serum alkaline phosphatase, ALT, AST, potassium. May decrease serum sodium. **Combo therapy:** May increase serum alkaline phosphatase, ALT, AST, amylase, creatinine, lipase. May decrease RBC, Hct, Hgb, lymphocytes, neutrophils, platelets; serum calcium, sodium, magnesium. May increase or decrease serum calcium, potassium.

AVAILABILITY (Rx)

Injection Solution: 40 mg/4 mL, 100 mg/10 mL, 120 mg/12 mL, 240 mg/24 mL vials.

ADMINISTRATION/HANDLING

 IV

Preparation • Visually inspect solution for particulate matter or discoloration. Solution should appear opalescent, colorless to pale yellow. Discard if solution is cloudy or contains particulate matter other than a few translucent to white proteinaceous particles. • Do not shake vial. • Withdraw required dose volume and dilute in 0.9% NaCl or D₅W. Final concentration will equal 1–10 mg/mL based on volume of diluent. • Mix by gentle inversion. • Do not shake. • Discard partially used or empty vials.

Rate of administration • Infuse over 30 min using sterile, nonpyrogenic, low protein-binding, 0.2- to 1.2-micron in-line filter. • Flush IV line upon completion.

Storage • Refrigerate diluted solution up to 7 days or store at room temperature for no more than 8 hrs (includes time of preparation and infusion). • Do not freeze.

🔬 IV INCOMPATIBILITIES

Do not infuse with other medications.

INDICATIONS/ROUTES/DOSAGE

cHL

IV: ADULTS, ELDERLY: (Single agent): 240 mg q2wks or 480 mg q4wks until disease progression or unacceptable toxicity.

CRC (Metastatic)

IV: ADULTS, ELDERLY, CHILDREN 12 YRS AND OLDER WEIGHING 40 KG OR MORE: (Single agent): 240 mg q2wks or 480 mg q4wks until disease progression or unacceptable toxicity. **(In combination with ipilimumab):** 3 mg/kg q3wks for 4 doses, then 240 mg q2wks or 480 mg q4wks (as a single agent) until disease progression or unacceptable toxicity. **CHILDREN 12 YRS AND OLDER WEIGHING LESS THAN 40 KG (Single agent):** 3 mg/kg q2wks until disease progression or unacceptable toxicity. **(In combination with ipilimumab):** 3 mg/kg q2wks for 4 doses, then 3 mg/kg q2wks (as a single agent) until disease progression or unacceptable toxicity.

Esophageal Cancer

IV: ADULTS, ELDERLY: (In combination with fluoropyrimidine- and platinum-containing chemotherapy): 240 mg q2wks or 480 mg q4wks until disease progression or unacceptable toxicity or up to 2 yrs. **(In combination with ipilimumab):** 3 mg/kg q2wks or 360 mg q3wks until disease progression, unacceptable toxicity, or up to 2 yrs. **Adjuvant treatment (resected esophageal or gastroesophageal junction cancer):**

240 mg q2wks or 480 mg q4wks until disease progression or unacceptable toxicity for up to 1 yr.

Gastric Cancer, Gastroesophageal Junction Cancer, Esophageal Adenocarcinoma

IV: ADULTS, ELDERLY: 240 mg q2wks (with chemotherapy q2wks) or 360 mg q3wks (with chemotherapy q3wks) until disease progression, unacceptable toxicity, or up to 2 yrs.

Hepatocellular Carcinoma

IV: ADULTS, ELDERLY: (In combination with ipilimumab): 1 mg/kg q3wks for 4 doses, then 240 mg q2wks or 480 mg q4wks (as a single agent) until disease progression or unacceptable toxicity.

Malignant Pleural Mesothelioma

IV: ADULTS, ELDERLY: (In combination with ipilimumab): 360 mg q3wks until disease progression, unacceptable toxicity, or up to 2 yrs in pts without disease progression.

Melanoma (Unresectable or Metastatic)

IV: ADULTS, ELDERLY, CHILDREN WEIGHING 40 KG OR GREATER: (Single agent): 240 mg q2wks or 480 mg q4wks until disease progression or unacceptable toxicity. **CHILDREN WEIGHING LESS THAN 40 KG:** 3 mg/kg q2wks or 6 mg/kg q4wks. **(In combination with ipilimumab): ADULTS, ELDERLY, CHILDREN WEIGHING 40 KG OR GREATER:** 1 mg/kg q3wks for a maximum of 4 doses or until unacceptable toxicity, whichever occurs first. After completing 4 doses of combination therapy, give 240 mg q2wks or 480 mg q4wks (as a single agent) **CHILDREN WEIGHING LESS THAN 40 KG:** 1 mg/kg, followed by ipilimumab 3 mg/kg on the same day q3wks for 4 doses, then 3 mg/kg q2wks or 6 mg/kg q4wks (as a single agent), until disease progression or unacceptable toxicity. **(Adjuvant treatment): ADULTS, ELDERLY, CHILDREN WEIGHING 40 KG OR GREATER:** 240 mg q2wks or 480 mg q4wks until disease progression or unacceptable toxicity for up to 1 yr. **CHILDREN WEIGHING LESS THAN 40 KG:** 3 mg/kg q2wks or 6 mg/kg q4wks until disease progression or unacceptable toxicity for up to 1 yr.

NSCLC

IV: ADULTS, ELDERLY: Metastatic: (Single agent): 240 mg q2wks or 480 mg q4wks until disease progression or unacceptable toxicity. **Metastatic NSCLC expressing PD-L1: (In combination with ipilimumab):** 360 mg q3wks until disease progression, unacceptable toxicity, or up to 2 yrs in pts without disease progression. **Metastatic or recurrent NSCLC: (In combination with ipilimumab and 2 cycles of histology-based platinum-doublet chemotherapy):** 360 mg q3wks until disease progression, unacceptable toxicity, or up to 2 yrs in pts without disease progression. **Neoadjuvant treatment of resectable NSCLC: (In combination with 3 cycles of histology-based platinum-doublet chemotherapy):** 360 mg q3wks. **Neoadjuvant and Adjuvant Treatment of resectable NSCLC:** 360 mg with platinum-doublet chemotherapy on the same day q3wks for up to 4 cycles, then continued as single-agent of 480 mg q4wks after surgery for up to 13 cycles (approx. 1 year).

RCC

IV: ADULTS, ELDERLY: (Single agent): 240 mg q2wks or 480 mg q4wks until disease progression or unacceptable toxicity. **(In combination with ipilimumab):** 3 mg/kg q3wks for 4 doses, then 240 mg q2wks or 480 mg q4wks (as a single agent) until disease progression or unacceptable toxicity. **(In combination with cabozantinib):** 240 mg q2wks or 480 mg q4wks until disease progression or unacceptable toxicity or up to 2 yrs.

SCCHN

IV: ADULTS, ELDERLY: (Single agent): 240 mg q2wks or 480 mg q4wks until disease progression or unacceptable toxicity.

Urothelial Carcinoma

IV: ADULTS, ELDERLY: Metastatic: (Single agent): 240 mg q2wks or 480 mg q4wks until disease progression or unacceptable toxicity. **(Adjuvant**

treatment): 240 mg q2wks or 480 mg q4wks until disease progression or unacceptable toxicity for up to 1 yr. **(First-line treatment of unresectable or metastatic urothelial carcinoma):** 360 mg q3wks (with cisplatin and gemcitabine) on the same day for up to 6 cycles, then 240 mg q2wks or 480 mg q4wks until disease progression or unacceptable toxicity, or up to 2 yrs from first dose.

Dose Modification

Based on Common Terminology Criteria for Adverse Events (CTCAE).

Withhold Treatment for Any of the Following Adverse Events

Grade 2 or 3 diarrhea or colitis; single-agent therapy–associated colitis; Grade 2 pneumonitis; serum AST or ALT greater than 3–5 times upper limit of normal (ULN) or serum bilirubin 1.5–3 times ULN; Grade 2 or 3 hypophysitis; Grade 2 adrenal insufficiency; serum creatinine greater than 1.5–6 times ULN; Grade 3 rash; first occurrence of any other Grade 3 adverse reaction. When nivolumab is administered in combination with ipilimumab and nivolumab is withheld, then ipilimumab should also be withheld.

Restarting Therapy

Resume when adverse reactions return to Grade 0 or 1.

Permanently Discontinue for Any of the Following Adverse Events

Combo-agent therapy (ipilimumab)–associated colitis; Grade 3 or 4 pneumonitis; serum AST or ALT greater than 5 times ULN or serum bilirubin 3 times ULN; pts with liver metastasis who begin treatment with baseline Grade 2 serum ALT or AST elevation who experience serum ALT or AST elevation greater than or equal to 50% from baseline that persists for at least 1 wk; Grade 4 hypophysitis; Grade 3 or 4 adrenal insufficiency; serum creatinine greater than 6 times ULN; Grade 4 rash; recurrence of any other Grade 3 adverse reaction; any life-threatening or Grade 4 adverse reaction; requirement for predniSONE 10 mg/day or greater (or equivalent) for more than 12 wks; persistent Grade 2 or 3 adverse reaction lasting longer than 12 wks.

Dosage in Renal Impairment

No dose adjustment.

Dosage in Hepatic Impairment

Mild to moderate impairment: No dose adjustment. **Severe impairment:** Not specified; use caution.

SIDE EFFECTS

Note: Percentage of side effects may vary depending on the use of single or combination therapy. **Frequent (50%–24%):** Fatigue, dyspnea, musculoskeletal pain, decreased appetite, cough, nausea, headache, constipation. **Occasional (19%–10%):** Vomiting, asthenia, diarrhea, edema, pyrexia, cough, dehydration, rash, abdominal pain, chest pain, arthralgia, decreased weight, blurred vision, pruritus, peripheral edema, generalized pain.

ADVERSE EFFECTS/TOXIC REACTIONS

Myelosuppression (anemia, lymphopenia, neutropenia, thrombocytopenia) is an expected response to therapy. May cause severe immune-mediated events including interstitial lung disease or pneumonitis (3%–10% of pts), colitis (21%–57% of pts), hepatitis (15%–28% of pts), hypophysitis (13% of pts), renal failure or nephritis (1%–2% of pts), hyperthyroidism (1% of pts), hypothyroidism (3%–19% of pts), rash (up to 37% of pts). Other adverse events including autoimmune nephropathy, demyelination, diabetic ketoacidosis, duodenitis, erythema multiforme, exfoliative dermatitis, facial and abducens nerve paresis, gastritis, iridocyclitis, motor dysfunction, pancreatitis, psoriasis, sarcoidosis, uveitis, vasculitis, ventricular arrhythmia, vitiligo reported in less than 2% of pts. Severe infusion-related reactions reported in less than 1% of pts. Occurrence of events is dependent on use of single or combination therapy. Upper respiratory tract infections including nasopharyngitis, pharyngitis, rhinitis reported in 11% of pts.

N

Immunogenicity (auto-nivolumab antibodies) occurred in 8.5% of pts.

NURSING CONSIDERATIONS

BASELINE ASSESSMENT

Obtain CBC, BMP, LFT, TSH; vital signs; urine pregnancy. Record weight in kg. Screen for history of arrhythmias, pituitary/pulmonary/thyroid disease, autoimmune disorders, diabetes, hepatic/renal impairment; allergy to predniSONE. Along with routine assessment, conduct full dermatologic exam, ophthalmologic exam/visual acuity. Receive full medication history and screen for interactions.

INTERVENTION/EVALUATION

Monitor CBC, LFT, serum electrolytes; thyroid panel if applicable. Diligently monitor for immune-mediated adverse events as listed in Adverse Effects/Toxic Reactions. Notify physician if any toxicities occur (see Appendix K) and initiate proper treatment. Obtain chest X-ray if interstitial lung disease, pneumonitis suspected. Screen for tumor lysis syndrome in pts with high tumor burden. Monitor I&O, daily weight. If predniSONE therapy is initiated for immune-mediated events, monitor capillary blood glucose and screen for corticosteroid side effects.

PATIENT/FAMILY TEACHING

• Serious adverse reactions may affect lungs, GI tract, kidneys, or hormonal glands; anti-inflammatory medication may need to be started. • Immediately contact physician if serious or life-threatening inflammatory reactions occur in the following body systems: colon (severe abdominal pain or diarrhea); kidney (decreased or dark-colored urine, flank pain); lung (chest pain, cough, shortness of breath); liver (bruising easily, dark-colored urine, clay-colored/tarry stools, yellowing of skin or eyes); pituitary (persistent or unusual headache, dizziness, extreme weakness, fainting, vision changes); thyroid (trouble sleeping, high blood pressure, fast heart rate [overactive thyroid]), (fatigue, goiter, weight gain [underactive thyroid]). • Use effective contraception to avoid pregnancy. Do not breastfeed.

nivolumab/relatimab-rmbw

nye-**vol**-ue-mab/rel-**at**-li-mab
(Opdualag)
Do not confuse nivolumab/relatlimab with dupilumab, leronlimab, nivolumab, or Opdualag with Opdivo.

FIXED COMBINATION(S)

Opdualag: nivolumab/relatimab-rmbw: 240 mg/80 mg.

◆CLASSIFICATION

PHARMACOTHERAPEUTIC: Programmed death receptor-1 (PD-1) blocking antibody, lymphocyte activation gene-3 (LAG-3) blocking antibody. Monoclonal antibody. **CLINICAL:** Antineoplastic.

USES

Treatment of adult and children 12 yrs of age or older with unresectable or metastatic melanoma.

PRECAUTIONS

Contraindications: Hypersensitivity to nivolumab/relatimab-rmbw. **Cautions:** Baseline cytopenias, diabetes, pts at risk for interstitial lung disease (e.g., COPD, sarcoidosis, connective disease disease); history of autoimmune disorders (Crohn's disease, demyelinating polyneuropathy, Guillain-Barré syndrome, Hashimoto's thyroiditis, hyperthyroidism, myasthenia gravis, rheumatoid arthritis, type 1 diabetes, vasculitis); hypothyroidism, pancreatitis; solid organ transplant, allogeneic hematopoietic stem cell transplantation.

ACTION

Nivolumab binds to programmed cell death ligand 1 (PD-L1), blocking interaction with PD-L1 and PD-L2. PD-L1 is an immune checkpoint protein expressed on tumor cells, which downregulates antitumor T-cell function. Relatlimab binds to LAG-3 receptor, blocking interaction with its ligands. LAG-3 pathway inhibition stimulates cytokine secretion and T-cell proliferation. **Therapeutic Effect:** Restores immune responses (including T-cell antitumor function), decreasing tumor growth and proliferation.

PHARMACOKINETICS

Widely distributed. Metabolism not specified. Steady-state of relatlimab reached in 16 wks. Excretion not specified. **Half-life:** (nivolumab): 26.5 days; (relatlimab): 26.2 days.

⧗ LIFESPAN CONSIDERATIONS

Pregnancy/Lactation: Avoid pregnancy; may cause fetal harm. Females of reproductive potential must use effective contraception during treatment and for at least 5 mos after discontinuation. Breastfeeding not recommended during treatment and for at least 5 mos after discontinuation. Human immunoglobulin G (IgG) is present in breast milk and known to cross the placenta. **Children:** Safety and efficacy not established in pts younger than 12 yrs or in children older than 12 yrs who weigh less than 40 kg. **Elderly:** No age-related precautions noted.

INTERACTIONS

DRUG: None significant. **HERBAL:** None significant. **FOOD:** None known. **LAB VALUES:** May increase serum alkaline phosphatase, ALT, AST, creatinine. May decrease Hgb, lymphocytes; serum sodium.

AVAILABILITY (Rx)

Fixed-Dose Combination, Injection Solution: 240 mg (nivolumab)/80 mg (relatlimab) per 20 mL (12 mg/4 mg/mL) in a single-dose vial.

ADMINISTRATION/HANDLING

 IV

Infusion guidelines • Compatible with di(2-ethylhexyl)phthalate (DEHP)–plasticized polyvinyl chloride (PVC), ethyl vinyl acetate (EVA), and polyolefin (PO) infusion bags. • Infuse via dedicated IV line using a sterile, nonpyrogenic, low-protein-binding, 0.2–1.2 micron in-line filter made of polyethersulfone (PES), nylon, or polyvinylidene (PVDF). • Flush IV line at the end of infusion. • May administer solution diluted or undiluted.

Preparation • Must be prepared by personnel trained in aseptic manipulations and admixing of cytotoxic drugs. • Visually inspect vials for particulate matter or discoloration. Solution should appear clear to opalescent, colorless to slightly yellow. Few translucent, proteinaceous particles may be present. Do not use if solution is cloudy, discolored, or particulate matter other than translucent-to-white particles is observed. • May dilute in 0.9% NaCl or D5W to a maximum infusion volume of 160 mL (adults and children 12 yrs or older weighing at least 40 kg) or 4 mg/mL (adults weighing less than 40 kg) to a final concentration of 3–12 mg/mL of nivolumab and 1–4 mg/mL of relatlimab.

Rate of administration • Infuse over 30 min. • Interrupt or slow rate of infusion if reactions occur.

Storage • Refrigerate unused vials in original carton. Protect from light. Do not freeze. • Diluted solution may be refrigerated for up to 24 hrs or stored at room temperature for up to 8 hrs (includes infusion time). • If refrigerated, allow diluted solution to warm to room temperature.

INDICATIONS/ROUTES/DOSAGE

Melanoma (Unresectable or Metastatic)
IV: ADULTS, CHILDREN 12 YRS AND OLDER WEIGHING AT LEAST 40 KGS: 480 mg/160 mg q4wks until disease progression or unacceptable toxicity.

Dose Modification
Based on Common Terminology Criteria for Adverse Events (CTCAE). No

dose reduction is required. Based on severity of adverse reactions, withhold treatment and consider starting corticosteroid therapy. Resume treatment if symptoms improve to Grade 1 or 0 after corticosteroid taper.

Withhold treatment for the following adverse reactions: Grade 2 pneumonitis, Grade 2 or 3 colitis, serum ALT/AST elevation 3–8 times upper limit of normal (ULN), serum bilirubin elevation 1.5–3 times ULN, Grade 2 or 3 nephritis with renal dysfunction, Grade 2 neurologic toxicity, Grade 3 or 4 endocrine toxicity; *suspected* Stevens-Johnson syndrome, toxic epidermal necrolysis, or drug reaction with eosinophilia and systemic symptoms (DRESS).

Permanently discontinue for the following adverse reactions: Grade 3 or 4 pneumonitis, Grade 4 colitis, serum ALT/AST elevation greater than 8 times ULN, serum bilirubin elevation greater than 3 times ULN, Grade 4 nephritis with renal dysfunction, Grade 3 or 4 neurologic toxicity, Grade 2–4 myocarditis, *confirmed* Stevens-Johnson syndrome, toxic epidermal necrolysis, or DRESS; Grade 3 or 4 infusion-related reactions; symptoms that do not improve to Grade 1 or 0 within 12 wks of starting corticosteroid therapy or unable to tolerate corticosteroid reduction to less than 10 mg predniSONE (or equivalent)/day. May consider permanent discontinuation for Grade 3 or 4 endocrine toxicity depending on severity.

Dosage in Hepatic/Renal Impairment

Mild to moderate impairment: No dose adjustment. **Severe impairment:** Not specified; use caution.

SIDE EFFECTS

Frequent (45%–24%): Musculoskeletal pain, fatigue, rash, pruritus, diarrhea.
Occasional (17%–15%): Nausea, headache, decreased appetite, cough, vitiligo.

ADVERSE EFFECTS/TOXIC REACTIONS

Anemia, lymphopenia are expected responses to therapy. May cause severe and/or fatal immune-mediated adverse reactions including acute kidney injury, nephritis; colitis, hepatitis, pancreatitis, pneumonitis; adrenal insufficiency, hypoparathyroidism, hyperthyroidism, hypophysitis, thyroiditis, type 1 diabetes mellitus including ketoacidosis; autoimmune neuropathy, encephalitis, Guillain-Barré syndrome, meningitis, myasthenia gravis, myelitis, nerve paresis; myocarditis, pericarditis, vasculitis; iritis, uveitis; myositis, polymyositis, rhabdomyolysis; aplastic anemia, hemolytic anemia, hemophagocytic lymphohistiocytosis, histiocytic necrotizing lymphadenitis, immune thrombocytopenic purpura; sarcoidosis, systemic inflammatory response syndrome. Immune-mediated adverse reactions can affect any organ at any time. Solid organ transplant rejection, allogeneic hematopoietic stem cell transplantation complications were reported. May cause cytomegalovirus infection/reactivation in pts with corticosteroid-refractory immune-related colitis. Dermatologic toxicities including Stevens-Johnson syndrome, toxic epidermal necrolysis may occur. DRESS, also known as multiorgan hypersensitivity, has been reported. DRESS may present with facial swelling, eosinophilia, fever, lymphadenopathy, and rash, which may be associated with other organ systems, such as hepatitis, hematologic abnormalities, myocarditis, nephritis. Life-threatening infusion reactions may occur.

NURSING CONSIDERATIONS

BASELINE ASSESSMENT

Obtain CBC, LFT, thyroid panel; pregnancy test in females of reproductive potential. Confirm compliance with effective contraception. Screen for history of autoimmune disorders, diabetes, pituitary/pulmonary/

thyroid disease. Perform full dermatologic exam; assess skin for moles, lesions, papillomas. Administer in an environment equipped to monitor for and manage infusion-related reactions. Question for previous infusion-related reactions prior to each infusion. Screen for active infection. Assess usual bowel movement patterns, stool characteristics. Offer emotional support.

INTERVENTION/EVALUATION

Monitor CBC, LFT, renal function, thyroid panel periodically. Assess for infusion reactions during each infusion. If reactions occur, interrupt or decrease rate of infusion. Immune-mediated reactions can affect any organ. Early detection and management are vital. Conduct a complete head-to-toe assessment frequently. Radiologic examination, blood sampling; treatment with corticosteroids should be considered if an immune-mediated reaction is suspected. Assess for eye pain/redness, visual changes at each office visit and at regular intervals. Monitor daily pattern of bowel activity, stool consistency. Assess skin for rash, lesions, dermatologic toxicities; symptoms of DRESS. Monitor blood glucose levels in pts treated with corticosteroids.

PATIENT/FAMILY TEACHING

• Immediately report symptoms of infusion-related reactions such as chills, cough, difficulty breathing, nausea, vomiting. • Report symptoms of drug-induced hypersensitivity syndrome (e.g., fever, swollen face/lymph nodes, skin rash/peeling/inflammation). • Serious adverse reactions may affect lungs, liver, intestines, kidneys, hormonal glands, nervous system (or any organ), which may require anti-inflammatory medication. • Immediately report any symptoms in the following body systems: colon (severe abdominal pain/swelling, diarrhea); eyes (pain, redness, vision problems), heart (chest pain, difficulty breathing), kidneys (decreased or dark-colored urine, flank pain); lung (chest pain, severe cough, shortness of breath); liver (bruising, dark-colored urine, clay-colored/tarry stools, nausea, yellowing of the skin or eyes); nervous system (confusion, difficulty breathing or swallowing; paralysis, weakness), pituitary (persistent or unusual headaches, dizziness, extreme weakness, fainting, vision changes); skin (blisters, bubbling, inflammation, rash), thyroid (trouble sleeping, high blood pressure, fast heart rate [overactive thyroid]; fatigue, goiter, weight gain [underactive thyroid]), vascular (low blood pressure, vein/artery pain or irritation). • Use effective contraception to avoid pregnancy. Do not breastfeed.

---

norepinephrine   `HIGH ALERT`

nor-ep-i-**nef**-rin
(Levophed)

■ **BLACK BOX ALERT** ■
Extravasation may produce severe tissue necrosis, sloughing. Using fine hypodermic needle, liberally infiltrate area with 10–15 mL saline solution containing 5–10 mg phentolamine.
Do not confuse Levophed with Levaquin or levoFLOXacin, or norepinephrine with EPINEPHrine.

◆CLASSIFICATION

PHARMACOTHERAPEUTIC: Alpha, beta agonist. **CLINICAL:** Vasopressor.

USES

Treatment of severe hypotension, cardiogenic shock, septic shock persisting after adequate fluid volume replacement.

PRECAUTIONS

Contraindications: Hypersensitivity to norepinephrine. Hypotension related to hypovolemia (except in emergency to maintain coronary/cerebral perfusion until volume replaced), mesenteric/peripheral vascular thrombosis (unless it is lifesaving procedure). **Cautions:** Concurrent use of MAOIs.

ACTION

Stimulates beta$_1$-adrenergic receptors, alpha-adrenergic receptors, increasing contractility, heart rate and producing vasoconstriction. **Therapeutic Effect:** Increases systemic B/P, coronary blood flow.

PHARMACOKINETICS

Route	Onset	Peak	Duration
IV	Rapid	1–2 min	N/A

Localized in sympathetic tissue. Metabolized in liver. Primarily excreted in urine.

⧗ LIFESPAN CONSIDERATIONS

Pregnancy/Lactation: Readily crosses placenta. May produce fetal anoxia due to uterine contraction, constriction of uterine blood vessels. **Children/Elderly:** No age-related precautions noted.

INTERACTIONS

DRUG: MAOIs (e.g., phenelzine, selegiline), antidepressants (tricyclic), SNRIs (e.g., DULoxetine), may increase concentration/effect. **HERBAL:** None significant. **FOOD:** None known. **LAB VALUES:** None significant.

AVAILABILITY (Rx)

Injection Solution: 1 mg/mL, 4 mg/250 mL, 8 mg/250 mL, 16 mg/250 mL.

ADMINISTRATION/HANDLING

 IV

Reconstitution • Add 4 mL (4 mg) to 250 mL D$_5$W (16 mcg/mL). **Maximum concentration:** 32 mL (32 mg) to 250 mL (128 mcg/mL).
Rate of administration • Closely monitor IV infusion flow rate (use infusion pump). • Monitor B/P q2min during IV infusion until desired therapeutic response is achieved, then q5min during remaining IV infusion. • Never leave pt unattended. • Maintain B/P at 90–100 mm Hg in previously normotensive pts, and 30–40 mm Hg below preexisting B/P in previously hypertensive pts. • Reduce

IV infusion gradually. Avoid abrupt withdrawal. • If using peripherally inserted catheter, it is imperative to check the IV site frequently for free flow and infused vein for blanching, hardness to vein, coldness, pallor to extremity. • If extravasation occurs, area should be infiltrated with 10–15 mL sterile saline containing 5–10 mg phentolamine (does not alter pressor effects of norepinephrine).
Storage • Do not use if solution is brown or contains precipitate. • Store at room temperature. Diluted solution stable for 24 hrs at room temperature.

▦ IV INCOMPATIBILITIES

Insulin.

▦ IV COMPATIBILITIES

Amiodarone, dexmedetomidine, diltiazem, heparin, nitroglycerin, potassium chloride, propofol, vasopressin.

INDICATIONS/ROUTES/DOSAGE

◀ALERT▶ If possible, blood, fluid volume depletion should be corrected before drug is administered. Recommend infusion via central venous access.

Acute Hypotension Unresponsive to Fluid Volume Replacement
IV infusion: ADULTS, ELDERLY: Initially, 0.05–0.15 mcg/kg/min. Titrate to goal mean arterial pressure (MAP). Usual dose range: 0.025–1 mcg/kg/min. **Maximum dose range for refractory shock:** 1–3.3 mcg/kg/min. **ADOLESCENTS, CHILDREN, INFANTS:** Initially, 0.05–0.1 mcg/kg/min; titrate to desired effect. **Maximum:** 2 mcg/kg/min.

Dosage in Renal/Hepatic Impairment
No dose adjustment.

SIDE EFFECTS

Norepinephrine produces less pronounced, less frequent side effects than EPINEPHrine. **Occasional (5%–3%):** Anxiety, bradycardia, palpitations. **Rare (2%–1%):** Nausea, anginal pain, shortness of breath, fever.

N

ADVERSE EFFECTS/TOXIC REACTIONS

Extravasation may produce tissue necrosis, sloughing. Overdose manifested as severe hypertension with violent headache (may be first clinical sign of overdose), arrhythmias, photophobia, retrosternal or pharyngeal pain, pallor, diaphoresis, vomiting. Prolonged therapy may result in plasma volume depletion. Hypotension may recur if plasma volume is not maintained.

NURSING CONSIDERATIONS

BASELINE ASSESSMENT

Monitor ECG; B/P q5–15 min (or per hospital guidelines). Be alert for sudden decrease in B/P. Infuse via a central venous line. Extravasation may occur if given via peripheral IV line. Assess for headache.

INTERVENTION/EVALUATION

Monitor IV flow rate diligently. Extravasation is characterized by blanching of skin over vein, coolness (results from local vasoconstriction); color, temperature of IV site extremity (pallor, cyanosis, mottling). Assess nailbed capillary refill. Monitor I&O; measure output hourly, report urine output less than 30 mL/hr. Once B/P parameter has been reached, IV infusion should not be restarted unless systolic B/P falls below 90 mm Hg.

N

obinutuzumab

oh-bi-nue-**tooz**-ue-mab
(Gazyva)

■ **BLACK BOX ALERT** ■ Hepatitis B virus reactivation, resulting in hepatic failure, fulminant hepatitis, and death have occurred. Screen all pts for hepatitis B virus infection before initiating treatment. Progressive multifocal leukoencephalopathy (PML) including fatal PML reported.

Do not confuse obinutuzumab with alemtuzumab, gemtuzumab, inotuzumab, polatuzumab, or trastuzumab.

◆CLASSIFICATION

PHARMACOTHERAPEUTIC: Anti-CD20 monoclonal antibody. **CLINICAL:** Antineoplastic.

USES

Treatment of previously untreated chronic lymphocytic leukemia (CLL), in combination with chlorambucil. Treatment of follicular lymphoma (FL) (in combination with bendamustine) and followed by obinutuzumab monotherapy in pts who relapsed after, or are refractory to, a riTUX-imab-containing regimen. In combination with chemotherapy, followed by obinutuzumab monotherapy in pts achieving at least a partial remission, for the treatment of adults with previously untreated stage II bulky, III, or IV follicular lymphoma. **OFF-LABEL:** CLL previously untreated as a single agent or in combination with acalabrutinib, ibrutinib, or venetoclax.

PRECAUTIONS

Contraindications: Hypersensitivity to obinutuzumab. **Cautions:** Baseline cytopenias, HBV infection, preexisting cardiac/pulmonary impairment; hematologic abnormalities (e.g., leukopenia, thrombocytopenia); electrolyte imbalance; conditions predisposing to infection (e.g., diabetes, renal failure, immunocompromised pts, open wounds).

ACTION

Targets CD20 antigen expressed on surface of B lymphocytes. Mediates B-cell lysis by activating complement-dependent cytotoxicity, antibody-dependent cellular cytotoxicity. **Therapeutic Effect:** Inhibits tumor cell growth and proliferation in CLL.

PHARMACOKINETICS

Metabolism and elimination not specified. **Half-life:** 28 days.

⌛ LIFESPAN CONSIDERATIONS

Pregnancy/Lactation: Avoid pregnancy. May cause transient peripheral B-cell depletion in neonates when used during pregnancy. Females of reproductive potential should use effective contraception during treatment and for at least 12 mos after initiation. Unknown if distributed in breast milk. **Children:** Safety and efficacy not established. **Elderly:** May have increased risk of adverse reactions.

INTERACTIONS

DRUG: May increase hypotensive effect of **ACE inhibitors (e.g., enalapril, lisinopril), angiotensin receptor blockers (e.g., losartan), beta blockers (e.g., metoprolol).** May decrease the therapeutic effect of **BCG (intravesical), vaccines (live).** May increase adverse effects of **natalizumab, vaccines (live). HERBAL:** Echinacea may diminish the therapeutic effect. **Herbals with hypotensive properties (e.g., garlic, ginger, ginkgo biloba)** may increase the hypotensive effect. **FOOD:** None known. **LAB VALUES:** May increase serum alkaline phosphatase, ALT, AST, bilirubin, creatinine, uric acid. May decrease albumin, Hgb, Hct, lymphocytes, neutrophils, platelets; serum potassium, sodium.

AVAILABILITY (Rx)

Injection Solution: 1,000 mg/40 mL (25 mg/mL) single-use vial.

ADMINISTRATION/HANDLING

◄**ALERT►** Administer via dedicated line. Do not administer IV push or bolus.

Withhold hypertensive medications at least 12 hrs before and 1 hr after administration. Do not mix with dextrose-containing fluids.

 IV

Reconstitution • Visually inspect for particulate matter or discoloration. • For 100-mg dose: withdraw 40 mL solution from vial and dilute only 4 mL (100 mg) in 100 mL 0.9% NaCl for immediate administration. Dilute remaining 36 mL (900 mg) into 250 mL 0.9% NaCl at same time and refrigerate for up to 24 hrs for cycle 1 day 2. For remaining infusions (day 8 and day 15 of cycle 1 and day 1 of cycles 2–6), dilute 40 mL (1,000 mg) solution in 250 mL NaCl infusion bag. • Gently mix by inversion. • Do not shake.

Rate of administration • **(CLL): Day 1 of cycle 1 (100 mg):** Infuse over 4 hrs (25 mg/hr). • Do not increase infusion rate. • **Day 2 of cycle 1 (900 mg):** Infuse at 50 mg/hr. • May increase by 50 mg/hr every 30 min to maximum rate of 400 mg/hr. • **Day 1 of cycles 2-6:** Infuse at 100 mg/hr. May increase rate q30 min to maximum rate of 400 mg/hr. • **(FL): Day 1 of cycle 1:** Infuse at 50 mg/hr. May increase by 50 mg/hr q30 min to maximum rate of 400 mg/hr. **Day 1 of cycles 2-6:** Infuse at 100 mg/hr. May increase rate q30 min to maximum rate of 400 mg/hr. • Increase rate based on tolerability.

Storage • Solution should appear clear, colorless to slightly brown. • May refrigerate diluted solution up to 24 hrs.

INDICATIONS/ROUTES/DOSAGE

Chronic Lymphocytic Leukemia (CLL)

◄ **ALERT** ► Premedicate with glucocorticoid, acetaminophen, and antihistamine to decrease severity of infusion reaction. Consider premedication with antihyperuricemics (allopurinol) 12–24 hrs for pts with high tumor burden or high circulating absolute lymphocyte count greater than 25×10^9/L. Recommend antimicrobial prophylaxis throughout treatment for pts with neutropenia.

IV: **ADULTS/ELDERLY:** Six treatment cycles of 28-day cycle. **Day 1 of cycle 1:** 100 mg. **Day 2 of cycle 1:** 900 mg. **Day 8 and Day 15 of cycle 1:** 1,000 mg. **Cycles 2–6:** 1,000 mg on day 1 of each subsequent 28-day cycle for 5 doses. Discontinue treatment if any severe to life-threatening infusion reactions occur.

Follicular Lymphoma (Relapsed/Refractory)

IV: **ADULTS, ELDERLY:** Six treatment cycles of 28 days (in combination with bendamustine). **Cycle 1:** 1,000 mg on days 1, 8, 15. **Cycles 2–6:** 1,000 mg on day 1 of each subsequent 28-day cycle for 5 doses. If achieves stable disease, complete or partial response, continue obinutuzumab (as monotherapy) 1,000 mg q2mos for 2 yrs.

Follicular Lymphoma (Previously Untreated)

IV: **ADULTS, ELDERLY:** **Cycle 1 (either in combination with bendamustine or with CHOP or CVP chemotherapy):** 1,000 mg wkly on days 1, 8, and 15. **Cycles 2–6 (in combination with bendamustine):** 1,000 mg on day 1 q28days for 5 doses. **Cycles 2–8 (in combination with CHOP):** 1,000 mg on day1 q21days for 5 doses (with CHOP), then 1,000 mg on day 1 q21 days for 2 doses (as monotherapy). **Cycles 2–8 (in combination with CVP):** 1,000 mg on day 1 q21days for 7 doses. **Then as monotherapy:** 1,000 mg q2mos for up to 2 yrs beginning approximately 2 mos after last induction phase.

Dosage in Renal/Hepatic Impairment

No dose adjustment.

SIDE EFFECTS

Frequent (69%): Infusion reactions (pruritus, flushing, urticaria). **Occasional (10%):** Pyrexia, cough.

ADVERSE EFFECTS/TOXIC REACTIONS

Myelosuppression (leukopenia, lymphopenia, neutropenia, thrombocytopenia) is

O

an expected response to therapy, but more severe reactions including bone marrow failure, febrile neutropenia, opportunistic infection may result in life-threatening events. Hepatitis B virus reactivation may occur. Infusion reactions including hypotension, tachycardia, dyspnea, bronchospasm, wheezing, laryngeal edema, nausea, vomiting, flushing, pyrexia may occur during infusion. Tumor lysis syndrome may present as acute renal failure, hypocalcemia, hyperuricemia, hyperphosphatemia within 12–24 hrs of infusion. Progressive multifocal leukoencephalopathy (PML) occurred rarely and may include weakness, paralysis, vision loss, aphasia, cognition impairment.

NURSING CONSIDERATIONS

BASELINE ASSESSMENT
Obtain CBC, BMP, uric acid; pregnancy test in females of reproductive potential. Screen for history of anemia, asthma, arrhythmias, COPD, diabetes, GI bleeding, hypertension, hepatitis B virus infection, hepatic/renal impairment, peripheral edema. Receive full medication history, esp. hypertension, anticoagulant medications. Perform baseline visual acuity. Offer emotional support.

INTERVENTION/EVALUATION
Monitor CBC, serum electrolytes, LFT, vital signs. Monitor for cardiovascular alterations, respiratory distress. If respiratory reactions occur, consider administration of oxygen, EPINEPHrine, albuterol treatments. Locate rapid-sequence intubation kit if respiratory compromise occurs. Monitor strict I&O, hydration status. If PML suspected, consult neurologist for proper management. Obtain ECG for palpitations, severe hypokalemia, hyponatremia. Monitor for infection (cough, fatigue, fever).

PATIENT/FAMILY TEACHING
• Treatment may depress your immune system and reduce your ability to fight infection. Report symptoms of infection such as body aches, chills, cough, fatigue, fever.

Avoid those with active infection. • Avoid alcohol. • Immediately report difficult breathing, severe coughing, chest tightness, wheezing. • Paralysis, vision changes, impaired speech, altered mental status may indicate life-threatening neurologic event. • Use effective contraception to avoid pregnancy.

ocrelizumab

ok-re-**liz**-ue-mab
(Ocrevus, Ocrevus Zunovo)
Do not confuse ocrelizumab with certolizumab, daclizumab, efalizumab, mepolizumab, natalizumab, or omalizumab.

◆CLASSIFICATION

PHARMACOTHERAPEUTIC: Anti-CD20 monoclonal antibody. **CLINICAL:** Multiple sclerosis agent.

USES
Treatment of adult pts with relapsing or primary progressive forms of multiple sclerosis (MS) including clinically isolated syndrome, relapsing-remitting disease, and active secondary progressive disease.

PRECAUTIONS
Contraindications: Life-threatening infusion reaction to ocrelizumab. Active hepatitis B virus (HBV) infection confirmed by positive results for hepatitis B surface antigen (HBsAg) and anti-HBV tests. **Cautions:** History of chronic opportunistic infections (esp. bacterial, invasive fungal, mycobacterial, protozoal, viral, tuberculosis); active infection, conditions predisposing to infection (e.g., diabetes, immunocompromised pts, renal failure, open wounds); intolerance to corticosteroids; history of depression, malignancies, breast cancer. Avoid administration of live or live attenuated vaccines during treatment and after discontinuation until B cells are no longer depleted.

ACTION

Monoclonal antibody that is directed against B cells, which express the cell surface antigen CD20 (thought to influence the course of MS through antigen presentation, autoantibody production, cytokine regulation, and formation of ectopic lymphoid aggregates in meninges). Binds to the cell surface to deplete CD20-expressing B cells. **Therapeutic Effect:** Reduces progression of MS.

PHARMACOKINETICS

Onset of action: Serum CD-19+ B-cell count reduced within 14 days. Duration of action: 72 wks (Range: 27–175 wks). Antibodies are primarily cleared by catabolism. **Half-life:** 26 days.

⌛ LIFESPAN CONSIDERATIONS

Pregnancy/Lactation: May cause transient peripheral B-cell depletion and lymphocytopenia in neonates when used during pregnancy. Immunoglobulins are known to cross the placenta. Females of reproductive potential must use effective contraception during treatment and up to 6 mos after discontinuation. Unknown if distributed in breast milk; however, immunoglobulin G (IgG) is present in breast milk. Breastfeeding not recommended. **Children:** Safety and efficacy not established. **Elderly:** No age-related precautions noted.

INTERACTIONS

DRUG: May increase concentration/effect of **BCG (intravesical)**. May alter concentration/effect of **vaccines (live)**. May increase adverse effects/toxicity of **natalizumab, tacrolimus. HERBAL:** Echinacea may diminish therapeutic effect. **FOOD:** None known. **LAB VALUES:** May decrease immunoglobulin A (IgA), immunoglobulin M (IgM), immunoglobulin G (IgG), neutrophils.

AVAILABILITY (Rx)

Injection Solution: 300 mg/10 mL (30 mg/mL). **Injection:** 920 mg ocrelizumab

and 23,000 units hyaluronidase per 23 mL (40 mg and 1,000 units per mL).

ADMINISTRATION/HANDLING

 IV

Preparation • Visually inspect for particulate matter or discoloration. Solution should appear clear to slightly opalescent, colorless to pale brown in color. • Do not use if solution is cloudy, discolored, or if visible particles are observed. • Withdraw proper dose from vial (10 mL for 300-mg dose; 20 mL for 600-mg dose) and dilute into 0.9% NaCl bag to a final concentration of approx. 1.2 mg/mL (300-mg dose in 250 mL 0.9% NaCl; 600-mg dose in 500 mL 0.9% NaCl). • Mix by gentle inversion. • Do not shake or agitate.

Rate of administration • First and second infusion: Start at 30 mL/hr via dedicated line using 0.2- or 0.22-micron in-line filter. If tolerated, increase rate by 30 mL/hr q30min to a maximum rate of 180 mL/hr for a duration of 2.5 hrs or longer. • **Subsequent infusions:** *(Option 1):* Start at 40 mL/hr via dedicated line using 0.2- or 0.22-micron in-line filter. If tolerated, increase rate by 40 mL/hr q30min to a maximum rate of 200 mL/hr for a duration of 3.5 hrs or longer. *(Option 2)* (without previous serious infusion reactions): Start infusion at 100 mL/hr for first 15 min, then increase to 200 mL/hr for the next 15 min. If no infusion reaction occurs, may increase to 250 mL/hr for the next 30 min, then increase to 300 mL/hr for the remaining 60 min (infusion duration) 2 hrs or longer. • **Mild infusion reactions:** Decrease rate by 50% and continue reduced rate for at least 30 min. If tolerated, may increase infusion rate as described above. • **Severe infusion reactions:** Interrupt infusion until symptoms resolve, then resume infusion at 50% of the initial infusion rate. • **Life-threatening infusion reaction:** Immediately stop infusion and permanently discontinue; do not restart.

Storage • May refrigerate diluted solution up to 24 hrs or store at room

O

temperature for up to 8 hrs (includes infusion time). • If diluted solution is refrigerated, allow to warm to room temperature before administration. • Discard solution if not administered within required time frame.

SQ

Note: OCREVUS ZUNOVO has different dosage and administration instructions than IV ocrelizumab. For SQ injection, use in the abdomen only.

Preparation • Allow vial to warm to room temperature. Do not use external heat sources. • Visually inspect solution for particulate matter or discoloration. Solution should appear clear to slightly opalescent, and colorless to slightly brown. Do not use if solution is cloudy, discolored, or if visible particles are observed. • Transfer the required injection volume needed for dose into SQ infusion set syringe containing 24- to 26-gauge needle. • Use infusion set with a priming volume that does not exceed 0.8 mL for administration. • Prime to eliminate air from line and stop before fluid reaches needle.

Administration • Insert needle subcutaneously into the abdomen (except for 2 inches [5 cm]) around navel. • Administer 23 mL of solution over approx. 10 min. • Do not inject into areas of active skin disease or injury such as sunburns, skin rashes, inflammation, skin infections, or active psoriasis. • Rotate injection sites. • Do not administer IV or IM.

Storage • Refrigerate unused vials in original carton to protect from light. Do not freeze. • Prepared syringe(s) may be refrigerated for up to 72 hrs, followed by storage at room temperature for up to 8 hrs. Protect from light. • If prepared syringe(s) are refrigerated, allow solutions to warm to room temperature before administration.

▓ IV INCOMPATIBILITIES

Do not dilute with other IV solutions. Do not mix or infuse with other medications.

INDICATIONS/ROUTES/DOSAGE

◄ALERT► Must be administered under the direct supervision of healthcare professionals with access to emergency medical supplies and who are trained to manage severe infusion reactions. If a dose is missed, administer as soon as possible; do not wait until the next regularly scheduled dose. Reset administration schedule so that the next subsequent infusion is 6 mos after the most recent dose. Subsequent doses must be separated by at least 5 mos.

Premedication
To reduce severity and frequency of infusion reaction, premedicate with methyl-PREDNISolone 100 mg (or equivalent) approx. 30 min prior to infusion and an antihistamine (e.g., diphenhydrAMINE) approx. 30–60 min prior to infusion. Consider an antipyretic (e.g., acetaminophen) based on previous infusion reactions.

Multiple Sclerosis
IV: ADULTS, ELDERLY: 300 mg once at wk 0 and wk 2, then 600 mg q6mos (beginning 6 mos after the first 300-mg dose). Observe pt for at least 1 hr after completion of infusion.
SQ: ADULTS, ELDERLY: 920 mg/23,000 units (920 mg ocrelizumab and 23,000 units of hyaluronidase) q6 mos.

Dosage in Renal/Hepatic Impairment
Mild impairment: No dose adjustment. **Moderate to severe impairment:** Not specified; use caution.

SIDE EFFECTS

Occasional (8%–5%): Back pain, cough, diarrhea, peripheral edema, extremity pain.

ADVERSE EFFECTS/TOXIC REACTIONS

Infusion-related reactions including bronchospasm, dizziness, dyspnea, erythema, fatigue, flushing, headache, hypotension, nausea, oropharyngeal pain, pharyngeal/laryngeal edema, pruritus, pyrexia, rash, tachycardia, throat irritation, urticaria was reported in 34%–40% of pts. Serious infusion reactions requiring hospitalization occurred in less than 1% of pts. Infections including upper respiratory tract infections (40%–49% of pts), lower respiratory tract infections (10% of pts), skin infections (16% of pts), herpes infection (6% of pts) may occur. Progressive multifocal leukoencephalopathy (PML), an opportunistic viral infection of the brain caused by the JC virus, has occurred in pts treated with other anti-CD20 antibodies; may result in progressive permanent disability and death. Symptoms of PML include altered mental status, aphasia, paralysis, vision loss, weakness. HBV reactivation was reported in pts treated with other anti-CD20 antibodies; may result in fulminant hepatitis, hepatic failure, death. May increase risk of malignancies including breast cancer.

NURSING CONSIDERATIONS

BASELINE ASSESSMENT

Assess baseline symptoms of MS (e.g., bladder/bowel dysfunction, cognitive impairment, depression, dysphagia, fatigue, gait disorder, numbness/tingling, pain, seizures, spasticity, tremors, weakness). Obtain vital signs. Question history of hypersensitivity reactions, infusion-related reactions. Ensure that proper resuscitative equipment, medical supplies are readily available (e.g., albuterol, antipyretics, antihistamines, EPINEPHrine, isotonic IV fluids, bag-valve mask, oxygen, rapid sequence intubation kit). Screen for active HBV. Pts who test negative for HBsAg and positive for anti-HBcAb+ should be referred to a hepatic specialist. If applicable, immunizations should be up-to-date according to guidelines at least 6 wks prior to initiation. Question history of chronic infections, herpes infection, depression, malignancies, breast cancer. Screen for active infection. Verify use of effective contraception in females of reproductive potential.

INTERVENTION/EVALUATION

Monitor vital signs. Diligently monitor for infusion-related reactions during infusion and for at least 1 hr after completion (esp. during initial infusions). If severe or life-threatening reactions occur, immediately stop infusion and provide appropriate medical support. Due to risk of respiratory compromise, pts with bronchospasm, dyspnea, hypoxia should be given immediate supplemental oxygen, hypersensitivity medications, hemodynamic support. If laryngeal or pharyngeal edema occurs, airway protection or possible intubation may be required. Mild to moderate infusion reactions may require interruption of infusion, decrease of infusion rate, symptom management. Closely monitor for HBV reactivation, symptoms of PML, new malignancies including breast cancer, infections. Conduct neurologic assessment. Assess for symptom improvement of MS.

PATIENT/FAMILY TEACHING

• Life-threatening infusion reactions, allergic reactions may occur during infusion and up to 24 hrs after completion of infusion. Immediately report difficulty breathing, chest pain, chest tightness, chills, dizziness, fast heart rate, fever, flushing, headache, hives, itching, low blood pressure, nausea, throat pain, or swelling, rash. • If applicable, vaccinations should be up to date at least 6 wks before starting treatment. Do not receive live vaccines. • Treatment may depress your immune system and reduce your ability to fight infection. Report symptoms of infection such as body aches, burning with urination, chills, cough, fatigue, fever. Avoid those with active infection. • Use effective contraception to avoid pregnancy. Do not breastfeed. • Due to pretreatment with a corticosteroid, pts with diabetes may experience a transient rise in blood sugar levels. • PML, an opportunistic viral infection of the brain, may cause progressive, permanent disabilities and death. Report symptoms of PML such as confusion, memory loss, paralysis, trouble speaking, vision loss, seizures, weakness. • Treatment may cause reactivation of HBV, depression, new cancers including breast cancer. • Notify physician if symptoms of MS do not improve.

O

octreotide

ock-**tree**-oh-tide
(Mycapssa, <u>SandoSTATIN</u>, <u>Sando</u>
<u>STATIN LAR Depot</u>)
**Do not confuse SandoSTATIN
with SandIMMUNE, SandoSTATIN
LAR, sargramostim, or simvas-
tatin.**

◆CLASSIFICATION

PHARMACOTHERAPEUTIC: Somatostatin analogue. **CLINICAL:** Secretory
inhibitory, growth hormone suppressant; antidiarrheal.

USES

Acromegaly: (Capsule): Long-term
maintenance treatment in pts with
acromegaly who have responded to and
tolerated treatment with octreotide or
lanreotide. **(Injection solution):** To
reduce blood levels of growth hormone
(GH) and insulin growth factor-1 in pts
having inadequate response to or cannot be treated with surgical resection,
pituitary irradiation, and bromocriptine mesylate at maximally tolerated
doses. **(LAR injection):** Long-term
maintenance therapy in pts having an
inadequate response to surgery and/
or radiotherapy, or for whom surgery
and/or radiotherapy, is not an option.
**Carcinoid tumors: (Injection solu-
tion):** Treatment of severe diarrhea
and flushing episodes associated with
metastatic carcinoid tumors. **(LAR
injection):** Long-term treatment of
severe diarrhea and flushing episodes
associated with metastatic carci-
noïd tumors. **Vasoactive intestinal
peptide tumors: (Injection solution):** Treatment of the profuse watery
diarrhea associated with vasoactive
intestinal peptide tumors (VIPomas)-
secreting tumors. **(LAR injection):**
Long-term treatment of the profuse
watery diarrhea associated with VIP-
secreting tumors.

PRECAUTIONS

Contraindications: Hypersensitivity to
octreotide. **Cautions:** Diabetic pts with
gastroparesis, renal failure, hepatic
impairment, HF, concomitant medications
altering heart rate or rhythm. Concurrent
use of medications that prolong QT interval, elderly.

ACTION

Suppresses secretion of serotonin, gastrin, VIP, insulin, glucagon, secretin,
pancreatic polypeptide. **Therapeutic Effect:** Prolongs intestinal transit
time. Decreases growth hormone in
acromegaly.

PHARMACOKINETICS

Route	Onset	Peak	Duration
SQ	N/A	N/A	Up to 12 hrs

Protein binding: 65%. Metabolized in
liver. Excreted in urine. Removed by
hemodialysis. **Half-life:** 1.7–1.9 hrs.

⧖ LIFESPAN CONSIDERATIONS

Pregnancy/Lactation: Unknown if distributed in breast milk. **Children:** Safety
and efficacy not established. **Elderly:** No
age-related precautions noted.

INTERACTIONS

DRUG: May decrease concentration/effect
of **cycloSPORINE, hormonal contraceptives. Glucagon, growth hormone,
insulin, oral antidiabetics (e.g., glipi-
ZIDE, metFORMIN)** may alter glucose
concentrations. **HERBAL: Herbals with
hypoglycemic properties (e.g., fenugreek), maitake** may increase hypoglycemic effect. **FOOD:** None known. **LAB
VALUES:** May decrease serum thyroxine
(T_4). May increase serum alkaline phosphatase, ALT, AST, GGT.

AVAILABILITY (Rx)

Capsules, Delayed-Release: 20 mg.
Injection Solution: 50 mcg/mL, 100
mcg/mL, 200 mcg/mL, 500 mcg/mL,
1,000 mcg/mL. **Injection Suspension:**

(SandoSTATIN LAR): 10-mg, 20-mg, 30-mg vials.

ADMINISTRATION/HANDLING

◀ **ALERT** ▶ SandoSTATIN may be given IV, IM, SQ. SandoSTATIN LAR Depot may be given only IM. Refrigerate.

IM
• Give immediately after mixing. • Administer deep IM in large muscle mass at 4-wk intervals. • Avoid deltoid injections.

SQ
• Do not use if discolored or particulates form. • Avoid multiple injections at same site within short periods.

 IV
• Dilute in 50–100 mL 0.9% NaCl or D₅W and infuse over 15–30 min. In emergency, may give IV push over 3 min. Following dilution, stable for 96 hrs at room temperature when diluted with 0.9% NaCl (24 hrs with D₅W). Infuse over 15–30 min.

PO
• Take at least 1 hr before or 2 hrs after meals. Administer whole; do not crush or break. Capsules cannot be chewed.

INDICATIONS/ROUTES/DOSAGE

Note: Schedule injections between meals (to decrease GI effects).

Carcinoid Tumor
IV, SQ: *(SandoSTATIN):* **ADULTS, ELDERLY:** Initial 2 wks, 100–600 mcg/day in 2–4 divided doses. Range: 50–750 mcg.
IM: *(SandoSTATIN LAR):* **ADULTS, ELDERLY:** Must be stabilized on SQ octreotide for at least 2 wks; 20 mg q4wks for 2 mos, then modify based on response. **Maximum:** 30 mg q4wks.

Vasoactive Intestinal Peptic-Secreting Tumor (VIPoma)
IV, SQ: *(SandoSTATIN):* **ADULTS, ELDERLY:** Initial 2 wks, 200–300 mcg/day in 2–4 divided doses. Titrate dose based on response/tolerance. **Usual range:** 150–450 mcg/day.
IM: *(SandoSTATIN LAR):* **ADULTS, ELDERLY:** Must be stabilized on SQ

octreotide for at least 2 wks; 20 mg q4wks for 2 mos, then modify based on response. **Maximum:** 30 mg q4wks.

Acromegaly
IV, SQ: *(SandoSTATIN):* **ADULTS, ELDERLY:** Initially, 50 mcg 3 times/day. Increase as needed. **Range:** 300–1,500 mcg/day. **Usual effective dose:** 100 mcg 3 times/day.
IM: *(SandoSTATIN LAR):* **ADULTS, ELDERLY:** Must be stabilized on SQ octreotide for at least 2 wks. 20 mg q4wks for 3 mos, then modify based on response. **Maximum:** 40 mg q4wks.
PO: **ADULTS, ELDERLY:** Initially, 20 mg twice daily. May adjust dose in 20 mg/day increments q2–4wks based on clinical response as follows: (60 mg/day): 40 mg every morning and 20 mg at night. (80 mg/day): 40 mg twice daily. **Maximum:** 80 mg/day.

Dosage in Renal/Hepatic Impairment
No dose adjustment.

SIDE EFFECTS

Frequent (10%–6%; 58%–30% in acromegaly pts): Diarrhea, nausea, abdominal discomfort, headache, injection site pain. **Occasional (5%–1%):** Vomiting, flatulence, constipation, alopecia, facial flushing, pruritus, dizziness, fatigue, arrhythmias, ecchymosis, blurred vision. **Rare (less than 1%):** Depression, diminished libido, vertigo, palpitations, dyspnea.

ADVERSE EFFECTS/TOXIC REACTIONS

Increased risk of cholelithiasis. Prolonged high-dose therapy may produce hypothyroidism. GI bleeding, hepatitis, seizures occur rarely.

NURSING CONSIDERATIONS

BASELINE ASSESSMENT
Establish baseline B/P, weight, thyroid function, serum glucose, electrolytes.

INTERVENTION/EVALUATION
Monitor serum glucose, electrolytes, thyroid function. In acromegaly, monitor growth hormone levels. Weigh every 2–3

O

days, report over 5-lb gain per wk. Monitor B/P, pulse, respirations periodically during treatment. Be alert for decreased urinary output, peripheral edema. Monitor daily pattern of bowel activity, stool consistency.

PATIENT/FAMILY TEACHING
• Therapy should provide significant improvement of severe, watery diarrhea.

ofatumumab

oh-fa-**tue**-mue-mab
(Kesimpta)

■ BLACK BOX ALERT ■ Hepatitis B virus (HBV) reactivation may occur, resulting in hepatitis, hepatic failure, death. Progressive multifocal leukoencephalopathy (PML) resulting in death may occur.
Do not confuse ofatumumab with omalizumab.

◆CLASSIFICATION
PHARMACOTHERAPEUTIC: Anti-CD20 monoclonal antibody. **CLINICAL:** Multiple sclerosis agent.

USES
Treatment of relapsing forms of multiple sclerosis in adults, including clinically isolated syndrome, relapsing-remitting disease, and active secondary progressive disease.

PRECAUTIONS
Contraindications: Hypersensitivity to ofatumumab. Active hepatitis B virus infection. **Cautions:** Conditions predisposing to infection (e.g., diabetes, renal failure, immunocompromised pts, open wounds).

ACTION
Binds to CD20 molecule, the antigen on surface of B-cell lymphocytes; leading to cell lysis. **Therapeutic Effect:** Reduces B-cell inflammation associated with neurodegeneration and accumulation of disability in MS.

PHARMACOKINETICS
Degraded into small peptides and amino acids by proteolytic enzymes. Eliminated through both a target-independent route and a B-cell–mediated route. **Half-life:** 16 days.

⧖ LIFESPAN CONSIDERATIONS
Note: In general, disease-modifying therapy is stopped prior to planned pregnancy and not initiated during pregnancy. **Pregnancy/Lactation:** Unknown if distributed in breast milk. **Children:** Safety and efficacy not established. **Elderly:** No age-related precautions noted.

INTERACTIONS
DRUG: May alter concentration/effect of **vaccines (live).** May increase concentration/effect of **natalizumab. HERBAL: Echinacea** may decrease therapeutic effect. **FOOD:** None known. **LAB VALUES:** May decrease neutrophils, platelets, blood immunoglobulin M.

AVAILABILITY (Rx)
Solution, Injection *(Sensoready Pen)*: 20 mg/0.4 mL in prefilled syringe.

ADMINISTRATION/HANDLING
SQ
Preparation • Remove syringe/Sensoready pen from refrigerator and allow solution to warm to room temperature (15–30 mins). • Visually inspect for particulate matter or discoloration. Solution should appear clear to slightly opalescent, colorless to slightly brownish-yellow. Do not use if solution is cloudy, discolored, or visible particles are observed.
Administration • Insert needle subcutaneously into abdomen (approx. 2 inches of navel), outer thigh, or upper arm and inject solution. • Do not inject into areas of active skin disease or injury such as sunburns, skin rashes, inflammation, skin infections, or active psoriasis. • Rotate injection sites. • Do not administer IV or intramuscularly.

Storage • Refrigerate syringe/Sensoready pen until time of use. • Do not freeze or expose to heating sources.

INDICATIONS/ROUTES/DOSAGE

Multiple Sclerosis (Relapsing)

Note: Administer all immunizations least 4 wks prior to initiation for live or live-attenuated vaccines, and at least 2 wks for inactivated vaccines.

SQ: ADULTS, ELDERLY: Initially, 20 mg once wkly for 3 doses (wks 0, 1, and 2). **Maintenance:** 20 mg once monthly starting at wk 4.

Dosage in Renal/Hepatic Impairment
No dose adjustment.

SIDE EFFECTS

Frequent (39%–14%): Upper respiratory tract infections, injection related-reactions (systemic). **Occasional (13%–5%):** Headache, injection site reactions (local), back pain.

ADVERSE EFFECTS/TOXIC REACTIONS

Most common serious adverse reactions were bacterial, viral, fungal infections (including pneumonia and sepsis), Progressive multifocal leukoencephalopathy may occur. Infections including urinary tract infections, upper respiratory tract infections may occur.

NURSING CONSIDERATIONS

BASELINE ASSESSMENT

Obtain CBC; pregnancy test in females of reproductive potential. Test for hepatitis B virus infection. Screen for active infection. Screen pts at high risk of hepatitis B virus. Assess baseline CBC prior to therapy. Offer emotional support.

INTERVENTION/EVALUATION

Monitor renal function, electrolytes. Monitor CBC for evidence of myelosuppression during therapy, and increase frequency of monitoring in pts who develop Grade 3 or 4 cytopenia. Monitor for blood dyscrasias (fever, sore throat,

signs of local infection, unusual bruising/bleeding from any site), symptoms of anemia (excessive fatigue, weakness). Closely monitor for infusion reactions.

PATIENT/FAMILY TEACHING

• Treatment may depress your immune system and reduce your ability to fight infection. Report symptoms of infection such as body aches, chills, cough, fatigue, fever. Avoid those with active infection. • Report symptoms of hepatitis (e.g., fatigue, yellow discoloration of skin/eyes).

OLANZapine

oh-**lan**-za-peen
(Apo-OLANZapine ✦, ZyPREXA, ZyPREXA Relprevv, ZyPREXA Zydis)

■ **BLACK BOX ALERT** ■
Elderly pts with dementia-related psychosis are at increased risk for mortality due to cerebrovascular events. Sedation (including coma), delirium reported following use of ZyPREXA Relprevv.
Do not confuse OLANZapine with olsalazine or QUEtiapine, or ZyPREXA with CeleXA or ZyrTEC.

FIXED-COMBINATION(S)

Symbyax: OLANZapine/FLUoxetine (an antidepressant): 6 mg/25 mg, 6 mg/50 mg, 12 mg/25 mg, 12 mg/50 mg.
Lybalvi: OLANZapine/samidorphan: 5 mg/10 mg, 10 mg/10 mg, 15 mg/10 mg, 20 mg/10 mg.

✦CLASSIFICATION

PHARMACOTHERAPEUTIC: Second-generation (atypical) antipsychotic. **CLINICAL:** Antipsychotic.

USES

Agitation/aggression: Treatment of acute agitation associated with schizophrenia and bipolar I mania. **Bipolar**

disorder: Treatment of acute mania, acute episodes with mixed features of bipolar I disorder (as monotherapy or in combination with lithium or valproate), and as maintenance treatment. **Major depressive disorder:** Treatment of bipolar depression in combination with FLUoxetine. Treatment of treatment-resistant depression in combination with FLUoxetine. **Schizophrenia:** Treatment of of schizophrenia. **OFF-LABEL:** Agitation/aggression associated with dementia, anorexia nervosa, acute hypomania, chemotherapy induced acute/delayed nausea or vomiting, delirium (ICU/non ICU), Huntington's disease associated chorea.

PRECAUTIONS

Contraindications: Hypersensitivity to OLANZapine. **Cautions:** Disorders in which CNS depression is prominent; cardiac disease, hemodynamic instability, prior MI, ischemic heart disease; hyperlipidemia, pts at risk for aspiration pneumonia, decreased GI motility, urinary retention, BPH, narrow-angle glaucoma, diabetes, elderly, pts at risk for suicide, Parkinson's disease, severe renal/hepatic impairment, predisposition to seizures.

ACTION

Antagonizes alpha$_1$-adrenergic, DOPamine, histamine, muscarinic, serotonin receptors. Produces anticholinergic, histaminic, CNS depressant effects. **Therapeutic Effect:** Diminishes psychotic symptoms through combined antagonism of DOPamine and serotonin receptors.

PHARMACOKINETICS

Widely distributed. Protein binding: 93%. Excreted in urine (57%), feces (30%). Not removed by dialysis. **Half-life:** 21–54 hrs.

⧗ LIFESPAN CONSIDERATIONS

Pregnancy/Lactation: Unknown if drug crosses placenta or is distributed in breast milk. **Children:** Safety and efficacy not established. **Elderly:** Use caution. Consider lower starting doses.

INTERACTIONS

DRUG: Alcohol, CNS depressants (e.g., LORazepam, morphine, zolpidem) may increase CNS depressant effects. **Anticholinergics (e.g., aclidinium, ipratropium, tiotropium, umeclidinium)** may increase anticholinergic effect. **QT-prolonging agents (e.g., amiodarone, haloperidol, moxifloxacin, sotalol)** may cause QT interval prolongation. **HERBAL:** Herbals with sedative properties (e.g., chamomile, kava kava, valerian) may increase CNS depression. **FOOD:** None known. **LAB VALUES:** May increase serum GGT, cholesterol, prolactin, ALT, AST.

AVAILABILITY (Rx)

Injection, Powder for Reconstitution: *(ZyPREXA):* 10 mg. **Suspension for IM Injection:** *(Relprevv):* 210 mg, 300 mg, 405 mg. **Tablets:** *(ZyPREXA):* 2.5 mg, 5 mg, 7.5 mg, 10 mg, 15 mg, 20 mg. **Tablets, Orally Disintegrating:** *(ZyPREXA Zydis):* 5 mg, 10 mg, 15 mg, 20 mg.

ADMINISTRATION/HANDLING

PO
• Give without regard to food.

Orally Disintegrating
• Remove by peeling back foil (do not push through foil). • Place in mouth immediately. • Tablet dissolves rapidly with saliva and may be swallowed with or without liquid.

IM (ZyPREXA Intramuscular)
• Reconstitute 10-mg vial with 2.1 mL Sterile Water for Injection to provide concentration of 5 mg/mL. • Use within 1 hr following reconstitution. • Discard unused portion.

IM (Relprevv)
• Dilute to final concentration of 150 mg/mL. • Shake vigorously to mix. • Store at room temperature for up to 24 hrs. For IM gluteal injection only.

---

underlined – top prescribed drug

INDICATIONS/ROUTES/DOSAGE

Schizophrenia

Note: Discontinue gradually to avoid withdrawal symptoms and reduce relapse.

PO: ADULTS, ELDERLY: Initially, 5–10 mg once daily. May increase to 10 mg/day within 5–7 days. If further adjustments are indicated, may increase by 5 mg/day at wkly or longer intervals. **Maintenance:** 10–20 mg/day. **Maximum:** 20 mg/day. **CHILDREN 13 YRS AND OLDER:** Initially, 2.5–5 mg/day. Titrate in 2.5- or 5-mg increments at wkly or longer intervals. Target dose: 10 mg. **Maximum:** 20 mg/day.

IM: *(Long-Acting [Relprevv]):* **ADULTS, ESTABLISHED ON 10 MG/DAY ORALLY:** 210 mg q2wks for 4 doses or 405 mg q4wks for 2 doses. **Maintenance:** 150 mg q2wks or 300 mg q4wks. **ESTABLISHED ON 15 MG/DAY ORALLY:** 300 mg q2wks for 4 doses. **Maintenance:** 210 mg q2wks or 405 mg q4wks. **ESTABLISHED ON 20 MG/DAY ORALLY:** 300 mg q2wks.

Depression Associated With Bipolar Disorder (With FLUoxetine)

PO: ADULTS, ELDERLY: Initially, 5 mg in evening. May increase dose in 5 mg increments at intervals of q1–7 days based on response and tolerability up to 15 mg/day (adjunctive therapy) or up to 20 mg/day (monotherapy).

Treatment-Resistant Depression (With FLUoxetine)

PO: ADULTS, ELDERLY: Initially, 5 mg in evening. May gradually increase dose based on response and tolerability up to 20 mg/day. Range: 5–20 mg/day.

Bipolar Mania

PO: ADULTS, ELDERLY: *(Monotherapy):* Initially, 10–15 mg/day. May increase by 5 mg/day at intervals of at least 24 hrs. **Range:** 5–20 mg/day. **Maximum:** 20 mg/day. *(In Combination With Lithium or Valproate):* Initially, 10 mg/day. **Range:** 5–20 mg/day. **CHILDREN 13 YRS OF AGE AND OLDER:** Initially, 2.5–5 mg/day. Adjust dose by 2.5–5 mg daily at wkly intervals to target dose of 10 mg/day. **Range:** 2.5–20 mg/day.

Agitation Associated With Schizophrenia and Bipolar I Mania

IM: ADULTS, ELDERLY: *(Short-Acting):* Initially, 5–10 mg. Additional doses (up to 10 mg) may be considered. However, allow at least 2 hrs (after initial dose) or 4 hrs (after second dose) to evaluate response. **Maximum:** 30 mg/day.

Dosage in Renal/Hepatic Impairment

No dose adjustment.

SIDE EFFECTS

Frequent (26%–10%): Drowsiness, agitation, insomnia, headache, nervousness, hostility, dizziness, rhinitis. **Occasional (9%–5%):** Anxiety, constipation, nonaggressive atypical behavior, dry mouth, weight gain, orthostatic hypotension, fever, arthralgia, restlessness, cough, pharyngitis, visual changes (dim vision). **Rare:** Tachycardia; back, chest, abdominal, or extremity pain; tremor.

ADVERSE EFFECTS/TOXIC REACTIONS

Rare reactions include seizures, neuroleptic malignant syndrome, a potentially fatal syndrome characterized by hyperpyrexia, muscle rigidity, irregular pulse or B/P, tachycardia, diaphoresis, cardiac arrhythmias. Extrapyramidal symptoms (EPS), dysphagia may occur. Overdose (300 mg) produces drowsiness, slurred speech.

NURSING CONSIDERATIONS

BASELINE ASSESSMENT

Obtain LFT, serum glucose, weight, lipid profile before initiating treatment. Assess behavior, appearance, emotional status, response to environment, speech pattern, thought content. Question history of suicidal ideation and behavior.

INTERVENTION/EVALUATION

Monitor B/P, serum glucose, lipids, LFT. Assess for tremors, changes in gait, abnormal muscular movements, behavior. Supervise suicidal-risk pt closely during early therapy (as depression lessens, energy level improves, increasing suicide potential). Assess for therapeutic response (interest in surroundings, improvement in self-care, increased ability to concentrate, relaxed facial expression). Assist with ambulation if dizziness occurs. Assess sleep pattern. Notify physician if extrapyramidal symptoms (EPS) occur.

PATIENT/FAMILY TEACHING

• Avoid dehydration, particularly during exercise, exposure to extreme heat, concurrent use of medication causing dry mouth, other drying effects. • Take medication as prescribed; do not stop taking or increase dosage. • Slowly go from lying to standing. • Avoid alcohol. • Avoid tasks that require alertness, motor skills until response to drug is established.

olaparib

oh-**lap**-a-rib
(Lynparza)

◆CLASSIFICATION

PHARMACOTHERAPEUTIC: PARP inhibitor. **CLINICAL:** Antineoplastic.

USES

Ovarian cancer: First-line maintenance treatment (in combination with bevacizumab) of advanced epithelial ovarian, fallopian tube, or primary peritoneal cancer in adults who are in complete or partial response to first-line, platinum-based chemotherapy and whose cancer is associated with homologous recombination deficiency (HRD)–positive status defined by a deleterious or suspected deleterious BRCA mutation, and/or genomic instability. Maintenance treatment of recurrent epithelial ovarian, fallopian tube, or primary peritoneal cancer in adults who are in complete or partial response to platinum-based

chemotherapy. Maintenance treatment of deleterious or suspected deleterious germline or somatic BRCA-mutated advanced epithelial ovarian, fallopian tube, or primary peritoneal cancer in pts who have complete or partial response to first-line platinum-based chemotherapy. **Breast cancer:** Treatment of adults with deleterious or suspected deleterious gBRCAm, HER2-negative metastatic breast cancer who have been treated with chemotherapy in the neoadjuvant, adjuvant, or metastatic setting. Adjuvant treatment of deleterious or suspected deleterious gBRCAm human epidermal growth factor receptor 2 (HER2)–negative high-risk early breast cancer in pts who have been treated with neoadjuvant or adjuvant chemotherapy. **Pancreatic cancer:** Maintenance treatment of adults with deleterious or suspected deleterious gBRCAm metastatic pancreatic adenocarcinoma whose disease has not progressed on at least 16 wks of first-line, platinum-based chemotherapy. **Prostate cancer:** Treatment of deleterious or suspected deleterious germline or somatic homologous recombination repair (HRR) gene–mutated metastatic castration-resistant prostate cancer in adults who have progressed following prior enzalutamide or abiraterone treatment. In combination with abiraterone and predniSONE or prednisoLONE for the treatment of adults with deleterious or suspected deleterious BRCA-mutated (BRCAm) metastatic castration-resistant prostate cancer (mCRPC). **OFF-LABEL:** Breast cancer (early, high risk), ovarian cancer (advanced, refractory).

PRECAUTIONS

Contraindications: Hypersensitivity to olaparib. **Cautions:** Baseline cytopenias, conditions predisposing to infection (e.g., diabetes, renal failure, immunocompromised pts, open wounds). History of pulmonary disease. Avoid concomitant use of strong or moderate CYP3A4 inhibitors, strong or moderate CYP3A4 inducers.

ACTION

Inhibits poly(ADP-ribose) polymerase (PARP) enzymes, involved in normal cellular hemostasis (e.g., DNA transcription, cell cycle regulation, and DNA repair). Disrupts cellular homeostasis, resulting in cell death. **Therapeutic Effect:** Inhibits tumor cell growth and metastasis.

PHARMACOKINETICS

Widely distributed. Metabolized in liver. Protein binding: 82%. Peak plasma concentration: 1–3 hrs. Steady-state concentration: 3–4 days. Excreted in urine (44%), feces (42%). **Half-life:** 11.9 hrs.

⏳ LIFESPAN CONSIDERATIONS

Pregnancy/Lactation: Avoid pregnancy; may cause fetal harm. Females of reproductive potential should use effective contraception during treatment and for at least 6 mos after discontinuation. Unknown if distributed in breast milk. **Children:** Safety and efficacy not established. **Elderly:** No age-related precautions noted.

INTERACTIONS

DRUG: Strong CYP3A4 inhibitors (e.g., **clarithromycin, ketoconazole, ritonavir**), moderate CYP3A inhibitors (e.g., **dilTIAZem, fluconazole, verapamil**) may increase concentration/effect. **Strong CYP3A4 inducers (e.g., carBAMazepine, phenytoin, riFAMpin),** moderate CYP3A4 inducers (e.g., **dexamethasone, modafinil, nafcillin**) may decrease concentration/effect. **HERBAL: Bitter orange** may increase concentration/effect. **FOOD: Grapefruit products** may increase concentration/effect. **LAB VALUES:** May increase mean corpuscular volume, serum creatinine. May decrease Hct, Hgb, lymphocytes, neutrophils, RBC.

AVAILABILITY (Rx)

🔖 **Tablets:** 100 mg, 150 mg.

ADMINISTRATION/HANDLING

PO

• Give without regard to food. • Administer tablet whole; do not break, cut, crush, or divide.

INDICATIONS/ROUTES/DOSAGE

Ovarian Cancer (Advanced, Germline or Somatic BRCA-Mutated), First-Line Maintenance Therapy (Monotherapy)

PO: ADULTS, ELDERLY: 300 mg twice daily until disease progression, unacceptable toxicity, or completion of 2 yrs of therapy. Pts with complete response at 2 yrs should discontinue treatment. Pts with evidence of disease at 2 yrs may continue treatment beyond 2 yrs.

Ovarian Cancer (Advanced, Recurrent)

PO: ADULTS, ELDERLY: 300 mg twice daily until disease progression or unacceptable toxicity.

Ovarian Cancer (Advanced HRD-Positive), First-Line Maintenance Therapy (Combination Therapy)

PO: ADULTS, ELDERLY: 300 mg twice daily (in combination with bevacizumab). Continue until disease progression, unacceptable toxicity, or completion of 2 yrs of therapy. Pts with a complete response at 2 yrs should discontinue olaparib. Pts with evidence of disease at 2 yrs may continue treatment (beyond 2 years). Bevacizumab duration is for a total of 15 mos.

Breast Cancer (Metastatic, HER2-Negative, BRCA-Mutated)

PO: ADULTS, ELDERLY: 300 mg twice daily. Continue until disease progression or unacceptable toxicity.

Breast Cancer (Adjuvant Treatment)

PO: ADULTS, ELDERLY: 300 mg twice daily for a total of 1 yr or until recurrence or unacceptable toxicity, whichever occurs first. Pts with hormone receptor positive HER2–negative breast cancer should continue concurrent treatment with endocrine therapy.

Pancreatic Cancer

PO: ADULTS, ELDERLY: 300 mg twice daily until disease progression or unacceptable toxicity.

Prostate Cancer (Metastatic, Castration-Resistant, Homologous Recombination Repair Gene-Mutated)

PO: ADULTS, ELDERLY: 300 mg twice daily until disease progression or unacceptable

O

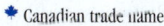 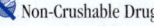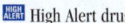

toxicity. Pts should also receive a gonado-tropin-releasing hormone analog or have had bilateral orchiectomy.

Prostate Cancer (BRCA-Mutated Metastatic Castration-Resistant)
Note: Pts should also receive a gonado-tropin-releasing hormone (GnRH) analog concurrently or should have had bilateral orchiectomy. **PO: ADULTS, ELDERLY:** 300 mg twice daily until disease progression or unacceptable toxicity.

Dose Modification
Dose Reduction for Adverse Reactions
PO: ADULTS, ELDERLY: Interrupt treatment until resolved. Then decrease to 200 mg twice daily. If further dose reduction is indicated, decrease to 100 mg twice daily.

Concomitant Use of Strong CYP3A4 Inhibitors
PO: ADULTS, ELDERLY: 150 mg twice daily.

Concomitant Use of Moderate CYP3A4 Inhibitors
PO: ADULTS, ELDERLY: 200 mg twice daily.

Dosage in Renal Impairment
Mild impairment: No dose adjustment. **Moderate to severe impairment:** Not specified; use caution.

Dosage in Hepatic Impairment
Not specified; use caution.

SIDE EFFECTS
Frequent (66%–21%): Fatigue, asthenia, nausea, vomiting, abdominal pain, diarrhea, dyspepsia, decreased appetite, headache, back pain, rash, myalgia, arthralgia, musculoskeletal pain, dysgeusia, cough.

ADVERSE EFFECTS/TOXIC REACTIONS
Myelodysplastic syndrome/acute myeloid leukemia reported in 2% of pts. Pneumonitis, including fatal cases, occurred in less than 1% of pts. Respiratory tract infections including nasopharyngitis, pharyngitis, upper respiratory tract infection occurred in 43% of pts.

NURSING CONSIDERATIONS
BASELINE ASSESSMENT
Obtain CBC. Do not initiate therapy until pts have recovered from hematologic toxicities caused by previous chemotherapy. Question history of pulmonary disease. Receive full medication history and screen for interactions. Offer emotional support.

INTERVENTION/EVALUATION
Monitor CBC monthly. For prolonged hematologic toxicities, interrupt treatment and monitor CBC wkly until recovery. If hematologic levels have not recovered to CTCAE Grade 1 or 0 after 4 wks of treatment interruption, consider hematology consultation for further investigations such as bone marrow analysis and blood sample for cytogenetics. Monitor for myelodysplastic syndrome/acute myeloid leukemia, pneumonitis. Monitor for infections (cough, fatigue, fever).

PATIENT/FAMILY TEACHING
• Treatment may depress your immune system and reduce your ability to fight infection. Report symptoms of infection such as body aches, burning with urination, chills, cough, fatigue, fever. Avoid those with active infection. • Report symptoms of bone marrow depression such as bruising, fatigue, fever, shortness of breath, weight loss; bleeding easily, bloody urine or stool. • Report new or worsening respiratory symptoms such as cough, difficulty breathing, fever, wheezing; may indicate severe lung inflammation. • Do not ingest grapefruit product, Seville oranges. • Do not take herbal products. • Use effective contraception to avoid pregnancy. Do not breastfeed.

olutasidenib
oh-**loo**-ta-**sid**-e-nib
(Rezlidhia)
■ **BLACK BOX ALERT** ■ Life-threatening and/or fatal differentiation syndrome with symptoms including fever, dyspnea, hypoxia, pulmonary

infiltrates, pleural or pericardial effusion, rapid weight gain or peripheral edema, hypotension, renal dysfunction may occur. Initiate corticosteroid therapy and hemodynamic monitoring in pts suspected of differentiation syndrome until symptoms resolve.

Do not confuse olutasidenib with ivosidenib or enasidenib.

◆CLASSIFICATION

PHARMACOTHERAPEUTIC: Isocitrate dehydrogenase-1 (IDH1) inhibitor. **CLINICAL:** Antineoplastic.

USES

Treatment of adults with relapsed or refractory acute myeloid leukemia (AML) with a susceptible isocitrate dehydrogenase-1 (IDH1) mutation.

PRECAUTIONS

Contraindications: Hypersensitivity to olutasidenib. **Cautions:** Hepatic impairment, uncontrolled hypertension, elderly. Avoid concomitant use of strong or moderate CYP3A4 inducers.

ACTION

Inhibits mutated IDH-1. In AML, IDH-1 mutants lead to increased levels of 2-hydroxyglutarate (2-HG) in leukemic cells. **Therapeutic Effect:** Causes remission and inhibition of mutant IDH-1 enzymatic activity, decreases 2-HG levels.

PHARMACOKINETICS

Widely distributed. Metabolized in liver. Protein binding: 93%. Peak plasma concentration: 4 hrs. Steady state reached in 14 days. Excreted in feces (75%), urine (17%). **Half-life:** 67 hrs.

⧗ LIFESPAN CONSIDERATIONS

Pregnancy/Lactation: Avoid pregnancy; may cause fetal harm. Recommendations for contraception not specified. Unknown if distributed in breast milk. Breastfeeding not recommended during treatment and for at least 2 wks after discontinuation. **Children:** Safety and efficacy not established. **Elderly:** May

have increased risk of hepatotoxicity, hypertension.

INTERACTIONS

DRUG: **Strong CYP3A4 inducers (e.g., carBAMazepine, phenytoin, rifAMPin), moderate CYP3A4 inducers (e.g., dexamethasone, modafinil, nafcillin)** may decrease concentration/effect; avoid use. May decrease concentration/effect of **CYP3A4 substrates (e.g., aripiprazole, atorvastatin, clonazepam, cyclosporine, dilTIAZem, QUEtiapine, zolpidem).** **HERBAL: St. John's wort** may decrease concentration/effect. **FOOD: High-fat meals** may increase concentration/effect. Administer on an empty stomach. **LAB VALUES:** May increase lymphocytes; serum alkaline phosphatase, ALT, AST, bilirubin, creatinine, lipase, uric acid. May decrease sodium, potassium.

AVAILABILITY (Rx)

Capsules: 150 mg.

ADMINISTRATION/HANDLING

PO
• Give at the same time each day on an empty stomach at least 1 hr before or 2 hrs after a meal. • Administer whole; do not cut, crush, or open capsule. • Capsule cannot be chewed. • If vomiting occurs after administration, give next dose at regularly scheduled time. • If a dose is missed, administer as soon as possible. Do not give a missed dose within 8 hrs of next dose.

INDICATIONS/ROUTES/DOSAGE

Acute Myeloid Leukemia (Relapsed or Refractory)
PO: **ADULTS, ELDERLY:** 150 mg twice daily for at least 6 mos or until disease progression or unacceptable toxicity.

Dose Modification
Differentiation Syndrome
Withhold treatment and start systemic corticosteroid therapy and hemodynamic monitoring until symptoms of differentiation syndrome improve and for a minimum of 3

days. May resume treatment at same dose when symptoms improve. If symptoms recur, restart systemic corticosteroid therapy and hemodynamic monitoring until symptoms of differentiation syndrome improve and for a minimum of 3 days. When symptoms improve, resume at a reduced frequency of 150 mg once daily for 7 days, then increase frequency to 150 mg twice daily.

Hepatotoxicity
Grade 3 Hepatotoxicity: Withhold treatment and obtain LFTs twice weekly until improved to Grade 1 or baseline, then resume at a reduced frequency of 150 mg once daily with continued monitoring of hepatic function. If hepatotoxicity improves to baseline within 28 days, increase frequency to 150 mg twice daily. Permanently discontinue if hepatotoxicity recurs at reduced frequency of 150 mg once daily. **Grade 4 Hepatotoxicity or Serum Alt, Ast Greater than 3 Times Upper Limit of Normal (Uln) with Total Bilirubin Greater than 2 Times Uln and Alkaline Phosphatase Less than 2 Time Uln (In The Absence Of Other Causes):** Permanently discontinue.

Noninfectious Leukocytosis
If indicated, treat with hydroxyurea per standard guidelines. Taper hydroxyurea after leukocytosis improves or resolves.

Other Adverse Reactions
Any Other Grade 3 Or 4 Adverse Reaction: Withhold treatment until improved to Grade 2 or less, then resume at a reduced frequency of 150 mg once daily. May increase frequency to 150 mg twice daily if symptoms improve to Grade 1 or less for at least 1 wk. Permanently discontinue if Grade 3 or 4 adverse reaction recurs at a reduced frequency of 150 mg once daily.

Dosage in Renal/Hepatic Impairment
Mild to moderate impairment: No dose adjustment. **Severe impairment:** Not specified; use caution.

SIDE EFFECTS

Frequent (38%–23%): Nausea, fatigue, malaise, arthralgia, bone/back/extremity/ neck pain, arthritis, joint effusion/swelling, constipation, pyrexia, dyspnea, rash, mucositis, gingivitis, oral ulceration, stomatitis, oral/oropharyngeal pain, pharyngitis, proctalgia, colitis. **Occasional (20%–10%):** Diarrhea, abdominal pain, edema, vomiting, cough, decreased appetite, headache, hypertension.

ADVERSE EFFECTS/TOXIC REACTIONS

Life-threatening and/or fatal differentiation syndrome, a condition with rapid proliferation and differentiation of myeloid cells, reported in 16% of pts. Differentiation syndrome may recur if treatment with corticosteroids and/or hydroxyurea is discontinued prematurely. Hepatotoxicity reported in 23% of pts. Median time to onset of hepatotoxicity was approx. 1 mo. May cause hypoxia, respiratory distress syndrome, decreased oxygen saturation. Gallbladder disorders, including biliary tract disorder, biliary colic, cholestasis cholangitis, were reported in less than 10% of pts. May prolong QT interval on ECG.

NURSING CONSIDERATIONS

BASELINE ASSESSMENT
Obtain CBC, BMP, LFT, B/P; pregnancy test in females of reproductive potential. Confirm presence of IDH-1 mutations in the blood or bone marrow. Receive full medication history (including herbal products) and screen for interactions. Question history of hepatic impairment, hypertension. Offer emotional support.

INTERVENTION/EVALUATION
Monitor LFT at least wkly for 2 mos, then every other week for the third month, then once for the fourth month, then every other month until discontinuation. Monitor B/P for hypertension. Monitor for symptoms of differentiation syndrome (dyspnea, fever, hypotension, hypoxia, pulmonary infiltrates, pleural or pericardial effusion, rapid weight gain or peripheral edema, renal dysfunction). If differentiation syndrome is suspected,

initiate corticosteroids and hemodynamic monitoring until symptoms resolve for at least 3 days. Monitor daily pattern of bowel activity, stool consistency. Ensure adequate hydration, nutrition.

PATIENT/FAMILY TEACHING
• Treatment may cause life-threatening differentiation syndrome within days of starting therapy. Report difficulty breathing, fever, low blood pressure, rapid weight gain, swelling of the hands or feet, decreased urine output. • Report liver problems (abdominal pain, bruising, clay-colored stool, amber or dark-colored urine, yellowing of the skin or eyes), skin reactions (rash, skin eruptions). • There is a high risk of interactions with other medications. Do not take newly prescribed medications unless approved by prescriber who originally started treatment. • Avoid herbal supplements (esp. St John's wort). • Report suspected pregnancy. Do not breastfeed. • Take at the same time each day on an empty stomach at least 1 hr before or 2 hrs after a meal.

---

omalizumab
TOP 100

oh-ma-**liz**-ue-mab
(Xolair)

■ **BLACK BOX ALERT** ■ Anaphylaxis (severe bronchospasm, hypotension, angioedema, syncope, urticaria) has occurred after first dose and in some cases after 1 yr of regular treatment.
Do not confuse omalizumab with ofatumumab.

◆CLASSIFICATION
PHARMACOTHERAPEUTIC: Monoclonal antibody. **CLINICAL:** Antiasthmatic.

USES
Asthma: Treatment of moderate to severe persistent asthma in adults and children 6 yrs of age and older reactive to perennial allergens and with symptoms inadequately controlled with inhaled corticosteroids. **Urticaria (chronic):** Chronic spontaneous urticaria in adults and children 12 yrs and older who remain symptomatic despite H1 antihistamine treatment. **Rhinosinusitis (chronic):** Add-on maintenance treatment of chronic rhinosinusitis with nasal polyps (CRSwNP) in adults with inadequate response to nasal corticosteroids. **Food allergy:** IgE-mediated food allergy in adults and pts 1 yr and older for the reduction of allergic reactions (type I), including anaphylaxisis, that may occur with accidental exposure to one or more foods.

PRECAUTIONS
Contraindications: Hypersensitivity to omalizumab. Do not use to treat acute bronchospasm, status asthmaticus. **Cautions:** Pts at risk for parasitic infections.

ACTION
Selectively binds to human immunoglobulin E (IgE). Inhibits binding of IgE on surface of mast cells, basophils. **Therapeutic Effect:** Prevents/reduces number of asthmatic attacks and corticosteroid use.

PHARMACOKINETICS
Absorbed slowly after SQ administration, with peak concentration in 7–8 days. Excreted primarily via hepatic degradation. **Half-life:** 26 days.

LIFESPAN CONSIDERATIONS
Pregnancy/Lactation: Because IgE is present in breast milk, omalizumab is expected to be present in breast milk. Use only if clearly needed. **Children:** Safety and efficacy not established in pts younger than 1 yr. **Elderly:** No age-related precautions noted.

INTERACTIONS
DRUG: May enhance the adverse/toxic effects of **loxapine**. **HERBAL:** None

---

significant. **FOOD:** None known. **LAB VALUES:** May increase serum IgE levels.

AVAILABILITY (Rx)

Injection, Prefilled Syringe: 75 mg/0.5 mL, 150 mg/mL. **Injection, Powder for Reconstitution:** 150 mg/1.2 mL after reconstitution.

ADMINISTRATION/HANDLING

SQ

Reconstitution • Use only Sterile Water for Injection to prepare for SQ administration. • Medication takes 15–20 min to dissolve. • Draw 1.4 mL Sterile Water for Injection into 3-mL syringe with 1-inch, 18-gauge needle; inject contents into powdered vial. • Swirl vial for approximately 1 min (do not shake) and again swirl vial for 5–10 sec every 5 min until no gel-like particles appear in the solution. • Do not use if contents do not dissolve completely within 40 min. • Invert vial for 15 sec (allows solution to drain toward the stopper). • Using new 3-mL syringe with 1-inch 18-gauge needle, obtain required 1.2-mL dose, replace 18-gauge needle with 25-gauge needle for SQ administration.
Rate of administration • SQ administration may take 5–10 sec to administer due to its viscosity.
Storage • Use only clear or slightly opalescent solution; solution is slightly viscous. • Refrigerate. • Reconstituted solution is stable for 8 hrs if refrigerated or within 4 hrs of reconstitution when stored at room temperature.

INDICATIONS/ROUTES/DOSAGE

◄**ALERT**► Give only under direct medical supervision. Should be administered in healthcare setting by health professionals. Dosage and frequency of administration are based upon total IgE levels and body weight (see table). IgE levels should be measured prior to initiating treatment and not during treatment. Pts should be observed a minimum of 2 hrs following each omalizumab treatment.

Asthma

SQ: **ADULTS, ELDERLY, CHILDREN 6 YRS AND OLDER:** 75–375 mg every 2 or 4 wks; dose and dosing frequency are individualized based on body weight and pretreatment IgE level (as shown in table). (Consult specific product labeling.)

Chronic Spontaneous Urticaria

SQ: **ADULTS, CHILDREN 12 YRS AND OLDER:** 150 mg or 300 mg q4wks. Dosing not dependent on IgE level or body weight.

Chronic Rhinosinusitis (With Nasal Polyps)

SQ: **ADULTS, ELDERLY:** 75–600 mg q2–4wks. Dose and frequency based on body weight and pretreatment total serum immunoglobulin E (IgE) levels (see manufacturer guidelines).

IgE-Mediated Food Allergy

SQ **ADULTS, ELDERLY, ADOLESCENTS, CHILDREN, INFANTS 1 YR AND OLDER:** 75 mg–600 mg q2–4 wks. Dose and frequency based on body weight and pretreatment total serum immunoglobulin E (IgE) levels (see manufacturer guidelines).

Dosage in Renal/Hepatic Impairment

No dose adjustment.

4-Wk Dosing Table

Pretreatment Serum IgE Levels (units/mL)	Weight 30–60 kg	Weight 61–70 kg	Weight 71–90 kg	Weight 91–150 kg
30–100	150 mg	150 mg	150 mg	300 mg
101–200	300 mg	300 mg	300 mg	See next table
201–300	300 mg	See next table	See next table	See next table

2-Wk Dosing Table

Pretreatment Serum IgE Levels (units/mL)	Weight 30–60 kg	Weight 61–70 kg	Weight 71–90 kg	Weight 91–150 kg
101–200	See preceding table	See preceding table	See preceding table	225 mg
201–300	See preceding table	225 mg	225 mg	300 mg
301–400	225 mg	225 mg	300 mg	Do not dose
401–500	300 mg	300 mg	375 mg	Do not dose
501–600	300 mg	375 mg	Do not dose	Do not dose
601–700	375 mg	Do not dose	Do not dose	Do not dose

SIDE EFFECTS

Frequent (45%–11%): Injection site ecchymosis, redness, warmth, stinging, urticaria, viral infection, sinusitis, headache, pharyngitis. **Occasional (8%–3%):** Arthralgia, leg pain, fatigue, dizziness. **Rare (2%):** Arm pain, earache, dermatitis, pruritus.

ADVERSE EFFECTS/TOXIC REACTIONS

Anaphylaxis, occurring within 2 hrs of first dose or subsequent doses, occurs in 0.1% of pts. Malignant neoplasms occur in 0.5% of pts.

NURSING CONSIDERATIONS

BASELINE ASSESSMENT

Obtain baseline serum total IgE level before initiation of treatment (dosage is based on pretreatment levels). Drug is not for treatment of acute exacerbations of asthma, acute bronchospasm, status asthmaticus.

INTERVENTION/EVALUATION

Monitor rate, depth, rhythm, type of respirations, quality/rate of pulse. Assess lung sounds for rhonchi, wheezing, rales. Observe lips, fingernails for cyanosis.

PATIENT/FAMILY TEACHING

• Increase fluid intake (decreases viscosity of pulmonary secretions). • Do not alter/stop other asthma medications. • Report allergic reactions (e.g., breathing difficulty, swelling of throat/tongue).

omega-3 acid- ethyl esters
TOP 100

oh-**may**-ga 3 as-id **eth**-il **es**-ters (Lovaza)
Do not confuse Lovaza with LORazepam.

◆CLASSIFICATION

PHARMACOTHERAPEUTIC: Omega-3 fatty acid. **CLINICAL:** Antilipemic agent.

USES

Dietary supplement for pts with early risk of CAD. **Lovaza:** Adjunct to diet to reduce very high (500 mg/dL or higher) serum triglyceride levels in adults. **OFF-LABEL:** Treatment of IgA nephropathy.

PRECAUTIONS

Contraindications: Hypersensitivity to omega-3 fatty acids. **Cautions:** Known sensitivity, allergy to fish.

ACTION

Reduces hepatic production of triglyceride-rich very low density lipoproteins (VLDL). **Therapeutic Effect:** Reduces serum triglyceride levels.

PHARMACOKINETICS

Widely distributed. Incorporated into phospholipids.

⧗ LIFESPAN CONSIDERATIONS

Pregnancy/Lactation: Unknown if distributed in breast milk. **Children:** Safety and efficacy not established in pts younger than 18 yrs. **Elderly:** No age-related precautions noted.

INTERACTIONS

DRUG: May increase concentration/effect of **antiplatelets (e.g., aspirin, clopidogrel), anticoagulants (e.g., warfarin).** **HERBAL:** None significant. **FOOD:** None known. **LAB VALUES:** May increase serum ALT, LDL.

AVAILABILITY (Rx)

Capsules: 300 mg, 500 mg, 1,000 mg.

ADMINISTRATION/HANDLING

PO
• *(Lovaza):* Give with food. Administer capsule whole (do not break, crush, dissolve, or allow chewing).

INDICATIONS/ROUTES/DOSAGE

◄ ALERT ► Before initiating therapy, pt should be on standard cholesterol-lowering diet for minimum of 3–6 mos. Continue diet throughout therapy.

Hypertriglyceridemia
PO: ADULTS, ELDERLY: *(Lovaza):* 4 g (4 capsules) once daily or 2 g (2 capsules) twice daily.

Dietary Supplement
PO: ADULTS, ELDERLY: 1–2 capsules 3 times/day.

Dosage in Renal/Hepatic Impairment
No dose adjustment.

SIDE EFFECTS

Occasional (5%–3%): Eructation, altered taste, dyspepsia. **Rare (2%–1%):** Rash, back pain.

ADVERSE EFFECTS/TOXIC REACTIONS

None known.

BASELINE ASSESSMENT
Assess serum triglyceride level, LFT. Obtain diet history, esp. fat consumption.

INTERVENTION/EVALUATION
Monitor serum triglyceride levels for therapeutic response. Monitor serum ALT, LDL periodically during therapy. Discontinue therapy if no response after 2 mos of treatment.

PATIENT/FAMILY TEACHING
• Continue to adhere to lipid-lowering diet (important part of treatment). • Periodic lab tests are essential part of therapy to determine drug effectiveness.

omeprazole TOP 100

oh-**mep**-ra-zole
(Losec , PriLOSEC, PriLOSEC OTC)
Do not confuse omeprazole with ARIPiprazole, pantoprazole, or esomeprazole, or PriLOSEC with Plendil, Prevacid, Prinivil, or PROzac.

FIXED-COMBINATION(S)

Konvomep: omeprazole/sodium bicarbonate (an antacid): 2 mg/84 mg/mL. **Yosprala:** omeprazole/aspirin (a platelet aggregation inhibitor): 40 mg/81 mg, 40 mg/325 mg. **Zegerid:** omeprazole/sodium bicarbonate (an antacid): 20 mg/1,100 mg, 40 mg/1,100 mg. **Zegerid Powder:** 20 mg/1,680 mg, 40 mg/1,680 mg.

◆ CLASSIFICATION

PHARMACOTHERAPEUTIC: Benzimidazole. **CLINICAL:** Proton pump inhibitor.

USES

Duodenal ulcer: Short-term treatment (usually within 4 wks) of active duodenal ulcer in adults. **Gastric ulcer:** Short-term treatment (4–8 wks) of active benign gastric ulcer in adults. **Gastroesophageal reflux**

disease (GERD): Treatment of symptomatic GERD (e.g., heartburn and other symptoms) for up to 4 wks in pts 1 yr of age and older. Short-term treatment (4–8 wks) of erosive esophagitis (EE) due to acid-mediated GERD that has been diagnosed by endoscopy in pts 1 yr of age and older. Maintenance healing of EE due to acid-mediated GERD in pts 1 yr of age and older. **Pathological hypersecretory conditions:** Long-term treatment of pathological hypersecretory conditions (e.g., Zollinger-Ellison syndrome, multiple endocrine adenomas, systemic mastocytosis) in adults. **OFF-LABEL:** Prevention/treatment of NSAID-induced ulcers, stress ulcer prophylaxis in critically ill pts. Barrett's esophagus, dyspepsia (functional). Eosinophilic esophagitis.

PRECAUTIONS

Contraindications: Hypersensitivity to omeprazole, other proton pump inhibitors. Concomitant use with products containing rilpivirine. **Cautions:** May increase risk of fractures, gastrointestinal infections. Hepatic impairment, pts of Asian descent.

ACTION

Inhibits hydrogen-potassium adenosine triphosphatase (H^+/K^+ ATP pump), an enzyme on the surface of gastric parietal cells. **Therapeutic Effect:** Increases gastric pH, reduces gastric acid production.

PHARMACOKINETICS

Route	Onset	Peak	Duration
PO	1 hr	2 hrs	72 hrs

Rapidly absorbed from GI tract. Protein binding: 95%. Primarily distributed into gastric parietal cells. Metabolized in liver. Primarily excreted in urine. Unknown if removed by hemodialysis. **Half-life:** 0.5–1 hr (increased in hepatic impairment).

⧗ LIFESPAN CONSIDERATIONS

Pregnancy/Lactation: Unknown if drug crosses placenta or is distributed in breast milk. **Children:** Safety and efficacy not established. **Elderly:** Use caution (bioavailability may be increased).

INTERACTIONS

DRUG: May decrease concentration/effects of **acalabrutinib, atazanavir, bosutinib, cefuroxime, clopidogrel, dasatinib, neratinib.** May increase concentration/effects of **escitalopram, voriconazole, oral anticoagulants (e.g., warfarin), phenytoin. HERBAL:** St. John's wort may decrease concentration/effects. **FOOD:** None known. **LAB VALUES:** May increase serum alkaline phosphatase, ALT, AST.

AVAILABILITY (Rx)

Oral Suspension: 2.5 mg/packet, 10 mg/packet.

🗨 **Capsules, Delayed-Release: (PriLO-SEC):** 10 mg, 20 mg, 40 mg. 🗨 **Tablets, Delayed-Release: (PriLOSEC OTC):** 20 mg.

ADMINISTRATION/HANDLING

PO

• Give 30–60 min before meals (breakfast preferred). • Give whole. Do not break, crush, dissolve, or divide delayed-release forms. • May open capsule, mix with applesauce, and give immediately.

PO (Suspension)

• Following reconstitution, allow to thicken (2–3 min). • Administer within 30 min.

INDICATIONS/ROUTES/DOSAGE

Duodenal Ulcer
PO: ADULTS, ELDERLY: 20 once daily for up to 4 wks.

Gastric Ulcer
PO: ADULTS, ELDERLY: 40 mg once daily for 4–8 wks.

GERD
PO: ADULTS, ELDERLY, CHILDREN 1–16 YRS OF AGE (20 KG OR GREATER): Symptomatic: 20 mg once daily for up to 4 wks. **10–19 KG:** 10 mg once daily. **5–9 KG:** 5 mg once daily. **EE due to Acid-Mediated GERD: ADULTS, ELDERLY, CHILDREN 1–16 YRS OF AGE (20 KG OR GREATER):** 20 mg once daily for 4–8 wks. **10–19 KG:** 10 mg once daily. **5–9 KG:** 5 mg once daily. **INFANTS 1 MOS TO LESS THAN 1 YR: 10 KG OR GREATER:** 10

mg for up to 6 wks. **5–9 KG:** 5 mg. **3–4 KG:** 2.5 mg. **Maintenance of Healing of EE due to Acid-Mediated GERD: ADULTS, ELDERLY, CHILDREN 1–16 YRS OF AGE (20 KG OR GREATER):** 20 mg once daily. **10–19 KG:** 10 mg once daily. **5–9 KG:** 5 mg once daily for 1 yr (studies do not extend beyond 1 yr).

Pathological Hypersecretory Conditions
PO: ADULTS, ELDERLY: Initially, 60 mg once daily. May increase up to 120 mg 3 times/day. Continue as long as clinically indicated.

H. pylori
PO: ADULTS, ELDERLY: Triple Therapy: 20 mg (with amoxicillin 1000 mg and clarithromycin 500 mg) twice daily for 10 days. Continue omeprazole for additional 18 days for ulcer healing/symptom relief. **Dual Therapy:** 40 mg once daily (clarithromycin 500 mg 3 times/day) for 14 days. Continue omeprazole for additional 14 days for ulcer healing/symptom relief.

OTC Use (Frequent Heartburn)
PO: ADULTS, ELDERLY: 20 mg/day for 14 days. May repeat after 4 mos if needed.

Dosage in Renal/Hepatic Impairment
No dose adjustment.

SIDE EFFECTS

Frequent (7%): Headache. **Occasional (3%–2%):** Diarrhea, abdominal pain, nausea. **Rare (2%):** Dizziness, asthenia, vomiting, constipation, upper respiratory tract infection, back pain, rash, cough.

ADVERSE EFFECTS/TOXIC REACTIONS

Pancreatitis, hepatotoxicity, interstitial nephritis occur rarely. May increase risk of *C. difficile* infection.

NURSING CONSIDERATIONS

INTERVENTION/EVALUATION

Evaluate for therapeutic response (relief of GI symptoms). Question if GI discomfort, nausea, diarrhea occurs.

PATIENT/FAMILY TEACHING

• Report headache, onset of black, tarry stools, diarrhea, abdominal pain. • Avoid alcohol. • Swallow capsules whole; do not chew, crush, dissolve, or divide. • Take before eating.

ondansetron

on-**dan**-se-tron
(Zofran, Zuplenz)
Do not confuse ondansetron with dolasetron, granisetron, or palonosetron, or Zofran with Zosyn.

◆CLASSIFICATION

PHARMACOTHERAPEUTIC: Selective 5-HT$_3$ receptor antagonist. **CLINICAL:** Antinausea, antiemetic.

USES

Prevention of nausea and vomiting (N/V) associated with highly emetogenic cancer chemotherapy, moderately emetogenic cancer chemotherapy, radiotherapy in pts receiving total body irradiation, single high-dose fraction to the abdomen, or daily fractions to the abdomen. Prevention of postoperative nausea and/or vomiting. **OFF-LABEL:** Gastroparesis (symptomatic N/V), nausea and/or vomiting (acute, severe), pregnancy associated N/V (severe/refractory).

PRECAUTIONS

Contraindications: Hypersensitivity to ondansetron, other HT$_3$ antagonists. Concomitant use of apomorphine. **Cautions:** Mild to moderate hepatic impairment, pts at risk for QT prolongation or ventricular arrhythmia (congenital long QT prolongation, QT interval–prolonging medications, hypokalemia, hypomagnesemia).

ACTION

Blocks serotonin, both peripherally on vagal nerve terminals and centrally in chemoreceptor trigger zone. **Therapeutic Effect:** Prevents nausea/vomiting.

PHARMACOKINETICS

Widely distributed. Protein binding: 70%–76%. Metabolized in liver. Primarily excreted in urine. Unknown if removed by hemodialysis. **Half-life:** 3–6 hrs (increased in hepatic impairment).

⏳ LIFESPAN CONSIDERATIONS

Pregnancy/Lactation: Unknown if drug crosses placenta or is distributed in breast milk. **Children:** Safety and efficacy not established in children younger than 1 mo. **Elderly:** No age-related precautions noted.

INTERACTIONS

DRUG: May increase concentration/effect of **apomorphine. QT interval–prolonging medications (e.g., amiodarone, azithromycin, ciprofloxacin, haloperidol)** may increase risk of QT interval prolongation, torsades de pointes. **HERBAL:** None significant. **FOOD:** None known. **LAB VALUES:** May transiently increase serum bilirubin, ALT, AST.

AVAILABILITY (Rx)

Film: 4 mg. **Injection Solution:** 2 mg/mL. **Oral Solution:** 4 mg/5 mL. **Tablets:** 4 mg, 8 mg, 24 mg. **Tablets, Orally Disintegrating:** 4 mg, 8 mg.

ADMINISTRATION/HANDLING

 IV

Reconstitution • May give undiluted. • For IV infusion, dilute with 50 mL D₅W or 0.9% NaCl before administration. **Rate of administration** • Give IV push over 2–5 min. • Give IV infusion over 15 min. **Storage** • Store at room temperature. • Stable for 48 hrs at room temperature following dilution.

IM
• Inject undiluted into large muscle mass.

PO
• Give without regard to food. Give 30 min prior to chemotherapy, 1–2 hrs before radiation, or 30–60 min prior to surgery.

Orally Disintegrating Tablets
• Do not remove from blister pack until needed. • Peel backing off; do not push through. • Place tablet on tongue; allow to dissolve. • Swallow with saliva.

🔲 IV COMPATIBILITIES

Acetaminophen, dexmedetomidine, magnesium sulfate, potassium chloride.

INDICATIONS/ROUTES/DOSAGE

Chemotherapy-Induced Nausea/Vomiting
IV: ADULTS, ELDERLY, CHILDREN 6 MOS AND OLDER: 3 doses of 0.15 mg/kg. **Maximum:** 16 mg. Give the first dose 30 min before the start of chemotherapy, then 4 and 8 hrs after the first dose.
PO: ADULTS, ELDERLY: Highly emetogenic: 24 mg as single dose 30 min before start of chemotherapy. **ADULTS, ELDERLY, CHILDREN 12–17 YRS OF AGE: Moderate emetogenic:** 8 mg 30 min before start of chemotherapy and 8 mg 8 hrs after the first dose. Then, 8 mg q12h for 1–2 days after completion of chemotherapy. **4–11 YEARS OF AGE:** 4 mg 30 min before the start of chemotherapy, with a subsequent 4-mg dose 4 and 8 hrs after the first dose, Then, 4 mg 3 times/day for 1–2 days after completion of chemotherapy.

Prevention of Postop Nausea/Vomiting
IV, IM: ADULTS, ELDERLY, CHILDREN OLDER THAN 12 YRS: 4 mg (undiluted) as a single dose. **CHILDREN 1 MO–12 YRS WEIGHING MORE THAN 40 KG:** 4 mg as a single dose. **CHILDREN 1 MO–12 YRS WEIGHING 40 KG OR LESS:** 0.1 mg/kg as a single dose. **PO: ADULTS, ELDERLY:** 16 mg 30–60 min before induction of anesthesia.

Prevention of Radiation-Induced Nausea/Vomiting
PO: ADULTS, ELDERLY: Total body radiotherapy: 8 mg 1–2 hrs before each fraction of radiotherapy each day. **Single**

 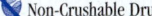

high-dose fraction radiotherapy of abdomen: 8 mg 1–2 hrs before radiotherapy, then 8–mg q8hrs after the first dose for 1–2 days after completion of radiotherapy. **Daily fractional radiotherapy to abdomen:** 8 mg 1–2 hrs before radiotherapy, then 8 mg q8hrs after the first dose for each day of radiotherapy.

Dosage in Renal Impairment
No dose adjustment.

Dosage in Hepatic Impairment
Mild to moderate impairment: No dose adjustment. **Severe impairment: Maximum daily dose:** 8 mg.

SIDE EFFECTS
Frequent (13%–5%): Anxiety, dizziness, drowsiness, headache, fatigue, constipation, diarrhea, hypoxia, urinary retention. **Occasional (4%–2%):** Abdominal pain, xerostomia, fever, feeling of cold, redness/pain at injection site, paresthesia, asthenia (loss of strength, energy). **Rare (1%):** Hypersensitivity reaction (rash, pruritus), blurred vision.

ADVERSE EFFECTS/TOXIC REACTIONS
Hypertension, acute renal failure, GI bleeding, respiratory depression, coma, extrapyramidal effects occur rarely. QT interval prolongation, torsades de pointes may occur.

NURSING CONSIDERATIONS

BASELINE ASSESSMENT
Assess degree of nausea, vomiting. Assess for dehydration if excessive vomiting occurs (poor skin turgor, dry mucous membranes, longitudinal furrows in tongue). Provide emotional support.

INTERVENTION/EVALUATION
Monitor ECG in pts with electrolyte abnormalities (e.g., hypokalemia, hypomagnesemia), HF, bradyarrhythmias, concurrent use of other medications that may cause QT prolongation, pts receiving high doses or frequent doses. Provide supportive measures. Assess mental status. Assess bowel sounds for peristalsis. Monitor daily pattern of bowel activity, stool consistency. Record time of evacuation.

PATIENT/FAMILY TEACHING
• Relief from nausea/vomiting generally occurs shortly after drug administration. • Avoid alcohol, barbiturates. • Report persistent vomiting. • Avoid tasks that require alertness, motor skills until response to drug is established (may cause drowsiness, dizziness).

---

oseltamivir

oh-sel-**tam**-i-veer
(Tamiflu)
Do not confuse Tamiflu with Thera-flu.

◆CLASSIFICATION
PHARMACOTHERAPEUTIC: Neuraminidase inhibitor. **CLINICAL:** Antiviral.

USES
Symptomatic treatment of uncomplicated acute illness caused by influenza A or B virus in adults and children 2 wks of age and older who are symptomatic no longer than 2 days. Prevention of influenza in adults, children 1 yr and older.

PRECAUTIONS
Contraindications: Hypersensitivity to oseltamivir. **Cautions:** Renal impairment.

ACTION
Selective inhibitor of influenza virus neuraminidase, an enzyme essential for viral replication. Acts against influenza A and B viruses. **Therapeutic Effect:** Suppresses spread of infection within respiratory system, reduces duration of clinical symptoms.

PHARMACOKINETICS

Widely distributed. Protein binding: 3%. Metabolized in liver. Primarily excreted in urine. **Half-life:** 6–10 hrs.

⧗ LIFESPAN CONSIDERATIONS

Pregnancy/Lactation: Unknown if distributed in breast milk. **Children:** Safety and efficacy not established in pts younger than 2 wks. **Elderly:** No age-related precautions noted.

INTERACTIONS

DRUG: May decrease concentration/effect of **influenza virus vaccine (live, attenuated). Probenecid** may increase concentration/effect. **HERBAL:** None significant. **FOOD:** None known. **LAB VALUES:** None significant.

AVAILABILITY (Rx)

Capsules: 30 mg, 45 mg, 75 mg. **Powder for Oral Suspension:** 6 mg/mL.

ADMINISTRATION/HANDLING

PO
• Give without regard to food (or may be given with food to improve tolerance). • May open capsules and mix with sweetened liquid. • Oral suspension stable for 10 days (room temperature) or 17 days (refrigerated) following reconstitution.

INDICATIONS/ROUTES/DOSAGE

Influenza
Note: Hospitalized pts may require longer treatment course. Initiate within 48 hrs of onset of symptoms. Consider duration longer than 5 days in pts with severe or complicated influenza.
PO: ADULTS, ELDERLY: 75 mg twice daily for 5 days. **ADOLESCENTS, CHILDREN WEIGHING MORE THAN 40 KG:** 75 mg twice daily for 5 days. **WEIGHING 23.1–40 KG:** 60 mg twice daily for 5 days. **WEIGHING 15.1–23 KG:** 45 mg twice daily for 5 days. **WEIGHING 15 KG OR LESS:** 30 mg twice daily for 5 days. **INFANTS AGES 2 WKS TO YOUNGER THAN 1 YR:** 3 mg/kg twice daily for 5 days.

Prevention of Influenza
Note: Initiate within 48 hrs of contact with an infected individual. Duration: 7–10 days (longer during community outbreaks).
PO: ADULTS, ELDERLY, CHILDREN 13 YRS AND OLDER: 75 mg once daily. **CHILDREN 1–12 YRS, WEIGHING MORE THAN 40 KG:** 75 mg once daily. **WEIGHING 23.1–40 KG:** 60 mg once daily. **WEIGHING 15.1–23 KG:** 45 mg once daily. **WEIGHING 15 KG simert:** 30 mg once daily.

Dosage in Renal Impairment
CrCl 31–60 mL/min: Treatment: 30 mg twice daily. Prevention: 30 mg once daily. **CrCl 11–30 mL/min:** Treatment: 30 mg once daily. Prevention: 30 mg every other day. **End-stage renal disease:** Not recommended.

Dosage in Hepatic Impairment
No dose adjustment.

SIDE EFFECTS

Frequent (10%–7%): Nausea, vomiting, diarrhea. **Rare (2%–1%):** Abdominal pain, bronchitis, dizziness, headache, cough, insomnia, fatigue, vertigo.

ADVERSE EFFECTS/TOXIC REACTIONS

Colitis, pneumonia, tympanic membrane disorder, fever occur rarely.

NURSING CONSIDERATIONS

BASELINE ASSESSMENT

Confirm test results of influenza A or B virus. Assess for symptoms of influenza (body aches, cough, congestion, dyspnea, fatigue, fever, headache). Educate importance of isolation precautions.

INTERVENTION/EVALUATION

Monitor for improvement of flu-like symptoms.

PATIENT/FAMILY TEACHING

• Begin as soon as possible from first appearance of flu symptoms (recommended within 2 days from symptom onset). • Treatment is not a cure, but it may shorten recovery time and reduce symptoms associated with influenza. • It is essential to complete the full course of treatment for the best therapeutic response. Do not prematurely stop treatment unless approved by prescriber. • Isolate from others to decrease spread of infection. • Not a substitute for a flu shot.

osimertinib

oh-sim-**er**-ti-nib
(Tagrisso)
Do not confuse osimertinib with afatinib, dasatinib, erlotinib, ibrutinib, imatinib, olaparib, or ospemifene, or Tagrisso with Targretin or Tasigna.

◆CLASSIFICATION

PHARMACOTHERAPEUTIC: Epidermal growth factor receptor (EGFR) inhibitor. Tyrosine kinase inhibitor. **CLINICAL:** Antineoplastic.

USES

Treatment of pts with metastatic epidermal growth factor receptor (EGFR) T790M mutation-positive non–small-cell lung cancer (NSCLC), as detected by FDA-approved test, who have progressed on or after EGFR tyrosine kinase inhibitor (TKI) therapy. First-line treatment of metastatic NSCLC in pts with EGFR exon 19 deletions or exon 21 L858R mutations. First-line treatment (in combination with pemetrexed and platinum-based chemotherapy) of adults with locally advanced or metastatic NSCLC whose tumors have EGFR exon 19 deletions or exon 21 L858R mutations. Adjuvant therapy after tumor resection for NSCLC in adults whose tumors have epidermal growth factor receptor (EGFR) exon 19 deletions or exon 21 L858R mutations. Treatment of adults with locally advanced, unresectable (stage III) NSCLC whose disease has not progressed during or following concurrent or sequential platinum-based chemoradiation therapy and whose tumors have EGFR exon 19 deletions or exon 21 L858R mutations.

PRECAUTIONS

Contraindications: Hypersensitivity to osimertinib. **Cautions:** Baseline cytopenias, COPD, heart disease (bradycardia, cardiomyopathy, heart block, HF, recent MI), conditions predisposing to infection (e.g., diabetes, renal failure, immunocompromised pts, open wounds), pts at risk for QTc interval prolongation or ventricular arrhythmia (congenital long QT syndrome, history for QT prolongation, medications that prolong QT interval, hypokalemia, hypomagnesemia); history of CVA, pulmonary embolism. Concomitant use of CYP3A4 inducers.

ACTION

Exhibits antitumor activity by irreversibly binding to mutant forms of EGFR. **Therapeutic Effect:** Inhibits tumor cell growth and metastasis.

PHARMACOKINETICS

Widely distributed. Metabolized in liver. Protein binding: Likely high. Peak plasma concentration: 3–24 hrs (median: 6 hrs). Steady state reached in 15 days. Excreted in feces (68%), urine (14%). Half-life: 48 hrs.

⧖ LIFESPAN CONSIDERATIONS

Pregnancy/Lactation: Avoid pregnancy; may cause fetal harm. Females of reproductive potential should use effective contraception during treatment and for at least 6 wks after discontinuation. Males with female partners of reproductive potential must use effective barrier methods during treatment and at least 4 mos after discontinuation. Unknown if distributed in breast milk. Breastfeeding not recommended during treatment and for up to 2 wks after discontinuation. May impair fertility in both females and males. **Children:** Safety and efficacy not established. **Elderly:** May have increased risk of Grade 3 or 4 adverse events. May require more frequent dose modifications.

INTERACTIONS

DRUG: QTc interval–prolonging medications (e.g., amiodarone, azithromycin, ciprofloxacin, haloperidol, methadone, tacrolimus) may increase risk of QTc prolongation. **Strong CYP3A4 inducers (e.g., carBAMazepine, phenytoin, rifAMPin)** may decrease concentration/effect. **Strong CYP3A4 inhibitors (e.g., clarithromycin, ketoconazole, ritonavir)** may increase concentration/risk of adverse effects. May decrease the therapeutic effect of **BCG (intravesical), vaccines (live)**. May increase adverse/toxic effects of **belimumab, natalizumab, vaccines (live)**. **HERBAL:** None significant. **FOOD:** None known. **LAB VALUES:** May decrease serum sodium, magnesium; Hgb, Hct, lymphocytes, neutrophils, platelets, RBCs. May decrease diagnostic effect of *Coccidioides immitis* skin test.

AVAILABILITY (Rx)

Tablets: 40 mg, 80 mg.

ADMINISTRATION/HANDLING

PO

• Tablets are hazardous; use cytotoxic precautions during handling and disposal. Recommend single gloving when handling intact tablets; double gloving, protective gown when handling liquid preparations. • Do not divide, crush, cut, or ultrasonicate tablets. • Give without regard to food. • If a dose is missed, skip missed dose and administer the next dose on schedule. • **Pts with dysphagia:** Disperse tablet in 60 mL of water (noncarbonated) only. • Stir until dissipated into small pieces (does not completely dissolve). • Deliver orally or via gastric tube. • Rinse container with 120–240 mL of water and administer any remaining drug residue. After oral administration of residue, instruct pt to thoroughly rinse mouth with water and swallow.

INDICATIONS/ROUTES/DOSAGE

Non–Small-Cell Lung Cancer (Adjuvant Therapy)
PO: ADULTS, ELDERLY: 80 mg once daily. Continue until disease progression or unacceptable toxicity, or for up to 3 yrs.

Non–Small-Cell Lung Cancer (Metastatic) (As Single Agent or In Combination Chemotherapy)
PO: ADULTS, ELDERLY: 80 mg once daily. Continue until disease progression or unacceptable toxicity.

Non–Small-Cell Lung Cancer (Locally Advanced or Metastatic)
Dose Modification
PO: ADULTS, ELDERLY: 80 mg once daily. Continue until disease progression or unacceptable toxicity.
Based on Common Terminology Criteria for Adverse Events (CTCAE).

Cardiac Toxicity
QTc interval greater than 500 msec on at least two separate ECGs: Withhold treatment until QTc interval is less than 481 msec or recovers to baseline. Once resolved, resume at 40 mg once daily. **QTc interval prolongation with symptoms of life-threatening arrhythmia:** Permanently discontinue. **Asymptomatic, absolute decrease in left ventricular ejection fraction (LVEF) of 10% from baseline and below 50%:** Withhold treatment for up to 4 wks. Resume treatment if improved to baseline. If not improved to baseline, permanently discontinue.

Pulmonary Toxicity
Interstitial lung disease/pneumonitis: Permanently discontinue.

Other Toxicities
Any Grade 3 or higher reaction: Withhold treatment for up to 3 wks. Resume treatment at 80 mg once daily or 40 mg once daily if improved to Grade 2 or lower within 3 wks. If not improved within 3 wks, permanently discontinue. **Concomitant use of strong CYP3A4 inducers:** Start dose at 160 mg once daily. May decrease dose to 80 mg once

daily if strong CYP3A4 inducer has been discontinued for at least 3 wks.

Dosage in Renal/Hepatic Impairment
Mild to moderate impairment: No dose adjustment. **Severe impairment:** Not specified; use caution.

SIDE EFFECTS

Frequent (42%–17%): Diarrhea, rash (generalized, erythematous, macular, maculopapular, papular, pustular), erythema, folliculitis, acne, dermatitis, acneiform dermatitis, dry skin, eczema, skin fissures, xerosis, nail disorders (inflammation, tenderness, discoloration, dystrophy, infection, ridging, onychoclasis, onycholysis, onychomadesis, paronychia), dry eye, blurry vision, keratitis, cataract, eye irritation, blepharitis, eye pain, increased lacrimation, vitreous floaters, nausea. **Occasional (16%–10%):** Decreased appetite, constipation, pruritus, cough, fatigue, back pain, stomatitis, headache.

ADVERSE EFFECTS/TOXIC REACTIONS

Myelosuppression (anemia, leukopenia, neutropenia, thrombocytopenia) is an expected response to therapy. Interstitial lung disease/pneumonitis reported in 3% of pts. May cause QTc interval prolongation (up to 3% of pts); cardiac toxicities including cardiomyopathy (1% of pts), decreased LVEF (2% of pts); other adverse effects including CVA, intracranial hemorrhage; pneumonia (4% of pts); venous thromboembolism including pulmonary embolism, jugular venous thrombosis, DVT (7% of pts).

NURSING CONSIDERATIONS

BASELINE ASSESSMENT
Obtain CBC, BMP, serum magnesium; vital signs; ECG. Confirm presence of T790M mutation in tumor specimen prior to initiation. Obtain pregnancy test in females of reproductive potential. Receive full medication history and screen for interactions. Question history of CVA, DVT, pulmonary embolism, pulmonary disease, cardiac disease. Obtain baseline echocardiogram to assess LVEF. Obtain visual acuity. Screen for active infection. Offer emotional support.

INTERVENTION/EVALUATION
Monitor CBC for cytopenias; BMP, serum magnesium for electrolyte abnormalities. Pts with cough, dyspnea, fever, worsening of respiratory status should be investigated for interstitial lung disease/pneumonitis. Pts with sudden chest pain, dyspnea, hypoxia, tachycardia should be evaluated for pulmonary embolism. Monitor for symptoms of DVT (leg or arm pain/swelling); CVA, intracranial hemorrhage (aphasia, altered LOC, facial droop, headache, hemiplegia, seizures). Assess LVEF by echocardiogram q3mos during therapy or more frequently in pts suspected of HF, congestive HF. Assess for eye pain, visual changes. Monitor for skin rash/toxicities, hypersensitivity reaction. Diligently monitor for infection. Monitor daily stool pattern, consistency.

PATIENT/FAMILY TEACHING
• Treatment may depress your immune system and reduce your ability to fight infection. Report symptoms of infection such as body aches, burning with urination, chills, cough, fatigue, fever. Avoid those with active infection. • Report symptoms of bone marrow depression such as bruising, fatigue, fever, shortness of breath, weight loss; bleeding easily, bloody urine or stool. • Report symptoms of abnormal heartbeats (dizziness, fainting, light-headedness, palpitations), heart failure (shortness of breath, fast or slow heart rate, exercise intolerance, swelling of the ankles or legs), severe lung inflammation (difficulty breathing, cough with fever, lung pain). • Use effective contraception to avoid pregnancy. Do not breastfeed. • Treatment may cause blood clots in the arms, legs, lungs, or brain. Immediately report symptoms of stroke (difficulty speaking, confusion, paralysis, vision loss), lung embolism (difficulty breathing, fast heart rate, chest pain), blood clots in the arms or legs (pain/swelling). • Do not take any newly prescribed medications unless

approved by doctor who originally started treatment. • Do not take herbal supplements.

oxaliplatin

ox-al-i-pla-tin

■ **BLACK BOX ALERT** ■
Anaphylactic-like reaction may occur within minutes of administration; may be controlled with EPINEPHrine, corticosteroids, antihistamines.

Do not confuse oxaliplatin with Aloxi, CARBOplatin, or CISplatin.

◆CLASSIFICATION
PHARMACOTHERAPEUTIC: Platinum-containing complex. Alkylating agent. **CLINICAL:** Antineoplastic.

USES
Colon cancer: Adjuvant treatment of stage III colon cancer after complete resection of primary tumor (in combination with infusional 5-fluorouracil and leucovorin); treatment of advanced colon cancer (in combination with infusional 5-fluorouracil and leucovorin). **OFF-LABEL:** Biliary tract cancer, chronic lymphocytic leukemia, esophageal cancer, gastric cancer, neuroendocrine tumors, non-Hodgkin lymphomas, ovarian cancer (advanced), pancreatic cancer (advanced/metastatic), testicular cancer (refractory).

PRECAUTIONS
Contraindications: History of allergy to oxaliplatin, other platinum compounds. **Cautions:** Previous therapy with other antineoplastic agents; radiation, renal impairment, pregnancy, immunosuppression, presence or history of peripheral neuropathy, elderly pts.

ACTION
Inhibits DNA replication and transcription by cross-linking with DNA strands. Cell cycle–phase nonspecific. **Therapeutic Effect:** Causes cellular death (apoptosis).

PHARMACOKINETICS
Widely distributed. Protein binding: 90%. Undergoes rapid, extensive nonenzymatic biotransformation. Excreted in urine. **Half-life:** 391 hrs.

⧗ LIFESPAN CONSIDERATIONS
Pregnancy/Lactation: If possible, avoid use during pregnancy, esp. first trimester. May cause fetal harm. Breastfeeding not recommended. **Children:** Safety and efficacy not established. **Elderly:** Increased incidence of diarrhea, dehydration, hypokalemia, fatigue.

INTERACTIONS
DRUG: Bone marrow depressants (e.g., cladribine) may increase myelosuppression, GI effects. **HERBAL:** None significant. **FOOD:** None known. **LAB VALUES:** May increase serum creatinine, bilirubin, ALT, AST, INR. May prolong prothrombin time.

AVAILABILITY (Rx)
Injection Solution: 5 mg/mL (10-mL, 20-mL vials).

ADMINISTRATION/HANDLING
◄**ALERT**► Wear protective gloves during handling of oxaliplatin. If solution comes in contact with skin, wash skin immediately with soap, water. Do not use aluminum needles or administration sets that may come in contact with drug; may cause degradation of platinum compounds.
◄**ALERT**► Pt should avoid ice, drinking cold beverages, touching cold objects during infusion and for 5 days thereafter (can exacerbate acute neuropathy).

▣ IV

Reconstitution • Dilute with 250–500 mL D_5W (never dilute with sodium chloride solution or other chloride-containing solutions).

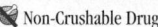

Rate of administration • Infuse over 2 hrs (extend to 6 hrs for acute toxicities).
Storage • Do not freeze. • Protect from light. • Store vials at room temperature. • After dilution, solution is stable for 6 hrs at room temperature, 24 hrs if refrigerated.

⚉ IV INCOMPATIBILITIES

Do not use a chloride-containing solution.

⚉ IV COMPATIBILITIES

Granisetron, ondansetron, palonosetron.

INDICATIONS/ROUTES/DOSAGE

Refer to individual protocols.
◄ ALERT ► Pretreat pt with antiemetics. Repeat courses should not be given more frequently than every 2 wks.

Colon Cancer, Advanced
IV: ADULTS: 85 mg/m^2 q2wks until disease progression or unacceptable toxicity (in combination with fluorouracil/leucovorin).

Colon Cancer, Stage III (Adjuvant Therapy)
IV: ADULTS: 85 mg/m^2 q2wks for up to 12 cycles (in combination with fluorouracil/leucovorin).

Dosage in Renal Impairment
CrCl less than 30 mL/min: Reduce dose to 65 mg/m^2.

Dosage in Hepatic Impairment
No dose adjustment.

SIDE EFFECTS

Frequent (76%–20%): Peripheral/sensory neuropathy (usually occurs in hands, feet, perioral area, throat but may present as jaw spasm, abnormal tongue sensation, eye pain, chest pressure, difficulty walking, swallowing, writing), nausea, fatigue, diarrhea, vomiting, constipation, abdominal pain, fever, anorexia. **Occasional (14%–10%):** Stomatitis, earache, insomnia, cough, difficulty breathing, backache, edema. **Rare (7%–3%):** Dyspepsia, dizziness, rhinitis, flushing, alopecia.

ADVERSE EFFECTS/TOXIC REACTIONS

Peripheral/sensory neuropathy can occur without any prior event by drinking or holding a glass of cold liquid during IV infusion. Pulmonary fibrosis (characterized as nonproductive cough, dyspnea, crackles, radiologic pulmonary infiltrates) may warrant drug discontinuation. Hypersensitivity reaction (rash, urticaria, pruritus) occurs rarely.

NURSING CONSIDERATIONS

BASELINE ASSESSMENT

Obtain CBC, renal function test. Question medical history as listed in Precautions. Offer emotional support.

INTERVENTION/EVALUATION

Monitor for decrease in WBC, platelets (myelosuppression is minimal). Monitor daily pattern of bowel activity, stool consistency. Monitor for diarrhea, GI bleeding (bright red, black tarry stool), neuropathy. Pt should avoid ice or drinking, holding glass of cold liquid during IV infusion and for 5 days following completion of infusion; may precipitate/exacerbate neuropathy (occurs within hrs or 1–2 days of dosing, lasts up to 14 days). Maintain strict I&O. Assess oral mucosa for stomatitis.

PATIENT/FAMILY TEACHING

• Promptly report fever, sore throat, signs of local infection, unusual bruising/bleeding from any site, persistent diarrhea, difficulty breathing. • Do not have immunizations without physician's approval (drug lowers resistance). • Avoid contact with those who have recently taken oral polio vaccine. • Avoid cold drinks, ice, cold objects (may produce neuropathy).

OXcarbazepine

ox-kar-**baz**-e-peen
(Oxtellar XR, <u>Trileptal</u>)
Do not confuse OXcarbazepine with carBAMazepine, or Trileptal with TriLipix.

◆CLASSIFICATION

PHARMACOTHERAPEUTIC: Carboxamide derivative, anticonvulsant. **CLINICAL:** Anticonvulsant.

USES

Immediate-release: Monotherapy or ad-junctive therapy in treatment of focal (partial) seizures in adults. Monotherapy of focal (partial) seizures in children 4 yrs and older, adjunctive therapy of focal (partial) seizures in children 2 yrs and older. **Extended-release:** Treatment of focal (partial) seizures in adults and children 6 yrs and older. **OFF-LABEL:** Trigeminal neuralgia.

PRECAUTIONS

Contraindications: Hypersensitivity to OXcarbazepine. **Cautions:** Renal impairment, sensitivity to carBAMazepine, pts at increased risk for suicide.

ACTION

Blocks sodium channels, stabilizing hyperexcited neural membranes, inhibiting repetitive neuronal firing, diminishing synaptic impulses. **Therapeutic Effect:** Prevents seizures.

PHARMACOKINETICS

Completely absorbed from GI tract. Metabolized in liver. Protein binding: 40%. Primarily excreted in urine. **Half-life:** 2 hrs; metabolite, 6–10 hrs.

⧖ LIFESPAN CONSIDERATIONS

Pregnancy/Lactation: Crosses placenta. Distributed in breast milk. **Children:** Safety and efficacy not established in children younger than 2 yrs. **Elderly:** Age-related renal impairment may require dosage adjustment.

INTERACTIONS

DRUG: Alcohol, CNS depressants (e.g., LORazepam, morphine, zolpidem) may have additive sedative effect. May decrease effectiveness of oral contraceptives, dolutegravir, doravirine, elvitegravir, rilpivirine, simeprevir, sofosbuvir, tenofovir alafenamide. May increase serotonergic effect of selegiline. **HERBAL:** None significant. **FOOD:** None known. **LAB VALUES:** May increase serum alkaline phosphatase, ALT, AST. May decrease serum sodium.

AVAILABILITY (Rx)

Oral Suspension: 300 mg/5 mL. **Tablets:** 150 mg, 300 mg, 600 mg.

🍒 **Tablets, Extended-Release:** 150 mg, 300 mg, 600 mg.

ADMINISTRATION/HANDLING

PO
• **(Immediate-Release):** Give twice daily without regard to food. • **(Extended-Release):** Give once daily on empty an stomach (1 hr before or 2 hrs after food). • Administer whole (do not cut, crush, or allow chewing).

INDICATIONS/ROUTES/DOSAGE

Adjunctive Treatment of Seizures
PO: ADULTS, ELDERLY, ADOLESCENTS: **(Immediate-Release):** Initially, 300–600 mg/day in 2 divided doses. May increase by 600 mg/day at wkly intervals. **Recommended dose:** 1,200 mg/day. **Maximum:** 2,400 mg/day. **ADOLESCENTS:** Initially, 300 mg twice daily. May increase in increments up to 600 mg/day at wkly intervals to a target dose of 1,200 mg/day in 2 divided doses. CHILDREN 4–16 YRS: Initially, 8–10 mg/kg in 2 divided doses. **Maximum:** 600 mg/day. Increase dose slowly over 2 wks. **Maintenance (based on weight):** CHILDREN WEIGHING MORE THAN 39 KG: 1,800 mg/day in 2 divided doses; CHILDREN WEIGHING 29.1–39 KG: 1,200 mg/day in 2 divided doses; CHILDREN WEIGHING 20–29 KG: 900 mg/day in 2 divided doses. CHILDREN 2–3 YRS: Initially, 8–10 mg/kg/day in 2 divided doses. **Maximum:** 600 mg/day in 2 divided doses. Increase dose slowly over 2–4 wks up to a **maximum** of 60 mg/kg/day in 2 divided doses.

O

(Extended-Release): ADULTS: Initially, 600 mg once daily. May increase by 600 mg/day at wkly intervals. **Maximum:** 2.4 g/day. ELDERLY: Initially, 300–450 mg/day. May increase by 300–450 mg/day at wkly intervals to desired clinical response. Range: Up to 2,400 mg/day.

Conversion to Monotherapy

PO: ADULTS, ELDERLY, ADOLESCENTS: **(Immediate-Release):** 600 mg/day in 2 divided doses (while decreasing concomitant anticonvulsant over 3–6 wks). May increase by 600 mg/day at wkly intervals up to 2,400 mg/day. CHILDREN 4–16 YRS: Initially, 8–10 mg/kg/day in 2 divided doses with simultaneous initial reduction of dose of concomitant antiepileptic over 3–6 wks. May increase by maximum of 10 mg/kg/day at wkly intervals (see below for recommended daily dose by weight).

Initiation of Monotherapy

PO: ADULTS, ELDERLY: **(Immediate-Release):** 600 mg/day in 2 divided doses. May increase by 300 mg/day every 3 days up to 1,200 mg/day. **(Extended-Release):** Initially, 600 mg once daily. May increase by 600 mg/day at wkly intervals up to 1,200–2,400 mg once daily. CHILDREN 4–16 YRS: **(Immediate-Release):** Initially, 8–10 mg/kg/day in 2 divided doses. Increase at 3-day intervals by 5 mg/kg/day to achieve maintenance dose by weight as follows:

Weight	Dosage
70+ kg	1,500–2,100 mg/day
60–69 kg	1,200–2,100 mg/day
50–59 kg	1,200–1,800 mg/day
41–49 kg	1,200–1,500 mg/day
35–40 kg	900–1,500 mg/day
25–34 kg	900–1,200 mg/day
20–24 kg	600–900 mg/day

Dosage in Renal Impairment

Mild to moderate impairment: No dose adjustment. **CrCl less than 30 mL/min:** Give 50% of normal starting dose, then titrate slowly to desired dose.

Dosage in Hepatic Impairment

Mild to moderate impairment: No dose adjustment. **Severe impairment:** Use caution with immediate-release; not recommended with extended-release.

SIDE EFFECTS

Frequent (22%–13%): Dizziness, nausea, headache. **Occasional (7%–5%):** Vomiting, diarrhea, ataxia (muscular incoordination), nervousness, dyspepsia, constipation. **Rare (4%):** Tremor, rash, back pain, epistaxis, sinusitis, diplopia.

ADVERSE EFFECTS/TOXIC REACTIONS

Clinically significant hyponatremia may occur, manifested as leg cramping, hypotension, cold/clammy skin, increased pulse rate, headache, nausea, vomiting, diarrhea. Suicidal ideation occurs rarely.

NURSING CONSIDERATIONS

BASELINE ASSESSMENT

Review history of seizure disorder (type, onset, intensity, frequency, duration, LOC). Receive full medication history and screen for interactions. Initiate seizure precautions.

INTERVENTION/EVALUATION

Assist with ambulation if dizziness, ataxia occur. Assess for visual abnormalities, headache. Monitor serum sodium. Assess for signs of hyponatremia (nausea, malaise, headache, lethargy, confusion). Assess for clinical improvement (decrease in intensity, frequency of seizures). Monitor for worsening depression, suicidal ideation.

PATIENT/FAMILY TEACHING

• Do not abruptly stop taking medication (may increase seizure activity). • Report if rash, nausea, headache, dizziness occurs. • May need periodic blood tests. • Avoid tasks that require alertness, motor skills until response to drug is established. • Avoid alcohol. • May decrease effectiveness of oral contraceptives. • Seek immediate medical attention if thoughts of suicide, new onset or worsening of anxiety, depression, or changes in mood occur.

oxyBUTYnin

ox-i-**bue**-ti-nin
(Ditropan XL, Gelnique, Oxytrol for Women)
Do not confuse oxyBUTYnin with OxyCONTIN.

◆CLASSIFICATION

PHARMACOTHERAPEUTIC: Anticholinergic. **CLINICAL:** Urinary antispasmodic.

USES

Immediate-release: Relief of symptoms (urgency, incontinence, frequency, nocturia, urge incontinence) associated with voiding in pts with unihibited or reflex neurogenic bladder in adults and children 5 yrs and older. **Extended-release (additional):** Treatment of symptoms associated with detrusor over-activity due to neurologic disorder (e.g., spina bifida) in adults and children 6 yrs and older.

PRECAUTIONS

Contraindications: Hypersensitivity to oxyBUTYnin. Uncontrolled narrow-angle glaucoma, urinary retention, gastric retention, or conditions with severely decreased GI motility. **Cautions:** Renal/hepatic impairment, bladder outflow obstruction, treated narrow-angle glaucoma, hyperthyroidism, coronary artery disease, HF, hypertension, arrhythmias, prostatic hyperplasia, myasthenia gravis, reduced GI motility, GI obstructive disorder, gastroesophageal reflux.

ACTION

Direct antispasmodic effect on smooth muscle; inhibits action of acetylcholine on smooth muscle. **Therapeutic Effect:** Increases bladder capacity, delays desire to void. Decreases urgency and frequency.

PHARMACOKINETICS

Route	Onset	Peak	Duration
PO	0.5–1 hr	3–6 hrs	6–10 hrs

Rapidly, well absorbed from GI tract. Metabolized in liver. Primarily excreted in urine. Unknown if removed by hemodialysis. **Half-life:** 1–2.3 hrs; metabolite, 7–8 hrs.

⧗ LIFESPAN CONSIDERATIONS

Pregnancy/Lactation: Unknown if drug crosses placenta or is distributed in breast milk. **Children:** No age-related precautions noted in pts older than 5 yrs. **Elderly:** May be more sensitive to anticholinergic effects (e.g., dry mouth, urinary retention).

INTERACTIONS

DRUG: Medications with anticholinergic action (e.g., aclidinium, ipratropium, tiotropium, umeclidinium) may increase anticholinergic effects. **HERBAL:** None significant. **FOOD:** None known. **LAB VALUES:** None significant.

AVAILABILITY (Rx)

Syrup: 5 mg/5 mL. **Tablets:** 2.5 mg, 5 mg. **Topical Gel (10%):** *(Gelnique):* 10% (1 g). **Transdermal:** *(Oxytrol for Women):* 3.9 mg/24 hrs.

🐢 **Tablets, Extended-Release:** 5 mg, 10 mg, 15 mg.

ADMINISTRATION/HANDLING

PO
• Give without regard to food. • Extended-release tablet must be swallowed whole; do not break, crush, dissolve, or divide.

Transdermal
• Apply patch to dry, intact skin on abdomen, hip, buttock. • Use new application

O

---

site for each new patch; avoid reapplication to same site within 7 days. • Normal exposure to water (e.g., bathing, swimming) should not affect patch.

Topical Gel
• **Gelnique:** Apply contents of 1 sachet once daily to dry, intact skin on abdomen, upper arms/shoulders, or thighs. • Do not bathe/shower until 1 hr after gel is applied.

INDICATIONS/ROUTES/DOSAGE

Neurogenic Bladder
PO: *(Immediate-Release):* **ADULTS:** 5 mg 2–3 times/day. May increase in 5-mg increments q2wks to 5 mg 4 times/day. **ELDERLY:** Initially, 2.5 mg 2–3 times/day. Increase cautiously. **CHILDREN OLDER THAN 5 YRS:** 5 mg twice daily. May increase to 5 mg 3 times/day.

PO: *(Extended-Release):* **ADULTS, ELDERLY:** 5–10 mg/day. May increase by 5-mg increments at 1–2 wk intervals. **Maximum:** 30 mg/day. **CHILDREN 6 YRS AND OLDER:** Initially, 5 mg once daily. May increase in 5 mg increments at wkly intervals. **Maximum:** 20 mg/day. **Transdermal: ADULTS:** 3.9 mg applied twice wkly. Apply every 3–4 days. Change patch on the same 2 days each wk. **Topical gel: ADULTS, ELDERLY:** 1 sachet (10%) 100 mg/g once daily.

Dosage in Renal/Hepatic Impairment
No dose adjustment.

SIDE EFFECTS
Frequent: Constipation, dry mouth, drowsiness, decreased perspiration. **Occasional:** Decreased lacrimation/salivation, impotence, urinary hesitancy/retention, suppressed lactation, blurred vision, mydriasis, nausea/vomiting, insomnia.

ADVERSE EFFECTS/TOXIC REACTIONS
Overdose produces CNS excitation (nervousness, restlessness, hallucinations, irritability), hypotension/hypertension, confusion, tachycardia, facial flushing, respiratory depression.

NURSING CONSIDERATIONS

BASELINE ASSESSMENT
Assess degree of dysuria, urgency, frequency, incontinence. Question medical history as listed in Precautions.

INTERVENTION/EVALUATION
Monitor for symptomatic relief. Monitor I&O; palpate bladder for urine retention. Monitor daily pattern of bowel activity, stool consistency.

PATIENT/FAMILY TEACHING
• Avoid alcohol. • May cause dry mouth (sugarless candy/gum may reduce effect). • Avoid tasks that require alertness, motor skills until response to drug is established (may cause drowsiness). • Avoid strenuous activity in warm environment.

---

oxyCODONE TOP 100 HIGH ALERT

ox-ee-**koe**-done
(Oxaydo, Oxy CONTIN, OxyIR, Roxicodone, RoxyBond, Supeudol, Xtampza ER)

■ **BLACK BOX ALERT** ■ OxyCONTIN **(controlled-release):** Not intended as an "as needed" analgesic or for immediate postop pain control. Extended-release should not be crushed, broken, or chewed (otherwise leads to rapid release and absorption of potentially fatal dose). Be alert to signs of abuse, misuse, and diversion. May cause potentially life-threatening respiratory depression. Prolonged use during pregnancy can cause neonatal withdrawal syndrome. Use of CYP3A4 inhibitors may increase effects/cause fatal respiratory depression. Concomitant use with benzodiazepines, other CNS depressants, may result in profound sedation, respiratory depression, coma, and death.

Do not confuse oxyCODONE with HYDROcodone, oxyBUTYnin, or oxyMORphone, OxyCONTIN with MS Contin or oxyBUTYnin, or Roxicodone with Roxanol.

FIXED-COMBINATION(S)

OxyCODONE/acetaminophen (a non-narcotic analgesic): 2.5 mg/325 mg; 5 mg/ 325 mg; 7.5 mg/ 325 mg; 10 mg/ 325 mg.

◆CLASSIFICATION

PHARMACOTHERAPEUTIC: Opioid agonist (Schedule II). **CLINICAL:** Analgesic.

USES

Immediate-release: Relief of acute or chronic, moderate to severe pain where the use of an opioid analgesic is appropriate and alternative treatments are inadequate. **Extended-release tablets (OxyCONTIN):** Management of pain requiring daily, around-the-clock, long-term treatment in adults and opioid-tolerant pts 11 yrs of age or older. **Capsules (Xtampza ER):** Indicated for adults only.

PRECAUTIONS

Contraindications: Hypersensitivity to oxyCODONE. Acute or severe bronchial asthma, hypercarbia, paralytic ileus (known or suspected), GI obstruction, significant respiratory depression. **Extreme Caution:** CNS depression, anoxia, hypercapnia, respiratory depression, seizures, acute alcoholism, shock, untreated myxedema, respiratory dysfunction. **Cautions:** Elevated ICP, hepatic/ renal impairment, coma, debilitated pts, head injury, biliary tract disease, toxic psychosis, acute abdominal conditions, hypothyroidism, prostatic hypertrophy, Addison's disease, urethral stricture, COPD, elderly, history of drug abuse and misuse, drug-seeking behavior, dependency.

ACTION

Binds with opioid receptors within CNS, causing inhibition of ascending pain pathway. **Therapeutic Effect:** Alters perception of and emotional response to pain.

PHARMACOKINETICS

Route	Onset	Peak	Duration
PO (immediate-release)	10–15 min	0.5–1 hr	3–6 hrs
PO (controlled-release)	10–15 min	0.5–1 hr	Up to 12 hrs

Widely distributed. Protein binding: 38%–45%. Metabolized in liver. Excreted in urine. Unknown if removed by hemodialysis. **Half-life:** 2–3 hrs (5 hrs controlled-release).

⧖ LIFESPAN CONSIDERATIONS

Pregnancy/Lactation: Readily crosses placenta. Distributed in breast milk. Respiratory depression may occur in neonate if mother received opiates during labor. Regular use of opiates during pregnancy may produce withdrawal symptoms in neonate (irritability, excessive crying, tremors, hyperactive reflexes, fever, vomiting, diarrhea, yawning, sneezing, seizures). **Children:** Paradoxical excitement may occur. Pts younger than 2 yrs are more susceptible to respiratory depressant effects. **Elderly:** Age-related renal impairment may increase risk of urinary retention. May be more susceptible to respiratory depressant effects.

INTERACTIONS

DRUG: **Alcohol, other CNS depressants (e.g., LORazepam, gabapentin, zolpidem)** may increase CNS effects, respiratory depression, hypotension. **Strong CYP3A4 inhibitors (clarithromycin, ketoconazole, ritonavir)** may increase concentration, toxicity. **Strong CYP3A4 inducers (carBAMazepine, phenytoin, rifAMPin)** may decrease concentration/effect. **MAOIs** may produce serotonin syndrome, a severe, sometimes fatal reaction. **HERBAL:** **Herbals with sedative properties (e.g., chamomile, kava kava, valerian)** may increase CNS depression. **FOOD:** **Grapefruit products** may increase potential for respiratory depression. **LAB VALUES:** May increase serum amylase, lipase.

AVAILABILITY (Rx)

◄**ALERT**► New formulation of controlled-release is intended to prevent medication from being cut, broken, chewed, crushed, or dissolved to reduce risk of overdose due to tampering, snorting, or injection.
Capsules: 5 mg. **Oral Concentrate:** 20 mg/mL. **Oral Solution:** 5 mg/5 mL. **Tablets:** 5 mg, 10 mg, 15 mg, 20 mg, 30 mg.

🖎 **Capsules, Extended-Release: Abuse Deterrent:** *(Xtampza):* 9 mg, 13.5 mg, 18 mg, 27 mg, 36 mg. **Tablets, Controlled-Release 12-Hour Abuse Deterrent:** *(Oxy-CONTIN):* 10 mg, 15 mg, 20 mg, 30 mg, 40 mg, 60 mg, 80 mg.

ADMINISTRATION/HANDLING

PO
• Give without regard to food. • **Controlled-release:** Swallow whole; do not break, crush, dissolve, or divide.

INDICATIONS/ROUTES/DOSAGE

Note: All doses should be titrated to desired effect. Do not abruptly discontinue in physically dependent pts. **Discontinuation:** When reducing the dose, discontinuing or tapering the dose should be done gradually (slow [10% reduction wkly or monthly] up to rapid [25%–50% reduction every few days]).

Analgesia
PO: *(Immediate-Release):* **ADULTS, ELDERLY:** Initially, 5 mg q4–6h PRN. **Usual dosage range:** 5–15 mg q4–6h. **INFANTS, CHILDREN, ADOLESCENTS: (50 KG OR GREATER):** 5–10 mg q4–6h prn. **(LESS THAN 50 KG):** Initially, 0.1–0.2 mg/kg/dose q4–6h as needed. **Usual dosage range:** 5–10 mg/dose.

Opioid Naive
PO: *(Controlled-Release):* **ADULTS, ELDERLY:** *(Tablets):* Initially, 10 mg q12h. *(Capsules):* Initially, 9 mg q12h.

◄**ALERT**► To convert from other opioids or nonopioid analgesics to oxy-CODONE controlled-release, refer to Oxy-CONTIN package insert. Dosages are reduced in pts with severe hepatic disease.

Dosage in Renal/Hepatic Impairment
Use caution. Titrate carefully.

SIDE EFFECTS

◄**ALERT**► Effects are dependent on dosage amount. Ambulatory pts, pts not in severe pain may experience dizziness, nausea, vomiting, hypotension more frequently than those in supine position or having severe pain. **Frequent:** Drowsiness, dizziness, hypotension (including orthostatic hypotension), anorexia. **Occasional:** Confusion, diaphoresis, facial flushing, urinary retention, constipation, dry mouth, nausea, vomiting, headache. **Rare:** Allergic reaction, depression, paradoxical CNS hyperactivity, nervousness in children, paradoxical excitement, restlessness in elderly, debilitated pts.

ADVERSE EFFECTS/TOXIC REACTIONS

Overdose results in respiratory depression, skeletal muscle flaccidity, cold/clammy skin, cyanosis, extreme drowsiness progressing to seizures, stupor, coma. Hepatotoxicity may occur with overdose of acetaminophen component of fixed-combination product. Tolerance to analgesic effect, physical dependence may occur with repeated use. **Antidote:** Naloxone (see Appendix H for dosage).

NURSING CONSIDERATIONS

BASELINE ASSESSMENT
Assess onset, type, location, duration of pain. Effect of medication is reduced if full pain recurs before next dose. Obtain vital signs before giving medication. If respirations are 12/min or less (20/min or less in children), withhold medication, contact physician. Assess for potential of abuse/misuse (e.g., drug-seeking behavior, mental health conditions, history of substance abuse).

INTERVENTION/EVALUATION

Palpate bladder for urinary retention. Monitor daily pattern of bowel activity, stool consistency. Initiate deep breathing, coughing exercises, esp. in pts with pulmonary impairment. Monitor pain relief, respiratory rate, mental status, B/P, level of consciousness. Screen for drug abuse and misuse, drug-seeking behavior

PATIENT/FAMILY TEACHING

• May cause dry mouth, drowsiness. • Avoid tasks that require alertness, motor skills until response to drug is established. • Avoid alcohol. • May be habit forming. • Do not chew, crush, dissolve, or divide controlled-release tablets. • Report severe constipation, absence of pain relief.

---

oxytocin   HIGH ALERT

ox-ee-**toe**-sin
(Pitocin)

■ **BLACK BOX ALERT** ■ Not to be given for elective labor induction, but can be used when there is a clear medical indication for induction.

Do not confuse Pitocin with Pitressin.

◆CLASSIFICATION

PHARMACOTHERAPEUTIC: Uterine smooth muscle stimulant. **CLINICAL:** Oxytocic agent.

USES

Indicated for the initiation or improvement of uterine contractions to achieve vaginal delivery in the following situations: induction of labor in pts with a medical indication (e.g., Rh problems, maternal diabetes, preeclampsia at or near term, when delivery is in the best interests of mother and fetus, or when membranes are prematurely ruptured and delivery is indicated). Stimulation or reinforcement of labor (e.g., selected cases of uterine inertia). Adjunctive therapy in the management of incomplete or inevitable abortion. **Postpartum:** To produce uterine contractions during third stage of labor and to control postpartum bleeding/hemorrhage.

PRECAUTIONS

Contraindications: Hypersensitivity to oxytocin. Adequate uterine activity that fails to progress, cephalopelvic disproportion, fetal distress without imminent delivery, grand multiparity, hyperactive or hypertonic uterus, obstetric emergencies that favor surgical intervention, prematurity, unengaged fetal head, unfavorable fetal position/presentation, when vaginal delivery is contraindicated (e.g., active genital herpes infection, invasive cervical cancer, placenta previa, cord presentation). **Cautions:** Induction of labor should be for medical, not elective, reasons. Generally not recommended in fetal distress, hydramnios, partial placental previa, predisposition to uterine rupture.

ACTION

Activates receptors that trigger increase in intracellular calcium levels in uterine myofibrils; increases prostaglandin production. **Therapeutic Effect:** Stimulates uterine contractions.

PHARMACOKINETICS

Route	Onset	Peak	Duration
IV	Immediate	N/A	1 hr
IM	3–5 min	N/A	2–3 hrs

Rapidly absorbed through nasal mucous membranes. Protein binding: 30%. Distributed in extracellular fluid. Metabolized in liver, kidney. Primarily excreted in urine. **Half-life:** 1–6 min.

⌧ LIFESPAN CONSIDERATIONS

Pregnancy/Lactation: Used as indicated, not expected to present risk of fetal abnormalities. Small amounts in breast milk. Breastfeeding not recommended. **Children/Elderly:** Not used in these pt populations.

0

INTERACTIONS

DRUG: Dinoprostone, misoprostol may increase concentration/effect. **HERBAL:** None significant. **FOOD:** None known. **LAB VALUES:** None significant.

AVAILABILITY (Rx)

Injection: *(Pitocin):* 10 units/mL. **Injection Solution:** 30 units/500 mL.

ADMINISTRATION/HANDLING

 IV

Reconstitution • Dilute 10–40 units (1–4 mL) in 1,000 mL of 0.9% NaCl, lactated Ringer's, or D$_5$W to provide concentration of 10–40 milliunits/mL solution.
Rate of administration • Give by IV infusion (use infusion device to carefully control rate of flow as ordered by physician).
Storage • Store at room temperature.

▓ IV COMPATIBILITIES

Heparin, insulin, potassium chloride.

INDICATIONS/ROUTES/DOSAGE

Induction or Stimulation of Labor
IV: ADULTS: 0.5–1 milliunit/min. May gradually increase in increments of 1–2 milliunits/min q30–60 minutes until desired contraction pattern is established. Rates greater than 9–10 milliunits/min are rarely required.

Abortion
IV: ADULTS: (Midterm elective abortion): 10–20 milliunits/min. **Maximum:** 30 units/12-hr dose. **(Incomplete, inevitable, or elective abortion):** 10 units as IV infusion after suction or a sharp curettage.

Control of Postpartum Bleeding
IV infusion: ADULTS: 5–10 units may be given initially and can be followed by a maintenance infusion of 10–40 units in 1,000 mL IV fluid at rate sufficient to sustain uterine contractions and control uterine atony.

IM: ADULTS: 10 units (total dose) after delivery.

Dosage in Renal/Hepatic Impairment
No dose adjustment.

SIDE EFFECTS

Occasional: Tachycardia, premature ventricular contractions, hypotension, nausea, vomiting. **Rare: Nasal:** Lacrimation/tearing, nasal irritation, rhinorrhea, unexpected uterine bleeding/contractions.

ADVERSE EFFECTS/TOXIC REACTIONS

Hypertonicity may occur with tearing of uterus, increased bleeding, abruptio placentae (i.e., placental abruption), cervical/vaginal lacerations. **Fetal:** Bradycardia, CNS/brain damage, trauma due to rapid propulsion, low Apgar score at 5 min, retinal hemorrhage occur rarely. Prolonged IV infusion of oxytocin with excessive fluid volume has caused severe water intoxication with seizures, coma, death.

NURSING CONSIDERATIONS

BASELINE ASSESSMENT
Assess baselines for vital signs, B/P, fetal heart rate. Determine frequency, duration, strength of contractions.

INTERVENTION/EVALUATION
Monitor B/P, pulse, respirations, fetal heart rate, intrauterine pressure, contractions (duration, strength, frequency) q15min. Notify physician of contractions that last longer than 1 min, occur more frequently than every 2 min, or stop. Maintain careful I&O; be alert to potential water intoxication. Check for blood loss.

PATIENT/FAMILY TEACHING
• Therapy will cause progression of labor. • If used for elective abortion, report increased abdominal pain, vaginal bleeding.

ozanimod

oh-zan-i-mod
(Zeposia)
Do not confuse ozanimod with fingolimod, ponesimod, or siponimod.

◆CLASSIFICATION

PHARMACOTHERAPEUTIC: Sphingosine 1-phosphate (S1P) receptor modulator. **CLINICAL:** Multiple sclerosis agent.

USES

Treatment of relapsing forms of multiple sclerosis (MS) in adults, including clinically isolated syndrome, relapsing-remitting disease, and active secondary progressive disease. Treatment of moderately to severely active ulcerative colitis in adults.

PRECAUTIONS

Contraindications: Hypersensitivity to ozanimod; recent (within 6 mos) MI; unstable angina; CVA; TIA; decompensated HF requiring hospitalization; NYHA class III/IV HF; sick sinus syndrome; Mobitz type II second- or third-degree AV block (unless pt has functioning pacemaker); severe, untreated sleep apnea; concomitant use of MAOIs. **Cautions:** Baseline lymphopenia; conditions predisposing to infection (e.g., diabetes, immunocompromised pts, renal failure, open wounds); baseline sinus bradycardia; hypertension; altered pulmonary function; pts at risk for developing AV block (congenital heart disease, ischemic heart disease, HF); pts at risk for macular edema (e.g., diabetes, history of uveitis); concomitant use of antiarrhythmics, beta blockers, calcium channel blockers. Not recommended with concomitant QT interval-prolonging medications, strong CYP2C8 inhibitors or inducers, breast cancer resistance protein (BCRP) inhibitors, adrenergic and serotonergic

drugs (e.g., SSRI, SNRI, opioids), foods containing high amounts of tyramine. Not recommended in pts with severe active infection, history of cardiac arrest, hepatic impairment, cerebrovascular disease, uncontrolled hypertension.

ACTION

Binds to S1P receptors 1 and 5, blocking capacity of lymphocytes to move out from lymph nodes, reducing the number of lymphocytes available to the CNS. **Therapeutic Effect:** May involve reduction of lymphocyte migration into the CNS, reducing inflammation.

PHARMACOKINETICS

Widely distributed. Metabolized in liver. Protein binding: 98%. Peak plasma concentration: 6–8 hrs. Excreted in feces (37%), urine (26%). **Half-life:** 21 hrs.

⧗ LIFESPAN CONSIDERATIONS

Pregnancy/Lactation: Avoid pregnancy; may cause fetal harm. Females of reproductive potential should use effective contraception during treatment and for at least 3 mos after discontinuation. Unknown if distributed in breast milk. **Children:** Safety and efficacy not established. **Elderly:** Not specified; use caution.

INTERACTIONS

DRUG: Beta-blockers (e.g., carvedilol, metoprolol), calcium channel blockers (e.g., dilTIAZem, verapamil), ceritinib, lacosamide may increase risk of AV block, bradycardia. **Class III antiarrhythmics (e.g., amiodarone, sotalol)** may increase risk of torsades de pointes in pts with baseline sinus bradycardia. **QT-interval prolonging agents (e.g., amiodarone, azithromycin, ciprofloxacin, haloperidol)** may enhance QT prolongation. May decrease therapeutic effect of **BCG (intravesical), vaccines (live) varicella vaccines**. **Strong CYP2C8 inhibitors (e.g., gemfibrozil)** may increase concentration/effect. **Strong CYP2C8 inducers (e.g., rifAMPin)**

0

may decrease concentration/effect. **MAOIs** (e.g., **phenelzine, selegiline**), **SSRIs** (e.g., **escitalopram, sertraline**), **SNRIs** (e.g., **DULoxetine, venlafaxine**) may increase risk of hypertensive crisis. **Alemtuzumab** may enhance immunosuppressive effect. **HERBAL:** Echinacea may decrease therapeutic effect. **FOOD:** **Foods or beverages containing high amounts of tyramine (e.g., aged cheese, pickled herring, red wine)** may cause release of norepinephrine, resulting hypertension. **LAB VALUES:** May increase serum ALT, AST, bilirubin. Expected to cause a dose-dependent reduction in peripheral lymphocyte count to 45% of baseline values.

AVAILABILITY (Rx)

Capsules: 0.23 mg, 0.46 mg, 0.92 mg.

ADMINISTRATION/HANDLING

PO

• Give without regard to meals. Administer capsule whole; do not break, cut, or crush. • If a dose is missed during the first 2 wks of therapy, reinitiate treatment starting with day 1 of titration regimen. If a dose is missed after the first 2 wks of therapy, continue maintenance regimen.

INDICATIONS/ROUTES/DOSAGE

Multiple Sclerosis

PO: ADULTS: Titration: 0.23 mg once daily on days 1–4, then increase to 0.46 mg once daily on days 5–7, then increase to 0.92 mg once daily on day 8. **Maintenance:** 0.92 mg once daily.

Ulcerative Colitis

PO: ADULTS: Initially, 0.23 mg once daily on days 1–4, then 0.46 mg once daily on days 5–7. **Maintenance:** 0.92 mg once daily starting on day 8.

Dosage in Renal Impairment

Mild to severe impairment: No dose adjustment.

Dosage in Hepatic Impairment

Mild to severe impairment: Not recommended.

SIDE EFFECTS

Rare (4%–2%): Orthostatic hypotension, back pain, hypertension, abdominal pain.

ADVERSE EFFECTS/TOXIC REACTIONS

Life-threatening infections (bronchitis, laryngitis, pharyngitis, upper respiratory tract infection, UTI) may occur. Fatal cases of cryptococcal meningitis, disseminated cryptococcal infections were reported. Herpes zoster infections reported in less than 1% of pts. Reactivation of herpes zoster infection may cause varicella zoster meningitis. Progressive multifocal leukoencephalopathy (PML), an opportunistic viral infection of the brain caused by the JC virus, may result in progressive permanent disability and death. Posterior reversible encephalopathy syndrome, a dysfunction of the brain that may evolve into an ischemic CVA or cerebral hemorrhage, may occur. Macular edema reported in less than 1% of pts. Pts with diabetes or history of uveitis are at an increased risk for developing macular edema. May result in transient bradycardia, AV conduction delays. Dose-dependent reductions of pulmonary function (absolute forced expiratory volume over 1 second) were reported. Hepatic injury (transaminitis) reported in 3%–5% of pts. Severe exacerbation of disability, including rebound disease, may occur after discontinuation. Malignancies including basal cell carcinoma, breast cancer, melanoma, seminoma may occur. Hypersensitivity reactions including rash, urticaria were reported.

NURSING CONSIDERATIONS

BASELINE ASSESSMENT

Obtain CBC, LFT, ECG. Assess baseline symptoms of MS (e.g., bladder/bowel dysfunction, cognitive impairment, depression, dysphagia, fatigue, gait disorder, numbness/tingling, pain, seizures, spasticity, tremors, weakness). Consultation with a cardiologist is advised in pts with QT interval prolongation greater than 450 msec in males or greater than 470 in females; arrhythmias requiring treatment with Class Ia or Class III antiarrhythmics; ischemic heart disease, HF, recent MI; history of Mobitz type II second- or third-degree AV block, sick sinus syndrome, sino-atrial heart block, cerebrovascular disease, uncontrolled hypertension. Pts without a documented history of vaccination against varicella zoster or a confirmed history of varicella infection (chickenpox) should be tested for antibodies prior to initiation. A full vaccination course for varicella in antibody-negative pts is recommended prior to initiation. If live attenuated vaccine immunization is required, give at least 1 mo prior to initiation. Receive full medication history and screen for interaction. Question history as listed in Precautions. Conduct ophthalmologic evaluation of the fundus (including the macula) prior to initiation. Withhold treatment in pts with active infection until resolved.

INTERVENTION/EVALUATION

Obtain LFT if hepatotoxicity (abdominal pain, clay-colored stool, amber or dark colored urine, jaundice, nausea) is suspected. During initiation, bradycardia and AV conduction delay is transient (initial effects lessened by titration). Conduct ophthalmic examination with any change of vision (or at regular intervals in pts with diabetes or history of uveitis). Pts with altered mental status, seizures, visual disturbances, unilateral weakness should be evaluated for cryptococcal meningitis, varicella zoster meningitis, posterior reversible encephalopathy syndrome, PML. Closely monitor for infections (body aches, cough, fever) during treatment and for at least 3 mos after discontinuation. If herpes zoster infection or other serious infection occurs, consider withholding treatment and initiate antimicrobial therapy. Closely monitor for adverse effects if other immunosuppressants are initiated within 3 mos after discontinuation. Monitor B/P for hypertension. Monitor for hypersensitivity reactions, new malignancies. Conduct neurological assessment. Assess for symptoms improvement of MS.

PATIENT/FAMILY TEACHING

• Treatment may depress your immune system and reduce your ability to fight infection. Report symptoms of infection such as body aches, burning with urination, chills, cough, fatigue, fever. Avoid those with active infection. Report travel plans to possible endemic areas. • Any changes of vision will require an immediate eye examination. • PML, an opportunistic viral infection of the brain, may cause progressive, permanent disabilities or death. Report symptoms of PML such as confusion, memory loss, paralysis, trouble speaking, loss of vision, seizures, weakness. • Posterior reversible encephalopathy syndrome, a condition resulting in brain swelling and narrowing of blood vessels, may lead to stroke; report confusion, severe headache, loss of vision, seizures, weakness. • Treatment may worsen high blood pressure or cause new cancers. • Report liver problems (abdominal pain, bruising, clay-colored stool, amber or dark colored urine, yellowing of the skin or eyes), lung problems (reduced lung function, shortness of breath), heart arrhythmias (chest pain, dizziness, fainting, palpitations, slow or rapid heart rate, irregular heart rate). • There is a high risk of interactions with other medications. Do not take newly prescribed medications unless approved by prescriber who originally started treatment. • Severe worsening of MS symptoms may occur after stopping treatment. • Avoid foods high in tyramine (aged, cured, fermented, pickled, smoked food).

PACLitaxel

HIGH ALERT

pak-li-**tax**-el
(Abraxane, Apo-**Pacl**itaxel)

■ **BLACK BOX ALERT** ■ Myelo-suppression is a major dose-limiting toxicity. Must be administered by certified chemotherapy personnel. Severe hypersensitivity reactions reported.

Do not confuse PACLitaxel with DOCEtaxel, PARoxetine, or Paxil.

◆CLASSIFICATION

PHARMACOTHERAPEUTIC: Taxane derivative, antimitotic agent. **CLINICAL:** Antineoplastic.

USES

Conventional: Breast cancer: Adjuvant treatment of node-positive breast cancer, metastatic breast cancer after failure of combination therapy or relapse within 6 mos of adjuvant therapy; subsequent therapy for advanced ovarian cancer or as first-line therapy (in combination with CISplatin). **Kaposi's sarcoma:** Treatment of AIDS-related Kaposi's sarcoma. **Non–small-cell lung cancer (NSCLC):** As first-line therapy (in combination with CISplatin) in pts who are not candidates for surgery or radiation therapy. **Ovarian cancer:** First-line therapy of advanced ovarian cancer (in combination with CISplatin). **Protein bound: Breast cancer:** Treatment of metastatic breast cancer after failure of combination chemotherapy or relapse within 6 mos of adjuvant chemotherapy. **Pancreatic cancer:** First-line treatment of metastatic adenocarcinoma of pancreas (in combination with gemcitabine). **NSCLC:** First-line treatment of locally advanced or metastatic NSCLC (in combination with CARBOplatin) in pts who are not candidates for curative surgery or radiation therapy. **OFF-LABEL:** Conventional: Anal cancer, bladder cancer, cervical cancer (advanced), esophageal cancer (metastatic), gastric cancer (metastatic), gestational trophoblastic neoplasia, head and neck cancer, melanoma (advanced/metastatic), testicular germ cell tumors, thyroid cancer (anaplastic). **Abraxane:** Biliary tract cancer, bladder cancer (metastatic), cervical cancer (advanced/recurrent), melanoma (metastatic), ovarian, fallopian tube or peritoneal cancer.

PRECAUTIONS

Contraindications: Hypersensitivity to PACLitaxel. Hypersensitivity to drugs developed with Cremophor EL (polyoxyethylated castor oil). Treatment of solid tumors with baseline neutrophil count less than 1,500 cells/mm^3; treatment of Kaposi's sarcoma with baseline neutrophil count less than 1,000 cells/mm^3. **Cautions:** Baseline cytopenias, cardiovascular disease, pulmonary disease, conditions predisposing to infection (e.g., diabetes, renal failure, immunocompromised pts, open wounds), hepatic impairment, concomitant use of strong CYP3A4 inhibitors, strong CYP3A4 inducers.

ACTION

Promotes microtubule assembly by enhancing action of tubulin dimers; stabilizes existing microtubules; inhibits their disassembly; interferes with late G_2 mitotic phase and inhibits cell lication. **Therapeutic Effect:** Inhibits cellular mitosis; suppresses cell proliferation, and modulates immune response.

PHARMACOKINETICS

Does not readily cross blood-brain barrier. Protein binding: 89%–98%. Metabolized in liver. Excreted in feces (71%), urine (14%). Not removed by hemodialysis. **Half-life:** 3-hr infusion: 13.1–20.2 hrs; 24-hr infusion: 15.7–52.7 hrs.

⧗ LIFESPAN CONSIDERATIONS

Pregnancy/Lactation: Avoid pregnancy; may cause fetal harm. Females of reproductive potential must use effective contraception during treatment and for at least 6 mos after discontinuation. Breastfeeding not recommended during treatment and for at least 2 wks after discontinuation. May impair fertility in both females and males. **Males:** Males with female partners of reproductive potential must use effective contraception during treatment and for at least 3 mos after discontinuation. **Children:** Safety and efficacy not established. **Elderly:** May have increased risk of adverse effects.

INTERACTIONS

DRUG: Strong CYP3A4 inhibitors (e.g., clarithromycin, ketoconazole, ritonavir) may increase concentration/effect. **Strong CYP3A4 inducers (e.g., carBAMazepine, phenytoin, rifAMPin)** may decrease effect. **Bone marrow depressants (e.g., cladribine)** may increase myelosuppression. **Strong CYP2C8 inhibitors (e.g., gemfibrozil)** may increase concentration/effect. **Vaccines (live)** may decrease concentration/effect. May increase concentration/effect of **vaccines (live)**. **HERBAL: Herbals with hypotensive properties (e.g., garlic, ginger, ginkgo biloba)** may increase effect. **Echinacea** may decrease therapeutic effect. **FOOD: Grapefruit products** may increase concentration/effect of paclitaxel (protein bound). **LAB VALUES:** May increase serum alkaline phosphatase, bilirubin, ALT, AST, triglycerides.

AVAILABILITY (Rx)

Injection, Powder for Reconstitution: *(Abraxane):* 100-mg vial. **Injection Solution:** 6 mg/mL (5-mL, 16.7-mL, 25-mL, 50-mL vials).

ADMINISTRATION/HANDLING

IV

◄**ALERT**► Wear gloves during handling; if contact with skin occurs, wash hands thoroughly with soap, water. If contact with mucous membranes occurs, flush with water.

PACLitaxel (Conventional)
Reconstitution • Dilute with 250–1,000 mL 0.9% NaCl, D$_5$W to final concentration of 0.3–1.2 mg/mL.
Rate of administration • Administer at rate per protocol (range: 1–96 hrs) through in-line filter not greater than 0.22 microns. • Monitor vital signs during infusion, esp. during first hour. • Discontinue administration if severe hypersensitivity reaction occurs.
Storage • Store unopened vials at room temperature. • Reconstituted solution is stable at room temperature for 72 hrs. • Store diluted solutions in bottles or plastic bags. Administer through polyethylene-lined administration sets (avoid plasticized PVC equipment or devices).

Abraxane (PACLitaxel—Protein Bound)
Reconstitution • Reconstitute each vial with 20 mL 0.9% NaCl to provide concentration of 5 mg/mL. • Slowly inject onto inside wall of vial; gently swirl over 2 min to avoid foaming. • Inject appropriate amount into empty PVC-type bag.
Rate of administration • Infuse over 30–40 min for pancreatic cancer. Do not use in-line filter.
Storage • Store unopened vials at room temperature. • Once reconstituted, use immediately but may refrigerate for up to 8 hrs.

▨ IV INCOMPATIBILITIES

◄**ALERT**► Data for Abraxane not known; avoid mixing with other medication.

▨ IV COMPATIBILITIES

Granisetron, ondansetron, palonesetron.

INDICATIONS/ROUTES/DOSAGE

Note: Premedication with dexAMETHasone, diphenhydrAMINE, and cimetidine, famotidine, or raNITIdine recommended. Refer to individual protocols.

P

PACLitaxel (Conventional)

Ovarian Cancer

IV: **ADULTS, ELDERLY:** **(Previously treated):** 135–175 mg/m^2/dose over 3 hrs q3wks. **(Previously untreated):** 175 mg/m^2 over 3 hrs q3wks (in combination with CISplatin) or 135 mg/m^2 over 24 hrs q3wks (in combination with CISplatin).

Breast Cancer (Adjuvant)

IV: **ADULTS, ELDERLY:** 175 mg/m^2 over 3 hrs q3wks for 4 cycles given sequentially to doxorubicin-containing combination chemotherapy.

Breast Cancer (Metastatic/Relapsed)

IV: **ADULTS, ELDERLY:** 175 mg/m^2 over 3 hrs q3wks (after failure of initial chemotherapy for metastatic disease or relapse within 6 mos of adjuvant chemotherapy).

Non–Small-Cell Lung Cancer

IV: **ADULTS, ELDERLY:** 135 mg/m^2 over 24 hrs q3wks followed by cisplatin, 75 mg/m^2.

Kaposi's Sarcoma (AIDS-Related)

IV: **ADULTS, ELDERLY:** 135 mg/m^2/dose over 3 hrs q3wks or 100 mg/m^2/dose over 3 hrs q2wks.

Dosage in Renal Impairment

No dose adjustment.

Dosage in Hepatic Impairment

Transaminase Level	Bilirubin	Dose
24-Hr Infusion		
Less than 2 times ULN	1.5 mg/dL or less	135 mg/m^2
2 to less than 10 times ULN	1.5 mg/dL or less	100 mg/m^2
Less than 10 times ULN	1.6–7.5 mg/dL or less	50 mg/m^2
3-Hr Infusion		
Less than 10 times ULN	1.25 mg/dL or less	175 mg/m^2
Less than 10 times ULN	1.26–2 times ULN	135 mg/m^2
Less than 10 times ULN	2.01–5 times ULN	90 mg/m^2
10 times ULN or greater	Greater than 5 times ULN	Avoid use

ULN: upper limit of normal

Dose Modification

Courses of PACLitaxel should be withheld until neutrophil count is 1,500 cells/mm^3 or more, and platelet count is 100,000 cells/mm^3 or more.

Abraxane (Protein Bound)

Breast Cancer (Metastatic)

IV infusion: **ADULTS, ELDERLY:** 260 mg/m^2 q3wks **or** 100 mg/m^2 on days 1, 8, 15 of a 28-day cycle (in combination with atezolizumab). Continue until disease progression or unacceptable toxicity.

Dose Modification

Severe neutropenia (ANC less than 500 cells/mm^3 for 1 wk or longer); severe sensory neuropathy: Reduce dose to 220 mg/m^2 for subsequent courses. **Recurrence of severe neutropenia, severe neuropathy:** Reduce dose to 180 mg/m^2 q3wks for subsequent courses. **CTCAE Grade 3 sensory neuropathy:** Hold until resolved to Grade 2 or 1, then reduce dose for subsequent courses. **Dosage of Abraxane for serum bilirubin greater than 1.5 mg/dL:** Dose unknown.

NSCLC (Locally Advanced or Metastatic)

IV: **ADULTS, ELDERLY:** 100 mg/m^2 on days 1, 8, 15 of each 21-day cycle (in combination with CARBOplatin) **or** 100 mg/m^2 on days 1, 8, 15 of a 28-day cycle (in combination with atezolizumab and CARBOplatin) for 4–6 cycles, followed by atezolizumab maintenance therapy **or** 100 mg/m^2 on days 1, 8, 15 of a 28-day cycle (in combination with pembrolizumab and CARBOplatin) for 4 cycles, followed by pembrolizumab maintenance therapy.

Adenocarcinoma of Pancreas (Metastatic) (in Combination With Gemcitabine)

IV: **ADULTS, ELDERLY:** 125 mg/m^2 on days 1, 8, 15 of each 28-day cycle (in combination with gemcitabine).

Dosage in Renal Impairment

No dose adjustment.

Dosage in Hepatic Impairment

	Mild Impairment (AST less than 10 times upper limit of normal [ULN], bilirubin 1.25 times ULN or less)	Moderate Impairment (AST less than 10 times ULN, bilirubin 1.26–2 times ULN)	Severe Impairment	
			(AST less than 10 times ULN, bilirubin 2.01–5 times ULN)	(AST more than 10 times ULN or bilirubin > 5 times ULN)
Breast cancer	No adjustment	Reduce dose to 200 mg/m²	Reduce dose to 130 mg/m² (may increase to 200 mg/m² in subsequent cycles)	Not recommended
NSCLC	No adjustment	Reduce dose to 75 mg/m²	Reduce dose to 50 mg/m² (may increase to 75 mg/m² in subsequent cycles)	Not recommended
Pancreatic	No adjustment	Not recommended	Not recommended	Not recommended

SIDE EFFECTS

Expected (90%–70%): Diarrhea, alopecia, nausea, vomiting. **Frequent (48%–46%):** Myalgia, arthralgia, peripheral neuropathy. **Occasional (20%–13%):** Mucositis, hypotension during infusion, pain/redness at injection site. **Rare (3%):** Bradycardia.

ADVERSE EFFECTS/TOXIC REACTIONS

Myelosuppression (anemia, neutropenia, thrombocytopenia) is an expected response to therapy, but more severe reactions including febrile neutropenia, sepsis may occur. Infections (candidiasis, respiratory tract infections, pneumonia) reported in 24% of pts. Pts with hepatic impairment may have increased risk of myelosuppression. Severe neuropathy was reported. Ocular toxicities (blurry vision, keratitis) reported in 10% of pts. Fatal interstitial lung disease (ILD), pneumonitis reported in 4% of pts. Severe hypersensitivity reactions, including anaphylaxis, may occur. Severe cardiovascular events (cardiac ischemia/infarction, chest pain, cardiac arrest, CVA, edema, hypertension, pulmonary embolism, SVT, transient ischemic attack, thrombosis) were reported.

NURSING CONSIDERATIONS

BASELINE ASSESSMENT

Obtain CBC, LFT prior to each course; pregnancy test in females of reproductive potential. Confirm compliance of effective contraception. Screen for active infection. Question history of cardiovascular disease, pulmonary disease, hepatic impairment. Receive full medication history and screen for interactions. Assess hydration status. Offer emotional support.

INTERVENTION/EVALUATION

Monitor CBC for myelosuppression; LFT for hepatotoxicity. Monitor for symptoms of hepatotoxicity (abdominal pain, jaundice, nausea, vomiting, weight loss) esp. in pts with hepatic impairment. Consider ABG, radiologic test if ILD/pneumonitis (excessive cough,

P

 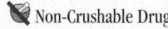

dyspnea, fever, hypoxia) is suspected. Consider treatment with corticosteroids if ILD/pneumonitis is confirmed. Monitor for infections (cough, fatigue, fever). Monitor daily pattern of bowel activity, stool consistency. Monitor for ocular toxicities, hypersensitivity reactions. Monitor for symptoms of DVT (leg or arm pain/swelling), CVA (aphasia, altered mental status, headache, hemiplegia, vision loss); MI (chest pain, dyspnea, syncope, diaphoresis, arm/jaw pain), PE (chest pain, dyspnea, tachycardia).

PATIENT/FAMILY TEACHING
• Treatment may depress your immune system response and reduce your ability to fight infection. Report symptoms of infection such as body aches, chills, cough, fatigue, fever. Avoid those with active infection. • Report symptoms of bone marrow depression (e.g., bruising, fatigue, fever, shortness of breath, weight loss; bleeding easily, bloody urine or stool). • Report symptoms of lung inflammation (excessive coughing, difficulty breathing, chest pain); liver problems (abdominal pain, bruising, clay-colored stool, amber- or dark-colored urine, yellowing of the skin or eyes). • Life-threatening blood clots may occur; report symptoms of DVT (swelling, pain, hot feeling in the arms or legs; discoloration of extremity), lung embolism (difficulty breathing, chest pain, rapid heart rate), stroke (confusion, one-sided weakness or paralysis, difficulty speaking), heart attack (chest pain, difficulty breathing, jaw pain, nausea, pain that radiates to the arm or jaw, sweating). • Use effective contraception to avoid pregnancy. Do not breastfeed. • Report any vision changes, eye redness. • Maintain proper hydration and nutrition. • Do not take newly prescribed medications unless approved by prescriber who originally started treatment. • Report allergic reactions of any kind.

palbociclib

pal-boe-**sye**-klib
(Ibrance)

◆CLASSIFICATION
PHARMACOTHERAPEUTIC: Cyclin-dependent kinase inhibitor. **CLINICAL:** Antineoplastic.

USES
Used in combination with an aromatase inhibitor (e.g., letrozole) for treatment of postmenopausal women and adult men with estrogen receptor–positive, human epidermal growth factor receptor 2 *(HER2)*–negative advanced breast cancer as initial endocrine-based therapy for metastatic disease or in combination with fulvestrant in women with disease progression following endocrine therapy.

PRECAUTIONS
Contraindications: Hypersensitivity to palbociclib. **Cautions:** Baseline cytopenias. History of pulmonary embolism. Avoid concomitant use of strong or moderate CYP3A4 inhibitors, strong or moderate CYP3A4 inducers.

ACTION
Reduces proliferation of breast cancer cell lines by preventing cellular progression from G1 into S phase of cell cycle. Combination with an aromatase inhibitor provides increased inhibition. **Therapeutic Effect:** Inhibits tumor cell growth and survival.

PHARMACOKINETICS
Widely distributed. Metabolized in liver. Protein binding: 85%. Peak plasma concentration: 6–12 hrs. Steady state reached in 8 days. Excreted in feces (74%), urine (18%). **Half-life:** 29 hrs.

⧗ LIFESPAN CONSIDERATIONS
Pregnancy/Lactation: Treatment is indicated for postmenopausal women. However, treatment may cause fetal harm

---

when administered during pregnancy. Females of reproductive potential should use effective contraception during treatment and up to 2 wks after discontinuation. Unknown if distributed in breast milk. **Children:** Safety and efficacy not established. Not indicated for this pt population. **Elderly:** No age-related precautions noted.

INTERACTIONS

DRUG: Strong CYP3A4 inhibitors (e.g., **clarithromycin, ketoconazole, ritonavir), moderate CYP3A4 inhibitors (e.g., dilTIAZem, fluconazole, verapamil)** may increase concentration/effect. **Strong CYP3A4 inducers (e.g., carBAMazepine, rifAMPin), moderate CYP3A4 inducers (e.g., nafcillin)** may decrease concentration/effect. May decrease the therapeutic effect of **vaccines (live)**. May increase adverse/toxic effects of **natalizumab, vaccines (live)**. **HERBAL:** St. John's wort may decrease concentration/effect. **Echinacea** may decrease therapeutic effect. **FOOD: Grapefruit products** may increase concentration/effect. **LAB VALUES:** May decrease Hgb, lymphocytes, neutrophils, platelets, WBC.

AVAILABILITY (Rx)

Tablets: 75 mg, 100 mg,125 mg.

 Capsules: 75 mg, 100 mg, 125 mg.

ADMINISTRATION/HANDLING

PO
• **Capsules:** Give with food. • Administer whole; do not break, crush, cut, or open capsule. • If vomiting occurs after dosing, do not readminister dose; give next dose at next scheduled time.
• **Tablets:** Give without regard to food.
• Administer tablet whole; do not break, crush, or split. Tablet cannot be chewed.

INDICATIONS/ROUTES/DOSAGE

Breast Cancer (Initial Endocrine-Based Therapy)
PO: ADULTS, ELDERLY: 125 mg once daily for 21 days, followed by a 7-day rest period to complete a 28-day cycle. Use in combination with an aromatase inhibitor (e.g., letrozole) once daily throughout 28-day cycle. For males, also consider treatment with leutinizing hormoneoreleasing hormone (LHRH) agonist. Continue until disease progression or unacceptable toxicity.

Breast Cancer (Disease Progression)
PO: ADULTS, ELDERLY: 125 mg once daily for 21 days, then 7 days off. Repeat q28 days (in combination with fulvestrant [and an LHRH agonist (e.g., goserelin) if pre- or perimenopausal]). Continue until disease progression or unacceptable toxicity.

Dose Reduction for Adverse Events

Dose Level	Dose
Recommended starting dose	125 mg/day
First dose reduction	100 mg/day
Second dose reduction	75 mg/day
Unable to tolerate 75 mg/ day	Permanently discontinue

Dose Modification
Based on Common Terminology Criteria for Adverse Events (CTCAE).

Hematologic Toxicities
Grade 1 or 2: No dose adjustment. **Grade 3 (except lymphopenia unless associated with clinical events [e.g., opportunistic infection]):** No dose adjustment. Withhold treatment until recovery to less than Grade 2. **Grade 3, ANC 500–1000 cells/mm³ plus fever that is greater than or equal to 38.5°C and/or active infection:** Interrupt treatment (and initiation of the next cycle) until recovery to Grade 2 or less. Resume at reduced dose upon starting.

Nonhematologic Toxicities
Grade 1 or 2: No dose adjustment. **Grade 3 or greater (if persistent despite optimal medical management):** Interrupt treatment until resolved to Grade 1 or less; Grade 2 or less if the event is not considered a serious medical risk. Resume at reduced dose upon starting.

P

Concomitant Use of Strong CYP3A4 Inhibitors

PO: ADULTS, ELDERLY: 75 mg once daily if unable to use alternative drug with minimal CYP3A4 inhibition. If CYP3A4 inhibitor is discontinued for 3–5 half-lives, increase palbociclib to the dose used prior to initiating strong CYP3A4 inhibitor.

Dosage in Renal Impairment

Mild to moderate impairment: No dose adjustment. **Severe impairment:** Not studied; use caution.

Dosage in Hepatic Impairment

Mild impairment: No dose adjustment. **Moderate to severe impairment:** Not studied; use caution.

SIDE EFFECTS

Frequent (41%–21%): Fatigue, nausea, alopecia, diarrhea. **Occasional (16%–13%):** Decreased appetite, vomiting, asthenia.

ADVERSE EFFECTS/TOXIC REACTIONS

Anemia, leukopenia, neutropenia, thrombocytopenia are expected responses to therapy. Grade 3 neutropenia reported in 57% of pts. The median onset of neutropenia was 15 days. Pulmonary embolism (5% of pts); upper respiratory tract infections including influenza, laryngitis, nasopharyngitis, pharyngitis, rhinitis, sinusitis (31% of pts); peripheral neuropathy (31% of pts); cheilitis, glossitis, glossodynia, mouth ulceration, stomatitis (25% of pts); epistaxis (11% of pts) were reported.

NURSING CONSIDERATIONS

BASELINE ASSESSMENT

Obtain ANC, CBC; pregnancy test in females of reproductive potential. Confirm estrogen receptor–positive, *HER2*-negative status. Screen for history of pulmonary embolism. Receive full medication history and screen for interactions. Assess hydration status. Screen for active infection. Offer emotional support.

INTERVENTION/EVALUATION

Monitor ANC, CBC at start of each cycle and on day 14 on the first two cycles. If any Grade 3 or 4 hematologic toxicity occurs, repeat CBC 7 days after interruption of therapy and at start of next cycle. If neutropenia occurs specifically, recommend treatment interruption, dose reduction, or delay in starting treatment for next cycle. Monitor for neurotoxicity (peripheral neuropathy), epistaxis. If chest pain, dyspnea, tachycardia occurs, provide supplemental O_2 and obtain radiologic testing to rule out pulmonary embolism.

PATIENT/FAMILY TEACHING

• Treatment may depress your immune system response and reduce your ability to fight infection. Report symptoms of infection such as body aches, chills, cough, fatigue, fever. Avoid those with active infection. • Report symptoms of bone marrow depression (e.g., bruising, fatigue, fever; shortness of breath, weight loss; bleeding easily, bloody urine or stool). • Immediately report chest pain, difficult breathing, fast heart rate, rapid breathing; may indicate life-threatening blood clot in the lungs. • Use effective contraception to avoid pregnancy. Do not breastfeed. • Drink plenty of fluids. • Do not ingest grapefruit products or herbal supplements.

---

paliperidone

pal-ee-**per**-i-done
(Invega, Invega Hafyera, Invega Sustenna, Invega Trinza)
Do not confuse Invega with Intuniv.

■ **BLACK BOX ALERT** ■ Elderly pts with dementia-related psychosis are at increased risk for mortality due to cerebrovascular events.

◆CLASSIFICATION

PHARMACOTHERAPEUTIC: Benzisoxazole derivative. **CLINICAL:** Second-generation (atypical) antipsychotic.

USES

Oral: Treatment of schizophrenia in adults and children 12 yrs and older. Treatment of schizoaffective disorder as monotherapy and as adjunct to mood stabilizers and/or antidepressants in adults. **Erzofri, Invega Sustenna:** Treatment of schizophrenia in adults. Treatment of schizoaffective disorder in adults as monotherapy and as adjunct to mood stabilizers or antidepressants. **Invega Trinza (3-month injection):** Treatment of schizophrenia in pts after adequate treatment with a 1-mo paliperidone extended-release injectable for at least 4 mos. **Invega Hafyera (6-month injection):** Treatment of schizophrenia in adults after adequate treatment with a 1 mo paliperidone extended-release injectable for at least 4 mos or a 3 mos paliperidone extended-release injectable for at least one 3 mos cycle. **OFF-LABEL:** Treatment of irritability associated with autistic disorder.

PRECAUTIONS

Contraindications: Sensitivity to paliperidone, risperiDONE. **Cautions:** History of cardiac arrhythmias, mild renal impairment (not recommended in moderate to severe impairment), HF, seizure disorder, predisposition to seizures, history of seizures, cardiovascular disease, pts at risk for QTc interval prolongation (congenital long QT syndrome, HF, medications that prolong QTc interval, hypokalemia, hypomagnesemia), pts at risk for aspiration pneumonia. May increase risk of stroke in pts with dementia-related psychosis. CNS depression, concomitant use of antihypertensives, hypovolemia or dehydration, high risk for suicide. Pts with breast cancer, other prolactin-dependent tumors; children, adolescents.

ACTION

May be a result of mixed central DOPamine and serotonin antagonism. **Therapeutic Effect:** Improves negative symptoms of psychosis; reduces incidence of extrapyramidal side effects.

PHARMACOKINETICS

Absorbed from GI tract. Metabolized in liver. Primarily excreted in urine. **Half-life:** 23 hrs.

⧗ LIFESPAN CONSIDERATIONS

Pregnancy/Lactation: Unknown if drug crosses placenta or is distributed in breast milk. **Children:** Safety and efficacy not established. **Elderly:** Potential for orthostatic hypotension. Age-related renal impairment may require dosage adjustment.

INTERACTIONS

DRUG: May decrease effects of **DOPamine agonists** (e.g., amantadine, pramipexole), **levodopa. Alcohol, CNS depressants** (e.g., **LORazepam, morphine, zolpidem**) may increase CNS depression. **Strong CYP3A4 inducers** (e.g., **carBAMazepine, phenytoin, rifAMPin**) may decrease concentration/effect. **QT interval–prolonging medications** (e.g., **amiodarone, azithromycin, ciprofloxacin, haloperidol, methadone, sotalol**) may increase risk of QTc interval prolongation. **HERBAL:** **St. John's wort** may decrease concentration/effect. **Herbals with sedative properties** (e.g., **chamomile, kava kava, valerian**) may increase CNS depression. **FOOD:** None known. **LAB VALUES:** May increase serum creatine phosphatase, uric acid, triglycerides, ALT, AST, prolactin. May decrease serum potassium, sodium, protein, glucose.

AVAILABILITY (Rx)

Injection Suspension: *(Invega Hafyera):* 1,092 mg/3.5 mL, 1,560 mg/5 mL. *(Erzofri, Invega Sustenna):* 39 mg/0.25 mL, 78 mg/0.5 mL, 117 mg/0.75 mL, 156 mg/mL, 234 mg/1.5 mL, 351 mg/2.25 mL. *(Invega Trinza):* 273 mg, 410 mg, 546 mg, 819 mg.

Tablets, Extended-Release: 1.5 mg, 3 mg, 6 mg, 9 mg

❧ Canadian trade name   ⧗ Non-Crushable Drug   **HIGH ALERT** High Alert drug

P

ADMINISTRATION/HANDLING

PO
• May give without regard to food.
• Do not crush, divide, or allow chewing.

IM
Monthly injection • Shake syringe for 10 sec to ensure homogenous suspension. Administer both initial injections (first injection on day 1 and the second injection 1 wk later) into deltoid muscle. • Monthly maintenance doses may be given in gluteal or deltoid muscle. **3-Month injection** • Shake syringe for 15 sec to ensure homogenous suspension. • Inject deep into deltoid or gluteal muscle. **6-Month injection** • Shake syringe for at least 15 sec to ensure homogenous suspension. • Inject deep into gluteal muscle.

INDICATIONS/ROUTES/DOSAGE

Schizophrenia
Note: Initial dose titration is not required. Increases should occur at intervals of more than 5 days.

PO: ADULTS, ELDERLY: Initially, 6 mg once daily. May increase dose in increments of 3 mg/day at intervals of more than 5 days. Range: 3–12 mg/day. **ADOLESCENTS 12–17 YRS WEIGHING 51 KG OR GREATER:** Initially, 3 mg/day. **Range:** 3–12 mg/day. **Maximum:** 12 mg/day. **LESS THAN 51 KG:** Initially, 3 mg/day. **Range:** 3–6 mg/day. **Maximum:** 6 mg/day.

IM: *(Erzofri):* ADULTS, ELDERLY: Initially, 351 mg, then 39–234 mg administered 4 wks after first injection. **Maximum:** 234 mg/mos. *(Invega Sustenna):* Note:* Overlap with oral antipsychotics is not necessary. **ADULTS, ELDERLY:** Initially, 234 mg on day 1 followed by 156 mg 1 wk later (second dose may be given 4 days before or after the wkly time point). **Maintenance:** 39–234 mg monthly starting 5 wks after initial dose (may adjust monthly based on response and tolerability). Monthly maintenance dose may be given 7 days before or after the monthly time point. *(Invega Trinza):* 273 mg to 819 mg q3mos (based on last dose of Invega Sustenna). Three-month IM used only after monthly IM dose established for at least 4 mos. The last 2 mos of monthly IM should be the same dosage strength before starting 3-mo injections. Adjustments can be made q3mos based on response and tolerability. *(Invega Hafyera):* FDA approved for schizophrenia only. 1,092–1,560 mg q6mos (based on Invega Sustenna for at least 4 mos or Invega Trinza for at least one 3 month cycle).

Schizoaffective Disorder
PO: ADULTS, ELDERLY: Initially, 6 mg once daily. May increase in increments of 3 mg/day at intervals of more than 4 days. **Range:** 3–12 mg/day. **Maximum:** 12 mg daily.

IM: *(Erzofri):* Initially, 351 mg, then 78–234 mg given 4 wks after first injection. **Maximum: 234 mg/mos. *(Invega Sustenna):* ADULTS, ELDERLY:** Initially, 234 mg on day 1, followed by 156 mg 1 wk later. **Maintenance:** 78–234 mg monthly, starting 5 wks after initial dose (may adjust monthly based on response and tolerability).

Dosage in Renal Impairment

Creatinine Clearance	Oral Dosage	IM Dosage
50–79 mL/min	Initially, 3 mg/d Maximum: 6 mg/d	Initially, 156 mg, then 117 mg 1 wk later, then 78 mg monthly
10–49 mL/min	Initially, 1.5 mg/d Maximum: 3 mg/d	Not recommended
Less than 10 mL/min	Not recommended	Not recommended

Dosage in Hepatic Impairment
No dose adjustment.

SIDE EFFECTS
Occasional (14%–4%): Tachycardia, headache, drowsiness, akathisia, anxiety, dizziness, dyspepsia, nausea.

ADVERSE EFFECTS/TOXIC REACTIONS
Neuroleptic malignant syndrome (NMS), hyperpyrexia, muscle rigidity, change

P

in mental status, unstable pulse or B/P, tachycardia, diaphoresis, cardiac arrhythmias, rhabdomyolysis, acute renal failure, tardive dyskinesia (protrusion of tongue, puffing of cheeks, chewing/puckering of mouth) may occur rarely. May prolong QT interval.

NURSING CONSIDERATIONS

BASELINE ASSESSMENT

Obtain renal function test. Assess behavior, appearance, emotional status, response to environment, speech pattern, thought content. Screen for comorbidities as listed in Precautions.

INTERVENTION/EVALUATION

Monitor B/P, heart rate, weight, renal function tests, ECG. Monitor for fine tongue movement (may be first sign of tardive dyskinesia). Supervise suicidal-risk pt closely during early therapy (as depression lessens, energy level improves, increasing suicide potential). Assess for therapeutic response (greater interest in surroundings, improved self-care, increased ability to concentrate, relaxed facial expression). Monitor for potential neuroleptic malignant syndrome (fever, muscle rigidity, unstable B/P or pulse, altered mental status).

PATIENT/FAMILY TEACHING

• Avoid tasks that may require alertness, motor skills until response to drug is established. • Use caution when changing position from lying or sitting to standing. • Report trembling in fingers, altered gait, unusual muscle/skeletal movements, palpitations, severe dizziness, fainting, swelling/pain in breasts, visual changes, rash, difficulty in breathing.

palonosetron

pal-oh-**noe**-se-tron
Do not confuse palonosetron with dolasetron, granisetron, or ondansetron.

FIXED-COMBINATION(S)

Akynzeo: palonosetron/netupitant (a substance P/neurokinin receptor antagonist): 0.5 mg/300 mg.

◆CLASSIFICATION

PHARMACOTHERAPEUTIC: Selective 5-HT$_3$ receptor antagonist. **CLINICAL:** Antiemetic.

USES

Prevention of acute and delayed nausea/vomiting associated with initial/repeated courses of moderately or highly emetogenic chemotherapy in adults, adolescents, children, infants 1 mo and older. Prevention of postop nausea/vomiting for up to 24 hrs following surgery in adults.

PRECAUTIONS

Contraindications: Hypersensitivity to palonosetron. **Cautions:** History of cardiovascular disease; pts at risk for QTc interval prolongation (congenital long QT syndrome, HF, medications that prolong QTc interval, hypokalemia, hypomagnesemia), pts at risk for ventricular arrhythmias.

ACTION

Antagonizes 5-HT$_3$ receptors, blocking serotonin on both peripheral and vagal nerve terminals in chemoreceptor trigger zone. **Therapeutic Effect:** Decreases episodes of nausea/vomiting associated with chemotherapy or postoperative recovery.

PHARMACOKINETICS

Protein binding: 52%. Metabolized in liver. Excreted in urine. **Half-life:** 40 hrs.

⏳ LIFESPAN CONSIDERATIONS

Pregnancy/Lactation: Unknown if distributed in breast milk. **Children:** Safety and efficacy not established in pts younger than 1 mo. **Elderly:** No age-related precautions noted.

INTERACTIONS

DRUG: SNRIs (e.g., DULoxetine, venlafaxine), SSRIs (e.g., citalopram,

P

FLUoxetine, sertraline), tricyclic antidepressants (e.g., amitriptyline, doxepin) may increase risk of serotonin syndrome. **HERBAL:** None significant. **FOOD:** None known. **LAB VALUES:** May transiently increase serum bilirubin, ALT, AST.

AVAILABILITY (Rx)

Injection Solution, Prefilled Syringe: 0.25 mg/5 mL.

ADMINISTRATION/HANDLING

 IV

Reconstitution • Give undiluted as IV push.
Rate of administration • Give IV push over 30 sec. Children: Infuse over 15 min. • Flush IV line with 0.9% NaCl before and following administration.
Storage • Store at room temperature. Solution should appear colorless, clear. Discard if cloudy precipitate forms.

INDICATIONS/ROUTES/DOSAGE

Chemotherapy-Induced Nausea/Vomiting
IV: ADULTS, ELDERLY: 0.25 mg as single dose 30 min before starting chemotherapy. **CHILDREN 1 MO TO YOUNGER THAN 17 YRS:** 20 mcg/kg as single dose 30 min before starting chemotherapy. **Maximum:** 1.5 mg.

Postop Nausea/Vomiting
IV: ADULTS, ELDERLY: 0.075 mg over 10 sec immediately before induction of anesthesia.

Dosage in Renal/Hepatic Impairment
No dose adjustment.

SIDE EFFECTS

Occasional (9%–5%): Headache, constipation. **Rare (less than 1%):** Diarrhea, dizziness, fatigue, abdominal pain, insomnia.

ADVERSE EFFECTS/TOXIC REACTIONS

Overdose may produce combination of CNS stimulation, depressant effects. May prolong QT interval. 5-HT$_3$ receptor antagonists are known to potentiate serotonin syndrome, esp. in pts taking serotonergic medications.

NURSING CONSIDERATIONS

BASELINE ASSESSMENT
Obtain BMP, serum magnesium in pts at risk for hypokalemia, hypomagnesemia, QT interval prolongation. Assess for signs of dehydration due to excessive vomiting (poor skin turgor, dry mucous membranes). Question history of cardiac disease, long QT syndrome, cardiac arrhythmias. Screen for concomitant home medications that prolong QT interval, increase risk of serotonin syndrome.

INTERVENTION/EVALUATION
Monitor BMP, serum magnesium; ECG in pts suspected of arrhythmia, QT interval prolongation. Monitor for nausea/vomiting. Assess for symptoms of serotonin syndrome (e.g., altered mental status, tachycardia, labile B/P, diaphoresis, hyperthermia, tremor, hyperreflexia, diarrhea, seizures). Monitor for hypersensitivity reaction.

PATIENT/FAMILY TEACHING
• Relief from nausea/vomiting generally occurs shortly after drug administration. • Report symptoms of serotonin overproduction such as confusion, excessive talking, fever, hallucinations, headache, hyperactivity, insomnia, racing thoughts, seizure activity, sexual dysfunction, tremors. • Report persistent vomiting. • Report palpitations, light-headedness, fainting; allergic reactions of any kind.

pamidronate

pam-id-roe-nate
Do not confuse pamidronate with alendronate, ibandronate, or risedronate.

◆CLASSIFICATION
PHARMACOTHERAPEUTIC: Bisphosphonate. **CLINICAL:** Hypocalcemic.

USES

Treatment of moderate to severe hypercalcemia associated with malignancy (with/without bone metastases). Treatment of moderate to severe Paget's disease. Treatment of osteolytic bone lesions of multiple myeloma or bone metastases of breast cancer. **OFF-LABEL:** Prevention of bone loss associated with androgen deprivation treatment in prostate cancer. Treatment of hyperparathyroidism.

PRECAUTIONS

Contraindications: Hypersensitivity to pamidronate, other bisphosphonates (e.g., risedronate, alendronate). **Cautions:** Baseline cytopenias, renal impairment, concurrent use with other nephrotoxic medications, history of thyroid surgery.

ACTION

Inhibits bone resorption, decreases mineralization by disrupting activity of osteoclasts. **Therapeutic Effect:** Lowers serum calcium concentration.

PHARMACOKINETICS

Route	Onset	Peak	Duration
IV	24–48 hrs	3–7 days	N/A

Rapidly absorbed by bone. Excreted in urine. Unknown if removed by hemodialysis. **Half-life:** 21–35 hrs.

⌛ LIFESPAN CONSIDERATIONS

Pregnancy/Lactation: Unknown if crosses placenta. Recommend discontinuation of drug as early as possible before a planned pregnancy. Unknown if fetal harm can occur. Unknown if distributed in breast milk. **Children:** Safety and efficacy not established. **Elderly:** May become overhydrated. Careful monitoring of fluid and electrolytes indicated; recommend dilution in smaller volume.

INTERACTIONS

DRUG: **NSAIDs (e.g., diclofenac, meloxicam, naproxen)** may increase adverse/toxic effects (e.g., increased risk of ulcer).

Proton pump inhibitors (e.g., omeprazole, pantoprazole) may decrease effect. **Aminoglycosides (e.g., gentamicin)** may increase risk of hypokalemia. **HERBAL:** None significant. **FOOD:** None known. **LAB VALUES:** None significant.

AVAILABILITY (Rx)

Injection, Powder for Reconstitution: 30 mg, 90 mg. **Injection Solution:** 3 mg/mL, 6 mg/mL, 9 mg/mL.

ADMINISTRATION/HANDLING

 IV

Reconstitution • Reconstitute each vial with 10 mL Sterile Water for Injection to provide concentration of 3 mg/mL or 9 mg/mL. • Allow drug to dissolve before withdrawing. • Dilute in 250–1,000 mL bag containing 0.45% or 0.9% NaCl or D₅W (1,000 mL for hypercalcemia of malignancy, 500 mL for Paget's disease, multiple myeloma, 250 mL for breast cancer).
Rate of administration • Adequate hydration is essential in conjunction with pamidronate therapy (avoid overhydration in pts with potential for HF). • Administer as IV infusion over 2–24 hrs for treatment of hypercalcemia; over 2 hrs for breast cancer; over 4 hrs for Paget's disease or multiple myeloma.
Storage • Store at room temperature. • Reconstituted vial is stable for 24 hrs if refrigerated; IV solution is stable for 24 hrs after dilution.

INDICATIONS/ROUTES/DOSAGE

Hypercalcemia of Malignancy

IV: ADULTS, ELDERLY: Moderate hypercalcemia (corrected serum calcium level 12–13.5 mg/dL): 60–90 mg as a single dose over 2–24 hrs. **Severe hypercalcemia (corrected serum calcium level greater than 13.5 mg/dL):** 90 mg as a single dose over 2–24 hrs.

Paget's Disease

IV: ADULTS, ELDERLY: 30 mg/day over 4 hrs for 3 consecutive days. May retreat if clinically indicated.

Osteolytic Bone Lesion (Multiple Myeloma)
IV: **ADULTS, ELDERLY:** 90 mg over 4 hrs once monthly.

Osteolytic Bone Metastases (Breast Cancer)
IV: **ADULTS, ELDERLY:** 90 mg over at least 2 hrs q3–4wks.

Dosage in Renal/Hepatic Impairment
Not recommended.

SIDE EFFECTS
Frequent (27%–18%): Temperature elevation (at least 1°C) 24–48 hrs after administration; erythema, swelling, induration, pain at catheter site in pts receiving 90 mg; anorexia, nausea, fatigue. **Occasional (10%–1%):** Constipation, rhinitis.

ADVERSE EFFECTS/TOXIC REACTIONS
Hypophosphatemia, hypokalemia, hypomagnesemia, hypocalcemia occur more frequently with higher dosages. Anemia, hypertension, tachycardia, atrial fibrillation, drowsiness occur more frequently with 90-mg doses. GI hemorrhage occurs rarely.

NURSING CONSIDERATIONS

BASELINE ASSESSMENT
Obtain CBC, serum calcium, ionized calcium, magnesium, phosphate; renal function test prior to therapy. Assess hydration status.

INTERVENTION/EVALUATION
Monitor serum calcium, ionized calcium, potassium, magnesium, creatinine, CBC. Provide adequate hydration; assess overhydration. Monitor I&O; assess lungs for crackles, dependent body parts for edema. Monitor B/P, temperature, pulse. Assess catheter site for redness, swelling, pain. Monitor food intake, daily pattern of bowel activity, stool consistency. Monitor for potential GI hemorrhage with 90-mg dosage.

PATIENT/FAMILY TEACHING
• Report symptoms of low blood calcium levels, including confusion, muscle twitching/cramps, numbness, seizures, tingling, jaw pain. • Immediately report GI bleeding.

panitumumab

pan-i-**toom**-ue-mab
(Vectibix)

■ **BLACK BOX ALERT** ■ 90% of pts experience dermatologic toxicities (dermatitis acneiform, pruritus, erythema, rash, skin exfoliation, skin fissures, abscess). Severe infusion reactions (anaphylaxis, bronchospasm, fever, chills, hypotension), fatal reactions have occurred.
Do not confuse panitumumab with daratumumab, necitumumab, ofatumumab.

◆CLASSIFICATION
PHARMACOTHERAPEUTIC: Epidermal growth factor receptor (EGFR) inhibitor, monoclonal antibody. **CLINICAL:** Antineoplastic.

USES
Treatment of wild-type RAS metastatic colorectal cancer either as first-line therapy in combination with FOLFOX or as monotherapy following disease progression after prior treatment with fluoropyrimidine-, oxaliplatin-, or irinotecan-based regimens.

PRECAUTIONS
Contraindications: Hypersensitivity to panitumumab. **Cautions:** Baseline electrolyte imbalance (esp. hypomagnesemia, hypokalemia), pulmonary disease, ocular disease, dehydration, skin disease (e.g., poorly healed wounds, skin fissures), elderly. Not indicated in pts with *RAS*-mutant metastatic colorectal cancer or for whom *RAS* mutation status is unknown.

P

ACTION

Binds specifically to epidermal growth factor receptor (EGFR) and competitively inhibits binding of epidermal growth factor. Blocks activation of intracellular tyrosine kinase. **Therapeutic Effect:** Inhibits tumor cell growth, survival, and proliferation.

PHARMACOKINETICS

Clearance varies by body weight, gender, tumor burden. **Half-life:** 3–10 days.

⧗ LIFESPAN CONSIDERATIONS

Pregnancy/Lactation: Avoid pregnancy; may cause fetal harm. Females of reproductive potential must use effective contraception during treatment and for at least 2 mos after discontinuation. Breastfeeding not recommended during treatment and for at least 2 mos after discontinuation. May impair fertility. **Children:** Safety and efficacy not established. **Elderly:** May have increased risk of adverse effects, severe diarrhea.

INTERACTIONS

DRUG: None significant. **HERBAL:** None significant. **FOOD:** None known. **LAB VALUES:** May decrease serum magnesium, calcium.

AVAILABILITY (Rx)

Injection Solution: 20 mg/mL vial (5-mL, 20-mL vials).

ADMINISTRATION/HANDLING

 IV

◄ALERT► Do not give by IV push or bolus. Use low protein-binding 0.2- or 0.22-micron in-line filter. Flush IV line before and after chemotherapy administration with 0.9% NaCl.

Reconstitution • Dilute in 100–150 mL 0.9% NaCl to provide concentration of 10 mg/mL or less. • Do not shake solution. Invert gently to mix. • Discard any unused portion.

Rate of administration • Infuse initial dose of 1,000 mg or less over 60 min.

If tolerated, give subsequent doses over 30 min. • Infuse doses greater than 1,000 mg over 90 min.

Storage • Refrigerate vials. • After dilution, solution may be stored for up to 6 hrs at room temperature, up to 24 hrs if refrigerated. • Discard if discolored, but solution may contain visible, translucent-to-white particulates (will be removed by in-line filter).

▦ IV INCOMPATIBILITIES

Do not mix with dextrose solutions or any other medications.

INDICATIONS/ROUTES/DOSAGE

◄ALERT► Stop infusion immediately in pts experiencing severe infusion reactions.

Metastatic Colorectal Cancer

IV infusion: ADULTS, ELDERLY: 6 mg/kg once q14 days as a single agent or in combination with FOLFOX (fluorouracil, leucovorin, and oxaliplatin). Continue until disease progression or unacceptable toxicity.

Dose Modification

Based on Common Terminology Criteria for Adverse Events (CTCAE).

Infusion Reactions

Mild to moderate reactions: Reduce infusion rate by 50% for remainder of infusion. **Severe reactions:** Discontinue infusion. Depending on severity, consider permanent discontinuation.

Skin Toxicity

For all Grade 3 skin toxicities, withhold treatment for 1–2 doses until improved to Grade 2 or less, then reduce dose as follows: **First occurrence of Grade 3:** Resume at same dose. **Second occurrence of Grade 3:** Reduce dose to 80% of initial dose. **Third occurrence of Grade 3:** Reduce dose to 60% of initial dose. **Fourth occurrence of Grade 3:** Permanently discontinue.

Dosage in Renal/Hepatic Impairment

No dose adjustment

 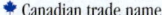

SIDE EFFECTS

Frequent (66%–17%): Erythema, pruritus, fatigue, nausea, rash, diarrhea, vomiting, dyspnea, pyrexia. **Occasional (15%–6%):** Cough, acne, dry skin, stomatitis, mucosal inflammation, growth of eyelashes.

ADVERSE EFFECTS/TOXIC REACTIONS

Dermatologic toxicities (acneiform dermatitis, erythema, paronychia, pruritus, rash, skin exfoliation, fissures) reported in 90% of pts. Fatal cutaneous or soft issue toxicities including abscesses, bullous mucocutaneous disease, necrotizing fasciitis, sepsis may occur. Sunlight/UV exposure may worsen dermatologic toxicities. May cause electrolyte depletion (hypomagnesemia, hypokalemia). Grade 3 or 4 infusion reactions (bronchospasm, chills, dyspnea, hypotension) reported in 4% of pts. Severe diarrhea may lead to dehydration, acute renal failure. Fatal interstitial lung disease (ILD), pneumonitis reported in 1% of pts. Ocular toxicities (keratitis, ulcerative keratitis, corneal perforation) may occur. Increased mortality/toxicity was reported when therapy used in combination with bevacizumab and chemotherapy.

NURSING CONSIDERATIONS

BASELINE ASSESSMENT

Obtain serum magnesium, potassium; pregnancy test in females of reproductive potential. Screen for active infection. Question history of pulmonary/ocular/skin disease. Conduct dermatologic exam. Review occurrence of prior infusion reactions prior to each dose. Assess usual bowel movement patterns, stool characteristics. Assess and correct hydration status. Offer emotional support. Assess *KRAS* mutational status in colorectal tumors and confirm the absence of a *RAS* mutation.

INTERVENTION/EVALUATION

Monitor serum magnesium, potassium periodically and for 8 wks after discontinuation. Monitor serum electrolytes if severe diarrhea occurs. Replete electrolytes as clinically indicated. Consider ABG, radiologic test if ILD/pneumonitis (excessive cough, dyspnea, fever, hypoxia) is suspected. Monitor daily pattern of bowel activity, stool consistency. Diarrhea must be treated promptly to reduce occurrence of severe dehydration, acute renal failure. Diligently assess for ocular toxicities (redness, pain of eye; dry eye, change of vision); skin for cutaneous and soft tissue toxicities.

PATIENT/FAMILY TEACHING

• Severe infusion reaction may occur; report chills, difficulty breathing, dizziness, fever. • Diarrhea may cause dehydration, electrolyte imbalance, low blood pressure, kidney injury, and may be life-threatening. Drink plenty of fluids. Report diarrhea or dehydration that does not improve with medical management. • Report toxic skin reactions (abscess, itching, peeling, rash, redness, sloughing, swelling); kidney problems (decreased urine output, flank pain, darkened urine), symptoms of lung inflammation (excessive coughing, difficulty breathing, chest pain); eye problems (redness, pain of eye; dry eye, change of vision). • Limit sunlight, UV exposure. Wear protective sunscreen, hats, clothing when outdoors. • Use effective contraception to avoid pregnancy. Do not breastfeed.

pantoprazole
TOP 100

pan-**toe**-pra-zole
(<u>Protonix</u>, Tecta)
Do not confuse pantoprazole with ARIPiprazole.

◆CLASSIFICATION

PHARMACOTHERAPEUTIC: Benzimidazole. **CLINICAL:** Proton pump inhibitor.

USES

Gastroesophageal reflux disease (GERD): Short-term treatment (up to 8 wks) of healing and symptomatic relief of erosive esophagitis (EE) in adults and children 5 yrs and older. Maintenance of healing of EE and reduction of relapse rates of heartburn symptoms in adults. **Hypersecretory conditions:** Long-term treatment of pathological hypersecretory conditions, including Zollinger-Ellison (ZE) syndrome in adults. **OFF-LABEL:** Barrett's esophagus, dyspepsia, eosinophillic esophagitis, *H. pylori* eradication, NSAID-induced ulcers, peptic ulcer disease, stress ulcer prophylaxis.

PRECAUTIONS

Contraindications: Hypersensitivity to pantoprazole, other proton pump inhibitors (e.g., lansoprazole, omeprazole). In combination with rilpivirine-containing products. **Cautions:** May increase risk of fractures, GI infections.

ACTION

Irreversibly binds to, inhibits hydrogen-potassium adenosine triphosphate, an enzyme on surface of gastric parietal cells. Inhibits hydrogen ion transport into gastric lumen. **Therapeutic Effect:** Increases gastric pH, reduces gastric acid production.

PHARMACOKINETICS

Route	Onset	Peak	Duration
PO	N/A	N/A	24 hrs

Primarily distributed into gastric parietal cells. Metabolized in liver. Protein binding: 98%. Primarily excreted in urine. Not removed by hemodialysis. **Half-life:** 1 hr.

⧖ LIFESPAN CONSIDERATIONS

Pregnancy/Lactation: Unknown if drug crosses placenta or is distributed in breast milk. **Children:** Safety and efficacy not established in pts younger than 5 yrs. **Elderly:** No age-related precautions noted.

INTERACTIONS

DRUG: May decrease concentration/effects of **acalabrutinib, cefuroxime, erlotinib, neratinib, pazopanib.**

Strong CYP2C19 inducers (e.g., FLUoxetine), strong CYP3A4 inducers (e.g., carBAMazepine, phenytoin, rifAMPin) may decrease concentration/effect. **HERBAL:** None significant. **FOOD:** None known. **LAB VALUES:** May increase serum creatinine, cholesterol, uric acid, glucose, lipoprotein, ALT.

AVAILABILITY (Rx)

Granules for Suspension: 40 mg/packet.
Injection, Powder for Reconstitution: 40 mg.

 Tablets, Delayed-Release: 20 mg, 40 mg.

ADMINISTRATION/HANDLING

IV

Reconstitution • Mix 40-mg vial with 10 mL 0.9% NaCl injection. • May be further diluted with 100 mL D₅W, 0.9% NaCl.
Rate of administration • Infuse 10 mL solution over at least 2 min. • Infuse 100 mL solution over at least 15 min. or as continuous infusion. • Flush IV line after administration.
Storage • Store vials at room temperature. • Once diluted with 10 mL 0.9% NaCl, stable for 6 hrs at room temperature; when further diluted with 100 mL, stable for 24 hrs at room temperature.

PO

Tablet • Preferably given before meals (can be given without regard to food). • Administer whole (do not split, cut, or allow chewing). • Administer oral suspension only in apple juice or applesauce. Best taken 30 min before a meal.

▦ IV COMPATIBILITIES

Insulin, norepinephrine, potassium chloride.

INDICATIONS/ROUTES/DOSAGE

Erosive Esophagitis (Treatment)
PO: ADULTS, ELDERLY: 40 mg/day for up to 8 wks. If not healed after 8 wks, may continue an additional 8 wks. **CHILDREN 5 YRS AND OLDER (WEIGHING 40 KG OR MORE):** 40

mg/day for up to 8 wks. **(WEIGHING 15–39 KG):** 20 mg/day for up to 8 wks.

IV: ADULTS, ELDERLY: 40 mg/day for 7–10 days.

Maintenance of Healing of Erosive Esophagitis

PO: ADULTS, ELDERLY: 40 mg once daily.

Hypersecretory Conditions

PO: ADULTS, ELDERLY: Initially, 80 mg twice daily. May titrate upward early in therapy. **Maintenance:** 40–200 mg/day. **Maximum:** 240 mg/day (as either 80 mg three times daily or 120 mg twice daily).

IV: ADULTS, ELDERLY: 80 mg twice daily. May increase to 80 mg q8h.

Prevention of Rebleeding in Peptic Ulcer Bleed (Unlabeled)

IV: ADULTS, ELDERLY: 80 mg followed by 8 mg/hr infusion for 72 hrs or 80 mg then 40 mg q12h for 72 hrs.

Dosage in Renal/Hepatic Impairment
No dose adjustment.

SIDE EFFECTS

Rare (less than 2%): Diarrhea, headache, dizziness, pruritus, rash.

ADVERSE EFFECTS/TOXIC REACTIONS

Symptomatic response to treatment does not preclude the presence of gastric malignancy. May increase risk of *C. difficile*–associated diarrhea; bone fractures of the hip, wrist, or spine. Hypersensitivty reactions, including anaphylaxis, were reported. Chronic use may cause atrophic gastritis, malabsorption of vitamin B12. May cause electrolyte abnormalities, including hypomagnesemia, which may lead to hypocalcemia, hypokalemia. IV injection may cause thrombophlebitis, abscess. IV form contains edate disodium, a metal ion chelator. Pts with zinc deficiency may require zinc supplementation. Due to risk of vial breakage, use of spiked system adapters is not recommended.

NURSING CONSIDERATIONS

BASELINE ASSESSMENT

Consider obtaining serum magnesium, calcium level periodically, esp. in pts at risk for hypocalcemia (hypomagnesemia, hypoparathyroidism, renal failure, vitamin D deficiency) or in pts receiving chronic therapy. Question history of pathological fractures, osteoporosis, osteopenia. Receive full medication history and screen for interactions/contraindications. Review diagnostic test results of esophagogastroduodenoscopy (EGD), biopsies, *H. Pylori* infection. Assess baseline symptoms of esophagitis, GERD, *H. Pylori* infection.

INTERVENTION/EVALUATION

Obtain serum magnesium as clinically indicated. Consider treatment with supplemental magnesium and/or calcium as needed. Monitor for hypomagnesemia (cardiac arrhythmias, muscle spasm, myalgia, paresthesia, QT interval abnormalities, seizures). Observe daily pattern of bowel activity, stool consistency (increased severity may indicate *C. difficile* infection). If frequent diarrhea occurs, obtain *C. difficile* toxin screen and initiate isolation precautions until test result is confirmed; manage hydration, electrolyte levels, protein intake. Evaluate for therapeutic response (relief of GI symptoms).

PATIENT/FAMILY TEACHING

• It is essential to complete drug therapy despite improvement of symptoms. Early discontinuation and noncompliance may cause return of esophagitis, GERD, *H. Pylori* infection, and associated symptoms. • Frequent, loose, foul-smelling stools; fever, abdominal discomfort, urgency may indicate infectious diarrhea that may be contagious to others. • Report symptoms of bone fractures (pain, deformity, changes in mobility). • Therapy may cause low levels of calcium, magnesium, vitamin B12 in the blood.

Report difficulty swallowing, fatigue, muscle cramps, muscle weakness, palpations, numbness, tingling, tremors. • There is a risk of interactions with other medications. Do not take newly prescribed medications unless approved by prescriber who originally started treatment.

PARoxetine

par-**ox**-e-teen
(Brisdelle, Paxil, Paxil CR, Pexeva)
■ **BLACK BOX ALERT** ■ Increased risk of suicidal thinking and behavior in children, adolescents, young adults 18–24 yrs with major depressive disorder, other psychiatric disorders.
Do not confuse PARoxetine with DULoxetine, FLUoxetine, piroxicam, pyridoxine, or vortioxetine, or Paxil with Doxil, Plavix, PROzac, or Taxol.

◆CLASSIFICATION

PHARMACOTHERAPEUTIC: Selective serotonin reuptake inhibitor (SSRI). **CLINICAL:** Antidepressant.

USES

Treatment of major depressive disorder (unipolar) (MDD). Treatment of panic disorder with or without agoraphobia, obsessive-compulsive disorder (OCD). Treatment of social anxiety disorder (SAD), generalized anxiety disorder (GAD), premenstrual dysphoric disorder (PMDD), posttraumatic stress disorder (PTSD). **Capsule:** Treatment of moderate to severe vasomotor symptoms associated with menopause. **OFF-LABEL:** Body dysmorphic disorder, self-injurious behavior.

PRECAUTIONS

Contraindications: Hypersensitivity to PARoxetine. Concurrent use of MAOIs with or within 14 days of MAOIs intended to treat psychiatric disorders, initiation in pts treated with linezolid or methylene blue; concomitant use with thioridazine, pimozide. **Capsule:** Pregnancy. **Cautions:** History of suicidal ideation and behavior; seizure disorder, hepatic/renal impairment, elderly, narrow-angle glaucoma, alcohol use. Avoid use in first trimester of pregnancy, alcohol use.

ACTION

Selectively blocks uptake of neurotransmitter serotonin at CNS neuronal presynaptic membranes, increasing its availability at postsynaptic receptor sites. **Therapeutic Effect:** Relieves depression, reduces obsessive-compulsive behavior, decreases anxiety.

PHARMACOKINETICS

Widely distributed. Metabolized in liver. Protein binding: 95%. Excreted in urine. Not removed by hemodialysis. **Half-life:** 24 hrs.

⬛ LIFESPAN CONSIDERATIONS

Pregnancy/Lactation: May impair reproductive function. Not distributed in breast milk. May increase risk of congenital malformations. **Children:** Safety and efficacy not established. **Elderly:** Age-related renal impairment may require dosage adjustment. Use caution.

INTERACTIONS

DRUG: Alcohol may increase adverse effects. **MAOIs (e.g., phenelzine, selegiline)** may increase the serotonergic effect. May increase concentration/effect of **NSAIDs (e.g., diclofenac, meloxicam, naproxen).** May decrease concentration/effect of **tamoxifen.** May increase adverse effects of **tricyclic antidepressants (e.g., amitriptyline). HERBAL: Glucosamine, herbals with anticoagulant/antiplatelet properties (e.g., garlic, ginger, ginkgo biloba)** may increase effect. **St. John's wort** may decrease concentra-

P

tion/effect. **FOOD:** None known. **LAB VALUES:** May decrease Hgb, Hct, WBC count.

AVAILABILITY (Rx)

Capsules: 7.5 mg. **Oral Suspension:** 10 mg/5 mL. **Tablets:** 10 mg, 20 mg, 30 mg, 40 mg.

Tablets, Controlled-Release: 12.5 mg, 25 mg, 37.5 mg.

ADMINISTRATION/HANDLING

PO

• Give without regard to food preferably in the morning (when used for vasomotor symptoms of menopause, give at bedtime). • Give with food, milk if GI distress occurs. • Do not crush, break, or allow chewing of controlled-release or immediate-release tablets.

INDICATIONS/ROUTES/DOSAGE

Depression
PO: *(Immediate-Release):* ADULTS: Initially, 10–20 mg/day. May increase by 10–20 mg/day at intervals of more than 1 wk. **Maximum:** 50 mg/day.
PO: *(Controlled-Release):* ADULTS: Initially, 25 mg/day. May increase by 12.5 mg/day at intervals of more than 1 wk. **Maximum:** 62.5 mg/day.

Generalized Anxiety Disorder (GAD)
PO: *(Immediate-Release):* ADULTS: Initially, 10 mg/day. May increase by 10 mg/day at intervals of more than 1 wk. **Range:** 20–50 mg/day.

Obsessive-Compulsive Disorder (OCD)
PO: *(Immediate-Release):* ADULTS: Initially, 20 mg/day. May increase by 10 mg/day at intervals of more than 1 wk. **Recommended dose:** 40–60 mg/day.

Panic Disorder
PO: *(Immediate-Release):* ADULTS: Initially, 10 mg/day. May increase by 10 mg/day at intervals of more than 1 wk. **Usual dose:** 20–40 mg/day. **Maximum:** 60 mg/day.
PO: *(Controlled-Release):* ADULTS, ELDERLY: Initially, 12.5 mg once daily. May increase by 12.5 mg/day at wkly intervals. **Maximum:** 75 mg/day.

Social Anxiety Disorder (SAD)
PO: *(Immediate-Release):* ADULTS: Initially, 10 mg/day. May increase by 10 mg/day at intervals of more than 1 wk. **Maximum:** 60 mg/day.
PO: *(Controlled-Release):* ADULTS, ELDERLY: Initially, 12.5 mg once daily. May increase by 12.5 mg/day at wkly intervals. **Maximum:** 37.5 mg/day.

Posttraumatic Stress Disorder (PTSD)
PO: *(Immediate-Release):* ADULTS: Initially, 20 mg/day. May increase by 10–20 mg/day at intervals of more than 1 wk. **Maximum:** 60 mg/day.

Premenstrual Dysphoric Disorder (PMDD)
PO: *(Controlled-Release):* ADULTS: Initially, 12.5 mg/day. May increase by 12.5 mg at wkly intervals. **Maximum:** 50 mg/day.

Vasomotor Symptoms
PO: ADULTS: *(Capsule):* 7.5 mg once daily at bedtime.

Usual Elderly Dosage
PO: Initially, 10 mg/day. May increase by 10 mg/day at intervals of more than 1 wk. **Maximum:** 40 mg/day.
PO: *(Controlled-Release):* Initially, 12.5 mg/day. May increase by 12.5 mg/day at intervals of more than 1 wk. **Maximum:** 50 mg/day (37.5 mg for SAD).

Dosage Renal/Hepatic Impairment
CrCl less than 30 mL/min, severe hepatic impairment: *(Immediate-Release):* Initially, 10 mg/day. May increase by 10 mg/dose at wkly intervals. **Maximum:** 40 mg/day. *(Extended-Release):* Initially, 12.5 mg/day. May increase by 12.5 mg/day at wkly intervals. **Maximum:** 50 mg/day. *(Brisdelle):* No dosage adjustment.

SIDE EFFECTS

Frequent (26%–8%): Nausea, drowsiness, headache, dry mouth, asthenia, constipation, dizziness, insomnia, diarrhea, diaphoresis, tremor. **Occasional (6%–3%):** Decreased appetite, respiratory disturbance (e.g., increased cough), anxiety, flatulence, paresthesia, yawning, decreased libido, sexual dysfunction, abdominal discomfort. **Rare:** Palpitations, vomiting, blurred vision, altered taste, confusion.

ADVERSE EFFECTS/TOXIC REACTIONS

Hyponatremia, seizures have been reported. Serotonin syndrome (agitation, confusion, diaphoresis, hallucinations, hyperreflexia) occurs rarely.

NURSING CONSIDERATIONS

BASELINE ASSESSMENT

Obtain LFT. Assess appearance, behavior, speech pattern, level of interest, mood. Question history of suicidal ideation and behavior.

INTERVENTION/EVALUATION

For pts on long-term therapy, CBC, LFT, renal function test should be performed periodically. Assess mental status for depression, suicidal ideation (esp. at beginning of therapy or change in dosage), anxiety, social functioning, panic attacks. Assess appearance, behavior, speech pattern, level of interest, mood.

PATIENT/FAMILY TEACHING

• Avoid alcohol, St. John's wort. • Therapeutic effect may take up to 4 wks. • Do not abruptly discontinue medication. • Avoid tasks that require alertness, motor skills until response to drug is established. • Seek immediate medical attention if thoughts of suicide, new onset or worsening of anxiety, depression, or changes in mood occur.

PAZOPanib

paz-**oh**-pa-nib
(Votrient)

■ **BLACK BOX ALERT** ■ Severe, fatal hepatotoxicity has been observed.

Do not confuse PAZOPanib with nintedanib, pegaptanib, tivozanib, or vandetanib.

CLASSIFICATION

PHARMACOTHERAPEUTIC: Vascular endothelial growth factor (VEGF) inhibitor. Tyrosine kinase inhibitor. **CLINICAL:** Antineoplastic.

USES

Treatment of advanced renal cell carcinoma (RCC), advanced soft-tissue sarcoma (STS) (in pts previously treated with chemotherapy). **OFF-LABEL:** Treatment of advanced thyroid cancer, desmoid tumors (progressive).

PRECAUTIONS

Contraindications: Hypersensitivity to PAZOPanib. **Cautions:** Baseline cytopenias, hepatic impairment, hypertension, cardiac disease (cardiomyopathy, HF), pulmonary disease, hypothyroidism, ocular disease, poorly healed wound, conditions predisposing to infection (e.g., diabetes, immunocompromised pts, renal failure, open wounds); history of thromboembolic events (CVA, DVT, MI, pulmonary embolism (PE). Pts at risk for GI perforation (e.g., Crohn's disease, diverticulitis, GI tract malignancies, peptic ulcers, peritoneal malignancies), tumor lysis syndrome (high tumor burden, dehydration), QTc interval prolongation, cardiac arrhythmias (congenital long QT syndrome, HF, QT interval–prolonging medications, hypokalemia, hypomagnesemia), bleeding (e.g., history of intracranial/GI/GU bleeding, coagulation disorders, recent trauma; concomitant use of anticoagulants, NSAIDs, antiplatelets). Do not initiate in pts with uncontrolled hypertension. Avoid use concomitant use of strong CYP3A4 inhibitors or inducers, gastric acid–reducing agents, QT interval–prolonging medications.

ACTION

Inhibits cell surface vascular endothelial growth factor receptors (VEGFR), platelet-derived growth factor receptors (PDGFR), fibroblast growth factor receptor (FGFR), cytokine receptor (cKIT), interleukin-2 receptor inducible T-cell kinase, lymphocyte-specific protein tyrosine kinase, and transmembrane glycoprotein receptor tyrosine kinase. **Therapeutic Effect:** Inhibits angiogenesis, blocks tumor growth.

PHARMACOKINETICS

Widely distributed. Metabolized in liver. Protein binding: greater than 99%. Peak plasma concentration: 2–4 hrs. Excreted primarily in feces, urine (4%). **Half-life:** 31 hrs.

⧗ LIFESPAN CONSIDERATIONS

Pregnancy/Lactation: Avoid pregnancy; may cause fetal harm. Females and males with female partners of reproductive potential must use effective contraception during treatment and for at least 2 wks after discontinuation. Breastfeeding not recommended during treatment and for at least 2 wks after discontinuation. May impair fertility in both female and males. **Children:** Safety and efficacy not established. **Elderly:** May have increased risk of adverse effects.

INTERACTIONS

DRUG: Antacids, H$_2$ antagonists (e.g., famotidine, raNITIdine), proton pump inhibitors (e.g., omeprazole, pantoprazole) may decrease concentration/effect. QT interval–prolonging medications (e.g., amiodarone, azithromycin, ciprofloxacin, haloperidol, methadone, sotalol) may increase risk of QTc interval prolongation. Strong CYP3A4 inhibitors (e.g., clarithromycin, ketoconazole, ritonavir) may increase concentration/effect. Strong CYP3A4 inducers (e.g., carBAMazepine, phenytoin, rifAMPin) may decrease concentration/effect. May decrease the therapeutic effect; increase adverse effects of **vaccines (live)**. **HERBAL:** Echinacea may decrease therapeutic effect. **FOOD:** Food may increase absorption/concentration. **Grapefruit products** may increase concentration/effect. **LAB VALUES:** May increase serum ALT, AST, bilirubin. May decrease serum magnesium, phosphate, potassium, sodium; leukocytes, lymphocytes, neutrophils, platelets. May increase or decrease serum glucose.

AVAILABILITY (Rx)

🖫 **Tablets:** 200 mg.

ADMINISTRATION/HANDLING

PO
• Give at least 1 hr before or 2 hrs after ingestion of food. • Give tablets whole; do not break, crush, dissolve, or divide.

INDICATIONS/ROUTES/DOSAGE

Renal Cell Carcinoma, Soft-Tissue Sarcoma
PO: **ADULTS, ELDERLY:** 800 mg once daily. Continue until disease progression or unacceptable toxicity.

Dose Reduction Schedule
Renal Cell Carcinoma
First reduction: 400 mg once daily. **Second reduction:** 200 mg once daily.

Soft Tissue Carcinoma
First reduction: 600 mg once daily. **Second reduction:** 400 mg once daily.

Dose Modification
Based on Common Terminology for Adverse Events.

Cardiac Toxicity
Symptomatic or Grade 3 left ventricular systolic dysfunction: Withhold treatment until improved to less than Grade 3, then resume if benefit outweighs risk. **Grade 4:** Permanently discontinue.

GI Fistula
Grade 2 or 3 GI fistula: Withhold treatment until improved, then resume if benefit outweighs risk. **Grade 4 GI fistula:** Permanently discontinue.

Hemorrhagic Events
Grade 2 hemorrhage: Withhold treatment until improved to Grade 1 or 0, then resume at reduced dose. **Grade 3 or 4**

P

hemorrhage; recurrence of Grade 2 hemorrhage: Permanently discontinue.

Hepatotoxicity
Serum ALT 3–8 times upper limit of normal ULN: Continue same dose and monitor LFT wkly until improved to Grade 1 or baseline. **Serum ALT greater than 8 times ULN:** Withhold treatment until improved to Grade 1 or baseline, then resume at no more than 400 mg daily if benefit outweighs risk. Continue to monitor LFT wkly for 8 wks. **Serum ALT greater than 3 times ULN with serum bilirubin greater than 2 times ULN; recurrence of serum ALT greater than 3 times ULN despite dose reduction:** Permanently discontinue.

Hypertension
Grade 2 or 3: Reduce dose and start antihypertensive therapy. Permanently discontinue if Grade 3 hypertension persists despite dose reduction and antihypertensive therapy. **Grade 4:** Permanently discontinue.

Proteinuria
24-hr urine protein 3 grams or greater: Withhold treatment until improved to Grade 1 or 0, then resume at reduced dose. Permanently discontinue if 24-hr urine protein does not improve or recurs. **Confirmed nephrotic syndrome:** Permanently discontinue.

Venous Thrombosis
Grade 3 venous thrombosis: Withhold treatment and manage for at least 1 wk, then resume at same dose. **Grade 4 venous thrombosis:** Permanently discontinue.

Other Events Requiring Permanent Discontinuation
Permanently discontinue if arterial thrombosis, thrombotic microangiopathy, GI perforation, ILD/pneumonitis, posterior reversible encephalopathy syndrome occur.

Concomitant Use of Strong CYP3A4 Inhibitors, Gastric Acid Reducers
If strong CYP3A4 inhibitor cannot be discontinued, reduced PAZOPanib dose to 400 mg. If gastric acid–reducing agents cannot be discontinued, consider short-acting antacid instead of proton pump inhibitor, H$_2$-receptor antagonist.

Dosage in Renal Impairment
No dose adjustment.

Dosage in Hepatic Impairment
Mild impairment: No dose adjustment. **Moderate impairment:** Reduce dose to 200 mg/day. **Severe impairment:** Not recommended.

SIDE EFFECTS
Note: Frequency and occurrence of side effects may vary depending on indicated treatment.
Frequent (69%–20%): Fatigue, diarrhea, nausea, decreased weight, hypertension, decreased appetite, change of hair color, vomiting, tumor pain, dysgeusia, headache, musculoskeletal pain, myalgia, abdominal pain, dyspnea. **Occasional (18%–5%):** Rash, cough, edema, mucositis, alopecia, dizziness, skin disorder, skin hypopigmentation, stomatitis, chest pain, insomnia, dysphonia, dyspepsia, dry skin, chills, vision blurred, nail disorder.

ADVERSE EFFECTS/TOXIC REACTIONS
Fatal hepatotoxicity may occur. Cardiac toxicities including QT interval prolongation, torsades de pointes; cardiac dysfunction (decreased left ventricular ejection fraction, HF) were reported. Fatal hemorrhagic events including epistaxis (8% of pts), mouth hemorrhage (3% of pts), rectal hemorrhage (2% of pts), Grade 4 hemorrhage (intracranial/subarachnoid/peritoneal hemorrhage), hemoptysis may occur. Fatal thromboembolism including CVA, DVT, MI, pulmonary embolism, transient ischemic attack was reported. Thrombotic microangiopathy including thrombotic thrombocytopenic purpura (TTP), hemolytic uremic syndrome reported in 1%–5% of pts. GI perforation or fistula reported in 1% of pts. Fatal interstitial lung disease (ILD), pneumonitis reported in less than 1% of

pts. Posterior reversible encephalopathy syndrome, a dysfunction of the brain that may evolve into an ischemic CVA or cerebral hemorrhage, may occur. Grade 3 hypertension reported in 1%–3% of pts. May impair healing of wounds. Tumor lysis syndrome may present as acute renal failure, hypocalcemia, hyperuricemia, hyperphosphatemia. Vascular disorders including arterial aneurysm, dissection, rupture may occur. Other reactions may include retinal changes/detachment, hypothyroidism, pancreatitis, pneumothorax, nephrotic syndrome.

NURSING CONSIDERATIONS

BASELINE ASSESSMENT

Obtain CBC, LFT; ECG; pregnancy test in females of reproductive potential. Confirm compliance of effective contraception. Assess LVEF by echocardiogram in pts with cardiomyopathy. Screen for active infection. Assess risk for bleeding. Assess usual bowel movement patterns, stool characteristics. Receive full medication history and screen for interactions. Assess skin for open wounds, surgical incisions. Assess adequate hydration prior to initiation due to increased risk of tumor lysis syndrome, diarrhea, vomiting. Question history as listed in Precautions. Offer emotional support.

INTERVENTION/EVALUATION

Monitor CBC for myelosuppression; LFT for hepatotoxicity; ECG for QT interval prolongation; urine protein level. Monitor for symptoms of hepatotoxicity (abdominal pain, jaundice, nausea, vomiting, weight loss) esp. in pts with hepatic impairment. Monitor B/P for hypertension. Consider ABG, radiologic test if ILD/pneumonitis (excessive cough, dyspnea, fever, hypoxia) is suspected. Consider treatment with corticosteroids if ILD/pneumonitis is confirmed. Assess LVEF by echocardiogram periodically if cardiomyopathy (dyspnea, extremity swelling, palpitations) is suspected. Monitor for infections (body aches, cough, fatigue, fever). Monitor daily pattern of bowel activity, stool consistency.

Ensure adequate hydration/nutrition. Monitor for ocular toxicities; symptoms of DVT (leg or arm pain/swelling); CVA, intracranial hemorrhage (aphasia, altered mental status, facial droop, hemiplegia, vision loss); MI (chest pain, diaphoresis, left arm/jaw pain, increased serum troponin, ST segment elevation), PE (chest pain, dyspnea, tachycardia). Bleeding of any kind can be life-threatening and must be treated immediately. Monitor serum uric acid level if tumor lysis syndrome (acute renal failure, electrolyte imbalance, cardiac arrhythmias, seizures) is suspected. Conduct neurological assessment. Pts with altered mental status, seizures, visual disturbances, unilateral weakness should be evaluated for posterior reversible encephalopathy syndrome. Assess for skin toxicities, poorly healed wounds.

PATIENT/FAMILY TEACHING

• Treatment may depress your immune system response and reduce your ability to fight infection. Report symptoms of infection such as body aches, chills, cough, fatigue, fever. Avoid those with active infection. • Report symptoms of bone marrow depression (e.g., bruising, fatigue, fever, shortness of breath, weight loss; bleeding easily, bloody urine or stool). • Report symptoms of lung inflammation (excessive coughing, difficulty breathing, chest pain); liver problems (abdominal pain, bruising, clay-colored stool, amber- or dark-colored urine, yellowing of the skin or eyes), eye problems (eye pain, change of vision), toxic skin reactions (rash, redness, sloughing, swelling). • Life-threatening blood clots may occur; report symptoms of DVT (swelling, pain, hot feeling in the arms or legs; discoloration of extremity), lung embolism (difficulty breathing, chest pain, rapid heart rate), stroke (confusion, one-sided weakness or paralysis, difficulty speaking), heart attack (chest pain, difficulty breathing, jaw pain, nausea, pain that radiates to the arm or jaw, sweating). • Life-threatening tumor lysis syndrome (a condition caused by the rapid breakdown of cancer cells), which can cause kidney failure, may occur. Report decreased urination, amber-colored urine;

confusion, difficulty breathing, fatigue, fever, muscle or joint pain, palpitations, seizures, vomiting. • Bleeding of any kind can be life-threatening. • Use effective contraception to avoid pregnancy. Do not breastfeed. • Drink plenty of fluids. • Do not take newly prescribed medications unless approved by prescriber who originally started treatment. • Treatment may affect the heart's ability to pump blood or alter the electrical conduction of the heart; report chest pain, difficulty breathing, dizziness, swelling of extremities, fainting, palpitations. • Take on empty stomach. • Treatment may worsen high blood pressure. • Immediately report severe or persistent abdominal pain, bloody stool, fever, vomiting blood; may indicate rupture in GI tract.

pegfilgrastim $\frac{TOP}{100}$

peg-fil-**gras**-tim
(Fulphila, Neulasta, Neulasta Onpro, Nyvepria, Udenyca, Udenyca Onbody, Stimufend, Ziextenzo)
Do not confuse Neulasta with Lunesta, Neumega, or Neupogen, or pegfilgrastim with filgrastim.

◆CLASSIFICATION

PHARMACOTHERAPEUTIC: Colony-stimulating factor. **CLINICAL:** Hematopoietic agent.

USES

Decreases incidence of infection (as manifested by febrile neutropenia) in pts with nonmyeloid malignancies receiving myelosuppressive chemotherapy associated with febrile neutropenia. To increase survival in pts acutely exposed to myelosuppressive doses of radiation.

PRECAUTIONS

Contraindications: Hypersensitivity to pegfilgrastim, filgrastim. **Cautions:** Any malignancy with myeloid characteristics, sickle cell disease. The 6-mg fixed dose should not be used in infants, children, or adolescents weighing less than

45 kg. Do not administer within 14 days before and 24 hrs after cytotoxic chemotherapy.

ACTION

Stimulates production, maturation, and activation of neutrophils within bone marrow. **Therapeutic Effect:** Increases phagocytic ability, antibody-dependent destruction; decreases incidence of infection.

PHARMACOKINETICS

Clearance is related to amount of circulating neutrophils. Serum concentration declines as neutropenia resolves. **Half-life:** 15–80 hrs.

⌛ LIFESPAN CONSIDERATIONS

Pregnancy/Lactation: Unknown if drug crosses placenta or is distributed in breast milk. **Children:** Safety and efficacy not established in children younger than 12 yrs. **Elderly:** No age-related precautions noted.

INTERACTIONS

DRUG: Pegloticase may decrease effect. May increase adverse/toxic effect of **bleomycin, tisagenlecleucel, topotecan. HERBAL:** None significant. **FOOD:** None known. **LAB VALUES:** May increase serum LDH, alkaline phosphatase, uric acid.

AVAILABILITY (Rx)

Injection Solution: *(Neulasta):* 6 mg/0.6 mL syringe. **Prefilled Syringe Kit:** *(Neulasta Onpro):* 6 mg/0.6 mL; dose delivers over 45 min time period about 27 hrs after application. **Prefilled Syringe:** *(Fulphila, Fylnetra, Nyvepria, Udenyca, Ziextenzo):* 6 mg/0.6 mL.

ADMINISTRATION/HANDLING
SQ

Preparation • Remove syringe from refrigerator and allow solution to warm to room temperature. • Visually inspect for particulate matter or discoloration. Do not use if solution is cloudy, discolored, or visible particles are observed. **Administration** • Insert needle subcutaneously into outer abdomen, upper arm, or outer thigh and inject solution. • Do not inject into areas of active skin disease or injury such as sunburns, skin rashes, inflammation, skin infections, or active psoriasis. • Rotate injection sites. • Do not administer IV or intramuscularly. **Storage** • Refrigerate in original carton until time of use. • Protect from light. • Do not shake. • Discard if left at room temperature for more than 48 hrs. • Avoid freezing. If accidentally frozen, may thaw in refrigerator. Discard if frozen more than once.

On Body Injector
• A healthcare provider must fill the injector prior to applying to pt's skin. Apply to intact, nonirritated skin on back of arms or abdomen. • Delivers pegfilgrastim over 45 min time period about 27 hrs after application. • May apply on same day as chemotherapy. Keep injector at least 4 inches away from electrical equipment.
Storage • Store in refrigerator until 30 min prior to use. • Kit should not be at room temperature for more than 12 hrs (including injecting time). Discard if at room temperature for more than 12 hrs.

INDICATIONS/ROUTES/DOSAGE

Note: Do not administer between 14 days before and 24 hours after administration of cytotoxic chemotherapy.
Neutropenia (Chemotherapy-Induced)
SQ: ADULTS, ELDERLY, CHILDREN 12–17 YRS, WEIGHING MORE THAN 45 KG: Give as single 6-mg injection once per chemotherapy cycle **31–44 KG:** 4 mg. **21–30 KG:** 2.5 mg. **10–20 KG:** 1.5 mg. **LESS THAN 10 KG:** 0.1 mg/kg.

Radiation Injury Syndrome
SQ: ADULTS, ELDERLY, CHILDREN WEIGHING 45 KG OR MORE: 6 mg once wkly for 2 doses. **31–44 KG:** 4 mg once wkly for 2 doses. **21–30 KG:** 2.5 mg once wkly for 2 doses. **10–20 KG:** 1.5 mg once wkly for 2 doses. **LESS THAN 10 KG:** 0.1 mg/kg once wkly for 2 doses.

Dosage in Renal/Hepatic Impairment
No dose adjustment.

SIDE EFFECTS

Frequent (72%–15%): Bone pain, nausea, fatigue, alopecia, diarrhea, vomiting, constipation, anorexia, abdominal pain, arthralgia, generalized weakness, peripheral edema, dizziness, stomatitis, mucositis, neutropenic fever.

ADVERSE EFFECTS/TOXIC REACTIONS

Capillary leak syndrome (hypoalbuminemia, hypotension, fluid overload, leukocytosis, hemoconcentration), glomerulonephritis, fatal splenic rupture may occur. Acute respiratory distress syndrome (ARDS) may occur in pts with sepsis. Serious hypersensitivity reactions including anaphylaxis, skin rash, urticaria, erythema, flushing may occur. Fatal sickle cell crisis may occur in pts with sickle cell disease. May act as growth factor stimulator for tumors of any type. Potential device failures of Neulasta Onpro may cause partial delivery of medication, increasing risk of neutropenia, febrile neutropenia. Abdominal pain, malaise, back pain, increased inflammatory markers (C-reactive protein, WBC) may indicate aortitis. Other reactions including Sweet syndrome (acute febrile neutrophic dermatosis), contact dermatitis, and local skin reactions may occur.

NURSING CONSIDERATIONS

BASELINE ASSESSMENT
Obtain CBC prior to initiation and routinely thereafter. Question history of sickle cell disease, glomerulonephritis, splenic disease, hypersensitivity reaction to acrylic adhesive on body (injector uses acrylic adhesive).

INTERVENTION/EVALUATION
Monitor neutrophil count for treatment effectiveness. Monitor for hypersensitivity reactions. Assess for hypoalbuminemia, peripheral edema, respiratory symptoms (cough, dyspnea) if weight has increased by 5% (or greater) and pt is hypotensive; may indicate capillary leak syndrome. Severe capillary leak syndrome should be treated with supportive measures (corticosteroids; monitoring of weight, B/P, al-

bumins levels) until resolution. Monitor Neulasta Onpro for device failures. Septic pts should be monitored for ARDS.

PATIENT/FAMILY TEACHING
• Drink plenty of fluids to maintain hydration. • Immediately report symptoms of capillary leak syndrome (dizziness, fatigue, sudden weight gain, shortness of breath, swelling of face or extremities). A delay in reporting symptoms may be life-threatening. • Fatal rupturing of the spleen can occur; report sudden abdominal pain or swelling, low blood pressure, fast heart rate. • Report chest pain, fever, palpitations, severe bone pain.

pembrolizumab

pem-broe-**liz**-ue-mab
(Keytruda)
Do not confuse pembrolizumab with atezolizumab, durvalumab, necitumumab, nivolumab, palivizumab, or panitumumab.

◆CLASSIFICATION

PHARMACOTHERAPEUTIC: Anti PD-1 monoclonal antibody. **CLINICAL:** Antineoplastic.

USES

BCG-unresponsive NMIBC: Treatment of patients with Bacillus Calmette-Guerin (BCG)–unresponsive, high-risk, non–muscle invasive bladder cancer (NMIBC) with carcinoma in situ (CIS), with or without papillary tumors, who are ineligible for or have elected not to undergo cystectomy. **Biliary tract cancer (BTC):** Treatment of pts with locally advanced unresectable or metastatic BTC (in combination with gemcitabine and cisplatin). **Cervical cancer:** In combination with chemotherapy, with or without bevacizumab, for the treatment of pts with persistent, recurrent, or metastatic cervical cancer whose tumors express PD-L1. As a single agent for the treatment of pts with recurrent or metastatic cervical cancer with disease progression on or

after chemotherapy whose tumors express PD-L1. In combination with chemoradiotherapy (CRT), indicated for treatment of pts with FIGO 2014 stage III-IVA cervical cancer. **Classical Hodgkin lymphoma (cHL):** Treatment of adults with relapsed or refractory cHL. Treatment of pediatric pts with refractory cHL or cHL that has relapsed after 2 or more lines of therapy. **Cutaneous squamous cell carcinoma (cSCC):** Treatment of pts with recurrent or metastatic cSCC or locally advanced cSCC that is not curable by surgery or radiation. **Endometrial carcinoma:** In combination with lenvatinib, for the treatment of pts with advanced endometrial carcinoma that is mismatch repair proficient (pMMR) or not MSI-H who have disease progression following prior systemic therapy in any setting and are not candidates for curative surgery or radiation. As a single agent, for the treatment of pts with advanced endometrial carcinoma that is MSI-H or dMMR who have disease progression following prior systemic therapy in any setting and are not candidates for curative surgery or radiation. In combination with carboplatin and paclitaxel, followed as a single agent, for treatment of adults with primary advanced or recurrent endometrial carcinoma. **Esophageal cancer:** Treatment of pts with locally advanced or metastatic esophageal or gastroesophageal junction (GEJ) (tumors with epicenter 1 to 5 cm above the GEJ) carcinoma that is not amenable to surgical resection or definitive chemoradiation either in combination with platinum- and fluoropyrimidine-based chemotherapy or as a single agent after one or more prior lines of systemic therapy for pts with tumors of squamous cell histology that express PD-L1. **Gastric cancer:** In combination with trastuzumab, fluoropyrimidine-, and platinum-containing chemotherapy, for the first-line treatment of pts with locally advanced unresectable or metastatic HER2-positive gastric or GEJ adenocarcinoma. First-line treatment of adults with locally advanced unresectable or metastatic HER2-negative gastric or gastroesophageal junction (GEJ) adenocarcinoma in com-

P

bination with chemotherapy. **Head and neck squamous cell cancer (HNSCC):** In combination with platinum and FU for the first-line treatment of pts with metastatic or unresectable, recurrent HNSCC. As a single agent for the first-line treatment of pts with metastatic or unresectable, recurrent HNSCC whose tumors express PD-L1. As a single agent for the treatment of pts with recurrent or metastatic HNSCC with disease progression on or after platinum-containing chemotherapy. **Hepatocellular carcinoma (HCC):** Treatment of pts with HCC who have been previously treated with sorafenib. **Melanoma:** Treatment of unresectable or metastatic melanoma. Adjuvant treatment of adults and children 12 yrs and older with Stage IIB, IIC, or III melanoma following complete resection. **Malignant pleural mesothelioma (MPM):** First-line treatment of adults with unresectable advanced or metastatic MPM (in combination with pemetrexed and platinum chemotherapy). **Merkel cell carcinoma (MCC):** Treatment of adults and children with recurrent locally advanced or metastatic MCC. **Microsatellite instability-high or mismatch repair deficient cancer:** Treatment of adults and children with unresectable or metastatic microsatellite instability-high (MSI-H) or mismatch repair deficient (dMMR) solid tumors that have progressed following prior treatment and who have no satisfactory alternative treatment options. **Microsatellite instability-high or mismatch repair deficient colorectal cancer (CRC):** Treatment of pts with unresectable or metastatic MSI-H or dMMR CRC. **Non–small-cell lung cancer (NSCLC):** In combination with pemetrexed and platinum chemotherapy, as first-line treatment of pts with metastatic nonsquamous NSCLC with no EGFR or ALK genomic tumor aberrations. In combination with CARBOplatin and either PACLitaxel or PACLitaxel protein-bound, as first-line treatment of pts with metastatic squamous NSCLC. As a single agent for the first-line treatment of pts with NSCLC expressing PD-L1 with no EGFR or ALK genomic tumor aberrations

and is Stage III where pts are not candidates for surgical resection or definitive chemoradiation, or metastatic. As a single agent for the treatment of pts with metastatic NSCLC whose tumors express PD-L1 with disease progression on or after platinum-containing chemotherapy. As a single agent, for adjuvant treatment following resection and platinum-based chemotherapy for adults with Stage IB (T2a 4 cm or greater), II, or IIIA NSCLC. Treatment of pts with resectable NSCLC (tumor 4 cm or greater or node positive) in combination with platinum-containing chemotherapy as neoadjuvant treatment, and continued as a single agent as adjuvant treatment after surgery. **Primary mediastinal large B-cell lymphoma (PMBCL):** Treatment of adult and children with refractory PMBCL or who have relapsed after 2 or more prior lines of therapy. **Renal cell carcinoma (RCC):** In combination with axitinib or lenvatinib, for the first-line treatment of adults with advanced RCC. Adjuvant treatment of pts with RCC at intermediate-high or high risk of recurrence following nephrectomy or following nephrectomy and resection of metastatic lesions. **Triple-negative breast cancer (TNBC):** Treatment of pts with high-risk early-stage TNBC in combination with chemotherapy as neoadjuvant treatment and then continued as a single agent as adjuvant treatment after surgery. In combination with chemotherapy, for the treatment of pts with locally recurrent unresectable or metastatic TNBC whose tumors express PD-L1. **Tumor mutational burden-high (TMB-H) cancer:** Treatment of adults and children with unresectable or metastatic TMB-H solid tumors that have progressed following prior treatment and who have no satisfactory alternative treatment options. **Urothelial carcinoma:** Treatment of pts with locally advanced or metastatic urothelial carcinoma who are not eligible for any platinum-containing chemotherapy or who have disease progression during or following platinum-containing chemotherapy, or within 12 mos of neoadjuvant or adjuvant treatment with platinum-containing chemotherapy. In combination with enfortumab vedotin for treatment of adults with locally advanced or metastatic urothelial carcinoma not eligible for CISplatin-containing chemotherapy. **OFF-LABEL:** Malignant pleural mesothelioma, mycosis fungoides.

PRECAUTIONS

Contraindications: Hypersensitivity to pembrolizumab. **Cautions:** Thyroid disease, hepatic/renal impairment, interstitial lung disease, electrolyte imbalance, hypertriglyceridemia.

ACTION

Inhibits programmed cell death-1 (PD-1) activity by binding to PD-1 receptors on T cell, blocking PD-1 ligands from binding, which inhibits the negative immune regulation caused by PD-1 signaling. **Therapeutic Effect:** Inhibits T-cell proliferation and cytokine production. Induces antitumor responses.

PHARMACOKINETICS

Metabolism not specified. Elimination not specified. Steady-state concentration: 18 wks. **Half-life:** 26 days.

⧗ LIFESPAN CONSIDERATIONS

Pregnancy/Lactation: Avoid pregnancy; may cause fetal harm. Unknown if distributed in breast milk. Females of reproductive potential must use effective contraception during treatment and up to 4 mos after discontinuation. **Children:** Safety and efficacy not established. **Elderly:** No age-related precautions noted.

INTERACTIONS

DRUG: None significant. **HERBAL:** None significant. **FOOD:** None known. **LAB VALUES:** May increase serum AST, glucose, triglycerides. May decrease albumin, serum calcium, sodium.

AVAILABILITY (Rx)

Injection Solution: 100 mg/4 mL.

ADMINISTRATION/HANDLING

🖱 **IV**

◀**ALERT**▶ Use 0.2–0.5-micron in-line filter.

Reconstitution • Withdraw required dose and mix into 0.9% NaCl infusion bag (diluent volume depends on dose required). • Final concentration of diluent bag should equal 1–10 mg/mL. • Allow refrigerated solution to warm to room temperature before infusing.

Rate of administration • Infuse via dedicated line over 30 min using a 0.2–0.5-micron filter.

Storage • Starting from the time of dilution, may refrigerate for 96 hrs or store at room temperature for up to 6 hrs. Store time should not exceed total combined time of reconstitution, dilution, storage, and infusion.

INDICATIONS/ROUTES/DOSAGE

BCG-Unresponsive NMIBC

IV: ADULTS, ELDERLY: 200 mg q3wks or 400 mg q6wks until persistent or recurrent high-risk NMIBC, disease progression, unacceptable toxicity, or up to 24 mos.

BTC

IV: ADULTS, ELDERLY: 200 mg q3wks or 400 mg q6wks until disease progression, unacceptable toxicity, or up to 24 mos. Administer prior to chemotherapy.

Cervical Cancer

IV: ADULTS, ELDERLY: 200 mg q3wks or 400 mg q6wks until disease progression, unacceptable toxicity, or up to 24 mos. Administer prior to chemoradiotherapy or chemotherapy with or without bevacizumab when given on the same day.

cSCC

IV: ADULTS, ELDERLY: 200 mg q3wks or 400 mg q6wks until disease progression, unacceptable toxicity, or up to 24 mos.

cHL, PMBCL

IV: ADULTS, ELDERLY: 200 mg q3wks or 400 mg q6wks. **CHILDREN 12 YRS AND OLDER:** 2 mg/kg (up to 200 mg) q3wks. Continue until disease recurrence, unacceptable toxicity, or up to 24 mos.

Endometrial Carcinoma

IV: ADULTS, ELDERLY: 200 mg q3wks or 400 mg q6wks until disease progression, unacceptable toxicity, or (for pembrolizumab) up to 24 mos (in combination with lenvatinib). **Single agent:** 200 mg q3wks or 400 mg

P

q6wks until disease progression, unacceptable toxicity, or up to 24 mos. **In combination with carboplatin and paclitaxel:** 200 mg q3wks or 400 mg q6wks until disease progression, unacceptable toxicity, or for pembrolizumab, up to 24 mos.

Esophageal Cancer
IV: ADULTS, ELDERLY: 200 mg q3wks or 400 mg q6wks until disease progression, unacceptable toxicity or up to 24 mos. Administer prior to chemotherapy when given on the same day.

Gastric Cancer
IV: ADULTS, ELDERLY: 200 mg q3wks or 400 mg q6wks until disease progression, unacceptable toxicity, or up to 24 mos. Administer prior to trastuzumab and chemotherapy when given on the same day.

HCC
IV: ADULTS, ELDERLY: 200 mg q3wks or 400 mg q6wks until disease progression, unacceptable toxicity, or up to 24 mos.

MPM
IV: ADULTS, ELDERLY: 200 mg q3wks or 400 mg q6wks (administer prior to chemotherapy when given on the same day).

HNSCC, NSCLC
IV: ADULTS, ELDERLY: 200 mg q3wks or 400 mg q6wks until disease progression, unacceptable toxicity, or up to 24 mos. Administer prior to chemotherapy when given on the same day.

NSCLC (Resectable)
IV: ADULTS, ELDERLY: 200 mg q3wks or 400 mg q6wks. Administer prior to chemotherapy when given on the same day. Neoadjuvant treatment in combination with chemotherapy for 12 wks or until disease progression that precludes definitive surgery or unacceptable toxicity, followed by adjuvant treatment as a single agent after surgery for 39 wks or until disease recurrence or unacceptable toxicity.

Melanoma (Unresectable or Metastatic):
IV: ADULTS, ELDERLY: 200 mg q3wks or 400 mgq6 wks until disease progression or unacceptable toxicity. **Adjuvant Treatment: ADULTS, ELDERLY:** 200 mg q3wks or 400 mg q6wks. **CHILDREN 12 YRS AND OLDER:** 2 mg/kg (up to 200 mg) q3wks.

Continue until disease recurrence, unacceptable toxicity, or up to 12 mos.

Microsatellite Instability-High or Mismatch Repair Deficient Cancer (MSI-H or dMMR), MSI-H, or dMMR Colorectal Cancer
IV: ADULTS, ELDERLY: 200 mg q3wks or 400 mg q6wks until disease progression, unacceptable toxicity, or up to 24 mos.

MCC
IV: ADULTS, ELDERLY: 200 mg q3wks or 400 mg q6wks. **CHILDREN 12 YRS AND OLDER:** 2 mg/kg (up to 200 mg) q3wks. Continue until disease recurrence, unacceptable toxicity, or up to 24 mos.

RCC
IV: ADULTS, ELDERLY: 200 mg q3wks or 400 mg q6wks until disease progression, unacceptable toxicity, or (for pembrolizumab) up to 24 mos (in combination with axitinib or lenvatinib). **Adjuvant treatment:** 200 mg q3wks or 400 mg q6wks.

TMB-H Cancer
IV: ADULTS, ELDERLY: 200 mg q3wks or 400 mg q6wks. **CHILDREN 12 YRS AND OLDER:** 2 mg/kg (up to 200 mg) q3wks. Continue until disease recurrence, unacceptable toxicity, or up to 24 mos.

TNBC
IV: ADULTS, ELDERLY: High-risk early-stage: Administer prior to chemotherapy when given on the same day. Neoadjuvant treatment in combination with chemotherapy for 24 wks (200 mg q3wks or 400 mg q6wks) or until disease progression or unacceptable toxicity, followed by adjuvant treatment as a single agent for up to 27 wks (200 mg q3wks or 400 mg q6wks) or until disease recurrence or unacceptable toxicity. **Locally recurrent:** 200 mg q3wks or 400 mg q6wks until disease progression, unacceptable toxicity, or up to 24 mos. Administer prior to chemotherapy when given on the same day.

Urothelial Carcinoma
IV: ADULTS, ELDERLY: 200 mg q3wks or 400 mg q6wks until disease progression, unacceptable toxicity, or up to 24 mos.

Dose Modification
Based on Common Terminology Criteria for Adverse Events (CTCAE).

Withhold treatment for any of the following adverse events: ALT or AST greater than 3–5 times upper limit of normal (ULN) or bilirubin 1.5–3 times ULN, Grade 2 or 3 colitis, Grade 3 hyperthyroidism, Grade 2 nephritis, Grade 2 pneumonitis, symptomatic hypophysitis; any Grade 3 treatment-related adverse reaction. **Permanently discontinue for any of the following adverse events:** ALT or AST greater than 5 times ULN or bilirubin 3 times ULN (or pts with liver metastasis who begin treatment with Grade 2 ALT, AST, if ALT or AST increases greater than or equal to 50% from baseline and lasts for at least 1 wk), Grade 3 or 4 infusion-related reaction, Grade 3 or 4 nephritis, Grade 3 or 4 pneumonitis; inability to reduce corticosteroid dose to 10 mg/day or less (or predniSONE equivalent) after last dose; persistent Grade 2 or 3 adverse reaction that does not recover to Grade 0–1 within 12 wks after last dose; any severe or Grade 3 treatment-related adverse reaction that recurs.

Dosage in Renal Impairment
No dose adjustment.

Dosage in Hepatic Impairment
Mild impairment: No dose adjustment. **Moderate to severe impairment:** Not studied, use caution.

SIDE EFFECTS

Frequent (47%–20%): Fatigue, nausea, cough, pruritus, rash, decreased appetite, constipation, diarrhea, arthralgia. **Occasional (18%–11%):** Dyspnea, extremity pain, peripheral edema, vomiting, headache, chills, insomnia, myalgia, abdominal pain, back pain, pyrexia, vitiligo, dizziness, upper respiratory tract infection.

ADVERSE EFFECTS/TOXIC REACTIONS

May cause severe immune-mediated events such as pneumonitis (2.9% of pts), colitis (1% of pts), hepatitis (0.5% of pts), hypophysitis (0.5% of pts), renal failure or nephritis (0.7% of pts), hyperthyroidism (1.2% of pts), hypothyroidism (8.3% of pts). Other reported events include adrenal insufficiency, arthritis, cellulitis, exfoliative dermatitis, hemolytic anemia, myositis, myasthenic syndrome, pancreatitis, partial seizures, pneumonia, optic neuritis, rhabdomyolysis, sepsis.

NURSING CONSIDERATIONS

BASELINE ASSESSMENT
Obtain CBC, BMP, LFT, TSH; pregnancy test in females of reproductive potential. Obtain weight in kg. Question history of adrenal/pituitary/pulmonary/thyroid disease, autoimmune disorders, hepatic/renal impairment, allergy to predniSONE. Conduct dermatologic exam, visual acuity. Offer emotional support.

INTERVENTION/EVALUATION
Monitor CBC, LFT, serum electrolytes; thyroid panel if applicable. Monitor for immune-mediated adverse events. Notify physician if any CTCAE toxicities occur and initiate proper treatment. Obtain chest X-ray if pneumonitis suspected. Screen for tumor lysis syndrome in pts with high tumor burden. Offer antiemetics if nausea, vomiting occurs. Monitor I&O, daily weight.

PATIENT/FAMILY TEACHING
• Serious adverse reactions may affect lungs, GI tract, kidneys, or hormonal glands, and predniSONE therapy may need to be started. • Immediately contact physician if serious or life-threatening inflammatory reactions occur in the following body systems: lung (chest pain, cough, shortness of breath); colon (severe abdominal pain or diarrhea); liver (bruising, clay-colored/tarry stools, yellowing of skin or eyes); pituitary (persistent or unusual headache, dizziness, extreme weakness, fainting, vision changes); kidney (decreased or dark-colored urine, flank pain); thyroid (insomnia, hypertension, tachycardia [overactive thyroid]), (fatigue, goiter, weight gain [underactive thyroid]). • Use effective contraception to avoid pregnancy. Do not breastfeed.

P

PEMEtrexed

pem-e-**trex**-ed
(<u>Alimta</u>, Pemfexy)
**Do not confuse PEMEtrexed with
methotrexate or PRALAtrexate.**

◆CLASSIFICATION

PHARMACOTHERAPEUTIC: Folate analog metabolic inhibitor. Antimetabolite. **CLINICAL:** Antineoplastic.

USES

Malignant pleural mesothelioma: Treatment of unresectable malignant pleural mesothelioma in combination with CISplatin whose disease is unresectable or who are otherwise not candidates for curative surgery. **Nonsquamous non–small-cell lung cancer (NSCLC):** Initial treatment of locally advanced or metastatic nonsquamous NSCLC (in combination with CISplatin). Initial treatment of metastatic, non-squamous NSCLC (in combination with platinum chemotherapy and pembrolizumab) in pts with no epidermal growth factor receptor (EGFR) or anaplastic lymphoma kinase (ALK) tumor aberrations. Maintenance treatment (single agent) of locally advanced or metastatic non-squamous NSCLC if no progression after 4 cycles of platinum-based first-line therapy. Single-agent treatment (after prior chemotherapy) of recurrent, metastatic non-squamous NSCLC. **OFF-LABEL:** Bladder cancer (metastatic), cervical cancer (recurrent), ovarian cancer (platinum-resistant), thymic malignancies.

PRECAUTIONS

Contraindications: Severe hypersensitivity to PEMEtrexed. **Cautions:** Hepatic/renal impairment, concurrent use of nephrotoxic medications, preexisting myelosuppression. Not indicated for squamous cell NSCLC.

ACTION

Inhibits biosynthesis of purine and thymidine nucleotides. Inhibits protein synthesis. **Therapeutic Effect:** Disrupts folate-dependent enzymes essential for cell replication.

PHARMACOKINETICS

Protein binding: 81%. Not metabolized. Excreted in urine. **Half-life:** 3.5 hrs.

LIFESPAN CONSIDERATIONS

Pregnancy/Lactation: Avoid pregnancy; may cause fetal harm. Females of reproductive potential must use effective contraception during treatment and for at least 6 mos after discontinuation. Unknown if distributed in breast milk. Breastfeeding not recommended during treatment and for at least 7 days after discontinuation. Males must use effective contraception during treatment and for at least 3 mos after discontinuation. **Children:** Safety and efficacy not established in pts younger than 18 yrs. **Elderly:** Higher incidence of fatigue, leukopenia, neutropenia, thrombocytopenia in pts 65 yrs and older.

INTERACTIONS

DRUG: Bone marrow depressants (e.g., cladribine) may increase risk of myelosuppression. May decrease concentration/therapeutic effects of **BCG (intravesical), vaccines (live).** May increase concentration/adverse effects of **vaccines (live).** May increase adverse/toxic effect of **natalizumab. HERBAL: Echinacea** may decrease therapeutic effect. **FOOD:** None known. **LAB VALUES:** May increase serum ALT, AST, creatinine.

AVAILABILITY (Rx)

Injection, Powder for Reconstitution: 100 mg; 500 mg.

ADMINISTRATION/HANDLING

⬚ **IV Infusion**

Reconstitution • Dilute 500-mg vial with 20 mL (4.2 mL to 100-mg vial) 0.9% NaCl to provide concentration of 25 mg/mL. • Gently swirl each vial until powder is completely dissolved. • Solution appears clear and ranges in color from colorless to yellow or green-yellow. • Dilute in 100 mL 0.9% NaCl.

Rate of administration • Infuse over 10 min.

Storage • Store at room temperature. • Refrigerate diluted solutions for up to 24 hr.

▦ IV INCOMPATIBILITIES

Use only 0.9% NaCl to reconstitute; flush line prior to and following infusion. Do not add any other medications to IV line.

INDICATIONS/ROUTES/DOSAGE

◀**ALERT**▶ Pretreatment with dexA-METHasone (or equivalent) will reduce risk, severity of cutaneous reaction; treatment with folic acid and vitamin B_{12} beginning 1 wk before treatment and continuing for 21 days after last PEMEtrexed dose will reduce risk of side effects. Do not begin new treatment cycles unless ANC 1,500 cells/mm³ or greater, platelets 100,000 cells/mm³ or greater, and CrCl 45 mL/min or greater.

Malignant Pleural Mesothelioma

IV: ADULTS, ELDERLY: 500 mg/m² on day 1 of each 21-day cycle in combination with CISplatin. Continue until disease progression or unacceptable toxicity.

Nonsquamous Non–Small-Cell Lung Cancer (NSCLC)

IV: ADULTS, ELDERLY: Initial treatment 500 mg/m² on day 1 of each 21-day cycle (administered after pembrolizumab and prior to CARBOplatin or CISplatin for up to 4 cycles) OR (administered prior to CISplatin up to 6 cycles) or until disease progression or unacceptable toxicity. **Maintenance or second-line treatment:** 500 mg/m² on day 1 of each 21-day cycle (as single agent). Continue until disease progression or unacceptable toxicity.

Dose Modification for Hematologic Toxicity
ANC less than 500 cells/mm³ and platelets 50,000 cells/mm³ or more: Reduce dose to 75% of previous dose. **Platelets less than 50,000 cells/mm³ without bleeding:** Reduce dose to 75% of previous dose. **Platelets less than 50,000 cells/**

mm³ **with bleeding:** Reduce dose to 50% of previous dose. **Nonhematologic toxicity Grade 3 or greater (excluding neurotoxicity):** Reduce dose to 75% of previous dose (excluding mucositis). **Grade 3 or 4 mucositis:** Reduce dose to 50% of previous dose.

Dosage in Renal Impairment
Not recommended with CrCl less than 45 mL/min.

Dosage in Hepatic Impairment
Grade 3 or 4 hepatic impairment: 75% of previous dose.

SIDE EFFECTS

Frequent (12%–10%): Fatigue, nausea, vomiting, rash, desquamation. **Occasional (8%–4%):** Stomatitis, pharyngitis, diarrhea, anorexia, hypertension, chest pain. **Rare (less than 3%):** Constipation, depression, dysphagia.

ADVERSE EFFECTS/TOXIC REACTIONS

Myelosuppression (anemia, neutropenia, thrombocytopenia) is an expected response to therapy. Severe, sometimes fatal renal toxicity may occur. Serious cutaneous events including bullous, blistering, and exfoliative skin toxicities, Stevens-Johnson syndrome, epidermal necrolysis may occur. Fatal cases of interstitial pneumonitis were reported. Radiation recall may occur in pts who have received radiation wks to yrs previously.

NURSING CONSIDERATIONS

BASELINE ASSESSMENT
Obtain CBC, BMP, LFT; pregnancy test in females of reproductive potential. Question history of hepatic/renal impairment. Receive full medication history and screen for interactions (esp. use of NSAIDs). Assess hydration status. Offer emotional support.

INTERVENTION/EVALUATION
Monitor CBC as clinically indicated; BMP, LFT periodically. Monitor for hemato-

P

logic toxicity (fever, sore throat, signs of local infection, unusual bruising/bleeding from any site), symptoms of anemia (excessive fatigue, weakness), renal toxicity. Assess skin for rash, lesions, dermatological toxicities. Obtain CXR if interstitial lung disease, pneumonitis suspected. Ensure adequate hydration.

PATIENT/FAMILY TEACHING

• Treatment may depress your immune system response and reduce your ability to fight infection. Report symptoms of infection such as body aches, chills, cough, fatigue, fever. Avoid those with active infection. • Use effective contraception to avoid pregnancy. Do not breastfeed. • Report unusual bruising or bleeding of any kind. • Treatment may cause severe lung inflammation; report cough, difficulty breathing, fever. • Report skin toxicities such as blistering, bubbling, sloughing of the skin; liver problems (bruising, confusion, amber- or orange-colored urine, abdominal pain, yellowing of the skin or eyes); kidney problems (decreased urine output, dark-colored urine, flank pain).

penicillin G potassium

pen-i-**sil**-in G po-**tas**-ee-um
(Pfizerpen-G)
Do not confuse penicillin with penicillAMINE.

◆CLASSIFICATION

PHARMACOTHERAPEUTIC: Penicillin. **CLINICAL:** Antibiotic.

USES

Treatment of severe infections including bacteremia, empyema, severe pneumonia, pericarditis, endocarditis, meningitis caused by penicillin G–susceptible microorganisms (streptococcal, pneumococcal, staphylococcal infections). **OFF-LABEL:** Lyme disease, osteomyelitis, prosthetic joint infection, skin/soft tissue infection (streptococcal).

PRECAUTIONS

Contraindications: Hypersensitivity to any penicillin. **Cautions:** Renal/hepatic impairment, seizure disorder, hypersensitivity to cephalosporins, asthma.

ACTION

Inhibits bacterial cell wall synthesis by binding to one or more of the penicillin-binding proteins of bacteria. **Therapeutic Effect:** Bactericidal.

PHARMACOKINETICS

Protein binding: 60%. Widely distributed (poor CNS penetration). Metabolized in liver. Primarily excreted in urine. **Half-life:** 0.5–1 hr (increased in renal impairment).

⧗ LIFESPAN CONSIDERATIONS

Pregnancy/Lactation: Readily crosses placenta; distributed in breast milk. **Children:** May delay renal excretion in neonates, young infants. **Elderly:** Age-related renal impairment may require dosage adjustment.

INTERACTIONS

DRUG: Probenecid may increase concentration/effect. **HERBAL:** None significant. **FOOD:** None significant. **LAB VALUES:** May cause positive Coombs' test. May increase serum ALT, AST, alkaline phosphatase, LDH. May decrease WBCs.

AVAILABILITY (Rx)

Injection, Powder for Reconstitution: 5 million units.

ADMINISTRATION/HANDLING

 IV

Reconstitution • After reconstitution, further dilute with 50–100 mL D_5W or 0.9% NaCl for final concentration of 100,000–500,000 units/mL (50,000 units/mL for infants, neonates).

Rate of administration • Infuse over 15–30 min.
Storage • Reconstituted solution is stable for 7 days if refrigerated.

▩ IV COMPATIBILITIES

Calcium gluconate, heparin, magnesium sulfate, potassium chloride.

INDICATIONS/ROUTES/DOSAGE

Usual Dosage

IV: ADULTS, ELDERLY: 12–24 million units/day in divided doses q4–6h. **INFANTS, CHILDREN, ADOLESCENTS:** 100,000–300,000 units/kg/day in divided doses q4–6h. **Maximum:** 24 million units/day. **NEONATES:** 50,000 units/kg/dose q8–12h.

Dosage in Renal Impairment

Dosage interval is modified based on creatinine clearance.

Creatinine Clearance	Dosage
Greater than 50 mL/min	No dose adjustment
10–50 mL/min	75% normal dose
Less than 10 mL/min	20%–50% normal dose
Hemodialysis	50%–100% normal dose q8–12h
Continuous renal replacement therapy	
Continuous venovenous hemofiltration	Loading dose 4 million units, then 2 million units q4–6h
Continuous venovenous hemodialysis	Loading dose 4 million units, then 2–3 million units q4–6h
Continuous venovenous hemodiafiltration	Loading dose 4 million units, then 2–4 million units q4–6h

Dosage in Hepatic Impairment

No dose adjustment.

SIDE EFFECTS

Occasional: Lethargy, fever, dizziness, rash, electrolyte imbalance, diarrhea, thrombophlebitis. **Rare:** Seizures, interstitial nephritis.

ADVERSE EFFECTS/TOXIC REACTIONS

Hypersensitivity reactions ranging from rash, fever, chills to anaphylaxis occur occasionally.

NURSING CONSIDERATIONS

BASELINE ASSESSMENT

Question for history of allergies, particularly penicillins, cephalosporins.

INTERVENTION/EVALUATION

Promptly report rash (hypersensitivity), diarrhea (with fever, abdominal pain, mucus, or blood in stool, may indicate antibiotic-associated colitis). Monitor I&O, urinalysis, electrolytes, renal function tests for nephrotoxicity.

pertuzumab

per-**tue**-zue-mab
(Perjeta)

■ **BLACK BOX ALERT** ■ Can result in embryo-fetal death, birth defects. Pts must be made aware of danger to fetus, need for effective contraception. May result in cardiac failure. Assess left ventricular ejection fraction.

◆ **CLASSIFICATION**

PHARMACOTHERAPEUTIC: *HER2* receptor antagonist. Monoclonal antibody. **CLINICAL:** Antineoplastic.

USES

Treatment of *HER2*-positive metastatic breast cancer in pts who have not received prior anti-*HER2* therapy or chemotherapy for metastatic disease in combination with trastuzumab and DOCEtaxel. Neoadjuvant treatment of pts with *HER2*-positive, locally advanced inflammatory, or early-stage breast cancer in combination with trastuzumab and chemotherapy. Adjuvant treatment of *HER2*-positive early breast cancer at high risk of recurrence (in combination with trastuzumab and chemotherapy).

◆ Canadian trade name   🗲 Non-Crushable Drug   **HIGH ALERT** High Alert drug

PRECAUTIONS

Contraindications: Hypersensitivity to pertuzumab. **Cautions:** Cardiomyopathy, HF, history of infusion-related reaction. Prior anthracycline therapy or irradiation. Conditions predisposing to infection (e.g., diabetes, immunocompromised pts, renal failure, open wounds), pts at risk for tumor lysis syndrome (high tumor burden).

ACTION

Targets human epidermal growth factor 2 (*HER2*), blocking ligand-initiated intercellular signaling, which can result in cell growth arrest and cell death. **Therapeutic Effect:** Inhibits cell growth and metastasis.

PHARMACOKINETICS

Peak plasma concentration reached after first maintenance dose. **Half-life:** 18 days.

⧖ LIFESPAN CONSIDERATIONS

Pregnancy/Lactation: Avoid pregnancy; may cause fetal harm. Females of reproductive potential must use effective contraception during treatment and for at least 7 mos after discontinuation. Unknown if distributed in breast milk. However, human immunoglobulin G (IgG) is present in breast milk and is known to cross the placenta. **Children:** Safety and efficacy not established. **Elderly:** No age-related precautions noted.

INTERACTIONS

DRUG: None significant. **HERBAL:** None significant. **FOOD:** None known. **LAB VALUES:** May decrease Hgb, Hct, leukocytes, neutrophils.

AVAILABILITY (Rx)

Injection Solution: 420 mg/14 mL (30 mg/mL) vial.

ADMINISTRATION/HANDLING

 IV

Reconstitution • Visually inspect for particulate matter or discoloration. Do not use if solution is cloudy, discolored, or if visible particles are observed. • Dilute in 250 mL 0.9% NaCl only (do not use D₅W). • Mix by gentle inversion. • Do not shake.

Rate of administration • Initial dose to be infused over 60 min. • Subsequent doses may be infused over 30–60 min.

Storage • Refrigerate unused vials in original carton. Protect from light. • May refrigerate diluted solution for up to 24 hrs. • Do not freeze.

▦ IV INCOMPATIBILITIES

Do not mix with any other medications.

INDICATIONS/ROUTES/DOSAGE

◀**ALERT**▶ Give as an IV infusion only. Do not give by IV push or bolus.

Breast Cancer (Metastatic)
IV infusion: ADULTS/ELDERLY: Initially, 840, followed by maintenance dose of 420 mg q3wks until disease progression or unacceptable toxicity (in combination with trastuzumab [or trastuzumab/hyaluronidase] and DOCEtaxel).

Breast Cancer (Adjuvant)
IV infusion: ADULTS, ELDERLY: 840 mg once, followed by maintenance dose of 420 mg q3wks for a total of 1 yr (up to 18 cycles) or until disease progression or unacceptable toxicity (as part of combination regimen containing trastuzumab [or trastuzumab/hyaluronidase] and standard anthracycline- and/or taxane-based therapy). Pertuzumab and trastuzumab (or trastuzumab/hyaluronidase) should begin on day 1 of the first taxane-containing cycle.

Breast Cancer (Neoadjuvant)
IV infusion: ADULTS, ELDERLY: 840 mg once, followed by 420 mg q3wks for 3–6 cycles. May be administered as one of the following regimens: 4 preoperative cycles of pertuzumab, trastuzumab (or trastuzumab/hyaluronidase), DOCEtaxel, then 3 postoperative cycles of 5-fluorouracil, epiRUBicin, and cycloPHOSphamide (FEC) **or** 3 or 4 preoperative cycles of FEC alone, then 3 or 4 preoperative

cycles of pertuzumab, trastuzumab (or trastuzumab/hyaluronidase), DOCEtaxel **or** 6 preoperative cycles of pertuzumab, trastuzumab (or trastuzumab/hyaluronidase), DOCEtaxel, and CARBOplatin **or** 4 preoperative cycles of dose-dense DOXOrubicin and cycloPHOSphamide alone, then 4 preoperative cycles of pertuzumab, trastuzumab (or trastuzumab/hyaluronidase), and PACLitaxel. **Note:** Continue trastuzumab (or trastuzumab/hyaluronidase) postoperatively to complete 1 yr of treatment.

Dosage in Renal/Hepatic Impairment
No dose adjustment.

SIDE EFFECTS

Frequent (67%–21%): Diarrhea, alopecia, nausea, fatigue, rash, peripheral neuropathy, anorexia, asthenia, mucosal inflammation, vomiting, peripheral edema, myalgia, nail disorder, headache. **Occasional (19%–12%):** Stomatitis, pyrexia, dysgeusia, arthralgia, constipation, increased lacrimation, pruritus, insomnia, dizziness. **Rare (10%–7%):** Nasopharyngitis, dry skin, paronychia.

ADVERSE EFFECTS/TOXIC REACTIONS

Myelosuppression (anemia, leukopenia, neutropenia) is an expected response to therapy, but more severe reactions including febrile neutropenia may be life-threatening. Upper respiratory tract infection occurs in 17% of pts. Pleural effusion occurred in 5% of pts. Tumor lysis syndrome may present as acute renal failure, hypocalcemia, hyperuricemia, hyperphosphatemia. Decreases in LVEF occurred in 4% of pts. Prior treatment with anthracyclines, chest radiotherapy may further increase risk of decreased LVEF.

NURSING CONSIDERATIONS

BASELINE ASSESSMENT

Obtain CBC. Assess left ventricular ejection fraction (LVEF) by echocardiogram. Negative pregnancy test must be confirmed before initiating treatment. Obtain *HER2* testing by an FDA-approved laboratory. Screen for active infection. Offer emotional support.

INTERVENTION/EVALUATION

Monitor ANC, CBC periodically. Assess LVEF at regular intervals. Monitor for symptoms of left ventricular dysfunction (arrhythmia, cough, dyspnea, peripheral edema). Monitor for infusion reactions, hypersensitivity reactions, anaphylaxis. If a significant infusion reaction occurs, slow or interrupt infusion and administer appropriate medical treatment. Observe pt closely for 60 min after the first infusion and for 30 min after subsequent infusions. Monitor for symptoms of tumor lysis syndrome (acute renal failure, hypocalcemia, hyperuricemia, hyperphosphatemia).

PATIENT/FAMILY TEACHING

• Treatment may depress your immune system response and reduce your ability to fight infection. Report symptoms of infection such as body aches, chills, cough, fatigue, fever. Avoid those with active infection. • Report symptoms of bone marrow depression such as bruising, fatigue, fever, shortness of breath, weight loss; bleeding easily, bloody urine or stool. • New-onset left heart dysfunction may occur; report shortness of breath, cough, swelling of ankles or feet, palpitations. • Therapy may cause life-threatening tumor lysis syndrome (a condition caused by the rapid breakdown of cancer cells), which can cause kidney failure. Report decreased urination, amber-colored urine; confusion, difficulty breathing, fatigue, fever, muscle or joint pain, palpitations, seizures, vomiting. • Use effective contraception to avoid pregnancy. Do not breastfeed.

 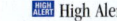

pertuzumab/ trastuzumab/ hyaluronidase-zzxf

per-**too**-zoo-mab/ tras-**tu**-zoo-mab/ **hye**-al-ure-**on**-i-dase
(Phesgo)

■**BLACK BOX ALERT**■ May cause cardiac failure; decreased left ventricular ejection fraction (LVEF), esp. in pts with anthracy-cline-containing chemotherapy regimens. Monitor LVEF prior to initiation and during treatment. Serious and fatal cases of interstitial lung disease (ILD), pneumonitis were reported. Symptoms usually occurred during or within 24 hrs of administration. Permanently discontinue if anaphylaxis, ILD, acute respiratory distress syndrome occurs. Treatment can result in embryo-fetal death and birth defects. Recommend effective contraception.

Do not confuse pertuzumab/ trastuzumab/hyaluronidase-zzxf with trastuzumab/hyaluronidase, ado-trastuzumab emtansine, fam-trastuzumab deruxtecan, pertuzumab, trastuzumab, or rituximab/hyaluronidase.

◆CLASSIFICATION

PHARMACOTHERAPEUTIC: *HER2* receptor antagonist, monoclonal antibody. **CLINICAL:** Antineoplastic.

USES

Neoadjuvant treatment of adults with human epidermal growth factor receptor 2 (*HER2*)-positive, locally advanced, inflammatory, or early-stage breast cancer (either greater than 2 cm in diameter or node positive) as a part of a complete treatment regimen for early breast cancer. Adjuvant treatment of adults with *HER2*-positive early breast cancer at high risk of recurrence. Treatment of *HER2*-positive metastatic breast cancer (in combination with DOCEtaxel) in adults who have not received prior anti-*HER2* therapy or chemotherapy for metastatic disease.

PRECAUTIONS

Contraindications: Hypersensitivity to pertuzumab, trastuzumab, hyaluronidase. **Cautions:** Baseline cytopenias, hepatic impairment, cardiovascular disease, HF, pulmonary disease, pts at risk for interstitial lung disease (e.g., COPD, sarcoidosis, connective disease disease); conditions predisposing to infection (e.g., diabetes, renal failure, immunocompromised pts, open wounds); treatment after anthracycline therapy.

ACTION

Pertuzumab targets the extracellular HER2 protein dimerization domain, inhibiting HER2 dimerization and blocking HER downstream. Trastuzumab binds to the extracellular domain of HER2. Hyaluronidase increases distribution and absorption of injected medications. **Therapeutic Effect:** Inhibits proliferation of tumor cells overexpressing HER2 protein.

PHARMACOKINETICS

Widely distributed. Peak plasma concentration: 3 days. Eliminated by parallel and nonlinear saturable target-mediated clearance. **Half-life:** Not specified.

⧖ LIFESPAN CONSIDERATIONS

Pregnancy/Lactation: Avoid pregnancy; may cause fetal harm. Females and males of reproductive potential should use effective contraception during treatment and for at least 7 mos after discontinuation. Unknown if distributed in breast milk. Breastfeeding not recommended during treatment and for at least 7 mos after discontinuation. **Children:** Safety and efficacy not established. **Elderly:** May have increased risk of cardiac dysfunction.

INTERACTIONS

DRUG: None significant. **HERBAL:** None significant. **FOOD:** None known. **LAB VALUES:** May increase serum ALT, AST, bilirubin, creatinine, potassium, sodium. May decrease serum albumin, glucose, potassium, sodium; absolute neutrophil count (ANC), Hgb, lymphocytes, neutrophils, platelets.

AVAILABILITY (Rx)

Injection Solution: (pertuzumab/trastuzumab/hyaluronidase-zzxf): 1,200 mg/600 mg/30,000 units/15 mL (80 mg, 40 mg/2,000 units/mL), 600 mg/600 mg/20,000 units per 10 mL (60 mg, 60 mg/2,000 units/mL).

ADMINISTRATION/HANDLING
SQ

Note: Must be administered only in the thigh. Do not give IV or IM. Combination regimen has different dosages and administration instructions than individual pertuzumab (IV), trastuzumab (IV or SQ). Do not substitute with ado-trastuzumab emtansine, fam-trastuzumab deruxtecan, pertuzumab, or trastuzumab. Pts may transition from IV pertuzumab and trastuzumab (see manufacturer guidelines). Must be administered by a healthcare professional. Consider premedication with analgesic, antipyretic, or antihistamine in pts with prior injection reactions.
Preparation • Visually inspect for particulate matter or discoloration. Solution should appear clear to opalescent, colorless to slightly brown. Do not use if solution is cloudy, discolored, or visible particles are observed. • Withdraw contents from vial into syringe. • To avoid clogging, immediately attach a 25- to 27-gauge hypodermic needle or subcutaneous infusion set to syringe.
Administration • Insert needle subcutaneously into thigh only, approx. 2.5 cm from previous injection sites. • Do not inject into areas of active skin disease or injury such as sunburns, skin rashes, inflammation, skin infections, or active psoriasis. • Rotate injection sites of right and left thigh.
Rate of administration • **Initial dose:** Inject over approx. 8 min. • **Maintenance dose:** Inject over approx. 5 min. Slow or pause injection if injection reaction occurs.

Storage • Refrigerate vials in original carton until time of use. Protect from light. Do not shake or freeze. • After vial is removed from refrigerator, use within 4 hrs. • May refrigerate syringe that contains solution for up to 24 hrs or store at room temperature for up to 4 hrs.

Treatment interruption/missed doses
• If treatment is interrupted or a dose is missed by less than 6 wks between injections, administer maintenance dose; do not wait until next dose. If treatment is interrupted or a dose is missed by more than 6 wks between injections, readminister initial dose, followed by maintenance doses at the usual intervals.

INDICATIONS/ROUTES/DOSAGE

Note: Give after completion of anthracycline therapy. If given for treatment of early breast cancer with DOCEtaxel or PACLitaxel, give DOCEtaxel or PACLitaxel after pertuzumab/trastuzumab/hyaluronidase-zzxf. If given for treatment of metastatic breast cancer with DOCEtaxel, give DOCEtaxel after pertuzumab/trastuzumab/hyaluronidase-zzxf.

Breast Cancer (*HER2*-Positive, Locally Advanced, Inflammatory, Early Stage) (Neoadjuvant Treatment)
SQ: ADULTS: Initially, 1,200 mg/600 mg/30,000 units as a single dose, then 600 mg/600 mg/20,000 units q3wks (in combination with chemotherapy). After surgery, continue pertuzumab/trastuzumab/hyaluronidase to complete 1 year of treatment (up to 18 cycles) or until disease progression or unacceptable toxicity.

Breast Cancer (*HER2*-Positive, Early Stage) (Adjuvant Treatment)
SQ: ADULTS: Initially, 1,200 mg/600 mg/30,000 units as a single dose, then 600 mg/600 mg/20,000 units q3wks for a total of 1 year (up to 18 cycles) or until disease progression or unacceptable toxicity as part of a complete regimen including anthracycline- and/or taxane-based chemotherapy. Start on day 1 of first taxane-containing cycle.

P

Breast Cancer (*HER2*-Positive, Metastatic)

SQ: ADULTS: Initially, 1,200 mg/600 mg/30,000 units as a single dose, then 600 mg/600 mg/20,000 units q3wks (in combination with DOCEtaxel 75–100 mg/m² IV q3wks based on tolerability) until disease progression or unacceptable toxicity.

Dose Modification
Cardiac Toxicity
Early breast cancer with baseline LVEF 55% or greater: Withhold treatment for at least 3 wks if a decrease in LVEF is less than 50% with a fall of greater than or equal to 10 percentage points below baseline. Resume if LVEF improves to either greater than or equal to 50% or less than 10 percentage points of baseline. **Metastatic breast cancer with baseline LVEF 50% or greater:** Withhold treatment for at least 3 wks for either a decrease in LVEF that is less than 40% or a decrease in LVEF of 40%–45% with a fall of greater than or equal to 10 percentage points below baseline. Resume if LVEF improves to either greater than or equal to 45% or 40%–45% with a fall of less than 10 percentage points below baseline.

Permanent Discontinuation
Discontinue treatment if LVEF has not improved, worsened, or pt has become symptomatic after 3 wks; severe hypersensitivity reaction (e.g., anaphylaxis) occurs.

Dosage in Renal Impairment
No dose adjustment.

Dosage in Hepatic Impairment
Not specified; use caution.

SIDE EFFECTS

Frequent (77%–29%): Alopecia, nausea, diarrhea, asthenia, fatigue. **Occasional (25%–6%):** Stomatitis, myalgia, arthralgia, constipation, dysgeusia, decreased appetite, insomnia, headache, peripheral neuropathy, dry skin, rash, cough, mucosal inflammation, injection site reaction, dyspepsia, pyrexia, dizziness, hot flush, decreased weight, back pain, paresthesia, dyspnea, nail discoloration, hemor-rhoids, erythema, abdominal pain, peripheral edema, dermatitis, nail disorder, rhinorrhea, malaise, bone pain, extremity pain, muscle spasm, musculoskeletal pain. **Rare (5%):** Increased lacrimation.

ADVERSE EFFECTS/TOXIC REACTIONS

Myelosuppression (anemia, lymphopenia, neutropenia, thrombocytopenia) is an expected response to therapy, but more severe reactions, including bone marrow depression, febrile neutropenia, may be life-threatening. May exacerbate chemotherapy-induced neutropenia. May cause cardiomyopathy, cardiac failure, and death. Other cardiac disorders may include arrhythmias, hypertension, asymptomatic decrease of LVEF; disabling HF. May increase risk of cardiac dysfunction in pts who receive anthracycline after stopping treatment. Pulmonary toxicities (acute respiratory distress syndrome, dyspnea, hypoxia, ILD, pulmonary edema, pneumonitis, pleural effusions, pulmonary fibrosis, pulmonary infiltrates, pulmonary insufficiency) were reported. Infections (upper respiratory tract infections, nasopharyngitis, paronychia, UTI, viral infections) were reported. Epistaxis reported in 12% of pts. Palmar-plantar erythrodysesthesia syndrome (PPES), a chemotherapy-induced skin condition that presents with skin redness, swelling, numbness, sloughing of the hands and feet, reported in 6% of pts. Severe hypersensitivity reactions, including anaphylaxis, may occur.

NURSING CONSIDERATIONS

BASELINE ASSESSMENT
Obtain CBC, BMP, LFT; pregnancy test in females of reproductive potential. Confirm compliance with effective contraception. Verify presence of HER2 protein overexpression or *HER2* gene amplification in tumor specimen. Administer in an environment equipped to monitor for and manage hypersensitivity reactions; verify emergency resuscitation equip-

ment/medications are readily available. Assess LVEF by echocardiogram or MUGA scan. A baseline LVEF of 50% or greater is required in pts after completion of anthracycline therapy. Question history of cardiovascular disease, HF, pulmonary disease, prior hypersensitivity reactions. Screen for active infection. Offer emotional support.

INTERVENTION/EVALUATION

Monitor CBC for myelosuppression; LFT for hepatotoxicity (bruising, jaundice, right upper abdominal pain, nausea, vomiting, weight loss) as clinically indicated. Diligently monitor for hypersensitivity reactions or injection reactions for at least 30 min after initial dose, then for at least 15 min after each maintenance dose. Severe reactions may require emergency resuscitation; early detection is vital. Consider ABG, radiologic test if pneumonitis (excessive cough, dyspnea, fever, hypoxia) is suspected. Consider treatment with corticosteroids if pneumonitis is confirmed. Assess LVEF by echocardiogram q3mos. If treatment is withheld due to change in LVEF, monitor LVEF at 3-wk intervals. After discontinuation, monitor LVEF q6mos for at least 2 yrs. Monitor for infections (body aches, cough, dysuria, fatigue, fever, urinary frequency). Monitor daily pattern of bowel activity, stool consistency. Assess skin for rash, erythema, toxicities.

PATIENT/FAMILY TEACHING

• Treatment may depress the immune system response and reduce ability to fight infection. Report symptoms of infection such as body aches, chills, cough, fatigue, fever. Avoid those with active infection. • Report symptoms of bone marrow depression (e.g., bruising, fatigue, fever, shortness of breath, weight loss; bleeding easily, bloody urine or stool). • Report symptoms of lung inflammation (excessive coughing, difficulty breathing, chest pain); heart failure (e.g., chest pain, difficulty breathing, palpitations,

swelling of extremities); liver problems (abdominal pain, bruising, clay-colored stool, amber or dark-colored urine, yellowing of the skin or eyes), UTI (fever, urinary frequency, burning during urination, foul-smelling urine). • Severe allergic reactions, including anaphylaxis, may occur. Difficulty breathing, dizziness, hives, rapid heart rate, rash, swelling of the face or tongue requires immediate medical attention. • Treatment may reduce the heart's ability to pump effectively; expect routine echocardiograms. • Use effective contraception to avoid pregnancy. Do not breastfeed. • Report bleeding of any kind. • Maintain proper hydration and nutrition.

phosphates potassium sodium

HIGH ALERT

fos-fates

◆CLASSIFICATION

PHARMACOTHERAPEUTIC: Electrolyte supplement. **CLINICAL:** Mineral.

USES

Prevention and treatment of hypophosphatemia.

PRECAUTIONS

Contraindications: **K-phosphate:** Hyperkalemia, hyperphosphatemia, hypocalcemia. **Na-phosphate:** Hypocalcemia, hypernatremia, hyperphosphatemia. **Cautions:** Renal impairment, concomitant use of potassium-sparing drugs, acid-base alteration, digitalized pts, cardiac disease, metabolic alkalosis.

ACTION

Active in bone deposition, calcium metabolism, utilization of B complex vitamins. Act as buffers in maintaining acid-base balance. Exert osmotic effect in small intestine. **Therapeutic Effect:** Correct hypophosphatemia, acidify urine, prevent calcium deposits in urinary tract, promote peristalsis in GI tract.

PHARMACOKINETICS

Poorly absorbed after PO administration. PO form excreted in feces; IV form excreted in urine.

⏳ LIFESPAN CONSIDERATIONS

Pregnancy/Lactation: Use caution in pregnant women with other medical conditions (e.g., preeclampsia). **Children:** Increased risk of dehydration in pts younger than 12 yrs. **Elderly:** No age-related precautions noted.

INTERACTIONS

DRUG: May increase concentration/effect of **angiotensin II receptor blockers (e.g., losartan, valsartan), ACE inhibitors (e.g., enalapril, lisinopril). NSAIDs (e.g., ibuprofen, meloxicam, naproxen)** may increase concentration/effect. **Antacids, calcium/magnesium salts, iron preparations** may decrease concentration/effect. **HERBAL:** None significant. **FOOD:** None known. **LAB VALUES:** None significant.

AVAILABILITY (Rx)

Injection Solution: *(Potassium Phosphate):* 3 mmol phosphate and 4.4 mEq potassium per mL. **Injection Solution:** *(Sodium Phosphate):* 3 mmol phosphate and 4 mEq sodium per mL.

ADMINISTRATION/HANDLING

 IV

Reconstitution • Must be diluted. In general, the dose, concentration, and rate of administration may be dependent on institution policy. In pts with renal dysfunction, slower rates (e.g., over 4–6 hrs) is recommended.
Rate of administration • Infuse over minimum of 4 hrs (usually over 6 hrs).
• **Maximum rate:** 0.06 mmol/kg/hr.
Storage • Store at room temperature.

INDICATIONS/ROUTES/DOSAGE

Note: *(K-Phosphate):* For each mmol of phosphate, 1.5 mEq of K will be given. *(Na-Phosphate):* For each mmol of phosphate, 1.3 mEq of Na will be given.

Hypophosphatemia
(Potassium Phosphate): **Phosphate level 2.3–3 mg/dL:** Initially, 0.08–0.16 mmol/kg over 4–6 hrs. **Phosphate level 1.6–2.2 mg/dL:** Initially, 0.16–0.32 mmol/kg over 4–6 hrs. **Phosphate level less than 1.5 mg/dL:** Initially, 0.32–0.64 mmol/kg over 4–6 hrs. *(Sodium phosphate):* **Phosphate level 2.3–3 mg/dL:** Initially, 0.16–0.32 mmol/kg over 4–6 hrs. **Phosphate level 1.6–2.2 mg/dL:** Initially, 0.32–0.64 mmol/kg over 4–6 hrs. **Phosphate level less 1.5 mg/dL or less:** Initially, 0.64–1 mmol/kg over 8–12 hrs.

SIDE EFFECTS

Frequent: Mild laxative effect (in first few days of therapy). **Occasional:** Diarrhea, nausea, abdominal pain, vomiting. **Rare:** Headache, dizziness, confusion, heaviness of lower extremities, fatigue, muscle cramps, paresthesia, peripheral edema, arrhythmias, weight gain, thirst.

ADVERSE EFFECTS/TOXIC REACTIONS

Hyperphosphatemia may produce extraskeletal calcification.

NURSING CONSIDERATIONS

BASELINE ASSESSMENT

Obtain BMP, serum phosphate, ionized calcium. Question history of renal impairment, cardiac disease. Assess hydration status.

INTERVENTION/EVALUATION

Monitor serum phosphate, potassium, calcium.

PATIENT/FAMILY TEACHING

• Report diarrhea, nausea, vomiting.

P

piperacillin/ tazobactam

pye-per-a-**sil**-in/tay-zoe-**bak**-tam
(Zosyn)
**Do not confuse Zosyn with
Zofran or Zyvox.**

◆CLASSIFICATION

PHARMACOTHERAPEUTIC: Penicillin. **CLINICAL:** Antibiotic.

USES

Intra-abdominal infections: Appendicitis (complicated by rupture or abscess) and peritonitis in adults and children 2 mos of age and older caused by β-lactamase–producing strains of *E. coli, Bacteroides fragilis, B. ovatus, B. thetaiotaomicron,* or *B. vulgatus.* **Pelvic infections:** Postpartum endometritis or pelvic inflammatory disease caused by β-lactamase–producing strains of *E. coli.* **Pneumonia:** Community-acquired pneumonia caused by β-lactamase–producing strains of *Haemophilus influenzae.* **Nosocomial pneumonia (moderate to severe):** Infections caused by β-lactamase–producing strains of *S. aureus* and susceptible *Acinetobacter baumanii, Haemophilus influenzae, Klebsiella pneumoniae,* and *P.aeruginosa.* **Skin and skin structure infections:** Including cellulitis, cutaneous abscesses, and ischemic/diabetic foot infections caused by β-lactamase producing strains of *S. aureus.*
OFF-LABEL: Bite wound infections, bloodstream infections (gram-negative bacteremia), cystic fibrosis, malignant (necrotizing) external otitis, neutropenic fever (high risk), sepsis/septic shock, UTIs (complicated).

PRECAUTIONS

Contraindications: Hypersensitivity to piperacillin/tazobactam, any penicillin. **Cautions:** History of allergies (esp. cephalosporins, beta-lactamase inhibitors), renal impairment, seizure disorder.

ACTION

Piperacillin: Inhibits bacterial cell wall synthesis by binding to PCN-binding proteins, which inhibit the final step of peptidoglycan synthesis. **Therapeutic Effect:** Bactericidal. **Tazobactam:** Inactivates bacterial beta-lactamase. **Therapeutic Effect:** Protects piperacillin from enzymatic degradation, extends its spectrum of activity, prevents bacterial overgrowth.

PHARMACOKINETICS

Widely distributed. Protein binding: 16%–30%. Primarily excreted unchanged in urine. Removed by hemodialysis. **Half-life:** 0.7–1.2 hrs (increased in hepatic cirrhosis, renal impairment).

⧗ LIFESPAN CONSIDERATIONS

Pregnancy/Lactation: Readily crosses placenta; appears in cord blood, amniotic fluid. Distributed in breast milk in low concentrations. May lead to allergic sensitization, diarrhea, candidiasis, skin rash in infants. **Children:** Dosage not established for pts younger than 12 yrs. **Elderly:** Age-related renal impairment may require dosage adjustment.

INTERACTIONS

DRUG: May decrease concentration/effects of **aminoglycosides (e.g., gentamicin, tobramycin).** May increase concentration, toxicity of **methotrexate. Probenecid** may increase concentration, risk of toxicity. **HERBAL:** None significant. **FOOD:** None known. **LAB VALUES:** May increase serum sodium, alkaline phosphatase, bilirubin, LDH, ALT, AST, BUN, creatinine, PT, PTT. May decrease serum potassium. May cause positive Coombs' test.

AVAILABILITY (Rx)

◄**ALERT►** Piperacillin/tazobactam is a combination product in an 8:1 ratio of piperacillin to tazobactam. **Injection Powder:** 2.25 g, 3.375 g, 4.5 g. **Premix Ready to Use:** 2.25 g (50 mL), 3.375 g (50 mL), 4.5 g (100 mL).

P

ADMINISTRATION/HANDLING

 IV

Reconstitution • Reconstitute each 1 g with 5 mL D₅W or 0.9% NaCl. Shake vigorously to dissolve. • Further dilute with at least 50 mL D₅W or 0.9% NaCl.

Rate of administration • Infuse over 30 min. Expanded infusion over 3–4 hrs.

Storage • Reconstituted vial is stable for 24 hrs at room temperature or 48 hrs if refrigerated. • After further dilution, stable for 24 hrs at room temperature or 7 days if refrigerated.

▦ IV COMPATIBILITIES

Acetaminophen, calcium gluconate, dexmedetomidine, heparin, magnesium sulfate, potassium chloride.

INDICATIONS/ROUTES/DOSAGE

Extended infusion: ADULTS, ELDERLY: 3.375–4.5 g over 4 hrs q8h.

Usual Dosage

IV: ADULTS, ELDERLY: (Mild to moderate infections): 3.375 g q6h. (Severe infections): 4.5 g q6-8h. (Coverage of *Pseudomonas aeruginosa*): 4.5 g q6h. **Maximum:** 18 g daily. **ADOLESCENTS, CHILDREN, INFANTS:** 240–300 mg piperacillin/kg/day divided in 3–4 doses. **Maximum daily dose:** 16 g/day. **NEONATES:** 80–100 mg piperacillin component/kg/dose q6–8h.

Creatinine Clearance	Dosage
20–40 mL/ min	2.25 g q6h (if usual dose is 3.375g q6h) or 4.5 g q8h or 3.375g q6h (if usual dose is 4.5 g q6h). Extended infusion over 4h (3.375g q8–12h).
Less than 20 mL/ min	2.25 g q8h (if usual dose is 3.375g q6h) or 4.5 g q12h or 2.25 g q6h (if usual dose is 4.5 g q6h). Extended infusion over 4h (3.375g q12h).

Dosage for Hemodialysis

IV: ADULTS, ELDERLY: 2.25 g q12h with additional dose of 0.75 g after each dialysis session.

Dosage for CRRT

CVVH	2.25–3.375 g q6–8h
CVVHD	2.25–3.375 g q6h
CVVHDF	3.375 g q6h

Dosage in Renal Impairment
Dosage and frequency are modified based on creatinine clearance.

Dosage in Hepatic Impairment
No dose adjustment.

SIDE EFFECTS

Frequent: Diarrhea, headache, constipation, nausea, insomnia, rash. **Occasional:** Vomiting, dyspepsia, pruritus, fever, agitation, candidiasis, dizziness, abdominal pain, edema, anxiety, dyspnea, rhinitis.

ADVERSE EFFECTS/TOXIC REACTIONS

Antibiotic-associated colitis, other superinfections (abdominal cramps, severe watery diarrhea, fever) may result from altered bacterial balance in GI tract. Overdose, more often with renal impairment, may produce seizures, neurologic reactions. Severe hypersensitivity reactions, including anaphylaxis, occur rarely.

NURSING CONSIDERATIONS

BASELINE ASSESSMENT

Obtain CBC; LFT in pts with hepatic impairment. Question for history of allergies, esp. to penicillins, cephalosporins.

INTERVENTION/EVALUATION

Monitor daily pattern of bowel activity, stool consistency; mild GI effects may be tolerable, but increasing severity may indicate onset of antibiotic-associated colitis. Be alert for superinfection: Fever, vomiting, diarrhea, anal/genital pruritus, oral mucosal changes (ulceration, pain, erythema). Monitor I&O, urinalysis. Monitor serum electrolytes, esp. potassium, renal function tests.

pirtobrutinib

pir-toe-**broo**-ti-nib
(Jaypirca)

Do not confuse pirtobrutinib with acalabrutinib, ibrutinib, or zanubrutinib, or Jaypirca with Adcirca.

◆CLASSIFICATION

PHARMACOTHERAPEUTIC: Bruton tyrosine kinase (BTK) inhibitor. **CLINICAL:** Antineoplastic.

USES

Mantle cell lymphoma (MCL): Treatment of adults with relapsed or refractory MCL after at least two lines of systemic therapy, including a BTK inhibitor. **Chronic lymphocytic leukemia or small lymphocytic lymphoma (CLL/SLL):** Treatment of adults with chronic CLL/SLL who have received at least two prior lines of therapy, including a BTK inhibitor and a BCL-2 inhibitor.

PRECAUTIONS

Contraindications: Hypersensitivity to pirtobrutinib. **Cautions:** Baseline cytopenias, hepatic/renal impairment, conditions predisposing to infection (e.g., diabetes, renal failure, immunocompromised pts, open wounds), chronic opportunistic infections (e.g., herpes virus infection, hepatitis B virus [HBV] infection, fungal infections), history of cardiac arrhythmia (e.g., atrial fibrillation/flutter, ventricular dysrhythmias); pts at risk for hemorrhage (e.g., history of intracranial/GI bleeding, coagulation disorders, recent trauma).

ACTION

A selective, noncovalent (reversible) BTK inhibitor that binds to Bruton tyrosine kinase (BTK), a signaling molecule that activates the pathways necessary for B-cell proliferation, trafficking, chemotaxis, and adhesion. **Therapeutic Effect:** Decreases malignant B-cell proliferation and tumor growth.

PHARMACOKINETICS

Widely distributed Metabolized in liver. Protein binding: 96%. Peak plasma concentration: 2 hrs. Steady-state reached in 5 days. Excreted in urine (57%), feces (37%). **Half-life:** 19 hrs.

⧗ LIFESPAN CONSIDERATIONS

Pregnancy/Lactation: Avoid pregnancy; may cause fetal harm. Females of reproductive potential must use effective contraception during treatment and for at least 7 days after discontinuation. Unknown if distributed in breast milk. Breastfeeding not recommended during treatment and for at least 1 wk after discontinuation. **Children:** Safety and efficacy not established. **Elderly:** May have increased risk of grade 3 or 4 adverse reactions.

INTERACTIONS

DRUG: **Strong CYP3A4 inhibitors (e.g., clarithromycin, ketoconazole, ritonavir)** may increase concentration/effect. **Strong CYP3A4 inducers (e.g., carBAMazepine, phenytoin, riFAMpin), moderate CYP3A4 inducers (e.g., dexamethasone, modafinil, nafcillin)** may decrease concentration/effect. **Anticoagulants (e.g., apixaban, heparin, warfarin), antiplatelets (e.g., aspirin, ticagrelor), chronic use of NSAIDS (e.g., diclofenac, indomethacin, meloxicam)** may increase risk of bleeding. May increase concentration/effects of **CYP3A4 substrates (e.g., busPIRone, tacrolimus, simvastatin), CYP2C8 substrates (e.g., amiodarone, carBAMazepine, rosiglitazone), CYP2C9 substrates (e.g., warfarin), P-gp substrates (e.g., dilTIAZem, tacrolimus).** **HERBAL:** **St. John's wort** may decrease concentration/effect. **Herbals with anticoagulant/antiplatelet properties (e.g., dong quai, feverfew, garlic, ginger, ginko biloba, white willow)** may increase risk of bleeding. **FOOD:** None known. **LAB VALUES:** May increase serum alkaline phosphatase, ALT, AST, creatinine, lipase. May decrease Hgb, lymphocytes, neutrophils,

P

platelets; serum calcium, sodium. May increase or decrease serum potassium.

AVAILABILITY (Rx)

Tablets: 50 mg, 100 mg.

ADMINISTRATION/HANDLING

PO

• Give without regard to food. • Administer tablet whole with water; do not break, cut, or allow chewing. • If a dose is missed by more than 12 hrs, skip the dose and follow the usual dosing schedule the following day.

INDICATIONS/ROUTES/DOSAGE

MCL (Relapsed or Refractory), CLL/SLL (Chronic)

PO: ADULTS: 200 mg once daily until disease progression or unacceptable toxicity.

Dose Modification

Based on Common Terminology Criteria for Adverse Events (CTCAE).

Grade 3 or 4 nonhematologic toxicities; absolute neutrophil count (ANC) 500-999 cells/mm³ with fever or infection; ANC less than 500 cell/mm³ lasting 7 days or more; platelet count 25,000–49,999 cell/mm³ with bleeding; platelet count less than 25,000 cell/mm³ **(First occurrence):** Withhold treatment until improved to grade 1 or baseline, then resume at 200 mg once daily. **(Second Occurrence):** Withhold treatment until improved to grade 1 or baseline, then resume at 100 mg once daily. **(Third occurrence):** Withhold treatment until improved to grade 1 or baseline, then resume at 50 mg once daily. **(Fourth occurrence):** Permanently discontinue.

Concomitant Use of Strong CYP3A4 Inhibitors

If use of a strong CYP3A4 inhibitor is unavoidable, reduce pirtobrutinib dose by 50 mg. If current dose is 50 mg once daily, withhold treatment until use of the strong CYP3A4 inhibitor is discontinued. If the strong CYP3A4 inhibitor is discontinued for 5 half-lives, resume pirtobrutinib dose prior to use of the strong CYP3A4 inhibitor.

Concomitant Use of Moderate CYP3A4 Inducers

If use of a moderate CYP3A4 inducer is unavoidable and current pirtobrutinib dose is 200 mg once daily, increase pirtobrutinib dose to 300 mg once daily. If current pirtobrutinib dose is 50 mg or 100 mg once daily, increase the dose by 50 mg.

Dosage in Renal Impairment

Mild to moderate impairment: No dose adjustment. **Severe impairment:** If current dose is 200 mg once daily, reduce dose to 100 mg once daily. Otherwise, reduce dose by 50 mg. If the current dosage is 50 mg once daily, permanently discontinue.

Dosage in Hepatic Impairment

No dose adjustment.

SIDE EFFECTS

Note: Frequency and occurrence of side effects vary based on indication of treatment. **Frequent (36%–21%):** Fatigue, bruising, cough, musculoskeletal pain, diarrhea, abdominal pain, dyspnea, dyspnea, edema, nausea. **Occasional (20%–10%):** Pyrexia, headache, rash, peripheral neuropathy, arthralgia, dizziness, constipation, insomnia, mucositis, hypertension, confusion, mental status change, decreased appetite, tachycardia.

ADVERSE EFFECTS/TOXIC REACTIONS

Myelosuppression (hemoglobinemia, lymphopenia, neutropenia, thrombocytopenia) is an expected response to therapy, but more severe reactions including febrile neutropenia, hemorrhagic thrombocytopenia may occur. Life-threatening bacterial, invasive fungal, viral; other opportunistic infections may occur. Grade

3 or 4 infections reported in 24% of pts. Life-threatening hemorrhagic events including intracranial hemorrhage, GI bleeding may occur. Grade 3 or 4 hemorrhage reported in 3% of pts. Grade 3 or 4 atrial fibrillation/atrial flutter reported in 2% of pts. New primary malignancies including non-melanoma skin cancer, melanoma, solid tumors (GU/breast cancers) have occurred. Life-threatening hepatotoxicity, hepatic injury may occur. Falls reported in 14% of pts. Renal insufficiency (renal failure, acute kidney injury) may occur.

NURSING CONSIDERATIONS

BASELINE ASSESSMENT

Obtain CBC; PT/INR (if on anticoagulation therapy); pregnancy test in female of reproductive potential. Confirm compliance of effective contraception. Assess risk for bleeding. Question history of atrial fibrillation, atrial flutter, cardiac disease; intracranial/GI/genitourinary bleeding, coagulation disorders, recent trauma; previous skin cancers. Assess usual bowel movement patterns, stool characteristics. Receive full medication history and screen for interactions. Screen for active infection. Consider prophylactic treatment of chronic or opportunistic infections. Due to increased risk of bleeding, weight the benefit-risk of withholding treatment for 3–7 days before or after surgery. Offer emotional support.

INTERVENTION/EVALUATION

Monitor CBC periodically for cytopenia. Monitor for infections (cough, fever, fatigue, nausea, vomiting), esp. respiratory tract infections, herpes virus infection, opportunistic infections, sepsis. If serious infection or sepsis occurs, initiate appropriate antimicrobial therapy. Monitor for HBV reactivation, new malignancies (skin and nonskin cancers). Obtain ECG if chest pain, dyspnea, palpitations occur.

Monitor for acute kidney injury (dark-colored urine, flank pain, decreased urine output, muscle aches), hemorrhagic events including intracranial hemorrhage (altered mental status, aphasia, blindness, facial drooping, hemiparesis, unequal pupils, seizures), GI bleeding (hematemesis, melena, rectal bleeding), genitourinary bleeding (hematuria), epistaxis. Monitor daily pattern of bowel activity, stool consistency. Monitor for drug toxicities if discontinuation or dose reduction of concomitant CYP3A4 inhibitor is unavoidable.

PATIENT/FAMILY TEACHING

• Treatment may depress your immune system and reduce your ability to fight infection. Report symptoms of infection such as body aches, burning with urination, chills, cough, fatigue, fever. Avoid those with active infection. • Report symptoms of bone marrow depression such as bruising, fatigue, fever, shortness of breath, weight loss; bleeding easily, bloody urine or stool. • Treatment may cause new cancers (skin and nonskin). • Report liver problems (abdominal pain, bruising, clay-colored stool, amber or dark colored urine, yellowing of the skin or eyes), kidney problems (decreased urine output, dark-colored urine, edema), heart arrhythmias (chest pain, dizziness, fainting, palpitations, slow or rapid heart rate, irregular heart rate); symptoms of hemorrhagic stroke (confusion, difficulty speaking, one-sided weakness or paralysis, loss of vision, seizures), bleeding of any kind. • Use effective contraception to avoid pregnancy. Do not breastfeed. • There is a high risk of interactions with other medications. Do not take newly prescribed medications unless approved by prescriber who originally started therapy. • Avoid herbal supplements. • Avoid tasks that require alertness, motor skills such as driving or operating machinery until response to drug is established.

pomalidomide

poe-ma-**lid**-oh-mide
(Pomalyst)

■ **BLACK BOX ALERT** ■ May cause life-threatening birth defects. Pregnancy contraindicated. Exclude pregnancy before initiating treatment. Females of reproductive potential must use two reliable forms of contraception or continuously abstain during treatment and for 4 wks after treatment. Deep vein thrombosis and pulmonary embolism may occur. Consider venous thromboembolism (VTE) prophylaxis during treatment.

◆**CLASSIFICATION**

PHARMACOTHERAPEUTIC: Angiogenesis inhibitor. **CLINICAL**: Antineoplastic.

USES

Multiple myeloma: Treatment of multiple myeloma (in combination with dexA-METHasone) in pts who have received at least two prior therapies including lenalidomide and a proteasome inhibitor and who have demonstrated disease progression on or within 60 days of completion of the last therapy. **Kaposi's sarcoma:** Treatment of adults with AIDS-related Kaposi sarcoma (KS) after failure of highly active antiretroviral therapy (HAART) or in pts with KS who are HIV negative.

PRECAUTIONS

◄**ALERT**► Do not donate blood products during therapy and for 1 month after therapy discontinuation; male pts must not donate sperm.
Contraindications: Hypersensitivity to pomalidomide. Pregnancy. **Cautions:** Anemia, HF, hepatic/renal impairment, smoking, breastfeeding, or prior history of CVA, MI, DVT, PE.

ACTION

Inhibits tumor cell proliferation and induces apoptosis (cell death) of hematopoietic cells. Enhances T-cell–and natural killer (NK) cell–mediated immunity. Inhibits proinflammatory cytokines. **Therapeutic Effect:** Inhibits tumor cell growth and metastasis.

PHARMACOKINETICS

Widely distributed. Metabolized in liver. Protein binding: 12%–44%. Peak plasma concentration: 2–3 hrs. Excreted in urine (73%), feces (15%). **Half-life:** 8–10 hrs.

⧗ LIFESPAN CONSIDERATIONS

Pregnancy/Lactation: Pregnancy/breastfeeding contraindicated. May cause fetal harm. Unknown if distributed in breast milk. Do not breastfeed. Must verify negative pregnancy status before initiation. Must use two reliable forms of birth control (intrauterine device [IUD], tubal ligation) plus barrier methods. Avoid pregnancy for at least 4 wks after discontinuation. **Males:** Must use condoms during treatment and up to 1 mo after treatment, despite prior history of vasectomy. Do not donate sperm. **Children:** Safety and efficacy not established. **Elderly:** May have increased risk of serious adverse effects, renal failure, electrolyte imbalance.

INTERACTIONS

DRUG: May decrease the therapeutic effect; increase adverse effects of **vaccines (live)**. **HERBAL: Echinacea** may decrease therapeutic effect. **FOOD:** None significant. **LAB VALUES:** May decrease Hgb, Hct, neutrophils, platelets, leukocytes, lymphocytes, serum calcium, potassium, sodium. May increase serum calcium, creatinine, glucose.

AVAILABILITY (Rx)

🖉 **Capsules:** 1 mg, 2 mg, 3 mg, 4 mg.

ADMINISTRATION/HANDLING

PO
• May be given without regard to food. • Administer whole with water. Do not break, open, or allow chewing.

INDICATIONS/ROUTES/DOSAGE

Multiple Myeloma

Note: Absolute neutrophil count (ANC) should be 500 cells/mm³ or greater and platelet count 50,000 cells/mm³ or greater prior to starting new cycles of therapy.

PO: ADULTS/ELDERLY: 4 mg once daily on days 1–21 of 28-day cycle (in combination with dexAMETHasone. Continue until disease progression or unacceptable toxicity.

Kaposi Sarcoma

PO: ADULTS: 5 mg once daily on days 1–21 of a 28-day cycle. Continue until disease progression or unacceptable toxicity. Continue HAART as HIV treatment in pts with AIDS-related Kaposi sarcoma.

Dose Modification

Neutropenia

ANC less than 500 cells/mm³ or febrile neutropenia: Withhold treatment until ANC is greater than 500 cells/mm³, then reduce dose to 3 mg once daily. **Any subsequent drop of ANC less than 500 cells/mm³ after prior reduction:** Withhold treatment until ANC is greater than 500 cells/mm³, then reduce dose by 1 mg less than previous dose. Discontinue if 1-mg dose is intolerable.

Thrombocytopenia

Platelet count less than 25,000 cells/mm³: Withhold treatment until platelet count greater than 50,000 cells/mm³, then reduce dose to 3 mg once daily. **Any subsequent platelet drop to less than 25,000 cells/mm³:** Withhold treatment until platelet count greater than 50,000 cells/mm³, then reduce dose by 1 mg less than previous dose. Discontinue if 1-mg dose is intolerable.

Dosage in Renal Impairment

Avoid use in pts with serum creatinine more than 3 mg/dL or CrCl less than 45 mL/min.

Dosage in Hepatic Impairment

Avoid use in pts with serum bilirubin more than 2 mg/dL and ALT, AST more than 3 times upper limit of normal (ULN).

SIDE EFFECTS

Frequent (55%–22%): Fatigue, constipation, nausea, diarrhea, dyspnea, back pain, peripheral edema, musculoskeletal chest pain, anorexia, rash. **Occasional (20%–7%):** Dizziness, pyrexia, muscle spasms, arthralgia, pruritus, vomiting, cough, weight loss, headache, bone pain, muscular weakness, anxiety, musculoskeletal pain, peripheral neuropathy, chills, dry skin, tremor, insomnia. **Rare (6%–1%):** Hyperhidrosis, extremity pain, back pain, night sweats, constipation.

ADVERSE EFFECTS/TOXIC REACTIONS

Myelosuppression (neutropenia, leukopenia, thrombocytopenia) is an expected outcome of therapy; may increase risk of infection such as pneumonia, upper respiratory tract infection, UTI. Neurologic events such as acute confusion, dizziness reported. Peripheral neuropathy occurred in 18% of pts. Venous thromboembolism including DVT, PE occurred in 3% of pts. Epistaxis occurred in 15% of pts. Increased risk of secondary malignancies reported. Acute renal failure reported in 16% of pts. Additional adverse events may include interstitial lung disease (ILD), neutropenic sepsis, *Pneumocystis jiroveci* pneumonia, respiratory syncytial virus infection, urinary retention, vertigo.

NURSING CONSIDERATIONS

BASELINE ASSESSMENT

Obtain CBC, BMP; pregnancy test in females of reproductive potential. Receive full medication history. Obtain baseline neurologic exam. Question history of diabetes mellitus, electrolyte imbalance,

 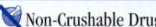

hepatic/renal impairment, pulmonary disease, thromboembolism, smoking.

INTERVENTION/EVALUATION

Monitor CBC, BMP. Obtain ECG for palpitations, chest pain, hypokalemia, hyperkalemia, hypocalcemia, bradycardia, ventricular arrhythmias. Immediately report dyspnea, chest pain, hypoxia, unilateral peripheral edema/pain (may indicate thromboembolic event). Perform routine neurologic assessments to screen for confusion, delirium. Monitor urine output, frequency.

PATIENT/FAMILY TEACHING

• Treatment may depress your immune system response and reduce your ability to fight infection. Report symptoms of infection such as body aches, chills, cough, fatigue, fever. Avoid those with active infection. • Report symptoms of bone marrow depression (e.g., bruising, fatigue, fever, shortness of breath, weight loss; bleeding easily, bloody urine or stool). • Do not donate blood. • Use effective contraception to avoid pregnancy. Do not breastfeed. • Go from lying to standing slowly (prevents postural hypotension, dizziness). Avoid tasks that require alertness, motor skills until response to drug is established. • Do not smoke. • Do not eat 2 hrs before or 2 hrs after dose. • Avoid alcohol. • Report difficulty breathing, chest pain, extremity pain or swelling, dizziness, confusion.

---

ponatinib

poe-**na**-ti-nib
(Iclusig)

■**BLACK BOX ALERT**■ Arterial occlusions have occurred, including CVA, fatal MI, large arterial vessel stenosis of the brain, severe peripheral vascular disease requiring revascularization. Events may occur in pts with or without cardiovascular risks, including pts younger than 50 yrs of age. Venous thromboembolism, serious HF, or left ventricular dysfunction were reported. Hepatotoxicity, including fatal hepatic failure, may occur.

Do not confuse ponatinib with afatinib, alectinib, dasatinib, bosutinib, gefitinib, imatinib, lapatinib, lenvatinib, neratinib, or tofacitinib.

◆**CLASSIFICATION**

PHARMACOTHERAPEUTIC: BCR-ABL tyrosine kinase inhibitor. **CLINICAL:** Antineoplastic.

USES

Philadelphia chromosome–positive acute lymphoblastic leukemia (Ph+ ALL): Newly diagnosed Ph+ ALL, in combination with chemotherapy. As monotherapy in Ph+ ALL for whom no other kinase inhibitors are indicated or T315I-positive Ph+ ALL. **Chronic myeloid leukemia (CML):** Chronic phase (CP) CML with resistance or intolerance to at least two prior kinase inhibitors. Accelerated phase (AP) or blast phase (BP) CML for whom no other kinase inhibitors are indicated. T315I-positive CML (chronic phase, accelerated phase, or blast phase). Not indicated for treatment of newly diagnosed chronic phase CML.

PRECAUTIONS

Contraindications: Hypersensitivity to ponatinib. **Cautions:** Baseline cytopenias; conditions predisposing to infection (e.g., diabetes, immunocompromised pts, open wounds), history of arterial/venous thrombosis (e.g., CVA, DVT, MI, PE), cardiac disease, cardiac conduction disorders, HF, hypertension; diabetes, electrolyte imbalance, glaucoma, hepatic impairment, hyperlipidemia, GI perforation, neuropathy (peripheral or cranial), ocular disorders, pancreatitis or alcohol abuse, history of ischemia, vascular stenosis; pts with high tumor burden; pts at risk for hemorrhage (e.g., history of intracranial/GI bleeding, coagulation disorders, recent trauma; concomitant use of anticoagulants, antiplatelets, NSAIDs).

ACTION

Inhibits viability of cells expressing native or mutant BCR-ABL tyrosine kinase, including T315I mutation, created by the Philadelphia chromosome abnormality. **Therapeutic Effect:** Inhibits tumor cell growth and metastasis.

PHARMACOKINETICS

Widely distributed. Metabolized in liver. Protein binding: Greater than 99%. Peak plasma concentration: 6 hrs or less. Excreted in feces (87%), urine (5%). **Half-life:** 24 hrs (**Range:** 12–66 hrs).

⧖ LIFESPAN CONSIDERATIONS

Pregnancy/Lactation: Avoid pregnancy; may cause fetal harm/malformations. Unknown if distributed in breast milk. Breastfeeding not recommended during treatment and for at least 6 days after discontinuation. Females of reproductive potential and males with female partners of reproductive potential should use effective contraception during treatment and for at least 3 wks after discontinuation. May impair fertility in females. **Children:** Safety and efficacy not established. **Elderly:** May have increased risk of adverse reactions/toxic effects. Use caution.

INTERACTIONS

DRUG: Strong **CYP3A4 inhibitors** (e.g., **clarithromycin, ketoconazole, ritonavir**) may increase concentration/effect. Strong **CYP3A4 inducers** (e.g., **carBAMazepine, phenytoin, rifAMPin**) may decrease concentration/effect. May decrease therapeutic effect of BCG **(intravesical), vaccines (live).**

HERBAL: Echinacea may decrease therapeutic effect. **FOOD: Grapefruit products** may increase concentration/effect. **LAB VALUES:** May increase serum alkaline phosphatase, amylase, ALT, AST, bilirubin, creatinine, lipase, triglycerides, uric acid. May decrease Hgb, Hct, leukocytes, lymphocytes, neutrophils, platelets; serum albumin, bicarbonate, phosphate. May increase or decrease serum calcium, glucose, potassium, sodium.

AVAILABILITY (Rx)

Tablets: 10 mg, 15 mg, 30 mg, 45 mg.

ADMINISTRATION/HANDLING

PO
• Give without regard to food. • Administer tablets whole; do not break, cut, or crush.

INDICATIONS/ROUTES/DOSAGE

Ph+ ALL (Newly Diagnosed)
PO: ADULTS, ELDERLY: Initially, 30 mg once daily, in combination with chemotherapy, with a reduction to 15 mg once daily upon achievement of MRD-negative (less than or equal to 0.01% BCR::ABL1/ABL1) CR at the end of induction.

Ph+ ALL (Monotherapy)
PO: ADULTS, ELDERLY: Initially, 45 mg once daily.

CP-CML
PO: ADULTS, ELDERLY: Initially, 45 mg once daily with a reduction to 15 mg once daily upon achievement of less than or equal to 1% BCR::ABL1.

AP-CML, BP-CML
PO: ADULTS, ELDERLY: Initially, 45 mg once daily.

Dose Modification
Based on Common Terminology for Adverse Events (CTCAE).

Hepatotoxicity
Grade 2 or greater serum ALT/AST elevation: Withhold treatment until

improved to Grade 1 or 0, then resume dose based on occurrence. **Occurrence at 45-mg dose:** Resume treatment at 30-mg dose. **Occurrence at 30-mg dose:** Resume treatment at 15-mg dose. **Occurrence at 15-mg dose:** Permanently discontinue. **Serum ALT/AST elevation greater than or equal to 3 times ULN with concurrent serum bilirubin elevation greater than 2 times ULN and serum alkaline phosphatase less than 2 times ULN:** Permanently discontinue.

Neutropenia/Thrombocytopenia
ANC less than 1,000 cells/mm³; platelet count less than 50,000 cells/mm³: Withhold treatment until ANC greater than or equal to 1,500 cells/mm³; or platelet count greater than or equal to 75,000 cells/mm³, then resume dose based on occurrence. **First occurrence:** Resume treatment at 45-mg dose. **Second occurrence:** Resume treatment at 30-mg dose. **Third occurrence:** Resume treatment at 15-mg dose.

Pancreatitis/Elevated Lipase
Asymptomatic Grade 1 or 2 serum lipase elevation: Consider withholding treatment or reducing dose. **Asymptomatic Grade 3 or 4 serum lipase elevation; asymptomatic radiologic pancreatitis (Grade 2 pancreatitis):** Withhold treatment until improved to Grade 1 or 0, then resume dose based on occurrence. **Occurrence at 45-mg dose:** Resume treatment at 30-mg dose. **Occurrence at 30-mg dose:** Resume treatment at 15-mg dose. **Occurrence at 15-mg dose:** Permanently discontinue. **Grade 4 pancreatitis:** Permanently discontinue.

Concomitant Use of Strong CYP3A4 Inhibitors
Reduce initial dose to 30 mg.

Dosage in Renal Impairment
Not specified; use caution.

Dosage in Hepatic Impairment
Mild to severe impairment: Reduce initial dose to 30 mg.

SIDE EFFECTS
Note: Percentages of side effects of chronic phase, accelerated phase, blast phase CML; Ph+ ALL may vary.
Frequent (69%–18%): Hypertension, abdominal pain, fatigue, asthenia, headache, dry skin, constipation, arthralgia, nausea, pyrexia, burning sensation, hyperesthesia, hypoesthesia, neuralgia, paresthesia, dysgeusia, muscular weakness, gait disturbance, areflexia, hypotonia, restless legs syndrome, myalgia, extremity pain, back pain, diarrhea, vomiting. **Occasional (17%–2%):** Dyspnea, dizziness, peripheral edema, cough, bone pain, musculoskeletal pain, mucositis, aphthous stomatitis, lip blister, mouth ulceration, mucosal eruption, oral pain, oropharyngeal pain, stomatitis, tongue ulceration, muscle spasm, conjunctival irritation, corneal abrasion/erosion, dry eye, hyperemia, eye pain, pruritus, decreased appetite, insomnia, decreased weight, generalized pain, erythema, alopecia, chills, blurry vision, tachycardia.

ADVERSE EFFECTS/TOXIC REACTIONS
Myelosuppression (anemia, leukopenia, neutropenia, thrombocytopenia) is an expected response to therapy, but more severe reactions including bone marrow failure, febrile neutropenia may be life-threatening. Fatal arterial occlusions including CVA, MI, stenosis of large arterial vessel of the brain, severe peripheral vascular disease requiring revascularization reported in 35% of pts; may occur within 2 wks of initiation (even at reduced doses of 15 mg/day). Coronary artery occlusion, MI occurred in 21% of pts. Venous thromboembolism (DVT, PE, superficial thrombophlebitis) occurred in 5%–9% of pts. Life-threatening events including cardiac bradyarrhythmias (requiring pacemaker implantation), complete heart block, sick sinus syndrome, atrial fibrillation with bradycardic pauses, atrial fibrillation, SVT, ventricular tachycardia; emergent hypertension (68% of pts), GI/intracranial hemorrhage (28% of

pts), hepatotoxicity (54% of pts), pancreatitis (6%), HF, left ventricular dysfunction (6% of pts); infections including cellulitis, nasopharyngitis, pneumonia, sepsis, upper respiratory tract infection, UTI; ocular toxicities including blindness, conjunctival hemorrhage, cataracts, periorbital edema, ocular hyperemia, iritis, iridocyclitis, ulcerative keratinitis; peripheral edema (31% of pts), pleural effusion (2% of pts), pericardial effusion (1% of pts); peripheral neuropathy, polyneuropathy, nerve compression (20% of pts) may occur. Tumor lysis syndrome may present as acute renal failure, hypocalcemia, hyperuricemia, hyperphosphatemia. Reversible posterior leukoencephalopathy may include aphasia, cognition impairment, paralysis, vision loss, weakness. Pts with newly diagnosed CML have an increased risk of severe toxicities. Improper wound healing, GI perforation may occur.

NURSING CONSIDERATIONS

BASELINE ASSESSMENT

Obtain CBC, BMP, LFT, serum ionized calcium, phosphate, uric acid; vital signs; weight. Obtain pregnancy test in females of reproductive potential. Receive full medication history including herbal products and screen for interactions. Question history as listed in Precautions. Screen for active infection. Conduct ophthalmologic, neurologic exam. Due to increased risk of tumor lysis syndrome, assess adequate hydration prior to initiation. Consider correcting electrolyte abnormalities prior to initiation. Obtain dietary consult. Screen for risk of bleeding; active infection. Assess skin for rash, lesions. Offer emotional support.

INTERVENTION/EVALUATION

Obtain ANC, CBC for myelosuppression q2wks for 3 mos, then monthly thereafter. Monitor serum lipase monthly; BMP, LFT, serum ionized calcium, phosphate, uric acid as indicated. Monitor ECG for cardiac arrhythmias. Due to extremely high risk for arterial occlusions, be vigilant when screening for CVA (aphasia, confusion, paresthesia, hemiparesis, seizures), MI (chest pain, diaphoresis, left arm/jaw pain, increased serum troponin, ST segment elevation), vascular compromise. Be alert for serious infection, opportunistic infection, sepsis. Monitor for GI perforation, hepatotoxicity, ocular disease, pancreatitis; symptoms of thromboembolism (arm/leg pain, swelling; chest pain, dyspnea, hypoxia, tachycardia), reversible posterior leukoencephalopathy, tumor lysis syndrome; other toxicities as listed in Adverse Reactions/Toxic Effects. Monitor daily pattern of bowel activity, stool consistency. Ensure adequate hydration, nutrition. Monitor weight, I&O.

PATIENT/FAMILY TEACHING

• Treatment may depress your immune system response and reduce your ability to fight infection. Report symptoms of infection such as body aches, chills, cough, fatigue, fever. Avoid those with active infection. • Report symptoms of bone marrow depression (e.g., bruising, fatigue, fever, shortness of breath, weight loss; bleeding easily, bloody urine or stool). • Life-threatening arterial blood clots may occur; report symptoms of heart attack (chest pain, difficulty breathing, jaw pain, nausea, pain that radiates to the left arm, sweating), stroke (blindness, confusion, one-sided weakness, loss of consciousness, trouble speaking, seizures). • Report symptoms of DVT (swelling, pain, hot feeling in the arms or legs), lung embolism (difficulty breathing, chest pain, rapid heart rate); liver problems (abdominal pain, bruising, clay-colored stool, amber or dark-colored urine, yellowing of the skin or eyes); HF (difficulty breathing, extremity swelling, sudden loss of breath, palpitations); inflammation of the pancreas (abdominal bruising; persistent, severe abdominal pain that radiates to the back [with or without vomiting]); eye problems (blindness, blurred vision, eye inflammation or bleeding, severe eye or head pain); heart arrhythmias (chest pain, dizziness, fainting, palpitations, slow or rapid heart rate, irregular heart rate); intestinal perforation

P

(severe abdominal pain, fever, nausea). • Use effective contraception to avoid pregnancy. Do not breastfeed. • Report planned surgical/dental procedures. • Immediately report bleeding of any kind. • Do not ingest grapefruit products, herbal supplements. • Do not take newly prescribed medications unless approved by the prescriber who originally started treatment.

ponesimod

poe-**nes**-i-mod
(Ponvory)
Do not confuse ponesimod with fingolimod, siponimod, or ozanimod.

◆CLASSIFICATION

PHARMACOTHERAPEUTIC: Sphingosine 1-phosphate (S1P) receptor-1 modulator. **CLINICAL:** Multiple sclerosis agent.

USES

Treatment of relapsing forms of multiple sclerosis (MS) in adults, including clinically isolated syndrome, relapsing-remitting disease, and active secondary progressive disease.

PRECAUTIONS

Contraindications: Hypersensitivity to ponesimod. Myocardial infarction, unstable angina, stroke, transient ischemic attack, decompensated heart failure requiring hospitalization, or Class III or IV heart failure in the last 6 mos. Sick sinus syndrome, Mobitz type II second- or third-degree AV block (unless pt has a functioning pacemaker). **Cautions:** Conditions predisposing to infection (e.g., diabetes, immunocompromised pts, renal failure, open wounds), baseline sinus bradycardia, hepatic impairment, hypertension, altered pulmonary function, pts at risk for developing AV block (e.g., congenital heart disease, ischemic heart disease, HF), pts at risk for macular edema (e.g., diabetes, history of uveitis). Concomitant use of antiarrhythmics, beta blockers, calcium channel blockers, immunosuppressants, immune modulators, antineoplastics, QT interval–prolonging medications. Not recommended in pts with severe active infection; history of cardiac arrest, cerebrovascular disease, uncontrolled hypertension; severe, untreated sleep apnea unless approved by a cardiologist.

ACTION

Binds with high affinity to S1P receptor, blocking capacity of lymphocytes to move out from lymph nodes, reducing the number of lymphocytes available to the CNS. **Therapeutic Effect:** May involve reduction of lymphocyte migration into the CNS, reducing inflammation.

PHARMACOKINETICS

Widely distributed. Metabolized in liver. Protein binding: 99%. Peak plasma concentration: 4 hrs. Excreted in feces (57%–80%), urine (10%–18%). Not removed by hemodialysis. **Half-life:** 33 hrs.

⧗ LIFESPAN CONSIDERATIONS

Pregnancy/Lactation: Avoid pregnancy; may cause fetal harm. Females of reproductive potential should use effective contraception during treatment and for 1 wk after the last ponesimod dose. Unknown if distributed in breast milk. **Children, Elderly:** Safety and efficacy not established.

INTERACTIONS

DRUG: Strong CYP3A4 inducers (e.g., carBAMazepine, phenytoin, rifAMPin) may decrease concentration/effect. **Beta-blockers (e.g., carvedilol, metoprolol)** may increase risk of AV block, bradycardia. **Class Ia antiarrhythmics (e.g., procainamide,**

quinidine), **Class III antiarrhythmics (e.g., amiodarone, sotalol)** may increase risk of torsades de pointes in pts with baseline sinus bradycardia. May increase QT interval–prolonging effect of **amiodarone, azithromycin, ciprofloxacin, haloperidol**. May decrease therapeutic effect of **vaccines (live)**. May increase toxic effect of **vaccines (live)**. May increase immunosuppressive effect of **alemtuzumab. HERBAL: Echinacea** may decrease therapeutic effect. **FOOD:** None known. **LAB VALUES:** May increase serum ALT, AST, cholesterol, C-reactive protein. Expected to cause a dose-dependent reduction in peripheral lymphocyte count from baseline values.

AVAILABILITY (Rx)

Tablets: 2 mg, 3 mg, 4 mg, 5 mg, 6 mg, 7 mg, 8 mg, 9 mg, 10 mg, 20 mg.

ADMINISTRATION/HANDLING

PO

• Give without regard to food. • Starter pack must be used as a 14-day titration prior to maintenance doses. • Interruption during titration is not recommended. If fewer than 4 consecutive doses are missed during titration, resume treatment with the first missed dose. If fewer than 4 consecutive doses are missed during maintenance, continue maintenance dose. If 4 or more consecutive doses are missed (titration or maintenance), restart titration with starter pack. • Administer tablet whole.

INDICATIONS/ROUTES/DOSAGE

Multiple Sclerosis (Relapsing)

PO: **ADULTS:** Titrate as follows: **Days 1–2:** 2 mg once daily. **Days 3–4:** 3 mg once daily. **Days 5–6:** 4 mg once daily. **Day 7:** 5 mg (single dose). **Day 8:** 6 mg (single dose). **Day 9:** 7 mg (single dose). **Day 10:** 8 mg (single dose). **Day 11:** 9 mg (single dose). **Days 12–14:** 10 mg once daily. **Maintenance:** 20 mg once daily starting on day 15.

Dosage in Renal Impairment
No dose adjustment.

Dosage in Hepatic Impairment
Mild impairment: No dose adjustment. **Moderate to severe impairment:** Not specified; use caution.

SIDE EFFECTS

Occasional (10%): Hypertension. **Rare (5%–2%):** Dyspnea, dizziness, cough, extremity pain, somnolence, pyrexia, vertigo.

ADVERSE EFFECTS/TOXIC REACTIONS

Life-threatening infections may occur. Fatal cases of cryptococcal meningitis, disseminated cryptococcal infections were reported. Herpes zoster infections reported in 5% of pts. Reactivation of herpes viral infection may cause herpes simplex encephalitis and varicella zoster meningitis. Progressive multifocal leukoencephalopathy (PML), an opportunistic viral infection of the brain caused by the JC virus, may result in progressive permanent disability and death. Respiratory tract infections, including bronchitis, laryngitis, pharyngitis, pneumonia, nasopharyngitis, sinusitis, tracheitis, reported in 37% of pts. Urinary tract infection (UTI) reported in 6% of pts. Posterior reversible encephalopathy syndrome, a dysfunction of the brain that may evolve into an ischemic CVA or cerebral hemorrhage, may occur. Macular edema reported in 2% of pts. Pts with diabetes or history of uveitis are at an increased risk for developing macular edema. AV conduction delays, bradycardia reported in 6% of pts. Dose-dependent reductions of pulmonary function (absolute forced expiratory volume over 1 second) reported in 4%–8% of pts. Hepatotoxicity reported in 5% of pts. Seizures reported in 2% of pts. May increase risk of hypertensive crisis. Cutaneous malignancies, including basal cell carcinoma, melanoma, squamous cell carcinoma, were reported. Rebound or severe exacerbation of MS symptoms may occur after discontinuation.

P

NURSING CONSIDERATIONS

BASELINE ASSESSMENT

Obtain CBC, LFT, ECG. Assess baseline symptoms of MS (e.g., bladder/bowel dysfunction, cognitive impairment, depression, dysphagia, fatigue, gait disorder, numbness/tingling, pain, seizures, spasticity, tremors, weakness). Consultation with a cardiologist is advised in pts with QT interval prolongation greater than 500 msec; arrhythmias requiring treatment with Class Ia or Class III antiarrhythmics; unstable ischemic heart disease, HF, uncontrolled hypertension, history of cardiac arrest, CVA or TIA (greater than 6 mos); history of Mobitz type II second- or third-degree AV block, sick sinus syndrome, sinoatrial heart block. First-dose monitoring is recommended in pts with preexisting cardiac conditions (baseline sinus bradycardia, first- or second-degree [Mobitz type I], history of MI [greater than 6 mos], HF) in a medical setting that can adequately treat symptomatic bradycardia. Pts without a documented history of vaccination against varicella zoster or a confirmed history of varicella infection (chickenpox) should be tested for antibodies prior to initiation. A full vaccination course for varicella in antibody-negative pts is recommended. Perform baseline ophthalmologic evaluation of the fundus (including the macula). Receive full medication history and screen for interaction (esp. antineoplastics, immunosuppressants; drugs known to cause bradycardia, AV conduction delay). Question history as listed in Precautions. Screen for active infection.

INTERVENTION/EVALUATION

Monitor LFT if hepatotoxicity (bruising, jaundice, right upper abdominal pain, nausea, vomiting, weight loss) is suspected. At initial treatment (within first 4–6 hrs after dose), therapy reduces heart rate, AV conduction. In pts with preexisting cardiac conditions, monitor for symptomatic bradycardia for at least 6 hrs after first dose with hourly pulse, B/P, then obtain ECG at the end of day 1. If heart rate is less than 45 beats/min, QTc interval is 500 msec or greater, or new-onset second-degree (or higher) AV block is present after first dose, continue monitoring until resolved. If intervention is required, continue heart monitoring overnight and repeat 4-hr monitoring after second dose. Conduct ophthalmic examination with any change of vision. Pts with altered mental status, seizures, visual disturbances, unilateral weakness should be evaluated for cryptococcal meningitis, varicella zoster meningitis, posterior reversible encephalopathy syndrome, PML. Persistent immunosuppressive effects may occur after discontinuation. Closely monitor for adverse effects if other immunosuppressants are initiated after discontinuation. Monitor for infections (cough, fatigue, fever, urinary frequency), esp. herpetic infections, respiratory tract infections, sepsis. Monitor B/P for hypertension. Assess skin for malignancies, new lesions. Conduct neurological assessment. Assess for improvement of MS symptoms.

PATIENT/FAMILY TEACHING

• Treatment may depress the immune system and reduce ability to fight infection. Report symptoms of infection such as body aches, burning with urination, chills, cough, fatigue, fever. Avoid those with active infection. • Any change of vision will require an immediate eye examination. • PML, an opportunistic viral infection of the brain, may cause progressive, permanent disabilities or death. Report symptoms of PML such as confusion, memory loss, paralysis, trouble speaking, vision loss, seizures, weakness. • Treatment may worsen high blood pressure or cause skin cancers. • Report liver problems (abdominal pain, bruising, clay-colored stool, amber or dark-colored urine, yellowing of the skin or eyes), lung problems (reduced lung function, shortness of breath), heart arrhythmias (chest pain, dizziness, fainting, palpitations, slow or irregular heart rate). • Posterior reversible encephalopathy syndrome, a dysfunction of the brain that may cause a stroke or bleeding in the brain, may occur. • Use effective contraception to avoid pregnancy. • Due to high risk of interactions, do not take newly prescribed medications unless approved by the prescriber who originally started treatment. • Do not receive live vaccines within 4 wks of initiation. • Avoid prolonged sun exposure/tanning beds. Use high SPF sunscreen, lip balm, clothing to protect against sunburn/skin irritation. • Severe worsening of MS symptoms may occur after stopping treatment.

---

potassium acetate

HIGH ALERT

potassium chloride

(Kaon-Cl, Klor-Con, <u>Klor-Con M10</u>, <u>Klor-Con M20</u>, Micro-K)
Do not confuse Micro-K with Macrobid or Micronase.

◆CLASSIFICATION

PHARMACOTHERAPEUTIC: Electrolyte. **CLINICAL:** Potassium replenisher.

USES

Potassium acetate: Treatment, prevention of hypokalemia when necessary to avoid chloride or acid/base imbalance (requires additional source of bicarbonate). **Potassium chloride:** Treatment of hypokalemia.

PRECAUTIONS

Contraindications: Acetate: Severe renal impairment, adrenal insufficiency, hyperkalemia. **Chloride:** Renal failure, hyperkalemia, conditions in which potassium retention is present. Solid oral dosage form in pts in whom there is structural, pathologic cause for delay in passage through GI tract. **Cautions:** Cardiac disease, acid-base disorders, potassium-altering disorders, digitalized pts, concomitant therapy that increases serum potassium (e.g., ACE inhibitors), renal impairment. Do not administer IV undiluted.

ACTION

Necessary for multiple cellular metabolic processes. Primary action is intracellular. **Therapeutic Effect:** Required for nerve impulse conduction, contraction of cardiac, skeletal, smooth muscle; maintains normal renal function, acid-base balance.

PHARMACOKINETICS

Well absorbed from GI tract. Enters cells by active transport from extracellular fluid. Primarily excreted in urine.

⧖ LIFESPAN CONSIDERATIONS

Pregnancy/Lactation: Unknown if drug crosses placenta or is distributed in breast milk. **Children:** No age-related precautions noted. **Elderly:** May be at increased risk for hyperkalemia. Age-related ability to excrete potassium is reduced.

INTERACTIONS

DRUG: May increase concentration/effect of **ACE inhibitors (e.g., enalapril, lisinopril), angiotensin II receptor blockers (e.g., losartan, valsartan), spironolactone, triamterene.** **HERBAL:** None significant. **FOOD:** None known. **LAB VALUES:** None known.

AVAILABILITY (Rx)

Potassium Acetate
Injection Solution: 2 mEq/mL.
Potassium Chloride
Injection Solution: 2 mEq/mL. **Oral Solution:** 20 mEq/15 mL, 40 mEq/15 mL. **Powder for Oral Solution:** 20 mEq/packet.
Capsules, Extended-Release: 8 mEq, 10 mEq. **Tablets, Extended-Release:** 8 mEq, 10 mEq, 15 mEq, 20 mEq.

ADMINISTRATION/HANDLING

 IV

Reconstitution • For IV infusion only, must dilute before administration, mix well, infuse slowly. • Avoid adding potassium to hanging IV.

Rate of administration • Routinely, give at concentration of no more than 40 mEq/L, no faster than 10 mEq/hr for peripheral infusion, 20–40 mEq/hr for central infusion. Refer to specific institution policy.

Storage • Store at room temperature. Use admixtures within 24 hrs.

PO
• Take with or after meals, with full glass of water (decreases GI upset). No more than 40 mEq should be given as single dose. • Liquids, powder, effervescent tablets: Mix, dissolve with juice, water before administering. • Do not break, crush, dissolve, or divide tablets; give whole.

▓ IV COMPATIBILITIES

Acetaminophen, calcium gluconate, clevidipine, dexmedetomidine, heparin, ibuprofen, magnesium sulfate, norepinephrine, propofol.

INDICATIONS/ROUTES/DOSAGE

Treatment of Hypokalemia
Note: Dosage is dependent on the age, weight, and clinical condition of the pt and laboratory determinations.
Potassium Acetate
IV: ADULTS, ELDERLY: Serum potassium 2.5–3.5 mEq/L: (maximum infusion rate): 10 mEq/hr; (maximum concentration): 40 mEq/L; **(Maximum):** 200 mEq/24h. **Serum potassium less than 2.5 mEq/L:** (maximum infusion rate): 40 mEq/hr (central line only).
INFANTS, CHILDREN, ADOLESCENTS: 0.5–1 mEq/kg/dose. (maximum infusion rate): 0.5 mEq/kg/hour or less. **(Maximum):** 40 mEq/dose.
Potassium Chloride
Note: Dosage is dependent on the age, weight, and clinical conditions of the pt and laboratory determinations.

PO: ADULTS, ELDERLY: Mild to moderate: (Serum potassium 3–3.4 mEq/L): Initially, 10–20 mEq given 2–4 times/day. (Maximum single dose): 40 mEq.
INFANTS, CHILDREN, ADOLESCENTS: 1–2 mEq/kg/day in divided doses. (Maximum single dose): 40 mEq.
IV: ADULTS, ELDERLY: 10 mEq/hr (or less); repeat as needed based on lab values. **INFANTS, CHILDREN, ADOLESCENTS:** 0.5–1 mEq/kg/dose **(Maximum:** 40 mEq); repeat as needed based on lab values.

Dosage in Renal/Hepatic Impairment
No dose adjustment. Use caution with potassium acetate (may increase serum aluminum and/or potassium).

SIDE EFFECTS

Occasional: Nausea, vomiting, diarrhea, flatulence, abdominal discomfort with distention, phlebitis with IV administration (particularly when potassium concentration of greater than 40 mEq/L is infused). **Rare:** Rash.

ADVERSE EFFECTS/TOXIC REACTIONS

Hyperkalemia (more common in elderly, pts with renal impairment) manifested as paresthesia, motor weakness, cold skin, hypotension, confusion, irritability, paralysis, cardiac arrhythmias. Too-rapid infusion may cause cardiac arrhythmia, ventricular fibrillation, cardiac arrest.

NURSING CONSIDERATIONS

BASELINE ASSESSMENT
Assess for hypokalemia (weakness, fatigue, polyuria, polydipsia). PO form should be given with food or after meals with full glass of water, fruit juice (minimizes GI irritation).

INTERVENTION/EVALUATION
Monitor serum potassium, calcium, phosphate. If GI disturbance occurs, dilute preparation further or give with meals. Monitor for decreased urinary output (may be indication of renal insufficiency). Check IV site closely

P

during infusion for evidence of phlebitis (heat, pain, red streaking of skin over vein, hardening of vein), extravasation (swelling, pain). Be alert to evidence of hyperkalemia (skin pallor/coldness, paresthesia, feeling of heaviness of lower extremities).

PATIENT/FAMILY TEACHING

• Report symptoms of high potassium levels (irregular heartbeat, muscle weakness, nausea, numbness, tingling).

pralsetinib

pral-**se**-ti-nib
(Gavreto)
Do not confuse pralsetinib with pazopanib, pemigatinib, pexidartinib, ponatinib, pralatrexate, ripretinib, or selpercatinib.

◆CLASSIFICATION

PHARMACOTHERAPEUTIC: *RET* kinase inhibitor. **CLINICAL:** Antineoplastic.

USES

Non–small-cell lung cancer (NSCLC): Treatment of adults with metastatic rearranged during transfection (RET) fusion-positive NSCLC. **Thyroid cancer:** Treatment of advanced or metastatic *RET* fusion-positive thyroid cancer in pediatric pts 12 yrs of age and older and adults who require systemic therapy and who are radioactive iodine–refractory (if radioactive iodine is appropriate).

PRECAUTIONS

Contraindications: Hypersensitivity to pralsetinib. **Cautions:** Baseline cytopenias, hepatic impairment, hypertension, conditions predisposing to infection (e.g., diabetes, immunocompromised pts, renal failure, open wounds); pts at risk for bleeding (e.g., history of intracranial/GI/GU bleeding, coagulation

disorders, recent trauma), interstitial lung disease (e.g., COPD, sarcoidosis, connective disease disease), tumor lysis syndrome (high tumor burden), poor wound healing (e.g., recent or planned surgery, chronic open wounds). Withhold treatment for at least 5 days prior to elective surgery or for at least 2 wks after major surgery and until wound is fully healed. Do not initiate in pts with uncontrolled hypertension. Avoid concomitant use of strong CYP3A4 inducers; combined P-gp and strong CYP3A4 inhibitors.

ACTION

Inhibits wild-type *RET*, oncogenic *RET* fusions, and *RET* mutations Certain activating point mutations in *RET* or chromosomal rearrangements involving in-frame fusions of *RET* can result in constitutively activated chimeric *RET* fusion proteins, which may act as oncogenic drivers, promoting tumor cell line proliferation. **Therapeutic Effect:** Demonstrates anti-tumor activity in cells harboring oncogenic *RET* fusions or mutations.

PHARMACOKINETICS

Widely distributed. Metabolized in liver. Protein binding: 97%. Peak plasma concentration: 2–4 hrs. Steady state reached in 3–5 days. Excreted in feces (73%), urine (6%). **Half-life:** 15.7 hrs.

⚕ LIFESPAN CONSIDERATIONS

Pregnancy/Lactation: Avoid pregnancy; may cause fetal harm. Females of reproductive potential must use effective, nonhormonal contraception during treatment and for at least 2 wks after discontinuation. Unknown if distributed in breast milk. Breastfeeding not recommended during treatment and for at least 2 mos after discontinuation. May impair fertility. **Males:** Males with female partners of reproductive potential must use effective contraception during treatment and for at least 1 wk after dis-

P

continuation. May impair fertility. **Children:** Safety and efficacy not established in pts younger than 12 yrs. **Elderly:** No age-related precautions noted.

INTERACTIONS

DRUG: **Strong CYP3A4 inhibitors (e.g., clarithromycin, ketoconazole, ritonavir), P-gp inhibitors (e.g., amiodarone, azithromycin, cyclosporine, dilTIAZem, verapamil)** may increase concentration/effect. **Strong CYP3A4 inducers (e.g., carBAMazepine, phenytoin, ri-fAMPin)** may decrease concentration/effect. **HERBAL:** None significant. **FOOD:** None known. **LAB VALUES:** May increase serum alkaline phosphatase, ALT, AST, bilirubin, creatinine, potassium. May decrease serum albumin, calcium, magnesium, phosphate, sodium; Hgb, lymphocytes, neutrophils, platelets.

AVAILABILITY (Rx)

 Capsules: 100 mg.

ADMINISTRATION/HANDLING

PO

• Give on empty stomach (no food for at least 2 hrs prior to or at least 1 hr after dose). • Administer capsules whole; do not break, cut, or crush. • Capsules cannot be chewed. • If a dose is missed, give as soon as possible on the same day. • If vomiting occurs after administration, give the next dose at regularly scheduled time (do not give additional dose).

INDICATIONS/ROUTES/DOSAGE

NSCLC (Metastatic RET Fusion-Positive), Thyroid Cancer (Advanced, Metastatic RET Fusion-Positive)
PO: ADULTS, CHILDREN 12 YRS OR OLDER: 400 once daily. Continue until disease progression or unacceptable toxicity.

Dose Reduction Schedule

First reduction: 300 mg once daily. **Second reduction:** 200 mg once daily. **Third reduction:** 100 mg once daily.

Unable to tolerate 100-mg dose: Permanently discontinue.

Dose Modification

Based on Common Terminology Criteria for Adverse Events (CTCAE).

Hepatotoxicity

Grade 3 or 4 hepatotoxicity: Withhold treatment until improved to Grade 1 or baseline, then resume at a reduced dose. Permanently discontinue if Grade 3 or 4 hepatotoxicity recurs.

Hemorrhagic Events

Grade 3 or 4 hemorrhage: Withhold treatment until improved to Grade 1 or 0. **Severe or life-threatening hemorrhage:** Permanently discontinue

Hypertension

Grade 3 hypertension (despite optimal hypertensive therapy): Withhold treatment until adequately controlled, then resume at reduced dose level. **Grade 4 hypertension:** Permanently discontinue.

Pulmonary Toxicity

Grade 1 or 2 ILD/pneumonitis: Withhold treatment until resolved, then resume at reduced dose. Permanently discontinue if ILD/pneumonitis recurs.

Other Toxicities

Any other Grade 3 or 4 toxicities: Withhold treatment until improved to Grade 2 or less, then resume at reduced dose level. Permanently discontinue if Grade 4 toxicity recurs.

Concomitant Use of Combined P-gp and Strong CYP3A4 Inhibitors

Note: If concomitant use of combined P-gp and strong CYP3A4 inhibitor is unavoidable, reduce pralsetinib dose as follows: **Current 400-mg dose:** Reduce dose to 200 mg once daily. **Current 300-mg dose:** Reduce dose to 200 mg once daily. **Current 200-mg dose:** Reduce dose to 100 mg once daily. If CYP3A4 inhibitor is discontinued for 3–5 half-lives, may resume dose prior to starting combined P-gp and strong CYP3A4 inhibitor.

Concomitant Use of Strong CYP3A4 Inducers

If concomitant use of strong CYP3A4 inducer is unavoidable, increase starting pralsetinib dose to double the current dose starting on day 7. If CYP3A4 inducer is discontinued for at least 14 days, may resume dose prior to starting strong CYP3A4 inducer.

Dosage in Renal Impairment
Not specified; use caution.

Dosage in Hepatic Impairment
Mild impairment: No dose adjustment. **Moderate to severe impairment:** Not specified; use caution.

SIDE EFFECTS

Note: Frequency and occurrence of side effects may vary based on treatment as monotherapy or in combination with other therapies.

Frequent (42%–22%): Musculoskeletal pain, constipation, hypertension, diarrhea, abdominal pain, dry mouth, stomatitis, mucosal inflammation, tongue ulceration, nausea, fatigue, asthenia, edema (eyelid, face, periorbital, peripheral), cough, headache, rash, eczema, migraine, pyrexia, dyspnea. **Occasional (20%–15%):** Peripheral neuropathy, dysesthesia, neuralgia, paresthesia, polyneuropathy, dizziness, vertigo, dysgeusia, decreased appetite.

ADVERSE EFFECTS/TOXIC REACTIONS

Myelosuppression (anemia, lymphopenia, neutropenia, thrombocytopenia) is an expected response to therapy. Life-threatening ILD/pneumonitis reported in 10% of pts. Grade 3 hypertension reported in 14% of pts. Serum ALT, AST elevation reported in 69% and 46% of pts, respectively. Serious hepatotoxicity reported in 2% of pts. Grade 3 or 4 hemorrhagic events reported in 3% of pts. Tumor lysis syndrome may present as acute renal failure, hypocalcemia,

hyperuricemia, hyperphosphatemia. May cause impaired wound healing or wound dehiscence requiring medical intervention. Pneumonia reported in 17% of pts. Palmar-plantar erythro-dysesthesia syndrome (PPES), a chemotherapy-induced skin condition that presents with skin redness, swelling, numbness, sloughing of the hands and feet, may occur.

NURSING CONSIDERATIONS

BASELINE ASSESSMENT
Obtain CBC, BMP, LFT, B/P; pregnancy test in females of reproductive potential. Confirm compliance of effective nonhormonal contraception. Verify presence of a *RET* gene fusion (NSCLC, thyroid cancer) or specific *RET* gene mutation (MTC) in tumor specimens or plasma. Due to increased risk of tumor lysis syndrome, routinely assess hydration. Conduct dermatological exam; assess for open wounds, lesions, surgical incisions. Question history of hepatic impairment, hemorrhagic events, hypertension, recent surgery. Receive full medication history and screen for interactions. Screen for active infection. Offer emotional support.

INTERVENTION/EVALUATION
Monitor CBC for myelosuppression periodically; LFT for hepatotoxicity (bruising, jaundice, right upper abdominal pain, nausea, vomiting, weight loss) q2wks for 3 mos, then monthly thereafter. If Grade 3 or 4 hepatotoxicity occurs, monitor LFT wkly until improved. Obtain serum uric acid level if tumor lysis syndrome (acute renal failure, electrolyte imbalance, cardiac arrhythmias, seizures) is suspected. Monitor B/P 1 wk after initiation, then at least monthly thereafter. If indicated, consider antihypertensive therapy. Monitor for infections (cough, fatigue, fever). Consider ABG, radiologic test if pneumonitis (excessive cough, dyspnea, fever, hypoxia) is suspected. Consider

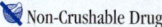

treatment with corticosteroids if pneumonitis is confirmed. Monitor for drug toxicities if discontinuation or dose reduction of concomitant CYP3A4 inhibitor, P-gp inhibitor is unavoidable. Assess skin for impaired wound healing, rash, PPES. Monitor daily pattern of bowel activity, stool consistency.

PATIENT/FAMILY TEACHING

• Treatment may depress the immune system response and reduce ability to fight infection. Report symptoms of infection such as body aches, chills, cough, fatigue, fever. Avoid those with active infection. • Report symptoms of bone marrow depression such as bruising, fatigue, fever, shortness of breath, weight loss; bleeding easily, bloody urine or stool. • Therapy may cause tumor lysis syndrome (a condition caused by the rapid breakdown of cancer cells), which can cause kidney failure and can be fatal. Report decreased urination, amber-colored urine; confusion, difficulty breathing, fatigue, fever, muscle or joint pain, palpitations, seizures, vomiting. • Report liver problems (abdominal pain, bruising, clay-colored stool, amber or dark-colored urine, yellowing of the skin or eyes), inflammation of the lung (excessive cough, difficulty breathing, chest pain), toxic skin reactions (sloughing, rash, poor healing of wounds). • Life-threatening bleeding may occur; report bloody stool, urine; rectal bleeding, nosebleeds, vomiting blood. • There is a high risk of interactions with other drugs. Do not take newly prescribed medications unless approved by prescriber who originally started treatment. Avoid grapefruit products, herbal supplements. • Use effective, nonhormonal contraception to avoid pregnancy. Do not breastfeed. Fertility may be impaired. • Notify physician before any planned surgeries/dental procedures. • Dose must be taken on an empty stomach.

pramipexole

pram-i-**pex**-ole
(Apo-Pramipexole ✶, Mirapex ER)
Do not confuse Mirapex with Mifeprex or MiraLax.

◆CLASSIFICATION

PHARMACOTHERAPEUTIC: DOPamine receptor agonist. **CLINICAL:** Antiparkinson agent.

USES

Immediate-release: Treatment of Parkinson's disease, moderate to severe primary restless legs syndrome. **Extended-release:** Treatment of Parkinson's disease.

PRECAUTIONS

Contraindications: Hypersensitivity to pramipexole. **Cautions:** History of orthostatic hypotension, pts at risk for hypotension, syncope, hallucinations, renal impairment (extended-release not recommended with CrCl less than 30 mL/min), concomitant use of CNS depressants, preexisting dyskinesia, elderly pts.

ACTION

Stimulates DOPamine receptors in striatum and substantia nigra. **Therapeutic Effect:** Relieves signs/symptoms of Parkinson's disease. Improves motor function.

PHARMACOKINETICS

Widely distributed. Protein binding: 15%. Steady-state concentrations achieved within 2 days. Primarily excreted in urine. Not removed by hemodialysis. **Half-life:** 8 hrs (12 hrs in pts older than 65 yrs).

⧗ LIFESPAN CONSIDERATIONS

Pregnancy/Lactation: Unknown if drug is distributed in breast milk. **Children:** Safety and efficacy not established. **Elderly:** Increased risk of hallucinations.

INTERACTIONS

DRUG: Antipsychotic agents (e.g., haloperidol) may decrease therapeutic effect. May increase concentration/effect of **levodopa-containing products. HERBAL: Herbals with hypotensive properties (e.g., garlic, ginger, ginkgo biloba)** may increase hypotensive effect. **Kava kava** may increase concentration/effect. **FOOD:** None known. **LAB VALUES:** None significant.

AVAILABILITY (Rx)

Tablets: 0.125 mg, 0.25 mg, 0.5 mg, 0.75 mg, 1 mg, 1.5 mg.

 Tablets, Extended-Release: (Mirapex ER): 0.375 mg, 0.75 mg, 1.5 mg, 2.25 mg, 3 mg, 3.75 mg, 4.5 mg.

ADMINISTRATION/HANDLING

PO

• Give without regard to food. Administer with food to decrease nausea. • **(Extended-Release):** Give once daily, without regard to food. • Give whole; do not break, crush, dissolve, or divide tablets.

INDICATIONS/ROUTES/DOSAGE

Parkinson's Disease

Note: When discontinuing, reduce dose by 0.75 mg/day until daily dose is 0.75 mg once daily, then reduce by 0.375 mg/day thereafter.

PO: (Immediate-Release): **ADULTS, ELDERLY:** Initially, 0.125 mg 3 times/day. Increase gradually (e.g., 0.125 mg/dose) no more frequently than every 5–7 days. **Usual dose:** 1.5–4.5 mg/day in divided doses. **Maximum:** 4.5 mg/day. **(Extended-Release):** Initially, 0.375 mg once daily. May increase by 0.375 mg no more frequently than 5–7 days. **Usual dose:** 1.5–4.5 mg once daily. **Maximum:** 4.5 mg once daily. **Note:** May switch overnight from immediate-release to extended-release at same daily dose.

Restless Legs Syndrome

Note: When discontinuing, gradually reduce dose q4–7 days.

PO: ADULTS, ELDERLY: (Immediate-Release): Initially, 0.125 mg once daily 2–3 hrs before bedtime. May increase to 0.25 mg after 4–7 days, then to 0.5 mg after 4–7 days (interval is 14 days in pts with renal impairment). **Maximum:** 0.75 mg/day.

Dosage in Renal Impairment

Dosage and frequency are modified based on creatinine clearance.

Parkinson's Disease

Immediate-Release

Creatinine Clearance	Initial Dosage	Maximum Dosage
30–50 mL/min	0.125 mg twice daily	0.75 mg 3 times/day
15–29 mL/min	0.125 mg once daily	1.5 mg once daily

Extended-Release

CrCl 30–50 mL/min: Initially, 0.375 mg every other day. May increase by 0.375 mg/day in 7 days or longer. **Maximum:** 2.25 mg once daily. **CrCl less than 30 mL/min:** Not recommended.

Dosage in Hepatic Impairment

No dose adjustment.

SIDE EFFECTS

Frequent: Early Parkinson's disease (28%–10%): Nausea, asthenia, dizziness, drowsiness, insomnia, constipation. **Advanced Parkinson's disease (53%–17%):** Orthostatic hypotension, extrapyramidal reactions, insomnia, dizziness, hallucinations. **Occasional: Early Parkinson's disease (5%–2%):** Edema, malaise, confusion, amnesia, akathisia, anorexia, dysphagia, peripheral edema, vision changes, impotence. **Advanced Parkinson's disease (10%–7%):** Asthenia, drowsiness, confusion, constipation, abnormal gait, dry mouth. **Rare: Advanced Parkinson's disease (6%–2%):** General edema, malaise, angina, amnesia, tremor, urinary frequency/incontinence, dyspnea, rhinitis, vision changes. **Restless legs syndrome: Frequent (16%):** Headache, nausea. **Occasional (13%–9%):** Insomnia, fatigue. **Rare (6%–3%):** Drowsiness, constipation, diarrhea, dry mouth.

ADVERSE EFFECTS/TOXIC REACTIONS

Vascular disease, atrial fibrillation, arrhythmias, pulmonary embolism, impulsive/compulsive behavior (pathological gambling, hypersexuality, binge eating) have been reported.

NURSING CONSIDERATIONS

BASELINE ASSESSMENT

Parkinson's disease: Assess for tremor, muscle weakness and rigidity, ataxia. **Restless legs syndrome:** Assess frequency of symptoms, sleep pattern.

INTERVENTION/EVALUATION

Assess for clinical improvement. Assist with ambulation if dizziness occurs. Assess for constipation; encourage fiber, fluids, exercise.

PATIENT/FAMILY TEACHING

• Hallucinations may occur, esp. in the elderly. • Go from lying to standing slowly. • Avoid tasks that require alertness, motor skills until response to drug is established. • If nausea occurs, take medication with food. • Avoid abrupt withdrawal. • Avoid alcohol. • Report new or increased impulsive/compulsive behaviors (e.g., gambling, sexual urges, compulsive eating or buying).

---

pravastatin

pra-va-sta-tin
Do not confuse pravastatin with atorvastatin, lovastatin, nystatin, pitavastatin, or simvastatin.

FIXED-COMBINATION(S)

Pravigard: pravastatin/aspirin (anticoagulant): 20 mg/81 mg, 40 mg/81 mg, 80 mg/81 mg, 20 mg/325 mg, 40 mg/325 mg, 80 mg/325 mg.

CLASSIFICATION

PHARMACOTHERAPEUTIC: Hydroxymethylglutaryl CoA (HMG-CoA) reductase inhibitor. **CLINICAL:** Antihyperlipidemic.

USES

Primary hypercholesterolemia: Adjunct to dietary therapy to reduce elevated total cholesterol (total-C), LDL-C, apoB, and triglyceride levels and to increase HDL-C in pts with primary hypercholesterolemia (heterozygous, familial and nonfamilial) and mixed dyslipidemia in adults. **Heterozygous familial hypercholesterolemia:** Adjunct to diet in children and adolescents aged 8 yrs of age and older with heterozygous familial hypercholesterolemia if LDL-C is 190 mg/dL or above or 160 mg/dL or above with family history of premature cardiovascular disease or presence of two or more cardiovascular risk factors. **Homozygous familial hypercholesterolemia:** Adjunct to other lipid-lowering treatments to reduce total-C and LDL-C in adults with homozygous familial hypercholesterolemia. **Prevention of atherosclerotic cardiovascular disease:** To reduce the risk of myocardial infarction (MI), stroke, revascularization procedures, and angina in adults with a history of coronary heart disease (CHD) and in adults without a history of CHD, but who have multiple CHD risk factors. **OFF-LABEL:** Transplantation (post heart or kidney). Certain immunosuppressives can induce or exacerbate hypercholesterolemia.

PRECAUTIONS

Contraindications: Hypersensitivity to pravastatin. Active hepatic disease or unexplained, persistent elevations of LFT results. Pregnancy, breastfeeding. **Cautions:** Hepatic impairment, substantial alcohol consumption. Withholding/discontinuing pravastatin may be necessary when pt is at risk for renal failure secondary to rhabdomyolysis, elderly.

ACTION

Interferes with cholesterol biosynthesis by preventing conversion of HMG-CoA

---

reductase to mevalonate, a precursor to cholesterol. **Therapeutic Effect:** Lowers LDL, VLDL cholesterol, plasma triglycerides; increases HDL.

PHARMACOKINETICS

Widely distributed. Protein binding: 50%. Metabolized in liver. Primarily excreted in feces. Not removed by hemodialysis. **Half-life:** 2–3 hrs. (Half-life including all metabolites: 77 hrs.)

⧗ LIFESPAN CONSIDERATIONS

Pregnancy/Lactation: Contraindicated in pregnancy (suppression of cholesterol biosynthesis may cause fetal toxicity) and lactation. Small amount is distributed in breast milk, but there is risk of serious adverse reactions in breastfeeding infants. Breastfeeding not recommended. **Children/Elderly:** No age-related precautions noted.

INTERACTIONS

DRUG: CycloSPORINE, clarithromycin, colchicine, erythromycin, gemfibrozil, niacin may increase concentration/effect. Bile acid sequestrants (e.g., cholestyramine) may decrease absorption. **HERBAL:** None significant. **FOOD:** Red yeast rice contains 2.4 mg lovastatin per 600 mg rice (may increase adverse effects). **LAB VALUES:** May increase serum creatine kinase (CK), transaminase.

AVAILABILITY (Rx)

Tablets: 10 mg, 20 mg, 40 mg, 80 mg.

ADMINISTRATION/HANDLING

PO

• Give without regard to food.

INDICATIONS/ROUTES/DOSAGE

◄**ALERT**► Prior to initiating therapy, pt should be on standard cholesterol-lowering diet for 3–6 mos. Low-cholesterol diet should be continued throughout pravastatin therapy.

Hyperlipidemia, Prevention of Coronary/Cardiovascular Events

PO: ADULTS, ELDERLY: 40–80 mg once daily.

Heterozygous Familial Hypercholesterolemia

PO: CHILDREN 14–18 YRS: 40 mg/day. **CHILDREN 8–13 YRS:** 20 mg/day.

Dose Modification

Dosage With Clarithromycin
Maximum: 40 mg/day.

Dosage With CycloSPORINE
ADULTS, ELDERLY: Initially, 10 mg/day. **Maximum:** 20 mg/day.

Dosage in Renal Impairment
For adults, give 10 mg/day initially. Titrate to desired response.

Dosage in Hepatic Impairment
See contraindications.

SIDE EFFECTS

Occasional (7%–4%): Nausea, vomiting, diarrhea, constipation, abdominal pain, headache, rhinitis, rash, pruritus. **Rare (3%–2%):** Heartburn, myalgia, dizziness, cough, fatigue, flu-like symptoms, depression, photosensitivity.

ADVERSE EFFECTS/TOXIC REACTIONS

Musculoskeletal effects, including myopathy, rhabdomyolysis, immune-mediated necrotizing myopathy, may occur. Pancreatitis, hepatitis, cholestatic jaundice, fatty liver, cirrhosis, fulminant hepatic necrosis, hepatoma, hepatic failure were reported. May increase fasting serum glucose, Hbg A1c. Cognitive impairment (memory loss, forgetfulness, amnesia, memory impairment, confusion) may occur.

NURSING CONSIDERATIONS

BASELINE ASSESSMENT

Obtain lipid panel, LFT; pregnancy test in females of reproductive potential. Obtain dietary history, esp. fat consumption.

INTERVENTION/EVALUATION

Monitor serum cholesterol, triglycerides for therapeutic response. Monitor LFT. Monitor daily pattern of bowel activity, stool consistency. Assess for rash, pruritus. Be alert for malaise, muscle cramping/

P

weakness; if accompanied by fever, may require discontinuation of medication.

PATIENT/FAMILY TEACHING

• Follow special diet (important part of treatment). • Report promptly any muscle pain/weakness, esp. if accompanied by fever, malaise. • Use effective contraception to avoid pregnancy. • Avoid direct exposure to sunlight.

prednisoLONE

pred-**niss**-oh-lone
(Millipred, Orapred ODT, Pred Forte, Pred Mild)
Do not confuse prednisoLONE with predniSONE or primidone.

FIXED-COMBINATION(S)

Blephamide: prednisoLONE/sulfacetamide (an anti-infective): 0.2%/10%.
Vasocidin: prednisoLONE/sulfacetamide: 0.25%/10%.

◆CLASSIFICATION

PHARMACOTHERAPEUTIC: Adrenal corticosteroid. **CLINICAL:** Anti-inflammatory, immunosuppressant.

USES

Systemic: Anti-inflammatory/immunosuppressant including allergic, autoimmune, endocrine, dermatologic, GI disease, hematologic, neoplastic, neurologic rheumatic, solid organ rejection. **Ophthalmic:** Treatment of conjunctivitis, corneal injury (from chemical/thermal burns, foreign body). **OFF-LABEL:** Bell's palsy, COPD (acute exacerbation), Duchenne muscular dystrophy, hepatitis (autoimmune), Kawasaki disease, myasthenia gravis (crises), pericarditis (acute/recurrent), *Pneumocystitis* pneumonia, urticaria (chronic spontaneous).

PRECAUTIONS

Contraindications: Hypersensitivity to prednisoLONE. Acute superficial herpes simplex keratitis, systemic fungal infections, varicella, live or attenuated virus vaccines. **Cautions:** Hyperthyroidism, cirrhosis, ocular herpes simplex, respiratory tuberculosis, untreated systemic infections, renal/hepatic impairment, diabetes, cataracts, glaucoma, seizure disorder, peptic ulcer disease, osteoporosis, myasthenia gravis, hypertension, HF, ulcerative colitis, thromboembolic disorders, elderly.

ACTION

Inhibits accumulation of inflammatory cells at inflammation sites, phagocytosis, lysosomal enzyme release/synthesis, release of mediators of inflammation. **Therapeutic Effect:** Prevents/suppresses cell-mediated immune reactions. Decreases/prevents tissue response to inflammatory process.

PHARMACOKINETICS

Protein binding: 65%–91%. Metabolized in liver. Excreted in urine. **Half-life:** 3.6 hrs.

⧖ LIFESPAN CONSIDERATIONS

Pregnancy/Lactation: Crosses placenta. Distributed in breast milk. Fetal cleft palate often occurs with chronic, first-trimester use. Breastfeeding not recommended. **Children:** Prolonged treatment or high dosages may decrease short-term growth rate, cortisol secretion. **Elderly:** May be more susceptible to developing hypertension or osteoporosis.

INTERACTIONS

DRUG: CYP3A4 inducers (e.g., carBAMazepine, phenytoin, rifAMPin) may decrease effects. May increase concentration/adverse effects of **vaccines (live), warfarin.** May decrease therapeutic effect of **aldesleukin, vaccines (live).** May increase hyponatremic effect of **desmopressin.** **HERBAL:** Echinacea may decrease ther-

P

apeutic effect. **FOOD:** None known. **LAB VALUES:** May increase serum glucose, lipids, sodium, uric acid. May decrease serum calcium, WBC, hypothalamic pituitary adrenal (HPA) axis function, potassium.

AVAILABILITY (Rx)

Solution, Ophthalmic: 1%. **Solution, Oral:** 15 mg/5 mL, 5 mg/5 mL, 10 mg/5 mL, 20 mg/5 mL, 25 mg/5 mL. **Suspension, Ophthalmic:** 1%, 0.12%. **Tablets:** 5 mg.

Tablets, Orally Disintegrating: 10 mg, 15 mg, 30 mg.

ADMINISTRATION/HANDLING
PO
* Give with food or fluids to decrease GI side effects.

Orally Disintegrating Tablets
* Do not break, crush, or divide tablets. * Remove from blister just prior to giving; place on tongue. * Pt may swallow whole or allow to dissolve in mouth with/without water.

Ophthalmic
* For ophthalmic solution, shake well before using. * Instill drops into conjunctival sac, as prescribed. * Avoid touching applicator tip to conjunctiva to avoid contamination.

INDICATIONS/ROUTES/DOSAGE
Usual Dosage
PO: ADULTS, ELDERLY: 10–60 mg/day as a single daily dose or in 2–4 divided doses. **(Low dose):** 2.5–10 mg/day. **(High dose):** 1–1.5 mg/kg/day (usually not to exceed 80–100 mg/day). **CHILDREN:** 0.1–2 mg/kg/day in divided doses 1–4 times/day.

Treatment of Conjunctivitis, Corneal Injury
Ophthalmic: ADULTS, ELDERLY, CHILDREN: *(Solution):* 1–2 drops every hr during day and q2h during night. After response, decrease dosage to 1 drop q4h, then 1 drop 3–4 times/day. *(Suspension):* 1–2 drops 2–4 times daily.

Dosage in Renal/Hepatic Impairment
No dose adjustment.

SIDE EFFECTS
Frequent: Insomnia, heartburn, nervousness, abdominal distention, diaphoresis, acne, mood swings, increased appetite, facial flushing, delayed wound healing, increased susceptibility to infection, diarrhea, constipation. **Occasional:** Headache, edema, change in skin color, frequent urination. **Rare:** Tachycardia, allergic reaction (rash, urticaria), psychological changes, hallucinations, depression. **Ophthalmic:** Stinging/burning, posterior subcapsular cataracts.

ADVERSE EFFECTS/TOXIC REACTIONS
Long-term therapy: Hypocalcemia, hypokalemia, muscle wasting (esp. arms, legs), osteoporosis, spontaneous fractures, amenorrhea, cataracts, glaucoma, peptic ulcer, HF, immunosuppression. **Abrupt withdrawal following long-term therapy:** Anorexia, nausea, fever, headache, severe/sudden joint pain, rebound inflammation, fatigue, weakness, lethargy, dizziness, orthostatic hypotension. Sudden discontinuance may be fatal.

NURSING CONSIDERATIONS

BASELINE ASSESSMENT
Question medical history as listed in Precautions. Obtain height, weight, B/P, serum glucose, electrolytes. Check results of initial tests (tuberculosis [TB] skin test, X-rays, ECG).

INTERVENTION/EVALUATION
Monitor B/P, weight, serum electrolytes, glucose, results of bone mineral density test, height, weight in children. Be alert to infection (sore throat, fever, vague symptoms); assess oral cavity daily for signs of *Candida* infection. Monitor for symptoms of adrenal insufficiency, immunosuppression.

P

PATIENT/FAMILY TEACHING

* Report fever, sore throat, muscle aches, sudden weight gain, swelling, loss of appetite, fatigue. * Avoid alcohol, limit caffeine. * Do not abruptly discontinue without physician's approval. * Avoid exposure to chickenpox, measles. * Long-term use may significantly increase risk of serious infections.

---

prednISONE

pred-ni-sone
(Apo-PredniSONE ✦, PredniSONE Intensol, Rayos, Winpred ✦)
Do not confuse prednISONE with methylPREDNISolone, prazosin, prednisoLONE, PriLOSEC, primidone, or promethazine.

◆CLASSIFICATION

PHARMACOTHERAPEUTIC: Adrenal corticosteroid. **CLINICAL:** Anti-inflammatory, immunosuppressant.

USES

Anti-inflammatory/immunosuppressant including allergic, autoimmune, endocrine, dermatologic, GI diseases, hematologic, neoplastic, neurologic rheumatic, solid organ rejection. **OFF-LABEL:** Alcoholic hepatitis, Bell's palsy, COPD (acute exacerbation), COVID-19, Duchenne muscular dystrophy, giant cell arteritis, graft-versus-host disease, hepatitis (autoimmune), Kawasaki disease, multiple myeloma (previously untreated), myasthenia gravis, prostate cancer (metastatic, castration-resistant), urticaria (chronic spontaneous).

PRECAUTIONS

Contraindications: Hypersensitivity to prednISONE. Acute superficial herpes simplex keratitis, systemic fungal infections, varicella, administration of live or attenuated virus vaccines. **Cautions:** Hyperthyroidism, cirrhosis, ocular herpes simplex, respiratory tuberculosis, untreated systemic infections, renal/hepatic impairment, following acute MI, cataracts, glaucoma, seizure disorder, peptic ulcer disease, osteoporosis, myasthenia gravis, hypertension, HF, ulcerative colitis, thromboembolic disorders, elderly, pts at risk for hyperglycemia (e.g., diabetes, recent surgery).

ACTION

Inhibits accumulation of inflammatory cells at inflammation sites, phagocytosis, lysosomal enzyme release/synthesis, release of mediators of inflammation. **Therapeutic Effect:** Prevents/suppresses cell-mediated immune reactions. Decreases/prevents tissue response to inflammatory process.

PHARMACOKINETICS

Widely distributed. Protein binding: 70%–90%. Metabolized in liver, converted to prednisoLONE. Primarily excreted in urine. Not removed by hemodialysis. **Half-life:** 2.5–3.5 hrs.

⧗ LIFESPAN CONSIDERATIONS

Pregnancy/Lactation: Crosses placenta. Distributed in breast milk. Fetal cleft palate often occurs with chronic, first trimester use. Breastfeeding not recommended. **Children:** Prolonged treatment or high dosages may decrease short-term growth rate, cortisol secretion. **Elderly:** May be more susceptible to developing hypertension or osteoporosis.

INTERACTIONS

DRUG: CYP3A4 inducers (e.g., carBAMazepine, phenytoin, rifAMPin) may decrease effects. May increase concentration/adverse effects of **vaccines (live)**, **warfarin**. May decrease therapeutic effects of **aldesleukin**, **vaccines (live)**. May increase hyponatremic effect of **desmopres-**

sin. **HERBAL:** **Echinacea** may decrease therapeutic effect. **FOOD:** None known. **LAB VALUES:** May increase serum glucose, lipids, sodium, uric acid. May decrease serum calcium, potassium, WBC, hypothalamic pituitary adrenal (HPA) axis function.

AVAILABILITY (Rx)

Solution, Oral: 1 mg/mL. **Solution, Oral Concentrate:** *(PredniSONE Intensol):* 5 mg/mL. **Tablets:** 1 mg, 2.5 mg, 5 mg, 10 mg, 20 mg, 50 mg.

 Tablet, Delayed-Release: *(Rayos):* 1 mg, 2 mg, 5 mg.

ADMINISTRATION/HANDLING

PO

• Administer after meals or with food or milk to decrease GI upset. • **Delayed-release**: Administer whole (do not break, divide, crush or allow chewing. • **Oral solution**: Only administer with calibrated dropper.

INDICATIONS/ROUTES/DOSAGE

Note: Dose dependent upon condition treated, pt response rather than by rigid adherence to age, weight, or body surface area.

Usual Dosage

PO: ADULTS, ELDERLY: 10–60 mg/day as a single daily dose or in 2–4 divided doses. **(Low dose):** 2.5–10 mg/day. **(High dose):** 1–1.5 mg/kg/day (usually not to exceed 80–100 mg/day). **CHILDREN:** 0.05–2 mg/kg/day in 1–4 divided doses.

Dosage in Renal/Hepatic Impairment

No dose adjustment.

SIDE EFFECTS

Frequent: Insomnia, heartburn, nervousness, abdominal distention, diaphoresis, acne, mood swings, increased appetite, facial flushing, delayed wound healing, increased susceptibility to infection, diarrhea, constipation. **Occasional:** Head-

ache, edema, change in skin color, frequent urination. **Rare:** Tachycardia, allergic reaction (rash, urticaria), psychological changes, hallucinations, depression.

ADVERSE EFFECTS/TOXIC REACTIONS

Long-term therapy: Muscle wasting (esp. in arms, legs), osteoporosis, spontaneous fractures, amenorrhea, cataracts, glaucoma, peptic ulcer, HF. **Abrupt withdrawal following long-term therapy:** Anorexia, nausea, fever, headache, rebound inflammation, fatigue, weakness, lethargy, dizziness, orthostatic hypotension. Sudden discontinuance may be fatal.

NURSING CONSIDERATIONS

BASELINE ASSESSMENT

Question medical history as listed in Precautions. Obtain height, weight, B/P, serum glucose, electrolytes. Check results of initial tests (tuberculosis [TB] skin test, X-rays, ECG).

INTERVENTION/EVALUATION

Monitor B/P, serum electrolytes, glucose, results of bone mineral density test, height, weight in children. Be alert to infection (sore throat, fever, vague symptoms); assess oral cavity daily for signs of *Candida* infection. Monitor for symptoms of adrenal insufficiency, immunosuppression.

PATIENT/FAMILY TEACHING

• Report fever, sore throat, muscle aches, sudden weight gain, swelling, loss of appetite, or fatigue. • Avoid alcohol, minimize use of caffeine. • Report symptoms of elevated blood sugar levels (blurred vision, headache, increased thirst, frequent urination). • Do not abruptly discontinue without physician's approval. • Avoid exposure to chickenpox, measles. • Long-term use may significantly increase risk of serious infections.

P

pregabalin

pre-**gab**-a-lin
(Lyrica, Lyrica CR)

◆CLASSIFICATION

PHARMACOTHERAPEUTIC: GABA analogue. **CLINICAL:** Anticonvulsant, antineuralgic, analgesic (Schedule V).

USES

Lyrica: Adjunctive therapy in treatment of focal (partial) onset seizures in adults and children 1 mo and older. Management of neuropathic pain associated with diabetic peripheral neuropathy or spinal cord injury. Management of postherpetic neuralgia. Management of fibromyalgia. **Lyrica CR:** Management of neuropathic pain associated with diabetic peripheral neuropathy, postherpetic neuralgia. **OFF-LABEL:** Chronic cough (refractory), generalized anxiety disorder (GAD), pruritus (chronic), social anxiety disorder (SAD), restless leg syndrome, vasomotor symptoms associated with menopause.

PRECAUTIONS

Contraindications: Hypersensitivity to pregabalin. **Cautions:** HF, renal impairment, cardiovascular disease, diabetes, history of angioedema, history of suicidal ideation and behavior. Concurrent use of thiazolidine antidiabetics (e.g., Actos).

ACTION

Binds to calcium channel sites in CNS tissue, inhibiting excitatory neurotransmitter release. Exerts antinociceptive, anticonvulsant activity. May affect descending noradrenergic and serotonergic pain transmission pathways from the brainstem to spinal cord. **Therapeutic Effect:** Decreases symptoms of painful peripheral neuropathy; decreases frequency of partial seizures.

PHARMACOKINETICS

Widely distributed. Excreted in urine unchanged. **Half-life:** 6 hrs.

⧗ LIFESPAN CONSIDERATIONS

Pregnancy/Lactation: Increased risk of fetal skeletal abnormalities. Unknown if distributed in breast milk. **Children:** Safety and efficacy not established in pts younger than 1 mo. **Elderly:** Age-related renal impairment may require dosage adjustment.

INTERACTIONS

DRUG: Alcohol, CNS depressants (e.g., LORazepam, morphine, zolpidem) may increase sedative effect. **HERBAL:** Herbals with sedative properties (e.g., chamomile, kava kava, valerian) may increase CNS depression. **FOOD:** None known. **LAB VALUES:** May increase CPK. May cause mild PR interval prolongation. May decrease platelet count.

AVAILABILITY (Rx)

Solution, Oral: 20 mg/mL.

Capsules: 25 mg, 50 mg, 75 mg, 100 mg, 150 mg, 200 mg, 225 mg, 300 mg.

Tablet, Extended-Release: 82.5 mg, 165 mg, 330 mg.

ADMINISTRATION/HANDLING

(Immediate-Release): • Give without regard to food. *(Extended-Release):* • Give once daily after evening meal. • Administer whole (do not split, crush, or allow chewing).

INDICATIONS/ROUTES/DOSAGE

Note: Discontinue gradually over at least 1 wk to minimize potential of increased seizure activity.

Focal (Partial) Onset Seizures

PO: **ADULTS, ELDERLY:** Initially, 150 mg/day in 2–3 divided doses. May increase at wkly intervals. **Maximum:** 600 mg/day. **ADOLESCENTS, CHILDREN, 4 YRS AND OLDER WEIGHING 30 KG OR MORE:** Initially, 2.5 mg/kg/day in 2 or 3 divided doses. May increase wkly based on clinical response and tolerability. **Maximum:** 10 mg/kg/day (not to exceed

---

P

600 mg/day). **LESS THAN 30 KG:** Initially, 3.5 mg/kg/day in 2 or 3 divided doses. May increase wkly based on clinical response and tolerability. **Maximum:** 14 mg/kg/day. **CHILDREN YOUNGER THAN 4 YRS, INFANTS WEIGHING LESS THAN 30 KG:** Initially, 3.5 mg/kg/day in 3 divided doses. May increase wkly based on response and tolerability. **Maximum:** 14 mg/kg/day.

Neuropathic Pain (Diabetes-Associated)
PO: *(Immediate-Release):* **ADULTS, ELDERLY:** Initially, 75–150 mg/day in 2–3 divided doses. May increase daily dose in increments of 75 mg/day q3 or more days based on response and tolerability. **Maximum:** 300–450 mg/day.
PO: *(Extended-Release):* **ADULTS, ELDERLY:** Initially, 165 mg once daily. May increase to 330 mg/day within 1 wk. **Maximum:** 330 mg/day.

Postherpetic Neuralgia, Neuropathic Pain Associated With Spinal Cord Injury
PO: *(Immediate-Release):* **ADULTS, ELDERLY:** Initially, 75 mg twice daily or 50 mg 3 times/day. May increase to 300 mg/day within 1 wk. May further increase to 600 mg/day after 2–4 wks. **Maximum:** 600 mg/day.
PO: *(Extended-Release):* **(Postherpetic neuralgia only): ADULTS, ELDERLY:** Initially, 165 mg once daily. May increase to 330 mg/day within 1 wk. May further increase to 660 mg once daily after 2–4 wks. **Maximum:** 660 mg/day.

Fibromyalgia
PO: ADULTS, ELDERLY: *(Immediate-Release):* Initially, 75 mg twice daily. May increase to 150 mg twice daily within 1 wk. **Maximum:** 225 mg twice daily.

Dosage in Renal Impairment

Creatinine Clearance	Daily Dosage
30–60 mL/min	75–300 mg in 2–3 divided doses
15–29 mL/min	25–150 mg in 1 or 2 doses
Less than 15 mL/min	25–75 mg once daily

Dosage for Hemodialysis
◄**ALERT**► Take supplemental dose immediately following dialysis.

Daily Dosage	Supplemental Dosage
25 mg	Single dose of 25 mg or 50 mg
25–50 mg	Single dose of 50 mg or 75 mg
75 mg	Single dose of 100 mg or 150 mg

Dosage in Hepatic Impairment
No dose adjustment.

SIDE EFFECTS
Frequent (32%–12%): Dizziness, drowsiness, ataxia, peripheral edema. **Occasional (12%–5%):** Weight gain, blurred vision, diplopia, difficulty with concentration, attention, cognition; tremor, dry mouth, headache, constipation, asthenia. **Rare (4%–2%):** Abnormal gait, confusion, incoordination, twitching, flatulence, vomiting, edema, myopathy.

ADVERSE EFFECTS/TOXIC REACTIONS
Abrupt withdrawal increases risk of seizure frequency in pts with seizure disorders; withdraw gradually over a minimum of 1 wk. May increase risk of suicidal thoughts and behavior.

NURSING CONSIDERATIONS

BASELINE ASSESSMENT
Seizure: Review history of seizure disorder (type, onset, intensity, frequency, duration, LOC). **Pain:** Assess onset, type, location, and duration of pain. Question history of suicidal ideation and behavior.

INTERVENTION/EVALUATION
Assess for seizure activity. Assess for clinical improvement; record onset of relief of pain. Assess for peripheral edema. Question for changes in visual acuity. Monitor weight.

PATIENT/FAMILY TEACHING
• Do not abruptly stop taking drug; seizure frequency may be increased. • Avoid

P

---

tasks that require alertness, motor skills until response to drug is established. • Avoid alcohol. • Seek immediate medical attention if thoughts of suicide, new-onset or worsening of anxiety, depression, or changes in mood occur.

---

propofol   `HIGH ALERT`

proe-poe-fol
(Diprivan, Fresenius Propoven, Propofol-Lipuro)
Do not confuse Diprivan with Diflucan or Ditropan, or propofol with fospropofol.

◆CLASSIFICATION

PHARMACOTHERAPEUTIC: Rapid-acting general anesthetic. **CLINICAL:** Sedative-hypnotic.

USES

Induction/maintenance of anesthesia. Continuous sedation in intubated and respiratory controlled adult pts in ICU. **OFF-LABEL:** Refractory status epilepticus.

PRECAUTIONS

Contraindications: Hypersensitivity to propofol, eggs, egg products, soybean or soy products. **Cautions:** Hemodynamically unstable pts, hypovolemia, severe cardiac/respiratory disease, elevated ICP, impaired cerebral circulation, preexisting pancreatitis, hyperlipidemia, seizure disorder, elderly, debilitated; peanut allergy.

ACTION

Causes CNS depression through agonist action of GABA receptors. **Therapeutic Effect:** Produces hypnosis rapidly.

PHARMACOKINETICS

Route	Onset	Peak	Duration
IV	40 sec	N/A	3–10 min

Rapidly, extensively distributed. Protein binding: 97%–99%. Metabolized in liver. Primarily excreted in urine. Unknown if removed by hemodialysis. Rapid awakening can occur 10–15 min after discontinuation. **Half-life:** 3–12 hrs.

⌛ LIFESPAN CONSIDERATIONS

Pregnancy/Lactation: Unknown if drug crosses placenta. Distributed in breast milk. Not recommended for obstetrics, breastfeeding mothers. **Children:** Safety and efficacy not established. FDA-approved for use in pts 2 mos and older. **Elderly:** No age-related precautions noted; lower dosages recommended.

INTERACTIONS

DRUG: Alcohol, **CNS depressants (e.g., LORazepam, morphine, zolpidem)** may increase CNS, respiratory depression, hypotensive effects. **Antihypertensive medications (e.g., amLODIPine, lisinopril, valsartan)** may increase hypotensive effects. **HERBAL:** Herbals with sedative properties (e.g., chamomile, kava kava, valerian) may increase CNS depression. **Herbals with hypotensive properties (e.g., garlic, ginger, ginkgo biloba)** may increase effect. **FOOD:** None known. **LAB VALUES:** May increase serum triglycerides.

AVAILABILITY (Rx)

Injection Emulsion: 10 mg/mL.

ADMINISTRATION/HANDLING

🖐 IV

◀**ALERT**▶ Do not give through same IV line with blood or plasma.
Reconstitution • May give undiluted, or dilute only with D_5W. • Do not dilute to concentration less than 2 mg/mL (4 mL D_5W to 1 mL propofol yields 2 mg/mL).
Rate of administration • Too-rapid IV administration may produce severe hypotension, respiratory depression, irregular muscular movements. • Observe for signs of extravasation (pain, discolored skin patches, white or blue

color to peripheral IV site area, delayed onset of drug action).

Storage • Store at room temperature. • Discard unused portions. • Do not use if emulsion separates. • Shake well before using.

▨ IV INCOMPATIBILITIES

Acetaminophen, calcium chloride.

▨ IV COMPATIBILITIES

Calcium gluconate, clevidipine, dexmedetomidine, heparin, insulin, magnesium sulfate, norepinephrine, potassium chloride.

INDICATIONS/ROUTES/DOSAGE

Anesthesia

IV infusion: ADULTS, ELDERLY: Induction, 2–2.5 mg/kg (approximately 40 mg q10sec until onset of anesthesia). **Maintenance:** Initially, 100–200 mcg/kg/min or 6–12 mg/kg/hr for 10–15 min. **Usual maintenance:** 50–100 mcg/kg/min or 3–6 mg/kg/hr. **CHILDREN 3–16 YRS:** Induction, 2.5–3.5 mg/kg over 20–30 sec, then infusion of 125–300 mcg/kg/min or 7.5–18 mg/kg/hr.

Sedation in ICU

IV infusion: ADULTS, ELDERLY: Initially, 5 mcg/kg/min; increase by increments of 5–10 mcg/kg/min q5–10 min until desired sedation level achieved. **Usual maintenance:** 5–50 mcg/kg/min. **Maximum:** 60–80 mcg/kg/min. Reduce dose after adequate sedation established, and adjust to response. Daily interruption with retitration (sedation vacation) recommended to minimize prolonged sedative effects. Generally, titrate down slowly to avoid rapid awakening.

Dosage in Renal/Hepatic Impairment

No dose adjustment.

SIDE EFFECTS

Frequent: Involuntary muscle movements, apnea (common during induc-

tion; often lasts longer than 60 sec), hypotension, nausea, vomiting, IV site burning/stinging. **Occasional:** Twitching, thrashing, headache, dizziness, bradycardia, hypertension, fever, abdominal cramps, paresthesia, coldness, cough, hiccups, facial flushing, green-tinted urine. **Rare:** Rash, dry mouth, agitation, confusion, myalgia, thrombophlebitis.

ADVERSE EFFECTS/TOXIC REACTIONS

Continuous infusion or repeated intermittent infusions of propofol may result in extreme drowsiness, respiratory depression, circulatory depression, delirium. Too-rapid IV administration may produce severe hypotension, respiratory depression, involuntary muscle movements. Pt may experience acute allergic reaction, characterized by abdominal pain, anxiety, restlessness, dyspnea, erythema, hypotension, pruritus, rhinitis, urticaria. May cause propofol infusion syndrome, a collection of metabolic disorders and organ system failures including metabolic acidosis, hyperkalemia, rhabdomyolysis, hepatomegaly; cardiac, renal failure.

NURSING CONSIDERATIONS

BASELINE ASSESSMENT

Resuscitative equipment, suction, O_2 must be available. Obtain vital signs before administration. Screen for hypersensitivity to egg or soy products.

INTERVENTION/EVALUATION

Observe for signs of wakefulness, agitation. Monitor respiratory rate, B/P, heart rate, O_2 saturation, depth of sedation, serum lipid, triglycerides (if used longer than 24 hrs). May change urine color to green. If continuous high-dose infusions do not properly induce sedation, consider additional sedatives (e.g., opioids, hypnotics, benzodiazepines) to achieve desired response.

P

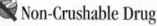

pyRIDostigmine

peer-id-oh-**stig**-meen
(Mestinon, Mestinon SR , Regonol)
**Do not confuse pyRIDostigmine
with PHYSostigmine, or Regonol
with Reglan or Renagel.**

◆CLASSIFICATION

PHARMACOTHERAPEUTIC: Anticholinesterase inhibitor. **CLINICAL:** Cholinergic muscle stimulant.

USES

Treatment of myasthenia gravis. **OFF-LABEL:** Postural orthostatic tachycardia syndrome.

PRECAUTIONS

Contraindications: Hypersensitivity to pyRIDostigmine. Mechanical, intestinal or urinary obstruction. **Cautions:** Bronchial asthma, COPD, bradycardia, seizure disorder, hyperthyroidism, cardiac arrhythmias, peptic ulcer, renal impairment.

ACTION

Prevents destruction of acetylcholine by inhibiting the enzyme acetylcholinesterase, enhancing impulse transmission across neuromuscular junction. **Therapeutic Effect:** Produces miosis; increases intestinal, skeletal muscle tone; stimulates salivary, sweat gland secretions.

PHARMACOKINETICS

Poorly absorbed from GI tract. Metabolized in liver. Excreted primarily unchanged in urine. **Half-life:** 1–2 hrs.

⧗ LIFESPAN CONSIDERATIONS

Pregnancy/Lactation: Unknown if drug crosses placenta or is distributed in breast milk. **Children:** Safety and efficacy not established. **Elderly:** No age-related precautions noted.

INTERACTIONS

DRUG: May increase concentration/effect of **fingolimod, ponesimod, siponimod. Corticosteroids (e.g., methylprednisolone, prednisone)** may increase concentration/effect. **HERBAL:** None significant. **FOOD:** None known. **LAB VALUES:** None significant.

AVAILABILITY (Rx)

Solution, Oral: 60 mg/5 mL. **Tablets:** 30 mg, 60 mg.

🐟 **Tablets: Extended-Release:** 180 mg.

ADMINISTRATION/HANDLING

PO
• Give with food, milk. • Tablets may be crushed. Do not chew, crush extended-release tablets (may be broken). • Give larger dose at times of increased fatigue (e.g., for those with difficulty in chewing, 30–45 min before meals).

🔳 IV INCOMPATIBILITIES

Do not mix with any other medications.

INDICATIONS/ROUTES/DOSAGE

Note: The following dosage ranges are for guidance only. Dosing is highly individualized.

Myasthenia Gravis
PO: ADULTS, ELDERLY: (Immediate-Release): Initially, 30–60 mg 3 times/day. May increase by 30 mg/dose q2–3 days up to 60–120 mg q3–4h while awake. Usual dose: 960 mg or less/day divided in 4–8 doses/day.
PO: (Sustained-Release): 180–360 mg once daily at bedtime (may be necessary to use immediate-release therapy in conjunction with sustained-release therapy). **ADOLESCENTS, CHILDREN, INFANTS: (Immediate-Release):** 0.5–1 mg/kg/dose (maximum single dose: 60 mg) q4h. **Maximum:** 7 mg/kg/day divided in 5–6 doses.

Dosage in Renal/Hepatic Impairment
No dose adjustment.

P

SIDE EFFECTS

Frequent: Miosis, increased GI/skeletal muscle tone, bradycardia, constriction of bronchi/ureters, diaphoresis, increased salivation. **Occasional:** Headache, rash, temporary decrease in diastolic B/P with mild reflex tachycardia, short periods of atrial fibrillation (in hyperthyroid pts), marked drop in B/P (in hypertensive pts).

ADVERSE EFFECTS/TOXIC REACTIONS

Overdose may produce cholinergic crisis, manifested as increasingly severe descending muscle weakness (appears first in muscles involving chewing, swallowing, followed by muscle weakness of shoulder girdle, upper extremities), respiratory muscle paralysis, followed by pelvis girdle/leg muscle paralysis. Requires withdrawal of all cholinergic drugs and immediate use of 1–4 mg atropine sulfate IV for adults, 0.01 mg/kg for infants and children younger than 12 yrs.

NURSING CONSIDERATIONS

BASELINE ASSESSMENT

Larger doses should be given at time of greatest fatigue. Assess muscle strength before testing for diagnosis of myasthenia gravis and following drug administration. Avoid large doses in pts with megacolon, reduced GI motility.

INTERVENTION/EVALUATION

Have facial tissues readily available at pt's bedside. Monitor respirations closely during myasthenia gravis testing or if dosage is increased. Assess diligently for cholinergic reaction, bradycardia in myasthenic pt in crisis. Coordinate dosage time with periods of fatigue and increased/decreased muscle strength. Monitor for therapeutic response to medication (increased muscle strength, decreased fatigue, improved chewing/swallowing functions).

PATIENT/FAMILY TEACHING

• Report nausea, vomiting, diarrhea, diaphoresis, profuse salivary secretions, palpitations, muscle weakness, severe abdominal pain, difficulty breathing.

P

QUEtiapine

kwet-**eye**-a-peen
(SEROquel, SEROquel XR)

■ **BLACK BOX ALERT** ■ Increased risk of suicidal ideation and behavior in children, adolescents, young adults 18–24 yrs with major depressive disorder, other psychiatric disorders. Elderly with dementia-related psychosis are at increased risk for death.
Do not confuse QUEtiapine with OLANZapine, or seroquel with seroquel XR or sinequan.

◆CLASSIFICATION

PHARMACOTHERAPEUTIC: Dibenzodiazepine derivative. **CLINICAL:** Second-generation (atypical) antipsychotic.

USES

Bipolar disorder: Acute treatment (monotherapy or adjunct to lithium or divalproex) of manic episodes associated with bipolar I disorder in adults and children 10 yrs and older. Acute treatment of depressive episodes associated with bipolar disorder in adults. Adjunct therapy for maintenance of bipolar I disorder in adults. **Major depressive disorder (unipoloar):** Adjunctive therapy in pts with an inadequate response to antidepressants for the treatment of major depressive disorder in adults. **Schizophrenia:** Treatment of schizophrenia in adults and children 13 yrs and older. **OFF-LABEL:** Autism, agitation/delirium in ICU, agitation/aggression/psychosis associated with dementia, generalized anxiety disorder (GAD), obsessive compulsive disorder (OCD), posttraumatic stress disorder (PTSD), psychosis in Parkinson's disease.

PRECAUTIONS

Contraindications: Hypersensitivity to QUEtiapine. **Cautions:** Renal/hepatic impairment, hyperlipidemia, pts at risk for aspiration pneumonia, cardiovascular disease (e.g., HF, history of MI), cerebrovascular disease, dehydration, hypovolemia, history of drug abuse/dependence, seizure disor-

der, hypothyroidism, pts at risk for suicide, Parkinson's disease, decreased GI motility, urinary retention, narrow-angle glaucoma, diabetes, visual problems, elderly, pts at risk for orthostatic hypotension. Avoid use in pts at risk for torsades de pointes (hypokalemia, hypomagnesemia, history of cardiac arrhythmias, congenital long QT syndrome, concurrent medications that prolong QT interval).

ACTION

Antagonizes DOPamine and serotonin (antipsychotic activity), histamine (somnolence), alpha$_1$-adrenergic (orthostatic hypotension) receptors. **Therapeutic Effect:** Diminishes symptoms associated with schizophrenia/bipolar disorders.

PHARMACOKINETICS

Widely distributed. Metabolized in liver. Protein binding: 83%. Primarily excreted in urine. **Half-life:** 6 hrs.

⧗ LIFESPAN CONSIDERATIONS

Pregnancy/Lactation: Unknown if drug is distributed in breast milk. Breastfeeding not recommended. **Children:** Safety and efficacy not established in children less than 10 yrs of age (bipolar mania) or less than 13 yrs of age (schizophrenia). **Elderly:** No age-related precautions noted, but lower initial and target dosages may be necessary.

INTERACTIONS

DRUG: QT interval–prolonging medications (e.g., **amiodarone, azithromycin, ciprofloxacin, haloperidol, methadone, sotalol**) may increase risk of QTc interval prolongation. **Alcohol, CNS depressants** (e.g., **LORazepam, morphine, zolpidem**) may increase CNS depression. May increase hypotensive effects of **antihypertensives. Strong CYP3A4 inducers** (e.g., **carBAMazepine, phenytoin, rifAMPin**) may decrease concentration/effect. **Strong CYP3A4 inhibitors** (e.g., **clarithromycin, ketoconazole**) may increase concentration/effect. **Anticholinergic agents** (e.g., **aclidinium, ipratropium, tiotropium, umeclidinium**) may increase anticholinergic effect. **HERBAL: Herbals with sedative properties (e.g., chamomile, kava kava, valerian)** may increase CNS depression. **St. John's wort** may decrease concentration/effect. **FOOD:** None known. **LAB VALUES:** May decrease total free thyroxine (T4) serum levels. May increase serum cholesterol, triglycerides, ALT, AST, WBC, GGT. May produce false-positive pregnancy test result.

AVAILABILITY (Rx)

Tablets: 25 mg, 50 mg, 100 mg, 200 mg, 300 mg, 400 mg.

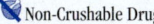 **Tablets, Extended-Release:** 50 mg, 150 mg, 200 mg, 300 mg, 400 mg.

ADMINISTRATION/HANDLING

PO

• Give immediate-release tablets without regard to food. • **Extended-release:** Administer whole. Do not break, crush, dissolve, or divide extended-release tablets. • Extended-release tablets should be given without regard to food or with a light meal in evening.

INDICATIONS/ROUTES/DOSAGE

• When restarting pts who have been off QUEtiapine for less than 1 wk, titration is not required, and maintenance dose can be reinstituted. • When restarting pts who have been off QUEtiapine for longer than 1 wk, follow initial titration schedule. • When discontinuing, gradual tapering recommended to avoid withdrawal symptoms and minimize risk of relapse.

Schizophrenia

PO: ADULTS, ELDERLY: *(Immediate-Release):* Initially, 25 mg twice daily, then increase in 25–50-mg increments divided 2–3 times/day on the second and third days; may further increase up to target dose of 300–400 mg/day in 2–3 divided doses by the fourth day. Further adjustments of 25–50 mg twice daily may be made at intervals of 2 days or longer. **Maintenance:** 400–800 mg/day. **Maximum:** 800 mg/day. *(Extended-Release):* Initially, 300 mg/day. May increase in increments of up to 300 mg/day at intervals as short as 1 day. **Range:** 400–800

mg/day in 1–3 divided doses. **Maximum:** 800 mg/day. **ADOLESCENTS:** *(Immediate-Release):* Initially, 25 mg twice daily on day 1, 50 mg twice daily on day 2, then increase by 100 mg/day to target dose of 200 mg twice daily on day 5. May further increase to 800 mg/day in increments of 100 mg or less daily. **Range:** 400–800 mg/day. **Maximum:** 800 mg. Total dose may be divided in 3 doses/day. *(Extended-Release):* Initially, 50 mg once daily on day 1, 100 mg on day 2, then increase in 100-mg increments each day until 400 mg once daily is reached on day 5. **Range:** 400–800 mg/day. **Maximum:** 800 mg/day.

Mania in Bipolar Disorder

PO: ADULTS, ELDERLY: *(Immediate-Release):* Initially, 100–200 mg once daily at bedtime or in 2 divided doses on day 1. May increase in increments of 100 mg/day to 200 mg twice daily on day 4. May further increase in increments of 200 mg/day to 800 mg/day **Maximum:** 800 mg/day; however, some pts may require dose up to 1,200 mg/day. *(Extended-Release):* Initially, 300 mg on day 1 in the evening; increase to 600 mg on day 2. Adjust dose base on response/tolerability. **Maximum:** 800 mg/day; however, some pts may require dose up to 1,200 mg/day. **CHILDREN 10 YRS AND OLDER:** *(Immediate-Release):* 25 mg twice daily on day 1, 50 mg twice daily on day 2, then 100 mg twice daily on day 3, 150 mg twice daily on day 4, then continue at target dose of 200 mg twice daily on day 5. **Usual range:** 200–300 mg twice daily. **Maximum:** 600 mg/day. *(Extended-Release):* 50 mg on day 1; 100 mg on day 2; then increase by 100 mg/day until target dose of 400 mg once daily on day 5. **Usual range:** 400–600 mg once daily. **Maximum:** 600 mg/day.

Depression in Bipolar Disorder

PO: ADULTS, ELDERLY: *(Extended-Release):* Initially, 50 mg on day 1 in the evening, 100 mg on day 2, 200 mg on day 3, 300 mg on day 4 and thereafter.

Adjunctive Therapy in MDD

PO: ADULTS, ELDERLY: *(Extended-Release):* Initially, 50 mg on days 1 and

2; then 150 mg on days 3 and 4; then 150–300 mg/day in 1–3 doses based on chosen formulation.

Dosage in Hepatic Impairment
(Immediate-Release): Initially, 25 mg/day. Increase by 25–50 mg/day to effective dose. *(Extended-Release):* Initially, 50 mg/day, increase by 50 mg/day until effective dose.

Dosage in Renal Impairment
No dose adjustment.

SIDE EFFECTS

Frequent (19%–10%): Headache, drowsiness, dizziness. **Occasional (9%–3%):** Constipation, orthostatic hypotension, tachycardia, dry mouth, dyspepsia, rash, asthenia, abdominal pain, rhinitis. **Rare (2%):** Back pain, fever, weight gain.

ADVERSE EFFECTS/TOXIC REACTIONS

May increase risk of death in elderly pts with dementia-related psychosis. Most deaths appeared to be cardiovascular (e.g., HF, sudden death) or infectious (e.g., pneumonia) in nature. May increase risk of life-threatening neuroleptic malignant syndrome (NMS). Symptoms of NMS may include hyperpyrexia, muscle rigidity, altered mental status, autonomic instability (irregular pulse/blood pressure, tachycardia, diaphoresis, cardiac arrhythmias); elevated CPK, rhabdomyolysis, acute renal failure. Tardive dyskinesia (potentially irreversible, involuntary, dyskinetic movements) has occurred. Metabolic changes including hyperglycemia, ketoacidosis, hyperosmolar coma, diabetes, dyslipidemia may occur. Agranulocytosis, leukopenia, neutropenia was reported. Cognitive and motor impairment reported in 24% of pts. Other effects may include body temperature dysregulation, cataracts, dysphagia, dystonia, extrapyramidal symptoms, orthostatic hypotension, falls, syncope, seizures. Overdose may cause heart block, hypotension, hypokalemia, tachycardia.

NURSING CONSIDERATIONS

BASELINE ASSESSMENT

Obtain CBC in pts with baseline leukopenia, neutropenia; pregnancy test in females of reproductive potential. Screen for active infection. Receive full medication history and screen for interactions. Question history as listed in Precautions. Assess risk of dysphagia, aspiration. Initiate fall precautions. Assess appearance, behavior, speech pattern, levels of interest. Offer emotional support.

INTERVENTION/EVALUATION

Monitor blood glucose in pts with diabetes; lipid profile after initiation and periodically thereafter. Monitor CBC, orthostatic vital signs frequently during the first mos of therapy. Monitor for hyperglycemia (blurred vision, confusion, excessive thirst, Kussmaul respirations, polyuria), infections (cough, fatigue, fever), body temperature dysregulation, dysphagia, dystonia, tardive dyskinesia, symptoms of NMS. Assess for therapeutic response (greater interest in surroundings, improved self-care, increased ability to concentrate, relaxed facial expression).

PATIENT/ FAMILY TEACHING

• Treatment may depress your immune system response and reduce your ability to fight infection. Report symptoms of infection such as body aches, chills, cough, fatigue, fever. Avoid those with active infection until response to drug is established. • Report symptoms of high blood sugar levels (e.g., blurred vision, excessive thirst/hunger, headache, frequent urination); nervous system changes (e.g., abnormal, involuntary movements [e.g., lip smacking, puckering, tongue protrusion or chewing, jaw movement, rapid blinking of the eye], difficulty swallowing, seizures, tremor; spasms of the neck, tongue, face). • Treatment may cause NMS (confusion, high fever, muscle rigidity, high or irregular B/P, heart arrhythmias), a life-threatening condition

Q

that can be confused with symptoms of severe infection. • Avoid tasks that require alertness, motor skills until response to drug is established. • Go slowly from lying to standing. • Do not take newly prescribed medications unless approved by prescriber who originally started treatment. • Avoid overheating, dehydration. • Seek immediate medical attention if thoughts of suicide, new onset or worsening of anxiety, depression, or changes in mood occur.

quinapril

kwin-a-pril
(Accupril)
■**BLACK BOX ALERT**■ May cause fetal injury, mortality. Discontinue as soon as possible once pregnancy detected.
Do not confuse Accupril with Accolate, Accutane, Aciphex, or Monopril.

FIXED-COMBINATION(S)

Accuretic: quinapril/hydroCHLORO-thiazide (a diuretic): 10 mg/12.5 mg, 20 mg/12.5 mg, 20 mg/25 mg.

◆CLASSIFICATION

PHARMACOTHERAPEUTIC: Angiotensin-converting enzyme (ACE) inhibitor. **CLINICAL:** Antihypertensive.

USES

Treatment of hypertension. Used alone or in combination with other antihypertensives. Adjunctive therapy in management of HF with reduced ejection fraction.

PRECAUTIONS

Contraindications: Hypersensitivity to quinapril. History of angioedema from previous treatment with ACE inhibitors, concomitant use with aliskiren in pts with diabetes. Concomitant use with neprilysin inhibitor (e.g., sacubitril) or within 36 hrs of switching to or from neprilysin inhibitor. **Cau-**

tions: Renal impairment, hypertrophic cardiomyopathy with outflow tract obstruction, major surgery, HF, hypovolemia, unstented bilateral renal artery stenosis, hyperkalemia, concurrent potassium supplements, severe aortic stenosis, ischemic heart disease, cerebrovascular disease.

ACTION

Suppresses renin-angiotensin-aldosterone system, preventing conversion of angiotensin I to angiotensin II, a potent vasoconstrictor. Lower angiotensin II causes an increase in plasma renin activity and decreased aldosterone secretion. **Therapeutic Effect:** Reduces peripheral arterial resistance, B/P.

PHARMACOKINETICS

Route	Onset	Peak	Duration
PO	1 hr	N/A	24 hrs

Widely distributed. Protein binding: 97%. Rapidly hydrolyzed to active metabolite. Primarily excreted in urine. Minimal removal by hemodialysis. **Half-life:** 1–2 hrs; metabolite, 3 hrs (increased in renal impairment).

⌛ LIFESPAN CONSIDERATIONS

Pregnancy/Lactation: Crosses placenta. Unknown if distributed in breast milk. May cause fetal, neonatal mortality or morbidity. **Children:** Safety and efficacy not established. **Elderly:** May be more sensitive to hypotensive effects.

INTERACTIONS

DRUG: Aliskiren may increase hyperkalemic effect. May increase potential for allergic reactions to **allopurinol. Angiotensin receptor blockers (e.g., losartan, valsartan)** may increase adverse effects. May increase adverse effects of **lithium, sacubitril. HERBAL:** Herbals with **hypertensive properties (e.g., licorice, yohimbe)** or **hypotensive properties (e.g., garlic, ginger, ginkgo biloba)** may alter effects. **FOOD:** None known. **LAB VALUES:** May increase serum BUN, alkaline phosphatase, bilirubin, creatinine, potassium, ALT, AST. May decrease serum sodium. May cause positive antinuclear antibody (ANA) titer.

AVAILABILITY (Rx)

Tablets: 5 mg, 10 mg, 20 mg, 40 mg.

ADMINISTRATION/HANDLING

PO
• Give without regard to food.

INDICATIONS/ROUTES/DOSAGE

Hypertension
PO: ADULTS: Initially, 10–20 mg/day. Evaluate response after 2–4 wks and titrate as needed up to 80 mg/day in one or two divided doses. **ELDERLY:** Initially, 10 mg once daily. Titrate to optimal response.

Adjunct to Manage HF
PO: ADULTS, ELDERLY: Initially, 5 mg twice daily. May titrate dose q1–2wks or longer. **Target dose:** 20 mg twice daily.

Dosage in Renal Impairment
Hypertension

Creatinine Clearance	Initial Dose
More than 60 mL/min	10 mg
30–60 mL/min	5 mg
10–29 mL/min	2.5 mg

HF

Creatinine Clearance	Initial Dose
Greater than 30 mL/min	5 mg
10–30 mL/min	2.5 mg

Dosage in Hepatic Impairment
No dose adjustment.

SIDE EFFECTS

Frequent (7%–5%): Headache, dizziness. **Occasional (4%–2%):** Fatigue, vomiting, nausea, hypotension, chest pain, cough, syncope. **Rare (less than 2%):** Diarrhea, cough, dyspnea, rash, palpitations, impotence, insomnia, drowsiness, malaise.

ADVERSE EFFECTS/TOXIC REACTIONS

Excessive hypotension ("first-dose syncope") may occur in pts with HF, those who are severely salt/volume depleted. Angioedema, hyperkalemia occur rarely. Agranulocytosis, neutropenia may occur in pts with collagen vascular disease (scleroderma, systemic lupus erythematosus), renal impairment. Nephrotic syndrome may occur in pts with history of renal disease.

NURSING CONSIDERATIONS

BASELINE ASSESSMENT
Obtain renal function test. Obtain B/P immediately before each dose in addition to regular monitoring (be alert to fluctuations). In pts with prior renal disease, urine test for protein by dipstick method should be made with first urine of day before beginning therapy and periodically thereafter. In pts with renal impairment, autoimmune disease, or taking drugs that affect leukocytes or immune response, CBC, differential count should be performed before beginning therapy and q2wks for 3 mos, then periodically thereafter.

INTERVENTION/EVALUATION
Monitor B/P for hypotension; renal function, serum potassium, WBC. Assist with ambulation if dizziness occurs.

PATIENT/FAMILY TEACHING
• Go slowly from lying to standing. • Full therapeutic effect may take 1–2 wks. • Report any sign of infection (sore throat, fever). • Skipping doses or voluntarily discontinuing drug may produce severe rebound hypertension. • Avoid tasks that require alertness, motor skills until response to drug is established. • Avoid alcohol.

quizartinib

kwiz-**ar**-ti-nib
(Vanflyta)

■ **BLACK BOX ALERT** ■ Life-threatening QT interval prolongation, torsades de pointes may occur, which may lead to cardiac arrest. Monitor QTc interval, serum electrolytes at baseline and during treatment. Do not initiate in pts with severe hypokalemia, hypomagnesemia; long QT syndrome, QTc interval greater than 450 msec. Concomitant use of QT interval-prolonging medications, moderate or strong CYP3A4 inhibitors may worsen QT interval prolongation. Reduce dose when given with strong CYP3A4 inhibitors.

Do not confuse quizartinib with baricitinib, ensartinib, osimertinib, or pexidartinib.

◆CLASSIFICATION

PHARMACOTHERAPEUTIC: Tyrosine kinase 3 (FLT3) inhibitor. **CLINICAL:** Antineoplastic.

USES

In combination with standard cytarabine and anthracycline induction and cytarabine consolidation, and as maintenance monotherapy following consolidation chemotherapy, for treatment of adults with newly diagnosed acute myeloid leukemia (AML) that is FLT3 internal tandem duplication (ITD) positive.

PRECAUTIONS

Contraindications: Hypersensitivity to quizartinib. Severe hypokalemia, hypomagnesemia; long QT syndrome; history of ventricular arrhythmias, torsades de pointes. **Cautions:** Baseline cytopenias, cardiac disease (controlled); conditions predisposing to infection (e.g., diabetes, renal failure, immunocompromised pts, open wounds); chronic opportunistic infections (e.g., herpes virus infection, hepatitis B or C virus infection, fungal

infections); pts at risk for QTc interval prolongation (hypokalemia, hypomagnesemia; concomitant use QT interval-prolonging medications). Avoid concomitant use of strong CYP3A4 inhibitors, strong or moderate CYP3A4 inducers, QT interval-prolonging medications. Avoid use in pts who are at significant risk of developing torsades de pointes (bradyarrhythmias, cardiac disease [uncontrolled or significant], HF, recent MI, high-degree atrioventricular block, severe aortic stenosis, tachyarrhythmias; uncontrolled hypertension, hypothyroidism; unstable angina). Not indicated as maintenance monotherapy after allogeneic hematopoietic stem cell transplantation (HSCT).

ACTION

Inhibits FLT3 kinase activity which prevents FLT3 receptor signaling. **Therapeutic Effect:** Blocks FLT3-ITD dependent cell proliferation.

PHARMACOKINETICS

Widely distributed. Metabolized in liver. Protein binding: 99% or greater. Peak plasma concentration: 4 hrs. Excreted in feces (76%), urine (2%). **Half-life:** 81 hrs.

⏳ LIFESPAN CONSIDERATIONS

Pregnancy/Lactation: Avoid pregnancy; may cause fetal harm. Females of reproductive potential must use effective contraception during treatment and for at least 7 mos after discontinuation. Unknown if distributed in breast milk. Breastfeeding not recommended during treatment and for at least 1 mo after discontinuation. May impair fertility. **Males:** Males with female partners of reproductive potential must use effective contraception during treatment and for at least 4 mos after discontinuation. May impair fertility. **Children:** Safety and efficacy not established. **Elderly:** No age-related precautions noted.

INTERACTIONS

DRUG: Strong CYP3A4 inhibitors (e.g., **clarithromycin, ketoconazole,**

 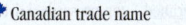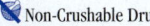

ritonavir) may increase concentration/effect. **Strong CYP3A4 inducers (e.g., carBAMazepine, phenytoin, riFAMpin), moderate CYP3A4 inducers (e.g., dexamethasone, modafinil, nafcillin)** may decrease concentration/effect. **QT interval-prolonging medications (e.g., amiodarone, azithromycin, ciprofloxacin, haloperidol, tacrolimus)** may increase risk of QT interval prolongation, torsades de pointes. **HERBAL:** St. John's wort may decrease concentration/effect. **FOOD:** None known. **LAB VALUES:** May increase serum alkaline phosphatase, ALT, AST, creatine phosphokinase, sodium. May decrease Hgb, lymphocytes, neutrophils, platelets; serum albumin, calcium, phosphate. May increase or decrease serum magnesium, potassium.

AVAILABILITY (Rx)

Tablets: 17.7 mg, 26.5 mg.

ADMINISTRATION/HANDLING

PO
• Give without regard to food at the same time each day. • Administer tablet whole; do not break, cut, or crush. Tablets cannot be chewed. • If a dose is missed, give as soon as possible, then give next dose at regularly scheduled time the following day. • If vomiting occurs after administration, give the next dose at the regularly scheduled time (do not give an additional dose). Do not give 2 doses on the same day.

INDICATIONS/ROUTES/DOSAGE

Note: Treatment course consists of up to 2 cycles (in combination with induction cytarabine and anthracycline), up to 4 cycles (in combination with high-dose cytarabine consolidation), and up to 36 cycles (with no break between cycles) as maintenance therapy. Start maintenance therapy after consolidation phase recovery of blood counts (absolute neutrophil count greater than 500 cells/mm³ and platelet count greater than 50,000 cells/mm³).

AML (FLT3 ITD-Positive)
PO: ADULTS: Induction *(7+3 regimen):* 35.4 mg once daily, starting on day 8, for days 8–21 of 28-day cycle (2 wks in each cycle). *(5 + 2 regimen as the second induction cycle):* Give on days 6–19 of 28-day cycle (2 wks in each cycle). **Consolidation:** 35.4 mg once daily, starting on day 6, for days 6-19 of 28-day cycle (2 wks in each cycle). **Maintenance:** 26.5 mg once daily on days 1–14 of first cycle if QTc interval is 450 msec or less. Increase to 53 mg once daily on day 15 of first cycle if QTc interval is 450 msec or less, or continue 26.5 mg once daily dose if QTc interval was greater than 500 msec during induction or consolidation.

Dose Reduction for Adverse Effects

Current Dose	Modified Dose
53 mg once daily	35.4 mg once daily
35.4 mg once daily	26.5 mg once daily
26.5 mg once daily	Withhold treatment
17.7 mg once daily	Withhold treatment

Dose Modification
Based on Common Terminology for Adverse Events (CTCAE).

Hematological Toxicities
Grade 4 neutropenia **or thrombocytopenia after achieving remission:** Reduce dose (see table above). Bone marrow evaluation is recommended.

Nonhematological Adverse Reactions
Grade 3 or 4 nonhematological adverse reactions: Withhold treatment until improved to grade 1 or less, then resume at previous dose. If adverse reaction improves to no less than grade 2, resume at reduced dose. If grade 3 or 4 adverse reaction does not improve after 28 days, permanently discontinue.

QTc Interval Prolongation
QTc interval 450–480 msec: Continue same dose. **QTc interval 481–500 msec:** Reduce dose without interrupting treatment. In the next cycle, resume at previous dose if QTC interval has decreased to less than 450 msec. Monitor

for QT interval prolongation during the first cycle at the increased dose. **QTc interval greater than 500 msec:** Withhold treatment until QTc interval returns to less than 450 msec, then resume at reduced dose. Continue 26.5 mg once daily dose during maintenance if QTc interval greater than 500 ms was observed during induction or consolidation. **Recurrent QTc interval greater than 500 msec:** If QTc interval greater than 500 ms recurs despite dose reduction and correction/elimination of other risk factors (e.g., serum electrolyte abnormalities, concomitant QT prolonging medications), permanently discontinue treatment.

Life-Threatening Arrhythmias
Torsades de pointes; polymorphic ventricular tachycardia; symptoms of life-threatening arrhythmias: Permanently discontinue.

Serum Electrolyte Abnormalities
Grade 3 or 4 hypokalemia, hypomagnesemia: Withhold treatment until hypokalemia, hypomagnesemia is corrected per institutional protocol. May resume at previous dose if adverse reaction improves to grade 2 or less without symptoms.

Concomitant Use of Strong CYP3A4 Inhibitor
If use of a strong CYP3A4 inhibitor is unavoidable, reduce dose as listed. If a strong CYP3A4 inhibitor is discontinued for 5 half-lives, may resume previous dose taken before use of a strong CYP3A inhibitor.

Current Dose	Modified Dose
53 mg once daily	26.5 mg once daily
35.4 mg once daily	17.7 mg once daily
26.5 mg once daily	17.7 mg once daily
17.7 mg once daily	Withhold treatment

Dosage in Renal/Hepatic Impairment
Mild to moderate impairment: No dose adjustment. **Severe impairment:** Not specified; use caution.

SIDE EFFECTS

Frequent (42%–25%): Diarrhea (colitis, enteritis, enterocolitis, gastroenteritis, neutropenic colitis), mucositis (anal inflammation, anal ulcer, anorectal discomfort, aphthous ulcer, laryngeal inflammation/pain, mucosal inflammation, edema mucosal, esophageal pain, esophageal ulcer, esophagitis oral disorder [blood blister, mucosa erosion, blistering, erythema, pain], pharyngeal inflammation, proctalgia, proctitis, stomatitis, tongue ulceration, vaginal ulceration, nausea, abdominal pain, headache, vomiting. **Occasional (17%–11%):** Decreased appetite, insomnia, dyspepsia, eye irritation (inflammation, irritation, pain, pruritus), foreign body sensation, keratitis, ulcerative keratitis, dry eye.

ADVERSE EFFECTS/TOXIC REACTIONS

Myelosuppression (anemia, neutropenia, thrombocytopenia) is an expected response to therapy, but more severe reactions including febrile neutropenia may be life-threatening. Life-threatening QT interval prolongation, torsades de pointes, cardiac arrest may occur. Life-threatening infections, including various bacterial/fungal/viral infection, herpes virus infection, opportunistic infections, pneumonia, sepsis, may occur. Severe diarrhea may cause dehydration, electrolyte imbalance, which can increase risk of cardiac arrhythmias. Life-threatening and/or fatal differentiation syndrome, a condition with rapid proliferation and differentiation of myeloid cells, was reported. Other adverse effects may include acute respiratory distress syndrome, cerebral infarction, neutrophilic dermatosis, pulmonary embolism, ventricular dysfunction.

NURSING CONSIDERATIONS

BASELINE ASSESSMENT

Obtain CBC, BMP, LFT, serum magnesium; ECG; pregnancy test in females of reproductive potential. Confirm compliance of effective contraception. Do not initiate in pts with QTc interval greater than 450 msec, severe hypokalemia, hy-

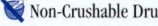

pomagnesemia; long QT syndrome; history of ventricular arrhythmias, torsades de pointes, or pts at significant risk of torsades de pointes. Correct electrolyte abnormalities prior to initiation. Assess risk for QT interval prolongation. Confirm presence of FLT3 ITD-positive mutation. Receive full medication history and screen for interactions. Screen for active infection. Consider prophylactic treatment of herpes simplex virus, chronic infections. Question history as listed in PRECAUTIONS. Offer emotional support.

INTERVENTION/EVALUATION

Monitor CBC for cytopenias; LFT for hepatotoxicity as clinically indicated. During induction and consolidation, obtain weekly ECGs (or more frequently if indicated). During maintenance, obtain weekly ECGs for at least 1 mo after initiation, with increase of dose, and as clinically indicated thereafter (severe hypokalemia, hypomagnesemia; chest pain, dyspnea, palpitations; concomitant use of QT interval-prolonging medications). Do not increase dose if QTc interval is greater than 450 msec. Closely monitor for infections (cough, fatigue, fever, nausea, vomiting), esp. respiratory tract infections, herpes virus infection, opportunistic infections, sepsis.
If serious infection occurs, interrupt or discontinue treatment and initiate appropriate antimicrobial therapy. Monitor for symptoms of differentiation syndrome (dyspnea, fever, hypotension, hypoxia, pulmonary infiltrates, pleural or pericardial effusion, rapid weight gain, peripheral edema, renal dysfunc-

tion, or concomitant febrile neutropenic dermatosis). If differentiation syndrome is suspected, initiate corticosteroids and hemodynamic monitoring until symptoms improve. Monitor for drug toxicities if discontinuation or dose reduction of concomitant CYP3A inhibitor is unavailable.

PATIENT/FAMILY TEACHING

* Treatment may depress your immune system response and reduce your ability to fight infection. Report symptoms of infection such as body aches, chills, cough, fatigue, fever. Avoid those with active infection. * Report symptoms of bone marrow depression such as bruising, fatigue, fever, shortness of breath, weight loss; bleeding easily, bloody urine or stool. * Treatment may cause life-threatening differentiation syndrome. Report difficulty breathing, fever, low blood pressure, rapid weight gain, swelling of the hands or feet; decreased urine output. * Life-threating heart arrhythmias may occur, which can be fatal. Report chest pain, dizziness, fainting, palpitations, shortness of breath, slow or rapid heart rate, irregular heart rate. Expect frequent electrocardiograms. * Report liver problems (abdominal pain, bruising, clay-colored stool, amber or dark colored urine, yellowing of the skin or eyes). * There is a high risk of interactions with other medications. Do not take newly prescribed medications unless approved by prescriber who originally started treatment. Do not take herbal products. * Do not receive live vaccines.

RABEprazole TOP 100

ra-**bep**-ra-zole
(<u>Aciphex</u>, Pariet ✦)
**Do not confuse Aciphex with
Accupril or Aricept, or RABEprazole with ARIPiprazole,
donepezil, lansoprazole, omeprazole, or raloxifene.**

◆CLASSIFICATION

PHARMACOTHERAPEUTIC: Proton
pump inhibitor. **CLINICAL:** Gastric
acid inhibitor.

USES

**Gastroesophageal reflux disease
(GERD):** Short-term treatment for healing and Short-term (4–8 wks) treatment
for healing and symptomatic relief of erosive or ulcerative GERD in adults. Maintainance healing and reduction in relapse
rates of symptoms in adults with erosive
or ulcerative GERD. Treatment of heartburn and other symptoms associated with
GERD for up to 4 wks in adults, for up to
8 wks in adolescents 12 yrs and older,
and children 1–11 yrs (sprinkle capsules
only) for up to 12 wks. **Duodenal
ulcers:** Short-term (up to 4 wks) treatment for healing and symptomatic relief
of duodenal ulcers in adults. ***H. pylori*
eradication:** Treatment of adults with *H.
pylori* infection and duodenal ulcer disease (active or history within the past 5
yrs) to eradicate *H. pylori* (in combination with amoxicillin and clarithromycin).
Hypersecretory conditions: Long-term
treatment of pathological hypersecretory
conditions (e.g., Zollinger-Ellison syndrome) in adults. **OFF-LABEL:** Barrett's
esophagus, functional dyspepsia, eosini-
philic esophagitis, NSAID-induced ulcers
(prevention).

PRECAUTIONS

Contraindications: Hypersensitivity to
RABEprazole, other proton pump inhibitors (e.g., omeprazole). Concomitant use
with rilpivirine-containing products. **Cautions:** Severe hepatic impairment,
osteoporosis.

ACTION

Suppresses gastric acid secretion by
inhibiting H^+/K^+–ATP pump. **Therapeutic Effect:** Increases gastric pH, reducing gastric acid production.

PHARMACOKINETICS

Rapidly absorbed after passing through
stomach relatively intact as delayed-
release tablet. Protein binding: 96%.
Metabolized in liver. Excreted in urine
(90%), feces. **Half-life:** 1–2 hrs
(increased with hepatic impairment).

⧗ LIFESPAN CONSIDERATIONS

Pregnancy/Lactation: Unknown if drug
crosses placenta or is distributed in breast
milk. **Children:** Safety and efficacy not
established in pts younger than 1 yr.
Elderly: No age-related precautions noted.

INTERACTIONS

DRUG: May decrease concentration/effects
of **acalabrutinib, cefuroxime, erlotinib, neratinib, pazopanib.** Strong
CYP2C19 inducers (e.g., **FLUoxetine**), strong CYP3A4 inducers
(e.g., **carBAMazepine, phenytoin,
rifAMPin**) may decrease concentra-
tion/effect. May decrease concentration
of **ketoconazole, clopidogrel, atazanavir. HERBAL:** None significant.
FOOD: None known. **LAB VALUES:** May
increase serum ALT, AST, thyroid-stimulating hormone (TSH).

AVAILABILITY (Rx)

🔻 **Tablets, Delayed-Release:** 20 mg.
Capsule, Sprinkle: 10 mg.

ADMINISTRATION/HANDLING

PO

Tablet • Give without regard to
food. • Administer whole (do not
crush, split, or allow chewing). • **Duodenal ulcer:** Give after a meal.

R

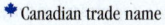 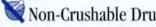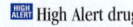

• **H. pylori eradication:** • Give with morning and evening meals.

Sprinkle

Capsule (sprinkle) • Administer 30 min before a meal. • Open capsule and sprinkle on soft food or a small amt of liquid (give within 15 min of preparation). • Do not administer capsule whole. Do not crush or allow chewing of granules.

INDICATIONS/ROUTES/DOSAGE

GERD (Treatment, Erosive/Ulcerative)
PO: ADULTS, ELDERLY: 20 mg once daily for 4–8 wks.

GERD (Maintenance Healing)
PO: ADULTS, ELDERLY: 20 mg once daily (duration up to 12 mos studied).

GERD (Symptomatic)
PO: ADULTS, ELDERLY: 20 mg once daily for up to 4 wks. **ADOLESCENTS 12 YRS AND OLDER**: 20 mg once daily for up to 8 wks. **CHILDREN 1–11 YRS WEIGHING 15 KG OR GREATER**: 10 mg once daily. **LESS THAN 15 KG**: Initially, 5 mg once daily. May increase to 10 mg once daily.

Duodenal Ulcer
PO: ADULTS, ELDERLY: 20 mg once daily before morning meal for up to 4 wks.

H. pylori Eradication
PO: ADULTS, ELDERLY: 20 mg (with amoxicillin and clarithromycin) twice daily with morning and evening meals for 7 days.

Hypersecretory Conditions
PO: ADULTS, ELDERY: Initially, 60 mg once daily. May titrate up to 100 mg once daily or 60 mg 2 times/day. Continue as long as clinical indicated.

Dosage in Renal Impairment
No dose adjustment.

Dosage in Hepatic Impairment
Mild to moderate impairment: No dose adjustment. **Severe impairment:** Use caution.

SIDE EFFECTS

Rare (less than 2%): Headache, nausea, dizziness, rash, diarrhea, malaise.

ADVERSE EFFECTS/TOXIC REACTIONS

Hyperglycemia, hypokalemia, hyponatremia, hyperlipemia occur rarely. May increase risk of bone fractures, *C. difficile*-associated colitis, fundic gland polyps, interstitial nephritis, vitamin B_{12} deficiency.

NURSING CONSIDERATIONS

BASELINE ASSESSMENT
Question history of GI disease, ulcers, GERD, hepatic impairment.

INTERVENTION/EVALUATION
Evaluate for therapeutic response (relief of GI symptoms). Question if GI discomfort, nausea, diarrhea, headache occurs. Assess skin for evidence of rash. Observe for evidence of dizziness; utilize appropriate safety precautions.

PATIENT/FAMILY TEACHING
• Swallow tablets whole; do not break, chew, dissolve, or divide tablets. • Report headache.

---

raloxifene

ra-**lox**-i-feen
(Evista)

■**BLACK BOX ALERT**■ Increases risk of deep vein thrombosis, pulmonary embolism. Women with coronary heart disease or pts at risk for coronary events are at increased risk for death due to stroke.
Do not confuse Evista with Avinza.

◆CLASSIFICATION

PHARMACOTHERAPEUTIC: Selective estrogen receptor modulator (SERM). **CLINICAL:** Osteoporosis preventive.

USES

Prevention/treatment of osteoporosis in post-menopausal women. Reduces risk of invasive breast cancer in postmenopausal women with osteoporosis and postmenopausal women at high risk for invasive breast cancer.

PRECAUTIONS

Contraindications: Hypersensitivity to raloxifene. Active or history of venous thromboembolic events, such as deep vein thrombosis (DVT), pulmonary embolism (PE), retinal vein thrombosis; women who are or may become pregnant, breastfeeding. **Cautions:** Cardiovascular disease, renal/hepatic impairment, pts at risk for thrombosis (immobility, indwelling venous catheter/access device, morbid obesity, genetic hypercoagulable conditions), unexplained uterine bleeding, elevated triglycerides in response to oral estrogen therapy.

ACTION

Selective estrogen receptor modulator (SERM) that binds to estrogen receptors, increasing bone mineral density. Blocks estrogen effects in breast/uterus. **Therapeutic Effect:** Reduces bone resorption, increases bone mineral density, reduces incidence of fractures.

PHARMACOKINETICS

Widely distributed. Protein binding: 95%. Metabolized in liver. Excreted primarily in feces. Unknown if removed by hemodialysis. **Half-life:** 27.7–32.5 hrs.

⌛ LIFESPAN CONSIDERATIONS

Pregnancy/Lactation: Unknown if distributed in breast milk. Contraindicated in pregnancy, breastfeeding. **Children:** Not used in this pt population. **Elderly:** No age-related precautions noted.

INTERACTIONS

DRUG: Bile acid sequestrants (e.g., cholestyramine) may decrease absorption/effect. May decrease absorption of **levothyroxine. HERBAL:** None significant. **FOOD:** None known. **LAB VALUES:** May lower serum total cholesterol, LDL. May decrease platelet count, serum inorganic phosphate, albumin, calcium, protein.

AVAILABILITY (Rx)

Tablets: 60 mg.

ADMINISTRATION/HANDLING

PO
• Give without regard to food.

INDICATIONS/ROUTES/DOSAGE

Note: Discontinue at least 72 hrs prior to and during prolonged immobilization (may increase risk for DVT/PE).
Prophylaxis/Treatment of Osteoporosis, Breast Cancer Risk Reduction
PO: ADULTS, ELDERLY: 60 mg/day.

Dosage in Renal/Hepatic Impairment
No dose adjustment.

SIDE EFFECTS

Frequent (25%–10%): Hot flashes, flu-like symptoms, arthralgia, sinusitis. **Occasional (9%–5%):** Weight gain, nausea, myalgia, pharyngitis, cough, dyspepsia, leg cramps, rash, depression. **Rare (4%–3%):** Vaginitis, UTI, peripheral edema, flatulence, vomiting, fever, migraine, diaphoresis.

ADVERSE EFFECTS/TOXIC REACTIONS

Thromboembolic events (DVT, pulmonary embolism, superficial thrombophlebitis) may occur, esp. in pts with immobility. May increase risk of uterine bleeding, hypertriglyceridemia; death due to stroke.

NURSING CONSIDERATIONS

BASELINE ASSESSMENT

Obtain lipid panel. Question history of thrombosis (CVA, DVT, PE). Question for possibility of pregnancy. Drug should be discontinued 72 hrs before and during prolonged immobilization (postop recovery, prolonged bed rest). Therapy may be resumed only after pt is fully ambulatory.

R

INTERVENTION/EVALUATION

Monitor serum total cholesterol, total calcium, phosphate, total protein, albumin, bone mineral density, platelet count. Diligently monitor for CVA (aphasia, blindness, confusion, paresthesia, hemiparesis, syncope), DVT (arm/leg pain, swelling), pulmonary embolism (chest pain, dyspnea, hypoxia, tachycardia).

PATIENT/FAMILY TEACHING

• Avoid prolonged restriction of movement during travel (increased risk of venous thromboembolic events). • Take supplemental calcium, vitamin D if daily dietary intake is inadequate. • Engage in regular weight-bearing exercise. • Modify, discontinue habits of cigarette smoking, alcohol consumption. • Report symptoms of DVT (swelling, pain, hot feeling in the arms or legs), lung embolism (difficulty breathing, chest pain, rapid heart rate), stroke (blindness, confusion, difficulty speaking, one-sided weakness, passing out).

---

ramelteon

ra-**mel**-tee-on
(Rozerem)
Do not confuse ramelteon with Remeron, or Rozerem with Razadyne or Remeron.

◆CLASSIFICATION

PHARMACOTHERAPEUTIC: Melatonin receptor agonist. **CLINICAL:** Hypnotic.

USES

Treatment of insomnia in pts who experience difficulty with sleep onset. **OFF-LABEL:** Delirium ICU (prevention).

PRECAUTIONS

Contraindications: Hypersensitivity to ramelteon. Concurrent fluvoxaMINE therapy, history of angioedema with previous ramelteon therapy. **Cautions:** Depression, other psychiatric conditions, alcohol consumption, other CNS depressants, moderate hepatic impairment, severe sleep apnea, COPD; concomitant strong CYP1A2 inhibitors (e.g., fluvoxaMINE).

ACTION

Selectively targets melatonin receptors thought to be involved in maintenance of circadian rhythm underlying normal sleep-wake cycle. **Therapeutic Effect:** Prevents insomnia characterized by difficulty with sleep onset.

PHARMACOKINETICS

Widely distributed. Protein binding: 82%. Metabolized in liver. Excreted in urine (84%), feces (4%). **Half-life:** 2–5 hrs.

⧖ LIFESPAN CONSIDERATIONS

Pregnancy/Lactation: Unknown if distributed in breast milk. Breastfeeding not recommended. **Children:** Safety and efficacy not established. **Elderly:** Age-related hepatic impairment may require dosage adjustment.

INTERACTIONS

DRUG: **CNS depressants (e.g., alcohol, morphine, oxyCODONE, zolpidem)** may increase CNS depression. **Strong CYP3A4 inducers (e.g., carBAMazepine, rifAMPin)** may decrease concentration/effect. **HERBAL:** **Herbals with sedative properties (e.g., chamomile, kava kava, valerian)** may increase CNS depression. **FOOD:** Onset of action may be reduced if taken with or immediately after a **high-fat meal.** **LAB VALUES:** May decrease serum cortisol, testosterone. May increase serum prolactin.

AVAILABILITY (Rx)

🔖 **Tablets, Film-Coated:** 8 mg.

ADMINISTRATION/HANDLING

PO

• Administer within 30 min before bedtime. • Do not give with, or immediately following, a high-fat meal. • Do not break, crush, dissolve, or divide tablet.

---

underlined – top prescribed drug

INDICATIONS/ROUTES/DOSAGE

Insomnia

PO: ADULTS, ELDERLY: 8 mg within 30 min before bedtime. **Maximum:** 8 mg.

Dosage in Renal Impairment

No dose adjustment.

Dosage in Hepatic Impairment

Mild to moderate impairment: No dose adjustment. **Severe impairment:** Not recommended.

SIDE EFFECTS

Frequent (7%–5%): Headache, dizziness, drowsiness (expected effect). **Occasional (4%–3%):** Fatigue, nausea, exacerbated insomnia. **Rare (2%):** Diarrhea, myalgia, depression, altered taste, arthralgia.

ADVERSE EFFECTS/TOXIC REACTIONS

Severe hypersensitivity reactions including anaphylaxis, angioedema, dyspnea, throat constriction may occur. Angioedema involving larynx, glottis, tongue can be fatal. Worsening of insomnia may indicate underlying psychiatric illness. May cause amnesic events including cooking, sleepwalking, sexual activity, sleep-driving. May increase risk of suicidal ideation and behavior. May affect reproductive hormones in adults (decreased testosterone levels, increased prolactin levels), resulting in unexplained amenorrhea, galactorrhea, decreased libido, impaired fertility.

NURSING CONSIDERATIONS

BASELINE ASSESSMENT

Assess B/P, pulse, respirations. Raise bed rails, provide call light. Provide environment conducive to sleep (quiet environment, low/no lighting, TV off). Do not give unless a full night of sleep is planned.

INTERVENTION/EVALUATION

Assess sleep pattern of pt. Evaluate for therapeutic response: rapid induction of sleep onset, decrease in number of nocturnal awakenings.

PATIENT/FAMILY TEACHING

• Take within 30 min before going to bed; confine activities to those necessary to prepare for bed. • Avoid tasks that require alertness, motor skills until response to drug is established. • Therapy may need to be discontinued if cooking, driving, sleepwalking, sexual activity occurs without recollection. • Do not take unless a full night of sleep is planned. • Avoid alcohol. • Do not take medication with or immediately after a high-fat meal.

ramipril

ram-i-pril
(Altace)

■ **BLACK BOX ALERT** ■ May cause fetal injury, mortality. Discontinue as soon as possible once pregnancy is detected.
Do not confuse Altace with alteplase, Amaryl, or Artane, or ramipril with enalapril or Monopril.

◆CLASSIFICATION

PHARMACOTHERAPEUTIC: Angiotensin-converting enzyme (ACE) inhibitor. **CLINICAL:** Antihypertensive.

USES

Hypertension: Treatment of hypertension. Used alone or in combination with other antihypertensives. **Heart failure:** Treatment of HF with reduced ejection fraction following MI. **Risk reduction of cardiovascular events:** Reduce risk of heart attack, stroke in pts 55 yrs and older at increased risk of developing major cardiovascular events. **OFF-LABEL:** Acute coronary syndrome (STEMI, non-STEMI), proteinuric chronic kidney disease (diabetic or nondiabetic).

R

PRECAUTIONS

Contraindications: Hypersensitivity to ramipril, other ACE inhibitors. History of ACE inhibitor–induced angioedema, concomitant use with aliskiren in pts with diabetes. Concomitant use or within 36 hrs of switching to or from a neprilysin inhibitor (e.g., sacubitril). **Cautions:** Renal impairment, elderly, collagen vascular disease, hyperkalemia, hypertrophic cardiomyopathy with outflow tract obstruction; unstented unilateral, bilateral renal artery stenosis; severe aortic stenosis; before, during, or immediately after major surgery; concomitant potassium supplements.

ACTION

Suppresses renin-angiotensin-aldosterone system. Blocks conversion of angiotensin I to angiotensin II, increases plasma renin activity, decreases aldosterone secretion. **Therapeutic Effect:** Reduces peripheral arterial resistance, decreasing B/P.

PHARMACOKINETICS

Route	Onset	Peak	Duration
PO	1–2 hrs	3–6 hrs	24 hrs

Widely distributed. Protein binding: 73%. Metabolized in liver. Primarily excreted in urine. Not removed by hemodialysis. **Half-life:** 5.1 hrs.

⧖ LIFESPAN CONSIDERATIONS

Pregnancy/Lactation: Crosses placenta. Distributed in breast milk. May cause fetal or neonatal mortality or morbidity. **Children:** Safety and efficacy not established. **Elderly:** May be more sensitive to hypotensive effects.

INTERACTIONS

DRUG: Aliskiren may increase hyperkalemic effect. May increase potential for allergic reactions to **allopurinol. Angiotensin receptor blockers** (e.g., **losartan, valsartan**) may increase adverse effects. May increase adverse effects of **lithium, sacubitril. HERBAL:** Herbals with hypertensive properties (e.g., **licorice,** yohimbe) or hypotensive properties (e.g., **garlic, ginger, ginkgo biloba**) may alter effects. **FOOD:** None known. **LAB VALUES:** May increase serum BUN, alkaline phosphatase, bilirubin, creatinine, potassium, ALT, AST. May decrease serum sodium. May cause positive antinuclear antibody (ANA) titer.

AVAILABILITY (Rx)

Capsules: 1.25 mg, 2.5 mg, 5 mg, 10 mg.

ADMINISTRATION/HANDLING

PO
• Give without regard to food. • Administer capsule whole (may open and mix with water, apple juice, or applesauce).

INDICATIONS/ROUTES/DOSAGE

Hypertension
PO: ADULTS, ELDERLY: Initially, 2.5 mg/day. Evaluate after 2–4 wks and titrate as needed up to 20 mg/day in 1 or 2 divided doses.

HF Following MI
PO: ADULTS, ELDERLY: Initially, 1.25–2.5 mg once daily. Increase dose (e.g., double dose) q1–2 wks or longer to a target dose of 10 mg once daily.

Risk Reduction for MI/Stroke
PO: ADULTS, ELDERLY: Initially, 2.5 mg/day for 7 days, then 5 mg/day for 21 days, then increase as tolerated to maintenance dose of 10 mg/day in 1–2 divided doses.

Dosage in Renal Impairment
CrCl equal to or less than 40 mL/min: 25% of normal dose.

Renal Failure and Hypertension
Initially, 1.25 mg/day titrated upward. **Maximum:** 5 mg/day. **Renal failure and HF:** Initially, 1.25 mg/day, titrated up to 2.5 mg twice daily.

Dosage in Hepatic Impairment
No dose adjustment. Discontinue for jaundice or marked elevation of hepatic enzymes.

SIDE EFFECTS

Frequent (12%–5%): Cough, headache. **Occasional (4%–2%):** Dizziness, fatigue, nausea, asthenia. **Rare (less than 2%):** Palpitations, insomnia, nervousness, malaise, abdominal pain, myalgia.

ADVERSE EFFECTS/TOXIC REACTIONS

Excessive hypotension ("first-dose syncope") may occur in pts with HF, severely salt or volume depleted. Angioedema, hyperkalemia occur rarely. Agranulocytosis, neutropenia may occur in pts with collagen vascular disease (scleroderma, systemic lupus erythematosus), renal impairment. Nephrotic syndrome may occur in pts with history of renal disease. May cause angioedema of the face, neck, throat, tongue. Cholestatic jaundice, fulminant hepatic necrosis may occur.

NURSING CONSIDERATIONS

BASELINE ASSESSMENT

Obtain B/P immediately before each dose, in addition to regular monitoring (be alert to fluctuations). Renal function tests should be performed before beginning therapy. Question history of hypersensitivity reaction, angioedema.

INTERVENTION/EVALUATION

In pts with prior renal disease, urine test for protein (by dipstick method) should be made with first urine of day before beginning therapy and periodically thereafter. In pts with renal impairment, autoimmune disease, or taking drugs that affect leukocytes or immune response, CBC, differential count should be performed before beginning therapy and q2wks for 3 mos periodically thereafter. Monitor B/P, renal function, serum potassium. Assess for cough (frequent effect). Assist with ambulation if dizziness occurs. Assess lung sounds for rales, wheezing in pts with HF. Monitor urinalysis for proteinuria. Monitor serum potassium in pts on concurrent diuretic therapy.

PATIENT/FAMILY TEACHING

• Do not discontinue medication without physician's approval. • Slowly go from lying to standing to minimize hypotensive effect. • Report palpitations, cough, chest pain. • Dizziness may occur in first few days. • Avoid alcohol. • Report swelling of the face, lips, or tongue.

ramucirumab

ra-mue-**sir**-ue-mab
(Cyramza)
Do not confuse ramucirumab with ranibizumab.

◆CLASSIFICATION

PHARMACOTHERAPEUTIC: Vascular endothelial growth factor (VEGF) inhibitor. Monoclonal antibody. **CLINICAL:** Antineoplastic.

USES

Gastric/gastroesophageal junction adenocarcinoma: As a single agent or in combination with PACLitaxel, for treatment of advanced or metastatic gastric or gastroesophageal junction adenocarcinoma with disease progression on or after prior fluoropyrimidine- or platinum-containing chemotherapy. **Non–small-cell lung cancer (NSCLC):** In combination with DOCEtaxel, for treatment of metastatic non–small-cell lung cancer with disease progression on or after platinum-based chemotherapy. In combination with erlotinib, for first-line treatment of metastatic NSCLC with epidermal growth factor receptor (EGFR) exon 19 deletions or exon 21 (L858R) mutations. **Colorectal cancer:** In combination with FOLFIRI, for treatment of metastatic colorectal cancer with disease progression on or after therapy with bevacizumab, oxaliplatin, and a fluoropyrimidine. **Hepatocellular carcinoma:** Treatment of advanced or relapsed/refractory hepatocellular carcinoma (as a single agent who have an alpha fetoprotein of greater than or

R

equal to 400 nanograms/mL and have been treated with sorafenib).

PRECAUTIONS

Contraindications: Hypersensitivity to ramucirumab. **Cautions:** History of arterial/venous thromboembolism (e.g., MI, cardiac arrest, CVA, cerebral ischemia), hepatic cirrhosis, electrolyte imbalance, hypertension, GI bleeding/perforation, chronic/unhealed wounds; baseline neutropenia, thrombocytopenia.

ACTION

Binds vascular endothelial growth factor (VEGF) receptor 2 and blocks binding of VEGF ligands, VEGF-A, VEGF-C, and VEGF-D. **Therapeutic Effect:** Inhibits/reduces tumor vascularity and growth.

PHARMACOKINETICS

Metabolism not specified. Elimination not specified.

⏳ LIFESPAN CONSIDERATIONS

Pregnancy/Lactation: May cause fetal harm. Females of reproductive potential should use effective contraception during treatment and up to 3 mos after discontinuation. Unknown if distributed in breast milk. **Children:** Safety and efficacy not established. **Elderly:** No age-related precautions noted.

INTERACTIONS

DRUG: None significant. **HERBAL:** None significant. **FOOD:** None known. **LAB VALUES:** May increase urine protein. May decrease neutrophils, serum sodium.

AVAILABILITY (Rx)

Injection Solution: 100 mg/10 mL, 500 mg/50 mL.

ADMINISTRATION/HANDLING

 IV

• Do not administer IV push or bolus. • Recommend premedication with IV histamine H_1 antagonist (e.g., diphenhydrAMINE) prior to each

infusion. Pts with prior Grade 1 or Grade 2 infusion reaction should also be premedicated with dexAMETHasone (or equivalent) and acetaminophen prior to each infusion. • Flush IV line with 0.9% NaCl upon infusion completion.

Reconstitution • Calculate dose, required solution volume, and number of vials needed using weight in kg. • Vials contain either 100 mg/10 mL or 500 mL/50 mL at concentration of 10 mg/mL. • Visually inspect for particulate matter. Discard if particulate matter or discoloration observed. • Using 250 mL 0.9% NaCl bag, withdraw and discard a volume equal to the total calculated volume of solution. • Slowly add required dose to diluent bag for final volume of 250 mL. Gently invert bag to mix; do not shake.

Rate of administration • Infuse over 60 min using 0.22-micron in-line filter via dedicated line if tolerated, may administer subsequent infusions over 30 min.

Storage • Refrigerate vials in original carton until time of use. • Do not freeze. • Diluted solution may be refrigerated up to 24 hrs or stored at room temperature for up to 4 hrs. • Protect from light.

🏵 IV INCOMPATIBILITIES

Do not dilute in dextrose-containing fluids or infuse concomitantly with other electrolytes or medications.

INDICATIONS/ROUTES/DOSAGE

Gastric Cancer (Advanced or Metastatic)
IV: ADULTS, ELDERLY: 8 mg/kg every 14 days, either as a single agent or in combination with wkly PACLitaxel. Continue until disease progression or unacceptable toxicity.

NSCLC
IV: ADULTS, ELDERLY: (Disease progression on or after platinum-based chemotherapy): 10 mg/kg on day 1 of a 21-day cycle in combination with DOCEtaxel. Continue until disease progression or unacceptable toxicity.

(First-line treatment): 10 mg/kg once q2wks (in combination with erlotinib). Continue until disease progression or unacceptable toxicity.

Colorectal Cancer
IV: ADULTS, ELDERLY: 8 mg/kg q2wks, in combination with FOLFIRI (irinotecan, leucovorin, 5-fluorouracil). Continue until disease progression or unacceptable toxicity.

Hepatocellular Carcinoma
IV: ADULTS, ELDERLY: 8 mg/kg q2wks (as single agent). Continue until disease progression or unacceptable toxicity

Dose Modification
Based on Common Terminology Criteria for Adverse Events (CTCAE).
Infusion-related reaction: Reduce infusion rate by 50% for Grade 1 or Grade 2 reaction. Permanently discontinue for Grade 3 or Grade 4 reaction. **Severe hypertension:** Interrupt treatment until controlled with medical management. Permanently discontinue for severe hypertension that is not controlled with antihypertensive therapy. **Proteinuria:** Interrupt treatment for urine protein level greater than or equal to 2 g/24 hrs. Restart treatment at reduced dose of 6 mg/kg every 14 days once urine protein level returns to less than 2 g/24 hrs. If level greater than or equal 2 g/24 hrs recurs, interrupt treatment and reduce dose to 5 mg/kg every 14 days once level returns to less than 2 g/24 hrs. Permanently discontinue for urine protein level greater than 3 g/24 hrs or in the setting of nephrotic syndrome. **Wound healing complications:** Interrupt treatment prior to scheduled surgery until wound is fully healed. **Arterial thromboembolic events, GI perforation, or Grade 3 or Grade 4 bleeding:** Permanently discontinue.

Dosage in Renal Impairment
No dose adjustment.

Dosage in Hepatic Impairment
Mild to moderate impairment: No dose adjustment. **Severe impairment:** Use caution

SIDE EFFECTS
Occasional (16%–9%): Hypertension, diarrhea, headache. **Ramucirumab plus PACLitaxel: Frequent (57%–20%):** Fatigue, diarrhea, peripheral edema, hypertension, stomatitis.

ADVERSE EFFECTS/TOXIC REACTIONS
Fatal hemorrhagic events including GI bleeding occurred in 3.4% of pts receiving single agent and in 4.3% of pts receiving combo therapy. GI perforations occurred in 0.7% of pts receiving single agent and in 1.2% of pts receiving combo therapy. Thromboembolic events including arterial thromboembolism, CVA, MI reported in 1.7% of pts. Severe hypertension occurred in 8% of pts receiving single agent and in 15% of pts receiving combo therapy despite medical management. Severe infusion-related reactions such as back pain/spasms, bronchospasm, chest pain, chills, dyspnea, flushing, hypotension, hypoxia, paresthesia, rigors/tremors, supraventricular tachycardia, wheezing occurred in 16% of pts. May cause ineffective wound healing or wound dehiscence requiring medical intervention. Reversible posterior leukoencephalopathy syndrome (RPLS) reported in less than 1% of pts. Proteinuria may indicate nephrotic syndrome. Clinical deterioration of hepatic cirrhosis, manifested by new-onset or worsening encephalopathy, ascites, or hepatorenal syndrome, was reported in pts receiving single agent. Other adverse reactions include epistaxis, intestinal obstruction, neutropenia, severe rash, thrombocytopenia.

NURSING CONSIDERATIONS

BASELINE ASSESSMENT
Obtain CBC, BMP, vital signs; pregnancy test in females of reproductive potential. Question history of CVA, hepatic impairment/cirrhosis, hypertension, MI, prior hypersensitivity reaction. Offer emotional support.

R

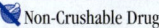

INTERVENTION/EVALUATION

Monitor CBC, serum electrolytes, vital signs. Persistent diastolic hypertension may indicate hypertensive emergency. Obtain ECG for arrhythmia, chest pain, palpitation. Consider RPLS in pts with altered mental status, confusion, headache, seizure, visual disturbances. Screen for GI bleeding, GI perforation. Notify physician if any CTCAE toxicities occur (see Appendix K). Monitor for hypersensitivity reaction. Once infusion is completed, IV access must be flushed with NS.

PATIENT/FAMILY TEACHING

• Treatment may cause severe allergic reaction or infusion-related reaction. • Use effective contraception to avoid pregnancy. Do not breastfeed. • Neurologic changes, including altered mental status, headache, seizures, trouble speaking, may indicate high blood pressure crisis or life-threatening brain swelling. • Immediately report abdominal pain, GI bleeding, vomiting blood. • Therapy may cause severe blood-clotting events such as heart attack or stroke.

rasagiline

ra-**sa**-ji-leen
(Azilect, Apo-Rasagiline ✦)
Do not confuse Azilect with Aricept.

◆CLASSIFICATION

PHARMACOTHERAPEUTIC: MAO type B inhibitor. **CLINICAL:** Antiparkinson agent.

USES

Treatment of signs/symptoms of Parkinson's disease as initial monotherapy or as adjunct therapy with or without levodopa.

PRECAUTIONS

Contraindications: Hypersensitivity to rasagiline. Concurrent use with methadone, traMADol, meperidine, MAOIs within 14 days of rasagiline, cyclobenzaprine, dextromethorphan, or St. John's wort. **Cautions:** Hepatic impairment (avoid use in moderate to severe impairment); cardiovascular, cerebrovascular disease, baseline hypotension. Avoid foods high in tyramine. Do not use within 5 wks of stopping FLUoxetine; do not start tricyclic, SSRI, or SNRI within 2 wks of stopping rasagiline. History of major psychotic disorder.

ACTION

Irreversibly and selectively inhibits monoamine oxidase type B, an enzyme that plays a major role in catabolism of DOPamine. Inhibition of DOPamine depletion reduces symptomatic motor deficits of Parkinson's disease. **Therapeutic Effect:** Reduces symptoms of Parkinson's disease; appears to delay disease progression.

PHARMACOKINETICS

Widely distributed. Protein binding: 88%–94%. Metabolized in liver. Excreted in urine (62%), feces (7%). **Half-life:** 1.3–3 hrs.

⏳ LIFESPAN CONSIDERATIONS

Pregnancy/Lactation: Unknown if distributed in breast milk. **Children:** Safety and efficacy not established. **Elderly:** No age-related precautions noted.

INTERACTIONS

DRUG: Alcohol may increase adverse effects. **MAOIs** (e.g., **phenelzine, selegiline), sympathomimetics** (e.g., **DOPamine)** may cause hypertensive crisis. **CNS stimulants** (e.g., **methylphenidate), strong CYP3A4 inhibitors** (e.g., **clarithromycin, ketoconazole, ritonavir), moderate CYP3A4 inhibitors** (e.g., **dilTIAZem, fluconazole, verapamil)** may increase concentration/effect. **Strong CYP3A4 inducers** (e.g., **carBAMazepine, phenytoin, rifampin), moderate CYP3A4 inducers** (e.g., **dexamethasone, modafinil,**

R

nafcillin) may decrease concentration/effect. **SSRIs (e.g. citalopram, fluoxetine), SNRIs (e.g., duloxetine, venlafaxine), tricyclic antidepressants (e.g., amitriptyline)** may increase risk of serotonin syndrome. **HERBAL: Herbals with hypotensive properties (e.g., black cohosh, garlic)** may increase effect. **St. John's wort** may decrease concentration/effect. **FOOD: Caffeine, foods/beverages containing tyramine** may result in hypertensive reaction, hypertensive crisis. **LAB VALUES:** May increase serum alkaline phosphatase, bilirubin, ALT, AST. May cause leukopenia.

AVAILABILITY (Rx)

Tablets: 0.5 mg, 1 mg.

ADMINISTRATION/HANDLING

PO
• Give without regard to food. • Avoid food, beverages containing tyramine (e.g., cheese, sour cream, yogurt, pickled herring, liver, figs, raisins, bananas, avocados, soy sauce, broad beans, yeast extracts, meat tenderizers, red wine, beer), excessive amounts of caffeine (e.g., coffee, tea).

INDICATIONS/ROUTES/DOSAGE

◄ALERT► When used in combination with levodopa, dosage reduction of levodopa should be considered.

Parkinson's Disease
PO: ADULTS, ELDERLY, MONOTHERAPY, ADJUNCTIVE THERAPY WITHOUT LEVODOPA: 1 mg once daily. **ADULTS, ELDERLY, ADJUNCTIVE THERAPY WITH LEVODOPA:** Initially, 0.5 mg once daily. If therapeutic response is not achieved, dose may be increased to 1 mg once daily.

Dose Modification
Concomitant use of CYP1A2 inhibitors, ciprofloxacin: 0.5 mg once daily.

Dosage in Hepatic Impairment
Mild impairment: 0.5 mg once daily. **Moderate to severe impairment:** Not recommended.

Dosage in Renal Impairment
No dose adjustment.

SIDE EFFECTS

Frequent (14%–12%): Headache, nausea. **Occasional (9%–5%):** Orthostatic hypotension, weight loss, dyspepsia, dry mouth, arthralgia, depression, hallucinations, constipation. **Rare (4%–2%):** Fever, vertigo, ecchymosis, rhinitis, neck pain, arthritis, paresthesia.

ADVERSE EFFECTS/TOXIC REACTIONS

Increase in dyskinesia (impaired voluntary movement), dystonia (impaired muscular tone) occurs in 18% of pts, angina occurs in 9%. Gastroenteritis, conjunctivitis reported in 3% of pts.

NURSING CONSIDERATIONS

BASELINE ASSESSMENT
Obtain LFT, B/P. Receive full medication history and screen for interactions. Question history of severe hepatic impairment, cardiovascular disease.

INTERVENTION/EVALUATION
Monitor B/P. Assess for clinical reversal of symptoms (improvement of tremor of head/hands at rest, mask-like facial expression, shuffling gait, muscular rigidity). If hallucinations or dyskinesia occurs, symptoms may be eliminated if levodopa dosage is reduced. Hallucinations generally are accompanied by confusion and, to a lesser extent, insomnia.

PATIENT/FAMILY TEACHING
• Orthostatic hypotension may occur more frequently after starting therapy. • Avoid tasks that require alertness, motor skills until response to drug is established. • Hallucinations may occur (more so in the elderly with Parkinson's disease), typically within first 2 wks of therapy. • Avoid foods that contain tyramine (cheese, sour cream, beer, wine, pickled herring, liver, figs, raisins, bananas, avocados, soy sauce, yeast extracts, yogurt, papaya, broad beans, meat

tenderizers), excessive amounts of caffeine (coffee, tea, chocolate), OTC preparations for hay fever, colds, weight reduction (may produce significant rise in B/P). • Do not take newly prescribed medications unless approved by prescriber who originally started therapy.

rasburicase

ras-**bure**-i-kase
(Elitek, Fasturtec ✦)

■ **BLACK BOX ALERT** ■ Severe hypersensitivity reactions including anaphylaxis reported. May cause severe hemolysis in pts with glucose-6-phosphate dehydrogenase (G6PD) deficiency. Screen pts at high risk for G6PD (African or Mediterranean descent) prior to therapy. Methemoglobinemia has been reported. Blood samples left at room temperature may interfere with uric acid measurements. Must collect blood samples in prechilled tubes containing heparin and immediately immerse in ice water bath. Assay plasma samples within 4 hrs of collection. Elitek enzymatically degrades uric acid in blood samples left at room temperature.

◆CLASSIFICATION

PHARMACOTHERAPEUTIC: Urate-oxidase enzyme. **CLINICAL:** Antihyperuricemic.

USES

Initial management of uric acid levels in pediatric and adult pts with leukemia, lymphoma, and solid tumor malignancies who are receiving chemotherapy expected to result in tumor lysis and subsequent elevation of plasma uric acid.

PRECAUTIONS

Contraindications: History of anaphylaxis or severe hypersensitivity to rasburicase. Prior rasburicase-associated drug reactions including hemolysis, methemoglobinemia. History of G6PD deficiency.

Cautions: Pts at high risk for G6PD deficiency (e.g., African, Mediterranean, or Southeast Asian descent).

ACTION

A urate-oxidase enzyme that converts uric acid into allantoin (an inactive metabolite of uric acid). Does not inhibit formation of uric acid. **Therapeutic Effect:** Decreases uric acid levels.

PHARMACOKINETICS

Half-life: 16–23 hrs.

⏳ LIFESPAN CONSIDERATIONS

Pregnancy/Lactation: Avoid pregnancy; may cause fetal harm. Unknown if distributed in breast milk. **Children/Elderly:** No age-related precautions noted.

INTERACTIONS

DRUG: None significant. **HERBAL:** None significant. **FOOD:** None known. **LAB VALUES:** May increase serum bilirubin, ALT. May decrease serum phosphate.

AVAILABILITY (Rx)

Injection, Powder for Reconstitution: 1.5 mg/vial, 7.5 mg/vial.

ADMINISTRATION/HANDLING

💉 IV

Reconstitution • Must use diluent provided in carton. • Reconstitute 1.5-mg vial with 1 mL of diluent or 7.5-mg vial with 5 mL of diluent to provide concentration of 1.5 mg/mL. • Gently swirl to mix. Do not shake. • Inspect for particulate matter or discoloration. • Dilute in 0.9% NaCl to achieve a final volume of 50 mL.
Rate of administration • Infuse over 30 min. • Do not use filter during reconstitution or infusion.
Storage • Refrigerate solution until time of use. • Discard after 24 hrs following reconstitution.

🔳 IV INCOMPATIBILITIES

Do not mix with other IV medications.

INDICATIONS/ROUTES/DOSAGE

Management of Hyperuricemia

IV: ADULTS, ELDERLY, CHILDREN: 0.2 mg/kg daily for up to 5 days. Dosing beyond 5 days or administration of more than 1 course is not recommended.

Dosage in Renal/Hepatic Impairment

No dose adjustment.

SIDE EFFECTS

Frequent (50%–46%): Vomiting, fever. **Occasional (27%–13%):** Nausea, headache, abdominal pain, constipation, diarrhea, mucositis, rash.

ADVERSE EFFECTS/TOXIC REACTIONS

Hypersensitivity reactions occurred in 4.3% of pts including injection irritation, peripheral edema, urticaria, pruritus. Anaphylaxis, hemolysis, methemoglobinemia occurred in less than 1%. Pulmonary hemorrhage, respiratory failure, supraventricular arrhythmias, ischemic coronary artery disorders, sepsis, abdominal, gastrointestinal infections occurred in greater than 2% of pts. Anti-rasburicase antibodies reported.

NURSING CONSIDERATIONS

BASELINE ASSESSMENT

Obtain uric acid level; pregnancy test in females of reproductive potential. Question for history of prior hypersensitivity reactions. Assess G6PD deficiency risk in potential candidates.

INTERVENTION/EVALUATION

Monitor uric acid levels. If hypersensitivity reaction occurs, stop infusion and immediately notify physician. Screen for clinical tumor lysis syndrome, hemolysis, methemoglobinemia. Follow strict procedure when collecting uric acid levels. Obtain ECG for chest pain/tightness, hyperkalemia, dyspnea. Assess skin for rash.

PATIENT/FAMILY TEACHING

* Report any allergic reaction, bronchospasm, chest pain or tightness, cough, difficulty breathing, dizziness, fainting, rash, or itching.

remdesivir

rem-**de**-si-vir
(Veklury)
Do not confuse remdesivir with oseltamivir, peramivir, or zanamivir.

◆**Classification**

PHARMACOTHERAPEUTIC: Nucleotide analog ribonucleic acid (RNA) polymerase inhibitor. **CLINICAL:** Antiviral.

USES

Treatment of coronavirus disease 2019 (COVID-19) in adults and pediatric pts (28 days of age and older and weighing at least 3 kg) with positive results of direct SARS-CoV-2 viral testing, who are hospitalized, or who are not hospitalized and have mild-to-moderate COVID-19 and are at high risk for progression to severe COVID-19.

PRECAUTIONS

Contraindications: Hypersensitivity to remdesivir. **Cautions:** Renal impairment, hepatic disease. Avoid concomitant use of chloroquine phosphate, hydroxychloroquine.

ACTION

Inhibits SARS-CoV-2 RNA-dependent RNA polymerase, essential for viral replication. Distributes into cells and metabolizes into active nucleoside triphosphate metabolite, which competes for incorporation into RNA chains, resulting in chain termination. **Therapeutic Effect:** Inhibits viral replication of coronavirus associated with COVID-19.

PHARMACOKINETICS

Widely distributed. Primarily metabolized by enzymatic activity into active metabolite (minimal hepatic metabolism). Protein binding: 88%–94%. Peak plasma

R

concentration: Less than 1 hr. Excreted in urine (49%), feces (less than 1%). **Half-life:** 1 hr.

⧗ LIFESPAN CONSIDERATIONS

Pregnancy/Lactation: Unknown if distributed in breast milk. **Children:** Safety and efficacy not established in pts younger than 28 days old or weighing less than 3 kg. **Elderly:** No age-related precautions noted.

INTERACTIONS

DRUG: Chloroquine, hydroxy-chloroquine may decrease antiviral/therapeutic effect. **Strong CYP3A4 inducers (e.g., carBAMazepine, phenytoin, rifAMPin)** may decrease concentration/effect. **HERBAL:** None significant. **FOOD:** None known. **LAB VALUES:** May increase serum ALT, AST, bilirubin, creatinine, glucose; prothrombin time. May decrease CrCl, estimated glomerular filtration rate (eGFR), Hgb, lymphocytes.

AVAILABILITY (Rx)

Injection, Powder for Reconstitution: 100 mg (for pediatric pts weighing 3–39 kg). **Injection Solution:** 100 mg/20 mL (5 mg/mL).

ADMINISTRATION/HANDLING

 IV

Note: Must be prepared and administered in the healthcare setting by a healthcare provider.
Reconstitution/Preparation • Reconstitute lyophilized powder with 19 mL Sterile Water for Injection. Discard vial if vacuum does not pull Sterile Water for Injection into vial. • Shake for 30 sec, then allow contents to settle for 2–3 min. Repeat until contents are completely dissolved (discard if not completely dissolved). • Reconstituted solution must be diluted in either 100 mL or 250 mL 0.9% NaCl infusion bag. Concentrated injection solution must be diluted in 250 mL 0.9% NaCl infusion bag only. • Visually inspect

for particulate matter or discoloration. Solution should appear clear, colorless to slightly yellow. Do not use if solution is cloudy or discolored or if visible particles are observed. • Withdraw and discard a volume from the infusion bag that is equal to the required volume of dose (40 mL for loading dose; 20 mL for maintenance dose). • Transfer required volume of dose to infusion bag. • Invert 20 times to mix. Do not shake.
Rate of administration • Infuse over 30–120 min based on tolerability.
Storage • Store unused vials containing lyophilized powder at controlled room temperature. Refrigerate unused vials containing concentrated injection solution or store at room temperature for up to 12 hrs. • May refrigerate diluted solution for up to 48 hrs or store at room temperature for up to 24 hrs. • Do not shake or freeze.

▦ IV INCOMPATABILITIES

Do not mix or infuse with other medications or solutions.
Note: Use lyophilized powder only in pts weighing 3–39 kg.

INDICATIONS/ROUTES/DOSAGE

COVID-19 Infection
Note: Treatment duration: Hospitalized pts requiring invasive mechanical ventilation and/or extracorporeal membrane oxygenation (ECMO) is 10 days; hospitalized pts not requiring invasive mechanical ventilation and/or ECMO is 5 days; nonhospitalized pts is 3 days.
IV: ADULTS, CHILDREN 12 YRS AND OLDER WEIGHING AT LEAST 40 KG: 200 mg on day 1, then 100 mg from day 2. **CHILDREN AGED 28 DAYS AND OLDER WEIGHING 3–39 KG:** 5 mg/kg on day 1, then 2.5 mg/kg from day 2. **Permanent discontinuation:** Discontinue in pts with hypersensitivity reactions, serum ALT greater than 10 times ULN, or serum ALT elevation associated with signs and symptoms of hepatic inflammation.

Dosage in Renal/Hepatic Impairment
No dose adjustment.

SIDE EFFECTS

Rare (5% to less than 1%): Nausea, injection site erythema.

ADVERSE EFFECTS/TOXIC REACTIONS

Hypersensitivity reactions including anaphylaxis, angioedema, bradycardia, diaphoresis, dyspnea, fever, hypertension, hypotension, hypoxia, nausea, rash, shivering, tachycardia wheezing have occurred. Grade 1 or 2 transaminase elevations were reported. Seizure activity, acute kidney occur rarely.

NURSING CONSIDERATIONS

BASELINE ASSESSMENT

Obtain vital signs, renal function test (BUN, serum creatinine; CrCl, eGFR), LFT. Confirm positive test for SARS-CoV-2. Question history of renal impairment, hepatic disease. Auscultate lung sounds. Assess for symptoms of COVID-19 (anosmia, cough, dysgeusia, dyspnea, fever, headache, muscle aches, respiratory failure, sepsis). Initiate isolation precautions.

INTERVENTION/EVALUATION

Monitor vital signs, eGFR, LFT. Assess for hypersensitivity reactions, esp. during initial doses. Monitor I&Os. Assess for acute kidney injury, esp. in critically ill pts (decreased urinary output, edema, flank pain, seizures); hepatic injury (abdominal pain, encephalopathy, fatigue, jaundice, nausea, vomiting). Monitor for worsening of COVID-19–related symptoms.

PATIENT/FAMILY TEACHING

• Treatment is not a cure, but it may shorten recovery time and reduce symptoms associated with COVID-19. • Severe allergic reactions, including anaphylaxis, can occur. If allergic reaction occurs, seek immediate medical attention. • Report symptoms of liver inflammation (abdominal pain, confusion, nausea, vomiting, yellowing of skin or eyes); kidney inflammation (decreased urine output, flank pain, darkened urine).

repotrectinib

re-poe-**trek**-ti-nib
(Augtyro)
Do not confuse repotrectinib with alectinib, entrectinib, or larotrectinib.

◆CLASSIFICATION

PHARMACOTHERAPEUTIC: Tyrosine-protein kinase ROS1 (ROS1) inhibitor; tropomyosin receptor tyrosine kinase (TRK) inhibitor. **CLINICAL:** Antineoplastic.

USES

Non–small-cell lung cancer (NSCLC): Treatment of adults with locally advanced or metastatic ROS1-positive NSCLC. **Solid tumors:** Treatment of adults and children 12 yrs and older with solid tumors that have a neurotrophic tyrosine receptor kinase (NTRK) gene fusion, are locally advanced or metastatic or where surgical resection is likely to result in severe morbidity, and have progressed following treatment or have no satisfactory alternative therapy.

PRECAUTIONS

Contraindications: Hypersensitivity to repotrectinib. **Cautions:** Baseline cytopenias, hepatic impairment, conditions predisposing to infection (e.g., diabetes, immunocompromised pts, renal failure, open wounds), pts at risk for interstitial lung disease (e.g., COPD, sarcoidosis, connective tissue disease); pts at risk for bone fractures (e.g., fall risk, osteoporosis, chronic use of corticosteroids); history of depression, mood disorder, psychiatric disorders; hyperuricemia,

R

gout. Avoid concomitant use of strong or moderate CYP3A inhibitors, strong or moderate CYP3A inducers, P-gp inhibitors.

ACTION

Inhibits the proto-oncogene tyrosine-protein kinase and the tropomysin receptor kinases (TRKs). **Therapeutic Effect:** Inhibits cancer cell proliferation.

PHARMACOKINETICS

Widely distributed. Metabolized in liver. Protein binding: 95%. Peak plasma concentration: 2–3 hrs after a single oral dose. Steady-state within 14 days of daily administration of 160 mg. Excreted in feces (89%), urine (5%). Half-life: 61 hrs (first dose), 40 hrs (steady state).

⧗ LIFESPAN CONSIDERATIONS

Pregnancy/Lactation: Avoid pregnancy; may cause fetal harm. Females of reproductive potential must use effective non-hormonal contraception during treatment and for at least 2 mos after discontinuation. Treatment may decrease effect of hormonal contraceptives. Unknown if distributed in breast milk. Breastfeeding not recommended during treatment and for at least 10 days after discontinuation. **Males:** Males with female partners of reproductive potential must use effective contraception during treatment and for at least 4 mos after discontinuation. **Children:** Safety and efficacy not established in pts with ROS1-positive NSCLC. Safety and efficacy not established in pts younger than 12 yrs with solid tumors who have *NTRK* gene fusion. **Elderly:** No age-related precautions noted.

INTERACTIONS

DRUG: **Strong CYP3A4 inhibitors (e.g., clarithromycin, ketoconazole, ritonavir), moderate CYP3A4 inhibitors (e.g., dilTIAZem, verapamil), P-gp inhibitors (e.g., amiodarone, azithromycin, carvedilol, cycloSPORINE)** may increase concentration/effect. **Strong CYP3A4 inducers (e.g., carBAMazepine, phenytoin, riFAMpin), moderate CYP3A4 inducers (e.g., dexamethasone, modafinil, nafcillin)** may decrease concentration/effect. May decrease concentration/effect of **CYP3A4 substrates (e.g., busPI-Rone, tacrolimus, simvastatin).** May decrease concentration/effect; decrease progestin or estrogen exposure of **hormonal contraceptives. HERBAL: St. John's wort** may decrease concentration/effect. **FOOD:** None known. **LAB VALUES:** May increase serum alkaline phosphatase, ALT, AST, gamma glutamyl transferase (GGT), glucose, sodium, uric acid. May decrease serum phosphate, potassium; Hgb, lymphocytes, neutrophils. May increase or decrease serum glucose. May increase aPTT, INR.

AVAILABILITY (Rx)

Capsules: 40 mg, 160 mg.

ADMINISTRATION/HANDLING

PO

• Give without regard to food at the same time each day. • Administer capsules whole; do not cut, dissolve, or open. Capsules cannot be chewed. • If a dose is missed or vomiting occurs after administration, skip the dose and give next dose at the regularly scheduled time.

INDICATIONS/ROUTES/DOSAGE

NSCLC (Locally Advanced or Metastatic, ROS1-Positive), Solid Tumors (Locally Advanced or Metastatic, NTRK gene fusion)

PO: ADULTS, CHILDREN 12 YRS AND OLDER: 160 mg once daily for 14 days, then increase to 160 mg twice daily. Continue until disease progression or unacceptable toxicity.

Dose Reduction Schedule

160 mg once daily: (First reduction): 120 mg once daily. **(Second reduction):** 80 once daily.

160 mg twice daily: (First reduction): 120 mg twice daily. **(Second reduction):** 80 twice daily.

Dose Modification
Based on Common Terminology Criteria for Adverse Events (CTCAE).

Central Nervous System (CNS) Toxicity
Intolerable grade 2 CNS effects: Withhold treatment until improved to grade 1 or baseline, then resume at same or reduced dose. Grade 3 CNS effects: Withhold treatment until improved to grade 1 or baseline, then resume at reduced dose. **Grade 4 CNS effects:** Permanently discontinue.

CPK Elevation
CPK elevation greater than 5 times upper limit of normal (ULN): Withhold treatment until improved to baseline or less than or equal to 2.5 times ULN, then resume at same dose.
CPK elevation greater than 10 times ULN or second occurrence of CPK elevation greater than 5 times ULN: Withhold treatment until improved to baseline or less than or equal to 2.5 times ULN, then resume at reduced dose.

Hepatotoxicity
Grade 3 hepatotoxicity: Withhold treatment until improved to grade 1 or baseline. Resume at same dose if resolved within 4 wks. **Recurrent grade 3 hepatotoxicity:** Withhold treatment until improved to grade 1 or baseline. Resume at reduced dose if resolved within 4 wks. **Grade 4 hepatotoxicity:** Withhold treatment until improved to grade 1 or baseline. Resume at reduced dose if resolved within 4 wks. Permanently discontinue if not resolved within 4 wks or if grade 4 hepatotoxicity recurs. **Serum ALT/AST greater than 3 times ULN with bilirubin greater than 1.5 times ULN (without cholestasis or hemolysis):** Permanently discontinue.

Hyperuricemia
Grade 3 or 4 elevated uric acid level: Withhold treatment until improved, then resume at same or reduced dose. Consider treatment with a urate-lowering medication.

Pulmonary Toxicity
Any grade interstitial lung disease (ILD)/pneumonitis: Withhold treatment if ILD/pneumonitis is suspected. Permanently discontinue if ILD/pneumonitis is confirmed.

Other Adverse Reactions
Any other intolerable grade 2–4 reaction: Withhold treatment until improved to grade 1 or baseline, then resume at same dose if resolved within 4 wks. Permanently discontinue if not resolved within 4 wks. **Recurrent grade 4 adverse reaction:** Permanently discontinue.

Concomitant Use of Strong or moderate CYP3A4 Inhibitors
Discontinue use of strong or moderate CYP3A inhibitors for 3–5 half-lives prior to initiating treatment.

Dosage in Renal Impairment
Mild to moderate impairment: No dose adjustment. **Severe impairment, ESRD on dialysis:** Not specified; use caution.

Dosage in Hepatic Impairment
Mild impairment: No dose adjustment. **Moderate to severe impairment:** Not specified; use caution.

SIDE EFFECTS
Frequent (65%–28%): Dizziness, vertigo, postural dizziness, dysgeusia, ageusia, anosmia, hypogeusia, constipation, dyspnea, fatigue, asthenia, ataxia, gait disturbance, incoordination. **Occasional (20%–11%):** Muscular weakness, nausea, headache, migraine, tension, headache, cough, edema, diarrhea, myalgia, myositis, musculoskeletal discomfort, musculoskeletal pain, vomiting, vision blurred, dry eye, visual impairment, visual field defect, cataract, conjunctivitis, eye pain, photophobia, photosensitivity reaction, visual acuity reduced, vitreous floaters,

R

blepharospasm, color blindness, diplopia, eye hematoma, eye swelling, eyelid disorder, eyelid injury, eyelid pruritus, glaucoma, night blindness, decreased appetite.

ADVERSE EFFECTS/TOXIC REACTIONS

Myelosuppression (anemia, lymphopenia, neutropenia) is an expected response to therapy. CNS adverse effects including altered mental status, aphasia, amnesia, ataxia, balance disorder, cognitive impairment, confusion, delirium, disturbance in attention, falls, hallucinations, memory impairment, peripheral neuropathy reported in 77% of pts. Mood disorders including affect lability, affective disorder, agitation, anxiety, depression, euphoria, irritability, mood swings, psychomotor dysfunction, reported in 6% of pts. Bone fractures of the acetabulum, feet/ankle, ribs, spine, sternum, reported in 2% of pts. ILD/pneumonitis reported in 3% of pts. May cause myalgia with/or without CPK elevation. Hyperuricemia reported in 5% of pts. Hepatotoxicity (transaminitis) reported in 38%–41% of pts. Respiratory tract infections, including pneumonia, aspiration pneumonia, lower respiratory tract infection, may occur.

NURSING CONSIDERATIONS

BASELINE ASSESSMENT

Obtain CBC, LFT, uric acid level; pregnancy test in females of reproductive potential. Confirm compliance of effective non-hormonal contraception. For pts with NSCLC, confirm presence of ROS1 rearrangement(s) in tumor specimens. For pts with solid tumors, confirm presence of an NTRK gene fusion. Question history of hepatic impairment, interstitial lung disease; depression, mood disorder, psychiatric disorders. Screen for active infection. Receive full medication history and screen for interactions. Discontinue strong or moderate CYP3A inhibitors for 3–5 half-lives prior to initiating treatment. Initiate fall precautions. Offer emotional support.

INTERVENTION/EVALUATION

Monitor CBC for myelosuppression (as clinically indicated); LFT for hepatotoxicity (bruising, jaundice, fatigue, right upper abdominal pain, nausea, vomiting, weight loss) q2wks for the first month, then monthly thereafter; CPK level q2wks for the first month, then as needed thereafter in pts with symptoms of CPK elevation (muscle pain/tenderness/weakness); serum uric acid level as clinically indicated. Diligently assess for new-onset or worsening of anxiety, depression, mood disorder. Consult a mental health professional if mood disorder is suspected. Consider ABG, radiologic test if ILD/pneumonitis (excessive cough, dyspnea, fever, hypoxia) is suspected. Consider treatment with corticosteroids if ILD/pneumonitis is confirmed. Monitor for symptoms of bone fractures (pain, deformity, changes in mobility), hyperuricemia (joint pain/inflammation/redness), myalgia (muscle pain/tenderness), infections (body aches, cough, fatigue, fever). If serious infection or sepsis occurs, initiate appropriate antimicrobial therapy. Monitor daily pattern of bowel activity, stool consistency.

PATIENT/FAMILY TEACHING

• Treatment may depress your immune system and reduce your ability to fight infection. Report symptoms of infection such as body aches, burning with urination, chills, cough, fatigue, fever. Avoid those with active infection. • Nervous system changes including altered memory, confusion, delirium, difficulty speaking, falls, gait disturbance, hallucinations, memory issues, numbness, tremors, other neurological effects, may occur. Avoid tasks that require alertness, motor skills until response to drug is established. • Report liver problems (abdominal pain, bruising, clay-colored stool, amber or dark colored urine, yellowing of the skin or eyes), inflammation of the lungs (excessive cough, difficulty breathing, chest pain), bone fractures (pain, deformity, changes in mobility), gout (pain, swelling, redness, warmth of the joint), muscle

---

R

pain/weakness. • Seek immediate medical attention if new-onset or worsening of anxiety, depression, or significant changes in mood occurs. • Use effective non-hormonal contraception to avoid pregnancy. Do not breastfeed. • There is a high risk of interactions with other medications. Do not take newly prescribed medications unless approved by prescriber who originally started treatment. Do not take herbal products.

reslizumab

res-li-**zoo**-mab
(Cinqair)
■ **BLACK BOX ALERT** ■
Anaphylaxis reported in less than 1% asthmatic pts, which usually occurred during or within 20 min of completion of infusion. Observe for appropriate period of time after administration.
Do not confuse reslizumab with certolizumab, daclizumab, eculizumab, efalizumab, mepolizumab, natalizumab, omalizumab, pembrolizumab, tocilizumab, or vedolizumab, or Cinqair with Cinryze, Cinolar, Cinobac, Sinemet, Singulair, or SINEquan.

◆CLASSIFICATION

PHARMACOTHERAPEUTIC: Interleukin-5 receptor antagonist. Monoclonal antibody. **CLINICAL:** Antiasthmatic.

USES

Add-on maintenance treatment of pts with severe asthma, aged 18 yrs and older, and with an eosinophil phenotype.

PRECAUTIONS

Contraindications: Hypersensitivity to reslizumab. **Cautions:** History of helminth (parasite) infection; long-term use of corticosteroids. Not indicated for treatment of other eosinophilic conditions; relief of acute bronchospasm, status asthmaticus, exercise-induced bronchospasm. History of anaphylaxis.

ACTION

Inhibits signaling of interleukin-5 cytokine, reducing production and survival of eosinophils responsible for asthmatic inflammation and pathogenesis. **Therapeutic Effect:** Prevents inflammatory process. Decreases number of asthma exacerbations.

PHARMACOKINETICS

Widely distributed. Degraded into small peptides and amino acids via proteolytic enzymes. Peak plasma concentration: reached by end of infusion. Excretion not specified. **Half-life:** 24 days.

⧗ LIFESPAN CONSIDERATIONS

Pregnancy/Lactation: Unknown if distributed in breast milk. However, human immunoglobulin G (IgG) is present in breast milk and is known to cross placenta. **Children:** Safety and efficacy not established. **Elderly:** No age-related precautions noted.

INTERACTIONS

DRUG: None known. **HERBAL:** None significant. **FOOD:** None known. **LAB VALUES:** May increase creatine phosphokinase (CPK).

AVAILABILITY (Rx)

Injection Solution: 100 mg/10 mL (10 mg/mL).

ADMINISTRATION/HANDLING

 IV

Preparation • Allow vial to warm to room temperature. • Visually inspect for particulate matter or discoloration. Solution should appear clear to slightly opalescent, colorless to pale yellow. • Proteinaceous particles may be present. • Air bubbles are expected and allowed. • Do not use if solution is cloudy or discolored or if foreign particles are observed. • Do not shake • Withdraw

R

proper dose volume from vial and dilute in 50 mL 0.9% NaCl bag. • Gently invert to mix. Do not shake (may cause foaming/precipitate formation). • Infuse via dedicated line. • After infusion is complete, flush IV line with 0.9% NaCl.

Rate of administration • Infuse over 20–50 min (depending on total volume of infusion), using an in-line, low protein-binding filter (pore size: 0.2 micron).

Storage • Refrigerate unused vials. • Do not freeze. • Diluted solution may be refrigerated or stored at room temperature for up to 16 hrs. • If refrigerated, allow diluted solution to warm to room temperature before use. • Protect from light.

▩ IV INCOMPATIBILITIES

Do not mix or infuse with other medications.

INDICATIONS/ROUTES/DOSAGE

Asthma (Severe)

IV: ADULTS, ELDERLY: 3 mg/kg once q4wks. To determine efficacy, treat for a minimum of 4 mos.

Dosage in Renal/Hepatic Impairment
Not specified; use caution.

SIDE EFFECTS

Rare (3%–1%): Oropharyngeal pain, myalgia.

ADVERSE EFFECTS/TOXIC REACTIONS

Life-threatening anaphylaxis reported in less than 1% of pts. Hypersensitivity reactions including bronchospasm, dyspnea, hypoxia, rash, urticaria, vomiting usually occurred during infusion or within 20 min after completion. Less than 1% of pts reported at least one malignant neoplasm within 6 mos of initiation. Unknown if treatment will influence the immunologic response to helminth (parasite) infection.

NURSING CONSIDERATIONS

BASELINE ASSESSMENT

Obtain serum CPK. Verify presence of eosinophil phenotype. Question his-

tory of hypersensitivity reaction. Therapy should be administered in a healthcare setting by medical professionals who are trained and prepared to readily manage anaphylaxis. Have anaphylactic medications (e.g., antihistamine, bronchodilator, corticosteroid, EPINEPHrine, H_2 receptor antagonist), intubation kit, supplemental oxygen readily available before initiation. Inhaled or systemic corticosteroids should not be suddenly discontinued upon initiation. Corticosteroids that are not gradually reduced may cause withdrawal symptoms or unmask conditions that were originally suppressed with corticosteroid therapy. Pts with preexisting helminth infection should be treated prior to initiation.

INTERVNTION/EVALUATION

Obtain serum CPK in pts complaining of myalgia. Diligently observe for hypersensitivity/anaphylactic reaction during infusion and directly after completion. If anaphylaxis occurs, discontinue infusion and provide immediate resuscitation support. Early detection is vital. Assess rate, depth, rhythm of respirations, oxygen saturation for therapeutic effectiveness. Assess lungs for wheezing, rales. Obtain pulmonary function test to assess disease improvement. Interrupt or discontinue therapy if helminth infection occurs, if worsening of asthma-related symptoms occurs (esp. in pts tapering off corticosteroids). Monitor for increased use of rescue inhalers; may indicate deterioration of asthma. Monitor for primary malignancies.

PATIENT/FAMILY TEACHING

• Treatment may cause life-threatening anaphylaxis. Immediately report allergic reactions such as difficulty breathing, hives, itching, low blood pressure, rash, swelling of the face or tongue, sudden coughing, vomiting, wheezing during infusion or immediately after infusion. • Therapy not indicated for relief of acute asthma or bronchospasm. • Have a rescue inhaler readily available. • Increased use of rescue inhalers may indicate worsening of asthma. • Seek

R

medical attention if asthma symptoms worsen or remain uncontrolled. • Do not stop corticosteroid therapy unless directed by prescriber. • Treatment may increase risk of new cancers or alter the body's immune response to parasite infections.

rezafungin

re-za-**fun**-jin
(Rezzayo)
Do not confuse rezafungin with anidulafungin, caspofungin, or micafungin or Rezzayo with Libtayo.

◆CLASSIFICATION

PHARMACOTHERAPEUTIC: Echinocandin antifungal. **CLINICAL:** Antifungal.

USES

Treatment in adults who have limited or no alternative options for the treatment of candidemia and invasive candidiasis.

PRECAUTIONS

Contraindications: Hypersensitivity to rezafungin or other echinocandins. **Cautions:** Hepatic impairment, pts with serious underlying medical conditions taking multiple concomitant medications. Not studied in pts with endocarditis, osteomyelitis, meningitis due to *Candida*.

ACTION

Inhibits synthesis of glucan (vital component of fungal cell formation), damaging fungal cell membrane. **Therapeutic Effect:** Causes lysis of fungal cells.

PHARMACOKINETICS

Widely distributed. Metabolism not specified. Protein binding: 86%–94%. Excreted in feces (74%), urine (26%). **Half-life:** 123–181 hrs.

⧗ LIFESPAN CONSIDERATIONS

Pregnancy/Lactation: Unknown if distributed in breast milk. **Children:** Safety and efficacy not established. **Males:** May decrease sperm motility, sperm numbers, and increased sperm with abnormal morphology. **Elderly:** No age-related precautions noted.

INTERACTIONS

DRUG: None significant. **HERBAL:** None significant. **FOOD:** None known. **LAB VALUES:** May increase serum ALT, AST. May decrease RBC.

AVAILABILITY (Rx)

Injection, Powder for Reconstitution: 200 mg.

ADMINISTRATION/HANDLING

 IV

Missed doses • If a dose is missed, administer as soon as possible if within 3 days of the scheduled infusion day. If a dose is missed by more than 3 days of the scheduled infusion day, revise the dosing schedule so there are at least 4 days before the next dose. A repeat loading dose of 400 mg should be given if a dose is missed by at least 2 wks.
Reconstitution • Reconstitute each vial (two vials for 400-mg dose or one vial for 200-mg dose) with 9.5 mL SWI to a final concentration of 20 mg/mL. • Swirl vial gently until powder is completely dissolved. Do not shake (minimizes foaming). • Visually inspect for particulate matter or discoloration. Solution should appear clear and pale yellow. Do not use if solution is cloudy, discolored, or visible particles are observed.
Dilution • Using a 250-mL infusion bag containing 0.9% NaCl, 0.45% NaCl, or D5W, withdraw and discard a volume that is equal to the volume of the reconstituted solution (20 mL for the 400-mg dose or 10 mL for the 200-mg dose). • Transfer dose from vial(s) to the infusion bag for a final volume of 250 mL. • Mix by gentle inversion. Do not shake or agitate.
Rate of administration • Infuse over 1 hr.

R

 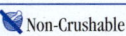

Infusion reactions • May decrease rate or interrupt infusion if infusion-related reactions occur.
Storage • Store unused vials at room temperature. • May refrigerate diluted solution for up to 48 hrs. Do not freeze.

INDICATIONS/ROUTES/DOSAGE

Candidemia, Invasive Candidiasis
IV: ADULTS, ELDERLY: 400 mg loading dose once, following by 200 mg once wkly. Safety beyond 4 wkly doses is not established.

Dosage in Renal/Hepatic Impairment
No dose adjustment.

SIDE EFFECTS

Occasional (12%–5%): Pyrexia, diarrhea, vomiting, nausea, abdominal pain, constipation. **Rare (3%):** Tremors.

ADVERSE EFFECTS/TOXIC REACTIONS

Infusion reactions, including chest tightness, flushing, nausea, urticaria, warming sensation, were reported. May cause photosensitivity. May increase hepatic enzymes. Pts with serious underlying medical conditions taking multiple concomitant medications may be at risk for clinically significant hepatic abnormalities.

NURSING CONSIDERATIONS

BASELINE ASSESSMENT

Obtain LFT. Obtain specimen culture and other laboratory data (e.g., histopathology, nonculture diagnostics) prior to initiation. Treatment may be initiated before cultures have resulted; however, antifungal therapy should be adjusted after specimen culture and laboratory data have resulted. Assess occurrence of infusion reactions prior to each dose. Administer in an environment equipped to manage infusion reactions. Question history of hepatic impairment. Obtain full medication history.

INTERVENTION/EVALUATION

Monitor LFT as clinically indicated. Check results of specimen culture and laboratory data to verify if continued treatment is warranted. Monitor for reactions during each infusion. Consider decreasing the rate or interrupting infusion if reactions occur.

PATIENT/FAMILY TEACHING

• Avoid prolonged sunlight exposure/tanning beds. Use high SPF sunscreen, lip balm, clothing to protect against sunburn, sun sensitivity. • Report liver problems (abdominal pain, bruising, clay-colored stool, amber or dark-colored urine, yellowing of the skin or eyes). • Avoid OTC medications (e.g., acetaminophen) that are toxic to the liver. • Report infusion-related reactions, such as chest tightness, flushing, nausea, urticaria, warming sensation.

ribociclib

rye-boe-**sye**-klib
(Kisqali)
Do not confuse ribociclib with palbociclib or riboflavin.

◆**CLASSIFICATION**

PHARMACOTHERAPEUTIC: Cyclin-dependent kinase inhibitor. **CLINICAL:** Antineoplastic.

USES

Treatment of adults with hormone receptor (HR)–positive, human epidermal growth factor receptor 2 (HER2)–negative advanced or metastatic breast cancer in combination with an aromatase inhibitor as initial endocrine-based therapy; or with fulvestrant as initial endocrine-based therapy or following disease progression on endocrine therapy in men or postmenopausal women. In combination with an aromatase inhibitor for the adjuvant treatment of adults with hormone receptor (HR)-positive, human epidermal growth factor receptor 2 (HER2)-negative stage II and III early breast cancer at high risk of recurrence.

PRECAUTIONS

Contraindications: Hypersensitivity to ribociclib. **Cautions:** Baseline cytopenias, hepatic impairment. Avoid concomitant use of strong CYP3A4 inhibitors, strong CYP3A4 inducers, QTc interval–prolonging medications. Avoid use in pts with or at risk for QTc prolongation (e.g., congenital long QT syndrome, hypokalemia, hypomagnesemia; uncontrolled, significant cardiac disease including MI, HF, unstable angina, bradyarrhythmias).

ACTION

Blocks retinoblastoma protein phosphorylation and prevents progression through cell cycle, resulting in arrest of G_1 phase. **Therapeutic Effect:** Inhibits tumor growth.

PHARMACOKINETICS

Widely distributed. Metabolized extensively in liver. Protein binding: 70%. Peak plasma concentration: 1–4 hrs. Excreted in feces (69%), urine (23%). **Half-life:** 30–55 hrs.

⏳ LIFESPAN CONSIDERATIONS

Pregnancy/Lactation: Indicated for postmenopausal women; however, may cause fetal harm/malformations when used during pregnancy. Females of reproductive potential should use effective contraception during treatment and for at least 3 wks after discontinuation. Unknown if distributed in breast milk. Breastfeeding not recommended during treatment and for at least 3 wks after discontinuation. **Children:** Safety and efficacy not established. **Elderly:** No age-related precautions noted.

INTERACTIONS

DRUG: Strong **CYP3A4 inhibitors** (e.g., **clarithromycin, ketoconazole, ritonavir**) may increase concentration/effect. Strong **CYP3A4 inducers** (e.g., car-**BAMazepine, phenytoin, rifAMPin**) may decrease concentration/effect. **QT interval–prolonging medications** (e.g., **amiodarone, azithromycin, ceritinib, haloperidol, moxifloxacin**) may increase risk of QT interval prolongation, torsades de pointes. May increase concentration/effect of **aprepitant, bosutinib, budesonide, pimozide, vaccines (live).** May decrease effect of **BCG (intravesical), vaccines**

(live). May increase adverse effects/toxicity of **natalizumab, pimecrolimus, tacrolimus. HERBAL: Echinacea, St. John's wort** may decrease concentration/effect. **FOOD: Grapefruit products** may increase concentration/effect. **LAB VALUES:** May increase serum ALT, AST, bilirubin. May decrease ANC, Hgb, lymphocytes, leukocytes, neutrophils, platelets; serum potassium, phosphate.

AVAILABILITY (Rx)

🐋 **Tablets:** 200 mg. **Blister Pack:** (21 tablets, 42 tablets, 63 tablets).

ADMINISTRATION/HANDLING

PO
• Give without regard to food. Administer tablet whole; do not break, cut, or crush. • Do not give if tablet is cracked, broken, or not intact. • Tablets cannot be chewed. If a dose is missed or vomiting occurs after administration, do not give extra dose. Administer next dose at regularly scheduled time.

INDICATIONS/ROUTES/DOSAGE

Breast Cancer (Advanced or Metastatic)
PO: ADULTS, ELDERLY: 600 mg once daily for 21 days, followed by 7 days off treatment of 28-day cycle. **In combination with an aromatase inhibitor:** Pre-/perimenopausal females, and males, should be treated with a luteinizing hormone–releasing hormone (LHRH) agonist (e.g., leuprolide). **In combination with fulvestrant:** Males should be treated with an LHRH agonist. Continue until disease progression or unacceptable toxicity.

Dose Reduction Schedule
First reduction: 400 mg/day. **Second reduction:** 200 mg/day. **Unable to tolerate 200 mg/day:** Permanently discontinue.

Early Breast Cancer
PO: ADULTS, ELDERLY: Initially, 400 mg once daily for 21 consecutive days, followed by 7 days off treatment. Dose reduction 200 mg/day. **Unable to tolerate 200 mg/day:** Permanently discontinue.

R

Dose Modification

Based on Common Terminology Criteria for Adverse Events (CTCAE).

Hepatotoxicity

Note: Defined as hepatotoxicity without total bilirubin greater than 2 times upper limit of normal (ULN). If serum ALT, AST elevation greater than 3 times ULN with total bilirubin greater than 2 times ULN, permanently discontinue. **Grade 1 serum ALT, AST elevation (up to 3 times ULN):** No dose adjustment. **Grade 2 serum ALT, AST elevation (greater than 3–5 times ULN) with baseline at less than Grade 2:** Withhold treatment until improved to baseline, then resume at same dose level. If baseline at less than Grade 2, do not withhold treatment. If Grade 2 serum ALT, AST elevation recurs, then resume at reduced dose level. **Grade 3 serum ALT, AST elevation (greater than 5–20 times ULN):** Withhold treatment until improved to baseline, then resume at reduced dose level. If Grade 3 serum ALT, AST elevation recurs, permanently discontinue. **Grade 4 serum ALT, AST elevation (greater than 20 times ULN):** Permanently discontinue.

Hematologic

Grade 1 or 2 neutropenia (ANC 1,000 cells/mm^3 to less than the lower limit of normal): No dose adjustment. **Grade 3 neutropenia (ANC 500 to less than 1,000 cells/mm^3:** Withhold treatment until recovery to Grade 2 or less, then resume at same dose level. If Grade 3 neutropenia recurs, withhold treatment until recovery to Grade 2 or less, then resume at reduced dose level. **Grade 3 febrile neutropenia:** Withhold treatment until recovery to Grade 2 or less, then resume at reduced dose level. **Grade 4 neutropenia (ANC less than 500 cells/mm^3):** Withhold treatment until recovery to Grade 2 or less, then resume at reduced dose level.

QTc Interval Prolongation

QTc interval prolongation greater than 480 msec: Withhold treatment until resolved to less than 481 msec, then resume at same dose level. If QTc interval prolongation greater than 480 msec recurs, withhold treatment until resolved to less than 481 msec, then resume at reduced dose level. **QTc interval prolongation greater than 500 msec:** Withhold treatment if QTc interval prolongation greater than 500 msec on at least two separate ECGs (within same visit). If QTc interval prolongation resolves to less than 481 msec after withholding treatment, resume at reduced dose level. **QTc interval prolongation greater than 500 msec (or greater than 60 msec from baseline) with torsades de pointes, polymorphic ventricular tachycardia, unexplained syncope, symptoms of serious arrhythmia:** Permanently discontinue.

Other Toxicities

Any other Grade 1 or 2 toxicities: No dose adjustment. **Any other Grade 3 toxicities:** Withhold treatment until resolved to Grade 1 or 0, then resume at same dose level. If Grade 3 toxicities recur, resume at reduced dose level. **Any other CTCAE Grade 4 toxicities:** Permanently discontinue.

Concomitant Use of Strong CYP3A4 Inhibitors

Reduce initial dose to 400 mg once daily if strong CYP3A4 inhibitor cannot be discontinued. If CYP3A4 inhibitor is discontinued for 3–5 half-lives, increase ribociclib to the dose used prior to initiating strong CYP3A4 inhibitor.

Dosage in Renal Impairment

Not specified; use caution.

Dosage in Hepatic Impairment

Mild impairment: No dose adjustment. **Moderate to severe impairment:** Reduce starting dose to 400 mg once daily.

SIDE EFFECTS

Frequent (52%–17%): Nausea, fatigue, diarrhea, alopecia, vomiting, constipation, headache, back pain, decreased appetite, rash. **Occasional (14%–11%):** Pruritus, pyrexia, insomnia, dyspnea, stomatitis, peripheral edema, abdominal pain.

ADVERSE EFFECTS/TOXIC REACTIONS

Myelosuppression (anemia, leukopenia, lymphopenia, neutropenia, thrombocytopenia) is an expected response to therapy, but more severe reactions, including febrile neutropenia, may be life-threatening. CTCAE Grade 3 or 4 neutropenia reported in 60% of pts. Severe hepatotoxicity reported in 10% of pts. QTc interval prolongation, infections including UTI may occur.

NURSING CONSIDERATIONS

BASELINE ASSESSMENT

Obtain ANC, CBC, BMP, LFT, vital signs, weight; pregnancy test in females of reproductive potential. Obtain ECG (note QTc interval). Initiate treatment only in pts with QTc interval less than 450 msec. Question history of cardiac disease, cardiac conduction disorders, hepatic impairment. Receive full medication history including herbal products and screen for interactions. Screen for risk of bleeding, QTc interval prolongation, active infection. Obtain dietary consult. Offer emotional support.

INTERVENTION/EVALUATION

Monitor ANC, CBC for myelosuppression; LFT for hepatotoxicity q2wks for the first 2 cycles, then prior to each subsequent cycle, then as clinically indicated. Monitor BMP, serum phosphate for electrolyte imbalance; consider correcting imbalances, esp. hypokalemia, hypomagnesemia (due to increased risk of cardiac arrhythmias, torsades de pointes). Obtain repeat ECG on day 14 of the first cycle and at the beginning of the second cycle, or more frequently if QTc interval prolongation occurs. Monitor daily pattern of bowel activity, stool consistency. Assess skin for rash, lesions. Monitor weight, I&O.

PATIENT/FAMILY TEACHING

• Treatment may depress your immune system and reduce your ability to fight infection. Report symptoms of infection such as body aches, burning with urination, chills, cough, fatigue, fever. Avoid those with active infection. • Report symptoms of bone marrow depression such as bruising, fatigue, fever, shortness of breath, weight loss; bleeding easily, bloody urine or stool. • Do not take newly prescribed medications unless approved by the prescriber who originally started treatment. • Report liver problems such as bruising, confusion, amber or dark-colored urine; right upper abdominal pain, yellowing of the skin or eyes; heart arrhythmias (chest pain, difficulty breathing, palpitations, passing out). • Therapy indicated for postmenopausal women; however, birth defects may occur when used during pregnancy. Use effective contraception to avoid pregnancy. Do not breastfeed. • Do not ingest grapefruit products, Seville oranges, starfruit, pomegranate, herbal supplements. • Report planned surgical/dental procedures. • Immediately report bleeding of any kind.

rimegepant

ri-**me**-je-pant
(Nurtec ODT)
Do not confuse rimegepant with ubrogepant.

◆ Classification

PHARMACOTHERAPEUTIC: Calcitonin gene–related peptide (CGRP) receptor antagonist. **CLINICAL:** Antimigraine.

USES

Treatment of migraines with or without aura in adults. Preventive treatment of episodic migraine in adults.

PRECAUTIONS

Contraindications: Hypersensitivity to rimegepant. **Cautions:** Not indicated for prevention of migraine.

ACTION

Binds to and inhibits calcitonin gene–related peptide (CGRP) receptor.

Therapeutic Effect: Relieves migraine headache.

PHARMACOKINETICS

Widely distributed. Metabolized in liver. Protein binding: 96%. Peak plasma concentration: 1.5 hrs. Excreted in urine (51%), feces (42%). **Half-life:** 11 hrs.

⌛ LIFESPAN CONSIDERATIONS

Pregnancy/Lactation: Unknown if distributed in breast milk. **Children:** Safety and efficacy not established. **Elderly:** Safety and efficacy not established.

INTERACTIONS

DRUG: Strong CYP3A4 inhibitors (e.g., clarithromycin, ketoconazole, ritonavir), moderate CYP3A4 inhibitors (e.g., dilTIAZem, fluconazole, verapamil), P-gp inhibitors (e.g., amiodarone, carvedilol, verapamil) may increase concentration/effect. **Strong CYP3A4 inducers (e.g., carBAMazepine, phenytoin, rifAMPin), moderate CYP3A4 inducers (e.g., bosentan, nafcillin)** may decrease concentration/effect. **HERBAL:** None significant. **FOOD:** None known. **LAB VALUES:** None known.

AVAILABILITY (Rx)

Tablets, Orally Disintegrating: 75 mg.

ADMINISTRATION/HANDLING

Orally Disintegrating Tablets
• Do not remove from blister pack until needed. • Peel backing off; do not push tablet through blister pack. • Place tablet on or under tongue; allow to dissolve. Swallow with saliva.

INDICATIONS/ROUTES/DOSAGE

Migraine Treatment (With or Without Aura)
PO: ADULTS: 75 mg once. Do not exceed 75 mg in a 24-hr period.

Migraine Prevention
PO: ADULTS, ELDERLY: 75 mg every other day.

Dose Modification
Concomitant Use of Strong/Moderate CYP3A4 Inhibitors
Avoid concomitant use of strong CYP3A4 inhibitors. Avoid second dose of rimegepant within 48 hrs of concomitant moderate CYP3A4 inhibitors.

Concomitant Use of Strong/Moderate CYP3A4 Inducers
Due to loss of efficacy, avoid concomitant use of strong or moderate CYP3A4 inducers.

Dosage in Renal Impairment
No dose adjustment.

Dosage in Hepatic Impairment
Mild to moderate impairment: No dose adjustment. **Severe impairment:** Avoid use.

SIDE EFFECTS

Rare (2%): Nausea.

ADVERSE EFFECTS/TOXIC REACTIONS

Hypersensitivity reactions including dyspnea, severe rash reported in less than 1% of pts.

NURSING CONSIDERATIONS

BASELINE ASSESSMENT
Question characteristics of migraine headaches (onset, location, duration, possible precipitating symptoms).

INTERVENTION/EVALUATION
Evaluate for relief of migraine headaches (photophobia, phonophobia, nausea, vomiting, pain, dizziness, fogginess). Monitor for hypersensitivity reactions.

PATIENT/FAMILY TEACHING
• Allergic reactions such as difficulty breathing, severe rash may occur. If allergic reaction occurs, seek immediate medical attention. • There is a high risk of interactions with other medications. Do not take newly prescribed medications unless approved by prescriber who originally started therapy.

underlined – top prescribed drug

risankizumab-rzaa

ris-an-**kiz**-ue-mab-rzaa
(Skyrizi)
**Do not confuse risankizumab
with ixekizumab.**

◆CLASSIFICATION

PHARMACOTHERAPEUTIC: Interleukin-23 antagonist. Monoclonal antibody. **CLINICAL:** Antipsoriatic agent.

USES

Treatment of moderate to severe plaque psoriasis in adults who are candidates for systemic therapy or phototherapy. Treatment of active psoriatic arthritis in adults. Treatment of moderately to severely active Crohn's disease in adults. Treatment of moderately to severely active ulcerative colitis in adults.

PRECAUTIONS

Contraindications: Hypersensitivity to risankizumab. **Cautions:** Conditions predisposing to infection (e.g., diabetes, immunocompromised pts, renal failure, open wounds), prior exposure to tuberculosis or use in pts who reside or travel to areas where TB is endemic. Avoid use during active infection. Concomitant use of live vaccines not recommended.

ACTION

Selectively binds to p19 subunit of interleukin-23 (IL-23) and inhibits interaction with IL-23 receptor. IL-23 is a cytokine that is involved in inflammatory and immune response. **Therapeutic Effect:** Alters biologic immune response; reduces inflammation of psoriatic lesions.

PHARMACOKINETICS

Widely distributed. Degraded into small peptides and amino acids via catabolic pathway. Peak plasma concentration: 3–14 days. Steady state reached in 16 wks. **Half-life:** 28 days.

⧗ LIFESPAN CONSIDERATIONS

Pregnancy/Lactation: Unknown if distributed in breast milk. However, human immunoglobulin G (IgG) is present in breast milk and is known to cross the placenta. **Children:** Safety and efficacy not established. **Elderly:** No age-related precautions noted.

INTERACTIONS

DRUG: None significant. **HERBAL:** Echinacea may decrease therapeutic effect. **FOOD:** None known. **LAB VALUES:** None known.

AVAILABILITY (Rx)

Injection Prefilled Syringe: 90 mg/mL, 150 mg/mL. **Injection, Prefilled Pen:** 150 mg/mL. **Injection, Prefilled Cartridge:** 180 mg/1.2 mL (150 mg/mL), 360 mg/2.4 mL (150 mg/mL). **Injection Solution:** 600 mg/10 mL (60 mg/mL).

ADMINISTRATION/HANDLING

SQ

Preparation • Remove prefilled syringe from refrigerator and allow solution to warm to room temperature (approx. 15–30 min) with needle cap intact. • Visually inspect for particulate matter or discoloration. Solution should appear clear to slightly opalescent, colorless to slightly yellow in color. Do not use if solution is cloudy or discolored or if visible particles are observed.

Administration • Insert needle subcutaneously into outer thigh or abdomen and inject solution. Injections to the outer arms may only be performed by a healthcare professional. • Do not inject into areas of active skin disease or injury such as sunburns, skin rashes, inflammation, skin infections, or active psoriasis. • Rotate injection sites. • Do not administer IV or intramuscularly. • If a dose is missed, administer as soon as possible, then give next dose at regularly scheduled time.

Storage • Refrigerate prefilled syringes in original carton until time of

R

use. • Protect from light. • Do not shake. • Do not freeze or expose to heating sources.

 IV

Preparation • Withdraw 10 mL from vial and dilute in 100 mL, 250 mL, or 500 mL D5W to a final concentration of 1.2–6 mg/mL. • Do not shake vial or diluted solution.

Rate of administration • Infuse over at least 1 hr for the 600 mg dose and at least 2 hrs for the 1,200 mg dose.

Storage • Refrigerate diluted solution for up to 20 hrs or store at room temperature for up to 4 hrs. • Protect from light. Do not freeze.

INDICATIONS/ROUTES/DOSAGE

Plaque Psoriasis, Psoriatic Arthritis
SQ: ADULTS, ELDERLY: 150 mg at wk 0 and wk 4, then q12wks thereafter. In pts with psoriatic arthritis, can be given alone or with nonbiologic disease-modifying antirheumatic drugs (DMARDs).

Crohn's Disease
ADULTS, ELDERLY: (Induction): 600 mg by IV infusion at wk 0, 4, and 8. **(Maintenance):** 180–360 mg by SQ injection at wk 12, then q8wks thereafter.

Ulcerative Colitis
ADULTS, ELDERLY: (Induction): 1,200 mg by IV infusion (over at least 2 hrs) at wks 0, 4, 8. **(Maintenance):** 180–360 mg by SQ injection at wk 12, and q8wks thereafter.

Dosage in Renal/Heptaic Impairment
Not specified; use caution.

SIDE EFFECTS

Rare (4%–2%): Headache, tension headache, sinus headache, fatigue, asthenia, injection site reactions (bruising, erythema, extravasation, hematoma, hemorrhage, infection, inflammation, irritation, pain, pruritus, swelling, warmth).

ADVERSE EFFECTS/TOXIC REACTIONS

Upper respiratory tract infections (bacterial, viral, unspecified) including nasopharyngitis, pharyngitis, rhinitis, sinusitis, tonsillitis reported in 13% of pts. Tinea infections reported in 1% of pts. Serious infections including cellulitis, herpes zoster, osteomyelitis, sepsis occurred in less than 1% of pts.

NURSING CONSIDERATIONS

BASELINE ASSESSMENT
Consider completion of age-appropriate immunizations prior to initiation. Pts should be evaluated for active tuberculosis and tested for latent infection prior to initiation and periodically during therapy. Induration of 5 mm or greater with tuberculin skin testing should be considered a positive test result when assessing if treatment for latent tuberculosis is necessary. Screen for active infection or chronic infections. Conduct dermatologic exam; record characteristics of psoriatic lesions. Assess pt's willingness to self-inject medication. Teach proper injection techniques.

INTERVENTION/EVALUATION
Assess skin for improvement of lesions. Monitor for symptoms of tuberculosis (cough, fatigue, hemoptysis, nocturnal sweating, weight loss), including those who tested negative for latent tuberculosis infection prior to initiating therapy. Interrupt or discontinue treatment if serious infection, opportunistic infection, or sepsis occurs.

PATIENT/FAMILY TEACHING
• Treatment may depress your immune system and reduce your ability to fight infection. Report symptoms of infection such as body aches, burning with urination, chills, cough, fatigue, fever; fungal infections. Avoid those with active infection. • Do not receive live vaccines. • Expect frequent tuberculosis screening. Report symptoms of tuberculosis such as cough, fatigue, night sweats, weight loss, or coughing up blood. • Report travel plans to possible endemic areas.

risedronate

ris-**ed**-roe-nate
(Actonel, Atelvia)
Do not confuse Actonel with Actos, or risedronate with alendronate.

FIXED-COMBINATION(S)

Actonel with Calcium: risedronate/calcium: 35 mg/6 × 500 mg.

◆CLASSIFICATION

PHARMACOTHERAPEUTIC: Bisphosphonate. **CLINICAL:** Calcium regulator.

USES

Actonel: Treatment of Paget's disease of bone. Treatment/prevention of osteoporosis in postmenopausal females, glucocorticoid-induced osteoporosis (daily dose 7.5 mg predniSONE or greater). Treatment of osteoporosis in males. **Atelvia:** Treatment of osteoporosis in postmenopausal women. **OFF-LABEL:** Prostate cancer (bone loss).

PRECAUTIONS

Contraindications: Hypersensitivity to risedronate, other bisphosphonates (e.g., alendronate); inability to stand or sit upright for at least 30 min; abnormalities of esophagus that delay esophageal emptying; hypocalcemia. **Cautions:** GI diseases (duodenitis, dysphagia, esophagitis, gastritis, ulcers [drug may exacerbate these conditions]), severe renal impairment (CrCl less than 30 mL/min).

ACTION

Inhibits bone resorption by action on osteoclasts or osteoclast precursors. **Therapeutic Effect: Osteoporosis:** Decreases bone resorption (indirectly increases bone mineral density). **Paget's disease:** Inhibition of bone resorption causes a decrease (but more normal architecture) in bone formation.

PHARMACOKINETICS

Rapidly absorbed. Bioavailability decreased when administered with food.

Protein binding: 24%. Not metabolized. Excreted unchanged in urine, feces. Not removed by hemodialysis. **Half-life:** 1.5 hrs (initial); 480 hrs (terminal).

⌛ LIFESPAN CONSIDERATIONS

Pregnancy/Lactation: Unknown if distributed in breast milk. **Children:** Not indicated for use in this pt population. **Elderly:** No age-related precautions noted.

INTERACTIONS

DRUG: Antacids containing aluminum, calcium, magnesium; may decrease absorption (avoid administration within 30 min of **risedronate**). Histamine H$_2$ receptor antagonists (e.g., famotidine), proton pump inhibitors (e.g., omeprazole, pantoprazole) may decrease concentration/effect. **HERBAL:** None significant. **FOOD:** None known. **LAB VALUES:** None significant.

AVAILABILITY (Rx)

Tablets: 5 mg, 30 mg, 35 mg, 75 mg, 150 mg. **Tablets, Delayed-Release:** 35 mg.

ADMINISTRATION/HANDLING

PO

• **(Actonel):** Administer 30–60 min before any food, drink, other oral medications to avoid interference with absorption. • Give on empty stomach with full glass of plain water (not mineral water). • Pt must avoid lying down for at least 30 min after swallowing tablet (assists with delivery to stomach, reduces risk of esophageal irritation). • Give whole; do not break, crush, dissolve, or divide tablet. • **(Atelvia):** Take in morning immediately following breakfast with at least 4 oz water (not mineral water). Administer table whole (do not cut, split, crush, or allow chewing). • Remain upright for 30 min after taking dose.

INDICATIONS/ROUTES/DOSAGE

Treatment/Prevention of Postmenopausal Osteoporosis
PO: ADULTS, ELDERLY: 5 mg once daily, or 35 mg once wkly, or 75 mg taken on

R

 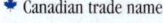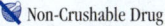

2 consecutive days for a total of 2 tablets each month or 150 mg once monthly.

Osteoporosis in Men to Increase Bone Mass
PO: ADULTS, ELDERLY: 35 mg once wkly.

Treatment/Prevention of Glucocorticoid-Induced Osteoporosis
PO: ADULTS, ELDERLY: 5 mg once daily.

Paget's Disease
PO: ADULTS, ELDERLY: 30 mg once daily for 2 mos. Retreatment may be considered (following post-treatment observation of at least 2 mos) if relapse occurs, or treatment fails to normalize serum alkaline phosphatase.

Dosage in Renal Impairment
Not recommended with CrCl less than 30 mL/min.

Dosage in Hepatic Impairment
No dose adjustment.

SIDE EFFECTS
Frequent (30%): Arthralgia. **Occasional (12%–8%):** Rash, diarrhea, constipation, nausea, abdominal pain, dyspepsia, flu-like symptoms, peripheral edema. **Rare (5%–3%):** Bone pain, sinusitis, asthenia, dry eye, tinnitus.

ADVERSE EFFECTS/TOXIC REACTIONS
Overdose produces hypocalcemia, hypophosphatemia, significant GI disturbances, osteonecrosis of jaw.

NURSING CONSIDERATIONS

BASELINE ASSESSMENT
Assess symptoms of Paget's disease (bone pain, bone deformities). Hypocalcemia, vitamin D deficiency must be corrected before therapy begins. Obtain baseline laboratory studies, esp. serum electrolytes, renal function. Verify pt is able to stand or sit upright for at least 30 min.

INTERVENTION/EVALUATION
Check serum electrolytes (esp. calcium, ionized calcium, phosphorus, alkaline phosphatase levels). Monitor I&O, BUN, creatinine in pts with renal impairment.

PATIENT/FAMILY TEACHING
• Expected benefits occur only when medication is taken with full glass (6–8 oz) of plain water first thing in the morning and at least 30 min before first food, beverage, medication of the day. Any other beverage (mineral water, orange juice, coffee) significantly reduces absorption of medication. • Do not lie down for at least 30 min after taking medication (potentiates delivery to stomach, reduces risk of esophageal irritation). • Report swallowing difficulties, pain when swallowing, chest pain, new/worsening heartburn. • Consider weight-bearing exercises; modify behavioral factors (cigarette smoking, alcohol consumption). • Report jaw pain, incapacitating bone, joint, or muscle pain.

risperiDONE

ris-**per**-i-done
(Perseris, RisperDAL, RisperDAL Consta, Risvan, Rykindo, Uzedy)

■ **BLACK BOX ALERT** ■ Increased risk of mortality in elderly pts with dementia-related psychosis, mainly due to pneumonia, HF.
Do not confuse RisperDAL with Restoril.

◆ **CLASSIFICATION**

PHARMACOTHERAPEUTIC: Benzisoxazole derivative. **CLINICAL:** Second-generation (atypical) antipsychotic. Antimanic agent.

USES
Schizophrenia: Treatment of schizophrenia in adults and adolescents 13–17 yrs of age. **Bipolar mania:** Monotherapy

treatment of acute manic or mixed episodes associated with bipolar I disorder in adults and adolescents 10–17 yrs of age. Adjunctive therapy (with lithium or valproate) for treatment of acute manic or mixed episodes associated with bipolar I disorder in adults. **Irritability associated with autistic disorder:** Treatment of irritability associated with autistic disorder, including symptoms of aggression towards others, deliberate self-injuriousness, temper tantrums, and quickly changing moods in children and adolescents 5–17 yrs of age. **OFF-LABEL:** Tourette's syndrome. Major depressive disorder, agitation/aggression associated with psychotic disorder or dementia, dilusional disorders, obsessive compulsive disorder (OCD).

PRECAUTIONS

Contraindications: Hypersensitivity to risperiDONE. **Cautions:** Renal/hepatic impairment, seizure disorder, cardiac disease, recent MI, breast cancer or other prolactin-dependent tumors, Parkinson's disease, elderly; pts at risk for aspiration, orthostatic hypotension; diabetes, decreased GI motility, urinary retention, BPH, xerostomia, visual problems, pts exposed to temperature extremes, preexisting myelosuppression, narrow-angle glaucoma; history of suicidal ideation and behavior.

ACTION

Antagonizes DOPamine, serotonin receptors in both CNS and periphery. **Therapeutic Effect:** Suppresses psychotic behavior.

PHARMACOKINETICS

Widely distributed. Protein binding: 90%. Metabolized in liver. Primarily excreted in urine. **Half-life:** 3–20 hrs; metabolite, 21–30 hrs (increased in elderly). **Injection:** 3–6 days.

LIFESPAN CONSIDERATIONS

Pregnancy/Lactation: Unknown if drug crosses placenta or is distributed in breast milk. Breastfeeding not recommended. **Children:** Safety and efficacy not established in children younger than 13 yrs for schizophrenia, 10 yrs for bipolar mania, and 5 yrs for autistic disorder. **Elderly:** More susceptible to postural hypotension. Age-related renal/hepatic impairment may require dosage adjustment.

INTERACTIONS

DRUG: **Alcohol, CNS depressants (e.g., LORazepam, morphine, zolpidem)** may increase CNS depression. **Strong CYP3A4 inducers (e.g., carBAMazepine, phenytoin, rifAMPin)** may decrease concentration/effect. **Anticholinergics (e.g., aclidinium, ipratropium, tiotropium, umeclidinium)** may increase anticholinergic effect. **HERBAL:** **Herbals with sedative properties (e.g., chamomile, kava kava, valerian)** may increase CNS depression. **FOOD:** None known. **LAB VALUES:** May increase serum prolactin, glucose, AST, ALT. May cause ECG changes.

AVAILABILITY (Rx)

Injection, Powder for Reconstitution: *(RisperDAL Consta):* 12.5 mg, 25 mg, 37.5 mg, 50 mg. **Oral Solution:** 1 mg/mL. **Syringe, Prefilled:** *(Perseris):* 90 mg, 120 mg. **Injectable Suspension, Extended-Release** *(Risvan):* 75 mg, 100 mg single-dose kits. *(Rykindo):* 12.5 mg/2 mL. *(Uzedy):* 50 mg/0.14 mL, 75 mg/0.21 mL, 100 mg/0.28 mL, 125 mg/0.35 mL, 150 mg/0.42 mL, 200 mg/0.56 mL, and 250 mg/0.7 mL. **Tablets:** 0.25 mg, 0.5 mg, 1 mg, 2 mg, 3 mg, 4 mg.

Tablets, Orally Disintegrating: 0.25 mg, 0.5 mg, 1 mg, 2 mg, 3 mg, 4 mg.

ADMINISTRATION/HANDLING

ALERT Do not administer via IV route.

IM (Risperdal Consta, Risvan)

Reconstitution • Use only diluent and needle supplied in dose pack. • Prepare suspension according to manufacturer's directions. • Administer immediately after reconstitution. • *(Risperdal Consta):* If 2 min pass between reconstitution and injection, shake upright vial vigorously back and forth to resuspend solution. • **(Risvan):** Administer within 15 min of reconstitution.

Rate of administration • Inject IM into upper outer quadrant of gluteus maximus or into deltoid muscle in upper arm (only gluteus for Rykindo).

Storage • Store at room temperature.

PO

• Give without regard to food. • May mix oral solution with water, coffee, orange juice, low-fat milk. Do not mix with cola, tea.

Orally Disintegrating Tablet

• Remove from blister pack immediately before administration. • Using gloves, place immediately on tongue. • Tablet dissolves in seconds. • Pt may swallow with or without liquid. • Do not split or chew.

SQ

Insert needle subcutaneously into abdomen only and inject solution. • Do not inject into areas of active skin disease or injury such as sunburns, skin rashes, inflammation, skin infections, or active psoriasis. • Rotate injection sites. • Do not rub injection site.

Storage • Refrigerate. Unopened package may be stored at room temperature for 30 days.

INDICATIONS/ROUTES/DOSAGE

Schizophrenia

PO: ADULTS, ELDERLY: Initially, 2 mg/day in 1–2 divided doses. May increase at intervals of 24 hrs or greater, in increments of 1–2 mg/day. **Recommended range:** 4–8 mg/day. **ADOLESCENTS:** Initially, 0.5 mg once daily (in morning or evening). May increase at intervals of 24 hrs or greater, in increments of 0.5–1 mg/day. **Recommended dose:** 3 mg/day. **IM: ADULTS, ELDERLY: (Risperdal Consta, Rykindo):** Initially, 25 mg q2 wks. May increase in increments of 12.5–25 mg q4wks. **Maximum:** 50 mg q2 wks. **(Risvan):** Initiate at 75 mg or 100 mg monthly. **SQ: ADULTS, ELDERLY: (Perseris):** Initially, 90–120 mg once monthly. Do not administer more than 1 dose (90 mg or 120

mg total). **(Uzedy):** Initiate as either once monthly or once q2mos the day after the last dose of oral therapy.

Uzedy
Dosage Recommendations for Switching from Daily Oral Risperidone

Prior Therapy	Monthly	q2 Mos
2 mg	50 mg	100 mg
3 mg	75 mg	150 mg
4 mg	100 mg	200 mg
5 mg	125 mg	250 mg

Bipolar Mania

PO: ADULTS, ELDERLY: Monotherapy/adjunctive therapy: Initially, 2–3 mg/day. May increase at intervals of 24 hrs or greater, in increments of 1 mg/day. **Recommended range:** 1–6 mg/day. **ADOLESCENTS, CHILDREN 10–17 YRS: Monotherapy:** Initially, 0.5 mg once daily (in morning or evening). May increase at intervals of 24 hrs or greater, in increments of 0.5–1 mg/day. **Recommended dose:** 1–2.5 mg per/day. **IM: ADULTS, ELDERLY: (Risperdal Consta, Rykindo):** Monotherapy/adjunctive therapy: 25 mg IM q2wks. May increase in increments of 12.5–25 mg q4wks. **Maximum:** 50 mg q2wks.

Irritability Associated with Autistic Disorder

PO: ADOLESCENT, CHILDREN 5–17 YRS WEIGHING 20 KG OR GREATER: Initially, 0.5 mg/day. After a minimum of 4 days, may increase to recommended dose of 1 mg/day. **LESS THAN 20 KG:** Initially, 0.25 mg/day. After a minimum of 4 days, may increase to recommended dose of 0.5 mg/day. Dose may be further increased at intervals of 2 wks or greater, in increments of 0.25 mg/day for pts less than 20 kg, or in increments of 0.5 mg/day for pts 20 kg or greater. **Dose range:** 0.5–3 mg/day.

Dosage in Renal/Hepatic Impairment

Mild to moderate impairment: No dose adjustment. **Severe impairment:** Initial dosage for adults, elderly pts is 0.5 mg twice daily. Dosage is titrated slowly to desired effect.

SIDE EFFECTS

Frequent (26%–13%): Agitation, anxiety, insomnia, headache, constipation. **Occasional (10%–4%):** Dyspepsia, rhinitis, drowsiness, dizziness, nausea, vomiting, rash, abdominal pain, dry skin, tachycardia. **Rare (3%–2%):** Visual disturbances, fever, back pain, pharyngitis, cough, arthralgia, angina, aggressive behavior, orthostatic hypotension, breast swelling.

ADVERSE EFFECTS/TOXIC REACTIONS

May cause tardive dyskinesia (characterized by tongue protrusion, puffing of the cheeks, chewing or puckering of mouth), neuroleptic malignant syndrome (hyperpyrexia, muscle rigidity, altered mental status, irregular pulse or B/P, tachycardia, diaphoresis, cardiac arrhythmias, rhabdomyolysis, acute renal failure). Hyperglycemia, life-threatening events such as ketoacidosis and hyperosmolar coma, death have been reported.

NURSING CONSIDERATIONS

BASELINE ASSESSMENT

Obtain LFT, renal function test. Assess behavior, appearance, emotional status, response to environment, speech pattern, thought content, baseline weight. Question history of suicidal ideation and behavior.

INTERVENTION/EVALUATION

Monitor B/P, heart rate, weight, LFT, ECG. Monitor for fine tongue movement (may be first sign of tardive dyskinesia, which may be irreversible). Monitor for suicidal ideation. Assess for therapeutic response (greater interest in surroundings, improved self-care, increased ability to concentrate, relaxed facial expression). Monitor for potential neuroleptic malignant syndrome: fever, muscle rigidity, irregular B/P or pulse, altered mental status. Monitor fasting serum glucose periodically during therapy. Diligently screen for suicidal ideation and behavior; new onset or worsening of anxiety, depression, mood disorder.

PATIENT/FAMILY TEACHING

• Seek immediate medical attention if thoughts of suicide, new onset or worsening of anxiety, depression, or changes in mood occur. • Avoid tasks that may require alertness, motor skills until response to drug is established (may cause dizziness/drowsiness). • Avoid alcohol. • Go from lying to standing slowly. • Report trembling in fingers, altered gait, unusual muscular/skeletal movements, palpitations, severe dizziness/fainting, swelling/pain in breasts, visual changes, rash, difficulty breathing.

---

riTUXimab

ri-**tux**-i-mab
(Riabni, Rituxan, Rituxan Hycela, Ruxience, Truxima)

■ **BLACK BOX ALERT** ■ Profound, occasionally fatal infusion-related reactions reported during first 30–120 min of first infusion. Tumor lysis syndrome leading to acute renal failure may occur 12–24 hrs following first dose. Severe, sometimes fatal, mucocutaneous reactions resulting in progressive multifocal leukoencephalopathy (PML) and death reported. Test all pts for hepatitis B virus (HBV) infection prior to initiation. HBV reactivation may cause fulminant hepatitis, hepatic failure, and death.
Do not confuse Rituxan with Remicade, or riTUXimab with bevacizumab, inFLIXimab, brentuximab, obinutuzumab, ofatumumab, ramucirumab, ruxolitinib.

◆CLASSIFICATION

PHARMACOTHERAPEUTIC: Anti-CD20 monoclonal antibody. **CLINICAL:** Disease-modifying antirheumatic drug (DMARD), antineoplastic, immunosuppressant.

USES

RiTUXimab: Non-Hodgkin's lymphomas: Treatment of CD20-positive non-Hodgkin's lymphomas (NHL): relapsed or refractory, low-grade, or follicular B-cell NHL; follicular B-cell NHL (previously untreated); nonprogressive,

R

 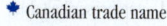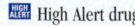

low-grade B-cell NHL; diffuse large B-cell NHL, previously untreated. **Chronic lymphocytic leukemia (CLL):** Treatment of CD20-positive CLL, in combination with fludarabine and cycloPHOSphamide (**Note:** Other medications have been approved with rituximab). **Rheumatoid arthritis (RA):** Treatment of adults with moderate to severe active RA, in combination with methotrexate, who have had an inadequate response to one or more TNF antagonists. **Polyangiitis:** Treatment of granulomatosis with polyangiitis GPA and microscopic polyangiitis (MPA) in adults and children 2 yrs and older. **Pemphigus vulgaris:** Treatment of moderate to severe pemphigus vulgaris. **OFF-LABEL:** Treatment of Burkitt's lymphoma, CNS lymphoma, Hodgkin's lymphoma graft vs host disease, multiple sclerosis, myasthenia gravis, immune thrombocytopenia. **Rituxan Hycela: Follicular lymphoma (FL):** Treatment of adults with relapsed or refractory follicular lymphoma as a single agent; previously untreated follicular lymphoma, in combination with first-line chemotherapy and, in pts achieving a complete or partial response to riTUXimab in combination with chemotherapy, as a single agent; nonprogressing (including stable disease) follicular lymphoma as a single agent after first-line cycloPHOSphamide, vinCRIStine and predniSONE chemotherapy. **Diffuse large B-cell lymphoma (DLBCL):** Treatment of adults with DLBCL in adults (previous untreated) in combination with cycloPHOSphamide, DOXOrubicin, vinCRIStine, predniSONE, or other anthracycline-based chemotherapy regimens. **Chronic lymphocytic leukemia (CLL):** Treatment of CLL, in combination with fludarabine and cycloPHOSphamide (previously untreated and previously treated CLL). Limitations: Only indicated in pts who have had at least one full dose of intravenous riTUXimab. Not indicated for treatment of nonmalignant conditions. **OFF-LABEL:** Acute lymphoblastic leukemia, Burkitt's lymphoma, dermatomyositis (refractory), graft-versus-host disease, hairy cell leukemia, Hodgkin's lymphoma, immune thrombocytopenia, multiple sclerosis, myasthenia gravis, Waldenström macroglobulinemia.

PRECAUTIONS

Contraindications: Hypersensitivity to ri-TUXimab. **Cautions:** Baseline cytopenias, active infection, conditions predisposing to infection (e.g., diabetes, renal failure, immunocompromised pts, open wounds); pts at risk for tumor lysis syndrome (high tumor burden), cardiac disease, elderly, pulmonary disease, renal impairment, hepatitis B virus (HBV) infection, hepatitis C virus (HCV) infection; pts at risk for GI perforation (Crohn's disease, diverticulitis, GI tract malignancies, peptic ulcers, peritoneal malignancies). Avoid administration of live or live attenuated vaccines during treatment and after discontinuation until B cells are no longer depleted.

ACTION

Binds to CD20, the antigen found on surface of B lymphocytes. Activates B-cell cytotoxicity. B cells may also play a role in development/progression of RA. Hyaluronidase increases the absorption rate of rituximab by increasing permeability of SQ tissue. **Therapeutic Effect:** Produces cytotoxicity, reduces tumor size. Signs/symptoms of rheumatoid arthritis are reduced; structural damage delayed.

PHARMACOKINETICS

Rapidly depletes B cells. **Half-life:** 59.8 hrs after first infusion, 174 hrs after fourth infusion.

⧖ LIFESPAN CONSIDERATIONS

Pregnancy/Lactation: May cause fetal harm due to fetal B-cell depletion and lymphocytopenia in neonates. Unknown if distributed in breast milk. Females of reproductive potential should use effective contraception during treatment and for at least 12 mos after discontinuation. Breastfeeding not recommended during treatment and for at least 6 mos after

---

R

discontinuation. **Children:** Safety and efficacy not established. **Elderly:** Increased risk of cardiac/pulmonary adverse reactions.

INTERACTIONS

DRUG: Denosumab, pimecrolimus may increase risk of adverse effects. May increase toxic effects of **leflunomide, natalizumab.** May alter concentration/effect of **vaccines (live). HERBAL: Echinacea** may decrease therapeutic effect. **FOOD:** None known. **LAB VALUES:** May increase serum creatinine, glucose; LDH. May decrease Hgb, Hct, leukocytes, lymphocytes, neutrophils, platelets, RBCs; B-cell counts, immunoglobulin concentrations. May diminish diagnostic effect of *Coccidioides immitis* skin test.

AVAILABILITY (Rx)

Injection Solution, IV: 10 mg/mL (10 mL, 50 mL). **Injection Solution, SQ:** *(Rituxan Hycela):* 1,400 mg/23,400 units, 1,600 mg/26,800 units.

ADMINISTRATION/HANDLING
🖉 IV

◀**ALERT**▶ Do not give by IV push or bolus. Must be administered by a healthcare professional who is experienced in management of severe infusion reactions.
Reconstitution • Dilute with 0.9% NaCl or D_5W to provide final concentration of 1–4 mg/mL in infusion bag.
Rate of administration • Initially infuse at rate of 50 mg/hr. If no hypersensitivity or infusion-related reaction, may increase infusion rate in 50 mg/hr increments q30min to maximum 400 mg/hr. • Subsequent infusion can be given at 100 mg/hr and increased by 100 mg/hr increments q30min to maximum 400 mg/hr.
Storage • Refrigerate vials. • Diluted solution is stable for 24 hrs if refrigerated or at room temperature.

SQ
Preparation • Visually inspect for particulate matter or discoloration.

Solution should appear clear to opalescent, colorless to slightly yellow in color. Do not use if solution is cloudy, discolored, or if visible particles are observed.
Administration • For 1,400 mg/23,400 unit dose (11.7 mL), insert needle subcutaneously into abdomen and inject solution over 5 min. • For 1,600 mg/26,800 unit dose (13.4 mL), insert needle subcutaneously into abdomen and inject solution over 7 min. • Do not inject into areas of active skin disease or injury such as sunburns, skin rashes, inflammation, skin infections, or active psoriasis. • If administration is interrupted, continue administering at the same site (or at different site) but only in the SQ abdomen. • Do not administer IV or intramuscular. • Rotate injection sites.
Storage • Refrigerate unused vials until time of use. • Protect from light. • Do not freeze or expose to heating sources. • Once transferred to syringe, may refrigerate for up to 48 hrs or store at room temperature for up to 8 hrs.

🔹 IV INCOMPATIBILITIES
Do not mix with any other medications.

INDICATIONS/ROUTES/DOSAGE
Note: All pts must receive at least one full dose of riTUXimab by IV infusion prior to receiving Rituxan Hycela SQ.

NHL (Relapsed/Refractory, Low-Grade or Follicular CD20-Positive B-Cell)
IV: ADULTS: 375 mg/m² wkly for 4 or 8 doses. **Retreatment:** 375 mg/m² once wkly for 4 doses.
SQ: ADULTS: 1,400 mg/23,400 units once wkly for 3 or 7 wks following full dose of IV rituximab at wk 1 (e.g., 4 or 8 wks total). **ADULTS: Retreatment:** 1,400 mg/23,400 units once wkly for 3 wks following full dose of IV riTUXimab at wk 1 (e.g., 4 wks total).

NHL (Diffuse Large B-Cell)
IV: ADULTS: 375 mg/m² on day 1 of each cycle up to 8 doses in combination with CHOP chemotherapy.
SQ: ADULTS: 1,400 mg/23,400 units on day 1 of cycles 2–8 of CHOP chemotherapy

R

for up to 7 cycles following full dose of IV riTUXimab at day 1, cycle 1 of CHOP therapy.

NHL (Follicular, CD20-Positive, B-Cell, Previously Untreated)

IV: ADULTS: 375 mg/m^2 on day 1 of each cycle up to 8 doses. **Maintenance (single agent):** 375 mg/m^2 q8wks for 12 doses.

SQ: ADULTS: 1,400 mg/23,400 units on day 1 of cycles 2–8 (q21 days), for up to 7 cycles following full dose of IV riTUXimab on day 1 of cycle 1 (e.g., up to 8 cycles total). In pts with partial or complete response, start maintenance therapy 8 wks after completion. Administer as single agent q8wks for 12 doses.

NHL (Nonprogressive, CD20-Positive, B-Cell Following 6–8 Cycles of CycloPHOSphamide, vinCRIStine, and PrednisoLONE [CVP therapy])

IV: ADULTS: 375 mg/m^2 once wkly for 4 doses q6mos. **Maximum:** 16 doses.
SQ: ADULTS: 1,400 mg/23,400 units once wkly for 3 wks (e.g., 4 wks total) at 6-mo intervals following completion of CVP therapy and a full dose of IV riTUXimab at wk 1. **Maximum:** 16 doses.

Rheumatoid Arthritis

IV: ADULTS: 1,000 mg every 2 wks times 2 doses (may give as monotherapy, with methotrexate, or with another DMARD). May repeat course q24wks (if needed, no sooner than 16 wks).

CLL

IV: ADULTS, CHILDREN: (Induction): 375 mg/m^2 in first cycle (on day prior to fludarabine/cycloPHOSphamide) and 500 mg/m^2 on day 1 in cycles 2–6, administered every 28 days.
SQ: ADULTS: 1,600 mg/26,800 units on day 1 of cycles 2–6 (q28 days) (in combination with fludarabine and cycloPHOSphamide) for a total of 5 cycles following full dose of IV riTUXimab on day 1 of cycle 1 (e.g., 6 cycles total).

GPA, MPA

IV: (Induction): ADULTS, CHILDREN: 375 mg/m^2 once wkly for 4 wks or 1 g q2wks for 2 doses (in combination with

methylPREDNISolone IV for 1–3 days, then daily predniSONE). **(Follow-up therapy):**
ADULTS: 500 mg as 2 infusions separated by 2 wks, then 500 mg or 1 g q4–6mos thereafter. **CHILDREN:** 250 mg/m2 q2wks for 2 doses, then 250 mg/m2 q6mos thereafter.

Pemphigus Vulgaris

IV: ADULTS, ELDERLY: 1,000 mg q2wks for 2 doses, then maintainance dose of 500 mg at months 12 and 18 and q6mos thereafter.

Dosage in Renal/Hepatic Impairment

No dose adjustment.

SIDE EFFECTS

Note: Side effects may vary depending on dose and indicated treatment. **Frequent (53%–14%):** Fever, chills, asthenia, constipation, nausea, headache, paresthesia, night sweats, pyrexia, rash, pruritus, abdominal pain, alopecia. **Occasional (13%–5%):** Cough, pain, rhinitis, peripheral neuropathy, back pain, bone pain, diarrhea, vomiting, dizziness, myalgia, arthralgia, hypotension, insomnia, erythema, throat irritation, urticaria, muscle spasm, dyspnea, hypertension, chest pain, flushing, anxiety, peripheral edema.

ADVERSE EFFECTS/TOXIC REACTIONS

Myelosuppression (anemia, leukopenia, lymphopenia, neutropenia, thrombocytopenia) is an expected response to therapy. Severe infusion reactions including anaphylaxis, angioedema, ARDS, bronchospasm, hypotension, hypoxia, pulmonary infiltrates were reported. Cardiac events including cardiogenic shock, MI, ventricular fibrillation may occur, particularly in pts with history of preexisting cardiac conditions. Severe, and sometimes fatal, mucocutaneous reactions including paraneoplastic pemphigus, Stevens-Johnson syndrome, lichenoid dermatitis, vesiculobullous dermatitis, toxic epidermal necrolysis may occur. Progressive multifocal leukoencephalopathy (PML), an opportunistic viral infection of the brain caused by the JC virus, may result in progressive permanent disability and death.

Infections including upper respiratory tract infection, pneumonia, pharyngitis, nasopharyngitis, bronchitis, UTI, sinusitis, conjunctivitis, influenza occurred in 15%–4% of pts. May cause HBV reactivation, resulting in fulminant hepatitis, hepatic failure, and death. Tumor lysis syndrome may present as acute renal failure, hypocalcemia, hyperuricemia, hyperphosphatemia. Fatal cases of bowel perforation/obstruction were reported.

NURSING CONSIDERATIONS

BASELINE ASSESSMENT

Obtain CBC; pregnancy test in females of reproductive potential; LFT in pts with history of HCV, HBV infection. Test all pts for hepatitis B virus infection. Initiate anti-HBV therapy if warranted. Recommend continuous ECG monitoring during initial infusions. Screen for active infection. Pretreatment with acetaminophen and diphenhydrAMINE before each infusion may prevent infusion-related effects. Confirm compliance of effective contraception. Conduct baseline dermatological exam and assess skin for open/unhealed wounds, lesions, moles. Receive full medication history and screen for interactions. Question history of cardiac disease, GI perforation, chronic infections, renal impairment. All pts planning to receive SQ must complete at least one full intravenous dose. Recommend prophylactic treatment for *Pneumocystis jiroveci* (PCP) and herpes virus infection in pts with CLL during treatment and for up to 12 mos after discontinuation. Offer emotional support.

INTERVENTION/EVALUATION

Monitor CBC at regular intervals. Monitor serum calcium, phosphate, uric acid if tumor lysis syndrome is suspected (acute renal failure, electrolyte imbalance, cardiac arrhythmias, seizures). Monitor for infections of any kind. Monitor for an infusion-related reaction; generally occurs within 30 min–2 hrs of beginning first infusion. Slowing infusion resolves symptoms. If given SQ, monitor pt at least 15 min following administration.

Pts who present with abdominal pain, fever, nausea, vomiting should be evaluated for bowel perforation/obstruction. Assess mouth for ulcerations; skin for cutaneous reactions. Closely monitor for exacerbation of hepatitis or HBV reactivation (amber- to orange-colored urine, fatigue, jaundice, nausea, vomiting). Due to risk of cardiovascular events, have emergency resuscitation equipment ready available. Offer antiemetic if nausea occurs, antidiarrheal if diarrhea occurs. Monitor daily pattern of bowel activity, stool consistency. Ensure adequate hydration, nutrition. Monitor weight, I&Os.

PATIENT/FAMILY TEACHING

• Treatment may depress the immune system and reduce the ability to fight infection. Report symptoms of infection such as body aches, burning with urination, chills, cough, fatigue, fever. Avoid those with active infection. • Report symptoms of bone marrow depression such as bruising, fatigue, fever, shortness of breath, weight loss; bleeding easily, bloody urine or stool. • Therapy may cause tumor lysis syndrome (a condition caused by the rapid breakdown of cancer cells), which can cause kidney failure and can be fatal. Report decreased urination, amber-colored urine, confusion, difficulty breathing, fatigue, fever, muscle or joint pain, palpitations, seizures, vomiting. • Use effective contraception to avoid pregnancy. Do not breastfeed. • PML, an opportunistic viral infection of the brain, may cause progressive, permanent disabilities and death. Report symptoms of PML, brain hemorrhage such as confusion, memory loss, paralysis, trouble speaking, vision loss, seizures, weakness. • Immediately report symptoms of infusion reactions (difficulty breathing, itching, hives, palpitations, rash, swelling of the face or tongue); severe mucocutaneous reactions (blisters, peeling of skin, ulceration of the mouth); HBV reactivation (fatigue, yellowing of the skin or eyes); bowel obstruction or perforation (abdominal pain, fever, nausea, vomiting); cardiovascular events (chest pain, cold/clammy skin, difficulty breathing, fainting,

R

◆ Canadian trade name   🦬 Non-Crushable Drug   🟥 High Alert drug

irregular heartbeat, palpitations, sweating). • Do not take newly prescribed medications unless approved by the prescriber who originally started treatment.

rivaroxaban

rye-va-**rox**-a-ban
(Xarelto)

■ **BLACK BOX ALERT** ■ Epidural/spinal hematomas may occur in pts receiving neuraxial anesthesia or spinal puncture, resulting in long-term or permanent paralysis. Factors increasing risk of epidural/spinal hematoma include indwelling epidural catheters, concomitant drugs such as NSAIDs, platelet inhibitors, other anticoagulants; history of traumatic or repeated spinal or epidural punctures, history of spinal deformity or spinal surgery. Monitor for signs and symptoms of neurologic impairment. Consider benefits and risks before neuraxial intervention in anticoagulated pts or planned thromboprophylaxis. Increased risk of stroke may occur in pts with atrial fibrillation when discontinuing for reasons other than bleeding.
Do not confuse rivaroxaban with argatroban.

◆CLASSIFICATION

PHARMACOTHERAPEUTIC: Factor Xa inhibitor. Direct oral anticoagulant. **CLINICAL:** Anticoagulant.

USES

Atrial fibrillation (nonvalvular) AF: Prevention of stroke and systemic embolism in adults with AF. **Coronary artery disease (CAD):** Risk reduction of major CV events in adults with CAD. **Risk reduction of recurrent DVT/PE:** Risk reduction in adults with continued risk following 6 mos or more of full anticoagulant treatment following DVT/PE. **Peripheral artery disease (PAD):** Risk reduction of major thrombotic events in adults with PAD. **Thromboprophylaxis:** Treatment of adults undergoing total hip/knee arthroplasty, adults hospitalized for acute medical illness who are at risk for thrombolic complications, children 2 yrs and older with congenital heart disease having undergone the Fontan procedure. **Venous thromboembolism (VTE):** Treatment of DVT/PE in adults, VTE, and risk reduction of VTE in pts less than 18 yrs of age after 5 or more days of initial parenteral anticoagulant treatment. **OFF-LABEL:** Acute coronary syndrome, heparin-induced thrombocytopenia (HIT), superficial vein thrombosis.

PRECAUTIONS

Contraindications: Hypersensitivity to rivaroxaban. Active major bleeding. **Cautions:** Renal/hepatic impairment, pts at increased risk of bleeding (e.g., thrombocytopenia, stroke, severe uncontrolled hypertension), elderly pts; avoid use with heparin, low molecular weight heparin (LMWH), aspirin, warfarin, NSAIDs. Pts with prosthetic heart valves or significant rheumatic heart disease.

ACTION

Selectively and reversibly blocks active site of factor Xa, a key factor in the intrinsic and extrinsic pathway of blood coagulation cascade. Inhibits platelet activation and fibrin clot formation. **Therapeutic Effect:** Inhibits blood coagulation.

PHARMACOKINETICS

Widely distributed. Peak plasma concentration: 2–4 hrs. Absorption dependent on site of drug release within GI tract. Avoid administration into small intestine due to reduced absorption. Protein binding: 92%–95%. Metabolized in liver. Excreted in urine (66%), feces (28%). **Half-life:** 5–9 hrs, 11–13 hrs (elderly pts).

⧗ LIFESPAN CONSIDERATIONS

Pregnancy/Lactation: Crosses placenta. Use during pregnancy should be avoided. Unknown if excreted in breast milk. **Children:** Safety and efficacy not established

---

in pts younger than 2 yrs. **Elderly:** May be at increased risk for bleeding due to age-related renal impairment. Use caution.

INTERACTIONS

DRUG: Strong CYP3A4 inhibitors (e.g., ketoconazole, clarithromycin, ritonavir) may increase concentration, risk of bleeding. **Strong CYP3A4 inducers (e.g., carBAMazepine, phenytoin, rifAMPin)** may decrease concentration/effect. **Anticoagulants (e.g., heparin, warfarin), antiplatelets (e.g., aspirin, clopidogrel), NSAIDs (e.g., ibuprofen, ketorolac, naproxen)** may increase bleeding risk. **Apixaban, dabigatran, edoxaban** may increase anticoagulant effect. **HERBAL: Herbals with anticoagulant/antiplatelet properties (e.g., garlic, ginger, ginkgo biloba)** may increase risk of bleeding. **FOOD: Grapefruit products** may increase risk of bleeding. **LAB VALUES:** May decrease platelets. May increase serum ALT, AST, bilirubin.

AVAILABILITY (Rx)

Tablets: 2.5 mg, 10 mg, 15 mg, 20 mg. **Oral Suspension:** 1 mg/mL (prepared by pharmacy).

ADMINISTRATION/HANDLING

PO
• Administer doses of 15 mg or greater with food; doses of 10 mg/day or less may be given without regard to food. • **Nonvalvular atrial fibrillation:** Give with evening meal. • Tablets may be crushed and mixed with applesauce immediately prior to use, then followed with food for doses 15 mg or more Only use the oral dosing syringe provided with oral suspension.

INDICATIONS/ROUTES/DOSAGE

Nonvalvular Atrial Fibrillation
PO: ADULTS, ELDERLY: (CrCl greater than 50 mL/min): 20 mg once daily with evening meal. **(CrCl 50 ml/min or less):** 15 mg daily with evening meal.

Coronary Artery Disease
PO: ADULTS, ELDERLY: 2.5 mg 2 times/day (plus aspirin 75–100 mg once daily).

Risk Reduction of Recurrent DVT/PE
PO: ADULTS, ELDERLY: (CrCl 15 mL/min or greater): 10 mg once daily (after at least 6 mos of standard anticoagulant treatment). **(CrCl less than 15 mL/min):** Avoid use.

Peripheral Artery Disease
PO: ADULTS, ELDERLY: 2.5 mg 2 times/day (plus aspirin 75–100 mg once daily).

Prophylaxis DVT/PE
PO: ADULTS, ELDERLY: Hip replacement: 10 mg once daily for 35 days (begin 6-10 hrs after surgery once hemostasis is established). **(CrCl less than 15 mL/min):** Avoid use. **Knee replacement:** 10 mg once daily for 12 days (begin 6-10 hrs after surgery once hemostasis established). **(CrCl less than 15 mL/min):** Avoid use. **Acute medically ill: (CrCl 15 mL/min or greater):** 10 mg once daily for recommended duration of 31–39 days. **CHILDREN 2 YRS AND OLDER:** Refer to manufacturer's prescribing information.

Treatment of DVT/PE
PO: ADULTS, ELDERLY: (CrCl 15 mL/min or greater): 15 mg 2 times/day. After 21 days, transition to 20 mg once daily. **(CrCl less than 15 mL/min):** Avoid use.

Dosage in Renal Impairment
See individual indications.

Dosage in Hepatic Impairment
Mild impairment: No dose adjustment. **Moderate to severe impairment:** Avoid use.

RECOMMENDED DOSAGE IN PEDIATRIC PTS

Treatment/Risk Reduction of Recurrent VTE (birth to less than 18 Yrs)
Note: Take with food to increase absorption.
PO: CHILDREN 50 KG OR GREATER: 20 mg once daily. **30–49.9 KG:** 15 mg once daily.

12–29.9 KG: 5 mg twice daily. **10–11.9 KG:** 3 mg 3 times/day. **9–9.9 KG:** 2.8 mg 3 times/day. **8–8.9 KG:** 2.4 mg 3 times/day. **7–7.9 KG:** 1.8 mg 3 times/day. **5–6.9 KG:** 1.6 mg 3 times/day. **4–4.9 KG:** 1.4 mg 3 times/day. **3–3.9 KG:** 0.9 mg 3 times/day. **2.6–2.9 KG:** 0.8 mg 3 times/day.

Thromboprophylaxis in Pediatric Pts With Congenital Heart Disease
Note: Give without regard to food.
PO: CHILDREN 50 KG OR GREATER: 10 mg once daily. **30–49.9 KG:** 7.5 mg once daily. **20–29.9 KG:** 2.5 mg twice daily. **12–19.9 KG:** 2 mg 2 times/day. **10–11.9 KG:** 1.7 mg 2 times/day. **8–9.9 KG:** 1.6 mg 2 times/day. **7–7.9 KG:** 1.1 mg 2 times/day.

SIDE EFFECTS

Rare (3%–1%): Wound secretion/oozing, extremity pain, muscle spasm, syncope, pruritus.

ADVERSE EFFECTS/TOXIC REACTIONS

Increased risk of bleeding/hemorrhagic events including retroperitoneal hemorrhage, cerebral hemorrhage, subdural hematoma, epidural/spinal hematoma (esp. with epidural catheters, spinal trauma). Serious reactions including jaundice, cholestasis, cytolytic hepatitis, Stevens-Johnson syndrome, hypersensitivity reaction, anaphylaxis reported.

NURSING CONSIDERATIONS

BASELINE ASSESSMENT

Obtain ECG for pts with a history of atrial fibrillation. Question for history of bleeding disorders, recent surgery, spinal punctures, intracranial hemorrhage, bleeding ulcers, open wounds, anemia, renal/hepatic impairment. Receive full medication history including herbal products.

INTERVENTION/EVALUATION

Be alert for complaints of abdominal/back pain, headache, confusion, weakness, vision change (may indicate hemorrhage). Question for increased menstrual bleeding/discharge. Assess peripheral pulses; skin for ecchymosis, petechiae. Check for excessive bleeding from minor cuts, scratches. Assess urine output for hematuria. Immediately report suspected pregnancy.

PATIENT/FAMILY TEACHING

• Do not take/discontinue any medication except on advice of physician. • Avoid alcohol, aspirin, NSAIDs. • Consult physician before surgery, dental work. • Use electric razor, soft toothbrush to prevent bleeding. • Report any unusual bleeding/bruising, spinal/epidural hematomas (e.g., tingling, numbness, muscular weakness). • Report if pregnant or planning to become pregnant. • Avoid grapefruit products.

rivastigmine

riv-a-**stig**-meen
(Exelon)

◆CLASSIFICATION

PHARMACOTHERAPEUTIC: Acetylcholinesterase inhibitor. **CLINICAL:** Anti-Alzheimer's dementia agent.

USES

PO: Treatment of mild to moderate dementia of Alzheimer's or mild to moderate dementia of Parkinson's disease. **Transdermal:** Treatment of mild, moderate, or severe dementia of the Alzheimer type. Treatment of mild to moderate dementia associated with Parkinson's disease. **OFF-LABEL:** Lewy body dementia, vascular dementia.

PRECAUTIONS

Contraindications: Hypersensitivity to rivastigmine, other carbamate derivatives (e.g., neostigmine), history of application site reactions with rivastigmine patch.

R

Cautions: Peptic ulcer disease, concurrent use of NSAIDs, sick sinus syndrome, bradycardia or supraventricular conduction defects, urinary obstruction, seizure disorders, asthma, COPD, body weight less than 50 kg.

ACTION

Increases acetylcholine in CNS by reversibly inhibiting hydrolysis by cholinesterase. **Therapeutic Effect:** Slows progression of symptoms of Alzheimer's disease, dementia of Parkinson's disease.

PHARMACOKINETICS

Widely distributed. Penetrates blood-brain barrier. Metabolized via cholinesterase-mediated hydrolysis. Excreted in urine (97%), feces (0.4%). **Half-life:** 1 hr (oral); 8–16 hrs (transdermal patch).

⧗ LIFESPAN CONSIDERATIONS

Pregnancy/Lactation: Unknown if distributed in breast milk. **Children:** Not indicated in this pt population. **Elderly:** No age-related precautions noted.

INTERACTIONS

DRUG: May interfere with **anticholinergics (e.g., dicyclomine, glycopyrrolate, scopolamine)** effects. May increase the bradycardic effect of **beta blockers (e.g., atenolol, carvedilol, metoprolol)**. May increase the adverse effects of **metoclopramide.** **HERBAL:** None significant. **FOOD:** None known. **LAB VALUES:** None significant.

AVAILABILITY (Rx)

Oral solution: 2 mg/mL. **Transdermal Patch:** 4.6 mg/24 hrs, 9.5 mg/24 hrs, 13.3 mg/24 hrs.

🐋 **Capsules:** 1.5 mg, 3 mg, 4.5 mg, 6 mg.

ADMINISTRATION/HANDLING

PO

• Give morning and evening doses with food. • Give capsule whole; do not break, cut, or open.

Oral Solution

• Using oral dosing syringe provided, withdraw the prescribed amount of solution from container. • May be swallowed directly from the syringe or mixed with a small glass of water, cold fruit juice, or soda (stir and administer the mixture).

Transdermal Patch

• May apply the day following the last oral dose. • Apply to upper or lower back, upper arm, or chest. • Avoid reapplication to same spot of skin for 14 days. • Do not apply to red, irritated, or broken skin. • Avoid eye contact. • After removal, fold patch to press adhesive together and discard.

INDICATIONS/ROUTES/DOSAGE

Alzheimer's Dementia (Mild to Moderate)

PO: ADULTS, ELDERLY: Initially, 1.5 mg twice daily. May increase by 3 mg (1.5 mg/dose) at intervals of at least 2 wks **Maximum:** 6 mg twice daily.

Transdermal: Initially, 4.6 mg/24 hrs. May increase at intervals of at least 4 wks to 9.5 mg/24 hrs and then to 13.3 mg/24 hrs.

Alzheimer's Dementia (Severe)

Transdermal: ADULTS, ELDERLY: Initially, 4.6 mg/24 hrs. May increase at intervals of at least 4 wks to 9.5 mg/24 hrs and then to 13.3 mg/24 hrs.

Parkinson's Dementia

PO: ADULTS, ELDERLY: Initially, 1.5 mg twice daily. May increase at intervals of at least 4 wks by 3 mg (1.5 mg/dose). **Maximum:** 6 mg twice daily.

Transdermal: Initially, 4.6 mg/24 hrs. May increase after 4 wks to 9.5 mg/24 hrs and then to 13.3 mg/24 hrs.

Dosage in Renal Impairment

No dose adjustment.

Dosage in Hepatic Impairment

PO: No dose adjustment.
Transdermal: **Maximum:** 4.6 mg/24 hrs.

SIDE EFFECTS

Frequent (47%–17%): Nausea, vomiting, dizziness, diarrhea, headache, anorexia.

R

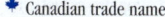 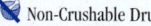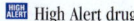

Occasional (13%–6%): Abdominal pain, insomnia, dyspepsia (heartburn, indigestion, epigastric pain), confusion, UTI, depression. **Rare (5%–3%):** Anxiety, drowsiness, constipation, malaise, hallucinations, tremor, flatulence, rhinitis, hypertension, flu-like symptoms, weight loss, syncope.

ADVERSE EFFECTS/TOXIC REACTIONS

Overdose can produce cholinergic crisis, characterized by severe nausea/vomiting, increased salivation, diaphoresis, bradycardia, hypotension, respiratory depression, seizures.

NURSING CONSIDERATIONS

BASELINE ASSESSMENT

Obtain vital signs. Assess history for peptic ulcer, urinary obstruction, asthma, COPD, cardiac disease. Assess cognitive, behavioral, functional deficits.

INTERVENTION/EVALUATION

Monitor for cholinergic reaction: GI discomfort/cramping, feeling of facial warmth, excessive salivation, diaphoresis, lacrimation, pallor, urinary urgency, dizziness. Monitor for nausea, diarrhea, headache, insomnia.

PATIENT/ FAMILY TEACHING

• Take with meals (at breakfast, dinner). • Swallow capsule whole. Do not break, chew, or divide capsules. • Report nausea, vomiting, diarrhea, diaphoresis, increased salivary secretions, severe abdominal pain, dizziness.

rizatriptan

rye-za-trip-tan
(Maxalt, Maxalt-MLT, Maxalt RPD ✦, Rizafilm)

◆CLASSIFICATION

PHARMACOTHERAPEUTIC: Serotonin 5-HT$_1$ receptor agonist. **CLINICAL:** Antimigraine.

USES

Treatment of acute migraine headache with or without aura in adults and children 6 yrs and older. **Rizafilm:** Acute treatment of migraine with or without aura in adults and in pts 12–17 yrs of age weighing 40 kg or more.

PRECAUTIONS

Contraindications: Hypersensitivity to rizatriptan. Basilar or hemiplegic migraine, history of stroke or transient ischemic attack; severe cardiovascular disease, coronary artery vasospasm, peripheral vascular disease, ischemic bowel disease, uncontrolled hypertension, use within 24 hrs of ergotamine-containing preparations or another serotonin receptor agonist, MAOI use within 14 days. **Cautions:** Mild to moderate renal/hepatic impairment, end-stage renal disease requiring dialysis, elderly, cardiovascular risks (e.g., hypertension, diabetes, hypercholesterolemia).

ACTION

Binds selectively to serotonin 5-HT$_1$ receptors in cranial arteries producing vasoconstriction. **Therapeutic Effect:** Relieves migraine headache.

PHARMACOKINETICS

Widely distributed. Protein binding: 14%. Crosses blood-brain barrier. Metabolized by liver. Excreted primarily in urine (82%), feces (12%). **Half-life:** 2–3 hrs.

⧗ LIFESPAN CONSIDERATIONS

Pregnancy/Lactation: Unknown if drug is distributed in breast milk. **Children:** Safety and efficacy not established in pts younger than 6 yrs. **Elderly:** No age-related precautions noted.

INTERACTIONS

DRUG: **Ergot derivatives** (e.g., ergotamine) may increase vasoconstrictive effect. **Strong CYP3A4 inhibitors** (e.g., clarithromycin, ketoconazole** may increase concentration/effect. **MAOIs** (e.g., phenelzine, selegiline), **propranolol** may dramatically increase concentration (avoid concurrent use). **HERBAL:** None significant. **FOOD: All foods** delay peak drug concentration by 1 hr. **LAB VALUES:** None significant.

AVAILABILITY (Rx)

Oral Film: 10 mg.
Tablets: 5 mg, 10 mg. **Tablets, Orally Disintegrating:** 5 mg, 10 mg.

ADMINISTRATION/HANDLING

PO

Tablet • Give without regard to food.

Oral disintegrating tablets (ODT) • Orally disintegrating tablet is packaged in individual aluminum pouch. • Open packet with dry hands. • Place tablet onto tongue, allow to dissolve, swallow with saliva. Administration with water is not necessary. **Film:** Place on tongue, where it will disintegrate within approximately 2 min and swallowed with saliva.

INDICATIONS/ROUTES/DOSAGE

Note: See interactions for caution with propranolol.

Acute Migraine Headache

PO: ADULTS OLDER THAN 18 YRS, ELDERLY: 5–10 mg. If significant improvement is not attained, dose may be repeated after 2 hrs. **Maximum:** 30 mg/24 hrs. (Use 5 mg/dose in pts taking propranolol with maximum of 15 mg/24 hrs.) **CHILDREN 6–17 YRS WEIGHING 40 KG OR MORE:** 10 mg as single dose. (Maximum 5 mg as single dose with propranolol.) **WEIGHING LESS THAN 40 KG:** 5 mg as a single dose. (Not recommended if taking propranolol.) *(Rizafilm):* **ADULTS 18 YRS AND OLDER, ELDERLY:** 10 mg. **Maximum:** 30 mg/24 hrs, with doses separated by at least 2 hrs. **12–17 YRS:** 10 mg times 1 dose administered on the tongue.

Dosage in Renal/Hepatic Impairment

No dose adjustment.

SIDE EFFECTS

Frequent (9%–7%): Dizziness, drowsiness, paresthesia, fatigue. **Occasional (6%–3%):** Nausea, chest pressure, dry mouth. **Rare (2%):** Headache; neck, throat, jaw pressure; photosensitivity.

ADVERSE EFFECTS/TOXIC REACTIONS

Cardiac reactions (ischemia, coronary artery vasospasm, MI), noncardiac vasospasm-related reactions (hemorrhage, CVA) may occur, esp. in pts with hypertension, diabetes, strong family history of coronary artery disease, obesity, smokers, males older than 40 yrs, postmenopausal women.

NURSING CONSIDERATIONS

BASELINE ASSESSMENT

Question for history of peripheral vascular disease, renal/hepatic impairment. Question pt regarding onset, location, duration of migraine, possible precipitating symptoms.

INTERVENTION/EVALUATION

Monitor for evidence of dizziness. Evaluate for relief of migraine headaches (photophobia, phonophobia, nausea, vomiting, pain, dizziness, fogginess).

PATIENT/FAMILY TEACHING

• Take single dose as soon as symptoms of an actual migraine headache appear. • Medication is intended to relieve migraine, not to prevent or reduce number of attacks. • Avoid tasks that require alertness, motor skills until response to drug is established. • Report immediately if palpitations, pain/tightness in chest/throat, pain/weakness of extremities occurs. • Do not remove orally disintegrating tablet from blister pack until just before dosing.

romosozumab-aqqg

roe-moe-**soz**-ue-mab
(Evenity)

■ **BLACK BOX ALERT** ■ May increase risk of myocardial infarction (MI), cerebrovascular accident (CVA), cardiovascular death. Do not initiate in pts with recent (within 1 yr)

R

MI, CVA. In pts with other cardio-vascular risks, consider whether the benefits of treatment outweigh the risks. Discontinue treatment in pts who develop MI, CVA.

Do not confuse romosozumab with atezolizumab, mepolizum-ab, pembrolizumab, trastuzum-ab, or vedolizumab, or Evenity with Emgality.

◆ CLASSIFICATION

PHARMACOTHERAPEUTIC: Sclerostin inhibitor. Monoclonal antibody. **CLINICAL:** Osteoporosis agent.

USES

Treatment of postmenopausal women with osteoporosis at high risk for frac-ture, defined as history of osteoporotic fracture, multiple risk factors for frac-ture, or pts who have failed or intolerant to other osteoporosis therapy.

PRECAUTIONS

Contraindications: Hypersensitivity to romosozumab-aqqg. Hypocalcemia prior to initiation. **Cautions:** Severe renal impair-ment (eGFR 15–29 mL/min) or receiving dialysis; pts at risk for osteonecrosis of the jaw (cancer, radiotherapy, poor oral hygiene, preexisting dental disease or infec-tion, anemia, coagulopathy, recent dental procedures, tooth extraction). History of MI, CVA, cardiovascular disease. Avoid use in pts with recent (within 1 yr) MI, CVA.

ACTION

Stimulates osteoblastic activity by inhib-iting sclerostin, a regulatory factor in bone metabolism. **Therapeutic Effect:** Increases bone mass, improves bone structure and strength, decreases bone reabsorption.

PHARMACOKINETICS

Widely distributed. Degraded into small peptides and amino acids via catabolic pathway. Peak plasma concentration: 5 days. Steady state reached in 3 mos. **Half-life:** 12.8 days.

⧖ LIFESPAN CONSIDERATIONS

Pregnancy/Lactation: Not indicated in female pts of reproductive potential. **Chil-dren:** Safety and efficacy not established. **Elderly:** No age-related precautions noted.

INTERACTIONS

DRUG: None significant. **HERBAL:** None significant. **FOOD:** None known. **LAB VAL-UES:** May decrease calcium.

AVAILABILITY (Rx)

Injection Solution, Prefilled Syringe: 105 mg/1.17 mL.

ADMINISTRATION/HANDLING
SQ

Preparation • Remove prefilled syringe from refrigerator and allow solu-tion to warm to room temperature (at least 30 min) with needle cap intact. • Visually inspect for particulate matter or discoloration. Solution should appear clear to opalescent, colorless to slightly yellow in color. Do not use if solution is cloudy or discolored or if vis-ible particles are observed.

Administration • Insert needle subcuta-neously into upper arm, outer thigh, or abdo-men and inject solution. • Do not inject into areas of active skin disease or injury such as sunburns, skin rashes, inflammation, skin infections, or active psoriasis. • Rotate injection sites. • Do not administer IV or intramuscularly. • If a dose is missed, administer as soon as possible, then give next dose at the date of last dose.

Storage • Refrigerate prefilled syringes in original carton until time of use. • Pro-tect from light. • Do not shake. • Do not freeze or expose to heating sources. • If not refrigerated, may store at room tem-perature (up to 77°F) for no more than 30 days. Discard if not used within 30 days.

INDICATIONS/ROUTES/DOSAGE
Postmenopausal Osteoporosis

SQ: ADULTS, ELDERLY: 210 mg (two 105-mg injections) once monthly for 12 mos. Give with supplemental calcium and vitamin D.

Dosage in Renal Impairment
No dose adjustment.

Dosage in Hepatic Impairment
Not specified; use caution.

SIDE EFFECTS

Occasional (13%–6%): Arthralgia, headache. **Rare (4%–2%):** Injection site reactions (pain, erythema), muscle spasms, peripheral edema, asthenia, neck pain, insomnia, paresthesia.

ADVERSE EFFECTS/TOXIC REACTIONS

MI, CVA, cardiovascular death reported in less than 1% of pts. Hypocalcemia reported in less than 1% of pts. Pts with severe renal impairment (eGFR 15–29 mL/min) or receiving dialysis have an increased risk of hypocalcemia. Hypersensitivity reactions including angioedema, erythema multiforme, dermatitis, rash, urticaria may occur. Symptomatic hypocalcemia reported in 7% of pts. Osteonecrosis of the jaw may present as mandibular pain, jaw bone erosion, periodontal/gingival infection or ulceration, osteomyelitis, slow healing of the mouth after dental procedures. Pts with cancer, radiotherapy, poor oral hygiene, preexisting dental disease or infection, anemia, coagulopathy may be at increased risk of developing osteonecrosis of the jaw. Atypical subtrochanteric and diaphyseal femoral fractures may occur with little or no trauma.

NURSING CONSIDERATIONS

BASELINE ASSESSMENT

Obtain serum calcium level. Hypocalcemia must be corrected prior to initiation. Calcium and vitamin D supplementation is recommended during treatment. Question history of MI, CVA, cardiovascular disease, renal impairment. Do not initiate in pts with recent (within 1 yr) MI, CVA. To assess the risk of osteonecrosis of the jaw, the prescriber should perform an oral examination prior to initiation. Question recent dental procedures or tooth extraction.

INTERVENTION/EVALUATION

Monitor serum calcium levels periodically, esp. in pts with severe renal impairment or receiving dialysis. Monitor for symptoms of CVA (aphasia, altered mental status, headache, hemiplegia, vision loss); MI (chest pain, dyspnea, syncope, diaphoresis, arm/jaw pain), osteonecrosis of the jaw (jaw pain/numbness, loosening of teeth, poor healing of the gums; hypocalcemia (muscle spasm, myalgia, paresthesia, seizures, QT interval prolongation, ventricular arrhythmias; Chvostek's sign, Trousseau's sign). A dull, aching thigh or groin pain should be evaluated for possible femoral fractures. Monitor for hypersensitivity reactions.

PATIENT/FAMILY TEACHING

• Report symptoms of heart attack (chest pain, difficulty breathing, jaw pain, nausea, pain that radiates to the arm or jaw, sweating), stroke (confusion, one-sided weakness, loss of consciousness, trouble speaking, vision loss); atypical leg fractures (dull, aching thigh or groin pain). • Treatment may cause low blood calcium levels; report difficulty swallowing, fatigue, muscle cramps, muscle weakness, palpations, paralysis, numbness, tingling, seizures. • Treatment may cause lack of blood supply to the jaw bone when the bone is exposed, which may lead to jaw necrosis. Report jaw pain or numbness, loosening of teeth, poor healing of the gums. Maintain proper oral hygiene. • Allergic reactions such as swelling of the face or tongue, rash, itching may occur.

rOPINIRole

roe-**pin**-i-role
Do not confuse rOPINIRole with RisperDAL.

◆CLASSIFICATION

PHARMACOTHERAPEUTIC: DOPamine agonist. **CLINICAL:** Antiparkinson agent.

USES

Treatment of signs/symptoms of Parkinson's disease. **Immediate-release only:** Treatment of moderate to severe primary restless legs syndrome (RLS).

PRECAUTIONS

Contraindications: Hypersensitivity to rOPINIRole. **Cautions:** History of orthostatic hypotension, cardiovascular or cerebrovascular disease, syncope, concurrent use of CNS depressants, preexisting dyskinesia, hepatic or severe renal dysfunction (end-stage renal disease [ESRD]), major psychotic disorder, elderly.

ACTION

Stimulates postsynaptic DOPamine receptors in caudate putamen in the brain. **Therapeutic Effect:** Relieves signs/symptoms of Parkinson's disease.

PHARMACOKINETICS

Widely distributed. Metabolized in liver. Protein binding: 40%. Steady state reached in 2 days. Excreted in urine. **Half-life:** 6 hrs.

⧗ LIFESPAN CONSIDERATIONS

Pregnancy/Lactation: Distributed in breast milk. Drug activity possible in breastfeeding infant. **Children:** Safety and efficacy not established. **Elderly:** No age-related precautions noted, but hallucinations may occur more frequently.

INTERACTIONS

DRUG: Alcohol, CNS depressants (e.g., LORazepam, morphine, zolpidem) may increase CNS depressant effects. **Antipsychotic agents (e.g., haloperidol)** may decrease therapeutic effect. **HERBAL: Herbals with hypotensive properties (e.g., garlic, ginger, ginkgo biloba)** may increase hypotensive effect. **Kava kava** may decrease concentration/effect. **FOOD: All foods** delay peak plasma levels by 1 hr but do not affect drug absorption. **LAB VALUES:** May increase serum alkaline phosphatase.

AVAILABILITY (Rx)

Tablets: 0.25 mg, 0.5 mg, 1 mg, 2 mg, 3 mg, 4 mg, 5 mg.

🐟 **Tablets, Extended-Release:** 2 mg, 4 mg, 6 mg, 8 mg, 12 mg.

ADMINISTRATION/HANDLING

PO
• May give without regard to food. • Do not break, crush, dissolve, or divide extended-release tablets.

INDICATIONS/ROUTES/DOSAGE

Parkinson's Disease
PO: *(Immediate-Release):* **ADULTS, ELDERLY:** Initially, 0.25 mg 3 times daily. May increase daily dose based on response and tolerability. **Doses up to 3 mg/day:** May increase daily dose by 0.75 mg q7 days. **Doses from 3–9 mg/day:** May increase daily dose by 1.5 mg q7 days. **Doses 9 mg/ day or more:** May increase daily dose by 3 mg q7 days. **Usual dose:** 12–16 mg/day. **Maximum:** 24 mg/day in 3 divided doses. *(Extended-Release):* Initially, 2 mg once daily for 1–2 wks. May increase by 2 mg/ day at 1 wk or longer interval. **Usual dose:** 12–16 mg/day. **Maximum:** 24 mg/day.

Discontinuation Taper
Gradually taper over 7 days as follows: Decrease frequency from 3 times/day to twice daily for 4 days, then decrease from twice daily to once daily for remaining 3 days.

Restless Legs Syndrome
PO: *(Immediate-Release):* **ADULTS, ELDERLY:** 0.25 mg once daily for days 1 and 2. May increase to 0.5 mg daily for days 3–7 and after 7 days to 1 mg daily. May further titrate upward in 0.5-mg increments q7days until reaching daily dose of 3 mg during wk 6. Daily dose may be increased to maximum of 4 mg beginning wk 7. Give all doses 1–3 hrs before bedtime. ESRD: 3 mg maximum.

Dosage in Renal/Hepatic Impairment
No dose adjustment. Use caution with severe renal impairment. Titrate cautiously in pts with hepatic impairment.

SIDE EFFECTS

Frequent (60%–40%): Nausea, dizziness, extreme drowsiness. **Occasional (12%–5%):** Syncope, vomiting, fatigue, viral infection, dyspepsia, diaphoresis, asthenia, orthostatic hypotension, abdominal discomfort, pharyngitis, abnormal vision, dry mouth, hypertension, hallucinations, confusion. **Rare (less than 4%):** Anorexia, peripheral edema, memory loss, rhinitis, sinusitis, palpitations, impotence.

ADVERSE EFFECTS/TOXIC REACTIONS

Dyskinesia, impulsive/compulsive behavior (pathologic gambling, hypersexuality, binge-eating) occur rarely.

NURSING CONSIDERATIONS

BASELINE ASSESSMENT

Parkinson's disease: Assess signs/symptoms (e.g., tremor, gait). **Restless legs syndrome:** Assess frequency of symptoms, sleep pattern.

INTERVENTION/EVALUATION

Assess for clinical improvement, clinical reversal of symptoms (improvement of tremors of head/hands at rest, mask-like facial expression, shuffling gait, muscular rigidity). Assist with ambulation if dizziness occurs. Monitor B/P, daytime alertness.

PATIENT/FAMILY TEACHING

• Drowsiness, dizziness may be an initial response. • Postural hypotension may occur more frequently during initial therapy. Slowly go from lying to standing. • Avoid tasks that require alertness, motor skills until response to drug is established. • If nausea occurs, take medication with food. • Hallucinations may occur, more so in the elderly than in younger pts with Parkinson's disease. • Report occurrence of falling asleep during activities of daily living, new or worsening symptoms, changes in B/P, fainting, unusual urges. • Avoid alcohol.

rosuvastatin

roe-**soo**-va-**sta**-tin
(Apo-Rosuvastatin ✦, <u>Crestor</u>, Ezallor Sprinkle)
Do not confuse rosuvastatin with atorvastatin, lovastatin, nystatin, pitavastatin, or simvastatin.

FIXED-COMBINATION(S)

Roszet: rosuvastatin/ezetimbe (an antihyperlipidemic): 5 mg/10 mg; 10 mg/10 mg; 20 mg/10 mg; 40 mg/10 mg.

◆CLASSIFICATION

PHARMACOTHERAPEUTIC: HMG-CoA reductase inhibitor. **CLINICAL:** Antihyperlipidemic.

USES

Risk reduction CV disease (primary prevention): Reduce risk of stroke, myocardial infarction, and arterial revascularization procedures in adults without coronary heart disease who are at an increased risk of cardiovascular (CV) disease based on age, hsCRP 2 mg/L or greater, and at least one additional CV risk factor. **(Secondary prevention):** Pts with established CV disease to reduce risk of MI, stroke, revascularization procedures, and angina. **Primary hyperlipidemia:** Adjunct to diet to reduce low-density lipoprotein-cholesterol (LDL-C) in adults with primary hyperlipidemia; reduce LDL-C and slow progression of atherosclerosis in adults. **Heterozygous familial hypercholesterolemia (HeFH):** Adjunct to diet to reduce LDL-C in adults and pts 8 yrs and older with HeFH. **Homozygous familial hypercholesterolemia (HoFH):** Adjunct to other LDL-C–lowering therapies to reduce LDL-C in adults and pts aged 7 yrs and older with homozygous familial hypercholesterolemia (HoFH). **OFF-LABEL:** Transplantation (post heart, kidney).

R

PRECAUTIONS

Contraindications: Hypersensitivity to rosuvastatin. Active hepatic disease, breastfeeding, pregnancy, unexplained, persistent elevations of hepatic enzymes. **Cautions:** Anticoagulant therapy, hepatic impairment, substantial alcohol consumption, elective major surgery, renal impairment, acute renal failure, uncontrolled hypothyroidism, elderly.

ACTION

Interferes with cholesterol biosynthesis by inhibiting conversion of the enzyme HMG-CoA to mevalonate, a precursor to cholesterol. **Therapeutic Effect:** Decreases LDL, VLDL, plasma triglyceride levels; increases HDL concentration.

PHARMACOKINETICS

Protein binding: 88%. Minimal hepatic metabolism. Primarily excreted in feces. **Half-life:** 19 hrs (increased in severe renal dysfunction).

⧖ LIFESPAN CONSIDERATIONS

Pregnancy/Lactation: Contraindicated in pregnancy (suppression of cholesterol biosynthesis may cause fetal toxicity), lactation. Risk of serious adverse reactions in breastfeeding infants. **Children:** Safety and efficacy not established in children younger than 7 yrs. **Elderly:** No age-related precautions noted.

INTERACTIONS

DRUG: Aluminum- and magnesium-containing antacids may decrease concentration/effects. Increased risk of myopathy with **colchicine, cyclo-SPORINE, fenofibrate, fenofibrate derivatives, gemfibrozil, niacin.** May increase anticoagulant effect of **warfarin. HERBAL:** None significant. **FOOD: Red yeast rice** contains 2.4 mg **lovastatin** per 600 mg rice. **LAB VALUES:** May increase serum alkaline phosphatase, bilirubin, creatinine phosphokinase, glucose, transaminases. May produce hematuria, proteinuria.

AVAILABILITY (Rx)

Capsule, Sprinkle: 5 mg, 10 mg, 20 mg, 40 mg. **Tablets:** 5 mg, 10 mg, 20 mg, 40 mg.

ADMINISTRATION/HANDLING

PO

Tablet • Give without regard to food. May give at any time of day. Administer tablet whole.

Capsule
• Administer whole (do not crush or allow chewing). • May open and sprinkle over soft food (should be swallowed within 60 min without chewing).

INDICATIONS/ROUTES/DOSAGE

Note: Dosing for pts of Asian descent: Initiate at 5 mg once daily. Consider the risks/benefits when pts of Asian descent are not adequately controlled at doses up to 20 mg/day.

Heterozygous Familial Hypercholesterolemia
PO: ADULTS, ELDERLY: Initially, 20–40 mg once daily. **CHILDREN 10 YRS AND OLDER, ADOLESCENTS:** 5–20 mg once daily. **Maximum:** 20 mg/day. **CHILDREN 8–9 YRS:** 5–10 mg once daily. **Maximum:** 10 mg/day.

Homozygous Familial Hypercholesterolemia
PO: ADULTS, ELDERLY: 40 mg once daily. **CHILDREN 7 YRS AND OLDER, ADOLES-CENTS:** 20 mg once daily.

Prevention of Atherosclerotic Cardiovascular Disease
PO: ADULTS, ELDERLY: *Primary Prevention:* (Moderate-intensity therapy): 5–10 mg once daily. (High-intensity therapy): 20–40 mg once daily. *Secondary Prevention:* (High-intensity therapy): 20-40 mg once daily.

Concurrent CycloSPORINE Use
PO: ADULTS, ELDERLY: 5 mg/day maximum.

Concurrent Gemfibrozil, Atazanavir/
Ritonavir, Lopinavir/Ritonavir or
Simeprevir Therapy

PO: ADULTS, ELDERLY: Initially, 5 mg/
day. 10 mg/day maximum.

**Dosage in Renal Impairment (CrCl less
than 30 mL/min)**

PO: ADULTS, ELDERLY: 5 mg/day; do not
exceed 10 mg/day.

Dosage in Hepatic Impairment

Contraindicated in active liver disease.

SIDE EFFECTS

Generally well tolerated. Side effects are
usually mild, transient. **Occasional (9%–
3%):** Pharyngitis, headache, diarrhea, dyspepsia, nausea, depression. **Rare (less than
3%):** Myalgia, asthenia, back pain.

ADVERSE EFFECTS/TOXIC REACTIONS

Potential for ocular lens opacities. Hypersensitivity reaction, hepatitis, rhabdomyolysis occur rarely.

NURSING CONSIDERATIONS

BASELINE ASSESSMENT

Obtain lipid panel, LFT; pregnancy test in
females of reproductive potential. Obtain
dietary history, esp. fat consumption.

INTERVENTION/EVALUATION

Monitor serum cholesterol, HDL, LDL, triglycerides for therapeutic response. Lipid
levels should be monitored within 2–4 wks
of initiation of therapy or change in dosage.
Monitor LFT at 12 wks following initiation
of therapy, at any elevation of dose, and
periodically (e.g., semiannually) thereafter.
Monitor CPK if myopathy is suspected. Assess for headache, sore throat. Be alert for
myalgia, weakness.

PATIENT/FAMILY TEACHING

* Use appropriate contraceptive measures. * Periodic lab tests are essential part
of therapy. * Maintain appropriate diet (important part of treatment). * Report unexplained muscle pain, tenderness, weakness,
esp. if associated with fever, malaise.

rucaparib

roo-**kap**-a-rib
(Rubraca)
**Do not confuse rucaparib with
neratinib, niraparib, olaparib.**

◆ CLASSIFICATION

PHARMACOTHERAPEUTIC: Poly (ADP-
ribose) polymerase (PARP) inhibitor. **CLINICAL:** Antineoplastic.

USES

Ovarian cancer: Maintenance treatment
of adults with a deleterious BRCA mutation (germline and/or somatic)–associated recurrent epithelial ovarian, fallopian
tube, or primary peritoneal cancer who
are in a complete or partial response to
platinum-based chemotherapy. **Prostate
cancer:** Treatment of adults with a deleterious BRCA mutation (germline and/or
somatic)–associated metastatic castration-
resistant prostate cancer (mCRPC) who
have been treated with androgen receptor-
directed therapy and a taxane-based chemotherapy. **OFF-LABEL:** Pancreatic cancer
(locally advanced or metastatic).

PRECAUTIONS

Contraindications: Hypersensitivity to
rucaparib. **Cautions:** Baseline cytopenias, hepatic impairment.

ACTION

Inhibits poly (ADP-ribose) polymerase
(PARP) enzymes (involved in DNA transcription, cell-cycle regulation, and DNA
repair). By inhibiting PARP, may cause
PARP DNA complexes resulting in DNA
damage and cancer cellular death.
Therapeutic Effect: Inhibits tumor cell
growth and metastasis.

PHARMACOKINETICS

Widely distributed. Metabolized in liver.
Protein binding: 70%. Peak plasma concentration: 1.9 hrs. Excretion not specified. **Half-life:** 17–19 hrs.

⌛ LIFESPAN CONSIDERATIONS

Pregnancy/Lactation: Avoid pregnancy; may cause fetal harm. Females of reproductive potential should use effective contraception during treatment and for at least 6 mos after discontinuation. Unknown if distributed in breast milk. Breastfeeding not recommended during treatment and for at least 2 wks after discontinuation. **Children:** Safety and efficacy not established. **Elderly:** No age-related precautions noted.

INTERACTIONS

DRUG: May decrease effect of **BCG (intravesical).** May alter concentration/effect of **lansoprazole, omeprazole, repaglinide, tiZANidine, warfarin. HERBAL:** None significant. **FOOD:** None known. **LAB VALUES:** May increase serum ALT, AST, cholesterol, creatinine. May decrease ANC, Hgb, absolute lymphocyte count, platelets.

AVAILABILITY (Rx)

Tablets: 200 mg, 250 mg, 300 mg.

ADMINISTRATION/HANDLING

PO
• Give without regard to food. • If a dose is missed or vomiting occurs after administration, do not give extra dose. Administer next dose at regularly scheduled time.

INDICATIONS/ROUTES/DOSAGE

Note: Administer only to pts with deleterious germline and/or somatic BRCA mutation.

Ovarian Cancer
PO: ADULTS, ELDERLY: 600 mg twice daily about 12 hrs apart. Continue until disease progression or unacceptable toxicity.

Prostate Cancer
PO: ADULTS, ELDERLY: 600 mg twice daily. Continue until disease progression or unacceptable toxicity. Pts should also receive a gonadotropin-releasing hormone analog or have had bilateral orchiectomy.

Dose Reduction Schedule
Starting dose: 600 mg twice daily. **First dose reduction:** 500 mg twice daily. **Second dose reduction:** 400 mg twice daily. **Third dose reduction:** 300 mg twice daily.

Dose Modification
Adverse Events, Nonhematologic Toxicity
Either withhold treatment or reduce dosage per dose reduction schedule.

Hematologic Toxicity
Withhold treatment until improved to Grade 1 or 0 and investigate cause. If myelodysplastic syndrome or acute myeloid leukemia confirmed, permanently discontinue.

Dosage in Renal Impairment
Mild to moderate impairment: No dose adjustment. **Severe impairment, ESRD:** Not specified; use caution.

Dosage in Hepatic Impairment
Mild impairment: No dose adjustment. **Moderate to severe impairment:** Not specified; use caution.

SIDE EFFECTS

Frequent (77%–21%): Nausea, asthenia, fatigue, vomiting, constipation, dysgeusia, decreased appetite, diarrhea, abdominal pain, dyspnea. **Occasional (17%–9%):** Dizziness, rash, pyrexia, photosensitivity reaction, pruritus.

ADVERSE EFFECTS/TOXIC REACTIONS

Myelosuppression (anemia, lymphopenia, neutropenia, thrombocytopenia) is an expected response to therapy. Myelodysplastic syndrome/acute myeloid leukemia reported in less than 1% of pts. Infections including nasopharyngitis, pharyngitis, upper respiratory tract infection occurred in 43% of pts. Febrile neutropenia reported in less than 1% of pts. Palmar-plantar erythrodysesthesia syndrome (PPES), a chemotherapy-induced skin condition, that presents with redness, swelling, numbness, skin sloughing of the hands and feet, was reported in 2% of pts.

NURSING CONSIDERATIONS

BASELINE ASSESSMENT
Obtain CBC, vital signs, weight. Do not initiate therapy until hematologic toxicities have recovered from previous chemotherapy. Obtain pregnancy test in females of reproductive potential. Question plans of breastfeeding. Question history of hepatic/renal impairment, hypercholesterolemia. Screen for risk of bleeding, active infection. Offer emotional support.

INTERVENTION/EVALUATION
Monitor CBC monthly; creatinine periodically. For prolonged hematologic toxicities caused by other chemotherapies, monitor CBC wkly until recovery. If hematologic levels have not recovered to CTCAE Grade 1 or 0 after 4 wks, consider hematology consultation for further investigations including bone marrow analysis, blood sample for cytogenetics. Diligently monitor for infection (cough, fatigue, fever). Monitor for myelodysplastic syndrome, acute myeloid leukemia. Assess skin for rash, lesions, sloughing. Monitor for decreased urine output, renal dysfunction.

PATIENT/FAMILY TEACHING
• Treatment may depress your immune system response and reduce your ability to fight infection. Report symptoms of infection such as body aches, chills, cough, fatigue, fever. Avoid those with active infection. • Report bleeding or easy bruising, bloody urine or stool, frequent infections, fatigue, shortness of breath, weakness, weight loss; may indicate acute bone marrow depression or acute leukemia. • Use effective contraception to avoid pregnancy. Do not breastfeed. • Do not take herbal supplements. • Report planned surgical/dental procedures.

rufinamide
rue-**fin**-a-myde
(Banzel)

◆CLASSIFICATION
PHARMACOTHERAPEUTIC: Triazole derivative. **CLINICAL:** Anticonvulsant.

USES
Adjunctive therapy in treatment of seizures associated with Lennox-Gastaut syndrome in adults and children 1 yr and older.

PRECAUTIONS
Contraindications: Hypersensitivity to rufinamide. Familial short QT syndrome. **Cautions:** Concomitant use of QT interval-shortening drugs, depression, pts at high risk for suicide, mild to moderate hepatic impairment (not recommended in pts with severe hepatic impairment), concurrent use with hormonal contraceptives.

ACTION
Modulates activity of sodium channels. Prolongs inactive state of the sodium channel in cortical neurons, limits sustained repetitive firing of sodium-dependent action potential, inhibiting excitatory neurotransmitter release. **Therapeutic Effect:** Decreases frequency/severity of seizure activity.

PHARMACOKINETICS
Widely distributed. Protein binding: 34%. Extensively metabolized via hydrolysis. Excreted primarily in urine. **Half-life:** 6–10 hrs.

⧗ LIFESPAN CONSIDERATIONS
Pregnancy/Lactation: May produce fetal skeletal abnormalities. May be distributed in breast milk. **Children:** Safety and efficacy not established in pts younger than 4 yrs. **Elderly:** Age-related renal, hepatic, or cardiac impairment may require initiation of therapy at low end of dosing range.

R

INTERACTIONS

DRUG: May increase concentration/ effect of **Fosphenytoin, lacosamide, lamoTRIgine, PHENobarbital, phenytoin.** May decrease concentration/ effect of **carBAMazepine. Valproate, lamoTRIgine** may increase concentration/effect. **Alcohol, CNS depressants (e.g., LORazepam, morphine, zolpidem)** may increase CNS depressant effect. **HERBAL:** None significant. **FOOD:** None known. **LAB VALUES:** May decrease WBCs.

AVAILABILITY (Rx)

Oral Suspension: 40 mg/mL. **Tablets:** 200 mg, 400 mg.

ADMINISTRATION/HANDLING

PO
• Give with food. • Tablets should be given whole, split in half, or crushed. • Shake oral suspension well before each dose; use bottle adapter and dosing syringes provided.

INDICATIONS/ROUTES/DOSAGE

Lennox-Gastaut Seizures
Note: Discontinue therapy gradually to minimize potential of increased seizure frequency (e.g., decrease by 25% q2days).
PO: ADULTS, ELDERLY: Initially, 400–800 mg/day, given in 2 equally divided doses. Dose should be increased by 400–800 mg/day every 2 days. **Maximum:** 3,200 mg/day, administered in 2 equally divided doses. **CHILDREN 1 YR AND OLDER:** Treatment should be initiated at a daily dose of 10 mg/kg/day, given in 2 equally divided doses. Increase by 10-mg/kg increments every other day to a target dose of 45 mg/kg/day or 3,200 mg/day, whichever is less, administered in 2 equally divided doses.

Dosage in Renal Impairment
No dose adjustment.

Dosage in Hepatic Impairment
Mild to moderate impairment: Use caution. **Severe impairment:** Not recommended.

SIDE EFFECTS

Children: Frequent (27%–11%): Headache, dizziness, fatigue, nausea, drowsiness, diplopia. **Occasional (6%–4%):** Tremor, nystagmus, blurred vision, vomiting. **Rare (3%):** Ataxia, upper abdominal pain, anxiety, constipation, dyspepsia, back pain, gait disturbance, vertigo. **Adults: Frequent (17%–7%):** Lethargy, vomiting, headache, fatigue, dizziness, nausea. **Occasional (5%– 4%):** Influenza, nasopharyngitis, anorexia, rash, ataxia, diplopia. **Rare (3%):** Bronchitis, sinusitis, psychomotor hyperactivity, upper abdominal pain, aggression, ear infection, inattention, pruritus.

ADVERSE EFFECTS/TOXIC REACTIONS

Suicidal ideation or behavior occurs rarely, noted as early as 1 wk after initiation of therapy and persisting for at least 24 wks. Shortening of the QT interval (up to 20 msec), hypersensitivity reaction (rash, fever, urticaria) have been noted. Abrupt withdrawal may precipitate seizure, status epilepticus.

NURSING CONSIDERATIONS

BASELINE ASSESSMENT

Obtain ECG. Review history of seizure disorder (intensity, frequency, duration, level of consciousness). Initiate seizure precautions. Question history of suicidal ideation and behavior.

INTERVENTION/EVALUATION

Provide safety measures as needed. Observe frequently for recurrence of seizure activity. Assess for clinical improvement (decrease in intensity, frequency of seizures). Assist with ambulation if drowsiness, lethargy occur. Question for evidence of headache. Monitor for suicidal ideation and behavior.

PATIENT/FAMILY TEACHING

• Do not abruptly withdraw medication (may cause seizures). • Avoid tasks that require alertness, motor skills until response to drug is established. • Strict maintenance of drug therapy is essential

underlined – top prescribed drug

for seizure control. • Avoid alcohol. • Use effective nonhormonal contraception to avoid pregnancy. • Seek immediate medical attention if thoughts of suicide, new onset or worsening of anxiety, depression, or changes in mood occur.

ruxolitinib

rux-oh-**li**-ti-nib
(Jakafi)

◆ CLASSIFICATION

PHARMACOTHERAPEUTIC: Janus-associated tyrosine kinase inhibitor. **CLINICAL:** Antineoplastic.

USES

Myelofibrosis: Treatment of intermediate or high-risk myelofibrosis, including primary myelofibrosis, post–polycythemia vera myelofibrosis, post–essential thrombocythemia myelofibrosis in adults. **Polycythemia vera:** Treatment of polycythemia vera in adults with an inadequate response to or intolerant of hydroxyurea. **Graft-versus-host disease (GVHD):** Treatment of steroid-refractory acute graft-versus-host disease (GVHD) in adults and children 12 yrs and older. Treatment of chronic graft-versus-host disease after failure of one or two lines of systemic therapy in adults and children 12 yrs and older.

PRECAUTIONS

Contraindications: Hypersensitivity to ruxolitinib. **Cautions:** Conditions predisposing to infection (e.g., diabetes, renal failure, immunocompromised pts, open wounds), chronic opportunistic infections (e.g., herpesvirus infection, hepatitis B virus [HBV] infection, fungal infections), renal/hepatic impairment, concomitant use of strong CYP3A4 inhibitors, history of bradycardia, conduction disturbances, ischemic heart disease, HF.

ACTION

Inhibits Janus-associated kinases (JAKs) JAK1 and JAK2, which mediates the signaling of cytokines and growth factor important for hematopoiesis and immune function. In myelofibrosis and polycythemia vera JAK1/2 activity is dysregulated. **Therapeutic Effect:** Modulates the affected JAK1/2 activity.

PHARMACOKINETICS

Widely distributed. Protein binding: 97%. Metabolized in liver. Excreted in urine (74%), feces (22%). **Half-life:** 3–5 hrs.

⧗ LIFESPAN CONSIDERATIONS

Pregnancy/Lactation: Unknown if distributed in breast milk. Not recommended in nursing mothers. Must either discontinue drug or discontinue breastfeeding. **Children:** Safety and efficacy not established. **Elderly:** No age-related precautions noted.

INTERACTIONS

DRUG: Strong CYP3A4 inhibitors (e.g., clarithromycin, ketoconazole) may increase concentration/effect. May increase adverse effects; decrease therapeutic effect of **vaccines (live).** May decrease therapeutic effect of **BCG (intravesical). HERBAL:** Echinacea may decrease therapeutic effect. **FOOD: Grapefruit products** may increase concentration. **LAB VALUES:** May decrease platelets, RBC, Hgb, Hct, WBC. May increase serum bilirubin, ALT, AST, cholesterol.

AVAILABILITY (Rx)

Tablets: 5 mg, 10 mg, 15 mg, 20 mg, 25 mg.

ADMINISTRATION/HANDLING
PO
• Give without regard to food.

Feeding Tube
• Suspend tablet in 40 mL water and stir for 10 min. • May administer suspension within 6 hrs after tablet has dispersed. • Flush with 75 mL water after administration.

R

INDICATIONS/ROUTES/DOSAGE

Myelofibrosis

PO: ADULTS: 20 mg twice daily if platelets greater than 200,000 cells/mm^3, or 15 mg twice daily if platelets 100,000–200,000 cells/mm^3, or 5 mg twice daily if platelets 50,000 to less than 100,000 cells/mm^3. Dose reduction based on platelet response. **Maximum:** 25 mg twice daily.

Polycythemia Vera

PO: ADULTS, ELDERLY: Initially, 10 mg bid. Doses titrated based on safety/efficacy.

GVHD (Acute)

PO: ADULTS, ELDERLY, CHILDREN 12 YRS AND OLDER: Initially, 5 mg twice daily. May increase to 10 mg twice daily after at least 3 days (if ANC and platelets have not decreased by 50% or greater from baseline).

GVHD (Chronic)

PO: ADULTS, ELDERLY, CHILDREN 12 YRS AND OLDER: 10 mg twice daily.

Dosage in Renal Impairment
Myelofibrosis

CrCl 15–59 mL/min	Platelets 100,000–150,000/mm^3	10 mg twice daily
CrCl 15–59 mL/min	Platelets 50,000 to less than 100,000/mm^3	5 mg once daily
CrCl 15–59 mL/min	Platelets less than 50,000/mm^3	Avoid use
End-stage renal disease (ESRD) on dialysis	Platelets 100,000–200,000/mm^3	15 mg after dialysis on days of dialysis
ESRD on dialysis	Platelets more than 200,000/mm^3	20 mg after dialysis on days of dialysis
ESRD not requiring dialysis		Avoid use

Polycythemia
CrCl 5–59 mL/min and any platelet count: 5 mg twice daily.
GVHD
CrCl 5–59 mL/min and any platelet count: 5 mg once daily. **ESRD on dialysis:** 5 mg once after dialysis. **ESRD not on dialysis:** Avoid use.

Dosage in Hepatic Impairment
Myelofibrosis

Hepatic impairment	Platelets 100,000–150,000/mm^3	10 mg twice daily
Hepatic impairment	Platelets 50,000 to less than 100,000/mm^3	5 mg once daily
Hepatic impairment	Platelets less than 50,000/mm^3	Avoid use

Polycythemia
Mild to severe and any platelet count: 5 mg twice daily.
GVHD
Stage 3 or 4 liver GVHD and any platelet count: 5 mg once daily.

SIDE EFFECTS

Frequent (23%–14%): Bruising, dizziness, vertigo, labyrinthitis, headache. **Occasional (9%–7%):** Weight gain, flatulence.

ADVERSE EFFECTS/TOXIC REACTIONS

May cause severe thrombocytopenia (70% of pts), anemia (96% of pts), neutropenia (18% of pts), which may improve with reduced dose or by temporarily withholding regimen. Anemic pts may require blood transfusions. Increased risk of developing opportunistic bacterial, mycobacterial, fungal, viral infections including herpes zoster, urinary tract infection, urosepsis, renal infection, pyuria. Increased risk of bleeding disorders including ecchymosis, hematoma, injection site hematoma, periorbital hematoma, petechiae, purpura.

NURSING CONSIDERATIONS

BASELINE ASSESSMENT

Obtain CBC, serum chemistries, renal function, LFT, urinalysis, cholesterol level. Assess recent vaccinations status. Receive full medication history including herbal products. Question for possibility of pregnancy, renal/hepatic impairment, HIV.

INTERVENTION/EVALUATION

Monitor CBC (every 2–4 wks until doses stabilized), serum chemistries, renal function, LFT, cholesterol. Obtain urinalysis with reflex culture for suspected UTI. Routinely assess vital signs, I&O, breath sounds, gait. Monitor temperature; be alert for fever, infectious process. Avoid IM injections, rectal temperatures, other traumas that induce bleeding. Assess skin for petechiae, hematoma, purpura.

PATIENT/FAMILY TEACHING

• Report any new bruising/bleeding, bloody stools or urine, fever, chills, rash, painful urination, suspected infection, fatigue, shortness of breath. • Do not breastfeed. • Avoid grapefruit products. • Open skin lesions, blisters may signal herpes infection. • Blood work will be routinely monitored; if on dialysis, take only following dialysis.

sacituzumab govitecan-hziy

sak-i-**tooz**-ue-mab goe-vi-**tee**-kan (Trodelvy)

■ **BLACK BOX ALERT** ■ Severe neutropenia may occur. Withhold treatment for absolute neutrophil count (ANC) less than 1,500 cells/mm³ or febrile neutropenia. Initiate antimicrobial therapy in pts with febrile neutropenia. Consider granulocyte colony-stimulating factor prophylaxis. Severe diarrhea may occur. If not contraindicated, administer atropine for early diarrhea of any severity. For onset of late diarrhea, evaluate for infectious processes.

Do not confuse sacituzumab govitecan with fam-trastuzumab deruxtecan, sarilumab, secukinumab.

◆ CLASSIFICATION

PHARMACOTHERAPEUTIC: Anti-Trop-2, antibody drug conjugate, topoisomerase I inhibitor. Monoclonal antibody. **CLINICAL:** Antineoplastic.

USES

Breast cancer: Treatment of unresectable, locally advanced or metastatic triple-negative breast cancer (mTNBC) in pts who have received 2 or more prior systemic therapies, at least one of them for metastatic disease. Treatment of unresectable, locally advanced or metastatic hormone receptor (HR)-positive, human epidermal growth factor receptor 2 (HER2)-negative (IHC 0, IHC 1+ or IHC 2+/ISH−) breast cancer in pts who have received endocrine-based therapy and at least 2 additional systemic therapies in the metastatic setting. **Urothelial cancer:** Treatment of locally advanced or metastatic urothelial cancer in adults who have previously received platinum-containing chemotherapy and either programmed death receptor-1 or programmed death-ligand 1 inhibitor.

PRECAUTIONS

Contraindications: Hypersensitivity to sacituzumab govitecan-hziy. **Cautions:** Baseline hematologic cytopenias, hepatic impairment, dehydration; conditions predisposing to infection (e.g., diabetes, renal failure, immunocompromised pts, open wounds), chronic opportunistic infections (e.g., herpesvirus infection, fungal infections). Do not substitute with other drugs containing irinotecan or its active metabolites. Pts who are homozygous for the UGT1A1*28 allele are at increased risk for neutropenia.

ACTION

An antibody drug conjugate consisting of a humanized antitrophoblast cell-surface antigen 2 (Trop-2) monoclonal antibody coupled to the topoisomerase I inhibitor SN-38. Trop-2 is overexpressed and is associated with cancer cell growth. Binds to Trop-2 and is internalized; SN-38 is released in tumors. **Therapeutic Effect:** Causes DNA damage, apoptosis, and cell death.

PHARMACOKINETICS

Widely distributed. Metabolized by UGT1A1 enzymes. Excretion not specified. **Half-life:** 16 hrs; (SN-38): 18 hrs.

⧗ LIFESPAN CONSIDERATIONS

Pregnancy/Lactation: Avoid pregnancy; may cause fetal harm. Females of reproductive potential should use effective contraception during treatment and for at least 6 mos after discontinuation. Unknown if distributed in breast milk. Breastfeeding not recommended during treatment and for at least 1 mo after discontinuation. May impair fertility. **Males:** Males with female partners of reproductive potential should use effective contraception during treatment and for at least 3 mos after discontinuation. **Children/Elderly:** Safety and efficacy not established.

INTERACTIONS

DRUG: UGT1A1 inhibitors (e.g., ata-zanavir, ketoconazole) may increase adverse effects. UGT1A1 inducers (e.g., carBAMazepine, phenytoin, ritonavir) decrease concentration/

effect. May decrease therapeutic effect of **BCG (intravesical), vaccines (live)**. **Irinotecan, pimecrolimus, tacrolimus (topical)** may enhance the adverse/toxic effects. **HERBAL:** Echinacea may decrease therapeutic effect. **FOOD:** None known. **LAB VALUES:** May increase activated partial thromboplastin time (aPTT), serum alkaline phosphatase, AST, ALT, magnesium. May decrease serum albumin, calcium, magnesium, potassium, phosphate, sodium; Hgb, leukocytes, neutrophils, platelets, RBCs. May increase or decrease serum glucose. May diminish diagnostic effect of *Coccidioides immitis* skin test.

AVAILABILITY (Rx)

Injection, Powder for Reconstitution: 180 mg.

ADMINISTRATION/HANDLING

 IV

Premedication • Give antipyretic, H_1 and H_2 blocker, antiemetic (either two- or three-drug combination) prior to each infusion. May give a corticosteroid in pts with prior infusion reaction.

Reconstitution • Must be prepared by personnel trained in aseptic manipulations and admixing of cytotoxic drugs. • Calculate the number of vials needed for reconstitution based on weight in kg at the beginning of each treatment cycle (or more frequently if body weight has changed by more than 10%). • Allow vial to warm to room temperature. • Reconstitute each vial with 20 mL of 0.9% NaCl to a final concentration of 10 mg/mL. • Swirl vial gently for up to 15 min until powder is completely dissolved. Do not shake or agitate. • Visually inspect for particulate matter or discoloration. Solution should appear clear and yellow in color. Do not use if solution is cloudy, discolored, or if visible particles are observed. • Dilute in an infusion bag containing 0.9% NaCl to a final concentration of 1.1–3.4 mg/mL (do not exceed 500 mL). Infusion bag must be made of polypropylene to minimize foaming.

Infusion guidelines • Do not administer as IV push or bolus. • Flush IV line with 20 mL of 0.9% NaCl after infusion is complete.

Rate of administration • **First infusion:** Infuse over 3 hrs. • **Subsequent infusions:** Infuse over 1–2 hrs if previously tolerated. May slow or interrupt infusion if infusion reactions occur.

Storage • Refrigerate unused vials in original carton. • May refrigerate diluted solution for up to 4 hrs. After refrigeration, diluted solution must be infused within 4 hrs (includes infusion time). • Protect from light. • Do not shake, agitate, or freeze.

IV INCOMPATABILITIES

Do not mix or infuse with other solutions or medications.

INDICATIONS/ROUTES/DOSAGE

Note: Withhold dose on day 1 of any cycle for ANC less than 1,500/mm³; withhold on day 8 of any cycle for ANC less than 1,000/mm³.

Breast Cancer (Triple-Negative)
IV: ADULTS: 10 mg/kg on days 1 and 8 of 21-day cycle. Continue until disease progression or unacceptable toxicity. **Maximum:** 10 mg/kg/dose.

Breast Cancer (HR+ HER2–)
IV: ADULTS: 10 mg/kg on days 1 and 8 of a 21-day cycle. Continue until disease progression or unacceptable toxicity. **Maximum:** 10 mg/kg/dose.

Urothelial Cancer (Locally Advanced or Metastatic)
IV: ADULTS, ELDERLY: 10 mg/kg on days 1 and 8 of a 21-day treatment cycle. Continue until disease progression or unacceptable toxicity. **Maximum:** 10 mg/kg/dose.

Dose Modification
Based on Common Terminology Criteria for Adverse Events (CTCAE).
Note: Do not re-escalate if a dose reduction is made.

S

Neutropenia

Grade 3 febrile neutropenia; Grade 4 neutropenia for 7 days or greater; Grade 3 or 4 neutropenia that delays dosing by 2 or 3 wks for recovery to less than or equal to Grade 1: For first occurrence, reduce dose by 25% and give granulocyte colony-stimulating factor. For second occurrence, reduce dose by 50%. For third occurrence, permanently discontinue. **Grade 3 or 4 neutropenia that delays dosing beyond 3 wks for recovery to less than or equal to Grade 1:** Permanently discontinue.

Severe Non-neutropenic Toxicity

Grade 4 nonhematologic toxicity of any duration; any Grade 3 or 4 treatment-induced nausea, vomiting, diarrhea (not controlled by antiemetics/antidiarrheal agents); other Grade 3 or 4 nonhematologic toxicity lasting greater than 48 hrs (despite medical management); Grade 3 or 4 non-neutropenic toxicity that delays dosing by 2 or 3 wks for recovery to less than or equal to Grade 1: For first occurrence, reduce dose by 25%. For second occurrence, reduce dose by 50%. For third occurrence, permanently discontinue. **Grade 3 or 4 non-neutropenia hematologic toxicity that does not improve to less than or equal Grade 1 within 3 wks:** Permanently discontinue.

Dosage in Renal Impairment

Mild impairment: No dose adjustment. **Moderate to severe impairment:** Not specified; use caution.

Dosage in Hepatic Impairment

Not specified; use caution.

SIDE EFFECTS

Frequent (69%–21%): Nausea, diarrhea, fatigue, vomiting, alopecia, constipation, rash, skin irritation/exfoliation, decreased appetite, abdominal pain/distension, headache, back pain, cough, dizziness, dyspnea. **Occasional (19%–11%):** Edema, pruritus, arthralgia, dry skin, mucositis, stomatitis, esophagitis, mucosal inflammation, pyrexia, insomnia, dehydration, dysgeusia, extremity pain.

ADVERSE EFFECTS/TOXIC REACTIONS

Myelosuppression (anemia, leukopenia, neutropenia, thrombocytopenia) is an expected response to therapy, but more severe reactions including severe neutropenia, febrile neutropenia may be life-threatening. Pts with uridine diphosphate-glucuronosyl transferase 1A1 (UGT1A1)*28 allele are at an increased risk of neutropenia, other adverse reactions. Diarrhea occurred in 63% of pts. Grade 3 or 4 diarrhea reported in 9% of pts. Life-threatening hypersensitivity reactions, including anaphylaxis, may occur. Grade 3 or 4 nausea and vomiting was reported. Pleural effusion reported in 2% of pts. Infections including bronchitis, influenza, pneumonia, respiratory syncytial virus infection, upper respiratory tract infection, UTI, viral infection were reported. Neuropathies including hypoesthesia, gait disturbance, muscular weakness, paresthesia, peripheral motor/sensorimotor neuropathy reported in 24% of pts.

NURSING CONSIDERATIONS

BASELINE ASSESSMENT

Obtain ANC, CBC, LFT; pregnancy test in females of reproductive potential. Confirm compliance of effective contraception. Confirm triple-negative breast cancer status. Obtain weight in kilograms. Verify status of UGT1A1*28 allele. Question occurrence of infusion reactions prior to each dose. Question history of hepatic impairment. Screen for active infection. Assess usual bowel movement patterns, stool characteristics. Assess and correct hydration status prior to each dose. Receive full medication history and screen for interactions. Offer emotional support.

INTERVENTION/EVALUATION

Monitor ANC, CBC for myelosuppression. Monitor for severe neutropenia, febrile neutropenia (esp. in pts with reduced UGT1A1 activity); infections (cough, fatigue, fever). If serious infection occurs, initiate appropriate antimicrobial therapy. Monitor for hypersensitivity reactions, infusion reactions during infusion and for at least 30 min after completion. If infusion-related reaction occurs, interrupt infusion and manage symptoms. Permanently discontinue if life-threatening infusion reaction, hypersensitivity reaction occurs. Diarrhea must be treated promptly. If diarrhea occurs, evaluate for infectious processes. If negative for infectious processes, recommend loperamide (antidiarrheal agent) 4 mg initially, then 2 mg with every episode of diarrhea up to a maximum of 16 mg/day. Discontinue antidiarrheal agent 12 hrs after diarrhea subsides. May give atropine for subsequent treatments in pts who exhibit excessive cholinergic response (e.g., abdominal cramping, diarrhea, salivation). Adequate fluid and electrolyte resuscitation should be considered. Offer antiemetics if nausea or vomiting occurs. Monitor I&Os, hydration status. Monitor for neuropathies.

PATIENT/FAMILY TEACHING

• Treatment may depress your immune system response and reduce your ability to fight infection. Report symptoms of infection such as body aches, chills, cough, fatigue, fever. Avoid those with active infection. • Report symptoms of bone marrow depression (e.g., bruising, fatigue, fever, shortness of breath, weight loss; bleeding easily, bloody urine or stool). • Severe allergic reactions, including anaphylaxis, can occur. If allergic reaction occurs, seek immediate medical attention. • Severe diarrhea may cause dehydration, electrolyte imbalance. Drink plenty of fluids. Report diarrhea that does not improve with medical management. Maintain proper hydration and nutrition. • Use effective contraception to avoid pregnancy. Do not breastfeed. • Nausea and vomiting is a common side effect. • Report nervous system changes (gait disturbance, pain, numbness, trouble walking); UTI (fever, urinary frequency, burning during urination, foul-smelling urine). • Do not take newly prescribed medications unless approved by the prescriber who originally started treatment.

sacubitril-valsartan

sak-**ue**-bi-tril
(Entresto)

■ **BLACK BOX ALERT** ■ May cause fetal harm, mortality. Discontinue as soon as pregnancy detected.

◆CLASSIFICATION

PHARMACOTHERAPEUTIC: Combination of sacubitril, a neprilysin inhibitor, and valsartan, an angiotensin II receptor blocker. **CLINICAL:** Reduces risk of complications in HF.

USES

To reduce the risk of cardiovascular death and hospitalization in pts with chronic HF (NYHA class II-IV) and reduced ejection fraction (benefits most evident with left ventricular ejection fraction below normal). Treatment of symptomatic HF with systemic left ventricular systolic dysfunction in pediatric pts 1 yr and older (reduces NT-proBNP and improves cardiovascular outcomes).

PRECAUTIONS

Contraindications: Hypersensitivity to sacubitril or valsartan; history of angioedema related to angiotensin-converting enzyme (ACE) inhibitor or angiotensin receptor blockers (ARB); concomitant use or within 36 hrs of ACE inhibitors; concomitant use of aliskiren in pts with diabetes. **Cautions:** Baseline anemia,

S

dehydration, hypovolemia, sodium depletion; concomitant use of potassium-sparing diuretics or potassium supplements; hepatic/renal impairment; unstented bilateral/unilateral renal artery stenosis; significant aortic/mitral stenosis. Pts with orthostatic hypotension.

ACTION

Sacubitril inhibits neprilysin, increasing peptide levels that are degraded by neprilysin (e.g., natriuretic peptides). Valsartan directly antagonizes angiotensin II receptors; blocks vasoconstrictor, aldosterone secreting effects of angiotensin II, inhibiting binding of angiotensin II to AT_1 receptors. **Therapeutic Effect:** Decreases risk of mortality in pts with chronic HF; produces vasodilation; decreases peripheral resistance; decreases B/P.

PHARMACOKINETICS

Widely distributed. Sacubitril is converted by esterases; not significantly metabolized after conversion. Valsartan is minimally metabolized in liver. Protein binding (both): 94%–97%. Peak plasma concentration: sacubitril: 30 min; valsartan: 1.5 hrs. Steady-state concentration: 3 days. Excretion: sacubitril: urine (52%–68%), feces (37%–48%); valsartan: feces (86%), urine (13%). Half-life: sacubitril: 1.4 hrs; valsartan: 9.9 hrs.

⏳ LIFESPAN CONSIDERATIONS

Pregnancy/Lactation: Avoid pregnancy; may cause fetal harm/mortality. Unknown if distributed in breast milk. Breastfeeding not recommended. **Children, Elderly:** No age-related precautions noted.

INTERACTIONS

DRUG: ACE inhibitors (e.g., enalapril, ramipril) may increase risk of angioedema (contraindicated). Potassium-sparing diuretics (e.g., spironolactone) may increase risk of hyperkalemia. May increase concentration/effect of NSAIDs

(e.g., **ibuprofen, naproxen**) May increase concentration/effect of **lithium**. **HERBAL:** Herbals with hypertensive properties (e.g., licorice, yohimbe) or hypotensive properties (e.g., garlic, ginger, ginkgo biloba) may alter effects. **FOOD:** None known. **LAB VALUES:** May increase serum BUN, creatinine, potassium. May decrease Hct, Hgb.

AVAILABILITY (Rx)

Fixed-Dose Combination Tablets: *(Sacubitril/valsartan):* 24 mg/26 mg, 49 mg/51 mg, 97 mg/103 mg. **Combination Oral Pellets:** 6 mg/6 mg, 15 mg/16 mg.

ADMINISTRATION/HANDLING

PO

Tablet • Give without regard to food.
Oral pellets: • Capsules cannot be swallowed. Oral pellets cannot be chewed or crushed. **•** Open the capsule and sprinkle onto 1–2 tsp of soft food (give immediately).

INDICATIONS/ROUTES/DOSAGE

HF

Note: Allow a 36-hr washout period when switching from or to an ACE inhibitor.

PO: ADULTS, ELDERLY: Tablets: Initially, 49 mg/51 mg twice daily. After approx. 2 wks, double the dose as tolerated to a maintenance dose of 97 mg/103 mg twice daily. **ADOLESCENTS, CHILDREN WEIGHING 50 KG OR GREATER: (Tablets):** Initially, 49 mg/51 mg twice daily for 2 wks, then increase to 72 mg/78 mg twice daily for 2 wks, then to 97 mg/103 mg twice daily. **WEIGHING 40–49 KG:** Initially, 24 mg/26 mg twice daily for 2 wks, then increase to 49 mg/51 mg twice daily for 2 wks, then to 72 mg/78 mg twice daily. **WEIGHING 40 KG OR LESS:** Initially 1.6 mg/kg/dose twice daily for 2 wks, then increase to 2.3 mg/kg/dose twice daily for 2 wks, then to 3.1 mg/kg/dose twice daily.

ADOLESCENTS, CHILDREN WEIGHING 50 KG OR GREATER: (Oral Pellets): 34–49 KG: Initially, 30 mg/32 mg/dose twice daily for 2 wks, then increase to 45 mg/48 mg/dose twice daily for 2 wks, then to 60 mg/64 mg/dose twice daily. **26–33 KG:** Initially, 24 mg/24 mg/dose twice daily for 2 wks, then increase to 30 mg/32 mg/dose twice daily for 2 wks, then to 45 mg/48 mg/dose twice daily. **19–25 KG:** Initially, 18 mg/18 mg/dose twice daily for 2 wks, then increase to 24 mg/24 mg/dose twice daily for 2 wks, then to 30 mg/32 mg/dose twice daily. **13–18 KG:** Initially, 12 mg/12 mg/dose twice daily for 2 wks, then increase to 18 mg/18 mg/dose twice daily for 2 wks, then to 24 mg/24 mg/dose twice daily. **Less than 13 KG:** Initially, 1.6 mg/kg/dose twice daily for 2 wks, then to 2.3 mg/kg/dose twice daily for 2 wks, then to 3.1 mg/kg/dose twice daily.

Dosage in Renal Impairment

Mild to moderate impairment: No dose adjustment. **Severe impairment:** Initially, 24 mg/26 mg twice daily. **Maintenance:** May double each dose every 2–4 wks up to 97 mg/103 mg twice daily based on tolerability.

Dosage in Hepatic Impairment

Mild impairment: No dose adjustment. **Moderate impairment:** Initially, 24 mg/26 mg twice daily. **Maintenance:** May double each dose every 2–4 wks up to 97 mg/103 mg twice daily based on tolerability. **Severe impairment:** Treatment not recommended.

SIDE EFFECTS

Occasional (9%): Cough, dizziness.

ADVERSE EFFECTS/TOXIC REACTIONS

Angioedema (less than 1% of pts), hypotension (18% of pts), orthostatic hypotension (2% of pts), impairment/decrease in renal function due to inhibition of renin-angiotensin-aldosterone system (5% of pts), elevation of serum creatinine greater than 50% from baseline (1.4% of pts), renal impairment including oliguria, azotemia, acute renal failure (5% of pts), hyperkalemia (12% of pts), serum potassium elevation greater than 5.5 mEq/L (4% of pts) have occurred.

NURSING CONSIDERATIONS

BASELINE ASSESSMENT

Obtain BMP; CBC in pts with baseline anemia. Obtain B/P, heart rate immediately before each dose, in addition to regular monitoring (be alert for fluctuations). Assess hydration status. Correct hydration/sodium depletion prior to initiation. Receive medication history and screen for interactions, esp. concomitant use of aliskiren, ACE inhibitors, ARBs, potassium-sparing diuretics, potassium supplements. Verify negative pregnancy status. Question history of hepatic/renal impairment, renal artery stenosis; angioedema, hypersensitivity reaction.

INTERVENTION/EVALUATION

Monitor renal function, serum potassium. Monitor for hyperkalemia, hypotension. If hypotension occurs, consider interrupting treatment or altering dose of diuretic, antihypertensive drugs and screen for dehydration/serum sodium depletion. If pt positive for dehydration, be cautious with PO/IV administration. Overhydration may exacerbate HF. Assist with ambulation if dizziness occurs. Monitor for hypersensitivity reaction, including angioedema. If angioedema occurs, interrupt treatment and institute therapy to protect airway patency.

PATIENT/FAMILY TEACHING

• Be cautious of fluid intake. Overhydration may lead to worsening of HF, while underhydration may lead to low blood pressure. • Report urine changes such as darkened urine, decreased output. • Immediately report allergic reactions such as difficulty breathing, itching, rash, tongue swelling; symptoms of high potassium levels such as extreme fatigue, muscle weakness, palpitations; suspected pregnancy. • Do not breastfeed. • Diuretics (water pills) may increase risk of low pressure or low potassium levels.

S

salmeterol

sal-**met**-er-all
(Serevent Diskus)

■ **BLACK BOX ALERT** ■ Long-acting beta₂-adrenergic agonists may increase risk of asthma-related deaths and asthma-related hospitalizations in pediatric and adolescent pts. Use only as adjuvant therapy in pts who are currently receiving but not adequately controlled on long-term asthma control medication.

Do not confuse salmeterol with Solu-Medrol, or Serevent with Atrovent, Combivent, Serentil, or Sinemet.

FIXED-COMBINATION(S)

Advair Diskus: salmeterol/fluticasone (a corticosteroid): 50 mcg/100 mcg, 50 mcg/250 mcg, 50 mcg/500 mcg. **Advair HFA:** salmeterol/fluticasone (a corticosteroid): 21 mcg/45 mcg, 21 mcg/115 mcg, 21 mcg/230 mcg.

◆CLASSIFICATION

PHARMACOTHERAPEUTIC: Beta₂-adrenergic agonist (long-acting). **CLINICAL:** Bronchodilator.

USES

Exercise-induced bronchospasm: Prevention of exercise-induced bronchospasm in pts 4 yrs of age and older (use with an inhaled corticosteroid [ICS] in pts with persistent asthma). **Asthma/bronchospasm:** treatment of asthma and prevention of bronchospasm (as combined therapy with ICS) in pts with reversible obstructive airway disease, including those with symptoms of nocturnal asthma in pts 4 yrs of age and older. **Chronic obstructive pulmonary disease (COPD):** Maintenance treatment of bronchospasm associated with COPD (including emphysema and chronic bronchitis).

PRECAUTIONS

Contraindications: Hypersensitivity to salmeterol. Treatment of status asthmaticus, acute episodes of asthma or COPD. Use as monotherapy in treatment of asthma without concomitant long-term asthma control medication (e.g., inhaled corticosteroids). **Cautions:** Not for acute symptoms; may cause paradoxical bronchospasm, severe asthma. Cardiovascular disorders (coronary insufficiency, arrhythmias, hypertension), seizure disorders, diabetes, hyperthyroidism, hepatic impairment, hypokalemia.

ACTION

Stimulates beta₂-adrenergic receptors in lungs, resulting in relaxation of bronchial smooth muscle. **Therapeutic Effect:** Relieves bronchospasm, reducing airway resistance.

PHARMACOKINETICS

Route	Onset	Peak	Duration
Inhalation (asthma)	30–45 min	2–4 hrs	12 hrs
Inhalation (COPD)	2 hrs	3.25–4.75 hrs	12 hrs

Low systemic absorption; acts primarily in lungs. Protein binding: 95%. Metabolized in liver. Excreted in urine (25%), feces (60%). **Half-life:** 5.5 hrs.

⧖ LIFESPAN CONSIDERATIONS

Pregnancy/Lactation: Unknown if distributed in breast milk. **Children:** No age-related precautions in pts older than 4 yrs. **Elderly:** Lower dosages may be needed (may be more susceptible to tachycardia, tremors).

INTERACTIONS

DRUG: Beta blockers (e.g., **carvedilol, metoprolol**) may reduce effect; may produce bronchospasm. **Strong CYP3A4 inhibitors (e.g., clarithromycin, ketoconazole, ritonavir), MAOIs (e.g., phenelzine, selegiline), tricyclic antidepressants (e.g., amitriptyline, doxepin)** may increase concentration/effects (wait 14 days after stopping MAOIs, tricyclic antidepressants before starting salmeterol). **HERBAL:** None significant. **FOOD:** None known. **LAB VALUES:** May

S

decrease serum potassium. May increase serum glucose.

AVAILABILITY (Rx)

Aerosol Powder Breath Activated, Inhalation: 50 mcg/inhalation.

ADMINISTRATION/HANDLING

Inhalation
• Remove from sealed pouch immediately prior to first use. Before inhaling the dose, breathe out fully (do not exhale into Diskus device). Activate and use only in level horizontal position. • Inhale quickly and deeply through Diskus. • Hold breath as long as possible before exhaling slowly. • Do not use a spacer or wash mouthpiece.

INDICATIONS/ROUTES/DOSAGE

Maintenance and Prevention Therapy for Asthma, Bronchospasm
Inhalation: ADULTS, ELDERLY, CHILDREN 4 YRS AND OLDER: 1 inhalation (50 mcg) q12h (used in combination with inhaled corticosteroids not as monotherapy).

Prevention of Exercise-Induced Bronchospasm
Inhalation: ADULTS, ELDERLY, CHILDREN 4 YRS AND OLDER: 1 inhalation at least 30 min before exercise. Additional doses should not be given for 12 hrs. Do not administer if already giving salmeterol twice daily.

Maintenance Therapy for COPD
Inhalation: ADULTS, ELDERLY: 1 inhalation (50 mcg) q12h.

Dosage in Renal/Hepatic Impairment
No dose adjustment.

SIDE EFFECTS

Frequent (28%): Headache. **Occasional (7%–3%):** Cough, tremor, dizziness, vertigo, throat dryness/irritation, pharyngitis. **Rare (less than 3%):** Palpitations, tachycardia, nausea, heartburn, GI distress, diarrhea.

ADVERSE EFFECTS/TOXIC REACTIONS

May prolong QT interval (can precipitate ventricular arrhythmias). Hypokalemia, hyperglycemia may occur.

NURSING CONSIDERATIONS

BASELINE ASSESSMENT
Question history of cardiac disease, hepatic impairment, seizure disorder. Screen for concomitant medications known to prolong QT interval. Assess lung sounds, vital signs.

INTERVENTION/EVALUATION
Monitor rate, depth, rhythm, type of respiration; quality/rate of pulse, B/P. Assess lungs for wheezing, rales, rhonchi. Periodically evaluate serum potassium levels.

PATIENT/FAMILY TEACHING
• Not for relief of acute episodes. • Keep canister at room temperature (cold decreases effects). • Do not stop medication or exceed recommended dosage. • Report chest pain, dizziness. • Wait at least 1 full min before second inhalation. • Administer dose 30–60 min before exercise when used to prevent exercise-induced bronchospasm. • Avoid excessive use of caffeine derivatives (coffee, tea, colas, chocolate).

sargramostim

sar-**gra**-moe-stim
(Leukine)
Do not confuse Leukine with leucovorin or Leukeran.

◆CLASSIFICATION

PHARMACOTHERAPEUTIC: Colony-stimulating factor. **CLINICAL:** Hematopoietic agent.

USES

Acute myelogenous leukemia (AML: following induction chemotherapy): Shortens time to neutrophil recovery and reduces incidence of severe and life-threatening infections and infections resulting in death following induction chemotherapy in adults 55 yrs and older. **Bone marrow transplant (BMT) (allogeneic or**

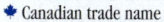 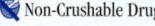

autologous): Treatment of delayed neutrophil recovery or graft failure after autologous or allogeneic BMT in adults and children 2 yrs and older. **Myeloid reconstitution:** Acceleration of myeloid reconstitution following autologous bone marrow or peripheral blood progenitor cell transplantation or following allogenic BMT in adults and children 2 yrs and older. **Peripheral stem cell transplant (allogeneic or autologous):** Mobilization of hematopoietic progenitor cells into peripheral blood for collection by leukapheresis and autologous transplantation in adults. **Hematopoietic radiation injury syndrome (acute):** Treatment to increase survival due to acute exposure to myelosuppressive radiation doses in adults and pts from birth to age 17 yrs. **OFF-LABEL:** Primary prophylaxis of neutropenia in pts receiving chemotherapy (outside transplant/AML) or at high risk for neutropenic fever. Neuroblastoma (refractory/relapsed).

PRECAUTIONS

Contraindications: Hypersensitivity to sargramostim. Concurrent (24 hrs preceding or following) myelosuppressive chemotherapy or radiation, pts with excessive leukemic myeloid blasts in bone marrow or peripheral blood (greater than 10%), known hypersensitivity to yeast-derived products. **Cautions:** Preexisting HF, fluid retention, cardiovascular disease, pulmonary disease (hypoxia, pulmonary infiltrates), renal/hepatic impairment.

ACTION

Stimulates proliferation/differentiation and functional activity of eosinophils, monocytes, neutrophils, and macrophages. **Therapeutic Effect:** Assists bone marrow in making new WBCs, increases their chemotactic, antifungal, antiparasitic activity. Increases cytoneoplastic cells, activates neutrophils to inhibit tumor cell growth.

PHARMACOKINETICS

Route	Onset	Peak	Duration
IV (increase WBCs)	7–14 days	N/A	1 wk

Detected in serum within 5 min after SQ administration. **Peak serum levels:** 1–3 hrs. **Half-life:** IV: 1 hr; SQ: 3 hrs.

⧖ LIFESPAN CONSIDERATIONS

Pregnancy/Lactation: Unknown if drug crosses placenta or is distributed in breast milk. **Children:** Safety and efficacy established in pediatric pts age 2 yrs and older for autologous peripheral blood progenitor cells and BMT, allogenic BMT, and treatment of delayed neutrophil recovery or graft failure. Safety and efficacy is also established in the setting of acute exposure to myelosuppressive doses of radiation among pediatric patients from birth to 17 yrs. **Elderly:** No age-related precautions noted.

INTERACTIONS

DRUG: May increase adverse effects of **tisagenlecleucel. Corticosteroids (e.g., dexA-METHasone, predniSONE)** may increase myeloproliferative effect. **HERBAL:** None significant. **FOOD:** None known. **LAB VALUES:** May increase serum ALT, AST, bilirubin, creatinine. May decrease serum albumin.

AVAILABILITY (Rx)

Injection, Powder for Reconstitution: 250 mcg.

ADMINISTRATION/HANDLING

SQ
• May be given without further dilution.

 IV

Reconstitution • Reconstitute with 1 mL Sterile Water for Injection (preservative free) or Bacteriostatic Water for Injection. Direct diluent to side of vial, gently swirl contents to avoid foaming; do not shake or agitate. • Dilute in 25–50 mL 0.9% NaCl to a concentration of 10 mcg/mL or greater. If final concentration less than 10 mcg/mL, 1 mg of human albumin per 1 mL of 0.9% NaCl should be added to provide a final albumin concentration of 0.1% (e.g., 1 mL 5% albumin per 50 mL 0.9% NaCl).

◄**ALERT**► Albumin is added before addition of sargramostim (prevents drug ad-

---

sorption to components of drug delivery system).

Rate of administration • Give each single dose over 30 min, 2 hr, 6 hr, or continuous infusion (indication specific).

Storage • Refrigerate powder, reconstituted solution, diluted solution for injection. • Do not shake. • Reconstituted solutions are clear, colorless. • Use within 6 hrs; discard unused portions. • Use 1 dose per vial; do not reenter vial.

INDICATIONS/ROUTES/DOSAGE

Neutrophil Recovery Following Chemotherapy in AML

IV: ADULTS 55 YRS OR OLDER: 250 mcg/m²/day (as 4-hr infusion) starting approximately 4 days following completion of induction chemotherapy (if day 10 bone marrow is hypoplastic with less than 5% blasts). Continue until ANC is greater than 1,500 cells/mm³ for 3 consecutive days or a maximum of 42 days. If WBC greater than 50,000 cells/mm³ and/or ANC greater that 20,000 cells/mm³, interrupt treatment or reduce dose by 50%.

Myeloid Recovery Following Bone Marrow Transplant (BMT), Myeloid Reconstitution After Autologous or Allogenic BMT

IV: ADULTS, ELDERLY, CHILDREN 2 YRS AND OLDER: Usual parenteral dosage: 250 mcg/m²/day (as 2-hr infusion). Begin 2–4 hrs after autologous bone marrow infusion and not less than 24 hrs after last dose of chemotherapy or last radiation treatment, when post marrow infusion ANC is less than 500 cells/mm³. Continue until ANC greater than 1,500 cells/mm³ for 3 consecutive days. If WBC greater than 50,000 cells/mm³ and/or ANC greater that 20,000 cells/mm³, interrupt treatment or reduce dose by 50%. Discontinue if blast cells appear or underlying disease progresses.

Bone Marrow Transplant Failure, Engraftment Delay

IV: ADULTS, ELDERLY, CHILDREN 2 YRS AND OLDER. 250 mcg/m²/day for 14 days. Infuse over 2 hrs. May repeat after 7 days off therapy if engraftment has not occurred. A third course with 500 mcg/m²/day for 14 days may be tried if engraftment still has not occurred.

Stem Cell Transplant, Mobilization

IV, SQ: ADULTS: 250 mcg/m²/day IV (as 24-hr infusion) or SQ once daily. Continue same dose throughout peripheral blood progenitor cell collection. If WBC greater than 50,000 cells/mm³, reduce dose by 50%.

Stem Cell Transplant, Posttransplant

IV, SQ: ADULTS, ELDERLY: 250 mcg/m²/day IV (as 24-hr infusion) or SQ once daily beginning immediately following infusion of progenitor cells. Continue until ANC greater than 1,500 cells/mm³ for 3 consecutive days.

Hematopoietic Radiation Injury Syndrome (Acute)

SQ: ADULTS, ELDERLY WEIGHING MORE THAN 40 KG: 7 mcg/kg once daily. Begin treatment as soon as possible after suspected or confirmed exposure to radiation doses greater than 2 Gy (gray). Do not delay if CBC not available. Continue until ANC remains greater than 1,000/cells mm³ for 3 consecutive CBCs (obtain q3days) or ANC exceeds 10,000/cells mm³ after radiation-induced nadir. **INFANTS, CHILDREN, ADOLESCENTS WEIGHING 40 KG OR GREATER:** (Weight-directed dosing): 7 mcg/kg once daily. **WEIGHING 15–39 KG:** 10 mcg/kg once daily. **WEIGHING LESS THAN 15 KG:** 12 mcg/kg once daily.

Dosage in Renal/Hepatic Impairment
No dose adjustment.

SIDE EFFECTS

Frequent: GI disturbances (nausea, diarrhea, vomiting, stomatitis, anorexia, abdominal pain), arthralgia or myalgia, headache, malaise, rash, pruritus. **Occasional:** Peripheral edema, weight gain, dyspnea, asthenia, fever, leukocytosis, capillary leak syndrome (fluid retention, irritation at local injection site, peripheral edema). **Rare:** Tachycardia, arrhythmias, thrombophlebitis.

S

ADVERSE EFFECTS/TOXIC REACTIONS

Pleural/pericardial effusion occurs rarely after infusion.

NURSING CONSIDERATIONS

BASELINE ASSESSMENT

Obtain CBC, BMP, LFT, vital signs. Question history of cardiac/pulmonary disease, renal/hepatic impairment.

INTERVENTION/EVALUATION

Monitor CBC with differential, serum renal/hepatic function, pulmonary function, vital signs, weight. Monitor for supraventricular arrhythmias during administration (particularly in pts with history of cardiac arrhythmias). Assess closely for dyspnea during and immediately following infusion (particularly in pts with history of lung disease). If dyspnea occurs during infusion, cut infusion rate by half. If dyspnea continues, stop infusion immediately. If neutrophil count exceeds 20,000 cells/mm³ or platelet count exceeds 500,000 cells/mm³, reduce dose by half, based on clinical condition of pt. Blood counts return to normal or baseline 3–7 days after discontinuation of therapy.

PATIENT/FAMILY TEACHING

• Report difficulty breathing, esp. during or immediately after infusion. • May increase risk of cardiac arrhythmias; report dizziness, fainting, palpitations. • Treatment may cause edema, fluid collection in the lungs or around the heart.

sarilumab

sar-**il**-ue-mab
(Kevzara)

■ **BLACK BOX ALERT** ■ Tuberculosis (TB), invasive fungal infections, other opportunistic infections leading to hospitalization and death were reported. Avoid use in pts with active infection. Withhold treatment until serious infection is controlled. Test for TB prior to and during treatment, regardless of initial result; if positive, start treatment for TB prior to initiation.
Do not confuse sarilumab with adalimumab, avelumab, belimumab, brodalumab, dupilumab, ipilimumab, nivolumab, or panitumumab.

◆CLASSIFICATION

PHARMACOTHERAPEUTIC: Interleukin-6 receptor antagonist. Monoclonal antibody. **CLINICAL:** Antirheumatic, disease modifying.

USES

Rheumatoid arthritis (RA): Treatment of adults with moderately to severely active rheumatoid arthritis who have had an inadequate response or intolerance to one or more DMARDs. May use as monotherapy or in combination with methotrexate (MTX) or other conventional DMARDs. **Polymyalgia rheumatica (PMR):** Treatment of adults with polymyalgia rheumatica (PMR) having an inadequate response to corticosteroids or cannot tolerate corticosteroid taper. **Polyarticular juvenile idiopathic arthritis (pJIA):** Treatment of pts weighing 63 kg or greater with active pJIA as monotherapy or in combination with conventional DMARDs. **OFF-LABEL:** COVID-19 infection (hospitalized) (alternative to tocilizumab).

PRECAUTIONS

Contraindications: Hypersensitivity to sarilumab. **Cautions:** Hyperlipidemia, hypertriglyceridemia, active hepatic disease or hepatic impairment; recent travel or residence in endemic TB or mycosis areas; history of chronic opportunistic infections (esp. bacterial, invasive fungal, mycobacterial, protozoal, viral, TB); conditions predisposing to infection (e.g., diabetes, immunocompromised pts, renal failure, open wounds); history of HIV, herpes zoster, hepatitis B virus (HBV) infection, malignancies; baseline neutropenia, thrombocytopenia; pts at risk for GI perforation (Crohn's disease, diverticulitis, GI tract malignancies, peptic ulcers, peritoneal malignancies). Not recommended in

S

pts with active infection, concomitant use of biological DMARDs; baseline ANC less than 2,000 cells/mm^3, platelet count less than 150,000 cells/mm^3, serum ALT, AST above 1.5 times upper limit of normal (ULN).

ACTION

Binds to interleukin-6 (IL-6) receptor, inhibiting signaling of IL-6, a cytokine involved in inflammatory and immune responses. **Therapeutic Effect:** Reduces inflammation of RA.

PHARMACOKINETICS

Widely distributed. Peak plasma concentration: 2–4 days. Excretion (200 mg dose): Linear, nonsaturable proteolytic pathway. (150 mg dose): Nonlinear, saturable target medicated pathway. **Half-life:** Concentration dependent: 200 mg q2wks (up to 10 days); 150 mg q2wks (up to 8 days).

⧗ LIFESPAN CONSIDERATIONS

Pregnancy/Lactation: Crosses the placental barrier, esp. during the third trimester. Unknown if distributed in breast milk; however, maternal immunoglobulin G (IgG) is present in breast milk. **Children:** Safety and efficacy not established. **Elderly:** Use caution (increased incidence of infections).

INTERACTIONS

DRUG: May decrease therapeutic effect of **BCG (intravesical), vaccines (live).** May increase adverse effects of **belimumab, natalizumab. HERBAL:** Echinacea may decrease therapeutic effect. **FOOD:** None known. **LAB VALUES:** May increase serum ALT, AST, cholesterol, LDL, HDL, triglycerides. May decrease leukocytes, neutrophils, platelets.

AVAILABILITY (Rx)

Injection Solution (Pen, Prefilled Syringe): 150 mg/1.14 mL, 200 mg/1.14 mL.

ADMINISTRATION/HANDLING

SQ

Preparation • Remove prefilled syringe from refrigerator and allow solution to warm to room temperature (approx. 30

min). • Visually inspect for particulate matter or discoloration. Solution should appear clear, colorless to slightly yellow in color. Do not use if solution is cloudy, discolored, or visible particles are observed.

Administration • Insert needle subcutaneously into upper arm, outer thigh, or abdomen and inject solution. • Do not inject into areas of active skin disease or injury such as sunburns, skin rashes, inflammation, skin infections, or active psoriasis. • Do not administer IV or intramuscularly. • Rotate injection sites. **Storage** • Refrigerate in original carton until time of use. • Protect from light. • May store at room temperature for up to 14 days. Once warmed to room temperature, do not place back into refrigerator. • Do not freeze or expose to heating sources. • Do not shake.

INDICATIONS/ROUTES/DOSAGE

Note: Do not initiate if ANC is less than 2,000 cells/mm^3; platelets less than 150,000 cells/mm^3; or serum ALT or AST greater than 1.5 times ULN.

Rheumatoid Arthritis

SQ: ADULTS, ELDERLY: 200 mg once q2wks (as monotherapy in combination with methotrexate).

PMR

SQ: ADULTS, ELDERLY: 200 mg q2wks (in combination with a tapering course of corticosteroids). May use as monotherapy following discontinuation of corticosteroids.

Dose Modification
Neutropenia
ANC greater than 1,000 cells/mm^3: No dose adjustment. **ANC 500–1,000 cells/mm^3:** Withhold treatment until ANC greater than 1000 cells/mm^3, then resume at 150 mg once q2wks. May increase to 200 mg once q2wks as clinically indicated. **ANC less than 500 cells/mm^3:** Permanently discontinue.

Hepatotoxicity
Serum ALT elevation up to 3 times ULN: Consider modifying dose of

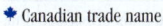 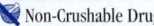
S

concomitant DMARDs. **Serum ALT elevation greater than 3–5 times ULN:** Withhold treatment until serum ALT less than 3 times ULN, then resume at 150 mg once q2wks. May increase to 200 mg once q2wks as clinically indicated. **Serum ALT elevation greater than 5 times ULN:** Permanently discontinue.

Serious Infection
Withhold treatment until serious infection is controlled, then resume as clinically indicated.

Thrombocytopenia
Platelet count 50,000–100,000 cells/mm³: Withhold treatment until platelet count greater than 100,000 cells/mm³, then resume at 150 mg once q2wks. May increase to 200 mg once q2wks as clinically indicated. **Platelet count less than 50,000 cells/mm³:** Permanently discontinue if confirmed by repeat testing.

Dosage in Renal Impairment
Mild to moderate impairment: No dose adjustment. **Severe impairment:** Not specified; use caution.

Dosage in Hepatic Impairment
Not specified; use caution.

SIDE EFFECTS

Rare (4%–2%): Injection site reactions (pain, erythema, pruritus).

ADVERSE EFFECTS/TOXIC REACTIONS

Serious, sometimes fatal, infections including aspergillosis, candidiasis, cellulitis, *Cryptococcus*, histoplasmosis, pneumonia, sepsis, tuberculosis; bacterial, mycobacterial, invasive fungal, opportunistic, viral infections were reported. Nasopharyngitis, upper respiratory tract infections, urinary tract infections occurred in 2–4% of pts. Neutropenia may increase risk of serious infection. GI perforation may occur, esp. in pts with history of diverticulitis or concomitant use of NSAIDs, corticosteroids. May increase risk for new malignancies. Hypersensitivity reactions including rash, urticaria reported in less than 1% of pts. May increase risk of HBV reactivation, which may result in fulminant hepatitis, hepatic failure, death.

NURSING CONSIDERATIONS

BASELINE ASSESSMENT
Obtain CBC, LFT, lipid panel. Assess onset, location, duration of pain, inflammation. Inspect appearance of affected joints for immobility, deformities. Pts should be evaluated for active tuberculosis and tested for latent infection prior to initiation and periodically during therapy. Induration of 5 mm or greater with tuberculin skin testing should be considered a positive test result when assessing if treatment for latent tuberculosis is necessary. Question history of chronic infections, opportunistic infections, herpes infection. Screen for active infection. Assess skin for open wounds. Question history of active hepatic disease, GI perforation, malignancies, HIV, HBV, hypersensitivity reactions. Receive full medication history and screen for interactions. Assess pt's willingness to self-inject medication.

INTERVENTION/EVALUATION
Assess for therapeutic response: relief of pain, stiffness, swelling; increased joint mobility; reduced joint tenderness; improved grip strength. Monitor neutrophil count, platelet count, LFT 4–6 wks after initiation, then q3mos thereafter. Monitor lipid panel 4–6 wks after initiation, then q6mos thereafter. Monitor for symptoms of tuberculosis, including those who tested negative for latent tuberculosis infection prior to initiating therapy. Interrupt or discontinue treatment if serious infection, opportunistic infection, or sepsis occurs and initiate appropriate antimicrobial therapy. Closely monitor for HBV reactivation.

PATIENT/FAMILY TEACHING
• Treatment may depress your immune system and reduce your ability to fight infection. Report symptoms of infection such as body aches, burning with urination, chills, cough, fatigue, fever. Avoid those with

S

active infection. • Do not receive live vaccines. • Expect frequent tuberculosis screening. Report travel plans to possible endemic areas. • A healthcare provider will show you how to properly prepare and inject medication. You must demonstrate correct preparation and injection techniques before using medication at home. • Report allergic reactions such as itching, hives, rash. • Immediately report severe or persistent abdominal pain, bloody stool, fever; may indicate rupture in GI tract. • Treatment may cause reactivation of HBV, new cancers. • Therapy may decrease platelet count, which may increase risk of bleeding. • Report liver problems such as bruising, confusion, amber or dark-colored urine; right upper abdominal pain; yellowing of the skin or eyes.

sAXagliptin

sax-a-**glip**-tin
(Onglyza)
Do not confuse sAXagliptin with SITagliptin or SUMAtriptan.

FIXED-COMBINATION(S)

Kombiglyze XR: sAXagliptin/met-FORMIN (an antidiabetic): 2.5 mg/1,000 mg, 5 mg/500 mg, 5 mg/1,000 mg.

◆ CLASSIFICATION

PHARMACOTHERAPEUTIC: DDP-4 inhibitor (gliptins). **CLINICAL:** Antidiabetic agent.

USES

Adjunctive treatment to diet and exercise to improve glycemic control in pts with type 2 diabetes as monotherapy or in combination with other antidiabetic agents.

PRECAUTIONS

Contraindications: Hypersensitivity to sAXagliptin. Type 1 diabetes, ketoacidosis. **Cautions:** Concurrent use of other glucose-lowering agents, moderate to severe renal impairment, end-stage renal disease requiring hemodialysis, concurrent use of strong CYP3A4 inhibitors (e.g., clarithromycin); history of pancreatitis.

ACTION

Slows the inactivation of incretin hormones by inhibiting DDP-4 enzyme. Incretin hormones increase insulin synthesis/release from pancreas and decrease glucagon secretion. **Therapeutic Effect:** Regulates glucose homeostasis.

PHARMACOKINETICS

Widely distributed. Metabolized in liver. Peak plasma concentration: 2 hrs. Excreted in urine (75%), feces (22%). **Half-life:** 2.5 hrs; metabolite, 3.1 hrs.

⌛ LIFESPAN CONSIDERATIONS

Pregnancy/Lactation: Unknown if distributed in breast milk. **Children:** Safety and efficacy not established. **Elderly:** Age-related renal impairment may require dosage adjustment.

INTERACTIONS

DRUG: May increase hypoglycemic effects of **insulin, sulfonylureas (e.g., glipiZIDE, glyBURIDE). Strong CYP3A4 inhibitors (e.g., clarithromycin, ketoconazole)** may increase concentration/effect. **Strong CYP3A4 inducers (e.g., carBAMazepine, phenytoin, rifAMPin)** may decrease concentration/effect. **HERBAL: Herbals with hypoglycemic properties (e.g., fenugreek)** may increase effect. **FOOD:** None significant. **LAB VALUES:** May slightly decrease WBCs, lymphocytes. May increase serum creatinine.

AVAILABILITY (Rx)

🐾 **Tablets:** 2.5 mg, 5 mg.

❖ Canadian trade name	🐾 Non-Crushable Drug	HIGH ALERT High Alert drug

ADMINISTRATION/HANDLING

PO
• May give without regard to food. • Administer whole. Do not break, crush, dissolve, or divide tablets.

INDICATIONS/ROUTES/DOSAGE

Type 2 Diabetes
PO: ADULTS, ELDERLY: 2.5 or 5 mg once daily. **Concurrent strong CYP3A4 inhibitors (e.g., ketoconazole):** 2.5 mg once daily. **Hemodialysis:** Give dose after dialysis.

Dosage in Renal Impairment
Mild impairment: No dose adjustment. **Moderate to severe impairment: CrCl less than 50 mL/min:** 2.5 mg once daily.

Dosage in Hepatic Impairment
No dose adjustment.

SIDE EFFECTS

Occasional (7%): Headache. **Rare (3%–1%):** Peripheral edema, sinusitis, abdominal pain, gastroenteritis, vomiting, rash.

ADVERSE EFFECTS/TOXIC REACTIONS

May cause HF, esp. in pts with cardiovascular disease. Concomitant use of hypoglycemic agents may increase risk of hypoglycemia. Pancreatitis reported in less than 1%. Hypersensitivity reactions including anaphylaxis, angioedema (tongue/lip swelling), exfoliative skin conditions. Other reactions include bullous pemphigoid, severe/disabling arthralgia. Infections including upper respiratory tract infection (8% of pts), UTI (7% of pts) may occur.

NURSING CONSIDERATIONS

BASELINE ASSESSMENT
Obtain blood glucose, hemoglobin A1c, renal function. Assess pt's understanding of diabetes management, routine home glucose monitoring. Receive full medication history and screen for interactions. Question history renal impairment, cardiovascular disease, pancreatitis.

INTERVENTION/EVALUATION
Monitor blood glucose, hemoglobin A1c level, renal function. Assess for hypoglycemia (diaphoresis, tremors, dizziness, anxiety, headache, tachycardia, perioral numbness, hunger, diplopia, difficulty concentrating), hyperglycemia (polyuria, polyphagia, polydipsia, nausea, vomiting, fatigue, Kussmaul breathing), hypersensitivity reactions. Concomitant use of beta blockers (e.g., carvedilol, metoprolol) may mask symptoms of hypoglycemia. Screen for glucose-altering conditions: Fever, increased activity or stress, surgical procedures. Obtain dietary consult for nutritional education. Severe abdominal pain, nausea may indicate pancreatitis.

PATIENT/FAMILY TEACHING
• Diabetes mellitus requires lifelong control. Diet and exercise are principal parts of treatment; do not skip or delay meals. Test blood sugar regularly. Monitor daily calorie intake. • When taking combination drug therapy or when glucose conditions are altered (excessive alcohol ingestion, insufficient carbohydrate intake, hormone deficiencies, critical illness), have a low blood sugar treatment available (e.g., glucagon, oral dextrose). • Persistent, severe abdominal pain that radiates to the back (with or without vomiting) may indicate acute pancreatitis. • Report joint pain; allergic reactions of any kind.

secukinumab

sek-ue-**kin**-ue-mab
(Cosentyx, Cosentyx Sensor Pen)
Do not confuse secuki-numab with canakinumab, ranibizumab, trastuzumab, ustekinumab

◆CLASSIFICATION

PHARMACOTHERAPEUTIC: Monoclonal antibody. Human interleukin-17A antagonist. **CLINICAL:** Antipsoriasis agent.

USES

Plaque psoriasis: Treatment of moderate to severe plaque psoriasis in pts 6 yrs of age and older and in adults who are candidates for systemic therapy or phototherapy. **Psoriatic arthritis (PsA):** Treatment of active PsA in pts 2 yrs of age and older. **Ankylosing spondylitis (AS):** Treatment of adults with active AS. **Nonradiographic axial spondyloarthritis (nr-axSpA):** Treatment of adults with active nr-axSpA with objective signs of inflammation. **Enthesitis-related arthritis (ERA):** Treatment of active ERA in pts 4 yrs of age and older. **Hidradenitis suppurativa (HS):** Treatment of adults with moderate to severe HS.

PRECAUTIONS

Contraindications: Hypersensitivity to secukinumab. **Cautions:** Elderly, active Crohn's disease, HIV infection, concomitant use of immunosuppressants; conditions predisposing to infections (e.g., diabetes, renal failure, immunocompromised pts, open wounds); hypersensitivity to latex (injector pen/prefilled syringe), preexisting or recent-onset CNS demyelinating disorders (e.g., multiple sclerosis, polyneuropathy); exposure to tuberculosis. Administration of live vaccines not recommended.

ACTION

Selectively binds to the interleukin-17A (IL-17A) cytokine, inhibiting its interaction with the IL-17 receptor. IL-17A is involved in inflammatory and immune responses. **Therapeutic Effect:** Inhibits release of proinflammatory cytokines.

PHARMACOKINETICS

Widely distributed. Degraded into small peptides and amino acids via catabolic pathway. Peak plasma concentration: 6 days. Steady state reached in 24 wks. Excretion not defined. **Half-life:** 22–31 days.

⧗ LIFESPAN CONSIDERATIONS

Pregnancy/Lactation: Unknown if distributed in breast milk. **Children:** Safety and efficacy not established in pts younger than 2 yrs. **Elderly:** No age-related precautions noted.

INTERACTIONS

DRUG: May increase concentration/effect of **baricitinib, BCG (intravesical), natalizumab. Belimumab, infliximab, vaccines (live)** may increase concentration/effect. **HERBAL: Echinacea** may decrease the therapeutic effect. **FOOD:** None known. **LAB VALUES:** None significant.

AVAILABILITY (Rx)

Injection for SQ Use: 300 mg/2 mL, 150 mg/mL solution, single-dose pen, single-dose prefilled syringe. 75 mg/0.5 mL solution, single-dose prefilled syringe. 150 mg, lyophilized powder in a single-dose vial for reconstitution. **Injector Pen:** 150 mg/mL solution. **Prefilled Syringe:** 150 mg/mL solution. **Injection for IV Use:** 125 mg/5 mL solution in a single-dose vial.

ADMINISTRATION/HANDLING

SQ

Reconstitution • Remove from refrigerator and allow vial to warm to room temperature for 15–30 min. • Inject 1 mL Sterile Water for Injection into vial. Do not shake or invert the vial. Allow vial to stand for approx. 10 min at room temperature to allow for dissolution.

Administration • Insert needle subcutaneously into upper arms, outer thigh, or abdomen and inject solution. • Do not inject into areas of active skin disease or injury such as sunburns, skin rashes, inflammation, skin infections, or active psoriasis. • Rotate injection sites.

Storage • Refrigerate until time of use. • Allow injector pen/prefilled syringe/vial or vial for reconstitution to warm to room temperature before use (15–30 min). • After reconstitution, use immediately or refrigerate for up to 24 hours. Do not freeze.

IV

Dilution • Before dilution, allow solution in vial(s) to sit for approx. 20 min at room temperature. • From infusion bag, withdraw a volume of 0.9% NaCl that

S

is equal to the calculated volume of solution required for dose. • Withdraw the calculated dose volume (mL) and add slowly into infusion bag. • Gently invert bag to mix. Do not shake.

Rate of Administration • Infuse over 30 min.

Storage • Refrigerate diluted solution for up to 24 hrs or store at room temperature for up to 4.5 hrs (includes start of the preparation to the completion of infusion.

INDICATIONS/ROUTES/DOSAGE

Note: IV dose only for adults with active nr-axSpA, AS, or PsA. **Loading dose:** 6 mg/kg given at Wk 0, followed by 1.75 mg/kg q4wks thereafter. **Without a loading dosage:** 1.75 mg/kg q4wks. **Maximum:** Maintenance dose 300 mg.

Ankylosing Spondylitis

SQ: ADULTS, ELDERLY (With a loading dose): 150 mg at wks 0, 1, 2, 3, and 4, then 150 mg q4wks. **May increase to 300 mg q4wks. (Without a loading dose):** 150 mg q4wks. May increase to 300 mg q4wks.

Axial Spondyloarthritis (Nonradiographic)

SQ: ADULTS, ELDERLY: (With a loading dose): 150 mg at wks 0, 1, 2, 3, and 4, then 150 mg q4wks. **(Without a loading dose):** 150 mg q4 wks. May increase to 300 mg q4wks.

Plaque Psoriasis

SQ: ADULTS, ELDERLY: 300 mg every wk for 5 doses, then 300 mg q4wks. (Some pts may only require 150 mg.) **CHILDREN 6 YRS AND OLDER WEIGHING 50 KG OR GREATER:** 150 mg once wkly at wks 0, 1, 2, 3, and 4, followed by 150 mg q4wks. **WEIGHING LESS THAN 50 KG:** 75 mg once wkly at wks 0, 1, 2, 3, and 4, then 75 mg q4wks.

Psoriatic Arthritis

Note: With coexistent plaque psoriasis, use dose for plaque psoriasis.
SQ: ADULTS, ELDERLY: (With a loading dose): 150 mg at weeks 0, 1, 2, 3, and 4, followed by 150 mg q4wks. May increase to 300 mg q4wks. **(Without a loading dose):** 150 mg q4wks. May increase to 300 mg q4wks. **CHILDREN 2 YRS AND OLDER WEIGHING 50 KG OR GREATER:** 150

mg once wkly at wks 0, 1, 2, 3, and 4, then 150 mg q4wks thereafter. **WEIGHING 15–49 KG:** 75 mg once wkly at wks 0, 1, 2, 3, and 4, then 75 mg q4wks thereafter.

Enthesitis-Related Arthritis

SQ: CHILDREN 4 YRS AND OLDER WEIGHING 50 KG OR GREATER: 150 mg once wkly at wks 0, 1, 2, 3, and 4, then 150 mg q4wks thereafter. **WEIGHING 15–49 KG:** 75 mg once wkly at wks 0, 1, 2, 3, and 4, then 75 mg q4wks thereafter.

Hidradenitis Suppurativa

SQ: ADULTS, ELDERLY: 300 mg at Wks 0, 1, 2, 3, and 4, then q4wks thereafter. If pt does not adequately respond, may increase to 300 mg q2wks.

Dosage in Renal/Hepatic Impairment

Not studied; use caution.

SIDE EFFECTS

Rare (4%–1%): Diarrhea, urticaria, rhinorrhea.

ADVERSE EFFECTS/TOXIC REACTIONS

May increase risk tuberculosis. Infections including nasopharyngitis (11% of pts), upper respiratory tract infection (2.5% of pts), mucocutaneous infection with *Candida* (1.2% of pts), rhinitis, pharyngitis, oral herpes (1% of pts) have occurred. May cause exacerbation of Crohn's disease. Hypersensitivity reactions including anaphylaxis were reported.

NURSING CONSIDERATIONS

BASELINE ASSESSMENT

Evaluate for active tuberculosis and test for latent infection prior to initiating treatment and periodically during therapy. Induration of 5 mm or greater with tuberculin skin testing should be considered a positive test result when assessing if treatment for latent tuberculosis is necessary. Antifungal therapy should be considered for those who reside or travel to regions where mycoses are endemic. Do not initiate therapy during active infection. Question history of active Crohn's disease, hepatitis B or C virus infection, HIV infection, demyelinating disorders, cardiovascular disease; concomitant use of immunosuppressive agents.

INTERVENTION/EVALUATION

Monitor skin for disease improvement. Monitor for symptoms of tuberculosis, including those who tested negative for latent tuberculosis infection prior to initiating therapy. Interrupt or discontinue treatment if serious infection, opportunistic infection, or sepsis occurs. Monitor for hypersensitivity reaction.

PATIENT/FAMILY TEACHING

• Treatment may depress your immune system response and reduce your ability to fight infection. Report symptoms of infection such as body aches, chills, cough, fatigue, fever. Avoid those with active infection. • Do not receive live vaccines. • Expect frequent tuberculosis screening. • Report travel plans to possible endemic areas. • Injector pen/prefilled syringe should not be used by pts with latex allergy. • Immediately report itching, hives, rash, swelling of the face or tongue; may indicate allergic reaction. • Treatment may cause worsening of Crohn's disease.

---

selegiline

se-**le**-ji-leen
(Emsam, Zelapar)

■ **BLACK BOX ALERT** ■ Antidepressants increase risk of suicidal thoughts and behavior in pediatrics and young adults. Monitor closely for changes in behavior, suicidal ideation. **Do not confuse Eldepryl with Elavil or enalapril, selegiline with Salagen, sertraline, or Stelazine, or Zelapar with Zaleplon, Zemplar, or ZyPREXA.**

◆CLASSIFICATION

PHARMACOTHERAPEUTIC: MAOI type B. **CLINICAL:** Antiparkinson agent, antidepressant.

USES

Oral: Adjunct to levodopa/carbidopa in treatment of Parkinson's disease. **Transdermal:** Treatment of major depressive disorder (MDD). **OFF-LABEL:** Treatment of early Parkinson's disease (monotherapy).

PRECAUTIONS

Contraindications: Hypersensitivity to selegiline. Concurrent use of meperidine. **Orally disintegrating tablet (additional):** Concomitant use or within 14 days of other MAOI, other drugs that are potent inhibitors of monoamine oxidase (e.g., linezolid), or opioids (e.g., meperidine, methadone, tramadol); concomitant use with cyclobenzaprine, dextromethorphan, or St. John's wort. **Transdermal (additional):** Pheochromocytoma; pts younger than 12 yrs of age; use of carBAMazepine, clomipramine, dextromethorphan, imipramine, meperidine, methadone, pentazocine, propoxyphene, serotonin reuptake inhibitors (SSRIs), tramadol (concomitantly or within 2 wks of selegiline discontinuation, or selegiline use within 4–5 half-lives [approximately 1 wk for most medications; 5 wks for fluoxetine] of discontinuation of contraindicated drug). **Cautions:** Renal/hepatic impairment, depression, elderly pts, major psychiatric disorder; pts at high risk of suicide; pts at high risk of hypotension (cerebrovascular disease, cardiovascular disease, hypovolemia).

ACTION

May increase dopaminergic activity by interfering with DOPamine reuptake at the synapse. **Therapeutic Effect:** Relieves signs/symptoms of Parkinson's disease (tremor, akinesia, posture/equilibrium disorders, rigidity). Improves mood with MDD.

PHARMACOKINETICS

Route	Onset	Peak	Duration
PO	1 hr	—	24–72 hrs

Widely distributed. Crosses blood-brain barrier. Protein binding: 90%. Metabolized in liver. Primarily excreted in urine. **Half-life: PO:** 10 hrs. **Transdermal:** 18–25 hrs.

⧖ LIFESPAN CONSIDERATIONS

Pregnancy/Lactation: Unknown if drug crosses placenta or is distributed in breast milk. **Children:** Safety and

S

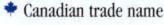 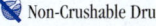

efficacy not established. **Elderly:** No age-related precautions noted.

INTERACTIONS

DRUG: Dextromethorphan, opioids (e.g., methadone, tramadol), SSRIs (e.g., escitalopram, sertraline), SNRIs (e.g., DULoxetine, venlafaxine) may increase serotonergic effect, increasing risk of serotonin syndrome; avoid use. **Alcohol** may increase adverse effects. **HERBAL: St. John's wort** may increase serotonergic effect. **Herbals with hypotensive properties (e.g., garlic, ginger, ginkgo biloba)** may increase hypotensive effect. **FOOD: Tyramine-rich foods** may produce hypertensive reactions. **LAB VALUES:** None significant.

AVAILABILITY (Rx)

Capsules: 5 mg. **Tablets:** 5 mg. **Tablets, Orally Disintegrating: (Zelapar):** 1.25 mg. **Transdermal: (Emsam):** 6 mg/24 hrs, 9 mg/24 hrs, 12 mg/24 hrs.

ADMINISTRATION/HANDLING
PO
• Give at breakfast and lunch. • Avoid tyramine-containing foods, large quantities of caffeine-containing beverages.

PO (Orally Disintegrating Tablets)
• Give in morning before breakfast and without liquid. • Peel off backing with dry hands (do not push tablets through foil). • Immediately place on top of tongue, allow to disintegrate. • Avoid food, liquids for 5 min before and after taking selegiline.

Transdermal
• Apply to dry, intact skin on upper torso or thigh, outer surface of upper arm. • Avoid exposure to external heat source. • Normal exposure to water unlikely to affect adhesion. • If patch becomes loose, press back into place. If patch falls off again, apply a new patch; follow same dose schedule. • Rotate application sites.

INDICATIONS/ROUTES/DOSAGE
Adjunctive Treatment of Parkinson's Disease
PO: ADULTS: (Capsule, Tablet): 5 mg at breakfast and lunch, given concomitantly with each dose of carbidopa and levodopa. **ELDERLY:** Initially, 5 mg in the morning. May increase up to 10 mg/day. **ADULTS, ELDERLY: (Orally Disintegrating Tablet):** Initially, 1.25 mg daily for at least 6 wks. May increase to maximum of 2.5 mg/day.

Major Depressive Disorder
Transdermal: ADULTS: Initially, 6 mg/24 hrs. May increase in 3 mg/24 hrs increments at minimum of 2 wks. **Maximum:** 12 mg/24 hrs. **ELDERLY: Maximum:** 6 mg/24 hrs.

Dosage in Renal/Hepatic Impairment
Orally disintegrating tablet: Not recommended in severe impairment. **Oral:** Use caution. **Transdermal:** No dose adjustment.

SIDE EFFECTS

Frequent (10%–4%): Nausea, dizziness, light-headedness, syncope, abdominal discomfort. **Occasional (3%–2%):** Confusion, hallucinations, dry mouth, vivid dreams, dyskinesia. **Rare (1%):** Headache, myalgia, anxiety, diarrhea, insomnia.

ADVERSE EFFECTS/TOXIC REACTIONS

Symptoms of overdose may vary from CNS depression (sedation, apnea, cardiovascular collapse, death) to severe paradoxical reactions (hallucinations, tremor, seizures). Impaired motor coordination, (loss of balance, blepharospasm, facial grimaces, feeling of heaviness in lower extremities), depression, nightmares, delusions, overstimulation, sleep disturbance, anger, hallucinations, confusion may occur.

NURSING CONSIDERATIONS

BASELINE ASSESSMENT
Receive full medication history and screen for contraindications/interactions. Question medical history as listed in Precautions. Assess current state of mental health.

INTERVENTION/EVALUATION
Be alert to neurologic effects (headache, lethargy, mental confusion, agitation). Moni-

tor for evidence of dyskinesia (difficulty with movement). Assess for clinical reversal of symptoms (improvement of tremors of head/hands at rest, mask-like facial expression, shuffling gait, muscular rigidity). Monitor for unusual behavior, worsening depression, suicidal ideation, especially at initiation of therapy or with changes in dosage.

PATIENT/FAMILY TEACHING

• Tolerance to dizziness, light-headedness develops during therapy. • Avoid tasks that require alertness, motor skills until response to drug is established. • Dry mouth, drowsiness, dizziness may be an expected response to drug. • Avoid alcohol. • Report worsening depression, unusual behavior, thoughts of suicide. • Avoid tyramine-rich foods. • Do not take newly prescribed medications unless approved by prescriber who originally started treatment. • Do not take herbal supplements.

selinexor

sel-i-nex-or
(Xpovio)
Do not confuse selinexor with Effexor or selegiline. Xpovio with Xeloda, Xgeva, Xtandi.

◆CLASSIFICATION

PHARMACOTHERAPEUTIC: Nuclear export inhibitor. **CLINICAL:** Antineoplastic.

USES

Multiple myeloma: Treatment of adults with relapsed or refractory multiple myeloma (in combination with dexAMETHasone) who have received at least four prior therapies and whose disease is refractory to at least two proteasome inhibitors, at least two immunomodulatory agents, and an anti-CD38 monoclonal antibody. Treatment of multiple myeloma (in combination with bortezomib and dexAMETHasone) in adults who have received at least 1 prior therapy. **Diffuse** large B-cell lymphoma: Treatment of adults with relapsed or refractory diffuse large B-cell lymphoma (DLBCL), not otherwise specified, including DLBCL arising from follicular lymphoma, after at least two lines of systemic therapy.

PRECAUTIONS

Contraindications: Hypersensitivity to selinexor. **Cautions:** Baseline cytopenias, hepatic impairment, optic disorders, uncorrected hyponatremia, fall risk, elderly, conditions predisposing to infection (e.g., diabetes, renal failure, immunocompromised pts, open wounds), chronic opportunistic infections (e.g., herpesvirus infection, fungal infections), pts at risk for bleeding (e.g., history of intracranial/GI/GU bleeding, coagulation disorders, recent trauma, concomitant use of anticoagulants, NSAIDs, antiplatelets).

ACTION

Reversibly inhibits nuclear export of tumor suppressor proteins, growth regulators, messenger RNA of oncogenic proteins by blocking protein exportin 1 (XPO1), leading to blockage of exportin 1. **Therapeutic Effect:** Reduces oncogenic proteins, causes cell cycle arrest and cancer cell apoptosis.

PHARMACOKINETICS

Widely distributed. Metabolized in liver. Protein binding: 95%. Peak plasma concentration: 4 hrs. Excretion not specified. **Half-life:** 6–8 hrs.

⧗ LIFESPAN CONSIDERATIONS

Pregnancy/Lactation: Avoid pregnancy; may cause fetal harm. Females and males with female partners of reproductive potential must use effective contraception during treatment and for at least 1 wk after discontinuation. Unknown if distributed in breast milk. Breastfeeding not recommended during treatment and for at least 1 wk after discontinuation. May impair fertility in females. **Children:** Safety and efficacy not established. **Elderly:** May have increased risk of serious or fatal adverse reactions.

S

INTERACTIONS

DRUG: May decrease therapeutic effect of **BCG (intravesical), vaccines (live).** Pimecrolimus, tacrolimus (topical) may enhance the adverse/toxic effects. May increase adverse effects of **natalizumab. HERBAL:** Echinacea may decrease therapeutic effect. **FOOD:** None known. **LAB VALUES:** May increase serum ALT, AST, bilirubin, creatine kinase, glucose, creatinine. May decrease serum albumin, calcium, sodium, magnesium, phosphate; absolute neutrophil count (ANC), Hgb, Hct, leukocytes, lymphocytes, neutrophils, platelets, RBCs. May increase or decrease serum potassium.

AVAILABILITY (Rx)

Tablets: 20 mg, 40 mg, 50 mg, 60 mg.

ADMINISTRATION/HANDLING

PO
• Give without regard to food. • Administer tablets whole with water; do not break, crush, or divide. Tablets cannot be chewed. • If a dose is missed or vomiting occurs after administration, give next dose at regularly scheduled time (do not give additional dose).

INDICATIONS/ROUTES/DOSAGE

Multiple Myeloma (Relapsed or Refractory)
PO: ADULTS: (Pts who have received at least 4 prior therapies): 80 mg on days 1 and 3 of each wk (in combination with dexAMETHasone. Continue until disease progression or unacceptable toxicity. (Pts who have received at least 1 prior therapy): 100 mg once wkly on day 1 of each wk (in combination with bortezomib and dexAMETHasone). Continue until disease progression or unacceptable toxicity.

DLBCL (Relapsed or Refractory)
PO: ADULTS: 60 mg on days 1 and 3 of each wk. Continue until disease progression or unacceptable toxicity.

Dose Reduction Schedule
Multiple myeloma: FIRST DOSE REDUCTION: 100 mg once wkly. **SECOND DOSE REDUCTION:** 80 once wkly. **THIRD DOSE REDUCTION:** 60 mg once wkly. **UNABLE TO TOLERATE 60-mg DOSE:** Permanently discontinue. **DLBCL: FIRST DOSE REDUCTION:** 40 mg on day 1 and 3 each of wk (80 mg total). **SECOND DOSE REDUCTION:** 60 once wkly. **THIRD DOSE REDUCTION:** 40 mg once wkly. **UNABLE TO TOLERATE 40-mg DOSE:** Permanently discontinue.

Dose Modification
Based on Common Terminology Criteria for Adverse Events (CTCAE).
Anemia
Multiple myeloma/DLBCL: HGB LESS THAN 8 mg/dL: Reduce one dose level. **Life-threatening anemia:** Withhold treatment until Hgb improves to 8 g/dL, then resume at reduced dose level.

Neutropenia
Multiple myeloma: ANC 500–1,000 cells/mm³ WITHOUT FEVER: Reduce one dose level. **ANC LESS THAN 500 cells/mm³ OR FEBRILE NEUTROPENIA:** Withhold treatment until ANC improves to 1,000 cells/mm³, then resume at reduced dose level. **DLBCL: ANC 500–1,000 cells/mm³ WITHOUT FEVER:** For first occurrence, withhold treatment until ANC improves to 1,000 cells/mm³, then resume at same dose. If recurs, reduce one dose level. **ANC LESS THAN 500 cells mm³ OR FEBRILE NEUTROPENIA:** Withhold treatment until ANC improves to 1,000 cells/mm³, then resume at reduced dose level.

Thrombocytopenia
Multiple myeloma: PLATELET COUNT 25,000–74,999 cells/mm³: Reduce one dose level. **PLATELET COUNT 25,000–74,999 cells/mm³ WITH BLEEDING:** Withhold treatment until bleeding resolves, then resume at reduced dose level. **PLATELET COUNT LESS THAN 25,000 cells/mm³:** Withhold treatment until platelet count improves to 50,000/mm³, then resume at one reduced dose level. **DLBCL: PLATELET COUNT 50,000–74,999 cells/mm³:** Interrupt one dose, then resume at same dose. **PLATELET COUNT 25,000–49,999 cells/mm³ WITHOUT BLEEDING:** For first occurrence, withhold treatment until platelet count improves

to greater than or equal to 50,000 cells/mm³, then resume at reduced dose level. **PLATELET COUNT 25,000–49,999 cells/mm³ *WITH* BLEEDING:** Withhold treatment until bleeding resolves and platelet count improves to 50,000 cells/mm³, then resume at reduced dose level. **PLATELET COUNT LESS THAN 25,000 cells/mm³:** Withhold treatment until platelet count improves to 50,000 cells/mm³, then resume at reduced dose level.

Diarrhea
Grade 2 diarrhea: For first occurrence, maintain dose. If recurs, reduce one dose level. **Grade 3 or 4 diarrhea:** Withhold treatment until improved to Grade 2 or less, then resume at reduced dose level.

Fatigue
Grade 2 fatigue (lasting longer than 7 days); Grade 3 fatigue: Withhold treatment until improved to Grade 1 or baseline, then resume at reduced dose level.

Hyponatremia
Serum sodium level 130 mmol/L or less: Withhold treatment until improved to greater than 130 mmol/L, then resume at reduced dose level.

Nausea/Vomiting
Grade 1 or 2 nausea/vomiting: Maintain dose. **Grade 3 nausea; Grade 3 or 4 vomiting:** Withhold treatment until improved to Grade 2 or less, then resume at one reduced dose level.

Ocular Toxicity
Grade 2 ocular toxicity (excluding cataract): Withhold treatment until improved to Grade 1 or baseline, then resume at one reduced dose level. **Grade 3 or 4 ocular toxicity:** Permanently discontinue. **Grade 2 (or higher) cataract:** Reduce one dose level.

Weight Loss/Anorexia
Weight loss of 10% to less than 20%; anorexia associated with significant weight loss or malnutrition: Withhold treatment until improved to more than 90% of baseline weight, then resume at one reduced dose level.

Other Nonhematologic Toxicity
Any other Grade 3 or 4 toxicity: Withhold treatment until improved to Grade 2 or lower, then resume at one reduced dose level.

Dosage in Renal Impairment
Mild to severe impairment: No dose adjustment. **ESRD, dialysis:** Not specified; use caution.

Dosage in Hepatic Impairment
Mild impairment: No dose adjustment. **Moderate to severe impairment:** Not specified; use caution.

SIDE EFFECTS

Note: Frequency and occurrence of side effects may vary based on indicated treatment. **Frequent (73%–24%):** Fatigue, asthenia, nausea, decreased appetite, decreased weight, diarrhea, vomiting, constipation, dyspnea. **Occasional (17%–10%):** Edema, cough, pyrexia, musculoskeletal pain, dizziness, insomnia, dehydration, dysgeusia, ageusia, vision blurred, reduced visual acuity, hypotension. headache, abdominal pain, peripheral neuropathy.

ADVERSE EFFECTS/TOXIC REACTIONS

Note: Frequency and occurrence of adverse reactions may vary based on indicated treatment.
Myelosuppression (anemia, leukopenia, lymphopenia, neutropenia, thrombocytopenia) is an expected response to therapy, but more severe reactions including febrile neutropenia, hemorrhagic thrombocytopenia may occur. Hemorrhagic events (corneal bleeding epistaxis, GI/rectal bleeding, hematoma, hematuria, subdural hematoma) reported in 10% of pts. GI toxicities (anorexia, diarrhea, nausea, vomiting, weight loss) reported in 80% of pts. Life-threatening hyponatremia reported in 39%–62% of pts. Serious and fatal infections (adenovirus, bronchitis, bronchiolitis, herpesvirus infection, pharyngitis, nasopharyngitis, parainfluenza,

S

pneumonia, respiratory syncytial virus infection, rhinitis, rhinovirus, sepsis, UTI) were reported. Life-threatening neurologic toxicities (amnesia, decreased level of consciousness, confusion, delirium, hallucinations) reported in 30% of pts. Falls reported in 8% of pts. Cardiac failure, cataracts reported in 3% of pts.

NURSING CONSIDERATIONS

BASELINE ASSESSMENT

Obtain ANC, CBC, BMP, body weight; pregnancy test in females of reproductive potential. Confirm compliance of effective contraception. Administer prophylactic antiemetic prior to each dose. Question history of hepatic impairment, herpesvirus infection, chronic opportunistic infections, optic disorders. Assess nutritional/hydration status. Obtain dietary consultation. Assess risk for bleeding. Screen for active infection. Initiate fall precautions. Assess usual bowel movement patterns, stool characteristics. Offer emotional support.

INTERVENTION/EVALUATION

Monitor ANC, CBC, BMP, body weight frequently during the first 3 mos of treatment, then as indicated. Diligently monitor for infections (cough, fever, fatigue), esp. respiratory tract infections, herpesvirus infection, sepsis. If serious infection or sepsis occurs, initiate appropriate antimicrobial therapy. Assess for symptoms of hyponatremia (coma, confusion, headache, lethargy, nausea, seizures, vomiting). Administer RBC transfusion per clinical guidelines if anemia occurs. Administer platelet transfusion per clinical guidelines if bleeding occurs in pts with thrombocytopenia. Consider growth colony-stimulating factor in pts with neutropenia. Withhold treatment 24 hrs before and 72 hrs after cataract surgery. Assess proper hydration/nutritional intake, I&Os. Offer antiemetics if nausea/vomiting occurs; antidiarrheal agent if diarrhea occurs. Monitor daily pattern of bowel activity, stool consistency. Monitor for neurologic toxicities (confusion, hallucinations, lethargy). Assess for visual changes at each office visit. If change

of vision occurs, consider referral to ophthalmologist. Monitor for GI/genitourinary bleeding, bloody stool; symptoms of intracranial bleeding (aphasia, blindness, confusion, facial droop, hemiplegia, seizures).

PATIENT/FAMILY TEACHING

• Treatment may depress your immune system and reduce your ability to fight infection. Report symptoms of infection such as body aches, burning with urination, chills, cough, fatigue, fever. Avoid those with active infection. • Report symptoms of bone marrow depression (e.g., bruising, fatigue, fever, shortness of breath, weight loss; bleeding easily, bloody urine or stool). • Report liver problems (abdominal pain, bruising, clay-colored stool, dark or amber-colored urine, yellowing of the skin or eyes), nervous system changes (confusion, delirium, difficulty speaking, dizziness, hallucinations, pain, paralysis, numbness), change of vision, fatigue, weight loss, bleeding of any kind. • Diarrhea, nausea, vomiting are common side effects that may cause dehydration, electrolyte imbalance, malnutrition. Drink plenty of fluids. Maintain proper caloric and nutritional intake. • Use effective contraception to avoid pregnancy. Do not breastfeed. • Avoid tasks that require alertness, motor skills until response to drug is established.

---

selpercatinib

sel-per-**ka**-tih-nib
(Retevmo)
Do not confuse selpercatinib with selinexor, selumetinib, or tucatinib.

◆CLASSIFICATION

PHARMACOTHERAPEUTIC: RET kinase inhibitor, tyrosine kinase inhibitor. **CLINICAL:** Antineoplastic.

USES

Non–small-cell lung cancer (NSCLC): Treatment of adults with locally advanced or metastatic NSCLC with a rearranged during transfection (RET) gene fusion. **Medullary thyroid cancer (MTC):** Treatment of adults and pts 2 yrs and older with advanced or metastatic MTC with a RET mutation. **Thyroid cancer:** Treatment of adults and pts 2 yrs and older with advanced or metastatic thyroid cancer with a RET gene fusion who require systemic therapy and who are radioactive iodine refractory (if radioactive iodine is appropriate). **Solid tumors:** Treatment of adults and pts 2 yrs and older with locally advanced or metastatic solid tumors with a RET gene fusion that has progressed on or following prior systemic treatment or have no alternative treatment options.

PRECAUTIONS

Contraindications: Hypersensitivity to selpercatinib. **Cautions:** Baseline cytopenias, hepatic impairment, hypertension, conditions predisposing to infection (e.g., diabetes, immunocompromised pts, renal failure, open wounds); pts at risk for QTc interval prolongation, cardiac arrhythmias (congenital long QT syndrome, HF, QT interval–prolonging medications, hypokalemia, hypomagnesemia); pts at risk for bleeding (e.g., history of intracranial/GI/GU bleeding, coagulation disorders, recent trauma, concomitant use of anticoagulants, NSAIDs, antiplatelets). Do not initiate in pts with uncontrolled hypertension.

ACTION

Inhibits wild-type RET, multiple mutated RET fusion proteins, vascular endothelial growth factor (VEGFR) 1 and VEGFR3 receptors, and fibroblast growth factor receptor (FGFR). Mutations in RET can result in activated RET fusion proteins, which can act as oncogenic drivers, promoting tumor cell line proliferation. **Therapeutic Effect:** Exhibits antitumor activity in cells with activation of RET proteins.

PHARMACOKINETICS

Widely distributed. Metabolized in liver. Protein binding: 97%. Peak plasma concentration: 2 hrs. Excreted in feces (69%), urine (24%). **Half-life:** 32 hrs.

⧗ LIFESPAN CONSIDERATIONS

Pregnancy/Lactation: Avoid pregnancy; may cause fetal harm. Females and males with female partners of reproductive potential must use effective contraception during treatment and for at least 1 wk after discontinuation. Unknown if distributed in breast milk. Breastfeeding not recommended during treatment and for at least 1 wk after discontinuation. May impair fertility in both females and males. **Children:** Safety and efficacy not established in pts younger than 2 yrs. **Elderly:** No age-related precautions noted.

INTERACTIONS

DRUG: Strong CYP3A4 inhibitors (e.g., **clarithromycin, ketoconazole, ritonavir), moderate CYP3A4 inhibitors (e.g., dilTIAZem, fluconazole, verapamil)** may increase concentration/effect. **Strong CYP3A4 inducers (e.g., carBAMazepine, phenytoin, rifAMPin), moderate CYP3A4 inducers (e.g., bosentan, nafcillin)** may decrease concentration/effect. **Histamine-2 receptor antagonists (e.g., famotidine); antacids containing magnesium, calcium, aluminum, bicarbonate; proton pump inhibitors (e.g., omeprazole, pantoprazole)** may reduce concentration/effect. **QT interval–prolonging medications (e.g., amiodarone, azithromycin, entrectinib, haloperidol, methadone, quetiapine, ribociclib)** may increase risk of QTc interval prolongation, cardiac arrhythmias. **HERBAL:** None significant. **FOOD:** None known. **LAB VALUES:** May increase serum alkaline phosphatase, ALT, AST, bilirubin, cholesterol (total), potassium. May decrease serum albumin, calcium, creatinine, magnesium, sodium; leukocytes, platelets. May increase or decrease serum glucose.

AVAILABILITY (Rx)

Capsules: 40 mg, 80 mg.

S

ADMINISTRATION/HANDLING

PO

• If concomitant use of proton pump inhibitor (e.g., pantoprazole) is unavoidable, give selpercatinib with food; otherwise, may give without regard to food. • Give 2 hrs before or 10 hrs after histamine-2 receptor antagonist (e.g., famotidine). • Give 2 hrs before or 2 hrs after locally acting antacid (e.g., magnesium-, calcium-, aluminum-, bicarbonate-containing antacids). • Administer capsules whole; do not break, cut, or open. • Capsules cannot be chewed. • Do not give a missed dose within 6 hrs of next dose. • If vomiting occurs after administration, give next dose at regularly scheduled time (do not give additional dose).

INDICATIONS/ROUTES/DOSAGE

NSCLC (Metastatic RET Fusion-Positive), MTC (Advanced or Metastatic RET-Mutant), Thyroid Cancer (Advanced, Metastatic RET Fusion-Positive), Solid Tumors (Advanced, Metastatic RET Fusion-Positive)

PO: ADULTS, CHILDREN 12 YRS AND OLDER: LESS THAN 50 KG: 120 mg twice daily. **50 KG OR GREATER:** 160 mg twice daily. Continue until disease progression or unacceptable toxicity. **CHILDREN 2 YRS TO LESS THAN 12 YRS:** $(1.53 \text{ m}^2 \text{ or greater})$: 160 mg twice daily. $(1.09–1.52 \text{ m}^2)$: 120 mg twice daily. $(0.66–1.08 \text{ m}^2)$: 80 mg twice daily. $(0.33–0.65 \text{ m}^2)$: 40 mg 3 times/day.

Dose Reduction Schedule

Dose Reduction for Adverse Reactions	Weighing less than 50 kg	Weighing 50 kg or greater
First reduction	80 mg twice daily	120 mg twice daily
Second reduction	40 mg twice daily	80 mg twice daily
Third reduction	40 mg once daily	40 mg twice daily

Permanently discontinue in pts unable to tolerate 3 dose reductions.

Dose Modification

Based on Common Terminology Criteria for Adverse Events (CTCAE).

Hepatotoxicity

Grade 3 or 4 hepatotoxicity: Withhold treatment and monitor serum ALT/AST wkly until improved to Grade 1 or baseline, then resume at a reduced dose by 2 dose levels. Continue to monitor serum ALT/AST wkly until 4 wks after reaching the dose prior to Grade 3 or 4 hepatotoxicity, then increase dose by 1 dose level (after at least 2 wks without recurrence), then increase to dose taken prior to Grade 3 or 4 hepatotoxicity (after at least 4 wks without recurrence).

Hemorrhagic Events

Grade 3 or 4 hemorrhage: Withhold treatment until improved to Grade 1 or 0. **Severe or life-threatening hemorrhage:** Permanently discontinue

Hypersensitivity Reactions

Any grade hypersensitivity reaction: Withhold treatment until resolved with corticosteroids, then resume at a reduced dose by 3 dose levels (while continuing corticosteroids). May increase dose by 1 dose level each wk until reaching the dose prior to hypersensitivity reaction, then taper corticosteroids.

Hypertension

Grade 3 hypertension (despite optimal hypertensive therapy): Withhold treatment until adequately controlled, then resume at reduced dose level. **Grade 4 hypertension:** Permanently discontinue.

QT Interval Prolongation

Grade 3 QT interval prolongation: Withhold treatment until improved to Grade 1 or 0 (or baseline), then resume at reduced dose level. **Grade 4 QT interval prolongation:** Permanently discontinue.

Other Toxicities

Any Grade 3 or 4 toxicities: Withhold treatment until improved to Grade 1 or 0, then resume at reduced dose level.

Concomitant Use of Strong CYP3A4 Inhibitor

Weighing 50 KG or Greater: Reduce dose to 80 mg twice daily. **Weighing Less Than 50 KG:** Reduce dose to 40 mg twice daily.

Concomitant Use of Moderate CYP3A4 Inhibitor
Weighing 50 KG or Greater: Reduce dose to 120 mg twice daily. **Weighing Less Than 50 KG:** Reduce dose to 80 mg twice daily.

Dosage in Renal Impairment
Mild to moderate impairment: No dose adjustment. **Severe impairment:** Not specified; use caution.

Dosage in Hepatic Impairment
Mild to moderate impairment: No dose adjustment. **Severe impairment:** Reduce dose to 80 mg twice daily.

SIDE EFFECTS
Frequent (39%–23%): Dry mouth, diarrhea, hypertension, fatigue, asthenia, malaise, edema (eye, eyelid, face, localized, lymph, peripheral, scrotal), rash, constipation, nausea, headache, abdominal pain. **Occasional (18%–16%):** Cough, dyspnea, vomiting.

ADVERSE EFFECTS/TOXIC REACTIONS
Leukopenia, thrombocytopenia are expected responses to therapy. Serious hepatotoxicity reported in 3% of pts. Serum ALT/AST elevation reported in 45% and 51% of pts, respectively. Grade 3 hypertension (17% of pts), Grade 4 hypertension (less than 1% of pts) has occurred. Concentration-dependent QT interval prolongation may occur, increasing risk of cardiac arrhythmias. Life-threatening hemorrhagic events (intraabdominal, GI, facial, genitourinary, intracranial, pulmonary, rectal, vaginal hemorrhage), ecchymosis, epistaxis, hematoma, hemoptysis, tracheal site hemorrhage may occur. Symptoms of hypersensitivity reactions including arthralgia, fever, myalgia, rash may occur with concurrent thrombocytopenia, transaminitis. May cause impaired wound healing.

NURSING CONSIDERATIONS

BASELINE ASSESSMENT
Obtain CBC, serum electrolytes, LFT, TSH, ECG, B/P; pregnancy test in females of reproductive potential. Confirm compliance of effective contraception. Verify presence of a RET gene fusion (NSCLC, thyroid cancer) or specific RET gene mutation (MTC) in tumor specimens or plasma. Withhold treatment at least 7 days prior to elective surgery. Do not administer for at least 2 wks after major surgery. Assess skin for open wounds, surgical incisions. Question history of hypertension, hepatic impairment, recent surgery. Assess risk for bleeding. Screen for active infection. Receive full medication history and screen for interactions.

INTERVENTION/EVALUATION
Monitor CBC, serum electrolytes, LFT, TSH, ECG periodically; LFT q2wks for the first 3 mos, then monthly thereafter (or wkly in pts with hepatotoxicity); B/P after 1 wk, then at least monthly thereafter. Manage hypersensitivity reactions with corticosteroids therapy. Assess for toxicities if concomitant use of CYP3A4 inhibitor is unavoidable. If concomitant use QT interval–prolonging medications is unavoidable, monitor ECG for QT interval prolongation, cardiac arrhythmias. Assess wounds/incisions for adequate healing following any surgery. Monitor daily pattern of bowel activity, stool consistency, I&Os. Monitor for bleeding of any kind; symptoms of intracranial bleeding (aphasia, blindness, confusion, facial droop, hemiplegia, seizures).

PATIENT/FAMILY TEACHING
• Treatment may depress your immune system and reduce your ability to fight infection. Report symptoms of infection such as body aches, burning with urination, chills, cough, fatigue, fever. Avoid those with active infection. • Report liver problems (abdominal pain, bruising, clay-colored stool, dark or amber-colored urine, yellowing of the skin or eyes), allergic reactions (rash, fever, muscle or joint pain), hemorrhagic stroke (confusion, difficulty speaking, one-sided weakness or paralysis, loss of vision), bleeding of any kind. • Use effective contraception to avoid pregnancy. Do not breastfeed. • Treatment may cause or worsen high blood pressure. • There is a high risk of interactions with

S

 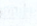

other medications. Do not take newly pre-scribed medications unless approved by prescriber who originally started treatment. Do not ingest grapefruit products or herbal supplements. Avoid use of acid-reducing medications. • Treatment may affect the electrical conduction of the heart, which may lead to arrhythmias; report chest pain, dizziness, fainting, palpitations. • Notify physician before any planned surgeries/dental procedures.

semaglutide

sem-a-**gloo**-tide
(Ozempic, Rybelsus, Wegovy)

■ **BLACK BOX ALERT** ■ Thyroid C-cell tumors have occurred in rodent studies with glucagon-like peptide-1 (GLP-1) receptor agonists; unknown if relevant in humans. Contraindicated in pts with a personal/family history of medullary thyroid carcinoma or in pts with multiple endocrine neoplasia syndrome type 2.
Do not confuse semaglutide with albiglutide, dulaglutide, liraglutide, or teduglutide.

◆**CLASSIFICATION**

PHARMACOTHERAPEUTIC: Glucagon-like peptide-1 (GLP-1) receptor agonist. **CLINICAL:** Antidiabetic.

USES

Ozempic, Rybelsus: Adjunct to diet and exercise to improve glycemic control in adults with type 2 diabetes mellitus. **Ozempic:** Risk reduction of major cardiovascular (CV) events in adults with type 2 diabetes mellitus and established cardiovascular disease. **Wegovy:** In combination with a reduced calorie diet and increased physical activity to reduce the risk of major adverse cardiovascular events (death, nonfatal myocardial infarction, or nonfatal stroke) in adults with established cardiovascular disease and either obesity or overweight. To reduce excess body weight and maintain weight reduction long term in adults and children 12 yrs and older with obesity and adults with overweight in the presence of at least one weight-related comorbid condition.

PRECAUTIONS

Contraindications: Hypersensitivity to sema-glutide. Personal/family history of medullary thyroid carcinoma (MTC). Pts with multiple endocrine neoplasia syndrome type 2 (MEN2). **Cautions:** Mild to moderate gastroparesis, renal impairment. History of pancreatitis. Not recommended in pts with severe GI disease, diabetic ketoacidosis, type 1 diabetes mellitus, or pancreatitis, or for use as first-line treatment regimen.

ACTION

Agonist of human glucagon-like peptide-1 (GLP-1). Increases glucose-dependent insulin secretion. Decreases inappropriate glucagon secretion. Slows gastric emptying. **Therapeutic Effect:** Augments glucose-dependent insulin secretion.

PHARMACOKINETICS

Widely distributed. Metabolized by proteolytic enzymes via protein degradation into small peptides, amino acids. Protein binding: greater than 99%. Peak plasma concentration: 1–3 days. Steady state reached in 4–5 wks. Excreted in urine (3% unchanged), feces. **Half-life:** 7 days.

⧖ LIFESPAN CONSIDERATIONS

Pregnancy/Lactation: Unknown if distributed in breast milk. Due to extended clearance period, recommend discontinuation of therapy at least 2 mos before planned pregnancy. **Children:** Safety and efficacy not established in pts younger than 12 yrs. **Elderly:** No age-related precautions noted.

INTERACTIONS

DRUG: May increase hypoglycemic effect of **insulins, sulfonylureas (e.g., glipiZIDE, glyBURIDE).** **HERBAL:** Herbals with **hypoglycemic properties (e.g., fenugreek, maitake)** may increase effect.

FOOD: None known. **LAB VALUES:** Expected to decrease serum glucose, Hgb A1c. May increase serum amylase, lipase.

AVAILABILITY (Rx)

Injection: *(Ozempic):* (Pen) 2 mg/3 mL (0.68 mg/mL) delivers 0.25 mg or 0.5 mg per injection; 2 mg/1.5 mL (1.34 mg/mL) delivers 0.25 mg or 0.5 mg per injection; 4 mg/3 mL (1.34 mg/mL) delivers 1 mg per injection; 8 mg/3 mL (2.68 mg/mL) delivers 2 mg per injection. *(Wegovy):* Single-dose pen delivers 0.25 mg, 0.5 mg, 1 mg, 1.7 mg, or 2.4 mg. **Tablets:** *(Rybelsus):* 3 mg, 7 mg, 14 mg.

ADMINISTRATION/HANDLING

PO

• Administer on an empty stomach, at least 30 min before the first food intake, beverage, or other oral medications of the day. • Take with 4 oz of plain water only. Eat 30–60 min after dose (may increase absorption). • Administer whole; do not break, cut, or crush. Tablets cannot be chewed.

SQ

Guidelines • Administer any time of the day, without regard to food, on the same day of each wk. May change administration day if the time between two doses is at least 2 days. • If dose is missed, administer within 5 days of missed dose. If more than 5 days pass after missed dose, wait until next regularly scheduled dose. **Preparation** • Visually inspect for particulate matter or discoloration. Solution should appear clear, colorless, and free of particles. Do not use if solution is cloudy, discolored, or visible particles are observed. **Administration** • Insert needle subcutaneously into abdomen, outer thigh, or upper arm, and inject solution. • Do not inject into areas of active skin disease or injury such as sunburns, skin rashes, inflammation, skin infections, or active psoriasis. • Do not administer IV or intramuscular. • Rotate injection sites. **Storage** • Refrigerate unused injector pens. • Once used, may refrigerate or store at room temperature for up to 56 days for Ozempic, 28 days for Wegovy. • Do not freeze. • Protect from sunlight.

INDICATIONS/ROUTES/DOSAGE

Type 2 Diabetes Mellitus, Risk Reduction of Major CV Events in Pts With Type 2 Diabetes Mellitus

Note: The lower initial dose (0.25 mg wkly) is intended to reduce GI symptoms. **SQ: ADULTS, ELDERLY:** Initially, 0.25 mg once wkly for 4 wks, then increase to 0.5 mg once wkly for at least 4 wks. If glycemic control is inadequate, increase to 1 mg wkly. May further increase dose to a maximum of 2 mg once wkly after at least 4 wks on the 1-mg dose. **PO: ADULTS, ELDERLY:** Initially, 3 mg once daily for 30 days, then increase to 7 mg once daily for at least 30 days. May further increase to 14 mg once daily. **Note:** The 3-mg dose is intended only for therapy initiation.

Weight Management (Chronic), Cardiovascular Risk Reduction

SQ: ADULTS, CHILDREN 12 YRS AND OLDER: Wks 1–4: 0.25 mg once wkly. **Wks 5–8:** 0.5 mg once wkly. **Wks 9–12:** 1 mg once wkly. **Wks 13–16:** 1.7 mg once wkly. **Wk 17 and thereafter (maintenance dose):** 2.4 mg once wkly. May decrease dose to 1.7 mg once wkly for up to 4 additional wks, then increase to 2.4 mg once wkly.

Dosage in Renal/Hepatic Impairment

Mild to severe impairment: No dose adjustment.

SIDE EFFECTS

Occasional (15%–5%): Nausea, vomiting, diarrhea, abdominal pain, constipation. **Rare (less than 1%):** Injection site reactions (pain, erythema), fatigue, dysgeusia, dizziness.

ADVERSE EFFECTS/TOXIC REACTIONS

May increase risk of acute renal failure or worsening of chronic renal impairment (esp. with dehydration), severe gastroparesis, pancreatitis, thyroid C-cell tumors. Hypersensitivity reactions including

S

✦ Canadian trade name   Non-Crushable Drug   HIGH ALERT High Alert drug anaphylaxis, angioedema were reported. May increase risk of hypoglycemia when used with other hypoglycemic agents, insulin. Diabetic retinopathy complications reported in 1% of pts. Worsening of diabetic retinopathy has been associated with rapid improvement of glucose control. Cholelithiasis reported in 2% of pts.

NURSING CONSIDERATIONS

BASELINE ASSESSMENT

Obtain glucose level, Hgb A1c. Obtain BUN, serum creatinine, eGFR, CrCl in pts with renal impairment. Question history of medullary thyroid carcinoma, multiple endocrine neoplasia syndrome type 2, hypersensitivity reaction, pancreatitis. Screen for use of other hypoglycemic agents, insulin. Assess pt's understanding of diabetes management, routine home glucose monitoring. Assess hydration status. Obtain dietary consult for nutritional education. Assess pt's willingness to self-inject medication.

INTERVENTION/EVALUATION

Monitor capillary blood glucose levels, Hgb A1c; renal function in pts with renal impairment reporting severe GI symptoms such as diarrhea, gastroparesis, vomiting. Monitor for hypersensitivity reaction. Screen for thyroid tumors (dysphagia, dyspnea, persistent hoarseness, neck mass). If tumor is suspected, consider endocrinologist consultation. Assess for hypoglycemia (anxiety, confusion, diaphoresis, diplopia, dizziness, headache, hunger, perioral numbness, tachycardia, tremors), hyperglycemia (confusion, fatigue, Kussmaul breathing, nausea, polyuria, vomiting). Screen for glucose-altering conditions: fever, stress, surgical procedures, trauma. Monitor for pancreatitis (severe, steady abdominal pain often radiating to the back [with or without vomiting]). Encourage fluid intake. Monitor I&Os.

PATIENT/FAMILY TEACHING

• A healthcare provider will show you how to properly prepare and inject medication. You must demonstrate correct preparation and injection techniques before using medication at home. • Diabetes mellitus requires lifelong control. Diet and exercise are principal parts of treatment; do not skip or delay meals. • Test blood sugar regularly. • Monitor daily calorie intake. • When taking additional medications to lower blood sugar or when glucose demands are altered (excessive alcohol ingestion, insufficient carbohydrate intake, hormone deficiencies, critical illness), have low blood sugar treatment available (glucagon, oral dextrose). • Therapy may increase risk of thyroid cancer; report lumps or swelling of the neck, hoarseness, shortness of breath, trouble swallowing. • Persistent, severe abdominal pain that radiates to the back (with or without vomiting) may indicate acute pancreatitis. • Report allergic reactions of any kind, esp. difficulty breathing, itching, rash, swelling of the face or throat. • Kidney injury or kidney failure may occur; report decreased urine output, amber-colored urine, flank pain.

sertraline

ser-tra-leen
(Zoloft)

■ **BLACK BOX ALERT** ■ Increased risk of suicidal ideation and behavior in children, adolescents, young adults 18–24 yrs with major depressive disorder, other psychiatric disorders.

Do not confuse sertraline with cetirizine, selegiline, Serentil, or Serevent, or Zoloft with Zocor.

◆CLASSIFICATION

PHARMACOTHERAPEUTIC: Selective serotonin reuptake inhibitor. **CLINICAL:** Antidepressant, anxiolytic, obsessive-compulsive disorder adjunct.

USES

Major depressive disorder (MDD) (unipolar): Treatment of MDD in adults. **Obsessive-compulsive disorder (OCD):** Treatment of OCD in adults and children 6 yrs and older. **Panic disorder:** Treatment of panic disorder with or without agoraphobia in adults. **Posttraumatic stress disorder (PTSD):** Treatment of PTDS in adults. **Premenstrual dysphoric disorder (PMDD):** Treatment of PMDD in adults. **Social anxiety disorder (SAD):** Treatment of SAD (social phobia) in adults. **OFF-LABEL:** Binge eating, body dysmorphic disorders, bulimia nervosa, generalized anxiety disorder (GAD).

PRECAUTIONS

Contraindications: Hypersensitivity to sertraline. MAOI use within 14 days (concurrently or within 14 days of stopping an MAOI or sertraline). Concurrent use of oral concentrate (contains alcohol) with disulfiram. Concurrent use with pimozide; initiation in pts treated with linezolid or methylene blue. **Cautions:** Seizure disorder, hepatic impairment, pts at risk for uric acid nephropathy, elderly, pts in third trimester of pregnancy, pts at high risk for suicide, family history of bipolar disorder or mania, pts with risk factors for QT prolongation (e.g., hypokalemia, hypomagnesemia), alcoholism. Pts in whom weight loss is undesirable.

ACTION

Blocks reuptake of the neurotransmitter serotonin at CNS neuronal presynaptic membranes, increasing availability at postsynaptic receptor sites. **Therapeutic Effect:** Relieves depression, reduces obsessive-compulsive behavior, decreases anxiety.

PHARMACOKINETICS

Widely distributed. Protein binding: 98%. Metabolized in liver. Excreted in urine (45%), feces (45%). Not removed by hemodialysis. **Half-life:** 26 hrs.

⌛ LIFESPAN CONSIDERATIONS

Pregnancy/Lactation: Unknown if drug crosses placenta or is distributed in breast milk. **Children:** Children and adolescents are at increased risk for suicidal ideation and behavior or worsening of depression, esp. during the first few mos of therapy. **Elderly:** No age-related precautions noted, but lower initial dosages recommended.

INTERACTIONS

DRUG: Alcohol, disulfiram may increase adverse effects. **Anticoagulants (e.g., heparin, rivaroxaban, warfarin), antiplatelets (e.g., aspirin, clopidogrel), NSAIDs (e.g., diclofenac, meloxicam, naproxen)** may increase risk of bleeding. **MAOIs (e.g., phenelzine, selegiline)** may cause neuroleptic malignant syndrome, serotonin syndrome. **Serotonergic drugs (e.g., busPIRone, carBAMazepine, linezolid, SNRIs [e.g., DULoxetine])** may cause serotonin syndrome. May increase concentration, toxicity of **tricyclic antidepressants (e.g., amitriptyline, doxepin). HERBAL:** Glucosamine, herbals with anticoagulant/antiplatelet **properties (e.g., garlic, ginger, ginkgo biloba, ginseng)** may increase concentration/effect. **St. John's wort** may increase concentration/effect. **FOOD:** Grapefruit products may increase concentration/effect. **LAB VALUES:** May increase total serum cholesterol, triglycerides, ALT, AST. May decrease serum uric acid.

AVAILABILITY (Rx)

Oral Concentrate: 20 mg/mL. **Tablets:** 25 mg, 50 mg, 100 mg.

🦫 **Capsules:** 150 mg, 200 mg.

ADMINISTRATION/HANDLING

PO
• Give with food, milk if GI distress occurs. • Oral concentrate must be diluted before administration. Mix with 4 oz water, ginger ale, lemon/lime soda, or orange juice only. Give immediately after mixing. • Administer capsules whole; do not open or crush. Capsule cannot be chewed.

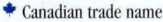 Canadian trade name   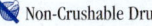 Non-Crushable Drug   High Alert drug

INDICATIONS/ROUTES/DOSAGE

Depression

PO: ADULTS: Tablets, oral solution: Initially, 50 mg/day. May increase by 25–50 mg/day at 7-day intervals up to 300 mg/day. **ELDERLY:** Initially, 25 mg/day. May increase by 25–50 mg/day at 7-day intervals up to 300 mg/day. **Capsules, usual dose:** 150–200 mg once daily. **Maximum:** 200 mg/day.

Obsessive-Compulsive Disorder (OCD)

PO: ADULTS, CHILDREN 13–17 YRS: Initially, 50 mg/day with morning or evening meal. May increase by 25–50 mg/day at 7-day intervals up to 200 mg/day. **ELDERLY, CHILDREN 6–12 YRS:** Initially, 25 mg/day. May increase by 25–50 mg/day at 7-day intervals. **Maximum:** 200 mg/day. **Capsules, usual dose:** 150–200 mg once daily. **Maximum:** 200 mg/day.

Panic Disorder

PO: ADULTS, ELDERLY: Initially, 25 mg once daily for 3–7 days. May increase to 50 mg/day. May further increase dose based on response and tolerability in increments of 25–50 mg at intervals of at least 1 wk. **Maximum:** 200 mg/day.

Posttraumatic Stress Disorder (PTSD)

PO: ADULTS, ELDERLY: Initially, 25–50 mg/day. May increase by 25–50 mg/day at 7-day intervals. Range: 50–200 mg/day. **Maximum:** 200 mg/day.

Premenstrual Dysphoric Disorder (PMDD)

PO: ADULTS: (Continuous daily dosing): Initially, 25 mg once daily. Over first month, increase to 50 mg once daily. In subsequent menstrual cycles, an increase up to 200 mg/day may be necessary. **(Luteal phase dosing):** Initially, 25 mg once daily during luteal phase. Over first month, increase to 50 mg once daily. In subsequent menstrual cycles, an increase up to 150 mg/day may be necessary.

Social Anxiety Disorder

PO: ADULTS, ELDELRY: Initially, 25–50 mg daily. After 6 wks, may increase in increments of 25–50 mg/day at intervals of 1 wk or longer. **Maximum:** 200 mg/day.

Dosage in Renal Impairment

No dose adjustment.

Dosage in Hepatic Impairment

Use caution.

SIDE EFFECTS

Frequent (26%–12%): Headache, nausea, diarrhea, insomnia, drowsiness, dizziness, fatigue, rash, dry mouth. **Occasional (6%–4%):** Anxiety, nervousness, agitation, tremor, dyspepsia, diaphoresis, vomiting, constipation, sexual dysfunction, visual disturbances, altered taste. **Rare (less than 3%):** Flatulence, urinary frequency, paresthesia, hot flashes, chills.

ADVERSE EFFECTS/TOXIC REACTIONS

Serotonin syndrome (seizures, arrhythmias, high fever), neuroleptic malignant syndrome (muscle rigidity, cognitive changes), suicidal ideation have occurred.

NURSING CONSIDERATIONS

BASELINE ASSESSMENT

Assess appearance, behavior, speech patterns, level of interest, mood. For pts on long-term therapy, CBC, renal function, LFT should be performed periodically. Question history of suicidal ideation and behavior.

INTERVENTION/EVALUATION

Assess mental status for depression, suicidal ideation (esp. at beginning of therapy or change in dosage), anxiety, social function, panic attack. Monitor daily pattern of bowel activity, stool consistency. Assist with ambulation if dizziness occurs.

PATIENT/FAMILY TEACHING

• Report headache, fatigue, tremor, sexual dysfunction. • Avoid tasks that require alertness, motor skills until response to drug is established (may cause dizziness, drowsiness). • Take with food if nausea occurs. • Avoid alcohol. • Do not take OTC medications without consulting physician. • Seek immediate medical attention if thoughts of suicide, new onset or worsening of anxiety, depression, or changes in mood occur.

S

sevelamer

se-**vel**-a-mer
(Renagel, Renvela)
**Do not confuse Renagel with
Reglan, Regonol, or Renvela, or
sevelamer with Savella.**

◆CLASSIFICATION

PHARMACOTHERAPEUTIC: Poly-
meric phosphate binder. **CLINICAL:**
Electrolyte modifier, antihyperphos-
phatemia agent.

USES

Control of serum phosphorus in pts with
chronic renal disease on hemodialysis.

PRECAUTIONS

Contraindications: Hypersensitivity to
sevelamer. Bowel obstruction. **Cautions:** Dysphagia, severe GI tract motility
disorders, major GI tract surgery.

ACTION

Binds with phosphate within the intestinal
lumen without altering calcium, aluminum,
or bicarbonate concentration. **Therapeutic Effect:** Inhibits phosphate absorption.
Decreases serum phosphate concentration.

PHARMACOKINETICS

Not absorbed systemically. Unknown if
removed by hemodialysis.

⧗ LIFESPAN CONSIDERATIONS

Pregnancy/Lactation: Not distributed
in breast milk. **Children:** Safety and efficacy not established. **Elderly:** No age-
related precautions noted.

INTERACTIONS

DRUG: May decrease concentration/
effect of **fluoroquinolones (e.g., levo-
FLOXacin), levothyroxine, mycophenolate. HERBAL:** None significant.
FOOD: May cause reduced absorption
of **vitamins D, E, K, folic acid. LAB
VALUES:** Expected to decrease serum
phosphate.

AVAILABILITY (Rx)

Powder for Oral Suspension: *(Renvela):*
0.8 g/pack, 2.4 g/pack.

Tablets: 400 mg, 800 mg.

ADMINISTRATION/HANDLING

PO

• Give with meals. • Space other medication by at least 1 hr before or 3 hrs
after sevelamer. • Give tablets whole;
do not break, crush, dissolve, or
divide. • **Oral suspension:** Mix 0.8 g
with 30 mL water (2.4 g with 60 mL
water). Stir vigorously to suspend (does
not dissolve) just prior to drinking.

INDICATIONS/ROUTES/DOSAGE

Hyperphosphatemia

PO: ADULTS, ELDERLY: 800–1,600 mg with
each meal, depending on severity of hyperphosphatemia (5.5–7.4 mg/dL: 800 mg 3
times/day; 7.5–8.9 mg/dL: 1,200–1,600 mg
3 times/day; 9 mg/dL or greater: 1,600 mg 3
times/day). *(Renvela):* **CHILDREN 6 YRS AND
OLDER:** (Pts not taking a phosphate binder):
BSA 0.75–1.1 m²: Initially, 800 mg 3 times
daily. Titrate as needed by 400 mg/dose at
2-wk intervals. **BSA greater than 1.1 m²:**
1,600 mg 3 times daily. Titrate as needed
by 800 mg/dose at 2-wk intervals. **Maintenance:** Based on serum phosphorus concentrations. Goal range: 3.5–5.5 mg/dL.

Serum Phosphorus Concentration	Dosage
Greater than 5.5 mg/dL	Increase by 400–800 mg per meal at 2-wk intervals
3.5–5.5 mg/dL	Maintain current dosage
Less than 3.5 mg/dL	Decrease by 400–800 mg per meal

Dosage in Renal/Hepatic Impairment
No dose adjustment.

SIDE EFFECTS

Frequent (20%–11%): Infection, pain,
hypotension, diarrhea, dyspepsia, nausea,
vomiting. **Occasional (10%–1%):** Headache, constipation, hypertension, increased
cough.

S

ADVERSE EFFECTS/TOXIC REACTIONS

Thrombosis occurs rarely.

BASELINE ASSESSMENT

Obtain serum calcium, phosphate. Question history of bowel obstruction, GI motility disorders.

INTERVENTION/EVALUATION

Monitor serum phosphate, calcium.

PATIENT/FAMILY TEACHING

• Take with meals, swallow tablets whole; do not chew, crush, dissolve, or divide tablets. • Report persistent headache, nausea, vomiting, diarrhea, hypotension.

simvastatin

sim-va-sta-tin
(FloLipid, Zocor)
Do not confuse simvastatin with atorvastatin, lovastatin, nystatin, pitavastatin, or pravastatin, or Zocor with Cozaar, Lipitor, Zoloft, or ZyrTEC.

FIXED-COMBINATION(S)

Vytorin: simvastatin/ezetimibe (a cholesterol absorption inhibitor): 10 mg/10 mg, 20 mg/10 mg, 40 mg/10 mg, 80 mg/10 mg.

◆CLASSIFICATION

PHARMACOTHERAPEUTIC: Hydroxymethylglutaryl-CoA (HMG-CoA) reductase inhibitor. **CLINICAL:** Antihyperlipidemic.

USES

Heterozygous familial hypercholesterolemia: To reduce elevated total cholesterol (total-C), LDL-C, apoB, and triglyceride levels and to increase HDL-C in pts with primary hypercholesterolemia. To reduce total-C, LDL-C, and apoB levels in males and postmenarche females 10–17 yrs of age with heterozygous familial hypercholesterolemia if LDL-C is 190 mg/dL or greater, or 160 mg/dL or greater with family history of premature cardiovascular disease, or presence of two or more cardiovascular risk factors. **Homozygous familial hypercholesterolemia:** To reduce total-C and LDL-C in pts with homozygous familial hypercholesterolemia as an adjunct to other lipid-lowering treatments. **Prevention of atherosclerotic cardiovascular disease: (Primary prevention):** To reduce the risk of myocardial infarction (MI), stroke, revascularization procedures, and angina in adults without a history of coronary heart disease (CHD), but who have multiple CHD risk factors. **(Secondary prevention):** To reduce the risk of myocardial infarction (MI), stroke, revascularization procedures, and angina in adults with a history of CHD. **OFF-LABEL:** Transplantation (kidney).

PRECAUTIONS

Contraindications: Hypersensitivity to simvastatin. Active hepatic disease or unexplained, persistent elevations of hepatic transaminases, pregnancy, breastfeeding, concurrent use of strong CYP3A4 inhibitors (e.g., clarithromycin, cycloSPORINE, gemfibrozil). **Cautions:** Hepatic disease, diabetes, severe renal impairment, substantial alcohol consumption. Withholding or discontinuing simvastatin may be necessary when pt is at risk for renal failure secondary to rhabdomyolysis. Concomitant use of other medications associated with myopathy.

ACTION

Interferes with cholesterol biosynthesis by inhibiting conversion of the enzyme HMG-CoA to mevalonate. **Therapeutic Effect:** Decreases LDL, cholesterol, VLDL, triglyceride levels; increase in HDL concentration.

PHARMACOKINETICS

Widely distributed. Protein binding: 95%. Metabolized in liver. Excreted in feces (60%), urine (13%). Unknown if removed by hemodialysis.

Route	Onset	Peak	Duration
PO (to reduce cholesterol)	3 days	14 days	N/A

⧖ LIFESPAN CONSIDERATIONS

Pregnancy/Lactation: Contraindicated in pregnancy (suppression of cholesterol biosynthesis may cause fetal toxicity), lactation. Risk of serious adverse reactions in breastfeeding infants. **Children:** Safety and efficacy not established in children less than 10 yrs of age or in premenarchal girls. **Elderly:** No age-related precautions noted.

INTERACTIONS

DRUG: CycloSPORINE, strong CYP3A4 inhibitors (e.g., clarithromycin, ketoconazole), amiodarone, calcium channel blockers (e.g., dilTIAZem, verapamil), colchicine, fibrates, gemfibrozil, niacin, ranolazine may increase risk of acute renal failure, rhabdomyolysis. Strong CYP3A4 inducers (e.g., carBAMazepine, phenytoin, rifAMPin) may decrease concentration/effect. **HERBAL:** St. John's wort may decrease concentration/effect. **FOOD:** Grapefruit products may increase concentration, toxicity. Red yeast rice contains 2.4 mg **lovastatin** per 600 mg rice. **LAB VALUES:** May increase serum creatine kinase (CK), transaminase.

AVAILABILITY (Rx)

Oral Suspension: 20 mg/5 mL, 40 mg/5 mL.
Tablets: 5 mg, 10 mg, 20 mg, 40 mg, 80 mg.

ADMINISTRATION/HANDLING

PO
• Give without regard to food. • Administer in evening for maximum efficacy. Shake suspension well for 20 sec before administering.

INDICATIONS/ROUTES/DOSAGE

Note: Limit 80-mg dose to pts taking simvastatin longer than 12 mos without evidence of myopathy.

Heterozygous Familial Hypercholesterolemia
PO: ADULTS, ELDERLY: 20–40 mg once daily in the evening.

Homozygous Familial Hypercholesterolemia
PO: ADULTS, ELDERLY: 20–40 mg once daily in the evening.

Prevention of Atherosclerotic Cardiovascular Disease
PO: ADULTS, ELDERLY: (Primary prevention): Moderate-intensity therapy: 20–40 mg once daily in the evening. **(Secondary prevention):** Moderate-intensity therapy: 20–40 mg once in the evening.

Heterozygous Familial Hypercholesterolemia (HeFH)
PO: CHILDREN 10–17 YRS: 10 mg once daily in evening. May increase to 20 mg once daily after 6 wks. May further increase to 40 mg once daily after additional 6 wks. **Maximum dose:** 40 mg/day.

Dosing Adjustment With Medications (CycloSPORINE, gemfibrozil): Do not exceed 10 mg/day. **(Amiodarone, amLODIPine, ranolazine):** Do not exceed 20 mg/day. **(DilTIAZem, dronedarone, verapamil):** Do not exceed 10 mg/day. **(Lomitapide):** Reduce simvastatin dose by 50% when initiating lomitapide. Do not exceed 20 mg/day.

Dosage in Renal Impairment
CrCl less than 30 mL/min: Initially, 5 mg/day.

Dosage in Hepatic Impairment
Contraindicated with active hepatic disease.

SIDE EFFECTS

Generally well tolerated. Side effects are usually mild and transient. **Occasional (3%–2%):** Headache, abdominal pain/cramps, constipation, upper respiratory tract infection. **Rare (less than 2%):** Diarrhea, flatulence, asthenia, nausea/vomiting, depression.

ADVERSE EFFECTS/TOXIC REACTIONS

May cause ocular lens opacities. Hypersensitivity reaction, hepatitis occur rarely. Myopathy (muscle pain, tenderness, weakness with elevated serum creatine kinase

S

[CK], sometimes taking the form of rhabdomyolysis) has occurred.

NURSING CONSIDERATIONS

BASELINE ASSESSMENT

Obtain lipid panel, LFT; urine pregnancy test in females of reproductive potential.

INTERVENTION/EVALUATION

Monitor serum cholesterol, triglyceride lab results for therapeutic response. Monitor LFT. Assess for headache, myopathy.

PATIENT/FAMILY TEACHING

• Use appropriate contraceptive measures. • Periodic lab tests are essential part of therapy. • Maintain appropriate diet. Avoid grapefruit products. • Report unexplained muscle pain, tenderness, weakness.

---

siponimod

si-**pon**-i-mod
(Mayzent)
Do not confuse siponimod with fingolimod or ozanimod.

◆CLASSIFICATION

PHARMACOTHERAPEUTIC: Sphingosine-1-phosphate receptor modulator.
CLINICAL: Multiple sclerosis agent.

USES

Treatment of relapsing forms of multiple sclerosis (MS), including clinically isolated syndrome, relapsing-remitting disease, and active secondary progressive disease, in adults.

PRECAUTIONS

Contraindications: Hypersensitivity to siponimod. Pts with CYP2C9*3/*3 genotype. Recent (within 6 mos) MI, unstable angina, CVA, TIA, decompensated HF requiring hospitalization, NYHA class III/IV HF, sick sinus syndrome, Mobitz type II second- or third-degree AV block (unless pt has functioning pacemaker). **Cautions:** Conditions predisposing to infection (e.g., diabetes,

immunocompromised pts, renal failure, open wounds), baseline sinus bradycardia, severe hepatic impairment, hypertension, altered pulmonary function, pts at risk for developing AV block (congenital heart disease, ischemic heart disease, HF), pts at risk for macular edema (e.g., diabetes, history of uveitis); history of syncope, thromboembolic events (CVA, pulmonary embolism, MI [more than 6 mos prior]). Concomitant use of antiarrhythmics, beta blockers, calcium channel blockers, immunosuppressants, immune modulators, antineoplastics, QT interval–prolonging medications. Not recommended in pts with severe active infection; history of cardiac arrest, cerebrovascular disease, uncontrolled hypertension, or severe, untreated sleep apnea unless approved by a cardiologist.

ACTION

Blocks capacity of lymphocytes to move out from lymph nodes, reducing the number of lymphocytes available to the CNS. **Therapeutic Effect:** May involve reduction of lymphocyte migration into the CNS, reducing inflammation.

PHARMACOKINETICS

Widely distributed. Metabolized in liver. Protein binding: 68%. Peak plasma concentration: 4 hrs. Steady state reached in 6 days. Excreted primarily in feces. **Half-life:** 30 hrs.

⌛ LIFESPAN CONSIDERATIONS

Pregnancy/Lactation: Avoid pregnancy; may cause fetal harm. Females of reproductive potential should use effective contraception during treatment and up to 10 days after discontinuation. Unknown if distributed in breast milk. **Children:** Safety and efficacy not established. **Elderly:** Age-related hepatic impairment may increase risk of adverse effects/hepatic injury.

INTERACTIONS

DRUG: Beta blockers (e.g., carvedilol, metoprolol), calcium channel blockers (e.g., dilTIAZem, verapamil), ceritinib, lacosamide may increase risk

---

of AV block, bradycardia. May decrease therapeutic effect of **BCG (intravesical)**, **live vaccines**. May increase toxic effect of **live vaccines**. **Fluconazole** may increase concentration/effect. **RifAMPin** may decrease concentration/effect. May increase toxic effects of **denosumab, leflunomide, natalizumab, tacrolimus (topical)**. May decrease therapeutic effect of **sipuleucel-T, tertomotide**. May increase immunosuppressive effect of **baricitinib, upadacitinib, tofacitinib, other immunosuppressants**. **HERBAL:** Echinacea may decrease therapeutic effect. **FOOD:** None known. **LAB VALUES:** May increase serum ALT, AST, bilirubin, GGT. Expected to cause a dose-dependent reduction in peripheral lymphocyte count to 20%–30% of baseline values.

AVAILABILITY (Rx)

Tablets: 0.25 mg, 1 mg, 2 mg.

ADMINISTRATION/HANDLING

PO
• Give without regard to meals. • Starter pack should be used in pts who titrate to 2 mg maintenance dose. Do not use starter pack in pts who titrate to 1 mg maintenance dose. • If one dose titration is missed for more than 24 hrs, reinitiate treatment starting with day 1 of titration regimen. • If treatment is interrupted for more than 4 consecutive days after initial titration is completed, reinitiate treatment starting with day 1 of titration regimen.

INDICATIONS/ROUTES/DOSAGE

Multiple Sclerosis (Relapsing)
PO: ADULTS, ELDERLY: (Pts with CYP2C9 genotypes *1/*1, *1/*2, or *2/*2): 0.25 mg on day 1, then 0.25 mg on day 2, then 0.5 mg on day 3, then 0.75 mg on day 4, then 1.25 mg on day 5. **Maintenance:** 2 mg once daily starting on day 6. **(Pts with CYP2C9 genotypes *1/*3 or *2/*3):** 0.25 mg on day 1, then 0.25 mg on day 2, then 0.5 mg on day 3, then 0.75

mg on day 4. **Maintenance:** 1 mg once daily starting on day 5.

Dosage in Renal Impairment
Mild to severe impairment: No dose adjustment.

Dosage in Hepatic Impairment
Mild to moderate impairment: No dose adjustment. **Severe impairment:** Use caution.

SIDE EFFECTS

Occasional (15%–6%): Headache, hypertension, peripheral edema, nausea, dizziness, diarrhea, extremity pain.

ADVERSE EFFECTS/TOXIC REACTIONS

Life-threatening infections (bronchitis, sinusitis, upper respiratory tract infection, fungal skin infection) reported in 3% of pts. Fatal cases of cryptococcal meningitis, disseminated cryptococcal infections were reported. Herpes zoster infections reported in 5% of pts. Reactivation of herpes viral infection may cause varicella zoster meningitis. Progressive multifocal leukoencephalopathy (PML), an opportunistic viral infection of the brain caused by the JC virus, may result in progressive permanent disability and death. Posterior reversible encephalopathy syndrome, a dysfunction of the brain that may evolve into an ischemic CVA or cerebral hemorrhage, may occur. Macular edema reported in 2% of pts. Pts with diabetes or history of uveitis are at an increased risk for developing macular edema. Bradycardia reported in 4% of pts. AV conduction delays reported in 5% of pts. Dose-dependent reductions of pulmonary function (absolute forced expiratory volume over 1 sec) reported in 3% of pts. Hepatic injury (transaminitis) reported in 10% of pts. Seizures reported in 2% of pts. Falls reported in 11% of pts. Rebound or severe exacerbation of disease may occur after discontinuation. May increase risk of hypertension, new malignancies. Fatal thromboembolic events including CVA, pulmonary embolism, MI reported in 3% of pts.

NURSING CONSIDERATIONS

BASELINE ASSESSMENT

Obtain CBC, LFT, ECG. Test all pts for CYP2C9 variants to determine CYP2C9 genotype. Assess baseline symptoms of MS (e.g., bladder/bowel dysfunction, cognitive impairment, depression, dysphagia, fatigue, gait disorder, numbness/tingling, pain, seizures, spasticity, tremors, weakness). Consultation with a cardiologist is advised in pts with QT interval prolongation greater than 500 msec; arrhythmias requiring treatment with Class Ia or Class III antiarrhythmic; ischemic heart disease, HF, history of cardiac arrest, recent MI; history of Mobitz type II second- or third-degree AV block, sick sinus syndrome, sinoatrial heart block. First-dose monitoring is recommended in pts with preexisting cardiac conditions (baseline sinus bradycardia, first- or second-degree [Mobitz type I], history of MI [more than 6 mos prior], HF) in a medical setting that can adequately treat symptomatic bradycardia. Pts without a documented history of vaccination against varicella zoster or a confirmed history of varicella infection (chickenpox) should be tested for antibodies prior to initiation. A full vaccination course for varicella in antibody-negative pts is recommended prior to initiation. Perform baseline ophthalmologic evaluation of the fundus (including the macula) prior to initiation. Receive full medication history and screen for interaction (esp. immunosuppressants; drugs known to bradycardia, AV conduction delay). Question history as listed in Precautions. Screen for active infection.

INTERVENTION/EVALUATION

At initial treatment (within first 4–6 hrs after dose), therapy reduces heart rate, AV conduction. In pts with preexisting cardiac conditions, monitor for symptomatic bradycardia for at least 6 hrs after first dose with hourly pulse, B/P, and then obtain ECG at the end of day 1. If heart rate is less than 45 beats/min, QTc interval is 500 msec or greater, or new-onset second-degree (or higher) AV block is present after 6 hrs of first dose, continue monitoring until resolved. If intervention is required, continue heart monitoring overnight and repeat 6-hr monitoring after second dose. Conduct ophthalmic examination with any change of vision. Pts with altered mental status, seizures, visual disturbances, unilateral weakness should be evaluated for cryptococcal meningitis, varicella zoster meningitis, posterior reversible encephalopathy syndrome, PML. Persistent immunosuppressive effects may occur for up to 3–4 wks after discontinuation. Closely monitor for adverse effects if other immunosuppressants are initiated within the first 3–4 wks after discontinuation. Monitor B/P for hypertension. Monitor for systemic or local infections, herpetic infections; symptoms of new malignancies. Conduct neurologic assessment. Assess for symptoms improvement of MS. Monitor for symptoms of MI (chest pain, diaphoresis, left arm/jaw pain, increased serum troponin, ST segment elevation), CVA (aphasia, altered mental status, facial droop, hemiplegia, vision loss), pulmonary embolism (chest pain, dyspnea, tachycardia).

PATIENT/FAMILY TEACHING

• Treatment may depress your immune system and reduce your ability to fight infection. Report symptoms of infection such as body aches, burning with urination, chills, cough, fatigue, fever. Avoid those with active infection. • Any change of vision will require an immediate eye examination. • PML, an opportunistic viral infection of the brain, may cause progressive, permanent disabilities or death. Report symptoms of PML such as confusion, memory loss, paralysis, trouble speaking, vision loss, seizures, weakness. • Treatment may worsen high blood pressure or cause new cancers. • Report liver problems (abdominal pain, bruising, clay-colored stool, amber or dark colored urine, yellowing of the skin or eyes), lung problems (reduced lung function, shortness of breath), heart arrhythmias (chest pain, dizziness, fainting, palpitations, slow or rapid heart rate, irregular heart rate). • Posterior reversible encephalopathy syndrome, a dysfunction of the brain that may cause a stroke or bleeding in the brain, may occur. • Treatment may cause life-threatening blood clots; report symptoms of heart attack (chest pain, difficulty breathing, jaw pain, nausea, pain that radiates to the left arm, sweating), lung embolism (difficulty breathing, chest pain, rapid heart rate), stroke (confusion, difficulty speaking, one-sided weakness or paralysis, loss of vision). • Use effective contraception to avoid pregnancy. Do not breast-feed. • Due to high risk of interactions, do not take newly prescribed medications unless approved by the provider who originally started treatment. • Do not receive live vaccines for at least 4 wks after last dose. • Severe worsening of MS symptoms may occur after stopping treatment.

sirolimus

sir-**oh**-li-mus
(Rapamune)
■ **BLACK BOX ALERT** ■ Increased susceptibility to infection and potential for development of lymphoma may result from immunosuppression. Not recommended for liver or lung transplant pts. Use only by physicians experienced in immunosuppressive therapy and management of transplant pts. **Do not confuse Rapamune with Rapaflo, or sirolimus with everolimus, pimecrolimus, tacrolimus, or temsirolimus.**

◆CLASSIFICATION

PHARMACOTHERAPEUTIC: mTOR kinase inhibitor. **CLINICAL:** Immunosuppressant.

USES

Prophylaxis of organ rejection of renal transplants in pts age 13 yrs and older at low- to high-immunologic risk (used initially with cyclosporine [CsA] and corticosteroids). Treatment of lymphangioleiomyomatosis. **OFF-LABEL:** Graft-versus-host disease (prevention, acute, chronic); heart, liver, and lung transplants (rejection prophylaxis); renal angiomyolipoma.

PRECAUTIONS

Contraindications: Hypersensitivity to sirolimus. **Cautions:** Cardiovascular disease (HF, hypertension); pulmonary disease, hepatic impairment, renal impairment, hyperlipidemia, perioperative period due to increased chance of surgical complications from impaired wound and tissue healing. Concurrent use with medications that may alter renal function.

ACTION

Inhibits T-lymphocyte activation and proliferation in response to antigenic and cytokine stimulation, and inhibits antibody production. **Therapeutic Effect:** Inhibits acute rejection of allografts and prolongs graft survival.

PHARMACOKINETICS

Widely distributed. Protein binding: 92%. Extensively metabolized in liver. Primarily excreted in feces (91%). **Half-life:** 57–63 hrs.

⧗ LIFESPAN CONSIDERATIONS

Pregnancy/Lactation: Unknown if crosses placenta or is distributed in breast milk. **Children:** Safety and efficacy not established in pts younger than 13 yrs. **Elderly:** No age-related precautions noted.

INTERACTIONS

DRUG: CYP3A4 inducers (e.g., **carBAMazepine, rifabutin, rifAMPin**) may decrease concentration/effect. **CYP3A4 inhibitors (e.g., clarithromycin, erythromycin, itraconazole, verapamil)** may increase concentration, toxicity. May increase concentration/effect of **cycloSPORINE** (take sirolimus 4 hrs after cycloSPORINE for renal transplant). May decrease

S

the therapeutic effect; increase adverse effects of **vaccines (live)**. **HERBAL:** Echinacea may decrease the therapeutic effect. **FOOD:** Grapefruit products may increase risk of myelotoxicity, nephrotoxicity. **LAB VALUES:** May increase serum ALT, AST, alkaline phosphatase, LDH, BUN, creatine phosphate, cholesterol, triglycerides, creatinine. May alter WBC, serum glucose, calcium. May decrease Hgb, Hct.

AVAILABILITY (Rx)

Oral Solution: 1 mg/mL.

Tablets: 0.5 mg, 1 mg, 2 mg.

ADMINISTRATION/HANDLING

• Doses should be taken 4 hrs after cycloSPORINE. • Take consistently with or without food. • Do not crush, split, or allow chewing of tablets. • Mix oral solution with only water or orange juice, stir vigorously, drink immediately.

INDICATIONS/ROUTES/DOSAGE

◄**ALERT**► Tablets and oral solution are not bioequivalent. (However, clinical equivalence shown at 2 mg dose.)

Prevention of Organ Transplant Rejection (Low to Moderate Risk)

PO: **ADULTS, CHILDREN 13 YRS AND OLDER WEIGHING MORE THAN 40 KG: Loading dose:** 6 mg on day 1. **Maintenance:** 2 mg/day. **ADULTS, CHILDREN 13 YRS AND OLDER WEIGHING LESS THAN 40 KG: Loading dose:** 3 mg/m² on day 1. **Maintenance:** 1 mg/m²/day.

Prevention of Organ Transplant Rejection (High Risk)

PO: **ADULTS: Loading dose:** Up to 15 mg on day 1. **Maintenance:** 5 mg/day. Obtain trough between 5–7 days. Continue therapy for 1 yr following transplantation. Further adjustments based on clinical status.

Lymphangioleiomyomatosis

PO: **ADULTS, ELDERLY:** Initially, 2 mg/day with dosage adjustment to maintain concentration between 5–15 ng/mL. Obtain serum trough level after 10–20 days. Once maintenance dose is adjusted,

further adjustments should be made at 7- to 14-day intervals. Once a stable dose is attained, serum trough levels should be assessed at least q3mos.

Dosage in Renal Impairment
No dose adjustment.

Dosage in Hepatic Impairment
Loading Dose: No change. **Maintenance Dose: MILD TO MODERATE IMPAIRMENT:** Reduce dose by 33%. **SEVERE IMPAIRMENT:** Reduce dose by 50%.

SIDE EFFECTS

Occasional: Hypercholesterolemia, hyperlipidemia, hypertension, rash. **High doses (5 mg/day):** Anemia, arthralgia, diarrhea, hypokalemia, peripheral edema, thrombocytopenia.

ADVERSE EFFECTS/TOXIC REACTIONS

Hepatotoxicity occurs rarely. Skin carcinoma (including basal cell, squamous cell, melanoma) has been observed.

NURSING CONSIDERATIONS

BASELINE ASSESSMENT

Obtain LFT; pregnancy test in females of reproductive potential. Question for medication usage (esp. cycloSPORINE, dilTIAZem, ketoconazole, rifAMPin). Determine if pt has chickenpox, herpes zoster, malignancy, infection.

INTERVENTION/EVALUATION

Monitor renal function, LFT periodically. Monitor serum cholesterol, triglycerides, platelets; Hgb. Obtain trough concentration 10–20 days after dose. Once maintenance dose is adjusted, make further adjustments at intervals of 7–14 days. Once stable dose is attained, assess trough concentration at least q3mos.

PATIENT/FAMILY TEACHING

• Avoid those with colds, other infections. • Avoid grapefruit products. • Avoid exposure to sunlight, artificial light

S

sources. • Strict monitoring is essential in identifying, preventing symptoms of organ rejection. • Do not chew, crush, dissolve, or divide tablets.

SITagliptin

sit-a-**glip**-tin
(Januvia)

Do not confuse Januvia with Enjuvia, Jantoven, or Janumet, or SITagliptin with sAXagliptin or SUMAtriptan.

FIXED-COMBINATION(S)

Janumet, Janumet XR: SITagliptin/metFORMIN (an antidiabetic): 50 mg/500 mg, 50 mg/1,000 mg.

◆CLASSIFICATION

PHARMACOTHERAPEUTIC: DPP-4 inhibitors (gliptins). **CLINICAL:** Antidiabetic agent.

USES

Adjunctive treatment to diet, exercise to improve glycemic control in pts with type 2 diabetes as monotherapy or in combination with other antidiabetic agents.

PRECAUTIONS

Contraindications: Hypersensitivity to SITagliptin. **Cautions:** Type 1 diabetes, diabetic ketoacidosis, renal impairment, end-stage renal disease, history of pancreatitis, angioedema with other DPP-4 inhibitors. Concurrent use of other glucose-lowering agents may increase risk of hypoglycemia.

ACTION

Inhibits DPP-4 enzyme, causing prolonged active incretin levels. Incretin regulates glucose homeostasis. **Therapeutic Effect:** Regulates glucose homeostasis. Increases synthesis and release of insulin from pancreatic cells; lowers glucagon secretion from pancreas, decreases hepatic glucose production.

PHARMACOKINETICS

Route	Onset	Peak	Duration
PO	N/A	1–4 hrs	24 hrs

Widely distributed. Protein binding: 38%. Excreted in urine (87%), feces (13%). **Half-life:** 12 hrs.

LIFESPAN CONSIDERATIONS

Pregnancy/Lactation: Unknown if distributed in breast milk. **Children:** Safety and efficacy not established. **Elderly:** No age-related precautions noted.

INTERACTIONS

DRUG: May enhance hypoglycemic effect of **insulin, sulfonylureas (e.g., glipiZIDE, glyBURIDE). HERBAL: Maitake** may increase hypoglycemic effect. **FOOD:** None known. **LAB VALUES:** May slightly increase WBCs, particularly neutrophil count. May increase serum creatinine.

AVAILABILITY (Rx)

Tablets: 25 mg, 50 mg, 100 mg.

ADMINISTRATION/HANDLING
PO
• May give without regard to food.

INDICATIONS/ROUTES/DOSAGE

Type 2 Diabetes
PO: ADULTS OVER 18 YRS, ELDERLY: 100 mg once daily.

Dosage in Renal Impairment
CrCl 30 mL/min to less than 50 mL/min: 50 mg once daily. **CrCl less than 30 mL/min, ESRD, dialysis:** 25 mg once daily.

Dosage in Hepatic Impairment
No dose adjustment.

SIDE EFFECTS

Occasional (5% and greater): Headache, nasopharyngitis. **Rare (3%–1%):** Diarrhea, abdominal pain, nausea.

S

ADVERSE EFFECTS/TOXIC REACTIONS

Hypersensitivity reactions including angioedema, Stevens-Johnson syndrome reported. Acute pancreatitis occurs rarely.

NURSING CONSIDERATIONS

BASELINE ASSESSMENT

Obtain renal function test, serum glucose; Hgb A1c. Assess pt's understanding of diabetes management, routine home glucose monitoring. Obtain dietary consult for nutritional education. Question history of renal impairment, type 1 diabetes, ketoacidosis, pancreatitis. Receive full medication history and screen for interactions.

INTERVENTION/EVALUATION

Monitor blood glucose, hemoglobin A1c level, renal function. Assess for hypoglycemia (diaphoresis, tremors, dizziness, anxiety, headache, tachycardia, perioral numbness, hunger, diplopia, difficulty concentrating), hyperglycemia (polyuria, polyphagia, polydipsia, nausea, vomiting, fatigue, Kussmaul breathing), hypersensitivity reaction. Concomitant use of beta blockers (e.g., carvedilol, metoprolol) may mask symptoms of hypoglycemia. Screen for glucose-altering conditions: fever, increased activity or stress, surgical procedures. Dietary consult for nutritional education. Severe abdominal pain, nausea may indicate pancreatitis.

PATIENT/FAMILY TEACHING

• Diabetes mellitus requires lifelong control. Diet and exercise is a principal part of treatment; do not skip or delay meals. Test blood sugar regularly. Monitor daily calorie intake. • When taking combination drug therapy or when glucose conditions are altered (excessive alcohol ingestion, insufficient carbohydrate intake, hormone deficiencies, critical illness), have a low blood sugar treatment available (e.g., glucagon, oral dextrose). • Persistent, severe abdominal pain that radiates to the back (with or without vomiting) may indicate acute pancreatitis. • Report joint pain; allergic reactions of any kind.

---

sodium bicarbonate

soe-dee-um bye-**kar**-boe-nate

FIXED-COMBINATION(S)

Konvomep: sodium bicarbonate/ omeprazole (PPI): 84 mg/2 mg/mL. **Zegerid:** 1,100 mg/20 mg, 1,100 mg/40 mg. **Zegerid Powder:** 1,680 mg/20 mg, 1,680 mg/40 mg.

◆CLASSIFICATION

PHARMACOTHERAPEUTIC: Alkalinizing agent. **CLINICAL:** Antacid, electrolyte supplement, urinary/systemic alkalinizer.

USES

Treatment of metabolic acidosis that can occur in severe renal disease, uncontrolled diabetes, circulatory insufficiency due to shock, anoxia, or severe dehydration. Treatment of certain drug intoxications, including poisoning by salicylates/methyl alcohol, in hemolytic reactions requiring alkalinization of the urine. **OFF-LABEL:** Prevention of contrast-induced nephropathy. Hyperkalemia (severe), metabolic acidosis (in pts with chronic kidney disease [CKD]).

PRECAUTIONS

Contraindications: Hypersensitivity to sodium bicarbonate. Hypernatremia, alkalosis, unknown abdominal pain, hypocalcemia, severe pulmonary edema. **Cautions:** HF, edematous states, renal insufficiency, cirrhosis.

ACTION

Dissociates to provide bicarbonate ion. **Therapeutic Effect:** Neutralizes hydrogen ion concentration, raises blood, urinary pH.

PHARMACOKINETICS

Route	Onset	Peak	Duration
PO	15 min	N/A	1–3 hrs

S

Route	Onset	Peak	Duration
IV	Immediate	N/A	8–10 min

Widely distributed. Sodium bicarbonate dissociates to sodium and bicarbonate ions. With increased hydrogen ion concentrations, bicarbonate ions combine with hydrogen ions to form carbonic acid, which then dissociates to CO_2, which is excreted by the lungs. Plasma concentration regulated by kidney (ability to form, excrete bicarbonate).

⧗ LIFESPAN CONSIDERATIONS

Pregnancy/Lactation: May cause hypernatremia, increase tendon reflexes in neonate or fetus whose mother is administered chronically high doses. May be distributed in breast milk. **Children:** No age-related precautions noted. Do not use as antacid in pts younger than 6 yrs. **Elderly:** Age-related renal impairment may require dosage adjustment.

INTERACTIONS

DRUG: May increase concentration, toxicity of **quiNIDine, quiNINE. HERBAL:** None significant. **FOOD: Milk, other dairy products** may result in milk-alkali syndrome. **LAB VALUES:** May increase serum, urinary pH.

AVAILABILITY (Rx)

Injection Solution (Rx): 0.5 mEq/mL, 1 mEq/mL.

ADMINISTRATION/HANDLING

IV

◀ALERT▶ For IV administration in neonates or infants, use 0.5 mEq/mL concentration.
Reconstitution • May give undiluted.
Rate of administration • For IV push, give up to 1 mEq/kg over 1–3 min for cardiac arrest. • For IV infusion, do not exceed rate of infusion of 1 mEq/kg/hr. • For children younger than 2 yrs, premature infants, neonates, administer by slow infusion, up to 10 mEq/min.
Storage • Store at room temperature.

PO
• Give 1–3 hrs after meals.

▦ IV INCOMPATIBILITIES
Calcium chloride.

▦ IV COMPATIBILITIES
DexmedeTOMIDine, heparin, insulin, potassium chloride.

INDICATIONS/ROUTES/DOSAGE

◀ALERT▶ May give by IV push, IV infusion, or orally. Dose individualized based on severity of acidosis, laboratory values, pt age, weight, clinical conditions. Do not fully correct bicarbonate deficit during the first 24 hrs (may cause metabolic alkalosis).

Cardiac Arrest

◀ALERT▶ Routine use not recommended.
IV: ADULTS, ELDERLY: Initially, 1 mEq/kg. May repeat based on arterial blood gases. **CHILDREN, INFANTS:** Initially, 0.5–1 mEq/kg. May repeat based on arterial blood gases.

Prevention of Contrast-Induced Nephropathy
IV infusion: ADULTS, ELDERLY: 154 mEq/L sodium bicarbonate in D_5W solution: 3 mL/kg/hr 1 hr immediately before contrast injection, then 1 mL/kg/hr during contrast exposure and for 6 hrs after procedure.

Metabolic Acidosis
IV: ADULTS, ELDERLY: Mild acidosis: 1–2 mEq/kg of body weight administered slowly. **More severe acidosis:** 2–5 mEq/kg of body weight administered over a 4–8 hr period. Subsequent therapy is dependent on the clinical response of the pt.

SIDE EFFECTS

Frequent: Abdominal distention, flatulence, belching.

ADVERSE EFFECTS/TOXIC REACTIONS

Excessive, chronic use may produce metabolic alkalosis (irritability, twitching, paresthesia, cyanosis, slow or shallow respirations, headache, thirst, nausea). Fluid overload results in headache, weakness, blurred vision, behavioral changes, incoordination, muscle twitching, elevated B/P, bradycardia, tachypnea, wheezing, coughing, distended neck veins. Extravasation may occur at the IV site, resulting in tissue necrosis, ulceration.

NURSING CONSIDERATIONS

BASELINE ASSESSMENT

Assess for symptoms of acidosis, alkalosis. Do not give PO medication within 1 hr of antacids.

INTERVENTION/EVALUATION

Monitor serum, urinary pH, CO_2 level, serum electrolytes, plasma bicarbonate levels. Monitor for metabolic alkalosis, fluid overload. Assess for clinical improvement of metabolic acidosis (relief from hyperventilation, weakness, disorientation). Monitor serum phosphate, calcium, uric acid levels. Assess for relief of gastric distress.

sofosbuvir/ velpatasvir

soe-**fos**-bue-vir/vel-**pat**-as-vir
(Epclusa)

■ BLACK BOX ALERT ■ Test all pts for hepatitis B virus (HBV) infection before initiation. HBV reactivation was reported in pts with hepatitis C virus (HCV)/HBV coinfection.

Do not confuse sofosbuvir with boceprevir, dasabuvir, fosamprenavir, or simeprevir, or velpatasvir with daclatasvir, grazoprevir, or paritaprevir.

◆ CLASSIFICATION

PHARMACOTHERAPEUTIC: Nucleotide analog NS5B polymerase inhibitor, NS5A inhibitor. **CLINICAL:** Antiviral.

USES

Treatment of chronic hepatitis C virus (HCV) genotype 1, 2, 3, 4, 5, or 6 infection in adults and pediatric pts 3 yrs and older without cirrhosis, or with compensated cirrhosis, or in combination with ribavirin in pts with decompensated cirrhosis.

PRECAUTIONS

Contraindications: Hypersensitivity to sofosbuvir, velpatasvir. If given with ribavirin, contraindications to ribavirin apply. **Cautions:** Anemia (when used with ribavirin), renal impairment, end-stage renal disease requiring hemodialysis, hepatic disease unrelated to HCV infection, HIV infection. Concomitant use of amiodarone (with or without beta blockers) in pts with underlying cardiac disease. Concomitant use of P-glycoprotein inducers, moderate CYP2B6 inducers, strong CYP2C8 inducers, moderate or strong CYP3A4 inducers not recommended.

ACTION

Sofosbuvir inhibits the HCV NS5B RNA-dependent RNA polymerase. Velpatasvir inhibits the VCV NS5A protein. **Therapeutic Effect:** Inhibits viral replication of HCV.

PHARMACOKINETICS

Widely distributed. Metabolized in liver. Protein binding: sofosbuvir: 61%–68%; velpatasvir: Greater than 99.5%. Peak plasma concentration: sofosbuvir: 0.5–1 hr; velpatasvir: 3 hrs. Excretion: sofosbuvir: urine (80%), feces (14%); velpatasvir: Feces (94%), urine (0.4%). **Half-life:** sofosbuvir: 0.5 hr; velpatasvir: 15 hrs.

⧗ LIFESPAN CONSIDERATIONS

Pregnancy/Lactation: When used with ribavirin, therapy is contraindicated in pregnant women and in men whose female partners are pregnant. Females and males with female partners of reproductive potential must use effective contraception for at least 6 mos following discontinuation (if therapy includes ribavirin). Unknown if distributed in

S

breast milk. **Children:** Safety and efficacy not established in pts younger than 3 yrs. **Elderly:** No age-related precautions noted.

INTERACTIONS

DRUG: Moderate or strong inducers of CYP2B6, CYP2C8, CYP3A4, P-glycoprotein (e.g., carBAMazepine, phenytoin, OXcarbazepine, rifampicin) may decrease concentration/effect of sofosbuvir/velpatasvir. **Amiodarone (with or without beta blockers** [e.g., carvedilol, metoprolol]) may significantly increase risk of symptomatic bradycardia. **Proton pump inhibitors** (e.g., omeprazole, pantoprazole) may decrease concentration/effect. **HERBAL:** None significant. **FOOD:** None known. **LAB VALUES:** May increase serum bilirubin (indirect), creatine phosphokinase (CPK), lipase.

AVAILABILITY (Rx)

Tablets, Fixed-Dose: sofosbuvir 400 mg/velpatasvir 100 mg, sofosbuvir 200 mg/velpatasvir 50 mg. **Oral Pellets:** sofosbuvir 200 mg/velpatasvir 50 mg, sofosbuvir 150 mg/velpatasvir 37.5 mg.

ADMINISTRATION/HANDLING

PO
• Give without regard to food. **Oral pellets:** • Pellets should not be chewed (causes bitter aftertaste). • Give without regard to food. In pediatric pts younger than 6 yrs of age, give oral pellets with food to increase tolerability related to palatability. • May sprinkle on 1 or more spoonfuls of non-acidic soft food (e.g., pudding, chocolate syrup, ice cream) at or below room temperature. Administer within 15 min of mixing with food.

INDICATIONS/ROUTES/DOSAGE

Hepatitis C Virus Infection
PO: **ADULTS, ELDERLY:** 400 mg/100 mg once daily. **CHILDREN 3 YRS AND OLDER: 30 KG OR GREATER:** 400 mg/100 mg once daily. **17–29 KG:** 200 mg/50 mg once daily. **WEIGHING LESS THAN 17 KG:** 150 mg/37.5 mg once daily.

Treatment Regimen and Duration
Pts without cirrhosis or pts with compensated cirrhosis (Child-Pugh A): 400 mg/100 mg once daily for 12 wks. **Pts with decompensated cirrhosis (Child-Pugh B or C):** 1 tablet once daily with ribavirin for 12 wks.

Dosage in Renal Impairment
Mild to moderate impairment: CrCl greater than or equal to 30 mL/min: No dose adjustment. **Severe impairment: CrCl less than 30 mL/min, end-stage renal disease:** Not specified; use caution.

Dosage in Hepatic Impairment
Mild to severe impairment: No dose adjustment.

SIDE EFFECTS

Frequent (22%–15%): Headache, fatigue. **Occasional (9%–5%):** Nausea, asthenia, insomnia, irritability. **Rare (2%):** Rash.

ADVERSE EFFECTS/TOXIC REACTIONS

Symptomatic bradycardia requiring pacemaker intervention was reported in pts taking amiodarone and sofosbuvir, in combination with daclatasvir or simeprevir. Cardiac arrest was reported in a pt taking amiodarone in combination with sofosbuvir and ledipasvir. Bradycardia usually occurred within hrs to days, but may occur up 2 wks after initiation (when used with amiodarone). Pts with underlying cardiac disease or advanced hepatic disease or taking concomitant beta blockers are at an increased risk for bradycardia when used concomitantly with amiodarone. Depression reported in 1% of pts.

NURSING CONSIDERATIONS

BASELINE ASSESSMENT
Obtain CBC (when used with ribavirin), renal function test, LFT, HCV-RNA level;

---

serum lipase; pregnancy test in female pts of reproductive potential. Confirm hepatitis C virus genotype. Question history of renal impairment, hepatic disease unrelated to HCV infection; HIV infection or use of antiretroviral therapy. Receive full medication history, and screen for interactions (esp. concomitant use of amiodarone).

INTERVENTION/EVALUATION

Monitor serum lipase, CPK. Periodically monitor HCV-RNA level for treatment effectiveness. If unable to discontinue amiodarone, recommend inpatient cardiac monitoring for at least 48 hrs, followed by outpatient or self-monitoring of HR for at least 2 wks after initiation. Cardiac monitoring is also recommended in pts who discontinue amiodarone just prior to initiation. Reinforce birth control compliance and obtain monthly pregnancy tests in female pts of reproductive potential taking concomitant ribavirin. Encourage nutritional intake.

PATIENT/FAMILY TEACHING

• Pts who take amiodarone during therapy may require inpatient and outpatient cardiac monitoring (and in some cases, pacemaker implantation) due to an increased risk of slow heartbeats or cardiac arrest. If amiodarone cannot be interrupted or discontinued, immediately report symptoms of slow heartbeat such as chest pain, confusion, dizziness, fainting, light-headedness, memory problems, palpitations, weakness. • Treatment may be used in combination with ribavirin. Inform pt of contraindications/adverse effects of ribavirin therapy. Use effective contraception to avoid pregnancy. Do not breastfeed. • Do not take newly prescribed medications unless approved by prescriber who originally started treatment. • Do not take herbal products. • Avoid alcohol. • Maintain proper nutritional intake.

solifenacin

sol-i-**fen**-a-sin
(VESIcare, VESIcare LS)

◆CLASSIFICATION

PHARMACOTHERAPEUTIC: Anticholinergic agent, muscarinic receptor antagonist. **CLINICAL:** Urinary antispasmodic.

USES

Treatment of overactive bladder with symptoms of urinary frequency, urgency, or urge incontinence. Treatment of neurogenic detrusor overactivity (NDO) in children 2 yrs and older.

PRECAUTIONS

Contraindications: Hypersensitivity to solifenacin. Gastric retention, uncontrolled narrow-angle glaucoma, urinary retention (tablet only). **Cautions:** Bladder outflow obstruction, GI obstructive disorders, decreased GI motility, controlled narrow-angle glaucoma, renal/hepatic impairment, pts at risk for QTc interval prolongation (congenital long QT syndrome, HF, medications that prolong QTc interval, hypokalemia, hypomagnesemia), hot weather and/or exercise.

ACTION

Inhibits muscarinic receptors. **Therapeutic Effect:** Decreases urinary bladder contractions, increases residual urine volume, decreases detrusor muscle pressure.

PHARMACOKINETICS

Widely distributed. Protein binding: 98%. Metabolized in liver. Excreted in urine (69%), feces (23%). **Half-life:** 40–68 hrs.

⧗ LIFESPAN CONSIDERATIONS

Pregnancy/Lactation: Unknown if drug crosses placenta or is distributed in breast milk. **Children:** Safety and efficacy not established. **Elderly:** No age-related precautions noted.

INTERACTIONS

DRUG: CYP3A4 inhibitors (e.g., keto-conazole, erythromycin, azole anti-fungals, clarithromycin) may increase concentration/effect. **Aclidinium, ipratropium, tiotropium, umeclidinium** may increase anticholinergic effect. **Strong CYP3A4 inducers (e.g., carBAMazepine, phenytoin, rifAMPin)** may decrease concentration/effect. **QT interval–prolonging medications (e.g., amiodarone, azithromycin, ciprofloxacin, haloperidol, methadone, sotalol)** may increase risk of QTc interval prolongation. **HERBAL:** None significant. **FOOD:** Grapefruit products may increase concentration/effect. **LAB VALUES:** None known.

AVAILABILITY (Rx)

Oral Suspension: 5 mg/5 mL. **Tablets:** 5 mg, 10 mg.

ADMINISTRATION/HANDLING

PO
• Give without regard to food. • Swallow tablets whole, with liquids. Do not crush or allow chewing.
Oral suspension • Shake well. Use oral syringe.

INDICATIONS/ROUTES/DOSAGE

Overactive Bladder
PO: **ADULTS, ELDERLY:** 5 mg/day; if tolerated, may increase to 10 mg/day.

NDO
PO: **CHILDREN (WEIGHING MORE THAN 60 KG):** 5 mg once daily. **Maximum:** 10 mg. **(46–60 KG):** 4 mg once daily. **Maximum:** 8 mg. **(31–45 KG):** 3 mg once daily. **Maximum:** 6 mg. **(16–30 KG):** 3 mg once daily. **Maximum:** 5 mg. **(9–15 KG):** 2 mg once daily. **Maximum:** 4 mg.

Dose Modification
Concomitant Use of Strong CYP3A4 Inhibitors
Maximum: 5 mg/day.

Dosage in Renal/Hepatic Impairment
Severe renal impairment (CrCl less than 30 mL/min) or moderate hepatic impairment: Maximum dosage is 5 mg/

day. Not recommended in severe hepatic impairment.

SIDE EFFECTS

Frequent (28%–13%): Dry mouth, constipation. **Occasional (5%–3%):** Blurred vision, UTI, dyspepsia, nausea. **Rare (2%–1%):** Dizziness, dry eyes, fatigue, depression, edema, hypertension, epigastric pain, vomiting, urinary retention.

ADVERSE EFFECTS/TOXIC REACTIONS

Angioneurotic edema, GI obstruction occur rarely. Overdose can result in severe anticholinergic effects (agitation, confusion, dysarthria, flushing, hyperthemia, pupil dilation).

NURSING CONSIDERATIONS

BASELINE ASSESSMENT
Assess symptoms of overactive bladder before beginning the drug. Question medical history as listed in Precautions. Screen for concomitant medications known to prolong QT interval. Obtain baseline ECG.

INTERVENTION/EVALUATION
Monitor I&O, anticholinergic effects, creatinine clearance. Assess for decrease in symptoms. Obtain bladder scan if urinary retention is suspected.

PATIENT/FAMILY TEACHING
• Avoid tasks requiring alertness, motor skills until response to drug is established. • Anticholinergic side effects include constipation, urinary retention, blurred vision, heat prostration in hot environment. • Use caution during exercise, exposure to heat.

somatropin

soe-ma-**troe**-pin
(Genotropin, Genotropin Miniquick, Humatrope, Norditropin FlexPro, Nutropin AQ NuSpin, Omnitrope, Saizen, Serostim, Zomacton, Zorbtive)
Do not confuse somatropin with SUMAtriptan.

S

◆CLASSIFICATION

PHARMACOTHERAPEUTIC: Polypeptide hormone. **CLINICAL:** Growth hormone.

USES

Pediatric pts: Growth hormone deficiency (GHD) due to inadequate secretion of endogenous growth hormone (GH). Growth failure secondary to chronic kidney failure associated with chronic kidney disease (CKD) up to the time of renal transplantation. Treatment of short stature associated with turner syndrome (TS). Treatment of Prader-Willi syndrome. Treatment of growth failure in children born small for gestational age who do not manifest catch-up growth by 2 yrs of age. Treatment of idiopathic short stature (ISS) defined by height standard deviation score 2.25 or lower, and associated with growth rates unlikely to permit attainment of adult height in the normal range, in pediatric pts whose epiphyses are not closed and for whom diagnostic evaluation excludes other causes associated with short stature. Treatment of short stature or growth failure associated with short stature hormone gene (SHOX) or associated with Noonan's syndrome. **Adult pts:** Replacement of endogenous GH in adults with GHD who meet either of the following two criteria: **(Adult onset):** Pts who have GHD, either alone or associated with multiple hormone deficiencies (hypopituitarism) as a result of pituitary disease, hypothalamic disease, surgery, radiation therapy, or trauma; **(Childhood onset):** GH deficiency during childhood as a result of congenital, genetic, acquired, or idiopathic causes. **HIV-associated wasting cachexia:** Treatment of pts with HIV-associated wasting or cachexia. **Short bowel syndrome:** Treatment of short bowel syndrome in pts receiving specialized nutritional support. **OFF-LABEL:** HIV adipose redistribution syndrome.

PRECAUTIONS

Contraindications: Hypersensitivity to growth hormone. Pts with Prader-Willi syndrome with growth hormone deficiency who are severely obese or have severe respiratory impairment, Prader-Willi syndrome who have a history of upper airway obstruction or sleep apnea, children with closed epiphyses, acute critical illness due to complications after open heart or abdominal surgery, multiple accidental trauma, acute respiratory failure, active neoplasia, diabetic retinopathy. Active malignancy, progression of active growing intracranial lesion or tumor. **Cautions:** Diabetes, elderly.

ACTION

Stimulates cartilaginous growth areas of long bones; increases number, size of skeletal muscle cells; influences size of organs; increases RBC mass by stimulating erythropoietin. Influences metabolism of carbohydrates (decreases insulin sensitivity), fats (mobilizes fatty acids), minerals (retains phosphorus, sodium, potassium by promotion of cell growth), proteins (increases protein synthesis). Exerts both insulin-like and diabetogenic effects. Enhances transmucosal transport of water, electrolytes, and nutrients across the gut. **Therapeutic Effect:** Stimulates growth.

PHARMACOKINETICS

Localized primarily in kidneys, liver. **Half-life:** **IV:** 20–30 min; **SQ, IM:** 3–5 hrs.

⌛ LIFESPAN CONSIDERATIONS

Pregnancy/Lactation: Unknown if drug is distributed in breast milk. **Children/Elderly:** No age-related precautions noted.

INTERACTIONS

DRUG: **Corticosteroids (e.g., hydrocortisone, predniSONE)** may inhibit growth response. **Oral estrogens** may decrease response to somatropin. **HERBAL:** None significant. **FOOD:** None known. **LAB VALUES:** May increase serum alkaline phosphatase, inorganic phosphorus, parathyroid hormone. May decrease glucose tolerance. May slightly decrease thyroid function.

AVAILABILITY (Rx)

Injection, Powder for Reconstitution: *(Genotropin):* 5 mg, 12 mg. *(Genotropin Miniquick):* 0.2 mg, 0.4 mg, 0.6 mg, 0.8 mg, 1 mg, 1.2 mg, 1.4 mg, 1.6 mg, 1.8 mg, 2 mg.

(Humatrope): 5 mg, 6 mg, 12 mg, 24 mg. *(Omnitrope):* 5.8 mg. *(Saizen):* 5 mg, 8.8 mg. *(Serostim):* 4 mg, 5 mg, 6 mg. *(Zomacton):* 5 mg, 10 mg. *(Zorbtive):* 8.8 mg. **Injection Solution:** *(Omnitrope):* 5 mg/1.5 mL, 10 mg/1.5 mL. *(Norditropin FlexPro Pen):* 5 mg/1.5 mL, 10 mg/1.5 mL, 15 mg/1.5 mL, 30 mg/3 mL. *(Nutropin AQ NuSpin):* 5 mg/2 mL, 10 mg/2 mL, 20 mg/2 mL.

ADMINISTRATION/HANDLING

◀ALERT▶ **Neonate:** Benzyl alcohol as a preservative has been associated with fatal toxicity (gasping syndrome) in premature infants. Reconstitute with Sterile Water for Injection only. Use only 1 dose per vial. Discard unused portion.

Reconstitution • *(Genotropin, Genotropin Miniquick):* Reconstitute with diluent provided. *(Humatrope):* Reconstitute with 1.5–5 mL diluent provided, swirl gently, do not shake. *(Humatrope Cartridge):* Dilute with solution provided with cartridge only. *(Nutropin):* Reconstitute each 5 mg with 1.5–5 mL diluent, swirl gently, do not shake. *(Omnitrope):* Reconstitute with diluents provided, swirl gently, do not shake. *(Saizen):* 5 mg: Reconstitute with 1–3 mL diluent provided, swirl gently, do not shake. 8.8 mg: Reconstitute with 2–3 mL diluent provided, swirl gently, do not shake. *(Serostim):* Reconstitute with Sterile Water for Injection. *(Zorbtive):* Reconstitute with 1–2 mL Bacteriostatic Water for Injection.

Storage • Long-term: Refrigerate all products except Zorbtive. Once reconstituted, Humatrope, Nutropin, Saizen, Zorbtive stable for 14 days, Genotropin for 21 days, Humatrope Cartridge for 28 days. *(Genotropin Miniquick):* Refrigerate, use within 24 hrs.

INDICATIONS/ROUTES/DOSAGE

Growth Hormone Deficiency

SQ: *(Genotropin, Omnitrope):* **ADULTS:** 0.04 mg/kg wkly divided into 6–7 equal doses/wk. May increase at 4- to 8-wk intervals to maximum of 0.08 mg/kg/wk. **CHILDREN:** 0.16–0.24 mg/kg wkly divided into equal doses 6 or 7 days/wk

SQ: *(Humatrope):* **ADULTS:** 0.006 mg/kg once daily. May increase to maximum of 0.0125 mg/kg/day. **CHILDREN:** 0.18–0.3 mg/kg wkly divided into alternate-day doses or 6 doses/wk.

SQ: *(Norditropin):* **ADULTS:** 0.004 mg/kg/day. May increase after 6 wks up to 0.016 mg/kg/day. **CHILDREN:** 0.17–0.24 mg/kg/wk divided into equal doses 6–7 days.wk.

SQ: *(Nutropin AQ):* **ADULTS:** 0.006 mg/kg once daily. May increase to maximum of 0.025 mg/kg/day (35 yrs or less) or 0.0125 mg/kg/day (older than 35 yrs). **CHILDREN:** 0.3 mg/kg wkly divided into equal daily doses.

SQ: *(Saizen):* **ADULTS:** 0.005 mg/kg/day. May increase up to 0.01 mg/kg/day after 4 wks. **CHILDREN:** 0.18 mg/kg/wk divided into equal daily doses 6–7 days/wk.

SQ: *(Zomacton):* **ADULTS:** 0.006 mg/kg/day. May increase up to 0.0125 mg/kg/day. **CHILDREN:** 0.18–0.3 mg/kg wkly divided into equal doses 6 or 7 days/wk.

Noonan Syndrome

SQ: *(Norditropin):* Up to 0.46 mg/kg wkly in equal doses 6–7 days/wk.

Chronic Renal Insufficiency

SQ: *(Nutropin, Nutropin AQ):* **CHILDREN:** 0.35 mg/kg wkly divided into equal daily doses. Continue until the time of renal transplantation.

Idiopathic Short Stature

SQ: *(Genotropin, Norditropin, Omnitrope):* Up to 0.47 mg/kg wkly divided into equal doses 6–7 times/wk. *(Humatrope):* Up to 0.37 mg wkly divided into equal doses 6–7 times/wk. *(Nutropin AQ):* Up to 0.3 mg/kg wkly divided into daily doses. *(Zomacton):* Up to 0.37 mg/kg wkly in equal doses 6–7 days/wk.

Turner's Syndrome

SQ: *(Humatrope, Nutropin AQ):* **CHILDREN:** 0.375 mg/kg wkly divided into equal doses 7 times/wk. *(Genotropin, Omnitrope):* 0.33 mg/kg wkly divided into 6–7 doses. *(Zomacton):* Up to 0.375 mg/kg/wk in equal doses 6–7 days/wk. *(Norditropin):* Up to 0.47 mg/kg/wk divided into equal dose 6–7 day/wk

S

AIDS-Related Wasting

SQ: *(Serostim):* **ADULTS WEIGHING MORE THAN 55 KG:** 6 mg once daily at bedtime. **ADULTS WEIGHING 45–55 KG:** 5 mg once daily at bedtime. **ADULTS WEIGHING 35–44 KG:** 4 mg once daily at bedtime. **ADULTS WEIGHING LESS THAN 35 KG:** 0.1 mg/kg once daily at bedtime.

Prader-Willi Syndrome

SQ: *(Genotropin, Omnitrope):* 0.24 mg/kg wkly divided into equal doses 6–7 times/wk.

Short Bowel Syndrome

SQ: *(Zorbtive):* **ADULTS:** 0.1 mg/kg/day for 4 wks. **Maximum:** 8 mg/day.

Dosage in Renal/Hepatic Impairment

No dose adjustment.

SIDE EFFECTS

Frequent: Otitis media, other ear disorders (with Turner's syndrome). **Occasional:** Carpal tunnel syndrome, gynecomastia, myalgia, peripheral edema, fatigue, asthenia. **Rare:** Rash, pruritus, visual changes, headache, nausea, vomiting, injection site pain/swelling, abdominal pain, hip/knee pain.

ADVERSE EFFECTS/TOXIC REACTIONS

May cause fluid retention, glucose tolerance, lipoatrophy. Intracranial hypertension may manifest as change of vision, headache, papilledema, nausea, vomiting. May increase risk of malignancy progression. Rapid growth may cause slipped capital femoral epiphyses. Hypersensitivity reactions including angioedema, anaphylaxis were reported.

NURSING CONSIDERATIONS

BASELINE ASSESSMENT

Obtain baseline lab chemistries, thyroid function, serum glucose, height, weight. Obtain full medical history (drug has multiple contraindications).

INTERVENTION/EVALUATION

Monitor bone growth, growth rate in relation to pt's age. Monitor serum calcium, glucose, phosphorus levels; renal, parathyroid, thyroid function. Observe for decreased muscle wasting in AIDS pts.

PATIENT/FAMILY TEACHING

• Follow correct procedure to reconstitute drug for administration and for safe handling/disposal of needles. • Regular follow-up with physician is important part of therapy. • Report development of severe headache, visual changes, pain in hip/knee, limping.

sonidegib

soe-ni-**deg**-ib
(Odomzo)

■ **BLACK BOX ALERT** ■ May cause embryo-fetal death/severe malformations when given during pregnancy. Verify pregnancy status before initiation. Female patients of reproductive potential must use effective contraception during treatment and for at least 20 mos after discontinuation. Due to the potential risk of exposure through semen, male patients must use condoms during sexual activity (even after a vasectomy) during treatment and for at least 8 mos after discontinuation. **Do not confuse sonidegib with vismodegib.**

◆CLASSIFICATION

PHARMACOTHERAPEUTIC: Hedgehog pathway inhibitor. **CLINICAL:** Antineoplastic.

USES

Treatment of adult pts with locally advanced basal cell carcinoma that has recurred following surgery or radiation therapy, or those who are not candidates for surgery or radiation.

PRECAUTIONS

Contraindications: Hypersensitivity to sonidegib. **Cautions:** Renal/hepatic impairment. Avoid concomitant use of strong or moderate CYP3A4 inhibitors, strong or moderate CYP3A4 inducers.

ACTION

Basal cell cancer is associated with mutation in Hedgehog pathway components, which can activate the pathway, causing nonrestrictive proliferation of skin basal cells. Binds to and inhibits smoothened homologue (SMO), the protein involved in Hedgehog signal transduction. **Therapeutic Effect:** Inhibits tumor cell growth and survival.

PHARMACOKINETICS

Poorly absorbed after PO administration (less than 10%). Metabolized in liver. Protein binding: greater than 97%. Peak plasma concentration: 2–4 hrs. Steady state reached in 4 mos. Excreted in feces (70%), urine (30%). **Half-life:** 28 days.

⌛ LIFESPAN CONSIDERATIONS

Pregnancy/Lactation: Avoid use; may cause fetal harm. Females of reproductive potential must use effective contraception during treatment and up to 20 mos after discontinuation. May impair fertility. **Males:** Males must use condoms during sexual activity (even after a vasectomy) during treatment and up to 8 mos after discontinuation. **Children:** Safety and efficacy not established. **Elderly:** May have increased risk of severe musculoskeletal adverse events (e.g., muscle spasms, myopathy).

INTERACTIONS

DRUG: Strong CYP3A4 inhibitors (e.g., clarithromycin, ketoconazole, ritonavir), moderate CYP3A4 inhibitors (e.g., dilTIAZem, fluconazole, verapamil) may increase concentration/effect. Strong CYP3A4 inducers (e.g., carBAMazepine, phenytoin, rifAMPin) may decrease concentration/effect. **HERBAL:** None significant. **FOOD:** High-fat meals may increase absorption/concentration. **LAB VALUES:** May increase serum ALT/AST, amylase, creatinine, CK, glucose, lipase. May decrease Hct, Hgb, lymphocytes.

AVAILABILITY (Rx)

Capsules: 200 mg.

ADMINISTRATION/HANDLING

PO
• Give on an empty stomach at least 1 hr before or 2 hrs after a meal.

INDICATIONS/ROUTES/DOSAGE

Basal Cell Carcinoma
PO: ADULTS, ELDERLY: 200 mg once daily. Continue until disease progression or unacceptable toxicity.

Dose Modification
Interrupt therapy for severe or intolerable musculoskeletal adverse reactions; first occurrence of serum CK level 2.5–10 times upper limit of normal (ULN); recurrent serum CK level 2.5–5 times ULN. Once resolved, resume at 200 mg once daily.

Discontinuation
Permanently discontinue for serum CK level greater than 2.5 times ULN with worsening renal function; serum CK level greater than 10 times ULN; recurrent serum CK level greater than 5 times ULN; recurrent severe or intolerable musculoskeletal adverse reactions.

Dosage in Renal Impairment
No dose adjustment.

Dosage in Hepatic Impairment
Mild impairment: No dose adjustment. **Moderate to severe impairment:** Not studied; use caution.

SIDE EFFECTS

Frequent (54%–23%): Muscle spasm, alopecia, dysgeusia, fatigue, nausea, diarrhea, musculoskeletal pain, decreased appetite. **Occasional (19%–10%):** Myalgia, abdominal pain, headache, generalized pain, vomiting, pruritus.

ADVERSE EFFECTS/TOXIC REACTIONS

Musculoskeletal events occurred in 68% of pts. Grade 3 or 4 musculoskeletal events (9% of pts) may require administration of muscle relaxants, analgesics/narcotics, magnesium supplementation, IV hydration. Serum CK level elevations

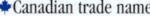 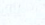

usually occur before musculoskeletal pain or spasms. Increased serum CK levels reported in 61% of pts. The median onset of serum CK elevation was approx. 12 wks. May increase risk of rhabdomyolysis. Amenorrhea lasting longer than 18 mos has occurred.

NURSING CONSIDERATIONS

BASELINE ASSESSMENT

Obtain CBC, BMP, LFT; pregnancy test in females of reproductive potential. Receive medication history and screen for interactions. Assess hydration status. Offer emotional support.

INTERVENTION/EVALUATION

Monitor renal function, serum CK levels periodically and with any musculoskeletal adverse events. If musculoskeletal adverse reactions occur with serum CK levels greater than 2.5 times ULN, obtain serum CK level at least wkly until resolution. Monitor urine color, output. Serum CK level elevation or worsening of renal function may indicate rhabdomyolysis. Monitor pregnancy status during therapy.

PATIENT/FAMILY TEACHING

• Treatment may cause severe muscle damage, which may cause kidney damage. • Report dark-colored urine or decreased urine output despite hydration. • Immediately report musculoskeletal symptoms such as muscle pain/spasms/tenderness/weakness. • Do not donate blood or blood products during treatment and up to 20 mos after discontinuation. • Use effective contraception to avoid pregnancy. Do not breastfeed. • Take on empty stomach at least 1 hr before or 2 hrs after a meal.

SORAfenib

soe-**raf**-e-nib
(NexAVAR)
Do not confuse NexAVAR with NexIUM, or SORAfenib with imatinib or SUNItinib.

◆**CLASSIFICATION**

PHARMACOTHERAPEUTIC: Vascular endothelial growth factor (VEGF) inhibitor. Tyrosine kinase inhibitor. **CLINICAL:** Antineoplastic.

USES

Renal cell carcinoma (RCC): Treatment of advanced RCC. **Hepatocellular carcinoma (HCC):** Treatment of unresectable HCC. **Differentiated thyroid carcinoma (DTC):** Treatment of locally recurrent or metastatic progressive differentiated thyroid carcinoma (DTC) refractory to radioactive iodine treatment. **OFF-LABEL:** Recurrent or metastatic angiosarcoma, resistant gastrointestinal stromal tumor.

PRECAUTIONS

Contraindications: Hypersensitivity to SORAfenib. Use in combination with CARBOplatin and PACLitaxel in pts with squamous cell lung cancer. **Cautions:** Uncontrolled hypertension, pulmonary disease, pts at risk for GI perforation (e.g., Crohn's disease, diverticulitis, GI tract malignancies, peptic ulcers, peritoneal malignancies), pts at risk for QTc interval prolongation (congenital long QT syndrome, HF, medications that prolong QTc interval, hypokalemia, hypomagnesemia), pts at risk for bleeding (e.g., history of intracranial/GI/genitourinary bleeding, coagulation disorders, recent trauma, concomitant use of anticoagulants, antiplatelets); unstable coronary artery disease, recent MI, HF, concurrent use with strong CYP3A4 inducers.

ACTION

Inhibits tumor cell proliferation by inhibiting intracellular Raf kinases and cell surface kinase receptors. **Therapeutic Effect:** Inhibits tumor growth and survival.

PHARMACOKINETICS

Metabolized in liver. Protein binding: 99.5%. Excreted in feces (77%), urine (19%). **Half-life:** 25–48 hrs.

⧗ LIFESPAN CONSIDERATIONS

Pregnancy/Lactation: Avoid use; may cause fetal harm. Females of reproductive

---

potential should use effective contraception during treatment and for at least 6 mos after discontinuation. Breastfeeding not recommended during treatment and for at least 2 wks after discontinuation. **Males:** Males with female partners of reproductive potential should use effective contraception during treatment and for at least 3 mos after discontinuation. May impair fertility. **Children:** Safety and efficacy not established. **Elderly:** No age-related precautions noted.

INTERACTIONS

DRUG: **Strong CYP3A4 inducers (e.g., carBAMazepine, PHENobarbital, rifAMPin)** may decrease concentration/effect. **QT interval–prolonging medications (e.g., amiodarone, azithromycin, ceritinib, haloperidol, moxifloxacin)** may increase risk of QT interval prolongation, cardiac arrhythmias. May increase anticoagulant effect of **warfarin.** **HERBAL:** None significant. **FOOD:** **High-fat meals** decrease effectiveness. **LAB VALUES:** May increase serum lipase, amylase, bilirubin, alkaline phosphatase, transaminases. May decrease serum phosphorus, lymphocytes, WBCs, Hgb, Hct.

AVAILABILITY (Rx)

 Tablets: 200 mg.

ADMINISTRATION/HANDLING

PO
• Give 1 hr before or 2 hrs after meal (high-fat meal reduces effectiveness). • Swallow tablet whole; do not break, crush, dissolve, or divide tablet.

INDICATIONS/ROUTES/DOSAGE

Renal Cell Carcinoma, Hepatocellular Carcinoma, Thyroid Carcinoma
PO: **ADULTS, ELDERLY:** 400 mg (2 tablets) twice daily without food. Continue until disease progression or unacceptable toxicity.

Dose Reduction Schedule
HCC/RCC: FIRST DOSE REDUCTION: 400 mg once daily. SECOND DOSE REDUCTION: 200 mg once daily or 400 mg every other day. **DTC:** FIRST DOSE REDUCTION: 400 mg once in the morning and 200 mg once

at night (12 hrs apart). SECOND DOSE REDUCTION: 200 mg twice daily. THIRD DOSE REDUCTION: 200 mg once daily

Dose Modification
Based on Common Terminology Criteria for Adverse Events (CTCAE).

Cardiac Toxicity
Grade 3 congestive HF: Withhold treatment until improved to Grade 1 or 0, then resume at reduced dose level. Permanently discontinue for Grade 3 congestive HF that does not improve within 30 days; Grade 4 congestive HF; Grade 2 or greater cardiac ischemia/infarction.

Dermatologic Toxicity
Note: If improved to Grade 1 or 0 from Grade 2 or 3 toxicity for at least 28 days, may increase dose by one dose level.
HCC/RCC: GRADE 2 TOXICITY: (First occurrence): Continue same dose and start topical therapy. (Not improved within 7 days; second or third occurrence): Withhold treatment until improved to Grade 1 or 0, then resume at reduced dose level. (Fourth occurrence): Permanently discontinue. GRADE 3 TOXICITY: (First or second occurrence): Withhold treatment until improved to Grade 1 or 0, then resume at reduced dose level. (Third occurrence): Permanently discontinue. DTC: GRADE 2 TOXICITY: (First occurrence): Reduce dose to 600 mg once daily. (Not improved within 7 days; second or third occurrence): Withhold treatment until improved to Grade 1, then reduce dose by one dose level (for second occurrence) or by two dose levels (for third occurrence). (Fourth occurrence): Permanently discontinue. GRADE 3 TOXICITY: (First occurrence): Withhold treatment until improved to Grade 1, then resume at reduced dose level. (Second occurrence): Withhold treatment until improved to Grade 1, then reduce dose by two dose levels. (Third occurrence): Permanently discontinue.

S

 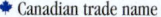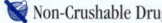

Hypertension

Grade 2 (symptomatic/persistent) hypertension; Grade 2 symptomatic increase greater than 20 mm Hg (diastolic); B/P greater than 140/90 mm Hg if previously within normal limits; Grade 3 hypertension: Withhold treatment until symptoms resolve and diastolic B/P is less than 90 mm Hg, then resume at reduced dose level. May further reduce if needed. **Grade 4 hypertension; more than 2 dose reductions are required:** Permanently discontinue.

Nonhematologic Toxicity

Any Grade 2 toxicity: Reduce dose by one dose level. **Any Grade 3 toxicity:** (FIRST OCCURRENCE): Withhold treatment until Grade 2 or less, then resume at reduced dose level. **(Not improved within 7 days; second or third occurrence):** Withhold treatment until Grade 2 or less, then reduce dose by two dose levels. (FOURTH OCCURRENCE): Withhold treatment until Grade 2 or less, then reduce dose by two dose levels for HCC and RCC, or 3 dose levels for DTC.

QT Interval Prolongation

QT interval greater than 500 msec; increase of 60 msec or greater from baseline: Withhold treatment and correct electrolyte abnormalities. May restart based on clinical judgment.

Permanent Discontinuation

Grade 2 or greater hemorrhage requiring medical intervention; any grade GI perforation; Grade 3 or 4 serum ALT elevation; serum ALT/ALT elevation greater than 3 times ULN with serum bilirubin 2 times ULN.

Dosage in Renal Impairment

No dose adjustment.

Dosage in Hepatic Impairment

Mild to moderate impairment: No dose adjustment. **Severe impairment:** Not specified.

SIDE EFFECTS

Frequent (43%–16%): Diarrhea, rash, fatigue, exfoliative dermatitis, alopecia, nausea, pruritus, hypertension, anorexia, vomiting. **Occasional (15%–10%):** Constipation, minor bleeding, dyspnea, sensory neuropathy, cough, abdominal pain, dry skin, weight loss, joint pain, headache. **Rare (9%–1%):** Acne, flushing, stomatitis, mucositis, dyspepsia, arthralgia, myalgia, hoarseness.

ADVERSE EFFECTS/TOXIC REACTIONS

Myelosuppression (anemia, leukopenia, neutropenia, thrombocytopenia) is an expected response to the therapy. Cardiac ischemia/MI reported in 3% of pts. Fatal hemorrhage (esophageal hemorrhage, bleeding from any site) was reported. Life-threatening cutaneous toxicities including Stevens-Johnson syndrome, toxic epidermal necrolysis, hand-foot skin reactions may occur. GI perforation reported in less than 1% of pts. May impair healing of wounds. An increased risk of mortality was reported in pts receiving other chemotherapeutic agents. May cause QT interval prolongation, thyroid-stimulating hormone (TSH) suppression, hepatotoxicity, neuropathy, intracranial hemorrhage, interstitial lung disease, pneumonitis, thrombotic microangiopathy, osteonecrosis of the jaw; arterial aneurysms, dissections, rupture.

NURSING CONSIDERATIONS

BASELINE ASSESSMENT

Obtain CBC, BMP, LFT, TSH, B/P; pregnancy test in females of reproductive potential. Screen for active infection. Question history as listed in Precautions. Receive full medication history and screen for interactions. Conduct dermatologic exam. Assess for poorly healed wounds/recent surgical wounds. Assess risk for QT interval prolongation. Offer emotional support.

INTERVENTION/EVALUATION

Monitor CBC, serum electrolytes, ECG; TSH (if applicable), LFT for hepatic injury (abdominal pain, jaundice, nausea, transaminitis, vomiting). Monitor B/P frequently. Diligently assess skin for cutaneous toxicities, impaired wound healing. Monitor for cardiac ischemia/infarction (chest pain, diaphoresis, left arm or jaw pain, ST segment elevation, serum troponin elevation), GI perforation (abdominal pain, fever, nausea, vomiting), infection (cough, fatigue, fever); neuropathy (gait disturbance, fine motor control difficulties, numbness); hypersensitivity reactions (anaphylaxis, urticaria), bleeding of any kind.

PATIENT/FAMILY TEACHING

• Treatment may depress your immune system response and reduce your ability to fight infection. Report symptoms of infection such as body aches, chills, cough, fatigue, fever. Avoid those with active infection. • Report symptoms of bone marrow depression (e.g., bruising, fatigue, fever, shortness of breath, weight loss; bleeding easily, bloody urine or stool). • Report symptoms of lung inflammation (excessive coughing, difficulty breathing, chest pain); liver problems (abdominal pain, bruising, clay-colored stool, dark or amber-colored urine, yellowing of the skin or eyes), toxic skin reactions (rash, redness, sloughing, swelling). • Life-threatening cardiac events may occur; report symptoms of heart attack (chest pain, difficulty breathing, jaw pain, nausea, pain that radiates to the arm or jaw, sweating). • Treatment may affect the heart's ability to pump blood or alter the electrical conduction of the heart, which may lead to HF, cardiac arrhythmias; report chest pain, difficulty breathing, dizziness, swelling of extremities, fainting, palpitations. • Bleeding of any kind can be life-threatening • Use effective contraception to avoid pregnancy. Do not breastfeed. • Do not take newly prescribed medications unless approved by prescriber who originally started treatment. • Treatment may worsen high blood pressure. • Immediately report severe or persistent abdominal pain, bloody stool, fever, vomiting blood; may indicate rupture in GI tract.

---

sotagliflozin

soe-ta-gli-**floe**-zin
(Inpefa)
Do not confuse sotagliflozin with bexagliflozin, canagliflozin, dapagliflozin, empagliflozin, or ertugliflozin.

◆CLASSIFICATION

PHARMACOTHERAPEUTIC: Sodium-glucose co-transporter 2 (SGLT2) inhibitor. **CLINICAL:** Cardiovascular agent.

USES

To reduce the risk of cardiovascular death; hospitalization for HF; and urgent HF visits in adults with HF or type 2 diabetes mellitus, chronic kidney disease, and other cardiovascular risk factors.

PRECAUTIONS

Contraindications: Hypersensitivity to sotagliflozin. **Cautions:** Hypovolemia/dehydration, elderly, pts at risk for lower leg amputation (diabetic foot ulcers, peripheral vascular disease); recent genital mycotic infection; pts at risk for diabetic ketoacidosis (insulin dose reduction, acute febrile illness, reduced calorie intake, surgery, alcohol abuse). Concomitant use of loop diuretics, other hypoglycemic agents (e.g., insulin, insulin secretagogues). Not recommended in pts with diabetic ketoacidosis, type 1 diabetes mellitus, moderate to severe hepatic impairment.

ACTION

Inhibits SGLT2 in proximal renal tubule, reducing reabsorption of filtered glucose and sodium, increasing delivery of sodium to the distal tubule. Inhibits SCLT1, reducing intestinal absorption of glucose and sodium. **Therapeutic Effect:** Reduces cardiac preload and afterload; downregulates sympathetic activity.

PHARMACOKINETICS

Widely distributed. Metabolized in liver. Protein binding: greater than 93%. Peak plasma concentration: 2.5–4 hrs. Excreted in urine (57%), feces (37%). **Half-life:** 21–35 hrs

S

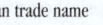 Canadian trade name   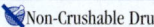 Non-Crushable Drug   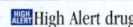 High Alert drug

⌛ LIFESPAN CONSIDERATIONS

Pregnancy/Lactation: Not recommended during second or third trimester. Unknown if distributed in breast milk. Breastfeeding not recommended. **Children:** Safety and efficacy not established. **Elderly:** May have increased risk for dehydration, hypotension, syncope related to volume depletion.

INTERACTIONS

DRUG: Insulin, insulin secretagogues (e.g., glyBURIDE) may increase risk of hypoglycemia. **UGT enzyme inducers** (e.g., carBAMazepine, lamoTRIgine, phenytoin, ritonavir) may decrease concentration/effect. **Loop diuretics** (e.g., furosemide) may increase risk of volume depletion and symptomatic hypotension. May decrease concentration/effect of lithium. May increase concentration/effect of digoxin. **HERBAL:** Herbals with hypoglycemic properties (e.g., fenugreek, flaxseed, ginseng, gotu kola) may increase risk of hypoglycemia. **FOOD:** None known. **LAB VALUES:** May decrease eGFR; serum creatinine. May interfere with 1,5-anhydrogluitol (1,5-AG) assay.

AVAILABILITY (Rx)

Tablets: 200 mg, 400 mg.

ADMINISTRATION/HANDLING

PO
• Give not more than 1 hr before the first meal of the day. • Administer tablet whole; do not break, cut, or crush. Tablet cannot be chewed. • If a dose is missed by more than 6 hrs, skip the dose and take the next dose at the regularly scheduled time. • If possible, withhold treatment for at least 3 days prior to surgery or procedures requiring NPO status. May resume treatment when oral intake is allowed and pt is clinically stable.

INDICATIONS/ROUTES/DOSAGE

Heart Failure (Risk Reduction)
PO: ADULTS, ELDERLY: Initially, 200 mg once daily for at least 2 wks, then increase to 400 mg once daily if tolerated.

Dosage in Renal Impairment
Note: During efficacy and safety studies, treatment was discontinued if eGFR fell below 15 mL/min. **eGFR 25–60 mL/min:** No dose adjustment. **eGFR less than 25 mL/min; pts on dialysis:** Not specified.

Dosage in Hepatic Impairment
Mild impairment: No dose adjustment. **Moderate to severe impairment:** Not recommended.

SIDE EFFECTS

Occasional (8%–7%): Diarrhea, hypoglycemia. **Rare (3%):** Dizziness.

ADVERSE EFFECTS/TOXIC REACTIONS

Symptomatic hypotension (orthostatic hypotension, postural dizziness, syncope) may occur, esp. in pts who are elderly, use concomitant loop diuretics, or have baseline systolic hypotension. Intravascular volume depletion may cause hypotension, syncope; acute kidney injury requiring dialysis. Hypoglycemic events were reported, esp. in pts using concomitant hypoglycemic medications. Fatal cases of ketoacidosis were reported. Infections including urosepsis, pyelonephritis, UTI, genital myocotic infections (male and female), upper respiratory tract infection may occur. May increase risk of lower limb amputations. Necrotizing fasciitis of the perineum (Fournier's gangrene), a life-threatening necrotizing infection of the genital and perineum region that requires urgent surgical intervention, has been reported. Hypersensitivity reactions including anaphylaxis, angioedema, urticaria were reported with other SGLT2 inhibitors.

NURSING CONSIDERATIONS

BASELINE ASSESSMENT

Obtain BUN, serum creatinine, eGFR, CrCl, B/P. Assess hydration status. Correct volume depletion prior to initiation.

Educate importance of maintaining a heart-healthy diet. Question history of renal/hepatic impairment, type 1 diabetes, ketoacidosis. Consider suspending treatment at least 3 days prior to any procedure requiring NPO status. Receive full medication history and screen for interactions. Screen for risks of lower limb amputation (e.g., peripheral vascular disease, diabetic foot ulcers). For pts with decompensated HF, treatment may begin when the pt is hemodynamically stable, including urgent outpatient treatment, during hospitalization, or immediately upon discharge from hospital.

INTERVENTION/EVALUATION

Monitor BUN, serum creatinine, eGFR, CrCl, B/P periodically. Monitor for hypoglycemia (anxiety, confusion, diaphoresis, diplopia, dizziness, headache, hunger, perioral numbness, tachycardia, tremors), hyperglycemia (fatigue, Kussmaul respirations, polyphagia, polyuria, polydipsia, nausea, vomiting), ketoacidosis (e.g., dehydration, confusion, extreme thirst, sweet-smelling breath, Kussmaul respirations, nausea). Pts presenting with metabolic acidosis should be screened for ketoacidosis, regardless of serum glucose levels. Concomitant use of beta blockers (e.g., carvedilol, metoprolol) may mask symptoms of hypoglycemia. Monitor for acute kidney injury (dark-colored urine, flank pain, decreased urine output, muscle aches), infections (cough, fatigue, fever), UTI (dysuria, fever, flank pain, malaise), mycotic infections, Fournier's gangrene (perineal necrosis). Screen for glucose-altering conditions: Fever, stress, surgical procedures, trauma. Monitor for hypersensitivity reactions (anaphylaxis, angioedema, urticaria). Encourage fluid intake. Monitor I&Os.

PATIENT/FAMILY TEACHING

• Eat a heart-healthy diet and limit intake of dietary sodium. • When taking combination blood sugar–lowering drug therapy or when glucose conditions are altered

(e.g., excessive alcohol ingestion, insufficient carbohydrate intake, hormone deficiencies, critical illness), have a low blood sugar treatment available (e.g., glucagon, oral dextrose). • Therapy may increase risk for dehydration and low blood pressure, which may cause low blood pressure, passing out, or kidney failure. Report decreased urination, amber-colored urine, flank pain, fatigue, swelling of the hands or feet. Drink enough fluids to maintain adequate hydration without exacerbating fluid overload. • Genital itching or discharge may indicate yeast infection. • Report symptoms of perineal necrosis (e.g., discoloration, pain, swelling of the scrotum, penis, or perineum). • Report symptoms of UTI, kidney infection (back pain, pelvic pain, burning while urinating, cloudy or foul-smelling urine). • Go slowly from lying to standing. • Do not breastfeed. • Treatment may need to be suspended 3 days before any procedure that requires no oral intake. • Allergic reactions such as anaphylaxis, hives; swelling of the face, lips, or tongue require immediate medical attention.

---

sotalol   HIGH ALERT

soe-ta-lol
(Betapace, Betapace AF, Sorine, Sotylize)

■ **BLACK BOX ALERT** ■ Initiation, titration to occur in a hospital setting with continuous ECG to monitor potential onset of life-threatening arrhythmias. Calculate CrCl prior to dosing. Adjust dose based on CrCl. Betapace should not be substituted for Betapace AF.
Do not confuse Betapace with Betapace AF, or sotalol with Stadol or Sudafed.

◆**CLASSIFICATION**

PHARMACOTHERAPEUTIC: Nonselective beta-adrenergic blocking agent.
CLINICAL: Antiarrhythmic Class II, Class III.

USES

Treatment of documented, life-threatening ventricular arrhythmias in ages 3 days and older and adults. Maintenance of normal sinus rhythm in adults and children aged 3 days and older with symptomatic atrial fibrillation/flutter who are currently in sinus rhythm. OFF-LABEL: Fetal tachycardia, treatment of supraventricular tachycardia.

PRECAUTIONS

Contraindications: Hypersensitivity to sotalol. Cardiogenic shock, congenital or acquired long QT syndrome, second- or third-degree heart block (unless functioning pacemaker is present), sinus bradycardia, uncontrolled HF, bronchial asthma or related bronchospastic conditions. Baseline QT interval greater than 450 msec, bronchospastic conditions, CrCl less than 40 mL/min, serum potassium less than 4 mEq/L, sick sinus syndrome. **Cautions:** Pts with history of ventricular tachycardia, ventricular fibrillation, cardiomegaly, compensated HF, diabetes mellitus, QT interval prolongation, concurrent medications that prolong QT interval, hypokalemia, hypomagnesemia, renal impairment, within first 2 wks post MI, peripheral vascular disease, Raynaud's syndrome, myasthenia gravis, psychiatric disease, bronchospastic disease. Concurrent use of digoxin, verapamil, dilTIAZem, history of severe anaphylaxis to allergens.

ACTION

Class II effects: Increases sinus cycle length, AV nodal refractoriness; decreases AV nodal conduction; slows heart rate. **Class III effects:** Prolongs atrial/ventricular action potentials, inducing effective refractory prolongation of atrial/ventricular muscle and atrial/ventricular accessory pathways. **Therapeutic Effect:** Produces antiarrhythmic activity.

PHARMACOKINETICS

Route	Onset	Peak	Duration
PO	1–2 hrs	2.5–4 hrs	8–16 hrs

Widely distributed. Primarily excreted unchanged in urine. Removed by hemodialysis. **Half-life:** 12 hrs (increased in elderly, renal impairment).

⧗ LIFESPAN CONSIDERATIONS

Pregnancy/Lactation: Crosses placenta. Distributed in breast milk. **Children:** Safety and efficacy not established in pts younger than 3 days. **Elderly:** Age-related peripheral vascular disease may increase susceptibility to decreased peripheral circulation. Age-related renal impairment may require dosage adjustment.

INTERACTIONS

DRUG: Strong CYP34A inhibitors (e.g., clarithromycin, ketoconazole, ritonavir) may increase concentration/effect. May mask symptoms of hypoglycemia, prolong hypoglycemic effects of **insulin, oral hypoglycemics (e.g., glipiZIDE, metFORMIN)**. QT-prolonging medications **(e.g., amiodarone, ciprofloxacin, fingolimod, haloperidol, ondansetron)** may increase risk of prolonged QT interval **Antacids** may decrease concentration/effect. **HERBAL: Herbals with hypotensive properties (e.g., garlic, ginger, ginkgo biloba)** may alter effects. **FOOD:** None known. **LAB VALUES:** May increase serum BUN, glucose, alkaline phosphatase, LDH, lipoprotein, ALT, AST, triglycerides, potassium, uric acid.

AVAILABILITY (Rx)

Solution, Intravenous: 150 mg/10 mL. **Solution, Oral:** 5 mg/mL. **Tablets:** 80 mg, 120 mg, 160 mg, 240 mg.

ADMINISTRATION/HANDLING

PO
• Give without regard to food. • Do not administer antacids within 2 hrs after dose.

INDICATIONS/ROUTES/DOSAGE

Note: Baseline QTc interval and CrCl must be determined before initiation.
Atrial Fibrillation/Flutter (Symptomatic)
Note: Initiation in pts with QTc interval greater than 450 msec is contraindicated.

PO: **ADULTS, ELDERLY:** Initially, 80 mg twice daily. May increase in increments of 80 mg/day q3days (if QTc interval is less than 500 msec). **Usual dose:** 120 mg twice daily. **Maximum:** 160 mg twice daily. **CHILDREN 2 YRS AND OLDER:** Initially, 1.2 mg/kg 3 times/day (3.6 mg/kg total daily dose). May titrate in at least 36-hr intervals to maximum of 2.4 mg/kg 3 times/day.

Ventricular Arrhythmias

PO: **ADULTS, ELDERLY:** Initially, 80 mg twice daily. May increase in increments of 80 mg/day q3days (if QTc interval is less than 500 msec). **Usual dose:** 160–320 mg/day in 2–3 divided doses. **CHILDREN 2 YRS AND OLDER:** Initially, 1.2 mg/kg 3 times/day (3.6 mg/kg total daily dose) May titrate in at least 36-hr intervals to maximum of 2.4 mg/kg 3 times a day.

Dosage in Renal Impairment

Dosage interval is modified based on creatinine clearance.

Atrial Fibrillation/Flutter

Creatinine Clearance	Dosage
Greater than 60 mL/min	12 hrs
40–60 mL/min	24 hrs
Less than 40 mL/min	Contraindicated

Ventricular Arrhythmias

Creatinine Clearance	Dosage
Greater than 60 mL/min	12 hrs
30–60 mL/min	24 hrs
10–29 mL/min	q36–48h

Dosage in Hepatic Impairment

No dose adjustment.

SIDE EFFECTS

Frequent: Diminished sexual function, drowsiness, insomnia, asthenia. **Occasional:** Depression, cold hands/feet, diarrhea, constipation, anxiety, nasal congestion, nausea, vomiting. **Rare:** Altered taste, dry eyes, pruritus, paresthesia of fingers, toes, scalp.

ADVERSE EFFECTS/TOXIC REACTIONS

Bradycardia, HF, hypotension, bronchospasm, hypoglycemia, prolonged QT interval, torsades de pointes, ventricular tachycardia, premature ventricular complexes may occur.

NURSING CONSIDERATIONS

BASELINE ASSESSMENT

QTc interval and CrCl must be determined prior to initiation. Pt must be on continuous cardiac monitoring upon initiation of therapy. Do not administer without consulting physician if pulse is 60 beats/min or less. Question medical history as listed in Precautions.

INTERVENTION/EVALUATION

Diligently monitor for arrhythmias. Assess B/P for hypotension, pulse for bradycardia. Assess for HF: Dyspnea, peripheral edema, jugular vein distention, increased weight, rales in lungs, decreased urinary output.

PATIENT/FAMILY TEACHING

• Do not discontinue, change dose without physician approval. • Avoid tasks requiring alertness, motor skills until response to drug is established (may cause drowsiness). • Periodic lab tests, ECGs are essential part of therapy. • Report rapid heartbeat, chest pain, swelling of ankles/legs, difficulty breathing.

sotorasib

soe-toe-**ras**-ib
(Lumakras)
Do not confuse sotorasib with sonidegib, sorafenib, sotalol, or sunitinib.

CLASSIFICATION

PHARMACOTHERAPEUTIC: KRAS inhibitor. **CLINICAL:** Antineoplastic.

USES

Treatment of adults with *KRAS G12C* mutated, locally advanced or metastatic non–small-cell lung cancer (NSCLC) who have received at least 1 prior systemic therapy.

PRECAUTIONS

Contraindications: Hypersensitivity to sotorasib. **Cautions:** Baseline cytopenias; history of hepatic impairment, interstitial lung disease (e.g., COPD, sarcoidosis, connective disease disease). Avoid concomitant use of strong CYP3A4 inducers, acid-reducing agents (e.g., proton pump inhibitors, H$_2$ antagonist, local antacids).

ACTION

Inhibits KRAS G12C (a tumor-restricted, mutant oncogenic form of KRAS) by forming an irreversible bond with KRAS G12C preventing downstream signaling without affecting wild-type KRAS. **Therapeutic Effect:** Blocks KRAS signaling, inhibits cell growth, promotes apoptosis in KRAS G12C cell lines only.

PHARMACOKINETICS

Widely distributed. Metabolized in liver. Protein binding: 89%. Peak plasma concentration: 1 hr. Steady state reached in 22 days. Excreted in feces (74%), urine (6%). **Half-life:** 5 hrs.

⌛ LIFESPAN CONSIDERATIONS

Pregnancy/Lactation: Unknown if distributed in breast milk. Breastfeeding not recommended during treatment and for at least 1 wk after discontinuation. **Children:** Safety and efficacy not established. **Elderly:** No age-related precautions noted.

INTERACTIONS

DRUG: Aluminum-, magnesium-, calcium-containing antacids, H$_2$ receptor antagonists (e.g., famotidine), proton pump inhibitors (e.g., omeprazole, pantoprazole), strong CYP3A4 inducers (e.g., carBAMazepine, phenytoin, rifAMPin) may decrease concentration/effect. May decrease concentration/effects of axitinib, bosutinib, encorafenib, finerenone, neratinib, olaparib vorapaxar, zanubrutinib. **HERBAL:** None significant. **FOOD:** None known. **LAB VALUES:** May increase serum alkaline phosphatase, ALT, AST; urine protein. May decrease Hgb, lymphocytes; serum albumin, calcium, sodium. May prolong activated partial thromboplastin time (aPPT).

AVAILABILITY (Rx)

Tablets: 120 mg, 240 mg, 320 mg.

ADMINISTRATION/HANDLING

PO

• Give without regard to food. • Administer tablet whole; do not break, cut, or crush. Tablets cannot be chewed. • If a dose is missed by more than 6 hrs, skip the dose and give at next regularly scheduled time. Do not give 2 doses at the same time to make up for a missed dose. • If vomiting occurs after administration, give the next dose at regularly scheduled time (do not give additional dose). • May disperse tablet into 120 mL (4 oz.) of noncarbonated water. Mix until small pieces are present (tablet will not completely dissolve) and administer within 2 hrs. Small pieces of tablet cannot be chewed. Rinse container with additional 120 mL of water and administer to ensure full dose was delivered. • Do not give 4 hrs before or 10 hrs after an acid-reducing agent.

INDICATIONS/ROUTES/DOSAGE

NSCLC (Locally Advanced or Metastatic)

PO: ADULTS: 960 mg once daily until disease progression or unacceptable toxicity.

Dose Reduction Schedule

First Reduction: 480 mg once daily. **Second Reduction:** 240 mg once daily. **Unable to Tolerate 240-mg Dose:** Permanently discontinue.

Dose Modification

Based on Common Terminology Criteria for Adverse Events (CTCAE).

Hepatotoxicity
Symptomatic Grade 2 Serum ALT/ AST Elevation; Grade 3 or 4 ALT/ AST Elevation: Withhold treatment until improved to Grade 1 or baseline, then resume at next lower dose level. Permanently discontinue if Grade 3 or 4 hepatotoxicity recurs. **Permanent Discontinuation:** Discontinue treatment for serum ALT/AST greater than 3 times upper limit of normal (ULN) with total bilirubin greater than 2 times ULN (not attributed to other causes).

Pulmonary Toxicity
Any Grade ILD/Pneumonitis: Withhold treatment if ILD/pneumonitis is suspected. Permanently discontinue if ILD/ pneumonitis is confirmed.

GI Toxicity
Grade 3 or 4 Nausea, Vomiting, or Diarrhea (Despite Supportive Therapy): Withhold treatment until improved to Grade 1 or baseline, then resume at next lower dose level.

Other Adverse Reactions
Any Other Grade 3 or 4 Reaction: Withhold treatment until improved to Grade 1 or baseline, then resume at next lower dose level.

Dosage in Renal Impairment
Mild to moderate impairment: No dose adjustment. **Severe impairment:** Not specified.

Dosage in Hepatic Impairment
Mild impairment: No dose adjustment. **Moderate to severe impairment:** Not specified.

SIDE EFFECTS

Frequent (42%–26%): Diarrhea, musculoskeletal pain, myalgia, fatigue, asthenia, nausea. **Occasional (20%–12%):** Cough, vomiting, constipation, dyspnea, abdominal pain, edema, arthralgia, decreased appetite, rash, dermatitis.

ADVERSE EFFECTS/TOXIC REACTIONS

Anemia, lymphopenia are expected responses to therapy. Serum ALT, AST elevation reported in 18% of pts. Hepatotoxicity may lead to liver injury and hepatitis. Life-threatening ILD/pneumonitis reported in 1% of pts. Pneumonia reported in 8% of pts.

NURSING CONSIDERATIONS

BASELINE ASSESSMENT
Obtain CBC, BMP, LFT; pregnancy test in females of reproductive potential. Verify presence of *KRAS G12C* mutation in plasma or tumor specimens. Question history of hepatic impairment, pulmonary disease. Screen for active infection. Receive full medication history and screen for interactions. Offer emotional support.

INTERVENTION/EVALUATION
Monitor LFT for hepatotoxicity (bruising, jaundice, right upper abdominal pain, nausea, vomiting, weight loss) q3wks for 3 mos, then monthly thereafter (or more frequently if hepatotoxicity occurs). Monitor for infections (cough, fatigue, fever). Consider ABG, radiologic test if pneumonitis (excessive cough, dyspnea, fever, hypoxia) is suspected. Consider treatment with corticosteroids if pneumonitis is confirmed. Assess skin for rash. Monitor daily pattern of bowel activity, stool consistency. GI side effects may require antiemetics, antidiarrheal agents. Ensure proper hydration.

PATIENT/FAMILY TEACHING
• Report symptoms of infection such as body aches, chills, cough, fatigue, fever. • Do not take 4 hrs before or 10 hrs after ingesting antacid medication. • Report liver problems (abdominal pain, bruising, clay-colored stool, amber or dark-colored urine, yellowing of the skin or eyes), inflammation of the lung (excessive cough, difficulty breathing, chest pain), rash. • There is a high risk of interactions with other medications. Do not take newly prescribed medications unless approved by prescriber who originally started therapy. • Treatment may cause diarrhea, nausea, and vomiting, which may require supportive care. Report worsening of GI symptoms or dehydration. Drink plenty of fluids.

 Canadian trade name   Non-Crushable Drug   High Alert drug

spironolactone

spir-**on**-oh-**lak**-tone
(Aldactone, CaroSpir)
Do not confuse Aldactone with Aldactazide.

FIXED-COMBINATION(S)
♦CLASSIFICATION

PHARMACOTHERAPEUTIC: Aldosterone receptor antagonist. **CLINICAL:** Potassium-sparing diuretic, antihypertensive.

USES

Ascites: Management of edema in cirrhotic pts when edema is unresponsive to fluid and sodium restriction. **HF with reduced ejection fraction:** Heart failure (NYHA class III–IV and reduced ejection fraction) to increase survival, manage edema, and to reduce need for hospitalization for HF. **Hypertension:** Management of hypertension (unresponsive to other therapies). **Primary hyperaldosteronism:** Treatment of primary hyperaldosteronism. Short-term preoperative treatment. Long-term maintenance therapy for pts with discrete aldosterone-producing adrenal adenomas who are not candidates for surgery. Long-term treatment for bilateral micro- or macronodular adrenal hyperplasia. **OFF-LABEL:**Female acne, female hirsutism. Hair loss (female pattern).

PRECAUTIONS

Contraindications: Hypersensitivity to spironolactone. Hyperkalemia, Addison's disease, concomitant use with eplerenone. **Cautions:** Dehydration, hyponatremia, concurrent use of supplemental potassium, elderly. Mild renal impairment, declining renal function, ACE inhibitors or angiotensin receptor blockers.

ACTION

Interferes with sodium reabsorption by competitively inhibiting action of aldosterone in distal tubule, promoting sodium and water excretion, increasing potassium retention. May decrease effect of aldosterone on arteriolar smooth muscle. **Therapeutic Effect:** Produces diuresis, lowers B/P.

PHARMACOKINETICS

Widely distributed. Protein binding: 91%–98%. Metabolized in liver to active metabolite. Primarily excreted in urine. Unknown if removed by hemodialysis. **Half-life:** 78–84 min.

⧗ LIFESPAN CONSIDERATIONS

Pregnancy/Lactation: Active metabolite excreted in breast milk. Breastfeeding not recommended. **Children:** No age-related precautions noted. **Elderly:** May be more susceptible to developing hyperkalemia. Age-related renal impairment may require dosage adjustment.

INTERACTIONS

DRUG: **ACE inhibitors (e.g., captopril, lisinopril), angiotensin receptor blockers (e.g., valsartan), eplerenone, potassium-containing medications, potassium supplements** may increase risk of hyperkalemia. **NSAIDs (e.g., ibuprofen, naproxen)** may decrease antihypertensive effect. **HERBAL:** **Herbals with hypertensive properties (e.g., licorice, yohimbe) or hypotensive properties (e.g., garlic, ginger, ginkgo biloba)** may alter effects. **FOOD:** **Food** increases absorption. **LAB VALUES:** May increase urinary calcium excretion, serum BUN, glucose, creatinine, magnesium, potassium, uric acid. May decrease serum sodium.

AVAILABILITY (Rx)

Oral Suspension: 25 mg/5 mL. **Tablets:** 25 mg, 50 mg, 100 mg.

ADMINISTRATION/HANDLING

PO
• Take with food to reduce GI irritation and increase absorption. **Suspension:**
• Shake well. • May give with or without food (give consistently with respect to food).

INDICATIONS/ROUTES/DOSAGE

Ascites (Due to Cirrhosis)
PO: ADULTS, ELDERLY: *(Tablet):* Initially, 100 mg/day as single dose. May titrate q3–5 days based on response and tolerability. **Maximum dose:** 400 mg once daily.

Hypertension
PO: ADULTS, ELDERLY: *(Tablet):* Initially, 12.5–25 mg once daily. May titrate q2wks as needed. **Maximum:** 100 mg. *(Suspension):* Initially, 20 mg/day in 1–2 divided doses. May titrate as needed q2wks up to 75 mg/day in 1–2 divided doses.

Primary Hyperaldosteronism
PO: ADULTS, ELDERLY: Initially, 12.5–25 mg once daily. Gradually titrate to the lowest effective dose. **Maximum dose:** 400 mg/day.

HF
PO: ADULTS, ELDERLY: *(Tablet):* Initially, 12.5–25 mg/day. May double the dose q4wks if serum potassium remains less than 5 mEq/L and renal function remains stable. **Maximum:** 50 mg/day. in 1 or 2 divided doses. *(Suspension):* Initially, 10–20 mg once daily. May titrate to 37.5 mg once daily if serum potassium remains less than 5 mEq/L and renal function remains stable.

Dosage in Renal Impairment
CrCl 50 mL/min or greater: Initially, 12.5–25 mg once daily. **Maintenance:** 25 mg once or twice daily. **CrCl 30–49 mL/min:** Initially, 12.5 mg once daily or every other day. **Maintenance:** 12.5–25 mg once daily. **CrCl less than 30 mL/min:** Not recommended.

Dosage in Hepatic Impairment
No dose adjustment.

SIDE EFFECTS
Frequent: Hyperkalemia (in pts with renal insufficiency, those taking potassium supplements), dehydration, hyponatremia, lethargy. **Occasional:** Nausea, vomiting, anorexia, abdominal cramps, diarrhea, headache, ataxia, drowsiness, confusion, fever. **Male:** Gynecomastia, impotence, decreased libido. **Female:** Menstrual irregularities (amenorrhea, postmenopausal bleeding), breast tenderness. **Rare:** Rash, urticaria, hirsutism.

ADVERSE EFFECTS/TOXIC REACTIONS
Severe hyperkalemia may produce arrhythmias, bradycardia, ECG changes (tented T waves, widening QRS complex, ST segment depression). May proceed to cardiac standstill, ventricular fibrillation. Cirrhosis pts at risk for hepatic decompensation if dehydration, hyponatremia occurs. Pts with primary aldosteronism may experience rapid weight loss, severe fatigue during high-dose therapy.

NURSING CONSIDERATIONS

BASELINE ASSESSMENT
Obtain serum electrolytes, renal function test, weight; B/P. Assess hydration status.

INTERVENTION/EVALUATION
Monitor serum electrolyte values, esp. for increased potassium, BUN, creatinine. Monitor B/P. Monitor for hyponatremia: mental confusion, thirst, cold/clammy skin, drowsiness, dry mouth. Monitor for hyperkalemia: colic, diarrhea, muscle twitching followed by weakness/paralysis, arrhythmias. Obtain daily weight. Note changes in edema, skin turgor.

PATIENT/FAMILY TEACHING
• Expect increase in volume, frequency of urination. • Therapeutic effect takes several days to begin and can last for several days when drug is discontinued. • Report irregular or slow pulse, symptoms of electrolyte imbalance (see previous Intervention/Evaluation). • Avoid foods high in potassium, such as whole grains (cereals), legumes, meat, bananas, apricots, orange juice, potatoes (white, sweet), raisins. • Avoid alcohol.

S

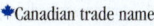 Canadian trade name   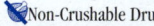 Non-Crushable Drug   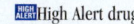 High Alert drug

sulfamethoxazole-trimethoprim

sul-fa-meth-**ox**-a-zole-trye-**meth**-oh-prim
(Bactrim, Bactrim DS, Sulfatrim)
Do not confuse Bactrim with bacitracin or Bactroban.

FIXED-COMBINATION(S)

Bactrim, Septra: sulfamethoxazole/trimethoprim: 5:1 ratio remains constant in all dosage forms (e.g., 400 mg/80 mg).

◆ CLASSIFICATION

PHARMACOTHERAPEUTIC: Sulfonamide derivative. **CLINICAL:** Antibiotic.

USES

Treatment of UTIs due to susceptible strains of *Escherichia coli, Klebsiella species, Enterobacter species, Morganella morganii, Proteus mirabilis,* and *Proteus vulgaris.* Treatment of acute exacerbations of chronic bronchitis, acute otitis media in pediatric pts due to susceptible strains of *Streptococcus pneumoniae* or *Haemophilus influenzae.* Treatment of enteritis caused by susceptible strains of *Shigella flexneri* and *S. sonnei.* Treatment of traveler's diarrhea due to susceptible strains of enterotoxigenic *E. coli.* Treatment of documented *Pneumocystis jirovecii* pneumonia, *P. jirovecii* pneumonia in individuals who are immunosuppressed and considered to be at an increased risk of developing *P. jirovecii* pneumonia. **OFF-LABEL:** Prosthetic joint infection, skin and soft tissue infections (cellulitis, impetigo), diabetic foot infection (MRSA), bacterial meningitis, intra-abdominal infection, intracranial abscess, osteomyelitis (MRSA), prostatitis, surgical prophylaxis.

PRECAUTIONS

Contraindications: Hypersensitivity to any sulfa medication, trimethoprim. History of drug-induced immune thrombocytopenia with sulfonamides or trimethoprim, infants younger than 4 wks, megaloblastic anemia due to folate deficiency, severe hepatic/renal impairment. Concomitant administration of dofetilide. **Cautions:** Pts with G6PD deficiency, hepatic/renal/thyroid impairment, porphyria, asthma, elderly, concurrent anticonvulsant therapy.

ACTION

Sulfamethoxazole: Interferes with bacterial folic acid synthesis and growth. **Trimethoprim:** Inhibits dihydrofolic acid reduction. **Therapeutic Effect:** Bactericidal in susceptible microorganisms.

PHARMACOKINETICS

Widely distributed. Protein binding: 45%–60%. Metabolized in liver. Excreted in urine. Minimally removed by hemodialysis. **Half-life:** sulfamethoxazole, 6–12 hrs; trimethoprim, 6–17 hrs (increased in renal impairment).

⧗ LIFESPAN CONSIDERATIONS

Pregnancy/Lactation: Contraindicated during pregnancy at term and during lactation. Readily crosses placenta. Distributed in breast milk. May produce kernicterus in newborn. **Children:** Contraindicated in pts younger than 2 mos; may increase risk of kernicterus in newborn. **Elderly:** Increased risk for severe skin reaction, myelosuppression, decreased platelet count.

INTERACTIONS

DRUG: May increase concentration/effects of **phenytoin, digoxin, oral hypoglycemics (e.g., glipiZIDE, metFORMIN), warfarin.** May increase adverse effects of **methotrexate. Strong CYP3A4 inducers (e.g., carBAMazepine, phenytoin, rifAMPin)** may decrease concentration/effect. **HERBAL:** **St. John's wort** may decrease concentration/effect. **Herbals with hypoglycemic properties (e.g., fenugreek)** may increase concentration/

effect. **FOOD:** None known. **LAB VALUES:** May increase serum BUN, creatinine, ALT, AST, bilirubin.

AVAILABILITY (Rx)

◀**ALERT**▶ All dosage forms have same 5:1 ratio of sulfamethoxazole (SMZ) to trimethoprim (TMP).
Injection Solution: SMZ 80 mg and TMP 16 mg per mL. **Oral Suspension:** SMZ 200 mg and TMP 40 mg per 5 mL. **Tablets:** *(Bactrim):* SMZ 400 mg and TMP 80 mg. **Tablets, Double Strength:** *(Bactrim DS):* SMZ 800 mg and TMP 160 mg.

ADMINISTRATION/HANDLING

 IV

Reconstitution • Dilute each 5 mL with 75–125 mL D$_5$W. • Do not mix with other drugs or solutions.
Rate of administration • Infuse over 60–90 min. Must avoid bolus or rapid infusion. • Do not give IM.
Storage • IV infusion (piggyback) stable for 2 hrs (5 mL/75 mL D$_5$W), 4 hrs (5 mL/100 mL D$_5$W), 6 hrs (5 mL/125 mL D$_5$W). • Discard if cloudy or precipitate forms.

PO
• Administer without regard to food. • Give with at least 8 oz water.

IV COMPATIBILITIES

DexmedeTOMIDine, magnesium sulfate.

INDICATIONS/ROUTES/DOSAGE

Usual Adult/Elderly Dosage Range
PO: 1–2 double-strength tablets q12–24h. **IV:** 8–20 mg/kg/day as trimethoprim in divided doses q6–12h.

Usual Dosage Range for Infants 2 Mos and Older, Children, Adolescents
PO/IV: 8–12 mg TMP/kg/day in divided doses q12h. **Maximum single dose:** 160 mg TMP.

Dosage in Renal Impairment

Creatinine Clearance	Dosage
15–30 mL/min	50% of usual dosage
Less than 15 mL/min	Not recommended
HD	2.5–10 mg/kg trimethoprim q24h (or 5–20 mg/kg 3 times/wk) (give after HD)
CRRT	2.5–7.5 mg/kg trimethoprim q12h

Dosage in Hepatic Impairment
No dose adjustment.

SIDE EFFECTS

Frequent: Anorexia, nausea, vomiting, rash (generally 7–14 days after therapy begins), urticaria. **Occasional:** Diarrhea, abdominal pain, pain/irritation at IV infusion site. **Rare:** Headache, vertigo, insomnia, seizures, hallucinations, depression.

ADVERSE EFFECTS/TOXIC REACTIONS

Rash, fever, sore throat, pallor, purpura, cough, shortness of breath may be early signs of serious adverse effects. Fatalities are rare but have occurred in sulfonamide therapy following Stevens-Johnson syndrome, toxic epidermal necrolysis, fulminant hepatic necrosis, agranulocytosis, aplastic anemia, other blood dyscrasias. Myelosuppression, decreased platelet count, severe dermatologic reactions may occur, esp. in the elderly.

NURSING CONSIDERATIONS

BASELINE ASSESSMENT

Obtain history for hypersensitivity to trimethoprim or any sulfonamide, sulfite sensitivity, bronchial asthma. Determine serum renal, hepatic, hematologic baselines.

INTERVENTION/EVALUATION

Monitor daily pattern of bowel activity, stool consistency. Assess skin for rash, pallor, purpura. Check IV site, flow rate. Monitor renal, hepatic, hematol-

S

---

ogy function. Assess I&O. Check for CNS symptoms (headache, vertigo, insomnia, hallucinations). Monitor for cough, shortness of breath. Assess for overt bleeding, ecchymosis, edema.

PATIENT/FAMILY TEACHING

• Continue medication for full length of therapy. • Take oral doses with 8 oz water and drink several extra glasses of water daily. • Report immediately any new symptoms, esp. rash, other skin changes, bleeding/bruising, fever, sore throat, diarrhea. • Avoid prolonged exposure to UV, direct sunlight.

SUMAtriptan

soo-ma-**trip**-tan
(Imitrex, Onzetra Xsail, Sumavel DosePro, Tosymra, Zembrace SymTouch)
Do not confuse SUMAtriptan with sAXagliptin, SITagliptin, somatropin, or ZOLMitriptan.

FIXED-COMBINATION(S)

Treximet: SUMAtriptan/naproxen (an NSAID): 85 mg/500 mg, 10 mg/60 mg.

◆CLASSIFICATION

PHARMACOTHERAPEUTIC: Serotonin 5-HT$_1$ receptor agonist. **CLINICAL:** Antimigraine.

USES

PO, SQ, intranasal: Acute treatment of migraine headache with or without aura. **SQ: (Excluding Zembrace):** Treatment of cluster headaches in adults as monotherapy or in combination with 100% oxygen. **OFF-LABEL:** Migraine-associated cyclic vomiting syndrome.

PRECAUTIONS

Contraindications: Hypersensitivity to SUMAtriptan. Management of hemiplegic or basilar migraine, peripheral vascular disease, CVA, ischemic heart disease (including angina pectoris, history of MI, silent ischemia, Prinzmetal's angina), severe hepatic impairment, transient ischemic attack, uncontrolled hypertension, MAOI use within 14 days, use within 24 hrs of ergotamine preparations or another 5-HT$_1$ agonist. Wolff-Parkinson-White syndrome or arrhythmias associated with other cardiac accessory conduction pathway disorders. **Cautions:** Mild to moderate hepatic impairment, seizure disorder, hypertension, elderly.

ACTION

Binds selectively to serotonin 5-HT$_1$ receptors in cranial arteries, producing vasoconstrictive effect on cranial blood vessels. **Therapeutic Effect:** Relieves migraine headache.

PHARMACOKINETICS

Route	Onset	Peak	Duration
Nasal	15 min	N/A	24–48 hrs
PO	30 min	2 hrs	24–48 hrs
SQ	10 min	1 hr	24–48 hrs

Widely distributed. Metabolized in liver. Protein binding: 10%–21%. Excreted in urine. **Half-life:** 2 hrs.

⌛ LIFESPAN CONSIDERATIONS

Pregnancy/Lactation: Unknown if distributed in breast milk. **Children:** Safety and efficacy not established. **Elderly:** No age-related precautions noted.

INTERACTIONS

DRUG: **Ergotamine-containing medications** may produce vasospastic reaction. **MAOIs (e.g., phenelzine, selegiline)** may increase concentration, half-life. **SSRIs (e.g., escitalopram, PARoxetine, sertraline)** and **SNRIs (e.g., DULoxetine, venlafaxine)** may increase risk of serotonin syndrome. **HERBAL:** None significant. **FOOD:** None known. **LAB VALUES:** None significant.

AVAILABILITY (Rx)

Injection, Prefilled Autoinjector: 3 mg/0.5 mL, 4 mg/0.5 mL, 6 mg/0.5 mL. **(Zembrace**

S

SymTouch): 3 mg/0.5 mL. **Injection Solution:** 6 mg/0.5 mL. *(Sumavel DosePro):* 6 mg/0.5 mL. **Nasal Powder.** *(Onzetra Xsail):* **Capsules:** 11 mg per nosepiece. **Nasal Solution:** *(Imitrex Nasal):* 5 mg/actuation, 20 mg/actuation. *(Tosymra):* 10 mg/actuation. **Tablets:** *(Imitrex):* 25 mg, 50 mg, 100 mg.

ADMINISTRATION/HANDLING

SQ

• Follow manufacturer's instructions for autoinjection device use. • Administer needleless (Sumavel DosePro) only to abdomen or thigh.

PO

• Swallow tablets whole. Do not break, crush, dissolve, or divide. • Take with full glass of water.

Nasal

• Unit contains only one spray—do not test before use. • Instruct pt to gently blow nose to clear nasal passages. • With head upright, close one nostril with index finger, breathe out gently through mouth. • Have pt insert nozzle into open nostril about one-half inch, close mouth and, while taking a breath through nose, release spray dosage by firmly pressing plunger. • Instruct pt to remove nozzle from nose and gently breathe in through nose and out through mouth for 10–20 sec; do not breathe in deeply.

INDICATIONS/ROUTES/DOSAGE

Acute Migraine Headache

PO: ADULTS, ELDERLY: 50–100 mg. Dose may be repeated after at least 2 hrs. **Maximum:** 100 mg/single dose; 200 mg/24 hrs.

SQ: ADULTS, ELDERLY: Initially, 6 mg once. May repeat a dose (usually same as first dose) after 1 hr. If 6-mg dose was not tolerated, subsequent doses of 1–5 mg may provide sufficient relief with better tolerability. **Maximum:** 6 mg/dose (12 mg/24 hrs).

Intranasal: ADULTS, ELDERLY: *(Solution):* Initially, 20 mg once (usual dose) in a single nostril. May repeat once after at least 2 hrs. **Maximum:** 40 mg/24h. *(Spray):* Initially,

10 mg once in one nostril. If initial dose was partially effective or headache recurs, may repeat dose once after at least 1 hr. **Maximum:** 30 mg/4 hrs. *(Nasal Powder):* (Breath-activated, using product specific device): Initially, a single dose of 22 mg (11 mg in each nostril). May repeat dose once after at least 2 hrs. **Maximum:** 44 mg/24 hrs separated by at least 2 hrs.

Cluster Headaches

SQ: ADULTS, ELDERLY: Initially, 6 mg. May repeat after 1 hr. **Maximum:** 6 mg/dose; 12 mg/24 hrs.

Dosage in Renal Impairment
No dose adjustment.

Dosage in Hepatic Impairment
Mild to moderate impairment: (maximum dose): 50 mg. **Severe impairment:** Contraindicated.

SIDE EFFECTS

Frequent: PO (10%–5%): Tingling, nasal discomfort. **SQ (greater than 10%):** Injection site reactions, tingling, warm/hot sensation, dizziness, vertigo. **Nasal (greater than 10%):** Altered taste, nausea, vomiting. **Occasional: PO (5%–1%):** Flushing, asthenia, visual disturbances. **SQ (10%–2%):** Burning sensation, numbness, chest discomfort, drowsiness, asthenia. **Nasal (5%–1%):** Nasopharyngeal discomfort, dizziness. **Rare: PO (less than 1%):** Agitation, eye irritation, dysuria. **SQ (less than 2%):** Anxiety, fatigue, diaphoresis, muscle cramps, myalgia. **Nasal (less than 1%):** Burning sensation.

ADVERSE EFFECTS/TOXIC REACTIONS

Excessive dosage may produce tremors, redness of extremities, reduced respirations, cyanosis, seizures, paralysis. Serious arrhythmias occur rarely, esp. in pts with hypertension, obesity, smokers, diabetes, strong family history of coronary artery disease. Serotonin syndrome may occur (agitation, confusion, hallucinations, hyperreflexia, myoclonus, shivering, tachycardia).

S

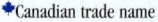 Canadian trade name   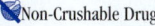 Non-Crushable Drug   **HIGH ALERT** High Alert drug

NURSING CONSIDERATIONS

BASELINE ASSESSMENT

Receive full medical history, medication history and screen for contraindications. Obtain pregnancy test in female pts of reproductive potential. Question regarding onset, location, duration of migraine, possible precipitating symptoms.

INTERVENTION/EVALUATION

Evaluate for relief of migraine headache and resulting photophobia, phonophobia (sound sensitivity), nausea, vomiting.

PATIENT/FAMILY TEACHING

• Follow proper technique for loading of autoinjector, injection technique, discarding of syringe. • Do not use more than 2 injections during any 24-hr period and allow at least 1 hr between injections. • Report immediately if wheezing, palpitations, skin rash, facial swelling, pain/tightness in chest/throat occur.

SUNItinib `HIGH ALERT`

soo-**nit**-in-ib
(Sutent)

■**BLACK BOX ALERT**■ Hepatotoxicity may be severe and/or result in fatal liver failure.
Do not confuse SUNItinib with imatinib or SORAfenib.

◆CLASSIFICATION

PHARMACOTHERAPEUTIC: Vascular endothelial growth factor (VEGF) inhibitor. Tyrosine kinase inhibitor.
CLINICAL: Antineoplastic.

USES

GI stromal tumor (GIST): Treatment of GIST after disease progression while on or demonstrating intolerance to imatinib. **Renal cell carcinoma (RCC):** Treatment of advanced RCC. Adjuvant treatment of adults at high risk of recurrent RCC following nephrectomy. **Pancreatic neuroendocrine tumor (PNET):** Treatment of progressive, well-differentiated PNET in adults with unresectable locally advanced or metastatic disease. **OFF-LABEL:** Soft tissue sarcoma (non-GIST), thyroid cancer (refractory).

PRECAUTIONS

Contraindications: Hypersensitivity to SUNItinib. **Cautions:** Cardiac dysfunction, bradycardia, electrolyte imbalance, bleeding tendencies, hypertension, history of prolonged QT interval, medications that prolong QT interval, hypokalemia, hypomagnesemia, concurrent use of strong CYP3A4 inducers or inhibitors, HF, renal/hepatic impairment, pregnancy.

ACTION

Inhibitory action against multiple receptor tyrosine kinases including growth factor receptors, vascular endothelial growth factors, colony-stimulating factor receptors, glial cell-line neurotrophic factor receptors. **Therapeutic Effect:** Prevents tumor cell growth, produces tumor regression, inhibits metastasis.

PHARMACOKINETICS

Widely distributed. Metabolized in liver. Protein binding: 95%. Excreted in feces (61%), urine (16%). **Half-life:** 40–60 hrs.

⊠ LIFESPAN CONSIDERATIONS

Pregnancy/Lactation: Has potential for embryotoxic, teratogenic effects. Breastfeeding not recommended. **Children:** Safety and efficacy not established. **Elderly:** No age-related precautions noted.

INTERACTIONS

DRUG: Strong **CYP3A4 inhibitors (e.g., clarithromycin, ketoconazole, ritonavir)** may increase concentration,

S

toxicity. **Strong CYP3A4 inducers (e.g., carBAMazepine, phenytoin, rifAMPin)** may decrease concentration/effects. May increase adverse effects of **bevacizumab**. May increase adverse effects; decrease therapeutic effect of **vaccines (live)**. **HERBAL:** St. John's wort may decrease concentration. **Herbals with hypoglycemic properties (e.g., fenugreek)** may increase hypoglycemic effect. **FOOD:** Grapefruit products may increase concentration/effect. **LAB VALUES:** May increase serum alkaline phosphatase, bilirubin, amylase, lipase, creatinine, ALT, AST. May alter serum potassium, sodium, uric acid. May produce thrombocytopenia, neutropenia. May decrease serum phosphate, thyroid function levels.

AVAILABILITY (Rx)

Capsules: 12.5 mg, 25 mg, 37.5 mg, 50 mg.

ADMINISTRATION/HANDLING

PO

• Give without regard to food. Avoid grapefruit products.

INDICATIONS/ROUTES/DOSAGE

GI Stromal Tumor, Renal Cell Carcinoma, RCC (Advanced Treatment)

PO: ADULTS, ELDERLY: 50 mg once daily for 4 wks, followed by 2 wks off in 6-wk cycle. Continue until disease progression or unacceptable toxicity.

Renal Cell Carcinoma (Adjuvant Treatment)

PO: ADULTS, ELDERLY: 50 mg once daily for 4 wks, followed by 2 wks off, for maximum of nine 6-wk cycles.

Pancreatic Neuroendocrine Tumor

PO: ADULTS, ELDERLY: 37.5 mg once daily continuously without a scheduled off-treatment period. Continue until disease progression or unacceptable toxicity.

Dose Modification

Note: Increase or decrease dosage in 12.5-mg increments is recommended based on safety and tolerability.

Concomitant Use of Strong CYP3A4 Inhibitors

Consider a dose reduction to a minimum of 37.5 mg/day (GIST, RCC) or 25 mg/day (PNET).

Concomitant Use of CYP3A4 Inducers

Consider a dose increase (monitor carefully for toxicity) to maximum of 87.5 mg/day (GIST, RCC) or 62.5 mg (PNET).

Dosage in Renal Impairment

No initial dose adjustment; subsequent adjustment may be needed.

Dosage in Hepatic Impairment

No dose adjustment initially; Grade 3 or 4 hepatotoxicity during treatment: withhold/discontinue if hepatotoxicity does not resolve.

SIDE EFFECTS

Stromal tumor: Common (42%–30%): Fatigue, diarrhea, anorexia, abdominal pain, nausea, hyperpigmentation. **Frequent (29%–18%):** Mucositis/stomatitis, vomiting, asthenia, altered taste, constipation, fever. **Occasional (15%–8%):** Hypertension, rash, myalgia, headache, arthralgia, back pain, dyspnea, cough. **Renal carcinoma: Common (74%–43%):** Fatigue, diarrhea, nausea, mucositis/stomatitis, dyspepsia, altered taste. **Frequent (38%–20%):** Rash, vomiting, constipation, hyperpigmentation, anorexia, arthralgia, dyspnea, hypertension, headache, abdominal pain. **Occasional (18%–11%):** Limb pain, peripheral/periorbital edema, dry skin, hair color change, myalgia, cough, back pain, dizziness, fever, tongue pain, flatulence, alopecia, dehydration.

ADVERSE EFFECTS/TOXIC REACTIONS

Palmar-plantar erythrodysesthesia syndrome (PPES) occurs occasionally (14%), manifested as blistering/rash/peeling of skin on palms of hands, soles of feet. Bleeding, decrease in left ventricular ejection fraction, deep vein thrombosis (DVT), pancreatitis, neutropenia, seizures occur rarely.

S

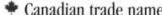

NURSING CONSIDERATIONS

BASELINE ASSESSMENT

Question possibility of pregnancy. Obtain baseline CBC, BMP, LFT before beginning therapy and prior to each treatment. Obtain baseline ECG, thyroid function tests. Question medical history as listed in Precautions.

INTERVENTION/EVALUATION

Assess eye area, lower extremities for early evidence of fluid retention. Offer antiemetics to control nausea, vomiting. Monitor daily pattern of bowel activity, stool consistency. Monitor CBC for evidence of neutropenia, thrombocytopenia; assess LFT for hepatotoxicity. Monitor for PPES. Monitor B/P.

PATIENT/FAMILY TEACHING

• Treatment may depress your immune system response and reduce your ability to fight infection. Report symptoms of infection such as body aches, chills, cough, fatigue, fever. Avoid those with active infection. • Avoid pregnancy; use effective contraceptive measures. • Promptly report fever, unusual bruising/bleeding from any site.

tacrolimus

ta-**kroe**-li-mus
(Astagraf XL, Envarsus XR, <u>Prograf</u>, Protopic)

■ **BLACK BOX ALERT** ■ Increased susceptibility to infection and potential for development of lymphoma. Extended-release associated with increased mortality in female liver transplant recipients. Topical form associated with rare cases of malignancy. Topical form should be used only for short-term and intermittent treatment. Not recommended in children younger than 2 yrs. Use only 0.03% ointment for children 2–15 yrs of age. Administer under supervision of physician experienced in immunosuppressive therapy.

Do not confuse Protopic with Protonix, or tacrolimus with everolimus, pimecrolimus, sirolimus, or temsirolimus.

◆CLASSIFICATION

PHARMACOTHERAPEUTIC: Calcineurin inhibitor. **CLINICAL:** Immunosuppressant.

USES

PO, injection: Prevention of organ rejection in adult and pediatric pts receiving kidney transplants (Prograf: kidney, heart, liver or lung transplants) in combination with other immunosuppressants. **Topical:** Moderate to severe atopic dermatitis in immunocompetent pts. **OFF-LABEL:** Myasthenia gravis, pancreas transplant, nephrotic syndrome.

PRECAUTIONS

Contraindications: Hypersensitivity to tacrolimus. **Cautions:** Hypersensitivity to HCO-60 polyoxyl 60 hydrogenated castor oil (used in solution for injection). Renal/hepatic impairment cardiac disease; history of chronic, opportunistic infections, concurrent use with other nephrotoxic drugs (e.g., cycloSPORINE), concurrent use of strong CYP3A4 inhibitors or induc-

ers. Avoid use of potassium-sparing diuretics, ACE inhibitors, potassium-based salt substitutes. Pts at risk for pure red cell aplasia (e.g., concurrent use of mycophenolate); pts at risk for QTc interval prolongation (congenital long QT syndrome, HF, medications that prolong QTc interval, hypokalemia, hypomagnesemia). **Topical:** Exposure to sunlight, UV light.

ACTION

Inhibits T-lymphocyte activation by binding to intracellular protein FKBP-12, forming a complex with calcineurin-dependent proteins, inhibiting calcineurin phosphatase activity. **Therapeutic Effect:** Suppresses immunological-mediated inflammatory response; prevents organ transplant rejection.

PHARMACOKINETICS

Variably absorbed after PO administration (food reduces absorption). Widely distributed. Protein binding: 99%. Metabolized in liver. Primarily excreted in feces. Not removed by hemodialysis. **Half-life:** 21–61 hrs.

⏳ LIFESPAN CONSIDERATIONS

Pregnancy/Lactation: Crosses placenta. Hyperkalemia, renal dysfunction noted in neonates. Distributed in breast milk. Breastfeeding not recommended. **Children:** May require higher dosages (decreased bioavailability, increased clearance). May make post-transplant lymphoproliferative disorder more common, esp. in pts younger than 3 yrs. **Elderly:** Age-related renal impairment may require dosage adjustment.

INTERACTIONS

DRUG: Aluminium-containing antacids may increase concentration/effect. **Strong CYP3A4 inhibitors (e.g., clarithromycin, ketoconazole, ritonavir), calcium channel blockers (e.g., dilTIAZem, verapamil)** may increase concentration/effect. **Strong CYP3A4 inducers (e.g., carBAMazepine, phenytoin, rifAMPin)** may decrease concentration/effect. **CycloSPORINE, foscarnet** may in-

 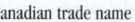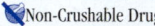

T

crease nephrotoxic effect. May decrease therapeutic effect; increase adverse effect of **vaccines (live)**. **Eplerenone, potassium-sparing diuretics (e.g., spironolactone)** may increase hyperkalemic effect. **QT interval–prolonging medications (e.g., amiodarone, azithromycin, ciprofloxacin, haloperidol, methadone, sotalol)** may increase risk of QTc interval prolongation. **HERBAL:** Echinacea may decrease therapeutic effect. **St. John's wort** may decrease concentration/effect. **FOOD:** None known. **Grapefruit products** may increase concentration, toxicity (potential for nephrotoxicity). **LAB VALUES:** May increase serum ALT, AST, amylase, bilirubin, BUN, cholesterol, creatinine, potassium, glucose, triglycerides. May decrease serum magnesium; Hgb, Hct, platelets. May alter leukocytes.

AVAILABILITY (Rx)

Capsules: *(Prograf):* 0.5 mg, 1 mg, 5 mg. **Injection Solution:** *(Prograf):* 5 mg/mL. **Ointment:** *(Protopic):* 0.03%, 0.1%. **Packet, Oral:** 0.2 mg, 1 mg.

Capsules, Extended-Release: *(Astagraf XL):* 0.5 mg, 1 mg, 5 mg. **Tablets, Extended-Release:** *(Envarsus XR):* 0.75 mg, 1 mg, 4 mg.

ADMINISTRATION/HANDLING

 IV

Reconstitution • Dilute with appropriate amount (250–1,000 mL, depending on desired dose) 0.9% NaCl or D_5W to provide concentration between 0.004 and 0.02 mg/mL.
Rate of administration • Give as continuous IV infusion (usually over 24 hrs). • Continuously monitor pt for anaphylaxis for at least 30 min after start of infusion. • Stop infusion immediately at first sign of hypersensitivity reaction.
Storage • Store diluted infusion solution in glass or polyethylene containers and discard after 24 hrs. • Do not store in PVC container (decreased stability, potential for extraction).

PO
• **Immediate-release:** Administer without regard to food. Be consistent with timing of administration. If dose is once daily, give in morning. If morning and evening doses differ, give larger dose in morning. • **Extended-release:** Give once daily in the morning on an empty stomach (at least 1 hr before or 2 hrs after a meal). Administer whole (do not chew, crush, or divide). A missed dose may be taken up to 14 hrs after usual scheduled time. • **Granules for oral suspension:** Mix with 15–30 mL of water (do not sprinkle on food). Granules will not completely dissolve. Give immediately after mixing. Add additional 15–30 mL of water to rinse cup and ensure all medication is taken.

Topical
• For external use only. • Do not cover with occlusive dressing. • Rub gently, completely onto clean, dry skin.

▓ IV COMPATIBILITIES
Heparin, insulin, potassium chloride.

INDICATIONS/ROUTES/DOSAGE
Note: Give initial postoperative dose no sooner than 6 hrs after liver or heart transplant and within 24 hrs of kidney transplant.

Prevention of Liver Transplant Rejection
PO: ADULTS, ELDERLY: *(Immediate-Release):* 0.1–0.15 mg/kg/day in 2 divided doses 12 hrs apart (in combination with corticosteroids). Titrate to target trough concentration. **CHILDREN:** 0.15–0.2 mg/kg/day (capsules) or 0.2 mg/kg/day (oral suspension) in 2 divided doses 12 hrs apart. Titrate to target trough concentration. **IV: ADULTS, ELDERLY, CHILDREN:** Initially, 0.03–0.05 mg/kg/day as continuous infusion.

Prevention of Kidney Transplant Rejection
PO: ADULTS, ELDERLY: *(Immediate-Release):* 0.2 mg/kg/day (in combination with azaTHIOprine) in 2 divided doses 12 hrs apart or 0.1 mg/kg/day (in combination with mycophenolate) in 2 divided doses 12 hrs apart. Titrate to target trough concentration. **CHILDREN:** 0.3

mg/kg/day (capsules or oral suspension) divided q12h. *(Extended-Release [Astagraf XL]): (With Basiliximab Induction):* (Prior to or within 48 hrs of transplant completion): 0.15–0.2 mg/kg once daily (in combination with corticosteroids and mycophenolate). Titrate to target trough concentration. **CHILDREN 4 YRS AND OLDER:** 0.3 mg/kg once daily. *(Without Basiliximab Induction):* **Pre-operative dose:** 0.1 mg/kg (administer within 12 hrs prior to reperfusion). **Post-operative dosing:** 0.2 mg/kg once daily (in combination with corticosteroids and mycophenolate). Give at least 4 hrs after pre-operative dose and within 12 hrs of reperfusion. Titrate to target trough concentration. *(Extended-Release [Envarsus XL]):* 0.14 mg/kg/day. **(Conversion from IV):** Administer first dose 8–12 hrs after discontinuing tacrolimus IV. **(Conversion from Immediate-Release):** Administer 70%–80% of total daily immediate-release tacrolimus dose. **IV: ADULTS, ELDERLY:** Initially, 0.03–0.05 mg/kg/day as continuous infusion.

Prevention of Heart Transplant Rejection
Note: Use in combination with an antimetabolite agent (e.g., azaTHIOprine, mycophenolate).
PO: ADULTS, ELDERLY: *(Immediate-Release):* Initially, 0.075 mg/kg/day in 2 divided doses 12 hrs apart. **CHILDREN:** 0.3 mg/kg/day (capsules or oral suspension) divided in 2 doses q12h. Titrate to target trough concentration.
IV: ADULTS, ELDERLY: Initially, 0.01 mg/kg/day as continuous infusion.

Lung Transplant
Note: Use in combination with an antimetabolite agent (e.g., azaTHIOprine, mycophenolate).
PO: ADULTS, ELDERLY: *(Immediate-Release):* Initially, 0.075 mg/kg/day in 2 divided doses, administered q12h. **CHILDREN:** 0.3 mg/kg/day (capsules or oral suspension) divided q12h. Titrate to target trough concentration.
IV: ADULTS, ELDERLY: Initially, 0.01–0.03 mg/kg/day as a continuous infusion.

Atopic Dermatitis
Topical: ADULTS, ELDERLY, CHILDREN 15 YRS AND OLDER: Apply 0.03% or 0.1% ointment to affected area twice daily. **CHILDREN 2–15 YRS:** Use 0.03% ointment twice daily. Continue treatment for 1 wk after symptoms have resolved. If no improvement within 6 wks, re-examine to confirm diagnosis.

SIDE EFFECTS

Frequent (greater than 30%): Headache, tremor, insomnia, paresthesia, diarrhea, nausea, constipation, vomiting, abdominal pain, hypertension. **Occasional (29%–10%):** Rash, pruritus, anorexia, asthenia, peripheral edema, photosensitivity.

ADVERSE EFFECTS/TOXIC REACTIONS

Hypersensitivity reactions, including anaphylaxis, were reported. Cardiac toxicities including myocardial hypertrophy, QT interval prolongation, torsades de pointes, MI, pericardial effusion, SVT, ventricular arrhythmias, may occur. May increase risk of new-onset diabetes after transplantation. May cause acute renal failure, GI perforation, hepatotoxicity, hyperkalemia, hypertension, myelosuppression (anemia, leukopenia, neutropenia, thrombocytopenia), new malignancies, pure red cell aplasia, thrombotic microangiopathy. Fatal infections including bacterial, fungal, protozoal, opportunistic, viral infections (including cytomegalovirus) were reported. Progressive multifocal leukoencephalopathy (PML), an opportunistic viral infection of the brain caused by the JC virus, may result in progressive permanent disability and death. Nephrotoxicity may occur with high doses. Neurotoxicities (e.g., confusion, depression, encephalopathy, myasthenia, myoclonus, neuralgia, neuropathy, paralysis, seizures) were reported.

NURSING CONSIDERATIONS

BASELINE ASSESSMENT

Obtain CBC, BMP, LFT; ECG; pregnancy test in females of reproductive potential. Question history of hepatic/renal impairment, cardiac disease, chronic opportunistic infections. Screen for active infection.

Receive full medication history and screen for interaction (esp. use of other immunosuppressants). Have aqueous solution of EPINEPHrine 1:1,000, O_2 available at bedside before beginning IV infusion.

INTERVENTION/EVALUATION

CBC should be performed wkly during first mo of therapy, twice monthly during second and third mos of treatment, then monthly throughout the first yr. Monitor BUN, serum creatinine, CrCl, eGFR pts with renal impairment. Monitor LFT periodically. Assess continuously for first 30 min following start of infusion and at frequent intervals thereafter. Monitor I&O closely. Monitor for infections (cough, fatigue fever), neurotoxicities, psychiatric symptoms. Monitor for cardiac ischemia/infarction (chest pain, diaphoresis, left arm or jaw pain, ST segment elevation, serum troponin elevation), GI perforation (abdominal pain, fever, nausea, vomiting), infection (cough, fatigue, fever); neuropathy (gait disturbance, fine motor control difficulties, numbness); hypersensitivity reactions (anaphylaxis, urticaria), bleeding of any kind.

PATIENT/FAMILY TEACHING

• Treatment may depress your immune system and reduce your ability to fight infection. Report symptoms of infection such as body aches, burning with urination, chills, cough, fatigue, fever. Avoid those with active infection. • Report lung problems (excessive coughing, difficulty breathing, chest pain); liver problems (abdominal pain, bruising, clay-colored stool, dark or amber-colored urine, yellowing of the skin or eyes), kidney problems (decreased urine output, flank pain, darkened urine), skin toxicities (rash, peeling); symptoms of heart attack (chest pain, difficulty breathing, jaw pain, nausea, pain that radiates to the left arm, sweating); bleeding of any kind. • Allergic reactions, including anaphylaxis, may occur. • Treatment may alter the electrical conduction of the heart, which may lead to cardiac arrhythmias; report chest pain, difficulty breathing, dizziness, swelling of extremities, fainting, palpitations. • Use effective contraception to avoid pregnancy. Do not breastfeed.

• Do not take newly prescribed medications unless approved by prescriber who originally started treatment. • Treatment may worsen high B/P. • Avoid exposure to sun, artificial light (may cause photosensitivity reaction). • Do not take within 2 hrs of taking antacids. • Do not ingest grapefruit products.

tafasitamab-cxix

ta-fa-**sit**-a-mab
(Monjuvi)
Do not confuse tafasitamab with basiliximab, naxitamab, rituximab, or trastuzumab.

◆CLASSIFICATION

PHARMACOTHERAPEUTIC: Anti-CD19, monoclonal antibody. **CLINICAL:** Antineoplastic.

USES

Treatment (in combination with lenalidomide) of adults with relapsed or refractory diffuse large B-cell lymphoma (DLBCL) not otherwise specified, including DLBCL arising from low-grade lymphoma and who are not eligible for autologous stem cell transplant.

PRECAUTIONS

Contraindications: Hypersensitivity to tafasitamab-cxix. Use of lenalidomide in pregnancy. **Cautions:**Baseline cytopenias, hepatic impairment, conditions predisposing to infection (e.g., diabetes, renal failure, immunocompromised pts, open wounds), chronic viral infections.

ACTION

Binds to CD19 antigen (expressed on the surface of pre-B and mature B lymphocytes and several B-cell malignancies, including DLBCL). Mediates B-cell lysis through apoptosis and immune effector mechanisms, including antibody-dependent cellular cytotoxicity and phagocytosis.

Therapeutic Effect: Causes cellular damage and death of malignant B cells.

PHARMACOKINETICS

Widely distributed. Metabolism not specified. Peripheral B-cell count reduced by day 8. Nadir reached within 16 wks. Excretion not specified. **Half-life:** 17 days.

⏳ LIFESPAN CONSIDERATIONS

Pregnancy/Lactation: Avoid pregnancy; may cause fetal harm due to fetal B-cell depletion and neonatal lymphopenia. Females of reproductive potential should use effective contraception during treatment and for at least 3 mos after discontinuation. Unknown if distributed in breast milk. However, human immunoglobulin G (IgG) is present in breast milk. **Children:** Safety and efficacy not established. **Elderly:** May have increased risk if adverse reactions.

INTERACTIONS

DRUG: May decrease therapeutic effect of **BCG (intravesical)**, **vaccines (live)**. May increase toxic effect of **cladribine**. May increase immunosuppressive effect of **baricitinib, tofacitinib, upadacitinib**. May increase the adverse/toxic effect of **natalizumab**. **HERBAL:** Echinacea may decrease therapeutic effect. **FOOD:** None known. **LAB VALUES:** May increase serum AST, creatinine, glucose, GGT, uric acid. May decrease serum albumin, calcium, magnesium, phosphate; Hgb, lymphocytes, neutrophils, platelets. May prolong activated partial thromboplastin (aPTT). May decrease diagnostic effect of *Coccidioides immitis* skin test.

AVAILABILITY (Rx)

Injection, Powder for Reconstitution: 200 mg.

ADMINISTRATION/HANDLING

🖱 IV

Premedication • Premedicate with acetaminophen, histamine H_1 or H_2 antagonist, and/or glucocorticosteroid 30 min to 2 hrs prior to initial infusion. If infusion reactions do not occur during the first 3 infusions, premedication is optimal for subsequent infusions. If infusion-related reaction occurs, administer premedication prior to each subsequent infusion.

Reconstitution • Must be prepared by personnel trained in aseptic manipulations and admixing of cytotoxic drugs. • Calculate the dose based on weight in kg. • While directing stream toward glass wall of vial, reconstitute each vial with 5 mL Sterile Water for Injection to a final concentration of 40 mg/mL. • Swirl vial(s) gently until powder is completely dissolved (up to 5 min). Do not shake or swirl aggressively. • Visually inspect for particulate matter or discoloration. Solution should appear colorless to slightly yellow. Do not use if solution is cloudy, discolored, or if visible particles are observed. • Dilute in 250 mL 0.9% NaCl infusion bag (final concentration of diluted solution should equal 2–8 mg/mL). • Mix by gentle inversion. Do not shake or agitate. • Discard used portions of vial(s).

Rate of administration • **Initial infusion:** Infuse via dedicated IV catheter at 70 mL/hr for 30 min, then increase to a rate so the infusion is completed within 1.5–2.5 hrs. • **Subsequent infusions:** Infuse within 1.5–2 hrs as tolerated.

Infusion-related reaction • **Grade 2 reaction:** Interrupt infusion and treat symptoms until improved to Grade 1, then resume infusion at no more than 50% of the infusion rate prior to interruption. If no further reactions occur within 1 hr and vital signs are stable, may increase infusion rate q30min to the rate prior to interruption. • **Grade 3 reaction:** Interrupt infusion and treat symptoms until improved to Grade 1, then resume infusion at no more than 25% of the infusion rate prior to interruption. If no further reactions occur within 1 hr and vital signs are stable, may increase infusion rate q30min to 50% of the infusion rate prior to interruption. Discontinue infusion if reaction recurs after escalating infusion rate. • **Grade 4 infusion reaction:** Discontinue infusion and permanently discontinue treatment.

Storage • Refrigerate unused vials in original carton. Protect from light. • May

 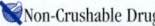

refrigerate or store reconstituted vials at room temperature for up to 12 hrs. • Diluted solution may be refrigerated for up to 18 hrs or stored at room temperature for up to 12 hrs. Protect from light. Do not freeze.

▨ IV INCOMPATABILITIES

Do not administer with other medications.

INDICATIONS/ROUTES/DOSAGE

Diffuse Large B-Cell Lymphoma (Relapsed or Refractory)

IV: ADULTS: 12 mg/kg (in combination with lenalidomide 25 mg for a maximum of 12 cycles) on treatment days (of 28-day cycle) as follows: **Cycle 1:** Days 1, 4, 8, 15, and 22. **Cycles 2 and 3:** Days 1, 8, 15, and 22. **Cycle 4 and thereafter:** Days 1 and 15. After 12 cycles, continue tafasitamab-cxix as a monotherapy until disease progression or unacceptable toxicity.

Dose Modification

Based on Common Terminology Criteria for Adverse Events (CTCAE).

Neutropenia

Neutrophil count 1,000 cells/mm³ or less for at least 7 days; neutrophil count 1,000 cells/mm³ or less with fever 100.4°F (38°C) or higher; neutrophil count less than 500 cells/mm³: Withhold treatment and lenalidomide until neutrophil count is 1,000 cells/mm³ or greater, then resume at same dose and reduce lenalidomide dose (see manufacturer guidelines).

Thrombocytopenia

Platelet count 50,000 cells/mm³ or less: Withhold treatment and lenalidomide until platelet count is 50,000 cells/mm³ or greater, then resume at same dose and reduce lenalidomide dose (see manufacturer guidelines).

Dosage in Renal Impairment

Mild to moderate impairment: No dose adjustment. **Severe impairment, ESRD:** Not specified; use caution.

Dosage in Hepatic Impairment

Mild impairment: No dose adjustment. **Moderate to severe impairment:** Not specified; use caution.

SIDE EFFECTS

Frequent (38%–22%): Fatigue, diarrhea, cough, pyrexia, peripheral edema, decreased appetite. **Occasional (19%–6%):** Back pain, constipation, abdominal pain, nausea, vomiting, muscle spasm, dyspnea, rash, pruritus, headache, arthralgia, extremity pain, paresthesia, dysgeusia. **Rare (5%–3%):** Decreased weight, nasal congestion, erythema, musculoskeletal pain, alopecia, hyperhidrosis.

ADVERSE EFFECTS/TOXIC REACTIONS

Myelosuppression (anemia, neutropenia, lymphopenia, thrombocytopenia) is an expected response to therapy, but more severe reactions, including febrile neutropenia, may be life-threatening. Infusion reactions, including chills, dyspnea, fever, flushing, hypertension, rash, may require emergent medical attention. Life-threatening infections, including bronchitis, nasopharyngitis, pneumonia, respiratory tract infection, sepsis, UTI, reported in 71% of pts. Grade 3 or 4 infections reported in 30% of pts. Progressive multifocal leukoencephalopathy (PML), an opportunistic viral infection of the brain caused by the JC virus, may result in progressive permanent disability and death. Exacerbation of COPD reported in 1% of pts.

NURSING CONSIDERATIONS

BASELINE ASSESSMENT

Obtain CBC; pregnancy test in females of reproductive potential. Verify use of effective contraception. Obtain weight in kg. Administer in an environment equipped to monitor for and manage infusion-related reactions; verify emergency resuscitation equipment/medications are readily available. Question history and severity of infusion reactions prior to each infusion. Screen for active infection. Offer emotional support.

INTERVENTION/EVALUATION

Monitor CBC for myelosuppression prior to each cycle. If neutrophil count is 1,000 cells/mm³ or less or platelet count is 50,000 cells/mm³ or less, monitor CBC wkly until improved. Consider granulocyte-stimulating factor in pts with neutropenia. Diligently monitor for infusion reactions during each infusion. Severe infusion reactions may require emergency resuscitation; early detection is vital. Monitor for infections (cough, fatigue, fever, urinary frequency/dysuria), symptoms of PML (confusion, dysarthria, paralysis, seizures). If serious infection occurs, initiate appropriate antimicrobial therapy. Monitor daily pattern of bowel activity, stool consistency.

PATIENT/FAMILY TEACHING

• Treatment may depress the immune system response and reduce ability to fight infection. Report symptoms of infection such as body aches, chills, cough, fatigue, fever. Avoid those with active infection. • Report symptoms of bone marrow depression (e.g., bruising, fatigue, fever, shortness of breath, weight loss; bleeding easily, bloody urine or stool). • Severe infusion reactions may occur. Immediately report infusion reactions of any kind. • PML, an opportunistic viral infection of the brain, may cause progressive, permanent disabilities and death. Report symptoms of PML, brain hemorrhage such as confusion, memory loss, paralysis, trouble speaking, vision loss, seizures. • Use effective contraception to avoid pregnancy. Do not breastfeed. • Maintain proper hydration and nutrition.

talazoparib

tal-a-**zoe**-pa-rib
(Talzenna)
Do not confuse talazoparib with niraparib, olaparib, or ruca-parib, or Talzenna with Senna.

◆CLASSIFICATION

PHARMACOTHERAPEUTIC: Poly (ADP-ribose) polymerase (PARP) inhibitor. **CLINICAL:** Antineoplastic.

USES

Breast cancer: Treatment of adults with deleterious or suspected deleterious germline BRCA-mutation *(gBRCAm)* HER2-negative locally advanced or metastatic breast cancer. **Prostate cancer:** In combination with enzalutamide for treatment of adults with HRR gene-mutated metastatic castration-resistant prostate cancer (mCRPC).

PRECAUTIONS

Contraindications: Hypersensitivity to talazoparib. **Cautions:** Baseline cytopenias, renal/hepatic impairment, conditions predisposing to infection (e.g., diabetes, renal failure, immunocompromised pts, open wounds); concomitant use of P-gp inhibitors. Do not initiate in pts who have not recovered from hematological toxicities related to prior chemotherapy.

ACTION

Inhibits poly (ADP-ribose) polymerase (PARP) enzymatic activity. PARP enzymes are involved in DNA transcription, cell cycle regulation and DNA repair. Inhibition causes cell death due to DNA damage. **Therapeutic Effect:** Inhibits tumor cell growth and survival.

PHARMACOKINETICS

Widely distributed. Metabolized by oxidation, dehydrogenation, and conjugation (with minimal hepatic metabolism). Protein binding: 74%. Peak plasma concentration: 1–2 hrs. Excreted in urine (69%), feces (20%). **Half-life:** 90 (±58) hrs.

⧗ LIFESPAN CONSIDERATIONS

Pregnancy/Lactation: Avoid pregnancy; may cause fetal harm. Females of reproductive potential must use effective contraception during treatment and for at least 7 mos after discontinuation. Unknown if distributed in breast milk.

T

Breastfeeding not recommended during treatment and for at least 1 mo after discontinuation. **Males:** Males with female partners of reproductive potential must use effective contraception during treatment and for at least 4 mos after discontinuation. May impair fertility. **Children:** Safety and efficacy not established. **Elderly:** No age-related precautions noted.

INTERACTIONS

DRUG: P-gp inhibitors (e.g., **amiodarone, azithromycin, captopril, carvedilol, cyclosporine, dilTIAZem, ketoconazole, ritonavir, verapamil**) may significantly increase concentration/effect. **Cladribine** may increase myelosuppression. **HERBAL:** None significant. **FOOD:** None known. **LAB VALUES:**May increase serum alkaline phosphatase, ALT, AST, glucose. May decrease Hgb, leukocytes, neutrophils, lymphocytes, platelets; serum calcium.

AVAILABILITY (Rx)

Capsules:0.1 mg, 0.25 mg, 0.35 mg, 0.5 mg, 0.75 mg, 1 mg.

ADMINISTRATION/HANDLING

PO
• Give without regard to meals. • Administer capsules whole; do not break, cut, or open. Capsules cannot be chewed. • If a dose is missed or vomiting occurs after administration, do not give extra dose. Administer next dose at regularly scheduled time.

INDICATIONS/ROUTES/DOSAGE

Note: Administer only to pts with germline BRCA mutation.

Breast Cancer
PO: ADULTS, ELDERLY: 1 mg once daily. Continue until disease progression or unacceptable toxicity.

mCRPC
Note: Pts should receive a gonadotropic-releasing hormone (GnRH) analog concurrently or have had bilateral orchiectomy. **PO: ADULTS, ELDERLY:** 0.5 mg once daily (in combination with enzalutamide).

Continue until disease progression or unacceptable toxicity.

Dose Reduction Schedule
First reduction: 0.75 mg once daily.
Second reduction: 0.5 mg once daily.
Third reduction: 0.25 mg once daily.
Unable to tolerate 0.25 mg dose: Permanently discontinue.

Dose Modification
Based on Common Terminology Criteria for Adverse Events (CTCAE).

Hematologic Toxicity
Hemoglobin less than 8 g/dL: Withhold treatment until improved to 9 g/dL (or greater), then resume at next reduced dose.
Platelet count less than 50,000 cells/mm³: Withhold treatment until improved to 75,000 cells/mm³ (or greater), then resume at next reduced dose.
Neutrophil count less than 1,000 cells/mm³: Withhold treatment until improved to 1,500 cells/mm³ (or greater), then resume at next reduced dose.

Nonhematologic Toxicity
Any Grade 3 or 4 adverse reaction: Withhold treatment until improved to Grade 1 or 0, then consider resuming at a reduced dose or discontinue.

Concomitant Use of P-gp Inhibitors
Reduce dose to 0.75 mg once daily. If P-gp inhibitor is discontinued for 3–5 half-lives, resume talazoparib dose to the dose used prior to starting P-gp inhibitor.

Dosage in Renal Impairment
Mild impairment: No dose adjustment. **Moderate impairment (CrCl 30–59 mL/min):** Reduce dose to 0.75 mg once daily. **Severe impairment:** Not specified; use caution.

Dosage in Hepatic Impairment
Mild impairment: No dose adjustment. **Moderate to severe impairment:** Not specified; use caution.

SIDE EFFECTS

Frequent (62%–21%): Fatigue, asthenia, nausea, headache, vomiting, alopecia, diarrhea, decreased appetite.

ADVERSE EFFECTS/TOXIC REACTIONS

Myelosuppression (anemia, leukopenia, neutropenia, thrombocytopenia) is an expected response to therapy. Grade 3 (or higher) anemia, neutropenia, thrombocytopenia reported in 39%–15% of pts. Acute myeloid leukemia, myelodysplastic syndrome was reported in pts who received prior chemotherapy with platinum agents and/or DNA-damaging agents.

NURSING CONSIDERATIONS

BASELINE ASSESSMENT

Obtain CBC; pregnancy test in females of reproductive potential. Obtain renal function test (BUN, serum creatinine, CrCl, eGFR) in pts with renal impairment; LFT in pts with hepatic impairment. Question history of hepatic/renal impairment, prior treatment with other chemotherapeutic agents. Receive full medication history and screen for interactions (esp. P-gp inhibitors). Screen for active infection. Do not initiate in pts who have not recovered from hematological toxicities related to prior chemotherapy. Offer emotional support.

INTERVENTION/EVALUATION

Monitor CBC monthly. If hematologic toxicities occur, monitor CBC wkly until blood counts recover. If blood counts do not recover, consider hematology consultation for further investigations such as bone marrow analysis and blood sample for cytogenetics. Monitor for acute myeloid leukemia, myelodysplastic syndrome (bleeding, bruising easily; fatigue, frequent infections, pyrexia, hematuria, melena, weakness, weight loss; cytopenias, increased requirements for blood transfusion). If acute myeloid leukemia or myelodysplastic syndrome occurs, discontinue treatment. If concomitant use of P-gp inhibitor is unavoidable, monitor for adverse reactions/drug toxicities.

Diligently screen for infections (cough, fatigue, fever). Monitor daily pattern of bowel activity, stool consistency. Encourage nutritional intake.

PATIENT/FAMILY TEACHING

• Treatment may depress your immune system and reduce your ability to fight infection. Report symptoms of infection such as body aches, burning with urination, chills, cough, fatigue, fever. Avoid those with active infection. • Treatment may cause severe bone marrow depression or new-onset myeloid leukemia; report bruising, fatigue, fever, frequent infections, shortness of breath, weight loss; bleeding easily, blood in urine or stool. • Use effective contraception to avoid pregnancy. Do not breastfeed. • Report liver problems (abdominal pain, bruising, clay-colored stool, amber- or dark-colored urine, yellowing of the skin or eyes). • Do not take newly prescribed medications unless approved by prescriber who originally started treatment.

---

tamoxifen HIGH ALERT

ta-**MOKS**-i-fen
(Nolvadex-D 🍁, Soltamox)

■ **BLACK BOX ALERT** ■ Serious, possibly life-threatening CVA, pulmonary emboli, uterine malignancy (endometrial adenocarcinoma, uterine sarcoma) have occurred. **Do not confuse tamoxifen with pentoxifylline, tamsulosin, or temazepam.**

◆CLASSIFICATION

PHARMACOTHERAPEUTIC: Selective estrogen receptor modulator (SERM). Estrogen receptor antagonist. **CLINICAL:** Antineoplastic.

USES

Breast cancer treatment: (Metastatic breast cancer): Treatment of adults with estrogen receptor-positive metastatic breast cancer. (**Adjuvant treatment of breast cancer**): Treatment of adults with early stage estrogen receptor–positive breast cancer; reduce occurrence of contralateral breast cancer. **Ductal carcinoma in situ (DCIS):** Reduce risk of invasive breast cancer in adult women with DCIS, following breast surgery and radiation. **Risk reduction:** Reduce the incidence of breast cancer in adult women at high risk for breast cancer. **OFF-LABEL:** Ovarian cancer (advanced and/or recurrent), treatment of endometrial cancer; gynecomastia, ovulation induction (breast cancer pts), idiopathic male infertility.

PRECAUTIONS

Contraindications: Hypersensitivity to tamoxifen. Concomitant warfarin therapy when used in treatment of breast cancer in high-risk women, history of deep vein thrombosis (DVT) or pulmonary embolism (in high-risk women for breast cancer and in women with DCIS). **Cautions:** Thrombocytopenia, pregnancy, history of thromboembolic events, hyperlipidemia, concomitant use of strong CYP2D6 inhibitors and/or moderate CYP2D6 inhibitors.

ACTION

Competitively binds to estrogen receptors on tumor, producing a complex. **Therapeutic Effect:** Inhibits DNA synthesis and estrogen effects. Slows tumor growth.

PHARMACOKINETICS

Well absorbed from GI tract. Metabolized in liver. Primarily excreted in feces. **Half-life:** 7 days.

⧗ LIFESPAN CONSIDERATIONS

Pregnancy/Lactation: Avoid pregnancy; may cause fetal harm. Nonhormonal contraceptives recommended during therapy and for at least 2 mos after discontinuation. Unknown if distributed in breast milk. Breastfeeding not recommended. **Children:** Safe and effective in girls 2–10 yrs with McCune-Albright syndrome, precocious puberty. **Elderly:** No age-related precautions noted.

INTERACTIONS

DRUG: Strong CYP3A4 inducers (e.g., carBAMazepine, phenytoin, rifAMPin) may decrease concentration/effect. **Strong CYP3A4 inhibitors (e.g., clarithromycin, ketoconazole)** may increase concentration/effect. May increase anticoagulant effect of **warfarin.** May decrease effect of **anastrozole, letrozole. Moderate/strong CYP2D6 inhibitors (e.g., FLUoxetine, sertraline)** may decrease efficacy and increase risk of breast cancer. **HERBAL:** None significant. **FOOD:** None known. **LAB VALUES:** May increase serum cholesterol, calcium, triglycerides, AST, ALT.

AVAILABILITY (Rx)

Solution, Oral: *(Soltamox):* 10 mg/5 mL.
Tablets: 10 mg, 20 mg.

ADMINISTRATION/HANDLING

PO
• Give without regard to food. • Use supplied dosing cup for oral solution.

INDICATIONS/ROUTES/DOSAGE

Metastatic Breast Cancer
PO: ADULTS, ELDERLY: 20 mg once daily. **Premenopausal:** Tamoxifen may be given (with ovarian suppression) in pts with no prior endocrine therapy or prior treatment with ovarian suppression and an AI. **Postmenopausal:** Tamoxifen may be given in pts with no prior endocrine therapy or prior endocrine therapy with an AI.

Breast Cancer Treatment
PO: ADJUVANT THERAPY (FEMALES), PREMENOPAUSAL WOMEN INITIATION: 20 mg once daily for 5 yrs. May continue for total of 10 yrs if premenopausal or perimenopausal after 5 yrs. If postmenopausal after 5 yrs, may continue for total of 10 yrs or switch to an AI up to total of 10 yrs of endocrine therapy. **POSTMENOPAUSAL WOMEN INITIATION:** Total duration of 10 yrs, or tamoxifen for an initial duration of 5 yrs, followed by an AI for up to 5 yrs (for total duration of 10 yrs) or

tamoxifen for 2–3 yrs, followed by an AI for up to 5 yrs (for a total duration of 7–8 yrs) or an AI for 5 yrs.

Ductal Carcinoma in Situ (DCIS)
PO: ADULTS, ELDERLY: 20 mg once daily for 5 yrs.

Breast Cancer Risk Reduction
PO: ADULTS, ELDERLY: 20 mg once daily for 5 yrs.

Dosage in Renal/Hepatic Impairment
No dose adjustment.

SIDE EFFECTS

Frequent: Women (greater than 10%): Hot flashes, nausea, vomiting. **Occasional:** Headache, nausea, vomiting, rash, bone pain, confusion, weakness, drowsiness. **Women (9%–1%):** Changes in menstruation, genital itching, vaginal discharge, endometrial hyperplasia, polyps. **Men:** Impotence, decreased libido.

ADVERSE EFFECTS/TOXIC REACTIONS

Retinopathy, corneal opacity, decreased visual acuity noted in pts receiving extremely high dosages (240–320 mg/day) for longer than 17 mos.

NURSING CONSIDERATIONS

BASELINE ASSESSMENT

Obtain CBC, serum calcium, estrogen receptor assay prior to therapy. Obtain baseline breast and gynecologic exams, mammogram results. Question history of thrombosis (DVT, PE).

INTERVENTION/EVALUATION

Obtain CBC, serum calcium periodically. Monitor for increased bone pain; ensure adequate pain relief. Monitor I&O, weight. Monitor for symptoms of DVT (leg or arm pain/swelling), PE (chest pain, dyspnea, tachycardia). Assess for hypercalcemia (increased urinary volume, excessive thirst, nausea, vomiting, constipation, hypotonicity of muscles, deep bone/flank pain, renal stones).

PATIENT/FAMILY TEACHING

• Report vaginal bleeding/discharge/itching, leg cramps, weight gain, shortness of breath, weakness. • May initially experience increase in bone, tumor pain (appears to indicate good tumor response). • Report persistent nausea, vomiting. • Report symptoms of DVT (e.g., swelling, pain, hot feeling in the arms or legs; discoloration of extremity), lung embolism (e.g., difficulty breathing, chest pain, rapid heart rate). • Nonhormonal contraceptives are recommended during treatment.

tamsulosin

tam-**soo**-loe-sin
(<u>Flomax</u>, Flomax CR✦)
Do not confuse Flomax with Flonase, Flovent, Foltx, Fosamax, or Volmax, or tamsulosin with tamoxifen or terazosin.

FIXED-COMBINATION(S)

Jalyn: tamsulosin/dutasteride (an androgen hormone inhibitor): 0.4 mg/0.5 mg.

◆CLASSIFICATION

PHARMACOTHERAPEUTIC: Alpha₁-adrenergic blocker. **CLINICAL:** Benign prostatic hyperplasia agent.

USES

Treatment of symptoms of benign prostatic hyperplasia (BPH). **OFF-LABEL:** Chronic prostatitis/pelvic pain (males), lower urinary tract symptoms (males), ureteral calculi expulsion/stent-related urinary symptoms.

PRECAUTIONS

Contraindications: Hypersensitivity to tamsulosin. **Cautions:** Concurrent use of phosphodiesterase (PDE5) inhibitors (e.g., sildenafil, tadalafil, vardenafil), baseline orthostatic hypotension. Not indicated for treatment of hypertension.

T

ACTION

Antagonist of alpha receptors in prostate. **Therapeutic Effect:** Relaxes smooth muscle in bladder neck and prostate; improves urinary flow, symptoms of prostatic hyperplasia.

PHARMACOKINETICS

Widely distributed. Protein binding: 94%–99%. Metabolized in liver. Primarily excreted in urine. Unknown if removed by hemodialysis. **Half-life:** 9–13 hrs.

⌛ LIFESPAN CONSIDERATIONS

Pregnancy/Lactation: Not indicated for use in women. **Children:** Not indicated in this pt population. **Elderly:** No age-related precautions noted.

INTERACTIONS

DRUG: Alpha-adrenergic blockers (e.g., doxazosin, prazosin, terazosin) may increase alpha-blockade effect. **Strong CYP3A4 inhibitors (e.g., clarithromycin, ketoconazole, ritonavir)** may increase concentration/effect. **Strong CYP3A4 inducers (e.g., carBAMazepine, phenytoin, rifAMPin)** may decrease concentration/effect. **HERBAL: Herbals with hypotensive properties (e.g., garlic, ginger, ginkgo biloba)** may alter effects. **St. John's wort** may decrease concentration/effect. **FOOD: Grapefruit products** may increase risk for orthostatic hypotension. **LAB VALUES:** None known.

AVAILABILITY (Rx)

 Capsules: 0.4 mg.

ADMINISTRATION/HANDLING

PO
• Give at same time each day, 30 min after the same meal. • Do not break, crush, or open capsule.

INDICATIONS/ROUTES/DOSAGE

Benign Prostatic Hyperplasia (BPH)
PO: ADULTS: 0.4 mg once daily, approximately 30 min after same meal each day. May increase dosage to 0.8 mg if inadequate response in 2–4 wks. If therapy discontinued or interrupted for several days, restart at 0.4 mg once daily.

Dosage in Renal/Hepatic Impairment
No dose adjustment.

SIDE EFFECTS

Frequent (9%–7%): Dizziness, drowsiness. **Occasional (5%–3%):** Headache, anxiety, insomnia, orthostatic hypotension. **Rare (less than 2%):** Nasal congestion, pharyngitis, rhinitis, nausea, vertigo, impotence.

ADVERSE EFFECTS/TOXIC REACTIONS

Orthostasis (dizziness, postural hypotension, vertigo) may occur upon initiation. Persistent, painful erection (priapism) occurs rarely. Intraoperative floppy iris syndrome was observed during cataract and glaucoma surgery, which may increase risk of eye complications during and after operation.

NURSING CONSIDERATIONS

BASELINE ASSESSMENT

Obtain vital signs. Assess history of prostatic hyperplasia (difficulty initiating urine stream, dribbling, sense of urgency, leaking). Question for sensitivity to other alpha-adrenergic blocking agents. Receive medication history and screen for interactions. Screen for presence of prostate caner.

INTERVENTION/EVALUATION

Monitor for orthostasis, especially upon initiation. Monitor for improvement of urinary symptoms. Priapism requires immediate medical attention.

PATIENT/FAMILY TEACHING

• Take at same time each day, 30 min after the same meal. • Go from lying to standing slowly. • Avoid tasks that require alertness, motor skills until response to drug is established. • Avoid grapefruit products. • Treatment may cause intraoperative floppy iris syndrome during eye surgery. Notify ophthalmologist of treatment with tamsulosin if glaucoma or cataract surgery is planned. • Seek medical attention if persistent, painful erection occurs. • Do not take newly prescribed medications unless approved by physician who originally started treatment.

teclistamab-cqyv

tek-**lis**-ta-mab
(Tecvayli)

■ **BLACK BOX ALERT** ■ Life-threatening cytokine release syndrome (CRS) was reported. Initiate treatment in a step-up dosing schedule. If CRS occurs, withhold treatment until resolved or permanently discontinue based on severity. Life-threatening neurotoxicities, including immune effector cell-associated neurotoxicity syndrome (ICANS), may occur. If ICANS occurs, withhold treatment until resolved or permanently discontinue based on severity.
Do not confuse teclistamab with amivantamab, tafasitamab, or talquetamab or Tecvayli with or Tivicay.

◆CLASSIFICATION

PHARMACOTHERAPEUTIC: Bispecific B-cell maturation antigen (BCMA)–directed CD3 T-cell engager. **CLINICAL:** Antineoplastic.

USES

Treatment of adults with relapsed or refractory multiple myeloma who have received at least four prior lines of therapy, including a proteasome inhibitor, an immunomodulatory agent, and an anti-CD38 monoclonal antibody.

PRECAUTIONS

Contraindications: Hypersensitivity to teclistamab-cqyv. **Cautions:** Baseline cytopenias, hepatic/renal impairment, conditions predisposing to infection (e.g., diabetes, renal failure, immunocompromised pts, open wounds), chronic opportunistic infections (e.g., herpes virus infection); history of cardiac arrhythmia (e.g., atrial fibrillation/flutter, ventricular dysrhythmias). Avoid administration of BCG (intravesical), live vaccines.

ACTION

A bispecific antibody, binds to two different targets at the same time: BCMA, a protein found on plasma cells and at higher levels on multiple myeloma cells, and CD3, a protein present on immune cells called T cells. **Therapeutic Effect:** By bringing myeloma cells and T cells together, helps the T cell to recognize and destroy the tumor cell.

PHARMACOKINETICS

Widely distributed. Metabolism not specified. Peak plasma concentration: 19–168 hrs. Steady state reached after 12 wkly doses. Excretion not specified. **Half-life:** 15 days.

⧗ LIFESPAN CONSIDERATIONS

Pregnancy/Lactation: Avoid pregnancy; may cause fetal harm (including B-cell lymphocytopenia). Females of reproductive potential must use effective contraception during treatment and for at least 5 mos after discontinuation. Unknown if distributed in breast milk. Human IgG is present in breast milk and is known to cross the placenta. Breastfeeding not recommended during treatment and for at least 3 mos after discontinuation. **Children:** Safety and efficacy not established. **Elderly:** No age-related precautions noted.

INTERACTIONS

DRUG: May increase concentration/effects of **CYP450 substrates (e.g., atorvastatin, fentaNYL, midazolam, phenytoin, theophylline, warfarin)**. May decrease therapeutic effect; increase adverse effects of **BCG (intravesical)**,

T

live vaccines. **Clozapine** may increase the risk and/or severity of hematologic toxicity. **HERBAL:** None significant. **FOOD:** None known. **LAB VALUES:** May increase serum alkaline phosphatase, ALT, AST, creatinine, GGT. May decrease Hgb, neutrophils, lymphocytes, platelets, RBC, WBC; serum albumin, calcium, gamma globulin, phosphorus, sodium.

AVAILABILITY (Rx)

Injection Solution: 30 mg/3 mL (10 mg/mL), 153 mg/1.7 mL (90 mg/mL).

ADMINISTRATION/HANDLING
SQ

Administration guidelines • Must be administered by a healthcare professional with medical support trained in the management of severe reactions including CRS, ICANS, and other neurological toxicities. • Preparation guidelines are highly specific based on pt's weight in kg. See manufacturer guidelines regarding the required injection volumes to obtain the total dose (may require one or two vials). • Do not combine different concentrations to obtain treatment dose. • Each injection volume should not exceed 2 mL. Doses requiring a volume greater than 2 mL should be divided equally into multiple syringes.

Premedication • Step-up doses and first full treatment dose: Premedicate with diphenhydrAMINE 50 mg PO or IV (or equivalent), acetaminophen 500–1,000 mg PO or IV, dexAMETHasone 16 mg PO or IV 1–3 hrs prior to each dose. • **Subsequent doses:** For pts who must reinitiate a step-up schedule following a dose delay or experience any grade CRS with any dose, continue premedication treatment.

Preparation • Must be prepared by personnel trained in aseptic manipulations and admixing of cytotoxic drugs. • Allow refrigerated vial(s) to warm to room temp (approx. 15 min). Do not use external heat sources. • After warming, gently swirl vial(s) for 10 sec; do not shake. • Visually inspect solution for particulate matter or discoloration. Solution should appear clear to slightly opalescent and colorless to light yellow. Do not use if solution is cloudy, discolored, or visible particles are observed. • Transfer the required injection volume needed for dose into syringe (see manufacturer guidelines).

Administration • Insert needle subcutaneously into the abdomen (preferred site) or outer thigh and inject solution. • Multiple injection sites must be at least 2 cm apart. • Do not inject into areas of active skin disease or injury such as sunburns, skin rashes, inflammation, skin infections, or active psoriasis. • Rotate injection sites. • Do not administer IV or intramuscularly.

Storage • Refrigerate unused vials in original carton until time of use. Protect from light. • Prepared syringes maybe refrigerated or stored at room temperature for up to 20 hrs. Protect from light.

INDICATIONS/ROUTES/DOSAGE

Note: Allow 2–4 days between first, second, and full treatment dose. If adverse reactions occur after any dose of the step-up phase, may withhold the subsequent dose up to 7 days to allow resolution of adverse reactions. If treatment is withheld for adverse reactions after the step-up schedule is completed, reinitiate the step-up schedule per manufacturer guidelines.

Multiple Myeloma (Relapsed or Refractory)

SQ: ADULTS, ELDERLY: (Step-up dosing schedule): (First dose): 0.06 mg/kg mg on day 1. **(Second dose):** 0.3 mg/kg on day 4. **(First full treatment dose):** 1.5 mg/kg on day 7. **Maintenance:** 1.5 mg/kg once wkly starting 7 days after the first full treatment dose. Pts achieving and maintaining complete response or better for a minimum of 6 mos may decrease dosing frequency to 1.5 mg/kg 2 qwks.

Dose Modification

Based on Common Terminology Criteria for Adverse Events (CTCAE).

CRS
Note: Admission to the intensive care unit (ICU) may be required for Grade 3 or 4 CRS or recurrent Grade 3 CRS.
Grade 1 CRS: Withhold treatment. Prior to next dose, verify CRS symptoms are resolved and premedicate per guidelines.
Grade 2 or 3 CRS: Withhold treatment. Prior to next dose, verify CRS symptoms are resolved and premedicate per guidelines. Pts should be hospitalized for 48 hrs after the next dose is given. **Recurrent Grade 3 CRS; Grade 3 CRS lasting 48 hrs or longer; Grade 4 CRS:** Permanently discontinue.

ICANS
Note: Neurology consultation should be considered for evaluation and management of any grade ICANS. Evaluate for other causes of neurologic symptoms. Seizure prophylaxis may be required. If indicated, give dexAMETHasone 10 mg IV q6hrs until symptoms improve to Grade 1 or 0, then taper. Admission to the ICU may be required for recurrent Grade 3 ICANS or Grade 4 ICANS.
Grade 1 ICANS: Withhold treatment until resolved. **Grade 2 ICANS:** Withhold treatment until resolved. Start dexAMETHasone therapy. Pts should be hospitalized for 48 hrs after the next dose is given. **Grade 3 ICANS: (First occurrence):** Withhold treatment until resolved. Start dexAMETHasone therapy. Pts should be hospitalized for 48 hrs after the next dose is given. **Recurrent Grade 3 ICANS:** Permanently discontinue treatment. Start dexAMETHasone therapy. **Grade 4 ICANS:** Permanently discontinue treatment. Start dexAMETHasone therapy or treat with methylPREDNISolone 1,000 mg IV daily for 2 or more days.

Neurologic Toxicity (Excluding ICANS)
Note: Neurology consultation should be considered for evaluation and management of any neurological toxicity. Evaluate for other causes of neurologic symptoms. Seizure prophylaxis may be required. Admission to the ICU may be required for recurrent Grade 3 neurologic toxicity or Grade 4 neurologic toxicity.
Grade 1 neurologic toxicity: Withhold treatment until resolved or stable. **Grade 2 neurologic toxicity; Grade 3 neurologic toxicity: (First occurrence):** Withhold treatment until improved to Grade 1 or 0. **Recurrent Grade 3 neurologic toxicity; Grade 4 neurologic toxicity:** Permanently discontinue treatment.

Infection
Note: Withhold treatment in pts with active infection during the set-up dosing schedule.
Grade 3–4 infection: Withhold treatment until improved to Grade 1 or 0. Consider permanent discontinuation if Grade 4 infection occurs.

Anemia
Hgb less than 8 g/dL: Withhold treatment until Hgb is 8 g/dL or greater.

Neutropenia
Absolute neutrophil count (ANC) less than 500 cells/mm³: Withhold treatment until ANC is 500 cells/mm³ or greater. **Febrile neutropenia:** Withhold treatment until ANC is 1,000 cells/mm³ or greater.

Thrombocytopenia
Platelet count less than 50,000 cells/mm³: Withhold treatment until platelets count is 50,000 cells/mm³ or greater.

Other Adverse Reactions
Any other Grade 3 adverse reactions: Withhold treatment until improved to Grade 1 or baseline. **Any other Grade 4 adverse reactions:** Withhold treatment until improved to Grade 1 or baseline, or consider permanent discontinuation.

Dosage in Renal Impairment
Mild to moderate impairment: No dose adjustment. **Severe impairment:** Not specified; use caution.

Dosage in Hepatic Impairment
Mild impairment: No dose adjustment. **Moderate to severe impairment:** Not specified; use caution.

SIDE EFFECTS

Frequent (76%–25%): Pyrexia, musculoskeletal pain, arthralgia, myalgia, extremity pain, injection site reactions (bruising, cellulitis, discomfort, edema, erythema, hematoma, induration, inflammation, pruritus, rash, swelling, fatigue, asthenia, headache, nausea). **Occasional (21%–11%):** Diarrhea, constipation, hypoxia, hypotension, motor dysfunction, rigidity, gait disturbance, muscle spasm, muscular weakness, bone pain, chills, cough, sensory neuropathy, tachycardia, pain (ear, flank, groin, oropharyngeal, jaw, tooth, tumor), edema, fluid retention, vomiting, hypertension, decreased appetite.

ADVERSE EFFECTS/TOXIC REACTIONS

Myelosuppression (anemia, leukopenia, lymphopenia, neutropenia, thrombocytopenia) is an expected response to therapy, but more severe reactions including bone marrow depression, febrile neutropenia may occur. CRS reported in 72% of pts, some of which were life-threatening. Symptoms of CRS may include fatigue, headache, hypotension, hypoxia, nausea, pyrexia, tachycardia; serious events may include acute respiratory distress syndrome, atrial fibrillation, capillary leak syndrome, disseminated intravascular coagulation (DIC), hepatocellular injury, hemophagocytic lymphohistiocytosis/macrophage activation syndrome (HLM/MAS), multiorgan dysfunction, pulmonary edema. Life-threatening neurological toxicities including ICANS, cerebral edema, Guillain-Barre syndrome, leukoencephalopathy, seizures may occur. Hepatotoxicity, including fatal cases, were reported. Life-threatening infections, including influenza, pneumonia, opportunistic infections, sepsis, upper respiratory tract infection, urinary tract infection reported in 17% of pts. Cardiac arrhythmias, including atrial flutter, bradycardia, cardiac arrest, supraventricular tachycardia, ventricular tachycardia, were reported. Acute kidney injury, renal impairment occurred in 11% of pts. Hemorrhagic events, including conjunctival hemorrhage, epistaxis, hematoma, hematuria, hemoperitoneum, hemorrhoidal hemorrhage, GI/GU/mouth bleeding, subdural hematoma, have occurred. Hypersensitivity reactions, including angioedema, reported in 1% of pts.

NURSING CONSIDERATIONS

BASELINE ASSESSMENT

Obtain CBC, BMP, LFT, pregnancy test in females of reproductive potential. Confirm compliance with effective contraception. Obtain weight in kilograms. Administer in an environment that is equipped to manage symptoms of CRS, ICANS, neurological toxicities. Pts may require hospitalization for management of adverse reactions. Premedicate all pts per administration guidelines. Question occurrence of adverse reactions prior to each dose. Question history of cardiac arrhythmias, hepatic/renal impairment, chronic opportunistic infections. Screen for active infection. Receive full medication history and screen for interactions. Consider antiviral prophylaxis to prevent herpes zoster reactivation. Conduct baseline neurological assessment. Offer emotional support.

INTERVENTION/EVALUATION

Monitor CBC for myelosuppression (bleeding, bruising, dyspnea, fever, petechiae, weakness); LFT for hepatotoxicity (bruising, jaundice, right upper abdominal pain, nausea, vomiting, weight loss) as clinically indicated. Diligently monitor for symptoms of CRS, ICANS, neurological toxicities throughout treatment, esp. during the step-up phase. Severe symptoms may require intensive care. Conduct routine neurological assessments. Aphasia, confusion, lethargy, tremor, seizures may indicate neurological toxicity, ICANS, which requires neurological consultation. Be alert for infections, esp. respiratory tract infections including pneumonia, bacterial/fungal/pneumococcal/viral pneumonia (cough, dyspnea, hypoxia, pleuritic chest pain), UTI (dysuria, fever, flank pain, malaise). If serious infection occurs, initiate appropriate antimicrobial therapy. Monitor daily pattern of bowel activity, stool consistency. Monitor for hemorrhagic events including intracranial hemorrhage (altered mental status, aphasia, blindness, hemiparesis, unequal pupils, seizures), GI/GU bleeding (hematemesis, melena, rectal bleeding), epistaxis.

PATIENT/FAMILY TEACHING

• Treatment may depress your immune system response and reduce your ability to fight infection. Report symptoms of infection such as body aches, chills, cough, fatigue, fever; burning while urinating, cloudy or foul-smelling urine. Avoid those with active infection. • Report symptoms of bone marrow depression such as bruising, fatigue, fever, shortness of breath, weight loss; bleeding easily, bloody urine or stool. • Treatment may cause life-threatening reactions that must be immediately treated. Report symptoms of CRS (chills, facial swelling, fever, low blood pressure, nausea, vomiting, or weakness), ICANS (confusion, difficulty speaking or slurred speech, loss of consciousness, loss of balance, or seizures). Severe symptoms may require hospitalization. • Avoid tasks that require alertness, motor skills such as driving or operating machinery until response to drug is established. • Pretreatment with acetaminophen, antihistamines, steroidal anti-inflammatories may help reduce treatment-related reactions. • Due to pretreatment with a corticosteroid, pts with diabetes may experience a transient rise in blood sugar levels. • Report liver problems (abdominal pain, bruising, clay-colored stool, amber or dark-colored urine, yellowing of the skin or eyes), kidney problems (decreased urine output, dark-colored urine), allergic reactions (difficulty breathing, hives, low blood pressure, rash, swelling of the face or tongue), heart problems (difficulty breathing, fainting, irregular heartbeats, palpitations, sweating). • Use effective contraception to avoid pregnancy. Do not breastfeed. • Life-threatening bleeding may occur; report bloody stool, urine; rectal bleeding, nosebleeds, or bleeding in the brain (confusion, difficulty speaking, weakness/paralysis, seizures, vision changes). • Treatment may cause reactivation of chronic viral infections.

tenapanor

ten-**a**-pa-nor
(Ibsrela, Xphozah)

◆CLASSIFICATION

PHARMACOTHERAPEUTIC: Sodium hydrogen exchanger 3 (NHE3) inhibitor (not a phosphate binder). **CLINICAL:** Phosphate-reducing agent. **Note:** Information on Ibsrela; see classification section Irritable Bowel Syndrome (IBS).

USES

Hyperphosphatemia: To reduce serum phosphorus in adults with chronic kidney disease (CKD) on dialysis as add-on therapy in pts who have an inadequate response to phosphate binders or who are intolerant of any dose of phosphate binder therapy.

PRECAUTIONS

Contraindications: Hypersensitivity to tenapanor. Children younger than 6 yrs of age; mechanical GI obstruction (known or suspected). **Cautions:** Diarrhea (discontinue if severe diarrhea occurs).

ACTION

NHE3 is an ion-exchange protein expressed on surface of intestinal epithelium that acidifies the epithelial cells. Decreases phosphate permeability through paracellular pathway. **Therapeutic Effect:** Decreases phosphate absorption/levels in pts with CKD on hemodialysis.

T

PHARMACOKINETICS

Minimal systemic absorption; mainly confined to GI tract. Absorbed tenapanor: Metabolized by CYP3A4. Protein binding: 99%. Excreted in feces (79%) and urine (9%).

⌛ LIFESPAN CONSIDERATIONS

Pregnancy/Lactation: Not distributed in breastmilk. **Children:** Contraindicated in pts younger than 6 yrs. **Elderly:** No age-related precautions noted.

INTERACTIONS

DRUG: May decrease absorption of **OATP2B1 substrates (e.g., enalapril). Sodium polystyrene sulfonate (SPS)** may decrease concentration/effect (binds to tenapanor in GI tract and should not be taken within 3 hrs of tenapanor). **HERBAL:** None significant. **FOOD:** None known. **LAB VALUES:** May decrease serum sodium. Expected to decrease serum phosphate.

AVAILABILITY (Rx)

Tablets: 10 mg, 20 mg, 30 mg.

ADMINISTRATION/HANDLING

Note: If a dose is missed, skip the missed dose and give the next dose at regularly scheduled time. Administration of sodium polystyrene sulfonate and tenapanor must be separated by 3 hrs.

PO
• Give with morning and evening meals.
• Do not to give immediately before hemodialysis (due to increased risk of diarrhea). Instead, give immediately before the next meal after hemodialysis.

INDICATIONS/ROUTES/DOSAGE

Note: Do not take before hemodialysis session. Instead, immediately take before the next meal after hemodialysis.

Hyperphosphatemia (Pts with CKD on Hemodialysis)
PO: ADULTS: 30 mg twice daily immediately before breakfast and dinner. May adjust dose based on phosphate levels.

Dosage in Renal/Hepatic Impairment
No dose adjustment.

SIDE EFFECTS

Frequent (53%–43%): Diarrhea (severe: 3%–5%).

ADVERSE EFFECTS/TOXIC REACTIONS

Severe diarrhea reported in 3%–5% of pts. Diarrhea resulting in dehydration and hyponatremia reported in less than 1% of pts.

NURSING CONSIDERATIONS

BASELINE ASSESSMENT

Obtain phosphate level in pts with CKD on hemodialysis. Questions history of severe GI tract motility disorders, major GI tract surgery. Question usual bowel movement patterns, stool characteristics. Assess hydration status. If concomitant use of OATP2B1 substrates (e.g., enalapril) is unavoidable, consider altering enalapril dose (monitor B/P, HR). Avoid stools softeners, laxatives.

INTERVENTION/EVALUATION

Monitor phosphate levels in pts with CKD on hemodialysis. Monitor for hypophosphatemia (altered mental status, dysphagia, decreased cardiac output, irritability, muscle weakness, respiratory depression). Closely monitor for diarrhea, dehydration.

PATIENT/FAMILY TEACHING

• Report severe diarrhea. Do not take stool softeners, laxatives. • Pts on hemodialysis should limit fluid intake as instructed by nephrology. • Securely store tablets away from children; life-threating diarrhea, dehydration may occur if accidentally ingested. • Report symptoms of low phosphate levels (difficulty swallowing, fatigue, muscle cramps, muscle weakness, palpations, paralysis, numbness, tingling). • Take immediately before breakfast and dinner. • Do not take before hemodialysis session (may increase risk of diarrhea). Instead, immediately take before the next meal after hemodialysis.

tenecteplase

ten-**eck**-te-plase
(TNKase)
Do not confuse TNKase with t-PA or tenecteplase with alteplase or Activase.

◆CLASSIFICATION

PHARMACOTHERAPEUTIC: Tissue plasminogen activator (tPA). **CLINICAL:** Thrombolytic.

USES

Management of ST-elevation myocardial infarction (STEMI) for lysis of thrombi to restore perfusion and reduce mortality. **OFF-LABEL:** Acute ischemic stroke, acute pulmonary embolism (hemodynamically stable, moderate to high risk; hemodynamically unstable, high risk; associated with cardiac arrest).

PRECAUTIONS

Contraindications: Hypersensitivity to tenecteplase. Active internal bleeding, cerebral aneurysm, AV malformation, bleeding diathesis, history of CVA, intracranial or intraspinal surgery or trauma within past 2 mos, intracranial neoplasm, severe uncontrolled hypertension. **Cautions:** Recent major surgery, GI or genitourinary (GU) bleeding, trauma, acute pericarditis, subacute bacterial endocarditis, pregnancy, severe hepatic impairment, hemorrhagic ophthalmic conditions, concurrent use of anticoagulants, elderly pts, cerebrovascular disease, hemostatic defects.

ACTION

Binds to fibrin in a thrombus and converts entrapped plasminogen to plasmin, initiating fibrinolysis. **Therapeutic Effect:** Degrades fibrin clots, fibrinogen, other plasma proteins.

PHARMACOKINETICS

Widely distributed. Metabolized in liver. **Half-life:** 90-130 min.

⧗ LIFESPAN CONSIDERATIONS

Pregnancy/Lactation: Unknown if distributed in breast milk. **Children:** Safety and efficacy not established. **Elderly:** May have increased risk of intracranial hemorrhage, stroke, major bleeding; caution advised.

INTERACTIONS

DRUG: Anticoagulants (e.g., apixaban, dabigatran, heparin, rivaroxaban, warfarin), antiplatelets (e.g., aspirin, clopidogrel) may increase risk of bleeding. May decrease effect of **tranexamic acid. HERBAL: Herbals with anticoagulant/antiplatelet properties (e.g., garlic, ginger, ginkgo biloba)** may increase risk of bleeding. **FOOD:** None known. **LAB VALUES:** Decreases plasminogen, fibrinogen levels during infusion, decreasing clotting time (confirms presence of lysis). May decrease Hgb, Hct.

AVAILABILITY (Rx)

Injection, Powder for Reconstitution: 50 mg.

ADMINISTRATION/HANDLING

💉 IV

Reconstitution • Add 10 mL Sterile Water for Injection without preservative to vial to a final concentration of 5 mg/mL. • Gently swirl until powder is dissolved. Do not shake. • If foaming occurs, leave vial undisturbed for several min. • Visually inspect for particulate matter or discoloration. Solution should appear clear, colorless to slightly yellow. Do not use if solution is cloudy, discolored, or if visible particles are observed.
Rate of administration • Administer as IV push over 5 sec.

T

 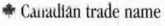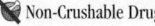

Storage • Unused vial may be refrigerated or stored at room temperature. • If possible, use immediately, but may refrigerate up to 8 hrs after reconstitution.

▧ IV INCOMPATIBILITIES

Do not mix with dextrose-containing solutions or any other medications.

INDICATIONS/ROUTES/DOSAGE

Give as single IV bolus over 5 sec. Precipitate may occur when given in IV line containing dextrose. Flush line with saline before and after administration.

Acute MI
IV: ADULTS: Dosage is based on pt's weight. Treatment should be initiated as soon as possible after onset of symptoms.

Weight (kg)	(mg)	(mL)
90 or more	50	10
80–less than 90	45	9
70–less than 80	40	8
60–less than 70	35	7
Less than 60	30	6

Dosage in Renal/Hepatic Impairment
No dose adjustment.

SIDE EFFECTS

Frequent: Bleeding (minor, 21.8%; major, 4.7%).

ADVERSE EFFECTS/TOXIC REACTIONS

Internal bleeding, including intracranial, retroperitoneal, GI, GU, respiratory sites, may occur. Lysis of coronary thrombi may produce atrial or ventricular arrhythmias, stroke.

NURSING CONSIDERATIONS

BASELINE ASSESSMENT

Obtain CBC, aPTT, fibrinogen level; ECG before initiation. Screen for contraindications.

INTERVENTION/EVALUATION

Monitor CBC, fibrinogen, aPTT per protocol. Monitor continuous ECG for arrhythmias, B/P, pulse, respirations q15min until stable, then hourly or per protocol. Asses peripheral pulses. Auscultate heart and lung sounds. Monitor for chest pain relief; notify physician of continuation/recurrence (note location, type, intensity). Monitor for bleeding of any kind, including symptoms of intracranial hemorrhage (altered mental status, aphasia, hemiparesis, unequal pupils, seizures, vision loss). Avoid any trauma that might increase risk of bleeding (e.g., injections, shaving). Assess neurologic status with vital signs.

---

tenofovir alafenamide (TAF) tenofovir disoproxil fumarate (TDF)

ten-**oh**-foe-veer (Vemlidy TAF, Viread TDF)

■ **BLACK BOX ALERT** ■ Serious, sometimes fatal, lactic acidosis and severe hepatomegaly with steatosis (fatty liver) have been reported. Severe exacerbations of hepatitis B virus (HBV) reported in pts coinfected with HIV-1 and HBV after discontinuation. If discontinuation of therapy occurs, monitor hepatic function for at least several mos. Reinitiate anti-HBV therapy if warranted.
Do not confuse tenofovir with adefovir, acyclovir, cidofovir, famciclovir, Retrovir, or valacyclovir.

FIXED-COMBINATION(S)

Atripla: tenofovir (TDF)/efavirenz/emtricitabine (antiretroviral agents): 300 mg/600 mg/200 mg. **Biktarvy:** tenofovir (TAF)/bictegravir/emtricitabine: 25 mg/50 mg/200 mg. **Cimduo:** tenofovir (TDF)/lamivudine 300 mg. **Complera:** tenofovir (TDF)/

emtricitabine/rilpivirine (antiretroviral agents): 300 mg/200 mg/25 mg. **Delstrigo:** tenofovir (TDF)/doravirine/lamivudine: 300 mg/100 mg/ 300 mg. **Descovy:** tenofovir (TAF)/emtricitabine: 25 mg/200 mg. **Genvoya:** tenofovir (TAF)/elvitegravir/ cobicistat/emtricitabine: 10 mg/150 mg/150 mg/200 mg. **Odefsey:** tenofovir (TAF)/emtricitabine/rilpivirine: 25 mg/200 mg/25 mg. **Stribild:** tenofovir (TDF)/elvitegravir (an integrase inhibitor)/cobicistat (a pharmacokinetic enhancer)/emtricitabine (a nucleoside reverse transcriptase inhibitor): 300 mg/150 mg/150 mg/200 mg. **Symtuza:** tenofovir (TAF)/darunavir/cobicistat/emtricitabine: 800 mg/150 mg/200 mg. **Symfi:** tenofovir (TDF)/efavirenz/lamivudine: 300 mg/600 mg/300 mg; 300 mg/400 mg/300 mg. **Truvada:** tenofovir (TDF)/emtricitabine (an antiretroviral agent): 300 mg/200 mg.

◆CLASSIFICATION

PHARMACOTHERAPEUTIC: Nucleotide analogue (reverse transcriptase inhibitor). **CLINICAL:** Antihepadnaviral, antiretroviral.

USES

Viread: Treatment of human immunodeficiency virus type 1 (HIV-1) infection, in combination with other antiretroviral agents, in adults and children 2 yrs of age and older weighing at least 10 kg. Treatment of chronic hepatitis B virus infection in adults and children 2 yrs of age and older and weighing at least 10 kg. **Vemlidy:** Treatment of chronic hepatitis B virus infection in adults and pts 6 yrs of age and older and weighing at least 25 kg with compensated liver disease. **OFF-LABEL: Viread:** HIV-1 postexposure prophylaxis (occupational/non-occupational).

PRECAUTIONS

Contraindications: Hypersensitivity to tenofovir. **Cautions:** Hepatic/renal impairment, elderly; history of pathological fractures, osteoporosis, osteopenia; depression.

ACTION

Inhibits HIV reverse transcriptase by interfering with HIV viral RNA–dependent DNA polymerase. Inhibits replication of hepatitis B virus (HBV) by inhibiting HBV polymerase. **Therapeutic Effect:** Slows HIV replication, reduces HIV RNA levels (viral load). Inhibits HBV replication.

PHARMACOKINETICS

Widely distributed. Not significantly metabolized. Protein binding: 0.7%–7.2%. Excreted in urine. Removed by hemodialysis. **Half-life:** 17 hrs.

⏳ LIFESPAN CONSIDERATIONS

Pregnancy/Lactation: Crosses placenta and is distributed in breast milk. Complete avoidance of breastfeeding by HIV-infected women is recommended to decrease potential transmission of HIV. **Children:** Safety and efficacy not established in children younger than 2 yrs. **Elderly:** No age-related precautions noted.

INTERACTIONS

DRUG: TDF may increase concentration/effect of **didanosine. TDF** may decrease concentration/effect of **atazanavir. CarBAMazepine, fosphenytoin, OXcarbazepine, PHENobarbital, primidone, rifAMPin, tipranavir** may decrease concentration/effect of TAF. **HERBAL: St. John's wort** may decrease concentration/effects of TAF. **FOOD: High-fat food** increases bioavailability. **LAB VALUES:** May increase serum amylase, ALT, AST, LDL-cholesterol, creatinine, creatine kinase, triglycerides; urine glucose.

AVAILABILITY (Rx)

Tablets: *(Vemlidy):* 25 mg. *(Viread):* 150 mg, 200 mg, 250 mg, 300 mg. **Oral Powder:** *(Viread):* 40 mg per 1 g of oral powder.

ADMINISTRATION/HANDLING

PO
• **Vemlidy:** Give with food. **Viread:** Give without regard to food. • Give oral powder with soft food. Do not mix in liquid; use only the supplied dosing scoop to measure powder.

INDICATIONS/ROUTES/DOSAGE

Hepatitis B

PO: *(Vemlidy):* ADULTS, ELDERLY: CHILDREN 6 YRS OF AGE AND OLDER AND WEIGHING AT LEAST 25 KG: 25 mg once daily with food. *(Viread):* ADULTS, ELDERLY, CHILDREN WEIGHING AT LEAST 35 KG: 300 mg once daily. **PTS WEIGHING AT LEAST 17 KG (able to swallow an intact tablet):** 28–34 KG: 250 mg; 22–27 KG: 200 mg; 17–21 KG: 150 mg once daily. CHILDREN WEIGHING AT LEAST 10 KG: **(unable to swallow a tablet):** *(Oral Powder):* 8 mg/kg/dose once daily. **Maximum:** 300 mg/day.

HIV (in Combination With Other Antiretroviral Agents)

PO: *(Viread):* ADULTS, ELDERLY, CHILDREN WEIGHING AT LEAST 35 KG: 300 mg once daily. **PTS WEIGHING AT LEAST 17 KG (able to swallow an intact tablet):** 28–34 KG: 250 mg; 22–27 KG: 200 mg; 17–21 KG: 150 mg once daily. CHILDREN 2 YRS AND OLDER and ADOLESCENTS WEIGHING 10 KG OR GREATER: **(unable to swallow a tablet):** *(Oral Powder):* 8 mg/kg/dose once daily. **Maximum:** 300 mg/day.

Dosage in Renal Impairment

Creatinine Clearance	Dosage
30–49 mL/min	300 mg q48h
10–29 mL/min	300 mg q72–96h
Hemodialysis	300 mg q7days or after approximately 12 hrs of dialysis

Dosage in Hepatic Impairment

Mild to severe impairment: No dose adjustment.

SIDE EFFECTS

Occasional: (11%–7%): Diarrhea, nausea, asthenia, pain (generalized). **Rare (5%–1%):** Headache, rash, abdominal pain, vomiting, decreased appetite, insomnia, dyspepsia, flatulence, sweating, myalgia, peripheral neuropathy, back pain, chest pain, fever, weight loss, dizziness.

ADVERSE EFFECTS/TOXIC REACTIONS

May cause new or worsening renal failure, including Fanconi syndrome (renal tubular injury, non-absorption of essential electrolytes, acids, buffers in renal tubules). Renal tubular injury may lead to rhabdomyolysis, osteomalacia, muscle weakness, myopathy. May decrease bone mineral density, leading to pathological fractures. May cause redistribution/accumulation of body fat (lipodystrophy). Fatal lactic acidosis, severe hepatomegaly with steatosis (fatty liver) was reported. If therapy is discontinued, pts coinfected with hepatitis B or C virus have an increased risk for viral replication, worsening of hepatic function, and may experience hepatic decompensation and/or failure. May induce immune recovery syndrome (inflammatory response to dormant opportunistic infections such as *Mycobacterium avium*, cytomegalovirus, PCP, tuberculosis or acceleration of autoimmune disorders, including Graves' disease, polymyositis, Guillain-Barre). Depression reported in 4% of pts.

NURSING CONSIDERATIONS

BASELINE ASSESSMENT

Obtain LFT, BUN, serum creatinine, CrCl, eGFR, CD4+ count, viral load, HIV-1 RNA level; urine glucose, urine protein; pregnancy test in females of reproductive potential. Obtain serum phosphate level in pts with renal impairment. Test all pts for HBV infection. Receive full medication history and screen for interactions. Question history of hepatic/renal impairment, hyperlipidemia, decreased mineral bone density, osteopenia, depression. Offer emotional support.

INTERVENTION/EVALUATION

Monitor CD4+ count, viral load, HIV-1 RNA level for treatment effectiveness. Monitor renal function as clinically indicated. An increase in serum creatinine greater than 0.4 mg/dL from baseline may indicate renal impairment. Obtain serum lactate level if lactic acidosis suspected. If concomitant medications were not discontinued or adjusted, closely monitor for adverse effects/toxic reactions. Assess for hepatic injury (bruising, hematuria, jaundice, right upper abdominal pain, nausea, vomiting, weight loss). If discontinuation of treatment occurs, monitor hepatic function for at least several months. Reinitiate anti-HBV therapy if warranted. Monitor for immune recovery syndrome, esp. after initiating treatment. Cough, dyspnea, fever, excess band cells on CBC may indicate acute infection (WBC may be unreliable in pts with uncontrolled HIV infection). Monitor daily pattern of bowel activity, stool consistency; I&Os.

PATIENT/FAMILY TEACHING

• Treatment does not cure HIV infection nor reduce risk of transmission. Practice safe sex with barrier methods or abstinence. • Drug resistance can form if treatment is interrupted; do not run out of supply. • As immune system strengthens, it may respond to dormant infections hidden within the body. Report any new fever, chills, body aches, cough, night sweats, shortness of breath. • Fatal cases of liver inflammation or failure have occurred; report abdominal pain, clay-colored stools, yellowing of skin or eyes, weight loss. • Report symptoms of kidney inflammation or disease (decreased urine output, flank pain, darkened urine); toxic skin reactions (rash, pustules, skin eruptions). • Report any psychiatric symptoms (agitation, delusions, depression, mood alteration, paranoia, suicidal ideation). • Breastfeeding not recommended. • Decreased bone density may lead to pathological fractures; report bone/extremity pain, suspected fractures. • Antiretrovirals may cause excess body fat in upper back, neck, breast, trunk, while also causing decreased body fat in legs, arms, face. • Do not take newly prescribed medications unless approved by prescriber who originally started treatment. • Do not take herbal products, esp. St. John's wort.

tepotinib

tep-**oh**-ti-nib
(Tepmetko)
Do not confuse tepotinib with capmatinib, crizotinib, erlotinib, nilotinib, talazoparib, tofacitinib, trametinib, or tucatinib or Tepmetko with Tabrecta.

◆CLASSIFICATION

PHARMACOTHERAPEUTIC: MET inhibitor; tyrosine kinase inhibitor. **CLINICAL:** Antineoplastic.

USES

Treatment of adults with metastatic non–small-cell lung cancer (NSCLC) harboring MET exon 14 skipping alterations.

PRECAUTIONS

Contraindications: Hypersensitivity to tepotinib. **Cautions:** Hepatic/renal impairment, pts at risk for interstitial lung disease (e.g., COPD, sarcoidosis, connective tissue disease), conditions predisposing to infection (e.g., diabetes, immunocompromised pts, renal failure, open wounds), history of effusion or edema (pleural effusion, generalized edema), thromboembolic events (including pulmonary embolism). Avoid concomitant use of combined P-glycoprotein (P-gp) and strong CYP3A4 inhibitors; P-gp substrates, strong CYP3A4 inducers.

ACTION

Selectively targets mesenchymal-epithelial transition (MET) (including mutant variant produced by exon 14 skipping). Inhibits hepatocyte growth factor–dependent and –independent MET phosphorylation and MET-dependent downstream signaling pathways. **Therapeutic Effect:** Inhibits tumor cell proliferation, anchorage-independent growth, and metastases of MET-dependent tumor cells.

PHARMACOKINETICS

Widely distributed. Metabolized in liver. Protein binding: 98%. Peak plasma

T

concentration: 8 hrs. Excreted in feces (85%), urine (14%). **Half-life:** 32 hrs.

⏳ LIFESPAN CONSIDERATIONS

Pregnancy/Lactation: Avoid pregnancy; may cause fetal harm. Females of reproductive potential and males with female partners of reproductive potential must use effective contraception during treatment and for at least 1 wk after discontinuation. Unknown if distributed in breast milk. Breastfeeding not recommended during treatment and for at least 1 wk after discontinuation. **Children:** Safety and efficacy not established. **Elderly:** No age-related precautions noted.

INTERACTIONS

DRUG: Combined strong CYP3A4 inhibitors (e.g., clarithromycin, ketoconazole, ritonavir) and P-gp inhibitors (e.g., amiodarone, azithromycin, cycloSPORINE, diltiazem, verapamil) may increase concentration/effect. **Strong CYP3A4 inducers (e.g., carBAMazepine, phenytoin, rifAMPin)** may decrease concentration/effect. May increase the serum concentration of **DOXOrubicin, PAZOPanib, topotecan. HERBAL:** None significant. **FOOD:** None known. **LAB VALUES:** May increase serum alkaline phosphatase, ALT, amylase, AST, creatinine, GGT, potassium. May decrease serum albumin, sodium; Hgb, lymphocytes, leukocytes.

AVAILABILITY (Rx)

Tablets: 225 mg.

ADMINISTRATION/HANDLING

PO
• Give with food (increases absorption).
• Administer tablet whole; do not break, cut, or crush. Tablets cannot be chewed.
• For pts having difficulty swallowing, may place tablet(s) in a glass containing 1 ox water. Stir, without crushing, until the tablet is dispersed into small pieces (tablets will not completely dissolve). Give immediately or within 1 hr.
• If a dose is missed, do not give within 8 hrs of next dose. • If vomiting occurs after administration, give the next dose at regularly scheduled time (do not give additional dose).

INDICATIONS/ROUTES/DOSAGE

NSCLC (Metastatic, MET Exon 14 Skipping Alterations)
PO: ADULTS, ELDERLY: 450 mg once daily until disease progression or unacceptable toxicity.

Dose Reduction Schedule
Reduction for adverse reaction: 225 mg once daily. **Unable to tolerate 225-mg dose:** Permanently discontinue.

Dose Modification
Based on Common Terminology Criteria for Adverse Events (CTCAE).

Serum ALT/AST Elevation
Grade 3 serum ALT/AST elevation without total bilirubin elevation: Withhold treatment until improved to baseline, then either resume at a same dose if serum ALT/AST elevation improves within 7 days or reduce dose if not improved within 7 days. **Grade 4 serum ALT/AST elevation without total bilirubin elevation:** Permanently discontinue.

Hyperbilirubinemia
Grade 3 total bilirubin elevation without serum ALT/AST elevation: Withhold treatment until improved to baseline, then either resume at a same dose if total bilirubin elevation improves within 7 days or permanently discontinue if not improved within 7 days. **Grade 4 total bilirubin elevation without serum ALT/AST elevation:** Permanently discontinue. **Total bilirubin elevation greater than 2 times with ALT/AST greater than 3 times ULN:** Permanently discontinue.

Pulmonary Toxicity
ILD/pneumonitis (any grade): Withhold treatment if ILD/pneumonitis is suspected. Permanently discontinue if ILD/pneumonitis is confirmed.

Other Adverse Reactions
Any other Grade 2 reactions: Continue same dose. If reaction is not tolerated, consider withholding treatment until resolved, then resume at reduced dose. **Any other Grade 3 reaction:** Withhold treatment until resolved, then resume at reduced dose. **Any other Grade 4 reaction:** Permanently discontinue.

Dosage in Renal/Hepatic Impairment
Mild to moderate impairment: No dose adjustment. **Severe impairment:** Not specified; use caution.

SIDE EFFECTS

Frequent (70%–20%): Edema (eye, face, general, genital, localized, periorbital, peripheral, scrotal), nausea, diarrhea, pain (back, bone, chest, extremity, musculoskeletal spine), arthralgia, arthritis, myalgia, fatigue, asthenia, dyspnea. **Occasional (16% to less than 10%):** Abdominal pain, constipation, decreased appetite, cough, vomiting, rash, pyrexia, dizziness, pruritus, headache.

ADVERSE EFFECTS/TOXIC REACTIONS

Myelosuppression (anemia, leukopenia, lymphopenia) is an expected response to therapy. Life-threatening LID/pneumonitis reported in 2% of pts. Serum ALT, AST elevation reported in 13% of pts. Grade 3 or 4 hepatotoxicity reported in 4% of pts. Pleural effusion reported in 13% of pts. Pneumonia reported in 11% of pts. Pulmonary embolism reported in 2% of pts.

NURSING CONSIDERATIONS

BASELINE ASSESSMENT
Obtain CBC, BMP, LFT; pregnancy test in females of reproductive potential. Confirm compliance of effective nonhormonal contraception. Verify presence of MET 14 skipping alterations in plasma or tumor specimens. Question history of hepatic/renal impairment, pulmonary disease, pleural effusion. Receive full medication history and screen for interactions. Assess for baseline edema. Offer emotional support.

INTERVENTION/EVALUATION
Monitor CBC for myelosuppression periodically; LFT for hepatotoxicity (bruising, jaundice, right upper abdominal pain, nausea, vomiting, weight loss) q2wks for 3 mos, then monthly thereafter (or more frequently if hepatotoxicity occurs). Monitor for infections (cough, fatigue, fever). Consider ABG, radiologic test if pneumonitis (excessive cough, dyspnea, fever, hypoxia) is suspected. Consider treatment with corticosteroids if pneumonitis is confirmed. If dyspnea occurs, obtain radiologic test to assess for pleural effusion. Monitor for symptoms of PE (chest pain, dyspnea, tachycardia). Monitor for edema (third spacing, dyspnea, weight gain). Monitor for toxicities if concomitant use with strong CYP3A4 inhibitors, P-gp inhibitors, or substrates is unavoidable. Monitor daily pattern of bowel activity, stool consistency.

PATIENT/FAMILY TEACHING
• Treatment may depress the immune system response and reduce ability to fight infection. Report symptoms of infection such as body aches, chills, cough, fatigue, fever. Avoid those with active infection. • Report liver problems (abdominal pain, bruising, clay-colored stool, amber or dark-colored urine, yellowing of the skin or eyes), inflammation of the lung (excessive cough, difficulty breathing, chest pain), kidney problems (decreased urine output, flank pain, darkened urine), symptoms of edema (shortness of breath, swelling of extremities, weight gain), lung effusion (chest pain, dry cough, shortness of breath); symptoms of lung embolism (difficulty breathing, chest pain, rapid heart rate). • Use effective contraception to avoid pregnancy. Do not breastfeed. • There is a high risk of interactions with other medications. Do not take newly prescribed medications unless approved by prescriber who originally started therapy.

teriflunomide

ter-i-**floo**-noe-myde
(Aubagio)

■ **BLACK BOX ALERT** ■ May result in major birth defects. Pregnancy must be excluded before initiating therapy and must be avoided during treatment or prior to completion of an accelerated elimination procedure. Severe hepatic injury may occur. Do not initiate in pts with acute/chronic liver disease or serum ALT greater than 2 times upper limit of normal.

Do not confuse teriflunomide with leflunomide.

◆**CLASSIFICATION**

PHARMACOTHERAPEUTIC: Pyrimidine synthesis inhibitor, immunomodulatory agent. **CLINICAL:** Multiple sclerosis agent.

USES

Treatment of relapsing forms of multiple sclerosis, including clinically isolated syndrome, relapsing-remitting disease, and active secondary progressive disease in adults.

PRECAUTIONS

Contraindications: Hypersensitivity to teriflunomide, leflunomide. Pregnant women or women of childbearing potential who are not using reliable contraception, severe hepatic impairment, concurrent use of leflunomide. **Cautions:** Baseline cytopenias, diabetes, pts older than 60 yrs, pulmonary disease, mild to moderate hepatic disease; conditions predisposing to infection (e.g., diabetes, renal failure, immunocompromised pts, open wounds); history of chronic opportunistic infections (esp. fungal/viral infections, TB); concomitant use of nephrotoxic medications. Not recommended in pts with severe immunodeficiency, bone marrow disease; severe, active infection. Do not initiate in pts with active or chronic infections until resolved.

ACTION

Inhibits pyrimidine synthesis, exhibiting anti-inflammatory and antiproliferative properties. **Therapeutic Effect:** May reduce number of activated lymphocytes in the CNS. May slow progression of multiple sclerosis.

PHARMACOKINETICS

Widely distributed. Peak concentration: 1–4 hrs. Protein binding: Greater than 99%. Metabolized by hydrolysis. Excreted in urine (23%), feces (38%). **Half-life:** 18–19 days.

⧖ LIFESPAN CONSIDERATIONS

Pregnancy/Lactation: Avoid pregnancy; may cause fetal harm. Females and males with female partners of reproductive potential must use effective contraception during treatment and until plasma drug concentrations are at least 0.02 mg/L following accelerated elimination procedure. Breastfeeding not recommended. **Children:** Safety and efficacy not established. **Elderly:** No age-related precautions noted.

INTERACTIONS

DRUG: May increase concentration/effects of **CYP2C8 substrates (e.g., repaglinide, PACLitaxel, rosuvastatin, topotecan).** May decrease concentration/effects of **warfarin, CYP1A2 substrates (e.g., DULoxetine, tiZANidine).** Concentration/effect may be altered by **vaccines (live).** **HERBAL: Echinacea** may decrease therapeutic effect. **FOOD:** None known. **LAB VALUES:** May increase serum potassium, ALT, AST, alkaline phosphatase, bilirubin. May decrease WBCs, neutrophil count.

AVAILABILITY (Rx)

Tablets: 7 mg, 14 mg.

ADMINISTRATION/HANDLING

PO
• Give without regard to food.

INDICATIONS/ROUTES/DOSAGE

Multiple Sclerosis
PO: ADULTS, ELDERLY: 7 mg or 14 mg once daily.

Adjustment of Toxicity
Serum ALT elevation greater than 3 times ULN: Discontinue teriflunomide and initiate drug elimination procedures: cholestyramine 8 g q8h for 11 days (if not tolerated, may decrease to 4 g q8h) or activated charcoal 50 g q12h for 11 days. **Note:** The 11 days do not need to be consecutive unless plasma concentration needs to be lowered rapidly.

Dosage in Renal Impairment
No dose adjustment.

Dosage in Hepatic Impairment
Mild to moderate impairment: No dose adjustment. **Severe impairment:** Contraindicated.

SIDE EFFECTS

Frequent (19%–6%): Headache, diarrhea, nausea, alopecia, paresthesia, upper abdominal pain. **Occasional (4%–3%):** Hypertension, oral herpes, anxiety, hypertension, toothache, musculoskeletal pain. **Rare (2%–1%):** Seasonal allergy, sciatica, burning sensation, carpal tunnel syndrome, blurred vision, acne, pruritus, myalgia, abdominal distention, conjunctivitis.

ADVERSE EFFECTS/TOXIC REACTIONS

Myelosuppression (lymphopenia, neutropenia, thrombocytopenia) was reported. Severe hepatic injury, hepatotoxicity may occur. Infections, opportunistic infections including aspergillosis, influenza, *Klebsiella* pneumonia, *Pneumocystis jiroveci* pneumonia, TB were reported (mainly occurring in pts taking concomitant immunosuppressive therapy). May increase risk of malignancies, proliferative disorders. Hypersensitivity reactions including angioedema, dyspnea, urticaria, and anaphylaxis may occur. May cause acute renal failure, peripheral neuropathy, hypertension, interstitial lung disease, pneumonitis, sudden cardiac death. Skin toxicities including Steven-Johnson syndrome, toxic epidermal necrolysis may occur.

NURSING CONSIDERATIONS

BASELINE ASSESSMENT
Obtain CBC, LFT; pregnancy test in females of reproductive potential. Assess baseline symptoms of MS (e.g., bladder/bowel dysfunction, cognitive impairment, depression, dysphagia, fatigue, gait disorder, numbness/tingling, pain, seizures, spasticity, tremors, weakness). Screen for active infection. Question history of hepatic/renal impairment, pulmonary disease, neuropathy; chronic, opportunistic infections. Evaluate for active TB and test for latent infection prior to and during treatment. Induration of 5 mm or greater with purified protein derivative (PPD) is considered a positive result when assessing for latent TB. Consider treatment with antimycobacterial therapy in pts with latent TB.

INTERVENTION/EVALUATION
Monitor CBC for myelosuppression; LFT for hepatotoxicity (abdominal pain, jaundice, nausea, transaminitis, vomiting) at least monthly for 6 mos. Conduct neurologic assessment. Assess for symptomatic improvement of MS. Monitor for neuropathy. Consider ABG, radiologic test if ILD/pneumonitis (excessive cough, dyspnea, fever, hypoxia) is suspected. Consider treatment with corticosteroids if ILD/pneumonitis is confirmed. Monitor for TB regardless of baseline PPD. Diligently monitor for acute infection (cough, fatigue, fever), opportunistic infections; reactivation of chronic infections. Monitor B/P for hypertension. Assess skin for cutaneous toxicities. Due to extended drug clearance (elimination may take up to 2 yrs), an accelerated elimination program may be needed (e.g., cholestyramine 8 g q8h for 11 days; activated charcoal 50 g q12h for 11 days).

T

PATIENT/FAMILY TEACHING

• Treatment may depress your immune system and reduce your ability to fight infection. Report symptoms of infection such as body aches, burning with urination, chills, cough, fatigue, fever. Avoid those with active infection. • Report symptoms of bone marrow depression (e.g., bruising, fatigue, fever, shortness of breath, weight loss; bleeding easily, bloody urine or stool). • Expect routine tuberculosis screening. Report any travel plans to possible endemic areas. • Do not receive live vaccines. • Report liver problems (abdominal pain, bruising, clay-colored stool, dark or amber-colored urine, yellowing of the skin or eyes), kidney problems (decreased urine output, flank pain, darkened urine); skin toxicities (rash, peeling, sloughing), nervous system pain/weakness/tingling. • Allergic reactions such as difficulty breathing, hives, rash, swelling of the face or tongue, can happen at any time. If allergic reaction occurs, seek immediate medical attention. • Treatment may worsen high blood pressure or cause new cancers. • Severe worsening of MS symptoms may occur after stopping treatment. • Use effective contraception to avoid pregnancy. Do not breastfeed.

T

teriparatide

ter-i-**par**-a-tide
(Forteo)

◆**CLASSIFICATION**

PHARMACOTHERAPEUTIC: Parathyroid hormone analog. **CLINICAL:** Osteoporosis agent.

USES

Treatment of postmenopausal women with osteoporosis who are at high risk for fracture (history of osteoporotic fracture or multiple risk factors for fracture) or have failed or intolerant to other available therapy. Reduces the risk of vertebral and nonvertebral fractures. Treatment to increase bone mass in men with primary or hypogonadal osteoporosis who are at high risk for fractures or have failed or are intolerant of other available osteoporosis therapy. Treatment of glucocorticoid-induced osteoporosis in men and women associated with chronic systemic glucocorticoids (e.g., 5 mg/day or more of predniSONE) at a high risk for fracture or have failed or intolerant of other available osteoporosis therapy.

PRECAUTIONS

Contraindications: Hypersensitivity to teriparatide. **Cautions:** Conditions that increase risk of osteosarcoma (e.g., Paget's disease, unexplained elevations of alkaline phosphatase level, children or young adults with open epiphyses, prior skeletal radiation therapy, implant therapy), hypercalcemia, hypercalcemic disorders (e.g., hyperparathyroidism), bone metastases, history of skeletal malignancies, metabolic bone diseases other than osteoporosis, cardiac disease, renal/hepatic impairment, pts at risk for orthostasis, active or recent urolithiasis.

ACTION

Stimulates osteoblast function by increasing gastrointestinal calcium absorption and increasing renal tubular reabsorption of calcium. **Therapeutic Effect:** Increases bone mineral density, bone mass/strength, reduces osteoporosis-related fractures.

PHARMACOKINETICS

Widely distributed. Metabolized in liver. Peak plasma concentration: 30 min. Excreted in urine. **Half-life:** 1 hr.

⧗ LIFESPAN CONSIDERATIONS

Pregnancy/Lactation: Unknown if drug crosses placenta or is distributed in breast milk. **Children:** Safety and efficacy not established. **Elderly:** No age-related precautions noted.

INTERACTIONS

DRUG: None known. **HERBAL:** None significant. **FOOD:** None known. **LAB VALUES:** May increase serum calcium (transient), uric acid.

AVAILABILITY (Rx)

Injection Solution: 600 mcg/2.4 mL (injector pen containing 28 daily doses of 20 mcg).

ADMINISTRATION/HANDLING

SQ
• Refrigerate, but minimize time out of refrigerator. Do not freeze; discard if frozen. • Administer into thigh, abdominal wall.

INDICATIONS/ROUTES/DOSAGE

Osteoporosis
SQ: ADULTS, ELDERLY: 20 mcg once daily into thigh, abdominal wall. Continue for up to 2 yrs (lifetime duration). Supplemental calcium and vitamin D are recommended if daily dietary intake is inadequate.

Dosage in Renal/Hepatic Impairment
No dose adjustment.

SIDE EFFECTS

Frequent (37%): Pain. **Occasional (10%–6%):** Arthralgia, asthenia, headache, dizziness, hypertension, cough, pharyngitis. **Rare (5%–2%):** Nausea, constipation, diarrhea, dyspepsia, rash, vertigo, vomiting, neck pain, dyspnea, leg cramps, GI disorder (unspecified), tooth disorder (unspecified), sweating.

ADVERSE EFFECTS/TOXIC REACTIONS

Angina pectoris has been reported. May increase risk of hypercalemia, kidney stones (urolithiasis). Orthostatic hypotension reported in 5% of pts. Pneumonia reported in 4% of pts.

NURSING CONSIDERATIONS

BASELINE ASSESSMENT

Obtain serum calcium, phosphate, PTH, bone mineral density. Question medical history as listed in Precautions.

INTERVENTION/EVALUATION

Monitor bone mineral density, serum calcium, phosphate, PTH. Observe for symptoms of hypercalcemia (anxiety, bradycardia, facial twitching; muscle cramps, spasm, weakness; seizures). Monitor B/P for hypotension, pulse for tachycardia.

PATIENT/FAMILY TEACHING

• Go from lying to standing slowly.
• Report persistent symptoms of hypercalcemia (nausea, vomiting, constipation, lethargy, asthenia).

---

testosterone

tes-**tos**-te-rone
(Androderm, AndroGel Pump, Aveed, Depo-Testosterone, Fortesta, Jatenzo, Kyzatrex, Natesto, Testim, Tlando, Testopel, Vogelxo, Xyosted)

■ **BLACK BOX ALERT** ■
Testosterone undecanoate and testosterone enanthate may cause an increase of blood pressure (B/P) that can increase the risk of life-threatening cardiovascular events, including CVA, MI, and cardiovascular death. Virilization in children and women may occur following secondary exposure to testosterone topical gel and solution. **Aveed:** Serious pulmonary oil microembolism reaction involving chest pain, dizziness, urge to cough, dyspnea, throat tightening, syncope; life-threatening hypersensitivity reactions, including anaphylaxis, reported during or immediately after administration.
Do not confuse testosterone with testolactone.

◆CLASSIFICATION

PHARMACOTHERAPEUTIC: Androgen. **CLINICAL:** Sex hormone.

USES

Hypogonadism: Treatment of testicular failure due to cryptorchidism, bilateral torsion, orchitis, vanishing testis syndrome, orchiectomy, Klinefelter syn-

---

 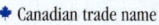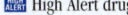

drome, chemotherapy, or toxic damage from alcohol or heavy metals; gonadotropin or luteinizing hormone–releasing hormone deficiency; or pituitary-hypothalamic injury from tumors, trauma, or radiation. **Delayed puberty:** To stimulate puberty in carefully selected males with delayed puberty. **OFF-LABEL:** Hormone therapy (transgender female to male).

PRECAUTIONS

Contraindications: Hypersensitivity to testosterone. Breastfeeding, pregnant or who may become pregnant, prostate (known or suspected) or breast cancer in males. **Depo-Testosterone (additional):** Severe cardiac/hepatic/renal disease. **Cautions:** Renal/hepatic/cardiac dysfunction, pts with history of MI or CAD; conditions influenced by edema (e.g., seizure disorder, migraines).

ACTION

Principal endogenous androgen promoting growth, development of male sex organs, maintains secondary sex characteristics in androgen-deficient males. **Therapeutic Effect:** Relieves androgen deficiency.

PHARMACOKINETICS

Widely distributed. Metabolized in liver. Protein binding: 98%. Primarily excreted in urine. Unknown if removed by hemodialysis. **Half-life:** 10–100 min.

⧗ LIFESPAN CONSIDERATIONS

Pregnancy/Lactation: Contraindicated in pregnant women, women who may become pregnant, or during lactation. **Children:** Safety and efficacy not established; use with caution. **Elderly:** May increase risk of hyperplasia, stimulate growth of occult prostate carcinoma.

INTERACTIONS

DRUG: May increase hepatotoxic effect of **cycloSPORINE**. May increase the anticoagulant effect of **warfarin**. **HERBAL:** None significant. **FOOD:** None known. **LAB VALUES:** May increase Hgb, Hct,

LDL, serum alkaline phosphatase, bilirubin, calcium, potassium, sodium, AST. May decrease HDL.

AVAILABILITY (Rx)

Capsule: *(Jatenzo):* 158 mg, 198 mg, 237 mg. *(Kyzatrex):* 100 mg, 150 mg, 200 mg. *(Tlando):* 112.5 mg. **Gel, Topical:** *(AndroGel):* 1.62%: packets containing 20.25 mg, 40.5% mg; pump 20.25 mg/actuation. *(Testim):* 50 mg of testosterone in a unit-dose tube. *(Vogelxo):* 50-mg packet or tube, 12.5 mg/actuation metered dose pump. *(Fortesta):* Metered-dose pump: 10 mg/actuation. **Injection:** *(Cypionate [Depo-Testosterone]):* 100 mg/mL, 200 mg/mL. *(Enanthate [Delatestryl]):* 200 mg/mL. *(Aveed [Undecanoate]):* 750 mg/3 mL. **Nasal Gel:** *(Natesto):* 5.5 mg/actuation. **Pellet for SQ Implantation:** *(Testopel):* 75 mg. **Solution, Topical:** 30 mg/activation. **Transdermal System Patch:** *(Androderm):* 2 mg/day or 4 mg/day. **Solution, Auto-injector:** *(Xyosted):* 50 mg/0.5 mL, 75 mg/0.5 mL, 100 mg/0.5 mL.

ADMINISTRATION/HANDLING

IM
• Give deep in gluteal muscle. • Do not give IV.

PO
• Give with morning and evening meals. • Administer capsule whole; do not break, cut, or crush. Capsule cannot be chewed.

Transdermal
• *(Androderm):* Apply to clean, dry area on skin on back, abdomen, upper arms, thighs. • Do not use tape to secure. Avoid bathing, swimming for at least 3 hrs after each application. • Do not apply to bony prominences (e.g., shoulder) or oily, damaged, irritated skin. Do not apply to scrotum. • Rotate application site with 7-day interval to same site.

Transdermal Gel
• *(AndroGel, Testim, Vogelxo):* Apply (morning preferred) to clean, dry,

T

intact skin of shoulder, upper arms. *(Foresta):* Apply to skin of front and inner thighs. • Upon opening packet(s), squeeze entire contents into palm of hand, immediately apply to application site. • Allow to dry. • Do not apply to genitals. • Avoid swimming, showering, or washing the administration site for a minimum of 2 hrs after application.

Topical Solution
• *(Axiron):* Apply using applicator to axilla at same time each morning. • Avoid washing site for 2 hrs after application.

Nasal Gel
• *(Natesto)* • Prime pump on first use by pumping 10 times into a sink. Follow steps according to manufacturer guidelines.

INDICATIONS/ROUTES/DOSAGE

Male Hypogonadism (Primary or Hypogonadotropic)
IM: ADULTS: *(Cypionate or Enanthate):* 75–100 mg/wk or 150–200 mg q2wks. *(Undecanoate):* 750 mg at initiation, 4 wks and q10 wks thereafter. **CHILDREN 12 YRS AND OLDER:** *(Cypionate or Enanthate):* Initiation of pubertal growth: 25–75 mg q3–4wks, gradually titrate q6–9mos to 100–150 mg. Duration: 3–4yrs. **Maintenance virilizing dose:** 200–250 mg q3–4wks. May convert to other testosterone replacement dosages once expected adult height and adequate virilization achieved.
PO: *(Jatenzo):* 237 mg twice daily in morning and evening. **Range:** 158–396 mg twice daily. *(Kyzatrex):* 200 mg in morning and evening. **Range:** 100–400 mg twice daily. *(Tlando):* 225 mg twice daily.
SQ: *(Pellets):* **ADULTS, CHILDREN 12 YRS AND OLDER:** 150–450 mg q3–6mos.
Topical gel: *(Fortesta):* 40 mg once daily in morning. **Range:** 10–70 mg. **Maximum:** 70 mg. *(Vogelxo):* 50 mg once daily (one tube or one packet or 4 pump actuations). **Range:** 50–100 mg/day.
Topical solution: ADULTS, ELDERLY: 60 mg once daily (1 pump activation of 30 mg to each axilla). **Range:** 30–120 mg.

Transdermal patch: *(Androderm):* **ADULTS, ELDERLY:** Start therapy with 4 mg/day patch applied at night. Apply patch to abdomen, back, thighs, upper arms. Dose adjustment based on testosterone levels. **Range:** 2–6 mg/day.
Transdermal gel: **ADULTS, ELDERLY:** *(AndroGel 1.62%):* Initial dose of 40.5 mg applied once daily in the morning to shoulder and upper arms. May increase to 81 mg. Further adjustments based on testosterone levels. *(Testim, Vogelxo):* **ADULTS, ELDERLY:** Initial dose of 5 g delivers 50 mg testosterone and is applied once daily to the shoulders, upper arms. May increase to 10 g (100 mg testosterone).
Nasal gel: *(Natesto):* **ADULTS ELDERLY:** 11 mg (2 actuations, 1 per each nostril) 3 times/day (6–8 hrs apart).

Delayed Male Puberty
IM: *(Enanthate):* **ADOLESCENTS:** 50–200 mg q2–4wks for limited duration (4–6 months).
SQ: *(Pellets):* **ADULTS:** 150–450 mg q3–6mos.

Dosage in Renal/Hepatic Impairment
Use caution.

SIDE EFFECTS
Frequent (37–10%): Increased blood pressure, skin blisters (transdermal), benign prostatic hypertrophy, increased hematocrit. *Topical:* skin reactions, itching, allergic contact dermatitis. **Occasional (10–3%):** Oily stools (due to IM injection oily solvent), injection site pain, application site erythema, edema, altered sense of smell, headache, acne, nausea (PO), diarrhea, back pain, nasopharyngitis (intranasal), rhinorrhea (intranasal), nose bleeding (intranasal). **Rare (less than 3%):** Fatigue, vertigo, insomnia, skin rash, weight gain, gynecomastia, increased appetite.

ADVERSE EFFECTS/TOXIC REACTIONS
Peliosis hepatitis (presence of blood-filled cysts in parenchyma of liver), hepatic neoplasms, hepatocellular carcinoma have been associated with pro-

longed high-dose therapy. Anaphylactic reactions occur rarely. Venous thromboembolism (e.g., DVT, PE) reported.

NURSING CONSIDERATIONS

BASELINE ASSESSMENT
Obtain CBC, BMP, LFT, lipid panel; weight, B/P. Wrist X-rays may be ordered to determine bone maturation in children. Question history of hepatic/renal impairment, seizure disorder, thromboembolism (CVA, MI, pulmonary embolism).

INTERVENTION/EVALUATION
Weigh daily, report wkly gain of more than 5 lb; evaluate for edema. Monitor B/P. Assess serum electrolytes, cholesterol, Hgb, Hct (periodically for high dosage), LFT, radiologic exam of wrist, hand (when using in prepubertal children). With breast cancer or immobility, check for hypercalcemia (anxiety, bradycardia, facial twitching; muscle cramps, spasm, weakness; seizures). Ensure adequate intake of protein, calories. Assess for virilization. Monitor sleep patterns. Monitor for CVA (aphasia, confusion, paresthesia, hemiparesis, seizures), MI (chest pain, diaphoresis, left arm/jaw pain, increased serum troponin, ST segment elevation), pulmonary embolism (chest pain, dyspnea, hypoxia, tachycardia).

PATIENT/FAMILY TEACHING
• Do not take any other medication without consulting physician. • Maintain diet high in protein, calories. • Weigh daily; report 5 lb/wk gain. • Report nausea, vomiting, acne, pedal edema. • **Females:** Promptly report menstrual irregularities, hoarseness, deepening of voice. • **Males:** Report frequent erections, difficulty urinating, gynecomastia. • Treatment may cause arterial or venous blood clots; report symptoms of heart attack (chest pain, difficulty breathing, jaw pain, nausea, pain that radiates to the left arm, sweating), stroke (blindness, confusion, one-sided weakness, loss of consciousness, trouble speaking, seizures); DVT (swelling, pain, hot feeling in the arms or legs), lung embolism (difficulty breathing, chest pain, rapid heart rate).

tezepelumab-ekko

tez-e-**pel**-ue-mab
(Tezspire)
Do not confuse tezepelumab with avelumab or lanadelumab.

◆CLASSIFICATION

PHARMACOTHERAPEUTIC: Thymic stromal lymphopoietin (TSLP) blocker. Immunoglobulin G2 monoclonal antibody. **CLINICAL:** Antiasthmatic.

USES
Add-on maintenance treatment of severe asthma in adult and pediatric pts 12 yrs of age and older.

PRECAUTIONS
Contraindications: Hypersensitivity to tezepelumab. **Cautions:** History of helminth (parasite) infection; long-term use of corticosteroids. Avoid concomitant use with live attenuated vaccines. Not indicated for relief of acute bronchospasm or status asthmaticus.

ACTION
Binds to human thymic stromal lymphopoietin (TSLP) preventing human TSLP from interacting with TSLP receptor. Reduces biomarkers and cytokines associated with inflammation, including blood eosinophils, immunoglobulin E, interleukin (IL)-5, and IL-13. **Therapeutic Effect:** Reduces asthma inflammatory cascade; relieves symptoms of asthma.

PHARMACOKINETICS
Widely distributed. Metabolism: undergoes proteolytic degradation via enzymes that are widely distributed in the body. Peak plasma concentration: 3–10 days. Steady-state reached in 12 wks. Eliminated via intracellular catabolism. **Half-life:** 26 days.

⧖ LIFESPAN CONSIDERATIONS

Pregnancy/Lactation: Unknown if distributed in breast milk. However, human immunoglobulin G is present in breast milk and is known to cross placenta. **Children:** Safety and efficacy not established in pts younger than 12 yrs. **Elderly:** No age-related precautions noted.

INTERACTIONS

DRUG: May increase adverse/toxicity of **vaccines (live)**. **HERBAL:** None significant. **FOOD:** None known. **LAB VALUES:** None known.

AVAILABILITY (Rx)

Injection Solution (Prefilled Pen, Prefilled Syringe, Single-Dose Glass Vial): 210 mg/1.91 mL (110 mg/mL).

ADMINISTRATION/HANDLING

SQ

Preparation • Remove prefilled syringe (or vial) from refrigerator and allow solution to warm to room temperature (approx. 1 hr) with needle cap intact. • Visually inspect for particulate matter or discoloration. Solution should appear clear to opalescent, colorless to slightly yellow. Do not use if solution is cloudy, discolored, or large visible particles are observed. Small air bubbles may be present.

Administration • Insert needle subcutaneously into upper arm, outer thigh, or abdomen (except for 2 inches around navel) and inject solution. If using prefilled syringe, push plunger down completely between the needle guard activation clips. Remove needle and release pressure on the plunger to engage the needle guard. • Do not inject into areas of active skin disease or injury such as sunburns, skin rashes, inflammation, skin infections, or active psoriasis. • Do not administer IV or intramuscularly. • Rotate injection sites.

Storage • Refrigerate unused prefilled syringes/vials in original carton. May store at room temperature for up to 30 days. • Protect from light. Do not shake. • Do not freeze or expose to heating sources. • Once warmed to room temperature, do not place back into refrigerator.

INDICATIONS/ROUTES/DOSAGE

Note: Prefilled pen can be administered by pts, caregivers, or healthcare providers.

Asthma (Severe)

SQ: ADULTS, CHILDREN 12 YRS AND OLDER: 210 mg once q4wks.

Dosage in Hepatic/Renal Impairment

Not studied; use caution.

SIDE EFFECTS

Rare (4%): Arthralgia, back pain, pharyngitis.

ADVERSE EFFECTS/TOXIC REACTIONS

Hypersensitivity reactions including allergic conjunctivitis, rash may occur within hrs to days after administration. Infections including bacterial/viral pharyngitis may occur. Unknown if treatment will influence the immunologic response to helminth (parasite) infection.

NURSING CONSIDERATIONS

BASELINE ASSESSMENT

Obtain pulse rate, oxygen saturation. Auscultate lung sounds. Question history of parasitic infection, hypersensitivity reaction. Pts with preexisting helminth (parasite) infection should be treated prior to initiation. Inhaled or systemic corticosteroids should not be suddenly discontinued upon initiation. Corticosteroids that are not gradually tapered may cause withdrawal symptoms or unmask conditions that were originally suppressed with corticosteroid therapy.

INTERVENTION/EVALUATION

Monitor rate, depth, rhythm of respirations. Assess lungs for wheezing. Monitor oxygen saturation. Interrupt or discontinue treatment if hypersensitivity reaction, worsening of asthma-related symptoms occurs (esp. in pts tapering off inhaled corticosteroids). Obtain pulmonary function test to assess clinical improvement. Monitor for in-

T

creased use of rescue inhalers; may indicate deterioration of asthma.

PATIENT/FAMILY TEACHING

• Treatment not indicated for relief of acute asthmatic episodes. Have a rescue inhaler readily available. Increased use of rescue inhaler may indicate worsening of asthma. Seek medical attention if asthma symptoms worsen or remain uncontrolled after starting therapy. • Report allergic reactions such as rash or allergic conjunctivitis. • Do not suddenly stop inhaled corticosteroid therapy. If appropriate, a gradual taper should be performed under medical supervision.

tiaGABine

tye-a-ga-been
(Gabitril)
Do not confuse tiaGABine with tiZANidine.

◆CLASSIFICATION

PHARMACOTHERAPEUTIC: Selective GABA reuptake inhibitor. **CLINICAL:** Anticonvulsant.

USES

Adjunctive therapy for treatment of focal (partial) onset seizures in adults and children 12 yrs or older.

PRECAUTIONS

Contraindications: Hypersensitivity to tiaGABine. **Cautions:** Hepatic impairment. Pts at risk for suicidal ideation and behavior.

ACTION

Enhances activity of gamma-aminobutyric acid (GABA), the major inhibitory neurotransmitter in the CNS. **Therapeutic Effect:** Inhibits seizure activity.

PHARMACOKINETICS

Widely distributed. Protein binding: 96%. Metabolized in liver. Primarily excreted in feces. **Half-life:** 2–5 hrs.

⧖ LIFESPAN CONSIDERATIONS

Pregnancy/Lactation: May cause fetal harm. Distributed in breast milk. **Children:** Safety and efficacy not established in pts younger than 12 yrs. **Elderly:** Age-related hepatic impairment may require dosage adjustment.

INTERACTIONS

DRUG: CNS depressants (e.g., alcohol, morphine, oxyCODONE, zolpidem) may increase CNS depression. **Strong CYP3A4 inducers (e.g., carBAMazepine, phenytoin, rifAMPin)** may decrease concentration/effect. **Strong CYP3A4 inhibitors (e.g., clarithromycin, ketoconazole)** may increase concentration/effect. **HERBAL:** Herbals with sedative properties (e.g., chamomile, kava kava, valerian) may increase CNS depression. None significant. **FOOD:** None known. **LAB VALUES:** None significant.

AVAILABILITY (Rx)

Tablets: 2 mg, 4 mg, 12 mg, 16 mg.

ADMINISTRATION/HANDLING

PO
• Give with food.

INDICATIONS/ROUTES/DOSAGE

Note: Pts not taking enzyme-inducing antiepileptic drugs (AEDs): Lower doses required and slower titration may be needed. Do not use a loading dose, rapid titration, and/or increase in large-dose increments.

Focal (Partial) Onset Seizures

PO: ADULTS, ELDERLY: Pts receiving enzyme-inducing AED regimens: Initially, 4 mg once daily. May increase by 4–8 mg/day at wkly intervals. **Maintenance:** 32–56 mg/day in 2–4 divided doses. **CHILDREN 12–18 YRS:**

Pts receiving enzyme-inducing AED regimens: Initially, 4 mg once daily for 1 wk. Then, 8 mg/day in 2 divided doses for 1 wk. Then, increase in 4–8 mg/day increments. Administer in 2–4 divided doses/day. **Maximum:** 32 mg/day in 2–4 divided doses.

Dosage in Renal Impairment
No dose adjustment.

Dosage in Hepatic Impairment
Use caution.

SIDE EFFECTS

Frequent (34%–20%): Dizziness, asthenia (loss of strength, energy), drowsiness, nervousness, confusion, headache, infection, tremor. **Occasional:** Nausea, diarrhea, abdominal pain, impaired concentration.

ADVERSE EFFECTS/TOXIC REACTIONS

Overdose characterized by agitation, confusion, hostility, weakness. Full recovery occurs within 24 hrs of discontinuation. Depression, suicidal ideation.

NURSING CONSIDERATIONS

BASELINE ASSESSMENT

Review history of seizure disorder (intensity, frequency, duration, level of consciousness). Observe frequently for recurrence of seizure activity. Initiate seizure precautions.

INTERVENTION/EVALUATION

For pts on long-term therapy, serum hepatic/renal function tests, CBC should be performed periodically. Assist with ambulation if dizziness occurs. Assess for clinical improvement (decrease in intensity, frequency of seizures). Monitor for depression, unusual behavior, suicidal ideation or thoughts.

PATIENT/FAMILY TEACHING

• Go from lying to standing slowly. • Avoid tasks that require alertness, motor skills until response to drug is established. • Avoid alcohol. • Seek immediate medical attention if thoughts of suicide,

new-onset or worsening of anxiety, depression, or changes in mood occur.

ticagrelor

tye-**ka**-grel-or
(Brilinta)

■ **BLACK BOX ALERT** ■ May cause significant, sometimes fatal bleeding. Do not use with active bleeding or history of intracranial bleeding. Do not initiate in pts planning urgent coronary artery bypass graft (CABG) surgery. Discontinue at least 5 days prior to any surgery. Suspect bleeding in any pt who is hypotensive and has had recent percutaneous coronary intervention (PCI), CABG, or other surgical procedures. If possible, manage bleeding without discontinuing therapy to decrease risk of cardiovascular events. Aspirin maintenance doses greater than 100 mg/day may reduce effectiveness and should be strictly avoided.

◆CLASSIFICATION

PHARMACOTHERAPEUTIC: $P2Y_{12}$ platelet aggregation inhibitor. **CLINICAL:** Antiplatelet.

USES

Reduce risk of cardiovascular death, MI, stroke in pts with acute coronary syndrome (ACS) or history of MI. Reduces risk of stent thrombosis in pts who have been stented for treatment of ACS. Coronary artery disease (stable) and high risk for ischemic cardiovascular events (primary prevention) to reduce risk of first MI or stroke in pts with coronary artery disease (CAD) at high risk for such events. To reduce risk of stroke in pts with acute ischemic stroke (NIH Stroke Scale score 5 or less) or high-risk transient ischemic attack (TIA).

PRECAUTIONS

Contraindications: Hypersensitivity to ticagrelor. History of intracranial hemor-

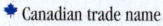 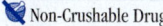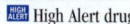

rhage, active pathologic bleeding, severe hepatic impairment. **Cautions:** Moderate hepatic impairment, renal impairment, history of hyperuricemia or gouty arthritis. Pts at increased risk of bradycardia, concurrent use of strong CYP3A4 inhibitors or inducers, elderly. (Recommend holding dose 5 days before planned surgery if applicable.) Pts with risk factors for bleeding (e.g., trauma, peptic ulcer disease).

ACTION
Reversibly inhibits platelet $P2Y_{12}$ ADP receptor to prevent signal transduction and platelet activation. **Therapeutic Effect:** Reduces platelet aggregation.

PHARMACOKINETICS
Widely distributed. Protein binding: 99%. Metabolized in liver. Primarily excreted in feces (58%), urine (26%). **Half-life:** 7–9 hrs.

⧗ LIFESPAN CONSIDERATIONS
Pregnancy/Lactation: Unknown if distributed in breast milk. **Children:** Safety and efficacy not established. **Elderly:** No age-related precautions noted.

INTERACTIONS
DRUG: **Strong CYP3A4 inhibitors** (e.g., clarithromycin, ketoconazole, ritonavir) may increase concentration/effect. **Strong CYP3A4 inducers** (e.g., carBAMazepine, phenytoin, rifAMPin) may decrease concentration/effect. **Anticoagulants** (e.g., warfarin), **antiplatelets** (e.g., aspirin, clopidogrel), **NSAIDs** (e.g., ibuprofen, ketorolac, naproxen) may increase risk of bleeding. May increase adverse effects of **apixaban, dabigatran, edoxaban, rivaroxaban.** May increase concentration/effect of **digoxin, simvastatin, lovastatin, rosuvastatin. HERBAL:** Herbals with anticoagulant/antiplatelet properties (e.g., **garlic, ginger, ginkgo biloba), glucosamine** may increase risk of bleeding. **FOOD: Grapefruit products**

may increase concentration/effect. **LAB VALUES:** May increase serum uric acid, creatinine.

AVAILABILITY (Rx)
Tablets: 60 mg, 90 mg.

ADMINISTRATION/HANDLING
PO
• Give without regard to food. • May be crushed, mixed with water, and drunk immediately (refill glass with water, stir and drink contents).

INDICATIONS/ROUTES/DOSAGE
Acute Coronary Syndrome
PO: ADULTS: Initially, 180 mg once, then 90 mg twice daily. (begin 12h after initial loading dose). Give in combination with aspirin. Continue for up to 12 mos, then decrease dose to 60 mg twice daily in combination with 75–100 mg aspirin.

CAD (With High Risk for Cardiovascular Events, Primary Prevention)
PO: ADULTS, ELDERLY: 60 mg twice daily (in combination with 75–100 mg aspirin). Continue indefinitely.

Minor Ischemic Stroke (NIHSS Score 5 or Less), High-Risk TIA
PO: ADULTS, ELDERLY: Initially, 180 mg once (in combination with 300–325 mg aspirin), then 90 mg twice daily in combination with 75–100 mg aspirin for 21–30 days, then continue long-term single antiplatelet therapy with 75–100 mg aspirin.

Dosage in Renal Impairment
No dose adjustment.

Dosage in Hepatic Impairment
Mild impairment: No dose adjustment. **Moderate impairment:** Use caution. **Severe impairment:** Avoid use.

SIDE EFFECTS
Occasional (13%–7%): Dyspnea, headache. **Rare (5%–3%):** Cough, dizziness, nausea, diarrhea, back pain, fatigue.

ADVERSE EFFECTS/TOXIC REACTIONS

Life-threatening events including intracranial bleeding, epistaxis, intrapericardial bleeding with cardiac tamponade, hypovolemic shock requiring vasopressive support or blood transfusion was reported. Pts with history of sick sinus syndrome, second- or third-degree AV block, bradycardic syncope have increased risk of bradycardia. May cause atrial fibrillation, hypotension, hypertension. Gynecomastia reported in less than 1% of men.

NURSING CONSIDERATIONS

BASELINE ASSESSMENT

Obtain CBC, renal function test. Question history of bleeding, stomach ulcers, colon polyps, head trauma, cardiac arrhythmias, unstable angina, recent MI, hepatic impairment, hypertension, stroke, pulmonary disease. Receive full medication history including herbal products.

INTERVENTION/EVALUATION

Routinely screen for bleeding. Assess skin for bruising, hematoma. Monitor renal function, uric acid, digoxin levels if applicable. Report hematuria, epistaxis, coffee-ground emesis, black/tarry stools.

PATIENT/FAMILY TEACHING

• It may take longer to stop bleeding during therapy. • Do not vigorously blow nose. • Use soft toothbrush, electric razor to decrease risk of bleeding. • Immediately report bloody stool, urine, or nosebleeds. • Report all newly prescribed medications. • Inform physician of any planned dental procedures or surgeries.

tigecycline

tye-gee-sye-kleen
(Tygacil)

■ **BLACK BOX ALERT** ■ An increase in all-cause mortality observed in Phase 3 and 4 clinical trials. Use is reserved when alternate treatment is not appropriate.

◆CLASSIFICATION

PHARMACOTHERAPEUTIC: Glycylcycline. **CLINICAL:** Antibiotic.

USES

Treatment of susceptible infections due to *E. coli, E. faecalis, S. aureus, S. agalactiae, S. anginosus* group (includes *S. anginosus, S. intermedius, S. constellatus), S. pyogenes, B. fragilis, Citrobacter freundii, E. cloacae, K. oxytoca, K. pneumoniae, B. thetaiotaomicron, B. uniformis, B. vulgatus, C. perfringens, Peptostreptococcus micros* including complicated skin/skin structure infections, complicated intra-abdominal infections, community-acquired bacterial pneumonia.

PRECAUTIONS

Contraindications: Hypersensitivity to tigecycline. **Cautions:** Hypersensitivity to tetracyclines; pregnancy, hepatic impairment, monotherapy for pts with intestinal perforation. Do not use for diabetic foot infections, healthcare (hospital)-acquired pneumonia, or ventilator-associated pneumonia.

ACTION

Inhibits protein synthesis by binding to ribosomal receptor sites of bacterial cell wall. **Therapeutic Effect:** Bacteriostatic effect.

PHARMACOKINETICS

Widely distributed. Metabolized in liver. Protein binding: 71%–89%. Excreted in feces (59%), urine (33%). **Half-life:** Single dose: 27 hrs; following multiple doses: 42 hrs.

⧗ LIFESPAN CONSIDERATIONS

Pregnancy/Lactation: May cause fetal harm. May be distributed in breast milk. Permanent discoloration of the teeth (brown-gray) may occur if used during tooth development. **Children:** Safety and efficacy not established in pts younger than 8 yrs. Use is reserved for when no effective alternative is available. **Elderly:** No age-related precautions noted.

INTERACTIONS

DRUG: May increase concentration/effect of **warfarin. HERBAL:** None significant. **FOOD:** None known. **LAB VALUES:** May increase serum alkaline phosphatase, amylase, BUN, bilirubin, glucose, LDH, ALT, AST. May decrease serum potassium; Hgb, leukocytes, platelets.

AVAILABILITY (Rx)

Injection, Powder for Reconstitution: *(Tygacil):* 50-mg vial.

ADMINISTRATION/HANDLING

 IV

Reconstitution • Reconstitute with 5.3 mL 0.9% NaCl or D_5W to a concentration of 10 mg/mL. Dilute in 100 mL 0.9% NaCl or D_5W.
Rate of administration • Infuse over 30–60 min. Flush IV line after infusion is complete.
Storage • Reconstituted solution may be stored at room temperature for up to 6 hrs (in vial) or 24 hrs if further diluted in NS or D5W (up to 48 hrs if refrigerated). • Reconstituted solution appears yellow to red-orange. • Discard if solution is discolored (green, black) or precipitate forms.

▓ IV COMPATIBILITIES

Heparin, norepinephrine, potassium chloride, propofol.

INDICATIONS/ROUTES/DOSAGE

Usual Dosage
IV: ADULTS OVER 18 YRS, ELDERLY: Initially, 100 mg, followed by 50 mg q12h for 5–14 days. **CHILDREN 12 YRS AND OLDER:** 50 mg q12h. **CHILDREN 8–11 YRS:** 1.2–2 mg/kg q12h. **Maximum:** 50 mg/dose.

Dosage in Renal Impairment
No dose adjustment.

Dosage in Hepatic Impairment
Mild to moderate impairment: No dose adjustment. **Severe impairment: IV: ADULTS OVER 18 YRS, ELDERLY:** Initially, 100 mg, followed by 25 mg q12h.

SIDE EFFECTS

Frequent (29%–13%): Nausea, vomiting, diarrhea. **Occasional (7%–4%):** Headache, hypertension, dizziness, increased cough, delayed healing. **Rare (3%–2%):** Peripheral edema, pruritus, constipation, dyspepsia, asthenia (loss of strength, energy), hypotension, phlebitis, insomnia, rash, diaphoresis.

ADVERSE EFFECTS/TOXIC REACTIONS

Dyspnea, abscess, pseudomembranous colitis (abdominal cramps, severe watery diarrhea, fever) ranging from mild to life-threatening may result from altered bacterial balance in GI tract.

NURSING CONSIDERATIONS

BASELINE ASSESSMENT
Obtain CBC, LFT. Question for history of allergies, esp. tetracyclines.

INTERVENTION/EVALUATION
Monitor daily pattern of bowel activity, stool consistency. Be alert for superinfection: fever, anal/genital pruritus, oral mucosal changes (ulceration, pain, erythema).

PATIENT/FAMILY TEACHING
• Report diarrhea, rash, mouth soreness, other new symptoms.

tiotropium

tye-oh-**trope**-ee-yum
(<u>Spiriva</u> HandiHaler, Spiriva Respimat)
Do not confuse Spiriva with Inspra, or tiotropium with ipratropium.

FIXED-COMBINATION(S)

Stiolto Respimat: tiotropium/olodaterol (a bronchodilator): 2.5 mcg/ 2.5 mcg.

◆CLASSIFICATION

PHARMACOTHERAPEUTIC: Anticholinergic (long-acting). **CLINICAL:** Bronchodilator.

USES

Long-term maintenance treatment of bronchospasm associated with COPD, including chronic bronchitis, emphysema, and for reducing COPD exacerbations. **Spiriva Respimat only:** Maintenance treatment of asthma in pts 6 yrs and older.

PRECAUTIONS

Contraindications: Hypersensitivity to tiotropium. History of hypersensitivity to ipratropium. **Cautions:** Narrow-angle glaucoma, prostatic hypertrophy, bladder neck obstruction, moderate to severe renal impairment, history of hypersensitivity to atropine, myasthenia gravis.

ACTION

Competitively and reversibly inhibits action of acetylcholine at muscarinic receptors in bronchial smooth muscle. **Therapeutic Effect:** Causes bronchodilation.

PHARMACOKINETICS

Binds extensively to tissue. Protein binding: 72%. Metabolized by oxidation. Excreted in urine. **Half-life:** 5–6 days.

⧗ LIFESPAN CONSIDERATIONS

Pregnancy/Lactation: Unknown if distributed in breast milk. **Children:** Safety and efficacy not established. **Elderly:** Higher frequency of dry mouth, constipation, UTI noted with increasing age.

INTERACTIONS

DRUG: Concurrent administration with **anticholinergics** (e.g., **aclidinium,** **umeclidinium, ipratropium**) may increase adverse effects. **Potassium chloride, potassium citrate** may increase risk of ulcers. **Pramlintide** may increase anticholinergic effect. **HERBAL:** None significant. **FOOD:** None known. **LAB VALUES:** None significant.

AVAILABILITY (Rx)

Inhalation Spray: (Spiriva Respimat): 1.25 mcg/actuation, 2.5 mcg/actuation. **Capsule, Inhalation: (Spiriva):** 18 mcg/capsule (in blister packs).

ADMINISTRATION/HANDLING

Inhalation
• **(Spiriva):** Open dustcap of HandiHaler by pulling it upward, then open mouthpiece. • Place capsule in center chamber and firmly close mouthpiece until a click is heard, leaving the dustcap open. • Hold HandiHaler device with mouthpiece upward, press piercing button completely in once, and release. • Instruct pt to breathe out completely before breathing in slowly and deeply but at rate sufficient to hear the capsule vibrate. • Have pt hold breath as long as it is comfortable until exhaling slowly. • Instruct pt to repeat once again to ensure full dose is received. • **(Spiriva Respimat):** See manufacturer guidelines.

Storage • Store at room temperature. Do not expose capsules to extreme temperature, moisture. • Do not store capsules in HandiHaler device. • Use immediately once foil is peeled back or removed.

INDICATIONS/ROUTES/DOSAGE

COPD (Maintenance Treatment, Reduction of COPD Exacerbations)

Inhalation: ADULTS, ELDERLY: (Spiriva): 18 mcg (1 capsule)/day via HandiHaler inhalation device. **(Spiriva Respimat [2.5 mcg/actuation]):** 2 inhalations (2.5 mcg/inhalation) once daily.

Asthma

Inhalation: ADULTS, ELDERLY, CHILDREN 6 YRS AND OLDER: (Spiriva Respimat

T

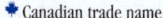 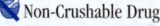

[1.25 mcg/actuation]): 2 inhalations of 1.25 mcg once daily. Maximum benefit may take up to 4–8 wks.

Dosage in Renal Impairment
CrCl 60 mL/min or less: Use caution in moderate to severe impairment.

Dosage in Hepatic Impairment
No dose adjustment.

SIDE EFFECTS

Frequent (16%–6%): Dry mouth, sinusitis, pharyngitis, dyspepsia, UTI, rhinitis. **Occasional (5%–4%):** Abdominal pain, peripheral edema, constipation, epistaxis, vomiting, myalgia, rash, oral candidiasis.

ADVERSE EFFECTS/TOXIC REACTIONS

Angina pectoris, depression, flu-like symptoms, glaucoma, increased intraocular pressure occur rarely.

NURSING CONSIDERATIONS

BASELINE ASSESSMENT
Question history of glaucoma, bladder outlet obstruction, renal impairment, myasthenia gravis. Auscultate lung sounds.

INTERVENTION/EVALUATION
Monitor rate, depth, rhythm, type of respiration; quality, rate of pulse. Assess lung sounds for rhonchi, wheezing, rales. Monitor ABGs. Observe for clavicular retractions, hand tremor. Evaluate for clinical improvement (quieter, slower respirations, relaxed facial expression, cessation of clavicular retractions).

PATIENT/FAMILY TEACHING
• Increase fluid intake (decreases lung secretion viscosity). • Do not use more than 1 capsule for inhalation in a 24-hr period. • Rinsing mouth with water immediately after inhalation may prevent mouth/throat dryness, thrush. • Avoid excessive use of caffeine derivatives (chocolate, coffee, tea, cola, cocoa). • Report eye pain/discomfort, blurred vision, visual halos.

---

tipiracil/trifluridine

trye-**flure**-i-deen/tye-**pir**-a-sil
(Lonsurf)
Do not confuse trifluridine with floxuridine, or tipiracil with tipifarnib or Pipracil.

◆CLASSIFICATION

PHARMACOTHERAPEUTIC: Antimetabolite/thymidine phosphorylase inhibitor. **CLINICAL:** Antineoplastic.

USES

Colorectal cancer: Treatment of pts with metastatic colorectal cancer as a single agent or in combination with bevacizumab who have been previously treated with fluoropyrimidine-, oxaliplatin-, and irinotecan-based chemotherapy, an anti-vascular endothelial growth factor (VEGF) biological therapy, and if RAS wild-type, an anti–epidermal growth factor (EGFR) therapy. **Gastric cancer:** Treatment of metastatic gastric or gastroesophageal junction adenocarcinoma previously treated with at least two prior lines of chemotherapy that included a fluoropyrimidine, a platinum, either a taxane or irinotecan, and if appropriate, HER2/neu-targeted therapy.

PRECAUTIONS

Contraindications: Hypersensitivity to trifluridine or tipiracil. **Cautions:** Baseline cytopenias, conditions predisposing to infection (e.g., diabetes, renal failure, immunocompromised pts, open wounds), pts at risk for tumor lysis syndrome (high tumor burden, dehydration), history of pulmonary embolism; pregnancy, moderate to severe hepatic impairment.

ACTION

Trifluridine (active cytotoxic component) interferes with DNA synthesis and cell proliferation of cancer cells. Tipiracil increases exposure of trifluridine by inhibiting metabolism via thymidine phos-

---

phorylase. **Therapeutic Effect:** Inhibits tumor cell growth and metastasis.

PHARMACOKINETICS

Widely distributed. Metabolized by thymidine phosphorylase (not metabolized in liver). Protein binding: trifluridine: 96%; tipiracil: 8%. Peak plasma concentration: 2 hrs. Excreted primarily in urine (50%). **Half-life:** trifluridine: 1.4 hrs (2.1 hrs at steady state); tipiracil: 2.1 hrs (2.4 hrs at steady state).

⧗ LIFESPAN CONSIDERATIONS

Pregnancy/Lactation: Avoid pregnancy; may cause fetal harm. Females and males with female partners of reproductive potential must use effective contraception during treatment and for at least 3 mo after discontinuation. Breastfeeding not recommended during treatment and for at least 1 day after discontinuation. **Children:** Safety and efficacy not established. **Elderly:** May have increased risk of neutropenia, thrombocytopenia.

INTERACTIONS

DRUG: May decrease therapeutic effect of **BCG (intravesical)**. **Cladribine** may increase immunosuppressive, myelosuppressive effect. May increase concentration/effects of **vaccines (live)**. **HERBAL:** Echinacea may decrease therapeutic effect. **FOOD:** None known. **LAB VALUES:** May decrease Hct, Hgb, platelets, neutrophils, RBC, WBC.

AVAILABILITY (Rx)

Fixed-Dose Combination Tablets: *(Trifluridine/Tipiracil):* 15 mg/6.14 mg, 20 mg/8.19 mg.

ADMINISTRATION/HANDLING

PO
• Give with morning and evening meals. Do not give on empty stomach.

INDICATIONS/ROUTES/DOSAGE

Note: Do not initiate the cycle until ANC is 1,500 cells/mm^3 or greater; febrile neutropenia is resolved; platelet count is 75,000 cells/mm^3 or greater; Grade 3 or 4 nonhematologic toxicity is resolved to Grade 1 or 0.

Colorectal, Gastric Cancer
Note: Refer to manufacturer prescribing information for calculated initial daily dose based on body surface area (BSA).
PO: ADULTS, ELDERLY: (Dose based on trifluridine component) 35 mg/m^2 (rounded to nearest 5-mg increment) twice daily on days 1–5 and days 8–12 of 28-day cycle. Continue until disease progression or unacceptable toxicity. **Maximum:** 80 mg/dose (based on trifluridine component).

Dose Modification
Based on Common Terminology Criteria for Adverse Events (CTCAE).

Hematologic/Nonhematologic Toxicity
Interrupt treatment for ANC less than 500 cells/mm^3; febrile neutropenia; platelet count less than 50,000 cells/mm^3; Grade 3 or 4 nonhematologic toxicity. Do not restart until ANC is 1,500 cells/mm^3 or greater; febrile neutropenia is resolved; platelet count is 75,000 cells/mm^3 or greater; Grade 3 or 4 nonhematologic toxicity is resolved to Grade 1 or 0 (except Grade 3 nausea and/or vomiting controlled by antiemetic therapy; Grade 3 diarrhea responsive to antidiarrheal medication). Once resolved, resume at decreased incremental dose of 5 mg/m^2 from previous dose. A maximum of 3 dose reductions is allowed to dosage minimum of 20 mg/m^2 twice daily. Do not increase dose after it has been reduced.

Dosage in Renal Impairment
Mild to moderate impairment: No dose adjustment. **Severe impairment:** Reduce dose to 20 mg/m^2 twice daily on days 1–5 and days 8–12 of a 28-day cycle. May further reduce dose to 15 mg/m^2 twice daily if unable to tolerate 20 mg/m^2 dose. Permanently discontinue if unable to tolerate 15 mg/m^2 dose.

Dosage in Hepatic Impairment
Mild impairment: No dose adjustment. **Moderate to severe impairment:** Avoid use.

SIDE EFFECTS

Frequent (52%–19%): Asthenia, fatigue, nausea, diarrhea, decreased appetite, vomiting, abdominal pain, pyrexia. **Occasional (8%–7%):** Stomatitis, dysgeusia, alopecia.

ADVERSE EFFECTS/TOXIC REACTIONS

Severe and/or life-threatening myelosuppression including anemia (77% of pts), Grade 3 anemia (18% of pts), neutropenia (67% of pts), Grade 3 or 4 neutropenia (27% and 11% of pts), thrombocytopenia (42% of pts), Grade 3 or 4 thrombocytopenia (5% and 1% of pts), febrile neutropenia (3.8% of pts) may occur. Infections including nasopharyngitis, UTI reported in 2%–4% of pts. Pulmonary embolism occurred in 2% of pts. Interstitial lung disease occurs rarely.

NURSING CONSIDERATIONS

BASELINE ASSESSMENT

Obtain CBC; pregnancy test in females of reproductive potential. Screen for active infection, history of pulmonary embolism. Assess hydration status. Question pt's usual stool characteristics (color, frequency, consistency). Offer emotional support.

INTERVENTION/EVALUATION

Follow proper handling and disposal procedures for cytotoxic drugs. Monitor ANC, CBC on day 15 of each cycle. If any Grade 3 or 4 hematologic toxicity occurs, repeat ANC, CBC more frequently. If chest pain, dyspnea, tachycardia occurs, provide supplemental O_2 and obtain radiologic testing to rule out pulmonary embolism. Diligently monitor for infection (cough, fatigue, fever). Monitor daily stool pattern, consistency. Encourage PO intake. Monitor for bleeding if thrombocytopenia occurs.

PATIENT/FAMILY TEACHING

• Treatment may depress your immune system response and reduce your ability to fight infection. Report symptoms of infection such as body aches, chills, cough, fatigue, fever. Avoid those with active infection. • Report symptoms of bone marrow depression (e.g., bruising, fatigue, fever, shortness of breath, weight loss; bleeding easily, bloody urine or stool). • Use effective contraception to avoid pregnancy. Do not breastfeed. • Immediately report chest pain, difficult breathing, fast heart rate, rapid breathing; may indicate life-threatening blood clot in the lungs. • Drink plenty of fluids. • Report diarrhea, nausea, vomiting that is not controlled by antinausea, antidiarrheal medication. • Report bleeding of any kind.

tirzepatide

tir-**zep**-a-tide
(Mounjaro, Zepbound)

■ **BLACK BOX ALERT** ■ Thyroid C-cell tumors have occurred in rodent studies with glucagon-like peptide-1 (GLP-1) receptor agonists. Contraindicated in pts with a personal/family history of medullary thyroid carcinoma or in pts with multiple endocrine neoplasia syndrome type 2. **Do not confuse tirzepatide with lixisenatide, plecanatide, or teriparatide.**

◆CLASSIFICATION

PHARMACOTHERAPEUTIC: GLP-1 receptor agonist. **CLINICAL:** Antidiabetic. Weight management.

USES

Mounjaro: Adjunct to diet and exercise to improve glycemic control in adults with type 2 diabetes mellitus. **Zepbound:** Adjunct to a reduced-calorie diet and increased physical activity for chronic weight management in adults with an initial body mass index (BMI) of: 30 kg/m² or greater or 27 kg/m² or greater in the presence of at least one weight-related comorbid condition (e.g., hypertension, dyslipidemia, type 2 diabetes mellitus, obstructive sleep apnea, or cardiovascular disease). Treatment of moderate to severe obstructive sleep apnea (OSA) in adults with obesity.

PRECAUTIONS

Contraindications: Hypersensitivity to tirzepatide. Personal/family history of medullary thyroid carcinoma. Pts with multiple endocrine neoplasia syndrome type 2. **Cautions:** Renal impairment, mild to moderate gastroparesis; history of pancreatitis. Not recommended in pts with severe GI disease, diabetic ketoacidosis, type 1 diabetes mellitus, pancreatitis, or use as first-line treatment regimen. Pulmonary aspiration in pts undergoing elective procedures requiring general anesthesia or deep sedation having residual gastric contents despite fasting.

ACTION

Activates GLP-1 receptors in pancreas, enhancing first- and second-phase insulin secretion and insulin sensitivity. Reduces glucagon secretion. Delays gastric emptying. **Therapeutic Effect:** Augments glucose-dependent insulin secretion, improving glycemic control.

PHARMACOKINETICS

Widely distributed. Metabolized by proteolytic cleavage of peptide backbone, beta-oxidation, and amide hydrolysis. Peak concentration: 8–72 hrs. Protein binding: 99%. Excreted in feces and urine as metabolites. **Half-life:** 5 days.

LIFESPAN CONSIDERATIONS

Pregnancy/Lactation: Nonoral contraceptives are recommended for 4 wks after initiation and with any increase in dosage. Oral contraceptives may be ineffective due to delayed gastric emptying (delay will diminish over time). Unknown if distributed in breast milk. **Children:** Safety and efficacy not established. **Elderly:** No age-related precautions noted.

INTERACTIONS

DRUG: **Insulin,** **metFORMIN,** **sulfonylureas** may increase hypoglycemic effect. May decrease therapeutic effect of **hormonal contraceptives, warfarin.** **HERBAL:** Herbals with hypoglycemic properties (e.g., **fenugreek, flaxseed, ginseng, gotu kola**) may increase risk of hypoglycemia. **FOOD:** None known. **LAB VALUES:** May increase serum amylase, lipase. Expected to decrease serum glucose; Hgb A1c.

AVAILABILITY (Rx)

Prefilled Injector Pen: 2.5 mg/0.5 mL, 5 mg/0.5 mL, 7.5 mg/0.5 mL, 10 mg/0.5 mL, 12.5 mg/0.5 mL, 15 mg/0.5 mL.

ADMINISTRATION/HANDLING
SQ

Guidelines • Administer any time of the day, without regard to meals, on the same day of each week. May change administration day if the time between 2 doses is at least 3 days (72 hrs). • If a dose is missed, administer within 4 days after missed dose. If more than 4 days pass after missed dose, wait until next regularly scheduled day. If insulin is also being used, injection sites should not be adjacent to each other.
Preparation • Visually inspect for particulate matter or discoloration. Solution should appear clear, colorless to slightly yellow. Do not use if solution is cloudy, discolored, or visible particles are observed.
Administration • Insert needle subcutaneously into abdomen, outer thigh, or upper arm and inject solution. • Do not inject into areas of active skin disease or injury such as sunburns, skin rashes, inflammation, skin infections, or active psoriasis. • Do not administer IV or intramuscularly. • Rotate injection sites.
Storage • Refrigerate unused injector pens in original carton. • Do not freeze. • Protect from light. • May store at room temperature for up to 21 days.

INDICATIONS/ROUTES/DOSAGE
Type 2 Diabetes Mellitus

SQ: **ADULTS, ELDERLY:** Initially, 2.5 mg once wkly for 4 wks, then increase to 5 mg once wkly. If glycemic response is inadequate, may further increase dose by 2.5-mg increments after at least 4 wks on current dose. **Maximum:** 15 mg once wkly.

Weight Management

SQ: ADULTS, ELDERLY: (Dose escalation): Initially, 2.5 mg once wkly for 4 wks, then increase to 5 mg once wkly. Dose may be increased in 2.5-mg increments, after at least 4 wks on the current dose. **Maintenance:** 5 mg, 10 mg, or 15 mg once wkly. **Maximum:** 15 mg once wkly.

OSA

SQ: ADULTS, ELDERLY: (Dose escalation): Initially, 2.5 mg once wkly for 4 wks, then increase to 5 mg once wkly. Dose may be increased in 2.5 mg increments, after at least 4 wks on the current dose. **Maintenance:** 10 mg or 15 mg once wkly. **Maximum:** 15 mg once wkly.

Dosage in Hepatic/Renal Impairment
No dose adjustment.

SIDE EFFECTS

Note: Frequency of side effects may escalate when dose is increased.
Occasional (12%–6%): Nausea, diarrhea, dyspepsia, constipation, abdominal pain. **Rare (5%–3%):** Vomiting, decreased appetite, injection site reactions.

ADVERSE EFFECTS/TOXIC REACTIONS

GLP-1 receptor agonists are associated with an increased risk of anaphylaxis, acute renal failure, or worsening of chronic renal impairment (esp. with dehydration); acute gallbladder disease, diabetic retinopathy, severe gastroparesis, pancreatitis, thyroid C-cell tumors. May increase risk of hypoglycemia when used with other hypoglycemic agents or insulin. Hypersensitivity reactions including eczema, urticaria reported in 3% of pts.

NURSING CONSIDERATIONS

BASELINE ASSESSMENT

Obtain fasting glucose level, Hgb A1c; BUN, serum creatinine, eGFR, CrCl in pts with renal impairment. Question history of medullary thyroid carcinoma, multiple endocrine neoplasia syndrome type 2, hypersensitivity reaction, pancreatitis, renal impairment, gastroparesis. Screen for use of other hypoglycemic agents, insulin; oral medications (esp. oral contraceptives). Assess pt's understanding of diabetes management, routine home glucose monitoring. Assess hydration status. Obtain dietary consult for nutritional education. Assess pt's willingness to self-inject medication.

INTERVENTION/EVALUATION

Monitor capillary blood glucose levels, Hgb A1c; renal function in pts with renal impairment reporting severe GI symptoms such as diarrhea, gastroparesis, vomiting. Monitor for hypersensitivity reaction. Screen for thyroid tumors (dysphagia, dyspnea, persistent hoarseness, neck mass). If tumor is suspected, consider endocrinologist consultation. Clinical significance of serum calcitonin level or thyroid ultrasound with GLP-1–associated thyroid tumors is debated/unknown. Assess for hypoglycemia (anxiety, confusion, diaphoresis, diplopia, dizziness, headache, hunger, perioral numbness, tachycardia, tremors), hyperglycemia (confusion, fatigue, Kussmaul breathing, nausea, polyuria, vomiting). Screen for glucose-altering conditions: Fever, stress, surgical procedures, trauma. Monitor for pancreatitis (severe, steady abdominal pain often radiating to the back [with or without vomiting]). Encourage fluid intake. Monitor I&Os.

PATIENT/FAMILY TEACHING

• A healthcare provider will show you how to properly prepare and inject medication. You must demonstrate correct preparation and injection techniques before using medication at home. • Diabetes mellitus requires lifelong control. Diet and regular exercise are principal parts of treatment; do not skip or delay meals. • Test blood sugar regularly. • Monitor daily calorie intake. • When taking additional medications to lower blood sugar (e.g., insulin, other oral hypoglycemic agents), have a low blood sugar treatment available (e.g., glucagon, oral dextrose). Be alert to conditions that alter glucose levels (e.g., fever, infection, stress, trauma). • Treatment may increase risk of thyroid cancer; report lumps or swelling of the neck; hoarseness, shortness of breath, trouble swallowing. • Persistent, severe abdominal pain that radiates to the back (with or without vomiting) may indicate acute pancreatitis. • Report allergic reactions of any kind, esp. difficulty breathing, itching, rash, swelling of the face or throat. • Kidney injury or kidney failure may occur; report decreased urine output, amber-colored urine, flank pain. • Oral contraceptives may be ineffective when treatment is started or after any increase of dosage.

tisotumab vedotin-tftv

tye-**sot**-ue-mab ve-**doe**-tin
(Tivdak)

■ **BLACK BOX ALERT** ■ Changes in corneal epithelium and conjunctiva may lead to severe vision loss, corneal ulcerations. Ophthalmic examination should be performed at baseline, prior to each dose, and as clinically indicated. To reduce risk of ocular toxicity, maintain premedication and proper eye care before, during, and after each infusion. Reduce dose, withhold, or permanently discontinue treatment based on clinical severity of ocular toxicity.
Do not confuse tisotumab vedotin with brentuximab vedotin, enfortumab vedotin, polatuzumab vedotin, or tivozanib, or Tivdak with Tivicay or tivozanib.

◆CLASSIFICATION

PHARMACOTHERAPEUTIC: Tissue factor (TF)–directed antibody drug conjugate (ADC). Antimicrotubular. Monoclonal antibody. **CLINICAL:** Antineoplastic.

USES

Treatment of adults with recurrent or metastatic cervical cancer with disease progression on or after chemotherapy.

PRECAUTIONS

Contraindications: Hypersensitivity to tisotumab vedotin-tftv. **Cautions:** Baseline cy-

topenias, mild hepatic impairment, severe renal impairment, interstitial lung disease (e.g., COPD, sarcoidosis, connective tissue disease), pts at risk for hemorrhage (e.g., history of severe hemorrhagic events, coagulation disorders, recent trauma; concomitant use of anticoagulants, antiplatelets); history of thromboembolism (e.g., DVT, pulmonary embolism); conditions predisposing to infection (e.g., diabetes, renal failure, immunocompromised pts, open wounds). Avoid use in pts with moderate to severe hepatic impairment.

ACTION

A TF-directed ADC (composed of anti-TF IgG1-kappa antibody conjugated to a microtubule-disrupting agent [monomethyl auristatin E, MMAE] via a protease-cleavable linker). Binds to TF-expressing cancer cells, followed by internalization of the ADC-TF complex and release of MMAE via proteolytic cleavage. MMAE disrupts microtubule network of active dividing cells, leading to cell cycle arrest. **Therapeutic Effect:** Causes apoptosis (cellular death) of tumor cells.

PHARMACOKINETICS

Widely distributed. Metabolized via catabolism into small peptides, amino acids, unconjugated MMAE, and unconjugated MMAE-related metabolites. Protein binding: 68%–82%. Peak plasma concentration: Near end of infusion. Steady state reached after 1 treatment cycle. Excretion: Not fully characterized. **Half-life:** (tisotumab vedotin): 2–7 days; (unconjugated MMAE): 2–4 days.

⏳ LIFESPAN CONSIDERATIONS

Pregnancy/Lactation: Avoid pregnancy; may cause fetal harm. Females of reproductive potential must use effective contraception during treatment and for at least 2 mos after discontinuation. Unknown if distributed in breast milk. Breastfeeding not recommended during treatment and for at least 3 wks after discontinuation. **Males:** Males with female partners of reproductive potential must use effective contraception during treatment and for at least 4 mos after discontinuation. May impair fertility. **Children:** Safety and efficacy not established. **Elderly:** May have increased risk of adverse effects/toxic reactions.

INTERACTIONS

DRUG: Strong CYP3A4 inhibitors (e.g., **clarithromycin, ketoconazole, itraconazole**) may increase concentration/effect. **Anticoagulants** (e.g., **heparin, warfarin**), **antiplatelets** (e.g., **aspirin, clopidogrel**) may increase risk of bleeding. **HERBAL:** Herbals with anticoagulant/antiplatelet properties (e.g., **garlic, ginger, ginkgo biloba**) may increase risk of bleeding. **FOOD:** None known. **LAB VALUES:** May increase serum alkaline phosphatase, ALT, AST, creatinine, creatinine kinase, lactate dehydrogenase, uric acid. May decrease serum albumin, glucose, magnesium, sodium; Hgb, leukocytes, lymphocytes, neutrophils, RBCs. May prolong activated partial thromboplastin time (aPPT); increase international normalized ratio (INR).

AVAILABILITY (Rx)

Injection, Powder for Reconstitution: 40 mg.

ADMINISTRATION/HANDLING
IV

Premedication • Prior to each infusion, administer topical corticosteroid eye drops, topical ocular vasoconstrictor drops after examination with a slit lamp.
Infusion guidelines • Infuse via a dedicated IV line using a sterile 0.2 micron in-line filter. • Do not administer as IV push or bolus. Protect IV solution from direct sunlight during administration.
Reconstitution • Must be prepared by personnel trained in aseptic manipulations and admixing of cytotoxic drugs. • Calculate the number of vials needed for reconstitution based on weight in kg. • Reconstitute each vial with 4 mL of Sterile Water for Injection to a final concentration of 10 mg/mL. • Swirl vial gently until powder is completely dissolved. Do not shake or agitate. • Visually inspect for particulate matter or discoloration.

Solution should appear clear to slightly opalescent, colorless to slightly brownish-yellow. Do not use if solution is cloudy, discolored, or if visible particles are observed. • Dilute in 0.9% NaCl, D_5W, or lactated Ringer's injection to a final concentration of 0.7–2.4 mg/mL. • Mix by gentle inversion. Do not shake or agitate. • Discard used portions of vial.
Rate of administration • Infuse over 30 min.
Storage • Refrigerate unused vials in original carton. • May refrigerate reconstituted vials for up to 24 hrs or store at room temperature for up to 8 hrs prior to dilution. • May refrigerate diluted solution containing: 0.9% NaCl for up to 18 hrs; D_5W for up to 24 hrs; lactated Ringer's injection for up to 12 hrs. • Do not freeze or expose unused vials, diluted solution to direct sunlight during preparation, transportation, administration, or storage.

⚏ IV INCOMPATABILITIES

Do not mix or infuse with other solutions or medications.

INDICATIONS/ROUTES/DOSAGE

Cervical Cancer (Recurrent or Metastatic)
IV: ADULTS: 2 mg/kg (up to maximum of 200 mg for pts 100 kg or greater) q3wks until disease progression or unacceptable toxicity.

Dose Reduction Schedule
First dose reduction: 1.3 mg/kg. **Second dose reduction:** 0.9 mg/kg. Permanently discontinue in pts unable to tolerate 0.9 mg/kg dose.

Dose Modification
Based on Common Terminology Criteria for Adverse Events (CTCAE).

Conjunctival Ulceration
Any ulceration: (First occurrence): Withhold treatment until complete conjunctival re-epithelialization, then resume at next lower dose. **(Second occurrence):** Permanently discontinue.
Conjunctival or Corneal Scarring or Symblepharon
Any scarring or symblepharon: Permanently discontinue.

Conjunctivitis, Other Ocular Reactions
Grade 1 conjunctivitis, other ocular reactions: Continue to monitor. **Grade 2 conjunctivitis, other ocular reactions: (first occurrence):** Withhold treatment until improved to Grade 1 or 0, then resume at same dose. **(Second occurrence):** Withhold treatment until improved to Grade 1 or 0, then resume at next lower dose. Permanently discontinue if not improved. **(Third occurrence):** Permanently discontinue. **Grade 3 or 4 conjunctivitis, other ocular reactions:** Permanently discontinue.

Keratitis
Superficial punctate keratitis (SPK): Monitor during treatment. **Confluent superficial keratitis: (First occurrence):** Withhold treatment until improved to SPK, then resume at next lower dose. **(Second occurrence):** Permanently discontinue. **Ulcerative keratitis or perforation:** Permanently discontinue.

Hemorrhage
Any grade pulmonary or central nervous system bleeding: Permanently discontinue. **Any other Grade 2 bleeding:** Withhold treatment until resolved, then resume at same dose. **Any other Grade 3 bleeding: (First occurrence):** Withhold treatment until resolved, then resume at same dose. **(Second occurrence):** Permanently discontinue. **Any other Grade 4 bleeding:** Permanently discontinue.

Peripheral Neuropathy
Grade 2 peripheral neuropathy (initial or worsening from baseline): Withhold treatment until improved to Grade 1 or 0, then resume at next lower dose. **Grade 3 or 4 peripheral neuropathy:** Permanently discontinue.

Pneumonitis
Grade 2 pneumonitis: Withhold treatment until improved to Grade 1 or 0 for persistent or recurrent pneumonitis, then consider resuming at next lower dose. **Grade 3 or 4 pneumonitis:** Permanently discontinue.

Dosage in Renal Impairment
Mild to moderate impairment: No dose adjustment. **Severe impairment, ESRD:** Not specified; use caution.

Dosage in Hepatic Impairment
Mild impairment: No dose adjustment. **Moderate to severe impairment:** Not recommended.

SIDE EFFECTS
Frequent (50%–21%): Fatigue, asthenia, nausea, alopecia, dry eye, lacrimation, diarrhea, rash, dermatitis, constipation, abdominal pain, myalgia, musculoskeletal pain. **Occasional (17%–12%):** Vomiting, decreased appetite, pyrexia, blepharitis, meibomianitis, eye pruritus, entropion, trichiasis, chalazion, meibomian dysfunction, arthralgia, pruritus, extremity pain, decreased weight.

ADVERSE EFFECTS/TOXIC REACTIONS
Myelosuppression (anemia, lymphopenia, leukopenia, neutropenia) is an expected response to therapy. Changes in corneal epithelium and conjunctiva may lead to severe vision loss, corneal ulcerations. Ocular toxicities, including corneal adverse effects, were reported in 60% of pts. Grade 3 ocular adverse effects, severe ulcerative keratitis, visual acuity changes to 20/50 (or worse) reported in up to 4% of pts. Peripheral neuropathy including hypoesthesia, hyperesthesia, gait disturbance, muscular weakness, paresthesia, peripheral motor/sensorimotor neuropathy, neuropathic pain demyelinating polyneuropathy reported in up to 42% of pts. Hemorrhagic events including GI/GU/oral/paranasal/rectal/vaginal hemorrhage, epistaxis, hemoptysis reported in up to 62% of pts. Life-threatening pneumonitis reported in 1% of pts. Urinary tract infections reported in 14% of pts. Venous thrombosis, pulmonary embolism occurred in 3% of pts.

NURSING CONSIDERATIONS

BASELINE ASSESSMENT

Obtain CBC, BMP, LFT; pregnancy test in females of reproductive potential. Verify use of effective contraception. Obtain weight in kg. Obtain ophthalmic exam at baseline and prior to each dose. Obtain visual acuity. Question history of hepatic/renal impairment, ocular disease, pulmonary disease, hemorrhagic events, thromboembolism (DVT, pulmonary embolism). Screen for active infection. Receive full medication history and screen for interactions. Offer emotional support.

INTERVENTION/EVALUATION

Monitor CBC, BMP, LFT as clinically indicated. Ophthalmic exams should be performed to monitor for eye toxicities. Monitor visual acuity. Apply ice packs over the eyes during infusion. Change cold packs as needed throughout infusion to ensure the eye areas remain cold. Continue administration of corticosteroid eye drops for 72 hrs after each infusion. Topical lubricating eye drops should be administered during treatment and for up to 30 days after discontinuation. Monitor for hemorrhagic events including GI/GU bleeding (hematemesis, hematuria, melena, oral/vaginal/rectal bleeding), epistaxis; symptoms of pulmonary embolism (chest pain, dyspnea, tachycardia), DVT (leg or arm pain/swelling), peripheral neuropathy (gait disturbance, incoordination, neuropathic pain, numbness, weakness). Consider ABG, radiologic test if pneumonitis (excessive cough, dyspnea, fever, hypoxia) is suspected. Consider treatment with corticosteroids if pneumonitis is confirmed. Monitor for infections (cough, fatigue, fever; urinary frequency, dysuria). Monitor daily pattern of bowel activity, stool consistency.

PATIENT/FAMILY TEACHING

• Treatment may depress your immune system response and reduce your ability to fight infection. Report symptoms of infection such as body aches, chills, cough, fatigue, fever. Avoid those with active infection. • Bleeding events may occur; report blood in stool or urine; nasal/oral/rectal/vaginal bleeding, vomiting up blood, or bleeding of any kind. • Blood clots may occur; report symptoms of DVT (swelling, pain, hot feeling in the arms or legs), lung embolism (difficulty breathing, chest pain, rapid heart rate). • Report liver problems (abdominal pain, bruising, clay-colored stool, amber- or dark-colored urine, yellowing of the skin or eyes), inflammation of the lung (excessive cough, difficulty breathing, fever, chest pain), nervous system changes (gait disturbance, lack of coordination; numbness, pain, trouble walking), rash; symptoms of UTI (fever, urinary frequency, burning with urination, foul-smelling urine). • Use effective contraception to avoid pregnancy. Do not breastfeed. • Treatment may cause severe eye toxicities, which may lead to severe vision loss, irritation, ulcers of the eye. Expect frequent eye examinations. It is essential to stay compliant with steroid eye drops and lubricating eye drops. Immediately report eye symptoms despite preventive care. Avoid wearing contact lenses.

tivozanib

tye-**voe**-zan-ib
(Fotivda)
Do not confuse tivozanib with axitinib, cabozantinib, lenvatinib, PAZOPanib, regorafenib, SORAfenib, SUNItinib, tepotinib, or tucatinib.

◆**CLASSIFICATION**

PHARMACOTHERAPEUTIC: Vascular endothelial growth factor receptor (VEGFR) inhibitor, kinase inhibitor. **CLINICAL:** Antineoplastic.

USES

Treatment of adults with relapsed or refractory advanced renal cell carcinoma (RCC) after 2 or more prior systemic therapies.

PRECAUTIONS

Contraindications: Hypersensitivity to tivozanib. **Cautions:** Baseline cytopenias, hepatic impairment, end-stage renal disease (ESRD), hypertension, cardiomyopathy, thyroid dysfunction (hyperthyroidism, hypothyroidism); recent (within 6 mos) CVA, MI, unstable angina, hemorrhagic events; pts at risk for hemorrhage (e.g., history of intracranial/GI/GU/pulmonary bleeding, coagulation disorders, recent trauma; concomitant use of anticoagulants, antiplatelets, chronic NSAIDs); history of arterial/venous thrombosis (e.g., CVA, DVT, MI, pulmonary embolism); pts at risk for thrombosis (immobility, indwelling venous catheter/access device, morbid obesity, genetic hypercoagulable conditions); recent or poorly healed wounds (e.g., recent or planned surgery, chronic open wounds, ulcers). Avoid use of strong CYP3A4 inducers.

ACTION

Inhibit phosphorylation of VEGFR-1, VEGFR-2, and VEGFR-3, preventing angiogenesis, vascular permeability, and tumor cell proliferation. **Therapeutic Effect:** Inhibits tumor growth.

PHARMACOKINETICS

Widely distributed. Metabolized in liver. Protein binding: greater than 99%. Peak plasma concentration: 10 hrs (range: 3–24 hrs). Steady state reached in 14 days. Excreted in feces (79%), urine (12%). **Half-life:** 111 hrs.

⧗ LIFESPAN CONSIDERATIONS

Pregnancy/Lactation: Avoid pregnancy; may cause fetal harm. Females of reproductive potential and males with female partners of reproductive potential must use effective contraception during treatment and for at least 1 mo after discontinuation. Unknown if distributed in breast milk. Breastfeeding not recommended during treatment and for at least 1 mo after discontinuation. May impair fertility in both females and males. **Children:** Safety and efficacy not established. **Elderly:** No age-related precautions noted.

INTERACTIONS

DRUG: **Anticoagulants (e.g., heparin, warfarin), antiplatelets (e.g., aspirin, clopidogrel), chronic use of NSAIDs (e.g., diclofenac, meloxicam, naproxen)** may increase risk of bleeding. **Strong CYP3A4 inducers (e.g., carBAMazepine, phenytoin, rifAMPin)** may decrease concentration/effect. **HERBAL:** **Herbals with anticoagulant/antiplatelet properties (e.g., garlic, ginger, ginkgo biloba)** may increase risk of bleeding. **FOOD:** None known. **LAB VALUES:** May increase serum alkaline phosphatase, ALT, amylase, AST, bilirubin, calcium, creatinine, glucose, lipase, potassium. May decrease serum magnesium, phosphate, sodium; lymphocytes, platelets. May increase or decrease Hgb. May prolong activated partial thromboplastin (aPTT).

AVAILABILITY (RX)

Capsules: 0.89 mg, 1.34 mg.

ADMINISTRATION/HANDLING

PO
• Give without regard to food (consistent administration regarding meals is recommended). • Capsules may be opened and sprinkled on food (absorption is increased by 20%).

INDICATIONS/ROUTES/DOSAGE

Renal Cell Carcinoma (Advanced, Relapsed, or Refractory)
PO: **ADULTS:** 1.34 mg once daily for 21 days, followed by a 7-day interruption,

of a 28-day cycle. Continue until disease progression or unacceptable toxicity.

Dose Reduction

If dose modification is required for an adverse reaction, reduce dose 0.89 mg once daily for 21 days, followed by a 7-day interruption, of a 28-day cycle.

Dose Modification

Based on Common Terminology Criteria for Adverse Events (CTCAE).

Cardiac Toxicity

Grade 3 cardiac failure: Withhold treatment until improved to Grade 1 or 0 (or baseline), then resume at reduced dose. Consider discontinuation based on severity.

Hypertension

Grade 3 hypertension (despite optimal hypertensive therapy): Withhold treatment until adequately controlled (Grade 2 or less), then resume at reduced dose level. **Grade 4 hypertension**: Permanently discontinue.

Proteinuria

Urine protein level greater than 2 g/24 hrs: Withhold treatment until urine protein level is less than 2 g/24 hrs, then resume at reduced dose. **Nephrotic syndrome**: Permanently discontinue.

Other Adverse Reactions

Any other persistent or intolerable Grade 2 or 3 adverse reaction; Grade 4 lab abnormality: Withhold treatment until improved to Grade 1 or 0 (or baseline), then resume at reduced dose. Any other Grade 4 adverse reaction: Permanently discontinue.

Permanent Discontinuation

Permanently discontinue in pts with Grade 3 or 4 hemorrhage; occurrence of arterial thromboembolism, reversible posterior leukoencephalopathy syndrome.

Dosage in Renal Impairment

Mild to severe impairment: No dose adjustment. **ESRD**: Not specified; use caution.

Dosage in Hepatic Impairment

Mild impairment: No dose adjustment. **Moderate impairment**: Reduce dose 0.89 mg once daily for 21 days, followed by a 7-day interruption, of a 28-day cycle. **Severe impairment**: Not specified; use caution.

SIDE EFFECTS

Frequent (67%–21%): Fatigue, asthenia, diarrhea, decreased appetite, nausea, dysphonia, cough, stomatitis. **Occasional (19% to less than 15%)**: Back pain, rash, dermatitis, eczema, erythema, photosensitivity reaction, pruritus, psoriasis, skin exfoliation/irritation, vomiting, decreased weight, dyspnea, delirium.

ADVERSE EFFECTS/TOXIC REACTIONS

Severe hypertension, hypertensive crisis may occur. Hypertension reported in 45% of pts with median onset occurring in 2 wks. Hypertensive crisis reported in 1% of pts. Life-threatening cardiac failure, cardiac ischemia reported in 2% and 3% of pts, respectively. Fatal arterial thrombosis, including CVA, has occurred. Life-threatening venous thromboembolism reported in 2% of pts. Hemorrhagic events, including epistaxis, hematuria, hemoptysis, contusion, intraocular hematoma, intracranial hemorrhage, GI/GU bleeding (hematemesis, melena, rectal bleeding), vaginal hemorrhage, were reported. Proteinuria may indicate acute renal injury or nephrotic syndrome. Thyroid dysfunction (hyperthyroidism, hypothyroidism) reported in 1% of pts. May cause impaired wound healing or wound dehiscence requiring medical intervention. Posterior reversible encephalopathy syndrome (PRLS), a dysfunction of the brain that may evolve into an ischemic CVA or cerebral hemorrhage, may occur. Palmar-plantar erythrodysesthesia syndrome (PPES), a chemotherapy-induced skin condition that presents with skin redness, swelling, numbness, sloughing of the hands and feet, may occur. Elevated hepatic enzymes (transaminitis) reported in 28%–30% of pts.

NURSING CONSIDERATIONS

BASELINE ASSESSMENT

Obtain BUN, serum creatinine, LFT, thyroid panel; B/P; pregnancy test in females of reproductive potential. Confirm compliance with effective contraception. Verify baseline hypertension is adequately controlled prior to initiation. Consider echocardiogram to asses LVEF in pts with cardiomyopathy. Question history of ESRD, hepatic impairment, hemorrhagic events, hypertension, recent surgery, thromboembolism (CVA, DVT, MI, pulmonary embolism), thyroid dysfunction. Assess risk for thrombosis. Receive full medication history and screen for interactions. Conduct dermatological exam; assess for open wounds, lesions, surgical incisions. Offer emotional support.

INTERVENTION/EVALUATION

Monitor renal function test, LFT, thyroid panel, urine protein periodically. If urine protein is greater than or equal to 2+ on dipstick, obtain 24-hr urine protein test. Monitor for decreased urine output, renal dysfunction, nephrotic syndrome. Monitor B/P after initiation, then at least monthly thereafter. Persistent diastolic hypertension may indicate hypertensive crisis. Medically manage diarrhea, nausea, vomiting prior to withholding treatment or dose reduction. Withhold treatment for at least 24 days prior to elective surgery or for at least 2 wks after major surgery and until wound is fully healed. Assess skin for impaired wound healing, new skin lesions, rash; symptoms of PPES. Monitor for MI (chest pain, diaphoresis, left arm/jaw pain, increased serum troponin, ST-segment elevation), CVA (aphasia, altered mental status, facial droop, hemiplegia, vision loss), pulmonary embolism (chest pain, dyspnea, tachycardia); cardiac failure (dyspnea, edema, palpitations, syncope); hemorrhagic events, including intracranial hemorrhage (altered mental status, aphasia, blindness, hemiparesis, unequal pupils, seizures), GI/GU bleeding (hematemesis, melena, rectal bleeding), epistaxis. RPLS should be considered in pts with altered mental status, confusion, headache, seizures, visual disturbances.

PATIENT/FAMILY TEACHING

• Life-threatening blood clots of the arteries and veins may occur; report symptoms of heart attack (chest pain, difficulty breathing, jaw pain, nausea, pain that radiates to the left arm, sweating), stroke (blindness, confusion, one-sided weakness, loss of consciousness, trouble speaking, seizures), DVT (swelling, pain, hot feeling in the arms or legs), lung embolism (difficulty breathing, chest pain, rapid heart rate). • Life-threatening bleeding may occur; report bloody stool, urine; rectal bleeding, nosebleeds, vomiting up blood, or bleeding of any kind. • Treatment may cause or worsen high blood pressure. Blurry vision, confusion, chest pain, headache, seizures may indicate life-threatening high blood pressure crisis. • Notify physician before any planned surgeries/invasive dental procedures. • Report liver problems (abdominal pain, bruising, clay-colored stool, amber- or dark-colored urine, yellowing of the skin or eyes), kidney problems (decreased urine output, flank pain, darkened urine), toxic skin reactions (sloughing, rash, poor healing of wounds). • Posterior reversible encephalopathy syndrome, a dysfunction of the brain that may cause a stroke or bleeding in the brain, may occur. • Treatment may reduce the heart's ability to pump effectively; report heart problems (difficulty breathing, fainting, palpitations, swelling of extremities). • Do not take newly prescribed medications unless approved by prescriber who originally started treatment.

T

✦ Canadian trade name   🐋 Non-Crushable Drug   🔺 High Alert drug

tiZANidine

tye-**zan**-i-deen
(Zanaflex)
Do not confuse tiZANidine with tiaGABine.

◆CLASSIFICATION

PHARMACOTHERAPEUTIC: Alpha$_2$-adrenergic agonist. **CLINICAL:** Antispastic.

USES

Acute and intermittent management of muscle spasticity (spasms, stiffness, rigidity), spasticity associated with multiple sclerosis or spinal cord injury. **OFF-LABEL:** Muscle spasm and/or musculoskeletal pain.

PRECAUTIONS

Contraindications: Hypersensitivity to tiZANidine. Concurrent use with strong CYP1A2 inhibitors (e.g., ciprofloxacin, fluvoxamine). **Cautions:** Renal/hepatic disease, pts at risk for severe hypotensive effects, cardiac disease, psychiatric disorders, elderly.

ACTION

Increases presynaptic inhibition of spinal motor neurons mediated by alpha$_2$-adrenergic agonists, reducing facilitation to postsynaptic motor neurons. **Therapeutic Effect:** Reduces muscle spasticity.

PHARMACOKINETICS

Metabolized in liver. Primarily excreted in urine. **Half-life:** 2 hrs.

INTERACTIONS

DRUG: Alcohol, other CNS depressants (e.g., **LORazepam, morphine, zolpidem**) may increase CNS depressant effects. **Strong CYP1A2 inhibitors (e.g., ciprofloxacin, fluvoxaMINE)** may increase concentration/adverse effects (contraindicated). **HERBAL: Herbals with hypotensive properties (e.g., garlic, ginger, ginkgo biloba)** may alter effects. **Herbals with sedative properties (e.g., chamomile, kava kava, valerian)** may increase CNS depression. **FOOD:** None known. **LAB VALUES:** May increase serum alkaline phosphatase, ALT, AST.

AVAILABILITY (Rx)

Capsules: 2 mg, 4 mg, 6 mg. **Tablets:** 2 mg, 4 mg.

ADMINISTRATION/HANDLING

PO
• Give without regard to food (consistent administration regarding meals is recommended). • Capsules may be opened and sprinkled on food (absorption is increased by 20%).

INDICATIONS/ROUTES/DOSAGE

Muscle Spasticity
PO: ADULTS, ELDERLY: Initially, 2 mg once daily at bedtime. May increase by 2–4 mg at intervals of 1–4 days. **Maximum:** 36 mg/day in 3–4 divided doses. **Discontinuation of therapy:** Gradually taper dose by 2–4 mg daily.

Dosage in Renal Impairment
May require dose reduction/less frequent dosing. **CrCl less than 25 mL/min:** Reduce dose by 50%. If higher doses needed, increase dose instead of frequency.

Dosage in Hepatic Impairment
Avoid use if possible. If used, monitor for adverse effects (e.g., hypotension).

SIDE EFFECTS

Frequent (49%–41%): Dry mouth, drowsiness, asthenia. **Occasional (16%–4%):** Dizziness, UTI, constipation. **Rare (3%):** Nervousness, amblyopia, pharyngitis, rhinitis, vomiting, urinary frequency.

ADVERSE EFFECTS/TOXIC REACTIONS

Hypotension may be associated with bradycardia, orthostatic hypotension, and, rarely, syncope. Risk of hypotension increases as dosage increases; hypotension is noted within 1 hr after administration. May cause visual hallucinations.

NURSING CONSIDERATIONS

BASELINE ASSESSMENT

Obtain LFT in pts with history of hepatic impairment. Record onset, type, location, duration of muscular spasm. Check for immobility, stiffness, swelling.

INTERVENTION/EVALUATION

Assist with ambulation at all times. For those on long-term therapy, serum hepatic/renal function tests should be performed periodically. Evaluate for therapeutic response (decreased intensity of skeletal muscle pain/tenderness, improved mobility, decrease in spasticity). Go from lying to standing slowly.

PATIENT/FAMILY TEACHING

• Avoid tasks that require alertness, motor skills until response to drug is established. • Avoid sudden changes in posture. • May cause hypotension, sedation, impaired coordination. • Avoid alcohol.

tobramycin

toe-bra-**mye**-sin
(TOBI, Tobrex)

■ **BLACK BOX ALERT** ■ May cause neurotoxicity, nephrotoxicity, ototoxicity. Ototoxicity usually is irreversible. Increased risk of neuromuscular blockade, including respiratory paralysis, particularly when given after anesthesia or muscle relaxants. May cause fetal harm.

Do not confuse tobramycin with vancomycin, or Tobrex with TobraDex.

FIXED-COMBINATION(S)

TobraDex: tobramycin/dexAMETHasone (a steroid): 0.3%/0.1% per mL or per g. **Zylet:** tobramycin/loteprednol: 0.3%/0.5%.

◆CLASSIFICATION

PHARMACOTHERAPEUTIC: Aminoglycoside. **CLINICAL:** Antibiotic.

USES

Systemic: Septicemia in children and adults: Caused by *P. aeruginosa, E. coli,* and *Klebsiella* species (spp). **Lower respiratory tract infections:** Caused by *P. aeruginosa, Klebsiella* spp, *Enterobacter* spp, *Serratia* spp, *E. coli,* and *S. aureus.* **Central nervous system infections (meningitis):** Caused by susceptible organisms. **Intra-abdominal infections, including peritonitis:** Caused by *E. coli, Klebsiella* spp., and *Enterobacter* spp. **Skin, bone, and skin structure infections:** Caused by *P. aeruginosa, Proteus* spp, *E. coli, Klebsiella* spp, *Enterobacter* spp, and *S. aureus.* **Complicated UTIs:** Caused by *P. aeruginosa, Proteus* spp (indole-positive and indole-negative), *E. coli, Klebsiella* spp, *Enterobacter* spp, *Serratia* spp, *S. aureus, Providencia* spp, and *Citrobacter* spp. **Ophthalmic:** Superficial eye infections: blepharitis, conjunctivitis, keratitis, corneal ulcers. **Inhalation:** Bronchopulmonary infections *(Pseudomonas aeruginosa)* in pts with cystic fibrosis. **OFF-LABEL: Systemic:** Peritonitis. **Inhalation:** Noncystic fibrosis bronchiectasis, pneumonia.

PRECAUTIONS

Contraindications: Hypersensitivity to tobramycin, other aminoglycosides (cross-sensitivity) and their components. **Cautions:** Renal impairment, auditory or vestibular impairment, conditions that depress neuromuscular transmission, Parkinson's disease, myasthenia gravis, hypocalcemia, pregnancy, elderly.

T

ACTION

Irreversibly binds to protein on bacterial ribosomes. **Therapeutic Effect:** Interferes with protein synthesis of susceptible microorganisms.

PHARMACOKINETICS

Widely distributed. Protein binding: Less than 30%. Excreted in urine. Removed by hemodialysis. **Half-life:** 2–4 hrs (increased in renal impairment, neonates; decreased in cystic fibrosis, febrile, or burn pts).

⌛ LIFESPAN CONSIDERATIONS

Pregnancy/Lactation: Readily crosses placenta; distributed in breast milk. May cause fetal nephrotoxicity. Ophthalmic form should not be used in breastfeeding mothers and only when specifically indicated in pregnancy. **Children:** Immature renal function in neonates, premature infants may increase risk of toxicity. **Elderly:** Age-related renal impairment may increase risk of toxicity; dosage adjustment recommended.

INTERACTIONS

DRUG: May decrease therapeutic effect of **BCG (intravesical), vaccine (live)**. **Foscarnet, mannitol** may increase concentration/effect. **Penicillin** may decrease concentration/effect. **HERBAL:** None significant. **FOOD:** None known. **LAB VALUES:** May increase serum BUN, bilirubin, creatinine, alkaline phosphatase, LDH, ALT, AST. May decrease serum calcium, magnesium, potassium, sodium. Therapeutic peak serum level: 5–20 mcg/mL; therapeutic trough serum level: 0.5–2 mcg/mL. Toxic peak serum level: greater than 20 mcg/mL; toxic trough serum level: greater than 2 mcg/mL.

AVAILABILITY (Rx)

Inhalation Powder: *(TOBI Podhaler):* 28 mg in a capsule. **Injection, Powder for Reconstitution:** 1.2 g. **Injection Solution:** 10 mg/mL, 40 mg/mL. **Ointment, Ophthalmic: *(Tobrex):*** 0.3%. **Solution, Nebulization: *(TOBI):*** 60 mg/mL. **Solution, Ophthalmic: *(Tobrex):*** 0.3%.

ADMINISTRATION/HANDLING

◀ **ALERT** ▶ Coordinate peak and trough lab draws with administration times.

 IV

Reconstitution • Dilute with 50–100 mL D₅W or 0.9% NaCl. Amount of diluent for infants, children depends on individual need.
Rate of administration • Infuse over 30–60 min.
Storage • Store vials at room temperature. • Solutions may be discolored by light or air (does not affect potency). • Refrigerate diluted solution for up to 96 hrs or store at room temperature for up to 24 hrs.

IM
• To minimize discomfort, give deep IM slowly. • Less painful if injected into gluteus maximus rather than lateral aspect of thigh.

Inhalation
• Refrigerate. • May store at room temperature up to 28 days after removing from refrigerator. • Do not use if cloudy or contains particulates. • **Podhaler:** Capsules must not be swallowed. • Doses should be as close as possible to 12 hrs apart and not less than 6 hrs apart. • Use Podhaler device supplied.

Ophthalmic
• Place gloved finger on lower eyelid, pull out until pocket is formed between eye and lower lid. • Place correct number of drops (1-2), ointment (half-inch ribbon) into pocket. • **Solution:** Apply digital pressure to lacrimal sac for 1–2 min (minimizes drainage into nose/throat, reducing risk of systemic effects). • **Ointment:** Instruct pt to close eye for 1–2 min, rolling eyeball (increases contact area of drug to eye). • Remove excess solution/ointment around eye.

▦ IV INCOMPATIBILITIES

Heparin, propofol.

T

⬚ IV COMPATIBILITIES

DexmedeTOMIDine, insulin, magnesium sulfate.

INDICATIONS/ROUTES/DOSAGE

◄ALERT► Space parenteral doses evenly around the clock. Dosage based on ideal body weight. Peak, trough levels determined periodically to maintain desired serum concentrations (minimizes risk of toxicity). Recommended peak level: 4–10 mcg/mL; trough level: 0.5–2 mcg/mL.

Usual Parenteral Dosage

IV: ADULTS, ELDERLY: 3–5 mg/kg/day in divided doses q8h. Once-daily dosing: 5–7 mg/kg every 24 hrs. **INFANTS, CHILDREN, ADOLESCENTS:** 6–7.5 mg/kg/day divided q6–8h. **NEONATES:**

Gestational Age	Postnatal Age	Dosage
Less than 30 wks	14 or less days	5 mg/kg/ dose q48h
	15 or more days	5 mg/kg/ dose q36h
30–34 wks	10 days or less	5 mg/kg/ dose q36h
	11–60 days	5 mg/kg/ dose q24h
35 wks or more	7 days or less	4 mg/kg/ dose q24h
	8–60 days	5 mg/kg/ dose q24h

Usual Ophthalmic Dosage

Ophthalmic ointment: ADULTS, ELDERLY, CHILDREN 2 MOS AND OLDER: Apply 1/2 inch to conjunctiva q8–12h (q3–4h for severe infections).

Ophthalmic solution: ADULTS, ELDERLY, CHILDREN 2 MOS AND OLDER: 1–2 drops in affected eye q4h (2 drops/hr for severe infections).

Usual Inhalation Dosage (Cystic Fibrosis)

Inhalation high dose: ADULTS, CHILDREN 6 YRS AND OLDER: 300 mg q12h 28 days on, 28 days off. *(Tobi Podhaler):* Four 28-mg capsules twice daily for 28 days followed by 28 days off.

Dosage in Renal Impairment

After loading dose of 1–2 mg/kg, maintenance dose and frequency are based on serum creatinine levels, creatinine clearance.

Creatinine Clearance	Dosing Interval
41–60 mL/min	q12h
21–40 mL/min	q24h
10–20 mL/min	q48h
Less than 10 mL/min	q72h
Hemodialysis	Loading dose 2–3 mg/kg, then 1–2 mg/kg q48–72h
Continuous renal replacement therapy	Loading dose 2–3 mg/kg, then 1–2.5 mg/kg q24–48h

Dosage in Hepatic Impairment

No dose adjustment.

SIDE EFFECTS

Occasional: IM: Pain, induration. **IV:** Phlebitis, thrombophlebitis. **Topical:** Hypersensitivity reaction (fever, pruritus, rash, urticaria). **Ophthalmic:** Tearing, itching, redness, eyelid swelling. **Rare:** Hypotension, nausea, vomiting.

ADVERSE EFFECTS/TOXIC REACTIONS

Nephrotoxicity (acute kidney injury, acute tubular necrosis, renal failure) may occur. Irreversible ototoxicity (dizziness, ringing/roaring in ears, hearing loss), neurotoxicity (headache, dizziness, lethargy, tremor, visual disturbances) occur occasionally. Risk increases with higher dosages or prolonged therapy or if solution is applied directly to mucosa. Superinfections, particularly fungal infections, may result from bacterial imbalance with any administration route. Anaphylaxis may occur.

NURSING CONSIDERATIONS

BASELINE ASSESSMENT

Dehydration must be treated before beginning parenteral therapy. Question for history of allergies, esp. aminoglycosides, sulfite (and parabens for topical, ophthalmic routes). Obtain baseline lab tests, esp. renal function.

T

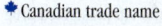 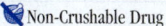

INTERVENTION/EVALUATION

Monitor I&O (maintain hydration), urinalysis, renal function. Monitor results of peak/trough blood tests. **Therapeutic serum level:** Peak: 5–20 mcg/mL; trough: 0.5–2 mcg/mL. **Toxic serum level:** Peak: Greater than 20 mcg/mL; trough: Greater than 2 mcg/mL. Be alert to ototoxic, neurotoxic symptoms. Evaluate IV site for phlebitis (heat, pain, red streaking over vein). Assess for rash. Monitor for superinfection, particularly anal/genital pruritus, changes of oral mucosa, diarrhea. When treating pts with neuromuscular disorders, assess respiratory response carefully. **Ophthalmic:** Assess for redness, swelling, itching, tearing.

PATIENT/FAMILY TEACHING

• Report any hearing, visual, balance, urinary problems, even after therapy is completed. • **Ophthalmic:** Blurred vision, tearing may occur briefly after application. • Report persistent tearing, redness, irritation.

tocilizumab

toe-si-**liz**-oo-mab
(Actemra, Actemra ACT Pen, Tofidence, Tyenne)

■ **BLACK BOX ALERT** ■ Tuberculosis, serious invasive fungal infections, other opportunistic infections have occurred. Test for tuberculosis prior to and during treatment, regardless of initial result. Consider treatment of latent TB prior to initiation.

◆CLASSIFICATION

PHARMACOTHERAPEUTIC: Interleukin (IL)-6 receptor inhibitor. **CLINICAL:** Antirheumatic, disease-modifying agent.

USES

Rheumatoid arthritis (RA): Treatment of moderate to severe RA in adults who had inadequate response to disease-modifying antirheumatic drugs (DMARDs). **Systemic juvenile idiopathic arthritis (SJIA):** Treatment of active SJIA in pts 2 yrs of age and older. **Polyarticular juvenile idiopathic arthritis (PJIA):** Treatment of active PJIA in pts 2 yrs and older. **Cytokine release syndrome (CRS):** Treatment of adults and children 2 yrs of age and older with chimeric antigen receptor (CAR) T-cell–induced severe or life-threatening **CRS giant cell arteritis (GCA):** Treatment of giant cell arteritis in adults. **Systemic sclerosis-associated interstitial lung disease (SSc-ILD):** To slow the rate of decline in pulmonary function in adults with SSc-ILD. **Coronavirus disease 2019 (COVID-19):** Hospitalized adults with COVID-19 who are receiving systemic corticosteroids and require supplemental oxygen, noninvasive or invasive mechanical ventilation, or extracorporeal membrane oxygenation (ECMO).

PRECAUTIONS

Contraindications: Hypersensitivity to tocilizumab. **Cautions:** Preexisting or recent-onset demyelinating disorders (e.g., multiple sclerosis), elderly, recent travel or residence in TB- or mycosis-endemic areas; history of chronic opportunistic infections (esp. bacterial, invasive fungal, mycobacterial, protozoal, viral, TB); history of HIV, herpes zoster, hepatitis B or C virus infection; conditions predisposing to infection (e.g., diabetes, renal failure, immunocompromised pts, open wounds), pts at risk for GI perforation (e.g., Crohn's disease, diverticulitis, GI tract malignancies, peptic ulcers, peritoneal malignancies). Do not initiate in pts with active infection; platelet count 100,000 cells/mm^3 or less, ANC less than 2,000 cells/mm^3; serum ALT, AST greater than 1.5 times ULN.

ACTION

Binds to IL-6 receptors, inhibiting signals of proinflammatory cytokines.

Therapeutic Effect: Inhibits/slows structural joint damage, improves physical function.

PHARMACOKINETICS

Distributed in steady state of plasma and tissue compartments. Undergoes biphasic elimination from circulation. **Half-life:** 11–13 days.

⧖ LIFESPAN CONSIDERATIONS

Pregnancy/Lactation: Unknown if distributed in breast milk; however, immunoglobulin G (IgG) is present in breast milk and is known to cross the placenta. **Children:** Safety and efficacy not established in conditions other than SJIA, severe or life-threatening CAR T-cell–induced cytokine release syndrome. **Elderly:** Cautious use due to increased risk of serious infections, malignancy.

INTERACTIONS

DRUG: May increase concentration/adverse effects of **baricitinib, natalizumab, tofacitinib, vaccines (live).** May decrease therapeutic effect of **vaccines (live).** May increase immunosuppressive effect of **anti-TNF agents (e.g., adalimumab, etanercept, infliximab).** **HERBAL:** Echinacea may decrease therapeutic effect. **FOOD:** None known. **LAB VALUES:** May increase serum ALT, AST, lipids. May decrease platelets, neutrophils.

AVAILABILITY (Rx)

Injection Solution: 20 mg/mL (80 mg/4 mL, 200 mg/10 mL, 400 mg/20 mL). **Syringe for SQ Administration:** 162 mg/0.9 mL. **Syringe Auto-injector:** 162 mg/0.9 mL.

ADMINISTRATION/HANDLING
◄**ALERT**► Do not infuse IV push or bolus.

 IV

Reconstitution • Dilute in 100 mL 0.9% NaCl (RA, GCA, COVID-19, CRS, PJIA, SJIA pts 30 kg or greater) or 50 mL 0.9% NaCl (PJIA, SJIA, and CRS in pts weighing less than 30 kg). • Prior to mixing, withdraw and discard volume of NaCl equal to

volume of patient-dosed solution. • Invert bag to avoid foaming. • Inject solution and dilute for mixture that equals 50 mL or 100 mL in NaCl bag.
Rate of administration • Infuse over 1 hr.
Storage • Refrigerate vials; do not freeze. • Diluted solutions may be stored for 24 hrs at room temperature or refrigerated. • Protect from light until time of use. • Solution appears colorless. Discard solution if it appears cloudy, discolored, or contains particulate.

SQ
Preparation • Visually inspect for particulate matter or discoloration. Solution should appear clear, colorless to pale yellow. Do not use if solution is cloudy, discolored, or visible particles are observed.
Administration • Insert needle subcutaneously and inject solution. • Do not inject into areas of active skin disease or injury such as sunburns, skin rashes, inflammation, skin infections, or active psoriasis. • Rotate injection sites. • Do not administer IV or intramuscularly. • If a dose is missed, administer as soon as possible, then adjust schedule to maintain dosing intervals.
Storage • Refrigerate prefilled syringes in original carton until time of use. • Protect from light. • Do not shake. • Do not freeze or expose to heating sources.

INDICATIONS/ROUTES/DOSAGE

Note: Do not infuse concomitantly in same IV line with other drugs. **RA, GCA, SSc-ILD, PJIA, and SJIA:** Do not begin if ANC less than 2,000 cells/mm^3, platelets less than 100,000 cells/mm^3, or ALT or AST more than 1.5 times ULN. **COVID-19:** Do not initiate in pts with an absolute neutrophil count (ANC) below 1,000 cells/mm^3, platelet count below 50,000 cells/mm^3, or serum ALT or AST above 10 times ULN.

Moderate to Severely Active Rheumatoid Arthritis
IV: ADULTS, ELDERLY: 4 mg/kg every 4 wks initially. May increase to 8 mg/kg every 4 wks. **Maximum:** 800 mg per dose.

T

SQ: ADULTS, ELDERLY WEIGHING 100 KG OR GREATER: 162 mg/wk. **WEIGHING LESS THAN 100 KG:** 162 mg every other wk. May increase to every wk based on clinical response.

Cytokine Release Syndrome

IV: ADULTS, CHILDREN WEIGHING 30 KG OR GREATER: 8 mg/kg. **PTS WEIGHING LESS THAN 30 KG:** 12 mg/kg. If no clinical improvement, 3 additional doses may be given with an interval of at least 8 hrs. **Maximum:** 800 mg/dose.

Giant Cell Arteritis

IV: ADULTS, ELDERLY: 6 mg/kg q4wks (in combination with tapering course of glucocorticoids). **Maximum:** 600 mg/dose. **SQ: ADULTS, ELDERLY:** 162 mg once every wk or every other wk (in combination with tapering course of glucocorticoid). May be given alone following discontinuation of glucocorticoid.

SSc-ILD

SQ: ADULTS, ELDERLY: 162 mg once weekly.

Dosage Modification (RA, GCA, SScILD)

Hepatic enzyme levels greater than ULN.

Lab Value	Recommendation
1–3 times ULN	Dose modify concomitant DMARDs or reduce dose to 4 mg/kg until ALT, AST normalized
Greater than 3–5 times ULN	Interrupt treatment until ALT, AST less than 3 times ULN, then follow guidelines for 1–3 times ULN
Greater than 5 times ULN	Discontinue treatment

Neutropenia

Low absolute neutrophil count (ANC) 500–1000 cells/mm³: Withhold dose. **ANC less than 500 cells/mm³:** Discontinue treatment.

Thrombocytopenia

Platelets 50,000–100,000 cells/mm³: Withhold dose. **Platelets less than 50,000 cells/mm³:** Discontinue treatment.

SJIA

IV: CHILDREN WEIGHING 30 KG OR MORE: 8 mg/kg q2wks. **CHILDREN WEIGHING LESS THAN 30 KG:** 12 mg/kg q2wks.

SQ: CHILDREN WEIGHING 30 KG OR MORE: 162 mg once every wk. **CHILDREN WEIGHING LESS THAN 30 KG:** 162 mg q2wks.

PJIA

IV: CHILDREN WEIGHING 30 KG OR MORE: 8 mg/kg q4wks. **CHILDREN WEIGHING LESS THAN 30 KG:** 10 mg/kg q4wks. **SQ: WEIGHING 30 KG OR MORE:** 162 mg q2wks. **WEIGHING LESS THAN 30 KG:** 162 mg q3wks.

COVID-19 Infection

IV: ADULTS, ELDERLY, CHILDREN 2 YRS OR OLDER WEIGHING 30 KG OR GREATER: 8 mg/kg. **CHILDREN 2 YRS OR OLDER WEIGHING LESS THAN 30 KG:** 12 mg/kg. If clinical symptoms worsen or do not improve after the first dose, one additional infusion may be given at least 8 hrs after the initial infusion. **Maximum:** 800 mg.

Dosage in Renal Impairment

Mild impairment: No dose adjustment. **Moderate to severe impairment:** Use caution (not studied).

Dosage in Hepatic Impairment

Not recommended.

SIDE EFFECTS

Occasional (8%–6%): Upper respiratory tract infection, nasopharyngitis, headache, hypertension. **Rare (5%–3%):** Infusion reaction, dizziness, bronchitis, rash, oral ulceration.

ADVERSE EFFECTS/TOXIC REACTIONS

Neutropenia may increase risk of infections. Fatal infections (bacterial arthritis, cellulitis, herpes zoster, pneumonia, UTI, gastroenteritis, diverticulitis), opportunistic infections (aspergillosis, candidiasis, *Cryptococcus*, pneumocystosis, TB) were reported. Serious hepatotoxicity may lead to liver transplantation or death. Hypersensitivity reactions (anaphylaxis, erythema, rash, urticaria) may occur. Demyelinating disorders (multiple sclerosis, chronic inflammatory demyelinating polyneuropathy) may occur. May increase risk of GI perforation, new malignancies. Other reactions may include Stevens-Johnson syndrome, pancreatitis.

NURSING CONSIDERATIONS

BASELINE ASSESSMENT

Obtain CBC, BMP, LFT, lipid panel; pregnancy test in females of reproductive potential. Assess onset, location, duration of pain, inflammation. Inspect appearance of affected joints for immobility, deformities. Evaluate for active TB and test for latent infection prior to and during treatment. An induration of 5 mm or greater with purified protein derivative (PPD) is considered a positive result when assessing for latent TB. Consider treatment with antimycobacterial therapy in pts with latent TB. Screen for active infection; history of chronic, opportunistic infections. Question history of hepatic impairment, malignancies; prior hypersensitivity reactions. Screen for concomitant use of other immunosuppressants.

INTERVENTION/EVALUATION

Monitor neutrophil, platelet count 4–8 wks after initiation, then q3mos thereafter. Monitor LFT for hepatic injury (abdominal pain, jaundice, nausea, transaminitis, vomiting) q4–8 wks for 6 mos after initiation, then q3mos thereafter. Obtain lipid panel 4–8 wks after initiation. Monitor for TB infection regardless of baseline PPD. Consider discontinuation if serious infection, opportunistic infection, sepsis occurs. Monitor for hypersensitivity reactions, demyelinating disorders, new malignancies. Report abdominal pain, GI hemorrhage, melena, hematemesis (may indicate GI perforation). Assess skin for cutaneous toxicities. Assess for therapeutic response: relief of pain, stiffness, swelling; increased joint mobility; reduced joint tenderness; improved grip strength.

PATIENT/FAMILY TEACHING

• Treatment may depress your immune system response and reduce your ability to fight infection. Report symptoms of infection such as body aches, chills, cough, fatigue, fever. Avoid those with active infection. • Expect routine tuberculosis screening. Report any travel plans to possible endemic areas. • Do not receive live vaccines. • Report liver problems (abdominal pain, bruising, clay-colored stool, dark or amber-colored urine, yellowing of the skin or eyes), skin reactions (rash, redness, swelling). • Immediately report severe or persistent abdominal pain, bloody stool, fever, vomiting blood; may indicate rupture in GI tract. • Treatment may cause reactivation of chronic viral infections; new cancers; demyelinating disorders such as MS. • Immediately report allergic reactions of any kind. • Other immunosuppressant drugs may increase risk of infection, bleeding.

tofacitinib

toe-fa-**sye**-ti-nib
(Xeljanz, Xeljanz XR)

■ **BLACK BOX ALERT** ■ Increased risk for developing bacterial, viral, invasive fungal, other opportunistic infections including tuberculosis, cryptococcosis, pneumocystosis that may lead to hospitalization or death; infections often occurred in combination with other immunosuppressants (methotrexate, corticosteroids). Closely monitor for development of infection. Test for latent tuberculosis prior to treatment and during treatment, regardless of initial result. Treatment for latent TB should be initiated before use. Malignancies including lymphoma, nonmelanoma skin cancer reported. Increased rate of Epstein-Barr virus–associated post-transplant lymphoproliferative disorder observed in renal transplant pts who are treated with tofacitinib and other immunosuppressive therapy drugs. Higher rate of all-cause mortality, including sudden cardiovascular death, was observed. Major adverse cardiovascular events (cardiovascular death, myocardial infarction, and stroke) observed in pts with at least one cardiovascular risk factor. Thrombosis, including pulmonary embolism, deep venous thrombosis, and arterial thrombosis, have occurred.
Do not confuse tofacitinib with tipifarnib or Xeljanz with Xeloda.

T

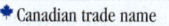 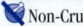

◆CLASSIFICATION

PHARMACOTHERAPEUTIC: Janus-associated kinase (JAK) inhibitor. **CLINICAL:** Antirheumatic, disease-modifying.

USES

Rheumatoid arthritis (RA): Treatment of adult pts with moderate to severe active RA who have had an inadequate response or intolerance to one or more TNF blockers. **Psoriatic arthritis (PsA):** Treatment of active PsA in pts who have had an inadequate response or intolerance to one or more TNF blockers. **Ulcerative colitis (UC):** Treatment of moderate to severe active in adults who have had an inadequate response or intolerance to one or more TNF blockers. **Polyarticular course juvenile idiopathic arthritis (pcJIA):** Treatment of active pcJIA in pts 2 yrs and older who have had an inadequate response or intolerance to one or more TNF blockers. **Ankylosing spondylitis (AS):** Treatment of adults with active who have had an inadequate response or intolerance to one or more TNF blockers. **OFF-LABEL:** Psoriasis, COVID-19 (hospitalized pts).

PRECAUTIONS

Contraindications: Hypersensitivity to tofacitinib. **Cautions:** Baseline cytopenias, hepatic/renal impairment, elderly, pulmonary disease, hyperlipidemia, pts who resided in or traveled to endemic areas; cardiac conduction abnormalities, HF; Asian ancestry, conditions predisposing to infection (e.g., diabetes, renal failure, immunocompromised pts, open wounds), pts at risk for GI perforation (e.g., Crohn's disease, diverticulitis, GI tract malignancies, peptic ulcers, peritoneal malignancies), history of chronic opportunistic infections (esp. bacterial, invasive fungal, mycobacterial, protozoal, viral infections including TB); thrombosis (arterial thrombosis, DVT, pulmonary embolism).

ACTION

Inhibits JAK enzymes, which are intracellular enzymes involved in stimulating hematopoiesis and immune cell functioning through a signaling pathway. **Therapeutic Effect:** Reduces inflammation, tenderness, swelling of joints; slows or prevents progressive joint destruction in rheumatoid arthritis (RA). Prevents cytokine or growth factor gene expression, reducing circulating natural killer cells and increasing B cells.

PHARMACOKINETICS

Widely distributed. Metabolized in liver. Protein binding: 40%. Peak plasma concentration: 30–60 min (instant-release); 4 hrs (extended-release). Steady state reached in 24–48 hrs. Excreted primarily in urine. **Half-life:** 3 hrs (instant-release); 6–8 hrs (extended-release).

⧗ LIFESPAN CONSIDERATIONS

Pregnancy/Lactation: Females of reproductive potential should use effective contraception during treatment. Breastfeeding not recommended during treatment and for at least 18 hrs after discontinuation. **Children:** Safety and efficacy not established in pts younger than 2 yrs. **Elderly:** Increased risk for serious infections, malignancy.

INTERACTIONS

DRUG: **Immunosuppressants (e.g., azaTHIOprine, cycloSPORINE)** may increase risk for added immunosuppression, infection. **Strong CYP3A4 inhibitors (e.g., clarithromycin, ketoconazole, ritonavir)** may increase concentration/effect. **Strong CYP3A4 inducers (e.g., carBAMazepine, phenytoin, rifAMPin)** may decrease concentration/effect. **Vaccines (live)** may alter concentration/effect. **HERBAL:** Echinacea may decrease the therapeutic effect. **FOOD:** None known. **LAB VALUES:** May increase ALT, AST, bilirubin, lipids, creatinine. May decrease Hgb, neutrophils, lymphocytes.

AVAILABILITY (Rx)

Tablets, *(Xeljanz):* 5 mg, 10 mg.

 (Xeljanz XR): 11 mg, 22 mg. **Oral Solution:** 1 mg/mL.

ADMINISTRATION/HANDLING

PO

Immediate-release, tablet, oral solution • Give without regard to food.
• Use provided bottle adapter to attach oral syringe.
Extended-release • Administer whole (do not crush, split, or allow chewing).
• XR tablet is not interchangeable or substitutable with oral solution.

INDICATIONS/ROUTES/DOSAGE

◄ALERT► Do not initiate treatment in pts with baseline active infection (systemic/localized), severe hepatic impairment, lymphocytes less than 500 cells/mm³, ANC less than 1,000 cells/mm³, Hgb less than 9 g/dL.

Rheumatoid Arthritis (Monotherapy or With Nonbiologic DMARD)

PO: ADULTS/ELDERLY: *(Xeljanz):* 5 mg twice daily. *(Xeljanz XR):* 11 mg once daily.

PsA (With Nonbiologic DMARD)

PO: ADULTS/ELDERLY: *(Xeljanz):* 5 mg twice daily. *(Xeljanz XR):* 11 mg once daily.

AS

PO: ADULTS, ELDERLY: *(Xeljanz):* 5 mg twice daily. *(Xeljanz XR):* 11 mg once daily.

UC

PO: ADULTS/ELDERLY: *(Xeljanz):* Induction: 10 mg twice daily for 8 wks. May transition to maintenance dose or continue 10 mg twice daily for additional 8 wks. Discontinue if 10 mg twice daily is ineffective after 4 mos. **Maintenance:** 5 mg twice daily. May increase to 10 mg twice daily for shortest duration. Use lowest effective dose to maintain response. *(Xeljanz XR):* **Induction:** 22 mg once daily for at least 8 wks. May continue for maximum of 16 wks or transition

to maintenance dose. Discontinue if 22 mg once daily dose is ineffective after 16 wks. **Maintenance:** 11 mg once daily. May increase to 22 mg once daily for shortest duration. Use lowest effective dose to maintain response.

pcJIA

PO: CHILDREN 2 YRS AND OLDER WEIGHING 10–19 KG: 3.2 mg (3.2 mL oral solution) twice daily. **20–39 KG:** 4 mg (4 mL oral solution) twice daily. **40 KG OR GREATER:** 5 mg (one 5-mg tablet or 5 mL oral solution) twice daily.

Dose Modification for RA/Psoriatic Arthritis

Hematologic Toxicity

ANC 500–1,000 cells/mm³: Withhold treatment until ANC is 1,000 cells/mm³, then resume previous dose based on response and tolerability. **ANC or lymphocyte count less than 500 cells/mm³:** Permanently discontinue. **Hgb less than 8 g/dL or a decrease of more than 2 g/dL:** Withhold treatment until Hgb level normalizes.

Concomitant Use of Strong/Moderate CYP3A4 Inhibitor, Strong CYPC19 Inhibitor
Reduce dose to 5 mg once daily (if taking 5 mg twice daily or 11 mg once daily).

Dose Modification for UC

Hematologic Toxicity

ANC 500–1,000 cells/mm³: *(Instant-Release):* Reduce dose to 5 mg twice daily (if taking 10 mg twice daily) or withhold treatment (if taking 5 mg twice daily) until ANC is greater than 1,000 cells/mm³, then resume previous dose based on response and tolerability. *(Extended-Release):* Reduce dose to 11 mg once daily (if taking 22 mg once daily) or withhold treatment (if taking 11 mg once daily) until ANC is greater than 1,000 cells/mm³, then resume previous dose based on response and tolerability. **ANC or lymphocyte count less than 500 cells/mm³:** Permanently discontinue. **Hgb less than 8 g/dL or a de-**

crease of more than 2 g/dL: Withhold treatment until Hgb level normalizes.

Concomitant Use of Strong/Moderate CYP3A4 Inhibitor, Strong CYPC19 Inhibitor (Instant-Release): Reduce dose to 5 mg twice daily (if taking 10 mg twice daily) or 5 mg once daily (if taking 5 mg twice daily). **(Extended-Release):** Reduce dose to 11 mg once daily (if taking 22 mg once daily) or 5 mg once daily (if taking 11 mg once daily).

Dose Modification for pcJIA
Hematologic Toxicity
ANC 500–1,000 cells/mm³: Withhold treatment until ANC is greater than 1,000 cells/mm³. **ANC or lymphocyte count less than 500 cells/mm³:** Permanently discontinue. **Hgb less than 8 g/dL or a decrease of more than 2 g/dL:** Withhold treatment until Hgb level normalizes.

Concomitant Use of Strong/Moderate CYP3A4 Inhibitor, Strong CYPC19 Inhibitor Reduce dose to 3.2 mg once daily (if taking 3.2 mg twice daily), or 4 mg once daily (if taking 4 mg twice daily), or 5 mg once daily (if taking 5 mg twice daily).

Dosage in Renal Impairment
Mild impairment: No dose adjustment. **Moderate to severe impairment: (RA/psoriatic arthritis):** Reduce dose to 5 mg once daily (if 5 mg twice daily or 11 mg once daily). **(UC):** **(Instant-Release):** If taking 10 mg twice daily, reduce to 5 mg twice daily. If taking 5 mg twice daily, reduce to 5 mg once daily. **(Extended-Release):** Reduce dose to 11 mg once daily (if taking 22 mg once daily) or 5 mg once daily (if taking 11 mg once daily). **(pcJIA):** Reduce dose to 3.2 mg once daily (if taking 3.2 mg twice daily), or 4 mg once daily (if taking 4 mg twice daily), or 5 mg once daily (if taking 5 mg twice daily).

Dosage in Hepatic Impairment
Mild impairment: No dose adjustment. **Moderate impairment: (RA/psoriatic arthritis):** Reduce dose to 5 mg once daily (if 5 mg twice daily or 11 mg once daily). **(UC):** **(Instant-Release):** If taking 10 mg twice daily, reduce to 5 mg twice daily. If taking 5 mg twice daily, reduce to 5 mg once daily. **(Extended-Release):** Reduce dose to 11 mg once daily (if taking 22 mg once daily) or 5 mg once daily (if taking 11 mg once daily). **(pcJIA):** Reduce dose to 3.2 mg once daily (if taking 3.2 mg twice daily), or 4 mg once daily (if taking 4 mg twice daily), or 5 mg once daily (if taking 5 mg twice daily). **Severe impairment:** Not recommended.

SIDE EFFECTS
Rare (4%–2%): Upper respiratory tract infection, diarrhea, nasopharyngitis, headache, hypertension.

ADVERSE EFFECTS/TOXIC REACTIONS
Neutropenia, lymphopenia may increase risk for infection. Serious infections may include aspergillosis, BK virus, cellulitis, coccidioidomycosis, *Cryptococcus*, cytomegalovirus, esophageal candidiasis, histoplasmosis, invasive fungal infections, listeriosis, pneumocystosis, pneumonia, tuberculosis, UTI, sepsis. May cause viral reactivation of herpes zoster infection. May increase risk of GI perforation, lymphoma, new malignancies (breast, lung, pancreatic, prostate cancer; melanoma, nonmelanoma skin cancer). Pts older than 50 yrs with at least one cardiovascular risk factor are at increased risk of sudden cardiac death if taking higher dose. Thrombotic events (arterial thrombosis, DVT, pulmonary embolism) have occurred. Hypersensitivity reactions (angioedema, urticaria) were reported. Hepatotoxicity reported in 1% of pts. Fatal interstitial lung disease may occur.

NURSING CONSIDERATIONS

BASELINE ASSESSMENT

Obtain CBC, BMP, LFT, lipid panel; pregnancy test in females of reproductive potential. Assess onset, location, duration of pain, inflammation. Inspect appearance of affected joints for immobility, deformities in pts with RA. Assess usual bowel movement patterns, stool characteristics in pts with UC. Evaluate for active TB and test for latent infection prior to and during treatment. An induration of 5 mm or greater with purified protein derivative (PPD) is considered a positive result when assessing for latent TB. Consider treatment with antimycobacterial therapy in pts with latent TB. Screen for active infection; history of chronic, opportunistic infections. Question history of hepatic/renal impairment, pulmonary disease, cardiovascular risk, thrombosis, malignancies; prior hypersensitivity reactions. Receive full medication history and screen for interactions.

INTERVENTION/EVALUATION

Monitor neutrophil, platelet count 4–8 wks after initiation, then q3mos thereafter. Monitor LFT for hepatic injury (abdominal pain, jaundice, nausea, transaminitis, vomiting) q4–8 wks for 6 mos after initiation, then q3mos thereafter. Obtain lipid panel 4–8 wks after initiation. Monitor for TB infection regardless of baseline PPD. Consider discontinuation if serious infection, opportunistic infection, sepsis occurs. Monitor for hypersensitivity reactions, new malignancies; symptoms of arterial thrombosis, DVT (leg or arm pain/swelling); PE (chest pain, dyspnea, tachycardia). Report abdominal pain, GI hemorrhage, melena, hematemesis (may indicate GI perforation). Monitor daily pattern of bowel activity, stool consistency. Consider ABG, radiologic test if ILD/pneumonitis (excessive cough, dyspnea, fever, hypoxia) is suspected. Consider treatment with corticosteroids if ILD/pneumonitis is confirmed. Assess for therapeutic response (arthritis): relief of pain, stiffness, swelling; increased joint mobility, improved grip strength; (UC): decreased abdominal pain, cramping, diarrhea; increased appetite, weight gain.

PATIENT/FAMILY TEACHING

• Treatment may depress your immune system response and reduce your ability to fight infection. Report symptoms of infection such as body aches, chills, cough, fatigue, fever. Avoid those with active infection. • Expect routine tuberculosis screening. Report any travel plans to possible endemic areas. • Do not receive live vaccines. • Report liver problems (abdominal pain, bruising, clay-colored stool, dark or amber-colored urine, yellowing of the skin or eyes), symptoms of lung inflammation (excessive coughing, difficulty breathing, chest pain); DVT (swelling, pain, hot feeling in the arms or legs; discoloration of extremity), lung embolism (difficulty breathing, chest pain, rapid heart rate). • Immediately report severe or persistent abdominal pain, bloody stool, fever, vomiting blood; may indicate rupture in GI tract. • Treatment may cause reactivation of chronic viral infections, new cancers. • Immediately report allergic reactions of any kind. • Avoid pregnancy. Do not breastfeed.

---

tolterodine

tol-**ter**-oh-deen
(Detrol, <u>Detrol LA</u>)
Do not confuse Detrol with Ditropan, or tolterodine with fesoterodine.

◆CLASSIFICATION

PHARMACOTHERAPEUTIC: Antimuscarinic agent. **CLINICAL:** Antispasmodic.

USES

Treatment of overactive bladder in pts with symptoms of urinary frequency, urgency, or urge incontinence.

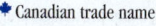 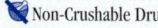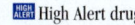

PRECAUTIONS

Contraindications: Hypersensitivity to tolterodine or fesoterodine. Gastric retention, uncontrolled narrow-angle glaucoma, urinary retention. **Cautions:** Renal impairment, bladder outflow obstruction (risk of urinary retention), GI motility disorders (e.g., pyloric stenosis [risk of gastric retention]), treated narrow-angle glaucoma, myasthenia gravis, pts risk for QTc interval prolongation (congenital long QT syndrome, HF, medications that prolong QTc interval, hypokalemia, hypomagnesemia), hepatic impairment, elderly.

ACTION

Antagonist of muscarinic receptors mediating urinary bladder contraction. Increases residual urine volume, reduces detrusor muscle pressure. **Therapeutic Effect:** Decreases urinary frequency, urgency.

PHARMACOKINETICS

Widely distributed. Protein binding: 96%. Metabolized in liver. Primarily excreted in urine. **Half-life:** Immediate-release: 2–10 hrs. Extended-release: 7–18 hrs.

⌛ LIFESPAN CONSIDERATIONS

Pregnancy/Lactation: Unknown if drug is distributed in breast milk. Breastfeeding not recommended. **Children:** Safety and efficacy not established. **Elderly:** No age-related precautions noted.

INTERACTIONS

DRUG: Strong CYP3A4 inhibitors (e.g., clarithromycin, ketoconazole, ritonavir) may increase concentration/effect. **Strong CYP3A4 inducers (e.g., carBAMazepine, phenytoin, rifAMPin)** may decrease concentration/effect. **Anticholinergics (e.g., aclidinium, ipratropium, tiotropium, umeclidinium)** may increase anticholinergic effect. **Strong CYP2D6 inhibitors (e.g., FLUoxetine, PARoxetine)** may increase concentration/effect. **QT interval–prolonging medications (e.g., amiodarone, azithromycin, ciprofloxacin, haloperidol, methadone, sotalol)** may increase risk of QTc interval prolongation. **HERBAL:** None significant. **FOOD:** None known. **LAB VALUES:** None known.

AVAILABILITY (Rx)

Tablets: 1 mg, 2 mg.

🔖 **Capsules, Extended-Release:** 2 mg, 4 mg.

ADMINISTRATION/HANDLING

PO
• May give without regard to food. • Give extended-release capsules whole; do not break, crush, or open.

INDICATIONS/ROUTES/DOSAGE

Overactive Bladder
PO: **ADULTS, ELDERLY: (Immediate-Release):** 1–2 mg twice daily. **With CYP3A4 inhibitors:** 1 mg twice daily. **(Extended-Release):** 2–4 mg once daily. **With CYP3A4 inhibitors:** 2 mg once daily.

Dosage in Renal/Hepatic Impairment
Mild to moderate impairment: (Immediate-Release): 1 mg twice daily. Use caution. **(Extended-Release):** 2 mg once daily. Use caution. **Severe impairment:** Not recommended.

SIDE EFFECTS

Frequent (40%): Dry mouth. **Occasional (11%–4%):** Headache, dizziness, fatigue, constipation, dyspepsia, upper respiratory tract infection, UTI, dry eyes, abnormal vision (accommodation problems), nausea, diarrhea. **Rare (3%):** Drowsiness, chest/back pain, arthralgia, rash, weight gain, dry skin.

ADVERSE EFFECTS/TOXIC REACTIONS

Hypersensitivity reactions (angioedema, airway obstruction, dyspnea, hypotension) resulting in hospitalization were reported. May cause gastric retention in pts with gastric motility disorders. Overdose can result in severe anticholinergic effects, including abdominal cramps, facial warmth, excessive salivation/lacrimation, diaphoresis, pallor, urinary urgency, blurred vision, prolonged QT interval.

NURSING CONSIDERATIONS

BASELINE ASSESSMENT

Assess degree of overactive bladder (urinary urgency, frequency, incontinence). Question history as listed in Precautions.

INTERVENTION/EVALUATION

Assist with ambulation if dizziness occurs. Question for visual changes. Monitor incontinence, postvoid residuals. Monitor ECG in pts at risk for QT interval prolongation.

PATIENT/FAMILY TEACHING

• May cause blurred vision, dry eyes/mouth, constipation. • Report any confusion, altered mental status. • Avoid tasks that require alertness, motor skills until response to drug is established.

---

topiramate

toe-**peer**-a-mate
(Eprontia, Qudexy XR, Topamax, Topamax Sprinkle, Trokendi XR)
Do not confuse Topamax or topiramate with Tegretol, Tegretol XR, or Toprol XL.

◆CLASSIFICATION

PHARMACOTHERAPEUTIC: Miscellaneous agent. **CLINICAL:** Anticonvulsant.

USES

Seizures: Monotherapy or adjunctive therapy for treatment of focal (partial) onset or primary generalized tonic-clonic seizures in pts 2 yrs and older (immediate-release, Qudexy XR) or 6 yrs and older (Trokendi XR). Adjunctive therapy for seizures associated with Lennox-Gastaut syndrome in pts 2 yrs and older (immediate-release,

Qudexy XR) or 6 yrs and older (Trokendi XR). **Migraine prevention:** Prevention of migraine headache in pts 12 yrs and older. **OFF-LABEL:** Alcohol use disorder, binge eating disorder, essential tremor, antipsychotic-induced weight gain, prophylaxis of cluster headaches, infantile spasms.

PRECAUTIONS

Contraindications: Hypersensitivity to topiramate. *(Extended-Release):* **Trokendi XR:** Recent alcohol use (within 6 hrs prior to or after). *(Qudexy XR):* Pts with metabolic acidosis who are taking metFORMIN. **Cautions:** Hepatic/renal impairment, elderly, respiratory impairment, strenuous exercise, heat exposure, concomitant use anticholinergic agents; history of congenital metabolism dysfunction, decreased mitochondrial activity; suicidal ideation and behavior.

ACTION

Blocks neuronal sodium channels, enhances GABA activity; antagonizes glutamate receptors and weakly inhibits carbonic anhydrase. **Therapeutic Effect:** Decreases seizure activity.

PHARMACOKINETICS

Widely distributed. Protein binding: 15%–41%. Metabolized in liver. Primarily excreted unchanged in urine. Removed by hemodialysis. **Half-life:** 21 hrs.

⧖ LIFESPAN CONSIDERATIONS

Pregnancy/Lactation: Unknown if distributed in breast milk. **Children:** Safety and efficacy not established in pts younger than 2 yrs. **Elderly:** Age-related renal impairment may require dosage adjustment.

INTERACTIONS

DRUG: Alcohol, CNS depressants (e.g., LORazepam, morphine, zolpidem) may increase CNS depression. **Strong CYP3A4 inducers (e.g., carBAMazepine, phenytoin, rifAMPin)** may decrease concentration/effect. **Carbonic anhydrase inhibitors** may increase risk of

 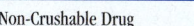

kidney stone formation and severity of metabolic acidosis. May decrease therapeutic effect of **oral contraceptives. Salicylates (e.g., aspirin), thiazide diuretics (e.g., hydrochlorothiazide)** may increase concentration/effect. **HERBAL:** Herbals with **sedative properties (e.g., chamomile, kava kava, valerian)** may increase CNS depression. **FOOD:** None known. **LAB VALUES:** May reduce serum bicarbonate, increase ALT, AST.

AVAILABILITY (Rx)

Capsules (Sprinkle): 15 mg, 25 mg.
Solution, Oral: *(Eprontia):* 25 mg/mL.
Tablets: *(Topamax):* 25 mg, 50 mg, 100 mg, 200 mg.

🐋 **Capsules, Extended-Release:** *(Trokendi XR):* 25 mg, 50 mg, 100 mg, 200 mg. *(Qudexy XR):* 25 mg, 50 mg, 100 mg, 150 mg, 200 mg.

ADMINISTRATION/HANDLING

PO

• Give without regard to food. Do not break, crush, dissolve, or divide tablets (bitter taste). • Sprinkle capsules may either be swallowed whole or contents sprinkled on teaspoonful of soft food and swallowed immediately; do not chew. • *(Trokendi XR):* Give whole. Do not sprinkle on food, chew, or crush. *(Qudexy XR):* Swallow whole; may open and sprinkle on spoonful of soft food. *(Eprontia):* Discard unused portion 60 days after first opening. • Use a calibrated measuring device.

INDICATIONS/ROUTES/DOSAGE

Note: Do not abruptly discontinue; taper gradually to prevent rebound effects.

Adjunctive Treatment of Focal (Partial) Onset Seizures, Lennox-Gastaut Syndrome (LGS), Tonic-Clonic Seizures
PO: ADULTS, ELDERLY, CHILDREN 17 YRS AND OLDER: *(Immediate-Release):* Initially, 25 mg once or twice daily for 1 wk. May increase by 25–50 mg/day at wkly intervals. **Usual maintenance dose:** 100–200 mg twice daily (focal [partial] onset) or 200 mg 2 times/day (primary tonic-clonic). **Maximum:** 400 mg/day. **CHILDREN 2–16 YRS:** Initially, 1–3 mg/kg/day to maximum of 25 mg at night for 1 wk. May increase by 1–3 mg/kg/day at wkly intervals given in 2 divided doses. **Maintenance:** 5–9 mg/kg/day in 2 divided doses. **Maximum:** 400 mg/day. **ADULTS, ELDERLY:** *(Extended-Release):* Initially, 25–50 mg/day. Increase by 25–50 mg/day at wkly intervals, up to 400 mg/day. **CHILDREN 2 YRS AND OLDER:** Initially, 25 mg (based on range of 1–3 mg/kg) once daily at bedtime for 1 wk. Increase dose by 1–3 mg/kg at 1–2 wk intervals up to 5–9 mg/kg once daily. **Maximum:** 400 mg/day.

Monotherapy With Focal (Partial) Onset, Tonic-Clonic Seizures
PO: ADULTS, ELDERLY, CHILDREN 10 YRS AND OLDER: *(Immediate-Release):* Initially, 25 mg twice daily. May increase at wkly intervals up to 400 mg/day according to the following schedule: Wk 1, 25 mg twice daily. Wk 2, 50 mg twice daily. Wk 3, 75 mg twice daily. Wk 4, 100 mg twice daily. Wk 5, 150 mg twice daily. Wk 6, 200 mg twice daily. **CHILDREN 2–9 YRS:** Initially, 25 mg once daily. Then 25 mg 2 times/day Wk 2; then increase by 25–50 mg/day at wkly intervals up to minimum dose. (See table below.) **ADULTS, ELDERLY, CHILDREN 10 YRS OR OLDER:** *(Extended-Release):* *(Qudexy XR, Trokendi XR):* Initially, 50 mg once daily for 1 wk. Increase by 50 mg/day at wkly intervals for first 4 wks, then by 100 mg/day for Wks 5 and 6, up to 400 mg once daily.

Wgt.	Minimum	Maximum
11 kg or less	150 mg/day in 2 divided doses	250 mg/day in 2 divided doses
12–22 kg	200 mg/day in 2 divided doses	300 mg/day in 2 divided doses
23–31 kg	200 mg/day in 2 divided doses	350 mg/day in 2 divided doses
32–38 kg	250 mg/day in 2 divided doses	350 mg/day in 2 divided doses
39 kg or greater	250 mg/day in 2 divided doses	400 mg/day in 2 divided doses

T

Migraine Prevention

PO: ADULTS, ELDERLY, CHILDREN 12 YRS AND OLDER: Initially, 25 mg/day. May increase by 25–50 mg/day at 7-day intervals up to a total daily dose of 100 mg/day in 1–2 divided doses.

Dosage in Renal Impairment

Reduce dose by 50% and titrate more slowly in pts who have CrCl less than 70 mL/min.

Dosage in Hepatic Impairment

Use caution.

SIDE EFFECTS

Frequent (30%–10%): Drowsiness, dizziness, ataxia, nervousness, nystagmus, diplopia, paresthesia, nausea, tremor. **Occasional (9%–3%):** Confusion, breast pain, dysmenorrhea, dyspepsia, depression, asthenia, pharyngitis, weight loss, anorexia, rash, musculoskeletal pain, abdominal pain, difficulty with coordination, sinusitis, agitation, flu-like symptoms. **Rare (3%–2%):** Mood disturbances (e.g., irritability, depression), dry mouth, aggressive behavior, impaired heat regulation.

ADVERSE EFFECTS/TOXIC REACTIONS

Psychomotor slowing, impaired concentration, language problems (esp. word-finding difficulties), memory disturbances occur occasionally. Metabolic acidosis, suicidal ideation occur rarely.

NURSING CONSIDERATIONS

BASELINE ASSESSMENT

Seizures: Review history of seizure disorder (intensity, frequency, duration, level of consciousness). Initiate seizure precautions. Provide quiet, dark environment. Question history of suicidal ideation and behavior; congenital metabolism dysfunction. **Migraine:** Assess pain location, duration, intensity. Assess renal function.

INTERVENTION/EVALUATION

Monitor renal function tests, LFT. Observe frequently for recurrence of seizure activity. Assess for clinical improvement (de-

crease in intensity/frequency of seizures). Diligently screen for suicidal ideation and behavior; new onset or worsening of anxiety, depression, mood disorder.

PATIENT/FAMILY TEACHING

• Avoid tasks that require alertness, motor skills until response to drug is established (may cause dizziness, drowsiness, impaired concentration). • Drowsiness usually diminishes with continued therapy. • Avoid use of alcohol, other CNS depressants. • Do not abruptly discontinue drug (may precipitate seizures). • Strict maintenance of drug therapy is essential for seizure control. • Maintain adequate fluid intake (decreases risk of renal stone formation). • Report blurred vision, eye pain. • Report suicidal ideation, depression, unusual behavior. • Use caution with activities that may increase core temperature (exposure to extreme heat, dehydration). • Oral contraceptives may become ineffective. Use other contraceptive measures to avoid pregnancy.

---

topotecan

toe-poe-**tee**-kan
(Hycamtin)

■ **BLACK BOX ALERT** ■ Severe myelosuppression may occur. Do not administer first cycle in pts with neutrophil count less than 1,500 cells/mm^3 and platelet count less than 100,000 cells/mm^3.

Do not confuse Hycamtin with Hycomine, Mycamine, or topotecan with irinotecan.

◆CLASSIFICATION

PHARMACOTHERAPEUTIC: Topoisomerase inhibitor. **CLINICAL:** Antineoplastic.

USES

Injection: (Cervical cancer): Treatment (in combination with CISplatin) of stage IVB, recurrent or persistent cervical cancer that is

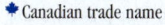 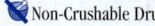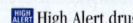

not amenable to curative treatment. (**Ovarian cancer**): Treatment of metastatic ovarian cancer (as a single agent) after disease progression on or after initial or subsequent chemotherapy. (**Small-cell lung cancer [SCLC]**): Treatment of SCLC (as a single agent) in pts with platinum-sensitive disease that has progressed at least 60 days after initiation of first-line chemotherapy. **Oral:** Treatment of relapsed SCLC in pts with a prior complete or partial response and who are at least 45 days from the end of first-line chemotherapy. **OFF-LABEL:** Treatment of Ewing's sarcoma, rhabdomyosarcoma, neuroblastoma, relapsed/refractory acute leukemias, osteosarcoma. CNS malignancy (relapsed/refractory), myelodysplastic syndromes, primary CNS lymphoma (relapsed/refractory).

PRECAUTIONS

Contraindications: Hypersensitivity to topotecan. Baseline neutrophil count less than 1,500 cells/mm^3 and platelet count less than 100,000 cells/mm^3, severe myelosuppression. **Cautions:** Mild myelosuppression, renal impairment, pulmonary disease, elderly, conditions predisposing to infection (e.g., diabetes, renal failure, immunocompromised pts, open wounds).

ACTION

Interacts with topoisomerase I, an enzyme that relieves torsional strain in DNA by inducing reversible single-strand breaks. Prevents relegation of DNA strand, resulting in damage to double-strand DNA, cell death. Acts at S phase of cell cycle. **Therapeutic Effect:** Produces cytotoxic effect.

PHARMACOKINETICS

Widely distributed. Metabolized via enzymatic hydrolysis. Protein binding: 35%. Excreted in urine (51%), feces (18%). **Half-life:** 2–3 hrs (increased in renal impairment).

⌛ LIFESPAN CONSIDERATIONS

Pregnancy/Lactation: Avoid pregnancy; may cause fetal harm. Females of reproductive potential must use effective contraception during treatment and for at least 6 mos after discontinuation. Breastfeeding not recommended during treatment and for at least 1 wk after discontinuation. May impair fertility in both females and males. **Males:** Males with female partners of reproductive potential must use effective contraception during treatment and for at least 3 mos after discontinuation. **Children:** Safety and efficacy not established. **Elderly:** Age-related renal impairment may require dosage adjustment.

INTERACTIONS

DRUG: May increase concentration/adverse effects; decrease concentration/therapeutic effects of **vaccines (live)**. **Bone marrow depressants (e.g., cladribine)** may increase risk of myelosuppression. **BCRP/ABCG2 inhibitors (e.g., omeprazole, verapamil)**, **P-glycoprotein/ABCB1 inhibitors (e.g., amLODIPine, digoxin)** may increase concentration/effect. **HERBAL:** None significant. **FOOD:** None known. **LAB VALUES:** May increase serum ALT, AST, bilirubin. May decrease Hgb, leukocytes, neutrophils, platelets, RBCs.

AVAILABILITY (Rx)

Injection, Powder for Reconstitution: 4 mg (single-dose vial). **Injection Solution:** 1 mg/mL (4 mL).

🌱 **Capsules:** 0.25 mg, 1 mg.

ADMINISTRATION/HANDLING

◄**ALERT**► Due to cytotoxic properties, handle with extreme care during preparation/administration.

PO
• Give without regard to food. • Administer whole; do not break, crush, dissolve, or divide capsule. • Do not give replacement dose if vomiting occurs. **Storage** • Refrigerate capsules.

 IV

Reconstitution *(Lyophylized powder):* • Calculate the number of vials needed for reconstitution based on body surface area. • Swirl vial gently until powder is completely dissolved. Do not shake or agitate. • Visually inspect for particulate matter or discoloration. Solution should appear light yellow to greenish in color. Dilute in 50–100 mL 0.9% NaCl or D_5W.

Rate of administration • Infuse over 30 min.

Storage • Store unused vials in original carton at room temperature. *(Solution for injection):* • Refrigerate vials. • May store diluted solution at controlled room temperature for no more than 24 hrs. • Protect from light.

▩ IV COMPATIBILITIES

Graniestron, ondansetron, palonosetron.

INDICATIONS/ROUTES/DOSAGE

◀ALERT▶ Do not give if baseline neutrophil count is less than 1,500 cells/mm^3 and platelet count is less than 100,000 cells/mm^3. For retreatment, neutrophils should be greater than 1,000 cells/mm^3, platelets greater than 100,000 cells/mm^3, and Hgb 9 g/dL or greater.

Ovarian Carcinoma
IV: ADULTS, ELDERLY: 1.5 mg/m^2/day for 5 consecutive days, beginning on day 1 of 21-day course. Continue until disease progression or unacceptable toxicity. **Neutrophils less than 500 cells/mm^3 or platelets less than 25,000 cells/mm^3:** Reduce dose to 1.25 mg/m^2/day for subsequent cycles.

Small-Cell Lung Cancer
PO: ADULTS, ELDERLY: 2.3 mg/m^2/day for 5 days; repeat q21days (dose rounded to nearest 0.25 mg). **Severe neutropenia or prolonged neutropenia, platelets less than 25,000 cells/mm^3, recovery from Grade 3 or 4 diarrhea:** Reduce dose by 0.4 mg/m^2/day for subsequent cycles.
IV: ADULTS, ELDERLY: 1.5 mg/m^2/day for 5 consecutive days q21days. **Neutrophils less than 500 cells/mm^3 or platelets**

less than 25,000 cells/mm^3: Reduce dose to 1.25 mg/m^2/day for subsequent cycles.

Cervical Cancer
IV: ADULTS, ELDERLY: 0.75 mg/m^2/day for 3 days (followed by CISplatin 50 mg/m^2 on day 1 only). Repeat q21days (baseline neutrophil count greater than 1,500 cells/mm^3 and platelet count greater than 100,000 cells/mm^3). **Severe febrile neutropenia (neutrophils less than 1,000 cells/mm^3 with temperature of 38°C) or platelet count less than 25,000 cells/mm^3:** Reduce dose to 0.6 mg/m^2/day for subsequent cycles. If necessary, further decrease dose to 0.45 mg/m^2/day. Continue for a maximum of 6 cycles (in nonresponders) or until disease progression or unacceptable toxicity.

Dosage in Renal Impairment
IV: No dosage adjustment in pts with mild renal impairment (CrCl 40–60 mL/min). **CrCl 20–29 mL/min:** 0.75 mg/m^2.
PO: CrCl 30–49 mL/min: 1.5 mg/m^2/day. May increase by 0.4 mg/m^2/day following first cycle if no GI/hematologic toxicities occur. **CrCl less than 30 mL/min:** Decrease dose to 0.6 mg/m^2/day. May increase by 0.4 mg/m^2/day following first cycle if no GI/hematologic toxicities occur.

Dosage in Hepatic Impairment
No dose adjustment.

SIDE EFFECTS

Frequent (77%–21%): Nausea, vomiting, diarrhea, total alopecia, headache, dyspnea. **Occasional (9%–3%):** Paresthesia, constipation, abdominal pain. **Rare:** Anorexia, malaise, arthralgia, asthenia, myalgia.

ADVERSE EFFECTS/TOXIC REACTIONS

Myelosuppression (anemia, neutropenia, thrombocytopenia) is an expected response to therapy, but more severe reactions including Grade 4 neutropenia, thrombocytopenia, Grade 3 or 4 anemia, febrile neutropenia, neutropenic enterocolitis may occur. Life-threatening sepsis

T

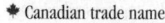 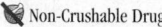

reported. Fatal interstitial lung disease, pneumonitis were reported. May cause severe extravasation and tissue injury. Hypersensitivity reactions including anaphylaxis, angioedema may occur.

NURSING CONSIDERATIONS

BASELINE ASSESSMENT

Obtain CBC (prior to each dose), LFT; pregnancy test in females of reproductive potential. Assess LVEF by echocardiogram. Question history pulmonary disease, renal impairment. Screen for active infection. Consider premedication with antiemetic at least 30 min before each dose. Due to high risk of extravasation and tissue injury with infusion, ensure patency of IV catheter. Assess hydration status. Offer emotional support.

INTERVENTION/EVALUATION

Monitor CBC for myelosuppression, LFT for hepatic injury (abdominal pain, jaundice, nausea, transaminitis, vomiting), renal function test in pts with renal impairment. Monitor for severe neutropenia, febrile neutropenia, infections (cough, fatigue, fever); thrombocytopenia-associated bleeding. Monitor daily pattern of bowel activity, stool consistency. Consider ABG, radiologic test if ILD/pneumonitis (excessive cough, dyspnea, fever, hypoxia) is suspected. Consider treatment with corticosteroids if ILD/pneumonitis is confirmed. Monitor for hypersensitivity reactions (anaphylaxis, angioedema).

PATIENT/FAMILY TEACHING

• Treatment may depress your immune system response and reduce your ability to fight infection. Report symptoms of infection such as body aches, chills, cough, fatigue, fever. Avoid those with active infection. • Report symptoms of bone marrow depression (e.g., bruising, fatigue, fever, shortness of breath, weight loss; bleeding easily, bloody urine or stool). • Seek immediate medical attention if severe allergic reactions (anaphylaxis, difficulty breathing; swelling of the face, tongue, throat) occur. • Report symptoms of lung inflamma-

tion (excessive coughing, difficulty breathing, chest pain); liver problems (abdominal pain, bruising, clay-colored stool, dark or amber-colored urine, yellowing of the skin or eyes). • Maintain proper hydration and nutrition. • Use effective contraception to avoid pregnancy. Do not breastfeed.

torsemide

tore-se-myde
(Soaanz)
Do not confuse torsemide with furosemide.

◆CLASSIFICATION

PHARMACOTHERAPEUTIC: Loop diuretic. **CLINICAL:** Antihypertensive, diuretic.

USES

Treatment of edema or volume overload.

PRECAUTIONS

Contraindications: Hypersensitivity to torsemide or any sulfonylurea. Anuria, hepatic coma. **Cautions:** Pts with cirrhosis, hypotension, hypokalemia.

ACTION

Enhances excretion of sodium, chloride, potassium, water at ascending limb of loop of Henle and distal renal tubules. Reduces plasma, extracellular fluid volume. **Therapeutic Effect:** Produces diuresis, relieves edema; lowers B/P.

PHARMACOKINETICS

Route	Onset	Peak	Duration
PO (diuresis)	30–60 min	1–2 hrs	6–8 hrs

Widely distributed. Protein binding: 97%–99%. Metabolized in liver. Primarily excreted in urine. Not removed by hemodialysis. **Half-life:** 2–4 hrs.

⌛ LIFESPAN CONSIDERATIONS

Pregnancy/Lactation: Unknown if drug is distributed in breast milk. **Chil-**

dren: Safety and efficacy not established. **Elderly:** No age-related precautions noted.

INTERACTIONS

DRUG: May increase concentration/effect of **NSAIDs (e.g., diclofenac, meloxicam, naproxen), aspirin** may increase risk of renal toxicity. **Bile acid sequestrants (e.g., cholestyramine)** may decrease absorption. May increase hyponatremic effect of **desmopressin**. May increase concentration/effect of **foscarnet**. **HERBAL:** Herbals with hypertensive properties (e.g., licorice, yohimbe) or hypotensive properties (e.g., garlic, ginger, ginkgo biloba) may alter effects. **Licorice** may increase hypokalemic effect. **FOOD:** None known. **LAB VALUES:** May increase serum BUN, creatinine, uric acid. May decrease serum calcium, chloride, magnesium, potassium, sodium.

AVAILABILITY (Rx)

Tablets: 5 mg, 10 mg, 20 mg, 40 mg, 60 mg, 100 mg.

ADMINISTRATION/HANDLING

PO
• Give without regard to food. Give with food to avoid GI upset, preferably with breakfast (prevents nocturia).

INDICATIONS/ROUTES/DOSAGE

Edema
PO: ADULTS, ELDERLY: Initially, 10–20 mg/day. May increase by approximately doubling dose until desired therapeutic effect is attained. **Maximum single dose:** 50–100 mg. **Maximum total daily dose:** 200 mg.

Dosage in Renal/Hepatic Impairment
No dose adjustment.

SIDE EFFECTS

Frequent (10%–4%): Headache, dizziness, rhinitis. **Occasional (3%–1%):** Asthenia, insomnia, nervousness, diarrhea, constipation, nausea, dyspepsia, edema, ECG

changes, pharyngitis, cough, arthralgia, myalgia. **Rare (less than 1%):** Syncope, hypotension, arrhythmias.

ADVERSE EFFECTS/TOXIC REACTIONS

Ototoxicity may occur with too-rapid IV administration or with high doses; must be given slowly. Overdose produces acute, profound water loss, volume/electrolyte depletion, dehydration, decreased blood volume, circulatory collapse.

NURSING CONSIDERATIONS

BASELINE ASSESSMENT

Obtain renal function test, serum electrolyte levels, esp. potassium. Obtain weight, B/P. Assess for peripheral edema. Assess lungs for crackles, signs of HF.

INTERVENTION/EVALUATION

Monitor B/P, renal function, serum electrolytes (esp. potassium), I&O, weight. Monitor for ototoxicity. Auscultate lungs for crackles. Check for signs of edema, particularly of dependent areas. Although less potassium is lost with torsemide than with furosemide, assess for signs of hypokalemia (change of muscle strength, tremor, muscle cramps, altered mental status, cardiac arrhythmias).

PATIENT/FAMILY TEACHING

• Take medication in morning to prevent excessive urination at night. • Expect increased urinary volume, frequency. • Report palpitations, muscle weakness, cramps, nausea, dizziness. • Do not take other medications (including OTC drugs) without consulting physician. • Eat foods high in potassium such as whole grains (cereals), legumes, meat, bananas, apricots, orange juice, potatoes (white, sweet), raisins.

tovorafenib

toe-voe-**raf**-en-ib
(Ojemda)
Do not confuse tovorafenib with dabrafenib, encorafenib,

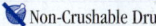

sorafenib, or, vemurafenib, or Ojemda with Ojjaara.

◆CLASSIFICATION

PHARMACOTHERAPEUTIC: Type II RAF kinase inhibitor. **CLINICAL:** Antineoplastic.

USES

Treatment of pts 6 mos of age and older with relapsed or refractory pediatric low-grade glioma (LGG) harboring a BRAF fusion or rearrangement or BRAF V600 mutation.

PRECAUTIONS

Contraindications: Hypersensitivity to tovorafenib. **Cautions:** Baseline cytopenias, hepatic/renal impairment, pts at risk for hemorrhage (e.g., history of GI bleeding, coagulation disorders, recent trauma; concomitant use of anticoagulants, antiplatelets, chronic NSAIDs). Avoid concomitant use of strong or moderate CYPP2C8 inhibitors, hormonal contraceptives, CYP3A4 substrates.

ACTION

A type II RAF kinase inhibitor of mutant BRAF V600E, wild-type BRAF, and wild-type CRAF kinases. **Therapeutic Effect:** Decreases cellular proliferation.

PHARMACOKINETICS

Widely distributed. Metabolized by aldehyde oxidase and CYPCC8. Protein binding: 97.5%. Peak plasma concentration: 3 hrs. Steady-state reached in 12 days. Excreted in feces (65%), urine (27%). **Half-life:** 56 hrs.

⌛ LIFESPAN CONSIDERATIONS

Pregnancy/Lactation: Avoid pregnancy; may cause fetal harm. Females of reproductive potential must use effective nonhormonal contraception during treatment and for at least 28 days after discontinuation. Unknown if distributed in breast milk. Breastfeeding not recommended during treatment and for at least 2 wks after discontinuation. May impair fertility. **Males:** Males with female partners of reproductive potential must use effective nonhormonal contraception during treatment and for at least 2 wks after discontinuation. May impair fertility. **Children:** Safety and efficacy not established in pts younger than 6 mos or a body surface area less than 0.3 m². **Elderly:** Not indicated in this population.

INTERACTIONS

DRUG: **Strong CYP2C8 inhibitors (e.g., clopidogrel, gemfibrozil, salmeterol), moderate CYP2C8 inhibitors** (e.g., irbesartan, **ritonavir, trimethoprim**) may increase concentration/effect. **Strong CYP2C8 inducers (e.g., phenytoin), moderate CYP2C8 inducers (e.g., riFAMpin)** may decrease concentration/effect. May decrease concentration/effect of **hormonal contraceptives, CYP3A4 substrates** (e.g., **busPIRone, tacrolimus, simvastatin.** **HERBAL:** None significant. **FOOD:** None known. **LAB VALUES:** May increase serum ALT, AST, bilirubin, creatine phosphokinase, LDH. May decrease Hgb, leukocytes; serum albumin, phosphate, potassium, sodium. May increase or decrease lymphocytes.

AVAILABILITY (Rx)

Tablets: 100 mg. **Powder for Oral Suspension:** 300 mg/12 mL (25 mg/mL).

ADMINISTRATION/HANDLING

PO

• Give without regard to food. • If a dose is missed by 3 days or less, administer as soon as possible. If a dose is missed by more than 3 days, skip the dose and give next dose at regularly scheduled time. • If vomiting occurs immediately after administration, repeat the dose. **Tablets** • Administer tablets whole with water (do not break, cut, crush or allow chewing). **Oral Suspension** • Reconstitute each bottle with 14 mL of room temperature water to a final concentration of 25 mg/mL. • Swirl until powder is completely resolved. • For doses greater than 300 mg, reconstitute 2 bottles and split the dose as equally as possible between the 2 bottles. Foaming after reconstitution reduces deliverable volume. • Use supplied syringe. • Discard if oral suspension if dose is not administered within 15 minutes after preparation.

INDICATIONS/ROUTES/DOSAGE

Low-Grade Glioma (Relapsed or Refractory)
PO: CHILDREN 6 MOS AND OLDER: 380 mg/m^2 once weekly (based on body surface area). **Maximum:** 600 mg once weekly. Continue until disease progression or intolerable toxicity.

Recommended Tablet Dosage

Body Surface Area (m^2)	Recommended Dosage
0.3–0.89 m^2	Administer oral suspension once weekly
0.9–1.12 m^2	400 mg once weekly
1.13–1.39 m^2	500 mg once weekly
1.40 m^2 or greater	600 mg once weekly

Recommended Dose for Oral Suspension

Body Surface Area (m^2)	Dose Volume (mL)	Recommended Dosage
0.3–0.35 m^2	5	125 mg once weekly
0.36–0.42 m^2	6	150 mg once weekly
0.43–0.48 m^2	7	175 mg once weekly
0.49–0.54 m^2	8	200 mg once weekly
0.55–0.63 m^2	9	225 mg once weekly
0.64–0.77 m^2	11	275 mg once weekly
0.78–0.83 m^2	12	300 mg once weekly
0.84–0.89 m^2	14	350 mg once weekly
0.9–1.05 m^2	15	375 mg once weekly
1.06–1.25 m^2	18	450 mg once weekly
1.26–1.39 m^2	21	525 mg once weekly
1.40 m^2 or greater	24	600 mg once weekly

Dose Modification
Based on Common Terminology Criteria for Adverse Events (CTCAE). See manufacturer guidelines for recommended dosage reduction for adverse events.

Hemorrhage
Intolerable grade 2 hemorrhage, grade 3 hemorrhage: Withhold treatment until improved to grade 1 or 0, then resume at reduced dose. If not improved, consider permanent discontinuation. **Grade 4 hemorrhage: First occurrence:** Withhold treatment until improved to grade 1 or 0, then resume at reduced dose, or permanently discontinue. **Recurrence:** Permanently discontinue.

Hepatotoxicity
Grade 3 hepatotoxicity: Withhold treatment until improved to grade 2 or less (or baseline). If improved within 8 days, resume at same dose. If not improved within 8 days, resume at reduced dose. **Grade 4 hepatotoxicity: First occurrence:** Withhold treatment until improved to grade 1 or 0, then resume at reduced dose, or permanently discontinue. **Recurrence:** Permanently discontinue.

Skin Toxicity Including Photosensitivity
Intolerable grade 2 skin toxicity, grade 3 or 4 skin toxicity: Withhold treatment until improved to Grade 1 or 0, then resume at reduced dose. If not improved, consider permanent discontinuation.

Other Adverse Reactions
Other intolerable grade 2 adverse reactions, other grade 3 adverse reactions: Withhold treatment until im-

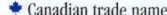 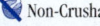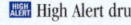

proved to grade 1 or 0, then resume at reduced dose. **Other grade 4 adverse reactions: First occurrence:** Withhold treatment until improved to grade 1 or 0, then resume at reduced dose, or permanently discontinue. **Recurrence:** Permanently discontinue.

Dosage in Renal Impairment

Mild to moderate impairment: No dose adjustment. **Severe impairment:** Not specified; use caution.

Dosage in Hepatic Impairment

Mild impairment: No dose adjustment. **Moderate to severe impairment:** Not specified; use caution.

SIDE EFFECTS

Frequent (77%–26%): Rash, skin exfoliation, eczema, drug eruption, hair color changes, fatigue, vomiting, pyrexia, dry skin, headache, constipation, nausea, dermatitis, abdominal pain, pruritus, edema (lip, periorbital, peripheral, face, vulva). **Occasional (22%–20%):** Diarrhea, colitis, enterocolitis, stomatitis, mouth ulceration, mucosal inflammation, aphthous ulcer, cheilitis.

ADVERSE EFFECTS/TOXIC REACTIONS

Myelosuppression (anemia, leukopenia, lymphopenia) is an expected response to therapy. Major, symptomatic hemorrhage in critical area or organ may occur. Hemorrhagic events may include tumor hemorrhage, subdural hemorrhage, epistaxis, hematemesis, hemoptysis; anal/GI/gingival/vaginal hemorrhage. Skin toxicities, including rash (67% of pts), dermatitis (26% of pts) were reported. Photosensitivity reactions occurred in 12% of pts. Hepatoxicity (transaminitis) reported in 42%–74% of pts. Mean time of onset of serum ALT/AST elevation was 14 days. Serum bilirubin elevation reported in 23% of pts. May cause reduction in growth velocity. May promote tumor growth in pts with NF1 tumors. Infections, including viral infection, upper respiratory tract infection, paronychia, may occur.

NURSING CONSIDERATIONS

BASELINE ASSESSMENT

Obtain LFT; pregnancy test in females of reproductive potential. Confirm compliance of effective nonhormonal contraception. Confirm presence of BRAF fusion or rearrangement, or BRAF V600 mutation in tumor specimen. Receive full medication history and screen for interactions. Question history of hepatic/renal impairment, prior hemorrhagic events. Offer emotional support.

INTERVENTION/EVALUATION

Monitor LFT for hepatotoxicity (abdominal pain, bruising, jaundice, nausea, vomiting, weight loss) 1 mo after initiation, then q3mos thereafter and as clinically indicated. Obtain CBC if serious bleeding occurs. Monitor for toxicities if discontinuation of strong or moderate CYP2C8 inhibitor is unavoidable. Closely monitor for epistaxis, hematemesis, hemoptysis; anal/GI/gingival/vaginal hemorrhage; symptoms of intracranial bleeding (aphasia, blindness, confusion, facial droop, hemiplegia, seizures), bleeding of any kind. Assess skin for rash, dermatitis, photosensitivity. Monitor for infections (body aches, cough, fatigue, fever). If serious infection or sepsis occurs, initiate appropriate antimicrobial therapy. Monitor daily pattern of bowel activity, stool consistency.

PATIENT/FAMILY TEACHING

• Treatment may depress your immune system and reduce your ability to fight infection. Report symptoms of infection such as body aches, burning with urination, chills, cough, fatigue, fever; fungal infections. Avoid with active infection. • Report liver problems (abdominal pain, bruising, clay-colored stool, amber or dark colored urine, yellowing of the skin or eyes); skin toxicities (rash, redness, inflammation). • Serious bleeding events may occur. Report nose bleeds, coughing up blood; symptoms of bleeding in the brain (confusion, difficulty speaking, one-sided weakness or paralysis, loss of vision, seizures), GI bleeding (bloody stools, rectal bleeding, vomiting up blood), bleeding of any kind. • Avoid prolonged sun exposure/tanning beds. Use high SPF sunscreen, lip balm, clothing to protect against sunburn. • There is a high risk of interactions with other medications. Do not take newly prescribed medications unless approved by prescriber who originally started therapy. • Use effective nonhormonal contraception to avoid pregnancy. Avoid breastfeeding.

traMADol

tram-a-dol
(Apo-TraMADol , ConZip, Qdolo)
■ **BLACK BOX ALERT** ■ May cause opioid addiction, abuse, misuse. Serious, life-threatening respiratory depression may occur. Extended-release tablets must be swallowed whole. Crushing, chewing, or dissolving of ER tablets can result in a fatal overdose. May cause neonatal opioid withdrawal syndrome. Concomitant use of alcohol, benzodiazepines, CNS depressants may cause profound sedation, respiratory depression, coma, or death. Use with any CYP3A4 inhibitor may result in increased concentration/effect, which may cause potentially fatal respiratory depression.
Do not confuse traMADol with tapentadol, Toradol, or Trandate, or Ultram with Ultracet.

FIXED-COMBINATION(S)

Ultracet: traMADol/acetaminophen (a non-narcotic analgesic): 37.5 mg/325 mg.

◆CLASSIFICATION

PHARMACOTHERAPEUTIC: Centrally acting synthetic opioid. **CLINICAL:** Analgesic.

USES

Immediate-release: Management of moderate to moderately severe pain. **Extended-release:** Around-the-clock management of moderate to moderately severe pain for extended period.

PRECAUTIONS

Contraindications: Hypersensitivity to traMADol, opioids. Pediatric pts under 12 yrs of age; postop management in pts under 18 yrs following tonsillectomy and/or adenoidectomy; severe respiratory depression; acute bronchial asthma in absence of appropriate monitoring; GI obstruction (paralytic ileus [known or suspected]). Concomitant use with or within 14 days following MAOI therapy. **Cautions:** CNS depression, anoxia, advanced hepatic cirrhosis, respiratory depression, elevated ICP, seizure disorder, hepatic/renal impairment, treatment of acute abdominal conditions, opioid-dependent pts, head injury, myxedema, hypothyroidism, hypoadrenalism, pregnancy. Avoid use in pts who are suicidal or addiction prone, emotionally disturbed, depressed, heavy alcohol users, elderly, debilitated.

ACTION

Binds to mu-opioid receptors in CNS, inhibiting ascending pain pathway. Inhibits reuptake of norepinephrine, serotonin, inhibiting descending pain pathways. **Therapeutic Effect:** Reduces pain.

PHARMACOKINETICS

Route	Onset	Peak	Duration
PO	Less than 1 hr	2–3 hrs	9 hrs

Widely distributed. Protein binding: 20%. Metabolized in liver (reduced in pts with advanced cirrhosis). Primarily excreted in urine. **Half-life:** 6–7 hrs (increased in renal/hepatic failure).

⧗ LIFESPAN CONSIDERATIONS

Pregnancy/Lactation: Crosses placenta. Distributed in breast milk. **Children:** Safety and efficacy not established in children younger than 17 yrs. **El-**

T

derly: Age-related renal impairment may require dosage adjustment.

INTERACTIONS

DRUG: Alcohol, CNS depressants (e.g., LORazepam, morphine, zolpidem) may increase CNS depression. Strong CYP3A4 inhibitors (e.g., clarithromycin, ketoconazole, ritonavir) may increase concentration/effect. May increase CNS depressant effect; decrease therapeutic effect of carBAMazepine. CarBAMazepine may decrease concentration/effect. Strong CYP2D6 inhibitors (e.g., FLUoxetine, PARoxetine) may decrease therapeutic effect. Linezolid, MAOIs (e.g., phenelzine, selegiline), ondansetron, SNRIs (e.g., DULoxetine, venlafaxine), SSRIs (e.g., escitalopram, PARoxetine, sertraline) may increase risk of serotonin syndrome, seizure activity. **HERBAL:** Herbals with sedative properties (e.g., chamomile, kava kava, valerian) may increase CNS depression. St. John's wort may decrease concentration/effect. Maitake may increase hypoglycemic effect. **FOOD:** None known. **LAB VALUES:** May increase serum creatinine, ALT, AST, urine protein. May decrease Hgb.

AVAILABILITY (Rx)

Tablets, Immediate-Release: 50 mg, 100 mg. **Solution, Oral:** *(Qdolo):* 5 mg/mL.

Capsules, Extended-Release: 100 mg, 200 mg, 300 mg. **Tablets, Extended-Release:** 100 mg, 200 mg, 300 mg.

ADMINISTRATION/HANDLING

PO
(Immediate-release): • Give without regard to meals. **Oral solution:** • Measure dose with a calibrated oral syringe. *(Extended-release):* • Administer whole (do not crush, dissolve, split. or allow chewing). **Capsule:** • Give without regard to meals. **Tablet:** Administer in a consistent manner of either with or without meals.

INDICATIONS/ROUTES/DOSAGE

Moderate to Moderately Severe Pain
PO: *(Immediate-Release):* ADULTS, ELDERLY, CHILDREN 17 YRS AND OLDER: 50 mg q4–6h as needed. May increase to 50–100 mg q4–6h as needed. **Maximum:** 400 mg/day for pts 75 yrs and younger; 300 mg/day for pts older than 75 yrs.
PO: *(Extended-Release):* ADULTS, ELDERLY, CHILDREN 18 YRS AND OLDER: Initially, 100 mg once daily. Titrate q5days in 100-mg/day increments. **Maximum:** 300 mg once daily.

Dosage in Renal Impairment
(Immediate-Release): For pts with CrCl less than 30 mL/min, increase dosing interval to q12h. **Maximum:** 200 mg/day. Do not use extended-release.

Dosage in Hepatic Impairment
(Immediate-Release): Cirrhosis: Dosage is decreased to 50 mg q12h. Do not use extended-release with severe hepatic impairment.

SIDE EFFECTS

Frequent (25%–15%): Dizziness, vertigo, nausea, constipation, headache, drowsiness. **Occasional (10%–5%):** Vomiting, pruritus, CNS stimulation (e.g., nervousness, anxiety, agitation, tremor, euphoria, mood swings, hallucinations), asthenia, diaphoresis, dyspepsia, dry mouth, diarrhea. **Rare (less than 5%):** Malaise, vasodilation, anorexia, flatulence, rash, blurred vision, urinary retention/frequency, menopausal symptoms.

ADVERSE EFFECTS/TOXIC REACTIONS

May cause seizure activity at usual dosages. Serotonin syndrome (altered mental status, autonomic instability, clonus, diaphoresis, hyperthermia, hyperreflexia, tremor) was reported. Hypersensitivity reactions (anaphylaxis, angioedema, bronchospasm), toxic skin reactions (Stevens-Johnson syndrome, toxic epidermal necrolysis), severe hypotension, respiratory depression, secondary hypogonadism, thyroid dysfunction, psychosis may occur. May increase risk of suicidal ideation and behavior.

NURSING CONSIDERATIONS

BASELINE ASSESSMENT

Assess onset, type, location, duration of pain. Receive full medication history (esp. serotonergic agents, CNS depressants). Question history as listed in Precautions. Assess risk of drug abuse and misuse.

INTERVENTION/EVALUATION

Monitor heart rate, B/P. Assist with ambulation if dizziness, vertigo occurs. Palpate bladder for urinary retention. Diligently screen for suicidal ideation and behavior; new onset or worsening of anxiety, depression, mood disorder. Screen for drug abuse and misuse, drug-seeking behavior. Monitor for seizure activity; symptoms of serotonin syndrome. Assess for clinical improvement, record onset of relief of pain. Monitor closely for misuse or abuse.

PATIENT/FAMILY TEACHING

• May cause physical dependence. • Pts with history of drug abuse are at increased risk for misuse or abuse. Take medication only as prescribed. • Avoid alcohol, other narcotics, sedatives. • Avoid tasks requiring alertness, motor skills until response to drug is established. • Report severe confusion, excessive sweating, difficulty breathing, excessive sedation, seizures, muscle weakness, tremors, chest pain, palpitations.

---

trametinib

tra-**me**-ti-nib
(Mekinist)
Do not confuse trametinib with imatinib or tipifarnib.

◆CLASSIFICATION

PHARMACOTHERAPEUTIC: MEK inhibitor. **CLINICAL:** Antineoplastic.

USES

Note: All indications in combination with dabrafenib.
Melanoma: Used as a single agent or in combination with dabrafenib for treatment of unresectable or metastatic melanoma with BRAF V600E or V600L mutations. Adjuvant treatment of melanoma, in combination with dabrafenib, in pts with BRAF V600E or BRAF V600K mutations and lymph node involvement, following complete resection. **Anaplastic thyroid cancer (ATC):** Treatment of locally advanced or metastatic ATC, in combination with dabrafenib, with BRAF V600E mutation and with no satisfactory locoregional treatment options. **Non–small-cell lung cancer (NSCLC):** Treatment of metastatic NSCLC, in combination with dabrafenib, in pts with BRAF V600E mutation. **Solid tumors:** Treatment of adults and children 1 yr of age and older with unresectable or metastatic solid tumors with BRAF V600E mutation who have progressed following prior treatment and have no satisfactory alternative treatment options. **Low-grade glioma (LGG):** Treatment of pts 1 yr of age and older with LGG, in combination with dabrafenib, with a BRAF V600E mutation requiring systemic therapy.

PRECAUTIONS

Contraindications: Hypersensitivity to trametinib. **Cautions:** Baseline cytopenias, cardiac disease (cardiomyopathy), diabetes, ocular disease, hepatic impairment, history of thromboembolic events (CVA, DVT, MI, pulmonary embolism [PE], pts at risk for GI perforation (e.g., Crohn's disease, diverticulitis, GI tract malignancies, peptic ulcers, peritoneal malignancies), interstitial lung disease (sarcoidosis, pulmonary fibrosis); conditions predisposing to infection (e.g., diabetes, immunocompromised pts, renal failure, open wounds).

ACTION

Reversibly and selectively inhibits mitogen-activated extracellular kinase

T

(MEK). MEK is a downstream effector of protein kinase Braf (BRAF). **Therapeutic Effect:** Decreases cellular proliferation; causes cell cycle arrest and apoptosis (cellular death).

PHARMACOKINETICS

Widely distributed. Protein binding: 97.4%. Peak plasma concentration: 1.5 hrs. Metabolized in liver. Excreted in feces (80%), urine (20%). **Half-life:** 3.9–4.8 days.

⧗ LIFESPAN CONSIDERATIONS

Pregnancy/Lactation: Avoid pregnancy; may cause fetal harm. Females and males with female partners of reproductive potential must use effective contraception during treatment and for at least 4 mos after discontinuation. Breastfeeding not recommended during treatment and for at least 4 mos after discontinuation. May impair fertility in females. **Males:** May decrease sperm count. **Children:** Safety and efficacy not established in pts younger than 1 yr. **Elderly:** May have increased risk of adverse effects, skin lesions, primary malignancies.

INTERACTIONS

DRUG: None significant. **HERBAL:** None known. **FOOD:** High-fat meals may decrease absorption/effect. **LAB VALUES: Single regimen:** May increase serum alkaline phosphatase, ALT, AST. May decrease serum albumin; Hgb, Hct. **Combination regimen:** May increase serum alkaline phosphatase, ALT, AST, bilirubin, calcium, creatinine, glucose, GGT, potassium. May decrease Hgb, Hct, leukocytes, lymphocytes, neutrophils, platelets; serum albumin, calcium, magnesium, phosphorus, potassium, sodium.

AVAILABILITY (Rx)

Oral Solution: 4.7 mg. **Tablets:** 0.5 mg, 2 mg.

ADMINISTRATION/HANDLING

PO

• Administer at least 1 hr before or 2 hrs after meal. • Do not crush or break tablets. • **Oral Solution:** After reconstitution, store in the original bottle below 25°C (77°F); do not freeze. **Concentration:** 0.05 mg/mL. • Discard solution after 35 days. • Do not take a missed dose within 12 hrs of the next dose.

INDICATIONS/ROUTES/DOSAGE

Melanoma (Metastatic or Unresectable)

PO: ADULTS/ELDERLY: 2 mg once daily (either as a single agent or in combination with dabrafenib). Continue until disease progression or unacceptable toxicity.

Melanoma (Adjuvant Treatment)

PO: ADULTS, ELDERLY: 2 mg once daily (in combination with dabrafenib). Continue for up to 1 yr in absence of disease progression or unacceptable toxicity.

Thyroid Cancer

PO: ADULTS, ELDERLY: 2 mg once daily (in combination with dabrafenib). Continue until disease progression or unacceptable toxicity.

NSCLC (Metastatic)

PO: ADULTS, ELDERLY: 2 mg once daily in combination with dabrafenib. Continue until disease progression or unacceptable toxicity.

Low-Grade Glioma, Solid Tumors

PO: CHILDREN 1 YR OF AGE AND OLDER: In combination with dabrafenib, dose is weight based. See tables below for dose of tablets and oral solution. Continue until disease progression or unacceptable toxicity.

Dosage for Tablets (Weight-Based)	Dosage for Oral Solution (Weight-Based)
26–37 kg: 1 mg	8 kg: 6 mL (0.3 mg)
38–50 kg: 1.5 mg	9 kg: 7 mL (0.35 mg)
	10 kg: 7 mL (0.35 mg)
51 kg or greater: 2 mg	11 kg: 8 mL (0.4 mg)
	12–13 kg: 9 mL (0.45 mg)
	14–17 kg: 11 mL (0.55 mg)
	18–21 kg: 14 mL (0.7 mg)
	22–25 kg: 17 mL (0.85 mg)
	26–29 kg: 18 mL (0.9 mg)
	30–33 kg: 20 mL (1 mg)
	34–37 kg: 23 mL (1.15 mg)
	38–41 kg: 25 mL (1.25 mg)
	42–45 kg: 28 mL (1.4 mg)
	46–50 kg: 32 mL (1.6 mg)
	≥51 kg: 40 mL (2 mg)

Dose Reduction Schedule

Trametinib regimen: FIRST DOSE REDUCTION: 1.5 mg once daily. **Second dose reduction:** 1 mg once daily. Discontinue if unable to tolerate 1-mg dose. **Dabrafenib combination regimen: FIRST DOSE REDUCTION:** 100 mg twice DAILY. **SECOND DOSE REDUCTION:** 75 mg twice daily. **THIRD DOSE REDUCTION:** 50 mg twice daily. Discontinue if unable to tolerate 50-mg dose.

Dose Modification

Based on Common Terminology Criteria for Adverse Events.

Cardiotoxicity
Asymptomatic decrease of left ventricular ejection fraction (LVEF) greater than 10% from baseline: Withhold trametinib up to 4 wks. If LVEF improved, resume at lower dose level. Discontinue if not improved. Do not modify dabrafenib dose. **Symptomatic HF or decrease of LVEF greater than 20% from baseline:** Discontinue trametinib. Withhold dabrafenib until improved, then resume at lower dose level.

Cutaneous Toxicity
Intolerable Grade 2 skin toxicity; Grade 3 or 4 skin toxicity: Withhold both regimens for up to 3 wks. If improved, resume both at lower dose level. Discontinue both regimens if not improved.

Febrile Events
Fever of 101.3°F–104°F (38.5°C–40°C): Do not modify trametinib dose. Withhold dabrafenib until fever resolved, then resume at either same dose or lower dose level. **Fever greater than 104°F (40°C) or complicated fever (dehydration, hypotension, renal failure):** Withhold trametinib until resolved, then resume at either same dose or lower dose level. Withhold dabrafenib until resolved, then resume at either lower dose level or discontinue.

New Primary Malignancies
Cutaneous: No changes required for either regimen. **Noncutaneous:** Do not change trametinib dose. Discontinue dabrafenib in pts who develop RAS mutation-positive malignancies.

Nonspecific Adverse Reactions
Other intolerable Grade 2 reactions; any other Grade 3 reactions: Withhold both regimens until resolved to Grade 0–1, then resume at lower dose level. Discontinue both regimens if not improved. **First occurrence of any other Grade 4 reaction:** Withhold both regimens until resolved to Grade 0–1, then resume at lower dose level or discontinue.

Ocular Toxicity
Grade 2 or 3 retinal pigment epithelial detachment: Withhold trametinib up to 3 wks. If improved to Grade 0–1, resume at lower dose level. Discontinue if not improved. Do not modify dabrafenib. **Retinal vein occlusion:** Discontinue trametinib. Do not modify dabrafenib. **Uveitis or iritis:** Do not modify trametinib. Withhold dabrafenib for up to 6 wks. If improved to Grade 0–1, then resume at same dose level. Discontinue if not improved.

T

Pulmonary Toxicity
Interstitial lung disease: Discontinue trametinib. Do not modify dabrafenib.

Venous Thromboembolism
Uncomplicated DVT/PE: Withhold trametinib for up to 3 wks. If improved to Grade 0–1, then resume at lower dose level. Discontinue if not improved. Do not modify dabrafenib. **Life-threatening PE:** Discontinue both regimens.

Dosage in Renal/Hepatic Impairment
No dose adjustment.

SIDE EFFECTS

Single Regimen
Frequent (57%–32%): Rash, diarrhea, lymphedema, peripheral edema. **Occasional (19%–10%):** Dermatitis acneiform, hypertension, stomatitis, mouth ulceration, mucosal ulceration, abdominal pain, dry skin, pruritus, paronychia, folliculitis, cellulitis, dizziness, dysgeusia, blurred vision, dry eye.

Combination Regimen
Frequent (71%–40%): Pyrexia, chills, fatigue, rash, nausea, vomiting. **Occasional (36%–11%):** Diarrhea, abdominal pain, peripheral edema, headache, cough, arthralgia, night sweats, myalgia, constipation, decreased appetite, back pain, dry skin, insomnia, dermatitis acneiform, dizziness, muscle spasm, extremity pain, actinic keratosis, erythema, oral/throat pain, pruritus, dry mouth, dehydration.

ADVERSE EFFECTS/TOXIC REACTIONS

Primary malignancies (basal or squamous cell carcinoma, keratoacanthoma, pancreatic adenocarcinoma, glioblastoma) were reported. DVT, PE reported in 9% of pts. May increase cell proliferation of wild-type BRAF melanoma or new malignant melanomas. Serious, sometimes fatal intracranial or GI bleeding occurred in 5% of pts. Other hemorrhagic events may include conjunctival/gingival/rectal/hemorrhoidal/vaginal bleeding, epistaxis, melena. Cardiomyopathy, HF, decreased LVEF reported in 7%–9% of pts. Ocular toxicities such as retinal vein occlusion, retinal detachment, vision loss, glaucoma, uveitis, iritis were reported. Cough, dyspnea, hypoxia, pleural effusion, infiltrates may indicate interstitial lung disease. Serious febrile reactions may lead to renal failure, severe dehydration, hypotension, rigors. Skin toxicities including palmar-plantar erythrodysesthesia syndrome (PPES), papilloma have occurred. Hyperglycemia reported in 2%–5% of pts. Other adverse effects may include hypertension, rhabdomyolysis, QT interval prolongation.

NURSING CONSIDERATIONS

BASELINE ASSESSMENT
Obtain CBC, BMP, LFT, ECG, vital signs; pregnancy test in females of reproductive potential. Confirm use of effective contraception. Verify BRAF V600E status. Obtain LVEF by echocardiogram. Assess skin for moles, lesions. Receive full medication history and screen for interactions. Screen for active infection. Question history as listed in Precautions. Offer emotional support.

INTERVENTION/EVALUATION
Monitor CBC for myelosuppression, LFT for hepatic injury (abdominal pain, jaundice, nausea, transaminitis, vomiting), ECG. Monitor for severe neutropenia, febrile neutropenia, infections (cough, fatigue, fever); symptoms of hyperglycemia (dehydration, confusion, extreme thirst, sweet-smelling breath, Kussmaul respirations, nausea); GI perforation (abdominal pain, fever, hematemesis). Assess skin for new lesion, toxicities q2mos. Assess LVEF for cardiomyopathy (dyspnea, edema, palpitations) by echocardiogram 1 mo after initiation, then q2–3mos thereafter. Obtain ophthalmologic exam for change of vision, eye irritation. Consider ABG, radiologic test if ILD/pneumonitis (excessive cough, dyspnea, fever, hypoxia)

is suspected. Consider treatment with corticosteroids if ILD/pneumonitis is confirmed. Monitor for ocular toxicities; symptoms of DVT (leg or arm pain/swelling), intracranial hemorrhage (aphasia, altered mental status, facial droop, hemiplegia, vision loss), PE (chest pain, dyspnea, tachycardia). Bleeding of any kind can be life-threatening and must be treated promptly.

PATIENT/FAMILY TEACHING

• Treatment may depress your immune system response and reduce your ability to fight infection. Report symptoms of infection such as body aches, chills, cough, fatigue, fever. Avoid those with active infection. • Report symptoms of bone marrow depression (e.g., bruising, fatigue, fever, shortness of breath, weight loss; bleeding easily, bloody urine or stool). • Report liver problems (abdominal pain, bruising, clay-colored stool, dark or amber-colored urine, yellowing of the skin or eyes), eye toxicities (eye redness, irritation; change of vision), heart problems (swelling of extremities, palpitations), symptoms of lung inflammation (excessive coughing, difficulty breathing, chest pain), DVT (swelling, pain, hot feeling in the arms or legs; discoloration of extremity), lung embolism (difficulty breathing, chest pain, rapid heart rate), high blood sugar levels (confusion, frequent urination, hunger, thirst). • Treatment may reduce the heart's ability to pump effectively; expect routine echocardiograms. • Use effective contraception to avoid pregnancy. Do not breastfeed. • New cancers may occur. • Immediately report severe or persistent abdominal pain, bloody stool, fever, vomiting blood; may indicate rupture in GI tract. • Bleeding may be life-threatening; report GI bleeding, symptoms of hemorrhagic stroke (confusion, one-sided weakness or paralysis, difficulty speaking).

trastuzumab

tras-**too**-zoo-mab
(Herceptin, Hercessi, Herzuma, Kanjinti, Ogivri, Ontruzant, Trazimera)

■ **BLACK BOX ALERT** ■ Subclinical and clinical HF (manifested as CHF, decreased left ventricular ejection fraction) may occur, esp. in pts receiving concomitant anthracycline therapy. Fatal infusion reactions and pulmonary toxicities may occur. Monitor for anaphylaxis, angioedema, interstitial pneumonitis, acute respiratory distress syndrome. Exposure during pregnancy may cause fetal harm and neonatal death.
Do not confuse trastuzumab with ado-trastuzumab, fam-trastuzumab (or biosimilars).

◆CLASSIFICATION

PHARMACOTHERAPEUTIC: HER2 receptor antagonist. Monoclonal antibody. **CLINICAL:** Antineoplastic.

USES

Adjuvant breast cancer: Treatment of HER2-overexpressing node-positive or node-negative breast cancer as part of a treatment regimen consisting of DOXOrubicin, cycloPHOSphamide, and either PACLitaxel or docetaxel; as part of a treatment regimen with DOCEtaxel and CARBOplatin; as a single agent following multimodality anthracycline-based therapy. **Metastatic breast cancer:** In combination with PACLitaxel for first-line treatment of HER2-overexpressing metastatic breast cancer; as a single agent for treatment of HER2-overexpressing breast cancer in pts having received one or more chemotherapy regimens for metastatic disease. **Metastatic gastric cancer:** In combination with CISplatin and capecitabine or 5-fluorouracil, for the treatment of pts with HER2-overexpressing metastatic gastric or gastroesophageal junction adenocarcinoma having not

 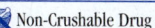

received prior treatment for metastatic disease. **OFF-LABEL:** Breast cancer (early stage, locally advanced or inflammatory neoadjuvant treatment), colorectal cancer (metastatic HER2+ with progression on conventional chemotherapy), endometrial cancer (advanced or recurrent HER2+).

PRECAUTIONS

Contraindications: Hypersensitivity to trastuzumab. **Cautions:** Baseline cytopenias, cardiac disease (cardiomyopathy, HF), pts at risk for interstitial lung disease (sarcoidosis, pulmonary fibrosis), tumor lysis syndrome (high tumor burden, dehydration); conditions predisposing to infection (e.g., diabetes, immunocompromised pts, renal failure, open wounds).

ACTION

Binds to extracellular domain of human epidermal growth factor receptor 2 (HER2) protein, inhibiting proliferation of tumor cells that overexpresss HER2 protein. **Therapeutic Effect:** Inhibits tumor cell growth and survival; mediates antibody-dependent cellular cytotoxicity.

PHARMACOKINETICS

Half-life: 11–23 days.

🕱 LIFESPAN CONSIDERATIONS

Pregnancy/Lactation: Females of reproductive potential should use effective contraception during treatment and for at least 7 mos after discontinuation. Unknown if distributed in breast milk. Breastfeeding not recommended. **Children:** Safety and efficacy not established. **Elderly:** Age-related cardiac dysfunction may require dosage adjustment.

INTERACTIONS

DRUG: May increase cardiotoxic effect of **anthracyclines** (e.g., **DOXOrubicin, epiRUBicin**). **HERBAL:** None significant. **FOOD:** None known. **LAB VALUES:** None significant.

AVAILABILITY (Rx)

Injection, Powder for Reconstitution: 150 mg in a single-dose vial for reconstitution.

ADMINISTRATION/HANDLING

 IV

Reconstitution • Reconstitute 150-mg vial with 7.4 mL Sterile Water for Injection to yield concentration of 21 mg/mL. • Gently swirl vial to mix. Do not shake. • If foaming appears, allow vial to stand for up to 5 min. • Visually inspect for particulate matter or discoloration. Solution should appear clear to slightly opalescent, colorless to pale yellow. Do not use if cloudy or discolored or if visible particles are observed. • Dilute in 250 mL 0.9% NaCl (do not dilute in D_5W). • Gently invert bag to mix.
Rate of administration • Do not give IV push or bolus. • Infuse loading dose (4 mg/kg) over 90 min. Infuse maintenance infusion (2 mg/kg) over 30–90 min.
Storage • Refrigerate unused vials. • May refrigerate diluted solution for up to 24 hrs. • Do not freeze.

✿ IV INCOMPATIBILITIES

Do not mix with D_5W or any other medications.

INDICATIONS/ROUTES/DOSAGE

Note: Do not substitute with ado-trastuzumab emtansine.
Breast Cancer (Adjuvant)
IV: ADULTS, ELDERLY: (With concurrent PACLitaxel or DOCEtaxel): Initially, 4 mg/kg (loading dose), then 2 mg/kg wkly for 12 wks, followed 1 wk later (when current chemotherapy completed) by 6 mg/kg q3wks for total therapy duration of 52 wks. **(With DOCEtaxel/CARBOplatin):** Initially, 4 mg/kg (loading dose), then 2 mg/kg wkly for a total of 18 wks, followed 1 wk later (when concurrent chemotherapy completed) by 6 mg/kg q3wks for total therapy duration of 52 wks. **(Following multimodality chemotherapy):** Initially, 8 mg/kg (loading dose), then 6 mg/kg q3wks for total of 52 wks.

Breast Cancer (Metastatic)
IV: ADULTS, ELDERLY: (Either as single agent or in combination with PAC-Litaxel): Initially, 4 mg/kg (loading dose), then 2 mg/kg wkly until disease progression.

Gastric Cancer
IV: ADULTS, ELDERLY: (In combination with CISplatin and either capecitabine or fluorouracil for 6 cycles, then as monotherapy): Initially, 8 mg/kg (loading dose), then 6 mg/kg q3wks until disease progression.

Dosage Adjustment in Cardiotoxicity
Left ventricular ejection fraction (LVEF) 16% or greater decrease from baseline WNL (within normal limits) or LVEF below normal limits and 10% or greater decrease from baseline: Hold treatment for 4 wks. Repeat LVEF q4wks. Resume therapy if LVEF returns to normal limits in 4–8 wks and remains at 15% or less decrease from baseline.

Dosage in Renal/Hepatic Impairment
No dose adjustment.

SIDE EFFECTS
Frequent (47%–18%): Generalized pain, asthenia, fever, nausea, chills, headache, cough, diarrhea, abdominal pain, dyspnea, rash. Occasional (14%–6%): Anorexia, insomnia, dizziness, peripheral edema, paresthesia, edema, nausea, vomiting, bone pain, arthralgia, accidental injury. Rare (5%–1%): Tachycardia, acne, peripheral neuritis, neuropathy.

ADVERSE EFFECTS/TOXIC REACTIONS
Myelosuppression (anemia, neutropenia, thrombocytopenia) is an expected response to therapy, but more severe reactions including febrile neutropenia may occur. May cause decrease in LVEF, cardiac arrhythmias, hypertension, HF, cardiomyopathy, cardiac death. Infusion reactions (asthenia, chills, fever, hypotension, nausea, vomiting, rash) have occurred, but more severe reactions including anaphylaxis, angioedema, hypoxia, severe hypotension can be fatal. Pulmonary toxicities (acute respiratory distress syndrome, dyspnea, interstitial pneumonitis, pulmonary infiltrates), infections (influenza, pharyngitis, rhinitis, sinusitis) were reported. Tumor lysis syndrome may present as acute renal failure, hypocalcemia, hyperuricemia, hyperphosphatemia.

NURSING CONSIDERATIONS

BASELINE ASSESSMENT
Obtain CBC, ECG; pregnancy test in females of reproductive potential. Assess LVEF by echocardiogram. Screen for active infection. Question for history of cardiac/pulmonary disease, infusion reactions. Offer emotional support.

INTERVENTION/EVALUATION
Monitor CBC for myelosuppression. Monitor for severe neutropenia, febrile neutropenia, infections (cough, fatigue, fever). Monitor serum uric acid level if tumor lysis syndrome (acute renal failure, electrolyte imbalance, cardiac arrhythmias, seizures) is suspected. Assess LVEF for cardiomyopathy (dyspnea, edema, palpitations) by echocardiogram q3mos (monthly if treatment is withheld for severe cardiomyopathy), then q6mos for 2 yrs after discontinuation. Diligently monitor infusion reactions. Have resuscitative equipment available if infusion reactions occur. Consider ABG, radiologic test if ILD/pneumonitis (excessive cough, dyspnea, fever, hypoxia) is suspected. Consider treatment with corticosteroids if ILD/pneumonitis is confirmed.

PATIENT/FAMILY TEACHING
• Treatment may depress your immune system response and reduce your ability to fight infection. Report symptoms of infection such as body aches, chills, cough, fatigue, fever. Avoid those with active infection. • Report symptoms of bone marrow depression (e.g., bruising, fatigue, fever, shortness of breath, weight loss; bleeding easily, bloody urine or

T

stool). • Treatment may reduce the heart's ability to pump effectively; expect routine echocardiograms. • Report heart problems (difficulty breathing, swelling of extremities, palpitations), kidney problems (decreased urine output, flank pain, darkened urine); symptoms of lung inflammation (excessive coughing, difficulty breathing, chest pain). • Use effective contraception to avoid pregnancy. Do not breastfeed. • Life-threatening infusion reactions may occur. Immediately report difficulty breathing, dizziness, rash; swelling of face, tongue, throat.

trastuzumab/ hyaluronidase

tras-**tu**-zoo-mab **hye**-al-ure-**on**-i-dase
(Herceptin Hylecta)

■ **BLACK BOX ALERT** ■ May cause cardiac failure, esp. in pts with anthracycline-containing chemotherapy regimens. Monitor left ventricular function prior to initiation and during treatment. Serious and fatal cases of interstitial lung disease (ILD), pneumonitis were reported. Symptoms usually occurred during or within 24 hrs of administration. Permanently discontinue if anaphylaxis, ILD, acute respiratory distress syndrome occurs. Treatment may cause fetal harm. Recommend effective contraception.
Do not confuse trastuzumab/ hyaluronidase with ado-trastuzumab emtansine, daratumumab/hyaluronidase, fam-trastuzumab deruxtecan, pertuzumab, trastuzumab (or biosimilars), or rituximab/hyaluronidase.

◆CLASSIFICATION

PHARMACOTHERAPEUTIC: Human epidermal growth factor receptor 2 (HER2) antagonist; monoclonal antibody. **CLINICAL:** Antineoplastic.

USES

Adjuvant breast cancer: Adjuvant treatment of adults with HER2-overexpressing node-positive or node-negative (estrogen receptor [ER]/progesterone receptor [PR]–negative or with one high-risk feature) breast cancer: As part of a treatment regimen consisting of DOXOrubicin, cycloPHOSphamide, and either PACLitaxel or DOCEtaxel; as part of a treatment regimen with DOCEtaxel and CARBOplatin; as a single agent following multimodal anthracycline-based therapy. **Metastatic breast cancer:** Treatment of adults as first-line therapy for HER2-overexpressing metastatic breast cancer (in combination with PACLitaxel); as a single agent for HER2-overexpressing breast cancer in pts who have received one or more chemotherapy regimens for metastatic disease.

PRECAUTIONS

Contraindications: Hypersensitivity to trastuzumab/hyaluronidase, trastuzumab-containing regimens. **Cautions:** Baseline cytopenias, active infection, pulmonary disorders (e.g., COPD, emphysema, pulmonary fibrosis), cardiovascular disease, HF, conditions predisposing to infection (e.g., diabetes, renal failure, immunocompromised pts, open wounds). Do not substitute with ado-trastuzumab or intravenous trastuzumab.

ACTION

Binds to extracellular domain of HER2 protein, inhibiting proliferation of HER2-overexpressing tumor cells. Mediates antibody-dependent cellular toxicity. Hyaluronidase increases dispersion and absorption of SQ injected medications by increasing permeability. **Therapeutic Effect:** Inhibits proliferation of cells overexpressing HER2 protein.

PHARMACOKINETICS

Widely distributed. Peak plasma concentration: 3 days. Eliminated by parallel and nonlinear saturable target mediated clearance. **Half-life:** Not specified.

⧗ LIFESPAN CONSIDERATIONS

Pregnancy/Lactation: Avoid pregnancy; may cause fetal harm. Females of reproductive potential should use effective contraception during treatment and for at least 7 mos after discontinuation. Breastfeeding not recommended during treatment and for at least 7 mos after discontinuation. **Children:** Safety and efficacy not established. **Elderly:** May have increased risk of cardiac dysfunction.

INTERACTIONS

DRUG: May increase cardiotoxic effects of **anthracyclines (e.g., DAUNOrubicin, DOXOrubicin, epirubicin).** Hyaluronidase may increase vasoconstricting effect of **phenylephrine. HERBAL:** None significant. **FOOD:** None known. **LAB VALUES:** May decrease Hgb, neutrophils, RBCs.

AVAILABILITY (Rx)

Injection Solution: trastuzumab 600 mg/hyaluronidase 10,000 units per 5 mL (120 mg/2,000 units/mL).

ADMINISTRATION/HANDLING

SQ

Preparation • Visually inspect for particulate matter or discoloration. Solution should appear clear to opalescent, colorless to yellow in color. Do not use if solution is cloudy or discolored or visible particles are observed. • Withdraw contents from vial into syringe. • To avoid clogging, immediately attach a hypodermic needle or subcutaneous infusion set to syringe.
Administration • Insert needle subcutaneously into left or right thigh (only), approx. 2.5 cm from previous injection sites. • Do not inject into areas of active skin disease or injury such as sunburns, skin rashes, inflammation, skin infections, or active psoriasis. • Rotate injection sites. • Do not administer IV or intramuscularly. • If a dose is missed, administer as soon as possible and adjustment schedule to maintain dosing intervals.
Rate of administration • Inject over 2–5 min.

Storage • Refrigerate vials in original carton until time of use. • Protect from light. • Do not shake or freeze. • After vial is removed from refrigerator, use within 4 hrs. • May store syringe containing solution at room temperature for up to 4 hrs or refrigerate for up to 24 hrs.

INDICATIONS/ROUTES/DOSAGE

Breast Cancer (HER2-Positive) (Adjuvant)
SQ: ADULTS: 600 mg/10,000 units q3wks (21-day cycle) for 52 wks or until disease recurrence (whichever occurs first). Extending treatment beyond 1 yr is not recommended. Give in combination with DOXOrubicin, cycloPHOSphamide, and either PACLitaxel or DOCEtaxel; or in combination with DOCEetaxel and CARBOplatin; or as a single agent following multimodality anthracycline-based therapy.

Breast Cancer (HER2-Positive, Metastatic)
SQ: ADULTS: 600 mg/10,000 units q3wks (21-day cycle) (in combination with PACLitaxel or as a single agent following one or more chemotherapy regimens for metastatic disease). Continue until disease progression or unacceptable toxicity.

Dose Modification
Cardiac Toxicity
Withhold treatment for 4 wks for an absolute decrease in left ventricular ejection fraction (LVEF) that is greater than or equal to 16% from baseline; absolute decrease in LVEF below institutional limits of normal and greater than or equal 10% from baseline. May resume if LVEF returns to normal limits and the absolute decrease from baseline is greater than or equal to 15% within 4–8 wks. Permanently discontinue if left ventricular dysfunction persists longer than 8 wks or treatment is withheld on more than three occasions for cardiac toxicity.

Dosage in Renal/Hepatic Impairment
Mild to severe impairment: Not specified; use caution.

T

SIDE EFFECTS

Frequent (33%–17%): Fatigue, diarrhea, arthralgia, injection site reactions (e.g., bruising, pain, dermatitis, discoloration, discomfort, erythema, fibrosis, hematoma, hemorrhage, induration, irritation, nodule, rash, ulcer), rash, myalgia. **Occasional (15%–6%):** Nausea, peripheral neuropathy, headache, flushing, edema, cough, extremity pain, pyrexia, nail disorder, abdominal pain, alopecia, erythema, constipation, hypertension, stomatitis, dyspnea, back pain, generalized pain, vomiting, insomnia, mucosal inflammation, pruritus, dizziness, paresthesia, nasal inflammation/discomfort.

ADVERSE EFFECTS/TOXIC REACTIONS

Myelosuppression (anemia, neutropenia) is an expected response to therapy. Cardiomyopathy reported in 5% of pts. Other cardiac disorders may include tachycardia, palpitations, congestive HF. Pulmonary toxicities (acute respiratory distress syndrome, dyspnea, hypoxia, ILD, noncardiogenic pulmonary edema, pneumonitis, pleural effusions, pulmonary fibrosis, pulmonary infiltrates, pulmonary insufficiency) were reported. Infections (upper respiratory tract infections, UTI, viral infections) were reported. Epistaxis reported in 6% of pts. Hypersensitivity reactions, including anaphylaxis, may occur.

NURSING CONSIDERATIONS

BASELINE ASSESSMENT

Obtain CBC; pregnancy test in females of reproductive potential. Confirm compliance of effective contraception. Verify presence of HER2 protein overexpression or HER2 gene amplification in tumor specimen. Assess LVEF by echocardiogram. Question history of cardiovascular disease, HF, hypersensitivity reactions, pulmonary disease. Screen for active infection. Offer emotional support.

INTERVENTION/EVALUATION

Monitor CBC periodically. Consider ABG, radiologic test if ILD/pneumonitis (excessive cough, dyspnea, fever, hypoxia) is suspected. Consider treatment with corticosteroids if ILD/pneumonitis is confirmed. Auscultate lung sounds. Monitor for symptoms of HF (chest pain, dyspnea, palpitations, swelling of extremities). Assess LVEF by echocardiogram q3mos. If treatment withheld due to change in LVEF, monitor LVEF at 4-wk intervals. If treatment is used as adjuvant therapy, assess LVEF q6mos for at least 2 yrs upon completion. Monitor for infections (cough, fatigue, fever). If serious infection occurs, initiate appropriate antimicrobial therapy. Monitor daily pattern of bowel activity, stool consistency. Offer antiemetic if nausea/vomiting occurs. Monitor for hypersensitivity reactions.

PATIENT/FAMILY TEACHING

• Treatment may depress your immune system response and reduce your ability to fight infection. Report symptoms of infection such as body aches, chills, cough, fatigue, fever. Avoid those with active infection. • Report symptoms of bone marrow depression (e.g., bruising, fatigue, fever, shortness of breath, weight loss; bleeding easily, bloody urine or stool). • Report symptoms of lung inflammation (excessive coughing, difficulty breathing, chest pain); heart failure (e.g., chest pain, difficulty breathing, palpitations, swelling of extremities); UTI (fever, urinary frequency, burning during urination, foul-smelling urine). • Treatment may reduce the heart's ability to pump effectively; expect routine echocardiograms. • Use effective contraception to avoid pregnancy. Do not breastfeed. • Nausea/vomiting is a common side effect. • Maintain proper hydration and nutrition. • Severe allergic reactions, including anaphylaxis, can occur. If allergic reaction occurs, seek immediate medical attention.

traZODone

traz-o-done
(Apo-TraZODone ✦)

◆CLASSIFICATION

PHARMACOTHERAPEUTIC: Serotonin reuptake inhibitor/antagonist. **CLINICAL:** Antidepressant.

USES

Treatment of major depressive disorder (MDD). **OFF-LABEL:** Insomnia, aggressive/agitated behavior associated with dementia.

PRECAUTIONS

Contraindications: Hypersensitivity to traZODone. Use of MAOIs (concurrently or within 14 days of discontinuing traZODone or MAOI); initiation in pt receiving linezolid or IV methylene blue. **Cautions:** Cardiac disease, cardiac conduction disorders, seizure disorder, elderly, hepatic/renal impairment, cerebrovascular disease; history of suicidal ideation and behavior, conditions predisposing to priapism (e.g., sickle cell disease), concomitant use of antihypertensives.

ACTION

Blocks reuptake of serotonin at neuronal presynaptic membranes, increasing its availability at postsynaptic receptor sites. **Therapeutic Effect:** Relieves depression.

PHARMACOKINETICS

Widely distributed. Protein binding: 85%–95%. Metabolized in liver. Primarily excreted in urine. **Half-life:** 5–9 hrs (increased in elderly).

☒ LIFESPAN CONSIDERATIONS

Pregnancy/Lactation: Crosses placenta; minimally distributed in breast milk. **Children:** Safety and efficacy not established in pts younger than 6 yrs. **Elderly:** More likely to experience sedative, hypotensive effects; lower dosage recommended.

INTERACTIONS

DRUG: Strong **CYP3A4 inhibitors (e.g., clarithromycin, ketoconazole)** may increase concentration/effect. May increase concentration/effect of **phenytoin. Strong CYP3A4 inducers (e.g., carBAMazepine, rifAMPin)** may decrease concentration/effect. May increase QT interval-prolonging effect of **clarithromycin. Linezolid, MAOIs (e.g., phenelzine, selegiline) venlafaxine** may increase serotonergic effect. **HERBAL:** Herbals with **sedative properties (e.g., chamomile, kava kava, valerian)** may increase toxic effect. **St. John's wort** may decrease concentration/effect. **FOOD:** None known. **LAB VALUES:** May decrease neutrophils, WBCs.

AVAILABILITY (Rx)

Tablets: 50 mg, 100 mg, 150 mg, 300 mg.

ADMINISTRATION/HANDLING

PO
• Give shortly after snack, meal (reduces risk of dizziness). • Give whole or as half-tablet by breaking along the score line.

INDICATIONS/ROUTES/DOSAGE

◄**ALERT**► Therapeutic effect may take up to 6 wks to occur.
Depression
PO: ADULTS: Initially, 50 mg twice daily. May increase in increments of 50 mg/day q3–7 days up to 75–150 mg twice daily. May further increase by 50–100 mg/day q2–4 wks. **Usual dosage range: 200 to 400 mg/day. Maximum:** 600 mg/day. **ELDERLY:** Initially, 25–50 mg at bedtime. May increase by 25–50 mg every 3–7 days. **Range:** 75–150 mg/day.

Dosage in Renal/Hepatic Impairment
Use caution.

T

 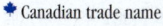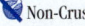

SIDE EFFECTS

Frequent   (9%–3%): Drowsiness, dry mouth, light-headedness, dizziness, headache, blurred vision, nausea, vomiting. **Occasional (3%–1%):** Nervousness, fatigue, constipation, myalgia/arthralgia, mild hypotension. **Rare:** Photosensitivity reaction.

ADVERSE EFFECTS/TOXIC REACTIONS

Priapism, altered libido, retrograde ejaculation, impotence occur rarely. Appears to be less cardiotoxic than other antidepressants, although arrhythmias may occur in pts with preexisting cardiac disease.

NURSING CONSIDERATIONS

BASELINE ASSESSMENT

Assess mental status, mood, behavior. For pts on long-term therapy, serum hepatic/renal function tests, blood counts should be performed periodically. Question history as listed in Precautions.

INTERVENTION/EVALUATION

Monitor for suicidal ideation (esp. at beginning of therapy or dosage change). Assess appearance, behavior, speech pattern, level of interest, mood. Assist with ambulation if dizziness, light-headedness occurs.

PATIENT/FAMILY TEACHING

• Immediately discontinue medication, consult physician if priapism occurs. • **Immediate-release:** May take after meal, snack. • **Extended-release:** Take on empty stomach. • May take at bedtime if drowsiness occurs. • Change positions slowly to avoid hypotensive effect. • Avoid tasks that require alertness, motor skills until response to drug is established. • Photosensitivity to sun may occur. • Report visual disturbances, worsening depression, suicidal ideation, unusual changes in behavior. • Do not abruptly discontinue medication.• Avoid alcohol.

tremelimumab-actl

tre-mel-**im**-ue-mab-actl
(Imjudo)
Do not confuse tremelimumab with adalimumab, belimumab, or ipilimumab.

◆CLASSIFICATION

PHARMACOTHERAPEUTIC: Cytotoxic T-lymphocyte-associated antigen 4 (CTLA-4)–blocking antibody. **CLINICAL:** Antineoplastic.

USES

Unresectable hepatocellular carcinoma (uHCC): Treatment of adults with uHCC in combination with durvalumab. **Non–small-cell lung cancer (NSCLC):** Treatment of adults with metastatic NSCLC with no sensitizing epidermal growth factor receptor (EGFR) mutations or anaplastic lymphoma kinase (ALK) genomic tumor aberrations in combination with durvalumab and platinum-based chemotherapy.

PRECAUTIONS

Contraindications: Hypersensitivity to tremelimumab-actl. **Cautions:** Baseline cytopenias, pts at risk for interstitial lung disease (e.g., COPD, sarcoidosis, connective tissue disease); history of autoimmune disorders (Crohn's disease, demyelinating polyneuropathy, Guillain-Barré syndrome, Hashimoto's thyroiditis, hyperthyroidism, myasthenia gravis, rheumatoid arthritis, type I diabetes, vasculitis); hypothyroidism, pancreatitis; solid organ transplant, allogeneic hematopoietic stem cell transplantation.

ACTION

A monoclonal antibody targeting activity of CTLA-4, a protein that inhibits T-cell activation and immune response to cancer, blocking the interaction of CTLA-4 with its ligands (CD80 and CD86). **Therapeutic Effect:** Removes inhibition of

T

immune response, promotes cancer cell death.

PHARMACOKINETICS

Widely distributed. Metabolism not specified. Steady state reached in 12 wks. Excretion not specified. **Half-life:** 16.9 days.

⧗ LIFESPAN CONSIDERATIONS

Pregnancy/Lactation: Avoid pregnancy; may cause fetal harm. Females of reproductive potential must use effective contraception during treatment and for at least 3 mos after discontinuation. Breastfeeding not recommended during treatment and for at least 3 mos after discontinuation. Human immunoglobulin G (IgG) is present in breast milk and known to cross the placenta. **Children:** Safety and efficacy not established. **Elderly:** No age-related precautions noted.

INTERACTIONS

DRUG: None known (see prescribing information for durvalumab and platinum-based chemotherapy). **HERBAL:** None significant. **FOOD:** None known. **LAB VALUES:** May increase serum alkaline phosphatase, amylase, ALT, AST, bilirubin, creatinine, GGT, glucose, lipase. May decrease Hgb, leukocytes, lymphocytes, neutrophils, platelets; serum albumin, calcium, magnesium. May increase or decrease serum potassium, sodium.

AVAILABILITY (Rx)

Injection Solution: 25 mg/1.25 mL (20 mg/mL), 300 mg/15 mL (20 mg/mL).

ADMINISTRATION/HANDLING

 IV

Infusion guidelines • Infuse via dedicated IV line using a sterile, low-protein-binding 0.2- or 0.22-micron, in-line filter. • Do not administer as IV push or bolus. • Use separate infusion bags for each product; do not combine tremelimumab-actl and durvalumab. • Administer each product separately on the same day (tremelimumab-actl first, then dur-

valumab, then platinum-based-therapy). • For cycle 1, infuse durvalumab 1–2 hrs after tremelimumb-actl, then infuse platinum-based therapy 1–2 hrs after durvalumab. If no infusion reaction occurred during cycle 1, subsequent cycles of durvalumab may be given immediately after tremelimumab-actl, and the start of infusion of platinum-based therapy can be reduced to 30 min. • See manufacturer guidelines regarding treatment with durvalumab, PEMEtrexed, and platinum-based therapy.

Preparation • Must be prepared by personnel trained in aseptic manipulations and admixing of cytotoxic drugs. • Visually inspect for particulate matter or discoloration. Solution should appear clear to slightly opalescent, colorless to slightly yellow. Do not use if solution is cloudy or discolored. • Dilute into an infusion bag containing D5W or 0.9% NaCl to a final concentration between 0.1 mg/mL and 10 mg/mL. • Mix by gentle inversion. Do not shake or agitate.

Rate of administration • Infuse over 60 min.

Infusion reactions • Grade 1 or 2 infusion reactions: Interrupt or slow infusion rate. **Grade 3 or 4 infusion reactions:** Permanently discontinue.

Storage • Refrigerate unused vials in original carton. Protect from light. Do not freeze or shake. • Diluted solution may be refrigerated or stored at room temperature for up to 24 hrs. Do freeze or shake.

INDICATIONS/ROUTES/DOSAGE

uHCC

IV: ADULTS, ELDERLY WEIGHING 30 KG AND GREATER: 300 mg once, followed by durvalumab 1,500 mg once on day 1 of cycle 1. **Maintenance:** After cycle 1 of combination therapy, continue durvalumab 1,500 mg (as a single agent) once q4wks until disease progression or unacceptable toxicity. **WEIGHING LESS THAN 30 KG:** 4 mg/kg once, followed by durvalumab 20 mg/kg on day 1 of cycle 1. **Maintenance:** After cycle 1 of combination ther-

T

---

apy, continue durvalumab 20 mg/kg (as a single agent) once q4wks until disease progression or unacceptable toxicity.

NSCLC (Metastatic)

Note: Continue durvalumab until disease progression or unacceptable toxicity. Starting cycle 5, dosing interval changes from q3wks to q4wks. If fewer than four cycles of platinum-based chemotherapy are given, the remaining cycles of tremelimumab-actl (up to a total of five) should be given after the platinum-based chemotherapy phase (in combination with durvalumab q4wks). Starting wk 12 of treatment, optional pemetrexed therapy may be given until disease progression or unacceptable toxicity.

IV: ADULTS, ELDERLY WEIGHING 30 KG OR GREATER: 75 mg q3wks (in combination with durvalumab 1,500 mg and platinum-based chemotherapy) for four cycles, then administer durvalumab 1,500 mg q4wks as a single agent with histology-based pemetrexed therapy q4wks, and a fifth dose of tremelimumab 75 mg in combination with durvalumab dose 6 at wk 16. **WEIGHING LESS THAN 30 KG:** 1 mg/kg q3wks in combination with durvalumab 20 mg/kg and platinum-based chemotherapy for four cycles, then administer durvalumab 20 mg/kg q4wks as a single agent with histology-based pemetrexed therapy q4wks, and a fifth dose of tremelimumab 1 mg/kg in combination with durvalumab dose 6 at wk 16.

Tumor Histology	Weight	Tremelimumab-actl Dose	Durvalumab Dose	Platinum-Based Chemotherapy Regimen
Nonsquamous NSCLC	30 kg or greater Less than 30 kg	75 mg 1 mg/kg	1,500 mg 20 mg/kg	CARBOplatin *and* nab-PACLitaxel **OR** CARBOplatin *or* CISplatin and PEMEtrexed
Squamous NSCLC	30 kg or greater Less than 30 kg	75 mg 1 mg/kg	1,500 mg 20 mg/kg	CARBOplatin *and* nab-PACLitaxel **OR** CARBOplatin *or* CISplatin and gemcitabine

Dose Modification

Based on Common Terminology Criteria for Adverse Events (CTCAE). No dose reduction is recommended. Based on severity of adverse reactions, withhold treatment or consider starting corticosteroid therapy. May resume treatment if symptoms improve to Grade 1 or 0 after corticosteroid taper.

Immune-Mediated Adverse Reactions

Withhold treatment for the following adverse reactions: Grade 2 pneumonitis; Grade 2 colitis; clinically unstable Grade 3 or 4 endocrinopathies; Grade 2 or 3 nephritis with renal dysfunction; Grade 2 neurological toxicities; *suspected* Stevens-Johnson syndrome (SJS), toxic epidermal necrolysis, or drug reaction with eosinophilia and systemic symptoms (DRESS); serum ALT/AST greater than 3–8 times ULN or total serum bilirubin greater than 1.5–3 times

ULN (hepatitis with no tumor involvement of the liver); baseline serum ALT/AST greater than 1–3 times ULN that increases to greater than 5–10 times ULN, or baseline serum ALT/AST greater than 3–5 times ULN that increases to greater than 8–10 times ULN (hepatitis with tumor involvement of the liver).

Permanently discontinue for the following adverse reactions: Grade 3 or 4 pneumonitis; Grade 3 or 4 colitis; clinically unstable Grade 3 or 4 endocrinopathies depending on severity; Grade 4 nephritis with renal dysfunction; Grade 3 or 4 neurologic toxicities; Grade 2–4 myocarditis; Grade 3 or 4 neurological toxicities; *confirmed* SJS, toxic epidermal necrolysis, or DRESS; serum ALT/AST greater than 8 times ULN or total serum bilirubin greater than 3 times ULN (hepatitis with no tumor involvement of the liver); serum ALT/AST greater than 10 times ULN or total serum bilirubin greater than 3 times ULN (hepatitis with tumor involvement of the liver); Grade 3 or 4 infusion-related reactions; recurrent Grade 3 immune-mediated reaction requiring immunosuppressive therapy; inability to reduce corticosteroid dose to 10 mg or less of prednisone (or equivalent)/day within 12 wks of starting corticosteroid therapy.

Dosage in Renal/Hepatic Impairment

Mild to moderate impairment: No dose adjustment. **Severe impairment:** Not specified; use caution.

SIDE EFFECTS

Note: Frequency and occurrence of side effects may vary based combined therapy regimen.
Frequent (32%–20%): Rash, diarrhea, fatigue, pruritus, musculoskeletal pain, abdominal pain. **Occasional (17%–10%):** Decreased appetite, pyrexia, nausea, insomnia.

ADVERSE EFFECTS/TOXIC REACTIONS

Myelosuppression (anemia, leukopenia, lymphopenia, thrombocytopenia) is an expected response to therapy. May cause severe and/or fatal immune-mediated adverse reactions including acute kidney injury, nephritis; colitis, hepatitis, pancreatitis, pneumonitis; adrenal insufficiency, hypoparathyroidism, hyperthyroidism, hypophysitis, thyroiditis, type I diabetes mellitus including ketoacidosis; autoimmune neuropathy, encephalitis, Guillain-Barré syndrome, meningitis, myasthenia gravis, myelitis, nerve paresis; myocarditis, pericarditis, vasculitis; iritis, uveitis; myositis, polymyositis, rhabdomyolysis; aplastic anemia, hemolytic anemia, hemophagocytic lymphohistiocytosis, histiocytic necrotizing lymphadenitis, immune thrombocytopenia; sarcoidosis, systemic inflammatory response syndrome. Immune-mediated adverse reactions can affect any organ at any time. May cause cytomegalovirus infection/reactivation in pts with corticosteroid-refractory immune-related coli-tis. Dermatologic toxicities including SJS, toxic epidermal necrolysis may occur. DRESS, also known as multiorgan hypersensitivity, has been reported. DRESS may present with facial swelling, eosinophilia, fever, lymphadenopathy, and rash, which may be associated with other organ systems, such as hepatitis, hematological abnormalities, myocarditis, nephritis. Life-threatening infusion reactions may occur.

NURSING CONSIDERATIONS

BASELINE ASSESSMENT

Obtain CBC, BMP, LFT, thyroid panel; pregnancy test in females of reproductive potential; vital signs. Confirm compliance with effective contraception. Obtain weight in kg on the day of each infusion. Confirm tumor histology in pts being treated for NSCLC. Screen for history of autoimmune disorders, diabetes, pituitary/pulmonary/thyroid disease. Administer in an environment equipped to monitor for and manage infusion-related reactions. Question for prior infusion reactions before administration of each product. Screen for active infection. Offer emotional support.

INTERVENTION/EVALUATION

Monitor CBC, LFT, renal function, thyroid panel as clinically indicated. Assess for infusion reactions during each infusion. If reactions occur, interrupt or decrease the infusion rate. Immune-mediated reactions can affect any organ. Early detection and management are vital. Conduct a complete head-to-toe assessment frequently. Radiological examination, blood sampling, and/or treatment with corticosteroids should be considered if an immune-mediated reaction is suspected. Assess for eye pain/redness, visual changes at each office visit and at regular intervals. Monitor daily pattern of bowel activity, stool consistency. Assess skin for rash, dermatological toxicities; symptoms of DRESS. Monitor blood glucose levels in pts treated with corticosteroids.

PATIENT/FAMILY TEACHING

• Immediately report symptoms of infusion-related reactions such as chills, cough, difficulty breathing, nausea, vomiting. • Report symptoms of drug-induced hypersensitivity syndrome (e.g., fever, swollen face/lymph nodes, skin rash/peeling/inflammation). • Serious adverse reactions may affect lungs, liver, intestines, kidneys, hormonal glands, nervous system (or any organ), which may require anti-inflammatory medication. Immediately report any symptoms in the following body systems: colon (severe abdominal pain/swelling, diarrhea); eyes (pain, redness, vision problems); heart (chest pain, difficulty breathing); kidneys (decreased or dark-colored urine, flank pain); lung (chest pain, severe cough, shortness of breath); liver (bruising, dark-colored urine, clay-colored/tarry stools, nausea, yellowing of the skin or eyes); nervous system (confusion, difficulty breathing or swallowing; paralysis, weakness); pituitary (persistent or unusual headaches, dizziness, extreme weakness, fainting, vision changes); skin (blisters, bubbling, inflammation, rash); thyroid (trouble sleeping, high blood pressure, fast heart rate [overactive thyroid]; fatigue, goiter, weight gain [underactive thyroid]); vascular (low blood pressure, vein/artery pain or irritation). • Use effective contraception to avoid pregnancy. Do not breastfeed.

trospium

tro-spee-um
(Trosec ✦)

FIXED-COMBINATION(S)

Cobenfy: trospium/xanomeline (muscarinic agonist): 20 mg/50 mg; 20 mg/100 mg; 30 mg/125 mg (indicated for the treatment of schizophrenia in adults).

◆CLASSIFICATION

PHARMACOTHERAPEUTIC: Anticholinergic. **CLINICAL:** Antispasmodic.

USES

Treatment of overactive bladder with symptoms of urge urinary incontinence, urgency, urinary frequency.

PRECAUTIONS

Contraindications: Hypersensitivity to trospium. Pts with or at increased risk of gastric retention, uncontrolled narrow-angle glaucoma, urinary retention. **Cautions:** Decreased GI motility, renal/hepatic impairment, obstructive GI disorders, ulcerative colitis, intestinal atony, myasthenia gravis, controlled narrow-angle glaucoma, bladder flow obstruction, Alzheimer's disease, hot weather/exercise, elderly.

ACTION

Antagonizes effect of acetylcholine on muscarinic receptors, producing parasympatholytic action. **Therapeutic Effect:** Reduces smooth muscle tone in bladder.

PHARMACOKINETICS

Minimally absorbed after PO administration. Protein binding: 50%–85%. Distributed in plasma. Excreted in feces (82%), urine (6%). **Half-life:** 20 hrs.

⧖ LIFESPAN CONSIDERATIONS

Pregnancy/Lactation: Unknown if drug crosses placenta or is distributed in breast milk. **Children:** Safety and efficacy not established. **Elderly:** Higher incidence of dry mouth, constipation, dyspepsia, UTI, urinary retention in pts 75 yrs and older.

INTERACTIONS

DRUG: Alcohol may increase CNS depression. **Anticholinergics (e.g., aclidinium, ipratropium, tiotropium, umeclidinium)** may increase anticholinergic effect. **HERBAL:** None significant. **FOOD: High-fat meals** may reduce absorption. **LAB VALUES:** None significant.

AVAILABILITY (Rx)

☙ **Tablets:** 20 mg. **Capsules, Extended-Release:** 60 mg.

ADMINISTRATION/HANDLING
PO
Immediate-release tablets • Administer with water on an empty stomach at least 1 hr prior to meals.
Extended-release capsules • Give whole (do not crush, break, or dissolve).
• Administer with water on empty stomach at least 1 hr before morning meal.

INDICATIONS/ROUTES/DOSAGE
Overactive Bladder
PO: ADULTS: *(Immediate-Release):* 20 mg twice daily. **ELDERLY 75 YRS AND OLDER:** 20 mg once daily. **ADULTS, ELDERLY:** *(Extended-Release):* 60 mg once daily in the morning.

Dosage in Renal Impairment
CrCl less than 30 mL/min: Immediate-release dose is reduced to 20 mg once daily at bedtime. Extended-release not recommended.

Dosage in Hepatic Impairment
Mild impairment: No dose adjustment. **Moderate to severe impairment:** Use with caution.

SIDE EFFECTS
Frequent (20%): Dry mouth. **Occasional (10%–4%):** Constipation, headache. **Rare (less than 2%):** Fatigue, upper abdominal pain, dyspepsia (heartburn, indigestion, epigastric pain), flatulence, dry eyes, urinary retention.

ADVERSE EFFECTS/TOXIC REACTIONS
Overdose may result in severe anticholinergic effects, characterized by nervousness, restlessness, nausea, vomiting, confusion, diaphoresis, facial flushing, hypertension, hypotension, respiratory depression, irritability, lacrimation. Supraventricular tachycardia and hallucinations occur rarely.

NURSING CONSIDERATIONS
BASELINE ASSESSMENT
Assess for dysuria, urinary urgency, frequency, incontinence.

INTERVENTION/EVALUATION
Monitor for symptomatic relief. Monitor I&O; palpate bladder for retention. Monitor daily pattern of bowel activity, stool consistency.

PATIENT/FAMILY TEACHING
• Report nausea, vomiting, diaphoresis, increased salivary secretions, palpitations, severe abdominal pain. **•** Swallow tablets, extended-release capsules whole. **•** Take 1 hr before meals.

ublituximab-xiiy

ue-bli-**tux**-i-mab
(Briumvi)
**Do not confuse ublituximab with
brentuximab, cetuximab, dinutuximab, isatuximab, margetuximab,
mirvetuximab, or rituximab.**

◆CLASSIFICATION

PHARMACOTHERAPEUTIC: CD20-di-
rected cytolytic monoclonal antibody.
CLINICAL: Multiple sclerosis agent.

USES

Treatment of adults with relapsing forms
of multiple sclerosis (MS), to include
clinically isolated syndrome, relapsing-
remitting disease, and active secondary
progressive disease.

PRECAUTIONS

Contraindications: Hypersensitivity to ubli-
tuximab-xiiy. Active hepatitis B virus (HBV)
confirmed by positive test for hepatitis B
surface antigen (HBsAg) and anti-HBV
tests. **Cautions:** Prior treatment-related infusion reactions. Pts who test positive for
hepatitis B core antibody (HBcAb+) or
are carriers of HBV (HBsAg+). Not recommended in pts with active infection.

ACTION

A CD20-directed cytolytic antibody that
targets CD20-expressing B cells (plays a
role in pathogenesis of MS) and binds to
them, triggering a series of immunological
reactions that ultimately lead to cell death,
removing them from circulation. **Therapeutic Effect:** Reduces progression of MS.

PHARMACOKINETICS

Widely distributed. Metabolized by proteolytic enzymes into small peptides and
amino acids. **Half-life:** 22 days.

⏳ LIFESPAN CONSIDERATIONS

Pregnancy/Lactation: Avoid pregnancy; may cause fetal harm (including
B-cell lymphocytopenia). Females of reproductive potential must use effective
contraception during treatment and for
at least 6 mos after discontinuation. Unknown if distributed in breast milk. **Children:** Safety and efficacy not established.
Elderly: Not specified.

INTERACTIONS

DRUG: May decrease therapeutic effect of
vaccines (live); increase adverse effects
of **vaccines (live). Corticosteroids
(e.g., predniSONE)** may increase immunosuppressive effect, risk of infection.
HERBAL: None significant. **FOOD:** None
known. **LAB VALUES:** May decrease neutrophils. Expected to decrease immunoglobulin levels.

AVAILABILITY (Rx)

Injection Solution: 150 mg/6 mL (25
mg/mL).

ADMINISTRATION/HANDLING
 IV

Infusion guidelines • Must be administered by a healthcare professional
trained in the management of infusion
reactions. • Administer via dedicated IV
line. • Monitor for infusion reactions for
at least 1 hr after completion of the first
two infusions (subsequent post-infusion
monitoring is at prescriber discretion). •
If a dose is missed, administer as soon as
possible (do not wait until next scheduled infusion), then reschedule the next
subsequent infusion 24 wks after the
missed dose. Subsequent infusions must
be separated by 5 mos. • If refrigerated,
diluted solutions should be allowed to
warm to room temperature before administration (approx. 2 hrs).
Premedication • Premedicate with
methylPREDNISolone 100 mg IV (or PO
equivalent) approx. 30 min prior to infusion; an antihistamine (e.g., diphenhydrAMINE) PO or IV approx. 30–60 min
prior to each infusion. An antipyretic
(e.g., acetaminophen) may also be considered.

U

Dilution • Visually inspect for particulate matter or discoloration. Solution should appear clear to opalescent, colorless to slightly yellow. Do not use if solution is cloudy or discolored. • Using a 250-mL 0.9% NaCl infusion bag, withdraw and discard a volume that is equal to the volume of the required dose (6 mL for 150-mg dose or 18 mL for 450-mg dose). • Transfer dose from vial into the infusion bag. • Mix by gentle inversion. Do not shake or agitate.

Rate of administration • First infusion: Infuse at 10 mL/hr for 30 min. If no infusion reactions occur, may increase to 20 mL/hr for 30 min, then 35 mL/hr for 1 hr, then 100 mL/hr for remaining 2 hrs. • **Second infusion; subsequent infusions:** Infuse at 100 mL/hr for 30 min. If no infusion reactions occur, may increase to 400 mL/hr for the remaining 30 min.

Infusion reactions • Mild to moderate reactions: Reduce infusion rate by 50% for at least 30 min. If reaction is tolerated, may re-escalate infusion rate. • **Severe reactions:** Interrupt infusion and treat symptoms. Once symptoms resolve, restart infusion at a reduced rate by 50% for at least 30 min. If tolerated, may re-escalate infusion rate.

Storage • Refrigerate unused vials in original carton. Protect from light. Do not freeze or shake. • Use immediately after dilution. May refrigerate diluted solution for up to 24 hrs. If refrigerated, allow to equilibrate to room temperature (about 2 hrs) and can be stored at room temperature for an additional 8 hrs (which includes time to warm to room temperature and infusion time).

INDICATIONS/ROUTES/DOSAGE

Multiple Sclerosis
IV: ADULTS, ELDERLY: **(Step-up dosing schedule):** 150 mg once, then 450 mg given 2 wks after first infusion, then 450 mg once 24 wks after first infusion (150 mg), then 450 mg once q24wks.

Dosage in Renal/Hepatic Impairment
Mild impairment: No dose adjustment.

Moderate to severe impairment: Not specified; use caution.

SIDE EFFECTS

Occasional (6%): Extremity pain, insomnia. **Rare (5%):** Fatigue.

ADVERSE EFFECTS/TOXIC REACTIONS

Life-threatening infections, including bacterial, fungal, viral infection, upper and lower respiratory tract infections, herpes virus infection, have occurred. Infections reported in 56% of pts. Infusion reactions, including anaphylaxis, chills, erythema, headache, influenza-like illness, nausea, pyrexia, tachycardia, throat irritation, may be life-threatening. HBV reactivation may occur, which may result in fulminant hepatitis, hepatic failure, death. Progressive multifocal leukoencephalopathy (PML), an opportunistic viral infection of the brain caused by the JC virus, may result in progressive permanent disability and death.

NURSING CONSIDERATIONS

BASELINE ASSESSMENT

Obtain pregnancy test in females of reproductive potential. Confirm compliance with effective contraception. Obtain HBV screening, quantitative serum immunoglobulin prior to initiation. For pts who are negative for HBsAg and positive for hepatitis B core antibody (HBcAb+) or are carriers of HBV (HBsAg+), consult hepatology prior to and during treatment. For pts with low serum immunoglobulins, consult immunology prior to initiation. Ensure all immunizations are up-to-date. If live-attenuated or live vaccine immunization is required, give at least 1 mo prior to initiation. Question history of herpes zoster infection, chronic infection. Administer in an environment equipped to monitor for and manage infusion reactions. Question for prior infusion reactions before each infusion. Screen for active infection. Offer emotional support.

U

INTERVENTION/EVALUATION

Assess for infusion reactions during each infusion. If reactions occur, interrupt or decrease the infusion rate. Early detection and management are vital. If anaphylactic reaction occurs, initiate supportive care (antipyretics, corticosteroids, oxygen therapy, IV hydration). Pts with altered mental status, seizures, visual disturbances, generalized or unilateral weakness should be evaluated for herpes zoster meningoencephalitis, PML. Monitor for infections (body aches, cough, fever, fatigue), herpes zoster, or hepatitis B virus reactivation. If serious infection or sepsis occurs, initiate appropriate antimicrobial therapy. Conduct routine neurological assessments. Monitor for improvement of MS symptoms.

PATIENT/FAMILY TEACHING

• Treatment may depress your immune system and reduce your ability to fight infection. Report symptoms of infection such as body aches, burning with urination, chills, cough, fatigue, fever. Avoid those with active infection. Report travel plans to possible endemic areas. • PML, an opportunistic viral infection of the brain, may cause progressive, permanent disabilities or death. Report symptoms of PML such as confusion, memory loss, paralysis, trouble speaking, vision loss, seizures, weakness. • Immediately report symptoms of infusion reactions such as chills, cough, difficulty breathing, itching, palpitations. If allergic reaction occurs, seek immediate medical attention. • Pretreatment with acetaminophen, antihistamines, steroidal anti-inflammatories may help reduce infusion reactions. • All vaccinations should be up-to-date prior to starting treatment. • Use effective contraception to avoid pregnancy. • Do not receive live vaccines within 4 wks of initiation.

ubrogepant

ue-**broe**-je-pant
(Ubrelvy)

Do not confuse ubrogepant with atogepant, rimegepant, or zavegepant.

◆**Classification**

PHARMACOTHERAPEUTIC: Calcitonin gene–related peptide (CGRP) receptor antagonist. **CLINICAL:** Antimigraine.

USES

Treatment of acute (moderate to severe) migraines with or without aura in adults.

PRECAUTIONS

Contraindications: Hypersensitivity to ubrogepant. Concomitant use of strong CYP3A4 inhibitors. **Cautions:** Hepatic/renal impairment. Not indicated for prevention of migraine. Avoid concomitant use of strong CYP3A4 inducers.

ACTION

Exact mechanism of action unknown. Binds to and inhibits calcitonin gene–related peptide (CGRP) receptor. **Therapeutic Effect:** Relieves migraine headache.

PHARMACOKINETICS

Widely distributed. Metabolized in liver. Protein binding: 87%. Peak plasma concentration: 1.5 hrs. Excreted in feces (42%), urine (6%). **Half-life:** 5–7 hrs.

⧗ LIFESPAN CONSIDERATIONS

Pregnancy/Lactation: May cause fetal harm. Unknown if distributed in breast milk. **Children:** Safety and efficacy not established. **Elderly:** No age-related precautions noted.

INTERACTIONS

DRUG: Strong CYP3A4 inhibitors (e.g., clarithromycin, ketoconazole, ritonavir), moderate CYP3A4 inhibitors (e.g., cycloSPORINE, fluconazole, verapamil), P-gp inhibitors (e.g., amiodarone, carvedilol, clarithromycin, itraconazole, verapamil) may increase concentration/

effect. **Strong CYP3A4 inducers (e.g., carBAMazepine, phenytoin, rifAMPin), moderate CYP3A4 inducers (e.g., dexamethasone, modafinil, nafcillin)** may decrease concentration/effect. **HERBAL:** **St. John's wort** may decrease concentration/effect. **FOOD:** None known. **LAB VALUES:** None known.

AVAILABILITY (Rx)

Tablets: 50 mg, 100 mg.

ADMINISTRATION/HANDLING

PO
• Give without regard to food.

INDICATIONS/ROUTES/DOSAGE

Migraine (With or Without Aura)
PO: ADULTS: 50 mg or 100 mg as a single dose. May repeat dose at least 2 hrs after initial dose. Do not exceed 200 mg in a 24-hr period.

Dose Modification

Concomitant Drug	Initial Dose	Second Dose (if Needed)
Moderate CYP3A4 inhibitors	50 mg	Avoid within 24 hrs
Weak CYP3A4 inhibitors	50 mg	50 mg
BCRP and/or P-gp only inhibitors	50 mg	50 mg
Strong CYP3A4 inducers	Avoid use	Avoid use
Weak or moderate CYP3A4 inducers	100 mg	100 mg

Dosage in Renal Impairment
Mild to moderate impairment: No dose adjustment. **Severe impairment: (CrCl 15–29 mL/min):** Initially, 50 mg. May repeat 50 mg dose at least 2 hrs after initial dose. **ESRD (CrCl less than 15 mL/min):** Avoid use.

Dosage in Hepatic Impairment
Mild to moderate impairment: No dose adjustment. **Severe impairment:**

Initially, 50 mg. May repeat 50 mg dose at least 2 hrs after initial dose.

SIDE EFFECTS

Rare (2%–1%): Nausea, somnolence, dry mouth.

ADVERSE EFFECTS/TOXIC REACTIONS

None known.

NURSING CONSIDERATIONS

BASELINE ASSESSMENT

Question characteristics of migraine headaches (onset, location, duration, possible precipitating symptoms). Receive full medication history and screen for interactions. Question history of hepatic/renal impairment.

INTERVENTION/EVALUATION

Evaluate for relief of migraine headaches (photophobia, phonophobia, nausea, vomiting, pain, dizziness, fogginess).

PATIENT/FAMILY TEACHING

• There is a high risk of interactions with other medications. Do not take newly prescribed medications unless approved by prescriber who originally started therapy. Do not take herbal products (esp. St. John's wort) or ingest grapefruit products. • Avoid tasks that require alertness, motor skills until response to drug is established.

umeclidinium

ue-**mek**-li-**din**-ee-um
(Incruse Ellipta)
Do not confuse umeclidinium with aclidinium or clidinium.

FIXED-COMBINATION(S)

Anoro Ellipta: umeclidinium/vilanterol (bronchodilator): 62.5 mcg/25 mcg. **Trelegy Ellipta:** umeclidinium/fluticasone (corticosteroid)/vilanterol (bronchodilator): 62.5 mcg/100 mcg/25 mcg.

U

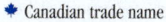 Canadian trade name    Non-Crushable Drug   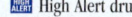 High Alert drug

◆CLASSIFICATION

PHARMACOTHERAPEUTIC: Anticholinergic. **CLINICAL:** Bronchodilator (long-acting).

USES

Long-term maintenance treatment of chronic obstructive pulmonary disease (COPD).

PRECAUTIONS

Contraindications: Hypersensitivity to umeclidinium. Severe hypersensitivity to milk proteins or any drug components. **Cautions:** Bladder neck obstruction, myasthenia gravis, narrow-angle glaucoma, prostatic hypertrophy, urinary retention. Not recommended in pts with acutely deteriorating COPD requiring emergent relief of acute symptoms.

ACTION

Inhibits muscarinic M_3 receptor in lungs, resulting in relaxation of bronchial smooth muscle. **Therapeutic Effect:** Relieves bronchospasm, reduces airway resistance, improves bronchodilation.

PHARMACOKINETICS

Rapidly absorbed following inhalation. Primarily metabolized by enzyme cytochrome P4502D6. Protein binding: 89%. Peak concentration: 5–15 min. Steady state reached within 14 days. **Half-life:** 11 hrs.

⧖ LIFESPAN CONSIDERATIONS

Pregnancy/Lactation: Unknown if distributed in breast milk. Must either discontinue drug or discontinue breastfeeding. **Children:** Not indicated in this pt population. **Elderly:** No age-related precautions noted.

INTERACTIONS

DRUG: Anticholinergics (e.g., aclidinium, ipratropium, tiotropium) may increase anticholinergic effect. **HERBAL:** None significant. **FOOD:** None known. **LAB VALUES:** None known.

AVAILABILITY (Rx)

Inhalation Powder, Breath-Activated: 62.5 mcg/capsule (in blister packs containing 7 or 30 doses).

ADMINISTRATION/HANDLING

Inhalation

Administration • Follow instructions for preparation according to manufacturer guidelines. • No need to shake the inhaler. Prior to inhaling dose, exhale fully (do not exhale into inhaler). Close lips tightly around inhaler and inhale (rapidly, steadily, and deeply). Do not breathe through nose or block air vent with fingers. • Remove mouthpiece and hold breath for 3–4 sec, then breathe out slowly and gently. Do not close container until medication has been inhaled. • Close lid cover.

Storage • Store at room temperature up to 6 wks after opening tray. • Do not refrigerate or freeze. • Protect from sunlight and moisture. • Discard after counter reaches 0. • Do not reuse inhaler.

INDICATIONS/ROUTES/DOSAGE

COPD

Inhalation: ADULTS, ELDERLY: One inhalation (62.5 mcg) once daily, at same time each day. **Maximum:** 1 inhalation/24 hrs.

Dose Modification
Deterioration of COPD: Discontinue treatment. Initiate short-acting bronchodilators and supportive pulmonary therapy.

Dosage in Renal Impairment
No dose adjustment.

Dosage in Hepatic Impairment
Mild to moderate impairment: No dose adjustment. **Severe impairment:** Use caution.

SIDE EFFECTS

Occasional (8%–5%): Nasopharyngitis, upper respiratory tract infection. **Rare (3%–1%):** Cough, arthralgia, viral respiratory tract infection, pharyngitis, myalgia, abdominal pain, toothache, tachycardia.

ADVERSE EFFECTS/TOXIC REACTIONS

Life-threatening asthma-related events, bronchospasm, worsening of COPD-related symptoms have been reported. Hypersensitivity reactions may occur (esp. in pts with undiagnosed severe milk protein allergy or allergy to products containing lactose). Worsening of narrow-angle glaucoma (eye pain, blurry vision, visual halos, colored images in association with red eyes from conjunctival congestion and corneal edema) may occur. May cause worsening of urinary retention, esp. in pts with prostatic hypertrophy or bladder neck obstruction.

NURSING CONSIDERATIONS

BASELINE ASSESSMENT

Obtain O_2 saturation, vital signs; pulmonary function test, if applicable. Assess respiratory rate, depth, rhythm. Assess lung sounds for wheezing. Screen for concomitant use of anticholinergic medications. Question history of asthma, BPH, bladder neck obstruction, glaucoma. Teach proper inhaler priming and administration techniques. Conduct ophthalmologic exam in pts with narrow-angle glaucoma.

INTERVENTION/EVALUATION

Routinely monitor O_2 saturation, vital signs. Auscultate lung sounds and monitor for symptom improvement. Recommend discontinuation of short-acting beta₂-agonists while on long-term therapy. Monitor for COPD deterioration, narrow-angle glaucoma, urinary retention/obstruction. Monitor for increased use of rescue inhaler; may indicate worsening of respiratory status.

PATIENT/FAMILY TEACHING

• Report fever, productive cough, body aches, paradoxical bronchospasm, difficulty breathing; may indicate lung infection, worsening of COPD. • Therapy not intended for acute COPD symptom relief, and extra doses are not advised. • Report symptoms of acute narrow-angle glaucoma, urinary retention, bladder distention. • Refill prescription when counter on left of inhaler reaches red area of scale. • Follow manufacturer guidelines for proper use of inhaler. • Drink plenty of fluids (decreases lung secretion viscosity). • Rinse mouth with water after inhalation to decrease mouth/throat irritation.

---

upadacitinib

ue-**pad**-a-**sye**-ti-nib
(Rinvoq)

■ **BLACK BOX ALERT** ■ Increased risk for developing bacterial, invasive fungal, viral, other opportunistic infections (including tuberculosis, herpes zoster, cryptococcosis, pneumocystosis), which may lead to hospitalization or death. Infections often occurred in combination with other immunosuppressants (methotrexate, other disease-modifying antirheumatic drugs). Closely monitor for infections. Test for latent tuberculosis prior to initiation and during treatment, regardless of initial result. Latent TB should be treated prior to initiation. Lymphomas, other malignancies were reported. Thromboembolic events, including deep vein thrombosis (DVT), pulmonary embolism (PE), arterial thrombosis, have occurred. Higher rate of all-cause mortality, including sudden cardiovascular death, was observed. Major adverse cardiovascular events (cardiovascular death, myocardial infarction, and stroke) were observed in pts with at least one cardiovascular risk factor.
Do not confuse upadacitinib with baricitinib or tofacitinib.

◆**CLASSIFICATION**

PHARMACOTHERAPEUTIC: Janus kinase (JAK) inhibitor. **CLINICAL:** Disease-modifying antirheumatic drug (DMARD).

USES

Active non-radiographic axial spondyloarthritis: Treatment of adults with active non-radiographic axial spondyloarthritis with objective signs of inflammation who have had an inadequate response or intolerance to TNF blocker therapy. **Ankylosing spondylitis:** Treatment of active ankylosing spondylitis in adults who have had an inadequate response or intolerance to one or more TNF blockers. **Atopic dermatitis:** Treatment of refractory, moderate-to-severe atopic dermatitis in adults and children 12 yrs of age and older weighing 40 kg whose disease is not adequately controlled with other systemic drug products, including biologics, or when use of those therapies is inadvisable. **Crohn's disease:** Treatment of adults with moderately to severely active Crohn's disease who had an inadequate response to or intolerance of one or more TNF blockers. **Polyarticular juvenile idiopathic arthritis (pJIA):** Treatment of pts age 2 yrs and older with active pJIA who have had an inadequate response or intolerance to one or more TNF blockers. **Psoriatic arthritis:** Treatment of active psoriatic arthritis in adults and children age 2 yrs and older who have had an inadequate response or intolerance to one or more TNF blockers. **Rheumatoid arthritis:** Treatment of moderately to severely active rheumatoid arthritis in adults who have had an inadequate response or intolerance to one or more TNF blockers. **Ulcerative colitis:** Treatment of moderately to severely active ulcerative colitis in adults who have had an inadequate response or intolerance to one or more TNF blockers.

PRECAUTIONS

Contraindications: Hypersensitivity to upadacitinib. **Cautions:** Baseline cytopenias, hepatic/renal impairment, elderly, uncontrolled hyperlipidemia; history of arterial or venous thrombosis (CVA, DVT, MI, PE); pts at risk for thrombosis (immobility, indwelling venous catheter/access device, morbid obesity, underlying atherosclerosis, genetic hypercoagulable conditions), recent travel or residence in TB- or mycosis-endemic areas; history of chronic opportunistic infections (bacterial, invasive fungal, mycobacterial, protozoal, viral, TB); infections including HIV, herpes zoster, hepatitis B or C virus; conditions predisposing to infection (e.g., diabetes, renal failure, immunocompromised pts, open wounds), pts at risk for GI perforation (e.g., Crohn's disease, diverticulitis, GI tract or abdominal malignancies, GI ulcers). Use of live, attenuated vaccines is not recommended.

ACTION

Inhibits JAK enzymes, which are intracellular enzymes involved in stimulating hematopoiesis and immune cell function via signaling pathway. **Therapeutic Effect:** Reduces inflammation, tenderness, swelling of joints; slows or prevents progressive joint destruction in rheumatoid arthritis (RA).

PHARMACOKINETICS

Widely distributed. Metabolized in liver. Protein binding: 52%. Peak plasma concentration: 2–4 hrs. Excreted in feces (38%), urine (24%). **Half-life:** 8–14 hrs.

LIFESPAN CONSIDERATIONS

Pregnancy/Lactation: Avoid pregnancy; may cause fetal harm. Females of reproductive potential must use effective contraception during treatment and for at least 4 wks after discontinuation. Unknown if distributed in breast milk. Breastfeeding not recommended during treatment and for at least 6 days after discontinuation. **Children:** Safety and efficacy not established. **Elderly:** No age-related precautions noted.

INTERACTIONS

DRUG: May decrease therapeutic effect of **vaccines (live), BCG (intravesical).** May increase adverse/toxic effects of **natalizumab, live vaccines. Strong CYP3A4 inhibitors** (e.g., **clarithro-**

mycin, **ketoconazole, ritonavir)** may increase concentration/effect. **Strong CYP3A4 inducers (e.g., rifAMPin, phenytoin, carBAMazepine, PHENobarbital)** may decrease concentration/effect. **HERBAL: Echinacea** may decrease therapeutic effect. **FOOD:** None known. **LAB VALUES:** May increase serum ALT, AST, creatine phosphokinase, low-density lipoprotein (LDL), high-density lipoprotein (HDL), total cholesterol. May decrease absolute lymphocyte count, absolute neutrophil count (ANC), Hgb.

AVAILABILITY (Rx)

Oral solution: 1 mg/mL.

 Tablets, Extended-Release: 15 mg, 30 mg, 45 mg.

ADMINISTRATION/HANDLING

PO

Tablets, extended-release • Give without regard to food. • Administer tablet whole; do not break, crush, or allow chewing.

Oral solution • Use the provided press-in bottle adapter and oral dosing syringe. **Note:** Not substitutable with extended-release tablets.

INDICATIONS/ROUTES/DOSAGE

◀ALERT▶ Do not initiate in pts with severe, active infection (systemic/localized), absolute lymphocyte count less than 500 cells/mm³, ANC less than 1,000 cells/mm³, Hgb less than 8 g/dL; severe hepatic impairment. Do not use in combination with other JAK inhibitors, biologic DMARDs, strong immunosuppressants (e.g., azathioprine, cycloSPORINE).

Active Non-Radiographic Axial Spondyloarthritis

PO: ADULTS, ELDERLY: 15 mg once daily.

Ankylosing Spondylitis

PO: ADULTS, ELDERLY: 15 mg once daily.

Atopic Dermatitis

PO: ADULT YOUNGER THAN 65 YRS, CHILDREN 12 YRS OF AGE AND OLDER WEIGHING 40 KG OR GREATER: 15 mg once daily. If response is inadequate, may increase to 30 mg once daily. **ADULTS 65 YRS AND OLDER.** 15 mg once daily.

Crohn's Disease

PO: ADULTS, ELDERLY: (Induction): 45 mg once daily for 12 wks. **(Maintenance):** 15 mg once daily (may increase to 30 mg for pts with refractory, severe, or extensive disease). Discontinue if an adequate therapeutic response is not achieved with the 30-mg dose.

pJIA

PO: CHILDREN WEIGHING 30 KG AND GREATER: 6 mg (6 mL oral solution) twice daily or 15 mg tablet once daily. **20–29 KG:** 4 mg (4 mL oral solution) twice daily. **10–19 KG:** 3 mg (3 mL oral solution) twice daily.

Psoriatic Arthritis

PO: ADULTS, ELDERLY: 15 mg once daily. **CHILDREN 30 KG AND GREATER:** 6 mg (6 mL oral solution) twice daily or 15 mg tablet once daily. **20–29 KG:** 4 mg (4 mL oral solution) twice daily. **10–19 KG:** 3 mg (3 mL oral solution) twice daily.

Rheumatoid Arthritis

PO: ADULTS: 15 mg once daily.

Ulcerative Colitis

PO: ADULTS, ELDERLY: (Induction): 45 mg once daily for 8 wks. **(Maintenance):** 15 mg once daily. May increase to 30 mg once daily in pts with refractory, severe, or extensive disease.

Dose Modification

Hematologic Toxicity

Hgb less than 8 g/dL: Withhold treatment until Hgb is greater than or equal to 8 gm/dL, then resume treatment. **Absolute lymphocyte count (ALC) less than 500 cells/mm³:** Withhold treatment until ALC is greater than or equal to 500 cells/mm³, then resume treatment. **ANC less than 1,000 cells/mm³:** Withhold treatment until ANC is greater than or equal to 1,000 cells/mm³, then resume treatment.

Hepatotoxicity

Withhold treatment until hepatotoxicity is resolved, then resume if clinically indicated.

Serious Infection

Withhold treatment until serious infection is resolved, then resume if clinically indicated

U

Dosage in Renal Impairment
Mild to severe impairment: No dose adjustment.

Dosage in Hepatic Impairment
Mild to moderate impairment: No dose adjustment. **Severe impairment:** Not recommended.

SIDE EFFECTS
Rare (4%–1%): Nausea, cough, pyrexia.

ADVERSE EFFECTS/TOXIC REACTIONS
Neutropenia, lymphopenia may increase risk of infection. Serious and sometimes fatal infections (bacterial, mycobacterial, invasive fungal, viral, other opportunistic infections) may occur. Serious infections may include cellulitis, cryptococcosis, esophageal candidiasis, herpes zoster, pneumonia, pneumocystosis, TB. Upper respiratory tract infections (laryngitis, nasopharyngitis, pharyngitis, pharyngotonsillitis, rhinitis, sinusitis, tonsillitis, viral infection) reported in 14% of pts. May cause viral reactivation of hepatitis B virus, herpes zoster. New nonmelanoma skin malignancies, lymphomas were reported. Thromboembolic events including DVT, pulmonary embolism, arterial thrombosis have occurred. May increase risk of GI perforation.

NURSING CONSIDERATIONS

BASELINE ASSESSMENT
Obtain CBC, LFT, lipid panel; pregnancy test in females of reproductive potential. Confirm compliance of effective contraception. Evaluate for active TB and test for latent TB infection. An induration of 5 mm or greater with purified protein derivative (PPD) is considered a positive result when assessing for latent TB. Consider treatment with antimycobacterial therapy in pts with latent TB. Screen for active infection. Question history of arterial/venous thrombosis, hepatic/renal impairment; chronic infections including HIV, hepatitis B or C virus, herpes zoster. Assess risk of GI perforation. Receive full medication history and screen for interactions. Recommend up-to-date vaccinations (non-live, attenuated), including prophylactic zoster vaccination, prior to initiation. Assess onset, location, duration of pain, inflammation. Inspect appearance of affected joints for immobility, deformities.

INTERVENTION/EVALUATION
Monitor CBC, LFT periodically; lipid panel 12 wks after initiation and as indicated thereafter. Monitor for TB regardless of baseline PPD. Diligently monitor for infections (cough, fatigue, fever). If severe acute infection, opportunistic infection occurs, withhold treatment and initiate appropriate antimicrobial therapy. Monitor for symptoms of GI perforation (abdominal pain, fever, melena, hematemesis); DVT (leg or arm pain/swelling), CVA (aphasia, altered mental status, hemiplegia, vision loss; seizures); MI (arm/jaw pain, chest pain, diaphoresis, dyspnea), PE (chest pain, dyspnea, tachycardia), hepatotoxicity (bruising, jaundice, right upper abdominal pain, nausea, vomiting, weight loss), viral infection reactivation. Assess for therapeutic response: relief of pain, stiffness, swelling; increased joint mobility; reduced joint tenderness; improved grip strength.

PATIENT/FAMILY TEACHING
• Treatment may depress your immune system response and reduce your ability to fight infection. Report symptoms of infection such as body aches, chills, cough, fatigue, fever. Avoid those with active infection. • Expect routine tuberculosis screening. Report any travel plans to possible endemic areas. • Do not receive live vaccines. • Report liver problems (abdominal pain, bruising, clay-colored stool, dark or amber-colored urine, yellowing of the skin or eyes; symptoms of DVT (swelling, pain, hot feeling in the arms or legs; discoloration of extremity). • Life-threatening arterial blood clots may occur; report symptoms of heart attack (chest pain, difficulty breathing, jaw pain, nausea, pain that radiates to the arm, sweating), lung embo-

lism (difficulty breathing, chest pain, rapid heart rate), stroke (confusion, difficulty speaking, one-sided weakness or paralysis, loss of vision). • Report severe or persistent abdominal pain, bloody stool, fever, vomiting; may indicate rupture in GI tract. • Treatment may cause reactivation of chronic infections, new cancers. • Use effective contraception to avoid pregnancy. Do not breastfeed.

ustekinumab
TOP 100

yoo-ste-**kin**-ue-mab
(Imuldosa, Otulfi, Pyzchiva, Stelara, Selarsdi, Steqeyma, Wezlana)
Do not confuse Stelara with Aldara, or ustekinumab with inFLIXimab or riTUXimab.

◆CLASSIFICATION
PHARMACOTHERAPEUTIC: Interleukin-12, interleukin-23 inhibitor, monoclonal antibody. **CLINICAL:** Antipsoriasis agent.

USES
Plaque psoriasis: Treatment of adults, children 6 yrs or older with moderate to severe plaque psoriasis who are candidates for systemic therapy or phototherapy. **Psoriatic arthritis:** Treatment of adults, children 6 yrs or older with active psoriatic arthritis. **Crohn's disease:** Treatment of adults with moderate to severe active Crohn's disease. **Ulcerative colitis:** Treatment of adults with moderate to severe active ulcerative colitis.

PRECAUTIONS
Contraindications: Hypersensitivity to ustekinumab. **Cautions:** Prior malignancies (esp. skin cancer), pts who resided or traveled to endemic areas; conditions predisposing to infection (e.g., diabetes, renal failure, immunocompromised pts, open wounds), history of chronic opportunistic infections (esp. bacterial, invasive fungal, mycobacterial, protozoal,

viral infections including herpes zoster, TB). Avoid use of live vaccines.

ACTION
Binds to and interferes with proinflammatory cytokines, interleukin-12, and interleukin-23, reducing these proinflammatory signalers. **Therapeutic Effect:** Shows clinical improvement of psoriasis, psoriatic arthritis.

PHARMACOKINETICS
Widely distributed. Degraded into small peptides and amino acids via catabolic pathways. Steady state reached in 28 wks. **Half-life:** 10–126 days.

⧖ LIFESPAN CONSIDERATIONS
Pregnancy/Lactation: Unknown if distributed in breast milk. **Children:** Safety and efficacy not established in pts younger than 6 yrs. **Elderly:** May have increased risk of infections.

INTERACTIONS
DRUG: May decrease therapeutic effect; increase adverse effects of **vaccines (live), BCG (intravesical).** May increase immunosuppressive effect of **baricitinib, inFLIXimab, upadacitinib. Belimumab, cladribine** may increase the immunosuppressive effect. May increase the toxic effect of **natalizumab. HERBAL: Echinacea** may decrease therapeutic effect. **FOOD:** None known. **LAB VALUES:** May increase lymphocyte count.

AVAILABILITY (Rx)
Injection Solution, Intravenous: 130 mg/26 mL. **Injection Solution, SQ (Prefilled Syringes):** 45 mg/0.5 mL, 90 mg/mL. **Injection Solution, SQ:** 45 mg/0.5 mL.

ADMINISTRATION/HANDLING
🖱 **IV**
Reconstitution • Calculate the number of vials needed for dose based on pt's weight. • Withdraw and discard a volume from 250-mL 0.9% NaCl infusion bag equal to the volume of vials needed for

dose. • Withdraw calculated dose from vial or vials and add to infusion bag to equal a final volume of 250 mL. • Visually inspect for particulate matter or discoloration. Do not use if solution is cloudy, discolored, or if visible particles are observed. **Rate of administration** • Infuse over at least 60 min. Use an in-line, low-protein-binding filter (0.2 microns).

Storage • Refrigerate unused vials in original carton until time of use. • Protect from light. • Keep vials upright. • Diluted solution may be stored at room temperature for up to 7 hrs.

SQ

Preparation • Visually inspect for particulate matter or discoloration. Solution should appear clear and colorless to slightly yellow in color. • Solution may contain a few small translucent or white particles.

Administration • Insert needle subcutaneously into upper arm, outer thigh, or abdomen and inject solution. • Do not inject into areas of active skin disease or injury such as sunburns, skin rashes, inflammation, skin infections, or active psoriasis. • Do not administer IV or intramuscular. • Rotate injection sites.

Storage • Refrigerate prefilled syringes in original carton until time of use. • Protect from light. • Do not freeze or expose to heating sources. • Do not shake.

INDICATIONS/ROUTES/DOSAGE

Plaque Psoriasis

SQ: ADULTS, ELDERLY WEIGHING 100 KG OR LESS: Initially, 45 mg, then 45 mg 4 wks later, followed by 45 mg every 12 wks. **WEIGHING MORE THAN 100 KG:** Initially, 90 mg, then 90 mg 4 wks later, followed by 90 mg every 12 wks. **Note:** 45 mg also efficacious; however, 90 mg is recommended due to greater efficacy. **CHILDREN 6 YRS AND OLDER WEIGHING MORE THAN 100 KG:** Initially, 90 mg, repeat in 4 wks, then q12 wks. **WEIGHING 60–100 KG:** Initially, 45 mg, repeat in 4 wks, then q12 wks. **WEIGHING 59 KG OR LESS:** Initially, 0.75 mg/kg, repeat in 4 wks, then q12 wks.

Psoriatic Arthritis

SQ: ADULTS, ELDERLY, CHILDREN 6–17 YRS WEIGHING 60 KG OR MORE: 45 mg repeated in 4 wks followed by 45 mg q12wks. **CHILDREN 6–17 YRS WEIGHING 59 KG OR LESS:** Initially, 0.75 mg/kg then repeat in 4 wks, then q12wks. **ADULTS, ELDERLY, CHILDREN 6–17 YRS WEIGHING 100 KG OR MORE WITH COEXISTENT MODERATE TO SEVERE PLAQUE PSORIASIS:** 90 mg repeated in 4 wks, then 90 mg q12wks. **WEIGHING 60–100 KG:** Initially, 45 mg, repeat in 4 wks, then q12 wks. **WEIGHING 59 KG OR LESS:** Initially, 0.75 mg/kg, repeat in 4 wks, then q12 wks.

Crohn's Disease

IV infusion: ADULTS, ELDERLY: Induction: (as a single dose) 520 mg (greater than 85 kg); 390 mg (56–85 kg); 260 mg (less than 56 kg). **SQ: Maintenance:** 90 mg q8wks beginning 8 wks following the IV induction dose.

Ulcerative Colitis

IV: ADULTS, ELDERLY WEIGHING MORE THAN 85 KG: Induction: 520 mg as single dose. **WEIGHING 56–85 KG:** 390 mg as single dose. **WEIGHING LESS THAN 56 KG:** 260 mg as single dose. **SQ: Maintenance:** 90 mg q8wks (starting 8 wks after IV induction dose).

Dosage in Renal/Hepatic Impairment
No dose adjustment.

SIDE EFFECTS

Occasional (8%–4%): Nasopharyngitis, upper respiratory tract infection, headache. **Rare (3%–1%):** Fatigue, diarrhea, back pain, dizziness, pruritus, injection site erythema, myalgia, depression.

ADVERSE EFFECTS/TOXIC REACTIONS

May increase risk of acute infections; reactivation of latent infections. Serious invasive and opportunistic bacterial, mycobacterial, fungal, viral infections (anal abscess, appendicitis, cellulitis, cholecystitis, diverticulitis, gastroenteritis, *Listeria* meningitis, listeriosis, ophthalmic herpes zoster, osteomyelitis, pneumonia, sepsis, TB, UTI, viral infections) requiring hospitalization were reported. May increase risk of new malignancies. Hypersensitivity reactions including angioedema, anaphylaxis were reported. Reversible posterior leukoencephalopathy syndrome (RPLS) may present as aphasia, altered mental status, paralysis, vision loss, weakness. Noninfectious pneumonias (interstitial/eosinophilic/cryptogenic-organizing pneumonia) were reported. Pts genetically deficient in IL-12/IL-23 are at an increased risk of disseminated infections from mycobacteria (non-tuberculosis, environmental mycobacterial), salmonella, BCG vaccines.

NURSING CONSIDERATIONS

BASELINE ASSESSMENT

Obtain pregnancy test in females of reproductive potential. Conduct dermatological exam; record characteristics of psoriatic lesions. Assess degree of abdominal pain, cramping; usual bowel movement patterns, stool characteristics in pts with UC. Evaluate for active TB and test for latent infection. An induration of 5 mm or greater with purified protein derivative (PPD) is considered a positive result when assessing for latent TB. Screen for active infection; history of chronic, opportunistic infections. Question history of prior malignancies. Consider completion of age-appropriate immunizations prior to initiation. BCG vaccines should not be given 1 yr prior to initiation or 1 yr after discontinuation.

INTERVENTION/EVALUATION

Obtain CBC if infection is suspected. Monitor for symptoms of TB (cough, fatigue, hemoptysis, nocturnal sweating, weight loss), including those who tested negative for latent TB infection. Monitor for infections (abdominal pain, cough, fatigue, fever). Interrupt or discontinue treatment if serious infection, opportunistic infection, or sepsis occurs. RPLS should be considered in pts with altered mental status, confusion, headache, seizures, visual disturbances. Assess skin for improvement of lesions in pts with psoriasis; decreased abdominal pain, cramping, diarrhea; increased appetite, weight gain in pts with UC.

PATIENT/FAMILY TEACHING

• Treatment may depress your immune system and reduce your ability to fight infection. Report symptoms of infection such as body aches, burning with urination, chills, cough, fatigue, fever; fungal infections. Avoid those with active infection. • Report travel plans to possible endemic areas. • Do not receive live vaccines, BCG vaccines. • Expect frequent TB screening. • Dormant or chronic viral, invasive fungal infections may become reactivated. • Nervous system changes including altered mental status, seizures, headache, blurry vision, high blood pressure, trouble speaking, one-sided weakness may indicate life-threatening brain dysfunction/swelling. • Treatment may cause new cancers. • Life-threatening allergic reactions (anaphylaxis, swelling of face, tongue, throat) must be reported immediately, regardless of the time the dose was administered.

U

valACYclovir

val-a-**sye**-kloe-veer
(Valtrex)
**Do not confuse valACYclovir
with acyclovir or valGANciclovir,
or Valtrex with Keflex or Valcyte.**

◆CLASSIFICATION

PHARMACOTHERAPEUTIC: Nucleoside analogue DNA polymerase inhibitor. **CLINICAL:** Antiviral.

USES

Cold sores (herpes labialis): Treatment of cold sores (herpes labialis) in adults and pts 12 yrs of age and older. **Genital herpes:** Treatment of the initial episode and recurrent episodes in immunocompetent adults. Chronic suppressive therapy of recurrent episodes in immunocompetent and in HIV-1–infected adults. Reduction of transmission of genital herpes in immunocompetent adults. **Herpes zoster:** Treatment of herpes zoster (shingles) in immunocompetent adults. **Chickenpox:** Treatment of chickenpox in immunocompetent pts aged 2 to less than 18 yrs. **OFF-LABEL:** Bell's palsy (new onset), cytomegalovirus (prevention in cell transplant pts), herpes simplex virus (prevention in immunocompromised pts), *Varicella* (chickenpox) treatment in adults, prevention in immunocompromised pts.

PRECAUTIONS

Contraindications: Hypersensitivity to acyclovir, valACYclovir. **Cautions:** Renal impairment, dehydration, elderly; concomitant use of nephrotoxic medications.

ACTION

Converted to acyclovir by intestinal/hepatic metabolism. Competes for viral DNA polymerase; inhibits incorporation into viral DNA. **Therapeutic Effect:** Inhibits DNA synthesis and viral replication.

PHARMACOKINETICS

Widely distributed to tissues, body fluids (including CSF). Protein binding: 13%–18%. Rapidly converted by hydrolysis to active compound acyclovir. Primarily excreted in urine. Removed by hemodialysis. **Half-life:** Acyclovir: 2.5–3.3 hrs (increased in renal impairment).

⧗ LIFESPAN CONSIDERATIONS

Pregnancy/Lactation: May cross placenta. May be distributed in breast milk. **Children:** Safety and efficacy not established in children younger than 2 yrs (chickenpox); younger than 12 yrs (cold sores). **Elderly:** Age-related renal impairment may require dosage adjustment.

INTERACTIONS

DRUG: Nephrotoxic medications (e.g., foscarnet) may increase risk of nephrotoxicity, renal impairment. May increase concentration/effect of **tiZANidine.** May decrease therapeutic effect of **cladribine.** **HERBAL:** None significant. **FOOD:** None known. **LAB VALUES:** None significant.

AVAILABILITY (Rx)

Tablets: 500 mg, 1,000 mg.

ADMINISTRATION/HANDLING

PO
• Give without regard to food. • If GI upset occurs, give with meals.

INDICATIONS/ROUTES/DOSAGE

Herpes Zoster (Shingles)
PO: ADULTS, ELDERLY: (Immunocompetent): 1 g 3 times/day for 7 days.

Herpes Simplex (Cold Sores)
PO: ADULTS, ELDERLY, CHILDREN 12 YRS AND OLDER: Immunocompetent: 2 g twice daily for 1 day.

Initial Episode of Genital Herpes
PO: ADULTS, ELDERLY: (Immunocompetent): 1 g twice daily for 10 days.

Recurrent Episodes of Genital Herpes
PO: ADULTS, ELDERLY: (Immunocompetent): 500 mg twice daily for 3 days.

Suppressive Therapy of Genital Herpes
PO: ADULTS, ELDERLY: (Immunocompetent): 1 g once daily in pts with normal immune function. In pts with a history of 9 or fewer recurrences/yr, an alternative dose is 500 mg once daily. In pts with HIV-1 with a CD4+ cell count greater than or equal to 100 cells/mm^3, 500 mg twice daily.

Reduction of Transmission
PO: ADULTS, ELDERLY: (Immunocompetent): In pts with a history of 9 or fewer recurrences/yr: 500 mg once daily for the source partner.

Chickenpox
PO: CHILDREN 2–17 YRS: (Immunocompetent): 20 mg/kg/dose 3 times/day for 5 days. **Maximum:** 1 g 3 times/day.

Dosage in Renal Impairment
Dosage and frequency are modified based on creatinine clearance. **Hemodialysis:** Give dose postdialysis.

Cold Sores/Herpes Zoster

Creatinine Clearance	Herpes Zoster	Cold Sores
30–49 mL/min	1 g q12h	1 g q12h × 2 doses
10–29 mL/min	1 g q24h	500 mg q12h × 2 doses
Less than 10 mL/min	500 mg q24h	500 mg as single dose

Genital Herpes

Creatinine Clearance	Initial Episode	Recurrent Episode	Suppressive Therapy
10–29 mL/min	1 g q24h	500 mg q24h	500 mg q24–48h
Less than 10 mL/min	500 mg q24h	500 mg q24h	500 mg q24–48h

Dosage in Hepatic Impairment
No dose adjustment.

SIDE EFFECTS

Frequent: Herpes zoster (17%–10%): Nausea, headache. **Genital herpes (17%):** Headache. **Occasional: Herpes zoster (7%–3%):** Vomiting, diarrhea, constipation (50 yrs and older), asthenia, dizziness (50 yrs and older). **Genital herpes (8%–3%):** Nausea, diarrhea, dizziness. **Rare: Herpes zoster (3%–1%):** Abdominal pain, anorexia. **Genital herpes (3%–1%):** Asthenia, abdominal pain.

ADVERSE EFFECTS/TOXIC REACTIONS

Thrombotic thrombocytopenic purpura/hemolytic uremic syndrome (TTP/HUS) was reported in pts with advanced HIV-1 disease and also allogenic bone marrow or renal transplant. Acute renal failure reported in elderly; pts with dehydration; history of renal impairment; concomitant use of nephrotoxic medications. Central nervous system effects, including agitation, encephalopathy, delirium, seizures, were reported.

NURSING CONSIDERATIONS

BASELINE ASSESSMENT
Tissue cultures for herpes zoster, herpes simplex should be obtained before giving first dose (therapy may proceed before results are known). Assess medical history, esp. HIV infection, bone marrow or renal transplantation, renal/hepatic impairment. Assess characteristics, frequency of lesions.

INTERVENTION/EVALUATION
Monitor CBC, LFT, renal function in pts requiring chronic treatment. Evaluate cutaneous lesions. Provide analgesics, comfort measures for herpes zoster (esp. exhausting to elderly). Encourage adequate hydration. Monitor for agitation, encephalopathy, delirium, seizures.

PATIENT/FAMILY TEACHING
• Drink plenty of fluids. • Do not touch lesions with fingers to avoid spreading infection to new site. • **Genital herpes:** Continue therapy for full length of treatment. • Avoid sexual intercourse during duration of lesions to prevent infecting partner. • ValACYclovir does not cure herpes. • Report if lesions recur or do not improve. • Pap smears should be done at least annually due to increased risk of cervical cancer in women with genital herpes. • Initi-

V

ate treatment at first sign of recurrent episode of genital herpes or herpes zoster (early treatment within first 24–48 hrs is imperative for therapeutic results).

valproic acid

val-**pro**-ick **as**-id
(Apo-Divalproex ✦, Depakote, Depakote ER, Depakote Sprinkle)

■ **BLACK BOX ALERT** ■ Fatal hepatic failure has occurred. Children younger than 2 yrs of age have an increased risk of developing fatal hepatotoxicity. May increase risk of valproate-induced acute hepatic failure and resultant deaths in pts with hereditary neurometabolic syndromes. May cause major congenital malformations, particularly neural tube defects (e.g., spina bifida). Life-threatening pancreatitis was reported. **Do not confuse Depakene with Depakote.**

◆ CLASSIFICATION

PHARMACOTHERAPEUTIC: Histone deacetylase inhibitor. **CLINICAL:** Anticonvulsant, antimanic, antimigraine.

USES

Bipolar disorder: Treatment of mania or acute mania with mixed features (with or without psychotic features) associated with bipolar disorder, as monotherapy or in combination with atypical antipsychotics. **Seizures:** Monotherapy or adjunctive therapy in pts with complex focal (partial) onset seizures and simple and complex absence seizures. Adjunctive therapy for pts with multiple seizure types that include absence seizures. **Migraine:** Prophylaxis of migraine headaches. **OFF-LABEL:** Refractory status epilepticus, bipolar major depression.

PRECAUTIONS

Contraindications: Hypersensitivity to valproic acid. Active hepatic disease, urea cycle disorders, known mitochondrial disorders caused by mutation in mitochondrial DNA polymerase gamma (POLG). Children under 2 yrs of age suspected of having POLG-related disorder. Migraine prevention in pregnant women and women of reproductive potential who are not using effective contraception. **Cautions:** Children younger than 2 yrs. Hepatic impairment, pts at risk for hepatotoxicity (e.g., cirrhosis, concomitant use of hepatotoxic medications), pts at high risk for suicide (e.g., history of ideation and behavior; depression), elderly, therapy requiring multiple anticonvulsants; congenital metabolic disorders, severe seizure disorders (accompanied by mental retardation), organic brain disease.

ACTION

Directly increases concentration of inhibitory neurotransmitter gamma-aminobutyric acid (GABA). **Therapeutic Effect:** Decreases seizure activity, stabilizes mood, prevents migraine headache.

PHARMACOKINETICS

Widely distributed. Protein binding: 80%–90%. Metabolized in liver. Primarily excreted in urine. Not removed by hemodialysis. **Half-life:** 9–16 hrs (may be increased in hepatic impairment, elderly pts, children younger than 18 mos).

⌛ LIFESPAN CONSIDERATIONS

Pregnancy/Lactation: Drug crosses placenta; is distributed in breast milk. **Children:** May have increased risk of hepatotoxicity. **Elderly:** May have increase incidence of insomnia.

INTERACTIONS

DRUG: Strong CYP3A4 inducers (e.g., carBAMazepine, phenytoin, rifAMPin) may decrease concentration/effect. May increase adverse effects of lamoTRIgine. Alcohol may increase CNS depression. **HERBAL:** Herbals with sedative properties (e.g., chamomile, kava kava, valerian) may increase concentration/effect. **Ginkgo biloba** may decrease concentration/effect. **FOOD:** None known. **LAB VALUES:** May increase serum LDH, bilirubin, ALT, AST. May cause false interpretation of urine ketone test. **Therapeutic serum level:** 50–100 mcg/mL; **toxic serum level:** Greater than 100 mcg/mL.

AVAILABILITY (Rx)

Capsules: Immediate-Release: 250 mg. **Capsules, Delayed-Release Sprinkle:** 125 mg. **Injection Solution:** 100 mg/mL. **Oral Solution:** 250 mg/5 mL.

 Tablets, Delayed-Release: 125 mg, 250 mg, 500 mg. **Tablets, Extended-Release:** 250 mg, 500 mg.

ADMINISTRATION/HANDLING

IV

Reconstitution • Dilute each single dose with at least 50 mL D_5W, 0.9% NaCl, or lactated Ringer's.
Rate of administration • Infuse over 60 min at rate of 20 mg/min or less. • Alternatively, single doses of up to 45 mg/kg given over 5–10 min (1.5–6 mg/kg/min).
Storage • Store vials at room temperature. • Diluted solutions stable for 24 hrs. • Discard unused portion.

PO

• Give without regard to food. Do not mix oral solution with carbonated beverages (may cause mouth/throat irritation). • May sprinkle capsule (Depakote Sprinkle) contents on applesauce and give immediately (do not chew sprinkle beads). • Give delayed-release/extended-release tablets whole. • Regular-release and delayed-release formulations usually given in 2–4 divided doses/day. Extended-release formulation (Depakote ER) usually given once daily.

INDICATIONS/ROUTES/DOSAGE

Seizures

PO: ADULTS, ELDERLY, CHILDREN 10 YRS AND OLDER: Initially, 10–15 mg/kg/day in 1–4 divided doses based on formulation selected. May increase by 5–10 mg/

kg/day at wkly intervals up to 60 mg/kg/day (therapeutic serum levels usually occur with daily doses of 1.5–2.5 g).
IV: ADULTS, ELDERLY, CHILDREN: Equivalent to total daily oral dose divided q6h.

Manic Episodes

PO: ADULTS, ELDERLY: Initially, 20–30 mg/kg/day in 1–4 divided doses based on selected formulation. After 2–3 days, adjust dose to reach desired clinical effect and therapeutic serum concentration. Therapeutic serum levels usually occur with daily doses of 1.5–2.5 g/day. **Maximum:** 60 mg/kg/day.

Prevention of Migraine Headaches

PO: ADULTS, ELDERLY, CHILDREN 17 YRS AND OLDER: Initially, 500 mg once daily (extended-release) or in 2 divided doses (delayed-release or extended-release), then increase in increments of 250 mg/day at intervals of 3 days (or more) up to 1 g/day in 1 or 2 divided doses based on chosen formulation.

Dosage in Renal Impairment
No dose adjustment.

Dosage in Hepatic Impairment
Mild to moderate impairment: Not recommended. **Severe impairment:** Contraindicated.

SIDE EFFECTS

Frequent: Epilepsy: Abdominal pain, irregular menses, diarrhea, transient alopecia, indigestion, nausea, vomiting, tremors, fluctuations in body weight. **Mania (22%–19%):** Nausea, drowsiness. **Occasional: Epilepsy:** Constipation, dizziness, drowsiness, headache, skin rash, unusual excitement, restlessness. **Mania (12%–6%):** Asthenia, abdominal pain, dyspepsia, rash. **Rare: Epilepsy:** Mood changes, diplopia, nystagmus, spots before eyes, unusual bleeding/bruising.

ADVERSE EFFECTS/TOXIC REACTIONS

Thrombocytopenia-associated bleeding, hyperammonemia, hypothermia were reported. Fatal hepatic failure may occur

V

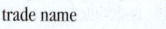

(particularly within the first 6 mos of treatment) and may be preceded by anorexia, facial edema, lethargy malaise, weakness, vomiting. Life-threatening pancreatitis may occur, which may include hemorrhage with rapid deterioration from initial symptoms to death. May increase risk of suicidal ideation and behavior. Drug reaction with eosinophilia and systemic symptoms (DRESS), also known as multiorgan hypersensitivity, has been reported. DRESS may present with facial swelling, eosinophilia, fever, lymphadenopathy, rash, which may be associated with other organ systems, such as hepatitis, hematologic abnormalities, myocarditis, nephritis.

NURSING CONSIDERATIONS

BASELINE ASSESSMENT

Obtain CBC, LFT. Question history of suicidal ideation and behavior. **Anticonvulsant:** Review history of seizure disorder (intensity, frequency, duration, level of consciousness). Initiate safety measures, quiet dark environment. **Antimanic:** Assess behavior, appearance, emotional status, response to environment, speech pattern, thought content. **Antimigraine:** Question characteristics of migraine headaches (onset, location, duration, possible precipitating symptoms).

INTERVENTION/EVALUATION

Monitor CBC, LFT, serum ammonia. Monitor for symptoms of DRESS. Diligently assess for suicidal ideation and behavior; new onset or worsening of anxiety, depression, mood disorder. **Anticonvulsant:** Observe frequently for recurrence of seizure activity. Assess skin for ecchymoses, petechiae. Monitor for clinical improvement (decrease in intensity/frequency of seizures). **Antimanic:** Assess for therapeutic response (interest in surroundings, increased ability to concentrate, relaxed facial expression). **Antimigraine:** Evaluate for relief of migraine headache and resulting photophobia, phonophobia, nausea, vomiting. **Therapeutic serum level:** 50–100

mcg/mL; **toxic serum level:** Greater than 100 mcg/mL.

PATIENT/ FAMILY TEACHING

• Do not abruptly discontinue medication after long-term use (may precipitate seizures). • Strict maintenance of drug therapy is essential for seizure control. • Avoid tasks that require alertness, motor skills until response to drug is established. • Drowsiness usually disappears during continued therapy. • Avoid alcohol. • Report liver problems such as nausea, vomiting, lethargy, altered mental status, weakness, loss of appetite, abdominal pain, yellowing of skin, unusual bruising/bleeding. • Seek immediate medical attention if thoughts of suicide, new onset or worsening of anxiety, depression, or changes in mood occur.

valsartan

val-**sar**-tan
(Apo-Valsartan ✦, Prexxartan, Diovan)
■ **BLACK BOX ALERT** ■ May cause fetal injury, mortality. Discontinue as soon as possible once pregnancy is detected.
Do not confuse Diovan with Zyban, or valsartan with losartan or Valstar.

FIXED-COMBINATION(S)

Diovan HCT: valsartan/hydroCHLOROthiazide (a diuretic): 80 mg/12.5 mg, 160 mg/12.5 mg, 160 mg/25 mg, 320 mg/12.5 mg, 320 mg/25 mg. **Exforge:** valsartan/amLODIPine (a calcium channel blocker): 160 mg/5 mg, 160 mg/10 mg, 320 mg/5 mg, 320 mg/10 mg.

◆CLASSIFICATION

PHARMACOTHERAPEUTIC: Angiotensin II receptor antagonist. **CLINICAL:** Antihypertensive.

USES

Hypertension: Treatment of hypertension alone or in combination with other antihypertensives in adults and children 1 yr and older. **Heart failure:** Treatment of HF (NYHA Class II–IV) in adults. **Post myocardial infarction:** Reduce mortality in high-risk pts (left ventricular failure/dysfunction) following MI. **OFF-LABEL:** Proteinuric chronic kidney disease.

PRECAUTIONS

Contraindications: Hypersensitivity to valsartan. Concomitant use with aliskiren in pts with diabetes. **Cautions:** Concurrent use of potassium-sparing diuretics or potassium supplements, mild to severe hepatic impairment, unstented bilateral/unilateral renal artery stenosis, renal impairment, significant aortic/mitral stenosis, elderly.

ACTION

Directly antagonizes angiotensin II receptors. Blocks vasoconstrictor, aldosterone-secreting effects of angiotensin II, inhibiting binding of angiotensin II to AT_1 receptors. **Therapeutic Effect:** Produces vasodilation, decreases peripheral resistance, decreases B/P.

PHARMACOKINETICS

Widely distributed. Food decreases peak plasma concentration. Protein binding: 95%. Metabolized in liver. Excreted in feces (83%), urine (13%). Unknown if removed by hemodialysis. **Half-life:** 6 hrs.

⧗ LIFESPAN CONSIDERATIONS

Pregnancy/Lactation: May cause fetal harm. Unknown if distributed in breast milk. **Children:** Safety and efficacy not established in pts younger than 1 yr. **Elderly:** No age-related precautions noted.

INTERACTIONS

DRUG: May increase concentration/effect of **ACE inhibitors** (e.g., **benazepril, lisinopril**), **potassium-sparing diuretics** (e.g., **spironolactone, triamterene**). **Potassium supplements, aliskiren** may increase serum potassium level. **HERBAL:** **Herbals with hypertensive properties** (e.g., **licorice, yohimbe**) **or hypotensive prop-**

erties (e.g., **garlic, ginger, ginkgo biloba**) may alter effects. **FOOD:** None known. **LAB VALUES:** May increase serum bilirubin, ALT, AST, BUN, creatinine, potassium. May decrease Hgb, Hct, WBC.

AVAILABILITY (Rx)

Solution, Oral: 4 mg/mL.
Tablets: 40 mg, 80 mg, 160 mg, 320 mg.

ADMINISTRATION/HANDLING

PO
• Give without regard to food. • Shake oral solution before using.

INDICATIONS/ROUTES/DOSAGE

Hypertension
PO: ADULTS, ELDERLY: Initially, 80–160 mg/day. Evaluate response after 2–4 wks and titrate dose as needed. **Maximum:** 320 mg/day. **CHILDREN 1–16 YRS:** Initially, 1 mg/kg/dose once daily (maximum initial daily dose: 40 mg/day). May increase up to 4 mg/kg/day. **Maximum:** 160 mg/day.

HF
PO: ADULTS, ELDERLY: Initially, 20–40 mg twice daily. May increase dose q1–2 wks based on response and tolerability up to target dose of 160 mg twice daily. **Maximum:** 320 mg/day.

Post-MI, Left Ventricular Dysfunction
PO: ADULTS, ELDERLY: May initiate as early as 12 hrs following MI. Initially, 20 mg twice daily. May titrate within 7 days to 40 mg twice daily, with subsequent titrations to a target maintenance dose of 160 mg twice daily, as tolerated.

Dosage in Renal Impairment
CrCl greater than 30 mL/min: No dose adjustment. **CrCl 30 mL/min or less: ADULTS:** Safety/efficacy not established. **CHILDREN 6–16 YRS:** Not recommended.

Dosage in Hepatic Impairment
No dose adjustment.

SIDE EFFECTS

Rare (2%–1%): Insomnia, fatigue, heartburn, abdominal pain, dizziness, headache, diarrhea, nausea, vomiting, arthralgia, edema.

V

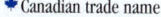 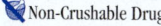

ADVERSE EFFECTS/TOXIC REACTIONS

Overdosage may manifest as hypotension, tachycardia. Bradycardia occurs less often. Viral infection, upper respiratory tract infection (cough, pharyngitis, sinusitis, rhinitis) occur rarely.

NURSING CONSIDERATIONS

BASELINE ASSESSMENT

Obtain renal function test; pregnancy in females of reproductive potential. Obtain B/P prior to each dose. Assess medication history (esp. diuretic). Question for history of hepatic/renal impairment, renal artery stenosis, severe HF.

INTERVENTION/EVALUATION

Monitor renal function, serum electrolytes periodically. Monitor B/P. Assess for for hypotension (dizziness, nausea, tachycardia, syncope, weakened pulse). Ensure adequate hydration.

PATIENT/ FAMILY TEACHING

• Use effective contraception to avoid pregnancy. • Report heart problems (difficulty breathing, palpitations, swelling of extremities), symptoms of low blood pressure (cold, clammy skin; dizziness, fast heart rate, sweating), kidney problems (decreased urine output, flank pain, darkened urine). • Drink plenty of fluids.

---

vancomycin

van-koe-**mye**-sin
(Firvanq, Vancocin)
Do not confuse vancomycin with clindamycin, gentamicin, tobramycin, or Vibramycin.

◆ CLASSIFICATION

PHARMACOTHERAPEUTIC: Tricyclic glycopeptide antibiotic. **CLINICAL:** Antibiotic.

USES

Systemic: Treatment of severe infections (e.g., bloodstream, bone, lower respiratory tract, skin, and skin structure) caused by susceptible strains of methicillin-resistant *staphylococcus aureus* (MRSA). Empiric therapy of infections when MRSA is suspected. **Infective endocarditis:** Treatment due to *Corynebacteria (diphtheroids), Enterococcal, Staphylococcal, Streptococcal* organisms. **PO:** Treatment of *C. difficile*–associated diarrhea. Treatment of enterocolitis caused by *S. aureus* (including MRSA). **OFF-LABEL:** *C. difficile* infection (prophylaxis), cystic fibrosis (acute exacerbation), diabetic foot infection, meningitis (bacterial), peritonitis, prosthetic joint infection, surgical prophylaxis.

PRECAUTIONS

Contraindications: Hypersensitivity to vancomycin. **Cautions:** Renal impairment, elderly, dehydration, pts at risk for extravasation (e.g., peripheral IV catheters, midline catheters, elderly, poor peripheral vasculature), concomitant use of other ototoxic, nephrotoxic medications.

ACTION

Binds to bacterial cell walls, altering cell membrane permeability, inhibiting RNA synthesis. **Therapeutic Effect:** Bactericidal.

PHARMACOKINETICS

PO: Poorly absorbed from GI tract. Primarily excreted in feces. **Parenteral:** Widely distributed (except CSF). Protein binding: 10%–50%. Primarily excreted unchanged in urine. Not removed by hemodialysis. **Half-life:** 4–11 hrs (increased in renal impairment).

⧖ LIFESPAN CONSIDERATIONS

Pregnancy/Lactation: Drug crosses placenta, distributed in breast milk following IV administration. **Children:** Close monitoring of serum levels recommended in premature neonates, young infants. **Elderly:** Age-related renal impairment may increase risk of ototoxicity, nephrotoxicity; dosage adjustment recommended.

INTERACTIONS

DRUG: May increase concentration/effects of **aminoglycosides (e.g., amikacin, gentamicin).** **HERBAL:** None significant. **FOOD:** None known. **LAB VALUES:** May increase BUN. **Therapeutic peak serum level:** (Not routinely obtained) 20–40 mcg/mL; **therapeutic trough serum level:** 10–20 mcg/mL. **Toxic peak serum level:** Greater than 40 mcg/mL; **toxic trough serum level:** Greater than 20 mcg/mL.

AVAILABILITY (Rx)

Capsules: 125 mg, 250 mg. **Infusion, Premix:** 750 mg/150 mL, 1 g/200 mL, 1,250 mg/250 mL, 1,500 mg/300 mL, 1,750 mg/350 mL. **Injection, Powder for Reconstitution:** 500 mg, 750 mg, 1 g. **Oral Solution:** 25 mg/mL, 50 mg/mL.

ADMINISTRATION/HANDLING

 IV

◄ALERT► Give by intermittent IV infusion (piggyback) or continuous IV infusion. Do not give IV push (may result in exaggerated hypotension or red man syndrome). Due to high risk of extravasation, consider infusion via central venous catheter.
Reconstitution • For intermittent IV infusion (piggyback), reconstitute each 500-mg vial with 10 mL Sterile Water for Injection (20 mL for 1-g vial) to provide concentration of 50 mg/mL. • Further dilute with D₅W or 0.9% NaCl to final concentration not to exceed 5 mg/mL.
Rate of administration • Administer over 60 min or longer (30 min for each 500 mg recommended). • Monitor B/P closely during IV infusion.
Storage • Refer to manufacturer labeling for appropriate storage conditions. • Discard if precipitate forms.

PO
• May give with food. • Powder for injection may be reconstituted and diluted for oral administration. Shake reconstituted oral solution well before each use.

▓ IV INCOMPATIBILITIES
Heparin, ibuprofen.

▓ IV COMPATIBILITIES
Acetaminophen, dexmedetomidine, insulin, magnesium sulfate, propofol.

INDICATIONS/ROUTES/DOSAGE
Note: Initial IV dosing in nonobese pts is based on actual body weight. Subsequent dosing is adjusted based on serum trough concentrations and renal function. Pt-specific dosing may be necessary to determine dose and interval (e.g., morbid obesity, critical illness, unstable renal function).

Usual Parenteral Dosage
Note: Initial dosing in nonobese pts should be based on actual body weight (obese pts on adjusted body weight). Subsequent dosing generally adjusted based on therapeutic monitoring.
IV: ADULTS, ELDERLY: Initially, 15–20 mg/kg/dose (rounded to nearest 250 mg) q8–12h. In seriously ill pts with documented/suspected MRSA infection, a loading dose of 20–35 mg/kg (maximum 3 g) may be considered. **ADOLESCENTS, CHILDREN, INFANTS:** Initially, 45–60 mg/kg/day divided q6–8h. Dose, frequency based on serum concentrations. **NEONATES:** Loading dose of 20 mg/kg; then 10–20 mg/kg/dose q12–48h.

Staphylococcal Enterocolitis, Antibiotic–Associated Pseudomembranous Colitis Caused by *Clostridium Difficile*
PO: ADULTS, ELDERLY: 125–500 mg 4 times/day for 10–14 days. **CHILDREN:** 40 mg/kg/day in 3–4 divided doses for 7–10 days. **Maximum:** 2 g/day.

V

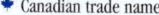

Dosage in Renal Impairment

After loading dose, subsequent dosages and frequency are modified based on creatinine clearance, severity of infection, and serum concentration of drug.

Dosage in Hepatic Impairment

No dose adjustment.

SIDE EFFECTS

Frequent: PO: Bitter/unpleasant taste, nausea, vomiting, mouth irritation (with oral solution). **Rare: Parenteral:** Phlebitis, thrombophlebitis, pain at peripheral IV site, dizziness, vertigo, tinnitus, chills, fever, rash, necrosis with extravasation. **PO:** Rash.

ADVERSE EFFECTS/TOXIC REACTIONS

Nephrotoxicity (acute kidney injury, acute tubular necrosis, renal failure), ototoxicity (temporary or permanent hearing loss) may occur. Too-rapid infusion may cause red man syndrome, a common adverse reaction characterized by pruritus, urticaria, erythema, angioedema, tachycardia, hypotension, myalgia, maculopapular rash (usually appears on face, neck, upper torso). Cardiovascular toxicity (cardiac depression, arrest) occurs rarely. Onset usually occurs within 30 min of start of infusion, resolves within hrs following infusion. May result from too-rapid rate of infusion. Extravasation may cause tissue necrosis. Infusions via peripheral IV or midline access may cause thrombophlebitis.

NURSING CONSIDERATIONS

BASELINE ASSESSMENT

Avoid other ototoxic, nephrotoxic medications if possible. Obtain culture, sensitivity test before giving first dose (therapy may begin before results are known). Consider placement of central venous line/PICC line.

INTERVENTION/EVALUATION

Monitor serum renal function tests, I&O. Assess skin for rash. Check hearing acuity, balance. Monitor B/P carefully during infusion. Monitor for red man syndrome. Evaluate IV site for phlebitis (heat, pain, red streaking over vein). Obtain vancomycin peak/trough level as ordered by physician or pharmacist. **Therapeutic serum level: Peak:** 20–40 mcg/mL; **trough:** 10–20 mcg/mL. **Toxic serum level: Peak:** Greater than 40 mcg/mL; **trough:** Greater than 20 mcg/mL.

PATIENT/ FAMILY TEACHING

• Continue therapy for full length of treatment. • Doses should be evenly spaced. • Report ringing in ears, hearing loss, changes in urinary frequency or consistency. • Lab tests are important part of total therapy.

vandetanib

van-**det**-a-nib
(Caprelsa)

■ **BLACK BOX ALERT** ■ Can prolong QT interval (torsades de pointes and sudden cardiac death reported). Do not use in pts with hypokalemia, hypocalcemia, hypomagnesemia, congenital long QT syndrome. Electrolyte imbalances must be corrected prior to initiating therapy. If medication that prolongs QT interval is needed, more frequent ECG monitoring is recommended. ECGs should be obtained during wks 2–4 and wks 8–12 after starting therapy and 3 mos thereafter. Pts with any dose reduction or interruption related to QT prolongation greater than 2 wks must have frequent ECG monitoring as noted above. Only certified prescribers and pharmacies with a restricted distribution program are able to prescribe and dispense.

◆CLASSIFICATION

PHARMACOTHERAPEUTIC: Epidermal growth factor receptor (EGFR) inhibitor. Vascular endothelial growth factor (VEGF) inhibitor. Tyrosine kinase inhibitor. **CLINICAL:** Antineoplastic.

USES

Treatment of symptomatic or progressive medullary thyroid cancer in pts with unresectable locally advanced or metastatic disease.

PRECAUTIONS

Contraindications: Hypersensitivity to vandetanib. Congenital long QT syndrome. **Cautions:** Baseline cytopenias, pts at risk for QTc interval prolongation (congenital long QT syndrome, HF, medications that prolong QTc interval, hypokalemia, hypomagnesemia), hypothyroidism, cerebrovascular disease, moderate to severe renal/hepatic impairment, hypertension, uncompensated HF, history of torsades de pointes.

ACTION

Inhibits tyrosine kinases including epidermal growth factor (EGF) and vascular endothelial growth factor (VEGF). Blocks intracellular signaling, angiogenesis, and cellular proliferation. **Therapeutic Effect:** Inhibits tumor cell growth and survival.

PHARMACOKINETICS

Widely distributed. Peak concentration: 4–10 hrs. Metabolized in liver. Protein binding: 90%. Excreted in feces (44%), urine (25%). **Half-life:** 19 days.

⏳ LIFESPAN CONSIDERATIONS

Pregnancy/Lactation: Avoid pregnancy; may cause fetal harm. Females of reproductive potential must use effective contraception during treatment and for at least 4 mos after treatment. Unknown if distributed in breast milk. **Children:** Safety and efficacy not established. **Elderly:** No age-related precautions noted.

INTERACTIONS

DRUG: QT interval–prolonging medications (e.g., amiodarone, azithromycin, ciprofloxacin, haloperidol, methadone, sotalol) may increase risk of QTc interval prolongation. **Strong CYP3A4 inducers (e.g., carBAMazepine, phenytoin, rifAMPin)** may decrease concentration/effect. **HERBAL: St. John's wort** may decrease concentration/effect. **FOOD: Grapefruit products** may increase risk of torsades de pointes, myelotoxicity. **LAB VALUES:** May decrease WBC, Hgb, neutrophils. May increase serum bilirubin, ALT, AST, creatinine; urine protein. May alter serum calcium, glucose, magnesium, potassium.

AVAILABILITY (Rx)

Tablets: 100 mg, 300 mg.

ADMINISTRATION/HANDLING

PO

• Give without regard to food. • Do not crush. • May disperse in 2 oz of noncarbonated water and stir for 10 min until tablet is evenly dispersed (will not completely dissolve). Administer dispersion immediately. Rinse residue in glass with 4 oz water and administer. Can be given via feeding tube. • Direct contact of crushed tablets with skin or mucous membranes should be strictly avoided. If contact occurs, wash thoroughly.

INDICATIONS/ROUTES/DOSAGE

Thyroid Cancer
Note: Do not begin unless QT_c interval is less than 450 msec. Maintain serum calcium and magnesium within normal limits. Maintain serum potassium at least 4 mEq/L or greater.
PO: ADULTS, ELDERLY: 300 mg once daily. Continue until disease progression or unacceptable toxicity.

Dose Modification
Dosage Adjustment for QT Prolongation or Toxicity
Interrupt therapy until resolved or improved, then restart at 100–200 mg once daily.

Dosage in Renal Impairment
CrCl less than 50 mL/min: 200 mg once daily. Closely monitor QT interval.

V

Dosage in Hepatic Impairment

Mild impairment: No dose adjustment. **Moderate to severe impairment:** Not recommended.

SIDE EFFECTS

Frequent   (57%–21%): Diarrhea/colitis, rash, dermatitis acneiform/acne, nausea, headache, fatigue, anorexia, abdominal pain. **Occasional (15%–10%):** Dry skin, vomiting, asthenia, photosensitivity, insomnia, nasopharyngitis, dyspepsia, cough, pruritus, weight decrease, depression.

ADVERSE EFFECTS/TOXIC REACTIONS

Prolonged QT interval resulting in torsades de pointes, ventricular arrhythmias, sudden cardiac death have been reported. Frequent diarrhea may result in electrolyte imbalances. Severe skin reactions, including Stevens-Johnson syndrome, have been reported. Interstitial lung disease (ILD) or pneumonitis reported (may result in respiratory-related death). Consider ILD in pts with hypoxia, pleural effusion, cough, dyspnea. Ischemic cerebrovascular events have been reported. Life-threatening events including hypertensive crisis, reversible posterior leukoencephalopathy syndrome (RPLS) have been noted. Adverse reactions resulting in death included respiratory failure/arrest, aspiration pneumonia, cardiac failure, sepsis, GI bleeding.

NURSING CONSIDERATIONS

BASELINE ASSESSMENT

Obtain CBC, BMP, LFT; ECG; pregnancy test in females of reproductive potential. Question for history of congenital long QT syndrome, HF, arrhythmias, hepatic/renal impairment, seizures, CVA, hemorrhagic events, HTN. Obtain full medication history and screen for interactions. Offer emotional support.

INTERVENTION/EVALUATION

Monitor CBC, serum electrolytes. Obtain ECG during wks 2–4, wks 8–12, then every 3 mos thereafter. Obtain ECG for palpitations, chest pain, hypokalemia, hyperkalemia, hypocalcemia, bradycardia, ventricular arrhythmias, syncope. Report any respiratory changes including dyspnea, cough (may indicate ILD). Reversible posterior leukoencephalopathy syndrome should be considered in pts with seizures, headache, visual disturbances, confusion, altered mental status. Ophthalmologic exams including slit lamp recommended in pts with visual disturbances.

PATIENT/FAMILY TEACHING

• Use effective contraception to avoid pregnancy. • Changes in mental status, seizures, headache, blurry vision, trouble speaking, one-sided weakness may indicate stroke, high blood pressure crisis, or life-threatening brain swelling. Immediately report any newly prescribed medications. • Limit exposure to sunlight. • Report any yellowing of skin or eyes, abdominal pain, bruising, black/tarry stools, dark urine, decreased urine output, skin changes. • Report palpitations, chest pain, shortness of breath, dizziness, fainting (may indicate arrhythmia).

varenicline

var-**en**-i-kleen
(Champix ✹, Tyrvaya)

◆ **CLASSIFICATION**

PHARMACOTHERAPEUTIC: Selective partial nicotine agonist. **CLINICAL:** Smoking deterrent.

USES

PO: Aid to smoking-cessation treatment. **Nasal spray:** Treatment of dry eye disease.

PRECAUTIONS

Contraindications: Hypersensitivity to varenicline. **Cautions:** Renal impairment, history of suicidal ideation or preexisting psychiatric illness, bipolar disorder, depression, schizophrenia, pts at risk for seizures (e.g., head trauma, seizure disorder).

ACTION

Prevents nicotine stimulation of mesolimbic dopamine system associated with nicotine addiction. **Therapeutic Effect:** Decreases desire to smoke.

PHARMACOKINETICS

Widely distributed. Absorption unaffected by food, time-of-day dosing. Peak plasma concentration: 3–4 hrs. Steady state reached within 4 days. Protein binding: 20%. Minimal metabolism. Removed by hemodialysis. Primarily excreted unchanged in urine. **Half-life:** 24 hrs.

⧗ LIFESPAN CONSIDERATIONS

Pregnancy/Lactation: Unknown if distributed in breast milk. **Children:** Not recommended. **Elderly:** Age-related renal impairment may require dosage adjustment.

INTERACTIONS

DRUG: May increase concentration/effect of **nicotine**. **HERBAL:** None significant. **FOOD:** None known. **LAB VALUES:** None significant.

AVAILABILITY (Rx)

Nasal Spray: 0.03 mg/actuation.

🐋 **Tablets:** 0.5 mg, 1 mg.

ADMINISTRATION/HANDLING

PO: • Give after meal and with full glass of water.

Nasal Spray
• Prime before using (7 sprays in the air away from face. If not used for more

than 5 days, re-prime with 1 spray).
• Do not shake. • Discard 30 days after opening bottle.

INDICATIONS/ROUTES/DOSAGE

◄**ALERT**► Therapy should start 1 wk before stopping smoking.
Smoking Deterrent
PO: ADULTS, ELDERLY: Days 1–3: 0.5 mg once daily. **Days 4–7:** 0.5 mg twice daily. **Day 8–end of treatment:** 1 mg twice daily. Therapy should last for total of 12 wks. Pts who have successfully stopped smoking at the end of 12 wks should continue with an additional 12 wks of treatment to increase likelihood of long-term abstinence.

Dosage in Renal Impairment
CrCl less than 30 mL/min: 0.5 mg once daily. **Maximum:** 0.5 mg twice daily. **End-stage renal disease, undergoing hemodialysis:** Maximum: 0.5 mg once daily.

Dry Eye
Nasal Spray: ADULTS, ELDERLY: 1 spray 2 times/day (approx. 12 hrs apart).

Dosage in Hepatic Impairment
No dose adjustment.

SIDE EFFECTS

Frequent (30%–13%): Nausea, insomnia, headache, abnormal dreams. **Occasional (8%–5%):** Constipation, abdominal discomfort, fatigue, dry mouth, flatulence, altered taste, dyspepsia, vomiting, anxiety, depression, irritability. **Rare (3%–1%):** Drowsiness, rash, increased appetite, lethargy, nightmares, gastric reflux, rhinorrhea, agitation, mood swings.

ADVERSE EFFECTS/TOXIC REACTIONS

Abrupt withdrawal may cause irritability, sleep disturbances in 3% of pts. Hypertension, angina pectoris, arrhythmia, bradycardia, coronary artery disease, gingivitis, anemia, lymphadenopathy occur rarely. May cause bizarre behavior, suicidal ideation. May increase risk for seizure activity.

V

 Canadian trade name   Non-Crushable Drug   High Alert drug

NURSING CONSIDERATIONS

BASELINE ASSESSMENT

Screen, evaluate for coronary heart disease (history of MI, angina pectoris), cardiac arrhythmias, suicidal ideation. Assess smoking pack/day history.

INTERVENTION/EVALUATION

Discontinue use if cardiovascular symptoms occur or worsen. Monitor for psychiatric symptoms (changes in behavior, mood, level of interest, appearance). Assess for cravings, noncompliance with cessation.

PATIENT/FAMILY TEACHING

• Initiate treatment 1 wk before quit-smoking date. • Take with food and with full glass of water. • Report persistent nausea, insomnia. • Seek immediate medical attention if thoughts of suicide, new onset or worsening of anxiety, depression, or changes in mood occur.

vasopressin

vay-soe-**pres**-in
(Vasostrict)
Do not confuse Pitressin with Pitocin.

◆CLASSIFICATION

PHARMACOTHERAPEUTIC: Posterior pituitary hormone. **CLINICAL:** Vasopressor, antidiuretic hormone analogue.

USES

Vasoconstriction: To increase blood pressure in adults with vasodilatory shock who remain hypotensive despite fluids and catecholamines. **OFF-LABEL:** Adjunct in treatment of acute massive GI hemorrhage or esophageal varices. Central diabetes insipidus, cadaveric organ recovery.

PRECAUTIONS

Contraindications: Hypersensitivity to vasopressin. **Cautions:** Seizure disorder, migraine, asthma, vascular disease, renal/cardiac disease, goiter (with cardiac complications), arteriosclerosis, nephritis, elderly.

ACTION

Stimulates a family of arginine vasopressin (AVP) receptors. **Therapeutic Effect:** Increases systemic vascular resistance and mean arterial BP; increases water permeability at renal tubules, causing a decreased urine volume and increased osmolality; causes smooth muscle contraction in GI tract.

PHARMACOKINETICS

Route	Onset	Peak	Duration
IV	N/A	N/A	0.5–1 hr
IM, SQ	1–2 hrs	N/A	2–8 hrs

Widely distributed. Metabolized in liver, kidney. Primarily excreted in urine. **Half-life:** 10–20 min.

⏳ LIFESPAN CONSIDERATIONS

Pregnancy/Lactation: Caution in giving to breastfeeding women. **Children/Elderly:** Caution due to risk of water intoxication/hyponatremia.

INTERACTIONS

DRUG: May increase concentration/effect of **desmopressin, fingolimod, ponesimod, siponimod.** Midodrine, **ozanimod** may increase concentration/effect. **HERBAL:** None significant. **FOOD:** None known. **LAB VALUES:** None significant.

AVAILABILITY (Rx)

Injection Solution: 20 units/mL. 0.2 units/mL (100 mL), 0.4 units/mL (100 mL). **Prefilled Syringe:** 5 units/5 mL.

V

ADMINISTRATION/HANDLING

 IV

Reconstitution • Dilute in D₅W or 0.9% NaCl to concentration of 0.1–1 unit/mL (usual concentration: 100 units/500 mL D₅W).
Rate of administration • Give as IV infusion.
Storage • Store at room temperature.

⚙ IV COMPATIBILITIES

Amiodarone, argatroban, dilTIAZem, heparin, insulin, milrinone (Primacor), nitroglycerin, norepinephrine.

INDICATIONS/ROUTES/DOSAGE

Vasodilatory Shock
IV infusion: ADULTS, ELDERLY: Initially, 0.03 units/min. Usual dosage range: 0.01–0.04 units/min.

Dosage in Renal/Hepatic Impairment
No dose adjustment.

SIDE EFFECTS

Frequent: Pain at injection site (with vasopressin tannate). **Occasional:** Abdominal cramps, nausea, vomiting, diarrhea, dizziness, diaphoresis, pale skin, circumoral pallor, tremors, headache, eructation, flatulence. **Rare:** Chest pain, confusion, allergic reaction (rash, urticaria, pruritus, wheezing, difficulty breathing, facial/peripheral edema), sterile abscess (with vasopressin tannate).

ADVERSE EFFECTS/TOXIC REACTIONS

Anaphylaxis, MI, water intoxication have occurred. Elderly, very young are at higher risk for water intoxication. May increase risk of ischemia (cardiac, mesenteric, limb, skin). Extravasation may cause tissue necrosis.

NURSING CONSIDERATIONS

BASELINE ASSESSMENT
Obtain serum electrolytes; urine specific gravity in pts with diabetes insipidus. Obtain B/P, heart rate.

INTERVENTION/EVALUATION
Monitor I&O closely, restrict intake as necessary to prevent water intoxication. Weigh daily if indicated. Check B/P, pulse frequently. Monitor serum electrolytes, urine specific gravity. Be alert for early signs of water intoxication (altered mental status, muscle cramping or twitching; seizures). Monitor for chest pain, tachycardia; hypersensitivity reactions.

PATIENT/FAMILY TEACHING
• Report headache, chest pain, shortness of breath, other symptoms. • Stress importance of I&O. • Avoid alcohol. • Report symptoms of water intoxication (e.g., confusion, cramping, nausea, muscle twitching, seizures, vomiting).

vedolizumab

ve-doe-**liz**-ue-mab
(Entyvio, Entivio Pen)
Do not confuse vedolizumab with certolizumab, eculizumab, natalizumab, omalizumab, tocilizumab.

◆CLASSIFICATION

PHARMACOTHERAPEUTIC: Selective adhesion molecule inhibitor. Monoclonal antibody. **CLINICAL:** GI agent.

USES

Treatment of moderate to severe active ulcerative colitis, moderate to severe active Crohn's disease.

PRECAUTIONS

Contraindications: Hypersensitivity to vedolizumab. **Cautions:** Hepatic impairment, pts who resided or traveled to endemic areas; conditions predisposing to infection (e.g., diabetes, renal failure, immunocompromised pts, open wounds), history of chronic opportunistic infections (esp. bacterial, invasive fun-

V

 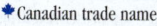 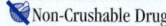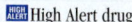

gal, mycobacterial, protozoal, viral infections including herpes zoster, TB), prior malignancies. Preexisting or recent-onset CNS demyelinating disorders including multiple sclerosis.

ACTION

Binds to T-lymphocyte integrin receptors and blocks the interaction with mucosal addressin cell adhesion molecule-1 (MAdCAM-1). Inhibits migration of memory T-lymphocytes across the endothelium into inflamed GI parenchymal tissue. **Therapeutic Effect:** Reduces chronic inflammation of colon.

PHARMACOKINETICS

Metabolism not specified. Excretion not specified. **Half-life:** 25 days.

⌛ LIFESPAN CONSIDERATIONS

Pregnancy/Lactation: Unknown if distributed in breast milk. Use caution when administering to nursing women. **Children:** Safety and efficacy not established. **Elderly:** No age-related precautions noted.

INTERACTIONS

DRUG: Anti-TNF agents (e.g., adalimumab, certolizumab, etanercept, infliximab) may increase adverse effects. May decrease the therapeutic effect; increase adverse effects of **vaccines (live)**. May decrease therapeutic effect of **BCG (intravesical)**. May increase toxic effect of **natalizumab**. **HERBAL: Echinacea** may decrease the therapeutic effect. **FOOD:** None known. **LAB VALUES:** May increase serum ALT, AST, bilirubin.

AVAILABILITY (Rx)

Lyophilized Powder for Injection: 300 mg.
Subcutaneous injection: 108 mg/0.68 mL single-dose prefilled syringe; single-dose prefilled pen.

ADMINISTRATION/HANDLING

 IV

Infusion guidelines • Do not administer IV push or bolus. • Reconstitute with Sterile Water for Injection and subsequently dilute with 0.9% NaCl only. • After infusion completed, flush IV line with 30 mL of 0.9% NaCl.

Reconstitution • Reconstitute with 4.8 mL Sterile Water for Injection. Direct stream toward glass wall to avoid excessive foaming. • Gently swirl contents for at least 15 sec until completely dissolved. • Do not shake or agitate. • Allow solution to sit at room temperature for up to 20 min to allow remaining foam to settle and powder to dissolve. If not fully dissolved after 20 min, allow additional 10 min for dissolution. Do not use if product is not dissolved within 30 min. • Visually inspect for particulate matter and discoloration. Do not use if discolored or if particulate matter is observed. • Prior to withdrawing solution, invert vial 3 times to ensure mixing. • Withdraw 5 mL and further dilute in 250 mL 0.9% NaCl bag. • Infuse immediately.

Rate of administration • Infuse over 30 min.

Storage • Reconstituted solution should appear clear to opalescent, colorless to light brownish yellow and free of particles. • May refrigerate reconstituted vials for 8 hrs; diluted solution in NS for 24 hrs. May store solutions diluted in NS at room temperature for 12 hrs.

SQ

Administration • Insert needle subcutaneously into outer thigh, abdomen, or upper arm and inject solution. • Do not inject into areas of active skin disease or injury such as sunburns, skin rashes, inflammation, skin infections, or psoriatic lesions. • Rotate injection sites at least 1 inch away from prior site. • Do not administer IV or intramuscularly.

Storage • Refrigerate until time of use. May store at room temperature for up to 7 days. • Do not freeze or expose to heating sources.

INDICATIONS/ROUTES/DOSAGE

Note: May switch to SQ injection at Wk 6. Discontinue in pts who do not show evidence of therapeutic benefit by wk 14.

V

Ulcerative Colitis and Crohn's Disease

IV: ADULTS, ELDERLY: 300 mg once at wk 0, wk 2, and wk 6, then q8 wks thereafter. **SQ: ADULTS, ELDERLY:** Following the first two IV doses, may switch to SQ injection on wk 6 to 108 mg q2wks.

Dosage in Renal/Hepatic Impairment

Not specified; use caution.

SIDE EFFECTS

Occasional (13%–4%): Nasopharyngitis, headache, arthralgia, nausea, pyrexia, upper respiratory tract infection, fatigue, cough, bronchitis, influenza, back pain. **Rare (3%):** Rash, pruritus, sinusitis, oropharyngeal pain, extremity pain.

ADVERSE EFFECTS/TOXIC REACTIONS

Infusion-related reactions, including anaphylaxis, characterized by bronchospasm, dyspnea, flushing, hypotension, laryngeal edema, nausea, pyrexia, tachycardia, wheezing, vomiting, reported in less than 1% of pts. May increase risk of severe infections such as anal abscess, cytomegaloviral colitis, giardiasis, *Listeria* meningitis, *Salmonella* sepsis, TB, UTI, which may lead to fatal sepsis. PML (weakness, paralysis, vision loss, aphasia, cognition impairment) has occurred rarely; however, immunocompromised pts are at increased risk for development. Hepatotoxicity with serum ALT, AST greater than 3 times upper limit of normal reported in less than 2% of pts. Malignancies including B-cell lymphoma, breast cancer, colon cancer, lung cancer of primary neuroendocrine carcinoma, lung neoplasm, malignant hepatic neoplasm, melanoma, renal cancer, squamous cell carcinoma, transitional cell carcinoma occur rarely.

NURSING CONSIDERATIONS

BASELINE ASSESSMENT

Obtain CBC, LFT; pregnancy test in females of reproductive potential. Screen for active infection; history of chronic, opportunistic infections. Question history of prior malignancies. Consider completion of age appropriate immunizations prior to initiation. Evaluate for active TB and test for latent infection prior to and during treatment. An induration of 5 mm or greater with tuberculin skin test should be considered a positive result when assessing for latent TB. Antifungal therapy should be considered for those who reside in or travel to regions where mycoses are endemic. Have supplemental oxygen, anaphylaxis kit readily available. Assess degree of abdominal pain, cramping; usual bowel movement patterns, stool characteristics.

INTERVENTION/EVALUATION

Monitor LFT. Obtain CBC if infection is suspected. Monitor for symptoms of TB (cough, fatigue, hemoptysis, nocturnal sweating, weight loss), including those who tested negative for latent TB infection. Monitor for infections (abdominal pain, cough, fatigue, fever). Interrupt or discontinue treatment if serious infection, opportunistic infection, or sepsis occurs. Monitor for hypersensitivity reaction. Infusion-related reactions generally occur within 2 hrs after infusion. Consider administration of antihistamine, antipyretic, and/or corticosteroid if mild to moderate hypersensitivity reaction occurs. If anaphylaxis occurs, provide immediate resuscitation support. Monitor for new onset or worsening of neurologic symptoms, esp. in pts with CNS disorders; may indicate PML.

PATIENT/FAMILY TEACHING

• Treatment may depress your immune system and reduce your ability to fight infection. Report symptoms of infection such as body aches, burning with urination, chills, cough, fatigue, fever; fungal infections. Avoid those with active infection. • Report travel plans to possible endemic areas. • Do not receive live vaccines. • Expect frequent TB screening. • Dormant or chronic viral, invasive fungal infections may become reactivated. • Treatment may cause new cancers. • Infusion may cause severe allergic reactions such as face/tongue swelling, hives, itching, low blood pressure, trouble breathing, or, in some cases, anaphylaxis. • Do not breastfeed. • Abdominal pain, bruising, clay-colored stools, dark-amber urine,

V

fatigue, loss of appetite, yellowing of skin or eyes may indicate liver problem. • Paralysis, vision changes, impaired speech, altered mental status may indicate life-threatening neurologic event called progressive multifocal leukoencephalopathy (PML).

vemurafenib

vem-ue-**raf**-e-nib
(Zelboraf)

◆**CLASSIFICATION**
PHARMACOTHERAPEUTIC: BRAF kinase inhibitor. **CLINICAL:** Antineoplastic.

USES
Melanoma: Treatment of unresectable or metastatic melanoma with a BRAF V600E mutation as detected by FDA-approved test. **Erdheim-Chester disease (ECD):** Treatment of ECD in pts with a BRAF V600E mutation. **OFF-LABEL:** Non–small-cell lung cancer with BRAF V600 mutation (refractory), melanoma metastatic or unresectable with BRAF V600K mutation.

PRECAUTIONS
Contraindications: Hypersensitivity to vemurafenib. **Cautions:** Hepatic impairment, pts at risk for QTc interval prolongation (congenital long QT syndrome, HF, medications that prolong QTc interval, hypokalemia, hypomagnesemia), elderly, prior radiation therapy.

ACTION
Inhibits kinase activity of certain mutated forms of BRAF. **Therapeutic Effect:** Blocks tumor cell proliferation in melanoma with the mutation.

PHARMACOKINETICS
Widely distributed. Protein binding: 99%. Minimally metabolized in liver. Primarily excreted in feces (94%). **Half-life:** 57 hrs. **Range:** 30–120 hrs.

⧗ LIFESPAN CONSIDERATIONS
Pregnancy/Lactation: Avoid pregnancy; may cause fetal harm. Females of reproductive potential must use effective contraception during treatment and for at least 2 mos after discontinuation. Unknown if distributed in breast milk. **Children:** Safety and efficacy not established. **Elderly:** May have increased risk of adverse reactions, side effects.

INTERACTIONS
DRUG: Strong **CYP3A4 inhibitors (e.g., clarithromycin, ketoconazole, ritonavir)** may increase concentration/effect. **Strong CYP3A4 inducers (e.g., carBAMazepine, phenytoin, rifAMPin)** may decrease concentration/effect. May increase concentration/effect of **digoxin**. QT interval–prolonging medications **(e.g., amiodarone, azithromycin, ciprofloxacin, haloperidol, methadone, sotalol)** may increase risk of QTc interval prolongation. **HERBAL:** None significant. **FOOD: Grapefruit products** may increase concentration/effect. **LAB VALUES:** May increase serum alkaline phosphatase, ALT, AST, gamma-glutamyl transferase (GGT), bilirubin.

AVAILABILITY (Rx)
🔖 **Film-Coated Tablets:** 240 mg.

ADMINISTRATION/HANDLING
PO
• Give without regard to food in the morning and evening, approx. 12 hrs apart with a full glass of water. • Administer tablets whole; do not break, crush, divide, or dissolve. • A missed dose can be taken up to 4 hrs prior to the next dose.

INDICATIONS/ROUTES/DOSAGE
Note: Management of adverse drug reactions may require dose reduction, treatment interruption, or discontinuation.

ECD, Melanoma
PO: ADULTS, ELDERLY: 960 mg twice daily (in morning and evening about 12

V

hrs apart). Continue until disease progression or unacceptable toxicity.

Dosage Modification

Based on Common Terminology Criteria for Adverse Events (CTCAE). **Grade 1 or Grade 2 (tolerable) toxicity:** No dose adjustment. **Grade 2 (intolerable) or Grade 3 toxicity: FIRST OCCURRENCE:** Interrupt treatment until toxicity returns to Grade 0 or 1, then resume at 720 mg twice daily. **SECOND OCCURRENCE:** Interrupt treatment, then resume at 480 mg twice daily. **THIRD OCCURRENCE:** Discontinue. **Grade 4 toxicity: FIRST OCCURRENCE:** Interrupt treatment, then resume at 480 mg twice daily. **SECOND OCCURRENCE:** Discontinue.

Dosage in Renal/Hepatic Impairment

Mild to moderate impairment: No dose adjustment. **Severe impairment:** Use with caution.

SIDE EFFECTS

Frequent (53%–33%): Arthralgia, alopecia, fatigue, rash, nausea. **Occasional (28%–11%):** Diarrhea, hyperkeratosis, headache, pruritus, pyrexia, dry skin, extremity pain, anorexia, vomiting, peripheral edema, erythema, dysgeusia, myalgia, constipation, asthenia. **Rare (8%–5%):** Maculopapular rash, actinic keratosis, musculoskeletal pain, back pain, cough, papular rash.

ADVERSE EFFECTS/TOXIC REACTIONS

Cutaneous squamous cell carcinoma (cuSCC) and keratoacanthomas reported in 24% of pts. Pts at increased risk of cuSCC include elderly pts, pts with prior skin cancer, chronic sun exposure. Hypersensitivity reactions including erythema, hypotension, anaphylaxis reported. Mild to severe photosensitivity was reported. Serious dermatologic reactions include Stevens-Johnson syndrome, toxic epidermal necrolysis. Ophthalmologic reactions including uveitis reported. Hepatotoxicity may lead to discontinuation.

NURSING CONSIDERATIONS

BASELINE ASSESSMENT

Obtain BMP; ECG; pregnancy test in females of reproductive potential. Confirm presence of BRAF V600E mutation. Review history for previous radiation therapy. Assess skin for moles, lesions, papilloma, and perform full dermatologic exam. Obtain ophthalmologic exam, visual acuity. Obtain full medication history (esp. QT interval–prolonging drugs) and screen for interactions. Offer emotional support.

INTERVENTION/EVALUATION

Monitor ECG 15 days after initiation, then monthly for first 3 mos, then q3mos thereafter. Routinely assess skin during treatment and for 6 mos after discontinuation. Immediately report any new skin lesions. Obtain ECG for palpitations, chest pain, syncope. Pruritus, difficulty breathing, erythema, hypotension may indicate anaphylaxis.

PATIENT/FAMILY TEACHING

• Treatment may cause new cancers. • Use effective contraception to avoid pregnancy. • Avoid sunlight exposure. • Report any skin changes, including new warts, sores, reddish bumps that bleed or do not heal, change in mole size or color. • Report yellowing of skin or eyes, abdominal pain, bruising, black/tarry stools, dark urine, decreased urine output, skin changes. • Report palpitations, chest pain, shortness of breath, dizziness, fainting (may indicate arrhythmia).

venetoclax

ven-**et**-oh-klax
(Venclexta)
Do not confuse venetoclax or Venclexta with Venelex.

◆CLASSIFICATION

PHARMACOTHERAPEUTIC: B-cell lymphoma 2 (BCL-2) inhibitor. **CLINICAL:** Antineoplastic.

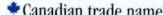 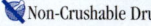

USES

Lymphocytic leukemia/small lymphocytic lymphoma (CLL/SLL): Monotherapy or in combination with riTUXimab or in combination with obinutuzumab for treatment of pts with chronic CLL/SLL with or without 17p deletion who have received at least one prior therapy. **Acute myeloid leukemia (AML):** Treatment of newly diagnosed AML in combination with azacitidine, or decitabine, or low-dose cytarabine in pts 75 yrs of age or older, or with co-morbidities precluding use of intensive induction chemotherapy. **OFF-LABEL:** Mantle cell lymphoma (relapsed/refractory), multiple myeloma (relapsed/refractory).

PRECAUTIONS

Contraindications: Hypersensitivity to venetoclax. Concomitant use of strong CYP3A4 inhibitors at initiation and during ramp-up phase. **Cautions:** Baseline cytopenias, concomitant use of moderate CYP3A4 inhibitors, P-gp inhibitors; conditions predisposing to infection (e.g., diabetes, renal failure, immunocompromised pts, open wounds), hepatic/renal impairment, electrolyte imbalance; history of gout; pts at high risk for tumor lysis syndrome (high tumor burden).

ACTION

Selectively binds to and inhibits anti-apoptotic protein BCL-2 overexpressed in CLL cells and AML cells, restoring process of apoptosis. **Therapeutic Effect:** Inhibits tumor cell growth and metastasis.

PHARMACOKINETICS

Widely distributed. Metabolized in liver. Protein binding: highly bound (unspecified). Peak plasma concentration: 5–8 hrs. Excreted in feces (greater than 99%). Half-life: 26 hrs.

⧗ LIFESPAN CONSIDERATIONS

Pregnancy/Lactation: Avoid pregnancy; may cause fetal harm/malformations. Females and males with female partners of reproductive potential should use effective contraception during treatment and for at least 30 days after discontinuation. Unknown if distributed in breast milk. Breastfeeding not recommended. May impair fertility in males. **Children:** Safety and efficacy not established. **Elderly:** No age-related precautions noted.

INTERACTIONS

DRUG: Strong CYP3A4 inhibitors (e.g., clarithromycin, ketoconazole), moderate CYP3A4 inhibitors (e.g., dilTIAZem, fluconazole, verapamil), P-gp inhibitors (e.g., cycloSPORINE, ranolazine, ticagrelor) may increase concentration/effect. Strong CYP3A4 inducers (e.g., carBAMazepine, phenytoin, rifAMPin) may decrease concentration/effect. May increase concentration/effect of **digoxin.** May decrease the therapeutic effect; increase adverse effects of **vaccines (live).** May increase immunosuppressive effect of **tofacitinib, upadacitinib.** **HERBAL: Bitter orange** may increase concentration/effect. **FOOD: Grapefruit products, seville oranges, star fruit** may increase concentration/effect. **LAB VALUES:** May decrease Hgb, Hct, neutrophils, platelets, RBCs; serum calcium, potassium. Tumor lysis syndrome may result in elevated serum phosphate, potassium, uric acid.

AVAILABILITY (Rx)

Tablets: 10 mg, 50 mg, 100 mg.

ADMINISTRATION/HANDLING

PO

• Give with food and water at same time each day. • Administer tablets whole; do not cut, crush, or divide. • If a dose is missed by no more than 8 hrs, administer as soon as possible. If dose is missed by more than 8 hrs or if vomiting occurs after dosing, skip dose and administer the next dose on schedule.

INDICATIONS/ROUTES/DOSAGE

CLL

PO: ADULTS, ELDERLY: Week 1: 20 mg once daily for 7 days. **Week 2:** 50 mg once daily for 7 days. **Week 3:** 100 mg once daily for 7 days. **Week 4:** 200 mg once daily for 7 days. **Week 5 and thereafter:** 400 mg once daily. Continue until disease progression or unacceptable toxicity. **In combination with riTUXimab:** Start riTUXimab administration after completing the 5-wk ramp-up dosing schedule for venetoclax and pt. has received 400 mg once daily for 7 days. Administer riTUXimab on day 1 of each 28-day cycle (at a dose of 375 mg/m² for cycle 1 and 500 mg/m² for cycles 2–6). Continue venetoclax 400 mg once daily for 24 mos from day 1 of cycle 1 of riTUXimab. **In combination with obinutuzumab:** Start obinutuzumab 100 mg on day 1 of cycle 1, then 900 mg on day 2 of cycle 1. Give 1,000 mg on days 8 and 15 of cycle 1 and on day 1 of each subsequent 28-day cycle for a total of 6 cycles. On day 22 of cycle 1, start venetoclax per the 5-wk ramp-up dosing schedule, completing the ramp-up phase on day 28 of cycle 2. Continue venetoclax 400 mg once daily from day 1 of cycle 3 until the last day of cycle 12.

AML

PO: ADULTS 75 YRS OR OLDER: Day 1: 100 mg once daily. **Day 2:** 200 mg once daily. **Day 3:** 400 mg once daily. **IN COMBINATION WITH AZACITIDINE OR DECITABINE: Day 4 and beyond:** 400 mg once daily. Continue until disease progression or unacceptable toxicity. **IN COMBINATION WITH LOW-DOSE CYTARABINE: Day 4 and beyond:** 600 mg once daily. Continue until disease progression or unacceptable toxicity.

Dose Modification

Based on Common Terminology Criteria for Adverse Events (CTCAE). For pts with dose interruption greater than 1 wk during 5-wk ramp-up phase or greater than 2 wks at 400 mg daily dose, reassess risk of tumor lysis syndrome to determine if reinitiation with a reduced dose is needed. Consider discontinuation in pts who require reduced dosage of less than 100 mg for more than 2 wks.

Dose Reduction Schedule

Note: During ramp-up phase, continue reduced dose for 1 wk before increasing dose.

Dose interruption at 400 mg: Resume at 300 mg. **Dose interruption at 300 mg:** Resume at 200 mg. **Dose interruption at 200 mg:** Resume at 100 mg. **Dose interruption at 100 mg:** Resume at 50 mg. **Dose interruption at 50 mg:** Resume at 20 mg. **Dose interruption at 20 mg:** Resume at 10 mg.

Tumor Lysis Syndrome

Any occurrence of blood chemistry abnormalities: Withhold next dose, then resume at same dose if resolved within 24–48 hrs of last dose. If not resolved within 48 hrs, resume at reduced dose. **Any event of tumor lysis syndrome:** Resume at reduced dose once resolved.

Grade 3 or 4 Nonhematologic Toxicity

First occurrence: Withhold treatment until resolved to Grade 1 or baseline, then resume at same dose. **Second and subsequent occurrences:** Withhold treatment until resolved, then follow dose reduction schedule (or reduce dose at prescriber's discretion).

Hematologic Toxicity

First occurrence of Grade 3 or 4 neutropenia with infection or fever; Grade 4 hematologic toxicity (except lymphopenia): Withhold treatment until resolved to Grade 1 or baseline, then resume at same dose. **Second and subsequent occurrences:** Withhold treatment until resolved, then follow dose reduction schedule (or reduce dose at prescriber's discretion).

Concomitant Use CYP3A4 Inhibitors, P-gp Inhibitors

Strong CYP3A4 inhibitors: Avoid inhibitor or reduce venetoclax dose by at least 75%. **Moderate CYP3A4 inhibitors or P-gp Inhibitors:** Avoid inhibitor or reduce venetoclax dose by at least 50%.

Dosage in Renal/Hepatic Impairment

Mild to moderate impairment: No dose adjustment. **Severe impairment:** Not specified; use caution.

 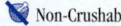

SIDE EFFECTS

Frequent (35%–14%): Diarrhea, nausea, fatigue, pyrexia, vomiting, headache, constipation. **Occasional (13%–10%):** Cough, peripheral edema, back pain.

ADVERSE EFFECTS/TOXIC REACTIONS

Myelosuppression (anemia, neutropenia, thrombocytopenia) is an expected response to therapy. Grade 3 or 4 neutropenia reported in 41% of pts. Pts with high tumor burden, renal impairment, concomitant use of strong or moderate CYP3A4 inhibitors, P-gp inhibitors may experience life-threatening tumor lysis syndrome, which mainly occurs during the 5-wk ramp-up phase and as early as 6–8 hrs after dose (hospitalization may be necessary). Tumor lysis syndrome may cause renal failure requiring emergent dialysis. Other reactions may include upper respiratory tract infection, pneumonia, autoimmune hemolytic anemia.

NURSING CONSIDERATIONS

BASELINE ASSESSMENT

Obtain ANC, CBC, BMP, renal function test; serum phosphate, calcium; vital signs prior to initiation and periodically thereafter. Obtain pregnancy test in female pts of reproductive potential. Question history of hepatic/renal impairment, gout. Assess all pts for high risk of tumor lysis syndrome and provide adequate hydration and antihyperuricemics (according to manufacturer guidelines) prior to first dose. Conduct tumor burden assessments including blood chemistries, radiologic testing (e.g., CT scan). Correct electrolyte imbalances prior to initiation. Receive full medication history (esp. CYP3A4 inhibitors, P-gp inhibitors, drugs with narrow therapeutic index). Screen for active infection. Offer emotional support.

INTERVENTION/EVALUATION

Monitor ANC, CBC for myelosuppression. Diligently monitor for tumor lysis syndrome (acute renal failure, electrolyte imbalance, cardiac arrhythmias, seizures). Monitor for infection and provide appropriate antimicrobial therapy if indicated. To reduce risk of neutropenia-associated infection, consider administration of granulocyte-colony stimulating factor (e.g., filgrastim). Monitor for toxicities if discontinuation of CYP3A4 inhibitors, P-gp inhibitors is unavoidable. Monitor I&O. Assess hydration status.

PATIENT/FAMILY TEACHING

• Treatment may depress your immune system and reduce your ability to fight infection. Report symptoms of infection such as body aches, chills, cough, fatigue, fever. Avoid those with active infection. • Therapy may cause tumor lysis syndrome (a condition caused by the rapid breakdown of cancer cells), which can cause kidney failure and may lead to death. Report decreased urination, amber-colored urine, confusion, difficulty breathing, fatigue, fever, muscle or joint pain, palpitations, seizures, vomiting. • Drink at least 6–8 glasses of water every day. • Use effective contraception to avoid pregnancy. Do not breastfeed. • Avoid grapefruit products, herbal supplements. • Do not take newly prescribed medications unless approved by prescriber who originally started therapy. • Do not receive live vaccines.

venlafaxine

ven-la-**fax**-een
(Effexor XR)

■ **BLACK BOX ALERT** ■ Increased risk of suicidal ideation and behavior in children, adolescents, young adults 18–24 yrs with major depressive disorder, other psychiatric disorders.

◆CLASSIFICATION

PHARMACOTHERAPEUTIC: Serotonin-norepinephrine reuptake inhibitor (SNRI). **CLINICAL:** Antidepressant.

USES

Treatment of major depressive disorder (unipolar). Treatment of generalized anxiety disorder (GAD), social anxiety disorder (SAD). Treatment of panic disorder, with or without agoraphobia. **OFF-LABEL:** Treatment of attention-deficit hyperactivity disorder (ADHD), obsessive-compulsive disorder (OCD), diabetic neuropathy, posttraumatic stress disorder (PTSD), episodic migraine prevention, narcolepsy, premenstrual dysphoric disorder, vasomotor symptoms associated with menopause.

PRECAUTIONS

Contraindications: Hypersensitivity to venlafaxine. Use of MAOIs intended to treat psychiatric disorders concurrently or within 14 days of discontinuing MAOI. Initiation of MAOI to treat psychiatric disorder within 7 days of discontinuing venlafaxine, initiation in pts receiving linezolid or IV methylene blue. **Cautions:** Seizure disorder, renal/hepatic impairment, pts at high risk for suicide, recent MI, mania, volume-depleted pts, narrow-angle glaucoma, HF, hyperthyroidism, abnormal platelet function, elderly.

ACTION

Potentiates CNS neurotransmitter activity by inhibiting reuptake of serotonin, norepinephrine, and, to lesser degree, DOPamine. **Therapeutic Effect:** Relieves depression.

PHARMACOKINETICS

Widely distributed. Protein binding: 25%–30%. Metabolized in liver. Primarily excreted in urine. Not removed by hemodialysis. **Half-life:** 3–7 hrs; metabolite, 9–13 hrs (increased in hepatic/renal impairment).

⧗ LIFESPAN CONSIDERATIONS

Pregnancy/Lactation: Unknown if distributed in breast milk. **Children:** Children, adolescents are at increased risk for suicidal ideation and behavior, worsening depression, esp. during first few mos of therapy. **Elderly:** Use caution.

INTERACTIONS

DRUG: **Strong CYP3A4 inhibitors (e.g., clarithromycin, ketoconazole, ritonavir)** may increase concentration/effect. **MAOIs (e.g., phenelzine, selegiline)** may cause neuroleptic malignant syndrome, autonomic instability (including rapid fluctuations of vital signs), extreme agitation, hyperthermia, altered mental status, myoclonus, rigidity, coma. **Strong CYP3A4 inducers (e.g., carBAMazepine, phenytoin, rifAMPin)** may decrease concentration/effect. **NSAIDs (e.g., diclofenac, meloxicam, naproxen), aspirin, warfarin** may increase risk of bleeding. **HERBAL:** **St. John's wort** may decrease concentration/effect. **Herbals with anticoagulant/antiplatelet properties (e.g., garlic, ginger, ginkgo biloba), glucosamine** may increase risk of bleeding. **FOOD: Grapefruit products** may increase concentration/effect. **LAB VALUES:** May increase serum cholesterol CPK, LDH, prolactin, GGT.

AVAILABILITY (Rx)

Tablets: 25 mg, 37.5 mg, 50 mg, 75 mg, 100 mg.

🐋 **Capsules, Extended-Release: (Effexor XR):** 37.5 mg, 75 mg, 150 mg. **Tablets, Extended-Release:** 37.5 mg, 75 mg, 112.5 mg, 150 mg, 225 mg.

ADMINISTRATION/HANDLING

PO

• Give with food. • Scored tablet may be crushed. • Do not break, crush, dissolve, or divide extended-release tablets. • May open capsule, sprinkle on applesauce. Give immediately without chewing and follow with full glass of water.

INDICATIONS/ROUTES/DOSAGE

Depression

PO: *(Immediate-Release):* **ADULTS, ELDERLY:** Initially, 75 mg/day in 2–3 divided doses with food. May increase in increments of up to 75 mg/day at intervals of no less than 4 days. Usual dose: 225–350 mg/day. **Maximum:** 375 mg/day in 3 divided doses.

V

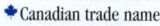 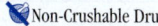

PO: *(Extended-Release):* **ADULTS, ELDERLY:** Initially, 37.5–75 mg/day as single dose with food. Pts initiated at 37.5 mg once daily may increase to 75 mg once daily after 4–7 days. Thereafter, may increase by 75 mg/day at intervals of 4 days or longer. Usual dose: 75–225 mg once daily. **Maximum:** 225 mg/day.

Generalized Anxiety Disorder (GAD)
PO: *(Extended-Release):* **ADULTS, ELDERLY:** Initially, 37.5–75 mg/day (pts initiated at 37.5 mg once daily may increase to 75 mg once daily after 4–7 days). May increase by 75 mg/day at 4-day intervals up to 225 mg/day.

Panic Disorder
PO: *(Extended-Release):* **ADULTS, ELDERLY:** Initially, 37.5 mg/day. May increase to 75 mg after 7 days followed by increases of 75 mg/day at 7-day intervals up to 225 mg/day.

Social Anxiety Disorder (SAD)
PO: *(Extended-Release):* **ADULTS, ELDERLY:** Initially, 75 mg/day given in a single dose. **Maximum:** 75 mg/day.

Dosage in Renal/Hepatic Impairment
Consider decreasing venlafaxine dosage by 50% in pts with moderate hepatic impairment, 25% in pts with mild to moderate renal impairment, 50% in pts on dialysis (withhold dose until completion of dialysis). When discontinuing therapy, taper dosage slowly over 2 wks.

SIDE EFFECTS

Frequent (greater than 20%): Nausea, drowsiness, headache, dry mouth. **Occasional (20%–10%):** Dizziness, insomnia, constipation, diaphoresis, nervousness, asthenia, ejaculatory disturbance, anorexia. **Rare (less than 10%):** Anxiety, blurred vision, diarrhea, vomiting, tremor, abnormal dreams, impotence.

ADVERSE EFFECTS/TOXIC REACTIONS

Sustained increase in diastolic B/P of 10–15 mm Hg occurs occasionally. Serotonin syndrome (agitation, confusion, hallucinations, hyperreflexia), neuroleptic malignant syndrome (muscular rigidity, fever, cognitive changes), suicidal ideation have occurred.

NURSING CONSIDERATIONS

BASELINE ASSESSMENT
Obtain weight, B/P. Assess appearance, behavior, speech pattern, level of interest, mood. Assess risk of suicide.

INTERVENTION/EVALUATION
Monitor signs/symptoms of depression, B/P, weight. Assess sleep pattern for evidence of insomnia. Check during waking hours for drowsiness, dizziness, anxiety; provide assistance as necessary. Assess appearance, behavior, speech pattern, level of interest, mood for therapeutic response. Monitor for suicidal ideation (esp. at initiation of therapy or changes in dosage).

PATIENT/ FAMILY TEACHING
• Take with food to minimize GI distress. • Do not increase, decrease, suddenly stop medication. • Avoid tasks that require alertness, motor skills until response to drug is established. • Report if breastfeeding, pregnant, or planning to become pregnant. • Avoid alcohol. • Seek immediate medical attention if thoughts of suicide, new onset or worsening of anxiety, depression, or changes in mood occur.

verapamil

ver-**ap**-a-mil
(Calan SR, Verelan, Verelan PM)
Do not confuse Verelan with Voltaren, or Calan with Colace or dilTIAZem.

FIXED-COMBINATION(S)

Tarka: verapamil/trandolapril (an ACE inhibitor): 240 mg/1 mg, 180 mg/2 mg, 240 mg/2 mg, 240 mg/4 mg.

◆ CLASSIFICATION

PHARMACOTHERAPEUTIC: Calcium channel blocker (nondihydropyridine). **CLINICAL:** Antihypertensive, antianginal, antiarrhythmic (class IV).

USES

Angina: Treatment of angina at rest (including chronic stable angina, vasospastic angina, unstable angina). **Atrial fibrillation/atrial flutter (Rate control):** *Oral:* Control of ventricular rate at rest and during stress in chronic atrial flutter and/or atrial fibrillation. *Parenteral:* Temporary control of rapid ventricular rate in atrial flutter/fibrillation (except when associated with accessory pathways). **Hypertension:** Management of hypertension. **Supraventricular tachycardia (SVT):** Prophylaxis of SVT (e.g., AV re-entrant tachycardia). Rapid conversion to sinus rhythm. **OFF-LABEL:** Cluster headache (prevention), migraine prevention, supraventricular tachycardia (acute), ventricular arrhythmias (idoiopathic left ventricular tachycardia, nonsustained ventricular tachycardia or ventricular premature beats).

PRECAUTIONS

Contraindications: Hypersensitivity to verapamil. Atrial fibrillation/flutter in presence of accessory bypass tract (e.g., Wolff-Parkinson-White, Lown-Ganong-Levine syndromes), severe left ventricular dysfunction, cardiogenic shock, second- or third-degree heart block (except with pacemaker), hypotension (SBP less than 90 mm Hg), sick sinus syndrome (except with pacemaker). **IV (additional):** Current use of IV beta-blocking agents, ventricular tachycardia. **Cautions:** Renal/hepatic impairment, concomitant use of beta blockers and/or digoxin, myasthenia gravis, elderly, hypertrophic cardiomyopathy. Avoid use in HF.

ACTION

Inhibits calcium ion entry across cardiac, vascular smooth-muscle cell membranes, dilating coronary arteries, peripheral arteries, arterioles. **Therapeutic Effect:** Decreases heart rate, myocardial contractility; slows SA, AV conduction. Decreases total peripheral vascular resistance by vasodilation.

PHARMACOKINETICS

Widely distributed. Protein binding: 90% (60% in neonates). Metabolized in liver. Primarily excreted in urine. Not removed by hemodialysis. **Half-life: Single dose:** 2–8 hrs; **multiple doses:** 4.5–12 hrs.

⌛ LIFESPAN CONSIDERATIONS

Pregnancy/Lactation: Drug crosses placenta; distributed in breast milk. Breastfeeding not recommended. **Children:** No age-related precautions noted. **Elderly:** Age-related renal impairment may require dosage adjustment.

INTERACTIONS

DRUG: May increase hypotensive effect of **angiotension-converting enzyme (ACE) inhibitors (e.g., enalapril, lisinopril), angiotensin II receptor blockers (e.g., valsartan), HCTZ, hydralazine.** May increase concentration/effects of **bosutinib, carBAMazepine, cyclosPORINE, dofetilide, eletriptan, lomitapide, neratinib, simvastatin, theophylline. HERBAL: Herbals with hypertensive properties (e.g., licorice, yohimbe) or hypotensive properties (e.g., garlic, ginger, ginkgo biloba)** may alter effects. **FOOD:** Grapefruit products may increase concentration/effect. **LAB VALUES:** ECG may show prolonged PR interval. **Therapeutic serum level:** 0.08–0.3 mcg/mL; **toxic serum level:** N/A.

AVAILABILITY (Rx)

Injection Solution: 2.5 mg/mL. **Tablets:** 40 mg, 80 mg, 120 mg.

�–¼ **Capsules, Extended-Release:** 100 mg, 120 mg, 180 mg, 200 mg, 240 mg,

V

300 mg, 360 mg. **Tablets, Extended-Release:** 120 mg, 180 mg, 240 mg.

ADMINISTRATION/HANDLING

 IV

Reconstitution • May give undiluted. **Rate of administration** • Administer IV push over 2 min for adults, children; give over 3 min for elderly. • Continuous ECG monitoring during IV injection is required for children, recommended for adults. • Monitor ECG for rapid ventricular rate, extreme bradycardia, heart block, asystole, prolongation of PR interval. Notify physician of any significant changes. • Monitor B/P q5–10min. • Pt should remain recumbent for at least 1 hr after IV administration. **Storage** • Store vials at room temperature.

PO
Immediate-release • May give without regard to food. **Extended-release** • May give without regard to food. Administer whole (do not crush or allow chewing). • Sustained-release capsules may be opened and sprinkled on applesauce, then swallowed immediately (do not chew).

▓ IV COMPATIBILITIES
Dexmedetomidine, propofol.

INDICATIONS/ROUTES/DOSAGE

Supraventricular Tachycardia (SVT)
IV: ADULTS, ELDERLY: Acute: Initially, 5 to 10 mg (0.075 to 0.15 mg/kg) over 2 min. **Repeat dose:** 10 mg (0.15 mg/kg) 30 min after initial dose. **PO: ADULTS, ELDERLY: (Chronic):** Initially, 40 mg 3–4 times daily. **Maximum:** 480 mg/day in 3–4 divided doses.

Angina
PO: *(Immediate-Release):* **ADULTS, ELDERLY:** Initially, 80–120 mg 3 times/day. May increase at 1- to 2-day intervals up to 480 mg/day in 3 divided doses. **Maximum:** 480 mg/day.

PO: *(Extended-Release):* Initially, 180 mg once daily. May increase at 7- to 14-day intervals up to 480 mg/day in 1–2 divided doses. **Maximum:** 480 mg/day.

Atrial Fibrillation (Ventricular Rate Control)
IV: ADULTS, ELDERLY: Acute: Initially, 0.075–0.15 mg/kg (usual: 5–10 mg) over 2 min. May repeat with 10 mg after 15–30 min. **PO:** *(Immediate-Release):* **Chronic:** Initially, 40 mg 3–4 times daily. To achieve rate control, may increase up to 480 mg/day in 3–4 divided doses.

Hypertension
PO: *(Immediate-Release):* **ADULTS, ELDERLY:** Initially, 40–80 mg 3 times daily. May increase at wkly intervals up to 480 mg/day in 3 divided doses. **Usual dose:** 120–360 mg/day in 3 divided doses. **Maximum:** 480 mg/day in 3 divided doses.

PO (Tablet): *(Extended-Release):* **ADULTS, ELDERLY:** Initially, 120–180 mg once daily. May increase at wkly intervals to 240 mg once daily, then 180 mg twice daily. **Usual dose:** 120–360 mg/day in 1 or 2 divided doses. **Maximum:** 480 mg/day in 1–2 divided doses.

PO (Capsule): *(Extended-Release):* **ADULTS, ELDERLY:** Initially, 100–200 mg once daily at bedtime. May increase dose at wkly intervals to 300 mg once daily, then 400 mg once daily maximum. **Usual dose:** 100–300 mg once at bedtime.

Dosage for Renal Impairment
CrCl less than 10 mL/min: Dose reduction (50%–75%) of normal dose recommended.

Dosage in Hepatic Impairment
Dose reduction (20%–50%) of normal dose recommended.

SIDE EFFECTS
Frequent (7%): Constipation. **Occasional (4%–2%):** Dizziness, light-headedness, headache, asthenia, nausea, peripheral edema, hypotension. **Rare (less than 1%):** Bradycardia, dermatitis, rash.

underlined – top prescribed drug

ADVERSE EFFECTS/TOXIC REACTIONS

Rapid ventricular rate in atrial flutter/fibrillation, marked hypotension, extreme bradycardia, HF, asystole, second- or third-degree AV block occur rarely.

NURSING CONSIDERATIONS

BASELINE ASSESSMENT

Obtain ECG, B/P, heart rate. Record onset, type (sharp, dull, squeezing), radiation, location, intensity, duration of anginal pain, precipitating factors (exertion, emotional stress).

INTERVENTION/EVALUATION

Assess pulse for quality, rate, rhythm. Monitor B/P. Monitor ECG for cardiac changes, particularly prolongation of PR interval. Assess for peripheral edema. For those taking oral form, monitor daily pattern of bowel activity, stool consistency. **Therapeutic serum level:** 0.08–0.3 mcg/mL; **toxic serum level:** N/A.

PATIENT/FAMILY TEACHING

• Do not abruptly discontinue medication. • Compliance with therapy regimen is essential to control anginal pain. • Go from lying to standing slowly. • Avoid tasks that require alertness, motor skills until response to drug is established. • Limit caffeine. • Avoid or limit alcohol. • Report continued, persistent angina pain, irregular heartbeats, shortness of breath, swelling, dizziness, constipation, nausea, hypotension. • Avoid grapefruit products.

---

vibegron

vye-**beg**-ron
(Gemtesa)
Do not confuse vibegron with mirabegron, vigabatrin, or vigadrone or Gemtesa with Gemzar.

◆CLASSIFICATION

PHARMACOTHERAPEUTIC: Beta-3 adrenergic receptor agonist. **CLINICAL:** Urinary antispasmodic.

USES

Treatment of overactive bladder in adults with symptoms of urge urinary incontinence, urgency, and urinary frequency. Treatment of overactive bladder with symptoms of urge urinary incontinence, urgency, and urinary frequency in adult males on pharmacological therapy for benign prostatic hyperplasia (BPH).

PRECAUTIONS

Contraindications: Hypersensitivity to vibegron. **Cautions:** Pts at risk for urinary retention (e.g., bladder outlet obstruction, concomitant use of muscarinic antagonists). Concomitant use of digoxin.

ACTION

Relaxes detrusor smooth muscle during bladder filling, increasing bladder capacity. **Therapeutic Effect:** Relives urinary incontinence, urgency, frequency.

PHARMACOKINETICS

Widely distributed. Metabolized in liver. Protein binding: 50%. Peak plasma concentration: 1–3 hrs. Steady state reached in 7 days. Excreted in feces (59%), urine (20%). **Half-life:** 30.8 hrs.

⧖ LIFESPAN CONSIDERATIONS

Pregnancy/Lactation: Unknown if distributed in breast milk. **Children:** Safety and efficacy not established. **Elderly:** No age-related precautions noted.

INTERACTIONS

DRUG: May increase concentration/toxic effect of **digoxin. HERBAL:** None significant. **FOOD:** None known. **LAB VALUES:** None significant.

AVAILABILITY (Rx)

Tablets: 75 mg.

ADMINISTRATION/HANDLING

PO

• Give without regard to food. • Administer tablet whole with water. Tablets may

V

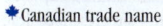 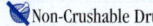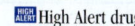

be crushed and mixed in applesauce and give immediately, followed by water.

INDICATIONS/ROUTES/DOSAGE
Overactive Bladder
PO: ADULTS: 75 mg once daily.

Dosage in Renal Impairment
Mild to severe impairment: No dose adjustment.

Dosage in Hepatic Impairment
Mild to moderate impairment: No dose adjustment. **Severe impairment:** Not specified; use caution.

SIDE EFFECTS
Rare (4%–2%): Headache, diarrhea, nausea, dry mouth, hot flush.

ADVERSE EFFECTS/TOXIC REACTIONS
Urinary retention may occur, esp. in pts with bladder outlet obstruction or taking concomitant muscarinic antagonist. Upper respiratory tract infection, including nasopharyngitis, may occur.

NURSING CONSIDERATIONS

BASELINE ASSESSMENT
Obtain digoxin level in pts taking digoxin. Assess severity of urinary incontinence, urgency, frequency. Screen for risk of urinary retention.

INTERVENTION/EVALUATION
Monitor for symptoms of urinary retention (abdominal pain, bladder distension, hesitancy). Obtain bladder scan in pts with urinary retention. Monitor digoxin levels (if applicable). Monitor for symptom improvement of overactive bladder.

PATIENT/FAMILY TEACHING
• Treatment may cause retention of urine. Report symptoms of urinary retention (abdominal pain, bladder distension, hesitancy). • Pts taking digoxin may require more frequent monitoring of digoxin levels. • Notify prescriber if symptoms of overactive bladder do not improve.

vilazodone

vil-**az**-oh-done
(Viibryd)
■ **BLACK BOX ALERT** ■ Increased risk of suicidal ideation and behavior in children, adolescents, and young adults 18–24 yrs of age with major depressive disorder, other psychiatric disorders.

◆ CLASSIFICATION
PHARMACOTHERAPEUTIC: Selective serotonin reuptake inhibitor. **CLINICAL:** Antidepressant.

USES
Treatment of major depressive disorder (unipolar) in adults.

PRECAUTIONS
Contraindications: Hypersensitivity to vilazodone. Use of MAOIs intended to treat psychiatric disorders (with or within 14 days of stopping vilazodone or MAOI), starting vilazodone in pts receiving linezolid or methylene blue. **Cautions:** Seizure disorder, pts at risk for suicide (history of ideation and behavior; depression), hepatic impairment, elderly.

ACTION
Enhances serotonergic activity in CNS by selectively inhibiting reuptake of serotonin. **Therapeutic Effect:** Relieves depression.

PHARMACOKINETICS
Widely distributed. Peak concentration: 4–5 hrs. Protein binding: 96%–99%. Metabolized in liver. **Half-life:** 25 hrs.

⌛ LIFESPAN CONSIDERATIONS
Pregnancy/Lactation: Unknown if drug crosses placenta or is excreted in breast milk. **Children:** Safety and efficacy not established. **Elderly:** No age-related precautions noted.

INTERACTIONS

DRUG: Alcohol may increase adverse effects. **Aspirin, NSAIDs** (e.g., **diclofenac, meloxicam, naproxen**), **warfarin** may increase risk of bleeding. **Strong CYP3A4 inhibitors** (e.g., **clarithromycin, ketoconazole**) may increase concentration. **BusPIRone, MAOIs** (e.g., **phenelzine, selegiline**) **SNRIs** (e.g., **venlafaxine**), **SSRIs** (e.g., **sertraline**), **traMADol** may increase risk of serotonin syndrome. **HERBAL: Herbals with anticoagulant/ antiplatelet properties** (e.g., **garlic, ginger, ginkgo biloba**), **glucosamine** may increase risk of bleeding. **St. John's wort, Syrian rue** may increase serotonergic effect. **FOOD:** None known. **LAB VALUES:** None significant.

AVAILABILITY (Rx)

Tablets: 10 mg, 20 mg, 40 mg.

ADMINISTRATION/HANDLING

PO

• Give with food (administration without food can result in inadequate drug concentration, may diminish effectiveness).

INDICATIONS/ROUTES/DOSAGE

Depression
PO: ADULTS, ELDERLY: Initially, 10 mg once daily for 7 days, followed by 20 mg once daily. May increase to 40 mg once daily after a minimum of 7 days. **Note:** When discontinuing treatment, reduce dose gradually. From 40 mg/day: Taper to 20 mg/day for 4 days, then 10 mg/day for 3 days. From 20 mg/day: Taper to 10 mg/day for 7 days.

Concomitant Use of Strong CYP3A4 Inhibitors
Do not exceed 20 mg once daily.

Concomitant Use of Strong CYP3A4 Inducers
May increase dose to 80 mg/day when used concomitantly for more than 14 days.

Dosage in Renal/Hepatic Impairment
No dose adjustment.

SIDE EFFECTS

Frequent (28%–23%): Diarrhea, nausea. **Occasional (9%–3%):** Dizziness, dry mouth, insomnia, vomiting, decreased libido, abnormal dreams, fatigue, sweating. **Rare (2%):** Dyspepsia, flatulence, paresthesia, restlessness, arthralgia, abnormal orgasm, delayed ejaculation, increased appetite, palpitations, tremor.

ADVERSE EFFECTS/TOXIC REACTIONS

Serotonin syndrome (agitation, confusion, hallucinations, hyperreflexia), neuroleptic malignant syndrome (fever, muscular rigidity, cognitive changes).

NURSING CONSIDERATIONS

BASELINE ASSESSMENT

Assess behavior, appearance, emotional status, response to environment, speech pattern, thought content, risk of suicide.

INTERVENTION/EVALUATION

Monitor B/P, heart rate, weight. Monitor for suicidal ideation (esp. at initiation of therapy or changes in dosage). Assess for therapeutic response (greater interest in surroundings, improved self-care, increased ability to concentrate, relaxed facial expression).

PATIENT/FAMILY TEACHING

• Avoid tasks that may require alertness, motor skills until response to drug is established (may cause dizziness). • Slowly go from lying to standing. • Take with food. • Do not suddenly stop taking medication; withdraw gradually. • Seek immediate medical attention if thoughts of suicide, new onset or worsening of anxiety, depression, or changes in mood occur. • Avoid alcohol.

viloxazine

vye-**lox**-a-zeen
(Qelbree)

■ **BLACK BOX ALERT** ■ May increase risk of suicidal thoughts and behavior. Monitor closely

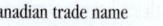 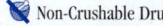

for emergence or worsening of symptoms.

Do not confuse viloxazine with vilazodone.

◆CLASSIFICATION

PHARMACOTHERAPEUTIC: Selective norepinephrine reuptake inhibitor. **CLINICAL:** Noradrenergic agent.

USES

Treatment of attention deficit hyperactivity disorder (ADHD) in adults and pediatric pts 6–17 yrs of age.

PRECAUTIONS

Contraindications: Hypersensitivity to viloxazine. Use or within 14 days after MAOI therapy. Concomitant use of *sensitive* CYP1A2 substrates or CYP1A2 substrates with a narrow therapeutic index. **Cautions:** Family history of suicide, psychiatric disorders. Personal history of hypertension, tachycardia, bipolar disorder, depression, psychosis, mania, other psychiatric illness. Pts at high risk for suicide ideation and behavior; concomitant use of CYP2D6 substrates, CYP3A4 substrates. Not recommended in pts with hepatic impairment; concomitant use of *moderate* CYP1A2 substrates.

ACTION

Blocks the reuptake of norepinephrine. The exact mechanism for the treatment of ADHD has not been fully elucidated. Appears to inhibit 5-HT$_{2B}$ receptors and activate 5-HT$_{2C}$ receptors. **Therapeutic Effect:** Increases motor acuity, attention span, mental alertness.

PHARMACOKINETICS

Widely distributed. Metabolized in liver. Protein binding: 76%–82%. Peak plasma concentration: approx. 5 hrs. Steady state reached in 2 days. Excreted in urine (90%), feces (1%). **Half-life:** 7 hrs (±4.74 hrs).

☒ LIFESPAN CONSIDERATIONS

Pregnancy/Lactation: Unknown if distributed in breast milk. May cause fetal harm. **Children:** Safety and efficacy not established in pts younger than 6 yrs. **Elderly:** Not indicated in elderly population.

INTERACTIONS

DRUG: **MAOIs (e.g., phenelzine, selegiline, tranylcypromine), potent inhibitors of monoamine oxidase (e.g., linezolid)** may increase risk of hypertensive crisis, serotonin syndrome. May increase adverse/toxic effects of **sensitive CYP1A2 substrates and CYP1A2 substrates with narrow therapeutic index (e.g., alosetron, DULoxetine, ramelteon, tiZANidine, theophylline), moderate CYP1A2 substrates (e.g., cloZAPine, pirfenidone), CYP2D6 substrates (e.g., desipramine, dextromethorphan, metoprolol, venlafaxine, risperiDONE, CYP3A4 substrates (e.g., busPIRone, midazolam, tacrolimus, tipranavir, simvastatin).** **HERBAL:** None significant. **FOOD:** None known. **LAB VALUES:** None significant.

AVAILABILITY (Rx)

🐦 **Capsules, Extended-Release:** 100 mg, 150 mg, 200 mg.

ADMINISTRATION/HANDLING

PO
• Give without regard to food. • Do not cut, crush, or allow chewing. • Administer whole or open and sprinkle on pudding or applesauce. Consume mixture without chewing (within 15 min for pudding or 2 hrs for applesauce). Do not store for future use.

INDICATIONS/ROUTES/DOSAGE

Note: If used long-term, periodically reevaluate necessity for treatment and adjust dose as needed.
ADHD
PO: CHILDREN 6–11 YRS: Initially, 100 mg once daily. May titrate in increments of 100 mg at wkly intervals based on response and tolerability. **Maximum:** 400

V

mg/day. **ADOLESCENTS 12–17 YRS:** Initially, 200 mg once daily. After 7 days, may increase dose to 400 mg once daily based on response and tolerability. **Maximum:** 400 mg/day. **ADULTS:** Initially, 200 mg once daily. May increase by 200 mg/day at wkly intervals. **Maximum:** 600 mg once daily.

Dosage in Renal Impairment
Mild to moderate impairment: No dose adjustment. **Severe impairment:** Reduce starting dose to 100 mg once daily. May titrate in increments of 50–100 mg at wkly intervals based on response and tolerability. **Maximum:** 200 mg/day.

Dosage in Hepatic Impairment
Mild to severe impairment: Not recommended.

SIDE EFFECTS

Occasional (16%–6%): Somnolence, lethargy, headache (migraine, tension headache), decreased appetite, fatigue. **Rare (5%–2%):** Abdominal pain, nausea, vomiting, insomnia, irritability, pyrexia.

ADVERSE EFFECTS/TOXIC REACTIONS

May increase risk of suicidal thoughts and behavior. Increased heart rate greater than or equal to 20 bpm reported in 22%–34% of pts. Increased diastolic blood pressure greater than or equal to 15 mm Hg reported in 13%–25% of pts. May cause manic or mixed episodes in pts with history of bipolar disorder. Respiratory tract infection reported in 7% of pts.

NURSING CONSIDERATIONS

BASELINE ASSESSMENT
Obtain B/P, heart rate, height/weight. Assess attention span, impulsivity, interaction with others, distractibility. Question for history of hepatic impairment, hypertension; anxiety; bipolar disorder, depression; family history of suicide, psy-

chiatric disorder. Receive full medication history and screen for interactions (esp. use of MAOIs, *sensitive* CYP1A2 substrates or CYP1A2 substrates with a narrow therapeutic index). Offer emotional support.

INTERVENTION/EVALUATION
Monitor B/P, heart rate periodically and during titration. Assess height/weight periodically. Diligently monitor for new-onset or worsening of agitation, anxiety, depression, mood disorder, panic attacks; manic behavior in pts with bipolar disorder (may be precursor for increased risk of suicidal thoughts and behavior), esp. during first few mos after initiation and during titration. Consult mental health professional if mood disorder is suspected. Monitor for toxicities if concomitant use of CYP2D6 substrates, CYP3A4 substrates is unavoidable. Assess for clinical improvement of ADHD.

PATIENT/FAMILY TEACHING
• Treatment may increase blood pressure and/or heart rate. • Seek immediate medical attention if new-onset or worsening of agitation, anxiety, depression, or changes in mood occur, esp. during the first few mos of therapy and during titration. • Avoid tasks that require alertness, motor skills until response to drug is established. • There is a high risk of interactions with other medications. Do not take newly prescribed medications unless approved by prescriber who originally started therapy. • Treatment affects weight and growth development.

V

vinBLAStine HIGH ALERT

vin-**blas**-teen

■ **BLACK BOX ALERT** ■ Must be administered by personnel trained in administration/handling of chemotherapeutic agents. For IV use only. Fatal if given intrathe-cally (ascending paralysis, death). Vesicant; avoid extravasation.

Do not confuse vinBLAStine with vinCRIStine or vinorelbine.

◆ CLASSIFICATION

PHARMACOTHERAPEUTIC: Antimi-crotubular. Vinca alkaloid. **CLINI-CAL:** Antineoplastic.

USES

Treatment of Hodgkin's lymphoma, Langerhans cell histiocytosis, advanced testicular carcinoma, Kaposi's sarcoma, Letterer-Siwe disease, choriosarcoma, mycosis fungoides. **OFF-LABEL:** Treatment of bladder, ovarian cancer; non–small-cell lung cancer; soft tissue sarcoma, melanoma.

PRECAUTIONS

Contraindications: Hypersensitivity to vin-BLAStine. Bacterial infection, significant granulocytopenia (unless as a result of condition being treated). **Cautions:** He-patic impairment, cardiovascular disease (e.g., cardiomyopathy, hypertension), pulmonary disease, baseline cytopenias, conditions predisposing to infection (e.g., diabetes, renal failure, immunocom-promised pts, open wounds); history of thrombosis (CVA, MI); pts at risk for ex-travasation (e.g., peripheral IV catheters, elderly, poor peripheral vasculature), recent exposure to radiation therapy, che-motherapy.

ACTION

Binds to tubulin, inhibiting microtubule formation; may interfere with nucleic acid, protein synthesis. **Therapeutic Ef-fect:** Inhibits cell division by disrupting mitotic spindle.

PHARMACOKINETICS

Does not cross blood-brain barrier. Pro-tein binding: 99%. Metabolized in liver. Excreted in urine (14%), feces (10%). **Half-life:** 24.8 hrs.

⧗ LIFESPAN CONSIDERATIONS

Pregnancy/Lactation: Avoid pregnancy; may cause fetal harm. Females of reproduc-tive potential must use effective contraception during treatment and for at least 6 mos after discontinuation. Breastfeeding not recom-mended during treatment and for at least 1 wk after discontinuation. May impair fertil-ity. **Males:** Males with female partners of reproductive potential must use effective contraception during treatment and for at least 3 mos after discontinuation. **Children/Elderly:** No age-related precautions noted.

INTERACTIONS

DRUG: Strong CYP3A4 inhibitors (e.g., clarithromycin, ketoconazole, rito-navir), moderate CYP3A4 inhibitors (e.g., dilTIAZem, fluconazole, vera-pamil) may increase concentration/effect. Strong CYP3A4 inducers (e.g., car-BAMazepine, phenytoin, rifAMPin), moderate CYP3A4 inducers (e.g., dexamethasone, modafinil, nafcillin) may decrease concentration/effect. May de-crease therapeutic effect of BCG (intraves-ical). Bone marrow depressants (e.g., cladribine) may increase myelosuppres-sion. Live virus vaccines may potentiate virus replication, increase vaccine side ef-fects, decrease pt's antibody response to vaccine. **HERBAL:** None significant. Echi-nacea may decrease the therapeutic effect. **FOOD:** None known. **LAB VALUES:** May increase serum uric acid.

AVAILABILITY (Rx)

Injection Solution: 1 mg/mL.

ADMINISTRATION/HANDLING

◄**ALERT**► May be carcinogenic, muta-genic, teratogenic. Handle with extreme care during preparation and administra-tion. Give by IV injection. Leakage from IV site into surrounding tissue may pro-duce extreme irritation. Avoid eye con-tact with solution (severe eye irritation, possible corneal ulceration may result). If eye contact occurs, immediately irri-gate eye with water.

V

IV

Note: In order to prevent inadvertent intrathecal administration, dispense as a piggyback (not a syringe).

Reconstitution • Using 1 mg/mL solution, further dilute in 25–50 mL D_5W or 0.9% NaCl.

Rate of administration • Infuse over 5–15 min. Prolonged administration time and/or increased volume may increase risk of vein irritation and extravasation.

Storage • Refrigerate unopened vials. • Solution appears clear, colorless. • Following dilution, solution is stable for up to 21 days if protected from light (consult manufacturer prescribing information). • Discard if solution is discolored or precipitate forms.

🞉 IV COMPATIBILITIES

Granisetron, ondansetron.

INDICATIONS/ROUTES/DOSAGE

◀ALERT▶ Dosage individualized based on clinical response, tolerance to adverse effects. When used in combination therapy, consult specific protocols for optimum dosage, sequence of drug administration. Strongly recommend dispensing in a minibag (not a syringe).

Usual Dosage

IV: ADULTS, ELDERLY: Initially, 3.7 mg/m^2 (adjust dose q7days based on WBC response) up to 5.5 mg/m^2 (second wk), 7.4 mg/m^2 (third wk), 9.25 mg/m^2 (fourth wk), and 11.1 mg/m^2 (fifth wk). **Maximum:** 18.5 mg/m^2. **CHILDREN:** 3–6 mg/m^2 q7–14days.

Dosage in Renal Impairment

Mild to severe impairment: No dose adjustment.

Dosage in Hepatic Impairment

Direct serum bilirubin 1.5–3 mg/dL: Reduce dose by 50%. **Greater than 3 mg/dL:** Avoid use.

SIDE EFFECTS

Frequent: Nausea, vomiting, alopecia. **Occasional:** Constipation, diarrhea, rectal bleeding, headache, paresthesia (occur 4–6 hrs after administration, persist for 2–10 hrs), malaise, asthenia, dizziness, pain at tumor site, jaw/face pain, depression, dry mouth. **Rare:** Dermatitis, stomatitis, phototoxicity, hyperuricemia.

ADVERSE EFFECTS/TOXIC REACTIONS

Myelosuppression (anemia, leukopenia) is an expected response to therapy. WBC reaches its nadir 4–10 days after initial therapy, recovers within 7–14 days (high dosage may require 21-day recovery period). Thrombocytopenia is usually mild and transient, with recovery occurring in a few days. Hepatic impairment may increase risk of toxicity. Acute shortness of breath, bronchospasm may occur, particularly when administered concurrently with mitoMYcin. Extravasation may cause severe tissue necrosis. Neurotoxicity (seizures, severe CNS damage), cardiovascular toxicities (angina pectoris, cardiomyopathy, CVA, hypertension, limb ischemia, MI, Raynaud's phenomenon), GI toxicities (hemorrhagic enterocolitis, GI bleeding, intestinal obstruction, paralytic ileus, toxic megacolon) may occur.

NURSING CONSIDERATIONS

BASELINE ASSESSMENT

Obtain CBC, LFT; pregnancy test in females of reproductive potential. Screen for active infection. Question history of cardiac/pulmonary disease, hepatic impairment. Assess patency of IV access. Offer emotional support.

INTERVENTION/EVALUATION

Monitor CBC for myelosuppression, LFT for hepatotoxicity (abdominal pain, jaundice, nausea, transamini-

V

---

tis, vomiting). Monitor for infections (cough, fatigue, fever), neurotoxicities (seizures, CNS effects), stomatitis, pulmonary toxicities (bronchospasm, dyspnea); symptoms of CVA (aphasia, altered mental status, facial droop, hemiplegia, vision loss); MI (chest pain, diaphoresis, left arm/jaw pain, increased serum troponin, ST segment elevation). Extravasation may result in cellulitis, phlebitis. Large amount of extravasation may result in tissue sloughing. If extravasation occurs, give local injection of hyaluronidase, apply warm compresses.

PATIENT/FAMILY TEACHING

• Treatment may depress your immune system response and reduce your ability to fight infection. Report symptoms of infection such as body aches, chills, cough, fatigue, fever. Avoid those with active infection. • Report symptoms of bone marrow depression (e.g., bruising, fatigue, fever, shortness of breath, weight loss; bleeding easily, bloody urine or stool). • Avoid pregnancy. Do not breastfeed. • Treatment may reduce the heart's ability to pump effectively. • Report heart problems (difficulty breathing, swelling of extremities, palpitations), liver problems (abdominal pain, bruising, clay-colored stool, dark or amber-colored urine, yellowing of the skin or eyes), skin reactions (rash, redness, swelling), seizures. • Life-threatening cardiovascular events may occur; report symptoms of heart attack (chest pain, difficulty breathing, jaw pain, nausea, pain that radiates to the arm or jaw, sweating), stroke (confusion, one-sided weakness or paralysis, difficulty speaking).

---

vinCRIStine

vin-**cris**-teen
(Marqibo)

■ **BLACK BOX ALERT** ■ Must be administered by personnel trained in administration/handling of chemotherapeutic agents. For IV use only. Fatal if given intrathecally (ascending paralysis, death). Vesicant; avoid extravasation. Marqibo and Vincasar are not interchangeable.
Do not confuse vinCRIStine with vinBLAStine.

◆CLASSIFICATION

PHARMACOTHERAPEUTIC: Antimicrotubular. Vinca alkaloid. **CLINICAL:** Antineoplastic.

USES

Treatment of acute lymphocytic leukemia (ALL), Hodgkin's lymphoma, advanced non-Hodgkin's lymphomas, neuroblastoma, rhabdomyosarcoma, Wilms tumor. **Marqibo:** Relapsed Philadelphia chromosome negative (Ph⁻) ALL in adults whose disease has progressed after 2 or more antileukemic therapies. **OFF-LABEL:** Treatment of multiple myeloma, chronic lymphocytic leukemia (CLL), brain tumors, small-cell lung cancer, Ewing's sarcoma, gestational trophoblastic tumors.

PRECAUTIONS

Contraindications: Hypersensitivity to vinCRIStine. Demyelinating form of Charcot-Marie-Tooth syndrome. Intrathecal administration. **Cautions:** Hepatic impairment, elderly, preexisting neuromuscular disorders, conditions predisposing to infection (e.g., diabetes, renal failure, immunocompromised pts, open wounds); pts at risk for extravasation (e.g., peripheral IV catheters, elderly, poor peripheral vasculature), recent exposure to radiation therapy, chemotherapy; pts at risk for tumor lysis syndrome (high tumor burden, dehydration); history of GI obstruction.

ACTION

Binds to tubulin, inhibiting microtubule formation; may interfere with nucleic

---

acid/protein synthesis. **Therapeutic Effect:** Inhibits cell division by disrupting mitotic spindle.

PHARMACOKINETICS

Does not cross blood-brain barrier. Protein binding: 75%. Metabolized in liver. Primarily excreted in feces by biliary system. **Half-life:** 24 hrs. **Marqibo:** 45 hrs.

⚠ LIFESPAN CONSIDERATIONS

Pregnancy/Lactation: If possible, avoid use during pregnancy, esp. first trimester. May cause fetal harm. Breastfeeding not recommended. **Children:** No age-related precautions noted. **Elderly:** More susceptible to neurotoxic effects.

INTERACTIONS

DRUG: Strong CYP3A4 inhibitors (e.g., clarithromycin, ketoconazole, ritonavir), moderate CYP3A4 inhibitors (e.g., dilTIAZem, fluconazole, verapamil) may increase concentration/effect. **Strong CYP3A4 inducers (e.g., carBAMazepine, phenytoin, rifAMPin), moderate CYP3A4 inducers (e.g., dexamethasone, modafinil, nafcillin)** may decrease concentration/effect. May decrease therapeutic effect of **BCG (intravesical). Live virus vaccines** may potentiate virus replication, increase vaccine side effects, decrease pt's antibody response to vaccine. **HERBAL: Echinacea** may decrease the therapeutic effect. **FOOD:** None known. **LAB VALUES:** May increase serum uric acid.

AVAILABILITY (Rx)

Injection Solution: 1 mg/mL. **Injection Suspension:** *(Marqibo):* 5 mg/31 mL.

ADMINISTRATION/HANDLING

Note: In order to prevent inadvertent intrathecal administration, dispense as a piggyback (not a syringe).

 IV

◄**ALERT**► May be carcinogenic, mutagenic, teratogenic. Handle with extreme care during preparation and administration. Use extreme caution in calculating, administering vinCRIStine. Overdose may result in serious or fatal outcome.

Injection Solution

Reconstitution • Dilute in 25–50 mL D_5W or 0.9% NaCl.

Rate of administration • Administer as 5–10 min infusion (preferred). • Do not infuse into extremity with impaired, potentially impaired circulation caused by compression or invading neoplasm, phlebitis, varicosity.

Storage • Refrigerate unopened vials. • Solution appears clear, colorless. • Discard if solution is discolored or precipitate forms.

Injection Suspension

• Calculate dose of vinCRIStine and remove volume equal to volume of intended solution from 100 mL 0.9% NaCl or D_5W infusion bag. Inject vinCRIStine into infusion bag (total volume: 100 mL).

Rate of administration • Administer over 60 min.

Storage • Must be administered within 12 hrs of preparation.

▦ IV COMPATIBILITIES

Granisetron, ondansetron.

INDICATIONS/ROUTES/DOSAGE

Note: Doses are almost always capped at 2 mg/dose/wk. Dosing and frequency may vary by protocol and/or treatment phase. Dispense in mini bag (not syringe).

Usual Dosage Injection Solution

IV: ADULTS, ELDERLY: 1.4 mg/m², frequency may vary based on protocol. **CHILDREN WEIGHING MORE THAN 10 KG:** 1.5–2 mg/m², frequency may vary based on protocol. **Maximum:** 2 mg/dose/wk. **CHILDREN WEIGHING LESS THAN 10 KG:** 0.05 mg/kg once wkly. **Maximum:** 2 mg.

Dosage in Renal Impairment
No dose adjustment.

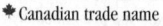 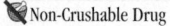
V

Dosage in Hepatic Impairment

Bilirubin	Dosage
Bilirubin greater than 3 mg/dL	50% of normal

ALL Injection Suspension
IV: **ADULTS, ELDERLY:** *(Marqibo):* 2.25 mg/m² q7days. Infuse over 1 hr.

Dosage in Renal/Hepatic Impairment
No dose adjustment.

SIDE EFFECTS

Expected: Peripheral neuropathy (occurs in nearly every pt; first clinical sign is depression of Achilles tendon reflex). **Frequent:** Peripheral paresthesia, alopecia, constipation/obstipation (upper colon impaction with empty rectum), abdominal cramps, headache, jaw pain, hoarseness, diplopia, ptosis/drooping of eyelid, urinary tract disturbances. **Occasional:** Nausea, vomiting, diarrhea, abdominal distention, stomatitis, fever.

ADVERSE EFFECTS/TOXIC REACTIONS

Myelosuppression (anemia, neutropenia, thrombocytopenia) is an expected response to therapy, but more severe reactions, including febrile neutropenia, may occur. Acute dyspnea, bronchospasm may occur, esp. when administered concurrently with mitoMYcin. Prolonged or high-dose therapy may produce foot/wrist drop, difficulty walking, slapping gait, ataxia, muscle wasting. Extravasation may cause severe tissue necrosis. Tumor lysis syndrome may present as acute renal failure, hypocalcemia, hyperuricemia, hyperphosphatemia. Paralytic ileus, bowel obstruction, colonic pseudo-obstruction may occur. Hepatotoxicity reported in 6%–11% of pts. Infections including pneumonia, sepsis, staphylococcal bacteremia may occur. Cardiac arrest reported in 5% of pts.

NURSING CONSIDERATIONS

BASELINE ASSESSMENT

Obtain CBC, LFT; pregnancy test in females of reproductive potential. Screen for active infection. Question history of hepatic impairment, neuromuscular disease. Assess risk of tumor lysis syndrome. Assess patency of IV access. Offer emotional support.

INTERVENTION/EVALUATION

Monitor CBC for myelosuppression; LFT for hepatotoxicity (abdominal pain, jaundice, nausea, transaminitis, vomiting). Monitor for infections (cough, fatigue, fever), sepsis, neurotoxicities, pulmonary toxicities (bronchospasm, dyspnea). Monitor serum uric acid level if tumor lysis syndrome (acute renal failure, electrolyte imbalance, cardiac arrhythmias, seizures) is suspected. Monitor for GI obstruction (abdominal pain, fever, nausea, vomiting). Extravasation produces stinging, burning, edema at injection site. Terminate injection immediately, locally inject hyaluronidase, apply heat (disperses drug, minimizes discomfort, cellulitis).

PATIENT/FAMILY TEACHING

• Immediately report any pain/burning at injection site during administration. • Treatment may depress your immune system response and reduce your ability to fight infection. Report symptoms of infection such as body aches, chills, cough, fatigue, fever. Avoid those with active infection. • Report symptoms of bone marrow depression (e.g., bruising, fatigue, fever, shortness of breath, weight loss; bleeding easily, bloody urine or stool). • Use effective contraception to avoid pregnancy. Do not breastfeed. • Report liver problems (abdominal pain, bruising, clay-colored stool, dark or amber-colored urine, yellowing of the skin or eyes), skin reactions (rash, redness, swelling). • Life-threatening tumor lysis syndrome (a condition caused by the rapid break-

V

down of cancer cells), which can cause kidney failure, may occur. Report decreased urination, amber-colored urine; confusion, difficulty breathing, fatigue, fever, muscle or joint pain, palpitations, seizures, vomiting. • Report abdominal pain, fever, nausea, vomiting; may indicate GI obstruction.

vinorelbine **HIGH ALERT**

vin-oh-**rel**-been
(Navelbine)

■ BLACK BOX ALERT ■ Must be administered by personnel trained in administration/handling of chemotherapeutic agents. Severe myelosuppression, resulting in serious infections, shock, death, may occur.
Do not confuse vinorelbine with vinBLAStine or vinCRIStine.

◆ CLASSIFICATION

PHARMACOTHERAPEUTIC: Antimicrotubular. Vinca alkaloid. **CLINICAL:** Antineoplastic.

USES

Single agent or in combination with CISplatin for treatment of unresectable, advanced or metastatic, non–small-cell lung cancer (NSCLC). **OFF-LABEL:** Refractory/recurrent solid tumors, Hodgkin's lymphoma, leukemias.

PRECAUTIONS

Contraindications: Hypersensitivity to vinorelbine. **Cautions:** Compromised marrow reserve due to prior chemotherapy/radiation therapy; hepatic impairment, neuropathy, pulmonary impairment.

ACTION

Binds to tubulin, inhibiting microtubule formation; may interfere with nucleic acid protein synthesis. **Therapeutic Effect:** Prevents cellular division by disrupting formation of mitotic spindle.

PHARMACOKINETICS

Widely distributed. Protein binding: 80%–90%. Metabolized in liver. Primarily excreted in feces by biliary system. **Half-life:** 28–43 hrs.

⧗ LIFESPAN CONSIDERATIONS

Pregnancy/Lactation: Avoid pregnancy; may cause fetal harm. Females of reproductive potential must use effective contraception during treatment and for at least 1 mo after discontinuation. Breastfeeding not recommended during treatment and for at least 9 days after discontinuation. May impair fertility in both females and males. **Males:** Males with female partners of reproductive potential must use effective contraception during treatment and for at least 3 mos after discontinuation. **Children:** Safety and efficacy not established. **Elderly:** No age-related precautions noted.

INTERACTIONS

DRUG: May increase immunosuppressive effect of **baricitinib, tofacitinib, upadacitinib. Cladribine** may increase myelosuppressive effect. May increase toxic effect of **natalizumab. CISplatin** may increase risk of granulocytopenia. May decrease concentration/therapeutic effect of **BCG intravesical vaccines (live).** May increase concentration/adverse effects of **vaccines (live). Strong CYP3A4 inhibitors (e.g., clarithromycin, ketoconazole)** may increase concentration/effects. **HERBAL:** Echinacea may decrease the therapeutic effect. **FOOD:** None known. **LAB VALUES:** May increase serum bilirubin, alkaline phosphatase, ALT, AST.

V

 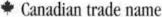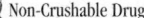

AVAILABILITY (Rx)

Injection Solution: 10 mg/mL (1 mL, 5-mL vials).

ADMINISTRATION/HANDLING

🖱 IV

◀**ALERT**▶ IV needle, catheter must be correctly positioned before administration. Leakage into surrounding tissue produces extreme irritation, local tissue necrosis, thrombophlebitis. Handle drug with extreme care during administration; wear protective clothing per protocol. If solution comes in contact with skin/mucosa, immediately wash thoroughly with soap, water.

Preparation • Must be diluted and administered via IV bag. • **IV Bag Dilution:** Dilute calculated vinorelbine dose with D$_5$W, 0.45% or 0.9% NaCl, 5% dextrose and 0.45% NaCl, Ringer's or lactated Ringer's to concentration of 0.5–2 mg/mL.

Rate of administration • Administer diluted vinorelbine over 6–10 min into side port of free-flowing IV closest to IV bag followed by flushing with 75–125 mL of one of the solutions. • If extravasation occurs, stop injection immediately; give remaining portion of dose into another vein.

Storage • Refrigerate unopened vials. • Protect from light. • Unopened vials are stable at room temperature for 72 hrs. • Do not administer if particulate has formed. • Diluted vinorelbine may be used for up to 24 hrs under normal room light when stored in polypropylene syringes or polyvinyl chloride bags at room temperature.

🔅 IV INCOMPATIBILITIES

Acyclovir (Zovirax), allopurinol (Aloprim), amphotericin B (Fungizone), amphotericin B complex (Abelcet, AmBisome, Amphotec), ampicillin (Omnipen), ceFAZolin (Ancef), cefTRIAXone (Rocephin), cefuroxime (Zinacef), 5-fluorouracil (5-FU), furosemide (Lasix), ganciclovir (Cytovene), methylPREDNISolone (SOLU-Medrol), sodium bicarbonate.

🔅 IV COMPATIBILITIES

Granisetron, ondansetron.

INDICATIONS/ROUTES/DOSAGE

◀**ALERT**▶ Dosage adjustments should be based on granulocyte count obtained on the day of treatment, as follows:

Granulocyte Count (cells/mm³) on Day of Treatment	Dosage
1,500 or higher	100% of starting dose
1,000–1,499	50% of starting dose
Less than 1,000	Do not administer

NSCLC Monotherapy
IV: **ADULTS, ELDERLY:** 30 mg/m^2 q7days.

NSCLC Combination Therapy With CISplatin
IV: **ADULTS, ELDERLY:** 25–30 mg/m^2 q7days.

Dosage in Renal Impairment
Mild to severe impairment: No dose adjustment. **ESRD requiring hemodialysis:** Decrease dose to 20 mg/m^2/wk given post-HD or on non-HD days.

Dosage in Hepatic Impairment

Serum Bilirubin	Dosage
2 mg/dL or less	100% of dose
2.1–3 mg/dL	50% of dose
Greater than 3 mg/dL	25% of dose

SIDE EFFECTS

Frequent (35%–12%): Asthenia, nausea, constipation, erythema, pain, vein discoloration at injection site, fatigue, peripheral neuropathy manifested as paresthesia, hyperesthesia, diarrhea, alopecia. **Occasional (10%–5%):** Phlebitis, dyspnea, loss of deep tendon reflexes. **Rare:** Chest pain, jaw pain, myalgia, arthralgia, rash.

ADVERSE EFFECTS/TOXIC REACTIONS

Myelosuppression (anemia, leukopenia, neutropenia, thrombocytopenia) is an expected response to therapy. Hemorrhagic cystitis, syndrome of inappropriate antidiuretic hormone reported in less than 1% of pts. Acute shortness of breath, severe bronchospasm occur infrequently, particularly in pts with preexisting pulmonary dysfunction. Hepatic toxicity may occur.

NURSING CONSIDERATIONS

BASELINE ASSESSMENT

Obtain CBC prior to each dose. Granulocyte count should be at least 1,000 cells/mm³ before vinorelbine administration. Granulocyte nadirs occur 7–10 days following dosing. Do not give hematologic growth factors within 24 hrs before administration of chemotherapy or earlier than 24 hrs following cytotoxic chemotherapy. Obtain pregnancy test in females of reproductive potential. Confirm compliance of effective contraception. Offer emotional support.

INTERVENTION/EVALUATION

Closely monitor injection site for swelling, redness, pain. Monitor CBC for myelosuppression during and following therapy (infection [fever, sore throat, signs of local infection], unusual bleeding/bruising, anemia [excessive fatigue, weakness]). Monitor pts developing severe granulocytopenia for evidence of infection, fever. Monitor daily pattern of bowel activity, stool consistency. Question for tingling, burning, numbness of hands/feet (peripheral neuropathy). Complaint of "walking on glass" is sign of hyperesthesia.

PATIENT/FAMILY TEACHING

• Treatment may depress your immune system response and reduce your ability to fight infection. Report symptoms of infection such as body aches, chills, cough, fatigue, fever. Avoid those with active infection. • Report symptoms of bone marrow depression (e.g., bruising, fatigue, fever, shortness of breath, weight loss; bleeding easily, bloody urine or stool). • Use effective contraception to avoid pregnancy. Do not breastfeed. • Report liver problems (abdominal pain, bruising, clay-colored stool, dark or amber-colored urine, yellowing of the skin or eyes), skin reactions (rash, redness, swelling). • Report new or worsening signs of neuropathy.

vismodegib

vis-moe-**deg**-ib
(Erivedge)

■ **BLACK BOX ALERT** ■ May result in embryo-fetal death or severe birth defects including missing digits, midline defects, irreversible malformations due to embryotoxic and teratogenic properties. Verify pregnancy status prior to initiation. Advise use of effective contraception in female pts. Advise male pts of potential exposure risk through seminal fluid.

◆CLASSIFICATION

PHARMACOTHERAPEUTIC: Hedgehog pathway inhibitor. **CLINICAL:** Antineoplastic.

USES

Treatment of adults with metastatic basal cell carcinoma, or with locally advanced basal cell carcinoma with recurrence after surgery, or pts who are not candidates for surgery or radiation.

PRECAUTIONS

◀**ALERT**▶ Do not donate blood products for at least 7 mos after discontinuation.

Contraindications: Hypersensitivity to vismodegib. **Cautions:** Hepatic impairment.

ACTION

Selectively inhibits Hedgehog pathway by binding to and inhibiting smoothened, a transmembrane protein involved in Hedgehog signal transduction. Hedgehog mutations associated with basal cell cancer can activate the pathway, resulting in proliferation of skin basal cells. **Therapeutic Effect:** Inhibits tumor cell growth and survival.

PHARMACOKINETICS

Metabolized in liver. Protein binding: 99%. Excreted in feces (82%), urine (4%). **Half-life:** 4 days (daily dosing), 12 days (single dose).

⧖ LIFESPAN CONSIDERATIONS

Pregnancy/Lactation: Avoid pregnancy; may cause fetal harm. Females of reproductive potential must use effective contraception during treatment and for at least 24 mos after discontinuation. Breastfeeding not recommended during treatment and for at least 24 mos after discontinuation. May impair fertility. **Males:** Males with female partners of reproductive potential must use effective contraception during treatment and for at least 3 mos after discontinuation. **Children:** Safety and efficacy not established. **Elderly:** Safety and efficacy not established.

INTERACTIONS

DRUG: None significant. **HERBAL:** None significant. **FOOD:** None known. **LAB VALUES:** May decrease potassium, sodium, GFR. May increase serum BUN, creatinine.

AVAILABILITY (Rx)

 Capsules: 150 mg.

ADMINISTRATION/HANDLING

PO

• Give without regard to food. • Give whole. Do not break, crush, or open capsule. If a dose is missed, resume dosing with the next scheduled dose.

INDICATIONS/ROUTES/DOSAGE

Advanced or Metastatic Basal Cell Carcinoma
PO: ADULTS/ELDERLY: 150 mg once daily. Continue until disease progression or unacceptable toxicity.

Dosage in Renal/Hepatic Impairment
No dose adjustment.

SIDE EFFECTS

Frequent (71%–40%): Muscle spasm, alopecia, dysgeusia, weight loss, fatigue. **Occasional (30%–11%):** Nausea, amenorrhea, diarrhea, anorexia, constipation, vomiting, arthralgia, loss of taste.

ADVERSE EFFECTS/TOXIC REACTIONS

Severe cutaneous reactions including Stevens-Johnson syndrome, toxic epidermal necrolysis. Drug reaction with eosinophilia and systemic symptoms (DRESS), also known as multiorgan hypersensitivity, has been reported. DRESS may present with facial swelling, eosinophilia, fever, lymphadenopathy, rash, which may be associated with other organ systems, such as hepatitis, hematologic abnormalities, myocarditis, nephritis.

NURSING CONSIDERATIONS

BASELINE ASSESSMENT

Obtain pregnancy test in females of reproductive potential. Question history of hepatic impairment. Offer emotional support.

INTERVENTION/EVALUATION

Monitor for skin toxicities; symptoms of DRESS.

PATIENT/FAMILY TEACHING

• Use effective contraception to avoid pregnancy. Do not breastfeed. • Do not donate blood for at least 2 yrs. • Toxic skin reactions (necrosis, redness, sloughing) may occur. • Severe multi-organ hypersensitivity reaction (DRESS) may cause life-threatening organ dysfunction; report chest pain, decreased urinary output, facial swelling, fever, rash, swelling of lymph nodes.

vitamin D (vitamin D analogues)

calcitriol

kal-si-**trye**-ole
(Calcijex ♣, Rocaltrol, Vectical)

doxercalciferol

dox-er-kal-**sif**-e-role
(Hectorol)

ergocalciferol

er-goe-kal-**sif**-e-role
(Drisdol)

paricalcitol

par-i-**kal**-si-tol
(Zemplar)

◆ CLASSIFICATION

PHARMACOTHERAPEUTIC: Fat-soluble vitamin. **CLINICAL:** Vitamin D analogue.

USES

Calcitriol: Management of hypocalcemia in pts with hypoparathyroidism or pseudohypoparathyroidism. Management of secondary hyperparathyroidism in pts with moderate to severe chronic kidney disease (CKD) not on dialysis. Management of hypocalcemia in pts on dialysis. **(Topical):** Treatment of mild to moderate plaque psoriasis in adults and children 2 yrs and older. **Doxercalciferol:** Treatment of secondary hyperparathyroidism in CKD on dialysis or in pts with stage 3 or 4 CKD not on dialysis. **Ergocalciferol:** Treatment of refractory rickets, familial hypophosphatemia, hypoparathyroidism. **Paricalcitol:** Treatment/prevention of secondary hyperparathyroidism associated with stage 3 and 4 CKD and stage 5 CKD pts on hemodialysis or peritoneal dialysis in adults and children 10 yrs and older. **OFF-LABEL: Calcitriol:** Vitamin D–dependent rickets. **Ergocalciferol:** Prevention/treatment of vitamin D deficiency in pts with CKD, osteoporosis prevention.

PRECAUTIONS

Contraindications: Hypersensitivity to cholecalciferol, ergocalciferol. Vitamin D toxicity, hypercalcemia. **Cautions:** Pts with malabsorption syndrome. Concurrent use with digoxin.

ACTION

Calcitriol: Binds to and activates the vitamin D receptor in kidney, parathyroid gland, intestine, and bone, stimulating intestinal calcium transport and absorption. Reduces parathyroid hormone (PTH) levels, improves calcium and phosphate homeostasis. **Doxercalciferol:** Controls intestinal absorption of dietary calcium, tubular reabsorption of calcium by the kidneys, and in conjunction with PTH, the mobilization of calcium from the skeleton. **Ergocalciferol:** Promotes active absorption of calcium and phosphorus, increasing serum levels to allow bone mineralization; mobilizes calcium and phosphate from bone, increases reabsorption of calcium and phosphate

V

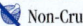

by renal tubules. **Paricalcitol:** Activates the vitamin D receptor in kidney, parathyroid gland, intestine and bone, reducing PTH levels and improving calcium and phosphate homeostasis. **Therapeutic Effect:** Essential for absorption, utilization of calcium, phosphate, control of PTH levels.

PHARMACOKINETICS

Calcitriol: Rapidly absorbed. Protein binding: 99.9%. Metabolized to active metabolite (ergocalciferol). Excreted in feces (49%), urine (16%). **Half-life:** 5–8 hrs. **Doxercalciferol:** Metabolized in liver. **Half-life:** 32–37 hrs. **Ergocalciferol:** Metabolized in liver. **Paricalcitol:** Readily absorbed. Protein binding: 99.8%. Metabolized in liver. Primarily excreted in feces. **Half-life:** 5–7 hrs.

⧗ LIFESPAN CONSIDERATIONS

Pregnancy/Lactation: Unknown if drug crosses placenta. Infant risk cannot be excluded. **Children/Elderly:** No age-related precautions noted.

INTERACTIONS

DRUG: Calcium-containing products, concurrent vitamin D (or derivatives) may increase risk of hypercalcemia. May increase **digoxin** toxicity due to hypercalcemia (may cause arrhythmias). May increase concentration/effect of **aluminum hydroxide, sucralfate. Bile acid sequestrants (e.g., cholestyramine)** may decrease absorption. **HERBAL:** None significant. **FOOD:** None known. **LAB VALUES:** May increase serum cholesterol, calcium, magnesium, phosphate, ALT, AST, BUN, creatinine.

AVAILABILITY (Rx)

Calcitriol
Capsules, Softgel: 0.25 mcg, 0.5 mcg.
Oral Solution: 1 mcg/mL. **Ointment:** 3 mcg/g (100 g).

Doxercalciferol
Capsules, Softgel: 0.5 mcg, 1 mcg, 2.5 mcg. **Injection Solution:** 4 mcg/2mL.

Ergocalciferol
Capsules: 50,000 units (1.25 mg).
Liquid, Oral: 8,000 units/mL (200 mcg/mL). **Tablets:** 10 mcg (400 units); 50 mg (2,000 units).

Paricalcitol
Capsules, Gelatin: 1 mcg, 2 mcg.

ADMINISTRATION/HANDLING

Calcitriol
PO
• May take without regard to food. • Administer with meals to reduce GI upset.

Doxercalciferol
PO
• May take without regard to food.

 IV
• May give as IV bolus via catheter at end of dialysis.

Ergocalciferol
PO
• May take without regard to food.

Paricalcitol
PO
• May take without regard to food. • For 3 times/wk dosing, give no more frequently than every other day.

INDICATIONS/ROUTES/DOSAGE

Calcitriol

Hypocalcemia on Chronic Renal Dialysis
PO: ADULTS, ELDERLY: Initially, 0.25 once daily or 3 times wkly. May increase by 0.25 mcg/day at 4- to 8-wk intervals. **Range:** 0.5–1 mcg/day.

Hypocalcemia in Hypoparathyroidism
PO: ADULTS, CHILDREN 6 YRS AND OLDER: Initially, 0.25 mcg/day. May increase at 2- to 4-wk intervals. **Range:** 0.5–2 mcg/day. **CHILDREN 1–5 YRS:** 0.25–0.75 mcg once daily.

V

Secondary Hyperparathyroidism Associated With Moderate to Severe CKD Not on Dialysis
PO: ADULTS, ELDERLY, CHILDREN 3 YRS AND OLDER: Initially, 0.25 mcg once daily or 3–4 times/wk. May increase to 0.5 mcg/day.

Plaque Psoriasis
Topical: ADULTS, ELDERLY, CHILDREN 2 YRS AND OLDER: Apply to affected area twice daily. **Maximum:** 200 g/wk (100 g/wk for children 2–6 yrs of age).

Doxercalciferol
Secondary Hyperparathyroidism (Dialysis)
PO: ADULTS, ELDERLY: Initially, 10 mcg 3 times wkly at dialysis (no more frequently than every other day). **Maximum:** 20 mcg 3 times/wk.
IV: ADULTS, ELDERLY: Initially, 4 mcg three times wkly at the end of dialysis (no more frequently than every other day). **Maximum:** 18 mcg/wk.

Secondary Hyperparathyroidism (Predialysis)
PO: ADULTS, ELDERLY: **Stage 3 or 4 CKD:** Initially, 1 mcg orally daily. **Maximum:** 3.5 mcg/day.

Ergocalciferol
Rickets
PO: ADOLESCENTS: 6,000 units for 3 or more mos, then 600 units daily. CHILDREN: 3,000–6,000 units for 3 or more mos, then 600 units daily. INFANTS: 2,000 units for 3 or more mos, then 400 units daily.

Hypoparathyroidism
PO: ADULTS, ELDERLY: 50,000–200,000 USP units daily concomitantly with calcium supplements.

Paricalcitol
Secondary Hyperparathyroidism in Stage 5 CKD
IV: ADULTS, ELDERLY: Initially, dose (mcg) = baseline iPTH (pg/mL) divided by 80. Administer 3 times/wk. **Titration:** Dose in mcg is based on most recent iPTH (pg/mL) divided by 80 with adjust-

ments based on serum calcium/phosphorous levels. Dose 3 times/wk. CHILDREN 10–16 YRS: Initially, dose (mcg) = baseline iPTH (pg/mL) divided by 120. Administer 3 times/wk. **Titration:** Increase each dose by 1 mcg 3 times/wk q4wks or decrease each dose by 2 mcg 3 times/wk at any time based on iPTH, serum calcium/phosphate level.

Secondary Hyperparathyroidism in Stages 3 and 4 CKD
Note: Initial dose based on baseline serum iPTH levels. Dose adjusted q2–4wks based on iPTH levels relative to baseline.
PO: ADULTS, ELDERLY: (iPTH 500 PG/ML OR LESS): 1 mcg/day or 2 mcg 3 times/wk. (iPTH GREATER THAN 500 PG/ML): 2 mcg/day or 4 mcg 3 times/wk. CHILDREN 10–16 YRS: Initially, 1 mcg 3 times/wk (no more frequently than every other day). Titrate q4wks by 1 mcg/dose.

Dosage in Renal/Hepatic Impairment
No dose adjustment.

SIDE EFFECTS
Frequencies not defined. **Calcitriol:** Cardiac arrhythmias, headache, pruritus, hypercalcemia, polydipsia, abdominal pain, metallic taste, nausea, vomiting, myalgia, soft tissue calcification. **Doxercalciferol:** Edema, pruritus, nausea, vomiting, headache, dizziness, dyspnea, malaise, hypercalcemia. **Ergocalciferol:** Hypercalcemia, hypervitaminosis D, decreased renal function, soft tissue calcification, bone demineralization, nausea, constipation, weight loss. **Paricalcitol:** Edema, nausea, vomiting, hypercalcemia.

ADVERSE EFFECTS/TOXIC REACTIONS
Early signs of overdose manifested as weakness, headache, drowsiness, nausea, vomiting, dry mouth, constipation, muscle/bone pain, metallic taste. Later signs of overdose evidenced by polyuria, polydipsia, anorexia, weight loss, noctu-

ria, photophobia, rhinorrhea, pruritus, disorientation, hallucinations, hyperthermia, hypertension, cardiac dysrhythmias.

NURSING CONSIDERATIONS

BASELINE ASSESSMENT
Obtain serum calcium, phosphate, PTH, vitamin D level (if indicated).

INTERVENTION/EVALUATION
Monitor serum calcium, phosphate, PTH, vitamin D level (if indicated); (therapeutic calcium level: 9–10 mg/dL). Estimate daily dietary calcium intake. Encourage adequate fluid intake. Monitor for signs/symptoms of vitamin D intoxication.

PATIENT/FAMILY TEACHING
• Adequate calcium intake should be maintained. • Dietary phosphorus may need to be restricted (foods high in phosphorus include beans, dairy products, nuts, peas, whole-grain products). • Oral formulations may cause hypersensitivity reactions. Avoid excessive doses. • Report signs/symptoms of hypercalcemia (headache, weakness, drowsiness, nausea, vomiting, dry mouth, constipation, metallic taste, muscle or bone pain). • Maintain adequate hydration. • Avoid changes in diet or supplemental calcium intake (unless directed by healthcare professional). • Avoid magnesium-containing antacids in pts with renal failure.

vonoprazan

von-**oh**-pra-zan
(Voquezna)
Do not confuse vonoprazan with pantoprazole or Sympazan.

◆ CLASSIFICATION

PHARMACOTHERAPEUTIC: Potassium-competitive acid blocker. **CLINICAL:** Potassium-competitive acid blocker

USES
Erosive esophagitis, relief of heartburn: Healing and maintenance of healing of all grades of erosive esophagitis and relief of heartburn associated with erosive esophagitis in adults. For relief of heartburn associated with nonerosive gastroesophageal reflux disease (GERD) in adults. *Helicobacter pylori* **Infection:** In combination with amoxicillin alone (dual therapy), or in combination with amoxicillin and clarithromycin (triple therapy), for treatment of *H. pylori* infection in adults.

PRECAUTIONS
Contraindications: Hypersensitivity to vonoprazon. Concomitant use of rilpivirine-containing medications. **Cautions:** Hepatic/renal impairment, recent *C. difficile* infection, pts at risk for hypocalcemia (e.g., hypomagnesemia, hypoparathyroidism, renal failure, vitamin D deficiency); history of fractures, osteoporosis, osteopenia. Avoid concomitant use of atazanavir, nelfinavir.

ACTION
Blocks final step of acid secretion in gastric parietal cells be competitively blocking binding of potassium to hydrogen-potassium adenosine triphosphate (ATPase). **Therapeutic Effect:** Suppresses gastric acid secretion.

PHARMACOKINETICS
Widely distributed. Metabolized in liver. Protein binding: 85%–88%. Peak plasma concentration: 1.5–2 hrs. Steady-state reached in 3–4 days. Excreted in urine (67%), feces (31%). Half-life: 7–8 hrs.

⧗ LIFESPAN CONSIDERATIONS
Pregnancy/Lactation: Unknown if distributed in breast milk. Breastfeeding not recommended. **Children:** Safety and efficacy not established. **Elderly:** No age-related precautions noted.

INTERACTIONS
DRUG: May decrease safety, efficacy of **rilpivirine-containing medications;**

use contraindicated. **Strong CYP3A4 inhibitors (e.g., clarithromycin, ketoconazole, ritonavir)** may increase concentration/effect. **Strong CYP3A4 inducers (e.g., carBAMazepine, phenytoin, riFAMpin), moderate CYP3A4 inducers (e.g., dexamethasone, modafinil, nafcillin)** may decrease concentration/effect. May increase concentration/effect of **CYP3A4 substrates (e.g., busPIRone, tacrolimus, simvastatin)**. May decrease concentration/effect of **CYP2C19 inhibitors (e.g., clopidogrel)**. **HERBAL:** None significant. **FOOD:** None known. **LAB VALUES:** May decrease serum calcium, magnesium, potassium, vitamin B12. May increase serum chromogranin A (CgA) levels, which may cause false-positive result in diagnostic investigations for neuroendocrine tumors.

AVAILABILITY (Rx)

Tablets: 10 mg, 20 mg.

ADMINISTRATION/HANDLING

PO
• Give without regard to food. • Administer tablet whole (do not cut, crush, or allow chewing).

INDICATIONS/ROUTES/DOSAGE

Note: Permanently discontinue treatment in pts who develop acute tubulointerstitial nephritis, toxic skin reactions, refractory hypocalcemia.

Healing of Erosive Esophagitis
PO: ADULTS: 20 mg once daily for 8 wks.

Maintenance of Healed Erosive Esophagitis
PO: ADULTS: 10 mg once daily for up to 6 mos.

Relief of Heartburn Associated With Nonerosive GERD
PO: ADULTS: 10 mg once daily for 4 wks.

H. pylori Infection
PO: ADULTS: Triple therapy: 20 mg twice daily (12 hrs apart), in combination with amoxicillin 1,000 mg and clarithromycin 500 mg each twice daily for 14 days. **Dual Therapy:** 20 mg twice daily (12 hrs apart), in combination with amoxicillin 1,000 mg 3 times/day for 14 days.

Dosage in Renal Impairment
Healing of erosive esophagitis
eGFR 30 ML/MIN OR GREATER: 20 mg once daily. **eGFR LESS THAN 30 ML/MIN:** 10 mg once daily.

Maintenance of healed erosive esophagitis; relief of heartburn associated with nonerosive GERD
MILD TO SEVERE IMPAIRMENT: No dose adjustment. **Treatment of H. Pylori infection: eGFR 30 ML/MIN OR GREATER:** 20 mg twice daily. **eGFR LESS THAN 30 ML/MIN:** Treatment not recommended.

Dosage in Hepatic Impairment
Healing of erosive esophagitis
MILD IMPAIRMENT: 20 mg once daily. **MODERATE TO SEVERE IMPAIRMENT:** 10 mg once daily.

Maintenance of healed erosive esophagitis; relief of heartburn associated with nonerosive GERD
MILD TO SEVERE IMPAIRMENT: No dose adjustment. **Treatment of H. Pylori infection: MILD IMPAIRMENT:** 20 mg twice daily. **MODERATE TO SEVERE IMPAIRMENT:** Treatment not recommended.

SIDE EFFECTS

Note: Frequency and type of side effects may vary based on indicated treatment, dosage, and combination use of amoxicillin, clarithromycin (see prescribing information). **Occasional (6%):** Gastritis. **Rare (4%–1% or less):** Abdominal pain, dyspepsia, hypertension, abdominal distension, constipation, diarrhea, nausea.

ADVERSE EFFECTS/TOXIC REACTIONS

Symptomatic response to treatment does not preclude the presence of gastric malignancy. May cause acute tubulointerstitial nephritis. May increase

V

risk of *C. difficile*–associated diarrhea; bone fractures of the hip, wrist, or spine. Severe cutaneous reactions, including Stevens-Johnson syndrome, toxic epidermal necrolysis were reported. Chronic use of acid-suppressing drugs may cause fundic polyps; malabsorption of vitamin B12 caused by hypo- or achlorhydria. May cause electrolyte abnormalities, including hypomagnesemia, which may lead to hypocalcemia, hypokalemia. May cause false-positive test result in diagnostic investigations for neuroendocrine tumors due to increased serum chromogranin A (CgA) levels.

NURSING CONSIDERATIONS

BASELINE ASSESSMENT

Obtain renal function test in pts with renal impairment; LFT in pts with hepatic impairment. Consider obtaining serum magnesium, calcium level periodically, esp. in pts at risk for hypocalcemia (hypomagnesemia, hypoparathyroidism, renal failure, vitamin D deficiency) or in pts receiving chronic therapy. Refer to manufacturer guidelines for amoxicillin, clarithromycin if treating with dual or triple therapy. Question history of hepatic/renal impairment; pathological fractures, osteoporosis, osteopenia. Receive full medication history and screen for interactions/contraindications. Review diagnostic test results of esophagogastroduodenoscopy, biopsies, *H. Pylori* infection. Withhold treatment at least 4 wks prior to diagnostic testing of CgA levels in pts being assessed for neuroendocrine tumors. Consider repeating test if initial CgA levels are elevated. Assess baseline symptoms of esophagitis, GERD, *H. Pylori* infection.

INTERVENTION/EVALUATION

Obtain serum magnesium, calcium as clinically indicated. Consider treatment with supplemental magnesium and/or calcium as needed. Monitor for hypocalcemia (cardiac arrhythmias, muscle spasm, myalgia, paresthesia, QT interval prolongation, Chvostek sign, Trousseau sign), Monitor for acute kidney injury, tubulointerstitial nephritis (dark-colored urine, flank pain, decreased urine output, muscle aches), toxic skin reactions (blisters, fever, rash, redness, inflammation, peeling, ulceration). If toxic reactions occur, consider a referral to a specialist. Observe daily pattern of bowel activity, stool consistency (increased severity may indicate *C. difficile* infection). If frequent diarrhea occurs, obtain *C. difficile* toxin screen and initiate isolation precautions until test result is confirmed; manage hydration, electrolyte levels, protein intake. Evaluate for therapeutic response (relief of GI symptoms).

PATIENT/FAMILY TEACHING

• It is essential to complete drug therapy despite improvement of symptoms. Early discontinuation and noncompliance may cause return of esophagitis, GERD, *H. Pylori* infection, and associated symptoms. • Frequent, loose, foul-smelling stools; fever, abdominal discomfort, urgency may indicate infectious diarrhea that may be contagious to others. • Report liver problems, severe skin reactions (blisters, fever, rash, redness, inflammation, peeling, ulcers), symptoms of bone fractures (pain, deformity, changes in mobility). • Therapy may cause low levels of calcium, magnesium, vitamin B12 in the blood. Report difficulty swallowing, fatigue, muscle cramps, muscle weakness, palpations, numbness, tingling, tremors. • There is a high risk of interactions with other medications. Do not take newly prescribed medications unless approved by prescriber who originally started treatment. Do not take herbal products. • Do not breastfeed. • Chronic use may cause gastric (stomach) polyps.

voriconazole

vor-i-**kon**-a-zole
(Vfend, Apo-Voriconazole)

Do not confuse voriconazole with fluconazole or Vfend with Venofer or Vimpat.

◆CLASSIFICATION

PHARMACOTHERAPEUTIC: Azole derivative. **CLINICAL:** Antifungal.

USES

Treatment of adults and children 2 yrs of age and older with invasive aspergillosis, , candidemia in non-neutropenics, and other deep tissue *Candida* infections (skin, abdomen, kidney, bladder wall, wounds), esophageal candidiasis, serious fungal infections caused by *Scedosporium apiospermum* and *Fusarium* species including *Fusarium solani*, in pts intolerant of, or refractory to, other therapy. **OFF-LABEL:** Neutropenic fever (empiric therapy), prophylaxis of invasive fungal infections, coccidioidomycosis (refractory).

PRECAUTIONS

Contraindications: Hypersensitivity to voriconazole. Concurrent administration of barbiturates (long acting), carBAMazepine, efavirenz (400 mg/day or greater), ergot alkaloids, pimozide, ivabradine, naloxegol, pimozide, quiNIDine (may cause prolonged QT interval, torsades de pointes), rifabutin, rifAMPin, ritonavir (800 mg/day or greater), sirolimus, St. John's wort tolvaptan, venetoclax (during initiation and titration in pts with chronic lymphocytic leukemia or small lymphocytic lymphoma). **Cautions:** Severe renal/hepatic impairment, hypersensitivity to other azole antifungal agents. Pts at risk for acute pancreatitis, pts with fructose intolerance, glucose-galactose malabsorption; concomitant nephrotoxic medications; pts at risk for QTc interval prolongation (congenital long QT syndrome, HF, medications that prolong QTc interval, hypokalemia, hypomagnesemia).

ACTION

Interferes with fungal cytochrome P450 activity, decreasing ergosterol synthesis, inhibiting fungal cell membrane formation. **Therapeutic Effect:** Damages fungal cell wall membrane.

PHARMACOKINETICS

Widely distributed. Protein binding: 58%. Metabolized in liver. Primarily excreted as metabolite in urine. **Half-life:** Variable, dose dependent.

⧗ LIFESPAN CONSIDERATIONS

Pregnancy/Lactation: May cause fetal harm. **Children:** Safety and efficacy not established in pts younger than 12 yrs. **Elderly:** No age-related precautions noted.

INTERACTIONS

DRUG: May increase concentration, risk of toxicity of **calcium channel blockers (e.g., dilTIAZem, verapamil), cycloSPORINE, ergot alkaloids, HMG-CoA reductase inhibitors (e.g., lovastatin), methadone, sirolimus, tacrolimus, warfarin.** Car-BAMazepine, rifabutin, rifAMPin may decrease concentration/effect. **QT interval–prolonging medications (e.g., amiodarone, azithromycin, ciprofloxacin, haloperidol, methadone, sotalol)** may increase risk of QTc interval prolongation. **HERBAL:** St. John's wort may significantly decrease concentration. **FOOD:** None known. **LAB VALUES:** May increase serum alkaline phosphatase, ALT, AST, bilirubin, creatinine. May decrease potassium.

AVAILABILITY (Rx)

Injection, Powder for Reconstitution: 200 mg. **Powder for Oral Suspension:** 200 mg/5 mL. **Tablets:** 50 mg, 200 mg.

V

ADMINISTRATION/HANDLING

 IV

Reconstitution • Reconstitute 200-mg vial with 19 mL Sterile Water for Injection to provide concentration of 10 mg/mL. Dilute in 0.9% NaCl or D_5W to provide concentration of 0.5–5 mg/mL.

Rate of administration • Infuse over 1–3 hrs at a rate not to exceed 3 mg/kg/hr. • Do not infuse concomitantly in same line with other drug infusions. • Do not infuse concomitantly even in separate lines with concentrated electrolyte solutions or blood products.

Storage • Store powder for injection at room temperature. • Use reconstituted solution immediately. • Do not use after 24 hrs when refrigerated.

PO
• Give 1 hr before or 1 hr after a meal.
• Do not mix oral suspension with any other medication or flavoring agent.
• Shake suspension for about 10 sec before use.

INDICATIONS/ROUTES/DOSAGE

Invasive Aspergillosis
IV: ADULTS, ELDERLY, ADOLESCENTS 15 YRS AND OLDER: Initially, 6 mg/kg q12h for 2 doses, then 4 mg/kg q12h. **CHILDREN 12–14 YRS WEIGHING 50 KG OR MORE:** 6 mg/kg q12h for 2 doses, then 4 mg/kg q12h. **WEIGHING LESS THAN 50 KG:** 9 mg/kg q12h for 2 doses, then 8 mg/kg q12h. **CHILDREN 2–11 YRS:** 9 mg/kg q12h for 2 doses, then 8 mg/kg q12h.
PO: ADULTS, ELDERLY, ADOLESCENTS 15 YRS AND OLDER: 200 mg q12h. **CHILDREN 12–14 YRS WEIGHING 50 KG OR MORE:** 200 mg q12h. **WEIGHING LESS THAN 50 KG:** 9 mg/kg q12h. **Maximum:** 350 mg/dose. **CHILDREN 2–11 YRS:** 9 mg/kg q12h. **Maximum:** 350 mg/dose.

Candidemia, Other Deep Tissue *Candida* Infections
IV: ADULTS, ELDERLY, ADOLESCENTS 15 YRS AND OLDER: Initially, 6 mg/kg q12h for 2 doses, then 3–4 mg/kg q12h. **CHILDREN 12–14 YRS WEIGHING 50 KG OR MORE:** 6 mg/kg q12h for 2 doses, then 3–4 mg/kg q12h. **WEIGHING LESS THAN 50 KG:** 9 mg/kg q12h for 2 doses, then 8 mg/kg q12h. **CHILDREN 2–11 YRS:** 9 mg/kg q12h for 2 doses, then 8 mg/kg q12h.
PO: ADULTS, ELDERLY, ADOLESCENTS 15 YRS AND OLDER: 200 mg q12h. **CHILDREN 12–14 YRS WEIGHING 50 KG OR MORE:** 200 mg q12h. **WEIGHING LESS THAN 50 KG:** 9 mg/kg q12h. **Maximum:** 350 mg/dose. **CHILDREN 2–11 YRS:** 9 mg/kg q12h. **Maximum:** 350 mg/dose.

Esophageal Candidiasis
PO: ADULTS, ELDERLY, ADOLESCENTS: 200 mg q12h. **CHILDREN 12–14 YRS WEIGHING 50 KG OR GREATER:** 200 mg q12h. **WEIGHING LESS THAN 50 KG:** 9 mg/kg q12h. **Maximum:** 350 mg/dose. **CHILDREN 2–11 YRS:** 9 mg/kg q12h. **Maximum:** 350 mg/dose.

Fusariosis
IV: ADULTS, EDLERLY: Initially, 6 mg/kg q12h for 2 doses, then 4 mg/kg q12h.
PO: (following improvement with initial IV therapy): 200 mg q12h.

Scedosporiosis
IV: ADULTS, ELDERLY: 6 mg/kg q12h for 2 doses, then 4 mg/kg q12h.
PO: 400 mg twice daily for 2 doses, then decrease to 200 mg q12h.

Dosage in Pts Receiving Phenytoin
IV: Increase maintenance dose to 5 mg/kg q12h.
PO: Increase 200 mg q12h to 400 mg q12h (pts weighing 40 kg or more) or 100 mg q12h to 200 mg q12h (pts weighing less than 40 kg).

V

Dosage in Pts Receiving Efavirenz
Increase dose to 400 mg q12h and reduce efavirenz to 300 mg/day.

Dosage in Renal Impairment
No dose adjustment. IV dosing not recommended in pts with CrCl 50 mL/min or less.

Dosage in Hepatic Impairment
Mild to moderate impairment: Reduce maintenance dose by 50%. **Severe impairment:** Use only if benefits outweigh risks. Monitor closely for toxicity.

SIDE EFFECTS
Frequent (20%–6%): Abnormal vision, fever, nausea, rash, vomiting. **Occasional (5%–2%):** Headache, chills, hallucinations, photophobia, tachycardia, hypertension.

ADVERSE EFFECTS/TOXIC REACTIONS
Hepatotoxicity (jaundice, hepatitis, hepatic failure), acute renal failure have occurred in severely ill pts.

NURSING CONSIDERATIONS

BASELINE ASSESSMENT
Obtain BMP, LFT; ECG. Correct electrolyte deficiencies prior to initiating treatment. Receive full medication history and screen for interactions. Question medical history as listed in Precautions.

INTERVENTION/EVALUATION
Monitor serum renal function, LFT. Monitor visual function (visual acuity, visual field, color perception) for drug therapy lasting longer than 28 days.

PATIENT/FAMILY TEACHING
• Take at least 1 hr before or 1 hr after a meal. • Avoid grapefruit products. • Report visual changes (blurred vision, photophobia, yellowing of skin/eyes). • Avoid performing hazardous tasks if changes in vision occur. • Avoid direct sunlight. • Women of childbearing potential should use effective contraception.

vortioxetine

vor-tye-ox-e-teen
(Trintellix)

■ **BLACK BOX ALERT** ■ Antidepressants have an increased risk of suicidal ideation and behavior in children, adolescents, and young adults. Monitor closely for worsening or emergence of suicidal thoughts and behaviors.
Do not confuse vortioxetine with FLUoxetine, PARoxetine, or venlafaxine.

◆ CLASSIFICATION
PHARMACOTHERAPEUTIC: Selective serotonin reuptake inhibitor (SSRI). **CLINICAL:** Antidepressant.

USES
Treatment of major depressive disorder (unipolar) in adults.

PRECAUTIONS
Contraindications: Hypersensitivity to vortioxetine. Use of monoamine oxidase inhibitors (MAOIs) intended to treat psychiatric disorders concurrently or within 21 days of stopping vortioxetine; do not use vortioxetine within 14 days of stopping an MAOI. Initiation of vortioxetine in pts receiving linezolid or intravenous methylene blue. **Cautions:** Dehydration, hepatic impairment, elderly, pts at risk for bleeding (e.g., history of intracranial/GI/genitourinary bleeding, coagulation disorders, recent trauma, concomitant use of anticoagulants, antiplatelets); history of suicidal ideation and behavior; family history of bipolar disorder, mania, hypomania.

ACTION
Blocks reuptake of neurotransmitter serotonin at CNS presynaptic membranes, increasing availability at postsynaptic receptor sites. **Therapeutic Effect:** Relieves depression.

V

PHARMACOKINETICS

Widely distributed. Metabolized in liver. Protein binding: 98%. Peak plasma concentration: 7–11 hrs. Steady state reached within 2 wks. Excreted in urine (59%), feces (26%). **Half-life:** 66 hrs.

⧖ LIFESPAN CONSIDERATIONS

Pregnancy/Lactation: May cause fetal harm when administered in third trimester. Unknown if distributed in breast milk. Exposed neonates are at increased risk of apnea, cyanosis, prolonged hospitalization, pulmonary hypertension, seizures, serotonin syndrome. **Children:** Safety and efficacy not established in pediatric population. **Elderly:** May have increased risk of dehydration, hyponatremia.

INTERACTIONS

DRUG: Strong CYP3A4 inducers (e.g., **carBAMazepine, phenytoin, rifAMPin**) may decrease concentration/effects. **Strong CYP2D6 inhibitors (e.g., buPROPion, FLUoxetine, PARoxetine)** may increase concentration/effect. **MAOIs** (e.g., **phenelzine, selegiline**) contraindicated; may cause malignant hyperthermia, hypertensive crisis, hyperreflexia, seizures, serotonin syndrome. **Alcohol** may increase adverse effects. **Serotonergic drugs (e.g., busPIRone, linezolid, traMADol)** may increase risk of serotonin syndrome. **Anticoagulants, antiplatelets, NSAIDs** may increase risk of bleeding. **HERBAL:** St. John's wort, Syrian rue may increase serotonergic effect. **Herbals with anticoagulant/antiplatelet properties (e.g., garlic, ginger, ginkgo biloba), glucosamine** may increase risk of bleeding. **FOOD:** None known. **LAB VALUES:** May decrease serum sodium.

AVAILABILITY (Rx)

Tablets: 5 mg, 10 mg, 20 mg.

ADMINISTRATION/HANDLING

PO
• Give without regard to food. May administer with milk or food if GI upset occurs.

INDICATIONS/ROUTES/DOSAGE

Major Depressive Disorder
PO: ADULTS/ELDERLY: Initially, 10 mg once daily. May increase to 20 mg as tolerated. May decrease to 5 mg/day for pts who do not tolerate higher doses. **Maintenance:** 5–20 mg once daily.

Dose Modification
Concomitant use of strong CYP2D6 inhibitors: Reduce dose by half of intended therapy. **Maximum:** 10 mg once daily. **Concomitant use of strong CYP inducers:** If coadministered for more than 14 days, consider increasing vortioxetine dose. **Maximum:** Do not exceed more than 3 times original dose. **CYP2D6 poor metabolizers: Maximum:** 10 mg once daily.

Discontinuation
Gradually taper dose to minimize incidence of withdrawal symptoms and to allow detection of re-emerging symptoms.

Dosage in Renal Impairment
No dose adjustment.

Dosage in Hepatic Impairment
Mild to moderate impairment: No dose adjustment. **Severe impairment:** Not recommended.

SIDE EFFECTS

Frequent (32%–22%): Nausea, sexual dysfunction. **Occasional (10%–3%):** Diarrhea, dizziness, dry mouth, constipation, vomiting, flatulence, abnormal dreams, pruritus.

ADVERSE EFFECTS/TOXIC REACTIONS

Life-threatening serotonin syndrome may include mental status changes (agitation, hallucinations, delirium, coma), autonomic instability (tachycardia, labile blood pressure, dizziness, sweating, flushing, hyperthermia), neuromuscular symptoms (tremor, rigidity, myoclonus [localized muscle twitching], hyperactive reflexes, incoordination), seizures, GI symptoms (nausea, vomiting, diarrhea). May increase risk of bleeding

V

events such as ecchymosis, hematoma, epistaxis (nosebleed), petechiae. Mania/hypomania may indicate baseline bipolar disorder. Syndrome of inappropriate antidiuretic hormone (SIADH), also known as water intoxication or dilutional hyponatremia, may induce seizures, coma, or death. Angioedema, dyspnea, rash may indicate allergic reaction. May increase risk of suicidal ideation and behavior once treatment is therapeutic. May alter sexual drive, ease of arousal, ease of reaching orgasm, or cause erectile dysfunction in men or decreased lubrication in women.

NURSING CONSIDERATIONS

BASELINE ASSESSMENT

Obtain serum electrolytes. Note serum sodium level. Assess appearance, behavior, speech pattern, level of interest, mood. Assess risk for bleeding. Receive full medication history including herbal products.

INTERVENTION/EVALUATION

Monitor serum sodium levels. Screen for signs of SIADH (confusion, seizures).

Diligently screen for suicidal ideation and behavior; new onset or worsening of anxiety, depression, mood disorder. Assess for improvement of depression (improved emotion, self-image, interest in activities; decreased agitation, loneliness, self-harm). Monitor for symptoms of serotonin syndrome, mania/hypomania. Monitor for allergic reactions.

PATIENT/FAMILY TEACHING

• Report neurologic changes: confusion, excessive talking, hallucinations, headache, hyperactivity, insomnia, racing thoughts, seizure-like activity, tremors; sexual dysfunction; fever; or any type of allergic reaction. • Avoid tasks that require alertness, motor skills until response to drug is established (may cause dizziness, drowsiness). • Seek immediate medical attention if thoughts of suicide, new onset or worsening of anxiety, depression, or changes in mood occur. • Report bleeding, bruising. • Severe allergic reaction may occur; report rash; swelling of the face, tongue, throat.

V

warfarin

war-far-in
(Jantoven)

■ **BLACK BOX ALERT** ■ May cause major or fatal bleeding. Risk factors include history of GI bleeding, hypertension, cerebrovascular disease, heart disease, malignancy, trauma, anemia, renal insufficiency, age 65 yrs and older, high anticoagulation factor (INR greater than 4). Consider cardiac/hepatic function, age, nutritional status, concurrent medications, risk of bleeding when dosing warfarin. Genetic variations have been identified as factors associated with dosage and bleeding risk. Genotyping tests are available. Perform regular monitoring of international normalized ratio (INR) on all pts during treatment.

Do not confuse Jantoven with Janumet or Januvia.

◆ CLASSIFICATION

PHARMACOTHERAPEUTIC: Vitamin K antagonist. **CLINICAL:** Anticoagulant.

USES

Prophylaxis and treatment of venous thrombosis and pulmonary embolism. Prophylaxis and treatment of thromboembolic complications associated with atrial fibrillation and/or cardiac valve replacement. Reduce risk of death, recurrent myocardial infarction (MI), and thromboembolic events (e.g., stroke, systemic embolization) following an MI.

PRECAUTIONS

Contraindications: Hypersensitivity to warfarin. Hemorrhagic tendencies (e.g., cerebral aneurysms, bleeding from GI tract), recent or potential surgery of eye or CNS, neurosurgical procedures, open wounds, severe uncontrolled or malignant hypertension, spinal puncture procedures, uncontrolled bleeding, ulcers, unreliable or noncompliant pts, unsupervised pts, blood dyscrasias, pericarditis or pericardial effusion, pregnancy (except in women with mechanical heart valves at high risk for thromboembolism), bacterial endocar-

ditis, threatened abortion. Major regional lumbar block anesthesia or traumatic surgery, eclampsia/preeclampsia. **Cautions:** Active tuberculosis, acute infection, diabetes, heparin-induced thrombocytopenia and deep vein thrombosis, pts at risk for hemorrhage, moderate to severe renal impairment, moderate to severe hypertension, thyroid disease, polycythemia vera, vasculitis, open wound, menstruating and postpartum women, indwelling catheters, trauma, prolonged dietary deficiencies, disruption of GI normal flora, history of peptic ulcer disease, protein C deficiency, elderly.

ACTION

Interferes with hepatic synthesis of vitamin K–dependent clotting factors, resulting in depletion of coagulation factors II, VII, IX, X. **Therapeutic Effect:** Prevents further extension of formed existing clot; prevents new clot formation, secondary thromboembolic complications.

PHARMACOKINETICS

Route	Onset	Peak	Duration
PO	1.5–3 days	5–7 days	2–5 days

Widely distributed. Protein binding: 99%. Metabolized in liver. Primarily excreted in urine. Not removed by hemodialysis. **Half-life:** 20–60 hrs.

⧗ LIFESPAN CONSIDERATIONS

Pregnancy/Lactation: Contraindicated in pregnancy (fetal, neonatal hemorrhage, intrauterine death). Crosses placenta; is not distributed in breast milk. **Children:** More susceptible to anticoagulant effect. **Elderly:** Increased risk of hemorrhage; lower dosage recommended.

INTERACTIONS

DRUG: **Amiodarone, azole antifungals (e.g., fluconazole), cimetidine, disulfiram, sulfamethoxazole-trimethoprim, levothyroxine, metroNIDAZOLE, NSAIDs (e.g., diclofenac, meloxicam, naproxen), omeprazole, platelet aggregation inhibitors (e.g., clopidogrel), salicylates (e.g.,**

W

aspirin), **thrombolytic agents** (e.g., **alteplase**), **thyroid hormones** (e.g., **levothyroxine**), may increase effect. **Strong CYP3A4 inducers** (e.g., **carBAMazepine, phenytoin, rifAMPin**), **nafcillin, oral contraceptives, sucralfate, vitamin K** may decrease effect. **HERBAL: Herbals with anticoagulant/antiplatelet properties** (e.g., **garlic, ginger, ginkgo biloba**), **fenugreek, glucosamine** may increase risk of bleeding. **FOOD: Foods rich in vitamin K** (e.g., **brussels sprouts, leafy greens, kale, spinach**) may decrease therapeutic effect. **Cranberry juice** may increase effect. **LAB VALUES:** None known.

AVAILABILITY (Rx)

Tablets: 1 mg, 2 mg, 2.5 mg, 3 mg, 4 mg, 5 mg, 6 mg, 7.5 mg, 10 mg.

ADMINISTRATION/HANDLING

PO

• Give without regard to food. Give with food if GI upset occurs. • Give at same time each day.

INDICATIONS/ROUTES/DOSAGE

◀**ALERT**▶ Initial dosing must be individualized with use of recommended institutional protocols. Response is influenced by numerous factors (e.g., age, organ function, genetic variations).

Anticoagulant

PO: ADULTS, ELDERLY: Initially, 5 mg once daily (for most pts). **Maintenance:** (Usual dose): 2–10 mg once daily. Once INR is therapeutic and stable, subsequent dosage may be guided by use of a maintenance dosing nomogram. INR should be checked wkly when out of range and approximately q4wks when stable and therapeutic.

Dosage in Renal/Hepatic Impairment

No dose adjustment. Closely monitor INR.

SIDE EFFECTS

Occasional: GI distress (nausea, anorexia, abdominal cramps, diarrhea). **Rare:** Hypersensitivity reaction (dermatitis, urticaria), esp. in those sensitive to aspirin.

ADVERSE EFFECTS/TOXIC REACTIONS

Hemorrhagic events including local ecchymoses to major hemorrhage (intracranial hemorrhage, GI/GU/nasal/oral/rectal bleeding) may occur. Hepatotoxicity, blood dyscrasias, necrosis, vasculitis, local thrombosis occur rarely. **Antidote:** Vitamin K. Amount based on INR, significance of bleeding. **Range:** 2.5–10 mg given orally or slow IV infusion (see Appendix H for dosage).

NURSING CONSIDERATIONS

BASELINE ASSESSMENT

Obtain CBC, PT/INR. Obtain genotyping prior to initiating therapy if available. Screen for major active bleeding, contraindications. Question recent history of bleeding, recent trauma, surgical procedures, epidural anesthesia.

INTERVENTION/EVALUATION

Obtain CBC, PT/INR daily until therapeutic level is achieved. When stabilized, follow with INR determination q4–6wks. Assess CBC for anemia; urine/stool for occult blood. Monitor for hypotension; complaints of abdominal/back pain, severe headache, confusion, seizures, hemiparesis, aphasia (may be sign of hemorrhage). Question for increase in amount of menstrual discharge. Assess for ecchymoses, petechiae. Check for excessive bleeding from minor cuts, scratches.

PATIENT/FAMILY TEACHING

• Blood levels will be monitored routinely. Do not take newly prescribed medications or discontinue treatment unless approved by prescriber who originally started treatment. • Avoid alcohol, aspirin, foods or supplements rich in vitamin K. • Consult with physician before surgery, dental work. • Urine may become orange. • Falls, subtle injuries, esp.

W

head or abdominal trauma, can be life-threatening. • Report bleeding, bruising, red or brown urine, black stools. • Use electric razor, soft toothbrush to prevent bleeding. • Report coffee-ground vomitus, blood-tinged mucus from cough. • Seek immediate medical attention for stroke-like symptoms (confusion, difficulty speaking, headache, one-sided weakness); bloody stool or urine.

zanamivir

zan-**am**-i-veer
(Relenza Diskhaler)

◆ CLASSIFICATION

PHARMACOTHERAPEUTIC: Neuraminidase inhibitor. **CLINI CAL:** Antiviral, anti-influenza.

USES

Treatment of uncomplicated acute illness due to influenza virus A and B in adults, children 7 yrs and older who have been symptomatic for no more than 48 hrs. Prevention of influenza A and B in adults and children 5 yrs and older.

PRECAUTIONS

Contraindications: Hypersensitivity to zanamivir. **Cautions:** Not recommended in pulmonary disease (e.g., COPD, asthma).

ACTION

Inhibits influenza virus enzyme neuraminidase, essential for viral replication. **Therapeutic Effect:** Prevents viral release from infected cells.

PHARMACOKINETICS

Widely distributed. Protein binding: Less than 10%. Not metabolized. Excreted unchanged in urine. **Half-life:** 2.5–5.1 hrs.

⌛ LIFESPAN CONSIDERATIONS

Pregnancy/Lactation: Unknown if drug crosses placenta or is distributed in breast milk. **Children:** Safety and efficacy not established in pts younger than 7 yrs (treatment) or younger than 5 yrs (prevention). **Elderly:** No age-related precautions noted.

INTERACTIONS

DRUG: May decrease levels/effect of **influenza virus vaccine (live/attenuated). HERBAL:** None significant. **FOOD:** None known. **LAB VALUES:** None significant.

AVAILABILITY (Rx)

Powder for Inhalation: 5 mg/blister.

ADMINISTRATION/HANDLING

Inhalation
• Instruct pt to use Diskhaler device provided, exhale completely; then, holding mouthpiece 1 inch away from lips, inhale and hold breath as long as possible before exhaling. • Rinse mouth with water immediately after inhalation (prevents mouth/throat dryness). • Store at room temperature.

INDICATIONS/ROUTES/DOSAGE

Treatment of Influenza Virus
Inhalation: ADULTS, ELDERLY, CHILDREN 7 YRS AND OLDER: 2 inhalations (one 5-mg blister per inhalation for total dose of 10 mg) twice daily (approximately 12 hrs apart) for 5 days. (Doses on first day should be separated by at least 2 hrs.)

Prevention of Influenza Virus
Inhalation: ADULTS, ELDERLY, CHILDREN 5 YRS AND OLDER: Postexposure prophylaxis (household exposure): Two inhalations (10 mg) once daily for 7 days after last known exposure. **(Institutional outbreak):** Two inhalations (10 mg) once daily for at least 2 wks and until approx. 7 days after identification of illness onset in the last pt.

Dosage in Renal/Hepatic Impairment
No dose adjustment.

SIDE EFFECTS

Occasional (3%–2%): Diarrhea, sinusitis, nausea, bronchitis, cough, dizziness, headache. **Rare (less than 1.5%):** Malaise, fatigue, fever, abdominal pain, myalgia, arthralgia, urticaria.

ADVERSE EFFECTS/TOXIC REACTIONS

May cause neutropenia. Bronchospasm may occur in pts with history of COPD, bronchial asthma. Neuropsychiatric events (e.g., confusion, seizures, hallucinations) have been reported.

Z

◆ Canadian trade name　　 Non-Crushable Drug　　**HIGH ALERT** High Alert drug

NURSING CONSIDERATIONS

BASELINE ASSESSMENT

Pts requiring an inhaled bronchodilator at same time as zanamivir should use the bronchodilator before zanamivir administration.

INTERVENTION/EVALUATION

Provide assistance if dizziness occurs. Monitor daily pattern of bowel activity, stool consistency.

PATIENT/FAMILY TEACHING

• Follow manufacturer guidelines for use of delivery device. • Avoid contact with those who are at high risk for influenza. • Continue treatment for full 5-day course. • In pts with respiratory disease, an inhaled bronchodilator should be readily available.

---

zanubrutinib

zan-ue-**broo**-ti-nib
(Brukinsa)
Do not confuse zanubrutinib with acalabrutinib or ibrutinib; Brukinsa with Imbruvica.

◆ CLASSIFICATION

PHARMACOTHERAPEUTIC: Bruton tyrosine kinase (BTK) inhibitor. **CLINICAL:** Antineoplastic.

USES

Mantle cell lymphoma (MCL): Treatment of adults with relapsed or refractory MCL who have received at least one prior therapy. **Waldenström macroglobulinemia:** Treatment of Waldenström macroglobulinemia in adults. **Marginal Zone lymphoma (MZL):** Treatment of adults with relapsed or refractory MZL who have received at least one anti–CD20-based regimen. **Chronic lymphocytic leukemia (CLL)/small lymphocytic lymphoma (SLL):** Treatment of adults with CLL/SLL. **Follicular lymphoma (FL):** Treatment of adults with relapsed or refractory FL, in combination with obinutuzumab, after 2 or more lines of systemic therapy.

PRECAUTIONS

Contraindications: Hypersensitivity to zanubrutinib. **Cautions:** Baseline cytopenias, hepatic/renal impairment, conditions predisposing to infection (e.g., diabetes, renal failure, immunocompromised pts, open wounds), chronic opportunistic infections (e.g., herpesvirus infection, hepatitis B virus [HBV] infection, fungal infections), pts at risk for bleeding (e.g., history of intracranial/GI/genitourinary bleeding, coagulation disorders, recent trauma, concomitant use of anticoagulants, antiplatelets); history of atrial fibrillation, atrial flutter, cardiac disease. Avoid concomitant use of strong or moderate CYP3A4 inducers.

ACTION

Highly selective BTK inhibitor that forms a covalent bond with a cysteine residue in the BTK active site, inhibiting activity of BKT. BKT is a signaling molecule of pathways necessary for B-cell proliferation. **Therapeutic Effect:** Inhibits malignant B-cell proliferation and reduces tumor growth.

PHARMACOKINETICS

Widely distributed. Metabolized in liver. Protein binding: 94%. Peak plasma concentration: 2 hrs. Excreted in feces (87%), urine (8%). **Half-life:** 2–4 hrs.

⌛ LIFESPAN CONSIDERATIONS

Pregnancy/Lactation: Avoid pregnancy; may cause fetal harm. Females of reproductive potential and males with female partners of reproductive potential must use effective contraception during treatment and for at least 1 wk after discontinuation. Unknown if distributed in breast milk. Breastfeeding not recommended during treatment and for at least 2 wks after discontinuation. **Children:** Safety and efficacy not established. **Elderly:** No age-related precautions noted.

INTERACTIONS

DRUG: May increase effect/adverse effects of **anticoagulants** (e.g., **heparin, warfarin**), **antiplatelets** (e.g., **aspirin, clopidogrel**), increasing risk of bleeding. **Strong CYP3A4 inhibitors** (e.g., **clarithromycin, ketoconazole, ritonavir**), **moderate CYP3A4 inhibitors** (e.g., **erythromycin, ciprofloxacin, dilTIAZem, fluconazole, verapamil**) may increase concentration/effect. **Strong CYP3A4 inducers** (e.g., **rifAMPin, phenytoin, carBAMazepine, PHENobarbital**), **moderate CYP3A4 inducers** (e.g., **dexamethasone, modafinil, nafcillin**) may decrease concentration/effect. May decrease effects of **BCG (intravesical), vaccines (live)**. May increase toxic effects **of natalizumab, live vaccines. Pimecrolimus, tacrolimus (topical)** may increase adverse/toxic effect. **HERBAL:** Echinacea may decrease therapeutic effect. **FOOD: Grapefruit products, seville oranges** may decrease concentration/effect. **LAB VALUES:** May increase serum ALT, bilirubin, uric acid. May decrease Hgb, leukocytes, lymphocytes, platelets, neutrophils, RBCs.

AVAILABILITY (Rx)

Capsules: 80 mg.

ADMINISTRATION/HANDLING

PO

• Give without regard to food. • Administer capsule whole; do not break, cut, or open. • If a dose is missed, administer as soon as possible on same day, then follow usual dosing schedule the following day.

INDICATIONS/ROUTES/DOSAGE

CLL, Macroglobulinemia, MCL, MZL, SLL, Waldenström

PO: ADULTS, ELDERLY: 160 mg twice daily or 320 mg once daily. Continue until disease progression or unacceptable toxicity.

Dose Modification

Based on Common Terminology Criteria for Adverse Events (CTCAE).

Grade 3 or 4 nonhematologic toxicity; Grade 3 thrombocytopenia *with* bleeding; Grade 4 thrombocytopenia (lasting more than 10 days); Grade 3 febrile neutropenia; Grade 4 neutropenia lasting more than 7 days: (**First occurrence**): Withhold treatment until improved to Grade 1 or 0 (or baseline), then resume at 160 mg twice daily or 320 mg once daily. (**Second occurrence**): Withhold treatment until improved to Grade 1 or 0 (or baseline), then resume at 80 mg twice daily or 160 mg once daily. (**Third occurrence**): Withhold treatment until improved to Grade 1 or 0 (or baseline), then resume at 80 mg once daily. (**Fourth occurrence**): Permanently discontinue.

Concomitant Use of CYP3A4 Inhibitors/Inducers

Strong CYP3A4 inhibitors: Reduce dose to 80 mg once daily. **Moderate CYP3A4 inhibitors:** Reduce dose to 80 mg twice daily. **Strong or moderate CYP3A4 inhibitors:** Avoid concomitant use.

Dosage in Renal Impairment

Mild to moderate impairment: No dose adjustment. **Severe impairment, hemodialysis:** Monitor for adverse reactions/toxic effects.

Dosage in Hepatic Impairment

Mild to moderate impairment: No dose adjustment. **Severe impairment:** Reduce dose to 80 mg twice daily.

SIDE EFFECTS

Frequent (36%–23%): Rash, diarrhea. **Occasional (14%–12%):** Bruising, musculoskeletal pain, myalgia, back pain, arthralgia, constipation, cough, hypertension. **Rare (4%):** Headache.

ADVERSE EFFECTS/TOXIC REACTIONS

Myelosuppression (anemia, leukopenia, lymphopenia, neutropenia, thrombocytopenia) is an expected response to therapy, but more severe reactions including febrile neutropenia, hemorrhagic thrombocytopenia may occur. Life-threatening hemorrhagic events including intracranial hemorrhage, GI bleeding, hematuria, hemothorax occurred in 2% of pts. Petechiae, purpura reported in 50% of pts. Life-threatening bacterial, invasive fungal, viral, other opportunistic infections; pneumonia may occur. Grade 3 infections reported in 23% of pts. Reactivation of HBV infection was reported. UTI reported in 11% of pts. New primary malignancies including basal cell carcinoma, squamous cell carcinoma (6% of pts), nonskin carcinomas (9% of pts) have occurred. Atrial fibrillation/atrial flutter reported in 2% of pts.

NURSING CONSIDERATIONS

BASELINE ASSESSMENT

Obtain CBC; PT/INR (if on anticoagulation therapy); pregnancy test in females of reproductive potential. Confirm compliance of effective contraception. Assess risk for bleeding. Question history of atrial fibrillation, atrial flutter, cardiac disease; intracranial/GI/genitourinary bleeding, coagulation disorders, recent trauma; previous skin cancers. Assess usual bowel movement patterns, stool characteristics. Receive full medication history and screen for interactions. Screen for active infection. Consider prophylactic treatment of herpes simplex virus, *Pneumocystis jirovecii* pneumonia, other infections. Offer emotional support.

INTERVENTION/EVALUATION

Monitor CBC periodically for cytopenias. Diligently monitor for infections (cough, fever, fatigue), esp. respiratory tract infections, herpesvirus infection, opportunistic infections, sepsis. If serious infection or sepsis occurs, initiate appropriate antimicrobial therapy. Monitor for HBV reactivation, new malignancies (skin and nonskin). Obtain ECG if chest pain, dyspnea, palpitations occur. Monitor for hemorrhagic events including intracranial hemorrhage (altered mental status, aphasia, blindness, hemiparesis, unequal pupils, seizures), GI bleeding (hematemesis, melena, rectal bleeding), genitourinary bleeding (hematuria),

epistaxis. Monitor daily pattern of bowel activity, stool consistency. Monitor for drug toxicities if discontinuation or dose reduction of concomitant CYP3A4 inhibitor is unavoidable.

PATIENT/FAMILY TEACHING

• Treatment may depress your immune system and reduce your ability to fight infection. Report symptoms of infection such as body aches, burning with urination, chills, cough, fatigue, fever. Avoid those with active infection. • Report symptoms of bone marrow depression such as bruising, fatigue, fever, shortness of breath, weight loss; bleeding easily, bloody urine or stool. • Treatment may cause new cancers; reactivation of HBV. • Report liver problems (abdominal pain, bruising, clay-colored stool, dark or amber-colored urine, yellowing of the skin or eyes), heart arrhythmias (chest pain, dizziness, fainting, palpitations, slow or rapid heart rate, irregular heart rate); symptoms of hemorrhagic stroke (confusion, difficulty speaking, one-sided weakness or paralysis, loss of vision, seizures). • Immediately report bleeding of any kind. • Use effective contraception to avoid pregnancy. Do not breastfeed. • There is a high risk of interactions with other medications. Do not take newly prescribed medications unless approved by prescriber who originally started therapy. • Avoid grapefruit products, herbal supplements (esp. St. John's wort).

zavegepant

za-**ve**-je-pant
(Zavzpret)
Do not confuse zavegepant with atogepant, rimegepant, or ubrogepant or Zavzpret with Zavesca.

◆CLASSIFICATION

PHARMACOTHERAPEUTIC: Calcitonin gene-related peptide (CGRP) receptor antagonist. **CLINICAL:** Antimigraine.

USES

Treatment of migraines with or without aura in adults.

PRECAUTIONS

Contraindications: Hypersensitivity to zavegepant. **Cautions:** Avoid concomitant use of organic anion transporting polypeptide 1B3 (OATP1B3) or sodium taurocholate co-transporting polypeptide (NTCP) transporters. Not recommended in pts with eGFR less than 30 mL/min. Avoid use in pts with severe hepatic impairment. Not indicated for prevention of migraine.

ACTION

Binds to and inhibits CGRP receptor. **Therapeutic Effect:** Relieves migraine headache.

PHARMACOKINETICS

Widely distributed. Peak concentration: 30 min. Metabolized in liver. Protein binding: 90%. Excreted in feces (80%), urine (11%). **Half-life:** 6.55 hrs.

⏳ LIFESPAN CONSIDERATIONS

Pregnancy/Lactation: Unknown if distributed in breast milk. **Children:** Safety and efficacy not established. **Elderly:** No age-related precautions noted.

INTERACTIONS

DRUG: **OATP1B3 inhibitors (e.g., clarithromycin, cyclosporine, ri-fAMPin), NTCP inhibitors (e.g., ezetimibe, irbesartan)** may increase concentration/effect. **OATP1B3 inducers, NTCP inducers, intranasal decongestants (e.g., oxymetazoline, phenylephrine)** may decrease concentration/effect. **HERBAL:** None significant. **FOOD:** None known. **LAB VALUES:** None significant.

AVAILABILITY (Rx)

Intranasal Spray: 10 mg single-use, unit-dose disposable device.

ADMINISTRATION/HANDLING

Intranasal
• Instruct pt to clear nasal passages as much as possible before use. • Tilt head slightly forward. • Insert spray tip into one nostril, away from nasal septum. • Pump medication into one nostril while pt holds other nostril closed, concurrently inspires through nose.

INDICATIONS/ROUTES/DOSAGE

Migraine (With or Without Aura)
Intranasal: ADULTS, ELDERLY: 10 mg (as a single spray) in one nostril as needed. **Maximum:** 10 mg/24 hrs.

Dosage in Renal Impairment
eGFR 30 mL/min or greater: No dose adjustment. **eGFR less than 30 mL/min:** Not recommended.

Dosage in Hepatic Impairment
Mild to moderate impairment: No dose adjustment. **Severe impairment:** Avoid use.

SIDE EFFECTS

Occasional (18%): Dysgeusia, ageusia. **Rare (4%–2%):** Nausea, nasal discomfort, vomiting.

ADVERSE EFFECTS/TOXIC REACTIONS

Hypersensitivity reactions, including facial swelling and urticaria, reported in less than 1% of pts.

NURSING CONSIDERATIONS

BASELINE ASSESSMENT
Question characteristics of migraine headaches (onset, location, duration, possible precipitating symptoms). Receive full medication history and screen for interactions. Question history of renal impairment.

INTERVENTION/EVALUATION
Evaluate for relief of migraine headache (photophobia, phonophobia, nausea,

Z

 Canadian trade name   🐢 Non-Crushable Drug   🔴 High Alert drug

vomiting, pain, dizziness, fogginess).
Monitor for hypersensitivity reactions.

PATIENT/FAMILY TEACHING

• Allergic reactions such as difficulty
breathing, severe rash may occur. If
allergic reaction occurs, seek immediate medical attention. • There is a risk
of interactions with other medications.
Do not take newly prescribed medications unless approved by prescriber
who originally started therapy. • Do not
use nasal decongestants within 1 hr of
zavegepant.

---

zidovudine

zye-**doe**-vue-deen
(Retrovir)

■ **BLACK BOX ALERT** ■ Neutropenia, severe anemia may occur.
Lactic acidosis, severe hepatomegaly with steatosis (fatty liver), including fatalities, have occurred.
Symptomatic myopathy, myositis
associated with prolonged use.

**Do not confuse Retrovir with
acyclovir or ritonavir.**

FIXED-COMBINATION(S)

Combivir: zidovudine/lamiVUDine
(an antiviral): 300 mg/150 mg.
Trizivir: zidovudine/lamiVUDine/
abacavir (an antiviral): 300 mg/150
mg/300 mg.

◆CLASSIFICATION

PHARMACOTHERAPEUTIC: Nucleoside reverse transcriptase inhibitors.
CLINICAL: Antiretroviral.

USES

Treatment of HIV infection in
combination with other antiretroviral
agents. Prevention of maternal/
fetal HIV transmission. **OFF-LABEL:**
HIV-1 nonoccupational postexposure
prophylaxis.

PRECAUTIONS

Contraindications: Potentially life-
threatening allergic reactions to
zidovudine or its components.
Cautions: Bone marrow compromise,
renal/hepatic impairment. Combination
with interferon with or without ribavirin in
HIV/hepatitis C virus (HCV) coinfection.

ACTION

Interferes with viral RNA-dependent
DNA polymerase, an enzyme necessary
for viral HIV replication. **Therapeutic
Effect:** Slows HIV replication, reducing
progression of HIV infection.

PHARMACOKINETICS

Widely distributed. Protein binding:
25%–38%. Metabolized in liver. Crosses
blood-brain barrier and is widely
distributed, including to CSF. Primarily
excreted in urine. **Half-life:** 0.5–3 hrs
(increased in renal impairment).

⧗ LIFESPAN CONSIDERATIONS

Pregnancy/Lactation: Unknown if
drug crosses placenta or is distributed
in breast milk. Unknown if fetal
harm or effects on fertility can occur.
Children: No age-related precautions
noted. **Elderly:** Information not available.

INTERACTIONS

DRUG: Cladribine, DOXOrubicin,
ganciclovir, interferons, valganciclovir
may increase concentration/effect.
HERBAL: None significant. **FOOD:** None
known. **LAB VALUES:** May increase mean
corpuscular volume (MCV).

AVAILABILITY (Rx)

Capsules: 100 mg. **Injection Solution:**
(Retrovir): 10 mg/mL. **Syrup:** 50 mg/5
mL. **Tablets:** 300 mg.

ADMINISTRATION/HANDLING

 IV

Reconstitution • Dilute in D₅W to a final
concentration no greater than 4 mg/mL.

Rate of administration • Infuse over 1 hr. May infuse over 30 min in neonates.

Storage • Refrigerate diluted solution for up to 24 hrs or store at room temperature for up to 8 hrs. • Do not use if solution is discolored or precipitate forms.

PO
• Give without regard to food. • Use a calibrated measuring device to accurately measure liquid dose.

▩ IV COMPATIBILITIES

Heparin, LORazepam (Ativan), morphine, potassium chloride.

INDICATIONS/ROUTES/DOSAGE

HIV Infection
PO: ADULTS, ELDERLY: 300 mg q12h. **CHILDREN 4 WKS TO 18 YRS WEIGHING 30 KG OR MORE:** 300 mg q12h. **WEIGHING 9–29 KG:** 9 mg/kg q12h or 6 mg/kg q8h. **WEIGHING 4–8 KG:** 12 mg/kg q12h or 8 mg/kg q8h.
IV: ADULTS, ELDERLY: 1 mg/kg/dose q4h around the clock. **NEONATES:** If unable to tolerate oral drugs, the IV dose should be 75% of the oral dose, using the same dosing interval.

Prevention of Maternal/Fetal HIV Transmission
Note: Pregnant women (greater than 14 wks of pregnancy): 100 mg PO 5 times/day until start of labor.
IV: DURING LABOR AND DELIVERY: 2 mg/kg loading dose, then IV infusion of 1 mg/kg/hr until clamping of the umbilical cord. **NEONATAL:** Begin within 12 hrs after birth and continue through 6 wks of age. **PO:** 2 mg/kg q6h. **IV:** 1.5 mg/kg infused over 30 min q6h.

Dosage in Renal Impairment
Adults, Elderly: CRCL LESS THAN 15 mL/min, INCLUDING HEMODIALYSIS OR PERITONEAL DIALYSIS: PO: 100 mg q8h or 300 mg once daily. **IV:** 1 mg/kg q6–8hr.

Infants Older than 6 Wks, Children, Adolescents: GFR 10 mL/min/1.73m² OR GREATER: No adjustment. **GFR LESS THAN 10 mL/min/1.73m²:** Administer 50% of dose q8h.

Dosage in Hepatic Impairment
No dose adjustment.

SIDE EFFECTS

Expected (46%–42%): Nausea, headache. **Frequent (20%–16%):** Abdominal pain, asthenia, rash, fever, acne. **Occasional (12%–8%):** Diarrhea, anorexia, malaise, myalgia, drowsiness. **Rare (6%–5%):** Dizziness, paresthesia, vomiting, insomnia, dyspnea, altered taste.

ADVERSE EFFECTS/TOXIC REACTIONS

Anemia (occurring most commonly after 4–6 wks of therapy), granulocytopenia may occur in pts with pretherapy low baselines. Neurotoxicity (ataxia, fatigue, lethargy, nystagmus, seizures) may occur.

NURSING CONSIDERATIONS

BASELINE ASSESSMENT
Obtain CBC, CD4 cell count, HIV RNA level, viral load. Obtain specimens for viral diagnostic tests before starting therapy (therapy may begin before results are obtained).

INTERVENTION/EVALUATION
Monitor CBC, CD4 cell count, HIV RNA levels. Monitor for bleeding. Assess for headache, dizziness. Monitor daily pattern of bowel activity, stool consistency. Evaluate skin for acne, rash. Monitor for opportunistic infections (fever, chills, cough, myalgia). Monitor I&O, serum renal function, LFT.

PATIENT/FAMILY TEACHING
• Treatment is not a cure for HIV infection, nor does it reduce risk of transmission to others. • Do not take any medications without physician's approval. • Bleeding from gums, nose, rectum may occur and should be

Z

reported to physician immediately. • Dental work should be done before therapy or after blood counts return to normal (often wks after therapy has stopped). • Inform physician if muscle weakness, difficulty breathing, headache, inability to sleep, unusual bleeding, rash, signs of infection occur.

ziprasidone

zi-**pras**-i-done
(<u>Geodon</u>, Zeldox ✦)

■ **BLACK BOX ALERT** ■ Increased risk of mortality in elderly pts with dementia-related psychosis, mainly due to pneumonia, HF.
Do not confuse ziprasidone with traZODone.

◆ CLASSIFICATION

PHARMACOTHERAPEUTIC: Second-generation (atypical) antipsychotic. **CLINICAL:** Antipsychotic.

USES

Schizophrenia: Treatment of schizophrenia in adults. **Bipolar I disorder:** Treatment of acute mania or mixed episodes associated with bipolar disorder with or without psychosis as monotherapy. Maintenance treatment of bipolar disorder as adjunct to lithium or valproic acid. **Agitation/aggression:** Acute treatment of agitation in schizophrenic pts in adults. **OFF-LABEL:** Agitation/aggression of bipolar disorder/substance intoxication, acute hypomania (monotherapy), delirium in the ICU (treatment), delusional infestation, major depressive disorder (treatment resistant). Tourette's syndrome, tic disorders, irritability associated with autism.

PRECAUTIONS

Contraindications: Hypersensitivity to ziprasidone. Conditions associated with risk of prolonged QT interval, congenital long QT syndrome, concurrent use of other QT-prolongation medications (e.g., amiodarone, moxifloxacin, tacrolimus, thioridazine). Uncompensated HF. Recent MI. **Cautions:** Pts with bradycardia, hypokalemia, hypomagnesemia may be at greater risk for torsades de pointes. History of MI or unstable heart disease, seizure disorder, cardiac arrhythmias, disorders in which CNS depression is a feature; pts at risk for aspiration pneumonia, hypotension, suicide; elderly, diabetes, hepatic impairment, Parkinson's disease, pts with breast cancer or other prolactin-dependent tumors.

ACTION

Antagonizes alpha-adrenergic, DOPamine, histamine, serotonin receptors; inhibits reuptake of serotonin, norepinephrine. **Therapeutic Effect:** Reduces symptoms of schizophrenia, depression.

PHARMACOKINETICS

Widely distributed. Food increases bioavailability. Protein binding: 99%. Metabolized in liver. Excreted in feces. Not removed by hemodialysis. **Half-life: (PO):** 7 hrs; **(IM):** 2–5 hrs.

⧗ LIFESPAN CONSIDERATIONS

Pregnancy/Lactation: Unknown if drug crosses placenta or is distributed in breast milk. **Children:** Safety and efficacy not established. **Elderly:** No age-related precautions noted. Use caution.

INTERACTIONS

DRUG: Alcohol, CNS depressants (e.g., LORazepam, morphine, zolpidem) may increase CNS depression. CarBAMazepine may decrease concentration. **QT interval–prolonging medications** (e.g., amiodarone, azithromycin, ciprofloxacin, haloperidol, methadone, sotalol) may increase risk of QTc interval prolongation. **HERBAL: Herbals with sedative properties (e.g., chamomile, kava kava, valerian)** may increase CNS depression. **FOOD: All foods** enhance bioavailability. **LAB VALUES:** May prolong QT interval. May increase serum glucose, prolactin levels.

AVAILABILITY (Rx)

Capsules: 20 mg, 40 mg, 60 mg, 80 mg. **Injection, Powder for Reconstitution:** 20 mg.

ADMINISTRATION/HANDLING

IM
• Store vials at room temperature; protect from light. • Reconstitute each vial with 1.2 mL Sterile Water for Injection to provide concentration of 20 mg/mL. • Reconstituted solution stable for 24 hrs at room temperature or 7 days if refrigerated.

PO
• Give with food. Administer capsules whole (do not open, crush, or allow chewing).

INDICATIONS/ROUTES/DOSAGE

◀ALERT▶ To discontinue therapy: Gradually discontinue to avoid withdrawal symptoms, minimize risk of relapses.

Schizophrenia
PO: ADULTS, ELDERLY: Initially, 20–40 mg twice daily with food. Titrate at intervals of no less than 2 days based on response and tolerability. **Maintenance:** 20–80 mg twice daily.

Acute Agitation (Schizophrenia)
IM: ADULTS, ELDERLY: 10 mg q2h or 20 mg q4h. **Maximum:** 40 mg/day. Switch to oral therapy as soon as possible.

Bipolar Disorder (Acute Episodes and Maintenance Treatment as Adjunct to Lithium or Valproate)
PO: ADULTS, ELDERLY (Acute): Initially, 40 mg twice daily. May increase to 60–80 mg twice daily on second day of treatment. **Maintenance:** 40–80 mg twice daily.

Dosage in Renal Impairment
Oral: No dose adjustment. **IM:** Use caution.

Dosage in Hepatic Impairment
Use caution.

SIDE EFFECTS

Frequent (30%–16%): Headache, drowsiness, dizziness. **Occasional:** Rash, orthostatic hypotension, weight gain, restlessness, constipation, dyspepsia. **Rare:** Hyperglycemia, priapism.

ADVERSE EFFECTS/TOXIC REACTIONS

Prolongation of QT interval (as seen on ECG) may produce torsades de pointes, a form of ventricular tachycardia.

NURSING CONSIDERATIONS

BASELINE ASSESSMENT
Obtain serum magnesium, potassium; ECG to assess risk for QT interval prolongation. Assess pt's behavior, appearance, emotional status, response to environment, speech pattern, thought content.

INTERVENTION/EVALUATION
Assess for therapeutic response (greater interest in surroundings, improved self-care, increased ability to concentrate, relaxed facial expression). Monitor weight.

PATIENT/FAMILY TEACHING
• Avoid tasks that require alertness, motor skills until response to drug is established. • Avoid alcohol. • Report chest pain, shortness of breathing, irregular heartbeats, fainting, palpitations.

ziv-aflibercept

ziv-a-**flib**-er-sept
(Zaltrap)
Do not confuse ziv-aflibercept with abatacept, Aricept, or etanercept.

Z

◆CLASSIFICATION

PHARMACOTHERAPEUTIC: Vascular endothelial growth factor (VEGF) inhibitor. **CLINICAL:** Antineoplastic.

USES

Treatment of metastatic colorectal cancer (mCRC) (in combination with 5-fluorouracil, leucovorin, irinotecan [FOLFIRI]) in pt resistant to or has progressed following an oxaliplatin-containing regimen. **OFF-LABEL:** Ascites (symptomatic) due to malignant ovarian cancer.

PRECAUTIONS

Contraindications: Hypersensitivity to ziv-aflibercept. **Cautions:** Baseline cytopenias, conditions predisposing to infection (e.g., diabetes, renal failure, immunocompromised pts, open wounds), pts at risk for bleeding (e.g., history of intracranial/GI/GU bleeding, coagulation disorders, recent trauma; concomitant use of anticoagulants, antiplatelet medication, NSAIDs), hypertension, elderly, history of arterial/venous thrombosis (e.g., CVA, DVT, MI, pulmonary embolism), GI perforation or hemorrhage.

ACTION

A recombinant fusion protein, comprising portions of binding domains of vascular endothelial growth factor (VEGF) receptors. Acts as a decoy receptor that prevents VEGF receptor binding/activation. **Therapeutic Effect:** Produces anti-angiogenesis/tumor regression.

PHARMACOKINETICS

Half-life: 6 days (**range:** 4–7 days).

⧖ LIFESPAN CONSIDERATIONS

Pregnancy/Lactation: Avoid pregnancy; may cause fetal harm. Females of reproductive potential and males should use effective contraception during therapy and for at least 3 mos after discontinuation. Unknown if distributed in breast milk. **Children:** Safety and efficacy not established. **Elderly:** May have increased risk of side effects, esp. diarrhea, dehydration, dizziness, weakness, weight loss.

INTERACTIONS

DRUG: May decrease therapeutic effect of **BCG (intravesical). Anticoagulants (e.g., heparin, warfarin), antiplatelets (e.g., aspirin, clopidogrel), NSAIDS (e.g., diclofenac, meloxicam, naproxen), thrombolytic therapy (e.g., alteplase)** may increase risk of bleeding in pts with treatment-induced thrombocytopenia. **Cladribine** may increase myelosuppressive effect. **HERBAL:** None significant. **FOOD:** None known. **LAB VALUES:** May increase serum ALT, AST, serum creatinine; urine protein. May decrease leukocytes, neutrophils, platelets.

AVAILABILITY (Rx)

Injection Solution: 100 mg/4 mL (25mg/mL), 200 mg/8mL (25 mg/mL).

ADMINISTRATION/HANDLING
💧 IV

Preparation • Visually inspect for particulate matter or discoloration. Solution should appear clear, colorless to pale yellow in color. Discard if solution is cloudy, discolored, or if visible particles are observed. • Withdraw proper dose from vial and dilute in 0.9% NaCl or D_5W to a final concentration of 0.6–8 mg/mL. Use polyvinyl chloride (PVC) infusion bags containing bis (2-ethyl-hexyl) phthalate (DEHP) or polyolefin. • Mix by gentle inversion. • Do not shake or agitate. • Discard unused portions.

Rate of administration • Infuse over 60 min via dedicated IV line using an in-line 0.2-micron polyethersulfone filter and an infusion set made of one of the following: Polypropylene, polyethylene-lined PVC, polyurethane, DEHP-free PVC-containing trioctyl-trimellitate (TOTM), PVC containing DEHP. • Do not use in-line filters made of polyvinylidene fluoride

---

Z

(PVDF) or nylon. • Do not administer as IV push or bolus.

Storage • Refrigerate unused vials. • Do not shake. • Protect from light. • May refrigerate diluted solution for up to 24 hrs or at controlled room temperature for up to 8 hrs.

⬛ IV INCOMPATIBILITIES

Do not infuse with other medications or solutions.

INDICATIONS/ROUTES/DOSAGE

Note: Delay treatment until ANC 1,500 cells/mm^3 or greater.

Metastatic Colorectal Cancer

IV: ADULTS, ELDERLY: 4 mg/kg (based on actual body weight) q2wks (in combination with FOLFIRI). Continue until disease progression or unacceptable toxicity.

Dose Modification

Hypertension (Treatment-Induced)

Severe hypertension, recurrent hypertension: Withhold treatment until hypertension is controlled, then permanently reduce to 2 mg/kg q2wks.

Proteinuria

Urine protein greater than or equal to 2 g/24 hrs: Withhold treatment until urine protein less than 2 g/24 hrs, then resume at previous dose. **Recurrent urine protein greater than 2 g/24 hrs:** Withhold treatment until urine protein less than 2 g/24 hrs, then resume with a permanent reduction to 2 mg/kg q2wks.

Permanent Discontinuation

Permanently discontinue if severe hemorrhage, GI perforation, impaired wound healing, fistula formation, hypertensive crisis, arterial thromboembolism, nephrotic syndrome, thrombotic microangiopathy, reversible posterior leukoencephalopathy occurs.

Dosage in Renal/Hepatic Impairment

No dose adjustment.

SIDE EFFECTS

Frequent (57%–24%): Diarrhea, fatigue, stomatitis, abdominal pain, decreased appetite. **Occasional (13%–9%):** Asthenia, dyspnea, headache. **Rare (3%–2%):** Skin hyperpigmentation, dystonia, oropharyngeal pain, dehydration, rhinorrhea, hemorrhoids, proctalgia.

ADVERSE EFFECTS/TOXIC REACTIONS

Myelosuppression (leukopenia, neutropenia, thrombocytopenia) is an expected response to therapy, but more severe reactions including bone marrow depression, febrile neutropenia may be life-threatening. Severe, sometimes fatal, hemorrhagic events including intracranial/ GI/GU/nasal/postprocedural hemorrhage may occur. GI perforations occurred in less than 1% of pts. May cause impaired wound healing or wound dehiscence requiring medical intervention, GI or non-GI fistula formation, severe hypertension, severe proteinuria, nephrotic syndrome, severe diarrhea, dehydration. Arterial thromboembolism including CVA, MI, TIA reported in up to 3% of pts. Reversible posterior leukoencephalopathy syndrome (RPLS) may present as aphasia, altered mental status, paralysis, vision loss, weakness. UTI reported in 6% of pts. Palmar-plantar erythrodysesthesia syndrome (PPES), a chemotherapy-induced skin condition that presents with redness, swelling, numbness, skin sloughing of the hands and feet, reported in 4% of pts.

NURSING CONSIDERATIONS

BASELINE ASSESSMENT

Obtain CBC, BUN, serum creatinine, LFT; urine protein; vital signs. Obtain pregnancy test in females of reproductive potential. Question for recent surgeries, dental procedures. Question history of thromboembolism (CVA, DVT, MI, pulmonary embolism), hypertension, hemorrhagic events. Screen for active infection. Screen for home medications that may increase risk of hemorrhage. Assess skin for open wounds, lesions, surgical incisions. Obtain dietary consult.

Z

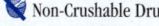

Assess hydration status. Offer emotional support.

INTERVENTION/EVALUATION

Monitor ANC, CBC for myelosuppression prior to each cycle; renal function test, LFT, urine protein periodically. Monitor B/P at least q2wks. Persistent diastolic hypertension may indicate hypertensive crisis. If urine dipstick proteinuria is greater than or equal to 2+, obtain 24-hr urine protein test. Withhold treatment for at least 4 wks prior to elective surgery or for at least 4 wks after major surgery and until wound is fully healed. Due to high risk for arterial occlusions, be vigilant when screening for CVA (aphasia, confusion, paresthesia, hemiparesis, seizures), MI (chest pain, diaphoresis, left arm/ jaw pain, increased serum troponin, ST segment elevation). RPLS should be considered in pts with altered mental status, confusion, headache, seizures, visual disturbances. Report abdominal pain, fever, hemoptysis, melena (may indicate GI perforation/fistula formation). Monitor skin for impaired wound healing, new skin lesions, rash, sloughing. Monitor for decreased urine output, renal dysfunction, nephrotic syndrome. Encourage fluid intake. Monitor daily pattern of bowel activity, stool consistency.

PATIENT/FAMILY TEACHING

• Life-threatening blood clots of the arteries and veins have occurred; report symptoms of heart attack (chest pain, difficulty breathing, jaw pain, nausea, pain that radiates to the left arm, sweating), stroke (blindness, confusion, one-sided weakness, loss of consciousness, trouble speaking, seizures), DVT (swelling, pain, hot feeling in the arms or legs), lung embolism (difficulty breathing, chest pain, rapid heart rate). Report liver problems (abdominal pain, bruising, clay-colored stool, amber or dark-colored urine, yellowing of the skin or eyes); skin changes (sloughing, rash, poor healing of wounds). • Life-threatening bleeding may occur; report bloody stool or urine, rectal bleeding, nosebleeds, vomiting up blood. • Treatment may depress your immune system response and reduce your ability to fight infection. Report symptoms of infection such as body aches, chills, cough, fatigue, fever. Avoid those with active infection. • Use effective contraception to avoid pregnancy. Do not breast-feed. • Nervous system changes, including altered mental status, seizures, headache, blurry vision, high blood pressure, trouble speaking, one-sided weakness, may indicate stroke, high blood pressure crisis, life-threatening brain dysfunction/swelling. • Notify physician before any planned surgeries/dental procedures. • Severe diarrhea may lead to dehydration; drink plenty of fluids.

---

zoledronic acid

zoe-le-**dron**-ik **as**-id
(Aclasta✦, Reclast)

◆CLASSIFICATION

PHARMACOTHERAPEUTIC: Bisphosphonate. **CLINICAL:** Calcium regulator, bone resorption inhibitor.

USES

Bone metastases (solid tumors): Treatment of documented bone metastases from solid tumors (in conjunction with neoplastic therapy). Prostate cancer that should have progressed following treatment with at least one hormonal therapy. **Hypercalcemia of malignancy:** Treatment of hypercalcemia of malignancy (albumin corrected serum calcium 12 mg/dL or greater). **Multiple myeloma:** Treatment of multiple myeloma. **Osteoporosis (fracture risk reduction):** Treatment and prevention of osteoporosis in postmenopausal females. To increase bone mass in males with osteoporosis. Treatment/prevention of glucocorticoid-induced osteoporosis.

Paget's disease: Treatment of Paget's disease of the bone. **OFF-LABEL:** Prevention of bone loss associated with aromatase inhibitor therapy in postmenopausal women with breast cancer or androgen deprivation therapy in men with prostate cancer. Adjuvant therapy in early-stage breast cancer in postmenopausal women.

PRECAUTIONS

Contraindications: Hypersensitivity to zoledronic acid, other bisphosphonates (e.g., alendronate, risedronate). **Reclast only:** CrCl less than 35 mL/min, acute renal impairment, hypocalcemia. **Cautions:** Elderly. **Oncology indications:** History of aspirin-sensitive asthma, mild to moderate renal impairment. **Non-oncology indications:** Pts with disturbances of calcium and mineral metabolism (e.g., hypoparathyroidism, malabsorption syndrome).

ACTION

Inhibits bone resorption by action on osteoclasts. Inhibits osteoclast activity/skeletal calcium release induced by tumors; inhibits osteoclast-mediated resorption. **Therapeutic Effect: Tumor:** Increases urinary calcium, phosphorus excretion; decreases serum calcium, phosphorus levels. **Osteoporosis:** Reduces bone turnover.

⧗ LIFESPAN CONSIDERATIONS

Pregnancy/Lactation: Unknown if drug crosses placenta or is distributed in breast milk. Recommend discontinuation of therapy as early as possible prior to a planned pregnancy. **Children:** Safety and efficacy not established. **Elderly:** Age-related renal impairment may require dosage adjustment.

INTERACTIONS

DRUG: Aminoglycosides (e.g., amikacin, gentamicin), calcitonin may increase concentration/effect. NSAIDs (e.g., diclofenac, meloxicam, naproxen) may increase concentration/effect. **Proton pump inhibitors (e.g., lansoprazole, pantoprazole)** may decrease therapeutic effect. **HERBAL:** None significant. **FOOD:** None known. **LAB VALUES:** May decrease serum magnesium, calcium, phosphate.

AVAILABILITY (Rx)

Injection Solution: 4 mg/5 mL vial, 4 mg/100 mL single-use ready-to-use bottle. 5 mg diluted in 100 mL ready-to-infuse solution.

ADMINISTRATION/HANDLING

◀**ALERT**▶ Pt should be adequately rehydrated before administration of zoledronic acid.

IV (Zometa)
Reconstitution • Dilute 4 mg (vial) in 100 mL 0.9% NaCl or D₅W.
Rate of administration • Infuse over at least 15 min.
Storage • Store unused vials at room temperature. • Infusion of solution must be completed within 24 hrs.

IV (Reclast)
• Infuse over at least 15 min. • Follow infusion with a 10-mL 0.9% NaCl flush of IV line.

🞗 IV INCOMPATIBILITIES

Do not mix with other medications.

INDICATIONS/ROUTES/DOSAGE

Hypercalcemia Malignancy (Zometa)
IV: ADULTS, ELDERLY: 4 mg infused over at least 15 min. Retreatment may be considered, but at least 7 days should elapse to allow for full response to initial dose.

Multiple Myeloma, Osteolytic Lesions, Bone Metastases From Solid Tumors (Zometa)
IV: ADULTS, ELDERLY: 4 mg q3–4wks.

Paget's Disease (Reclast)
IV: ADULTS, ELDERLY: 5 mg as a single dose. (Retreatment): A repeated dose of 5

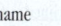 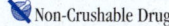

mg may be considered after 12 mos in pts with biochemical relapse (e.g., elevated serum alkaline phosphatase), radiographic progression of disease, or recurrent pain.

Osteoporosis (Fracture Risk Reduction)
IV: ADULTS: *(Reclast):* **(Males/ postmenopausal women): (High risk):** 5 mg once q12mos. **(Low risk):** 5 mg q2yrs.

Treatment/Prevention of Glucocorticoid-Induced Osteoporosis (Reclast)
IV: ADULTS, ELDERLY: 5 mg once yearly.

Dosage in Renal Impairment
(Reclast): **CrCl less than 35 mL/ min:** Contraindicated.
(Zometa): Multiple myeloma, metastatic bone lesions of solid tumors.

Creatinine Clearance	Dosage
50–60 mL/min	3.5 mg
40–49 mL/min	3.3 mg
30–39 mL/min	3 mg
Less than 30 mL/min	Not recommended

(Zometa): Hypercalcemia of malignancy. **Mild to moderate impairment:** No adjustment. **Severe impairment: (SCr greater than 4.5 mg/dL):** Use caution only after considering risk versus benefit.

Dosage in Hepatic Impairment
No dose adjustment.

SIDE EFFECTS
Frequent (44%–26%): Fever, nausea, vomiting, constipation. **Occasional (15%–10%):** Hypotension, anxiety, insomnia, flu-like symptoms (fever, chills, bone pain, myalgia, arthralgia). **Rare:** Conjunctivitis.

ADVERSE EFFECTS/TOXIC REACTIONS
Renal toxicity may occur if IV infusion is administered in less than 15 min.

NURSING CONSIDERATIONS

BASELINE ASSESSMENT
Obtain renal function test; serum calcium, phosphate. Assess hydration status (adequate hydration is essential to reduce renal injury). Obtain dental exam for pts at risk for osteonecrosis.

INTERVENTION/EVALUATION
Monitor renal function; serum calcium, phosphate. Assess vertebral bone mass (document stabilization, improvement). Assess for fever. Monitor food intake, daily pattern of bowel activity, stool consistency. Check I&O, serum BUN, creatinine in pts with renal impairment.

ZOLMitriptan

zole-mi-**trip**-tan
(<u>Zomig</u>, Zomig Rapimelt ✦)
Do not confuse ZOLMitriptan with almotriptan, rizatriptan or SUMAtriptan.

◆ **CLASSIFICATION**
PHARMACOTHERAPEUTIC: Serotonin 5-HT$_1$ receptor agonist. **CLINICAL:** Antimigraine.

USES
Oral: Treatment of acute migraine attack with or without aura in adults. **Nasal:** Treatment of acute migraine with or without aura in adults and children 12 yrs and older. **OFF-LABEL:** Short-term prevention of menstrual migraines. Treatment of cluster headaches.

PRECAUTIONS
Contraindications: Hypersensitivity to ZOLMitriptan. Arrhythmias associated with conduction disorders (e.g., Wolff-Parkinson-White syndrome), basilar or hemiplegic migraine, coronary artery disease, ischemic heart disease (including angina pectoris, history of MI, silent ischemia, Prinzmetal's angina), uncontrolled hypertension, use within 24 hrs of ergotamine-containing preparations

Z

or another serotonin receptor agonist, MAOI used within 14 days. **Additional for nasal spray:** Cerebrovascular syndromes (e.g., stroke), peripheral vascular disease. **Cautions:** Hepatic impairment, cardiovascular risks (e.g., hypertension, hypercholesterolemia, smoking, obesity, diabetes), elderly.

ACTION

Binds selectively to serotonin receptors, producing vasoconstrictive effect and reducing inflammation on cranial blood vessels. **Therapeutic Effect:** Relieves migraine headache.

PHARMACOKINETICS

Widely distributed. Protein binding: 25%. Metabolized in liver. Excreted in urine (60%), feces (30%). **Half-life:** 2.8–3.7 hrs.

⧗ LIFESPAN CONSIDERATIONS

Pregnancy/Lactation: Unknown if drug is distributed in breast milk. **Children:** Safety and efficacy not established in pts younger than 12 yrs. **Elderly:** No age-related precautions noted.

INTERACTIONS

DRUG: May increase concentration/effect of **ergot derivatives** (e.g., **ergotamine**), **MAOIs** (e.g., **phenelzine, selegine**). **Bromocriptine** may increase concentration/effect. **HERBAL:** None significant. **FOOD:** None known. **LAB VALUES:** None significant.

AVAILABILITY (Rx)

Nasal Spray: 2.5 mg, 5 mg. **Tablets:** 2.5 mg, 5 mg.

 Tablets, Orally Disintegrating: 2.5 mg, 5 mg.

ADMINISTRATION/HANDLING

PO
• Give without regard to food. Tablets may be broken in half to achieve a smaller initial dose.

Orally Disintegrating Tablet (ODT)
• Give whole; do not break, crush, cut. • Place on pt's tongue; allow to dissolve. • Not necessary to administer with liquid.

Nasal
• Instruct pt to clear nasal passages as much as possible before use. • With head upright, pt should close one nostril with index finger, breathe out gently through mouth. • Instruct pt to insert nozzle into open nostril about one-half inch, close mouth, and while taking a breath through nose, release spray dosage by firmly pressing plunger. • Have pt remove nozzle from nose, gently breathe in through nose and out through mouth for 5–10 sec. Tell pt to avoid breathing in deeply.

INDICATIONS/ROUTES/DOSAGE

Acute Migraine Attack
PO: ADULTS, ELDERLY, CHILDREN OLDER THAN 18 YRS: Initially, 1.25–2.5 mg (**Maximum:** 5 mg). If headache returns, may repeat dose after 2 hrs. **Maximum:** 10 mg/24 hrs.

Orally disintegrating tablet: ADULTS, ELDERLY: Initially, 2.5 mg (**Maximum:** 5 mg) at onset of migraine headache. If headache returns, may repeat dose after 2 hrs. **Maximum:** 10 mg/24 hrs.

Intranasal: ADULTS, ELDERLY, CHILDREN 12 YRS AND OLDER: Initially, 2.5–5 mg as a single dose (**Maximum:** 5 mg). If headache returns, may repeat dose after 2 hrs. **Maximum:** 5 mg/dose, 10 mg/24 hrs.

Dosage in Renal Impairment
No dose adjustment.

Dosage in Hepatic Impairment
Nasal/ODT: MILD IMPAIRMENT: No dose adjustment. **MODERATE TO SEVERE IMPAIRMENT:** Not recommended. **Tablet: MILD IMPAIRMENT:** No dose adjustment. **MODERATE TO SEVERE IMPAIRMENT:** Initially, 1.25 mg. **Maximum daily dose:** 5 mg in severe impairment.

Z

SIDE EFFECTS

Frequent (8%–6%): PO: Dizziness, paresthesia, neck/throat/jaw pressure, drowsiness. **Nasal:** Altered taste, paresthesia. **Occasional (5%–3%): PO:** Warm/hot sensation, asthenia, chest pressure. **Nasal:** Nausea, drowsiness, nasal discomfort, dizziness, asthenia, dry mouth. **Rare (2%–1%):** Diaphoresis, myalgia.

ADVERSE EFFECTS/TOXIC REACTIONS

Cardiac events (ischemia, coronary artery vasospasm, MI), noncardiac vasospasm-related reactions (hemorrhage, stroke) occur rarely, particularly in pts with hypertension, diabetes, strong family history of coronary artery disease; pts who are obese; smokers; males older than 40 yrs; postmenopausal women.

NURSING CONSIDERATIONS

BASELINE ASSESSMENT

Question for history of peripheral vascular disease, coronary artery disease, renal/hepatic impairment, MAOI use. Question characteristics of migraine headaches (onset, location, duration, possible precipitating symptoms).

INTERVENTION/EVALUATION

Monitor for evidence of dizziness. Monitor B/P, esp. in pts with hepatic impairment. Evaluate for relief of migraine headaches (photophobia, phonophobia, nausea, vomiting, pain, dizziness, fogginess).

PATIENT/FAMILY TEACHING

• Take single dose as soon as symptoms of actual migraine attack appear. • Medication is intended to relieve migraine, not to prevent or reduce number of attacks. • Avoid tasks that require alertness, motor skills until response to drug is established. • Report chest pain; palpitations; tightness in throat; edema of face, lips, eyes; rash; easy bruising; blood in urine or stool; pain or numbness in arms or legs.

zolpidem

zole-**pi**-dem
(Ambien, Ambien CR, Edluar, Sublinox ✦, Zolpimist)
■ **BLACK BOX ALERT** ■ Complex sleep behaviors, including sleep-walking, sleep-driving, and engaging in other activities while not fully awake, may occur. Some of these events may cause serious injuries, including death.
Do not confuse Ambien with Abilify, Ativan, or zolpidem with LORazepam, zaleplon, or Zyloprim.

◆CLASSIFICATION

PHARMACOTHERAPEUTIC: Hypnotic, miscellaneous (Schedule IV). **CLINICAL:** Sedative-hypnotic.

USES

Ambien, Edluar, Zolpimist: Short-term treatment of insomnia (with difficulty of sleep onset). **Ambien CR:** Treatment of insomnia (with difficulty of sleep onset and/or sleep maintenance). **Sublingual (generic):** Treatment of insomnia characterized by middle-of-the-night awakening followed by difficulty returning to sleep in pts with 4 or more hrs of sleep time remaining.

PRECAUTIONS

Contraindications: Hypersensitivity to zolpidem. Pts who experience complex sleep behaviors after use. **Cautions:** Hepatic impairment, obstructive sleep apnea, debilitated, elderly, respiratory disease (e.g., COPD, emphysema), myasthenia gravis, depressive disorders; history of drug abuse and misuse.

ACTION

Enhances action of inhibitory neurotransmitter gamma-aminobutyric acid (GABA). Increases chloride conduction, neuronal hyperpolarization; inhibits action potential and decreases neuronal ex-

Z

citability. **Therapeutic Effect:** Induces sleep with fewer nightly awakenings, improves sleep quality.

PHARMACOKINETICS

Route	Onset	Peak	Duration
PO	30 min	N/A	6–8 hrs

Widely distributed. Protein binding: 92%. Metabolized in liver; excreted in urine. Not removed by hemodialysis. **Half-life:** 1.4–4.5 hrs (increased in hepatic impairment).

⏳ LIFESPAN CONSIDERATIONS

Pregnancy/Lactation: Drug crosses placenta and is distributed in breast milk. **Children:** Safety and efficacy not established. **Elderly:** More likely to experience falls or confusion; decreased initial doses recommended. Age-related hepatic impairment may require dosage adjustment.

INTERACTIONS

DRUG: Alcohol, CNS depressants (e.g., gabapentin, LORazepam, morphine) may increase CNS depression. **Strong CYP3A4 inducers (e.g., carBAMazepine, phenytoin, rifAMPin)** may decrease concentration/effect. **Strong CYP3A4 inhibitors (e.g., clarithromycin, ketoconazole)** may increase concentration/effect. **HERBAL:** Herbals with sedative properties (e.g., chamomile, kava kava, valerian) may increase CNS depression. **FOOD:** None known. **LAB VALUES:** None significant.

AVAILABILITY (Rx)

Capsules: 7.5 mg. **Oral Solution:** 5 mg/actuation. **Tablets:** 5 mg, 10 mg. **Tablets, Sublingual:** 1.75 mg, 3.5 mg, 5 mg, 10 mg. 🔷 **Tablets, Extended-Release:** 6.25 mg, 12.5 mg.

ADMINISTRATION/HANDLING

PO

• For faster sleep onset, do not give with or immediately after a meal. • Give extended-release tablets whole; do not break, crush, dissolve, or divide. • Ed-

luar sublingual tablets to be placed under tongue and allowed to disintegrate. Do not give with water or allow pt to swallow tablet. • Spray Zolpimist directly into mouth over tongue.

INDICATIONS/ROUTES/DOSAGE

Note: Dosage adjustment is recommended for female pts.

Sleep-Onset Insomnia

PO: *(Tablet [Immediate-Release], Spray, Sublingual Tablet):* **ADULTS:** 5–10 mg (males), 5 mg (females) immediately before bedtime. **ELDERLY, DEBILITATED:** 5 mg immediately before bedtime. **PO:** *(Extended-Release):* **ADULTS:** 6.25–12.5 mg (males), 6.25 mg (females) immediately before bedtime. **ELDERLY, DEBILITATED:** 6.25 mg immediately before bedtime.

Sleep Maintenance Insomnia (Awakening With 4 Hrs of Planned Sleep)

PO: ADULTS: *(Sublingual):* 3.5 mg (males), 1.75 mg (females), taken once in middle of night with 4 or more hrs of expected sleep.

Dosage in Renal Impairment

No dose adjustment.

Dosage in Hepatic Impairment

Mild to moderate impairment: *(Immediate-Release Tablet, Spray, Sublingual Tablet):* 5 mg. *(Extended-Release Tablet):* 6.25 mg. *(Intermezzo):* 1.75 mg. **Severe impairment:** Avoid use.

SIDE EFFECTS

Occasional (7%): Headache, change in appetite. **Rare (less than 2%):** Dizziness, nausea, diarrhea, muscle pain, sleepwalking.

ADVERSE EFFECTS/TOXIC REACTIONS

Overdose may produce severe ataxia (clumsiness, unsteadiness), bradycardia, diplopia, severe drowsiness, nausea, vomiting, difficulty breathing, unconsciousness. Abrupt withdrawal following long-term use

Z

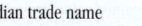 ✦ Canadian trade name   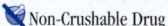 Non-Crushable Drug   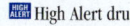 High Alert drug

may produce weakness, facial flushing, diaphoresis, vomiting, tremor. Drug tolerance/dependence may occur with prolonged use. May cause amnesic events that include cooking, sleepwalking, sexual activity, driving.

NURSING CONSIDERATIONS

BASELINE ASSESSMENT

Assess vital signs, mental status, sleep patterns. Raise bed rails, provide call light. Provide environment conducive to sleep (back rub, quiet environment, low lighting). Do not give unless a full night of sleep is planned. Initiate fall precautions.

INTERVENTION/EVALUATION

Monitor sleep pattern. Evaluate for therapeutic response to insomnia: Decrease in number of nocturnal awakenings, increase in length of sleep. Monitor daytime alertness, respiratory rate, behavior profile.

PATIENT/FAMILY TEACHING

• Do not abruptly discontinue medication after long-term use. • Avoid alcohol and tasks that require alertness, motor skills until response to drug is established. • Tolerance, dependence may occur with prolonged use. • Do not break, chew, crush, dissolve, or divide extended-release tablets; swallow whole. • Therapy may need to be discontinued if cooking, driving, sleepwalking occurs without recollection. • Do not take unless a full 8 hrs of sleep is planned.

---

zonisamide

zoe-**nis**-a-mide
(Zonegran, Zonisade)
Do not confuse zonisamide with lacosamide.

◆ CLASSIFICATION

PHARMACOTHERAPEUTIC: Anticonvulsant, miscellaneous. **CLINICAL:** Anticonvulsant.

USES

Adjunctive therapy in treatment of focal (partial) onset seizures in adults and pts 16 yrs and older. **OFF-LABEL:** Binge eating disorder.

PRECAUTIONS

Contraindications: Hypersensitivity to zonisamide. Allergy to sulfonamides. **Cautions:** Renal/hepatic impairment, metabolic acidosis (e.g., severe respiratory disease); history of suicidal ideation and behavior.

ACTION

May stabilize neuronal membranes, suppress neuronal hypersynchronization by blocking sodium, calcium channels. **Therapeutic Effect:** Reduces seizure activity.

PHARMACOKINETICS

Widely distributed. Metabolized in liver. Extensively bound to RBCs. Protein binding: 40%. Primarily excreted in urine. **Half-life:** 63 hrs (plasma), 105 hrs (RBCs).

⧗ LIFESPAN CONSIDERATIONS

Pregnancy/Lactation: Crosses placenta. Unknown if distributed in breast milk. **Children:** Safety and efficacy not established in pts younger than 16 yrs. **Elderly:** No age-related precautions noted, but lower dosages recommended.

INTERACTIONS

DRUG: Alcohol, CNS depressants (e.g., **LORazepam, morphine, zolpidem**) may increase sedative effect. **Strong CYP3A4 inducers** (e.g., **carBAMazepine, phenytoin, rifAMPin**) may increase metabolism, decrease effect. **HERBAL: Herbals with sedative** properties (e.g., **chamomile, kava kava, valerian**) may increase CNS depression. **FOOD:** None known. **LAB VALUES:** May increase serum BUN, creatinine.

AVAILABILITY (Rx)

Oral Suspension: 100 mg/5 mL.

🖫 **Capsules:** 25 mg, 50 mg, 100 mg.

ADMINISTRATION/HANDLING

PO
• Give without regard to food. • Give capsules whole; do not break, cut, or crush. Shake suspension well before every administration. • Do not give to pts allergic to sulfonamides.

INDICATIONS/ROUTES/DOSAGE

Note: Do not use if CrCl is less than 50 mL/min. Discontinue gradually to minimize the potential of increased seizure activity and withdrawal symptoms.

Focal (Partial) Onset Seizures
PO: ADULTS, ELDERLY, CHILDREN 16 YRS AND OLDER: Initially, 100 mg/day in 1 or 2 divided doses. Based on clinical response and tolerability, may increase by 100 mg daily q2wks to 400 mg daily. **Maximum:** 600 mg/day.

Dosage in Renal Impairment
Not recommended with CrCl less than 50 mL/min.

Dosage in Hepatic Impairment
Use with caution.

SIDE EFFECTS

Frequent (17%–9%): Drowsiness, dizziness, anorexia, headache, agitation, irritability, nausea. **Occasional (8%–5%):** Fatigue, ataxia, confusion, depression, impaired memory/concentration, insomnia, abdominal pain, diplopia, diarrhea, speech difficulty. **Rare (4%–3%):** Paresthesia, nystagmus, anxiety, rash, dyspepsia, weight loss.

ADVERSE EFFECTS/TOXIC REACTIONS

Overdose characterized by bradycardia, hypotension, respiratory depression, coma. Leukopenia, anemia, thrombocytopenia occur rarely.

NURSING CONSIDERATIONS

BASELINE ASSESSMENT
Review history of seizure disorder (intensity, frequency, duration, level of consciousness). Initiate seizure precautions. CBC, LFT should be performed before therapy begins and periodically during therapy.

INTERVENTION/EVALUATION
Observe frequently for recurrence of seizure activity. Assess for clinical improvement (decrease in intensity, frequency of seizures). Assist with ambulation if dizziness occurs.

PATIENT/FAMILY TEACHING
• Strict maintenance of drug therapy is essential for seizure control. • Avoid tasks that require alertness, motor skills until response to drug is established. • Avoid alcohol. • Report if rash, back/abdominal pain, blood in urine, fever, sore throat, ulcers in mouth, easy bruising occur. • Seek immediate medical attention if thoughts of suicide, new onset or worsening of anxiety, depression, or changes in mood occur.

Z

CORRECT USE OF ORAL INHALERS FOR ASTHMA AND COPD

An **inhaler** is a medical device used for delivering medication into the lungs through the work of a person's breathing. There are a wide variety of inhalers, and they are primarily used in the treatment of asthma and COPD.

Common types of inhalers include metered-dose inhalers (MDI), dry powder inhalers, and soft mist inhalers. The various inhalation devices for asthma and COPD are likely to be equally effective in delivering medication to the lungs when used correctly. Choosing an inhaler should be based on the pt's ability to use it properly (e.g., cognition, dexterity, strength), pt preference, and cost of inhaler.

Metered-dose inhalers (MDIs) consist of a pressurized canister containing medication that fits into a boot-shaped plastic mouthpiece. MDIs usually require good hand-breath coordination (although the use of a spacer may help with this). A spacer is a device that is placed on the mouthpiece of the inhaler, allowing the medicine to break into smaller droplets, which can move easier and deeper into the lungs. The purpose of a spacer is to hold medication in a tube between the inhaler and mouth after release and to improve inhaled medication delivery to the lungs, which decreases potential side effects (e.g., candidiasis [thrush] and dysphonia [hoarseness]). A valved holding chamber (VHC) spacer is a one-way valve at the mouthpiece that traps and holds the medicine. This helps regulate the flow of medication, allowing the pt to take a slow, deep breath. Many VHC spacers are lined with an antistatic coating, which helps keep medication from sticking to the sides of the chamber.

Dry powder Inhalers do not require a propellant, but usually contain a chamber in which the powdered medication is deposited prior to each dosage. The powder can then be inhaled by breathing a deep, fast breath. These inhalers require less hand-breath coordination than MDIs but require adequate strength of inhalation (e.g., difficult for very young children). There are multiple-dose devices that hold more than 1 dose and single-dose devices, which are filled with a capsule prior to each treatment.

Soft mist inhalers (SMIs) release a light mist containing medication without the need for a propellant/suspension. Upon pressing a button, the inhaler creates a mist of medication, allowing for inhalation into the lungs. This inhaler requires less coordination when using and may be helpful for young patients or patients who have difficulty with MDI inhalers.

Smart inhalers will automatically update an application (program) with information that includes the time of day, air quality, and number of uses through device sensor technology. This information is sent via Bluetooth to a mobile device app and is later shared with the pt's physician to determine what kind of things can trigger issues with asthma and other problems.

METERED-DOSE INHALERS (MDIs)

General Instructions	Products
• Prime inhaler before use (if needed). • Shake inhaler for 10 seconds. • If using a spacer, attach the spacer to the inhaler. • Exhale fully, away from the inhaler. • Close lips around the mouthpiece of the inhaler or, if using a spacer, around the spacer. • Press the canister down and inhale deeply and slowly through the mouth at the same time. • Remove the inhaler (or spacer) from the mouth. • Hold breath for about 10 sec or as long as comfortable. • Wait about 60 sec before administering another inhalation of medicine. • Rinse with water and spit it out.	Advair HFA (fluticasone/salmeterol)
	Aerospan (flunisolide)
	Alvesco (ciclesonide)
	Asmanex HFA (mometasone)
	Atrovent HFA (ipratropium)
	Bevespi Aerosphere (glycopyrrolate/formoterol)
	Breztri Aerosphere (glycopyrrolate/formoterol/budesonide)
	Dulera (mometasone/formoterol)
	Flovent HFA (fluticasone propionate)
	ProAir HFA (albuterol)
	Proventil HFA (albuterol)
	Symbicort (budesonide/formoterol)
	Ventolin HFA (albuterol)
	Xopenex HFA (levalbuterol)

METERED DOSE INHALER (MDI), BREATH-ACTUATED: REDIHALER

General Instructions	Products
• Hold inhaler upright and open cap. • Exhale fully, away from mouthpiece. • Close lips around mouthpiece. • Breathe in deeply. • Remove inhaler and hold breath for 10 sec. • Exhale slowly, away from the inhaler. • Click the cap closed to prep inhaler for next inhalation. • Cap must be closed before each inhalation or dose will not be delivered. If the cap remains open for more than 2 min, or it is left in the open position, close the cap before use. • Rinse with water and spit it out.	Qvar RediHaler (beclomethasone dipropionate)

SOFT-MIST INHALER: RESPIMAT

General Instructions	Products
• Prime inhaler by turning the base in direction of arrows, opening the cap and pressing the button. Do this 3 times or until a mist comes out of the mouthpiece. No need to prime inhaler again. • Put mouthpiece in the mouth and tighten lips around the end without covering the air vents. • While inhaling deeply and steady through the mouth, press the dose release button. • Hold breath for 10 sec, then breathe out slowly. • Close cap of the inhaler.	Combivent Respimat (albuterol/ipratropium)
	Spiriva Respimat (tiotropium)
	Stiolto Respimat (tiotropium/olodaterol)
	Striverdi Respimat (olodaterol)

DRY-POWDER INHALER (DPI): DIGIHALER

General Instructions	Products
• Hold upright and open the cap fully until it clicks (this prepares the dose). • Exhale fully, away from the mouthpiece. • Put mouthpiece in the mouth and tighten lips around it. • Do not the block air vents with fingers or lips. • Breathe in quickly and deeply through the mouth. • Remove inhaler from mouth and hold breath for 10 sec. • Close cap firmly over the mouthpiece. • Rinse with water and spit it out.	AirDuo Digihaler (fluticasone/salmeterol)
	Armonair Digihaler (fluticasone)
	Proair Digihaler (albuterol)

DRY-POWDER INHALER (DPI): DISKUS

General Instructions	Products
• Open inhaler with thumb grip, pushing it away until mouthpiece shows and snaps into place. • Hold inhaler flat and level with mouthpiece toward you and slide the lever away from the mouthpiece until it clicks. • Breathe out fully through the mouth, away from the inhaler. • Put the mouthpiece in the mouth and tighten the lips around it. • Breathe in quickly and deeply through the mouth. • Remove device from the mouth and hold breath for 10 sec, then breathe out slowly. • Close inhaler by sliding the thumb grip until it clicks, covering the mouthpiece. • Rinse with water and spit it out.	Advair Diskus (fluticasone/salmeterol) Flovent Diskus (fluticasone) Serevent Diskus (salmeterol)

DRY-POWDER INHALER (DPI): ELLIPTA

General Instructions	Products
• Slide inhaler cover down to reveal mouthpiece. • Breathe out fully through the mouth, away from the inhaler. • Put mouthpiece between lips and close mouth firmly around it. Do not block the air vents with fingers. • Breathe in quickly and deeply through the mouth. • Remove inhaler from the mouth and hold breath for 5 sec. • Breathe out slowly and gently. • Close inhaler by sliding cover up and over the mouthpiece. • Rinse with water and spit it out.	Anoro Ellipta (umeclidinium/vilanterol) Arnuity Ellipta (fluticasone) Breo Ellipta (fluticasone/vilanterol) Incruse Ellipta (umeclidinium) Trelegy Ellipta (fluticasone/umeclidinium/vilanterol)

DRY-POWDER INHALER (DPI): FLEXHALER

General Instructions	Products
• Hold inhaler upright and remove cap. • Holding the inhaler in the middle, twist the grip as far as it will go in one direction, then back in the other direction until it clicks. • Breathe out fully through the mouth, away from the inhaler. • Put mouthpiece in the mouth and tighten lips around it. • Breathe in rapidly and deeply through the mouth and hold breath for 10 sec. • Remove the inhaler from the mouth and exhale slowly. • Rinse with water and spit it out.	Pulmicort Flexhaler (budesonide)

DRY-POWDER INHALER (DPI): PRESSAIR

General Instructions	Products
• Remove protective cap and hold inhaler with mouthpiece facing the mouth and button on the top. • Press button all the way down (to load dose) and release. If the control window does not turn green, then repeat. • Breathe out completely through the mouth, away from the inhaler. • Place mouthpiece in the mouth, tighten lips around it, and take a strong, deep breath through the mouth, until the lungs are filled. • Remove inhaler from the mouth and hold breath for as long as is comfortably possible. • Make sure the control window is now red (means inhalation was done correctly).	Duaklir Pressair (aclidinium bromide/formoterol fumarate) Tudorza Pressair (aclidinium bromide)

DRY-POWDER INHALER (DPI): RESPICLICK

General Instructions	Products
• Hold inhaler upright and open the cap fully, until it clicks.	AirDuo RespiClick (fluticasone/salmeterol)
• Breathe out completely through the mouth, away from the inhaler.	ProAir RespiClick (albuterol)
• Place the mouthpiece in the mouth and tighten lips around it. Do not block the vent above the mouthpiece.	
• Breathe in quickly and deeply through the mouth, until the lungs are filled.	
• Remove inhaler from the mouth and hold breath for 10 sec.	
• Rinse with water and spit it out.	

DRY-POWDER INHALER (DPI): TWISTHALER

General Instructions	Products
• Hold inhaler upright and remove the cap by twisting it in a counterclockwise direction.	Asmanex Twisthaler (mometasone)
• Breathe out fully through the mouth, away from the inhaler.	
• Place the mouthpiece in the mouth and tighten lips around it, holding the inhaler horizontally.	
• Do not cover the ventilation holes; take a fast, deep breath through the mouth.	
• Remove inhaler from the mouth and hold breath for 10 sec.	
• Replace the cap, turning it in a clockwise direction and gently press it down until a click is heard.	
• Rinse with water and spit it out.	

WOUND CARE

A wound is any process that disrupts the normal structure and function of tissues. Wounds can be closed (e.g., bruise, sprain, deep tissue injury) or open (e.g., abrasion, surgical wound). The most common chronic wounds are nonhealing surgical wounds, pressure ulcers, diabetic foot ulcers, and venous ulcers.

COMMON TYPES OF WOUNDS

Skin tears: Caused by mechanical forces such as shear, friction, or blunt force. Usually occurs in the fragile, nonelastic skin of older adults (e.g., can be caused by the simple mechanical force used to remove a bandage or from friction as the skin brushes against a surface). Skin tears occur in the epidermis and dermis but do not extend through the subcutaneous layer.

Venous ulcers: Caused by lack of blood return to the heart, leading to pooling of fluid in the veins of the lower legs. Usually occurs on the medial lower leg and has irregular edges due to maceration.

Arterial ulcers: Caused by lack of blood flow and oxygenation to tissues. Usually occurs in the distal areas of the body (e.g., feet, heels, and toes).

Diabetic ulcers: Commonly present in pts with diabetes. Usually develops on the plantar aspect of the feet and toes of a pt with diabetes due to lack of sensation of the pressure or injury.

Pressure injuries: Localized damage to the skin or underlying soft tissue, usually over a bony prominence, as a result of intense and prolonged pressure in combination with shear. Factors putting a pt at risk for developing pressure injuries include nutrition, mobility, sensation, and moisture. Pressure injuries commonly occur on the sacrum, heels, ischial tuberosity, and coccyx. Pressure injuries are staged from 1 to 4 based on the extent of tissue damage.

Stage 1: Intact skin with a localized area of nonblanched erythema where prolonged pressure has occurred.

Stage 2: Partial-thickness loss of skin with exposed dermis. The wound may appear like an intact or ruptured blister. Stage 2 pressure injuries heal by re-epithelialization.

Stage 3 Full-thickness tissue loss in which fat is visible, but cartilage, tendon, ligament, muscle, and bone are not exposed. The depth of tissue damage varies by anatomic location.

Stage 4: Full-thickness tissue loss and also exposed cartilage, tendon, ligament, muscle, or bone. Osteomyelitis (bone infection) may be present.

WOUND HEALING

Wound healing is a complex process resulting in restored cell structure and tissue layers after an injury. When skin is damaged, it begins to heal from the bottom layer up and from the outside inward. Wound healing involves cellular, physiologic, biochemical, and molecular processes. They are interdependent and overlapping. An acute wound usually heals within several wks, whereas chronic wounds take 6 wks or longer to heal. Additionally, other factors can delay the healing process. These include trauma/edema, infection, necrosis, lack of oxygen delivery to the tissues, advanced age, obesity, chronic diseases (e.g., diabetes, anemia), vascular insufficiency, immobility, pressure necrosis, and immunodeficiency.

WOUND HEALING

Hemostasis (blood clotting): Immediately after the injury, blood vessels constrict, and clotting factors are activated. Within the first few minutes of injury, platelets in the blood begin to stick to the injured site, changing into a shape more suitable for clotting, and release chemical signals to promote clotting. This results in the activation of fibrin, which forms a mesh and acts as a "glue" to bind platelets to each other. The clot plugs the break in the blood vessel, slowing and preventing further bleeding.

Inflammation: Vasodilation occurs that allows white blood cells to move into the wound. Damaged and dead cells are cleared out, along with bacteria and other pathogens or debris. This happens through the process of phagocytosis (white blood cells engulf debris and destroy it). Platelet-derived growth factors are released into the wound causing the migration and division of cells during the proliferative phase. The inflammatory process appears as edema, erythema, and exudate.

Proliferation (growth of new tissue): Includes epithelialization, angiogenesis, collagen formation, and wound contraction. **Epithelialization** is the development of new epidermis and granulation tissue. Granulation tissue is new connective tissue with new, fragile, thin-walled capillaries. **Angiogenesis** is the process of vascular endothelial cells forming new blood vessels. Capillaries begin to develop within the wound 24 hrs after injury. **Collagen formation** provides strength and integrity to the wound. **Wound contraction**, initiated by myofibroblasts, decreases the size of the wound by gripping the wound edges and contracting using a mechanism that resembles that in smooth muscle cells.

Maturation phase (remodeling): During maturation and remodeling, collagen continues to be created to strengthen the wound and prevent it from reopening.

WOUND DRESSINGS

Dressings play a major role in wound management. They protect the wound, keeping it moist, and thus promote healing (only diabetic, dry, gangrenous toes require a moisture-free environment for effective healing).

Hydrocolloid, hydrogel, film, and foam dressing can handle large amounts of exudate and promote auto-debridement. Alginate and collagen-based dressings promote granulation of tissue. Silver and iodine dressings are used to avoid infections, which may delay wound healing.

WOUND CARE PRODUCTS

Description	General Uses	Comments
Alginate dressings: Spun fibers of brown seaweed that act as ion exchange mechanisms to absorb serous fluid or exudate, forming a gel-like covering that conforms to the shape of the wound.	Full-thickness burns, surgical wounds, split-thickness graft donor sites, refractory decubitis, chronic ulcers.	Can be left in place until soaked with exudate. Do not moisten prior to use. Nonadhesive, nonocclusive; not recommended for dry or minimally exudative wounds.

Continued

Description	General Uses	Comments
Collagenase ointment: Sterile enzymatic débriding ointment that possesses the ability to digest collagen in necrotic tissue. **Products:** Santyl.	Débriding chronic dermal ulcers and severely burned areas	May apply directly to the wound or to a sterile gauze pad, which is then applied to the wound and properly secured. Discontinue when granulation tissue is well established. Optimal pH for enzymatic action is 6–8. Avoid acidic agents for cleansing; avoid detergents and agents containing heavy metal (e.g., mercury or silver), which may adversely affect enzymatic activity.
Trypsin, castor oil, Peru balsam: Trypsin is a mild débriding agent that helps shed damaged skin cells. **Castor oil** acts as a lubricant to protect tissue. **Peru balsam** increases blood flow to a wound area, reduces wound odor.	Promotes healing/ treatment of decubitus ulcers, varicose ulcer, and dehiscent wounds.	Promotes healing and relieves pain caused by bed sores and other skin ulcers.
Hydrophilic polyurethane foam: Also called open cell foam dressings. Sheets of foamed solutions of polymers containing variably sized open cells that can hold wound exudate away from wound bed. Maintains moist wound environment.	Wounds with at least a moderate amount of exudate, including abrasions, incisions, lacerations, pressure ulcers, infected wounds, draining peristomal wounds.	For partial- or full-thickness wounds having moderate or more drainage. Not recommended for wounds with little to no exudate or when tunneling is present. Good for cavitating wounds. Highly absorbent, semiocclusive dressing.
Hydrocolloids: Active surface of the dressing is coated with a cross-linked adhesive mass containing a dispersion of gelatin, pectin, and carboxymethyl cellulose together with other polymers that form a flexible wafer. Absorbs water and swells, forming a gel. Moist conditions produced under the dressing promote fibrinolysis, angiogenesis, and wound healing.	Minimal to moderate exudate in partial and full thickness wounds. Cuts and abrasions. First- and second-degree burns. Pressure ulcers. Stasis ulcers.	Not for wounds producing heavy exudate, infected wounds, dry eschar-covered wounds. May provide pain relief. Good for chronic wounds that are epithelializing. Can be left in place for up to 7 days. Can shower while wearing.

Description	General Uses	Comments
Hydrogels: Glycerin- or water-based dressings designed to hydrate the wound (promotes autolytic debridement or provides for a moist wound healing promoting granulation and epithelialization). May absorb small amounts of exudate.	Partial and full thickness wounds. Dry to minimal exudate. Cuts and abrasions. First- and second-degree burns. Pressure ulcers. Stasis ulcers.	Not for wounds producing moderate to heavy exudate. May provide pain relief. Good for wounds that are debriding. Good for keeping a dry wound moist. Can be left in place for 1–3 days.
Iodine compounds: Cadexomer iodine: Iodine is complexed with a polymeric cadexomer starch vehicle, forming a topical gel or paste. The cadexomer moiety absorbs exudate and debris and releases iodine for antimicrobial activity.	Chronic nonhealing, exuding wounds including pressure or leg ulcers and exuding, infected wounds.	Requires use of a secondary dressing. Contraindicated in pts with iodine sensitivity, Hashimoto's thyroiditis, nontoxic nodular goiter, children. Dressing to be changed when it turns white, indicating that the iodine has been depleted. Do not use on dry necrotic tissue.
Silver compounds Silver sulfadiazine cream: Silver possesses bactericidal properties. Has been shown to reduce bacterial density, vascular margination, migration of inflammatory cells. Enhances rate of re-epithelialization.	Prevent infection in second- and third-degree burns. Prevent or treat infection in chronic wounds.	May have cytotoxic effects that could delay wound healing. Allergic reactions may occur. Avoid use with collagenase- or trypsin-containing debriding agents.
Film dressings: Polyurethane sheets coated on one side with an adhesive that is inactivated by moisture and will not adhere to a moist surface such as the wound bed. Have no absorbent capacity and are impermeable to fluids and bacteria but are semipermeable to oxygen and water vapor.	Superficial wounds with minimal or no exudate. Wounds on elbows, heels, or flat surfaces; covering of blisters; and retention of primary dressing. Minor burns, lacerations, stage I and II pressure ulcers.	Prevents wound desiccation and contamination by bacteria. Not recommended for use on wounds with moderate to heavy exudate. Promotes autolysis of necrotic tissue in the wound; maintains moist environment. Avoid in arterial ulcers and infected wounds requiring frequent monitoring. Do not use as primary dressing on wounds with depth or tunneling. May provide pain relief. Usually changed up to 3 times/wk.

Continued

Description	General Uses	Comments
Becaplermin gel: Recombinant formulation of platelet-derived growth factor that promotes cell mitogenesis and proliferation of cells involved in wound repair. Enhances formation of granulation tissue. **Products:** Regranex.	Diabetic foot ulcers that extend into subcutaneous tissue or beyond and have an adequate blood supply.	Usually applied daily. Adequate blood supply and absence of necrotic tissue are needed for efficacy. Repeated use (3 or more tubes) may increase risk of cancer-related death. Use cautiously in pts with known malignancy.

Appendix C

DRUGS OF ABUSE

Substance	Brand/Street Names	Administered	Comments
Amphet-amines	*Adderall, Dexedrine, Vyvanse, Desoxyn.* Bennies, Black Beauties, Crank, Ice, Speed, Uppers	Oral Injection Smoking	Psychosis (paranoia, picking at the skin, preoccupation with one's own thoughts, auditory and visual hallucinations) Increased BP and HR, insomnia, loss of appetite, physical exhaustion **Overdose:** Agitation, increased body temperature, hallucinations, convulsions, possible death
Barbiturates	*Amytal, Seconal.* Barbs, Block Busters, Christmas Trees, Goof Balls, Pinks, Red Devils, Reds and Blues, Yellow Jackets	Oral Injection	Mild euphoria, lack of restraint, relief of anxiety, sleepiness, impairment of memory, judgment, and coordination; irritability, paranoid and suicidal ideation **Overdose:** CNS depression, decreased respiration, increased HR, decreased BP, decreased urine production, decreased body temperature, coma, possible death
Benzodiaze-pines	*Ativan, Klonopin, Valium, Xanax.* Benzos, Downers, Xannies.	Oral Snort	Amnesia, hostility, irritability, vivid or disturbing dreams. **Overdose:** Extreme drowsiness, confusion, impaired coordination, decreased reflexes, respiratory depression, coma, possible death

Continued

Substance	Brand/Street Names	Administered	Comments
Cocaine	Blow, Coca, Coke, Crack, Flake, Snow, Soda Cot	Snort Injection Smoking	Euphoria, increased alertness and excitation, restlessness, irritability, anxiety, increased BP and HR, dilated pupils, insomnia, loss of appetite **Overdose:** Irregular heartbeat, ischemic heart conditions, sudden cardiac arrest, palpitations, convulsions, stroke, death
Dextromethorphan	Found in some cough and cold medications. Poor man's PCP, velvet, Robo, Triple C	Oral	Impaired motor, function, feeling of being separated from one's body and environment, euphoria, slurred speech, confusion, dizziness, distorted visual perceptions
Fentanyl	*Duragesic.* Apache, China Girl, China Town, Dance Fever, Friend, Goodfellas, Great Bear, He-Man, Jackpot, King Ivory, Murder 8, Tango and Cash.	Injection Snort Smoking Oral Spiked onto blotter paper.	Relaxation, euphoria, pain relief, sedation, confusion, drowsiness, dizziness, nausea, vomiting, urinary retention, pupillary constriction, respiratory depression **Overdose:** Stupor, changes in pupillary size, cold and clammy skin, cyanosis, coma, respiratory failure leading to death
Flunitrazepam	*Rohypnol.* Circles, Forget Pill, Forget-Me-Pill, La Rocha, Lunch Money Drug, Pingus, R2, Reynolds, Roach, Roach 2, Roaches, Roachies, Roapies, Robutal, Rochas Dos, Rohypnol, Roofies, Rophies, Ropies, Roples, Row-Shay, Ruffies, Wolfies	Oral Snort	Drowsiness, sleep, decreased anxiety, amnesia (no memory of events while under the influence of the substance), increased or decreased reaction time, impaired mental functioning and judgment, confusion, aggression, excitability, slurred speech, loss of motor coordination, weakness, headache, respiratory depression **Overdose:** Severe sedation, unconsciousness, slow HR, suppression of respiration

Substance	Brand/Street Names	Administered	Comments
GHB	Easy Lay, G, Georgia Home Boy, GHB, Goop, Grievous Bodily Harm, Liquid Ecstasy, Liquid X, Scoop	Oral	Euphoria, drowsiness, decreased anxiety, confusion, memory impairment, unconsciousness, seizures, slowed HR, greatly slowed breathing, lower body temperature, vomiting, nausea **Overdose:** Coma, death
Heroin	Big H, Black Tar, China, Hell Dust, Horse, Negra, Smack, Thunder	Injection Snort Smoking	Feeling a surge of euphoria or "rush" followed by a twilight state of sleep and wakefulness, drowsiness, respiratory depression, constricted pupils, nausea, warm flushing of the skin, dry mouth, heavy extremities **Overdose:** Slow and shallow breathing, blue lips and fingernails, clammy skin, convulsions, coma, possible death
Hydromor-phone	D, Dillies, Dust, Footballs, Juice, Smack	Oral Injection	Feelings of euphoria, relaxation, sedation, reduced anxiety, constipation, pupillary constriction, urinary retention, nausea, vomiting, respiratory depression, dizziness, impaired coordination, loss of appetite, rash, slow or rapid heartbeat, and changes in BP **Overdose:** Severe respiratory depression, drowsiness progressing to stupor or coma, lack of skeletal muscle tone, cold and clammy skin, constricted pupils, reduction in BP and HR

Continued

Substance	Brand/Street Names	Administered	Comments
Inhalants	Gluey, Huff, Rush, Whippets	Inhaling	Cognitive abnormalities (mild impairment to severe dementia), slurred speech, inability to coordinate movements, euphoria, dizziness, weight loss, muscle weakness, disorientation, inattentiveness, lack of coordination, irritability, depression, damage to the nervous system **Overdose:** Loss of consciousness and/or death
Ketamine	Cat Tranquilizer, Cat Valium, Jet K, Kit Kat, Purple, Special K, Special La Coke, Super Acid, Super K, Vitamin K	Injection Snort Smoking	Hallucinations, distorts perceptions of sight and sound, makes the user feel disconnected and not in control, increase BP and HR, involuntarily rapid eye movement, dilated pupils, salivation, tear secretions, stiffening of the muscles **Overdose:** Unconsciousness, dangerously slowed breathing
LSD	Acid, Dots, Mellow Yellow, Window Pane	Oral	Dilated pupils, higher body temperature, increased heart rate and blood pressure, sweating, loss of appetite, sleeplessness, dry mouth, tremors, extreme changes in mood, impaired depth and time perception accompanied by distorted perception of the shape and size of objects, movements, colors, sound, touch, and the user's own body image **Overdose:** Intense "trip" episodes, psychosis, possible death

Substance	Brand/Street Names	Administered	Comments
Marijuana	Aunt Mary, BC Bud, Blunts, Boom, Chronic, Dope, Gangster, Ganja, Grass, Hash, Herb, Hydro, Indo, Joint, Kif, Mary Jane, Mota, Pot, Reefer, Sinsemilla, Skunk, Smoke, Weed, Yerba Vaping: E-cigs, e-hookahs, mods, vape pens, vapes, tank systems, Juuls, Juuling	Smoking	Problems with memory and learning, distorted perception, difficulty in thinking and problem-solving, loss of coordination, sedation, bloodshot eyes, increased heart rate, coughing from lung irritation, increased appetite, and increased BP **Overdose:** No deaths reported
MDMA/(ecstasy)	Adam, Beans, Clarity, Disco Biscuit, E, Ecstasy, Eve, Go, Hug Drug, Lover's Speed, MDMA, Peace, STP, X, XTC, Molly	Oral	Euphoria, feelings of closeness, empathy, sexuality, confusion, anxiety, depression, paranoia, sleep problems, drug craving, muscle tension, tremors, involuntary teeth clenching, muscle cramps, nausea, faintness, chills, sweating, blurred vision **Overdose:** Hyperthermia; liver, kidney, cardiovascular system failure; death
Mescaline	Buttons, Cactus, Mesc, Peyoto	Oral Smoking	Intense nausea, vomiting, dilation of the pupils, increased HR and BP, rise in body temperature (causes heavy perspiration), headaches, muscle weakness, impaired motor coordination, illusions, hallucinations, altered perception of space and time, altered body image **Overdose:** No deaths reported

Continued

Substance	*Brand*/Street Names	Administered	Comments
Methadone	Amidone, Chocolate Chip Cookies, Fizzies with MDMA, Wafer	Oral Injection	Psychological dependence, sweating, itchy skin, sleepiness, withdrawal symptoms (anxiety, muscle tremors, nausea, diarrhea, vomiting, abdominal cramps) **Overdose:** Slow/shallow breathing, blue fingernails and lips, stomach spasms, clammy skin, convulsions, weak pulse, coma, possible death
Methamphetamine	*Desoxyn.* Batu, Bikers Coffee, Black Beauties, Chalk, Chicken Feed, Crank, Crystal, Glass, Go-Fast, Hiropon, Ice, Meth, Methlies Quick, Poor Man's Cocaine, Shabu, Shards, Speed, Stove Top, Tina, Trash, Tweak, Uppers, Ventana, Vidrio, Yaba, Yellow Bam	Oral Injection Snort Smoking	Violent behavior, anxiety, confusion, insomnia, psychotic features (e.g., paranoia, aggression, visual/auditory hallucinations, mood disturbances, delusions), increased wakefulness, increased physical activity, decreased appetite, rapid breathing and HR, irregular heartbeat, increased BP, hyperthermia **Overdose:** Death from stroke, heart attack, or multiple organ problems
Morphine	*MS-Contin, Oramorph SR, MSIR, Roxanol, Kadian, RMS.* Dreamer, Emsel, First Line, God's Drug, Hows, M.S., Mister Blue, Morf, Morpho, Unkie	Oral Injection	Euphoria, relief of pain, decrease in hunger, inhibition of cough reflex **Overdose:** Cold and clammy skin, lowered BP, sleepiness, slowed breathing, slow pulse rate, coma, possible death

Substance	Brand/Street Names	Administered	Comments
Oxycodone	*OxyContin, OxyIR.* Hillbilly Heroin, Kicker, OC, Ox, Roxy, Percs, Oxy	Oral Injection Snort	Euphoria, feelings of relaxation, pain relief, sedation, respiratory depression, constipation, papillary constriction, cough suppression **Overdose:** Extreme drowsiness, muscle weakness, confusion, cold/clammy skin, pinpoint pupils, shallow breathing, slow HR, fainting, coma, possible death
Psilocybin	Magic Mushrooms, Mushrooms, Shrooms	Oral	Nausea, vomiting, muscle weakness, lack of coordination, hallucinations, inability to discern fantasy from reality, panic reactions **Overdose:** Longer, more intense "trip" episodes, psychosis, possible death
Xylazine	Horse Anesthetic	Injection Oral Smoking Inhaled through nose	Associated with severe respiratory and CNS depression; potential disfiguring, life-threatening skin ulcers **Overdose:** Sedation, dry mouth, hyporeflexia, disorientation, hypothermia, hyperglycemia

HERBALS: COMMON NATURAL MEDICINES

The use of herbal therapies is increasing in the United States. Because of the rise in the use of herbal therapy, the following is presented to provide some basic information on some of the more popular herbs. Please note this is not an all-inclusive list, which is beyond the scope of this handbook. **NOTE:** Using herbals can be unsafe in certain health conditions or taking certain medications. Always consult a doctor before taking herbal supplements.

Herbal Supplement	Common Uses	Side Effects
Aloe vera	Acne, skin injuries (e.g., burns), psoriasis, digestive problems	**PO:** abdominal pain, cramps **TOPICAL:** burning itching, contact dermatitis
Ashwagandha	Manage perimenopausal symptoms, anxiety, stress, depression, insomnia, sexual function, fatigue; improve mental alertness; aid in weight loss; combat inflammation and pain	Vomiting, diarrhea, nausea, altered hepatic enzymes, hepatic toxicity
Bilberry	Improves visual acuity (e.g., cataracts, dry eyes, night vision), atherosclerosis, chronic fatigue, venous insufficiency,	Nausea, abdominal discomfort; may lower blood sugar levels
Bitter orange	Indigestion, dyspepsia, constipation, diarrhea	When combined with caffeine, may increase BP, HR
Black cohosh	Menopausal conditions, painful menstruation, uterine spasms, and vaginitis	Breast pain, mild weight gain, cramping, headache, muscle pain, rash, upset stomach
Chamomile	Mild sedative, relaxant, sleeping aid	Mild skin rash, itching, drowsiness, vomiting (large amounts)
Chasteberry	Menstrual irregularities (e.g., dysmenorrhea, amenorrhea, metrorrhagia)	Headache, menstrual bleeding, upset stomach, weight gain, rash, dizziness
Coenzyme Q-10	Heart failure, angina, diabetes, hypertension, fertility, reduce headaches	Abdominal pain, loss of appetite, nausea, vomiting, headache, dizziness, insomnia, fatigue; may reduce effects of warfarin
Cranberry	Prevention of UTI, neurogenic bladder, lower BP, improve eyesight, cardiovascular health	Large amounts may cause stomach upset, increase risk of developing kidney stones, alter effects of warfarin
Echinacea	Strengthens the body's immune system, prevention against colds and flu	Nausea, vomiting, diarrhea, abdominal pain; may exacerbate autoimmune diseases (e.g. multiple sclerosis, rheumatoid arthritis)

Herbal Supplement	Common Uses	Side Effects
Evening primrose	Reduces symptoms of arthritis and premenstrual syndrome (PMS)	Upset stomach, headache, may increase risk of seizures, bleeding with antiplatelets/anticoagulants
Feverfew	Migraine headaches, menstrual cramps	Heartburn, nausea, diarrhea, abdominal pain, bloating; may increase bleeding with blood thinning supplement or medications
Garlic	Cardiovascular conditions, including high cholesterol and triglyceride levels associated with the risk of atherosclerosis	Breath/body odor, GI burning/irritation, heartburn, flatulence, nausea, vomiting, diarrhea; may increase effects of antiplatelets or anticoagulants
Ginger	Pain relief (menstrual cramps, arthritis-based conditions), improves blood glucose regulation, reduces nausea	High doses (5 g or more) may cause abdominal discomfort, heartburn, diarrhea, mouth irritation; may increase effects of antiplatelets or anticoagulants
Ginkgo biloba	Conditions associated with aging, including poor circulation and memory loss	Headache, dizziness, heart palpitations, upset stomach, constipation, allergic reactions, may increase effects of antiplatelets or anticoagulants; may interfere in managing diabetes, large amounts may cause seizures
Ginseng	General tonic to increase overall body tone, helpful in elevating energy levels and improving resistance to stress	Insomnia, nausea, headache, hypertension, digestive problems, vaginal bleeding, breast pain, dizziness; may decrease effect of warfarin
Goldenseal	Healing properties and antiseptic, or germ-stopping, qualities, used for colds and flu, soothing the nose lining when it is inflamed or sore	Excitability, hallucinations, constipation, skin irritation, digestive disorders, increase sensitivity to sunlight
Glucosamine	Improves eye health, reduce joint pain/inflammation, improve bone health	Nausea, heartburn, diarrhea, constipation, may increase risk of bleeding with warfarin
Gotu kola	Boosts cognitive function, varicose veins, venous insufficiency, reduces anxiety	Nausea, stomach pain, may have additive sedative effects with CNS depressants (e.g., zolpidem)
Grapefruit	Boosts immune system, weight management, reduce risk of kidney stones	May increase concentration/effects of benzodiazepine, calcium channel blockers, carbamazepine, estrogens, statins

Continued

Herbal Supplement	Common Uses	Side Effects
Green tea	Combats fatigue, prevents arteriosclerosis, lowers cholesterol, aids in weight loss	Nausea, vomiting, abdominal bloating, dyspepsia, flatulence; may increase effects of caffeine, stimulants
Hawthorn	Heart-related conditions (e.g., angina, atherosclerosis, heart failure, and high blood pressure)	Well tolerated; most common: Dizziness; may cause nausea, GI complaints, fatigue, sweating, rash
Kava kava	Reduces anxiety, calm nerves, help to sleep	Drowsiness, headache, indigestion, nausea, loss of appetite, enlarged pupils, allergic skin reactions; may increase drowsiness with alcohol, benzodiazepines, other CNS depressants
L-carnitine	Possibly effective for angina, heart failure, hyperlipidemia, kidney failure, male infertility, increase ovulation, weight loss, improve blood glucose levels	Nausea, vomiting, abdominal cramps, heartburn, gastritis, diarrhea, seizures, body odor
Licorice	Ulcer treatment/prevention, weight reduction, decrease cough, sore throat	Excessive amounts can cause pseudohyperaldosteronism (sodium, water retention; hypokalemia; alkalosis); may reduce effects of antihypertensives, warfarin; may increase BP, cause edema, arrhythmias
Melatonin	Jet lag, insomnia, shift-work disorder	Headache, dizziness, nausea, drowsiness; may increase drowsiness with alcohol, benzodiazepines, other CNS depressants; may increase effects of antiplatelets or anticoagulants
Milk thistle	Liver disorders, bone health, diabetes management, prevention of decline in brain function, acne control	Well tolerated; nausea, diarrhea, itching, bloating
Nettle	Reduces joint pain/inflammation, manages blood glucose, seasonal allergies, minor respiratory conditions, benign prostatic hyperplasia,	Well tolerated; upset stomach, sweating, allergic skin reactions; may decrease effects of warfarin
Passion flower	Anxiety, restlessness, insomnia, symptoms of menopause	Dizziness, drowsiness, loss of coordination, confusion, allergic reaction; may increase drowsiness with alcohol, benzodiazepines, other CNS depressants

Herbal Supplement	Common Uses	Side Effects
Peppermint	Eases headaches, fatigue; boosts energy; supports digestion, memory; reduces gut spasms, common cold; relieves menstrual cramps	Heartburn, dry mouth, nausea, vomiting; may increase concentration/side effects of cyclosporine
Red yeast	Improves blood circulation, lowers cholesterol, lowers stroke risk	Abdominal discomfort, heartburn, flatulence, dizziness, headache; may increase risk of myopathy with cyclosporine
SAMe	Osteoarthritis, pain of fibromyalgia	Nausea, diarrhea, constipation, mild insomnia, dizziness, anxiety, irritability, sweating; may increase risk of serotonin syndrome with antidepressants, antipsychotics, amphetamines, dextromethorphan, St John's wort; may decrease effect of levodopa
Saw palmetto	Enlarged prostate	Dizziness, headache, nausea, diarrhea; may increase effects of antiplatelets or anticoagulants; may decrease effects of contraceptives
St. John's wort	Treatment of mental disorders, mild to moderate depression	Agitation, anxiety, dizziness, diarrhea, constipation, stomach discomfort, dry mouth, headache; may decrease effect of alprazolam, bupropion, tacrolimus, cyclosporine, simvastatin, oral contraceptives, omeprazole, phenytoin, protease inhibitors, NNRTIs, warfarin, voriconazole; may increase serotonin effects with antidepressants, dextromethorphan, triptans
Turmeric	Lessens inflammation, reduces pain of osteoarthritis, improves memory, lowers risk of heart disease, depression	Well tolerated; upset stomach, nausea, dizziness, diarrhea; may increase effects of antiplatelets or anticoagulants; may increase risk of hypoglycemia with antidiabetic medications, decrease BP with antihypertensives
Valerian	Insomnia, anxiety-associated restlessness, sleeping disorders	Headache, dizziness, drowsiness, upset stomach, vivid dreams, mental dullness; may increase drowsiness with alcohol, benzodiazepines, other CNS depressants

LIFESPAN, CULTURAL ASPECTS, AND PHARMACOGENOMICS OF DRUG THERAPY

LIFESPAN

Drug therapy is unique to pts of different ages. Age-specific competencies involve understanding the development and health needs of the various age groups. Pregnant pts, children, and elderly people represent different age groups with important considerations during drug therapy.

CHILDREN

In pediatric drug therapy, drug administration is guided by the age of the child, weight, level of growth and development, and height. The dosage ordered is to be given either by kilogram of body weight or by square meter of body surface area, which is based on the height and weight of the child. Many dosages based on these calculations must be individualized based on pediatric response.

If the oral route of administration is used, often syrup or chewable tablets are given. Additionally, sometimes medication is added to liquid or mixed with foods. Remember to never force a child to take oral medications because choking or emotional trauma may ensue.

If an intramuscular injection is ordered, the vastus lateralis muscle in the midlateral thigh is used because the gluteus maximus is not developed until walking occurs and the deltoid muscle is too small. For intravenous medications, administer very slowly in children. If given too quickly, high serum drug levels will occur with the potential for toxicity.

PREGNANCY

Females of childbearing years should be asked about the possibility of pregnancy before any drug therapy is initiated. Advise a patient who is either planning a pregnancy or believes she may be pregnant to inform her physician immediately. During pregnancy, medications given to the mother pass to the fetus via the placenta. Teratogenic (fetal abnormalities) effects may occur. Breastfeeding while the mother is taking certain medications may not be recommended due to the potential for adverse effects on the newborn.

The choice of drug ordered for pregnant females is based on the stage of pregnancy because the fetal organs develop during the first trimester. Cautious use of drugs in females of reproductive age who are sexually active and who are not using contraceptives is essential to prevent the potential for teratogenic or embryotoxic effects.

ELDERLY

Elderly people are more likely to experience an adverse drug reaction owing to physiologic changes (e.g., visual, hearing, mobility changes, chronic diseases) and cognitive changes (short-term memory loss or alteration in the thought process) that may lead to multiple medication dosing. In chronic disease states such as hypertension, glaucoma, asthma, or arthritis, the daily ingestion of multiple medications increases the potential for adverse reactions and toxic effects.

Decreased renal or hepatic function may lower the metabolism of medications in the liver and reduce excretion of medications, thus prolonging the half-life of the drug and the potential for toxicity. Dosages in elderly people should initially be smaller than for the general adult population and then slowly titrated based on patient response and therapeutic effect of the medication.

CULTURE

The term *ethnopharmacology* was first used to describe the study of medicinal plants used by indigenous cultures. More recently, it is being used as a reference to the action and effects of drugs in people from diverse racial, ethnic, and cultural backgrounds. Although there are insufficient data from investigations involving people from diverse backgrounds that would provide reliable information on ethnic-specific responses to all medications, there is growing evidence that modifications in dosages are needed for some members of racial and ethnic groups. There are wide variations in the perception of side effects by pts from diverse cultural backgrounds. These differences may be related to metabolic differences that result in higher or lower levels of the drug, individual differences in the amount of body fat, or cultural differences in the way individuals perceive the meaning of side effects and toxicity. Nurses and other healthcare providers need to be aware that variations can occur with side effects, adverse reactions, and toxicity so that pts from diverse cultural backgrounds can be monitored.

Some cultural differences in response to medications include the following:

African Americans: Generally, African Americans are less responsive to beta blockers (e.g., propranolol [Inderal]) and angiotensin-converting enzyme (ACE) inhibitors (e.g., enalapril [Vasotec]).

Asian Americans: On average, Asian Americans have a lower percentage of body fat, so dosage adjustments must be made for fat-soluble vitamins and other drugs (e.g., vitamin K used to reverse the anticoagulant effect of warfarin).

Hispanic Americans: Hispanic Americans may require lower dosages and may experience a higher incidence of side effects with tricyclic antidepressants (e.g., amitriptyline).

Native Americans: Alaskan Natives (Inuit) may experience prolonged muscle paralysis with the use of succinylcholine when administered during surgery.

There has been a desire to exert more responsibility over one's health and, as a result, a resurgence of self-care practices. These practices are often influenced by folk remedies and the use of medicinal plants. In the United States, there are several major ethnic population subgroups (White, Black, Hispanic, Asian, and Native Americans). Each of these ethnic groups has a wide range of practices that influence beliefs and interventions related to health and illness. At any given time, in any group, treatment may consist of the use of traditional herbal therapy, a combination of ritual and prayer with medicinal plants, customary dietary and environmental practices, or the use of Western medical practices.

AFRICAN AMERICANS

Many African Americans carry the traditional health beliefs of their African heritage. Health denotes harmony with nature of the body, mind, and spirit, whereas illness is seen as disharmony that results from natural causes or divine punishment. Common practices to the art of healing include treatments with herbals and rituals known empirically to restore health. Specific forms of healing include using home remedies, obtaining medical advice from a physician, and seeking spiritual healing.

Examples of healing practices include the use of hot baths and warm compresses for rheumatism, the use of herbal teas for respiratory illnesses, and the use of kitchen condiments in folk remedies. Lemon, vinegar, honey, saltpeter, alum, salt, baking soda, and Epsom salt are common kitchen ingredients used. Goldenrod, peppermint, sassafras, parsley, yarrow, and rabbit tobacco are a few of the herbals used.

HISPANIC AMERICANS

The use of folk healers, medicinal herbs, magic, and religious rituals and ceremonies are included in the rich and varied customs of Hispanic Americans. This ethnic group believes that God is responsible for allowing health or illness to occur. Wellness may be viewed as good luck, a reward for good behavior, or a blessing from God. Praying, using herbals and spices, wearing religious objects such as medals, and maintaining a balance in diet and physical activity are methods considered appropriate in preventing evil or poor health.

Hispanic ethnopharmacology is more complementary to Western medical practices. After the illness is identified, appropriate treatment may consist of home remedies (e.g., use of vegetables and herbs), use of over-the-counter patent medicines, and use of physician-prescribed medications.

ASIAN AMERICANS

For Asian Americans, harmony with nature is essential for physical and spiritual well-being. Universal balance depends on harmony among the elemental forces: fire, water, wood, earth, and metal. Regulating these universal elements are two forces that maintain physical and spiritual harmony in the body: the *yin* and the *yang*. Practices shared by most Asian cultures include meditation, special nutritional programs, herbology, and martial arts.

Therapeutic options available to traditional Chinese physicians include prescribing herbs, meditation, exercise, nutritional changes, and acupuncture.

NATIVE AMERICANS

The theme of total harmony with nature is fundamental to traditional Native American beliefs about health. It is dependent on maintaining a state of equilibrium among the physical body, the mind, and the environment. Health practices reflect this holistic approach. The method of healing is determined traditionally by the medicine man, who diagnoses the ailment and recommends the appropriate intervention.

Treatment may include heat, herbs, sweat baths, massage, exercise, diet changes, and other interventions performed in a curing ceremony.

EUROPEAN AMERICANS

Europeans often use home treatments as the front-line interventions. Traditional remedies practiced are based on the magical or empirically validated experience of ancestors. These cures are often practiced in combination with religious rituals or spiritual ceremonies.

Household products, herbal teas, and patent medicines are familiar preparations used in home treatments (e.g., saltwater gargle for sore throat).

PHARMACOGENOMICS

Traditionally, medications are prescribed using a "one size fits all" philosophy. In general, the genetic makeup is similar in all humans, regardless of race or sex. However, people inherit variations in their genes, which can affect the way a person responds to a medication. A genetic variation may make a medication stay in the body longer, causing serious side effects, or a variation may make the medication less potent.

For example, two people taking the same cancer medication may have very different responses. One may have severe, life-threatening side effects, whereas the second may have few, if any, side effects. The drug may shrink a tumor in one person but not in another.

Pharmacogenomics examines how a person's genetic makeup affects response to medications. Although widespread application still lies in the future, pharmacogenomics has the potential to personalize medical therapies. Physicians eventually will be able to prescribe medications based on an individual's genotype, thereby maximizing effectiveness and minimizing side effects.

Pharmacogenomics is an expanding field that explores the effect of interindividual genetic differences on pharmacokinetics, pharmacodynamics, drug efficiency, and safety of drug treatments. Pharmacogenomic biomarkers (proteins) can provide predictive tools for improving drug response and reducing adverse drug reactions. These biomarkers mainly originate from genes encoding drug-metabolizing enzymes, drug transporters, drug targets, and human leukocyte antigens. Currently, more than 100 drugs contain pharmacogenomic information in the package labeling. The goal is to develop personalized genetic-based strategies that will optimize therapeutic outcomes.

Personalized treatments are especially warranted when prescribing medications with a narrow therapeutic index or when toxicity can be life-threatening. Antineoplastics, anticoagulants, and anti-HIV therapies are often administered at maximum tolerated doses. This approach can result in toxicity and/or produce a poor response to therapy. Severe adverse drug reactions are one of the most common reasons for hospital admissions. Genetic testing for drug responses is expected to decrease hospitalizations by as much as 30%.

Carbamazepine (Tegretol) has been linked to dose-dependent side effects and life-threatening adverse effects. It is metabolized by enzymes encoded by the CYP3A4 gene to its active metabolite. An association has been found between the HLA-B*1502 allele and risk of Stevens-Johnson syndrome/toxic epidermal necrolysis, particularly in Asians. Before initiating carbamazepine treatment in high-risk patients, genetic testing for the HLA-B*1502 allele is recommended by the Food and Drug Administration (FDA).

Tumor cells carry the same genetic polymorphisms of normal cells. However, malignant cells are genetically unstable and can produce genetic changes that can alter disposition of active drug at the tumor site. Genetic analysis of tumors can help predict therapeutic benefit (or lack thereof) of targeted biologics such as **trastuzumab (Herceptin)** for ERBB2 *(HER2)*-amplified breast cancers or **erlotinib (Tarceva)** for epidermal growth factor receptor (EGFR)-overexpressing lung cancers.

Genetic mutations in tumors can also predict resistance to treatment, as noted in colorectal cancers, where activating mutations in *KRAS* are known to be a predictive marker for resistance to the EGFR-specific monoclonal antibodies **cetuximab (Erbitux)** and **panitumumab (Vectibix).**

By utilizing the information provided by pharmacogenomic testing, drug therapy is changing to a more individualized approach. Anticipated benefits of pharmacogenomics include creation of better vaccines, safer medications targeted to specific diseases, and more appropriate dosing of medications at the onset of therapy. Ultimately, we may see a decrease in healthcare costs due to more efficient clinical trials, reduced adverse drug reactions, and less time needed to find effective therapy for patients.

LABORATORY TEST REFERENCE RANGES

NOTE: The reference values provided should be used as a guideline only. Reference values vary based on demographics of the healthy population from which specimens are obtained and specific methods and/or instruments used to assay specimens. Results are based on the reference value of the laboratory in which the test was done.

Laboratory Test	Reference Range
Albumin, serum	3.5–5.5 g/dL
Activated partial thromboplastin time (aPTT)	25–35 seconds
Aminotransferase, serum alanine (ALT, SGPT)	10–40 units/L
Aminotransferase, serum aspartate (AST, SGOT)	10–40 units/L
Alkaline phosphatase, serum	30–120 units/L
Amylase, serum	25–125 units/L
Bilirubin, serum (total)	0.3–1 mg/dL
Bilirubin, serum (direct)	0.1–0.3 mg/dL
Blood urea nitrogen (BUN), serum or plasma	8–20 mg/dL
Calcium, ionized, serum	1.12–1.23 mmol/L
Calcium, serum	8.6–10.2 mg/dL
Chloride, serum	98–106 mEq/L
Cholesterol, serum (total)	Less than 200 mg/dL
Cholesterol, serum (HDL)	Female: Less than 50 mg/dL; male: Less than 40 mg/dL
Cholesterol, serum (LDL)	Less than 100 mg/dL
Creatinine clearance, urine	90–140 mL/min/1.73 m²
Creatinine, serum	Female: 0.5–1.1 mg/dL; male: 0.7–1.3 mg/dL
Creatine kinase, serum (total)	Female: 30–135 Units/L; male: 55–170 Units/L
Erythrocyte count	4.2–5.9 million/μL
Ferritin, serum	Female: 24–307 ng/mL; male: 24–336 ng/mL
Glucose, plasma (fasting)	70–99 mg/dL
Hematocrit, blood	Female: 37%–47%; male: 42%–50%
Hemoglobin A1C	4%–5.6%
Hemoglobin, blood	Female: 12–16 g/dL; male: 14–18 g/dL
Iron, serum	50–150 mcg/dL
Iron-binding capacity, serum (total)	250–310 mcg/dL
Lactate dehydrogenase (LDH), serum	80–225 units/L
Leukocyte count	4000–11,000/microliter

Laboratory Test	Reference Range
Leukocyte differential count	
Segmented neutrophils	50%–70%
Band forms	0%–5%
Lymphocytes	30%–45%
Monocytes	0%–6%
Basophils	0%–1%
Eosinophils	0%–3%
Lipase, serum	10–140 units/L
Magnesium, serum	1.6–2.6 mEq/L
Mean corpuscular hemoglobin (MCH)	28–32 pg
Mean corpuscular hemoglobin concentration (MCHC)	33–36 g/dL
Mean corpuscular volume	80–98 fL
Osmolality, serum	275–295 mOsm/kg H_2O
Oxygen saturation, arterial blood	95% or greater
pH, urine	4.5–8
Partial thromboplastin time (activated) (aPTT)	25–35 seconds
Phosphorus, serum	3–4.5 mg/dL
Platelet count	150,000–450,000/microliter
Potassium, serum	3.5–5 mEq/L
Proteins, serum (total)	5.5–9 g/dL
Prothrombin time, plasma	11–13 seconds
Sodium, serum	136–145 mEq/L
Thyroid-stimulating hormone (TSH), serum	0.5–4 milliunits/L
Transferrin, serum	200–400 mg/dL
Triglycerides, serum (fasting)	Optimal: Less than 100 mg/dL Normal: Less than 150 mg/dL
Urea nitrogen, blood	8–20 mg/dL
Uric acid, serum	3–7.0 mg/dL

DRUG INTERACTIONS

OVERVIEW

A drug interaction is a situation in which a substance (e.g., another drug, food, or herbal) can affect the activity of a drug when administered together. This action can be synergistic (drug effect is increased) or antagonistic (drug effect is decreased). Drugs that increase the concentration of another drug can lead to an increase in side effects or even a drug overdose. Drugs that decrease the concentration of another drug may decrease the therapeutic effect.

Factors that may contribute to drug interactions include:

- Old age: Liver metabolism, renal function, nerve transmission decrease with age. Also a sensory decrease increases the chance of errors in drug administration.
- Polypharmacy: As the number of medications taken increases, the potential that some of them will interact is more likely.
- Genetic factors: Genes synthesize enzymes that metabolize drugs. Some races have genotypic variations that may decrease or increase the activity of these enzymes. This is seen in variations in the isozymes of cytochrome P450.
- Hepatic or renal diseases: Blood concentrations of drugs that are metabolized in the liver and/or eliminated by the kidneys may be altered if these organs are not functioning correctly.

Drug interactions may be the result of various processes. These processes may include alterations in the pharmacokinetics of the drug such as in the absorption, distribution, metabolism, and excretion or the result of pharmacodynamics properties of the drug (e.g., coadministration of a receptor antagonist and an agonist for the same receptor).

PHARMACOKINETIC INTERACTIONS

Modifying the effect of a drug may be caused by differences in absorption, distribution, metabolization, or excretion of one or both of the drugs compared with the expected behavior of each drug when taken individually.

ABSORPTION

Changes in motility: Some drugs such as the prokinetic agents increase the speed that a substance passes through the intestines. If a drug is present in the digestive tract's absorption zone for less time, its blood concentration will decrease. The opposite will occur with drugs that decrease intestinal motility.

Certain drugs require an acid stomach pH for absorption while others require the basic pH of the intestines. Modification in the pH could change this absorption. In the case of antacids, an increase in pH can alter the absorption of other drugs.

Drug solubility—Food: Absorption of some drugs can be reduced if administered together with food (e.g., warfarin and avocado).

Formation of nonabsorbable complexes:

- Chelation: The presence of di- or trivalent cations can cause the chelation of certain drugs, making them harder to absorb (e.g., tetracyclines or fluoroquinolones and dairy products).

- Binding with proteins: Some drugs (e.g., sucralfate) bind to proteins, and for this reason, sucralfate is contraindicated in enteral feeding.
- Drugs that are retained in the intestinal lumen can form large complexes that impede their absorption. This can occur with cholestyramine if associated with drugs such as digoxin or warfarin.

Action on the P-glycoprotein of the enterocytes appears to be one of the mechanisms promoted by consumption of grapefruit juice in increasing the bioavailability of various drugs.

DISTRIBUTION

The main interaction mechanism is competition for plasma protein transport. The drug that arrives first binds with the plasma protein, leaving the second drug dissolved in plasma, which modifies its concentration (e.g., displacement of bilirubin from albumin binding site by ceftriaxone increases the risk of kernicterus in neonates).

METABOLISM

Most drugs are eliminated from the body, at least in part, by being changed chemically to a less lipid-soluble product (i.e., metabolized) and thus more likely to be excreted from the body via the kidney or bile. Drugs may go through two different metabolic processes: phase 1 and phase 2 metabolism.

In phase 1 metabolism, hepatic microsomal enzymes found in the endothelium of liver cells metabolize drugs via hydrolysis and oxidation and reduction reactions. These chemical reactions make the drug more water soluble. In phase 2 metabolism, large water-soluble substances (e.g., glucuronic acid, sulfate) are attached to the drug, forming inactive, or significantly less active, water-soluble metabolites. Phase 2 processes include glucuronidation, sulfation, conjugation, acetylation, and methylation.

Virtually any of the phase 1 and phase 2 enzymes can be inhibited, and some of these enzymes can be induced by drugs. Inhibiting the activity of metabolic enzymes results in increased concentrations of the drug (substrate), whereas inducing metabolic enzymes results in decreased concentrations of the drug (substrate).

The term "cytochrome P450" (CYP enzymes) refers to a family of more than 100 enzymes in the human body that modulate various physiologic functions. First identified in the 1950s, the CYP enzyme system contains two large subgroups: Steroidogenic and xenobiotic enzymes. Only the xenobiotic group is involved in the metabolism of drugs. The xenobiotic group includes four major enzyme families: CYP1, CYP2, CYP3, and CYP4. The primary role of these families is the metabolism of drugs. These families are further subdivided into subfamilies designated by a capital letter and given a specific enzyme number (1, 2, 3, etc.) according to the similarity in amino acid sequence it shares with other enzymes (e.g., CYP1A2).

The key CYP450 enzymes include CYP1A2, CYP2C9, CYP2C19, CYP2D6, and CYP3A4 and may be responsible for metabolism of 75% of all drugs, with the CYP3A subfamily responsible for nearly half of this activity.

The CYP enzymes are found in the endoplasmic reticulum of cells in a variety of human tissue but are primarily concentrated in the liver and intestine. CYP enzymes can be both inhibited and induced, leading to increased or decreased serum concentration of the drug (along with its effects).

The following tables of CYP substrates, inhibitors, and inducers provide a perspective on drugs that are affected by, or affect, cytochrome P450 (CYP) enzymes.

CYP substrate includes drugs reported to be metabolized, at least in part, by one or more CYP enzymes. **CYP inhibitor** includes drugs reported to inhibit one or more CYP enzymes. **CYP inducer** contains drugs reported to induce one or more CYP enzymes.

P450 ENZYMES: SUBSTRATES, INHIBITORS, INDUCERS
CYP1A2 ENZYME

CYP1A2 SUBSTRATES	CYP1A2 INHIBITORS	CYP1A2 INDUCERS
Clozapine (Clozaril)	Cimetidine (Tagamet)	Barbiturates
Mirtazapine (Remeron)	Ciprofloxacin (Cipro)	Carbamazepine (Tegretol)
Olanzapine (Zyprexa)	Fluvoxamine	Rifampin (Rifadin)
Ramelteon (Rozerem)		Smoking
Ropinirole (Requip)		
Tizanidine (Zanaflex)		

- CYP1A2 enzyme is increasingly involved in drug interactions.
- More potent inhibitors include cimetidine, ciprofloxacin, and fluvoxamine.
- Smoking is the most important inducer, but rifampin and barbiturates also can increase enzyme activity.
- Example of reaction: Tizanidine plasma concentrations increased more than 30-fold when the inhibitor fluvoxamine was given concurrently.

CYP2C9 ENZYME

CYP2C9 SUBSTRATES	CYP2C9 INHIBITORS	CYP2C9 INDUCERS
Candesartan (Atacand)	Amiodarone (Cordarone)	Barbiturates
Celecoxib (Celebrex)	Clopidogrel (Plavix)	Carbamazepine (Tegretol)
Diclofenac (Voltaren)	Fluconazole (Diflucan)	Rifampin (Rifadin)
Glipizide (Glucotrol)	Metronidazole (Flagyl)	St. John's wort
Glyburide (DiaBeta)	Sulfamethoxazole	
Ibuprofen (Advil, Motrin)	Valproic acid (Depakote)	
Irbesartan (Avapro)		
Meloxicam (Mobic)		
Warfarin (Coumadin)		

- More potent inhibitors include amiodarone, metronidazole, and sulfamethoxazole.
- All of the inducers can substantially increase enzyme activity.
- Both warfarin and oral hypoglycemics are of serious concern with regard to drug interactions. Substrates warranting attention include warfarin and oral hypoglycemics.

CYP2C19 ENZYME

CYP2C19 SUBSTRATES	CYP2C19 INHIBITORS	CYP2C19 INDUCERS
Citalopram (Celexa)	Cimetidine (Tagamet)	Barbiturates
Diazepam (Valium)	Clopidogrel (Plavix)	Carbamazepine (Tegretol)
Escitalopram (Lexapro)	Esomeprazole (Nexium)	Rifampin (Rifadin)
Omeprazole (Prilosec)	Fluconazole (Diflucan)	St. John's wort
Pantoprazole (Protonix)	Fluvoxamine	
Sertraline (Zoloft)	Modafinil (Provigil)	

- Inhibition by itself does not frequently cause adverse effects compared with other CYP enzymes because many of the substrates do not have serious toxicity.
- Inhibition or induction of the enzyme nonetheless may result in an adverse drug interaction.
- Racial background is important in the likelihood of being deficient in this enzyme (e.g., 3%–5% of Caucasians and 12%–23% of Asians are poor metabolizers of this enzyme).

CYP2D6 ENZYME

CYP2D6 SUBSTRATES	CYP2D6 INHIBITORS	CYP2D6 INDUCERS
Amitriptyline (Elavil)	Amiodarone (Cordarone)	See comment below
Duloxetine (Cymbalta)	Bupropion (Wellbutrin)	
Fluoxetine (Prozac)	Fluoxetine (Prozac)	
Metoclopramide (Reglan)	Paroxetine (Paxil)	
Metoprolol (Lopressor)		
Paroxetine (Paxil)		
Risperidone (Risperdal)		
Tamoxifen (Nolvadex)		
Tolterodine (Detrol)		
Tramadol (Ultram)		
Venlafaxine (Effexor)		

- Potent inhibitors include fluoxetine and paroxetine.
- Evidence suggests that this enzyme is not very susceptible to enzyme induction.
- Genetics, rather than drug therapy, account for most ultra-rapid metabolizers (e.g., Greeks, Portuguese, Saudis, and Ethiopians have high enzyme activity).

CYP3A4 ENZYME

CYP3A4 SUBSTRATES	CYP3A4 INHIBITORS	CYP3A4 INDUCERS
Alfuzosin (Uroxatral)	Amiodarone (Cordarone)	Carbamazepine (Tegretol)
Alprazolam (Xanax)	Clarithromycin (Biaxin)	Efavirenz (Sustiva)
Budesonide (Entocort EC)	Diltiazem (Cardizem)	Phenobarbital
Carbamazepine (Tegretol)	Fluconazole (Diflucan)	Rifampin (Rifadin)
Cyclosporine (Neoral)	Fluoxetine (Prozac)	St. John's wort
Fluticasone (Flovent)	Itraconazole (Sporanox)	
Lovastatin (Mevacor)	Ketoconazole (Nizoral)	
Sildenafil (Viagra)	Verapamil (Calan, Isoptin)	
Simvastatin (Zocor)		

- This enzyme metabolizes about half of all medications on the market.
- Drug toxicity of CYP3A4 substrates due to inhibition of CYP3A4 is relatively common.
- This enzyme is very sensitive to induction, tending to lower plasma concentrations of substrates, resulting in reduced efficacy of the substrate.
- Most potent inhibitors include clarithromycin, itraconazole, and ketoconazole.

- Rifampin is a potent inducer and may reduce serum concentrations of substrates by as much as 90%.

EXCRETION

RENAL EXCRETION

Only the free fraction of a drug that is dissolved in the blood is removed via the kidneys. Drugs that are tightly bound to proteins are not available for renal excretion, as long as they are not metabolized when they may be excreted as metabolites. Creatinine clearance is used as a measure of kidney function.

BILE EXCRETION

Bile excretion always involves energy in active transport across the epithelium of the bile duct against a concentration gradient. Bile excretion of drugs mainly occurs when their molecular weight is greater than 300 and contain both polar and lipophilic groups. Glucuronidation of the drug in the kidney will also enhance bile excretion.

PHARMACODYNAMIC INTERACTIONS

PHARMACOLOGIC RECEPTORS

- **Pure agonists:** Drugs bind to the main locus of the receptor, causing a similar effect to that of the main drug. For example, fentanyl and midazolam can lead to increased sedation, or vancomycin and an aminoglycoside can lead to increased potential for nephrotoxicity.
- **Partial agonists:** Drugs bind to one of the receptor's secondary loci, having the same effect to that of the main drug but with lower intensity.
- **Antagonists:** Drugs bind directly to the receptor's main locus but their effect is opposite to that of the main drug. For example, an opioid and naloxone cause a decreased effect of the opioid, reversal of sedation, respiratory depression, and hypotension.

SIGNAL TRANSDUCTION MECHANISMS

These are processes that commence after the interaction of the drug with the receptor. For example, hypoglycemia produces a release of catecholamines, which triggers compensation mechanisms that increase blood glucose levels. For example, if a patient is taking both insulin (which reduces glucose) and also a beta blocker for heart disease, the beta blocker will block the catecholamine receptors. This will block the reaction triggered by the catecholamines if hypoglycemia occurs, with an increased risk of a serious reaction.

Appendix H

ANTIDOTE/REVERSAL AGENTS

Agent	Antidote/Reversal Agents	Dosage
Acetaminophen	Acetylcysteine (Acetadote, Mucomyst)	PO: ADULTS, CHILDREN: Loading dose: 140 mg/kg, then 70 mg/kg q4h for a total of 18 doses. IV: ADULTS, CHILDREN: Loading dose: 150 mg/kg over 60 min, then 50 mg/kg over 4 hrs, then 100 mg/kg over 16 hrs.
Anticholinergic agents (e.g., atropine)	Physostigmine	IM/IV: ADULTS: Initially, 0.5–2 mg, then repeat q10–30min until response occurs or adverse effects occur. IM/IV: INFANTS, CHILDREN, ADOLESCENTS: Initially, 0.02 mg/kg (Max: 0.5 mg/dose). May repeat after 15–20 min to maximum total dose of 2 mg, or until response occurs or adverse cholinergic effects occur.
Vitamin K antagonist (VKA) (e.g., warfarin)	Balfaxar, Kcentra Prothrombin Complex concentrate (Factors II, VII, IX, X, Protein C, Protein S)	Dose based on pre-dose INR, expressed in units of factor IX activity. (Give with Vitamin K) **INR 2 to <4:** 25 units/kg. **Maximum:** 2,500 units. **INR 4–6:** 35 units/kg. **Maximum:** 3,500 units. **INR >6:** 50 units/kg. **Maximum:** 5,000 units.
Apixaban (Eliquis)/ rivaroxaban (Xarelto)	Andexanet alfa (Andexxa)	**Low Dose:** Apixaban (5 mg or less)/rivaroxaban (10 mg or less): 400 mg IV bolus at a rate of 30 mg/min then 4 mg/min for up to 120 min. **High Dose:** Apixaban (more than 5 mg)/rivaroxaban (more than 10 mg): 800 mg IV bolus, at a rate of 30 mg/min then 8 mg/min for up to 120 min.
Arsenic	Dimercaprol (BAL in oil)	Mild Poisoning IM: ADULTS, CHILDREN: 2.5 mg/kg/dose q6h for 2 days, then q12h for 1 day, then once daily for 10 days. Severe Poisoning IM: ADULTS, CHILDREN: 3 mg/kg/dose q4h for 2 days, then q6h for 1 day, then q12h for 10 days.
Benzodiazepines (e.g., midazolam)	Flumazenil (Romazicon)	IV: ADULTS: 0.2 mg over 30 sec. May give 0.3-mg dose after 30 sec if desired LOC not obtained. Additional doses of 0.5 mg can be given over 30 sec at 1-min intervals up to cumulative dose of 3 mg. CHILDREN: Initial dose: 0.01 mg/kg (**maximum:** 0.2 mg) over 15 sec with repeat dose of 0.01 mg/kg (**maximum:** 0.2 mg) after 45 sec, then given every minute to maximum total cumulative dose of 1 mg.
Beta blockers (e.g., propranolol)	Glucagon	IV: ADULTS: 3–10 mg over 3–5 min, followed by infusion of 3–5 mg/hr.

Continued

Agent	Antidote/ Reversal Agents	Dosage
Calcium channel blockers (e.g., verapamil)	Glucagon	IV: ADULTS: 3–10 mg over 3–5 min, followed by infusion of 3–5 mg/hr.
Carbamate pesticides	Atropine	IV: ADULTS: Mild-moderate symptoms: Initially, 1–2 mg bolus. Repeat by doubling dose q3–5min. Severe symptoms: Initially 3–5 mg. Repeat by doubling dose q3–5min. IV INFUSION: ADULTS: 10%–20% total cumulative IV bolus as continuous infusion/hr. IM: ADULTS (Mild symptoms): 2 mg. If severe symptoms develop after first dose, 2 additional doses should be repeated in 10 min. (Severe symptoms): Immediately administer three 2-mg doses. IV/IM: CHILDREN: 0.05–0.1 mg/kg. Repeat q3–5 min as needed. IM (Atro-Pen 0.25 mg). (Mild symptoms): 1 injection. If severe symptoms develop, give 2 additional injections given in rapid succession 10 min after receiving first injection. Severe symptoms: Administer three 0.25-mg doses.
Dabigatran (Pradaxa)	Idarucizumab (Praxbind)	IV: 5 g (give as 2 separate 2.5 g doses no more than 15 minutes apart).
Digoxin (Lanoxin)	Digoxin immune FAB (Digibind)	**ADULTS** **Acute ingestion unknown amount:** IV: Initially, 10 vials. If needed, a second dose of 10 vials (20 vials adequate to treat most life-threatening ingestions. **Chronic toxicity (serum concentration unavailable):** IV: 6 vials adequate to reverse most cases of toxicity.
Edoxaban (Savaysa)	See apixaban (Eliquis)	See apixaban (Eliquis)
Ethylene glycol	Fomepizole (Antizol)	IV: ADULTS, CHILDREN: Loading dose 15 mg/kg, then 10 mg/kg q12h for 4 doses, then 15 mg/kg q12h thereafter until ethylene glycol levels reduced to less than 20 mg/dL and patient is asymptomatic with normal pH.
Extravasation vasoconstrictive agents (e.g., dopamine)	Phentolamine (Regitine)	ADULTS, CHILDREN: Infiltrate area with small amount of solution made by diluting 5–10 mg in 10 mL 0.9% NaCl within 12 hrs of extravasation.
Heparin	Protamine	IV: ADULTS, CHILDREN: Dosage is determined by most recent dosage of heparin 1 mg protamine neutralizes approximately 100 units of heparin units of heparin. **Maximum:** 50 mg. If aPTT remains elevated, may repeat 0.5 mg protamine for every 100 units of heparin
Hyperkalemia	Sodium polystyrene sulfonate (Kayexalate, SPS)	PO: ADULTS, ELDERLY: 15 g 1–4 times/day. CHILDREN: 1g/kg q6h. Maximum dose: 15 g.

Agent	Antidote/Reversal Agents	Dosage
Hypoglycemia	Glucagon (Baqsimi, GlucaGen, Gvoke, Zegalogue)	**Baqsimi: 4 yrs and older:** 3 mg intranasally once. May repeat in 15 min. **GlucaGen: 6 yrs and older weighing 25 kg or greater or with unknown weight 6 yrs and older:** 1 mg (1 mL) SQ or IM once. May repeat in 15 min. **Pts weighing less than 25 kg or pts with unknown weight less than 6 yrs of age:** 0.5 mg SQ or IM once. May repeat in 15 min. **Gvoke: 2 yrs or older or 45 kg or greater:** 1 mg SQ once. May repeat in 15 min. **2–12 yrs and less than 45 kg:** 0.5 mg SQ once. May repeat in 15 min. **Zegalogue: 6 yrs and older:** 0.6 mg SQ once. May repeat in 15 min.
Ifosfamide	Mesna (Mesnex)	Mesna dose (IV) equal to 20% of daily ifosfamide dose at 0 hr, followed by 2 mesna doses (PO), each equal to 40% of daily ifosfamide dose, given 2 and 6 hrs after ifosfamide dose.
Iron	Deferoxamine (Desferal)	Acute IM: ADULTS: Initially, 1,000 mg, then 500 mg q4h for 2 doses. Additional doses of 0.5 g q4–12h. **Maximum:** 6 g/24 hrs. CHILDREN 3 YRS AND OLDER: 90 mg/kg/dose then 45 mg/kg/dose q4–12h as needed. **Maximum:** 6 g/24 hrs. IV: ADULTS, CHILDREN: 15 mg/kg/hr. **Maximum:** 6 g/24 hrs. Chronic IM: ADULTS: 500–1,000 mg/day. IV: ADULTS, CHILDREN: 15 mg/kg/hr. Standard dose: ADULTS: 40–50 mg/kg/day. CHILDREN: 20–40 mg/kg/day.
Isoniazid	Pyridoxine (vitamin B_6)	IV: ADULTS, CHILDREN: Total dose of pyridoxine equal to amount of isoniazid ingested as first dose of 1–4 g IV, at rate of 0.5–1 g/min. If acute ingestion not known, give 5 g at rate of 1 g/min. May repeat q5–10min.
Lead	Calcium EDTA	Recommended dose for blood lead level less than 70 mcg/dL but greater than 20 mcg/dL is 1,000 mg/m2/day given IV or IM.
Lead	Dimercaprol (BAL in oil)	Mild IM: ADULTS, CHILDREN: 3–4 mg/kg q4h for 3–5 days. Begin calcium EDTA with second dose. Severe and Lead Encephalopathy IM: ADULTS, CHILDREN: 4 mg/kg/dose q4h for 5 days. Begin calcium EDTA with second dose.

Continued

Agent	Antidote/Reversal Agents	Dosage
Methanol	Fomepizole (Antizol)	IV: ADULTS, CHILDREN: Loading dose 15 mg/kg, then 10 mg/kg q12h for 4 doses, then 15 mg/kg q12h thereafter until ethylene glycol levels reduced to less than 20 mg/dL and patient is asymptomatic with normal pH.
Opioids (e.g., morphine)	Nalmefene Zurnai Opvee	IV: Initially, 0.25 mcg/kg followed by 0.25 mcg/kg incremental doses at 2- to 5-min intervals. Total dose above 1 mcg/kg does not provide additional therapeutic effect. **Zurnai: Adults, pts 12 yrs and older:** 1.5 mg IM or SQ into the anterolateral aspect of the thigh (through clothing if necessary). **Opvee:** 2.7 mg intranasally into one nostril. Additional doses can be given q2–5min in alternating nostrils.
Opioids (e.g., morphine)	Naloxone	**Naloxone:** IV, IM, SQ: 0.4–2 mg. May repeat q2–3min up to a total of 10 mg. **Zimhi:** IM, SQ: 5 mg. May repeat q2–3min until pt responds or emergency personnel arrive. **Evzio:** IM, SQ: 2 mg. May repeat q2–3min until pt responds or emergency personnel arrive. **Narcan:** 4 mg intranasally. May repeat q2–3min until pt responds or emergency personnel arrive. **Kloxxado:** 8 mg intranasally. May repeat q2–3min until pt responds or emergency personnel arrive.
Organophosphate pesticides	Atropine	See carbamate pesticides.
Organophosphate pesticides	Pralidoxime (Protopam)	IV: ADULTS: 1–2 g. Repeat in 1–2 hrs if muscle weakness has not been relieved, then at 10- to 12-hr intervals if cholinergic signs recur. CHILDREN: 20–50 mg/kg/dose. Repeat in 1–2 hrs if muscle weakness is not relieved, then at 10- to 12-hr intervals if cholinergic signs recur. IM: ADULTS, CHILDREN 40 KG OR MORE: (Mild symptoms): 600 mg, repeat q15min to maximum dose of 1,800 mg. (Severe symptoms): 600 mg repeated twice rapidly to total dose of 1,800 mg.
Rivaroxaban (Xarelto)	See apixaban (Eliquis)	See apixaban (Eliquis).
Warfarin (Coumadin)	Phytonadione (vitamin K)	PO/IV/SQ: ADULTS: 2.5–10 mg/dose. May repeat in 12–48 hrs if given PO, 6–12 hrs if given by IV or SQ route. CHILDREN: 0.5–5 mg depending on need for further anticoagulation, severity of bleeding.

PREVENTING MEDICATION ERRORS AND IMPROVING MEDICATION SAFETY

Medication safety is a high priority for the healthcare professional. Prevention of medication errors and improved safety for the pt are important, esp. in today's healthcare environment when today's pt is older and sometimes sicker and the drug therapy regimen can be more sophisticated and complex.

A medication error is defined by the National Coordinating Council for Medication Error Reporting and Prevention (NCC MERP) as "any preventable event that may cause or lead to inappropriate medication use or pt harm while the medication is in the control of the health care professional, pt, or consumer."

Most medication errors occur as a result of multiple, compounding events as opposed to a single act by a single individual.

Use of the wrong medication, strength, or dose; confusion over sound-alike or look-alike drugs; administration of medications by the wrong route; miscalculations (esp. when used in pediatric pts or when administering medications intravenously); and errors in prescribing and transcription all can contribute to compromising the safety of the pt. The potential for adverse events and medication errors is definitely a reality and is potentially tragic and costly in both human and economic terms.

Healthcare professionals must take the initiative to create and implement procedures to prevent medication errors from occurring and implement methods to reduce medication errors. The first priority in preventing medication errors is to establish a multidisciplinary team to improve medication use. The goal for this team would be to assess medication safety and implement changes that would make it difficult or impossible for mistakes to occur. Some important criteria in making improved medication safety successful include the following:

• Promote a nonpunitive approach to reducing medication errors.
• Increase the detection and the reporting of medication errors, near misses, and potentially hazardous situations that may result in medication errors.
• Determine root causes of medication errors.
• Educate about the causes of medication errors and ways to prevent these errors.
• Make recommendations to allow organization-wide, system-based changes to prevent medication errors.
• Learn from errors that occur in other organizations and take measures to prevent similar errors.

Some common causes and ways to prevent medication errors and improve safety include the following:

Handwriting: Poor handwriting can make it difficult to distinguish between two medications with similar names. Also, many drug names sound similar, esp. when the names are spoken over the telephone, poorly enunciated, or mispronounced.

• Take time to write legibly.
• Keep phone or verbal orders to a minimum to prevent misinterpretation.

1259

- Repeat back orders taken over the telephone.
- When ordering a new or rarely used medication, print the name.
- Always specify the drug strength, even if only one strength exists.
- Express dosages for oral liquids only in metric weights or volumes (e.g., mg or mL), not by teaspoon or tablespoon.
- Print generic and brand names of look-alike or sound-alike medications.

Zeros and decimal points: Hastily written orders can present problems even if the name of the medication is clear.

- Never leave a decimal point "naked." Place a zero before a decimal point when the number is less than a whole unit (e.g., use 0.25 mg or 250 mcg, **not** .25 mg).
- Never have a trailing zero following a decimal point (e.g., use 2 mg, **not** 2.0 mg).

Abbreviations: Errors can occur because of a failure to standardize abbreviations. Establishing a list of abbreviations that should never be used is recommended.

- Never abbreviate unit as "U"; spell out "unit."
- Do not abbreviate "once daily" as OD or QD or "every other day" as QOD; spell it out.
- Do not use D/C, as this may be misinterpreted as either discharge or discontinue.
- Do not abbreviate drug names; spell out the generic and/or brand names.

Ambiguous or incomplete orders: These types of orders can cause confusion or misinterpretation of the writer's intention. Examples include situations when the route of administration, dose, or dosage form has not been specified.

- Do not use slash marks—they may be read as the number one (1).
- When reviewing an unusual order, verify the order with the person writing the order to prevent any misunderstanding.
- Read over orders after writing.
- Encourage that the drug's indication for use be provided on medication orders.
- Provide complete medication orders—do not use "resume preop" or "continue previous meds."
- Provide the age and, when appropriate, the weight of the pt.

High-alert medications: Medications in this category have an increased risk of causing significant pt harm when used in error. Mistakes with these medications may or may not be more common but may be more devastating to the pt if an error occurs. A list of high-alert medications can be obtained from the Institute for Safe Medication Practices (ISMP) at www.ismp.org.

Technology available today that can be used to address and help solve potential medication problems or errors includes the following:

- Electronic prescribing systems—This refers to computerized prescriber order entry systems. Within these systems is the capability to incorporate medication safety alerts (e.g., maximum dose alerts, allergy screening). Additionally, these systems should be integrated or interfaced with pharmacy and laboratory systems to provide drug-drug and drug-disease interactions alerts and include clinical order screening capability.
- Bar codes—These systems are designed to use bar-code scanning devices to validate identity of pts, verify medications administered, document administration, and provide safety alerts.

- "Smart" infusion pumps—These pumps allow users to enter drug infusion protocols into a drug library along with predefined dosage limits. If a dosage is outside the limits established, an alarm is sounded and drug delivery is halted, informing the clinician that the dose is outside the recommended range.
- Automated dispensing systems; point-of-use dispensing system—These systems should be integrated with information systems, esp. pharmacy systems.
- Pharmacy order entry system—This should be fully integrated with an electronic prescribing system with the capability of producing medication safety alerts. Additionally, the system should generate a computerized medication administration record (MAR), which would be used by the nursing staff while administering medications.

Medication reconciliation: Medication errors generally occur at transition points in the pt's care (admission, transfer from one level of care to another [e.g., critical care to general care area], and discharge). Incomplete documentation can account for up to 60% of potential medication errors. Therefore it becomes necessary to accurately and completely reconcile medication across the continuum of care. This includes the name, dosage, frequency, and route of medication administration.

Medication reconciliation programs are a process of identifying the most accurate list of all medications a pt is taking and using this list to provide correct medications anywhere within the healthcare system. The focus is on not only compiling a list but also using the list to reduce medication errors and provide quality pt care.

Additional Strategies to Reduce Medication Errors

The ISMP, Food and Drug Administration (FDA), and other agencies have identified high-risk areas associated with medication errors. They include the following:

At-risk population: At-risk populations primarily include pediatric and geriatric pts. For both, this risk is due to altered pharmacokinetic parameters with little published information regarding medication use in these groups. Additionally, in the pediatric population, the risk is due to the need for calculating doses based on age and weight, lack of available dosage forms, and concentrations for smaller children.

In a USP report, more than one third of medication errors reaching the pt occurred in pts 65 yrs of age and older. Almost 40% of people 60 yrs and older take at least five medications. More than 50% of fatal hospital medication errors involve seniors. In the senior population, age-related physiologic changes (e.g., decreased renal function, reduced muscle mass) increase the risk for adverse events.

Avoid abbreviations and nomenclature: The confusion caused by abbreviations has prompted the ISMP to develop a list of abbreviations that should be avoided (see back cover of handbook).

Recognize prescription look-alike and sound-alike medications: The ISMP has developed an extensive list of confused drug names (see www.jointcommission.org). See individual monographs for **DO NOT CONFUSE** information.

Focus on high-alert medications: High-alert medications are medications that bear a heightened risk of causing significant pt harm if incorrectly used. High-alert medications in the handbook have a colored background for the entire monograph.

Look for duplicate therapies and interactions: Drug interactions and duplicate therapies can increase risk of adverse reactions. Refer to individual monographs for significant interaction information (drug, herbal, food).

Report errors to improve process: This action plays an important role in preventing further errors. The intent is to identify system failures that can be altered to prevent further errors.

PARENTERAL FLUID ADMINISTRATION

Replacing fluids in the body is based on body fluid needs. Water comprises approximately 60% of the adult body. Approximately 40% is intracellular fluid, and 20% is extracellular fluid, of which 15% is interstitial (tissues) and 5% is intravascular. The walls separating these compartments are porous, allowing water to move freely between them. Small particles such as sodium and chloride can pass through the walls, but larger molecules such as proteins and starches usually are unable to pass through the walls.

Hydrostatic and osmotic pressures are forces that move water and regulate the body's water. Intravenous fluid manipulates these two pressures. Hydrostatic pressure reflects the weight and volume of water. The greater the volume, the higher the blood pressure.

Effects of Osmotic Pressure: *Osmosis* is the diffusion of water across a semipermeable membrane from an area of high concentration to an area of low concentration (water moves into the compartment of higher concentration of particles, or solute). This is similar to the action of a sponge soaking up water. This pull is referred to as *osmotic pressure*. It is the number of particles in each compartment that keeps water where it is supposed to be. By administering fluids with more (or fewer) particles than blood plasma, fluid is pulled into the compartment where it is needed the most.

How do we know where the water is needed? To assess water balance, measure the *osmolality* of blood plasma (number of particles [osmoles] in a kilogram of fluid). *Osmolarity* is the number of particles in a liter of fluid. Normal serum osmolality is approximately 300 milliosmoles (mOsm) per liter.

Crystalloids are made of substances that form crystals (e.g., sodium chloride) and are small, so easy movement between compartments is possible. Crystalloids are categorized by their tonicity (a synonym for osmolality). An isotonic solution has the same number of particles (osmolality) as plasma and will not promote a shift of fluids into or out of cells. Examples of isotonic crystalloid solutions are 0.9% sodium chloride and lactated Ringer's solution. Dextrose 5% in water is another isotonic crystalloid. However, it is quickly metabolized, and the fluid quickly becomes hypotonic. Hypotonic solutions (e.g., D_5W, 0.45% sodium chloride) are a good source of free water, causing a shift out of the vascular bed and into cells by way of osmosis. Hypotonic solutions are given to correct cellular dehydration and hypernatremia. Hypertonic solutions have more particles than body water and pull water back into the circulation, which can shrink cells.

SODIUM CHLORIDE
USES

- Extracellular fluid replacement when chloride loss is greater than or equal to sodium loss
- Treatment of metabolic alkalosis in the presence of fluid loss; chloride ions cause a compensatory decrease of bicarbonate ions
- Sodium depletion, extracellular fluid volume deficit with sodium deficit
- Initiation and termination of blood transfusion, preventing hemolysis of RBCs (occurs with Dextrose in Water solutions)

SIDE EFFECTS/ABNORMALITIES

- Hypernatremia
- **Acidosis:** 0.9% sodium chloride contains one-third more chloride ions than is present in extracellular fluid; excess chloride ions cause loss of bicarbonate, resulting in acidosis
- **Hypokalemia:** Increased potassium excretion at the same time extracellular fluid is increasing, which further decreases potassium concentration in extracellular fluid
- Circulatory overload

DEXTROSE (GLUCOSE)

EFFECTS

- Provides calories for essential energy
- Improves hepatic function because it is converted into glycogen
- Spares body protein, preventing unnecessary breakdown of protein tissue
- Prevents ketosis
- Stored in the liver as glycogen, causing a shift of potassium from extracellular to intracellular fluid compartment

USES

- Dehydration
- Hyponatremia
- Hyperkalemia
- Vehicle of drug delivery and nutrition

Note: Once infused, dextrose is rapidly metabolized to water and carbon dioxide, becoming hypotonic rather than isotonic.

SIDE EFFECTS/ABNORMALITIES

- Dehydration: Osmotic diuresis occurs if dextrose is given faster than the pt's ability to metabolize it
- Hypokalemia (see Effects)
- Hyperinsulinism due to rapid infusion of hypertonic solution
- Water intoxication due to an imbalance based on increase in extracellular fluid volume from water alone

SELECTED PARENTERAL FLUIDS

Solution	Comments
Dextrose 5% in Water (D5W)	Supplies approximately 170 cal/L and free water to aid in renal excretion of solutes Avoid excessive volumes in pts with increased antidiuretic hormone activity or to replace fluids in hypovolemic pts
0.9% Sodium chloride (0.9% NaCl)	Isotonic fluid commonly used to expand extracellular fluid in presence of hypovolemia Can be used to treat mild metabolic alkalosis

Solution	Comments
0.45% Sodium chloride (0.45% NaCl)	Hypotonic solution that provides sodium, chloride, and free water; sodium and chloride allow kidneys to select and retain needed amounts Free water is desirable as aid to kidneys in elimination of solutes
3% Sodium chloride	Used only to treat severe hyponatremia
Lactated Ringer's solution	Isotonic solution that contains sodium, potassium, calcium, and chloride in approximately the same concentrations as found in plasma Used to treat hypovolemia, burns, and fluid loss as bile or diarrhea

COMMON TERMINOLOGY CRITERIA FOR ADVERSE EVENTS (CTCAE)

The Common Terminology Criteria for Adverse Events (CTCAE) is descriptive terminology used for reporting an adverse event (AE) in a concise and standardized manner. It is supported by the U.S. Department of Health and Human Services, National Institutes of Health, and National Cancer Institute. An AE term is a unique representation of a specific event that can be used for medical documentation and scientific analyses. Along with cancer medications, other drugs may use the CTCAE system for dose and treatment modifications.

CTCAE terms are grouped by system organ classes, such as *Blood/lymphatic, GI, Nervous, Renal,* and *Respiratory* disorders. Within each system organ class, AEs are listed and accompanied by a brief description. A grading scale is then provided for each AE term, and each grade refers to a specific severity.

The CTCAE grading scale displays Grades 1–5 with particular descriptions and/ or recommendations. The severity for each AE is based on the following generalized guidelines: **Grade 1**: Asymptomatic or mild symptoms; clinical or diagnostic observations only; intervention not indicated. **Grade 2**: Moderate; symptoms, minimal, local, or noninvasive intervention indicated; limiting age-appropriate instrumental activity of daily living (ADL). **Grade 3**: Severe or medically significant symptoms, but not immediately life-threatening; hospitalization or prolonged hospitalization may be indicated; disabling; limiting self-care ADL. **Grade 4**: Life-threatening consequences; urgent intervention indicated. **Grade 5**: Death related to AE.

CTCAE EXAMPLES

Adverse Event	Grade				
	1	2	3	4	5
Blood/ Lymphatic **Anemia**	Hgb < lower limit of normal– 10 g/dL	Hgb 8–10 g/dL	Hgb <8 g/dL; transfusion indicated	Life-threatening consequences Urgent intervention indicated	Death
Gastrointes-tinal **Diarrhea**	Increase of <4 stools/ day over baseline Mild ostomy output	Increase of 4–6 stools/day over baseline Moderate ostomy output	Increase of 7 stools/day over baseline Severe ostomy output Hospitalization required	Life-threatening consequences Urgent intervention indicated	Death
General **Fever**	38–39°C (100.4– 102.2°F)	>39–40°C (102.3– 104°F)	>40°C (>104° F) for less than 24 hrs	>40°C (>104°F) for more than 24 hrs	Death

Adverse Event	Grade				
	1	2	3	4	5
Infections **UTI**	N/A	Localized; local intervention indicated (topical, antifungal, antiviral)	IV antibiotic, antifungal, antiviral intervention indicated. Radiologic or surgical intervention indicated	Life-threatening consequences Urgent intervention indicated	Death
Investigations **Lipase increased**	>ULN–1.5 times ULN	>1.5–2 times ULN	>2–5 times ULN	>5 times ULN	N/A
Metabolism/ Nutrition **Hyperkalemia**	>ULN–5.5 mmol/L	>5.5–6 mmol/L	>6–7 mmol/L	>7 mmol/L; life-threatening consequences	Death
Nervous System **Intracranial hemorrhage**	Asymptomatic; clinical or diagnostic observations only; intervention not indicated	Moderate symptoms; intervention indicated	Ventriculostomy, ICP monitoring, intraventricular thrombolysis, or invasive intervention indicated; hospitalization	Life-threatening consequences; urgent intervention indicated	Death
Respiratory **Pneumonitis**	Asymptomatic; clinical or diagnostic observations only; intervention not indicated	Symptomatic; medical intervention indicated; limiting instrumental ADLs	Severe symptoms; limiting self-care, ADLs; oxygen indicated	Life-threatening respiratory compromise; urgent intervention indicated (e.g., tracheotomy or intubation)	Death
Vascular Disorders **Thromboembolism**	Medical intervention not indicated (e.g., superficial thrombosis)	Medical intervention Indicated	Urgent medical intervention indicated (e.g., pulmonary embolism or intracardiac thrombus	Life-threatening consequences with hemodynamic or neurologic instability	Death

ULN, Upper limit of normal.

CONTRACEPTION CHOICES

IMPLANTS

The implant is a long-acting reversible contraceptive (LARC) that is a highly effective and safe contraceptive option for pts. *Nexplanon* is the only contraceptive implant available in the United States and is currently approved for up to 3 yrs. *Nexplanon* is a matchstick-sized rod containing 68 mg of the progestin etonogestrel (ENG). It is inserted into the underside of the non-dominant arm by a healthcare provider. It releases 60-70 mcg/day of etonogestrel initially, 30-40 mcg/day at the end of the second yr, and 25-30 mcg/day at the end of the third yr.

Advantages of the ENG implant include its reversibility, effectiveness, and long-term use. Once removed, there is a rapid return of fertility, typically within two menstrual cycles. Minor procedure-related risks include localized bleeding, redness, swelling, bruising, and discomfort. If the implant is inserted greater than 5 days after the onset of menses, a backup non-hormonal contraceptive should be used for 7 days.

Adverse effects: Decreased libido, headache, weight gain, acne, breast pain, changes in mood, vaginitis, gastrointestinal issues.

INTRAUTERINE DEVICES (IUDS)

IUDs are the most commonly used LARC, with continued increase in use due to their high efficacy and safety. Differences among IUDs are the active ingredient, copper (Cu) versus progestin levonorgestrel (LNG), and their effect on menstrual bleeding. IUDs are inserted directly through the cervix into the uterus by a healthcare provider. Five IUDs are currently available, each made from a T-shaped polyethylene frame with barium sulfate, allowing for x-ray imaging. *Paragard*, the Cu-IUD, is the only hormone-free option and is FDA approved for 10 yrs. The hormonal IUDs each contain LNG. *Mirena* and *Liletta* have the same size frame containing 52 mg of LNG with approval for 8 yrs. *Kyleena* and *Skyla* have smaller frames that contain 19.5 and 13.5 mg of LNG with approval for 5 and 3 yrs, respectively. The primary advantage of IUDs is their high efficacy. Similar to the implant, there is a rapid return of fertility after IUD removal, typically within two menstrual cycles. Insertion is commonly associated with pain, discomfort, dizziness, and nausea. Following placement, pts may experience cramping. If an LNG-IUD is placed greater than 7 days after the start of menstrual bleeding, a backup non-hormonal contraceptive should be used for 7 days. The Cu-IUD does not require a backup non-hormonal contraceptive after placement.

Adverse Effects: (LNG IUD): Nausea, headache, acne, ovarian cysts, irregular bleeding (first 3-6 mos). **(Cu IUD):** Irregular heavy bleeding, dysmenorrhea.

INJECTION

Depo-Provera (medroxyprogesterone acetate [MPA]) is an injectable hormonal contraceptive administered either intramuscularly (IM) or subcutaneously (SQ). It is administered q3mos by a healthcare provider (IM) or the patient (SQ). Two MPA products are currently available: SQ (*Depo-SubQ Provera* 104; MPA-SQ) and IM (*Depo-Provera*; MPA-IM). *Depo-SubQ Provera* 104 contains 104 mg of MPA administered SQ in the upper anterior thigh or abdomen q12-14 wks. *Depo-Provera* contains 150 mg of PMA administered IM in the gluteal or deltoid muscle q11–13 wks. The MPA injection is associated with significant gynecological bleeding, (highest during the first yr), including irregular/unpredictable bleeding, spotting, and heavy or prolonged bleeding. The MPA injection is associated with significant weight gain. It may reduce bone mineral density (BMD) with the most significant impact occurring after 2 yrs of use (calcium and vitamin D supplementation are recommended). Compared with all other contraceptives, the injection is associated with the longest delay in return of normal fertility (6–12 mos). If MPA is started greater than 7 days after the start of menstrual bleeding, a backup non-hormonal contraceptive should be used for 7 days.

ORAL (COMBINED AND PROGESTIN-ONLY)

Most oral contraceptives contain the estrogen ethinyl estradiol and a progestin. Monophasic oral contraceptives contain fixed doses of estrogen and progestin in each active pill. In multiphasic oral contraceptives, the amount of one or both hormones varies throughout the 28-day cycle. Older oral contraceptive formulations contain 21 active tablets and 7 placebo or iron tablets (causes 13 scheduled withdrawal bleeds/yr). Regimens with fewer hormone-free days or continuous or extended cycles have fewer withdrawal bleeds/yr and are more commonly used. Progestin-only pills (POPs) or minipills contain norethindrone or drospirenone and are taken orally once daily (taking norethindrone at the same time each day is crucial for preventing pregnancy and breakthrough bleeding). Compared with the implant, IUDs, and injection, COCs and minipills have reduced efficacy. Both COCs and minipills have a relatively quick return of normal fertility, roughly three menstrual cycles.

Benefits: COCs may improve premenstrual dysphoric disorder symptoms, hirsutism, and acne (decreases free testosterone concentration), reduce risk of endometrial and epithelial ovarian cancer, reduce bleeding volume and dysmenorrhea, lower incidence of ectopic pregnancy and benign breast disease, increase hemoglobin concentration.

Adverse effects: (COC): Breast tenderness/enlargement, unscheduled bleeding/spotting; increased risk of stroke, acute MI, peripheral artery disease in females with hypertension; increased risk of venous thromboembolism (VTE) (higher risk in females 40 yrs of age and older, obese, inherited thrombophilia, or history of VTE). **(Progestin only):** Irregular bleeding, norethindrone can worsen acne.

Contraindications to estrogen-containing contraceptives include females aged greater than 35 years who smoke tobacco; history of venous thromboembolism (VTE), stroke, coronary artery disease (CAD), hypercoagulable state, or thrombosis of heart valves; history of liver, breast, or ovarian cancer; liver disease; headaches with focal neurological symptoms; uncontrolled hypertension; and diabetes with vascular disease.

Contraindications to progestin-containing contraceptives include breast, liver, or progestin-sensitive cancer and liver disease.

TRANSDERMAL PATCH

Patch contraceptives are combination hormonal contraceptives (CHCs) containing both estrogen and progestin. Each patch should be replaced weekly for 3 wks followed by a patch-free wk to allow for menses. Patches should be applied to clean, dry, intact skin on the back, abdomen, buttocks, or upper arm. Currently available contraceptive patches *(Xulane, Zafemy)* deliver an average daily dose of 35 mcg of ethinyl estradiol (EE) and 150 mcg norelgestromin. *Twila* delivers an average daily dose of 30 mcg EE and 120 mcg of levonorgestrel. The patch can improve acne, dysmenorrhea, irregular menses, and heavy bleeding. Contraceptive patches can be easily applied by the patient and offer convenience, considering they are applied once per week. The patch may be removed at any time and takes approximately four menstrual cycles for normal fertility to return. If the patch is applied greater than 24 hours after the start of menstrual bleeding, a backup non-hormonal contraceptive should be used for 7 days.

If detachment occurs or delayed application exceeds 2 days, a backup non-hormonal contraceptive should be used for 7 days.

Benefits: Same as combination oral contraceptives.

Adverse effects: Skin irritation, nausea, irregular bleeding, headache, weight fluctuations, changes in mood, fatigue.

The efficacy of the patches may be reduced in overweight or obese females. Their use is contraindicated in patients with a BMI greater than or equal to 30 kg/m^2 due to increased risk of VTE.

VAGINAL RING CONTRACEPTIVES

Vaginal ring contraceptives are CHCs consisting of a latex-free, flexible ring that is inserted vaginally. The ring is inserted by the patient and remains in place for 3 wks, followed by a 1-wk ring-free period to allow for menses, after which a new ring is placed. Contraceptive rings currently available in the U.S.-*EluRyng, NuvaRing,* and *Haloette* delivers an average daily dose of ethinyl estradiol (EE) 15 mcg/etonogestrel 0.12 mg and *Annovera* delivers an average daily dose of EE 13 mcg/segesterone acetate 0.15 mg. *NuvaRing* and *EluRyng* may be left in place for 4 wks (extended-cycle) to avoid monthly menses. The vaginal ring offers convenient dosing and can be inserted and removed by the pt in the privacy of her home. The ring may be removed at any time and takes approximately three cycles for normal fertility to return. If *Annovera* is inserted greater than 5 days or *EluRyng, NuvaRing,* or *Haloette* are inserted greater than 24 hours after the start of menstrual bleeding, a backup non-hormonal contraceptive should be used for 7 days. It is important for patients to replace the ring as soon as it is remembered. If the vaginal ring is displaced or insertion is delayed greater than 2 hours for *Annovera* or greater than 3 hours for *EluRyng, NuvaRing,* and *Haloette,* a backup non-hormonal contraceptive should be used for 7 days.

Benefits: Ring can improve acne, dysmenorrhea, irregular menses, heavy bleeding.

Adverse effects: Nausea, irregular bleeding or spotting, headache, breast tenderness.

BARRIER METHODS

Barrier contraceptives are commonly used and are the least effective method due to the need for correct and consistent use. Spermicide can be used alone or with another barrier contraceptive to improve efficacy.

Barrier contraceptives include male and female condoms, cervical caps, diaphragms, and select nonoxynol-9-containing spermicides (sponges, gels, and foams). Diaphragms and cervical caps require a prescription, while all other products are available OTC. Barrier contraceptives are cost effective, and are readily available without a prescription (e.g., condoms, spermicides, and sponges). Male latex condoms offer the best protection, though non-latex male condoms made of polyurethane or polyisoprene may be recommended for patients who are allergic to latex. Barrier contraceptives offer excellent options for individuals who are unable to tolerate or use other contraceptives.Patients must be cognizant of which lubricants are compatible with condoms to decrease risk of weakening or breakage. Additionally, sponges, cervical caps, and diaphragms should not be used during menses or by patients with history of toxic shock syndrome (TSS). Depending on the product, potential side effects include TSS, vaginal burning and irritation, and urinary tract infections. Pts who have recently given birth are required to wait at least 6 wks prior to inserting a new sponge, cervical cap, or diaphragm. Patients allergic to latex, polyurethane, or silicone could have a potential reaction to condoms or cervical caps.

EMERGENCY CONTRACEPTIVES (EC)

ECs are used after unprotected intercourse to prevent unintended pregnancy. Common indications include contraceptive failure or lack of use. ECs should not be used as routine contraception, do not protect against STIs, and cannot terminate an existing pregnancy. Four EC options are available: the Cu-IUD and three emergency contraception pills (ECPs). The common-practice ECPs are ulipristal (UPA) 30 mg taken as a single dose and LNG 1.5 mg taken as a single dose or 0.75 mg taken twice 12 hours apart. Less commonly, *Yuzpe* (EE 100 mcg/LNG 0.5 mg) taken twice 12 hours apart can also be utilized.

The Cu-IUD is highly effective (99.9%) when used within 120 hours (5 days) of ovulation following unprotected intercourse. Efficacy of ECPs decreases as time from intercourse increases. When taken correctly, UPA possesses the highest efficacy followed by LNG. Compared with other ECs, LNG is accessible to patients given its availability over the counter. UPA and the Cu-IUD methods are not impacted by patient weight. Use of an ECP does not negatively affect a patient's ability to conceive at a later time. LNG is affected by body weight and may be less effective for patients with a BMI greater than or equal to 30 kg/m^2.

Adverse effects: Nausea, vomiting, headache, abdominal pain, fatigue, dizziness, breast tenderness.

COMPARISON OF ORAL CONTRACEPTIVES AND ALTERNATIVES

Products	Estrogen	Progestin
Monophasic Pills		
Apri **Cyred EQ**	EE 30 mcg × 21 days	Desogestrel 0.15 mg × 21 days
Ocella **Yasmin**	EE 30 mcg × 21 days	Drospirenone 3 mg × 21 days
Beyaz **Yaz**	EE 20 mcg × 24 days	Drospirenone 3 mg × 24 days
Nextstellis	Estetrol 14.2 mg × 24 days	Drospirenone 3 mg × 24 days
Kelnor 1/35 **Zovia 1/35**	EE 35 mcg × 21 days	Ethynediol diacetate 1 mg × 21 days
Altavera **Marlissa** **Portia**	EE 30 mcg × 21 days	Levonorgestrel 0.15 mg × 21 days
Iclevia **Jolessa** **Seasonale**	EE 30 mcg × 84 days	Levonorgestrel 0.15 mg × 84 days
Afirmelle **Larissia** **Lessina**	EE 20 mcg × 21 days	Levonorgestrel 0.1 mg × 21 days
Amethyst **Dolishale**	EE 20 mcg × 28 days (continuous, no pill-free interval)	Levonorgestrel 90 mcg × 28 days (continuous, no pill-free interval)
Balziva **Briellyn**	EE 35 mcg × 21 days	Norethindrone 0.4 mg × 21 days
Necon **Nortrel 0.5/35**	EE 35 mcg × 21 days	Norethindrone 0.5 mg × 21 days

Continued

Products	Estrogen	Progestin
Generess Fe (chewable) *Kaitlib Fe* (chewable) *Layolis Fe* (chewable)	EE 25 mcg × 24 days	Norethindrone 0.8 mg × 24 days
Alyacen 1/35 *Dasetta 1/35* *Nortrel 1/35-21*	EE 35 mcg × 21 days	Norethindrone 1 mg × 21 days
Junel Fe 1/20 *Loestrin Fe 1/20*	EE 20 mcg × 21 days	Norethindrone acetate 1 mg × 21 days
Junel Fe 24 *Loestrin 24 Fe* *Mibelas 24 Fe* (chewable) *Femlyv* (oral disintegrating tablet)	EE 20 mcg × 24 days	Norethindrone acetate 1 mg × 24 days
Junel Fe 1.5/30 *Loestrin Fe 1.5/30* *Microgestin Fe 1.5/30*	EE 30 mcg × 21 days	Norethindrone acetate 1.5 mg × 21 days
Estarylla *Nymyo*	EE 35 mcg × 21 days	Norgestimate 0.25 mg × 21 days
Cryselle *Elinest* *Lo/Ovral*	EE 30 mcg × 21 days	Norgestrel 0.3 mg × 21 days
BIPHASIC PILLS		
Kariva *Mircette* *Simliya* *Viorele*	EE 20 mcg × 21 days, placebo × 2 days, 10 mcg × 5 days	Desogestrel 0.15 mg × 21 days
Camrese Lo *LoJaimiess* *LoSeasonique*	EE 20 mcg × 84 days, 10 mcg × 7 days	Levonorgestrel 0.1 mg × 84 days
Amethia *Daysee* *Seasonique*	EE 30 mcg × 84 days, 10 mcg × 7 days	Levonorgestrel 0.15 mg × 84 days
Lo Loestrin Fe	EE 10 mcg × 26 days	Norethindrone acetate 1 mg × 24 days
Triphasic Pills		
Caziant *Velivet*	EE 25 mcg × 21 days	Desogestrel 0.1 mg × 7 days, 0.125 mg × 7 days, 0.15 mg × 7 days
Enpresse *Levonest* *Trivora*	EE 30 mcg × 6 days, 40 mcg × 5 days, 30 mcg × 10 days	Levonorgestrel 0.05 mg × 6 days, 0.075 mg × 5 days, 0.125 mg × 10 days
Aranelle *Leena*	EE 35 mcg × 21 days	Norethindrone 0.5 mg × 7 days, 1 mg × 9 days, 0.5 mg × 5 days
Alyacen 7/7/7 *Nortrel 7/7/7* *Pirmella 7/7/7*	EE 35 mcg × 21 days	Norethindrone 0.5 mg × 7 days, 0.75 mg × 7 days, 1 mg × 7 days

COMPARISON OF ORAL CONTRACEPTIVES AND ALTERNATIVES—cont'd

Products	Estrogen	Progestin
Estrostep Fe *Tilia Fe* *Tri-Legest Fe-28*	EE 20 mcg × 5 days, 30 mcg × 7 days, 35 mcg × 9 days	Norethindrone acetate 1 mg × 21 days
Tri-Lo-Estarylla *Tri-Lo-Marzia* *Tri-Lo-Sprintec* *Tri-VyLibra Lo*	EE 25 mcg × 21 days	Norgestimate 0.18 mg × 7 days, 0.215 mg × 7 days, 0.25 mg × 7 days
Tri-Estarylla *Tri-Sprintec* *Tri-VyLibra*	EE 35 mcg × 21 days	Norgestimate 0.18 mg × 7 days, 0.215 mg × 7 days, 0.25 mg × 7 days

QUADRIPHASIC PILLS

Natazia	Estradiol valerate 3 mg × 2 days, then 2 mg × 22 days, then 1 mg × 2 days, then 2-day pill-free interval	Dienogest none × 2 days, then 2 mg × 5 days, then 3 mg × 17 days, then none × 4 days
Fayosim *Quartette* *Rivelsa*	EE 20 mcg × 42 days, 25 mcg × 21 days, 30 mcg × 21 days, 10 mcg × 7 days	Levonorgestrel 0.15 mg × 84 days

Progestin-Only Pills ("mini-pill")

Drospirenone *(chewable)*	Not applicable	Drospirenone 3.5 mg × 24 days
Slynd	Not applicable	Drospirenone 4 mg × 24 days
Camila *Incassia* *Jencycla* *Nora-BE*	Not applicable	Norethindrone 0.35 mg × 28 days (continuous, no pill-free interval)
Opill	Not applicable	Norgestrel 0.075 mg × 28 days (continuous, no pill-free days)

Emergency Contraception

Aftera *AfterPill* *E-Con* *EContra One-Step* *Her Style* *Julie* *Levonorgestrel* *My Choice* *My Way* *New Day* *Opcicon One-Step* *Option 2* *Preventeza* *React* *Take Action* *Plan B One-Step*	Not applicable	Levonorgestrel 1.5 mg tablet × 1
Ella	Not applicable	Ulipristal 30 mg tablet × 1 (progesterone receptor modulator)

Continued

NONORAL ALTERNATIVES TO ORAL CONTRACEPTION

Brand NameDose/ Route	Comments	Estrogen	Progestin
Annovera	Vaginal ring inserted and left in for 3 wks, then removed for 1 wk. Ring should be washed and can be reused for up to 13 cycles.	Ethinyl estradiol 13 mcg/day	Segesterone acetate 150 mcg/day
Depo-Provera	IM injection (gluteal or deltoid muscle) once q3mos.	None	Medroxyprogesterone acetate 150 mg
Depo-SubQ Provera 104	SQ injection into the anterior thigh or abdomen, once q3mos (12–14 wks).	None	Medroxyprogesterone acetate 104 mg
Kyleena (IUD)		None	Levonorgestrel 17.5 mcg/day (after first 24 days of insertion), then reduces to 7.4 mcg/day after 5 yrs. Remove by the end of the fifth year.
Liletta (IUD)		None	Levonorgestrel ~20 mcg/day initially, then reduces to about 6.5 mcg/day after 8 yrs. Remove by the end of the eighth year.
Mirena (IUD)		None	Levonorgestrel 21 mcg/day (after 24 days, reduces to about 11 mcg/day after 5 yrs and about 7 mcg/day after 8 yrs). Remove after 8 yrs.
Nexplanon (implant)	Implanted subdermally just under the skin at the inner side of the nondominant arm.	None	Etonogestrel 60–70 mcg/day (after about 5–6 wks), then reduces to about 35–45 mcg/day at the end of the first yr to about 30–40 mcg/day at the end of the second yr, and to about 25–30 mcg/day at the end of the third yr. Must be removed by the end of the third year.

NONORAL ALTERNATIVES TO ORAL CONTRACEPTION—cont'd

Brand NameDose/ Route	Comments	Estrogen	Progestin
NuvaR- ing, EluRyng	Vaginal ring inserted and left in for 3 wks and removed for 1 wk.	Ethinyl estradiol 15 mcg/day	Etonogestrel (active form of desogestrel) 0.12 mg/ day
ParaGard (IUD)		Nonhormonal, copper IUD. Must be removed after 10 yrs.	
Phexxi (vaginal gel)	One full applicator up to 1 hr before each episode of vaginal intercourse. Can be used during menstrual cycle.	Nonhormonal, lactic acid, citric acid, and potassium bitartrate vaginal gel.	
Skyla (IUD)		None	Levonorgestrel 14 mcg/day (after first 24 days of insertion and declines to 5 mcg/day after 3 yrs). Remove by the end of the third yr.
Twirla (transdermal patch)	Applied wkly (for 3 wks, then wk 4 is patch-free)	Ethinyl estradiol 30 mcg/day	Levonorgestrel 120 mcg/day
Xulane, Zafemy (transdermal patch)	Applied wkly (for 3 wks, then wk 4 is patch-free)	Ethinyl estradiol 35 mcg/day	Norelgestromin (active form of norgestimate) 150 mcg/day

HORMONES

USES

Functions of the body are regulated by two major control systems: the nervous system and the endocrine (hormone) system. Together they maintain homeostasis and control different metabolic functions in the body.

Hormones are concerned with control of different metabolic functions in the body (e.g., rates of chemical reactions in cells, transporting substances through cell membranes, cellular metabolism [growth/secretions]). By definition, a hormone is a chemical substance secreted into body fluids by cells and has control over other cells in the body.

Hormones can be local or general:

- *Local hormones* have specific local effects (e.g., acetylcholine, which is secreted at parasympathetic and skeletal nerve endings).
- *General hormones* are mostly secreted by specific endocrine glands (e.g., epinephrine/norepinephrine are secreted by the adrenal medulla in response to sympathetic stimulation), transported in the blood to all parts of the body, causing many different reactions.

Some general hormones affect all or almost all cells of the body (e.g., thyroid hormone from the thyroid gland increases the rate of most chemical reactions in almost all cells of the body); other general hormones affect only specific tissue (e.g., ovarian hormones are specific to female sex organs and secondary sexual characteristics of the female).

ACTION

Endocrine hormones almost never directly act intracellularly affecting chemical reactions. They first combine with hormone receptors either on the cell surface or inside the cell (cell cytoplasm or nucleus). The combination of hormone and receptors alters the function of the receptor, and the receptor is the direct cause of the hormone effects. Altered receptor function may include the following:

Altered cell permeability, which causes a change in protein structure of the receptor, usually opening or closing a channel for one or more ions. The movement of these ions causes the effect of the hormone.

Activation of intracellular enzymes immediately inside the cell membrane (e.g., hormone combines with receptor that then becomes the activated enzyme adenyl cyclase, which causes formation of cAMP).

◄ ALERT ► cAMP has effects inside the cell. It is not the hormone but cAMP that causes these effects.

Regulation of hormone secretion is controlled by an internal control system, the negative feedback system:

- Endocrine gland oversecretes.
- Hormone exerts more and more of its effect.
- Target organ performs its function.
- Too much function in turn feeds back to endocrine gland to decrease secretory rate.

The endocrine system contains many glands and hormones. A summary of the important glands and their hormones secreted are as follows:

The pituitary gland (hypophysis) is a small gland found in the sella turcica at the base of the brain. The pituitary is divided into two portions physiologically: the anterior pituitary (adenohypophysis) and the posterior pituitary (neurohypophysis). Six important hormones are secreted from the anterior pituitary and two from the posterior pituitary.

Anterior pituitary hormones:
* Growth hormone (GH)
* Adrenocorticotropin (corticotropin)
* Thyroid-stimulating hormone (thyrotropin) (TSH)
* Follicle-stimulating hormone (FSH)
* Luteinizing hormone (LH)
* Prolactin

Posterior pituitary hormones:
* Antidiuretic hormone (vasopressin)
* Oxytocin

Almost all secretions of the pituitary hormones are controlled by hormonal or nervous signals from the hypothalamus. The hypothalamus is a center of information concerned with the well-being of the body, which in turn is used to control secretions of the important pituitary hormones just listed. Secretions from the posterior pituitary are controlled by nerve signals originating in the hypothalamus; anterior pituitary hormones are controlled by hormones secreted within the hypothalamus. These hormones are as follows:
* Thyrotropin-releasing hormone (TRH) releasing thyroid-stimulating hormone
* Corticotropin-releasing hormone (CRH) releasing adrenocorticotropin
* Growth hormone–releasing hormone (GHRH) releasing growth hormone and growth hormone inhibitory hormone (GHIH) (same as somatostatin)
* Gonadotropin-releasing hormone (GnRH) releasing the two gonadotropic hormones, LH and FSH
* Prolactin inhibitory factor (PIF) causing inhibition of prolactin and prolactin-releasing factor

ANTERIOR PITUITARY HORMONES

All anterior pituitary hormones (except growth hormone) have as their principal effect stimulating target glands.

GROWTH HORMONE (GH)

Growth hormone affects almost all tissues of the body. GH (somatotropin) causes growth in almost all tissues of the body (increases cell size, increases mitosis with increased number of cells, and differentiates certain types of cells). Metabolic effects include increased rate of protein synthesis, mobilization of fatty acids from adipose tissue, decreased rate of glucose utilization.

THYROID-STIMULATING HORMONE (TSH)

Thyroid-stimulating hormone controls secretion of the thyroid hormones. The thyroid gland is located immediately below the larynx on either side of and anterior to the trachea and secretes two significant hormones, thyroxine (T_4) and triiodothyronine (T_3), which have a profound effect on increasing the metabolic rate of the body. The thyroid gland also secretes calcitonin, an important hormone for calcium metabolism. Calcitonin promotes deposition of calcium in the bones, which decreases calcium concentration in the extracellular fluid.

ADRENOCORTICOTROPIN

Adrenocorticotropin causes the adrenal cortex to secrete adrenocortical hormones. The adrenal glands lie at the superior poles of the two kidneys. Each gland is composed of two distinct parts, the adrenal medulla and the cortex. The adrenal medulla, related to the sympathetic nervous system, secretes the hormones epinephrine and norepinephrine. When stimulated, they cause constriction of blood vessels, increased activity of the heart inhibitory effects on the GI tract, and dilation of the pupils. The adrenal cortex secretes corticosteroids, of which there are two major types: mineralocorticoids and glucocorticoids. Aldosterone, the principal mineralocorticoid, primarily affects electrolytes of the extracellular fluids. Cortisol, the principal glucocorticoid, affects glucose, protein, and fat metabolism.

LUTEINIZING HORMONE

Luteinizing hormone plays an important role in ovulation and causes secretion of female sex hormones by the ovaries and testosterone by the testes.

FOLLICLE-STIMULATING HORMONE

Follicle-stimulating hormone causes growth of follicles in the ovaries before ovulation and promotes formation of sperm in the testes.

Ovarian sex hormones are estrogens and progestins. Estradiol is the most important estrogen; progesterone is the most important progestin.

Estrogens mainly promote proliferation and growth of specific cells in the body and are responsible for development of most of the secondary sex characteristics. Primarily cause cellular proliferation and growth of tissues of sex organs/other tissue related to reproduction. Ovaries, fallopian tubes, uterus, vagina increase in size. Estrogen initiates growth of breast and milk-producing apparatus, external appearance.

Progesterone stimulates secretion of the uterine endometrium during the latter half of the female sexual cycle, preparing the uterus for implantation of the fertilized ovum. Decreases the frequency of uterine contractions (helps prevent expulsion of the implanted ovum). Progesterone promotes development of breasts, causing alveolar cells to proliferate, enlarge, and become secretory in nature.

Testosterone is secreted by the testes and formed by the interstitial cells of Leydig. Testosterone production increases under the stimulus of the anterior pituitary gonadotropic hormones. It is responsible for distinguishing characteristics of the masculine body (stimulates the growth of male sex organs and promotes the development of male secondary sex characteristics, e.g., distribution of body hair; effect on voice, protein formation, and muscular development).

PROLACTIN

Prolactin promotes the development of breasts and secretion of milk.

POSTERIOR PITUITARY HORMONES
ANTIDIURETIC HORMONE (ADH) (VASOPRESSIN)

ADH can cause antidiuresis (decreased excretion of water by the kidneys). In the presence of ADH, the permeability of the renal-collecting ducts and tubules to water increases, which allows water to be absorbed, conserving water in the body. ADH in higher concentrations is a very potent vasoconstrictor, constricting arterioles everywhere in the body, increasing B/P.

OXYTOCIN

Oxytocin contracts the uterus during the birthing process, esp. toward the end of the pregnancy, helping expel the baby. Oxytocin also contracts myoepithelial cells in the breasts, causing milk to be expressed from the alveoli into the ducts so that the baby can obtain it by suckling.

PANCREAS

The pancreas is composed of two tissue types: *acini* (secrete digestive juices in the duodenum) and *islets of Langerhans* (secrete insulin/glucagons directly into the blood). The islets of Langerhans contain three cells: alpha, beta, and delta. Alpha cells secrete glucagon, beta cells secrete insulin, and delta cells secrete somatostatin.

Insulin promotes glucose entry into most cells, thus controlling the rate of metabolism of most carbohydrates. Insulin also affects fat metabolism.

Glucagon effects are opposite those of insulin, the most important of which is increasing blood glucose concentration by releasing it from the liver into the circulating body fluids.

Somatostatin (same chemical as secreted by the hypothalamus) has multiple inhibitory effects: depresses secretion of insulin and glucagon, decreases GI motility, decreases secretions/absorption of the GI tract.

NUTRITION: ENTERAL

Enteral nutrition (EN), also known as *tube feedings,* provides food/nutrients via the GI tract using special formulas, delivery techniques, and equipment. All routes of EN consist of a tube through which liquid formula is infused.

INDICATIONS

Tube feedings are used in pts with major trauma, burns; those undergoing radiation and/or chemotherapy; pts with hepatic failure, severe renal impairment, physical or neurologic impairment; preop and postop to promote anabolism; prevention of cachexia, malnutrition; dysphagia, pts requiring mechanical ventilation.

ROUTES OF ENTERAL NUTRITION DELIVERY

NASOGASTRIC (NG):

INDICATIONS: Most common for short-term feeding in pts unable or unwilling to consume adequate nutrition by mouth. Requires at least a partially functioning GI tract.

ADVANTAGES: Does not require surgical intervention and is fairly easily inserted. Allows full use of digestive tract. Decreases abdominal distention, nausea, vomiting that may be caused by hyperosmolar solutions.

DISADVANTAGES: Temporary. May be easily pulled out during routine nursing care. Has potential for pulmonary aspiration of gastric contents, risk of reflux esophagitis, regurgitation.

NASODUODENAL (ND), NASOJEJUNAL (NJ):

INDICATIONS: Pts unable or unwilling to consume adequate nutrition by mouth. Requires at least a partially functioning GI tract.

ADVANTAGES: Does not require surgical intervention and is fairly easily inserted. Preferred for pts at risk for aspiration. Valuable for pts with gastroparesis.

DISADVANTAGES: Temporary. May be pulled out during routine nursing care. May be dislodged by coughing, vomiting. Small lumen size increases risk of clogging when medication is administered via tube, more susceptible to rupturing when using infusion device. Must be radiographed for placement, frequently extubated.

GASTROSTOMY:

INDICATIONS: Pts with esophageal obstruction or impaired swallowing; pts in whom NG, ND, or NJ not feasible; when long-term feeding indicated.

ADVANTAGES: Permanent feeding access. Tubing has larger bore, allowing noncontinuous (bolus) feeding (300–400 ml over 30–60 min q3–6h). May be inserted endoscopically using local anesthetic (procedure called *percutaneous endoscopic gastrostomy* [PEG]).

DISADVANTAGES: Requires surgery; may be inserted in conjunction with other surgery or endoscopically (see **ADVANTAGES**). Stoma care required. Tube may be inadvertently dislodged. Risk of aspiration, peritonitis, cellulitis, leakage of gastric contents.

JEJUNOSTOMY:

INDICATIONS: Pts with stomach or duodenal obstruction, impaired gastric motility; pts in whom NG, ND, or NJ not feasible; when long-term feeding indicated.

ADVANTAGES: Allows early postop feeding (small bowel function is least affected by surgery). Risk of aspiration reduced. Rarely pulled out inadvertently.

DISADVANTAGES: Requires surgery (laparotomy). Stoma care required. Risk of intraperitoneal leakage. Can be dislodged easily.

INITIATING ENTERAL NUTRITION

With continuous feeding, initiation of isotonic (about 300 mOsm/L) or moderately hypertonic feeding (up to 495 mOsm/L) can be given full strength, usually at a slow rate (30–50 ml/hr) and gradually increased (25 ml/hr q6–24h). Formulas with osmolality greater than 500 mOsm/L are generally started at half strength and gradually increased in rate, then concentration. Tolerance is increased if the rate and concentration are not increased simultaneously.

SELECTION OF FORMULAS

Protein: Has many important physiologic roles and is the primary source of nitrogen in the body. Provides 4 kcal/g protein. Sources of protein in enteral feedings: sodium caseinate, calcium caseinate, soy protein, dipeptides.

Carbohydrate (CHO): Provides energy for the body and heat to maintain body temperature. Provides 3.4 kcal/g carbohydrate. Sources of CHO in enteral feedings: corn syrup, cornstarch, maltodextrin, lactose, sucrose, glucose.

Fat: Provides concentrated source of energy. Referred to as *kilocalorie dense* or *protein sparing*. Provides 9 kcal/g fat. Sources of fat in enteral feedings: corn oil, safflower oil, medium-chain triglycerides.

Electrolytes, vitamins, trace elements: Contained in formulas (not found in specialized products for renal/hepatic insufficiency).

All products containing protein, fat, carbohydrate, vitamin, electrolytes, trace elements are nutritionally complete and designed to be used by pts for long periods.

COMPLICATIONS

MECHANICAL: Usually associated with some aspect of the feeding tube.

Aspiration pneumonia: Caused by delayed gastric emptying, gastroparesis, gastroesophageal reflux, or decreased gag reflex. May be prevented or treated by reducing infusion rate, using lower-fat formula, feeding beyond pylorus, checking residuals, using small-bore feeding tubes, elevating head of bed 30–45 degrees during and for 30–60 min after intermittent feeding, and regularly checking tube placement.

Esophageal, mucosal, pharyngeal irritation, otitis: Caused by using large-bore NG tube. Prevented by use of small bore whenever possible.

Irritation, leakage at ostomy site: Caused by drainage of digestive juices from site. Prevented by close attention to skin/stoma care.

Tube, lumen obstruction: Caused by thickened formula residue, formation of formula-medication complexes. Prevented by frequently irrigating tube with clear water (also before and after giving formulas/medication), avoiding instilling medication if possible.

GASTROINTESTINAL: Usually associated with formula, rate of delivery, unsanitary handling of solutions or delivery system.

Diarrhea: Caused by low-residue formulas, rapid delivery, use of hyperosmolar formula, hypoalbuminemia, malabsorption, microbial contamination, or rapid GI transit time. Prevented by using fiber supplemented formulas, decreasing rate of delivery, using dilute formula, and gradually increasing strength.

Cramps, gas, abdominal distention: Caused by nutrient malabsorption, rapid delivery of refrigerated formula. Prevented by delivering formula by continuous methods, giving formulas at room temperature, decreasing rate of delivery.

Nausea, vomiting: Caused by rapid delivery of formula, gastric retention. Prevented by reducing rate of delivery, using dilute formulas, selecting low-fat formulas.

Constipation: Caused by inadequate fluid intake, reduced bulk, inactivity. Prevented by supplementing fluid intake, using fiber-supplemented formula, encouraging ambulation.

METABOLIC: Fluid/serum electrolyte status should be monitored. Refer to monitoring section. In addition, the very young and very old are at greater risk of developing complications such as dehydration or overhydration.

MONITORING

Daily: Estimate nutrient intake, fluid intake/output, weight of pt, clinical observations.

Weekly: Serum electrolytes (potassium, sodium, magnesium, calcium, phosphorus), blood glucose, BUN, creatinine, hepatic function tests (e.g., AST, ALT, alkaline phosphatase), 24-hr urea and creatinine excretion, total iron-binding capacity (TIBC) or serum transferrin, triglycerides, cholesterol.

Monthly: Serum albumin.

Other: Urine glucose, acetone (when blood glucose is greater than 250), vital signs (temperature, respirations, pulse, B/P) q8h.

DRUG THERAPY: DOSAGE FOR SELECTION/ADMINISTRATION:

Drug therapy should not have to be compromised in pts receiving enteral nutrition:
* Temporarily discontinue medications not immediately necessary.
* Consider an alternate route for administering medications (e.g., transdermal, rectal, intravenous).
* Consider alternate medications when current medication is not available in alternate dosage forms.

ENTERAL ADMINISTRATION OF MEDICATIONS:

Medications may be given via feeding tube with several considerations:
* Tube type
* Tube location in the GI tract
* Site of drug action
* Site of drug absorption
* Effects of food on drug absorption
* Use of liquid dosage forms is preferred whenever possible; many tablets may be crushed; contents of many capsules may be emptied and given through large-bore feeding tubes.
* Many oral products should not be crushed (e.g., sustained-release, enteric coated, capsule granules).
* Some medications should not be given with enteral formulas because they form precipitates that may clog the feeding tube and reduce drug absorption.
* Feeding tube should be flushed with water before and after administration of medications to clear any residual medication.

NUTRITION: PARENTERAL

Parenteral nutrition (PN), also known as *total parenteral nutrition* (TPN) or *hyperalimentation* (HAL), provides required nutrients to pts by IV route of administration. The goal of PN is to maintain or restore nutritional status caused by disease, injury, or inability to consume nutrients by other means.

INDICATIONS

Conditions when pt is unable to use alimentary tract via oral, gastrostomy, or jejunostomy route. Impaired absorption of protein caused by obstruction, inflammation, or antineoplastic therapy. Bowel rest necessary because of GI surgery or ileus, fistulas, or anastomotic leaks. Conditions with increased metabolic requirements (e.g., burns, infection, trauma). Preserve tissue reserves (e.g., acute renal failure). Inadequate nutrition from tube feeding methods.

COMPONENTS OF PN

To meet IV nutritional requirements, six essential categories in PN are needed for tissue synthesis and energy balance.

Protein: In the form of crystalline amino acids (CAA), primarily used for protein synthesis. Several products are designed to meet specific needs for pts with renal failure (e.g., NephrAmine), hepatic disease (e.g., Hepat Amine), stress/trauma (e.g., Aminosyn HBC), use in neonates and pediatrics (e.g., Aminosyn PF, TrophAmine). Calories: 4 kcal/g protein.

Energy: In the form of dextrose, available in concentrations of 5%–70%. Dextrose less than 10% may be given peripherally; concentrations greater than 10% must be given centrally. Calories: 3.4 kcal/g dextrose.

IV fat emulsion: Available in 10% and 20% concentrations. Provides a concentrated source of energy/calories (9 kcal/g fat) and is a source of essential fatty acids. May be administered peripherally or centrally.

Electrolytes: Major electrolytes (calcium, magnesium, potassium, sodium; also acetate, chloride, phosphate). Doses of electrolytes are individualized, based on many factors (e.g., renal/hepatic function, fluid status).

Vitamins: Essential components in maintaining metabolism and cellular function; widely used in PN.

Trace elements: Necessary in long-term PN administration. Trace elements include zinc, copper, chromium, manganese, selenium, molybdenum, iodine.

Miscellaneous: Additives include insulin, albumin, heparin, and H_2 blockers (e.g., cimetidine, ranitidine, famotidine). Other medication may be included, but compatibility for admixture should be checked on an individual basis.

ROUTE OF ADMINISTRATION

PN is administered via either peripheral or central vein.

Peripheral: Usually involves 2–3 L/day of 5%–10% dextrose with 3%–5% amino acid solution along with IV fat emulsion. Electrolytes, vitamins, trace elements are added according to pt needs. Peripheral solutions provide about 2,000 kcal/day and 60–90 g protein/day.

ADVANTAGES: Lower risks vs. central mode of administration.

1283

DISADVANTAGES: Peripheral veins may not be suitable (esp. in pts with illness of long duration); more susceptible to phlebitis (due to osmolalities greater than 600 mOsm/L); veins may be viable only 1–2 wks; large volumes of fluid are needed to meet nutritional requirements, which may be contraindicated in many pts.

Central: Usually utilizes hypertonic dextrose (concentration range of 15%–35%) and amino acid solution of 3%–7% with IV fat emulsion. Electrolytes, vitamins, trace elements are added according to pt needs. Central solutions provide 2,000–4,000 kcal/day. Must be given through large central vein with high blood flow, allowing rapid dilution, avoiding phlebitis/thrombosis (usually through percutaneous insertion of catheter into subclavian vein, then advancement of catheter to superior vena cava).

ADVANTAGES: Allows more alternatives/flexibility in establishing regimens; allows ability to provide full nutritional requirements without need of daily fat emulsion; useful in pts who are fluid restricted (increased concentration), those needing large nutritional requirements (e.g., trauma, malignancy), or those for whom PN indicated more than 7–10 days.

DISADVANTAGES: Risk with insertion, use, maintenance of central line; increased risk of infection, catheter-induced trauma, and metabolic changes.

MONITORING

May vary slightly from institution to institution.

Baseline: CBC, platelet count, prothrombin time (PT), weight, body length/head circumference (in infants), serum electrolytes, glucose, BUN, creatinine, uric acid, total protein, cholesterol, triglycerides, bilirubin, alkaline phosphatase, lactate dehydrogenase (LDH), AST, albumin, prealbumin, other tests as needed.

Daily: Weight, vital signs (temperature, pulse, respirations [TPR]), nutritional intake (kcal, protein, fat), serum electrolytes (potassium, sodium chloride), glucose (serum, urine), acetone, BUN, osmolarity, other tests as needed.

2–3 times/wk: CBC, coagulation studies (PT, partial thromboplastin time [PTT]), serum creatinine, calcium, magnesium, phosphorus, acid-base status, other tests as needed.

Weekly: Nitrogen balance, total protein, albumin, prealbumin, transferrin, hepatic function tests (AST, ALT), serum alkaline phosphatase, LDH, bilirubin, Hgb, uric acid, cholesterol, triglycerides, other tests as needed.

COMPLICATIONS

Mechanical: Malfunction in system for IV delivery (e.g., pump failure; problems with lines, tubing, administration sets, catheter). Pneumothorax, catheter misdirection, arterial puncture, bleeding, hematoma formation may occur with catheter placement.

Infectious: Infections (pts often more susceptible to infections), catheter sepsis (e.g., fever, shaking, chills, glucose intolerance where no other site of infection is identified).

Metabolic: Includes hyperglycemia, elevated serum cholesterol and triglycerides, abnormal serum hepatic function tests.

Fluid, electrolyte, acid-base disturbances: May alter serum potassium, sodium, phosphate, magnesium levels.

Nutritional: Clinical effects seen may be due to lack of adequate vitamins, trace elements, essential fatty acids.

DRUG THERAPY/ADMINISTRATION METHODS:

Compatibility of other intravenous medications pts may be administered while receiving parenteral nutrition is an important concern.

Intravenous medications usually are given as a separate admixture via piggyback to the parenteral nutrition line, but in some instances may be added directly to the parenteral nutrition solution. Because of the possibility of incompatibility when adding medication directly to the parenteral nutrition solution, specific criteria should be considered:

- Stability of the medication in the parenteral nutrition solution
- Properties of the medication, including pharmacokinetics that determine if the medication is appropriate for continuous infusion
- Documented chemical and physical compatibility with the parenteral nutrition solution

In addition, when medication is given via piggyback using the parenteral nutrition line, important criteria should include the following:

- Stability of the medication in the parenteral nutrition solution
- Documented chemical and physical compatibility with the parenteral nutrition solution

Index

---

bold page # – main drug entry

Bold – generic drug name   regular type – trade name

---

bold page # – main drug entry

---

bold page # – main drug entry

---

bold page # – main drug entry

COMMONLY USED ABBREVIATIONS

ABG(s)—arterial blood gas(es)
ACE—angiotensin-converting enzyme
ADHD—attention-deficit hyperactivity disorder
AIDS—acquired immunodeficiency syndrome
ALT—alanine aminotransferase, serum
ANC—absolute neutrophil count
aPTT—activated partial thromboplastin time
ARB—angiotensin receptor blocker
AST—aspartate aminotransferase, serum
AV—atrioventricular
bid—twice per day
BMP—basic metabolic panel
B/P—blood pressure
BSA—body surface area
BUN—blood urea nitrogen
CAD—coronary artery disease
CBC—complete blood count
CrCl—creatinine clearance
CNS—central nervous system
CKD—chronic kidney disease
CO—cardiac output
COPD—chronic obstructive pulmonary disease
CPK—creatine phosphokinase
CSF—cerebrospinal fluid
CT—computed tomography
CVA—cerebrovascular accident
D_5W—dextrose 5% in water
DBP—diastolic blood pressure
dl—deciliter
DNA—deoxyribonucleic acid
DVT—deep vein thrombosis
ECG—electrocardiogram
ECHO—echocardiogram
EEG—electroencephalogram
g—gram
GGT—gamma glutamyl transpeptidase
GI—gastrointestinal
GU—genitourinary
Hct—hematocrit
HDL—high-density lipoprotein
HF—heart failure
Hgb—hemoglobin
HIV—human immunodeficiency virus
HMG-CoA—3-hydroxy-3-methylglutaryl-coenzyme A (HMG-CoA; statins)
HTN—hypertension
I&O—intake and output
ICP—intracranial pressure
IgA—immunoglobulin A
IM—intramuscular
IOP—intraocular pressure
IV—intravenous
IVP—intravenous push
IVPB—intravenous piggyback
K—potassium
kg—kilogram
LDH—lactate dehydrogenase
LDL—low-density lipoprotein
LFT—liver function test
LOC—level of consciousness
MAC—*Mycobacterium avium* complex
MAOI—monoamine oxidase inhibitor
mcg—microgram
mEq—milliequivalent
mg—milligram
MI—myocardial infarction
mo/mos—month/months
NKA—no known allergies
Na—sodium
NaCl—sodium chloride
NG—nasogastric
NSAID(s)—nonsteroidal anti-inflammatory drug(s)
OD—right eye
OS—left eye
OTC—over the counter
OU—both eyes
PCP—*Pneumocystis jiroveci* pneumonia
PO—orally, by mouth
prn—as needed
PSA—prostate-specific antigen
PT—prothrombin time
PTCA—percutaneous transluminal coronary angiography
qid—four times a day
RBC—red blood cell count
REM—rapid eye movement
RNA—ribonucleic acid
SA—sinoatrial node
SBP—systolic blood pressure
subQ—subcutaneous
SSRI—selective serotonin reuptake inhibitor
tbsp—tablespoon
tid—three times daily
TNF—tumor necrosis factor
tsp—teaspoon
UTI—urinary tract infection
VLDL—very-low-density lipoprotein
WBC—white blood cell count